Current Genitourinary Cancer Surgery

Second Edition

CURRENT GENITOURINARY CANCER SURGERY

Second Edition

EDITED BY

E. David Crawford, M.D.

Professor of Surgery
Chairman, Division of Urology
Director, Clinical Cancer Center
Associate Director, University of Colorado Cancer Center
University of Colorado Health Sciences Center
Attending Physician
Denver Veterans Administration Medical Center
Rose Medical Center
Denver, Colorado

Sakti Das, M.B.B.S., M.S.

Chairman, Department of Urology
Kaiser Permanente Medical Center
Walnut Creek, California
Associate Clinical Professor of Urology
University of California School of Medicine
Davis, California

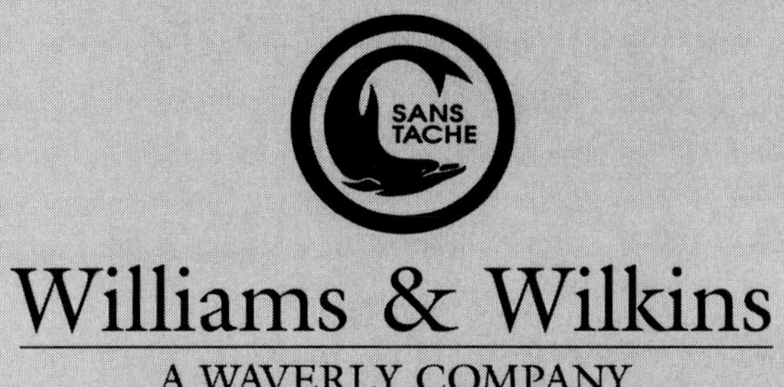

Williams & Wilkins

A WAVERLY COMPANY

BALTIMORE • PHILADELPHIA • LONDON • PARIS • BANGKOK
BUENOS AIRES • HONG KONG • MUNICH • SYDNEY • TOKYO • WROCLAW

Editor: Carroll C. Cann
Managing Editor: Susan Hunsberger
Production Coordinator: Cindy Park
Copy Editor: Christiane Odyniec
Book Project Editor: Kathy Gilbert
Designer: Karen Klinedinst
Cover Designer: Karen Klinedinst
Typesetter: Maryland Composition Co., Inc.
Printer: R. R. Donnelley
Binder: R. R. Donnelley

ISBN 0-683-02185-0

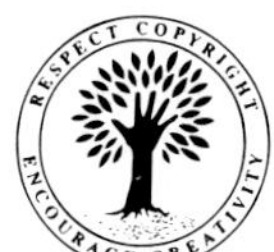

Rose Tree Corporate Center
1400 North Providence Road
Building II, Suite 5025
Media, Pennsylvania 19063-2043 USA

Accurate indications, adverse reactions and dosage schedules for drugs are provided in this book, but it is possible that they may change. The reader is urged to review the package information data of the manufacturers of the medications mentioned.

Printed in the United States of America

First Edition,

Library of Congress Cataloging-in-Publication Data

Current Genitourinary cancer surgery / edited by E. David Crawford. Sakti Das.
  —2nd ed.
    p.   cm.
   Rev. ed. of: Current genitourinary cancer surgery. 1990.
   Includes bibliographical references and index.
   ISBN 0-683-02185-0
   1. Genitourinary organs—Cancer—Surgery. I. Crawford, E. David.
II. Das, Sakti, III. Current genitourinary cancer surgery.
  [DNLM: 1. Urogenital Neoplasms—surgery. WJ 160 G3306 1996]
  RD670.G52 1996
  616.99′46059—dc20
  DNLM/DLC
  for Library of Congress   96-8186
                                   CIP

The publishers have made every effort to trace the copyright holders for borrowed material. If they have inadvertently overlooked any, they will be pleased to make the necessary arrangements at the first opportunity.

To purchase additional copies of this book, call our customer service department at **(800) 638-0672** or fax orders to **(800) 447-8438.** For other book services, including chapter reprints and large quantity sales, ask for the Special Sales department.

Canadian customers should call **(800) 268-4178,** or fax **(905) 470-6780.** For all other calls originating outside of the United States, please call **(410) 528-4223** or fax us at **(410) 528-8550.**

Visit Williams & Wilkins on the Internet: **http://www.wwilkins.com** or contact our customer service department at **custserv@wwilkins.com.** Williams & Wilkins customer service representatives are available from 8:30 am to 6:00 pm, EST, Monday through Friday, for telephone access.

97 98 99
1 2 3 4 5 6 7 8 9 10

To

The memory of
Willet F. Whitmore, Jr.

Foreword

Today we are at the crossroads of significant changes in the diagnosis and treatment of all urologic malignancies. For instance, the ongoing discoveries at the molecular level are placing at the fingertips of all practicing urologists diagnostic and therapeutic modalities that require an understanding of concepts that were within the domain of lab scientists only a short period of time ago. The practice of urologic oncology is a complex, multidisciplinary endeavor, and its understanding requires not only mastering the field of urologic surgery, but also a knowledge and familiarity of the role of our medical and radiation oncology associates. In addition, it is common to utilize the talents of our colleagues in other disciplines of medicine. An example that comes to mind is the teamwork required with cardiothoracic surgeons who are an integral part of the surgical approach for resection of renal cell carcinomas with extensive caval thrombi when circulatory arrest is indicated. When to consult with others for the benefit of patients in our charge is frequently a therapeutic strategy that the astute urologist must utilize.

To assemble the leaders in various fields, and then to get them to present their techniques and data in a scholarly yet succinct manner is no easy task. However, the editors of *Current Genitourinary Cancer Surgery* have risen to the challenge. The wealth of new information presented in this latest edition, when added to the time-honored techniques used by the contributors, gives the reader information of substance to take to the bedside.

This relevant textbook is useful for the urologist in the day-to-day problem solving of what is often the controversial nature of our profession. The rapidly evolving guidelines and emergence of managed care place an added burden on the practitioner, and *Current Genitorurinary Cancer Surgery* gives the reader a point of reference as he or she struggles with the changing paradigms of medicine in general and urology in particular.

The bibliographies have been compiled to provide the most current references rather than an encyclopedic review of the literature. In this regard the reader will have access to articles to buttress the information by leaders in all aspects of urologic surgery. As mentioned, it is the focus of this book to concentrate on surgical approaches along with all aspects of care for patients with urologic malignancies. In summary, this edition of *Current Genitourinary Cancer Surgery* builds on the precedents of the previous edition, and positions the reader for forthcoming editions as new discoveries require future updates.

David G. McLeod, M.D.
Chief, Urology Service
Walter Reed Army Medical Center,
Washington, DC, and Professor of
Surgery, Uniformed Services University
of the Health Sciences, Bethesda, MD

Preface

More than half a decade has elapsed since the publication of the first edition of *Current Genitourinary Cancer Surgery.* The phenomenal evolution in the various spheres of urologic oncology during this interval has compelled us to embark upon this new second edition. The perennial outpouring of new ideas and controversies makes us feel like we are in a phase of transition in perpetuity. Yet scientific understanding can only blossom in the compost of skepticism and controversy. Urologists at large are unavoidably involved in this process of learning by constantly sifting through available information. Urologic oncology constitutes a major segment of our practice because genitourinary cancers account for more than 25% of all cancers in the United States. With escalating life expectancy, public awareness and interest in screening and early detection of cancers, urologic oncology will demand more attention.

The continual new developments from molecular understanding to sophisticated diagnostic and therapeutic strategies pose an enchanting as well as challenging affront. From the tremendous excitement engendered by the virtually curative potential of combined modality therapeutic approach in the management of testicular tumors, to the unresolved debates around prostatic cancer issues, the practicing urologist is challenged to keep abreast of a wide spectrum of therapeutic options including radiation therapy, chemotherapy and hormonal manipulations, while at the same time maintaining his or her surgical expertise with refinements in newer surgical nuances.

In this second edition we have assembled international stalwarts offering their didactic views and practical guidance in a systematic manner encompassing surgical approaches, diagnostic modalities, nonsurgical therapies as well as addressing areas of continuing and supportive care. Organ specific neoplasms are discussed in individual chapters preceded by a comprehensive overview section. Surgical therapy of genitourinary cancers is elaborated through stepwise illustrations to guide urologists regardless of their level of preparation and training. The spectrum of surgical recommendations encompasses traditional as well as recent techniques that generate healthy controversy and scientific curiosity. Modern surgical approaches, such as laparoscopic extirpative surgeries, newer continent urinary diversion, improved technical nuances for radical retropubic and perineal prostatectomies and nerve sparing retroperitoneal lymphadenectomy to preserve ejaculatory function, are discussed from the perspectives of enhancement of traditional surgical procedures. Alternative and adjuvant approaches to the managemet of genitourinary tumors are presented by radiation therapists and medical oncologists. The management of genitourinary malignancies is often a multidisciplinary process. Therefore, chemotherapy, immunotherapy and hormonal therapy are presented from the perspective of urologic oncologists as well as those of medical oncologists. It is imperative that all practicing urologists develop a working knowledge of chemotherapy and biologic response modification because exquisite sensitivity has been demonstrated by genitourinary cancers to a number of conventional and investigative agents. We conclude with a chapter on the genetic basis for urologic malignancy, looking at the nascent vista that may soon unravel the fundamental mystery of genetic implications in genitourinary neoplasms.

We deeply appreciate and thank the contributors for the time and effort they have devoted to sharing their expertise with the readers of this text. The generous support of our staff at the Department of Surgery and the Cancer Center at the University of Colorado Health Sciences Center and the Department of Urology at Kaiser Permanente Medical Center, Walnut Creek is gratefully acknowledged. Our special thanks to our publishing staff for their patient help, accommodation and versatility at every step of the production. Through the collective efforts of these friends and the constant encouragement, good wishes, help and forbearance of many others who remain in the background, once again our dream of producing an improved second edition has materialized.

We thank you all in earnest sincerity.

E. David Crawford, M.D.
Denver, Colorado

Sakti Das, M.B.B.S., M.S.
Walnut Creek, California

Contributors

JOHN B. ADAMS, II, M.D.
Assistant Professor of Urology
Medical College of Georgia
Augusta, Georgia

JAN ADOLFSSON, M.D.
Associate Professor
Department of Urology, 60500
Karolinska Hospital
Stockholm, Sweden

ROBERT J. AMATO, M.D.
Associate Professor of Medicine
Department of Genitourinary Oncology
University of Texas
MD Anderson Cancer Center
Houston, Texas

ROBERT A. BADALAMENT, M.D.
Clinical Associate Professor
School of Public Health
Ohio State University
Columbus, Ohio

DUKE K. BAHN, M.D.
Clinical Associate Professor
Department of Radiation Oncology
Wayne State University School of Medicine
Detroit, Michigan

ZORAN L. BARBARIC, M.D.
Professor of Radiology
Department of Radiology
U.C.L.A. School of Medicine
Los Angeles, California

LAURENCE S. BASKIN, M.D.
Assistant Professor of Urology and Pediatrics
University of California, San Francisco
San Francisco, California

MARC BEAGHLER, M.D.
Chief Resident
Department of Urology
Loma Linda University Medical Center
Loma Linda, California

ARIE S. BELLDEGRUN, M.D.
Professor, Division of Urology
U.C.L.A. School of Medicine
Los Angeles, California

NABIL K. BISSADA, M.D.
Professor and Chief of Urologic Oncology
Department of Urology
Medical University of South Carolina
Charleston, South Carolina

DAVID A. BLOOM, M.D.
Professor, Division of Urology
University of Michigan Medical School
Ann Arbor, Michigan

STUART D. BOYD, M.D.
Professor of Urology
Department of Urology
University of Southern California Medical Center
Los Angeles, California

ELY BRAND, M.D.
Department of OB/GYN
University of Colorado Health Sciences Center
Denver, Colorado

PETER R. CARROLL, M.D.
Professor and Chairman, Division of Urology
University of California San Francisco
San Francisco, California

JEFFREY K. COHEN, M.D.
Associate Professor
Division of Urology
Medical College of Pennsylvania
Pittsburgh, Pennsylvania

R. LEE COX, M.D.
Instructor in Urology
University of Colorado Health Sciences Center
Denver, Colorado

E. DAVID CRAWFORD, M.D.
Professor and Chairman, Division of Urology
University of Colorado Health Sciences Center
Denver, Colorado

KENNETH B. CUMMINGS, M.D.
Professor and Chairman
Department of Urology
Robert Wood Johnson Medical School
New Brunswick, New Jersey

SAKTI DAS, M.D.
Clinical Associate Professor of Urology
University of California School of Medicine
Davis, California

MARK L. DAVIDNER, M.D.
Associate Clinical Professor of Medicine
University of Missouri-Kansas City
Kansas City, Missouri

MARILYN DAVIS, R.N., M.S.
Schering Corporation
Hyattsville, Maryland

EDWARD P. DEANTONI, PH.D.
Assistant Professor of Urology
University of Colorado Health Sciences Center
Denver, Colorado

ALFRED A. deLORIMIER, M.D.
Professor of Surgery
Department of Pediatric Surgery
University of California San Francisco
San Francisco, California

JOHN P. DONOHUE, M.D.
Distinguished Professor Emeritus
Department of Urology
Indiana University Hospital
Indianapolis, Indiana

ROBERT E. DONOHUE, M.D.
Professor of Urology
University of Colorado Health Sciences Center
Denver, Colorado

MARIE DUCLOS, M.D.
Fellow
Department of Radiation Oncology
Wayne State University School of Medicine
The Detroit Medical Center
Detroit, Michigan

MARILYN H. DUNCAN, M.D.
Associate Professor Pediatric Oncology Program
Department of Pediatrics
University of New Mexico School of Medicine
Albuquerque, New Mexico

MARIO A. EISENBERGER, M.D.
Associate Professor of Urology and Oncology
Johns Hopkins University Medical School
Baltimore, Maryland

PAMELA I. ELLSWORTH, M.D.
Fellow in Pediatric Urology
Division of Urology
University of Florida College of Medicine
Gainesville, Florida

DONALD A. ELMAJIAN, M.D.
Fellow, Genitourinary Oncology
University of Southern California Medical Center
Los Angeles, California

RICHARD G. EVANS, M.D.
Professor and Chairman
Department of Radiation Oncology
University of Kansas Medical Center
Kansas City, Kansas

ROBERT A. FIGLIN, M.D.
Professor of Medicine
Department of Medicine, Division of Oncology
UCLA School of Medicine
Los Angeles, California

ROBERT C. FLANIGAN, M.D.
Professor and Chairman
Department of Urology
Loyola University Medical Center
Maywood, Illinois

JEFFREY D. FORMAN, M.D.
Professor and Associate Chairman
Department of Radiation Oncology
Wayne State University School of Medicine
Detroit Medical Center-Harper Hospital
Detroit, Michigan

FUAD S. FREIHA, M.D.
Professor of Surgery and Chief, Urologic Oncology
Stanford University Medical Center
Stanford, California

VISWANATHAN GAJENDRAN, M.D.
Fellow in Urology
University of Florida College of Medicine
Gainesville, Florida

INDERBIR S. GILL, M.D.
Associate Professor
Division of Urology
University of Nebraska Medical Center
Omaha, Nebraska

SETH H. GLICK, M.D.
Chief Resident
Department of Urology
University of California School of Medicine
Davis, California

EDMOND T. GONZALES, JR. M.D.
Professor and Chief
Pediatric Urology
Baylor College of Medicine
Houston, Texas

H. BARTON GROSSMAN, M.D.
Professor of Urology and Cell Biology
University of Texas M.D. Anderson Cancer Center
Houston, Texas

H. ROGER HADLEY, M.D.
Professor and Chairman, Department of Urology
Loma Linda University Medical Center
Loma Linda, California

STEVEN L. HANCOCK, M.D.
Associate Professor
Department of Radiation Oncology
Stanford University Medical Center
Stanford, California

RICHARD K. HEPPE, M.D.
Assistant Clinical Professor
Division of Urology
University of Colorado Health Sciences Center
Denver, Colorado

ROBERT R. ISACKSEN, M.D.
Chief Resident
Department of Urology
Loyola University Medical Center
Maywood, Illinois

MICHAEL A.S. JEWETT, M.D.
Professor and Chairman, Division of Urology
University of Toronto
Toronto, Ontario, Canada

BYRON D. JOYNER, M.D.
Chief Resident
Department of Urology
Massachusetts General Hospital
Harvard Medical School
Boston, Massachusetts

LOUIS R. KAVOUSSI, M.D.
Associate Professor of Urology
Johns Hopkins University School of Medicine
Baltimore, Maryland

LONNIE T. KLEIN, M.D.
Senior Resident
Department of Urology
Columbia University College of Physicians & Surgeons
New York, New York

MARTIN A. KOYLE, M.D.
Professor of Urology
Department of Urology
University of Colorado Health-Sciences Center
Denver, Colorado

JAGDEESH N. KULKARNI, M.D.
Head
Division of Urologic Oncology
Tata Memorial Hospital
Bombay, India

FRED LEE, M.D.
Clinical Professor
Department of Radiation Oncology
Wayne State University School of Medicine
Detroit, Michigan

SETH P. LERNER, M.D.
Assistant Professor
Scott Department of Urology
Baylor College of Medicine
Houston, Texas

JOHN LEUNG, M.D.
Resident, Department of Radiation Oncology
Wayne State University School of Medicine
The Detroit Medical Center
Detroit, Michigan

S. LAWRENCE LIBRACH, M.D.
Director, Division of Palliative Medicine, Mount Sinai Hospital
Associate Professor, Department of Family and Community Medicine
University of Toronto
Toronto, Ontario, Canada

GARY LIESKOVSKY, M.D.
Professor of Urology
Department of Urology
University of Southern California School of Medicine
Los Angeles, California

CHRISTOPHER J. LOGOLHÉTIS
Professor of Medical Oncology
University of Texas MD Anderson Cancer Center
Houston, Texas

FRANKLIN C. LOWE, M.D.
Clinical Associate Professor
Department of Urology
Columbia University College of Physicians & Surgeons
New York, New York

MICHAEL J. MANYAK, M.D.
Associate Professor
Department of Urology
George Washington University Medical Center
Washington, D.C.

W. SCOTT McDOUGAL, M.D.
Professor and Chairman
Department of Urology
Massachusetts General Hospital
Harvard Medical School
Boston, Massachusetts

LORI MERLOTTI, M.D.
Allegheny General Hospital
Medical College of Pennsylvania
Pittsburgh, Pennsylvania

HRAIR-GEORGE O. MESROBIAN, M.D.
Associate Professor
Chief, Division of Pediatric Urology
Medical College of Wisconsin
Milwaukee, Wisconsin

RALPH J. MILLER, JR. M.D.
Assistant Professor
Division of Urology
Medical College of Pennsylvania
Pittsburgh, Pennsylvania

ROBERT P. MYERS, M.D.
Professor of Urology
Department of Urology
Mayo Clinic
Rochester, Minnesota

HARMESH NAIK, M.D.
Senior Fellow, Medical Oncology
Wayne State University
Harper Hospital
Detroit, Michigan

PERINCHERY NARAYAN, M.D.
Professor and Chairman
Department of Urology
University of Florida College of Medicine
Gainesville, Florida

MARK J. NOBLE, M.D.
Associate Professor of Surgery
Department of Urology
University of Kansas Medical Center
Kansas City, Kansas

JAMES T. PARSONS, M.D.
Professor of Radiation Oncology
University of Florida Shands Cancer Center
Gainesville, Florida

PAUL C. PETERS, M.D.
Professor of Urology
Department of Urology
University of Texas Southwestern Medical Center
Dallas, Texas

KENNETH J. PIENTA, M.D.
Associate Professor of Medicine
University of Michigan Medical Center
Ann Arbor, Michigan

ARTHUR T. PORTER, M.D.
Professor and Chairman
Department of Radiation Oncology
Wayne State University
Detroit, Michigan

JOSEPH C. PRESTI, M.D.
Assistant Professor
Department of Urology
University of California San Francisco Medical Center
San Francisco, California

ROBERT A. READ, M.D., PH.D.
Department of Surgery
University of Colorado Health Sciences Center
Denver, Colorado

ESCHWAR REDDI, M.D.
Associate Professor of Radiation Oncology
University of Kansas Medical Center
Kansas City, Kansas

JOHN F. REDMAN, M.D.
Professor and Chairman
Department of Urology
University of Arkansas College of Medicine
Little Rock, Arkansas

JEROME P. RICHIE, M.D.
Professor and Chairman
Department of Urology
Brigham and Women's Hospital
Boston, Massachusetts

HERBERT C. RUCKLE, M.D.
Associate Professor
Department of Urology
Loma Linda University Medical Center
Loma Linda, California

MICHAEL F. SAROSDY, M.D.
Professor and Chairman
Division of Urology
University of Texas Health Sciences Center
San Antonio, Texas

PETER T. SCARDINO, M.D.
Professor and Chairman
Scott Department of Urology
Baylor College of Medicine
Houston, Texas

MICHAEL J. SCHUTZ, M.D.
Assistant Professor
Department of Urology
University of Arkansas School of Medical Sciences
Little Rock, Arkansas

JOHN D. SEIGNE, M.B.
Junior Faculty Associate
Department of Urology
University of Texas MD Anderson Cancer Center
Houston, Texas

KATSUTO SHINOHARA, M.D.
Assistant Adjunct Professor
Department of Urology
University of California, San Francisco Medical Center
San Francisco, California

BARRY A. SHUMAN, M.D.
Assistant Professor
Division of Urology
Medical College of Pennsylvania
Pittsburgh, Pennsylvania

DONALD G. SKINNER, M.D.
Professor and Chairman
Department of Urology
University of Southern California Medical Center
Los Angeles, California

STEPHEN R. SMALLEY, M.D.
Clinical Professor
Department of Radiation Oncology
University of Kansas Medical Center
Kansas City, Kansas

ROBERT B. SMITH, M.D.
Professor
Department of Urology
UCLA School of Medicine
Los Angeles, California

Susan M. Smith, M.D.
Clinical Instructor
Department of Radiation Oncology
University of Kansas Medical Center
Kansas City, Kansas

Joseph A., Smith, Jr., M.D.
Professor and Chairman
Department of Urology
Vanderbilt University Medical Center
Nashville, Tennessee

Mitchell H. Sokoloff, M.D.
Resident, Division of Urology
UCLA School of Medicine
Los Angeles, California

Richard W. Sutherland, M.D.
Assistant Professor
Pediatric Urology
Baylor College of Medicine
Houston, Texas

Samir S. Taneja, M.D.
Chief Resident
Department of Urology
UCLA Medical Center
Los Angeles, California

Rodney J. Taylor, M.D.
Professor and Chairman
Division of Urology
University of Nebraska Medical Center
Omaha, Nebraska

Ian M. Thompson, M.D.
Chief
Urology Service
Brooke Army Medical Center
Fort Sam Houston, Texas

J. Brantley Thrasher, M.D.
Assistant Clinical Professor of Surgery
University of Washington School of Medicine
Tacoma, Washington

Greg Van Stiegman, M.D.
Professor of Surgery
Department of Surgery
University of Colorado Health Sciences Center
Denver, Colorado

Thomas S. Vates, M.D.
Clinical Instructor
Department of Pediatric Urology
Wayne State University
Children's Hospital of Michigan
Detroit, Michigan

Steve W. Waxman, M.D.
Fellow in Urology
University of Colorado Health Sciences Center
Denver, Colorado

Vernon E. Weldon, M.D.
Chief
Department of Urology
Marin General Hospital
San Rafael, California

Ralph W. deVere White, M.D.
Professor and Chairman, Division of Urology
University of California School of Medicine
Davis, California

Stuart S. Winter, M.D.
Assistant Professor
Pediatric Oncology Program; Department of Pediatrics
University of New Mexico School of Medicine
Albuquerque, New Mexico

Kirk J. Wojno, M.D.
Assistant Professor
Department of Pathology
University of Michigan Medical School
Ann Arbor, Michigan

Marc Wolach, M.D.
Assistant Clinical Professor
Department of Urology
University of Colorado Health Sciences Center
Denver, Colorado

David P. Wood, M.D.
Associate Professor
Division of Urology
University of Kentucky Medical Center
Lexington, Kentucky

Robert A. Zlotecki, M.D., Ph.D.
Assistant Professor of Radiation Oncology
University of Florida Shands Cancer Center
Gainesville, Florida

Contents

ANATOMY

An Anatomic Approach to the Kidneys and Retroperitoneum

John F. Redman

I began to investigate the transversalis fascia. I sought it in books, where its descriptions were vague and unconvincing; in anatomy departments which had no dissection to offer; and in the human body where I failed entirely to find it.

DENIS BROWNE (1)

Any surgeon who has pursued the detailed aspects of anatomy has shared Denis Browne's frustrations. Although the transversalis fascia is a vital component in extirpative cancer surgery, many of its aspects have been difficult to define. Anatomy that seemed clear in the dissecting room or in surgical texts can become confused through a developing incision in an actual surgical procedure. This chapter details a careful, thorough anatomic approach to the kidneys and retroperitoneum that can eliminate much of that confusion.

RETROPERITONEAL CONNECTIVE TISSUE

The basis for an understanding of the retroperitoneum is a knowledge of the retroperitoneal connective tissue. There has been much confusion in the literature regarding what lies between the peritoneum, aptly described by Browne as a "membrane hardly thicker than a soap-bubble (1)," and the lining muscles of the abdominal cavity. This tissue is more complex than just "packing material" between the osteomuscular wall and the peritoneum.

A brief description of its embryologic origins should help in understanding the retroperitoneal connective tissue. Hayes gives a clear description, and his conclusions coincide with what is seen surgically in regard to anatomic findings and planes of dissection (2). The retroperitoneal connective tissue is derived from three separate embryologic origins.

1. A parietal layer, from the young mesenchymal tissue intimately associated with the developing musculature of the abdominal wall.
2. A visceral layer, from loose mesenchymal tissue distributed between the developing intrinsic fascia of the muscles.
3. The coelomic epithelium.

The parietal layer becomes the transversalis fascia, which is the intrinsic investing fascia of the muscular abdominal wall. The coelomic epithelium becomes the peritoneum, which is backed by a thin supportive tissue containing nutrient vessels. The intermediate layer derived from loose mesenchyme is intimately related to the supportive backing of the peritoneum. As it grows within this intermediate layer of connective tissue, the enlarging kidney compresses the tissue to form a limiting fascial-like structure (Gerota's fascia). In a similar manner, the ureter and spermatic vessels are surrounded by this tissue and thus are held to the serosal surface. This intermediate retroperitoneal connective tissue has been loosely termed the subserosal layer.

The retroperitoneal connective tissue becomes more complex by virtue of what Hayes has termed "fusion fascia." One should recall that the primitive gut, with the structures arising in its mesentery (the pancreas), at one time was covered with peritoneum over most of its circumference as well as its mesentery. With rotation of the gut, the duodenum and pancreas, as well as the ascending and descending colon, come to rest on the primitive coelomic epithelium. The colonic mesentery in part comes to rest against the serosal covering of the duodenum and pancreas. With obliteration of the peritoneum per se, a firm fascia is produced.

Tobin described three "dissectable strata" of the retroperitoneal connective tissue.

1. An inner stratum associated intimately with the peritoneum and with the digestive system with its nerve blood supply.

2. An intermediate stratum embedding the adrenals, urogenital system, and the great vessels.
3. An outer stratum, which is the intrinsic fascia of the components of the body wall (Fig. 1.1) (3, 4).

In the region of the kidneys, the intermediate stratum (particularly in obese individuals) may be in the form of two laminae, with local thickenings of the ventral lamina forming the renal (Gerota's) fascia with its contained perirenal fat. The dorsal lamina forms the perirenal fat and the areolar tissue between the ventral (Gerota's) lamina and the transversalis fascia (Fig. 1.2). In thinner individuals, the intermediate stratum caudal to the region of the kidney will not be laminated.

In keeping with Tobin's belief that "a knowledge of the fascial strata of the abdomen and pelvis is a great asset to the surgeon who operates in these regions," it may be stated that cleavage planes exist theoretically

1. Between the transversalis fascia and the intermediate stratum (subserosal layer),
2. Between the intermediate stratum and the inner stratum (supporting connective tissue of the peritoneum),

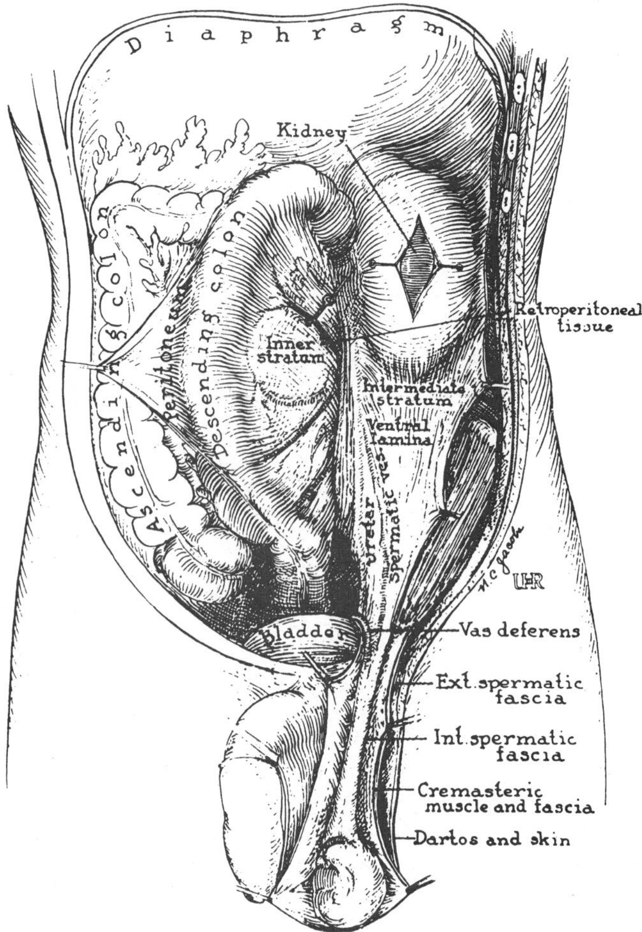

Fig. 1.2.   Intermediate stratum of the retroperitoneal tissue in the region of the kidney. (From Tobin CE, Benjamin JA, Wells JC. Continuity of the fasciae lining the abdomen, pelvis, and spermatic cord. Surg Gynecol Obstet 1946;83:575. By permission of Surgery, Gynecology & Obstetrics.)

3. Between the intermediate stratum and the colon and its mesentery, and
4. Between the intermediate stratum and the pancreas and duodenum (Fig. 1.3) (3).

Graphic evidence that these planes exist is provided by radiographic studies of extraperitoneal effusions and by the identification of planes of dissection of retroperitoneal abscesses (5, 6).

SURGICAL APPROACHES TO THE KIDNEY AND RETROPERITONEUM

The incisions used to gain access to the kidneys and retroperitoneum fall basically into four groups: midline abdominal, transverse abdominal, flank, and thoracoabdominal incisions. The placement and execution of the incisions of the body wall are well described in several excellent urologic surgical texts (7, 8). The following descriptions of the surgical approaches deal primarily with the location and development of retroperitoneal tissue planes.

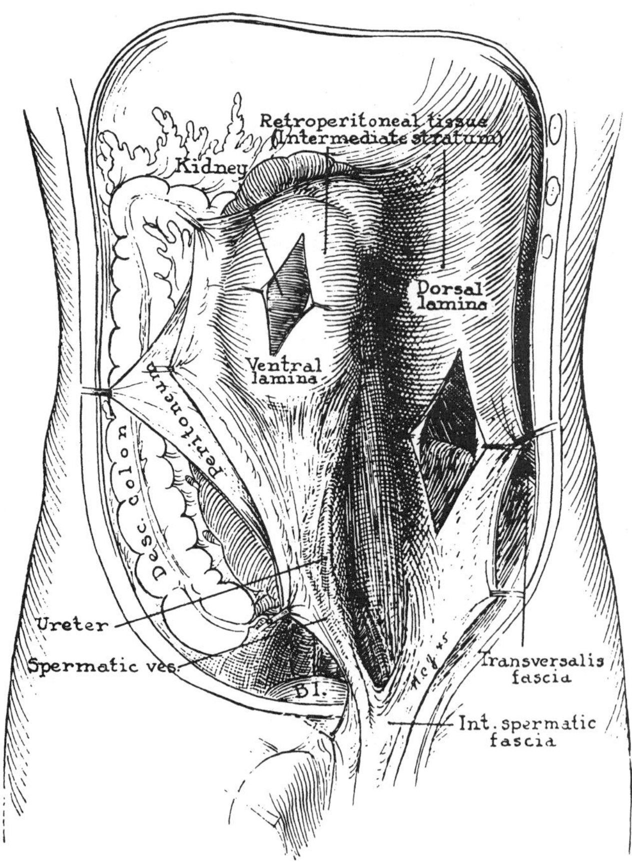

Fig. 1.1.   Strata of the retroperitoneal connective tissue. (From Tobin CE, Benjamin JA, Wells JC. Continuity of the fasciae lining the abdomen, pelvis, and spermatic cord. Surg Gynecol Obstet 1946;83:575. By permission of Surgery, Gynecology & Obstetrics.)

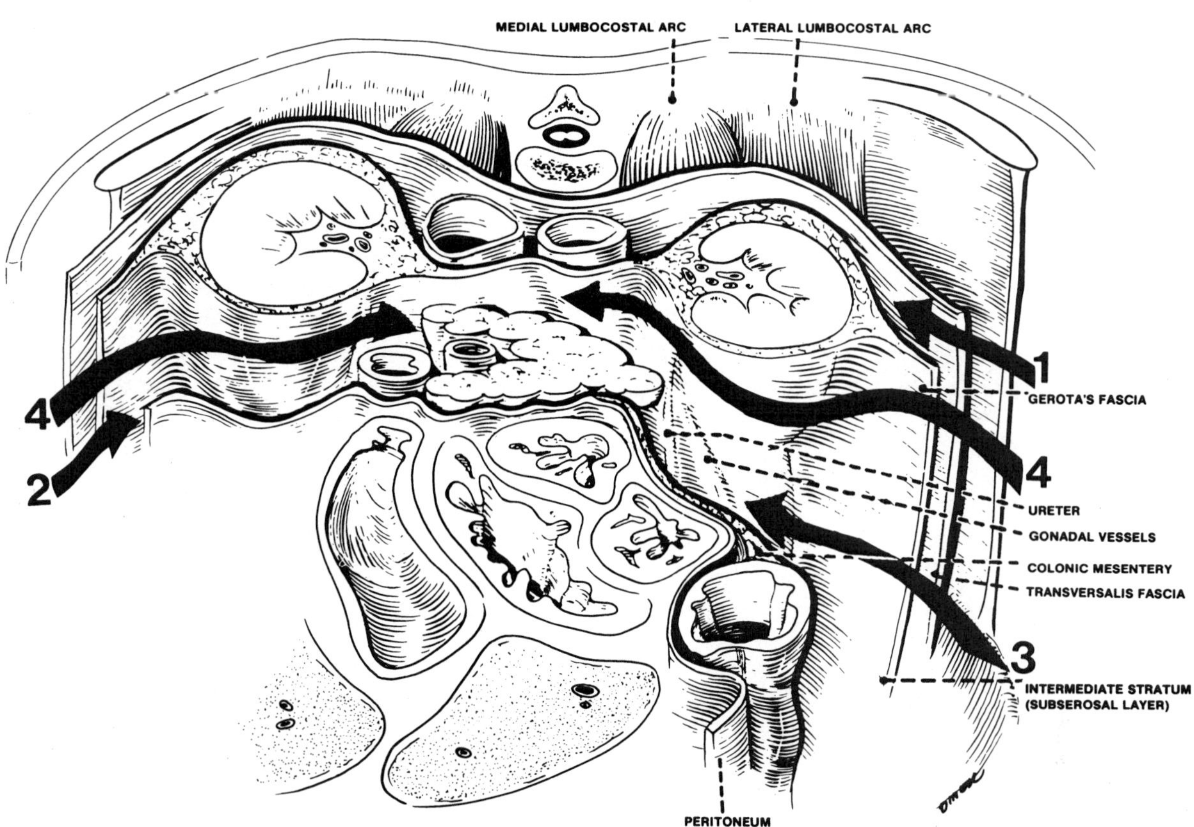

Fig. 1.3. Anatomic cleavage planes (1) between the transversalis fascia and the intermediate stratum (subserosal layer), (2) between the intermediate stratum and the inner stratum (supporting connective tissue of the peritoneum), (3) between the intermediate stratum and the colon and colonic mesentery, and (4) between the intermediate stratum and the pancreas and duodenum.

Midline and Transverse Abdominal Transperitoneal Approaches

This section reviews the salient anatomic points for an incision that gives wide exposure to the retroperitoneum without disturbing the investments of the kidney, presumably the approach most preferred by the surgeon.

From within the peritoneal cavity, on exposure of the tissue just lateral to the lateral border of the ascending colon, it may be noted that the peritoneum, along with the thin but adherent underlying tissue containing small vessels, can be moved freely over an underlying layer. This layer can be seen through the thin peritoneum and its supporting layer. The underlying tissue is the subserosal layer of retroperitoneal connective tissue.

An incision through the peritoneum and its underlying connective tissue along the colonic border opens a tissue plane (fusion fascia) that may be carried medially between the colon per se and the underlying intermediate stratum of retroperitoneal connective tissue and its condensation (Gerota's fascia). On the right side, if the peritoneal incision is carried around the hepatic flexure of the colon and around the cecum, the plane may be developed as it is carried dorsal to the mesentery of the colon. The plane may be further developed by carrying the dissection dorsal to the duodenum (fusion fascia).

Gerota's fascia is contiguous across the midline over the vena cava and aorta, extending over the renal vessels of the left side. If the peritoneal incision is carried cranially from the cecum to the level where the duodenum emerges from its retroperitoneal position, the entirety of the ascending colon and small bowel may be displaced from the abdominal cavity.

The right kidney, as well as the right ureter, the gonadal vessels, and the aorta and vena cava, will remain undisturbed, covered with an intact Gerota's fascia. The lymphatics and lymph nodes should also be visible and undisturbed.

On the left side, a similar plane of dissection may be achieved by incision of the peritoneum and its supporting connective tissue on the lateral aspect of the descending colon. The peritoneal incision may be carried around the splenic flexure of the colon. Exposure of the peritoneum that lies between the caudal border of the pancreas and the cranial margin of the transverse colon will be enhanced by division of the omentum to separate the stomach from the transverse colon. With incision of the peritoneum between the transverse colon and the pancreas, the cleavage plane over Gerota's fascia is developed.

The duodenum may be elevated by pursuing the cleavage plane dorsal to that structure. Division of the inferior mesenteric vein as it joins the splenic vein gives even wider exposure. As one moves cranially, the pancreas may be elevated off the intermediate stratum to reveal the left kidney and adrenal and the renal vasculature, which usually can be seen clearly through the thin overlying Gerota's fascia. On the left side, the stomach, pancreas, and spleen may be rolled to the right side of the abdomen by continuation of the peritoneal incision around the lateral aspect of the tail of the pancreas and parietal peritoneal attachment of the greater curvature of the stomach.

Extraperitoneal Transverse Abdominal and Subcostal Flank Exposures

These two incisions are basically the same as those just described. However, instead of being directed through the abdominal and flank musculature directly into the peritoneal cavity, the incisions are deepened through the muscle without incision of the dorsal investing fascia of the transversus abdominis muscle. The aponeurosis of the transversus abdominis may be incised laterally in the direction of its fibers. If the incision is to approach or cross the midline, the posterior rectus sheath may be incised after the rectus itself has been incised. If the midline is not crossed, the rectus may merely be retracted medially.

The further development of the incision along anatomic planes is accomplished more easily if approached in a lateral-to-medial direction. The layer immediately underlying the aponeurosis of the transversus abdominis muscle, the dorsal investing fascia of the transversus abdominis, is the transversalis fascia. A plane may be developed between the intermediate stratum and the transversalis fascia if one moves in a lateral-to-medial direction. As the intermediate stratum and underlying peritoneum are reflected, the transversalis fascia can be progressively incised.

From the lateral border of the rectus to the midline, the amount of extraperitoneal connective tissue becomes more scant, and in some individuals the peritoneum becomes frankly adherent to the transversalis fascia. In some, the plane of dissection can be carried between the transversalis fascia and the posterior rectus sheath across the midline. In others, the adherence is so dense that a plane cannot be established.

To gain access to the other side, the surgeon should incise the peritoneum as close to the midline as possible, with closure of the peritoneum once the plane is gained on the contralateral side. Caudally, the peritoneal envelope, surrounded by its retroperitoneal connective tissue, may be swept medially. The correct plane of dissection can be ascertained by examination of the dorsal aspect of the transversus abdominis muscle. If bare muscle fibers are noted, the surgeon may assume that the incision is not deep enough. Identification of fascia over the muscle confirms the correct plane. Laterally, sweeping the retroperitoneal connective tissue from the transversalis fascia becomes more difficult at times because of the adherence of one structure to the other, particularly laterally at the level of the midaxillary line and at the lateral apposition of the transversus abdominis to the quadratus lumborum.

A similar situation occurs over the psoas muscle. If the surgeon observes bare muscle fibers over the quadratus or psoas muscle, it is necessary only to sharply incise the fibrous tissue that is being swept medially to regain the plane between transversalis fascia and the retroperitoneal connective tissue. At first, this may seem risky because of the grossly similar appearance of these glistening surfaces to peritoneum, colon, or dilated ureter. The peritoneal envelope, surrounded by its retroperitoneal connective tissue that encases the ureter and spermatic vessels, can be swept from the posterior abdominal wall, the lateral abdominal wall, and the anterior abdominal wall toward the midline. The only adherence of the peritoneum occurs deep in the pelvis, where it is tethered at the level of the internal ring by the remnants of the patent processus vaginalis peritonei. Cranially, the retroperitoneal connective tissue can be separated from the posterolateral abdominal wall.

At times, the retroperitoneal connective tissue adheres to the fibrous tissue arcs over the quadratus lumborum muscle (lateral lumbocostal arc) and over the psoas muscle (medial lumbocostal arc), which represents the point of insertion of the diaphragm over the surface of these muscles. The retroperitoneal connective tissue is scant between the peritoneum and transversalis fascia on the undersurface of the diaphragm. At times, it is necessary to pursue a plane between the transversalis fascia and the diaphragm to maintain an extraperitoneal cleavage plane.

Generally, in the course of freeing the retroperitoneal connective tissue from the diaphragm, numerous penetrating vessels will be noted. These should be sealed (preferably by electrocautery) to prevent staining of the tissue, which makes the identification of anatomic cleavage planes more difficult. The surgeon should remember that in the case of neoplasms, these vessels may be greatly enlarged.

Following the freeing of the peritoneal envelope with its adherent retroperitoneal connective tissue, a plane of dissection can be started by incising along the lateral border of the colon to obtain the cleavage plane between the colon and its mesentery and the subserosal layer. This plane of dissection can be carried across the midline. To obtain access to the renal vasculature or to the vena cava or aorta, the intermediate stratum must be incised over the vessels. The only major vessels that penetrate this subserosal layer from the dorsal to the ventral aspect occur in the midline; these are the inferior mesenteric artery, superior mesenteric artery, and celiac axis.

12th-Rib Flank Exposure

Attention to detail is essential for a true subperiosteal resection of the tip of the 12th rib. To gain a subperiosteal plane of dissection, it is generally easiest to sharply reflect the periosteum from the caudal keel of the rib with a periosteal elevator. Excursions with the periosteal elevator at right angles to the keel penetrate the periosteum in the same manner as if one were to incise the periosteum with a knife. The rib edge is sharp, and to remove the periosteum, one must carefully follow the contours of this edge. Once the inner aspect of the rib has been exposed, it is easy to strip the periosteum from it.

It is usually possible to identify a muscular layer immediately under the periosteum. This muscle is the diaphragm. If pleura is present, it will be located between the periosteum and the diaphragm. If the pleura extends beyond the periosteum of the 12th rib, the incision is best developed from the more medial aspect where transversalis fascia has been incised, and the diaphragm is best exposed from its inner aspect. With incision of the diaphragmatic attachments caudal to the 12th rib, one can usually strip the pleura from the inner aspect of the periosteum of the 12th rib using the snowshoe principle, peeling the pleura away much as one would peel away a hernia sac from the spermatic cord. An attempt to perform this dissection from the periosteal side generally allows access to the pleural cavity.

11th-Rib Extraperitoneal Flank Exposure

Great lengths of the 11th rib may be resected and the exposure maintained extrapleurally if attention is given to detail, which is even more important in the case of 11th-rib incision than in 12th-rib exposure. Almost without exception, the pleura will be seen extending under the periosteum of the 11th rib. With progression to the medial aspect of the incision, the retroperitoneal connective tissue is swept from the transversalis fascia and the diaphragm can be freed at the level of the lateral lumbocostal arc, i.e., the insertion of the diaphragm over the quadratus lumborum. This incision may be carried caudally and laterally to free the diaphragmatic attachments. The pleura can then be swept from the underside of the periosteum of the 11th rib with broad-based traction (snowshoe principle).

Thoracoabdominal Transpleural Exposure

Any of the ribs, as high as the seventh, may be chosen for this incision. The incision usually begins at the midaxillary line over the body of the rib and is carried along the axis of the rib. The incision may be carried down to the midline if the exposure is to be transpleural and transperitoneal; if the incision is to be transpleural but extraperitoneal, a paramedian incision may be used. The rib is resected subperiosteally. The pleural cavity is entered with incision through the periosteum.

Before incision of the diaphragm at the costochondral junction, if the surgeon wishes to remain extraperitoneal, the caudal portion of the incision should be developed in the manner already described for extraperitoneal exposures. Because of the scant amount of retroperitoneal connective tissue between the peritoneum and its supporting connective tissue and the transversalis fascia overlying the diaphragm, an incision made from the cranial aspect of the diaphragm may well enter directly into the peritoneum if the peritoneum is not freed from the caudal aspect of the diaphragm before this maneuver.

The entire peritoneal envelope, with its supporting connective tissue, may be mobilized from the retroperitoneum as described for the extraperitoneal transverse abdominal and sub-costal flank exposures. If the procedure is carried out intraperitoneally on the right side, the liver can be rotated medially for further exposure by careful incision of the right triangular ligament, which represents the reflection of the peritoneum onto the hepatic surface.

Dorsolumbar Flap Incision for Thoracoabdominal Extrapleural Exposure

This incision allows similar exposure to that gained with a transpleural transthoracic exposure. The anatomic key to this incision is the division of the lateral lumbocostal arc of the diaphragm, i.e., the attachment of the diaphragm to the quadratus lumborum muscle. The diaphragm can then be retracted upward with the pleural reflection (costophrenic sinus). Nagamatsu et al. state that, "if this is performed with care and deliberation, it is entirely possible to avoid pleural injury (9)." Because the ribs are resected at the costal arc, the adherence of the pleura to the periosteum of the ribs is not disturbed; thus, there is less opportunity for injury to the pleura. The remainder of the dissection is carried out as in the previously mentioned extrapleural exposures.

Lumbodorsal Incision

Anatomically, this incision is simple. With the correct placement of the incision, only the lumbodorsal fascia is incised in the direction of the skin incision, along with the latissimus dorsi and the serratus posterior inferior muscle ventrally. The quadratus lumborum is noted in the medial aspect of the incision and is reflected medially, and the iliohypogastric nerve is preserved. With incision of the transversalis fascia, the extraperitoneal connective tissue is visible.

REFERENCES

1. Browne D, Sydney MB. Some anatomical points in the operation for undescended testicle. Lancet 1933;224:460.
2. Hayes MA. Abdominopelvic fasciae. Am J Anat 1950;87:119.
3. Tobin CE, Benjamin JA, Wells JC. Continuity of the fasciae lining the abdomen, pelvis and spermatic cord. Surg Gynecol Obstet 1946;83:575.
4. Tobin CE. The renal fascia and its relation to the transversalis fascia. Anat Rec 1944;89:295.
5. Meyers MA, Whalen JP, Peelle K, et al. Radiologic features of extraperitoneal effusions. Radiology 1972;104:249.
6. Stevenson EOS, Ozeran RS. Retroperitoneal space abscesses. Surg Gynecol Obstet 1969;128:1202.
7. Hinman F. Atlas of urosurgical anatomy. Philadelphia: WB Saunders, 1993.
8. Kabalin JN. Surgical anatomy of the genitourinary tract: anatomy of the retroperitoneum and kidney. In: Walsh PC, Retik AB, Stamey TA, et al., eds. Campbell's urology. 6th ed. Philadelphia: WB Saunders, 1992:3.
9. Nagamatsu GR, Lerman PH, Berman MH. The dorsolumbar flap incision in urologic surgery. J Urol 1952;67:787.

Adrenal

Surgery of the Adrenal Gland

John P. Donohue

Any discussion of surgery of the adrenal gland is best preceded by a review of the diagnosis and pathophysiology of its surgical diseases according to their origin from either the cortex or medulla. Details of the surgical approach may then follow in the same logical sequence.

DIAGNOSIS OF SURGICALLY TREATABLE ADRENAL DISORDERS

Adrenal Cortex

Adrenocortical lesions are classified according to their distinctive hormonal manifestation resulting from the hyperfunction of the specialized cells of the zona glomerulosa, zona fasciculata, and zona reticularis of the adrenal cortex.

Aldosteronism

Primary aldosteronism is characterized by hypertension secondary to inappropriate excessive production of aldosterone by the zona glomerulosa of the adrenal cortex. As a result, it is associated with suppression of plasma renin activity, hypokalemia, and metabolic alkalosis. Although primary aldosteronism here refers to the functional adrenal adenoma, it can also be caused by bilateral micronodular hyperplasia of zona glomerulosa cells. This condition is believed to occur in about 20% of the patients with chemical aldosteronism (1).

Diagnosis. A major clinical feature is benign hypertension, usually in the absence of severe vascular disease. Urinary aldosterone and potassium excretion are elevated; likewise, plasma aldosterone is elevated, but serum potassium is reduced. Although relative hypervolemia exists (secondary to increased sodium resorption at the proximal tubules in exchange for potassium), hypernatremia is only mild and metabolic alkalosis is often not severe. Both normokalemic and nonalkalotic forms have also been recognized. Patients are usually between 30 and 60 years of age. Few children have been reported as having aldosteronism. The most common symptom is relative muscle weakness, and the most common sign is hypertension.

The key to establishing the diagnosis is finding elevated urinary and plasma aldosterone together with unprovoked hypokalemia. The other major criterion for diagnosis is suppression of renal renin production. The two most reliable tests for primary aldosteronism are:

1. Failure to suppress aldosterone output during sodium loading (saline suppression test, i.e., 2 L over 2 to 3 hours), and
2. Failure to stimulate plasma renin activity, even in the presence of sodium deprivation (negative furosemide stimulation test) (Table 2.1).

Therefore, the sine qua non of the diagnosis of primary aldosteronism is failure to suppress plasma aldosterone after saline loading (2 L in 3 hours) and failure of plasma renin activity to be stimulated by salt and volume depletion (40 mg furosemide every 8 hours, 10 meq sodium diet for 24 hours, and 2 hours of ambulation). These rigid criteria positively identified some 125 patients with primary aldosteronism and surgically removed adrenal adenomas.

Once the diagnosis of aldosteronism is confirmed by a negative saline (aldosterone) suppression test and a negative furosemide (renin) stimulation test, the next step is localization of the disease. In the author's experience, the two best localizing techniques are adrenal venous blood collections for aldosterone (with cortisol levels as a check on the accuracy of the sample) and adrenal venography (2).

Treatment. Surgical treatment is best reserved for those patients whose conditions are diagnosed as unilateral disease (3). The differential adrenal venous sampling and venography can provide diagnostic accuracy in more than 90% of patients. Those with bilateral hyperplasia (excessive aldosterone production from both adrenals in the absence of any adenoma noted on venography) are best treated medically with spironolactone orally, ranging from 100 to 400 mg a day.

Cushing's Syndrome

Cushing's syndrome is a general term referring to the clinical presentation of corticosteroid excess. This condition can be pro-

Table 2.1.   Tests for Diagnosis of Adrenal Surgical Diseases

TESTS	ALDOSTERONISM	CUSHING'S SYNDROME	VIRILIZATION	PHEOCHROMOCYTOMA	NEUROBLASTOMA	1°/2° CARCINOMA	INCIDENTAL ADENOMA
Plasma renin activity (PRA)	+						−
Lasix stimulation (PRA, Aldo)	−						−
Serum electrolytes (K$^+$, CO$_2$)	+						−
Plasma aldosterone (PA)	+						−
Urine aldosterone (UA)	+						−
Differential adrenal venous samples (diff. adr. VV)	+	±					−
Isotopic scan (19-iodo cholesterol)	+	+					+
Isotopic scan (M-BIG)				+			
Computed tomography (CT scan)	+	+	+	+	+	+	+
Magnetic resonance imaging (MRI)				+			
Plasma cortisol (OHC)		+	+				−
Plasma 17-ketosteroids (17-Ketos)			+				
Serum testosterone (T)			+				
Fractionated ketosteroids (Fr. Ketos)			+				
Pregnanetriols (S. Pregnt.)			+				−
Clonidine suppression test				+			−
Catecholamines (VMA, HVA)				+			−
Serum norepinephrine (NE)				+	+		−
Serum epinephrine (E)				+	+		−
Urine norepinephrine (U/NE)				+	+		−
Urine epinephrine (U/E)				+	+		−
Selective venous IVC/SVC samples				+			
Whole lung tomography (WLTs)					+	+	
Skull, sella x-ray incl. CT scan		+					
Bone scan, incl. skeletal survey					+	+	
Angiography		+		+			
Selective basilar venous samples (ACTH)		+					
Serum ACTH		+					−
Dexamethasone suppression		+					−

duced by the administration of glucocorticoid or can occur naturally from several pathologic dysfunctional states (3–6). A basophilic pituitary adenoma was originally described by Harvey Cushing as the cause of the syndrome (7). However, this adenoma is responsible for about 75 to 80% of the syndrome presentations. Other causes include adrenal tumors producing excess cortisol and other benign or malignant tumors producing adrenocorticotropic hormone (ACTH) (8–12).

Diagnosis. The clinical presentation is classic. Prominent findings are truncal obesity with peripheral extremity muscle wasting out of keeping with the central obesity. Plethora, hypertension, and increased bruising and striae are also distinctive features. In women, hirsutism and amenorrhea may be present. On physical examination, the classic moon facies and buffalo hump are well known. The moon facies is caused by an increased size of cheek fat pads. Because the changes are often subtle, old photographs are helpful in recognizing them. Hypertension is almost always present. Renin profiles are generally low because vascular volume is expanded. Major problems with long-term corticosteroid excess are infections and cardiovascular accidents from chronic hypertension.

Laboratory findings vary with the cause of the syndrome. Cushing's syndrome, caused by pituitary adenoma, is associated with elevated plasma ACTH (normal, 95 ± 12 pg/mL). In Cushing's disease, these values are roughly doubled to 164 ± 19 pg/mL. Elevated fasting blood sugar is seen late in the disease, but a diabetic-type glucose tolerance curve is commonly present due to excess production of glucocorticoid. Adrenal computed tomography (CT) scans reveal bilateral symmetric enlargement of the adrenals. Confirmation of pituitary Cushing's syndrome requires demonstration of increased production of corticosteroids by the adrenals and increased production of ACTH from the anterior pituitary. This can be proved by demonstration of increased urinary and plasma cortisol, increased plasma ACTH and corticosteroid suppression with synthetic corticosteroids such as dexamethasone, and administration of blockers of corticosteroid synthesis such as metyrapone (13). Failure to suppress corticosteroids with low-dose dexamethasone (1 mg), but successful suppression with high-dose dexamethasone (4 mg) can be taken as evidence of pituitary-dependent Cushing's disease. The ability of metyrapone to inhibit the synthesis of corticosteroid by blocking 11-hydroxylation also makes it a useful diagnostic tool. As 11-hydroxylation is blocked, substance "S" is produced instead of cortisol. Patients with Cushing's disease of pituitary origin have an increased production of substance "S" because of their hyperplastic glands. They also have an increased ability to produce corticosteroids when stimulated by ACTH. The metyrapone stimulation test is useful in discriminating the pituitary-dependent Cushing's disease when there is a hyperactive response from adrenal tumors with a failure to respond (14). Patients with ectopic ACTH production also fail to respond to metyrapone stimulation. A single-dose test is carried out by administering 30 mg/kg at midnight and measuring plasma levels of substance "S," cortisol, and ACTH at 8:00 AM the following morning (14).

Cushing's syndrome caused by benign adenomas is best proved by measuring elevated plasma cortisol values with loss of diurnal curve, i.e., persistently elevated plasma values even in the afternoon and evening. In patients with a primary adrenal disorder, i.e., glucocorticoid excess secondary to tumor, ACTH is suppressed. Furthermore, failure to suppress plasma cortisol with both the 1- and 4-mg doses of dexamethasone is a characteristic feature of the adrenal tumor. Once these chemical values are confirmed, further diagnostic studies should include arteriography (many of these tumors can be quite large with massive and variable blood supply), administration of radioactive cholesterol (^{131}I-C19), ultrasonograms, and CT scans. Usually, differential venous collections and venography are not necessary to localize these tumors. CT scans are helpful in localizing small adrenal adenomas in the 2-cm range. Most secretory adrenocortical adenomas are associated with hyperaldosteronism. Of 85 cases reviewed, 13 were associated with Cushing's syndrome, 65 with aldosteronism, and 7 with inappropriate virilization (15). In one series, 149 patients with Cushing's syndrome were analyzed (16); 121 of these cases were associated with bilateral hyperplasia and presumably extra-adrenal pituitary stimulation, 13 were caused by primary adrenal adenoma, and 15 by adrenal carcinoma. Therefore, about 20% of patients with Cushing's syndrome will have primary adrenal tumors, either adenoma or carcinoma.

Treatment. The treatment of this condition is directed toward the primary dysfunction. Adrenalectomy is indicated in the 20% of cases that are caused by primary adrenal tumors. It is very important to identify and localize the source of excess corticosteroid production. Localization techniques that are most practical are CT scan, radioisotopic study with C-19 ^{131}I, and arteriography (in the event of a large tumor).

Virilizing Tumors

Adrenal hirsutism and virilization may come from a variety of causes including congenital deficiencies in steroid production (congenital adrenal hyperplasia), adrenal tumors, Cushing's syndrome secondary to increased ACTH production by the pituitary, ovarian tumors, polycystic ovaries, or ill-defined variants thereof. Hirsutism is most commonly idiopathic (17).

Diagnosis. Virilizing adrenal tumors in women are characterized by amenorrhea, hirsutism, deep voice, increased muscle mass, enlargement of the clitoris, and sometimes a decrease in breast size. In prepubertal boys, such tumors may produce precocious puberty, early-onset prostatic enlargement, pubic axillary hair, and beard growth. The testes remain small. In the more adult male, tumors may be recognized only as space-occupying lesions or by their metastases. These tumors must be differentiated from congenital adrenal hyperplasia, idiopathic hirsutism, Cushing's syndrome, and other ovarian diseases.

Generally, adrenal tumors do not produce much testosterone, but ovarian tumors do. Fractionated ketosteroids and measurement of dehydroepiandrosterone elevations are helpful. Testosterone elevations are more likely to be gonadal in origin. In addition, other major androgen precursors, such as delta-5-pregnenolone, progesterone, and 17-hydroxyprogesterone, may be elevated. Most virilizing adrenal tumors are not suppressible by administration of dexamethasone. They also fail to increase secretion in response to ACTH administration. Localization by adrenal radioisotope scanning (18), CT scans, and sometimes venography, arteriography, and ultrasonography is useful. Usually, if a solitary benign tumor can be located and removed, the prognosis is good. Large tumors are often malignant, however, and prognostic advice to the patient should be guarded.

Adrenal Medulla

Pheochromocytoma

Pheochromocytomas have been found along the distribution of chromaffin tissue, which is laid down during fetal development and has mostly disappeared by late childhood. The largest accumulations of chromaffin tissue are in the adrenal medulla and in the organ of Zuckerkandl at the origin of the inferior mesenteric artery. Most pheochromocytomas are located between the diaphragm and pelvic floor (19–22). In the sporadic, nonfamilial pheochromocytoma, about 80% of tumors involve a single adrenal, 10% are extra-adrenal, and 10% are malignant. For this reason, they are sometimes referred to as the "10% tumors" (23). In children, they may be called the "30% tumors" (24). The catecholamines norepinephrine (NE) and epinephrine (E) are synthesized from the precursor amino acid tyrosine. The enzyme phenylethylamine *N*-methyl transferase (PNMT) converts NE to E; this is almost exclusively a property of the adrenal medulla (85% of adrenal catecholamine is epinephrine). Although most pheochromocytomas arise in the adrenal medulla, most tumors secrete primarily NE. If, however, it is determined that there is predominant secretion of E, then the tumor is almost invariably located in the adrenal. A purely E-secreting tumor is extremely uncommon and difficult to diagnose because hypertension is minimal; in fact, the presenting symptom in some patients is shock.

The variable complex of symptoms experienced by a patient with a pheochromocytoma probably mostly reflects the proportion of NE to E secreted. Symptoms stem more from secretion of E, whereas NE determines the level of hypertension. Nearly all patients have troublesome headaches; excessive sweating is almost as common. Other symptoms are palpitations, episodes of uneasiness or anxiety, pallor, flushing, weakness, nausea, tremor, chest pain, shortness of breath, and abdominal cramps. As is well known, any one patient's combination of symptoms occurs in "spells," which may appear related to precipitating events such as smoking, sexual intercourse, pressure on the abdomen, and defecation. Symptoms precipitated by micturition denote a urinary bladder location for the pheochromocytoma. Although the hypertension is famous for its paroxysmal nature, probably more than 50% of patients have sustained hypertension. An orthostatic decrease in blood pressure in an untreated hypertensive patient suggests the diagnosis of pheochromocytoma. (This finding is also suggestive of primary aldosteronism.) In some patients, the single clue to the existence of a pheochromocytoma is a hypertensive crisis associated with pregnancy, the administration of a general anesthetic, surgery, or the use of certain drugs. Drugs like morphine, ACTH, parenteral guanethidine, or parenteral methyldopa may release catecholamines from the tumor, whereas propranolol may increase the pressor response to circulating E.

Diagnosis. The diagnosis of pheochromocytoma is made from outpatient biochemical tests. Three kinds of measurements are made in urine: vanillylmandelic acid (VMA), total metanephrines (normetanephrine and metanephrine), and free catecholamines. These tests provide meaningful information, are available to any physician, and are nearly equal in their sensitivity and specificity. If all three are carried out simultaneously, 95% of pheochromocytomas will be detected. The urine must be kept acidic by prior addition of hydrochloric acid or acetic acid to the collection container.

The quantitation of catecholamines in plasma was formerly carried out by fluorometric methods, procedures that required meticulous technique and large plasma samples and that frequently provided inaccurate results. A major advance in this area was the development of the radioenzymatic assay for measurement of catecholamines. Plasma is incubated with an enzyme that transfers a ^{3}H-containing methyl group from S-adenosylmethionine (SAM) to the catecholamine. The radiolabeled catecholamine is then isolated, and the radioactivity is counted. The radioenzymatic assay used at Indiana University School of Medicine (developed by D. P. Henry) uses the enzyme PNMT to transfer a ^{3}H-methyl group from SAM to NE to produce ^{3}HE. Using this assay at the same institution, researchers have taken measurements of plasma NE and the urinary excretion of NE, including excretion measured in an easily collected morning urine sample ("sleep NE"), and have clearly delineated patients with pheochromocytoma from other hypertensive patients. NE can be measured in plasma samples from multiple sites of venous drainage to find a tumor whose location has been elusive (25).

The radioenzymatic assay is having an important effect on investigative studies of the sympathoadrenal system, and it appears that it may in part revise our approach to the diagnosis of pheochromocytoma. Similar assays are under evaluation from important metabolites of catecholamines in plasma, which may further increase our diagnostic accuracy (26, 27).

The clonidine suppression test is another useful aid in the diagnosis of pheochromocytoma (28). Plasma catecholamines are normally increased through the activation of the sympathetic nervous system. In pheochromocytoma, however, they arise through synthesis by the tumor itself. The excess diffusion into the plasma bypasses normal storage and release mecha-

nisms. Clonidine decreases resting plasma catecholamines by inhibition of centrally mediated adrenergic influences. Because of this central blocking effect, clonidine does not suppress catecholamine release in pheochromocytoma. This fact is useful when making a diagnosis in patients with essential hypertension whose catecholamine release is thought to be neurogenically mediated but not mediated by tumor. Clonidine should suppress the catecholamine release in essential hypertensives by blocking the central neurogenic release mechanisms. This phenomenon is particularly helpful because clonidine suppression does not occur (i.e., plasma epinephrine and norepinephrine values are not suppressed) in patients with pheochromocytoma. This test is fairly specific (i.e., few false-positive results). It is an adjunctive test that is useful in patients with elevated catecholamines who need to be distinguished from those with essential hypertension.

When the diagnosis of pheochromocytoma is firmly established, the next step is to try to find its location. Occasionally, an intravenous pyelogram shows the tumor. In the author's experience, CT scans can delineate most adrenal pheochromocytomas. In the past, the tumor was located by arteriography. (This procedure has been replaced, however, by the safer isotopic scanning with 131-MIBG) (26, 27). Knowing where the tumor resides and the anatomy of its blood supply may allow the surgeon to plan the approach in a more efficient manner.

Arteriography is not particularly dangerous when carried out by an experienced radiologist and when patients are pretreated with phenoxybenzamine, an alpha-adrenergic receptor-blocking drug that has contributed greatly to the management of patients with pheochromocytoma. The dosage of phenoxybenzamine is determined by the antihypertensive response, and treatment should continue for at least 1 week before adequate receptor blockade is achieved. Total protection against spikes in blood pressure is not possible. During arteriography and surgery, preparations should be made for the administration of intravenous phenoxybenzamine (and propranolol if problematic tachycardia or arrhythmias occur). Use of propranolol should be limited to situations where alpha blockade has already been established.

Improved CT techniques have greatly simplified the diagnosis (i.e., localization) of pheochromocytoma. Despite these improvements, multiple, asymptomatic, or metastatic pheochromocytomas have remained difficult to locate because prior imaging techniques were nonspecific. The advent of the radiopharmaceutic agent 131-MIBG permits scintigraphic localization based on functional principles. This agent resembles norepinephrine in molecular structure; it is thought to enter adrenergic tissue by the same mechanism as the pressor amine itself. Incorporation in medullary tissue metabolic pathways localizes the isotope effectively for scanning. It has special value in localizing multiple, metastatic, or asymptomatic tumors.

Familial Pheochromocytomas

The characteristics of familial pheochromocytomas differ in some ways from those of the more common sporadic type. Fifty percent of familial tumors are bilateral, yet extra-adrenal locations almost never occur. The familial pheochromocytoma is more likely to secrete epinephrine. In some instances, this may be the only biochemical abnormality, which can make the condition difficult to diagnose. These tumors usually occur as part of well-recognized syndromes.

Multiple endocrine adenomatosis type II (MEA-II) or Sipple's syndrome consists of pheochromocytoma, medullary thyroid carcinoma, and primary hyperparathyroidism. Pheochromocytoma is not associated with MEA-I (pituitary, pancreatic, and parathyroid tumors); only hyperparathyroidism is common to MEA-I and MEA-II. A small percentage of patients with von Recklinghausen's neurofibromatosis and von Hippel-Lindau's cerebellar hemangioblastomatosis will have pheochromocytomas.

Neuroblastoma

This tumor, although often adrenal in origin, is the subject of Chapter 44.

Primary Adrenal Carcinoma

Primary adrenocortical carcinoma is relatively uncommon, with a frequency of about 2 per 1,000,000 per year. Although these tumors carry a generally poor prognosis, cure can be achieved with complete surgical resection in those who present early enough without metastases. Five-year cure rates of 25 to 40% are seen in those patients with the primary tumor thought to be completely resected.

Staging has three levels. Stage I refers to tumor confined to the adrenal gland with no evidence of local or distant spread. Stage II refers to direct extension of tumor into adjacent tissues or spread to the regional lymph nodes. Stage III indicates distant metastases. The most common sites of metastases are liver, lung, peritoneum or pleura, lymph nodes, and renal and venous (i.e., renal venous or vena cava) involvement. Other common points of involvement are bone, pancreas, brain, and direct extension into diaphragm, pancreas, or small intestine.

About 50% of patients who present with low-stage primary adrenal carcinoma have their tumors completely resected surgically. The remaining patients do less well. The 5-year survival rate for stage I is about 50%, for stage II about 15%, and for stage III about 5%.

Adrenal carcinoma is associated with several hormonal presentations, which are about evenly distributed. One of the common presentations is Cushing's syndrome with corticosteroid excess. Inappropriate secretion of ketogenic steroids is also well known in carcinomas.

There is no useful chemotherapeutic program for this disease. Although some considered Orthopara-DDD for metastatic disease because of its destructive effect on the adrenal cortex, its clinical usefulness has largely been unproven.

Secondary adrenal carcinomas result from metastatic hematogenous spread, generally from breast or lung. Renal cell carcinoma can directly involve the adrenal, as does a rare case of ureteral or even testicular carcinoma. These are usually postmortem discoveries. Occasionally, a clinical decision must be made for a person who has had a single primary tumor treated successfully some years earlier. In such a case, it is appropriate to remove the adrenal if this is the only clinically evident tumor.

Incidental Tumors

Nonfunctioning adenomas represent one of the more interesting clinical situations in recent years. Their management is based on evidence of functional activity that is excessive. Critical tests relate to ruling out aldosteronism and Cushing's disease. It is also reasonable to screen for ketogenic steroid excess, although this condition would rarely be present. Table 2.1 indicates the appropriate screening studies, for which all results will be negative.

One of the important considerations in the nonfunctioning adenoma is the relationship of size and clinical behavior. In general, adenomas smaller than 2 cm that are nonfunctional can be followed safely with serial ultrasound and CT examina-

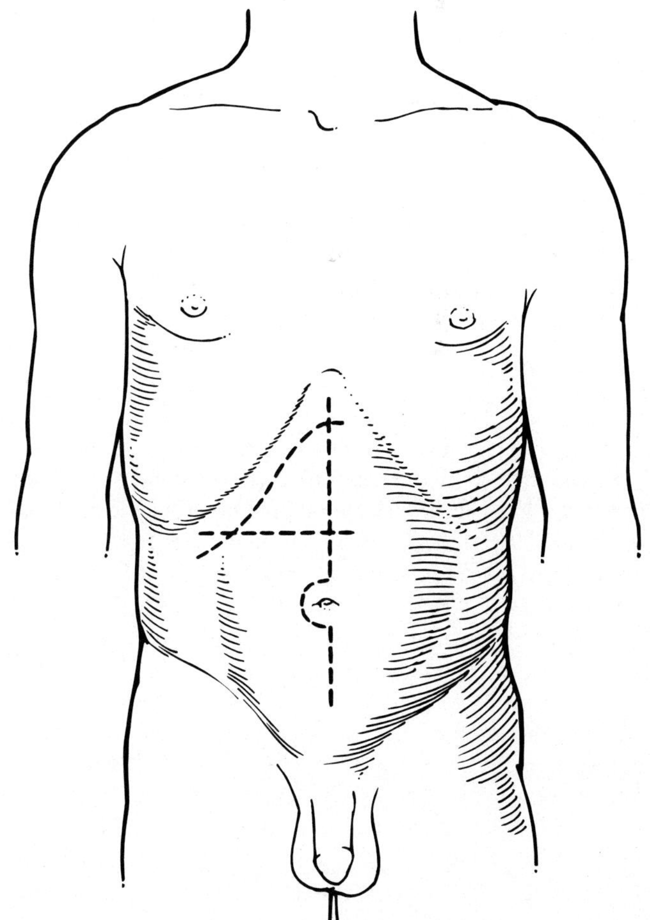

Fig. 2.1. Midline, transverse, or subcostal incisions are suitable for approach to retroperitoneal tumors including adrenal tumors.

tions. If there is evidence of any rapid growth exceeding 3 cm, adrenal resection is indicated. On the other hand, it is known that most will remain stable and, if there is no evidence of growth or functional activity, such patients can be followed safely. It is well known from Conn's early work (29), and that derived from the Thorndike Laboratories, that about 5% of postmortem examinations will reveal some adrenal corticoadenomatous growth; hence, the rather exaggerated predictions by Conn many years ago about the true instance of aldosteronism.

There is an interesting parallel between the renal corticoadenoma and the adrenal corticoadenoma. Growth kinetics suggest that beyond a certain critical mass, tumors must be considered malignant although they may well have a similar histologic appearance when grossly smaller. A 1-cm renal cortical adenoma may well have the same histologic features as a well-differentiated renal carcinoma. The same extrapolation holds true for the adrenal. A 1-cm cortical adenoma is invariably benign, yet a 10-cm cortical tumor is invariably malignant. The change from a well-differentiated smaller tumor to a usually poorly differentiated large tumor involves many deregulation factors currently under study. In any case, the nonfunctioning adenoma that is less than 2 cm is generally followed expectantly, and a patient with any tumor larger than 2.5 cm is considered a reasonable candidate for surgery (30).

SURGICAL APPROACHES AND TECHNIQUES

Surgery for Aldosteronism

In the usual case, the approach is dorsal. With the patient in the prone position, the pyelograms are reviewed and the suitable rib is chosen for subperiosteal excision. Usually this is the 12th rib, or the 11th rib in a large patient, particularly on the left. The rib is removed as proximal as possible near its articulation to facilitate exposure (Figs. 2.1, 2.2, and 2.3).

A key point in exposure of the adrenal through the dorsal route is the caudal mobilization of the kidney and adrenal without entering Gerota's fascia. With a hand or sponge stick placed medial and caudad in the apex of the wound, the kidney and other contents within Gerota's fascia can be drawn posteriorly and laterally. Such posterolateral retraction of the kidney allows separation of the superior aspect of the adrenal from the diaphragm and hepatic structures on the right and the pancreas on the left. Very gentle dissection with forceps is satisfactory before Harrington or malleable retractors are placed on the liver or pancreas. Narrow or broad Deaver retractors are sometimes useful medially. Vascular clips and silk ligatures are used for proximal traction on the adrenal. The structures are tied in continuity with 2-0 black silk on the proximal or gland side (Fig. 2.4). Vascular clips are used on the body wall or renal

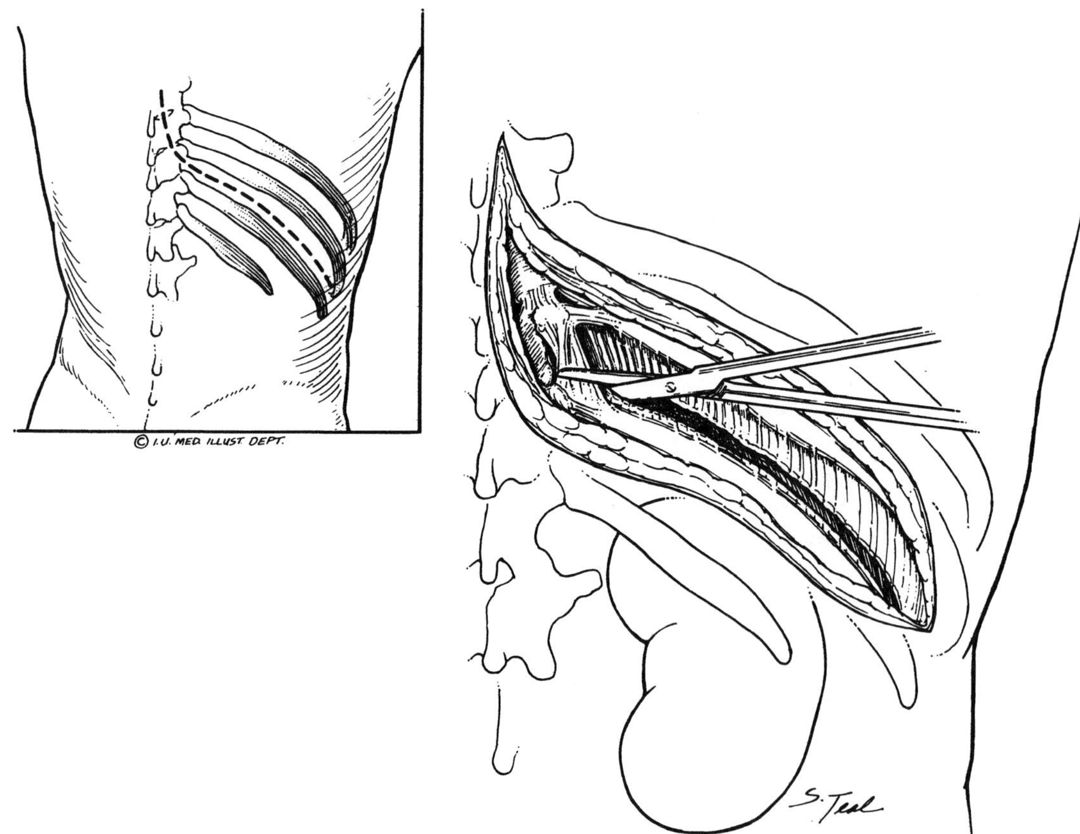

Fig. 2.2.   A key component of the dorsal approach is incision of the costovertebral ligament. This incision can be done under vision or blindly by palpation, incising medially on the superior surface of the rib to the level of the vertebra. The key is to stay on the superior and dorsal aspect of the rib and to divide the ligamentous attachments sharply with heavy scissors or a diathermic blade.

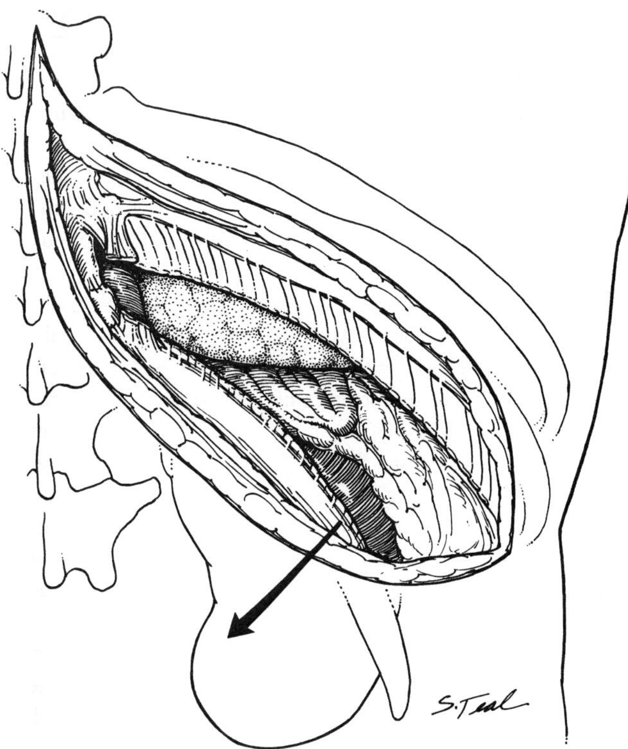

Fig. 2.3. The rib can be retracted inferiorly with ease once the costovertebral ligaments have been divided. This approach greatly widens the aperture necessary for good retraction and exposure.

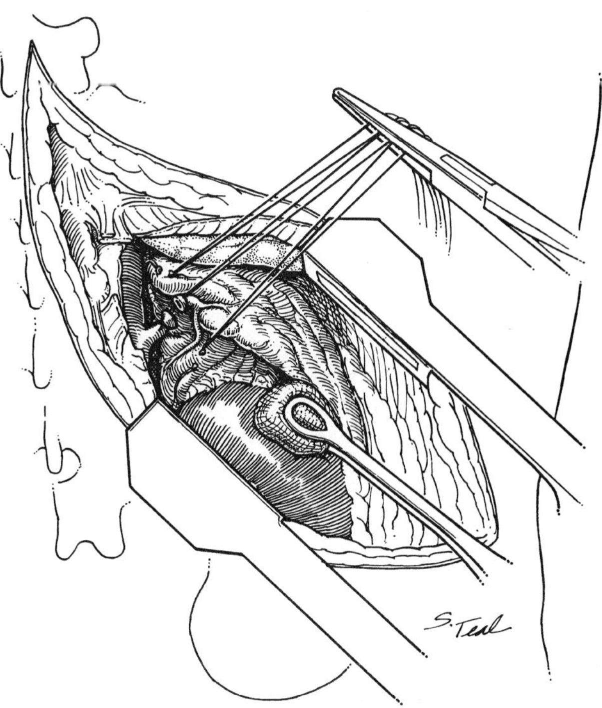

Fig. 2.4. After placement of a self-retaining retractor, the kidney is retracted caudad with a sponge stick. Ties can be placed on the medial, i.e., adrenal aspect and cut and divided on the great vessel side of the dissection. This is a useful method for manipulation of the gland through this small incision.

side. This technique allows meticulous dissection without blood loss. Every effort must be made not to manipulate the gland itself. Any rough movements can cause swelling within the gland and subsequent difficulty identifying adenomas. Even slight spillage of blood into tissue planes may obscure the edges of the gland. If spillage occurs, copious irrigation can be used to clean off tissue planes.

The common adrenal vein is often the last portion of the dissection, particularly when one is mobilizing the right adrenal. Once the gland has been fully mobilized, the common right adrenal vein is secured between 2-0 silk ligatures. When the vein is more apical, its early division and removal provide better glandular mobilization. Should venous length be a problem, one can doubly clip the venous structures on either side and divide between them. Usually, with gentle elevation, one can achieve enough length for double ligatures (Fig. 2.4).

If the pleural cavity has been entered, both the parietal and diaphragmatic closures are made with nonabsorbable sutures. Air in the pleural space is evacuated through a small red rubber catheter. During positive pressure lung inflation, the tube is removed. Normally a chest tube is not necessary postoperatively. The only special consideration postoperatively is the need to follow serum potassium determinations twice a day for the first several days. Hyperkalemia secondary to suppression of the contralateral zona glomerulosa is rare. For the same reason, replacement therapy with mineralocorticoids has not been necessary. More than 80% of patients become normotensive within

several weeks postoperatively. When a unilateral adenoma is clearly localized, a good result can be expected from surgery (3–6).

Surgery for Cushing's Disease

Once the diagnosis has been established and a primary adrenocortical tumor has been revealed as the cause of excess cortisol secretion (as opposed to pituitary tumor with excess ACTH production with bilateral adrenocortical hyperplasia), removal of the tumor-bearing adrenal is the treatment of choice.

It must be emphasized that preoperative preparation requires tissue fixation of corticosteroids. Therefore, cortisone acetate, 50 mg 4 times a day, is recommended for at least 1 if not 2 days preoperatively. The rate of return of adrenal secretion by the contralateral suppressed adrenal cortex is variable. Therefore, intraoperative corticosteroids are essential, and gradual tapering over 1 week to a base level of 30 mg of cortisol per day maintenance is a reasonable therapeutic trial. Then gradual tapering to levels as low as 10 to 15 mg a day can be attempted. Weakness, fatigue, hypotension, and hyponatremia are clues that replacement is inadequate.

Technique

The small adrenal adenoma producing Cushing's syndrome can be treated by the dorsal approach as described earlier for primary aldosteronism. However, larger tumors, if localized to one side, are best approached through a transverse upper abdominal or thoracoabdominal incision (12).

Transabdominal approach. Most surgeons prefer a transverse incision extending across both rectus muscles to the tip of the 12th rib or resecting the distal 12th rib. To expose the right adrenal, the liver and gallbladder are retracted cephalad. The distal stomach, duodenum, and hepatic flexure of the colon are retracted medially. Occasionally hepatic and colonic adhesions must be divided. The posterior peritoneum can be reflected medially after incising the mesocolon and separating it from the anterior aspect of Gerota's fascia (Fig. 2.5). Retraction of the duodenum and head of the pancreas medially (Kocher maneuver) is helpful in gaining exposure of the right adrenal (Fig. 2.6). Gentle caudad retraction of the upper pole of the kidney aids in the dissection of the right adrenal gland. The key to the dissection is thorough mobilization of the inferior vena cava and right renal venous structures so that the adrenal gland can be mobilized from the vena cava to obtain superior exposure. The vena cava can be retracted medially in this area using vein retractors. Clips and silk ligatures are useful in dividing fatty nerve or small arterial structures surrounding the gland. Ligatures on the proximal glandular side assist in gentle traction, and the cava can be retracted medially to expose the common

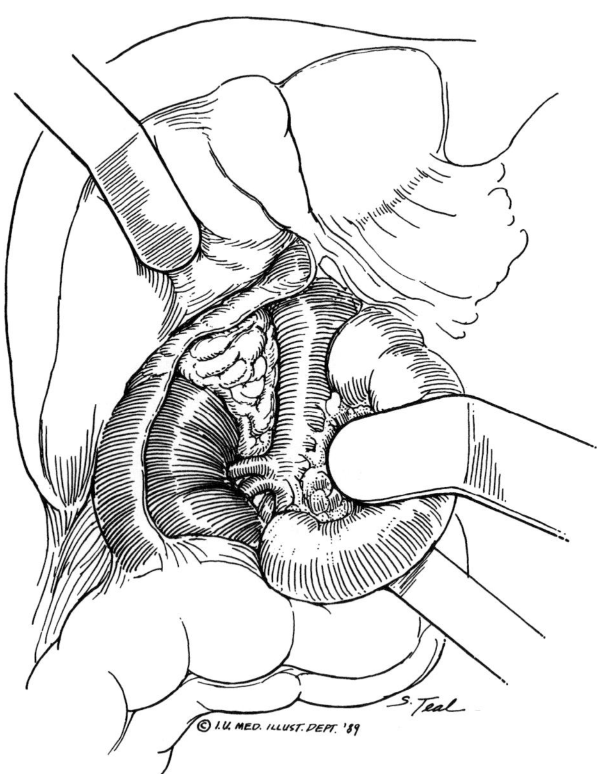

Fig. 2.6. The Kocher maneuver permits mobilization of the duodenum and the head of the pancreas (pictured in the retractor) medially. This exposes the vena cava and the hilar aspect of the kidney and adrenal.

right adrenal vein. In larger tumors, exposure of the common right adrenal vein may require dissection of the caudate lobe of the liver. Deep Harrington retractors are useful in this hepatic retraction when necessary.

The left adrenal is more accessible when approached through the abdomen. One approach is to incise the mesentery of the transverse colon to the left of the middle colic artery and then to expose the left renal vein just below this (Fig. 2.7). This procedure is useful if the patient is thin and the tumor is not large. However, in larger patients or in those with big tumors, if one is working transabdominally, it is better either to reflect the colon, spleen, and pancreas medially (Fig. 2.8) or to simply incise the gastrocolic ligament and enter the lesser peritoneal sac. The posterior peritoneum is then incised, exposing the adrenal directly below. The adrenal vasculature can then be easily divided between clips or ligatures as the gland is displaced laterally and medially. If the gastrocolic approach is used, the stomach and pancreas must be retracted medially and cephalad, the duodenum medially, and the colon laterally and inferiorly. For larger tumors it is safer if the mesocolon and lineophrenic ligaments are divided all the way around, sometimes even as high and medial as the gastroesophageal hiatus. This approach allows the spleen, colon, and pancreas to be reflected medially and anteriorly off Gerota's fascia to expose any large tumor below. In addition, this approach gives excellent exposure of the upper abdominal aorta, medial diaphragm,

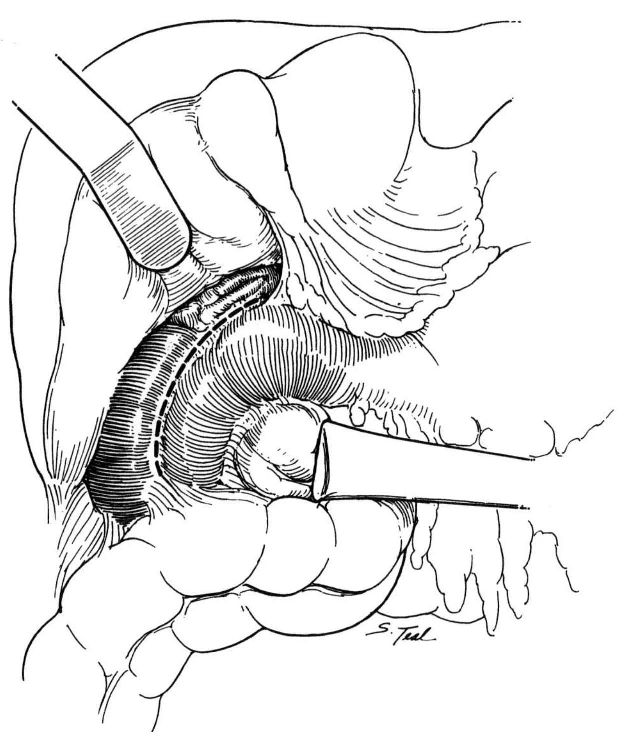

Fig. 2.5. The line of incision for the Kocher maneuver is lateral to the duodenum. The hepatic flexure of the colon is first retracted medially to demonstrate the first and second portions of the duodenum. The posterior incision begins at the foramen of Winslow and is carried down to the turn of the duodenum in its third portion.

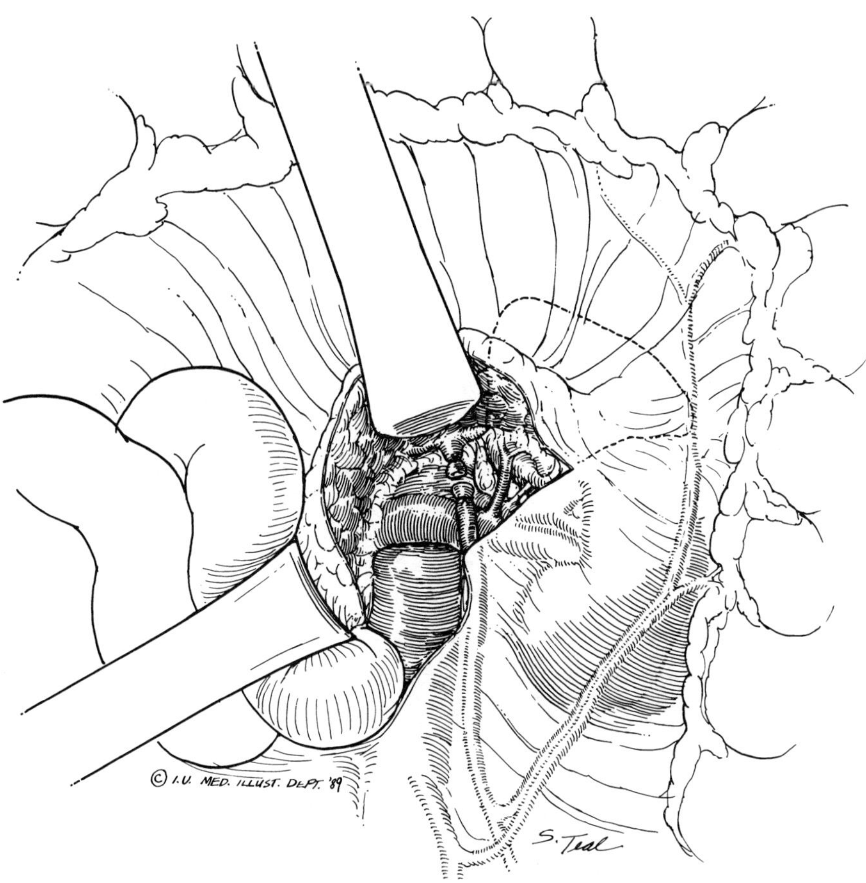

Fig. 2.7.   Approach through the root of the small bowel with division of the inferior mesenteric vein to better expose the left renal hilum and adrenal vessels. This technique has long been used to facilitate suprahilar dissection in retroperitoneal lymphadenectomies done through the anterior approach.

celiac and superior mesenteric vessels, and crus of the diaphragm. Vascular control is more secure with this technique.

Thoracoabdominal approach.   Another approach to the adrenal tumor is the lumbar extraperitoneal or thoracoabdominal incision (Fig. 2.9). An incision is made at the level of the 11th or 12th rib and the diaphragm and pleura are incised. On the left side, the spleen and colon are mobilized medially in their peritoneal envelope using blunt and sharp dissection. Then Gerota's fascia is exposed and the renal vein is identified. On the left, the common adrenal vein can usually be secured early and the tumor mobilized between clips or ligatures off the kidney and medial aspect of the diaphragm (Fig. 2.10). Various crural attachments and the inferior phrenic vascular supply are easily mobilized and divided. Some direct aortic or renal arterial communications are also encountered, but these are usually small and well visualized in advance, provided the usual care is taken with exposure. After removal, the area is irrigated thoroughly and the peritoneal sac is simply dropped over the kidney, which has been allowed to resume its normal position. The wound is usually closed in layers with interrupted nonabsorbable suture material. The same principles apply on the right side. However, retraction of the liver off the anterior aspect of

Gerota's fascia below may require more careful sharp and blunt dissection. Usually we prefer to enter the abdomen rather than to remain extraperitoneal in right adrenal surgery simply because this approach facilitates the exposure of the high vena cava and posterior venous vascular contributions of the adrenal gland itself. The location of the adrenal on each side is more central than lateral. Therefore, there is little reason to try to remain extraperitoneal, particularly on the right side.

Surgery for Virilizing Tumors

Before any operative procedure for a virilizing adrenal tumor, the differential diagnostic steps to rule out idiopathic and/or iatrogenic cause must be taken (see the section on diagnosing virilizing tumors in this chapter). A good medical and family history is essential. Then differential chemistries and imaging studies can be done to rule out an ovarian cause as noted earlier. If the only lesion is an adrenal tumor, unilateral adrenalectomy is indicated.

The surgical approach to these tumors is the same as for the adrenal tumor causing Cushing's disease. Smaller tumors can be approached dorsally or by the lumbar routes. Larger tumors are best approached with large upper transverse incisions. Care

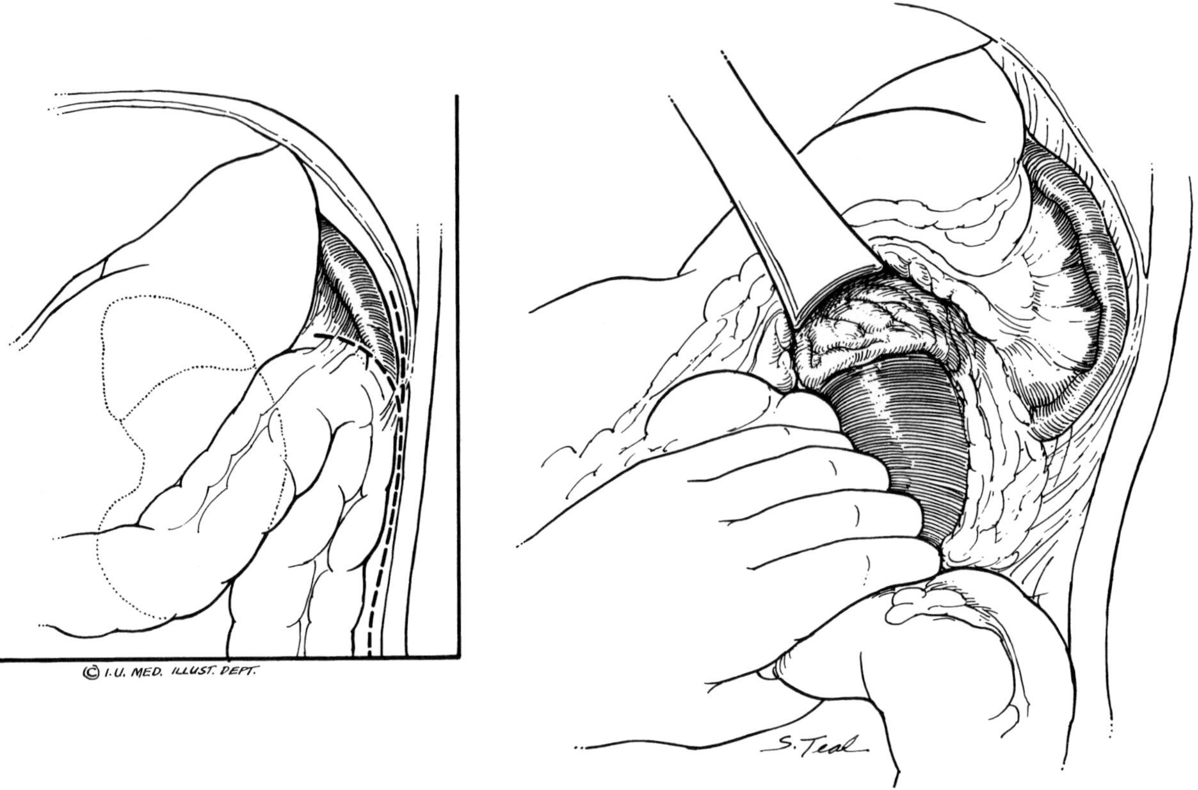

Fig. 2.8. Lateral approach to the left adrenal and the lines of paracolic incision, including lineocolic and lineophrenic attachments (inset). This approach permits retraction of the colon medially and retraction of the pancreas medially and cephalad to expose the underlying adrenal.

must be taken to obtain central vascular exposure using transabdominal techniques as noted earlier.

Surgery for Pheochromocytoma

Preparation for Surgery

In the operating room, a team approach consisting of internist, surgeon, and anesthesiologist is required. Preoperative treatment with phenoxybenzamine dampens or may even abolish the hypertensive episodes that can be associated primarily with induction of anesthesia and with handling of the tumor.

The adrenergic blockade created by phenoxybenzamine relieves the vasoconstrictor state produced by the excessive secretion of catecholamines and provides time before surgery for expansion of the vascular space.

Thus, the profound hypotension that may immediately follow removal of the pheochromocytoma is, for the most part, prevented. The management of the pheochromocytoma patient from the stage of tumor localization and throughout the perioperative period is not simple. It is the author's strong recommendation that these procedures be performed in hospitals where several similar cases are handled annually.

Surgical Approach

The transabdominal approach. The author's preference is a high abdominal transverse incision, the so-called chevron incision, extending from the tip of the 12th rib bilaterally up along the costal margins. Most bilateral adrenal exposures together with paravertebral examination are obtained with this approach.

To expose the right adrenal, the liver and gallbladder are retracted cephalad and the stomach and duodenum are drawn medially, after incision of the posterior peritoneum and development of the Kocher maneuver (Figs. 2.2 and 2.3). It is important to gently draw the kidney caudad and to develop and retract the inferior cava medially to obtain control of the right adrenal vein. It is also useful to identify and clip the small right adrenal arterial vessels as they arise from the origin of the right renal artery below the cava or directly from the aorta in this area.

The left adrenal gland may be exposed in the event of a small tumor by incising the posterior peritoneum and ligament of Treitz and ligating the inferior mesenteric vein and dividing it. This approach allows cephalad retraction of the body of the pancreas in a deep Harrington retractor. The adrenal is easily visualized just lateral to the superior mesenteric artery and medial to the upper pole of the left kidney. In most instances, the left adrenal vein is easily secured through this approach (Fig. 2.7, incision of the root of the small bowel and mobilization of the pancreas). If the left adrenal tumor is large, most prefer to incise the mesocolon and to divide the lineocolic and lineorenal attachments and again to mobilize the pancreas ceph-

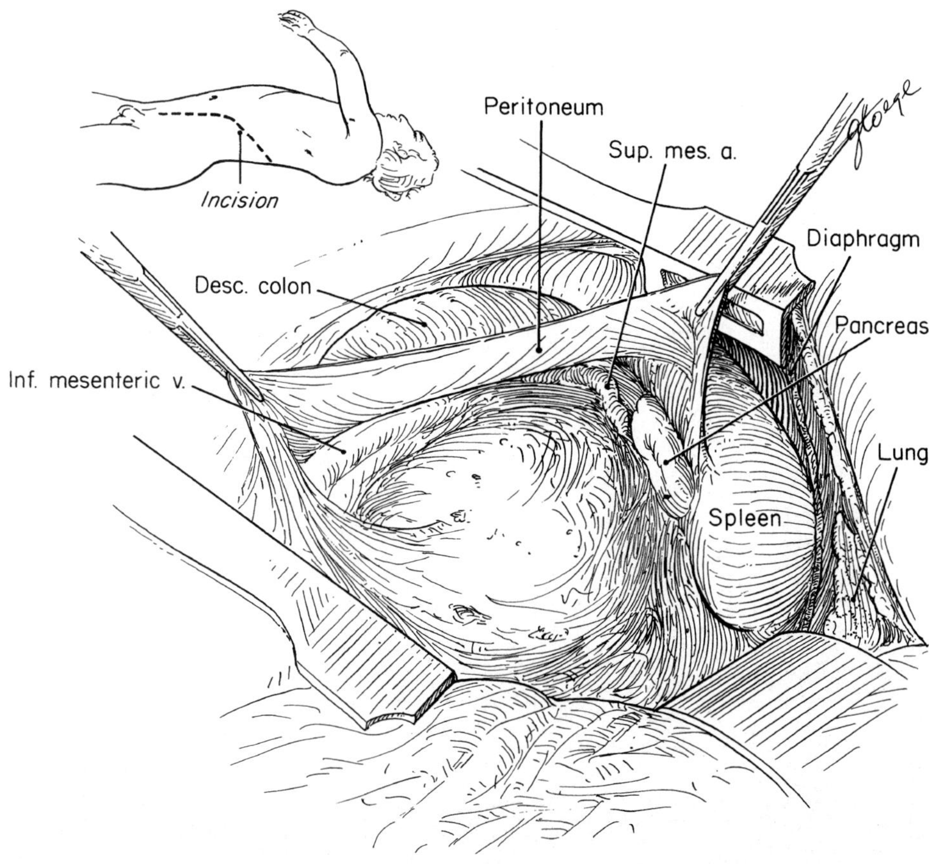

Fig. 2.9. Mobilization of the peritoneum off the underlying Gerota's fascia. The relationship of the inferior mesenteric artery, pancreas, and spleen is also shown. This approach is viewed from the left flank incision (inset).

alad (Fig. 2.8). If the left adrenal tumor is quite large, it is sometimes best to continue the incision of the mesocolon cephalad to include the lineophrenic attachments. Exposure is facilitated by continuing the posterior peritoneal incision above the spleen to the gastroesophageal hiatus. Then the spleen and pancreas can be mobilized in continuity cephalad and medially, thus exposing the entire upper retroperitoneal space. Occasionally, division of the short gastric vessels may be necessary to mobilize the adrenal completely out of the left upper quadrant (Figs. 2.7, 2.8).

Once exposed, the tumor is removed, with great care devoted to minimal manual pressure on the tumor itself. Ligatures and clips are preferred if possible, with gentle traction on proximal ligatures providing elevation of the tumor mass. With preoperative alpha blockade using phenoxybenzamine, this is somewhat less critical than it formerly was; nonetheless, it is still an important consideration to ensure stable blood pressure throughout the operation. Every effort is made to tie the adrenal vein first. Opportunities to clip and divide small adrenal artery branches early in the angle between the crus of the diaphragm and the renal artery should be encouraged. Once the essential vascular tributaries are divided and ligated, the tumor is gently elevated out of the wound. One should attempt to stay wide around the tumor capsule, even taking adjacent nodes and fat

to a moderate degree. Because 10% of these lesions are malignant, the author believes that wide excision is better than capsular or subcapsular enucleation.

Closure of the wound is generally with 0 nonabsorbable suture material. The author prefers running sutures to the peritoneum and transversalis and the posterior rectus sheath, which is included. Several interrupted 0 sutures are placed at the midline in figure-of-eight fashion. The anterior rectus sheath is closed with interrupted 0 nonabsorbable sutures as are the internal oblique and external oblique. The subcutaneous tissue is closed with interrupted 3-0 chromic catgut, and the skin is closed with vertical interrupted skin staples.

Postoperative considerations include careful monitoring of the central venous pressure. The author prefers a Swan-Ganz catheter for optimal central wedge pressure and also uses intra-arterial lines from the moment of surgical induction to 1 or 2 days postoperatively. Hypotension is a rare occurrence because these patients are generally well blocked for 2 weeks preoperatively with phenoxybenzamine. Some surgeons avoid preoperative blockade, preferring to transfuse patients postoperatively with whole blood and colloid to manage the pressure drops in unblocked patients. Their rationale is that the palpation for other tumors is more effective in the unblocked patient. Because this is only a 10% factor and CT scanning is highly

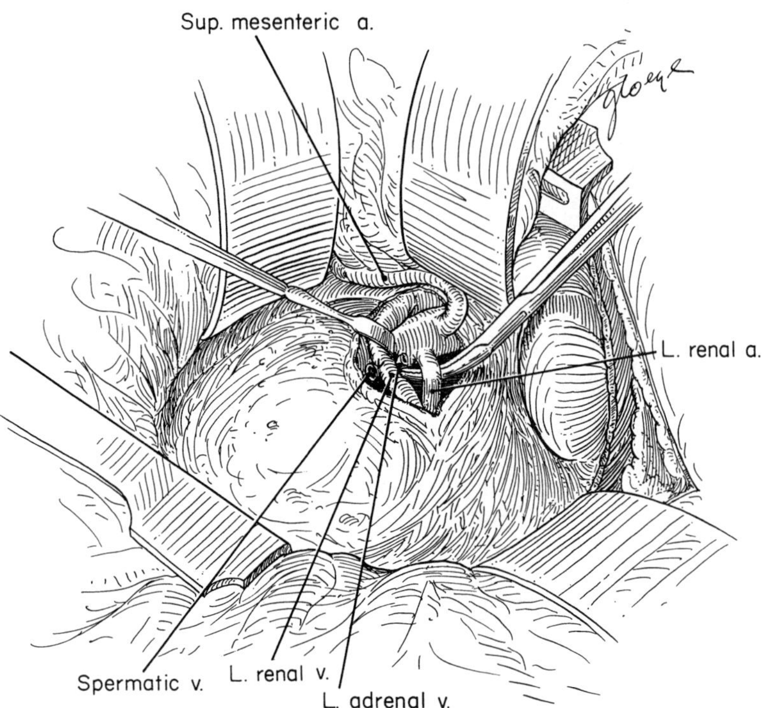

Fig. 2.10.   After the peritoneum and pancreas are retracted medially, the renal and adrenal vessels are mobilized by dividing Gerota's fascia, which overlies them.

effective in localizing retroperitoneal tumors, we have avoided the uncertainties of this approach with its attendant risk of hepatitis and pressure swings.

LAPAROSCOPIC ADRENALECTOMY

There have been a few reports of adrenal neoplasms resected via laparoscopic approach (31). There are anatomic features that favor this approach. The adrenal adenoma is usually small and the gland itself lies in the retroperitoneal suprarenal space, which can be insufflated without morbidity. Visualization of the gland with adenoma should be feasible. With the recent impetus for minimal invasiveness, more experience with this approach will accumulate.

Finally, a team approach cannot be overemphasized. Internists, anesthesiologists, and urologic surgeons, all with an endocrine background and experience, are the ideal combination for preoperative and postoperative patient management.

REFERENCES

1. Donohue JP. Primary aldosteronism. In: Kaufman JJ, ed. Current urologic therapy. 2nd ed. Philadelphia: WB Saunders, 1986:5.
2. Weinberger MH, et al. Primary aldosteronism: diagnosis, localization and treatment. Ann Intern Med 1979;90:386.
3. Hunt TK, Schambelan M, Biglieri EG. Selection of patients and operative approach in primary aldosteronism. Ann Surg 1975;182:353.
4. Nelson DH. The adrenal cortex: physiological function and disease. In: Smith LH Jr, ed. Major problems in internal medicine: Cushing's syndrome. Philadelphia: WB Saunders, 1980:153.
5. Glenn JF, Peterson RE, Mannix H Jr. Cushing's disease. In: Surgery of the adrenal gland. New York: MacMillan, 1968.
6. Donohue JP. Cushing syndrome and Cushing disease. In: Seidman EJ, Hanno PM, eds. Current urologic therapy. 3rd ed. Philadelphia: WB Saunders, 1994:10.
7. Cushing H. The pituitary body and its disorders. Philadelphia: JB Lippincott, 1912.
8. Hutter AM, Kayhoe DE. Adrenal cortical carcinoma: clinical features of 138 patients. Am J Med 1966;41:572.
9. Neville AM, Mackay, AM. The structure of the human adrenal cortex in health and disease. Clin Endocrinol Metab 1972;1: 361.
10. Lewinsky BS, Grigor KM, Sympington T. The clinical and pathologic features of "non-hormonal" adrenocortical tumors. Cancer 1975;33:778.
11. Singer W, et al. Ectopic ACTH syndrome: clinicopathological correlations. J Clin Pathol 1978;31:591.
12. Egdahl RH. Surgery of the adrenal gland. N Engl J Med 1968;278:939.
13. Liddle GW. Tests of pituitary-adrenal suppressibility in the diagnosis of Cushing's syndrome. J Clin Endocrinol Metab 1960;20:1539.
14. Jubiz W, et al. Single dose metyrapone test. Arch Intern Med 1970;125:472.
15. Neville AM. The nodular adrenal. Invest Cell Pathol 1978;1: 99.
16. Scott HW Jr, et al. Surgical experience with Cushing's disease. Ann Surg 1977;185:524.

17. Givens JR. Hirsutism and hyperandrogenism. Adv Intern Med 1976;21:221.
18. Freitas JE, Beierwaltes WH, Nishiyama RH. Adrenal hyperandrogenism: detection by adrenal scintigraphy. J Endrocrinol Invest 1978;1:59.
19. Frankel F. Ein fall von Doppelseitigem, vollig latent verlaufenen nebennieren-tumor und gleichzeitiger nephritis mit veranderun-gen and circulations apparat und retinitis. Arch Pathol Anat Phys 1886;103:244.
20. Mayo C. Paroxysmal hypertension with tumor of retroperitoneal nerve. JAMA 1927;89:1047.
21. Pincoffs MC. A case of paroxysmal hypertension associated with suprarenal tumor. Trans Assoc Am Physicians 1929;44:295.
22. Shipley AM. Paroxysmal hypertension associated with tumor of the suprarenal. Ann Surg 1929;90:742.
23. Hume DM. Pheochromocytoma and hypertension: an analysis of 207 cases. Int Abstr Surg 1960;99:458.
24. Stackpole RH, Melicow MM, Uson AC. Pheochromocytoma in children. J Pediatr 1963;66:315.
25. Ganguly A, et al. Diagnosis and localization of pheochromocytoma. Am J Med 1979;67:21.
26. Sisson JC, et al. Scintigraphic localization of pheochromocytoma. N Engl J Med 1981;305:12.
27. Yazaki T, et al. Usefulness of scintigraphic imaging using 131 iodine-metaiodobenzylguanidine in localization of asymptomatic pheochromocytoma. J Urol 1985;134:107.
28. Bravo EL, et al. Clonidine-suppression test. N Engl J Med 1981;305:623.
29. Conn JW. Presidential address. Painting background: primary aldosteronism, a new clinical syndrome. J Lab Clin Med 1955;45:3.
30. Bodie B, et al. Cleveland clinic experience with adrenal cortical carcinoma. J Urol 1989;141:257.
31. Suzuki K, Kageyama S, Ueda D, et al. Laparoscopic surgery for adrenal tumors. In: Das S, Crawford DE, eds. Urologic laparoscopy. Philadelphia: WB Saunders, 1994:211.

KIDNEY-RENAL CELL CARCINOMA

Primary Renal Cell Carcinoma

An Overview

Seth H. Glick and Ralph W. deVere White

Renal cell carcinoma is a relatively rare malignancy, accounting for 2 to 3% of all cancers. Its incidence has been slowly rising over the past few decades, with approximately 23,000 cases diagnosed annually (1). The peak incidence of renal cell carcinoma is in the sixth to seventh decade of life with a male-to-female predominance of approximately 2 to 1 (2). It can be expected that with the increase in imaging studies being performed for nonurologic disease, a higher percentage of renal cell carcinomas will be discovered incidentally. This should increase the detection of surgically curable disease, thus helping to improve survival rates. It also may be argued that many of these cancers will be of lower malignant potential at the time of detection, further supporting those who favor nephron-sparing surgery.

Heredity does play a role in the development of renal cell carcinoma. Patients with von Hippel-Lindau disease are at risk for developing tumors at multiple sites, including renal cell carcinoma. These tumors are often small, are multifocal, and may be bilateral. A gene found on the short arm of chromosome 3 has been linked to von Hippel-Lindau disease (3). Patients with a translocation between the short arm of chromosome 3 and chromosomes 6 and 8 are predisposed to renal cell carcinoma as well, not related to von Hippel-Lindau disease (4, 5). Many authors have found a consistent region of chromosome 3 that is deleted in a majority of renal cell cancers (6, 7). They hypothesize that this may be the region of a tumor suppressor gene (6). There may be other hereditary factors involved with renal cell carcinoma. Zbar et al. reported a family with nine members over three generations who had a papillary form of renal cell carcinoma (8). This was not linked to the von Hippel-Lindau gene or a chromosome 3 translocation. Currently, the genetic determining factor has not been found in this family. A recent article has associated mutations of the tumor suppressor gene p53 with metastatic disease and poor outcome in renal cell carcinoma (9). Staining for the mutated p53 was found in 49 of 175 renal tumors (28%), with 11 of 13 metastatic lesions (85%) staining positively.

HISTOPATHOLOGY

The origin of renal cell carcinoma is thought to be cells from the proximal convoluted tubules. Oberling et al., using electron microscopy and immunohistochemistry, have found a relationship between epithelial cells of the proximal convoluted tubule and those of renal cancers (10).

The gross size of renal cell carcinomas is quite variable. They are most commonly unilateral, from 5 to 10 cm in diameter. However, 5% of patients have multiple, unilateral tumors (11). Bilateral tumors occur in 0.5 to 1.5% of patients (often associated with other systemic diseases such as cystic disease or von Hippel-Lindau) (12).

There is some controversy about whether small tumors should be considered malignant. Certain authors have advocated that tumors less than 3 cm be considered as renal adenomas because they rarely metastasize (13, 14). However, most urologists believe that these small tumors are not intrinsically benign, they are just early in their development and have not had the time to spread. There are multiple reports of small renal cell carcinomas that have already metastasized.

Grossly, these tumors are often irregular and are not encapsulated. Color may vary according to whether there is any fibrosis, necrosis, or hemorrhage. About 20% have a large cystic component (15).

Microscopically, there are two predominant cell types seen in renal cell carcinoma (15). Most common is the clear cell variant, with sheets of large, clear cells separated by fibrous septae. These cells are clear secondary to their abundance of glycogen and lipid. Granular cells are found less frequently. They have a granular, eosinophilic cytoplasm. Although one cell type may be predominant, both of these cell variants are often found in the foci of cancer. There does not appear to be any prognostic significance in which cell type predominates. Recently, a third rare cell type, chromophobe cell carcinoma, has been described (16). All these cell types may be found in a predominantly solid glandular pattern or less commonly in a papillary pattern (15). A sarcomatoid variant is found infrequently, with sheets of spindle-shaped cells. This form of renal cell carcinoma has a worse prognosis (17).

Usually, renal cell carcinomas are quite uniform, with little pleomorphism or nuclear atypia. Grading of these tumors depends mainly on nuclear morphology (15). High-grade lesions have larger, more irregular nuclei with large nucleoli. Although grade does have some prognostic importance, tumor stage is a much better predictor of outcome in patients with renal cell carcinoma (18).

DNA ploidy analysis of these tumors has been disappointing. Nakano et al. reviewed the DNA ploidy status of 72 patients with renal cell carcinoma (19). They found aneuploidy in 50% of patients, which correlated with tumor grade. However, ploidy status did not correlate with tumor stage or survival. They also found heterogeneity in ploidy when several samples were taken from the same patient. There are other authors who feel that ploidy does give prognostic information (20, 21). However, ploidy is not currently a standard part of the evaluation of patients with renal cell carcinoma.

STAGING/PROGNOSIS

Although the histology of renal cell carcinoma does give important prognostic information, the most important information regarding survival of these patients is the tumor stage and thus the ability of the tumor to be totally surgically resected. Historically, the staging system most commonly used is Robson's modification of the Flocks and Kadesky system (22). In summary, this system designates tumor confined within the renal capsule as stage I, tumor confined within Gerota's fascia as stage II, tumor within the renal vein, inferior vena cava, or regional lymphatics as stage III, and tumor involving adjacent organs or distant metastases as stage IV. This system has fallen out of favor relative to the TNM system due to its lack of consistent prognostic information in stage III. It has been shown in multiple studies that tumor thrombus extending into the renal vein or inferior vena cava without lymph node involvement does not worsen survival (23, 24). Conversely, patients with positive lymph nodes have similar survival rates to those with distant metastases, with overall 5-year survival rate less than 20% (25).

The TNM staging system allows for separation of nodal involvement from vascular invasion (Fig. 3.1) (26). A review of this classification by Bassil et al. found that the primary tumor stage in this classification was prognostically important (27). They showed 5-year survival rates of 100%, 91%, 72%, 56%, 30%, and 25% for TNM stage T1, T2, T3a, T3b, T3c, and T4, respectively.

Surgical removal of the entire tumor is generally accepted

PRIMARY TUMOR

TN	Primary tumor cannot be assessed
T0	No evidence of primary tumor
T1	Tumor 2.5 cm or less in greatest dimension limited to the kidney
T2	Tumor more than 2.5 cm in greatest dimension limited to the kidney
T3	Tumor extends into major veins or invades adrenal gland or perinephric tissues but not beyond Gerota's fascia
	T3a Tumor invades adrenal gland or perinephric tissues but not beyond Gerota's fascia
	T3b Tumor grossly extends into renal vein(s) or vena cava
T4	Tumor invades beyond Gerota's fascia

REGIONAL LYMPH NODES (N)

NX	Regional lymph nodes cannot be assessed
N0	No regional lymph node metastasis
N1	Metastasis in a single lymph node, 2 cm or less in greatest dimension
N2	Metastasis in a single lymph node, more than 2 cm but not more than 5 cm in greatest dimension, or multiple lymph nodes, none more than 5 cm in greatest dimension
N3	Metastasis in a lymph node more than 5 cm in greatest dimension

DISTANT METASTASIS (M)

MX	Presence of distant metastasis cannot be assessed
M0	No distant metastasis
M1	Distant metastasis

STAGE GROUPING

Stage I	T1	N0	M0
Stage II	T2	N0	M0
Stage III	T1	N1	M0
	T2	N1	M0
	T3a	N0, N1	M0
	T3b	N0, N1	M0
Stage IV	T4	Any N	M0
	Any T	N2, N3	M0
	Any T	Any N	M1

HISTOPATHOLOGIC TYPE

The histopathologic types are:
Renal cell carcinoma
   Adenocarcinoma
   Renal papillary adenocarcinoma
   Tubular carcinoma
   Granular cell carcinoma
   Clear cell carcinoma (hypernephroma)
The predominant cancer is adenocarcinoma; subtypes are clear-cell and granular-cell carcinoma. A grading system as below is recommended when feasible. The staging system does not apply to sarcomas of the kidney. A separate classification is published for nephroblastomas.

HISTOPATHOLOGIC GRADE (G)

GX	Grade cannot be assessed
G1	Well differentiated
G2	Moderately well differentiated
G3–4	Poorly differentiated/undifferentiated

Fig. 3.1.   TNM classification of primary renal cell carcinoma. (26)

Table 3.1. Survival Rates by Stage (28)

	STAGE	5-YEAR SURVIVAL (%)	10-YEAR SURVIVAL (%)
A[a]	I	60–82	56–60
	II	47–80	20–67
	III	15–35	17–38
	IV	0–5	0–3
	Skinner		
B[b]	I + RV alone	66	49
	+ IVC alone	55	43
	II + IVC alone	50	33
	III + LN and IVC	0	0

[a] Adapted from Johnson et al. (29), McNichols and Segura (30), Skinner et al. (31), Robson et al. and deKernion and Berry (32).
[b] Skinner et al. (24).
RV, renal vein involvement; IVC, inferior vena caval involvement; LN, lymph node.

as the best chance for cure in these patients. Couillard et al. reviewed several series of patients treated by radical nephrectomy for primary renal cell carcinoma (Table 3.1) (28). Although the 5-year survival rate for patients with stage I disease (60 to 82%) was similar to that for stage II disease (47 to 80%), 10-year survival was much less (56 to 60% versus 20 to 67%). Patients with lymph node involvement had significantly worse prognoses. Pizzocaro, in a review of the literature, found 5-year survival rates for node-positive disease to be between 8 and 35% (33). Involvement of adjacent organs is a grave prognostic sign as well. Even if the primary tumor appears to be completely excised, there is a less than 5% 5-year survival rate. The question of prognosis in patients with involvement of the inferior vena cava has been debated in the past. Skinner et al. have shown that involvement of the inferior vena cava has similar survival rates to that of stage II tumors in the absence of metastatic disease (24). However, patients with caval involvement do have a greater chance of having metastatic disease at the time of presentation. Invasion of the tumor into the renal pelvis has little prognostic importance (34).

CLINICAL PRESENTATION

Renal cell carcinoma may present with a wide range of signs and symptoms. The classic triad of flank pain, gross hematuria, and flank mass is only found in approximately 10% of patients, usually those with more advanced disease.

Hematuria, either gross or microscopic, is the most common presenting feature in this disease. Skinner et al., in a review of 309 patients with renal cell carcinoma who underwent nephrectomy, found some form of hematuria in 59% (31). Usually the hematuria is total, gross, and painless. However, with hemorrhage into these tumors, they may become acutely painful. Clot colic secondary to ureteral obstruction is common. A flank or abdominal mass was found in 45% of patients, and pain was found in 41%. Weight loss was another common symptom, seen in 28% of patients.

Renal cell carcinomas are increasingly being found as incidental findings on imaging studies of the abdomen for nonurologic problems. About 20% of tumors in one study were found incidentally (35). They were usually smaller, of lower stage, and thus had better prognoses.

The sudden appearance of a varicocele, usually left sided, has been the presenting sign in 2 to 11% of cases (31, 36). This is caused by obstruction of the left gonadal vein by tumor thrombus in the left renal vein. Less frequently, vena caval thrombus will obstruct the right gonadal vein causing an acute right-sided varicocele.

The wide variety of presenting symptoms in renal cell carcinoma is due to the paraneoplastic syndromes often associated with this malignancy. These are a collection of symptoms that masquerade as other systemic illnesses but are actually due to humoral and local effects of renal cell cancer. Anemia is the most common of these findings (41%) (15). The anemia is out of proportion to any blood loss secondary to hematuria. It is normocytic and normochromic but associated with decreased serum iron and iron-binding capacity. It may be related to a decrease in erythropoietin production by the kidney (37). However, there is a small percentage of patients who present with erythrocytosis due to an erythropoietin-secreting tumor. Hypertension is common and may be renin mediated (38, 39). Hyperpyrexia is found in 15 to 20% of patients secondary to production of endogenous pyrogen by the tumor (38, 39). Hypercalcemia is found in 5 to 20% of patients (40). This may be due to either osseous metastases or production of a parathyroid-like hormone by the tumor. Elevation of prostaglandins has also been thought to contribute to the hypercalcemia. Hepatic dysfunction related to renal cell carcinoma is known as Stauffer syndrome (41). Elevated liver function test results, alkaline phosphatase, and prothrombin time are found and are sometimes associated with hepatosplenomegaly. The cause is unknown. Liver function should return to normal after removal of the tumor. Persistence of liver abnormalities after nephrectomy bodes for poor prognosis (42). Other, less common systemic manifestations of renal cell carcinoma include amyloidosis, protein-losing enteropathy, and polyneuromyopathy. An increase of human chorionic gonadotropin has been found that may lead to symptoms of decreased libido or gynecomastia (43).

DIAGNOSTIC IMAGING

The intravenous pyelogram (IVP) with nephrotomography is often the initial study used to detect renal cell carcinoma. This is because most of these patients present with either flank pain or hematuria, and the IVP is used to evaluate for function, anatomy, and obstruction of the kidney and ureter. The IVP will show a mass effect that usually warrants further diagnostic workup. This mass effect can be seen as distortion of the calices, lack of visualization of part of the collecting system, or distortion of the renal outline.

For certain cases (e.g., intravenous dye allergy or renal failure), renal ultrasound may be the initial diagnostic test. Ultrasound has been found to be highly accurate in the detection of solid renal masses, with a sensitivity of 97% and specificity of 97% (44). Ultrasonic criteria for simple cystic mass include a smooth wall with lack of septation, absence of internal echoes, good sound transmission, a round or oval shape, and acoustic shadowing at the edges of the cyst (45). A complex mass is considered neoplastic unless proven otherwise. Cyst aspiration with injection of contrast material can help to differentiate a simple cyst from a cyst with tumor. Simple cysts will be smooth walled and contain clear fluid without malignant cells that are low in protein and lactate dehydrogenase (46). A computed tomography (CT) scan is often performed to confirm the diagnosis.

The CT scan has become the most common means of staging the primary tumor and has essentially replaced angiography except in rare settings (see below). Multiple studies have shown an increase in the accuracy of staging with CT versus angiography (47–49). Limitations of the CT scan include a tendency to overread the local extent of disease. It is also limited in assessing tumor spread to regional nodes unless the nodal disease is of adequate size. False-positive readings of enlarged lymph nodes have occurred; thus, such readings should be confirmed with needle biopsy (45). CT is also relatively accurate in the diagnosis of renal vein and vena caval involvement with tumor thrombus; however, it lacks in the ability to diagnose the extent of caval involvement.

Magnetic resonance imaging (MRI) is being used increasingly in the workup of solid renal masses. CT scanning does seem to be more accurate in staging the primary renal lesion, especially if the mass is less than 3 cm (50). However, MRI has the advantages over CT of being able to image the tumor in multiple planes. It is also more accurate in determining the presence and level of tumor invasion into vascular structures. A recent study comparing the efficacy of CT versus real-time ultrasound versus MRI versus venacavography showed that MRI and venacavography were 100% sensitive in detecting caval thrombus, with CT and ultrasound less sensitive (79% and 59%, respectively) (47).

Ultrasound with color Doppler flow imaging has recently been used to assess the extent of vascular tumor thrombus. It appears to be similar to MRI in the ability to predict tumor thrombus, with sensitivity of 89%, but may be limited in patients with bulky tumors (51).

Further metastatic workup includes the chest radiograph and certain laboratory tests including liver function tests and alkaline phosphatase. At one time, the radionucleotide bone scan was part of the preoperative evaluation. However, multiple reviews have shown that bone scans are warranted only in patients with elevated serum alkaline phosphatase or bone pain (52, 53). There is a significant incidence of false-positive scan readings that can obscure accurate staging.

TREATMENT OF LOCALIZED RENAL CELL CARCINOMA

The treatment of localized renal cell carcinoma is complete surgical excision. Results with chemotherapy, immunotherapy,

and radiation therapy have not even approached those attained with surgical excision (28). A radical nephrectomy is the procedure of choice, with removal of the kidney, perinephric fat, Gerota's fascia, and ipsilateral adrenal gland en bloc. A case might be made for leaving the adrenal behind if the tumor is not in the upper pole of the kidney and the adrenal looks normal on CT scan. The authors agree with Roby and Schellhammer, who advocate leaving the adrenal in these cases because adrenal metastases are so rare (54). However, the radical nephrectomy classically involves removal of the ipsilateral adrenal.

There is not much controversy in performing a radical nephrectomy versus simple nephrectomy. Although no randomized study has been performed recently comparing these two surgical procedures, it is logical to assume that if simple nephrectomy is performed, a certain percentage of patients with T3 lesions will not be cured, whereas they would have been cured had radical nephrectomy been performed. There is no real benefit to leaving Gerota's fascia, and as the two procedures are similar in terms of operative time and difficulty, radical nephrectomy remains the standard of care for treatment of localized renal cell carcinoma.

There are some who advocate renal-sparing local excision of small renal cell carcinomas in patients with a normal contralateral kidney (55, 56). They believe that smaller tumors, which tend to be of lower grade and stage, can be removed by enucleation or partial nephrectomy with a very low incidence of local recurrence. A similar survival rate has been shown for T1 and T2 tumors after local excision compared with radical nephrectomy (57, 58). However, this approach has been questioned for many reasons. Although small tumors do have a tendency toward lower grade and stage, there are small tumors that have a higher malignant potential and have metastasized (59). Smaller sites of cancer not detectable by imaging studies have been found pathologically in the ipsilateral kidney in 20% of cases (60). Although they are improving quite rapidly, imaging studies are still lacking when compared with pathologic staging of the tumor. Thus, radical nephrectomy is still the mainstay of treatment for renal cell cancer in the presence of a normal contralateral kidney.

Locally advanced disease is often difficult to assess preoperatively. In approximately 10% of patients, the cancer extends into adjacent organs (22, 61). These are usually large tumors that are symptomatic. Patients with adrenal invasion (T3a) may be cured with radical nephrectomy. However, with T4 disease (tumor extending beyond Gerota's fascia) prognosis is poor (62). Thus, resection in these patients should be limited to those with significant symptoms.

The use of regional lymph node dissection along with radical nephrectomy is controversial. Approximately 20% of patients will have nodal disease without evidence of other metastatic sites (25). However, even with node dissection, survival rates for these patients remain poor. In a review of the literature, Pizzocaro found 5-year survival rates between 8 and 35% with positive nodes after radical nephrectomy (33). Hulten et al. found that no patients survived at 5 years with nodal disease

(63). No benefit has been found in performing extended lymphadenectomy (64). Although it may not be beneficial in terms of survival benefit, local node dissection is helpful in determining prognosis and can be performed with minimal morbidity.

Many authors have shown that survival for patients with renal vein and vena cava tumor thrombus approaches that for patients with stage II disease if the tumor thrombus can be removed (23, 24, 65, 66). Caval thrombus is found in approximately 8 to 15% of patients, more commonly on the right side, and is directly related to the size of the primary tumor (29, 67). Accurate preoperative evaluation is essential in determining the approach to these tumors. As has already been discussed, MRI and color Doppler flow imaging are the least invasive and most informative imaging studies in assessing the extent of the thrombus. Venacavography has similar efficacy but with increased morbidity and is being used less frequently. Tumors in the renal vein only can be removed with minimal morbidity. If the thrombus extends over the edge of the renal vein, it can usually be milked back into the vein before ligation with minimal risk of tumor embolization. The surgical approach to the removal of tumor thrombus in the inferior vena cava depends on the level to which the thrombus extends. Caval thrombi have been divided into three groups: type I (50%) are subhepatic, type II (40%) are intrahepatic, and type III (10%) are atrial (24, 68). The surgical approaches in removing these thrombi will be discussed in later chapters.

The treatment of patients with bilateral renal cell carcinoma or renal cell carcinoma in a solitary kidney will often require some difficult decisions. However, renal-sparing surgical procedures can be performed with minimal morbidity and mortality relative to radical nephrectomy. Given the alternative of dialysis, with its multiple complications and associated decrease in life span, the risk of recurrence is often well worth it in these patients.

The incidence of bilateral renal cell carcinoma is 1.8 to 3.0% (11, 69). Wickham has reported that patients with bilateral, synchronous renal tumors did not live beyond 5 months without surgical intervention (70). Surgical options for patients with bilateral synchronous disease include the following:

1. Unilateral partial nephrectomy followed by contralateral nephrectomy,
2. Bilateral partial nephrectomies, and
3. Bilateral radical nephrectomy.

The goal is to preserve as much functioning renal parenchyma as possible while removing the entire cancer. In most cases, one kidney will be involved to a greater degree than the other. In this case, a partial nephrectomy can be performed on the side with the smaller tumor, followed by nephrectomy of the more diseased side. If there is a problem with the partial nephrectomy that requires total nephrectomy, then a parenchymal-sparing operation may still be able to be performed on the other, more involved side. It has been suggested that these two procedures be performed in a staged manner (26, 71). This would allow assessment of renal function in the partial nephrec-

tomy side before contralateral nephrectomy. However, others believe that renal function can be adequately assessed before the initial operation so that both procedures can be performed at the same time (28). A preoperative angiogram is mandatory in determining vascular anatomy to preserve the most renal parenchyma. Local recurrence rates of 10% for stage I tumors are reasonable (12, 56–58, 72–74). The 5-year survival rate is approximately 70 to 80% for synchronous, bilateral renal cell carcinoma after surgery (73).

Patients with von Hippel-Lindau disease have a 30 to 40% chance of renal cell carcinoma development (75). These tumors are usually small, bilateral, and of lower malignant potential. They also have a propensity to recur. Thus, renal-sparing procedures of enucleation or partial nephrectomy should be performed, with nephrectomy reserved for only dire cases with the kidney totally replaced with tumor. These cancers tend to have a thick capsule surrounding them, making enucleation easy. However, Marshall et al. have found microsopic extension through this capsule (76). Thus, an attempt should be made to remove the capsule, and margin biopsies should be used to aid in removing all the cancer while preserving as much functioning parenchyma as possible.

Similar thought processes must go into the treatment of renal cell carcinoma in a solitary kidney. Most often a partial nephrectomy will suffice. However, in cases where there is a large renal tumor in the midpole of the kidney, more advanced techniques might be necessary to save the patient from dialysis. Bench surgery with autotransplantation or in situ surgery may be necessary. In situ hypothermia via a variety of techniques (77, 78) may be necessary if ischemia times of greater than 30 minutes are anticipated (79).

Treatment of Metastatic Renal Cell Carcinoma

In general, results of treatment of metastatic renal cell carcinoma with systemic therapy or radiation therapy have been poor. However, trials are currently underway to evaluate different forms of immunotherapy. Early results show some promise for these new forms of immunomodulation. Surgical treatment is largely reserved for palliation of symptoms. However, patients with solitary metastases may benefit from radical nephrectomy with resection of metastatic disease.

Approximately 2 to 4% of patients with metastatic renal cell carcinoma present with a solitary metastasis (80–82). Survival rates for metastatic renal cell carcinoma are quite poor, with minimal 5-year survival (Table 3.2). However, several studies have shown an improvement in 5-year survival with surgery (Table 3.3). This improvement does not appear to hold for multiple metastases. Neves et al. reported a 3-year survival rate of 19% for solitary metastasis versus 4.3% for multiple metastases after surgical removal of all cancer (92). It has been suggested that the best results are obtained in patients with solitary metastasis to the lung (86). Thus, in appropriate surgical candidates, surgery for solitary metastases does appear to prolong survival. In view of the lack of efficacious systemic

Table 3.2. Survival Rates of Patients With Distant Metastases (28)

	SURVIVAL (%)		
	NO. OF PATIENTS	1-YEAR	5-YEAR
Boxer et al. (83)	34	68	8
Johnson et al. (84)	93	26	—
Klugo et al. (85)	101	26	6
Maldazys and deKernion (86)	32	21	—
Middleton (80)	141	10	0
Montie et al. (87)	78	18	—
Patel and Lavengood (88)	41	17	2
Rafla (89)	24	13	0
Selli et al. 1983	20	34	—
Skinner et al. (31)	77	—	8
Thompson et al. (90)	65	22	—

therapy, this may be the best option. However, the percentage of patients with metastatic renal cell carcinoma who are cured by surgery is quite low.

Surgery for patients with multiple metastases is mainly limited to palliation of symptoms. Surgical bebulking of renal tumors has not been found to prolong survival (Table 3.4). deKernion et al. have compared the survival of patients with metastatic renal cell carcinoma who had adjunctive nephrectomy to those who did not undergo surgery. Their survival curves were the same (62). This is mainly because most patients with metastatic renal cell carcinoma die of their metastatic disease and not bulky local disease (93). If certain forms of immunotherapy do prove to be of significant benefit to patients with metastatic renal cell carcinoma, then debulking of the primary tumor may become the standard of care. The incidence of spontaneous regression is less than 1% (31, 94–96). This is independent of surgery and often limited to pulmonary metastases.

Radiation therapy has not been shown to be beneficial in treatment of renal cell carcinoma except for palliation of metastases to bone. Some reports in the early 1970s indicated a possible neoadjuvant role for radiation therapy (97). However, a subsequent randomized study by van der Werf-Messing showed no improvement in survival with neoadjuvant radiation therapy

Table 3.3. Survival Rates After Excision of Solitary Metastases (28)

	SURVIVAL (%)		
	NO. OF PATIENTS	3-YEAR	5-YEAR
Middleton (80)	59	45	34
Tolia and Whitmore (82)	—	—	35
Klugo et al. (85)	10	60	50
O'Dea (81)	44	27	16
Golimbu et al. (91)	21	43	25
Dineen 1988	29	41	13

Table 3.4. Median Survival (Months) With and Without Nephrectomy in Metastatic Renal Cell Carcinoma (28)

	NEPHRECTOMY	NO NEPHRECTOMY
Johnson et al. (84)	11	8
Klugo et al. (85)	15	5
Montie et al. (87)	6	1
Rafla (89)	8	7

and nephrectomy versus nephrectomy alone (98). The use of radiation therapy as an adjuvant treatment of metastatic renal cell carcinoma has not been successful in improving survival (99).

Similarly, the results with chemotherapy have been quite poor. Yagoda reviewed the literature and found minimal responses that were usually short lived in 39 agents reviewed (100). The reason for the lack of response of renal cell carcinoma may be related to the multidrug resistance gene (101, 102). This gene encodes for p-glycoprotein, a 170-kd transmembrane protein that is involved in actively pumping drugs out of cells. It remains to be seen whether other genes related to programmed cell death can be used to elucidate resistance to chemotherapy.

Hormonal therapy with progestational agents had been advocated as a treatment option for renal cell carcinoma. Efficacy in treating estrogen-induced clear cell tumor in a Syrian hamster by Kirtman et al. in 1949 is the basis for this treatment (103). Bloom reviewed the literature in 1973 and found a 15% response rate of metastatic renal cell carcinoma to hormonal therapy (104). However, in a review of their experience, deKernion et al. found no response to progestational agents (62).

Immunotherapy with biologic response modifiers is currently being investigated. Interferon alpha has been shown to produce a response in 15 to 20% of patients in nonrandomized phase II trials (105–107). However, responses were often short (8 to 10 months) and usually in patients with indicators of more responsive disease (good performance status, prior nephrectomy, long disease-free interval, and lung predominant metastatic disease) (108). Interleukin-2 has been studied, and response rates of up to 15% have been tempered by toxic side effects and high cost (109). Combination therapy with interferon alpha and interleukin-2 has not shown an increase in response rate over interleukin-2 alone (45). However, preliminary studies with low-dose interferon alpha/interleukin-2 combination have shown similar short-term efficacy but with a decrease in toxicity so that this regimen can be given in an outpatient setting (45). Other forms of immunotherapy, such as autolymphocyte therapy, have shown some efficacy in early clinical trials. An ongoing clinical trial (Cellcor 93-C-02) is evaluating response to interferon alpha versus autolymphocyte therapy with cimetidine.

REFERENCES

1. Boring CC, Squires TS, Tong T. Cancer statistics, 1992. CA Cancer J Clin 1992;1:30.

2. Kantor AF. Current concepts in the epidemiology and etiology of primary renal cell carcinoma. J Urol 1977;117:415.

3. Hosoe S, Brauch H, et al. Localization of the von Hippel-Lindau disease gene to a small region of chromosome 3. Genomics 1990;8:634.

4. Cohen AJ, Li FP, et al. Hereditary renal cell carcinoma associated with a chromosomal translocation. N Engl J Med 1979;301:592.

5. Kovacs G, Brusa P, DeRiese W. Tissue-specific expression of a constitutional 3;6 translocation: development of multiple bilateral renal cell carcinomas. Int J Cancer 1989;43:422.

6. Carroll PR, Murty VVS, et al. Abnormalities at chromosome region 3p12014 characterize clear cell renal carcinoma. Cancer Genet Cytogenet 1987;27:253.

7. Zbar B, Brauch H, Talmadge C, et al. Loss of alleles of loci on the short arm of chromosome 3 in renal cell carcinoma. Nature 1987;327:721.

8. Zbar B, Tory K, et al. Hereditary papillary renal cell carcinoma. J Urol 1994;151:561.

9. Uhlman DO, Nguyen PL, et al. Association of immunohistochemical staining for p53 with metastatic progression and poor survival in patients with renal cell carcinoma. J Natl Cancer Inst 1994;86:1470.

10. Oberling C, Riviere M, Magrenau F. Ultrastructure of the clear cells in renal carcinomas and its importance for the demonstration of their renal origin. Nature 1960;186:402.

11. Moertal CG, Dockerty MB, Baggenstoss AH. Multiple primary malignant neoplasm III. Tumors of multicentric origin. Cancer 1961;14:238.

12. Jacobs SC, Berg SI, Lawson RK. Synchronous bilateral renal cell carcinoma: total surgical excision. Cancer 1980;46:2341.

13. Bell ET. Renal diseases. 2nd ed. Philadelphia: Lea & Febiger, 1950.

14. Hicks WK. Benign tubular adenoma with malignant transformation. J Urol 1954;71:162.

15. Brodsky GL, Garnick MB. Renal tumors in the adult patient. In: Tisher CC, Brenner BM, eds. Renal pathology. 2nd ed. Philadelphia: JB Lippincott, 1994;2:1540.

16. Thoenes W, Storkel S, et al. Chromophobe cell renal carcinoma and its variants: a report on 32 cases. J Pathol 1988;155:277.

17. Tomera KV, Farrow GM, Lieber MD. Sarcomatoid renal carcinoma. J Urol 1983;130:657.

18. Mostofi FK. Pathology and spread of renal cell carcinoma. In: King JS Jr, ed. Renal neoplasia. Boston: Little, Brown, & Co., 1967:41.

19. Nakano E, Kondoh M, et al. Flow cytometric analysis of nuclear DNA content of renal cell carcinoma correlated with histologic and clinical features. Cancer 1993;72:1319.

20. Klöppel G, et al. Prognosis of renal cell carcinoma related to nuclear grade, DNA content, and Robson stage. Eur Urol 1986;12:426.

21. Ljungberg B, Stenling R, Roos G. Prognostic value of DNA content in metastatic renal cell carcinoma. J Urol 1986;136:801.

22. Robson CJ, Churchill BM, Anderson W. Results of radical nephrectomy for renal cell carcinoma. J Urol 1969;101:297.

23. Cherrie RJ, Goldman DG, Lindner A, et al. Prognostic implications of vena caval extension of renal cell carcinoma. J Urol 1982;128:910.

24. Skinner DG, Pfister RF, Colvin R. Extension of renal cell carcinoma into the vena cava: the rationale for aggressive surgical management. J Urol 1972;107:711.

25. deKernion JB. Lymphadenectomy for renal cell carcinoma: therapeutic implications. Urol Clin North Am 1980;7:697.

26. Das S. Primary renal-cell carcinoma: an overview. In: Crawford ED, Das S, eds. Current genitourinary cancer surgery. 1st ed. Philadelphia: Lea & Febiger, 1990:22.

27. Bassil B, Dosoretz DE, Prout GR Jr. Validation of the tumor, nodes, and metastases classification of renal cell carcinoma. J Urol 1985;134:450.

28. Couillard DR, deVere White RW. Surgery of renal cell carcinoma. Urol Clin North Am 1993;20:263.

29. Johnson DE, Swanson DA, Von Eschenback AC. Tumors of the genitourinary tract. In: Smith DR, ed. General urology. Los Altos: Appleton-Lange, 1984.

30. McNichols DW, Segura JW, deWeerd JH. Renal cell carcinoma: long-term survival and late recurrence. J Urol 1981;2126:17.

31. Skinner DG, Colvin RB, Vermillion CD, et al. Diagnosis and management of renal cell carcinoma: a clinical and pathologic study of 309 cases. Cancer 1971;28:1165.

32. deKernion JB, Berry D. The diagnosis and treatment of renal cell carcinoma. Cancer 1980;45:1947.

33. Pizzocaro G. Lymphadenectomy in renal adenocarcinoma. In: deKernion JB, Pavone-Macaluso M, eds. Tumor of the kidney: international perspective in urology. Baltimore: Williams & Wilkins. 1986;13:75.

34. Siminovitch JMP, Montie JE, Stratton RA. Prognostic indicators in renal adenocarcinoma. J Urol 1983;130:20.

35. Thompson IM, Peck M. Improvement in survival of patients with renal cell carcinoma: role of serendipitously detected tumor. J Urol 1988;140:487.

36. Pinals RS, Krane SK. Medical aspects of renal carcinoma. Postgrad Med J 1962;38:507.

37. Chisholm GD, Roy RR. The systemic effects of malignant renal tumors. Br J Urol 1971;43:687.

38. Hollifield JW, et al. Renin-secreting clear-cell carcinoma of the kidney. Arch Intern Med 1975;135:859.

39. Sufrin G, et al. Hormones in renal cancer. J Urol 1977;117:433.

40. Lytton B, Rosof B, Evans J. Parathyroid hormone-like activity in a renal carcinoma producing hypercalcemia. J Urol 1965;93:127.

41. Stauffer MH. Nephrogenic hepatosplenomegaly. Gastroenterology 1961;40:694.

42. Boxer RJ, et al. Non-metastatic hepatic dysfunction associated with renal carcinoma. J Urol 1978;119:468.

43. Turkington RW. Ectopic production of prolactin. N Engl J Med 1971;285:1455.

44. Smith EH, Bennett AH. The usefulness of ultrasound in the evaluation of renal masses in adults. J Urol 1975;113:525.

45. deKernion JB, Belldegrum A. Renal tumors. In: Walsh PC, Retik AB, Stamey TA, et al., eds. Campbell's urology. 6th ed. Philadelphia: WB Saunders, 1992;2:1068.

46. Lang EK. Asymptomatic space occupying lesions of the kidney: a programmed sequential approach and its impact on quality and cost of health care. South Med J 1977;70:277.

47. Kallman DA, King BF, et al. Renal vein and inferior vena cava tumor thrombus in renal cell carcinoma: CT, US, MRI, and venacavography. J Comput Assist Tomogr 1992;16:240.

48. Lang E. Comparison of dynamic and conventional computed tomography, angiography, and ultrasonography in the staging of renal cell carcinoma. Cancer 1984;54:2205.

49. Richie JP, et al. Computerized tomography scan for diagnosis and staging of renal cell carcinoma. J Urol 1983;129:1114.

50. Hricak H, Thoeni RF, et al. Detection and staging of renal neoplasms: a reassessment of MR imaging. Radiology 1988; 166:643.

51. McGahan JP, Blake LC, et al. Color flow sonographic mapping of intravascular extension of malignant renal tumors. J Ultrasound Med 1993;12.

52. Atlas Il, Kwan D, Stone N. Value of serum alkaline phosphatase and radionuclide bone scans in patients with renal cell carcinoma. Urology 1991;38:220.

53. Lindner A, Goldman DG, deKernion JB. Cost effective analysis of prenephrectomy radioisotope scans in renal cell carcinoma. Urology 1983;22:127.

54. Roby EL, Schellhammer PF. Adrenal gland and renal cell carcinoma: is ipsilateral adrenalectomy a necessary component of radical nephrectomy? J Urol 1986;135:453.

55. Carini M, et al. Conservative surgical treatment of renal cell carcinoma: clinical experience and reappraisal of indications. J Urol 1988;140:725.

56. Marberger M, et al. Conservative surgery of renal cell carcinoma: the EIRSS experience. Br J Urol 1981;53:528.

57. Novick AC, Stream S, Montie JE. Conservative surgery for renal cell carcinoma: a single center experience with 100 patients. J Urol 1989;141:835.

58. Zinke H, Engen DE, Henning KM. Treatment of renal cell carcinoma by in situ partial nephrectomy and extracorporeal operation with autotransplantation. Mayo Clin Proc 1985;60: 651.

59. Talamo TS, Shomard JW. Small renal adenocarcinoma with metastasis. J Urol 1980;124:132.

60. Mukamel E, et al. Incidental small renal tumors occupying clinical overt renal cell carcinoma. J Urol 1988;140:22.

61. Williams RD. Renal, perirenal, and ureteral neoplasms. In: Gillenwater JY, Grayhack JT, Howards SS, et al., eds. Adult and pediatric urology. Chicago: Year Book, 1987;1:534.

62. deKernion JB, Ramming KP, Smith RB. Natural history of metastatic renal cell carcinoma: a computer analysis. J Urol 1978;120:148.

63. Hulten L, et al. Occurrence and localization of lymph node metastases in renal carcinoma. Scand J Urol Nephrol 1969;3: 129.

64. Siminovitch JP, Montie JE, Stratton RA. Lymphadenectomy in renal adenocarcinoma. J Urol 1982;127:1090.

65. deKernion JB, Mukamel E. Selection of initial therapy for renal cell carcinoma. Cancer 1987;60:539.

66. Kearney GP, Waters WB, Klein LA, et al. Results of inferior vena cava resection for renal cell carcinoma. J Urol 1981;125: 769.

67. Gancharenko V, Gerlock JA Jr, Kadir S, et al. Incidence and distribution of venous extension in 70 hypernephromas. AJR 1979;133:263.

68. Pritchett TR, Lieskovsky G, Skinner DG. Extension of renal cell carcinoma into the vena cava: clinical review and surgical approach. J Urol 1986;135:460.

69. Abeshouse BS, Weinberg T. Malignant renal neoplasms: a clinical and pathological study. Arch Surg 1945;50:46.

70. Wickham JEA. Conservative renal surgery for adenocarcinoma: the place of bench surgery. Br J Urol 1975; 47:25.

71. Novick AC. Partial nephrectomy for renal cell carcinoma. Urol Clin North Am 1987;14:419.

72. Bazeed MA, et al. Synchronous bilateral renal cell carcinoma: total surgical excision. Eur Urol 1986;12:238.

73. Smith RB, et al. Bilateral renal cell carcinoma and renal cell carcinoma in the solitary kidney. J Urol 1984;132:450.

74. Topley M, Novick AC, Montie JE. Long-term results following partial nephrectomy for localized renal adenocarcinoma. J Urol 1984;131:1050.

75. Bernstein SM, Koyle MA, Gittes RF. Partial nephrectomy, extracorporeal surgery, and autotransplantation for renal cell carcinoma. In: Crawford ED, Das S, eds. Current genitourinary cancer surgery. 1st ed. Philadelphia: Lea & Febiger, 1990:50.

76. Marshall FF, Taxy JB, Fishman EK, et al. The feasibility of surgical enucleation for renal cell carcinoma. J Urol 1986; 135:231.

77. Fowler JE. Nephrectomy in renal cell carcinoma. Urol Clin North Am 1987;14:749.

78. Mathur UK, Ramsey EW. Comparison of methods for preservation of renal function during ischemic renal surgery. J Urol 1983;129:163–165.

79. Novick AC, Cosgrove DM. Surgical approach for the removal of renal cell carcinoma extending into the vena cava and the right atrium. J Urol 1980;123:947.

80. Middleton RG. Surgery for metastatic renal cell carcinoma. J Urol 1967;97:973.

81. O'Dea MJ, Zinke H, Utz DC, et al. The treatment of renal cell carcinoma with solitary metastases. J Urol 1978;120:540.

82. Tolia BM, Whitmore WF Jr. Solitary metastases from renal cell carcinoma. J Urol 1975;114:836.

83. Boxer RJ, Waisman J, Lieber MM, et al. Renal carcinoma: computer analysis of 96 patients treated by nephrectomy. J Urol 1979;122:598.

84. Johnson DE, Kaesler KE, Samuels ML. Is nephrectomy justified with metastatic renal carcinoma? J Urol 1975;114: 27.

85. Klugo RC, Detmers M, Stiles RE, et al. Aggressive versus conservative treatment of stage IV renal cell carcinoma. J Urol 1977;118:244.

86. Maldazys JD, deKernion JB. Prognostic factors in renal cell carcinoma. J Urol 1986;136:376.

87. Montie JE, Stewart BH, Strafton RA, et al. The role of adjuvant nephrectomy in patients with metastatic renal cell carcinoma. J Urol 1977;117:272.

88. Patel NP, Lavengood RW. Renal cell carcinoma: natural history and results of treatment. J Urol 1978;119:722.

89. Rafla S. Renal cell carcinoma: natural history and results of treatment. Cancer 1970;25:26.

90. Thompson IM, Shannon H, Ross G Jr, et al. An analysis of factors affecting survival in 150 patients with renal carcinoma. J Urol 1975;114:694.

91. Golimbu M, Joshi P, Sperber A, et al. Renal cell carcinoma: survival and prognostic factors. Urology 1986;27:291.

92. Neves RJ, Zinke H, Taylor WF. Metastatic renal cell cancer and radical nephrectomy: identification of prognostic factors and patient survival. J Urol 1988;139:1173.

93. Geboers ADH, Debruyne FMJ. Limitations of surgical curability in renal cell carcinoma. Winter Urologic Forum, Streamboats Springs, Colorado, 1987.

94. Lokich JJ, Harrison JH. Renal cell carcinoma: natural history and chemotherapeutic experience. J Urol 1975;114:371.

95. Mims MM, Christenson B, Schlumberger FC, et al. A ten year evaluation of nephrectomy for extensive renal cell carcinoma. J Urol 1966;95:10.

96. Wagle DG, Scal DR. Renal cell carcinoma: a review of 256 cases. J Surg Oncol 1970;2:23.

97. Cox CE, Lacy SJ, Montgomery WG, et al. Renal adenocarcinoma: a 28 year review with emphasis on rationale and feasibility of preoperative radiotherapy. J Urol 1970;104:53.

98. van der Werf-Messing B. Carcinoma of the kidney. Cancer 1973;32:1056.

99. Peeling WB, Martell B, Shepheard BG. Postoperative irradiation in the treatment of renal cell carcinoma. Br J Urol 1969;41:23.

100. Yagoda A. Chemotherapy of renal cell carcinoma. Semin Urol 1989;7:199.

101. Fojo AT, et al. Intrinsic drug resistance in kidney cancers is associated with expression of a human multidrug resistance gene. J Clin Oncol 1987;5:1922.

102. Kakehi Y, et al. Measurement of multidrug resistance messenger RNA in urogenital cancers: elevated expression in renal cell carcinoma is associated with intrinsic drug resistance. J Urol 1988;139:862.

103. Kirtman M, Bacon RC. Renal adenomas and carcinomas in diethylstilbesterol-treated male golden hamsters. Anat Rec 1949;103:475.

104. Bloom MJ. Hormone-induced and spontaneous regression in metastatic renal cancer. Cancer 1973;32:1006.

105. Figlin RA, deKernion JB, et al. Recombinant interferon alpha-2A in metastatic renal cell carcinoma: assessment of antitumor activity and anti-interferon antibody formation. J Clin Oncol 1988;6:1604.

106. Kirkwood JM, et al. A randomized study of low and high doses of leukocyte alpha-interferon in metastatic renal cell carcinoma: the American Cancer Society collaborative trial. Cancer Res 1985;45:863.

107. Muss HB. Interferon therapy for renal cell carcinoma. Semin Oncol 1987;13(Suppl):36.

108. Sarna G, Figlin R, deKernion J. Interferon in renal cell carcinoma: the UCLA experience. Cancer 1987;59:610.

109. Rosenberg SA, Lotze MT, et al. Prospective randomized trial of high-dose interleukin-2 alone or in conjunction with lymphokine-activated killer cells for the treatment of patients with advanced cancer. J Natl Cancer Inst 1993;85:622.

SUGGESTED READINGS

Bennington JL, Beckwith JB. Tumors of the kidney, renal pelvis and ureter. In: Firminger HI, ed. Atlas of the tumor pathology. 2nd series, fascicle 12. Washington: AFIP, 1975.

Bodney GP. Current status of chemotherapy in metastatic renal cancer. In: Johnson DE, Samuels ML, eds. Cancer of the genitourinary tract. New York: Raven Press, 1979:67.

Boring CC, Squires TS, Bottinger LE. Prognosis in renal carcinoma. Cancer 1970;26:780.

Clarke BG, Goode WJ Jr. Fever and anemia in renal cancer. N Engl J Med 1956;354:107.

Cockett ATK, Davis RS, et al. Intrarenal and in situ kidney work bench surgery under hypothermia. Urology 1980;15:112.

Cummings KB, Li W, Ryan JA, et al. Intraoperative management of renal cell carcinoma with supradiaphragmatic caval extension. J Urol 1979;122:829.

deKernion JB, Lindner A. Treatment of advanced renal cell carcinoma. In: Kuss R, Murphy G, Khoury S, eds. Proceedings of the First International Symposium of Kidney Tumors. New York: Alan R. Liss, 1982:641.

Demas BE, Stafford SA, Hricak H. Kidneys. In: Stark DD, Bradley WG, eds. Magnetic resonance imaging. St. Louis: CV Mosby, 1988:1187.

Droller MJ, ed. Surgical management of urologic disease: an anatomical approach. St. Louis: Mosby Year Book, 1992:343.

Fallon B. Renal parenchymal tumors B: clinical and diagnostic features. In: Culp DA, Loening SA, eds. Genitourinary oncology. Philadelphia: Lea & Febiger, 1985:202.

Fernando AR, Armstrong DMG, Griffiths JR, et al. Protective effect of inosine on the canine kidney during ischemia at 37 degrees centigrade. Transplantations 1977;23:504.

Gibbons RP, Correa JR, et al. Surgical management of renal lesions using in situ hypothermia and ischemia. J Urol 1976;115:12.

Gittes RF. Partial nephrectomy: in situ or extracorporeal. In: Walsh PC, Gittes RF, Perlmutter AD, et al., eds. Campbell's urology. 5th ed. Philadelphia: WB Saunders, 1986;3:2454.

Glenn JF, ed. Urologic surgery. Philadelphia: JB Lippincott, 1991:22.

Harris DT. Hormonal therapy and chemotherapy of renal cell carcinoma. Semin Oncol 1983;10:422.

Hatcher PA, Anderson EE, Paulson DF, et al. Surgical management and prognosis of renal cell carcinoma invading the vena cava. J Urol 1991;145:20.

Krane RJ, deVere White RW, Davis Z, et al. Removal of renal cell carcinoma extending into the right atrium using cardiopulmonary bypass, profound hypothermia, and circulatory arrest. J Urol 1984;131:945.

Leach G, Lieber MM. Partial nephrectomy: Mayo Clinic experience 1957–1977. Urology 1980;15:219.

Metzner PF, Boyce WH. Simplified hypothermia: an adjunct to conservative renal surgery. Br J Urol 1972;44:76.

Novick AC, Zincke H, Neves RJ, et al. Surgical enucleation for renal cell carcinoma. J Urol 1986;135:235.

Richie EW. The place of radiotherapy in the management of parenchymal carcinoma. J Urol 1966;95:313.

Richie JP, Garnick MG. Primary renal and ureteral cancer. In: Rieseback RE, Garnick MB, eds. Cancer and the kidney. Philadelphia: Lea & Febiger, 1982:683.

Robson CJ. Radical nephrectomy for renal cell carcinoma. J Urol 1963;89:37.

Schefft P, et al. Surgery for renal cell carcinoma extending into the inferior vena cava. J Urol 1978;120:128.

Schrier RW, et al. protection of mitochondrial function by
mannitol in ischemic renal failure. Am J Physiol 1984;247:
F365.

Swanson DA, Johnson DE. The management of renal carcinoma.
Weekly Urology Update Series. 1978;1:2(lesson 36).

Sznol M, Parkinson DR. Clinical applications of IL-2. Oncology
1994;8:61.

Tannenbaum M. Ultrastructural pathology of human renal cell
tumors. Pathol Annu 1971;6:259.

Timmons SL, Ward R, deVere White RW. In situ renal perfusion.
World J Urol 1990;8:55.

Wickham JEA, Mathur VK. Hypothermia in conservative renal
surgery of renal disease. Br J Urol 1971;39:727.

Wickham JEA, Hanley HF, Jockes AM. Regional renal
hypothermia. Br J Urol 1967;39:727.

Wilhelm E, Schrott JM, et al. Transvenous perfusion cooling of the
kidney: a new technique of local renal hypothermia. Invest Urol
1978;16:87.

4

Radical Nephrectomy

Thoracoabdominal Extrapleural Approach

Sakti Das

HISTORICAL PERSPECTIVES

Erastus Wolcott of Milwaukee performed the first reported nephrectomy in 1861, which was chronicled in brilliant detail by Charles Stoddard (1). This serendipitous nephrectomy, of what was presumed preoperatively to be a hepatic cyst, was accomplished through an anterior transperitoneal approach.

Because of their deep thoracoabdominal location, the kidneys have been approached through a variety of incisions. The lumbar approach of Gustav Simon, for the first deliberately planned nephrectomy in 1869, had a significant limitation of exposure (2). In 1876, Kocher advocated the anterior transperitoneal route to remove a "sarcomatous" kidney (3). The transperitoneal approach, although providing better access to the pedicle and allowing examination of the contralateral kidney (of utmost importance in the period before pyelography), nonetheless became unpopular because of the increased mortality rate due to peritonitis and shock.

The oblique flank incision described by Kuster in 1883 pioneered the development of a number of variations and modifications in the flank approach, allowing better access to the kidney without violation of the pleura or peritoneum (4). In 1926, Bernard Fey reported his extrapleural abdominothoracic incision along the 11th rib, which continued downward and medially toward the epigastrium, with resection or downward displacement of the 11th rib (5). Use of this incision has had sporadic resurgence, with more recent modifications by Presman, Turner-Warwick, and others (6–8).

SURGICAL OBJECTIVES AND RATIONALE

Ideal extirpative surgery for renal cell carcinoma is accomplished by the following:

1. Early ligation of the renal pedicle before any manipulation or mobilization of the neoplasm,
2. Removal of the renal neoplasm with intact surrounding Gerota's fascia, and
3. Regional lymphadenectomy.

The incision or approach used should also allow an adequate intraperitoneal exploration for intra-abdominal metastases.

Advocates of the anterior transperitoneal and the thoracoabdominal intrapleural approaches have claimed that these incisions provide better access to the renal pedicle and the suprahilar regions, respectively, compared with the conventional flank incision. However, use of the 10th-intercostal-space or 11th-rib supracostal extrapleural transperitoneal approach makes the early control of the renal pedicle, a thorough laparotomy, and excellent exposure of the suprahilar retroperitoneum feasible. When exploration of the thoracic cavity is not needed, the supracostal incision can provide adequate exposure while preventing the additional morbidity of thoracotomy.

The preference of radical nephrectomy over simple nephrectomy for the management of renal carcinoma has been championed by Robson (9). Despite the lack of prospective studies comparing the two modalities, improved results of radical nephrectomy compared with those reported earlier reaffirm the importance of removing the intact Gerota's fascia with its contents, the kidney, and the adrenal gland. Many of these tumors, especially large or peripherally located ones, spread through the capsule into the perinephric fat, enhancing the chances of local recurrence and dissemination if Gerota's fascia is not excised. One might make a case for not removing the ipsilateral adrenal gland in renal carcinoma involving the lower half of the kidney, especially if the adrenal appears normal on computed tomography scan. The incidence of adrenal metastases in such instances is extremely rare (10).

The therapeutic value of lymphadenectomy for renal cell carcinoma, however, has not been unequivocally established. Rarely, a patient with micrometastases to one or two proximal nodes may be cured by lymphadenectomy, but involvement of the lymph nodes is usually an important prognostic determinant indicating disseminated disease. Currently, lymphadenectomy is mainly considered an important staging procedure that allows for the selection of patients who may need adjuvant therapy (11).

An extensive bilateral retroperitoneal lymphadenectomy, similar to that performed for testicular tumors, is not warranted for renal cell carcinoma. To reduce the morbidity from such a procedure while accomplishing the objectives of lymphadenectomy, we limit regional lymphadenectomy to the clearing of the nodal tissues of the aortocaval area and the area around the ipsilateral great vessel (the aorta in the case of a tumor on the left side, and the vena cava for a tumor on the right side), from the level of the diaphragmatic crus above to the inferior mesenteric artery at the distal limit. The contralateral renal hilar region and the posterolateral aspect of the contralateral great vessel are not dissected.

INDICATIONS AND CONTRAINDICATIONS

Most radical nephrectomies can be conveniently performed through the modified high-flank or extrapleural thoracoabdominal approach. The location or the size of the tumor is not a contraindication. The following situations, however, make alternative incisions more pragmatically desirable.

1. A few patients cannot be placed in the flank position because of a spinothoracic deformity or because they have circulatory decompensation in the lateral position.
2. If bilateral renal surgery is contemplated, an anterior transperitoneal incision is ideal.
3. In the case of tumors in a solitary kidney, either in situ or ex vivo (bench surgery), excision of the neoplasm is necessary. Ex vivo surgery is performed through the anterior approach; otherwise, the patient must be repositioned in the supine position to obtain better access to the hypogastric artery or the iliac vessels for autotransplantation.
4. If thrombus extraction from the renal vein or vena cava is contemplated for renal carcinoma on the left side, an anterior approach is again preferred because adequate control of the inferior vena cava is difficult to achieve through a left-flank incision.
5. An intrapleural thoracoabdominal incision may be necessary for diagnostic exploration of pulmonary metastasis or for therapeutic excision of the metastasis with radical nephrectomy.
6. Thoracotomy is also mandatory when better access to the proximal portion of the inferior vena cava or the right atrium is necessary to extract a tumor thrombus.

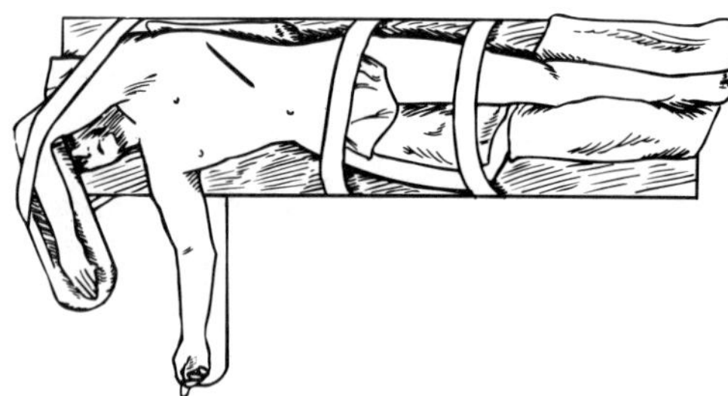

Fig. 4.1. The patient is positioned midway between supine and true lateral decubitus. The incision is made from angle of the eleventh rib along its upper border toward epigastrium across midline (left-sided position).

SURGICAL PROCEDURE

The patient is placed about midway between the full lateral and supine positions. This position is often achieved by placing the patient in the true lateral position; the upper torso is then allowed to roll backward. A small sandbag is placed near the scapula. Sequential compression devices are applied to both the lower extremities below the knee to prevent venous thromboembolism. The ipsilateral lower extremity is extended over the flexed opposite leg with a pillow between. The table is flexed, and wide adhesive tapes are applied across the iliac crest to the table to stabilize the patient (Fig. 4.1). The position of the 11th rib is indelibly marked before skin preparation. An 18-French Foley catheter is inserted for intraoperative and postoperative monitoring of urine output. We prefer to stand on the right side of the patient for both right and left radical nephrectomy.

Incision

The incision begins near the angle of the 11th rib at the posterior axillary line and continues along the upper costal margin toward the epigastrium. The anterior rectus sheath, external oblique, latissimus dorsi, and more posteriorly, part of the serratus posterior inferior muscles are divided with cutting diathermy. The rectus abdominis muscle is transected, and the internal oblique and transversus abdominis are divided up to the tip of the 11th rib (Fig. 4.2A).

The intercostal muscles of the 10th interspace are exposed and carefully dissected off the upper margin of the 11th rib, and the underlying diaphragm is thereby exposed (Fig. 4.2B). This part of the dissection requires caution because the thin linear margin of the pleural reflection becomes apparent near the middle of the interspace.

Identification of the pleura is aided and its integrity confirmed when the anesthetist expands the lung, whereby the inferior pulmonary margin descends to occupy the pleural space. By blunt finger dissection, the pleura is pushed away from the inner surface of the lower rib (Fig. 4.2C). The pleura, if opened inadvertently, can be closed with mattress or continuous sutures of 3-0 chromic catgut, taking bites through the adjacent diaphragm for a secure hold. The suture is tied while the anesthetist expels the pneumothorax by positive pressure ventilation.

Further posteriorly, the sharp margin of the costovertebral ligament is encountered at the upper edge of the rib. The overlying latissimus dorsi and erector spinae muscles are strongly retracted, and the ligament is divided, allowing the rib to be hinged downward.

The exposed diaphragm is now incised parallel to the rib approximately 2 cm below the pleural reflection. The incised upper edge of the diaphragm is wrapped around the upper (10th) rib and sutured to the serratus posterior inferior and, more anteriorly, to the deeper fibers of the latissimus dorsi (Fig. 4.2D). This modification by Witherington deters inadvertent pleural injury from retraction at later stages of the dissection (8).

Anteromedially, the posterior rectus sheath and the peritoneum are opened widely, and a careful laparotomy is performed to detect any metastases or other associated disease. A self-retaining retractor is applied between the ribs in the posterior aspect of the wound.

Left Radical Nephrectomy

The descending colon is held up, and the peritoneum of the lateral paracolic gutter is incised (Fig. 4.3). Superiorly, this incision is carried through the anterior lamella of the splenocolic ligament, thereby allowing inferomedial mobilization of the splenic flexure. Care must be taken not to injure the inferior pole of the spleen at this stage. The splenic flexure and the descending colon, with their mesentery, are bluntly mobilized from the underlying Gerota's fascia and retroperitoneum. The hand inside the abdomen, lifting the colon with its peritoneal attachment and blood supply, is an excellent guide to the proper plane anterior to the Gerota's fascia. Generous mobilization of this posterior peritoneum and wide exposure of the retroperitoneum make subsequent dissection easy to perform. At this stage, the anteromedial aspect of the vena cava should be visible medially, as should the origin of the superior mesenteric artery superiorly and the posterior surface of the pancreas with the splenic vessels anterosuperiorly.

If the mesentery of the descending colon adheres to the

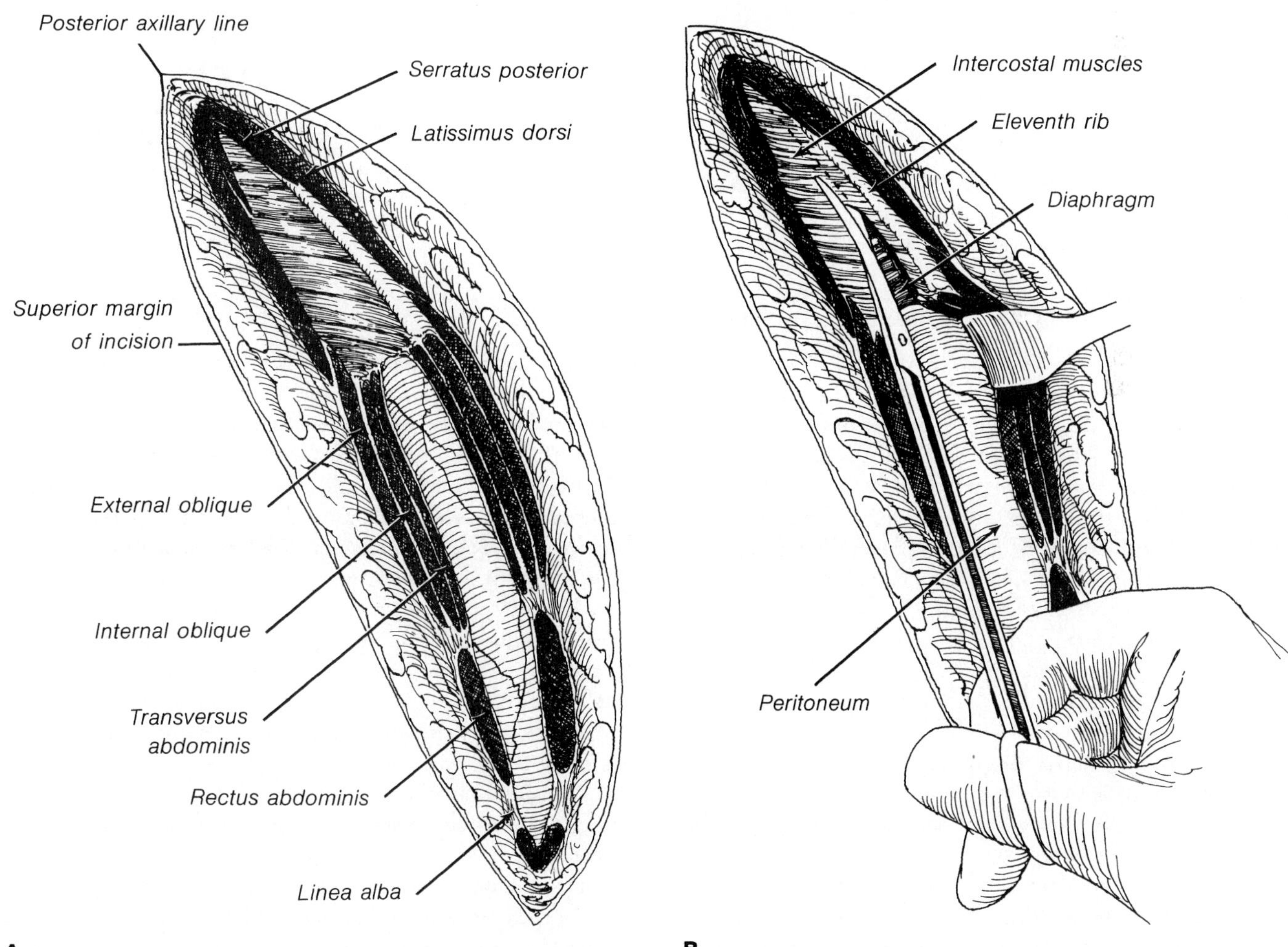

Fig. 4.2. **A.** Division of parietal muscle layers, exposing intercostal muscles of tenth interspace (view of left-sided incision from patient's right side). **B.** Division of intercostal muscles, exposing underlying diaphragm.

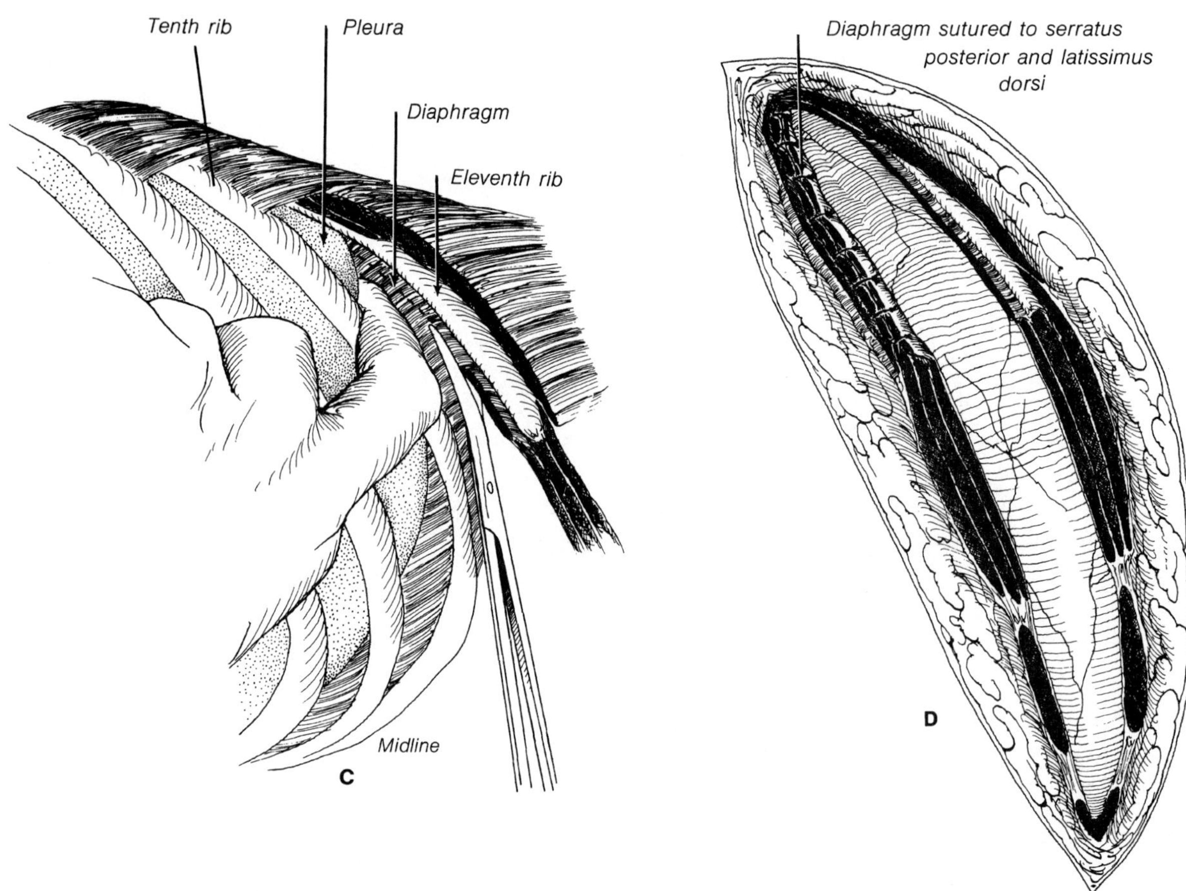

Fig. 4.2. *(continued)* **C.** Pleura is reflected superiorly by blunt dissection away from eleventh rib and diaphragm. Diaphragm is incised below pleural reflection (view of left-sided incision from patient's right side). **D.** Superior edge of incised diaphragm is wrapped around tenth rib and sutured to serratus posterior inferior and latissimus dorsi.

tumor, the area in doubt should be circumscribed and left with the Gerota's fascia for en bloc removal. Ischemic injury to the colon is unlikely as long as its marginal arcades are preserved. The tumor must not be manipulated during this stage.

The large left renal vein coursing medially across the aorta is now easily identified (Fig. 4.4). As the diaphanous medial extension of the Gerota's fascia over the renal vein is dissected, the left adrenal vein is seen near the renal hilum. The adrenal vein is divided between ligatures of 2-0 silk to avoid tearing while retracting the renal vein. The renal artery lies directly posterosuperior to the renal vein. The renal vein is retracted downward, allowing palpation and dissection of the renal artery.

The superior mesenteric artery and the renal artery must be identified as separate entities before any attempt at arterial ligation is made. The grave error of ligating the superior mesenteric artery has been known to occur, especially with large and medially encroaching tumors. The renal artery is ligated in continuity with 1-0 silk (Fig. 4.5A) and is not divided at this stage. Accessory renal arteries are palpated for at this stage and ligated similarly if detected. The renal vein is ligated and divided where it terminates at the inferior vena cava. The distal stump of the divided renal vein is held up by its ligature, and any lumbar vein must be sought entering the renal vein from behind (Fig. 4.5B). Such a lumbar vein must be divided between ligatures in case it tears and retracts into the paravertebral muscles, causing troublesome hemorrhage. The renal artery already ligated is now further dissected up to its origin, where it is doubly ligated and divided (Fig. 4.5C).

Starting below the divided renal vessels, the surgeon pushes the Gerota's fascia laterally away from the psoas major. At the lower extent of the wound, the ureter is divided between ligatures of 1-0 chromic catgut near the pelvic brim. The gonadal vessels are ligated with 2-0 silk and divided at about the same level (Fig. 4.6A). The kidney, ensheathed by Gerota's fascia, is now held medially and separated from the psoas major and quadratus lumborum muscles on its posterolateral aspect (Fig. 4.6B). A few large collateral vessels require ligature and division.

Dissection is continued superiorly, stripping the thin layer of Gerota's fascia around the adrenal gland from the inferior surface of the diaphragm. Medially and above, the small adrenal branches from the aorta and phrenic arteries are divided between hemostatic clips (Fig. 4.7). The kidney harboring the

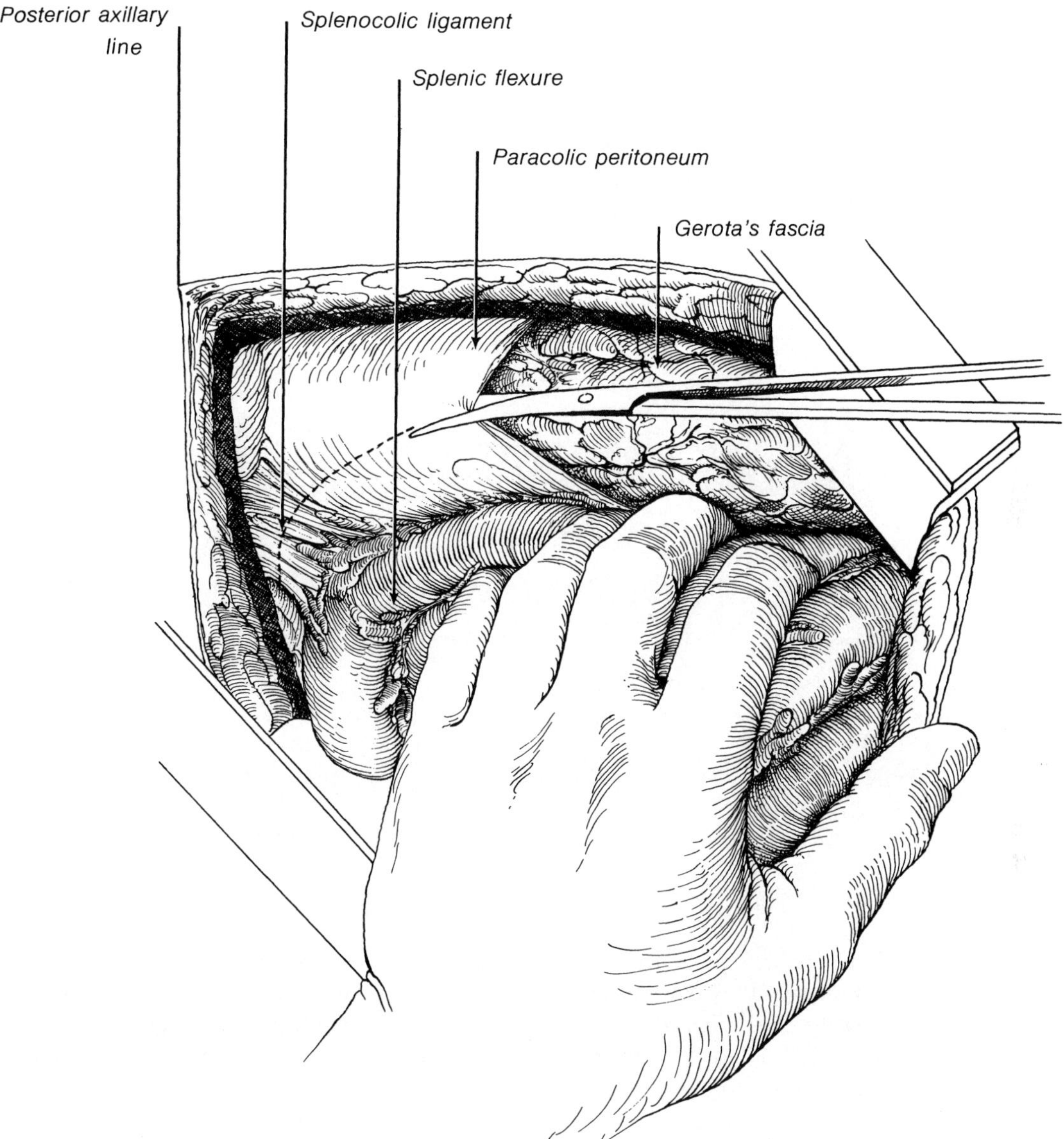

Fig. 4.3. Incision of lateral paracolic peritoneum is carried above and medially through splenocolic ligament.

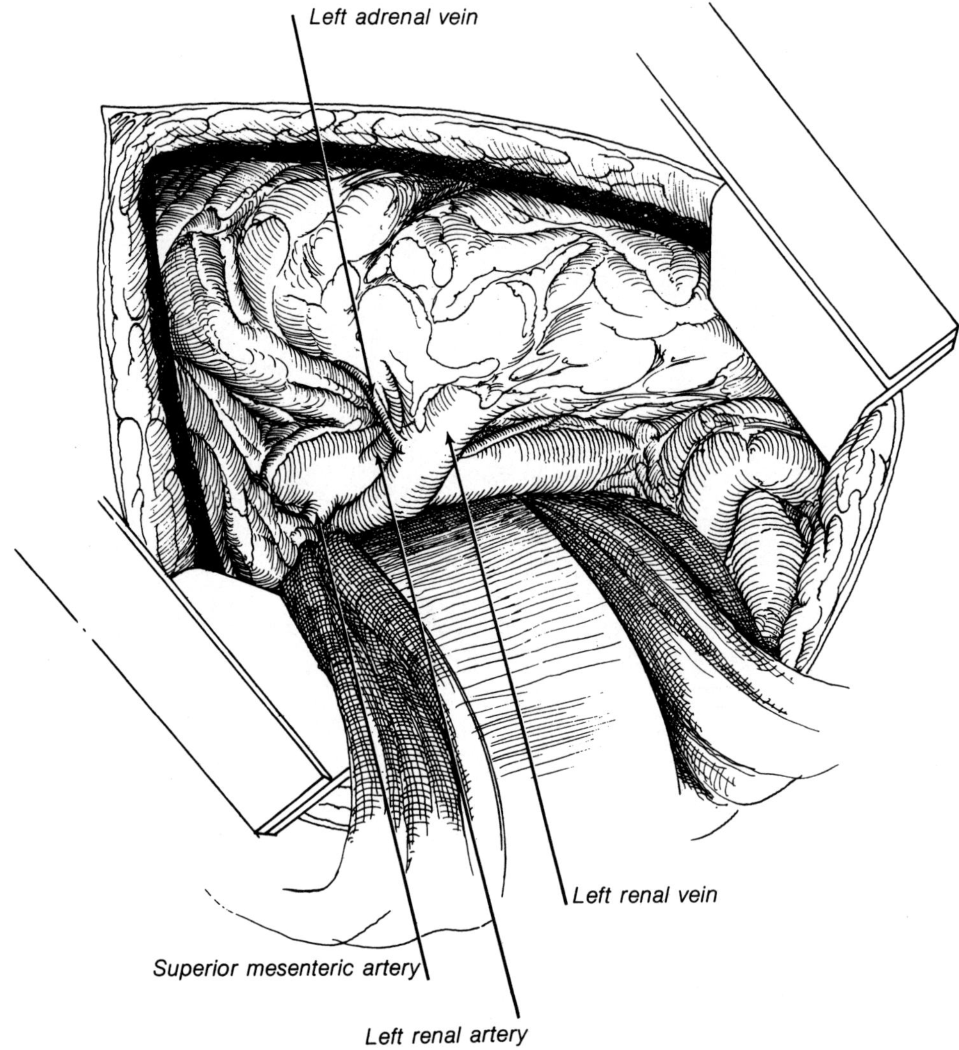

Fig. 4.4.   Medial reflection of descending colon, exposing retroperitoneal structures.

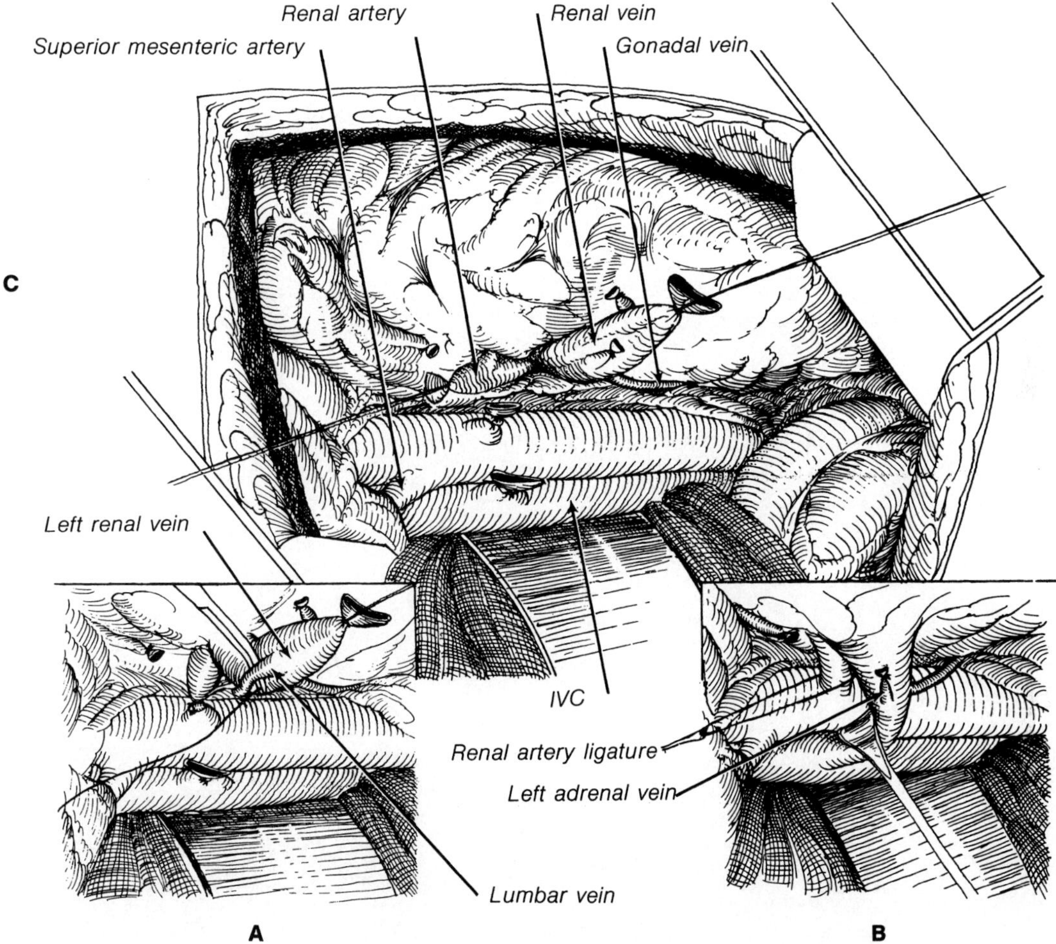

Fig. 4.5. **A.** Left renal vein is retracted downward after division of left adrenal vein. Renal artery is ligated in continuity. **B.** Distal stump of left renal vein is held up, and any lumbar vein entering from behind is sought. **C.** Left renal vein and artery have been doubly ligated and divided.

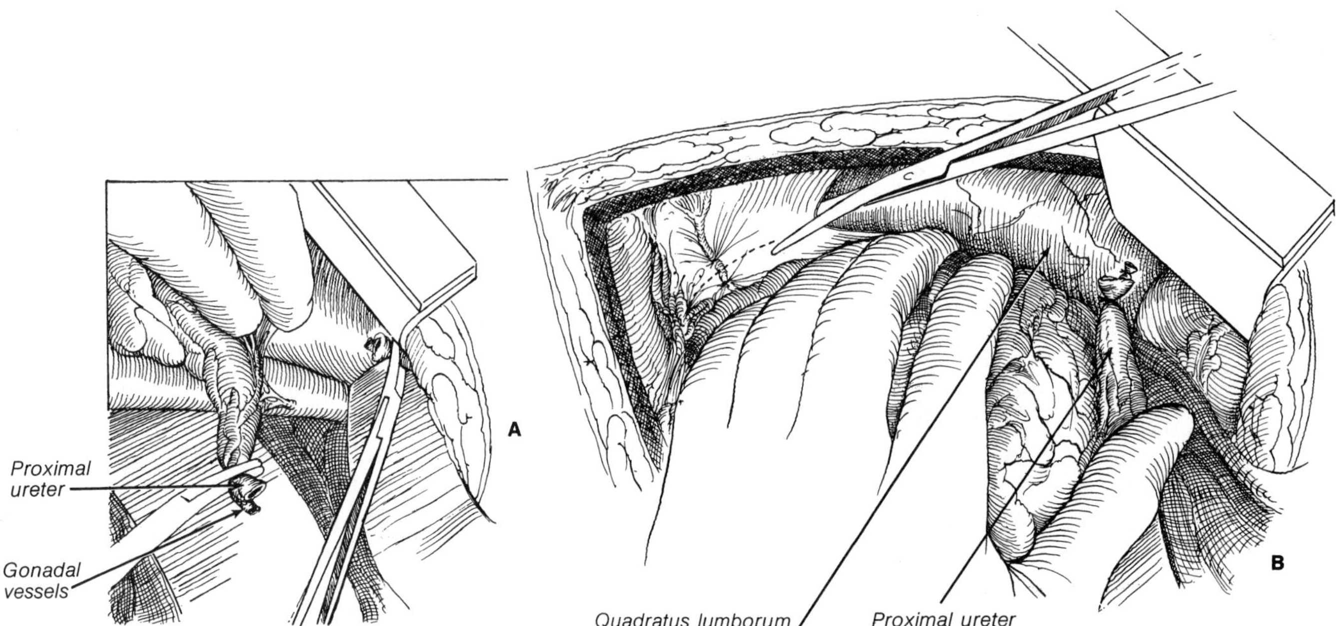

Fig. 4.6.   A. Ureter and gonadal vessels are ligated and divided near pelvic brim. **B.** Kidney enclosed by Gerota's fascia is dissected away from quadratus lumborum and psoas major muscles on posterolateral aspect.

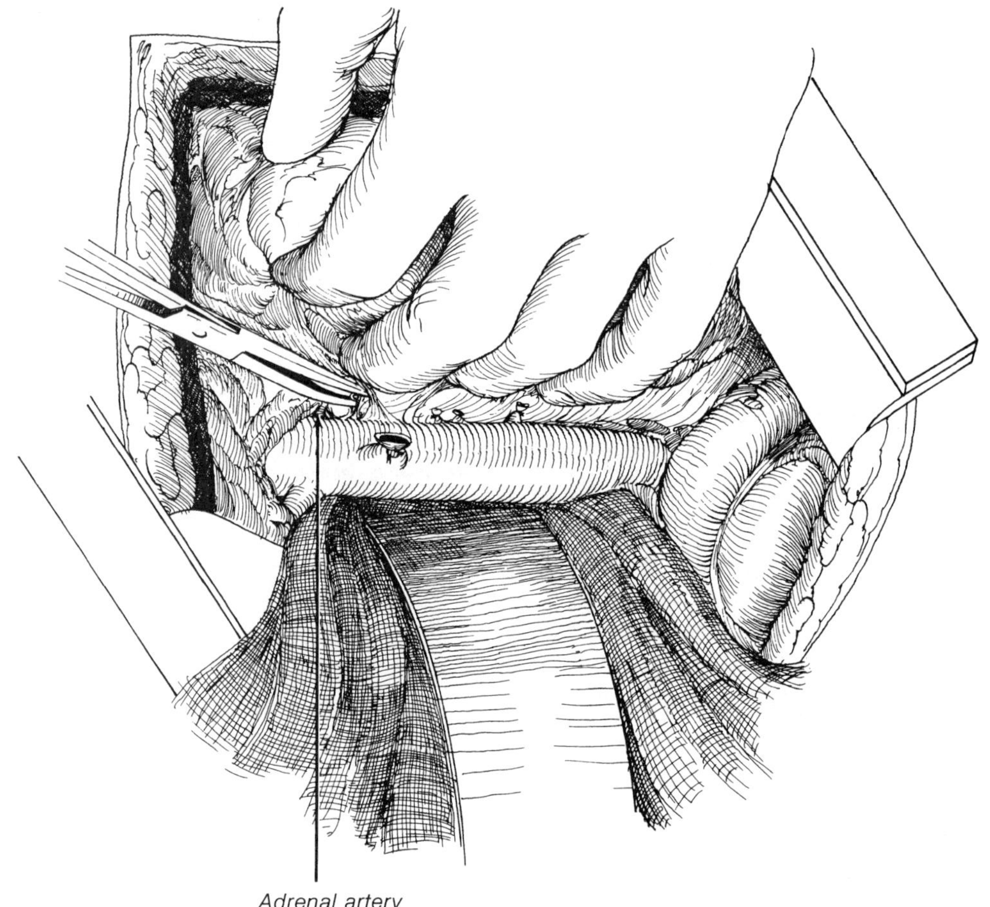

Fig. 4.7.   Dissection is continued on superior and medial aspects. Adrenal branches from aorta are divided between hemostatic clips.

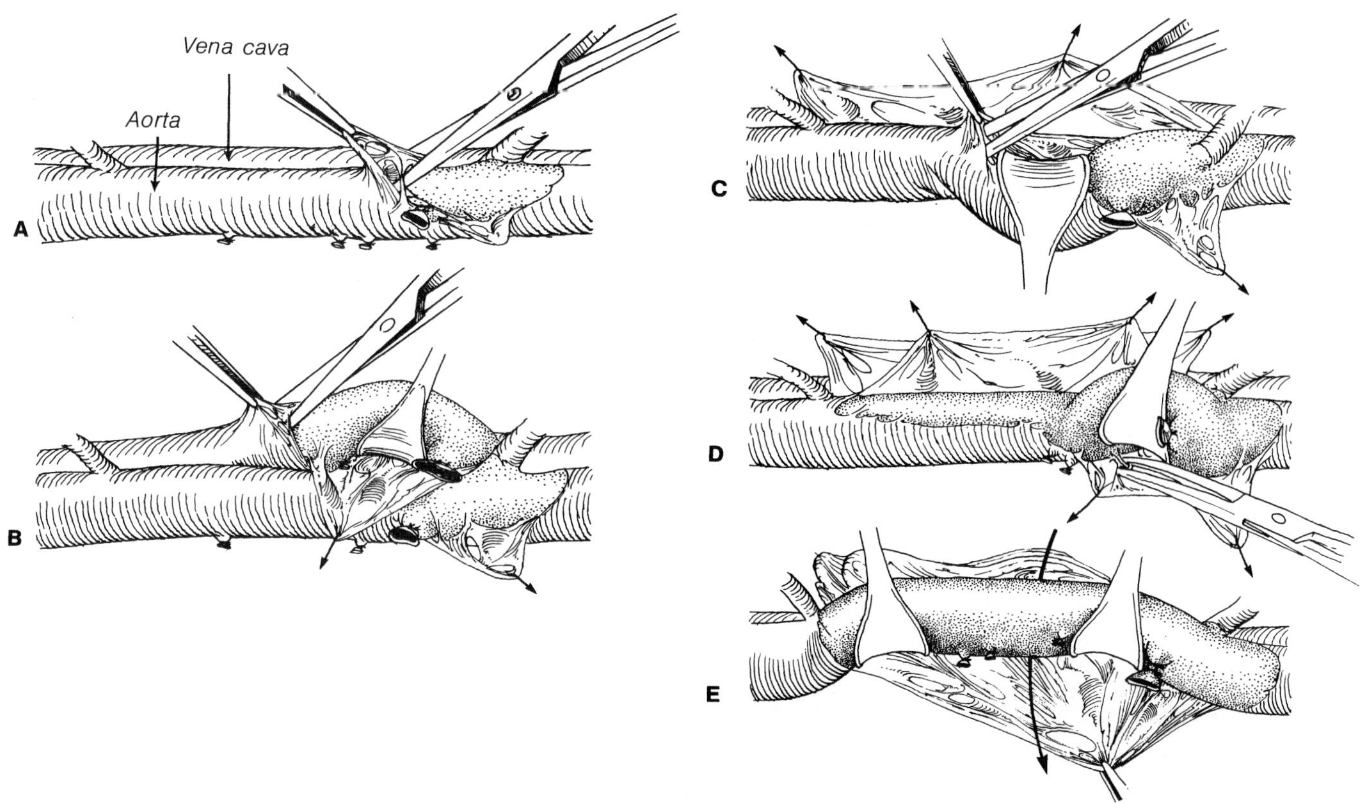

Fig. 4.8. **A.** Suprahilar dissection, stripping tissues from front of diaphragmatic crus and aorta to below renal vessels. **B.** Anteromedial aspect of vena cava is dissected away from aortocaval tissues. **C.** Anteromedial aspect of aorta is dissected away from aortocaval tissues. **D.** Lateral para-aortic tissues are dissected away from aorta. **E.** Aorta is held up on retractors; lateral para-aortic and aortocaval tissues are pulled out en bloc behind aorta.

tumor and the adrenal gland with the covering Gerota's fascia are removed en bloc.

Regional lymphadenectomy is now carried out, unless the nephrectomy is being performed as a palliative measure or the patient's age and general condition preclude further extensive surgery. Dissection is begun at the suprahilar region, bringing down the tissues in front of the diaphragmatic crus lateral to the aorta. The node-bearing fibrofatty tissue is pushed medially over the aorta. As dissection continues along the subadventitial plane, the tissues in front of the aorta are brought downward, skirting the origins of the celiac and superior mesenteric artery up to below the origins of the renal arteries (Fig. 4.8A).

Similar dissection up and down the anteromedial surface of the vena cava separates the aortocaval nodal tissues away from the vena cava (Fig. 4.8B). A few lumbar veins require ligature and division. The adventitia in front of the aorta is split down to the origin of the inferior mesenteric artery. The medial leaf of adventitia with the aortocaval tissues is separated from the aorta dividing the lumbar arteries (Fig. 4.8C). The lateral aspect of the aorta is then dissected away from the para-aortic nodal tissue on the left side (Fig. 4.8D). As the lumbar arteries in this area are divided, the aorta can be held up on vein retractors.

The lateral para-aortic nodal envelope is now grasped with the fingers. As it is pulled out, the dissected aortocaval nodal tissues are pushed behind the aorta and removed in continuity, exposing the anterior spinal ligaments (Fig. 4.8E).

Hemostatic clips must be used generously throughout the procedure to prevent postoperative lymph leakage or collection. The wound is copiously irrigated with distilled water. General hemostasis and, in particular, the integrity of the spleen are checked. Most of the inadvertent splenic tears can be managed by applying microfibrillar purified bovine corium collagen (Avitene; Alcon, Humacao, Puerto Rico), and splenectomy is rarely necessary. The wound is closed in layers without drains.

Right Radical Nephrectomy

On the right side, the inferior margin of the right lobe of the liver often encroaches on the posterior part of the wound after the 11th-rib supracostal incision. The avascular right triangular ligament is divided, and the inferior surface of the liver is carefully retracted upward. The incision of the lateral paracolic peritoneum is continued upward and medially to the front of the vena cava above the duodenum (Fig. 4.9). The second part of the duodenum is reflected medially to expose the entire width of the inferior vena cava.

The thin adventitial layer in front of the vena cava is dissected to expose the termination of the renal veins. The left renal vein and the medial margin of the vena cava are retracted to expose the right renal artery in a more posterior plane. The right renal artery is ligated in continuity at this site between

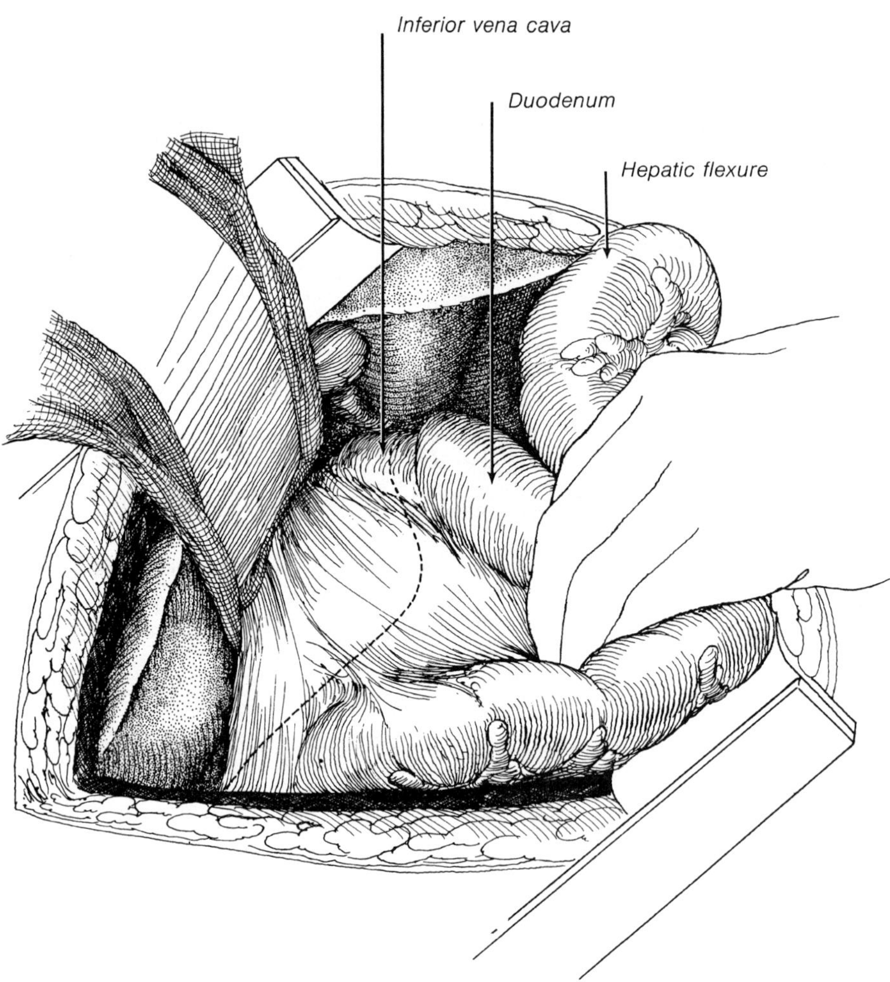

Fig. 4.9. Incision of paracolic peritoneum on right side is carried across front of inferior vena cava above duodenum.

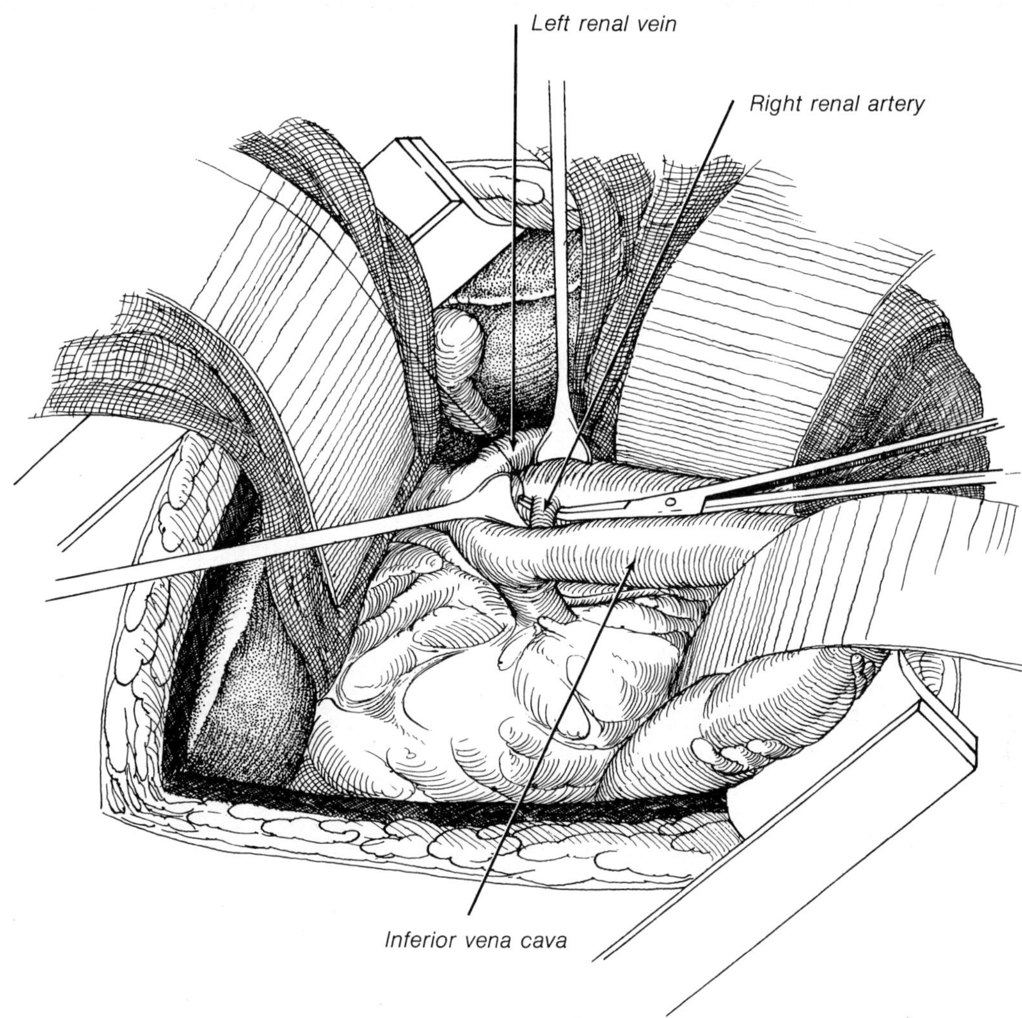

Fig. 4.10.   Right renal artery is dissected between vena cava and aorta and ligated near origin of artery.

the aorta and the vena cava (Fig. 4.10). The right renal vein is ligated and divided. The artery is then religated twice and is divided between the proximal two and distal single ligature.

On the right side, there are usually several adrenal veins with a short, direct course into the vena cava. They must be sought carefully along the lateral aspect of the vena cava behind the right lobe of the liver and divided between ligatures. The remainder of the procedure is similar to that described for the left side.

Regional lymphadenectomy is then carried out. The surgeon dissects the node-bearing tissues around the vena cava and the aortocaval area down to the level of the inferior mesenteric artery.

POSTOPERATIVE CARE

A chest radiograph is routinely done in the recovery room. Management of any inadvertent pleural injuries that escaped notice during the surgical procedure depends on the degree of the resultant pneumothorax. Minor pneumothorax (less than

10%) is absorbed within a few days and does not require intervention. Major pneumothorax must be immediately drained via a needle introduced into the second intercostal space in the midclavicular line. The needle is connected to an underwater-sealed container and is removed as soon as no further air bubbles are expelled. Prompt expansion of the underlying lung is confirmed by a repeated chest radiograph.

Nasogastric suction is continued until postoperative ileus is resolved and intestinal peristalsis is resumed. Parenteral fluid replacement must take into account the large protein-rich transudate loss from the renal fossa and retroperitoneum. Partial colloid replacement with plasma or albumin is often necessary for the first few days. Vigorous pulmonary care and early ambulation are mandatory.

REFERENCES

1. Stoddard CL. Case of encephaloid disease of the kidney removal. Med Surg Reporter 1861;7:126.
2. Simon G. Uber die Zulassigkeit der einseitigen Nephrotomie bei Harnleiterbauchfisteln: (Vortrag. gehalten im

Operationssaal der chirurgischen Klinik unmittelbar border Operation.) In: Chirurgie der Nieren. Erlangen, Ferdinand Enke, 1871;1.

3. Kocher T. Eine Nephrotomie wegen Nierensarkom. Dtsch Z Chir 1878;9:312.
4. Kuster E. Uber einen Fall von Nierenextirpation mit Demonstration. (Wird in extenso verkoffentlicht werden.) Discussion. Berl Klin Wschr. 1883;20:604.
5. Fey B. L'abord du rein par la voie thoraco-abdominale. Arch Urol Clin Necker 1926;5:169.
6. Presman D. Eleventh intercostal space incision for renal surgery. J Urol 1955;74:578.
7. Turner-Warwick RT. The supracostal approach to the renal area. Br J Urol 1965;37:671.
8. Witherington R. Improving the supracostal loin incisions. J Urol 1980;124:73.
9. Robson CJ. Radical nephrectomy for renal cell carcinoma. J Urol 1963;89:37.
10. Roby EL, Schellhammer PF. Adrenal gland and renal cell carcinoma: is ipsilateral adrenalectomy a necessary component of radical nephrectomy? J Urol 1986;135:453.
11. deKernion JB. Radical nephrectomy. In: Ehrlich RM, ed. Modern technics in surgery (urologic surgery). Mount Kisco, NY: Futura, 1980.

5

Radical Nephrectomy

Thoracoabdominal Intrapleural Approach

Richard K. Heppe and E. David Crawford

Renal cell carcinoma has been poorly responsive to treatment with radiation, chemotherapy, and immunotherapy. The only chance for successful management of this disease is complete surgical extirpation. To this end, removal of the kidney with its investing Gerota's fascia and the adrenal gland has become the preferred treatment.

Radical nephrectomy can be accomplished through a variety of approaches. The intrapleural thoracoabdominal approach is one that we have found most useful. Because this method ensures wide exposure of the kidney, renal vessels, aorta, and vena cava, this incision is ideal for use with large or upper pole lesions, adrenal tumors, large retroperitoneal masses, and retroperitoneal lymph node dissection. In addition, this approach may be advantageously used in renal transplantation, donor nephrectomy, partial nephrectomy, and nephroureterectomy for renal pelvic and ureteral tumors. When one is performing the operation for renal cell carcinoma, the intrapleural approach allows for palpation of the ipsilateral lung for metastases and, on the right side, for control of the vena cava in the chest in the event of a caval thrombus.

HISTORICAL PERSPECTIVES

One of the first descriptions of renal cell carcinoma was made in 1613, when Daniel Sennert described a "hard tumor" of a kidney and believed that it was an incurable disease resulting in cachexia or dropsy (1). Confusion existed in the late 1800s concerning the origin of these tumors. Grawitz observed that tumors of the kidney had a histologic structure similar to that of adrenal tissue and contended that these tumors developed from aberrant adrenal rests (2). The term "hypernephroma" was used in an attempt to describe the adrenal origin of these tumors.

The first tumor nephrectomy was performed accidentally in 1861 by Walcott, who thought the mass removed was a cyst of the liver (3). However, it was found to be a renal neoplasm. Simon performed the first planned nephrectomy in 1869 on a

46-year-old woman whose left ureter had been damaged during a partial hysterectomy, resulting in urinary fistulas with drainage from the vagina and the abdominal scar (4). The operation was successful and the fistulas were cured.

In the early period after Simon's operation the mortality rate was high, but subsequent improvements in the surgical technique significantly reduced the postoperative complications. Most of the early nephrectomies were performed via the lumbar extraperitoneal or transperitoneal route. The need for improved exposure eventually led to the introduction of incisions through the lower thoracic cage. Fey first described the thoracoabdominal incision in 1926 (5). In 1946, Marshall found a 10th-rib thoracoabdominal incision valuable in the surgical repair of war injuries and envisioned the possibility of its use in civilian cases as well (6). This approach incorporated many of the advantages of the transperitoneal and rib-resecting flank approaches.

SELECTION OF PATIENTS

Renal cell carcinoma is often referred to as the "internists' tumor" because of the bizarre pattern of metastases; therefore, a detailed history should be obtained and a careful physical examination performed to detect any unusual metastases. Patients considered for radical nephrectomy should have localized disease (stage A, B, or C). Preoperative evaluation should encompass those areas most commonly involved with metastases. Chest radiographs, chest computed tomography scans, bone scans with spot films of abnormal areas, angiograms with selective and flush studies, liver function studies, hematologic parameters including clotting profile, and renal function tests are often part of the standard evaluation.

Vena caval studies should be performed in selected patients. Ultrasound is useful in detecting and defining the extent of vena caval thrombi (7). We do not routinely use angioinfarction of the renal artery. When one is confronted with metastatic disease, it is unrealistic to remove the primary tumor in the hope that the metastases will regress. Distant metastases are already present at the time of diagnosis in about one third of patients with renal cell carcinoma. Palliative nephrectomy may be justified in patients with a reasonable life expectancy who have severe symptoms secondary to a primary lesion, such as local pain, hemorrhage, or endocrinopathy. However, these symptoms are rarely severe enough to require nephrectomy and can usually be controlled by other means. An occasional patient with one or two isolated metastases amenable to surgical resection may undergo nephrectomy. Palliative nephrectomy may also be considered when a response to a chemotherapeutic drug or other modality, such as immunotherapy, has occurred. Angioinfarction followed by nephrectomy may lead to regression of metastasis in a small number of patients. A study by the Southwest Oncology group, however, found no benefit from this treatment in 30 patients with metastatic renal cell carcinoma (8).

PREOPERATIVE PREPARATION

Preoperative preparation for radical nephrectomy is standard to most other major operative procedures. An intravenous infusion of Ringer's lactate is begun the evening before surgery to ensure adequate preoperative hydration. Patients who have large tumors or evidence of contiguous organ involvement should also undergo a standard bowel preparation.

The role of preoperative percutaneous transaortic occlusion of the renal artery remains uncertain, but one of the main advantages of this procedure is that it allows division of the renal vein without the need to first dissect out and divide the artery. Further delay of surgery after infarction allows for shrinkage

of caval tumor thrombus, resolution of arteriovenous shunting, and improvement of the patient's nutritional status (9). However, infarction may also induce severe pain, fever, and nausea and may compromise the patient's ability to tolerate an extensive operation. In patients who have a vena caval thrombus, this procedure may be helpful in minimizing disturbance of the tumor thrombus while the surgeon is attempting to obtain arterial control. However, we have not found infarction particularly useful in large tumors when attempting to decrease the amount of operative hemorrhage because there is generally collateral circulation to the kidney.

SURGICAL PROCEDURE

After adequate presurgical preparation, the patient is brought to the operating room and general endotracheal anesthesia is administered. A central venous line is placed in most patients, especially in those who are at high operative risk. An indwelling catheter is inserted in the bladder.

Position

One of the crucial initial aspects of the operation is the patient's position, which should be supervised by the operating surgeon. The patient is moved to the ipsilateral side of the operating table, and a large towel or sandbag is positioned under the back (Fig. 5.1). The break in the operating table should be located just above the iliac crest. The leg in contact with the table is flexed 90° and the pelvis is nearly supine. The ipsilateral shoulder is positioned approximately 30° off the horizontal,

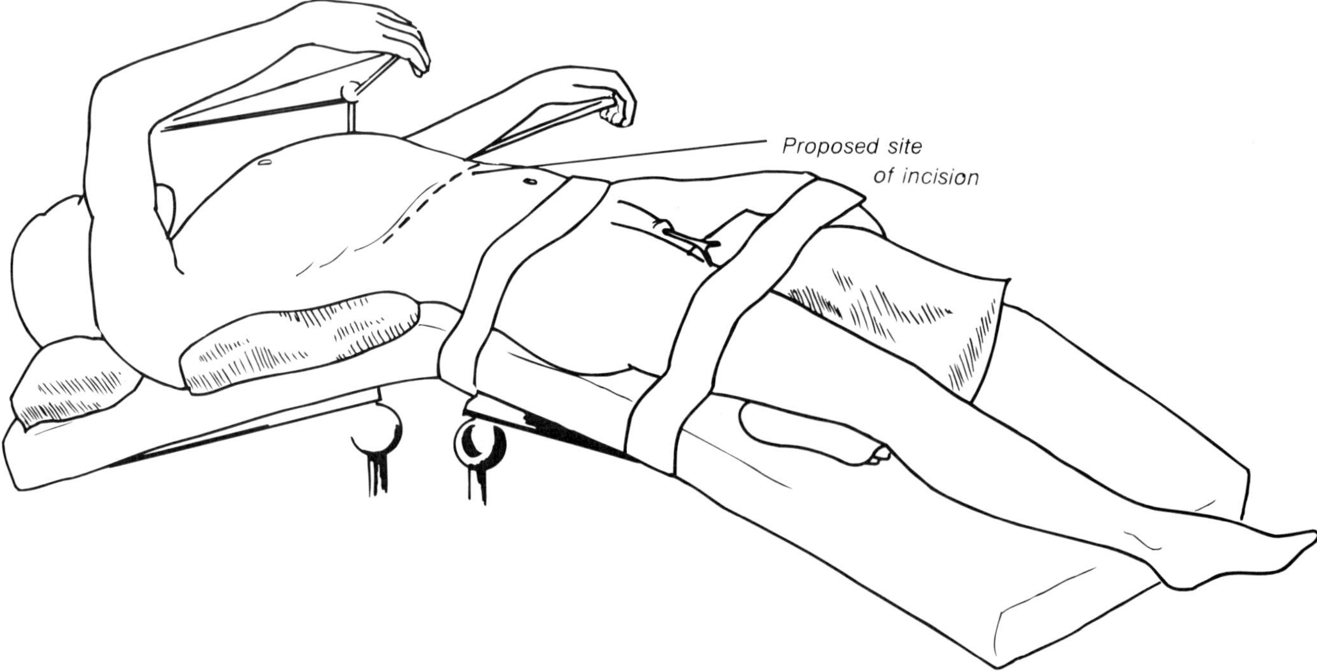

Fig. 5.1.   The patient is positioned on the ipsilateral side of the operating table, with the break in the table located just above the iliac crest. The ipsilateral shoulder is positioned approximately 30° off the horizontal, and the arm is extended across the chest and placed on a Mayo stand or adjustable armrest.

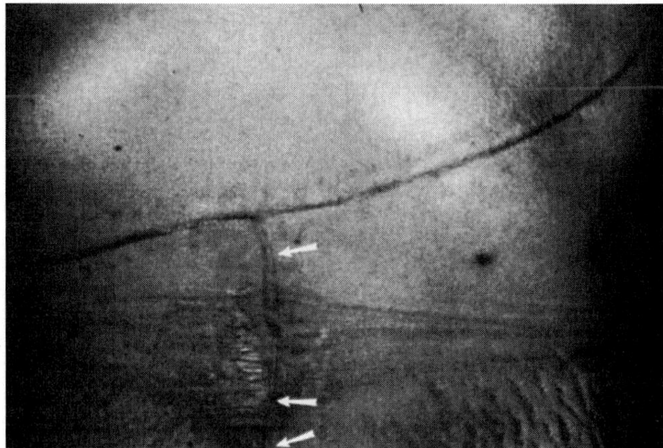

Fig. 5.2. Postoperative photograph of a left thoracoabdominal incision showing "T" dropped as a perpendicular in the midline (arrows). An 8-lb renal tumor was removed via this incision.

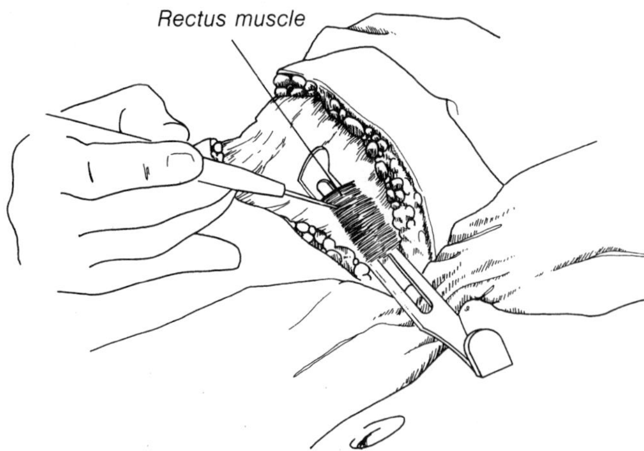

Fig. 5.4. An Army-Navy retractor is passed under the rectus muscle, and the muscle is divided with the electrocautery unit. After the costochondral junction is divided, the peritoneal cavity is entered.

and the arm is brought across the chest and placed on a Mayo stand or an adjustable armrest. An axillary pad is positioned, and the patient is secured to the table with wide adhesive tape placed over the shoulders and hips. In the final position, the pelvis is nearly horizontal to the operating table.

Incision

The choice of a rib for resection depends on the nature of the primary renal tumor. In general, lower-pole tumors can be approached through a 10th-rib incision. However, in patients with large upper-pole tumors or with right-sided tumors and vena caval thrombi, the best approach is through an eighth- or ninth-rib incision. The incision is begun at the midaxillary line, is extended across the costochondral junction, and is curved slightly downward onto the abdominal wall to avoid injury to the intercostal nerves.

The medial extent of the incision is determined by the extent of the tumor and the size of the patient; if necessary, it may even be extended across the epigastrium to the contralateral side. For extremely large tumors, the incision may be in a "T" form and may be carried inferiorly as a midline incision. (Figure 5.2 is an 8-week postoperative photograph of a 41-year-old woman who had an 8-lb renal tumor removed from such an incision.) The latissimus dorsi muscle is divided, and after division of the overlying muscle, the distal two thirds of the rib are resected subperiosteally (Fig. 5.3). The incision is carried medially, and the anterior rectus sheath is incised.

Technique

An Army–Navy retractor is passed under the rectus abdominis, and the muscle itself is divided with an electrocautery unit (Fig. 5.4). The superior epigastric vessels encountered are either fulgurated or ligated with 3-0 chromic catgut sutures. The costochondral junction is divided sharply with Mayo scissors.

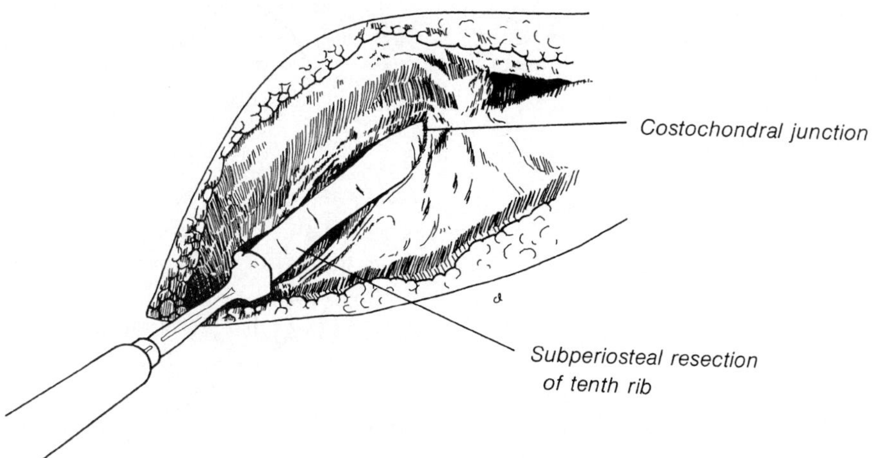

Fig. 5.3. Tenth rib is resected in a subperiosteal fashion. Posterior to the rib are the periosteum and pleura, which are sharply incised to enter the pleural cavity. Care should be exercised not to damage the lung during this maneuver.

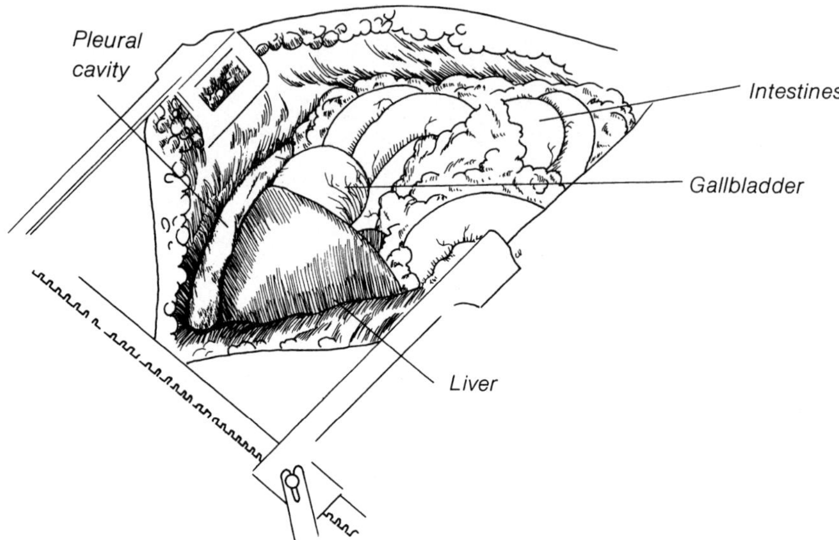

Fig. 5.5. Finochietto retractor is placed in the wound between the divided costal cartilage, exposing the abdominal contents.

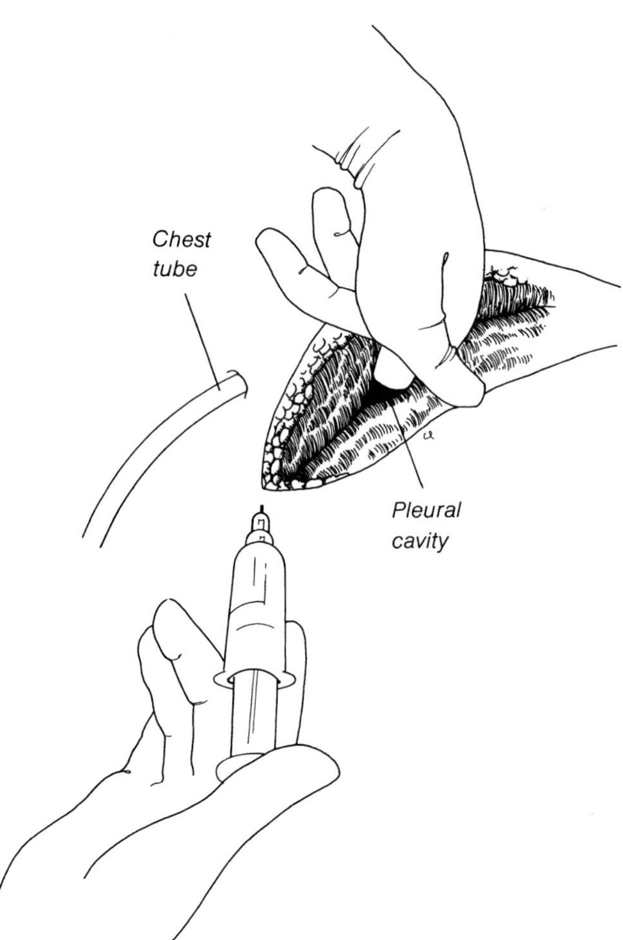

Fig. 5.6. Percutaneous injection of bupivacaine hydrochloride into the neurovascular bundle of the resected rib. Two interspaces above and below, as well as the chest tube site, are injected. The index finger is placed into the chest cavity to direct the position of the needle.

The peritoneal cavity is entered after incising the posterior rectus sheath. The pleural cavity is entered through the posterior periosteum, and the diaphragm is divided for a distance of 10 to 15 cm dorsolaterally in the direction of its fibers; the lower edge of the lung must be protected while the diaphragmatic pleura and diaphragm are being incised. A Finochietto retractor is placed in the wound and positioned between the divided costal cartilages (Fig. 5.5).

The retractor is spread as wide as possible; because of the patient's position, the abdominal contents will fall to the contralateral side. The remainder of the procedure for radical nephrectomy is described in Chapter 4.

After en bloc removal of the kidney, the wound is carefully inspected for any bleeding, but the incision is not drained unless postoperative bleeding is a concern. We have not found it necessary to close the lateral paracolic incisions, but the omentum should be pulled over the loops of intestine whenever possible to prevent the formation of any adhesions. A no. 32 chest tube is positioned in the pleural cavity through a separate stab wound at the posterior axillary line and is secured with a no. 1 braided silk suture (Fig. 5.6).

At the conclusion of the procedure, we have found it helpful to inject 5 mL of 0.75% solution of bupivacaine hydrochloride into the intercostal space of the incision and two interspaces above and below as well as into the chest tube site (10). The percutaneous injection is performed by placing a finger within the thorax to ensure proper needle placement. The syringe should be aspirated before each injection to prevent an inadvertent intravascular injection. The use of this solution reduces the postoperative analgesic requirement.

Closure

The diaphragm is closed in two layers (Fig. 5.7), the first layer consisting of interrupted 2-0 polyglactin (Vicryl; Ethicon,

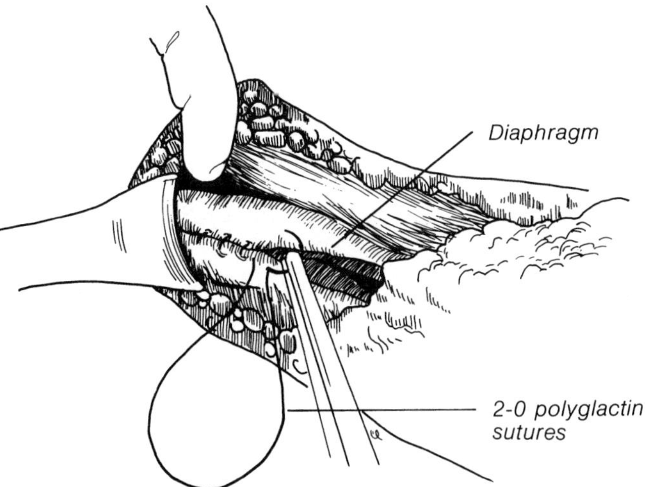

Fig. 5.7. The diaphragm is closed in two layers. The first layer consists of interrupted 2-0 polyglactin (Vicryl) sutures placed so that the knots are tied on the posterior surface of the diaphragm. A running 2-0 Vicryl suture is used on the pleural surface.

Sommerville, NJ) sutures placed so that the knots are tied on the posterior surface of the diaphragm. A running 2-0 Vicryl suture is used on the pleural surface. The thoracic part of the incision is closed with interrupted figure-of-eight no. 1 Vicryl sutures through all the muscle layers of the chest wall (Fig. 5.8). It is important to include the diaphragm medially in the last one or two sutures. The sutures are then tied, starting with the most posterior stitch. The posterior rectus fascia and muscle layers are approximated with no. 0 Vicryl sutures. The previously placed thoracic sutures are secured, and the subcutaneous tissue is approximated with 2-0 Vicryl sutures. The method of skin closure depends on the surgeon's preference.

POSTOPERATIVE CARE AND COMPLICATIONS

Postoperative care for radical nephrectomy is similar to that for most extensive surgical procedures. We observe the patient in the intensive care unit for at least 24 hours after the surgical procedure. The chest tube is connected to suction drainage for

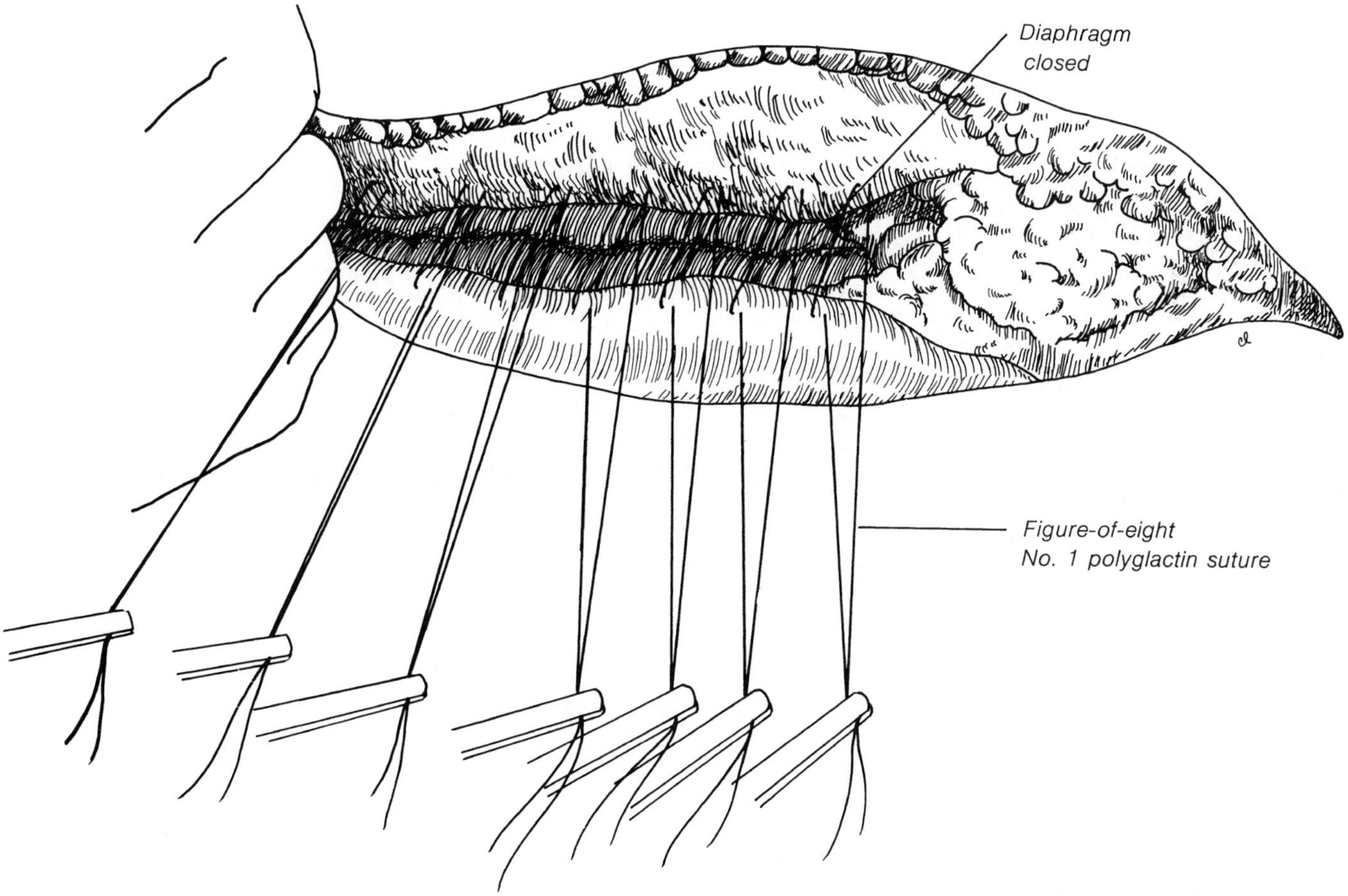

Fig. 5.8. Figure-of-eight no. 1 Vicryl sutures are placed through all muscular layers of the chest wall. It is important to include the diaphragm medially in the last one or two sutures. The sutures are not tied until all have been placed.

24 hours or until significant drainage ceases and there is no evidence of an air leak. The tube is then connected to a water seal for 4 hours. An expiratory chest radiograph is taken; if there is no evidence of a pneumothorax, the chest tube may be removed. If a possible air leak is still a significant concern after 4 hours of water seal, despite a negative chest radiograph, the tube may be clamped proximal to any connectors. Another chest radiograph should be taken in 4 hours. Under these circumstances, with a negative expiratory chest radiograph, one can be certain of a completely expanded lung with no air leak. As mentioned, postoperative pain can be significantly reduced by the routine use of an intercostal nerve block. A nasogastric tube is left in place, and fluid intake is withheld until adequate bowel sounds are present and flatus is passed.

Some of the postoperative complications that may occur include secondary hemorrhage, pneumothorax, wound dehiscence, and intercostal neuralgia. Other less common complications include cerebrovascular accidents, precipitation of congestive heart failure, myocardial infarction, pulmonary embolus, atelectasis, and pneumonia. Proper selection of patients, adequate preoperative preparation, and good postoperative care and ambulation will prevent many of these problems.

REFERENCES

1. Sennert D. Medicinae practicae. Venice, 1641;1.
2. Grawitz PA. Die Entstehung von Nierentumoren aus Nebennierengewebe. Verh Disch Ges Chir 1884;13:28.
3. Murphy LJT. Renal tumors. In: The history of urology. Murphy LJT, ed. Springfield, IL: Charles C. Thomas, 1972.
4. Simon G. Exstirpation eine Niere an Menschen. Dtsch Klin 1870;22:137.
5. Fey B. L'abord du rein par la voie thoraco-Abdominale. Arch Urol Clin Necker 1926;5:169.
6. Marshall DF. Urogenital wounds in an evacuation hospital. J Urol 1946;55:119.
7. Crawford ED, Rogers HC, Mettler FA, et al. Ultrasonic detection of renal tubular carcinoma extending into the inferior vena cava. J Urol 1980;124:538.
8. Gottesman JE, Crawford ED, Grossman HB, et al. Infarction-nephrectomy for metastatic renal carcinoma: Southwest Oncology Group Study. Urology 1985;25:248.
9. Wettlaufer JN, Kumpe DA, Redmond PL. Preoperative ethanol renal embolization and planned delayed nephrectomy in select patients with poor risk renal cell carcinoma. 84th annual meeting of AUA, Dallas, May 1989. Abstract no. 386.
10. Crawford ED, Skinner DG, Capparell DB. Intercostal nerve block with thoracoabdominal incision. J Urol 1979;121:290.

6

Radical Nephrectomy

Anterior Subcostal Transperitoneal Approach

Paul C. Peters

DEFINITION OF THE APPROACH

The subcostal transperitoneal approach allows early access to the renal pedicle, permitting ligation and division. This early ligation serves to diminish further blood loss and prevent tumor dissemination via the renal vein. The most important pathologic characteristic of renal cell carcinoma is its tendency to invade its own venous system. We define radical nephrectomy as the removal of the kidney and adrenal with surrounding Gerota's fascia intact (Fig. 6.1). The ureter and ipsilateral gonadal vein are removed to the level of the common iliac artery. Retrograde metastases via the gonadal vein to the apex of the vagina have been reported. Regional nodes are removed from the crus of the diaphragm to the bifurcation of the common iliac artery on the ipsilateral side, including any nodes seen anterior to the aorta and cava at the hilus of the kidney.

PREPARATION OF THE PATIENT

Preparatory tests include cardiorespiratory evaluation, renal and liver function tests, and bone scan. It is essential that the variables that may be encountered within the abdomen, including the possibility of postoperative dialysis support when a solitary kidney is tumor bearing, be discussed with the patient. An abdominal computed tomography scan is helpful to exclude metastatic disease, and magnetic resonance imaging and sonography are of particular help in evaluating extension into the venous system. Preoperative baseline electrolyte and blood gas determinations, hemogram, bleeding and clotting times, partial thromboplastin time, prothrombin time, and platelet count are also valuable. Typing and cross-matching for 4 units of blood should be completed before the surgical procedure.

Angioinfarction of the renal mass is rarely used. It is considered when the tumor is large (i.e., greater than 17 cm) and crosses the midline. It is very important that the colon be completely empty at the time of surgery. This increases the flexibility in its displacement for needed exposure of the retroperitoneal mass. The colon may be cleansed by a strict liquid diet for 3 days preoperatively. Our current method is to have the patient consume a clear liquid diet for 2 days before hospital admission and then drink a gallon of an osmotically active agent (Golytely; Braintree Laboratories, Braintree, MA) in a 4- or 5-hour period the afternoon before morning surgery. Cleansing enemas are used only if the stool remains brown or rectal examination reveals persistent stool in the rectum. Antibiotic preparation of the bowel is done only when there is a suggestion from the preoperative studies that invasion of the bowel may be present and that en bloc resection of the renal tumor and adjacent bowel (large or small) may be necessary. Our preferred bowel preparation consists of neomycin given orally, starting 24 hours before surgery in the dose of 1 g each hour for 4 hours and then 1 g every 4 hours until the patient is nil per os for surgery. In addition, the patient receives 1 g of erythromycin given 4 times in the 24 hours before surgery. The patient may take 1 ounce of water to facilitate swallowing the pills. An alternative protocol is 1 g of neomycin and 1 g of metronidazole given orally at 6:30 PM and 11:30 PM the day before surgery (1).

SURGICAL PROCEDURE

General endotracheal anesthesia is used. The assumption is made here that the costal arch of the patient is wide enough to allow the use of a subcostal incision from the tip of the 11th rib one to two fingers below the rib margin, crossing the ipsilateral rectus just below the xiphoid cartilage and extending 2 cm into the opposite rectus or more if needed. A chevron incision as shown in Figure 6.2 is used for bilateral lesions.

The skin is incised with a knife, and an electrocautery tool is used to cut through the other layers into the peritoneal cavity. The operator should protect the underlying layers with one hand and use the electrocautery tool for cutting the fascia and for hemostasis. The author prefers to enter the peritoneal cavity in the midline and extend the incision laterally from this point

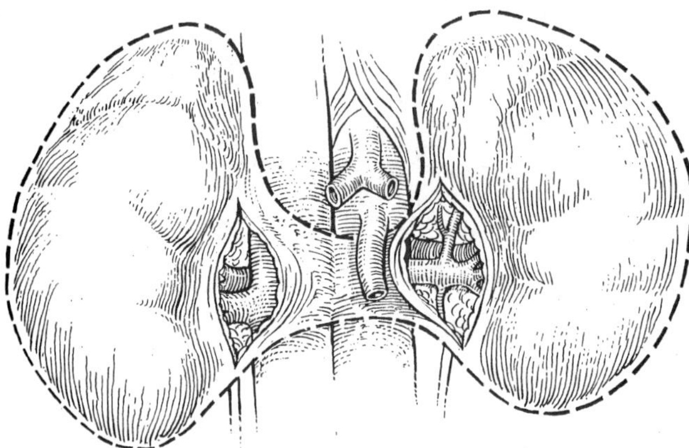

Fig. 6.1. Concept of the letter H or barbell configuration of Gerota's fascia surrounding the kidneys and enveloping the renal pedicles. The adrenal may be left in place or removed as desired.

using the protecting hand (Fig. 6.2). An assistant finds it useful to grasp bleeding points with a tonsil hemostat just before fulguration. The falciform (ligamentum teres) ligament is then divided between clamps and suture ligated with 2-0 or 3-0 silk. General access to the peritoneal cavity is thus obtained (Fig. 6.2). At this point, the abdominal contents are thoroughly explored. The liver, gallbladder, small and large bowel, and stomach are carefully examined. Diverticula of the colon are noted. Metastases to the colon and small bowel are sought. Mobility of the kidney is tested. Internal genitalia are palpated in the pelvis, and the position of the balloon catheter in the bladder is verified.

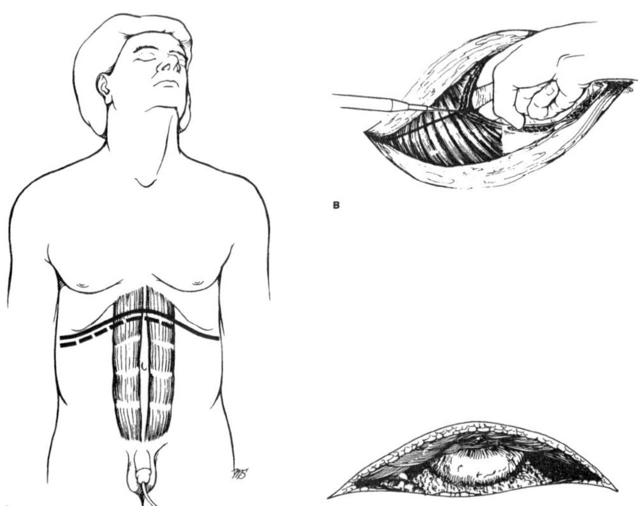

Fig. 6.2. Subcostal approach to renal cancer. **A.** Incision on right side going into rectus on left a short distance. Patient is supine with table flexed 20° in center. **B.** Incision of muscle layers with electrocautery using other hand to protect underlying structures. **C.** Ligamentum teres divided between suture ligatures. Peritoneal cavity is open and ready for exploration. Bookwalter retractor will be inserted.

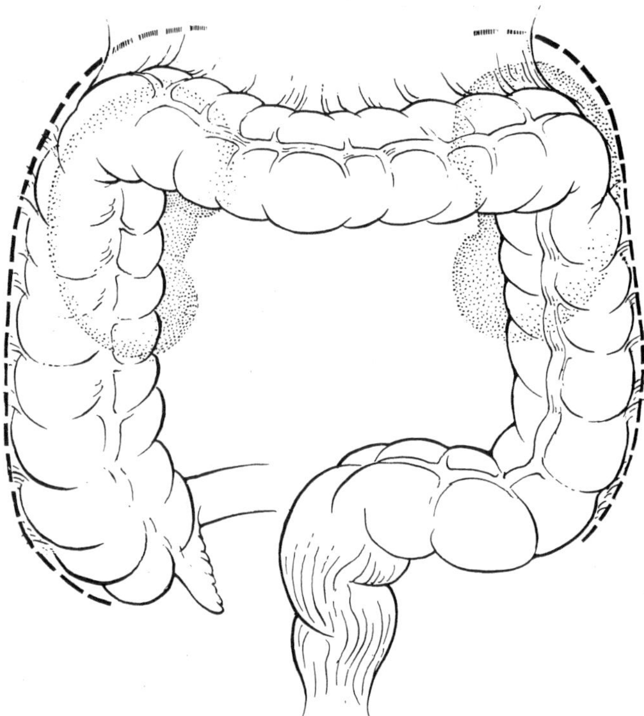

Fig. 6.3. Line of incision is seen in the posterior parietal peritoneum to reflect colon medially on either side to expose the kidney surrounded by Gerota's fascia.

Technique

A few points are emphasized in our technique for radical nephrectomy. Use of the Bookwalter retractor has negated the need for more than one assistant in most circumstances. It has also allowed the inclusion of retractors as needed to give excellent exposure and has replaced the use of multiple retractors and large superior retractors, which required much effort by the assistant. The Bookwalter retractor is also adjustable and may be changed in position. Retractors may be added or removed as needed during the procedure.

On the left side (Fig. 6.3), the posterior parietal peritoneal incision, made lateral to the colon after the abdomen is opened, is carried well above the splenic flexure. On large upper pole tumors, the incision may be carried around the splenic pedicles and superiorly and medially to the aorta near its diaphragmatic hiatus. This allows safe medial retraction of the spleen and tail of the pancreas and gives excellent exposure for dissection of the renal artery and left adrenal gland (2).

Variables such as the size of the tumor or extensive vascular invasion may influence the method of handling the pedicle. Preoperative angioinfarction may help considerably by decreasing the volume of collateral circulation around the tumor, particularly in tumors that are large enough to cross the midline. It also offers the advantage of allowing the surgeon to ligate the renal vein before exposing the artery immediately beneath it, particularly when the renal vein is large and filled with tumor.

When the tumor has extended into the vena cava, control is obtained of all venous tributaries in the area, as well as the vena cava proximally and distally, before extraction of the tumor thrombus. The cava is mobilized proximally and distally to place vascular tapes around it so that angled vascular clumps may be used for temporary occlusion proximal and distal to the tumor thrombus. The entry point of the left renal vein must also be mobilized so that it can be temporarily occluded if a cavotomy is necessary.

In addition, the right gonadal vein should be divided between ligatures in right-sided tumors. On the right side, a large lumbar tributary commonly enters the cava posteriorly near the orifice of the renal vein. Preferably, this tributary is ligated at the time of proximal and distal mobilization of the inferior vena cava. By elevating the vascular tapes, one can reduce flow in the cava temporarily and gently palpate the tumor thrombus to determine its extent. One can often milk it back into the renal vein so that a partial occlusion of the vena cava by a curved Satinsky or DeBakey vascular clamp will suffice to allow removal of the specimen with the thrombus included. The cava can be inspected to be certain there is no thrombus adherent to or invading the caval wall and can then be closed with a running 4-0 or 5-0 nonabsorbable polypropylene suture. In other circumstances, the tumor can be milked back below the diaphragm and removed via cavotomy, with the cava and renal tributaries temporarily occluded as described earlier.

When the tumor extends into the heart, cardiac surgery consultants provide cardiac bypass or intrapericardial occlusion of the inferior vena cava, if necessary, for complete removal of tumor thrombus. This is dramatic surgery and does not often result in long-term survival. We advise thoracic surgery consultation in such cases and strongly recommend that the operation be carried out in the room usually used for open heart surgery so that equipment needed by the thoracic surgeon in an urgent manner is readily available. When the inferior vena cava is extensively involved above and below the renal vein, it may be removed. On the left side, one may safely ligate the left renal vein in the case of a right-sided tumor, relying on established collateral branches and the gonadal and adrenal veins to effectively drain the left kidney. If the tumor has been obstructing the cava return for some time, good collateral drainage is usually present (3). When the right kidney is the one to be saved, autotransplantation or renal-portal anastomosis is suggested if the entire cava must be removed. One could consider an end-to-end superior anastomosis of the renal vein to the caval stump at the level of resection. Venous substitution prostheses are not recommended because they tend to thrombose. In the unusual circumstance resulting in one having to remove the abdominal vena cava and left kidney (left renal tumor involving abdominal vena cava diffusely), one can facilitate the anastomosis of the right renal vein to the vena cava superiorly by using autogenous superficial femoral vein for the interposition. Vascular surgery consultation is advised in this circumstance (preferably preoperatively). Clagett et al. and Vaughan et al. (3, 4) have reported the successful use of superficial or deep femoral vein in more

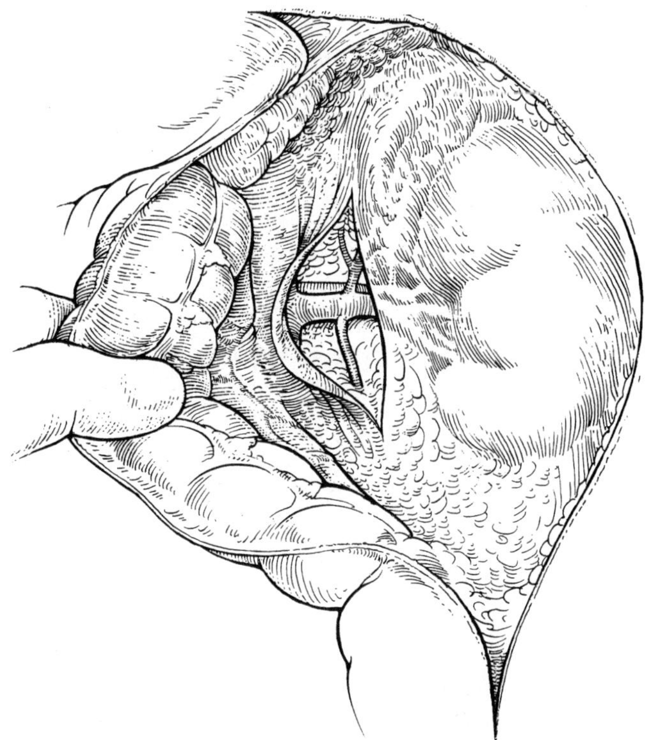

Fig. 6.4. The colon is reflected medially on the left side. The incision in Gerota's fascia shows renal vessels, permitting early ligation of pedicle.

than 20 cases when a large vessel is needed to substitute for aorta, vena cava, or renal vein.

After the artery has been controlled and divided between 0-silk ligatures, and a suture ligature of 3-0 silk has been placed distal to the ligature on the artery, the vein can be treated in a similar manner if it has not been previously divided. The ureter is divided between 2-0 silk ligatures at the point where it crosses the common iliac artery. Gerota's fascia is then dissected (Fig. 6.4). Clips and silk ligatures are used as necessary as one frees the superior attachments of Gerota's fascia from the diaphragm and from the posterior muscles of the abdomen and also as one clips or ligates any small adrenal branches that may be encountered. The kidney is then removed en bloc, and nodes along the renal pedicle are dissected from the interaortocaval area from the crus of the diaphragm to the bifurcation of the common iliac artery on the ipsilateral side.

The therapeutic advantage of lymphadenectomy has yet to be demonstrated in a prospective randomized study. In a series of 352 cases from Dallas hospitals, 16% of patients who underwent lymphadenectomy were classified as having stage C disease by the finding of positive nodes. These tumors would have been understaged had the lymphadenectomy not been performed. Six percent of those having the lymphadenectomy had microscopic nodal involvement only and these surely would have been missed. In addition, our data show a 25% 5-year survival rate for those who had nodes and a lymphadenectomy; the 5-year survival rate was only 9% for those who had positive nodes without lymphadenectomy. We prefer to remove the gonadal vein as well on the ipsilateral side, although one infrequently finds microscopic involvement of this vessel.

On the left side, cases of renal cell carcinoma have been reported in which the tumor extended retrograde along the gonadal vein, manifested clinically by vaginal bleeding due to involvement of the apex of the vagina by metastatic disease. Figure 6.3 shows the extension of the incision in the posterior parietal peritoneum to the aortic hiatus of the diaphragm to allow one to mobilize the spleen and pancreas medially. The plane between Gerota's fascia and the peritoneum is easily defined in these cases to expose the pedicle before manipulation of the mass, as described previously (Fig. 6.4).

We do not use copious irrigation of the tumor bed. An effort has been made to reperitonealize the posterior parietal peritoneum in each case with a running 2-0 chromic gut suture, with care taken to place the sutures approximately 1 cm apart to prevent herniation of the bowel through the posterior parietal peritoneum in the postoperative course. No drains are used. A layered closure is completed with nonabsorbable sutures after hemostasis is secured by cautery and by ligation with silk sutures. Nasogastric suction and parenteral fluids are used until the passage of flatus is observed postoperatively.

REFERENCES

1. Peters PC. Radical nephrectomy—anterior transabdominal approach. In: Crawford ED, Das S, eds. Current genitourinary cancer surgery. Philadelphia: Lea & Febiger, 1990:45.
2. Skinner DG. Surgical approach to renal cancer. In: Urological cancer. Orlando, FL: Grune & Stratton, 1983:429.
3. Clagett PG, et al. Creation of a neo-aortoiliac system (NAIS) from lower extremity deep and superficial veins. Ann Surg 1993;218:239.
4. Vaughan WG, Clagett PG, Lopez-Viego, M. Acute renal failure following a renal vein ligation and division: a case of successful thrombectomy and renal vein reconstruction. Perspect Vasc Surg 1993;6:111.

7

Nephron-Sparing Surgery for Renal Cell Carcinoma

Steve W. Waxman and Martin A. Koyle

INTRODUCTION

In the late 1800s, partial nephrectomy was first applied to the treatment of renal tumors; however, complications including urinary fistulae, excessive bleeding, and excessive postoperative mortality led to its abandonment (1). Although Gregoire first proposed the concept of a radical nephrectomy for renal cell cancer in 1905, it was Robson's reports in 1963 and 1969 of improved survival after radical nephrectomy for renal cell carcinoma that increased enthusiasm for this technique (2). The concept of nephron-sparing surgery for the treatment of renal cell carcinoma received newfound interest through the experience of Semb in 1955 and Puigvert in 1966, following the work of Seldinger, who showed the potential benefits and clarified the selection factors for segmental nephrectomy (3, 4).

The pioneering techniques of renal transplantation and vascular surgery described originally by Carrel at the turn of the century did not achieve widespread use until the first successful cases of renal allotransplantation performed in Boston and Paris in 1954 (5). The application of such principles allowing autotransplantation was extended to bench surgery, which further added to the surgical methods to perform nephron-sparing surgery for the treatment of renal cell carcinoma (6, 7).

Improvements in imaging technology, beginning with renal angiography and continuing with ultrasonography, computed tomography (CT), and magnetic resonance imaging (MRI), have all added to the improved diagnosis of renal cell carcinoma. These technologies have also facilitated the application of in vivo nephron-sparing surgery to the treatment of renal tumors.

INDICATIONS FOR NEPHRON-SPARING SURGERY

Approximately 28,000 new cases of renal cell carcinoma are detected each year in the United States. It is estimated that there will be 11,000 deaths due to renal cell carcinoma in the United States in 1995 (8). The number of new cases of renal cell carcinoma detected annually in the United States has increased over the past several years (9). There are increasing numbers of smaller renal lesions being detected as incidental findings due to the increased use of standard noninvasive imaging techniques, improved definition, improved techniques, and newer imaging modalities, including the helical CT scanner (10–12). These early detected lesions tend to be smaller and more localized and are the most amenable to nephron-sparing surgery.

Radiographic imaging can help delineate a variety of lesions in kidneys; however, it is not always possible to distinguish among renal cell carcinoma, adenoma, sarcoma, and oncocytoma with the existing imaging modalities (13). After surgical excision, approximately 10 to 15% of small CT-enhancing renal masses presumed to be cancers preoperatively will prove to be benign adenomas or oncocytomas (14).

Nephron-sparing surgery has been shown to be a successful form of therapy for cases of localized renal cell carcinoma in which there is a need to preserve renal parenchyma. This need is most obvious in patients with bilateral renal cell carcinoma, masses of uncertain cause, or renal cell carcinoma involving a solitary functioning kidney and in those patients with compromised renal function. In a review of the recent literature, nephron-sparing surgery for renal cell carcinoma compares favorably with radical nephrectomy. The 5-year disease-specific survival rates have been reported by Thrasher et al. (15). Their summary of seven prior series showed a 5-year survival rate of 66 to 79% for radical nephrectomy versus 78 to 90.5% for conservative surgery (2, 15–20). Nephron-sparing surgery has been shown to provide good surgical treatment of stage I disease, with a local recurrence rate of about 10% (19–28). Bilateral renal cell carcinoma is found in 1 to 2% of cases, with synchronous and asynchronous lesions occurring approximately equally. Jacobs et al. have shown that patients with bilateral disease do as well as those with unilateral renal cell carcinoma when matched stage for stage (22).

Patients with von Hippel-Lindau disease present a special dilemma; renal cell carcinoma will develop in 35 to 40% of patients, and the majority will have bilateral recurrent tumors. Many of these tumors occur within the wall of an otherwise benign-appearing renal cyst; therefore, the method of nephron-sparing surgery becomes a matter of some controversy in light of the high expected occurrence of future lesions. Whether a partial nephrectomy or simple enucleation is performed, it is generally agreed that nephron-sparing surgery should be attempted in patients with von Hippel-Lindau disease because results are superior to bilateral radical nephrectomy with subsequent dialysis and allotransplantation (29).

A further indication for nephron-sparing surgery includes renal cell carcinoma in patients with impaired contralateral renal function. This impairment is usually secondary to benign disorders including calculus disease, glomerulonephritis, pyelonephritis, obstruction, or vascular insufficiency. In patients with bilateral synchronous renal cell carcinoma amenable to nephron-sparing surgery, most would approach the problem as staged procedures (1). Staged partial nephrectomy in bilateral synchronous renal cell carcinoma may allow for the contralateral kidney to maintain renal function should there be acute tubular necrosis involving the operative kidney, thus reducing the need for temporary dialysis. In bilateral synchronous renal cell carcinoma with a large tumor on one side, precluding a partial nephrectomy, it is best to perform the partial nephrectomy first on the less-involved side followed by a radical nephrectomy on the opposite side at a later date. This again potentially decreases the need for temporary dialysis if acute tubular necrosis ensues postoperatively. In cases of a small tumor burden bilaterally, simultaneous partial nephrectomies can be performed.

The main controversy regarding nephron-sparing surgery involves its use in localized renal cell carcinoma with a normal contralateral kidney (13, 30). Novick and colleagues have shown that in single, small (less than 4 cm) kidney tumors with a normal contralateral kidney, nephron-sparing surgery is as safe and effective as radical nephrectomy (1, 13). There is concern, however, about the 10 to 20% incidence of multicentricity in serially sectioned kidneys, thus potentially increasing the chances for surgical failure after partial nephrectomy (31–33). Long-term follow-up for those undergoing nephron-sparing surgery for renal cell carcinoma with a normal contralateral kidney is necessary to assess the ultimate benefits of nephron-sparing procedures.

A final area in which nephron-sparing surgery can be valuable is in the indeterminate renal lesion. If ultrasound, CT scan, MRI, or arteriogram is unable to exclude a complex cystic or solid mass, then exploration, assessment, and resection (if necessary) are indicated. Should the lesion prove to be benign, it would be beneficial to undertake a partial rather than a radical nephrectomy. Although rare, it is currently not recommended to biopsy percutaneously or aspirate complex cystic or solid masses due to the possibility of seeding the tract with malignant cells should renal cell carcinoma be present (34, 35).

PREOPERATIVE PREPARATION

The diagnosis and staging of solid or complex cystic renal masses must be as complete and precise as possible to prepare adequately for nephron-sparing surgery. Whether the renal lesion or lesions have been discovered through workup of urinary tract signs or symptoms or incidentally, specific radiographic studies are essential to planning the procedure. There have

been significant improvements in ultrasound, CT, and MRI scanning so that angiography has been precluded in selected instances. After the lesions have been identified and localized and metastatic disease has been ruled out, selective renal arteriography can be used to delineate the renal vasculature, particularly in midrenal, large, and bilateral tumor situations. For smaller, especially polar lesions, we believe that angiography is not mandatory (Figs. 7.1 and 7.2).

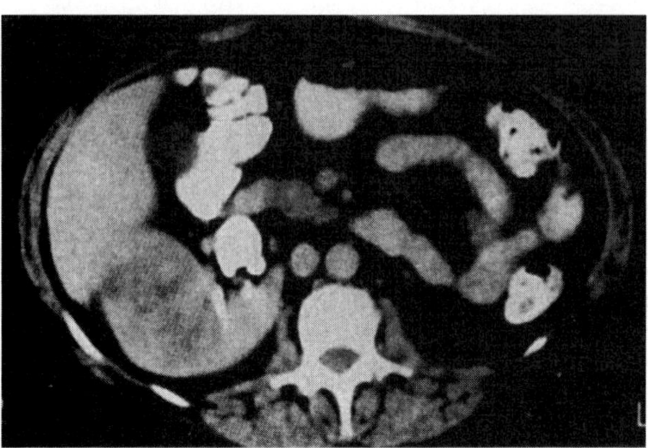

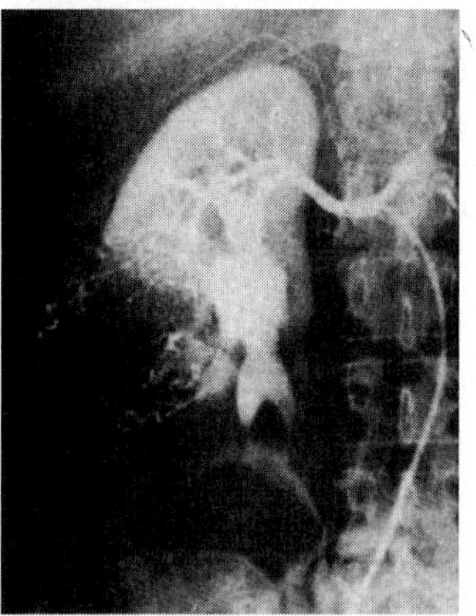

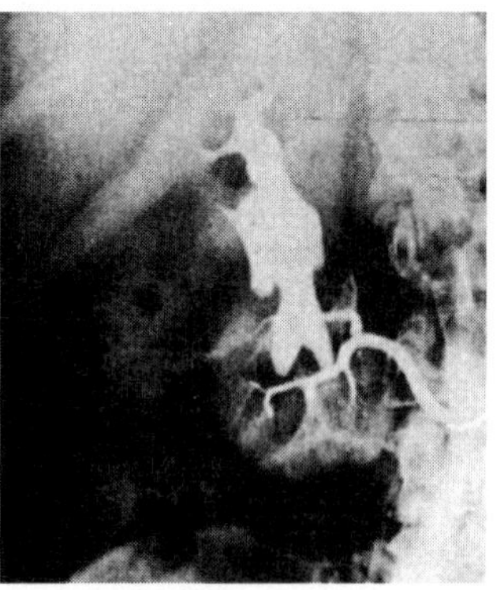

Fig. 7.1. A 63-year-old woman who had her left kidney removed for benign disease (infection) was seen to evaluate fevers. **A.** A CT scan demonstrated a large mass in the midportion of her solitary right kidney. Angiography (**B&C**) demonstrated separate major renal arteries to the upper and lower poles, suggesting that partial nephrectomy was feasible. (CT scans and angiograms courtesy of LTI Medica and Bristol-Myers Company. Copyright 1986 by Learning Technology Inc.)

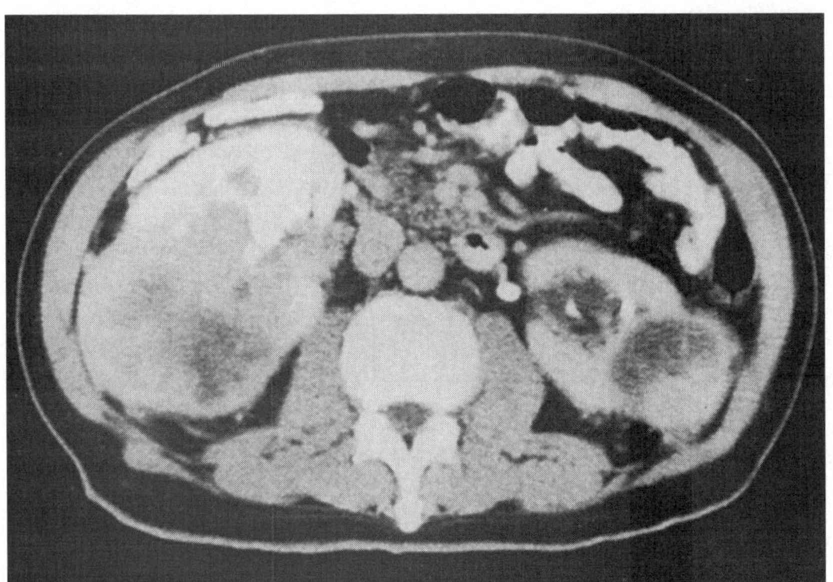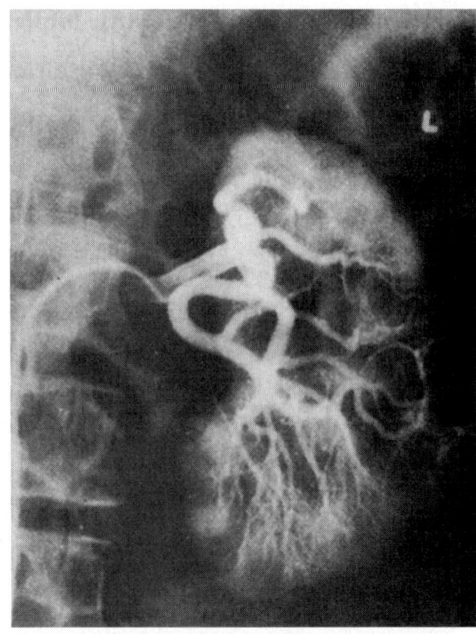

Fig. 7.2.   Right flank and upper quadrant pain, weight loss, and anorexia developed in a 68-year-old man. **A.** The CT scan revealed a large right renal tumor and a smaller tumor on the left. A right radical nephrectomy was performed. **B.** Selective angiography of the left kidney confirmed a midportion 5-cm tumor, amenable to renal-sparing surgery. (CT scans and angiograms courtesy of LTI Medica and Bristol-Myers Company. Copyright 1986 by Learning Technology Inc.)

Selective renal venography is used less frequently with improved noninvasive techniques, particularly with MRI and ultrasound. However, venography is useful in patients with large, centrally located tumors for which there is a possibility of intrarenal venous thrombosis, which may imply a more advanced local tumor stage and increase the technical complexity of the tumor excision (30).

Nuclear renal scans are appropriate in cases in which the contribution to function of each kidney is necessary.

SURGICAL MANAGEMENT

Blood products are made available for large and centrally located tumors. For lesser lesions, a type and screen only is done. The patient is vigorously hydrated preoperatively to assure adequate renal perfusion.

After general anesthesia has been induced, a Foley catheter is placed to dependent drainage, and the appropriate venous and arterial lines are placed depending on the patient's medical status and the anticipated procedure.

Many nephron-sparing procedures have been described, including simple and modified enucleations, polar segmental, wedge resection, major transverse resection, and extracorporeal bench surgery with autotransplantation. Although the surgical approach to the kidney is influenced by the location and number of lesions, along with prior surgery, body habitus, and physician preference, basic surgical principles must be adhered to for a successful result and to avoid complications. These basic surgical principles include the following.

1. Early vascular control.
2. Preservation of renal function with no or minimal ischemia.
3. Complete tumor excision with negative surgical margins.
4. Watertight closure of the collecting system if it is entered.
5. Meticulous hemostasis.
6. Closure of the renal defect (36).

Technical points that help reduce the chances of renal ischemia include the following.

1. Maintaining adequate hydration and blood pressure in the operative and perioperative periods.
2. Minimally manipulating the renal artery.
3. Administering mannitol and furosemide 5 minutes before and just after release of arterial occlusion.
4. Surface cooling of the kidney with ice slush in cases where large or multiple tumors may require more than 30 minutes of operative time (Fig. 7.3).
5. Clamping of the renal artery but not the renal vein.
6. Avoiding intermittent arterial clamping.
7. Adding calcium channel blockers and low (renal) doses of inotropic pressors. This has reportedly been advantageous in maintaining perfusion and reducing ischemic insults (37).

Attempts to decrease the effects of warm ischemia on the kidney or decrease the number of oxygen free radicals following reperfusion have been investigated (38). Efforts to decrease free radicals by using allopurinol, a xanthine oxidase inhibitor, have also been tried to improve renal function after ischemia (39).

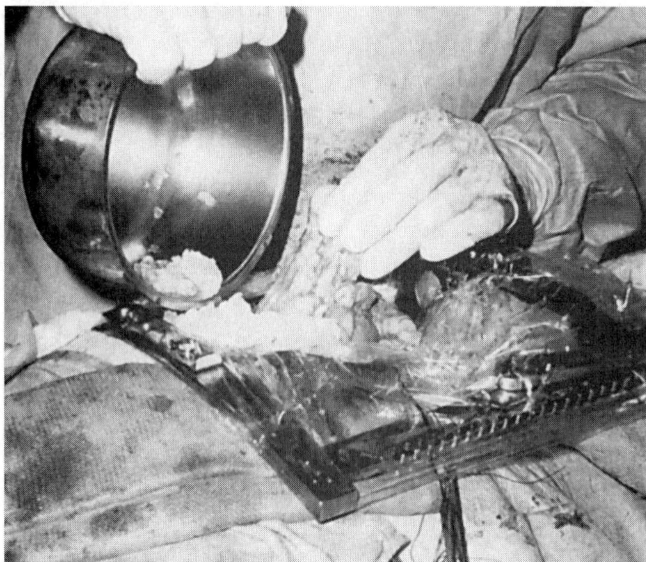

Fig. 7.3. Renal preservation is satisfactorily accomplished in most cases of partial nephrectomy using surface cooling methods. After the kidney is mobilized, it is wrapped in a Lahey bag and covered with iced slush. (Surgical photography by Lester V. Bergman, courtesy LTI Medica and Bristol-Myers Company. Copyright 1986 by Learning Technology Inc.)

Free radical scavengers such as glutathione have also been evaluated for their protection of renal function after ischemia (40). Calcium channel blockers such as verapamil have been shown to produce vasodilation and diuresis when infused into the renal artery. This may help inhibit postischemic smooth muscle vascular spasm and establish a diuresis in the postclamping period, thus protecting against ischemic injury (41–44). Energy-providing compounds such as ATP-magnesium chloride have been studied for their ability to provide protection against warm ischemia and enhance recovery following clamping of the renal artery (45, 46).

Intraoperative ultrasound can be very useful in locating lesions that are small, multiple, and/or deep within the renal parenchyma (47). Methods used to improve and achieve hemostasis after partial nephrectomy include the application of perirenal fat, hemostatic fibers, wafers, or sponges and Argon Beam Coagulation (Valley Lab, Boulder, CO) to "paint" the raw cut parenchymal surface. The Cavitron Device can be used to dissect the renal parenchyma without cutting across vessels, thus allowing their ligation before division and lessening blood loss from the procedure (48). The neodymium:YAG laser has also been used by some authors in conjunction with partial nephrectomy to aid in both dissection and hemostasis. The tumor and adjacent tissue are photocoagulated with the laser before excision. Once the tumor has been excised, the parenchyma defect can be laser coagulated (49). Fibrin Glue, made from the patient's own blood, has also been used to fill parenchymal defects and aid in hemostasis (50).

In Situ Partial Nephrectomy

Although nephron-sparing surgery can be performed in many different ways and for multiple indications, in situ partial ne-

phrectomy remains the most popular and most commonly used form. Simple enucleation, segmental polar nephrectomy, wedge resection, and major transverse resection are included in this technique. The most common incision for in situ nephrectomy is an extraperitoneal flank incision through the bed of either the 11th or 12th rib. The operation can be performed through a transabdominal or thoracoabdominal incision as well.

Simple Enucleation

Surgical enucleation for kidney tumors was first described by Vermooten in 1950 (51). Since that time, numerous authors have described their techniques and results for single or multiple enucleations for renal cell carcinoma. In cases of familial renal cell carcinoma, von Hippel-Lindau disease, or multiple tumors, simple enucleation is necessary to preserve the remaining parenchyma. The drawbacks of this procedure are the reportedly high rates of residual disease due to microscopic capsular invasion of the pseudocapsule around the tumor, vascular invasion, and multicentric tumors. Even with the removal of a rim of normal parenchyma around the pseudocapsule, there have been reports of residual tumor following modified simple enucleation. If the tumor is in an apical, basilar, or superficial location, wedge resection or segmental polar nephrectomy is preferable to simple enucleation when performing nephron-sparing surgery on sporadic renal cell carcinoma (51–62).

Operative technique. In patients who require bilateral simple enucleations, a chevron or midline abdominal incision can be performed to provide access to both kidneys. If only one kidney is going to be operated on, a flank or modified chevron incision can be used. Most superficial renal cell carcinomas have a distinct pseudocapsule surrounding them; however, as has been reported, there is frequently capsular invasion by tumor cells. Therefore, a rim of normal parenchyma should be kept with the tumor to decrease the chance of positive margins. Usually, a circumferential incision of the normal renal capsule and parenchyma is performed, and then the plane is developed with sharp and blunt dissection. The handle of the scalpel is helpful to use for blunt dissection. In most enucleations for peripheral tumors it is not necessary to occlude the renal artery, and the small vessels transected during the enucleation can be suture ligated with 4-0 chromic sutures or coagulated.

In large tumors or those involving the hilum of the kidney, which have a fairly extensive blood supply and require more extensive dissection, either segmental or main renal artery occlusion followed by surface cooling may be necessary before enucleation. The base and sides of the surface defects should be sampled and frozen section analysis should be performed to assure clear margins. Hemostasis should be attained, and either perirenal fat or other hemostatic substance placed into the defect and sutured into place to provide complete hemostasis. In cases in which there is doubt concerning the complete encasement of the tumor by pseudocapsule on arteriography and CT scanning, a wedge resection should be performed with an adequate margin of normal-appearing parenchyma. In patients with familial renal cell carcinoma or von Hippel-Lindau disease, simple modified enucleation maintains the maximum amount of functional renal parenchyma with a minimal degree of dissection and renal manipulation; however, the high reported rates of residual disease must be recognized when performing this procedure (60).

Segmental Polar Nephrectomy

A segmental polar nephrectomy is the procedure of choice when performing nephron-sparing surgery for a renal cell carcinoma in the upper or lower pole of the kidney. Ligation of the apical or basilar segmental artery will not only allow for visual identification of the demarcation between these zones and the rest of the kidney, but will also maintain perfusion to the remainder of the kidney. If the line of demarcation is not plainly visible, methylene blue can be injected distally into the segmental branch to outline it more clearly (Fig. 7.4). Once the area of demarcation is identified, the main renal artery is occluded and surface cooling begun. After 15 minutes of cooling, the partial nephrectomy can be done by incising the renal capsule at the line of demarcation. This incision should be at least 1 to 2 cm from visible tumor. Using sharp and blunt dissection, the cortex and medulla are dissected, thus excising the polar segment. It is likely that the collecting system will be entered and thus will need to be closed using interrupted or continuous 4-0 chromic suture, ensuring a water-tight closure. Any small vessels that have been transected during the dissection must be

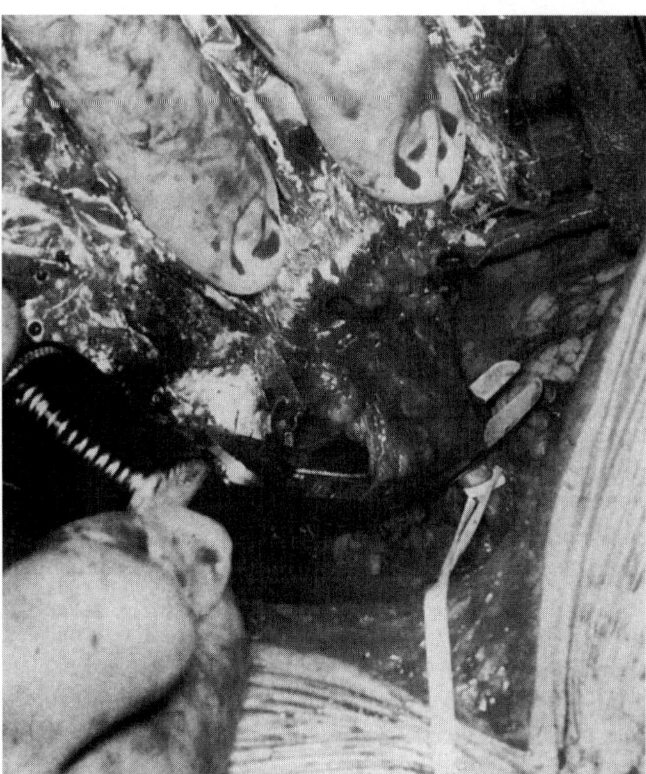

Fig. 7.5. A noncrushing vascular bulldog clamp has been placed across both renal artery and vein. (Surgical photography by Lester V. Bergman, courtesy of LTI Medica and Bristol-Myers Company. Copyright 1986 by Learning Technology Inc.)

suture ligated with 4-0 chromic figure-of-eight sutures. The renal artery is unclamped, and the cut surface of the kidney is checked for hemostasis. After hemostasis has been achieved, the cut surface is then closed over either Oxycel or another hemostatic agent using bolster sutures through the renal capsule. If the defect is too large to close primarily, a piece of perirenal fat may be incorporated into the closure with bolster sutures of 2-0 or 3-0 chromic. The perinephric space is drained with either a Penrose drain or a closed suction drainage system.

This technique has the advantage of being an anatomic dissection with removal of only that tissue which is supplied by the apical or basilar segmental artery branches. It is important not to stretch the indications in attempting to resect a large apical or basilar lesion that encroaches on the border of the line of demarcation. It is much better to obtain a 1- to 2-cm safety margin of normal parenchyma when performing a polar nephrectomy rather than risk leaving behind residual disease. In the larger apical or basilar lesions, a major transverse resection is the best method when selecting nephron-sparing surgery. Whenever the collecting system is entered, care should be taken not only to perform a meticulous closure that is water tight, but also to provide adequate coverage with renal parenchyma or other tissue during the closure so as to decrease the chances for urinary fistula formation. When the collecting system has been opened, one may wish to place an internal ureteral stent (Figs. 7.5, 7.6, 7.7, 7.9 and 7.10).

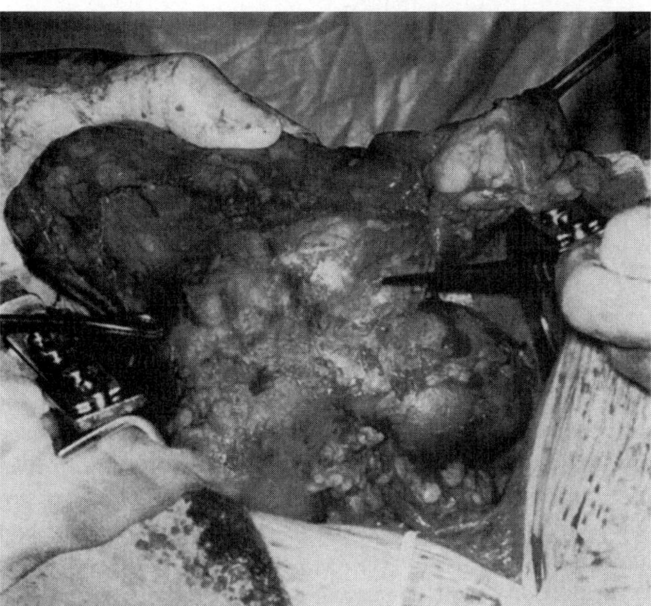

Fig. 7.4. Gerota's fascia and the perinephric fat have been dissected off the normal renal portion but will be removed with the segmental nephrectomy specimen. (Surgical photography by Lester V. Bergman, courtesy of LTI Medica and Bristol-Myers Company. Copyright 1986 by Learning Technology Inc.)

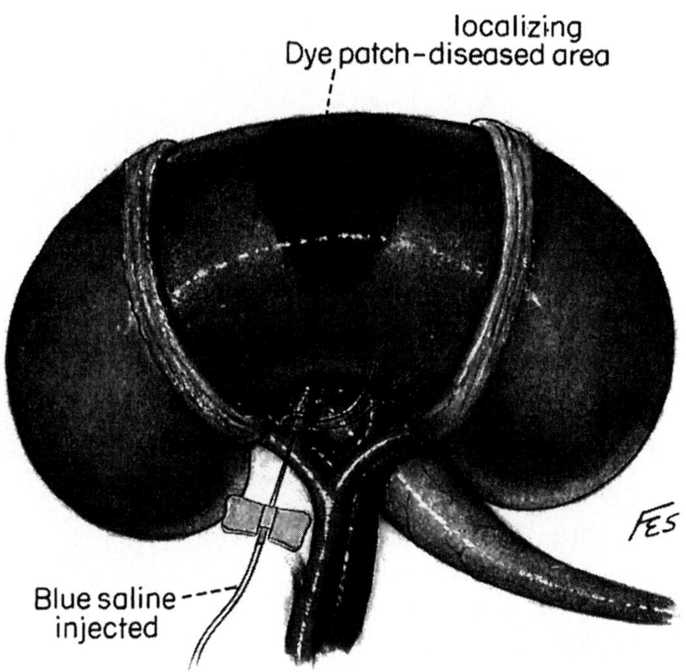

Fig. 7.6. The injection of a segmental vessel with dilute indigo carmine stains the corresponding renal segment and allows vessels to be sacrificed appropriately and safely. (From Gittes RF. Partial Nephrectomy and Bench Surgery: Techniques and Applications. In: Libertino EJ, Zinman LA, eds. Reconstructive Urologic Surgery: Pediatric and Adult. Baltimore: Williams & Wilkins, 1977.)

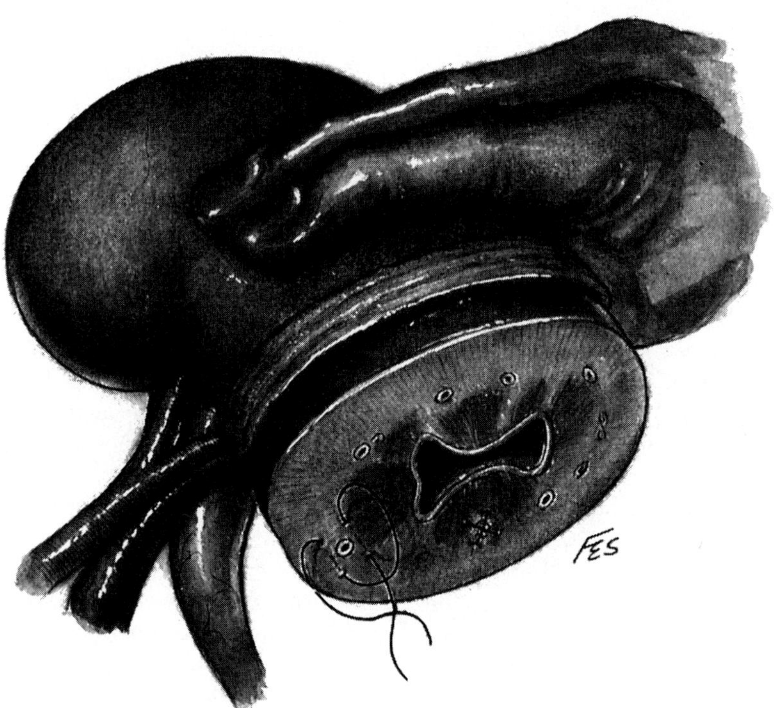

Fig. 7.7. In partial nephrectomy, individual vessels are identified and ligated using a figure-of-eight suture of 4-0 chromic catgut or polyglycolic acid (PGA). (From Gittes RF. Partial Nephrectomy and Bench Surgery: Techniques and Applications. In: Libertino EJ, Zinman LA, eds. Reconstructive Urologic Surgery: Pediatric and Adult. Baltimore: Williams & Wilkins, 1977.)

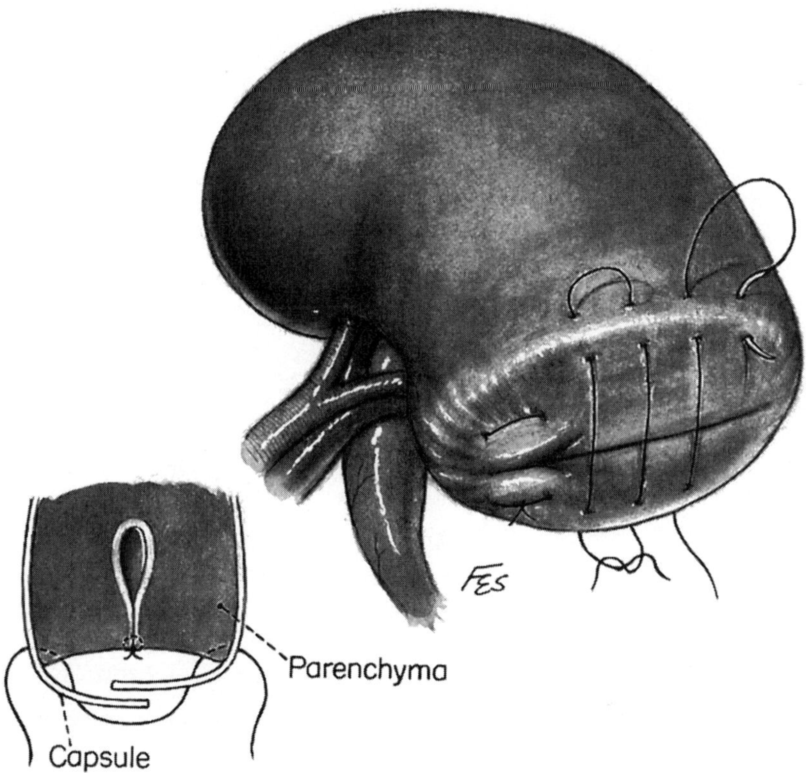

Fig. 7.8. If there is any available capsule after partial nephrectomy, it can be used to cover the raw parenchyma. It is secured with horizontal mattress sutures of 2-0 or 3-0 absorbable suture. (From Gittes RF. Partial Nephrectomy and Bench Surgery: Techniques and Applications. In: Libertino EJ, Zinman LA, eds. Reconstructive Urologic Surgery: Pediatric and Adult. Baltimore: Williams & Wilkins, 1977.)

Wedge Resection

Wedge resection finds its greatest use in larger surface lesions or those surface lesions with questionable capsule integrity. When these tumors are large, they may encompass more than one renal segment. A drawback to this procedure is its association with possible heavier bleeding than the more anatomical polar segmental nephrectomy. These patients require renal artery occlusion with surface cooling before dissection and excision.

Operative technique. Once the kidney has been mobilized and the fascia opened (except for the portion directly overlying the lesion), the renal artery is occluded and the kidney is cooled for 15 minutes in ice slush. The renal capsule is then incised circumferentially, leaving an approximately 1- to 2-cm margin of normal parenchyma. Dissection is then carried down in a wedge shape using sharp and blunt dissection. If the collecting system is entered, it is closed with 4-0 chromic continuous or interrupted suture. If a large portion of parenchyma is excised, then an internal ureteral stent should be considered if the collecting system is opened (Fig. 7.10). All vessels transected during the excision are suture ligated with 4-0 chromic figure-of-eight sutures. If there is any question of tumor involvement of the surgical margins, frozen section analysis can be performed. Once hemostasis has been achieved with the chromic suture

ligatures, the renal defect is then closed by approximation of the cut margins after placing oxycel in the defect and closing over with bolster sutures of 2-0 or 3-0 chromic. If the defect is too large, then perirenal fat, peritoneum, fascia, or muscle can be inserted into the defect and bolster sutures of 2-0 or 3-0 chromic placed (Figs. 7.8). After the defect has been closed, the renal artery can be unclamped, and a Penrose drain or closed suction system used to drain the perirenal space.

Major Transverse Resection

In very large polar tumors involving more than one renal segment, a transverse "guillotine" partial nephrectomy can be performed. If possible before occluding the main renal artery, the segmental branches supplying the pole involving the tumor should be ligated. Once the renal artery is occluded and the kidney cooled for 15 minutes in iced saline, the renal capsule is then incised in a transverse fashion approximately 1 to 2 cm from the tumor. Sharp and blunt dissection are then performed, with the collecting system most often being entered. After the tumor has been resected, an indwelling double "J" ureteral stent is placed, and the collecting system closed with 4.0 chromic interrupted or continuous sutures (Fig. 7.10). All transected vessels are suture ligated with 4.0 chromic figure-of-eight sutures. The renal defect can then be closed just as with the wedge resection. The renal artery is then unclamped, and

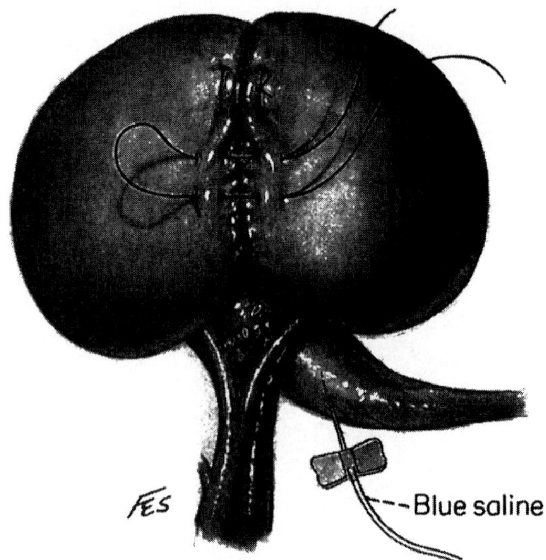

Fig. 7.9. Injection of blue saline to confirm watertight integrity of the collecting system. (From Gittes RF. Partial Nephrectomy and Bench Surgery: Techniques and Applications. In: Libertino EJ, Zinman LA, eds. Reconstructive Urologic Surgery: Pediatric and Adult. Baltimore: Williams & Wilkins, 1977.)

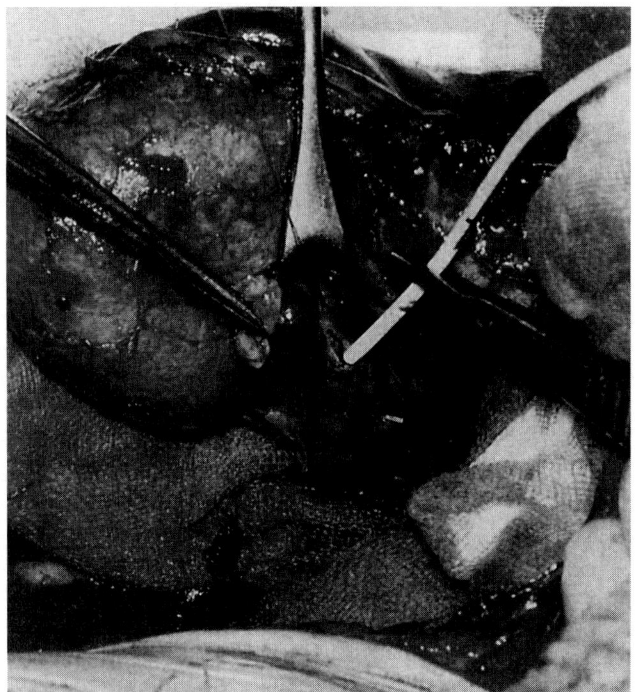

Fig. 7.10. Nephrostomy tubes and Silastic internal stents are often helpful in cases requiring extensive dissection of the collecting system. (Surgical photography by Lester V. Bergman, courtesy of LTI Medica and Bristol-Myers Company. Copyright 1986 by Learning Technology Inc.)

the wound is drained with either a Penrose or closed suction system. An alternative form of hemostasis in the performance of partial nephrectomy for a polar lesion is a kidney tourniquet composed of rubber tubing that provides polar temporary hemostasis by constriction (63).

After the renal defect has been closed and renal artery circulation has been restored, the patient is given a second bolus of intravenous mannitol and furosemide. The kidney should resume function promptly and be allowed to rewarm. Any bleeding after restoration of arterial flow is promptly controlled with direct compression, hemostatic agents, or suture ligature. It is important to continue a brisk diuresis and maintain adequate fluid volume following partial nephrectomy. After placement of the drain, the muscle, fascia, and skin are closed in the usual manner. With advances in laparoscopic techniques, nephron-sparing surgery using an endoscopic wedge resection method has been reported; however, its clinical appropriateness remains controversial (64).

Extracorporeal Partial Nephrectomy and Autotransplantation

The first partial nephrectomy and autotransplantation for renal cancer was performed by Calne in 1971 (65). This technique is technically more challenging than in situ partial nephrectomy and carries with it greater risk and a higher complication rate. The procedure should be reserved for that relatively select group of patients with large central tumors that are not amenable to in situ excision. Although the advantages of working with optimal exposure, a bloodless field, and ability to conserve the maximum amount of parenchyma are afforded by this method, its risk and complication rate are much higher than those for in situ partial nephrectomy. Disadvantages of bench surgery with autotransplantation include the increased risk of ischemic damage to the kidney, prolonged operating time, increased complexity of the technique, and the need for arterial, venous, and ureteral anastomoses with all their attendant risks. The disease-free survival rate for renal cell carcinoma after bench surgery has not been proven to be greater than that for in situ partial nephrectomy (19, 24, 66).

Operative Technique

Extracorporeal partial nephrectomy and autotransplantation can be performed through a flank, chevron, or midline abdominal incision. After the patient is given mannitol and furosemide, the kidney is removed by a standard radical nephrectomy with or without division of the ureter. Following kidney removal, it is flushed with 500 mL of chilled University of Wisconsin renal transplant solution. The perinephric fat is removed from the kidney to appreciate the full extent of the tumor. The kidney is submerged in ice slush of saline. If it is at all possible to leave the ureter intact, the extracorporeal partial nephrectomy can be performed on the abdominal wall, thus decreasing the chance of ureteral ischemia due to compromise of its blood

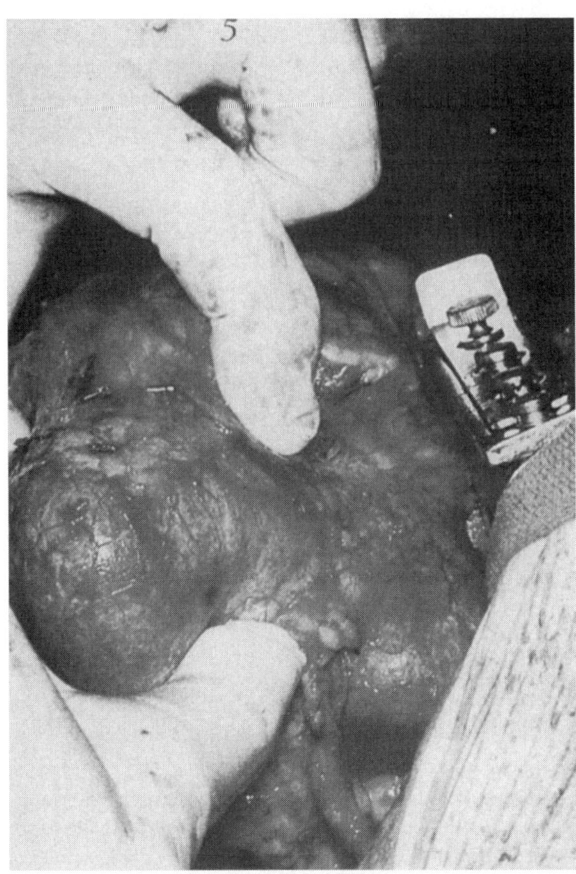
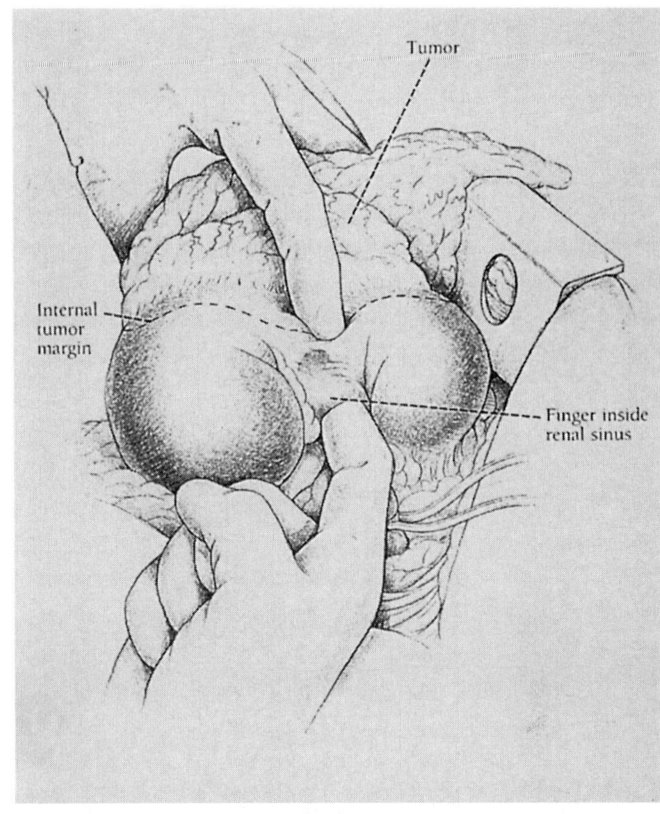

Fig. 7.11. Bimanual palpation of the kidney allows more accurate definition of the extent of tumor involvement. (Surgical photography by Lester V. Bergman, and drawing by William B. Westwood, courtesy LTI Medica and Bristol-Myers Company. Copyright 1986 by Learning Technology Inc.)

supply following excision of large hilar or lower pole renal tumors.

With the aid of optical magnification, excision of the tumor is begun at the renal hilus, with all the segmental arteries and veins to the region of the tumor identified. Those vessels that clearly are involved with the tumor are ligated and divided. The tumor is excised by making an incision through the renal capsule approximately 1 to 2 cm from the tumor border. All transected blood vessels on the cut renal surface are suture ligated with 4-0 chromic suture. The collecting system is entered and then closed with 4-0 chromic interrupted or running suture. Frozen sections of the margins are obtained to assure that the kidney is free of tumor. The parenchymal defects are then closed with absorbable sutures using bolsters as necessary (Figs. 7.11 and 7.12).

Autotransplantation into the iliac fossa is then performed using the same vascular techniques performed in renal allotransplantation. Alternatively, if a midline incision has been used for the nephrectomy, the incision can be extended caudally to allow access to the iliac vessels. If the ureter is left intact during the extracorporeal partial nephrectomy, the autotransplantation may be accomplished by flipping the kidney over or keeping it in its normal orientation with the vessels lying anteriorly and anastomosing the renal artery and vein to the

iliac vessels (57). Once the iliac vessels are dissected free, the renal vein is anastomosed to the external iliac vein in an end-to-side fashion while the artery is anastomosed either end-to-side to the external iliac artery or end-to-end with the hypogastric artery. The venous anastomosis is performed with 5-0 nonabsorbable vascular sutures, and the arterial anastomosis uses 5-0 or 6-0 sutures. After the anastomoses are complete, the venous clamps are released first, followed by the arterial clamps. Manual compression is usually adequate to stop any parenchymal oozing. If the ureter has been transected for the extracorporeal partial nephrectomy, it is reimplanted into the bladder with a ureteral neocystostomy using either an extravesical or intravesical approach. We prefer, however, to leave the ureter in continuity if possible. An internal ureteral stent may be left in place, and the perinephric space may be drained with a closed suction system (1).

Postoperative Complications

The complication rate after partial nephrectomy is in the range of 15 to 20% (20, 67, 68). The overall operative mortality rate is 1 to 1.5%.

The most common complications after partial nephrectomy are urinary fistulae and acute renal failure. Novick et al. found

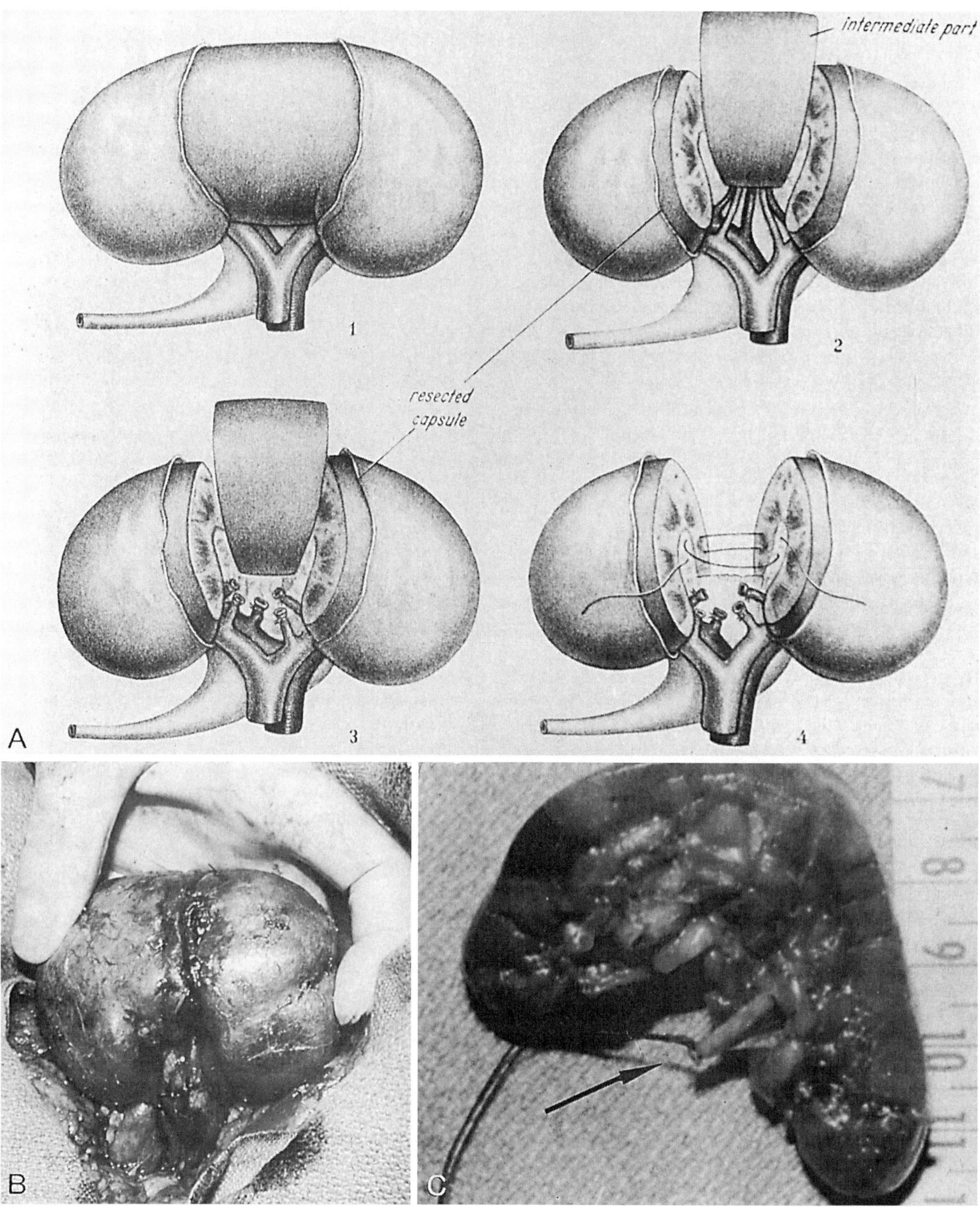

Fig. 7.12.   A. Technique for excision and closure of midportion lesions. **B.** Anastomosis of upper and lower poles has been performed after midportion nephrectomy. **C.** The arrow identifies a ligated calyx containing a cortical rest. (From Gittes RF, Elliot ML. Renal cortical rest and chronic hematuria. A syndrome treated by mid-kidney partial nephrectomy. J Urol 1973;109:14.)

that a fistula was more likely to develop if the tumor was larger than 4 cm, required major reconstruction on the collecting system, or required bench surgery (68). Renal failure was more likely to develop in patients requiring extracorporeal partial nephrectomy compared with in situ operations. Most investigators are finding that nephron-sparing surgery can almost always be done in situ, thus obviating the more complex ex vivo surgery with its attendant complications.

CONCLUSIONS

Nephron-sparing surgery continues to undergo change in its indications and applications to renal cell carcinoma. In those patients with familial renal cell carcinoma, von Hippel-Lindau disease, multiple renal tumors, or renal cell carcinoma in a solitary kidney, partial nephrectomy provides the best option for treatment. In patients with bilateral renal cell carcinoma or renal cell carcinoma in a solitary kidney, 5-year cause-specific survival rates of 85 to 90% have been reported. Local tumor recurrence rates of 4 to 9% are also reported over the same time (20, 60). Most recently, Novick et al. reported cancer-specific survival rates of 100% in patients with unilateral, stage I tumors smaller than 4 cm that were treated with nephron-sparing surgery (68). In patients with "imperative" indications, such as bilateral renal cell carcinoma or renal cell carcinoma in a solitary kidney, nephron-sparing surgery has a definite advantage over radical nephrectomy, which would leave the patient anephric, in need of dialysis, and with its attendant morbidities. It is in the area of "elective" indications, such as renal cell carcinoma with a normal contralateral kidney, where controversy still exists about the advisability of nephron-sparing surgery.

In its favor, partial nephrectomy spares healthy renal parenchyma, which may be crucial in the future for patients with deterioration in contralateral renal function. It also may be protective in patients who require future partial nephrectomy in the contralateral kidney, thus leaving the patient with less than half of one kidney, resulting in possible hyperfiltration injury (69). Nephron-sparing surgery also has a special use in the management of the indeterminate renal lesion. If CT scan, ultrasound, and arteriography are unable to exclude a complex cyst, oncocytoma, or adenoma, partial nephrectomy may allow for excision of the lesion while sparing healthy renal parenchyma. Improvements in technique, indications, and application of nephron-sparing surgery have allowed it to attain its rightful place in the treatment of localized renal cell carcinoma.

REFERENCES

1. Novick AC. Partial nephrectomy for renal cell carcinoma. Urol Clin North Am 1987;14:419.
2. Robson CJ, Churchill BM, Anderson W. The results of radical nephrectomy for renal cell carcinoma. J Urol 1969;101:297.
3. Semb C. Partial resection of the kidney: operative technique. Acta Chir Scand 1955;109:360.
4. Puigvert A. Partial nephrectomy for renal lithiasis: experience with 208 cases. Int Surg 1966;461:555.
5. Bernstein SM, Koyle MA, Gittes RF. Partial nephrectomy, extracorporeal surgery, and autotransplantation for renal cell carcinoma. In: Crawford DE, Das S. Current genitourinary cancer surgery. Philadelphia: Lea & Febiger, 1990:50.
6. Hardy JD. High ureteral injuries, management by autotransplantation of the kidney. JAMA 1963;184:97.
7. Serrallach-Mila N, Paravisini J, Mayd-Valls, et al. Renal autotransplantation. Lancet 1965;2:1130.
8. Wingo TA, Tong T, Bolden S. Cancer statistics: 1995. CA Cancer J Clin 1995;45:8.
9. Smith SJ, Bosniak MA, Megibow AJ, et al. Renal cell carcinoma: earlier discovery and increased detection. Radiology 1989;170:699.
10. Konnack JW, Grossman HB. Renal cell carcinoma as an incidental finding. J Urol 1985;134:1094.
11. Tsukamoto T, Kumamoto Y, Yamazahi K, et al. Clinical analysis of incidentally found renal cell carcinoma. Eur Urol 1991;19:109.
12. Thompson IM, Peak M. Improvement in survival of patients with renal cell carcinoma: the role of serendipitously detected tumor. J Urol 1988;140:487.
13. Butler BP, Novick AC, Miller DP, et al. Management of small unilateral renal cell carcinomas: radical vs. nephron-sparing surgery. Urology 1995;45:34.
14. Bosniak MA. Problems in the radiologic diagnosis of renal parenchymal tumors. Urol Clin North Am 1993;20:217.
15. Thrasher JB, Robertson JE, Paulson DF. Expanding indications for conservative renal surgery and renal carcinoma. Urology 1994;43:165.
16. Skinner DG, Colvin RB, Vermilon CD, et al. Diagnosis and management of renal cell carcinoma: a clinical and pathologic study of 309 cases. Cancer 1971;28:1165.
17. Lieber MM, Tomera FM, Taylor WF, et al. Renal adenocarcinoma in young adults: survival and variables affecting prognosis. J Urol 1981;125:164.
18. Marberger M, Pugh RCB, Auvert J, et al. Conservative surgery of renal carcinoma: the EIRSS experience. Br J Urol 1981;53:528.
19. Novick AC, Stream S, Montie JE, et al. Conservative surgery for renal cell carcinoma: a single-center experience with 100 patients. J Urol 1989;141:835.
20. Morgan WR, Zincke H. Progression and survival after renal-conserving surgery for renal cell carcinoma: experience in 104 patients in extended follow-up. J Urol 1990;144:852.
21. Bazeed MA, Scharfe T, Becht E, et al. Synchronous bilateral renal cell carcinoma: total surgical excision. Eur Urol 1986;12:238.
22. Jacobs SC, Berg SI, Lawson RD. Synchronous bilateral renal cell carcinoma: total surgical excision. Cancer 1980;46:2341.
23. Schiff M Jr, Bagley DH, Litton B. Treatment of solitary and bilateral renal carcinomas. J Urol 1979;121:581.
24. Smith RB, et al. Bilateral renal cell carcinoma and renal cell carcinoma in the solitary kidney. J Urol 1984;132:450.
25. Topley M. Partial nephrectomy for kidney tumors. Urol Newsletter 1983;1:1.
26. Topley M, Novick AC, Montie JE. Long-term results following nephrectomy for localized renal adenocarcinoma. J Urol 1984;131:1050.

27. Zinke H, Swanson SK. Bilateral renal cell carcinoma: influence of synchronous and asynchronous occurrence on patient survival. J Urol 1982;128:913.

28. Zinke H, Engen DE, Henning KM, et al. Treatment of renal cell carcinoma by in situ partial nephrectomy and extracorporeal operation with autotransplantation. Mayo Clin Proc 1985;60:651.

29. Specs EK, et al. Transplantation in patients with a history of renal cell carcinoma: long-term results and clinical considerations. Surgery 1982;91:282.

30. Licht MR, Novick AC. Nephron sparing surgery for renal cell carcinoma. J Urol 1993;145:1.

31. Muakmel E, Konichezky M, Englestein D, et al. Incidental small renal tumors accompanying clinically overt renal cell carcinoma. J Urol 1988;140:22.

32. Cheng WS, Farrow GM, Zinke H. Incidence of multicentricity in renal cell carcinoma. J Urol 1991;146:1221.

33. Lee SE, Kim HH. Validity of kidney-preserving surgery for localized renal cell carcinoma. Eur Urol 1994;25:204.

34. Amis ES, Cronan JJ, Pfister RC. Needle puncture of cystic renal masses: a survey of the Society of Uroradiology. AJR 1987;148:297.

35. Shenoy PD, Lakhkar MK, Ghosh MK, et al. Cutaneous seeding of renal carcinoma by Chiba needle aspiration biopsy. Acta Radiol 1991;32:50.

36. Novick AC. Renal sparing surgery for renal cell carcinoma. Urol Clin North Am 1987;14:419.

37. Swanson DA. Surgical issues and the management of localized renal cell carcinoma. South Central Section Seminar. 1995; 13:1.

38. Schrier RW, et al. Protection of mitochondrial function by mannitol in ischemic acute renal failure. Am J Physiol 1984; 247:F365.

39. Hansson R, et al. Effect of xanthine oxidase inhibition on renal circulation after ischemia. Transplant Proc 1982;14:51.

40. Paller MS, Hoidal JR, Ferris TF. Oxygen free radicals in ischemic acute renal failure in the rat. J Clin Invest 1984;74: 1156.

41. Ichikawa I, Miele JF, Brenner BM. Reversal of renal cortical actions of angiotensin II by verapamil and manganese. Kidney Int 1979;16:137.

42. McCrorey HL, et al. Effect of calcium transport inhibitors on renal hemodynamics and electrolyte excretion in the dog. In: Lichardus B, Schrier RW, Ponce J, eds. Hormonal regulation of sodium excretion. New York: Elsevier/North Holland Biomechanical Press, 1980:113.

43. Wait RB, White G, Davis JH. Beneficial effects of verapamil on postischemic renal failure: accelerated recovery with adenosine triphosphate-magnesium chloride infusion. Arch Surg 1977;112:729.

44. Malis CD, et al. Effects of verapamil in models of ischemic acute renal failure in the rat. Am J Physiol 1983;245:F735.

45. Oslas MB, et al. Postischemic renal failure: accelerated recovery with adenosine triphosphate-magnesium chloride infusion. Arch Surg 1977;112:729.

46. Siegel NJ, et al. Enhanced recovery from acute renal failure by the postischemic infusion of adenine nucleotides and magnesium chloride in rats. Kidney Int 1980;17:338.

47. Marshall FF, Holdford SS, Hamper UM. Intraoperative sonography of renal tumors. J Urol 1992;1393.

48. Chopp RT, Shah BB, Addonizio JC. Use of ultrasonic surgical aspirator in renal surgery. Urology 1983;22:157.

49. Malloy TR, Shultz RE, Wein AJ, et al. Renal preservation utilizing neodymium: YAG laser. Urology 1986;27:99.

50. Levinson AK, Swanson DA, Johnson DE, et al. Fibrin glue for partial nephrectomy. Urology 1991;38:314.

51. Vermooten V. Indications for conservative surgery and certain renal tumors: a study based on the growth pattern of the clear cell carcinoma. J Urol 1956;64:200.

52. Graham SD Jr, Glenn JF. Enucleative surgery for renal malignancy. J Urol 1979;122:546.

53. Novick AC, Zinke H, Neves RJ, et al. Surgical enucleation for renal cell carcinoma. J Urol 1986;135:235.

54. Jaeger N, Weissbach L, Vahlensieck W. Value of enucleation of tumor in solitary kidneys. Eur Urol 1985;11:369.

55. Bazeed MA, Scharfe T, Becht E, et al. Conservative surgery of renal cell carcinoma. Eur Urol 1986;12:238.

56. Marberger M. Conservative surgery for renal adenocarcinoma. In: deKernion JB, Pavone-Macaluso M, eds. Tumors of the kidney: international perspectives on urology. section 2. Baltimore: Williams & Wilkins, 1986;13:157.

57. Lieber MM. Renal cell carcinoma: new developments. Mayo Clin Proc 1985;60:715.

58. Morse MJ, Sloan JW. Partial nephrectomy and renal cell carcinoma: part II. J Urol 1986;135:165. Abstract no. 245.

59. Rosenthal CL, Kraft R, Zingg EJ. Organ preserve in surgery and renal cell carcinoma: tumor enucleation vs. partial kidney resection. Eur Urol 1984;10:222.

60. Marshall FF, Taxy JB, Fishman EK, et al. The feasibility of surgical enucleation for renal cell carcinoma. J Urol 1986;135: 231.

61. Blackley SK, Ladaga L, Woolfitt RA, et al. In situ study of the effectiveness of enucleation in patients with renal cell carcinoma. J Urol 1988;140:6.

62. Stephens R, Graham S. Enucleation of tumor vs. partial nephrectomy as conservative treatment of renal cell carcinoma. Cancer 1990;12:2663.

63. Goldwasser BZ, Carson CC, Shalaby NF, et al. Kidney tourniquet: a new instrument for regional blood control and partial nephrectomy. Urology 1988;32:6.

64. McDougal EM, Clayman RV, Anderson K. Laparoscopic wedge resection of a renal tumor: initial experience. J Laparoendosc Surg 1993;3:577.

65. Calne RY. Tumor in a single kidney: nephrectomy, excision, and autotransplantation. Lancet 1971;2:761.

66. Stormont TJ, Bilhartz DL, Zincke H. Pitfalls of "bench surgery" and autotransplantation for renal cell carcinoma. 1992;67:621.

67. Steinbach F, Stockle M, Mueller SC, et al. Conservative surgery of renal cell tumors in 140 patients: 21 years of experience. J Urol 1994;148:24.

68. Licht MR, Novick AC, Gormastic M. Nephron sparing surgery in incidental versus suspected renal cell carcinoma. J Urol 1994;152:39.

69. Herr HW. Partial nephrectomy for renal cell carcinoma with a normal opposite kidney. Cancer 1994;73:160.

8

Surgical Management of Renal Cell Carcinoma with Vena Caval Extension

Thomas S. Vates and Kenneth B. Cummings

INTRODUCTION

Renal cell carcinoma (RCC) is the third most common urologic malignancy, with approximately 27,000 new cases and 10,900 deaths estimated on an annual basis (1). RCC is predominantly a hypervascular tumor, and invasion of the intrarenal veins is a common event, with subsequent tumor extension into the renal veins occurring in 30% of cases (2, 3). The incidence of intraluminal inferior vena caval extension ranges from 4 to 10%, with the incidence of extension into the right atrium ranging from 0.4 to 1% (4, 5). Tumor propagation in the renal vein is by direct extension, with the tumor thrombus carrying its own blood supply parasitized from the renal artery. Propagation of tumor growth within the lumen of the inferior vena cava is cephalad, in the direction of venous flow. However, a "bland" thrombus that does not have a component of tumor cells can also form but will propagate in the caudad direction. Because of the relative shortness of the right renal vein, inferior venal caval thrombi occur more frequently with right-sided tumors (6).

The insidious natural history of intraluminal growth may be appreciated from Kaufman's report of the value of inferior venacavograms, in which he noted that 50% of patients with complete caval occlusion had no associated symptoms (7). The growth rate in these cases obviously permitted the development of sufficient collateral venous return to the heart from the lower torso via the lumbar and azygous system to obviate symptoms referable to caval obstruction. Clayman and Gonzalez have presented an excellent review of the anatomic and radiologic development of collateral venous drainage that can occur during caval obstruction (8).

RATIONALE FOR AGGRESSIVE SURGICAL EXTIRPATION

Initial reports of inferior vena caval extension from RCC reflected a uniformly poor prognosis (6, 9, 10). In 1970, Marshall et al. reported on 11 such patients, 8 of whom were dead or dying 1 year postoperatively (4). However, in 1972 Skinner et al. reported a 55% 5-year survival rate (6 of 11 patients) and a 43% 10-year survival rate (4 of 11 patients) for patients with RCC and vena caval extension (11). Several contemporary series have reported 5-year survival rates ranging from 55 to 69% for patients whose conditions were diagnosed as RCC and intraluminal inferior vena caval extension. These long-term survivors showed no documented metastatic disease preoperatively and underwent complete tumor and thrombus removal in the absence of positive regional nodes and lack of contiguous organ spread (12–16). Some series have reported less optimistic 5-year survival rates ranging from 5 to 50% (17–20).

The operative mortality rate for radical nephrectomy and caval tumor thrombectomy is approximately 5 to 10% (21). However, several factors can affect the long-term survival of patients with intraluminal tumor thrombi. Some of these factors are as follows.

1. Evidence of metastatic disease documented preoperatively.
2. Incomplete removal of tumor thrombi.
3. Involvement of contiguous organs.
4. Positive regional lymph nodes.

All of these factors result in significantly decreased survival rates.

As expected, patients with metastatic disease diagnosed preoperatively had the worst outcome. Cherrie et al. noted only 5% of patients with distant metastases survived 2 years and none survived 5 years (17). Suggs et al. reported that of five patients with evidence of metastatic disease before surgical treatment, none survived beyond 12 months (16). More optimistic 2-year and 5-year survival rates of 37.5% and 12.5%, respectively, for patients with known preoperative metastases were reported by Neves and Zincke (13).

Regional lymph node involvement significantly shortens survival time. Skinner et al. reported no survivors when the renal vein and regional nodes were involved (22). Novick et al. noted a 10.9% 3-year survival rate for patients with either regional lymph node involvement or distant metastases. In addition, there was no significant difference in survival between patients with regional lymph node metastasis compared with patients with distant metastasis (23). The mean survival time of patients with nodal disease but with no evidence of preoperative metastasis was 15 months, as reported by Neves and Zincke (13).

Unfortunately, the effect on survival of perinephric fat invasion and the extent of rostral spread of the tumor thrombus is more difficult to assess. With respect to perinephric fat invasion, Schefft et al. reported that if there were no tumor present in the perinephric fat, there would be an increase in survival (24). Sosa et al. combined patients with both positive regional lymph nodes and perinephric fat invasion into one group and reported a mean survival time of 17 months, with only three patients surviving 2 years (20). Montie et al. noted that although there was a trend toward decreased survival with perinephric fat invasion, this was not statistically significant (21). In two separate clinical series reported by Swierzewski et al. and Novick et al., both noted that among patients with localized RCC, there was no significant difference in survival rates between those patients with or without perinephric fat invasion (15, 23).

The issue of rostral spread of tumor thrombus is even more perplexing. In an early study of six patients and a review of the literature, Clayman et al. noted that the level of cephalad extent of tumor thrombus apparently had no bearing on survival (8). Sosa et al. noted a distinct inverse correlation between survival and extent of tumor thrombus. They also noted a higher likelihood of finding tumor in the regional nodes and/or perinephric fat invasion in patients with tumor thrombi above the hepatic veins, with a subsequent decreased survival time in patients with extensive thrombi (20). Skinner et al. reported a 0% 5-year survival rate for patients with tumor thrombi extending into the right atrium (25). The data from a study conducted by Montie et al. suggest that a statistically significant effect on survival was seen in patients with extension of the tumor thrombus into the right atrium (21).

However, several studies have shown that the extent of thrombus propagation has no significant effect on survival. Cherrie et al. noted a subjective impression that supradiaphragmatic extension of a vena caval thrombus has a negative effect on survival; however, this was unsupported by any test of statistical significance (17). Unlike Sosa's series, Novick's series noted that a significantly greater proportion of intra-atrial thrombi was observed in patients with localized RCC. Surprisingly, the 3-year survival rate for patients with intra-atrial thrombi (56%) was better than that for patients with retrohepatic thrombi (46%). However, this difference was not statistically significant (23, 26). Recently, Glazer and Novick evaluated the long-term follow-up of patients with atrial thrombi who underwent extirpative surgery. They noted a 4-year survival rate of 70% with a median survival time of 5.1 years if the tumor did not penetrate the renal capsule. If the tumor

did penetrate the capsule, the 4-year survival rate was 13% with a median survival time of 1 year (27).

The role of radical nephrectomy and inferior vena caval thrombectomy for patients with metastatic disease identified preoperatively is limited. If a patient is to participate in a protocol with biologic response modifiers, this procedure can be considered in rare instances (16). Additionally, radical nephrectomy with tumor thrombectomy may be contemplated for patients with an isolated metastatic lesion that is easily resectable (21).

DIAGNOSTIC IMAGING OF INFERIOR VENA CAVAL TUMOR THROMBI

Detailed imaging studies are necessary to define the limits of vena caval tumor thrombi and are essential in the planning of successful surgical extirpation. There are several imaging modalities available to evaluate patients with tumor thrombus, including ultrasound with color Doppler flow, computed tomography (CT) scan, magnetic resonance imaging (MRI), venacavography, transesophageal echocardiography (TEE), and intraoperative ultrasound (IOUS). Recognizing the strengths and limitations of each of these modalities will allow for an appropriate surgical approach.

CT scans have become the cornerstone in the initial evaluation of patients with renal tumors (Fig. 8.1) (28). CT scans are highly accurate and have a reported staging accuracy of 67 to 90% for the detection of intravascular tumor thrombi (29, 30). With the application of dynamic thin-section CT scan, Zeman et al. reported a 90% accuracy rate in detecting the presence of tumor thrombi (29). It is important that the tumor thrombus be visualized when using CT scan because renal vein enlargement and actual tumor propagation are often independent processes. Although early studies assessing the use of CT scans in the evaluation of patients with tumor thrombi merely used

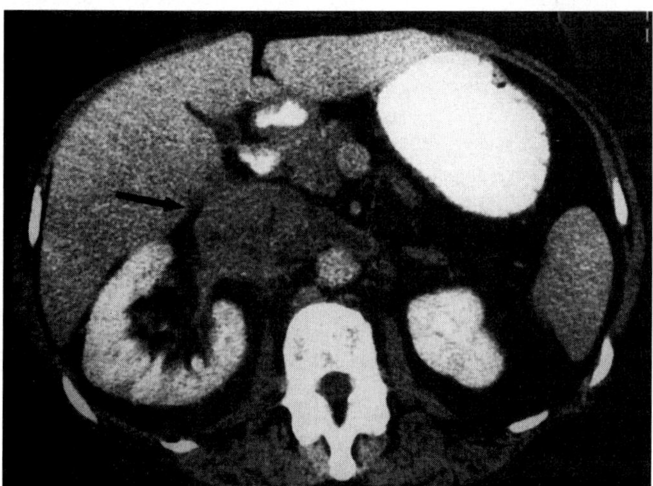

Fig. 8.1. CT scan demonstrating tumor thrombus within the inferior vena cava with extension into left renal vein.

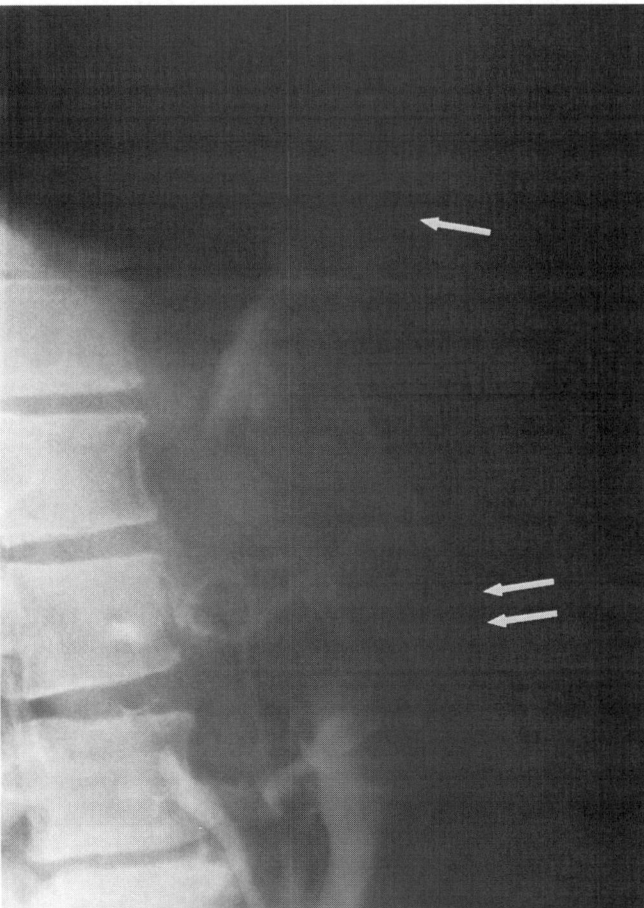

Fig. 8.2. Lateral inferior venacavogram demonstrating intraluminal tumor thrombus. Single arrow marks supradiaphragmatic thrombus; double arrow marks infradiaphragmatic thrombus.

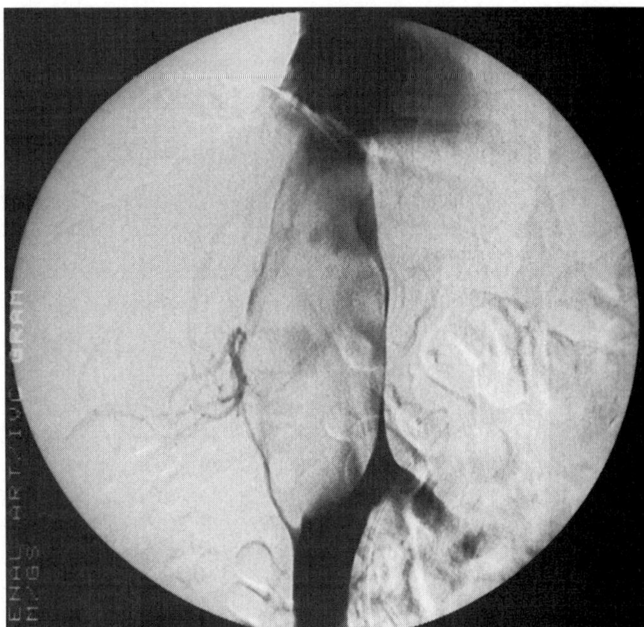

Fig. 8.3. PA view of digital subtraction inferior venacavogram revealing intraluminal tumor thrombus.

the presence of renal vein dilatation as the criterion for tumor extension, Zeman et al. warn against this; three patients in their series had a tumor thrombus without dilatation (29). Other sources of error seen when using CT scans include under-opacification, streaming, streak artifacts, and layering caused by the greater physical density of the contrast material (31). Most authors believe that CT scanning is done primarily as a staging procedure to assess the local extent of tumor, regional adenopathy, and intra-abdominal metastasis and to identify vena caval involvement. After inferior vena caval involvement has been detected, additional studies to assess the extent and level of caval involvement are performed.

Inferior venacavography was the standard imaging modality for evaluating intravascular extension of RCC (Figs. 8.2 and 8.3). Venacavography also provides superior demonstration of the collateral circulation (Fig. 8.4). However, inferior venacavography is an invasive procedure and requires the use of iodinated contrast. In addition, if there is total occlusion of the inferior vena cava, then either a superior venacavogram or right heart catheterization may need to be performed to assess the rostral spread of the tumor thrombus (Fig. 8.5A and B).

The role of MRI is still evolving with respect to evaluating patients with vena caval tumor thrombi; however, it has shown promising results in determining both the presence and level of spread of caval thrombi (Figs. 8.6 and 8.7). In an early report on the use of MRI in assessing caval thrombi, Pritchett et al. reported that MRI correctly staged the level of tumor thrombus

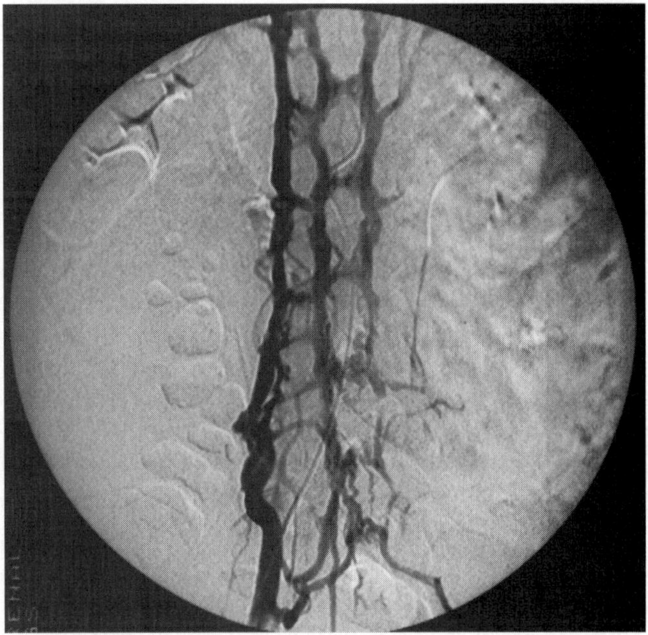

Fig. 8.4. Digital subtraction inferior venacavogram showing complete caval occlusion and development of collateral circulation via the azygous and hemiazygous system.

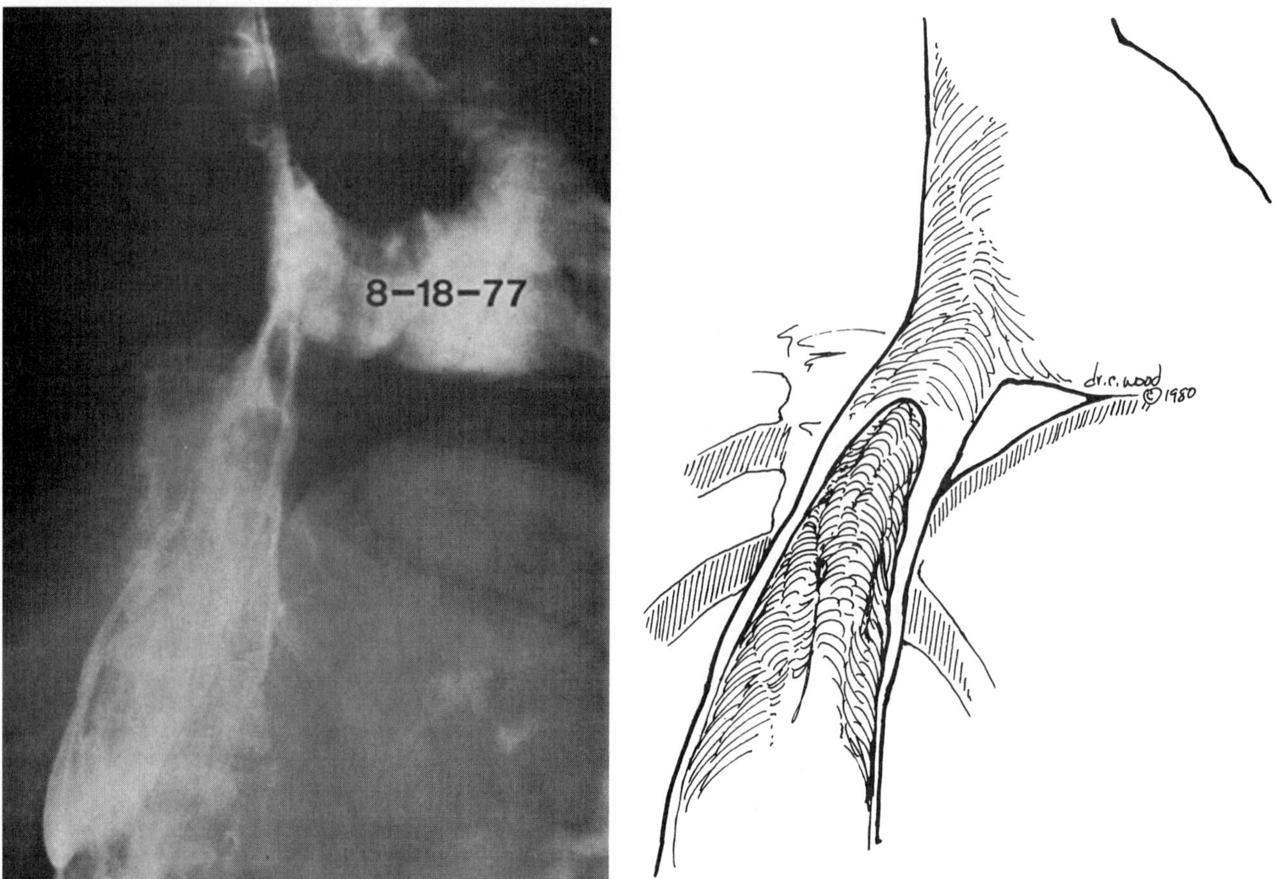

Fig. 8.5. Right heart catheterization for visualization of tumor thrombus apex.

in four of five patients and missed the presence of right atrial extension in one patient (32). In a prospective study of 44 patients (11 with inferior vena caval involvement and 17 with renal vein involvement), venacavography and MRI correctly identified 9 of 11 patients (82%) with inferior vena caval

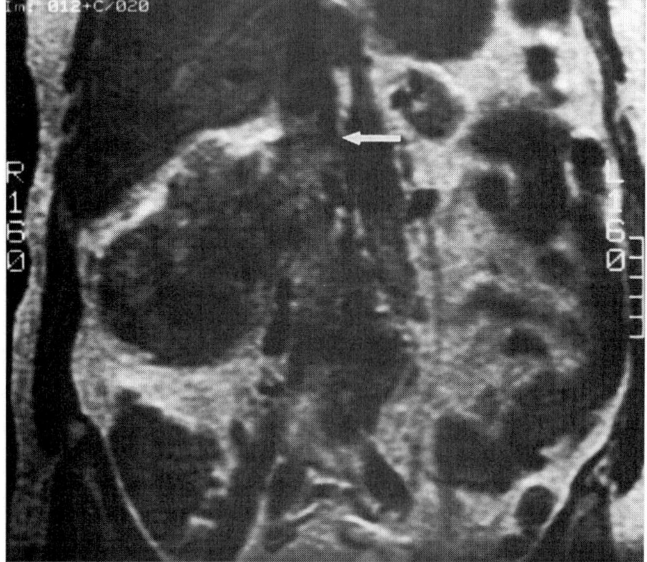

Fig. 8.6. T-1 weighted post gadolinium coronal MRI of right renal cell carcinoma with intraluminal caval thrombus.

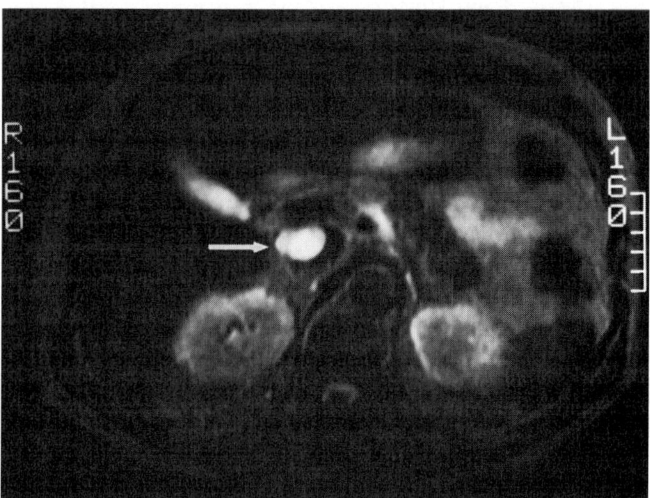

Fig. 8.7. T-2 weighted MRI with vena caval thrombus.

thrombi. When both tests were combined, all 11 cases of vena caval extension were identified.

Venacavography was slightly more sensitive (71%) in identifying the presence of renal vein thrombi than MRI (65%), but this difference was not statistically significant (31). Several recent studies have shown that MRI has a 100% sensitivity rate for detecting vena caval tumor thrombi (30, 33–35).

Goldfarb et al. noted that MRI delineated the presence and extent of a caval thrombus with 100% sensitivity. Venacavography was only 94% sensitive, and 50% of the patients in this series required both antegrade and retrograde studies to define the full extent of caval thrombi (34). When comparing MRI and venacavography with CT scans, Goldfarb et al. noted that although CT scans demonstrated the presence of a caval thrombus in all patients, the cephalad extent could only be determined in 33% of patients (34). Kallman et al. also reported a sensitivity rate of 100% for MRI in the detection of tumor thrombus. However, the specificity was 85% due to three false-positive results, which were accounted for by flow artifacts. Several factors other than slow flow can compromise the images obtained with MRI. These include extrinsic caval compression, respiratory motion, and cardiac motion.

New MRI pulse sequences with short repetition times, including flat low-angle shot (FLASH) and gradient recalled acquisition in steady state (GRASS), have been developed to attempt to define vascular extension of tumor growth in a better manner (36, 37). In these pulse sequences, flowing blood appears bright because fully magnetized protons continually enter the selected section while adjacent tissues (thrombus) become partly saturated. Lowering their relative signal intensity, GRASS imaging has excellent sensitivity to flow and is not compromised by respiratory motion artifact when performed with breath-holding techniques. Roubidoux et al. demonstrated that MRI using GRASS imaging techniques correctly identified 100% of patients (13 of 13) with caval thrombus, 88% of patients (23 of 26) with renal vein thrombus, and 80% of patients (4 of 5) with atrial thrombus (35). Extrinsic caval compression, which can significantly affect the quality of images obtained with cavography and CT, does not interfere with detection of thrombi using GRASS MRI. Roubidoux et al. recommend using cine GRASS to eliminate cardiac motion artifact. The single false-negative case of atrial extension in this study was not depicted with cine cardiac GRASS (35). However, MRI cannot be used for all patients, specifically patients with claustrophobia, cardiac pacemakers, certain intracerebral vascular clips, cochlear implants, and intraocular foreign bodies (34, 35).

Some authors believe that MRI should be the imaging modality of choice if the CT scan demonstrates vena caval involvement; they also believe that venacavography should be limited to those patients who are not candidates for MRI or in whom the MRI is equivocal (34, 35, 38, 39). However, Straton et al. reported on one patient who underwent a noncardiac gated MRI with images judged to be of satisfactory quality that failed to demonstrate right atrial extension, which was subsequently confirmed on venacavography (40). We believe that the imaging modality should be the one that the surgeon and radiologist feel most comfortable in interpreting. As experience is gained with GRASS MRI, it will assume a role of importance in the evaluation of these patients, with venacavography being held in reserve for difficult situations.

Transabdominal ultrasound can also be used to evaluate patients preoperatively for the presence of renal or caval tumor thrombus. Unfortunately, its accuracy depends on the skill and experience of the ultrasonographer and the patient's body habitus. It had been estimated that the renal vein and inferior vena cava are not completely visualized in 12.5% and 43.5% of cases, respectively (41). However, certain modifications of real-time ultrasound have increased the ability to detect tumor thrombi. McGahan et al. reported an overall 95% sensitivity in detecting venous involvement with tumor thrombus with color Doppler flow imaging (42). IOUS has also been used to supplement preoperative imaging studies. Harris et al., using a 7-MHz probe, performed IOUS on five patients in whom the presence or extension of an inferior vena caval thrombus was equivocal. IOUS provided excellent dynamic images of the thrombus or was able to definitively rule out the presence of a thrombus (43). They concluded that IOUS is beneficial in the following situations:

1. Cases in which the presence of renal vein or inferior vena cava involvement is equivocal on preoperative imaging.
2. Cases in which there is a question intraoperatively about the extent of a known thrombus (43).

TEE has also been used to assess patients with caval thrombi. Treiger et al. described five patients with caval thrombi who were assessed with TEE. The authors performed TEE intraoperatively and found that three of five patients had tumor thrombi extending further than was expected based on the preoperative imaging studies (44). Additionally, TEE provides information about possible residual tumor and intraoperative myocardial function. TEE also allows one to determine if intracardiac air is present after closure of the right atrium (44, 45, 46).

CLASSIFICATION OF INFERIOR VENA CAVAL TUMOR THROMBI

There are several classification schemes for vena caval thrombi. Pritchett et al. divided tumor thrombi into three groups—subhepatic, intrahepatic, and atrial (47). Neves and Zincke classified caval thrombi into four groups—renal, infrahepatic, intrahepatic, and atrial (13). We prefer the classification in Figure 8.8, which organizes caval thrombi based on the level of involvement and the surgical approach necessary—supradiaphragmatic (intracardiac, intrapericardial) and infradiaphragmatic (retrohepatic, infrahepatic).

SURGICAL CONSIDERATIONS

Systemic vascular control is essential for the prevention of intraoperative complications (tumor embolization to the lungs, un-

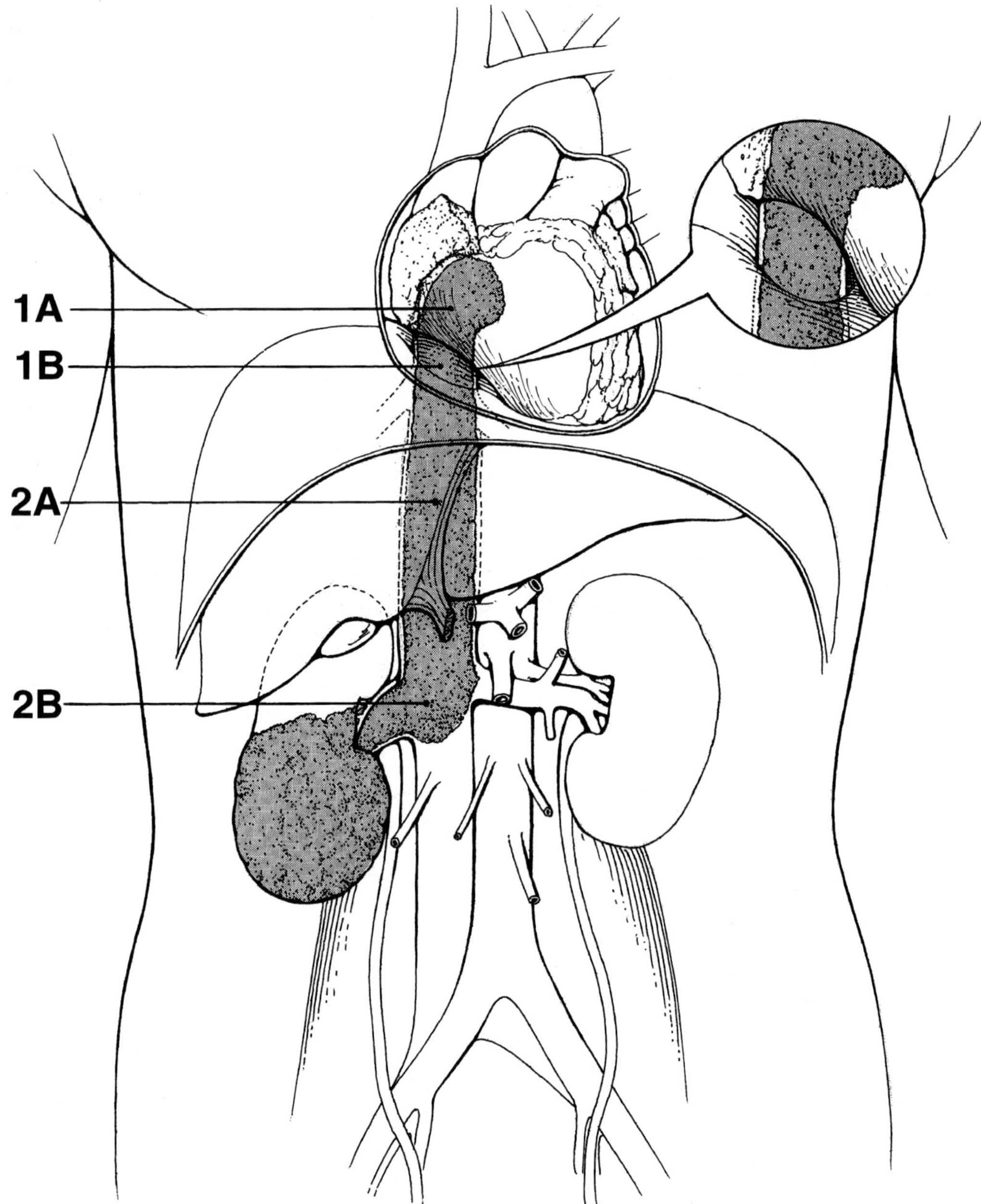

Fig. 8.8.   Vena caval tumor thrombus classification. 1: Supradiaphragmatic; A: intracardiac; B: intrapericardial; 2: infradiaphragmatic; A: retrohepatic; B: infrahepatic.

controlled hemorrhage, and failure to perform a complete tumor thrombectomy). The facts gleaned from imaging studies both classify the intracaval thrombi with respect to the location and provide information regarding the collateral venous return. These studies permit anticipation of patient tolerance of proximal caval occlusion. The absence of significant collateral venous return predicts the need for achieving circulatory arrest of the lower torso by cross-clamping the aorta or, alternatively, by performing a cardiopulmonary bypass. The principles of the surgical procedure and the technical considerations in extirpation of caval thrombi are best described by using the established classification as a basis.

SUPRADIAPHRAGMATIC-INTRAPERICARDIAL (IB) AND INFRADIAPHRAGMATIC-RETROHEPATIC (IIA) EXTENSION

A tumor thrombus that extends intraluminally in the vena cava to the level of the hepatic veins (retrohepatic) or is supradiaphragmatic but does not extend into the heart requires the same surgical approach. It is necessary to gain caval control intrapericardially above the apex of the tumor thrombus. Technical variation is dictated by the kidney involved and the magnitude of the collateral venous return. Significant venous collaterals rarely develop in patients who do not have complete caval obstruction either by tumor thrombus or by bland thrombus, which forms below the tumor thrombus (infrarenally). In such patients, intrapericardial interruption of the inferior vena caval return results in significant diminution of venous return, diminution of cardiac output, and profound hypotension. This condition can be prevented by temporary circulatory arrest to the lower torso, which effectively divides the circulating blood volume, with resulting perfusion of the upper torso at normal pressure and flow (48).

Caval thrombi emanating from a left renal tumor are best approached through a midline incision with the patient in a supine position. Caval thrombi emanating from a right-sided tumor may alternatively be approached through a high (eighth to ninth rib) thoracoabdominal incision with the patient in the modified flank position with torque of the lower torso (49). With the patient in a supine position, we use a midline abdominal incision with a median sternotomy to permit IB vascular control of the inferior vena cava (Fig. 8.9).

The sites and sequence of vascular interruption for an IB intrapericardial-extracardiac right renal tumor thrombus are shown in Figure 8.10.

Surgical Technique

An intra-arterial and Swan-Ganz catheter are placed before exploratory laparotomy. The abdomen is explored, and a careful examination for evidence of metastatic disease is completed. The right and transverse colon, small bowel mesentery, and duodenum are mobilized to the left with interruption of the inferior mesenteric vein if this structure impedes adequate mo-

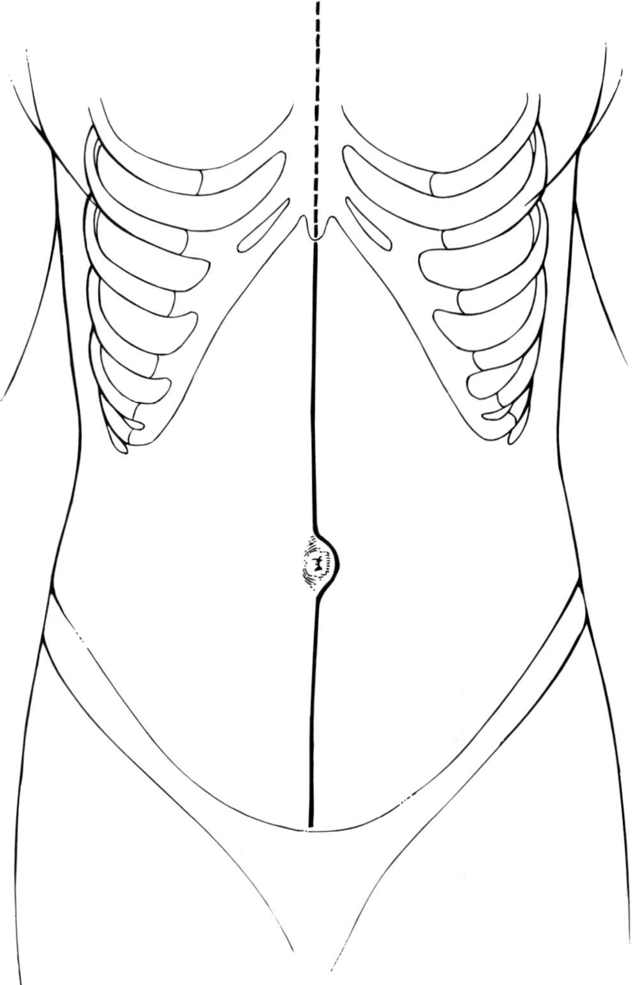

Fig. 8.9. Midline incision with median sternotomy to allow cardiopulmonary bypass.

bilization. The bowel is then placed in a Lahey bag and retracted in a cephalad direction to expose the retroperitoneum, right renal tumor, and retroperitoneal vessels. The renal hilum is then explored carefully (Fig. 8.11). Any suspicious nodes are excised and submitted for frozen section study. If the patient is considered to be a suitable surgical candidate, the renal artery is ligated using two ligatures of silk (Fig. 8.12). Ligation of the renal artery may result in shrinkage of the tumor thrombus.

The abdominal incision is extended in a cephalad direction with a median sternotomy. Bone wax is applied to the incised surface of the sternum to control bleeding. The pericardium is opened, and its edges are secured to the drapes at the wound margins with interrupted 2-0 silk sutures (Fig. 8.13). Palpation of the intrapericardial inferior vena cava reveals the apex of the tumor thrombus. A cardiac tourniquet loop is used to secure the inferior vena cava proximal to the thrombus. Temporary occlusion of the inferior vena cava is performed, and the vital signs are observed. When collateral circulation is not adequate (as shown by a significant drop in systemic blood pressure), it

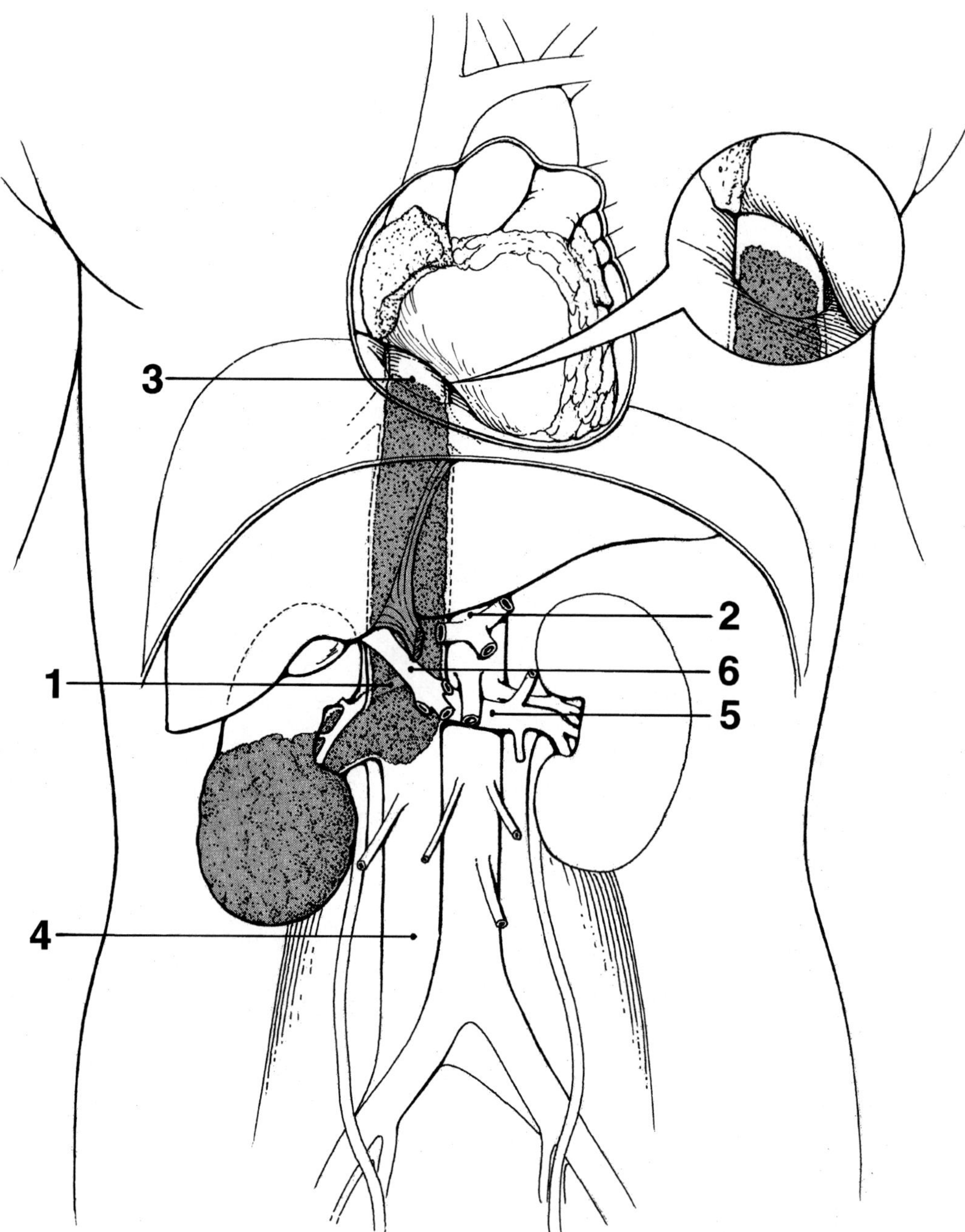

Fig. 8.10. Sequence of vascular interruption for a IB intrapericardial right renal tumor. 1: right renal artery; 2: proximal aorta; 3: proximal IVC; 4: distal IVC; 5: left renal vein; 6: etpasis.

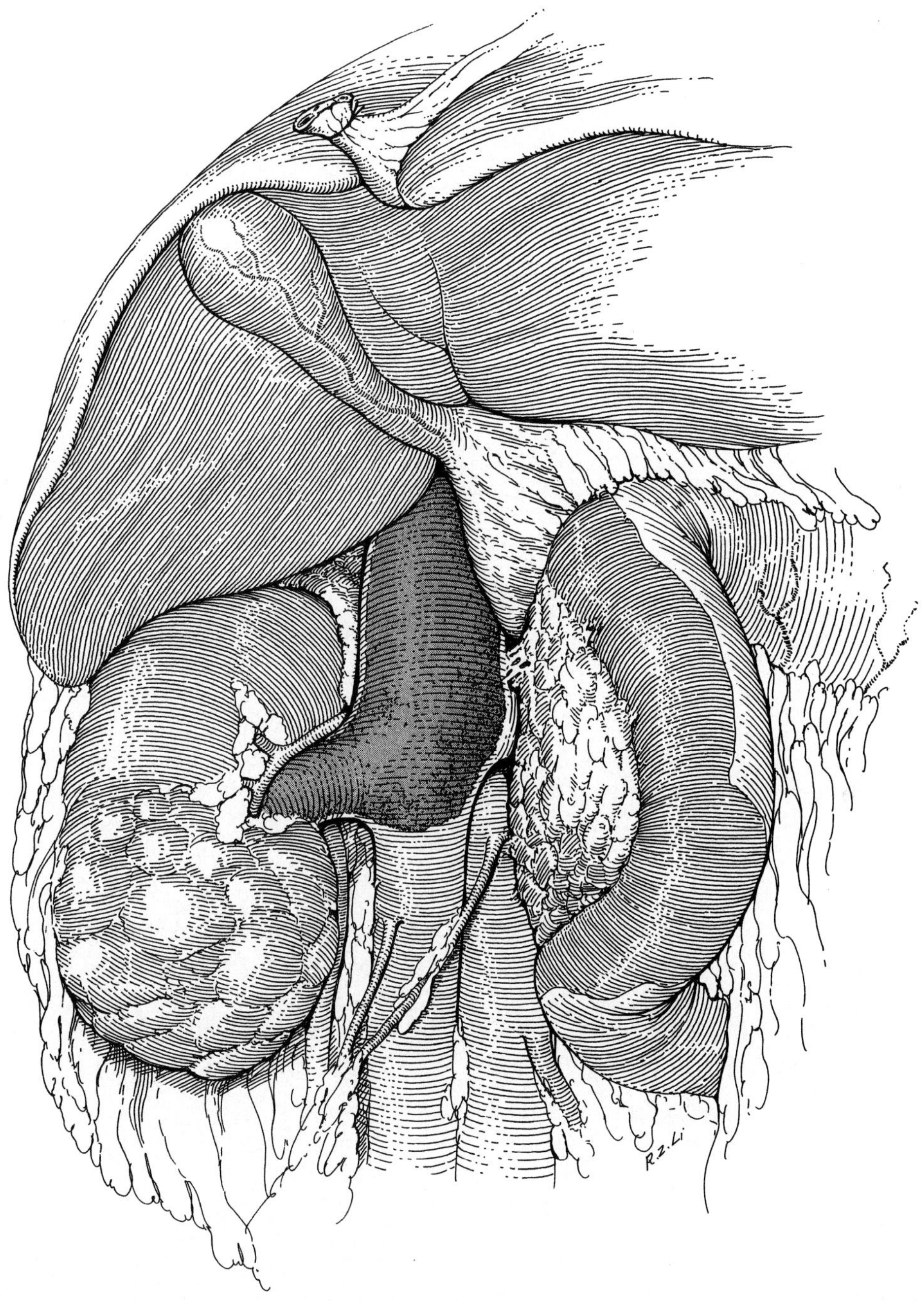

Fig. 8.11.   Retroperitoneal mobilization of the surgical field in preparation for removal of a right renal cell carcinoma with a caval thrombus.

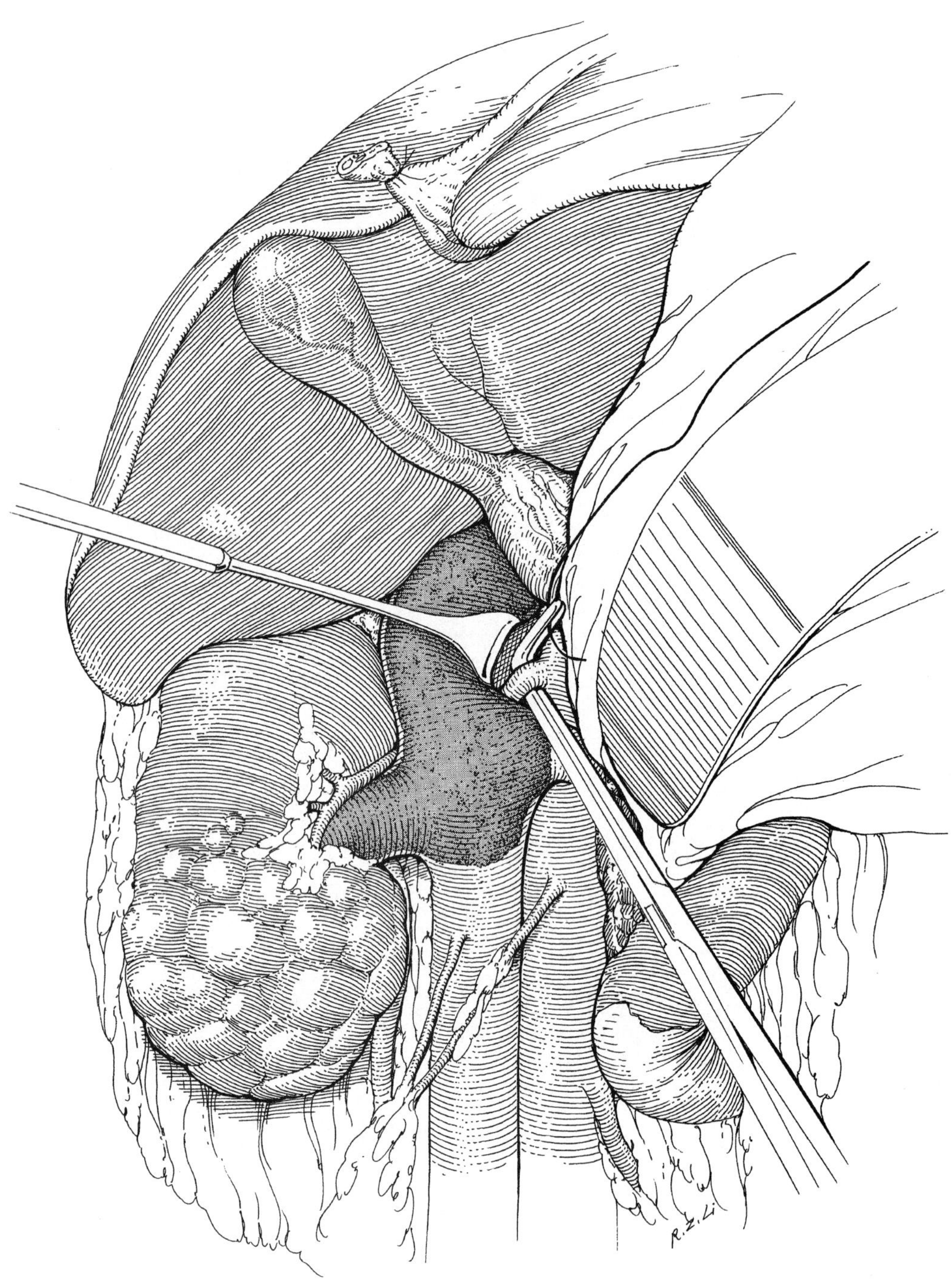

Fig. 8.12.   Isolation of the right renal artery.

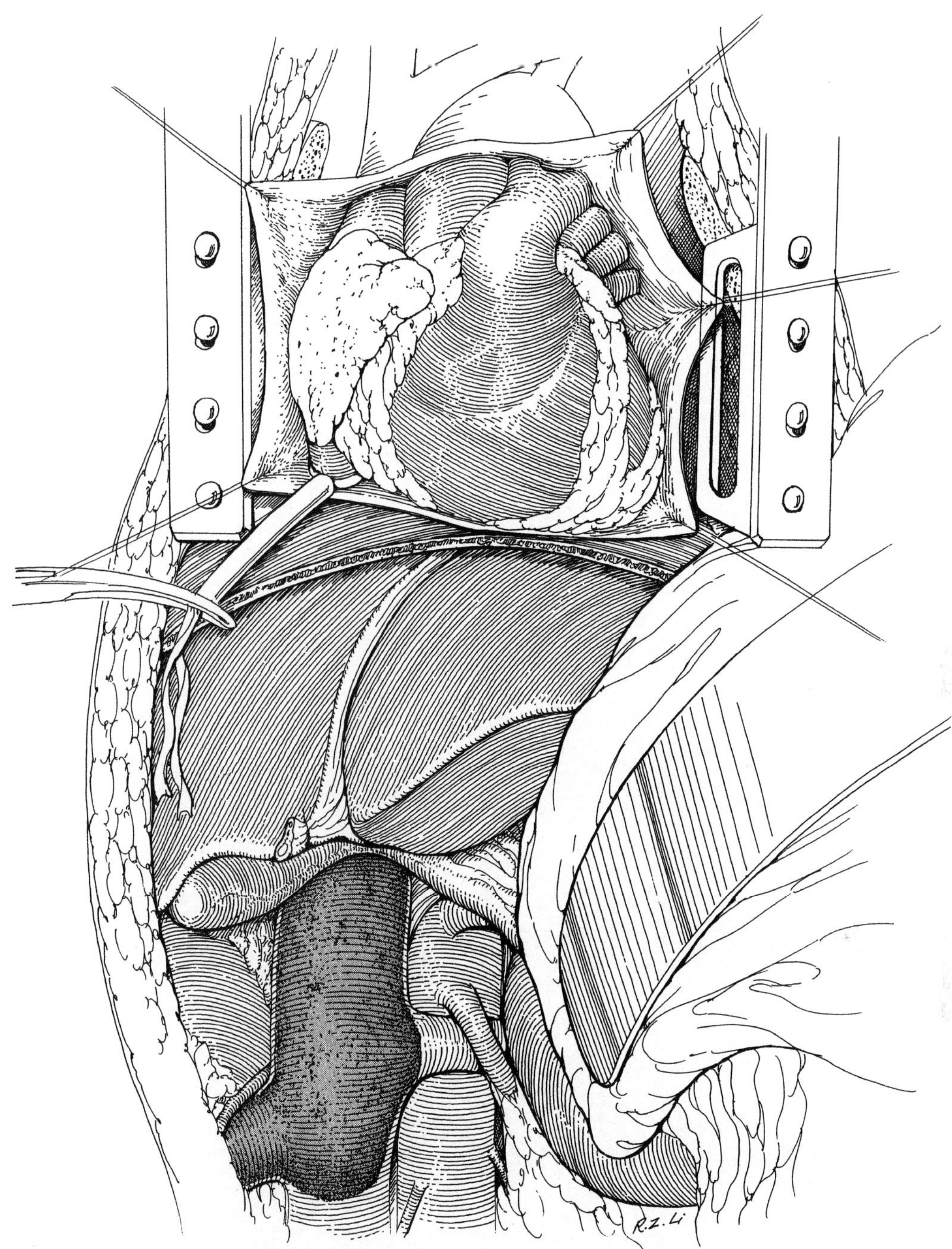

Fig. 8.13. Intrapericardial control of the inferior vena cava.

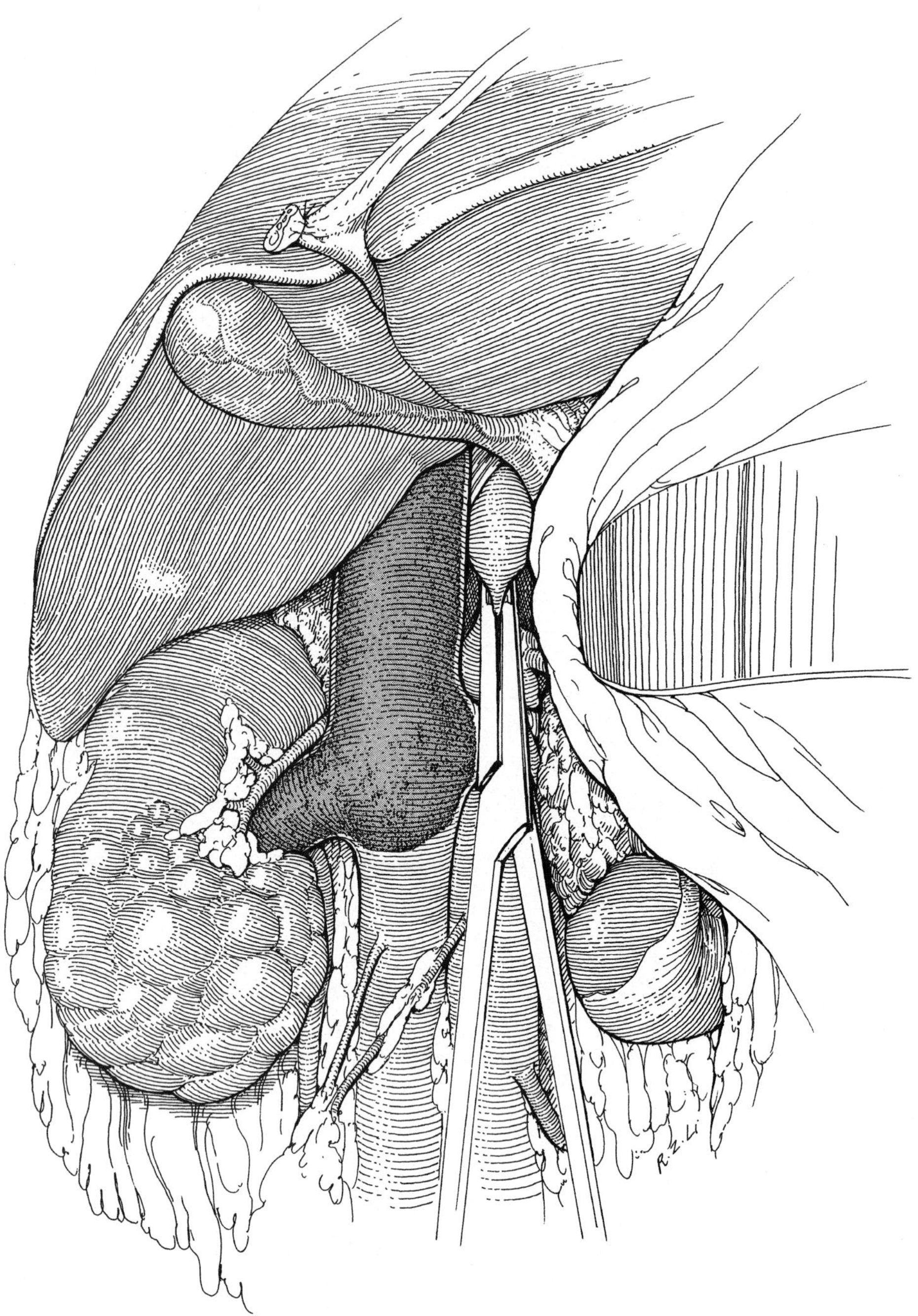

Fig. 8.14.   Aortic cross-clamp at the diaphragmatic hiatus.

is necessary to cross-clamp the aorta at the diaphragmatic hiatus above the celiac axis (Fig. 8.14).

When this decision has been made, attention is returned to the abdomen, and the operative field is prepared for execution of thrombectomy from the inferior vena cava and radical nephrectomy. The liver is then delivered free of its diaphragmatic attachments (coronary and triangular ligaments) by incising these and exposing the bare area of the liver (Fig. 8.15) (50). This exposure is further facilitated by the previously performed median sternotomy. The liver is now rotated medially to expose the retrohepatic vena cava (Fig. 8.16). Caudad to the main hepatic veins there are usually several small hepatic veins that are best interrupted, thus providing better exposure and facilitating tumor thrombectomy.

The proximal lumbar veins are identified and interrupted with care to prevent disruption in the continuity of the intraluminal caval thrombus. When caval obstruction by tumor thrombus is complete, lumbar veins may serve to communicate via the azygos and hemiazygos systems with the remaining patent inferior vena cava. Under such circumstances, lumbar

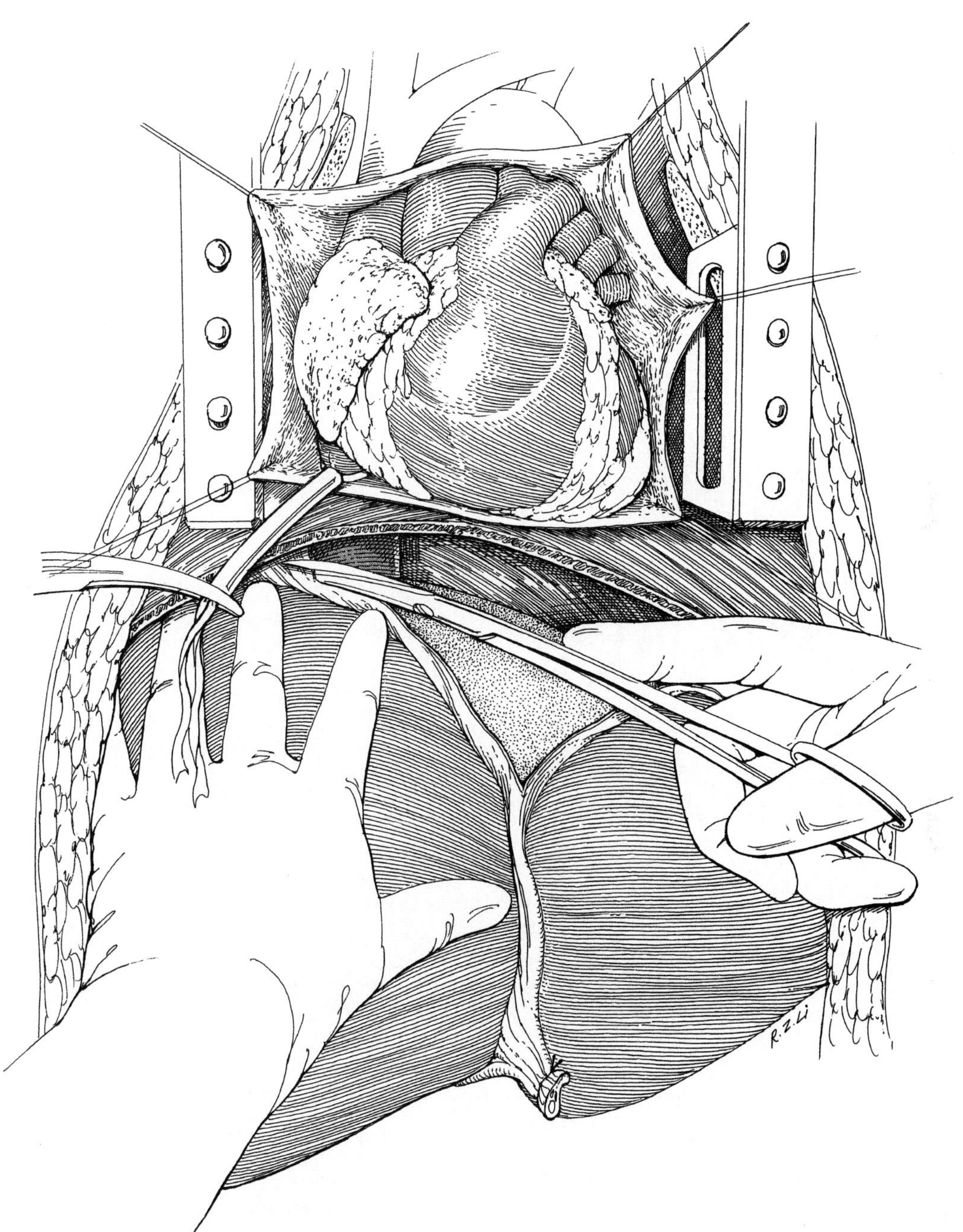

Fig. 8.15. Mobilization of the ligamentous attachments of the liver.

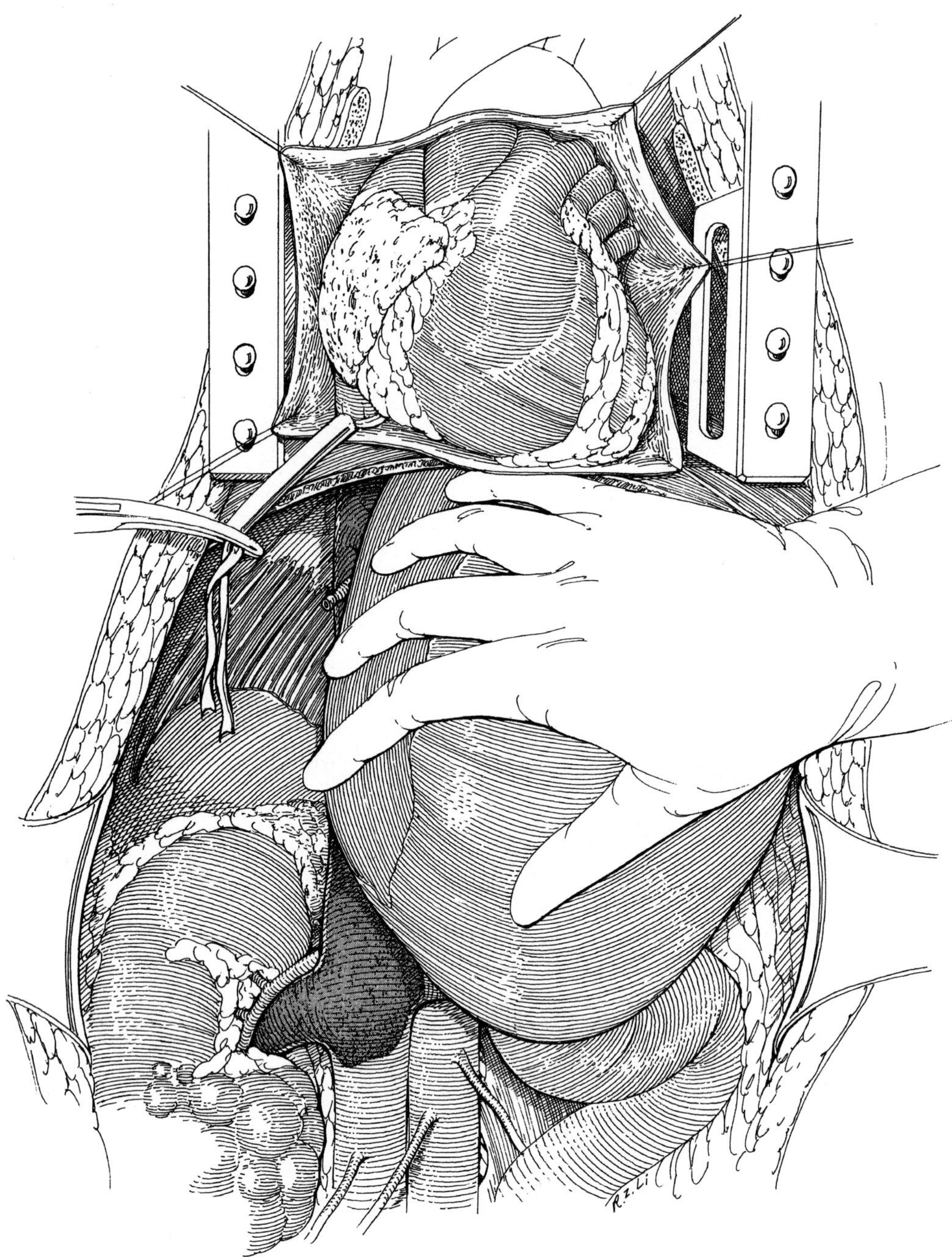

Fig. 8.16. Surgical exposure of the retrohepatic cava.

veins may approach the size of the external iliac veins and are best occluded with a Rummel tourniquet rather than sacrificed. The inferior vena cava is then further exposed, and a Rummel tourniquet is passed around the distal vena cava just above the bifurcation. Prior palpation will define the presence of distal bland thrombus and its extent. When a bland thrombus extends below the bifurcation of the vena cava into the iliac veins, it is necessary to gain venous control distal to the limits of the bland thrombus. A Rummel tourniquet is then placed around the left renal vein and left loosely in position (Fig. 8.17). If it

is unnecessary to cross-clamp the aorta, it is advisable to place a vascular tape around the left renal artery. This tape may be used to secure the renal artery in the event that collateral venous drainage (left adrenal and left gonadal) is inadequate to prevent venous engorgement of the left kidney when the main left renal vein is occluded.

It has been estimated that 25% of the inferior vena caval return is from the hepatic veins and, despite aortic cross-clamping, venous bleeding from the portal vascular bed via the hepatic veins will impair adequate visualization of the interior of

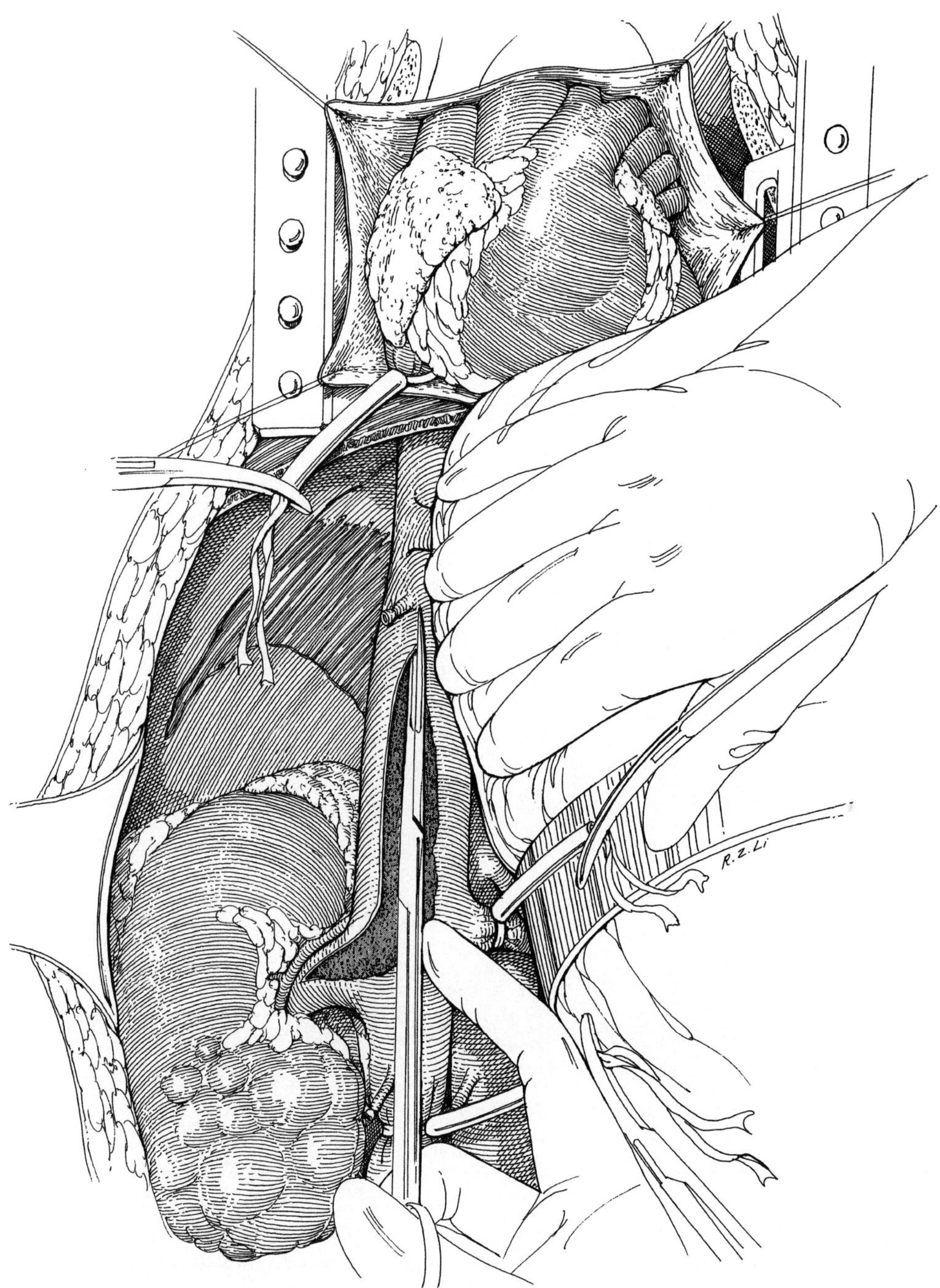

Fig. 8.17. Complete vascular isolation of the inferior vena cava and initiation of the cavotomy.

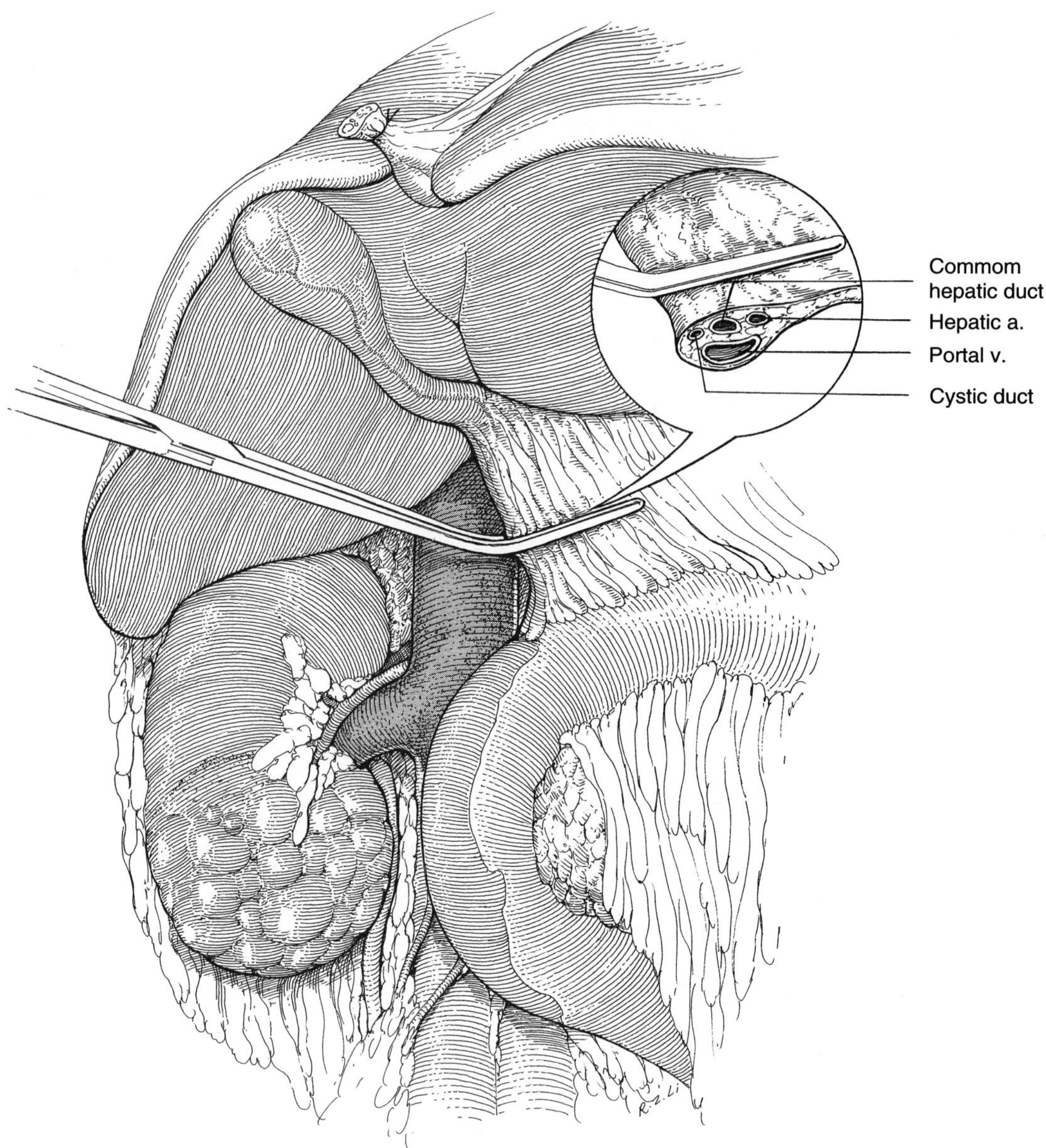

Fig. 8.18. Vascular control of the porta hepatis.

the vena cava at the time of thrombectomy (51). This can be significantly reduced by using Pringel's maneuver (cross-clamping the porta hepatis) (52). At the foramen of Winslow, the porta hepatis is easily defined between the index finger and thumb (Fig. 8.18). An alternative to cross-clamping the porta hepatis in its entirety is to dissect the vascular structures (portal vein and hepatic artery) and to secure these with vascular tapes. This method has a theoretical advantage of preventing crush injury to the common bile duct, but we consider it an unnecessary step. The aorta is then sufficiently exposed at the diaphragmatic hiatus above the celiac axis to permit occlusion with an aneurysm clamp under direct vision (Fig. 8.14).

Before vascular isolation of the inferior vena cava from the right atrium to the pelvis, it is advisable to administer 25 g of mannitol intravenously and to give a single dose of heparin.

This protects against renal and hepatic injury as well as thrombotic phenomena in the lower torso should circulatory arrest be prolonged due to extended cross-clamping. The patient is then placed in a 20° Trendelenburg position. The aorta is cross-clamped (Fig. 8.14). When the pulmonary wedge pressure increases to 15 mm Hg and systolic blood pressure is 120 mm Hg, the intrapericardial inferior vena cava is occluded (Fig. 8.17). Occlusion of the abdominal aorta and the intrapericardial inferior vena cava effectively divides the circulating blood volume in half. Attention to the systemic arterial and left ventricular filling pressures allows precise sequential clamping of the aorta and vena cava to avoid upper torso hypervolemia or hypovolemia. Venous return from the lower extremities constitutes a major source of blood loss at the time of cavotomy and is eliminated next by distal caval occlusion (Fig. 8.17). An atraumatic occlusive clamp is then applied to the porta hepatis (Fig. 8.18), and the remaining Rummel tourniquet on the left renal vein is occluded (Fig. 8.17).

The incision in the vena cava is initiated with a scimitar (no. 12 blade) and is continued with Pott-Smith scissors proximally to a level just below the hepatic veins (Fig. 8.17). A no. 20 Foley catheter with a 30-mL balloon is used for tumor thrombus extraction and is found to be less traumatic than a Fogarty catheter (48, 53). The catheter is advanced through the cavotomy until its tip can be palpated above the apex of the tumor thrombus within the pericardium. The tumor thrombus is usually delivered intact with gentle downward traction on the catheter and manual caval compression (Figs.

8.19 and 8.20). If the tumor thrombus cannot be delivered intact, it can be removed in a piecemeal manner. Montie et al. reported on the piecemeal removal of the tumor thrombus in 20 of 48 patients and noted no differences in survival (21).

Bleeding from the cavotomy results from the uncontrolled lumbar veins and blood remaining in the liver draining via the hepatic veins. Ordinary disposable suction allows for clear visualization of the inferior vena cava and thereby permits precise rapid removal of the thrombus. The tumor thrombus often adheres loosely to the intima of the vena cava, and actual mural invasion of the caval wall is a rare event (54). Kitner dissection of the thrombus from the intima of the cava may be necessary. In case the thrombus appears more densely adherent, insertion

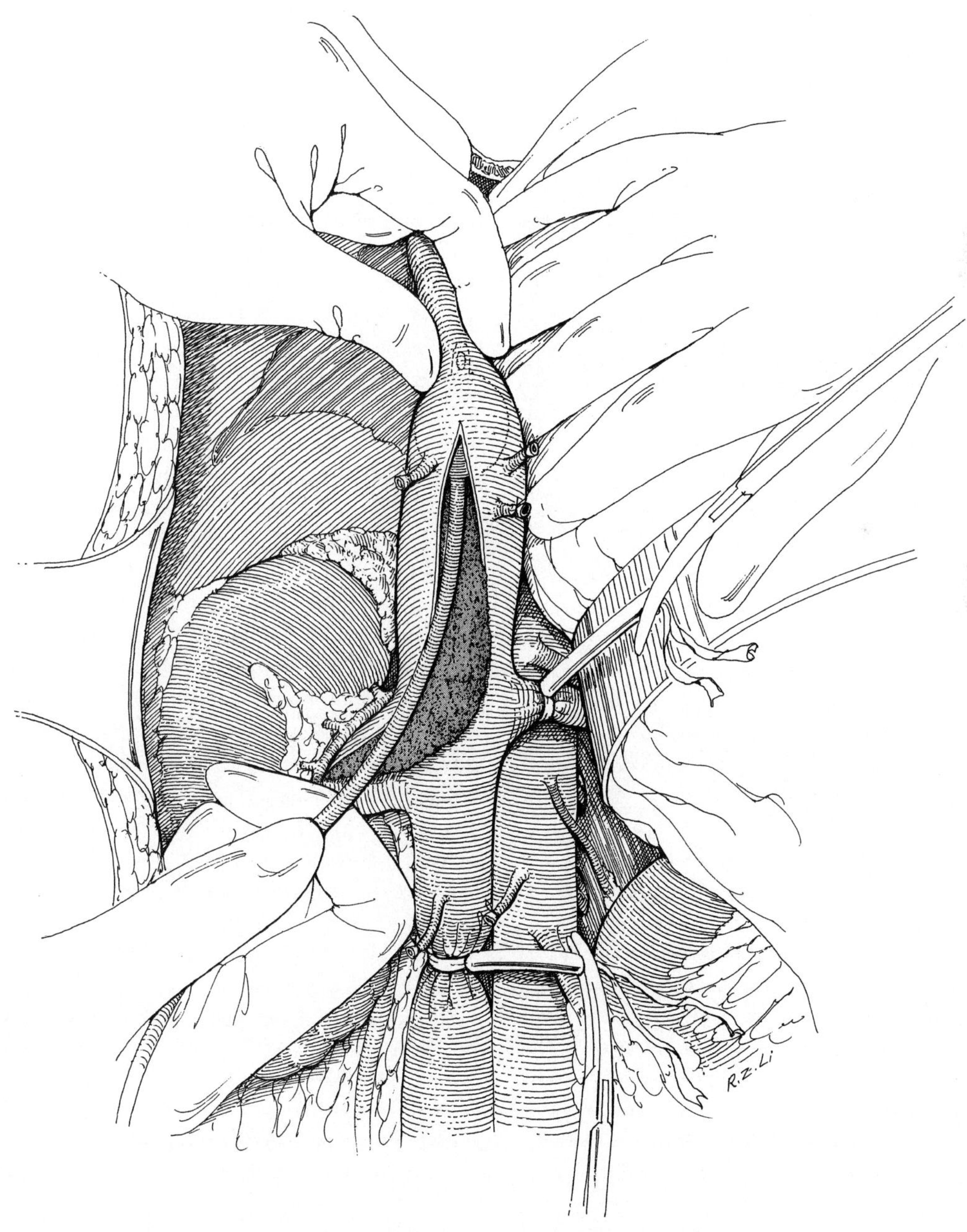

Fig. 8.19. Technique for extraction of a tumor thrombus from the inferior vena cava.

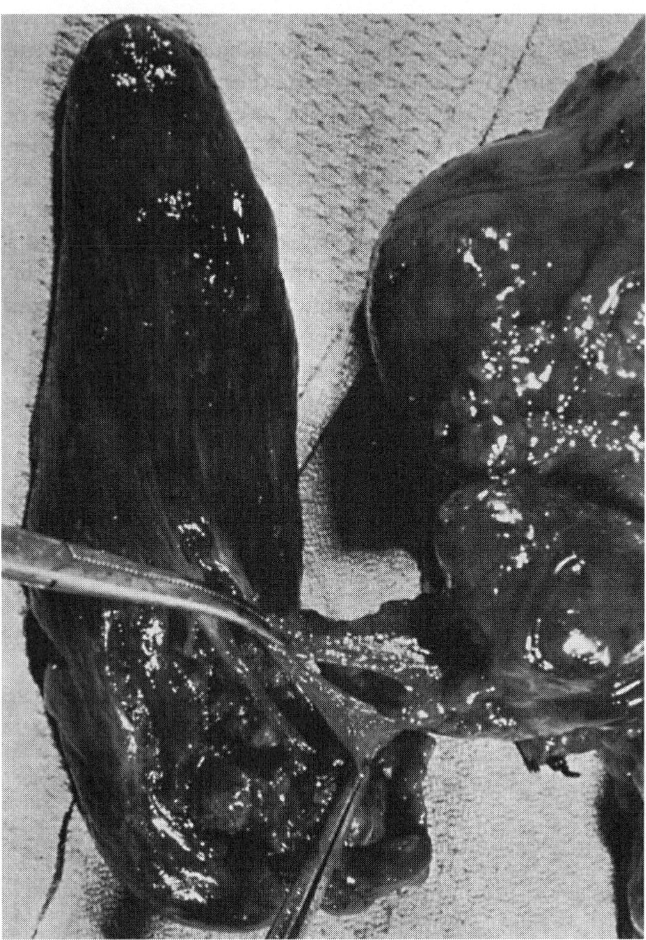

Fig. 8.20.   Extracted tumor thrombus.

of the index finger into the cavotomy below the hepatic veins enables most surgeons to reach the level of the right atrium and to free any attached thrombi fragments. The inferior vena cava is next flushed vigorously with sterile water. Rarely, we have used an endarterectomy curette to detach any visible "presumed tumor" remaining within the vena cava. However, on subsequent pathologic analysis, no viable tumor was detected in this material.

A Satinsky clamp is then placed across the cavotomy (Fig. 8.21). The remaining posterior wall of the renal vein is transected, and its proximal end is secured. The sequence of removal of the various vascular clamps is important to allow evacuation of air and debris before systemic circulation is restored and to avoid hypotension (Fig. 8.22). The left renal vein tourniquet is released first, followed by removal of the clamp on the porta hepatis. The Satinsky clamp is briefly vented, with the caval edges secured with Allis clamps to ensure adequate replacement of the clamp subsequent to the escape of trapped air. The position of the patient (20° Trendelenburg) protects against air embolization and promotes egress through the cavotomy as the isolated cava fills with blood. The aortic cross-clamp is then released, followed by the occlusive tourniquets at the distal and

proximal ends of the vena cava. The cavotomy is closed with a running suture of 5-0 polypropylene (Fig. 8.21).

Radical nephrectomy and regional lymphadenectomy are then performed. In patients with significant collateral circulation via the azygos and phrenic veins, care must be taken during mobilization of the posterior and subphrenic portions of the kidney. Accessory venous tributaries from the involved kidney frequently communicate with this venous network and may be transected. After delivery of the kidney, the renal bed should be carefully explored for venous bleeding. These veins in the retroperitoneum and beneath the diaphragm may bleed vigorously and are best secured with carefully placed figure-of-eight ligatures (Fig. 8.23).

IIA tumor thrombi should be approached in the same fashion because it is impossible, in adults, to gain proximal caval control above the hepatic veins extrapericardially (Fig. 8.24) (55).

Cross-clamping times have ranged from 14 to 30 minutes and have not been associated with hepatic or renal injury. Normothermic vascular isolation of the liver during hepatic resection is tolerated for up to 30 minutes (55, 56). If collateral venous return is sufficient to obviate cross-clamping the aorta, consideration must the prevention of venous engorgement of the normal kidney and viscera. When the left kidney is involved with tumor, it is best to secure the right renal artery with a vascular tape during the period of right renal venous occlusion (Fig. 8.25). Marshall et al. reported a case in which renal failure lasted for 24 days after occlusion of the left renal vein for only 30 minutes (4). Other authors have advocated the occlusion of the superior mesenteric artery at the time of venous occlusion of the porta hepatis (Pringel's maneuver) to prevent vascular engorgement of the bowel (52). This technique is appropriate when the aorta is not cross-clamped.

Rarely, thrombus extension into the hepatic veins has occurred with an associated Budd-Chiari syndrome. The normal venous effluent from the hepatic veins probably accounts for the rarity of this event. However, should intraluminal extension into the hepatic veins pose difficulty in complete extirpation of the tumor thrombus, the occlusive clamp on the porta hepatis should be released. Venous hemorrhage with this maneuver is brisk and should aid in the removal of residual intraluminal tumor thrombi within the hepatic veins. Using a dental mirror to aid in visualization has permitted the successful use of an endarterectomy curette.

Alternative Techniques for IB and IIA Extension

In elderly patients and in patients with recognized atherosclerosis of the aorta, it may be inappropriate to cross-clamp the aorta. It has been our recent policy to routinely include a member from the cardiac surgery department on our operative team. The midline abdominal incision with median sternotomy is used. When the intrapericardial inferior vena cava is occluded,

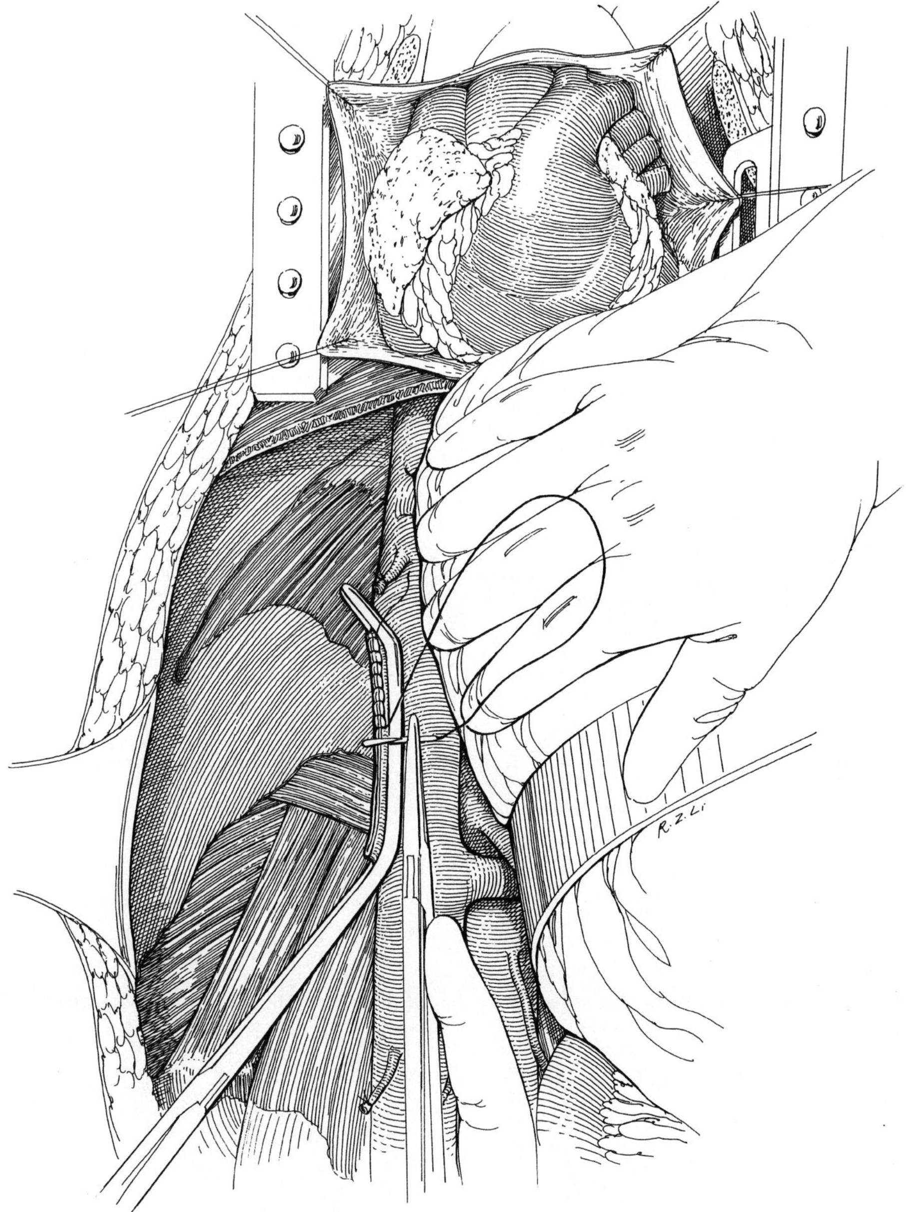

Fig. 8.21.   Vena caval closure.

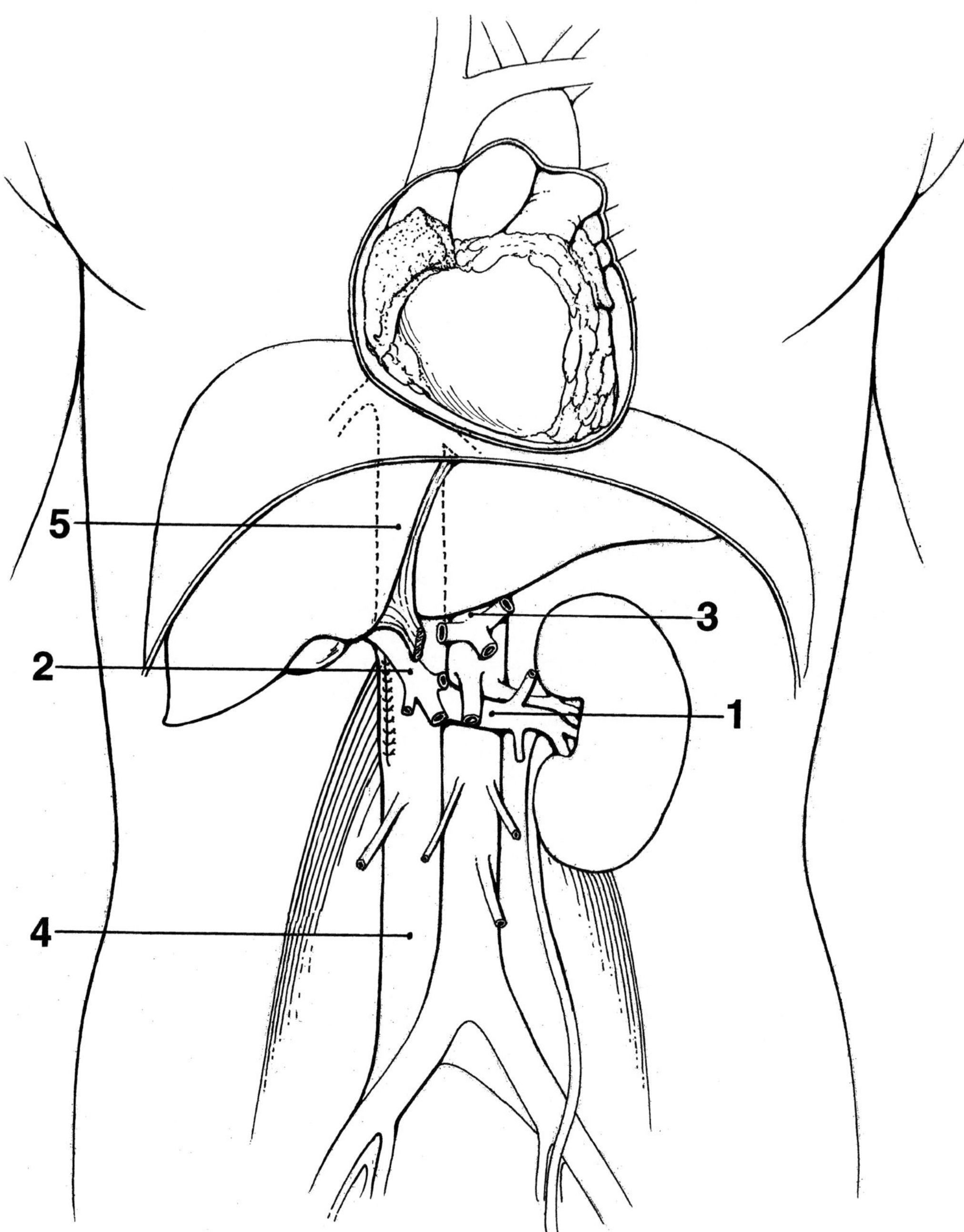

Fig. 8.22. Sequence of vascular restoration for Type IB and IIA tumor thrombi. I: Left renal vein; 2: porta hepatis; 3: aorta; 4: distal IVC; 5: proximal IVC.

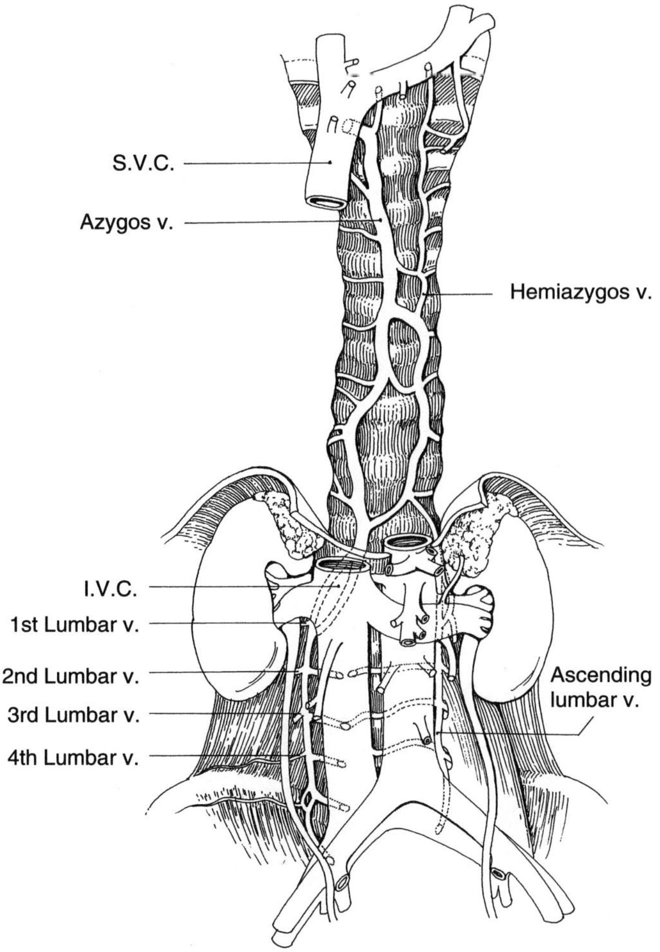

Fig. 8.23. Retroperitoneal anatomy of the venous system.

the patient is observed to determine if collateral venous return will provide an adequate cardiac output. In the event that cardiac output fails and systemic blood pressure drops, a cardiac bypass is performed. The systemic administration of heparin required for such a procedure contributes significantly to the ultimate blood loss but is unavoidable. Those aspects previously described in detail for the management of IB tumor thrombi (other than aortic cross-clamping) are followed. Important variations include distal caval control before initiating bypass and consideration of occlusion of the superior mesenteric artery. The first is necessary because one component of cardiac bypass includes cannulation of the iliac veins. When bypass is initiated, the risk of retrograde tumor flow is real. The second prevents vascular congestion of the bowel during the period of portal venous occlusion.

In the event that the required cavotomy is of such length to preclude occlusion with a Satinsky clamp, it may be sewn from cephalad to caudad after flushing. Before final caval closure is completed, an occlusive clamp is placed, caval inflow is restored, and the cava is vented.

INFRADIAPHRAGMATIC-INFRAHEPATIC (IIB) EXTENSION

Incision

We prefer a thoracoabdominal incision for intraluminal caval thrombi extension at this level. The intraluminal caval extension here is less apt to obstruct the vena cava, and in this clinical situation the vena cava may be controlled below the hepatic veins. Venous return via the hepatic veins is estimated to represent 25% of the total inferior vena caval cardiac return and is sufficient to sustain adequate cardiac output in most patients (51). With significant hypotension, the aorta may be cross-clamped.

Technique

The sequence of vascular control for this level of involvement is illustrated in Figure 8.26. When proximal caval exposure is inadequate to permit its occlusion by placement of a vascular tourniquet, the liver is best mobilized as previously described. Interruption of the lumbar veins reduces blood loss and improves visualization at the time of cavotomy. Alternatively, a vena cava clip may be placed just above the tumor thrombus. However, because the approach prevents only gross embolization of tumor thrombi, we prefer the former approach.

The sequence of vascular control for right-sided tumors is as follows:

1. Right renal artery,
2. Subhepatic vena cava,
3. Distal vena cava above the bifurcation, and
4. Left renal vein.

If collateral venous drainage of the left kidney is not sufficient to prevent venous engorgement, the left renal artery may be secured with the previously placed vascular tape. Cavotomy and thrombus extension are carried out as previously described.

Cavectomy has been advocated by certain authors and can be safely performed (50). For right renal tumors, this procedure can be performed without significantly jeopardizing the remaining left kidney, but cavectomy for left renal tumors requires management of the venous drainage from the right kidney. An end-to-side renal portal vein anastomosis has been successfully used (50). Cavectomy should rarely be used because of the rarity with which direct caval invasion occurs. Furthermore, in those cases in which caval invasion has been documented, the dismal survival rates have not been improved with cavectomy (50).

SUPRADIAPHRAGMATIC-INTRACARDIAC (IA) EXTENSION (FIG. 8.27)

Tumor thrombi that have reached this level require cardiopulmonary bypass with, alternatively, hypothermia and cardiac arrest. When the right atrial extension is modest, it is reasonable to displace the tumor apex manually into the intrapericar-

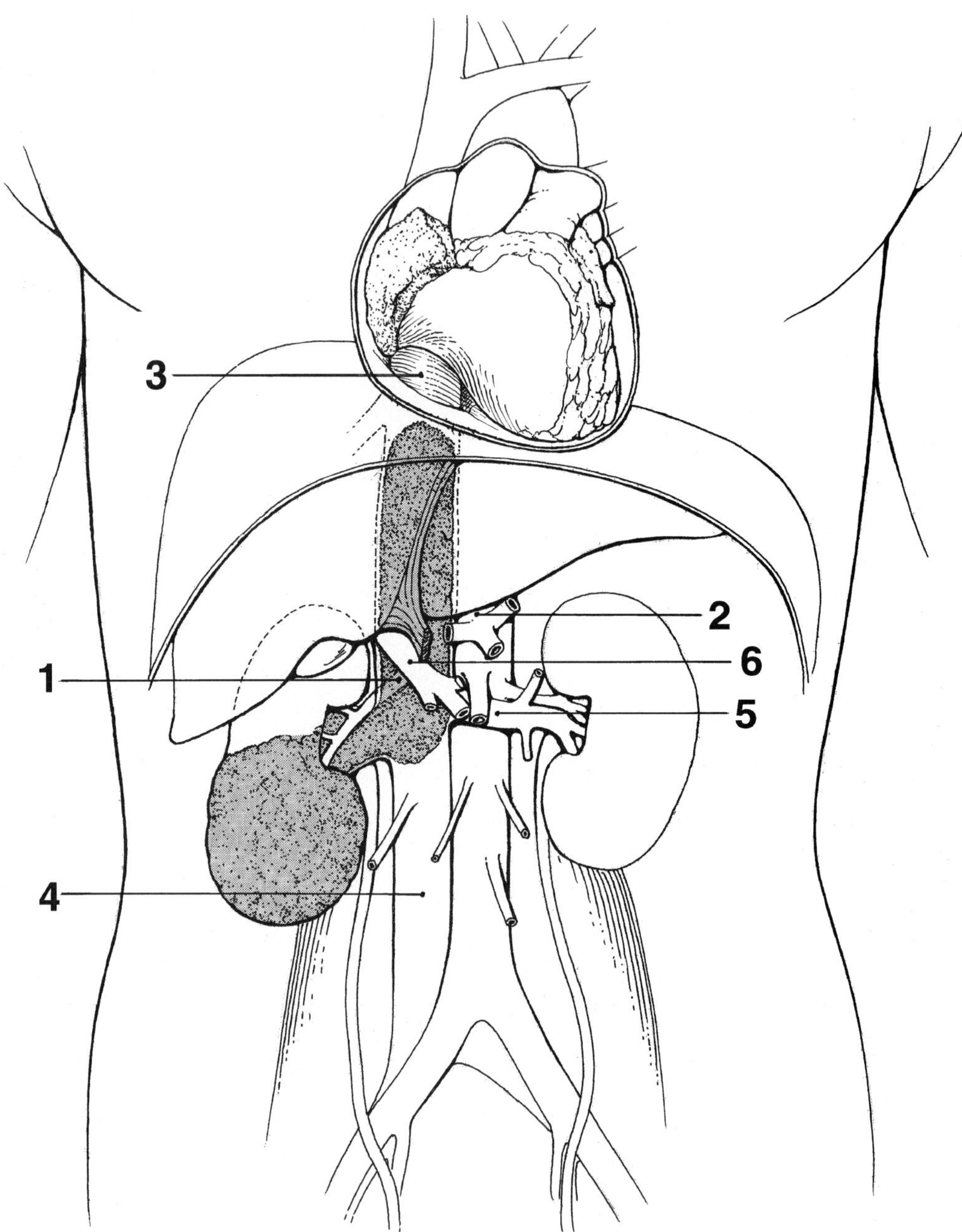

Fig. 8.24.   Sequence of vascular interruption for IIA tumor thrombus. 1: Right renal artery; 2: proximal aorta; 3: proximal IVC; 4: distal IVC; 5: left renal vein; 6: porta hepatis.

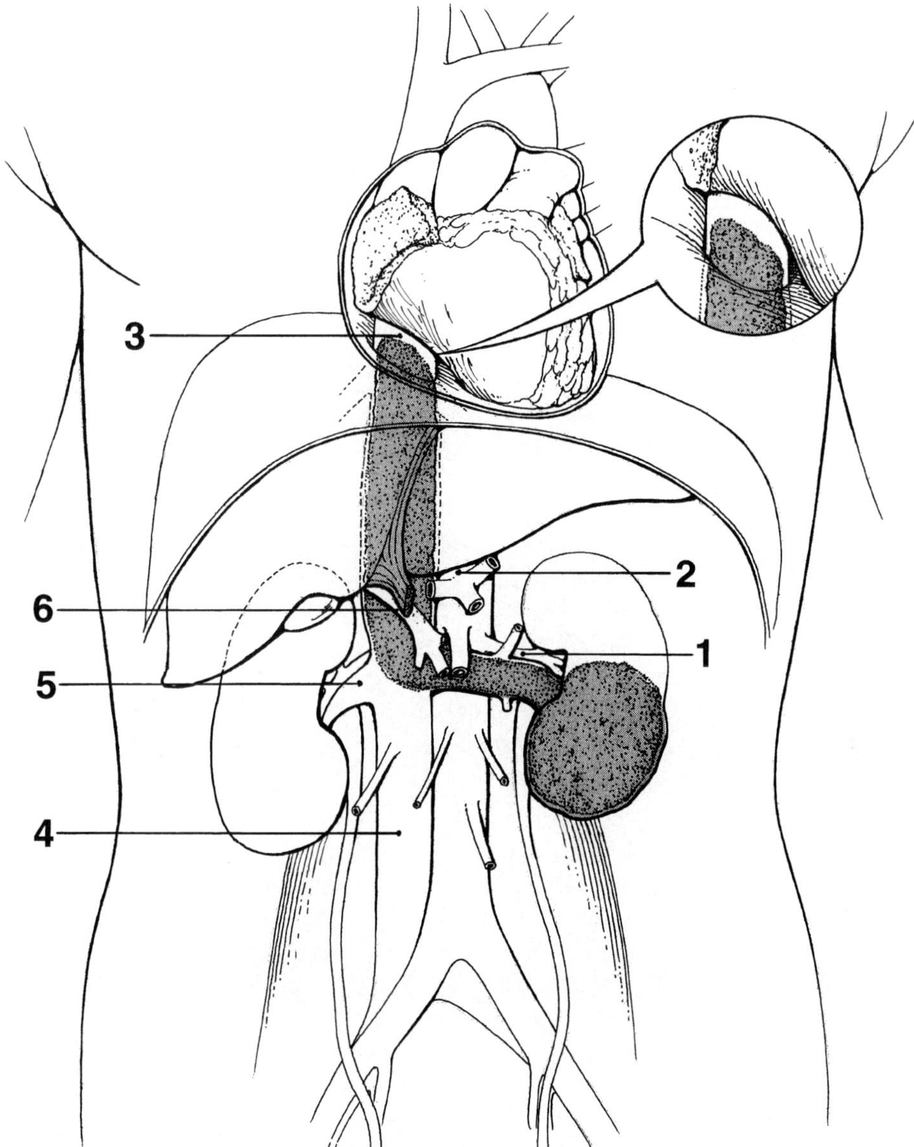

Fig. 8.25. Sequence of vascular interruption for IB left renal tumor thrombus. 1: Left renal artery; 2: proximal aorta; 3: proximal IVC; 4: distal IVC; 5: right renal vein; 6: porta hepatis.

dial inferior vena cava or to provide occlusion above this level. In such circumstances, the remainder of the procedure is performed as previously described with cardiac bypass.

In the event that cardiac extension is significant, the heart is opened and the tumor is extracted (Fig. 8.28). Such patients initially undergo bypass with the skull packed in ice. Core body temperature is reduced to 19.5°C, and the circulation is arrested. The operation is then performed as indicated in a bloodless field. After closure of the atriotomy and vena cavotomy, cardiopulmonary bypass circulation is reinstituted and the heart is defibrillated when core temperature is warmed to 36°C.

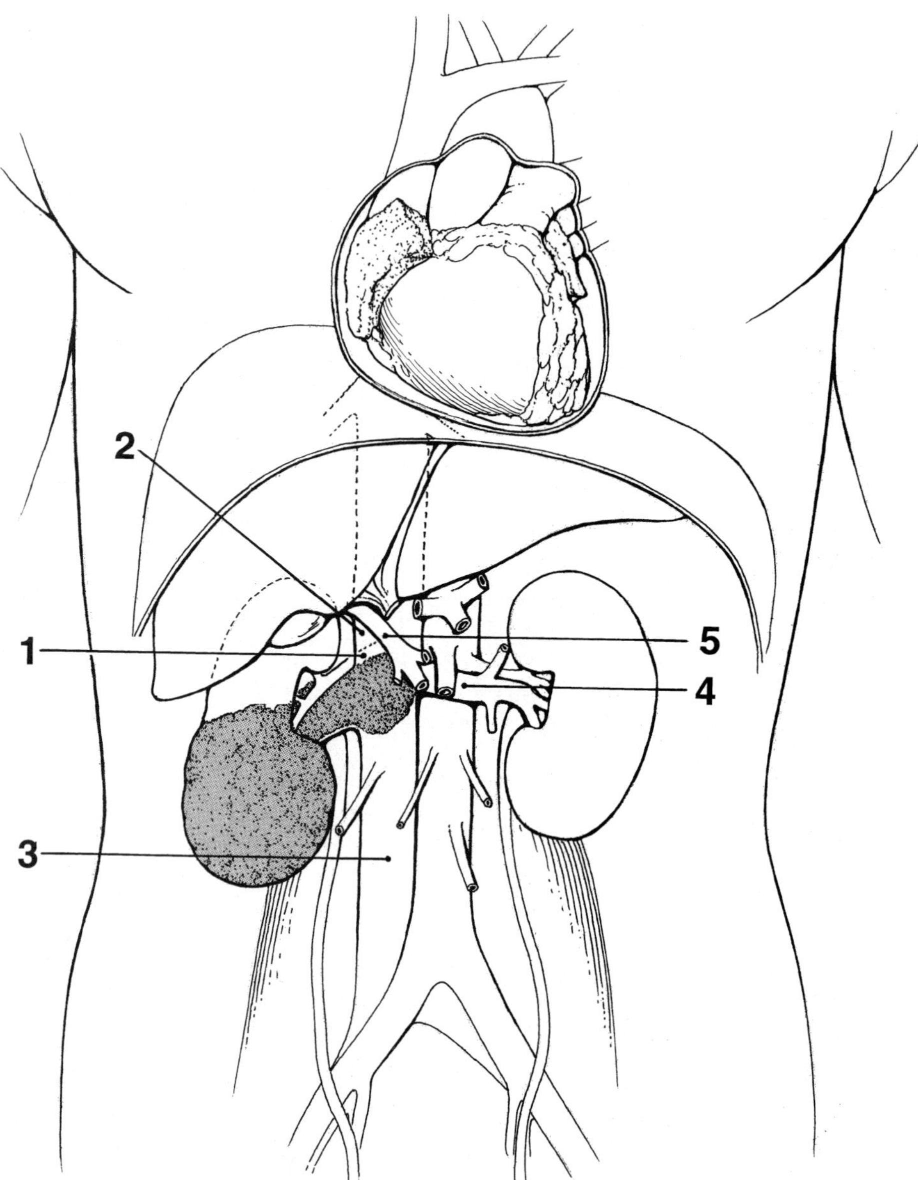

Fig. 8.26. Sequence of vascular interruption for an IIB tumor thrombus. 1: Right renal artery; 2: proximal IVC; 3: distal IVC; 4: left renal vein: 5: porta hepatis.

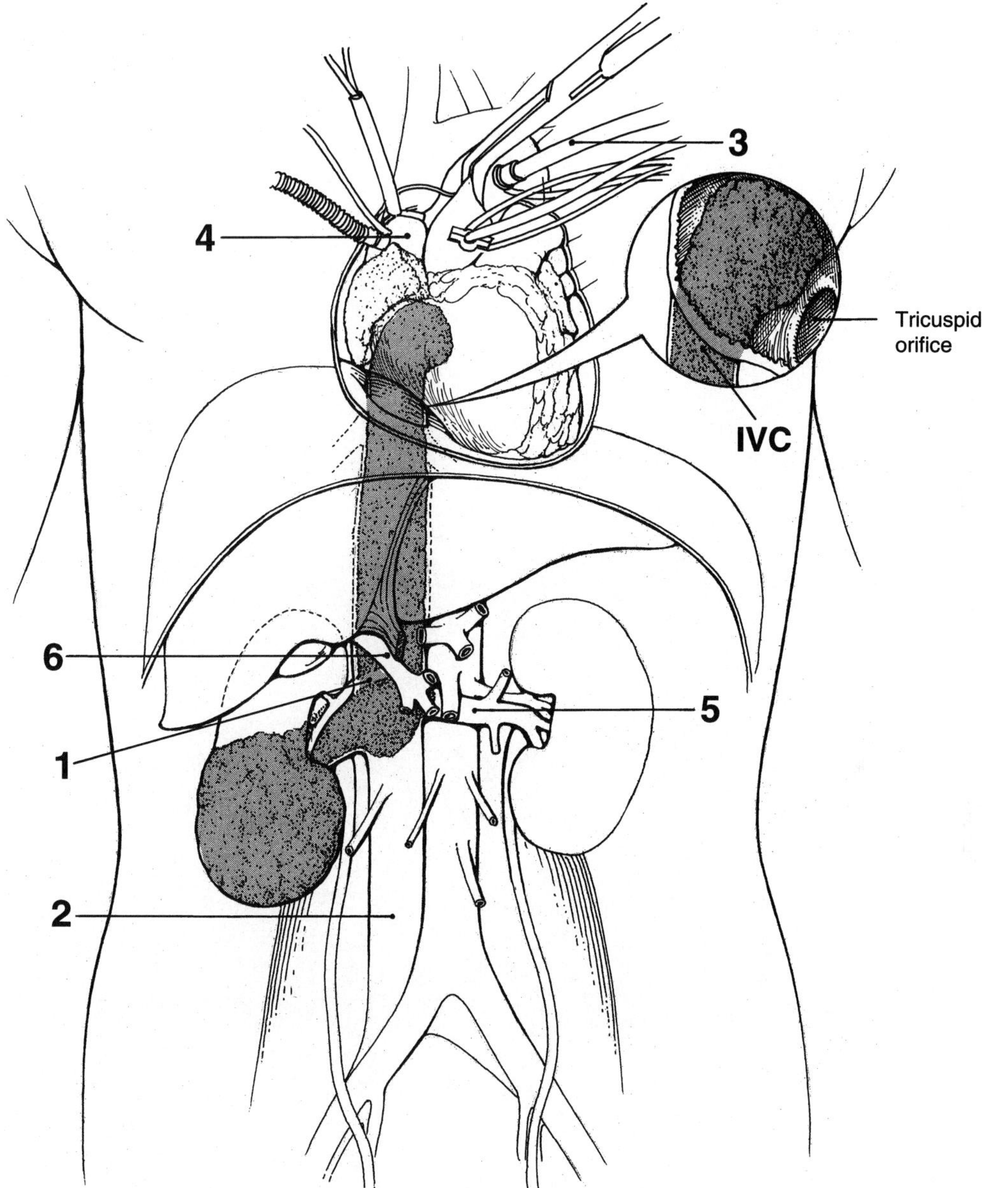

Fig. 8.27.   Sequence of vascular interruption for IA right renal tumor thrombus. 1: Right renal artery; 2: distal IVC; 3: cardiopulmonary bypass; 4: proximal IVC; 5: left renal vein; 6: porta hepatis.

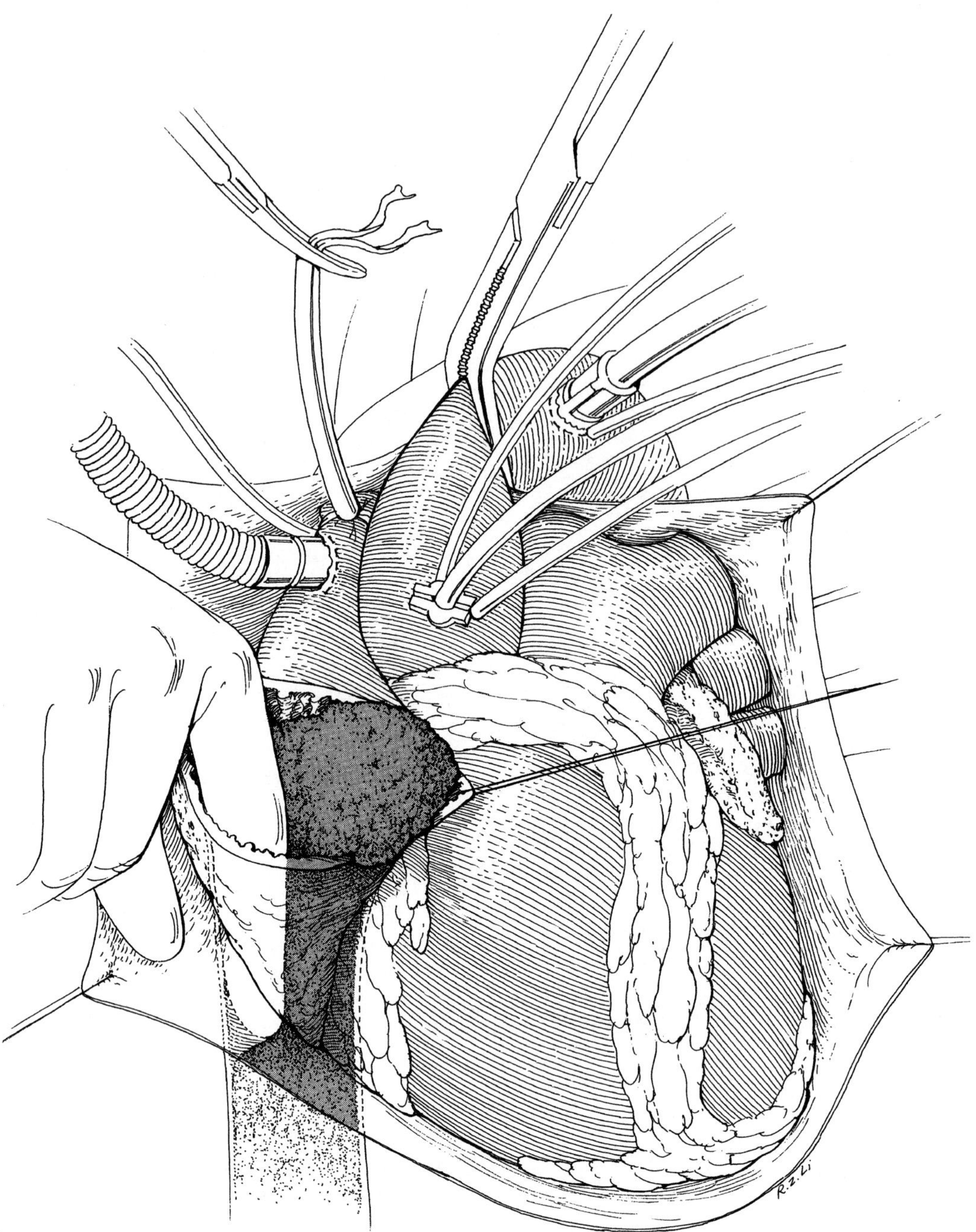

Fig. 8.28. Atriotomy and manual dissection of tumor thrombus.

CONCLUSION

Current surgical techniques have made extirpation of intraluminal caval extension from RCC relatively safe. Because of the variability in vascularization of the tumor thrombi, a neat extraction as depicted in Figure 8.20 is not always possible. Tumor thrombi that have lost their vascular supply vary in appearance from gritty yellow and friable to necrotic curd. The intraluminal tumor extraction in these situations is technically more difficult, time-consuming, and often performed piecemeal.

In those cases in which the girth of the extrahepatic vena cava has been dramatically increased, we have excised an appropriate longitudinal strip of caval wall, performing "cavaplasty" at the time of caval closure.

When resection of the intraluminal extension is complete and performed as outlined without dissemination, prognosis depends on known factors related to tumor extension and nodal involvement. The procedure is not warranted in patients with gross nodal disease or known metastatic disease.

REFERENCES

1. Guinan PD, Vogelzang NJ, Fremgen AM, et al. Renal cell carcinoma: tumor size, stage and survival. J Urol 1995;153:901.
2. Angervall L, Carlstrom E, Wailqvist L, et al. Effects of clinical and morphological variables on spread of renal carcinoma in an operative series. Scand J Urol Nephrol 1969;3:124.
3. Robson CL, Churchill BN, Anderson W. The results of radical nephrectomy for renal cell carcinoma. J Urol 1969;101:297.
4. Marshall VF, Middleton RD, Hallsway GR, et al. Surgery for renal cell carcinoma in the vena cava. J Urol 1970;103:414.
5. Svine S. Tumor thrombus of the inferior vena cava resulting from renal cell carcinoma. Scand J Urol Nephrol 1969;3:245.
6. Nis C. Thrombosis of the inferior vena cava associated with malignant renal tumors. J Urol 1946;55:583.
7. Kaufman JJ, Burke DE, Goodwin WE. Abdominal venography in urological disease. J Urol 1956;75:160.
8. Clayman RV, Gonzalez R, Fraley, EE. Renal cell cancer invading the inferior vena cava: clinical review and anatomical approach. J Urol 1980;123:157.
9. Riches EW, Griffiths IH, Thackray AC. New growths of the kidney and ureter. Br J Urol 1951;23:297.
10. Myers GH, Fehrenbaker IG, Kelalis PP. Prognostic significance of renal vein invasion by hypernephroma. J Urol 1968;100:420.
11. Skinner DG, Peister RF, Colvin R. Extension of renal cell carcinoma into the vena cava: the rationale for aggressive surgical management. J Urol 1972;107:711.
12. Vaislic CD, Puel P, Grondon P, et al. Cancer of the kidney invading the vena cava and heart. J Thorac Cardiovasc Surg 1986;91:604.
13. Neves RJ, Zincke H. Surgical treatment of renal cancer with vena cava extension. Br J Urol 1987;59:390.
14. Hatcher PA, Anderson EE, Paulson DF, et al. Surgical management and prognosis of renal cell carcinoma invading the vena cava. J Urol 1991;145:20.
15. Swierzewski DJ, Swierzewski MJ, Libertino JA. Radical nephrectomy in patients with renal cell carcinoma with venous, vena caval and atrial extension. Am J Surg 1994;168:205.
16. Suggs WD, Smith RB, Dodson TF, et al. Renal cell carcinoma with inferior vena caval involvement. J Vasc Surg 1991;14:413.
17. Cherrie RJ, Goldman DG, Lindner A, et al. Prognostic implications of vena caval extension of renal cell carcinoma. J Urol 1982;128:910.
18. Steinberg GD, Reitz BA, Marshall FF. Surgical treatment of renal cell carcinoma with extension into the vena cava. World J Urol 1991;9:193.
19. Belis JA, Kandzari SJ. Five-year survival following excision of renal cell carcinoma extension into inferior vena cava. Urology 1990;35:228.
20. Sosa RE, Muecke EC, Vaughan ED, et al. Renal cell carcinoma extension into the inferior vena cava: the prognostic significance of the level of vena caval involvement. J Urol 1984;132:1097.
21. Montie JE, Pontes JE, Novick AC, et al. Resection of inferior vena cava tumor thrombi from renal cell carcinoma. Am Surg 1991;57:56.
22. Skinner DG, Vermillion CD, Colvin RB. The surgical management of renal cell carcinoma. J Urol 1972;107:705.
23. Novick AC, Kaye MC, Cosgrove DM, et al. Experience with cardiopulmonary bypass and deep hypothermic circulatory arrest in the management of retroperitoneal tumors with large vena caval thrombi. Ann Surg 1990;212:472.
24. Schefft P, Novick AC, Straffon RA, et al. Surgery for renal cell carcinoma extending into the inferior vena cava. J Urol 1977;120:28.
25. Skinner DG, Pritchett TR, Lieskovsky G, et al. Vena caval involvement by renal cell carcinoma. Ann Surg 1989;210:387.
26. Klein EA, Kaye MC, Novick AC. Management of renal cell carcinoma with vena caval thrombi via cardiopulmonary bypass and deep hypothermic circulatory arrest. Urol Clin North Am 1991;18:445.
27. Glazer AA, Novick AC. Long term follow-up after surgical treatment for renal cell carcinoma extending into the right atrium. J Urol 1995;153:314A.
28. Marks WN, Korobkin M, Callen PW, et al. CT diagnosis of tumor thrombus of the renal vein and inferior vena cava. AJR 1978;131:843.
29. Zeman RK, Cronan JJ, Rosenfield AT, et al. Renal cell carcinoma: dynamic thin-section CT assessment of vascular invasion and tumor vascularity. Radiology 1985;167:393.
30. Kaliman DA, King BF, Hattery RR, et al. Renal vein and inferior vena cava tumor thrombus in renal cell carcinoma: CT, US, MRI, and venacavography. J Comput Assist Tomogr 1992;16:240.
31. Horan JJ, Robertson CN, Choyke PL, et al. The detection of renal carcinoma extension into the renal vein and inferior vena cava: a prospective comparison of venacavography and magnetic resource imaging. J Urol 1989;142:943.
32. Pritchett TR, Raval JK, Benson RC, et al. Preoperative magnetic resonance imaging of vena caval tumor thrombi: experience with 5 cases. J Urol 1987;138:1220.
33. Amendola MA, King LR, Pollack HM, et al. Staging of renal carcinoma using magnetic resonance imaging at 1.5 tesla. Cancer 1990;66:40.
34. Goldfarb DA, Novick AC, Lorig R, et al. Magnetic resonance imaging for assessment of vena caval tumor thrombi: a comparative study with venacavography and computerized tomography scanning. J Urol 1990;144:1100.
35. Roubidoux MA, Dunnick NR, Sostman HD, et al. Renal carcinoma: detection of venous extension with gradient-echo MRImaging. Radiology 1992;182:269.
36. Bradley WF. When should GRASS be used? Radiology 1988;169:574.
37. Haase A, et al. FLASH imaging: rapid NMR imaging using low flip angle pulses. J Magn Reson Imaging 1986;67:258.
38. Hockley NM, Foster RS, Bihrle R, et al. Use of magnetic resonance imaging to determine surgical approach to renal cell carcinoma with caval extension. Urology 1990;36:55.
39. Myneni L, Hricak H, Carroll PR. Magnetic resonance imaging of renal carcinoma with extension into the vena cava: staging accuracy and recent advances. Br J Urol 1991;68:571.
40. Straton CS, Libertino JA, Larsen CR. Is magnetic resonance

imaging alone accurate enough in staging renal cell carcinoma. Urology 1992;40:351.

41. Schwerk WB, Schwerk WN, Rodeck G. Venous renal tumor extension: a prospective US evaluation. Radiology 1985;156:491.

42. McGahan JP, Blake LC, White R, et al. Color flow sonographic mapping of intravascular extension of malignant renal tumors. J Ultrasound Med 1993;12:403.

43. Harris DD, Ruckle HC, Gaskill DM, et al. Intraoperative ultrasound: determination of the presence and extent of vena caval tumor thrombus. Urology 1994;44:189.

44. Treiger BFG, Humphrey LS, Peterson CV, et al. Transesophageal echocardiography in renal cell carcinoma: an accurate diagnostic technique for intracaval neoplastic extension. J Urol 1991;145:1138.

45. Allen G, Klingman R, Ferraris VA, et al. Transesophageal echocardiography in the surgical management of renal cell carcinoma with intracardiac extension. J Cardiovasc Surg 1991;32:833.

46. Hasnain JU, Watson RJN. Transesophageal echocardiography during resection of renal cell carcinoma involving the inferior vena cava. South Med J 1994;87:273.

47. Pritchett TR, Lieskovsky G, Skinner DG. Extension of renal cell carcinoma into the vena cava: clinical review and surgical approach. J Urol 1986;135:460.

48. Cummings KB, Li Wei, Ryan JA, et al. Intraoperative management of renal cell carcinoma with supradiaphragmatic caval extension. J Urol 1979;122:829.

49. Goodwin WE. Ileal ureter. In: Cooper P, ed. The craft of surgery. Boston: Little, Brown & Co., 1971.

50. McCullough DL, Gittes RF. Vena cava resection for renal cell carcinoma. J Urol 1974;112:162.

51. Leiter E. Inferior vena caval thrombosis in malignant renal tumors. JAMA 1966;198:1167.

52. Pringel JH. Notes on the arrest of hepatic hemorrhage due to trauma. Ann Surg 1908;48:541.

53. Freed SZ, Gurdman NR. The removal of renal cell carcinoma thrombus extending into the right atrium. J Urol 1975;113:163.

54. Skinner DG, deKernion JB. Clinical manifestations and treatment of renal parenchymal tumors. In: Skinner DG, deKernion JB, eds. Genitourinary cancer. Philadelphia: WB Saunders, 1978.

55. Heaney JP, et al. An improved technique for vascular isolation of the liver: experimental study and case reports. Ann Surg 1966;163:237.

56. Albo D Jr, Christianson C, Rasmussen BL. Massive liver trauma involving the suprarenal vena cava. Am J Surg 1969;118:1960.

IV

RENAL PELVIS AND URETER

9

Primary Carcinoma of the Upper Urinary Urothelium

An Overview

John D. Seigne and H. Barton Grossman

INTRODUCTION

Primary carcinomas of the renal pelvis and ureter are unusual neoplasms that account for 5 to 6% of all urothelial tumors. Renal pelvic tumors comprise between 5 and 10% of all renal tumors and are 3 to 4 times more common than ureteral tumors (1, 2). The classification used by the National Center for Health Statistics includes renal pelvic tumors with all other tumors of the kidney. Therefore, specific epidemiologic data on renal pelvic tumors are difficult to obtain. Ureteral tumors are classified separately, resulting in more reliable data regarding this site. In the 1987 statistical review, ureteral tumors were twice as common in men compared with women. The peak incidence occurred in white men in their sixties (10 cases per 100,000 population per year (3)).

ETIOLOGY

The renal pelvis, ureter, and bladder have a similar embryologic origin and are all lined by transitional cell epithelium. Because the entire urothelium is bathed in the same urinary carcinogens, upper tract tumors share many common etiologic factors with their more frequent bladder counterparts.

The most important etiologic agent in the development of transitional cell carcinoma is tobacco smoke. In the United States, it is estimated that cigarette smoking causes 70% of upper tract tumors in men and 40% in women (4). A dose-response relationship has been documented, with heavier smokers being at higher risk than the average smoker. The dose-response relationship appears to be steeper for upper tract tumors than bladder tumors, with heavy smokers having a 2.5 times greater risk of upper tract tumor development than bladder tumor development (5).

An increased risk of bladder cancer in textile workers ex-posed to synthetic dyes was first noted by Rehn in 1895. Subsequently, Heuper et al. showed that bladder cancer developed in dogs after oral ingestion of betanaphthylamine, thereby demonstrating that arylamines were the carcinogens causing bladder cancer in the DuPont dye workers (6). Occupational exposure to arylamines, especially betanaphthylamine and benzidine, has been associated with a 20-fold increased risk of bladder cancer development (7, 8). The risk of upper tract tumor development is also increased, but to a lesser extent, after occupational exposure to these carcinogens. Workers in the textile, dye, rubber, plastic, tanning, and printing industries appear to be at increased risk (9).

The heavy use of nonsteroidal analgesics, especially those containing phenacetin, reportedly leads to a twofold to fourfold greater risk of upper tract tumor development. The reason for this increased risk is unknown (10). It has been postulated that the orthoaminophenol metabolites of phenacetin are carcinogenic to the urothelium because these metabolites have some structural similarity to the known industrial carcinogen betanaphthylamine (11). However, a recent report analyzing p53 gene mutations in a series of phenacetin-induced tumors found a spectrum of mutations rather than the specific type of mutations that would be suggestive of carcinogen-induced DNA damage (12).

An increased incidence of papillary carcinomas of the renal pelvis has been reported in association with Balkan nephropathy. Balkan nephropathy is a form of chronic interstitial nephritis that is found in certain areas of Bulgaria, Romania, and Serbia. All affected geographic areas lie within the central Danube basin. The cause of Balkan nephropathy is unknown but thought to be an environmental toxin. Renal pelvic tumors comprise 40% of all renal malignancies in the endemic regions, and bilateral tumors occur in approximately 10% of the affected patients (13).

Upper tract urothelial tumors have also been associated with a history of cyclophosphamide therapy (14). Chronic infection or chronic irritation from stone disease has been associated with the development of tumors of the squamous cell type (15). Historically, several cases of renal pelvic carcinoma have been reported after retrograde pyelography using Thorotrast (16).

LOCATION AND DISSEMINATION

Urothelial tumors develop 3 to 4 times more often in the renal pelvis than in the ureter. Of ureteral tumors, 75% occur in the distal ureter, 20% in the midureter, and 5% in the upper ureter (17). Bilateral upper tract tumors are rare, occurring synchronously in 1.5 to 2% of cases and metachronously in 6 to 8% of cases. In patients with primary carcinoma of the bladder, subsequent upper tract tumor formation is uncommon, with an incidence of 3% or less (18). The reverse is not the case; bladder tumors occur in 30 to 50% of patients after treatment of a prior upper tract tumor (1, 19). Classically, the subsequent bladder tumors form close to the ureteral orifice on the side in which the primary upper tract tumor developed. The high incidence and the pattern of subsequent bladder tumor formation, combined with the low incidence of contralateral tumor growth, support the theory that tumor cells disseminate by way of the urine. Further support for this dissemination theory is provided by experimental animal models of tumor implantation (20) and by molecular analysis of synchronous and metachronous tumors (21). An alternative theory holds that tumor multifocality can be explained by an epithelial field defect that affects the entire urothelium. In support of this theory are the occurrence of contralateral tumors, the fact that metachronous tumors may form many years after definitive treatment of the primary tumor (these two findings, although infrequent, are difficult to explain in the urinary dissemination theory), and the common findings of separate areas of carcinoma and carcinoma in situ in the same cystectomy specimens. In all likelihood, a combination of both of these mechanisms explains subsequent multifocal tumor formation after definitive treatment of an upper tract tumor.

High-grade ureteral tumors have an increased propensity to invade the muscular wall of the ureter and its surrounding structures. High-grade renal pelvic tumors are more likely to invade the renal parenchyma than adjacent organs (22). The lymphatics of the kidney and ureter drain to the paracaval, para-aortic, and pelvic nodes. The degree of lymph node involvement depends on the grade, stage, and site of the primary tumor (23). Upper tract tumors may invade the renal hilum and involve the renal vein in a similar fashion to renal cell carcinoma (24). The most common sites for hematogenous metastases are the liver, bone, and lung (25).

PATHOLOGY

Most upper tract tumors are papillary. Tumors may be single or multiple (Fig. 9.1). In some patients, the tumors give rise

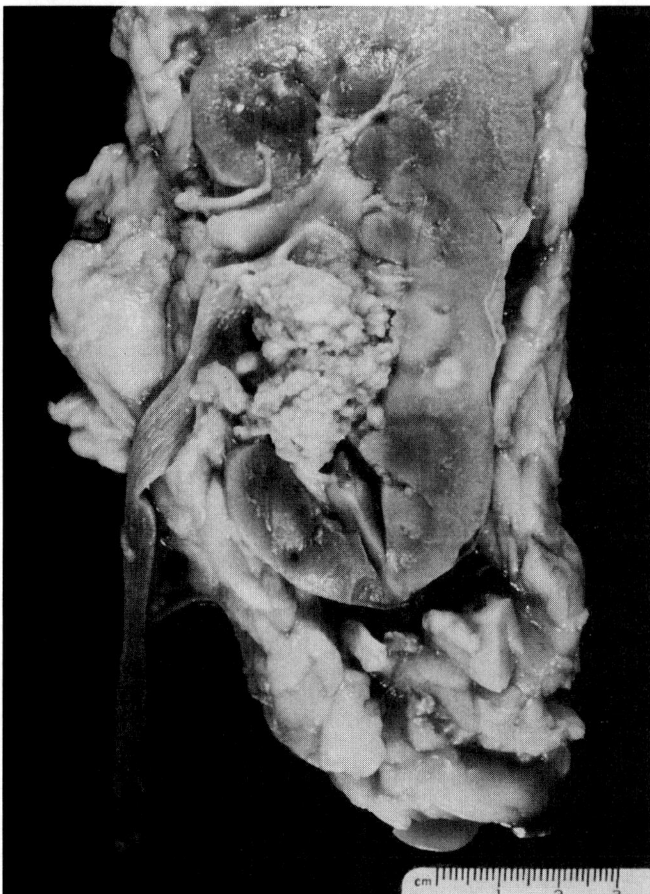

Fig. 9.1. Photograph of a transected nephroureterectomy specimen showing a papillary transitional cell carcinoma occupying the lower portion of the renal pelvis and inferior calyces. (Courtesy of Dr. Patricia Troncoso.)

to urinary tract obstruction with subsequent hydronephrosis, pyonephrosis, and stone formation. Carcinoma in situ of the upper tracts is seldom symptomatic and rarely found without a prior diagnosis of a urothelial cancer. Carcinoma in situ is found in the distal ureter in 7 to 25% of patients undergoing cystectomy for primary bladder cancer (26).

Histologically, three main types of tumor occur—transitional cell carcinoma, squamous cell carcinoma, and adenocarcinoma. Transitional cell carcinomas are by far the most frequent histologic type, accounting for 90% of tumors. Squamous carcinoma follows as a distant second, at 7%, and is usually associated with chronic inflammation, such as that from a staghorn calculus. Adenocarcinomas occur less than 1% of the time, with the remaining 2% of tumors being small cell or unclassified carcinomas (17).

Transitional cell carcinomas of the upper tract are graded in a similar fashion to bladder cancer. The most commonly used grading system for transitional cell carcinomas is based on the degree of cellular anaplasia. This system groups tumors into three grades corresponding to well (grade 1), moderately (grade 2), and poorly (grade 3) differentiated (27). Grade 1 tumors, which comprise approximately 20% of upper tract tumors, are papillary and well differentiated. Grade 2 tumors are predominantly papillary and account for the majority of tumors (60%). Grade 3 tumors, which comprise 20% of tumors, are solid or infiltrating in 50% of cases and histologically anaplastic. The grade of the tumor has substantial prognostic importance. In a review of 60 patients with ureteral cancer at the Massachusetts General Hospital, the 5-year survival rate of patients with grade 1 tumors was 100%; for grade 2 tumors it was 81% (P < 0.05), and for grade 3 tumors it was 29% (P < 0.01) (Fig. 9.2) (28).

DNA ploidy and S-phase fraction have been examined as potential prognostic indicators in upper tract tumors. As expected, high-grade tumors are largely aneuploid or tetraploid and have a high labeling index. Low-grade tumors are the opposite. Tumors that are aneuploid or have a high labeling index are associated with poor survival in most case series. However, on multivariate analysis, both ploidy and S-phase fraction are less informative than either stage or grade. There is some suggestion in the literature that these methods may be useful in predicting disease progression and survival in grade 2 and stage T2 tumors, thus allowing identification of patients for conservative therapy. However, both DNA ploidy and S-phase fraction lack the necessary sensitivity and specificity to apply to individual patients (29, 30).

Mutations of the tumor suppressor genes Rb and p53 have been found to be important prognostic factors in both superficial and invasive bladder cancer (31, 32). No studies examining

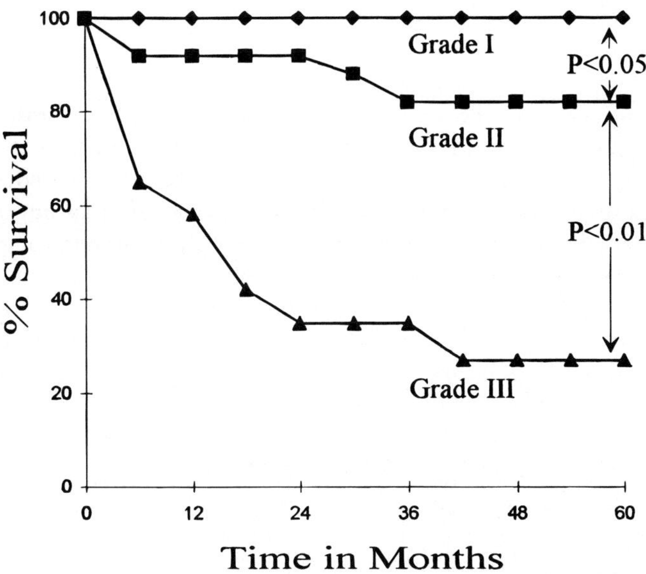

Fig. 9.2. Survival, in months, of 60 patients with transitional cell carcinoma of the ureter according to tumor grade. Statistically significant differences in survival are noted between patients with grade 1 and grade 2 tumors, and between patients with grade 2 and grade 3 tumors. (From Heney NM, Nocks BN, Daly JJ, et al. Prognostic factors in carcinoma of the ureter. J Urol 1981;125:632–636. Used with permission from Williams & Wilkins.)

Table 9.1. A Comparison of the TNM and Grabstald Staging Systems for Tumors of the Renal Pelvis and Ureter

CLINICOPATHOLOGIC FINDINGS	TNM SYSTEM	GRABSTALD SYSTEM
Carcinoma in situ	Tis	0
Papillary, noninvasive tumor	Ta	
Tumor invades submucosa	T1	A
Tumor invades muscularis	T2	B
Tumor invades periureteral tissue or renal parenchyma	T3	C
Tumor invades adjacent organs or perinephric fat	T4	C
Single regional lymph node involved, less than 2 cm	N1	D
Multiple nodes involved or greater than 2 cm	N2–3	D
Distant metastasis	M1	D

the significance of tumor suppressor gene mutations in upper tract tumors have been reported to date.

STAGING

Two staging systems are regularly used to classify upper tract tumors. The more commonly used system is that of Grabstald et al., which is a modification of the Jewett-Strong-Marshall classification developed for bladder cancer (33). The alternative TNM system developed by the American Joint Committee on Cancer and The Union Internationale Contre Le Cancer (AJCC-UICC) provides a more precise classification of these tumors (34). The classification systems are outlined in Table 9.1.

Clinical stage has been demonstrated to have a significant correlation to survival for both the Grabstald and the TNM systems (1, 28) (Fig. 9.3). A criticism of the TNM system has been that stage T3 understages ureteral cancer and overstages renal pelvic cancer. A review of 611 patients in Illinois suggested that the renal parenchyma acted as a relative anatomic barrier to tumor spread. In this series, the patients whose renal pelvic tumors invaded the kidney parenchyma (T3) had better prognoses than the patients whose ureteral tumors invaded the periureteral tissues (T3) (22).

DIAGNOSIS

Clinical Presentation

The median age at which patients present with upper tract tumors is 60 years, with a range of 29 to 80 years. Upper tract tumors occur twice as often in men as in women. Hematuria is the most common presentation, occurring in 60 to 70% of patients. The hematuria classically occurs throughout urination and is associated with vermiform or wormlike clots (casts of the ureter). Flank pain occurs in 30% of patients. The pain may be dull, due to low-grade ureteral obstruction, or severe (e.g., when passing an obstructing clot). Irritative voiding

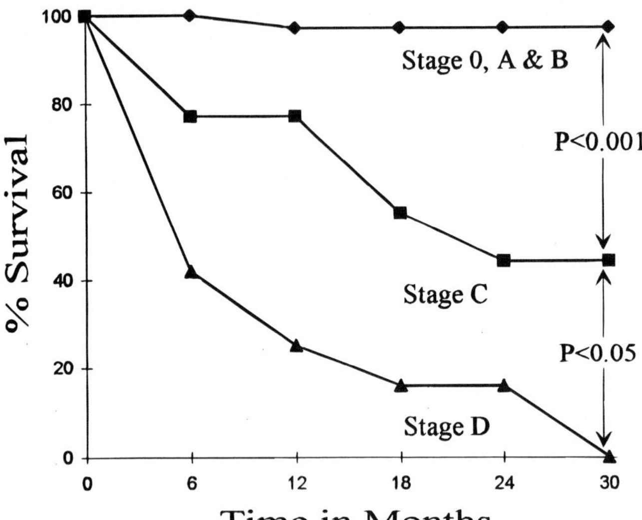

Fig. 9.3. Survival, in months, of 60 patients with transitional cell carcinoma of the ureter according to tumor stage. A statistically significant difference in survival is noted between low-stage (0, A, and B) and high-stage (C) tumors. Patients with nodal or distant metastatic disease (Stage D) had the worst prognosis. (From Heney NM, Nocks BN, Daly JJ, et al. Prognostic factors in carcinoma of the ureter. J Urol 1981;125:632–636. Used with permission from Williams & Wilkins.)

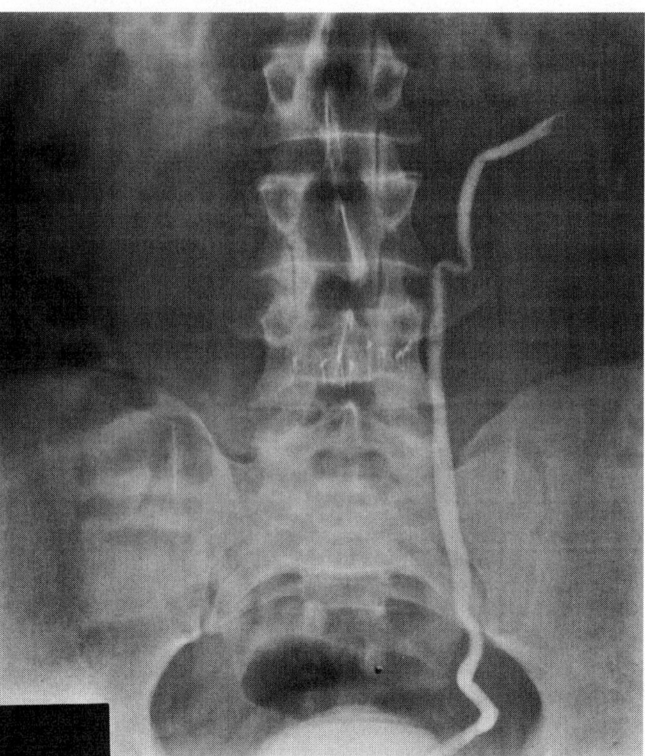

Fig. 9.4. Retrograde urogram showing a filling defect occupying the left renal pelvis. The filling defect was confirmed to be a papillary transitional cell carcinoma on nephroureterectomy. (Courtesy of Dr. Ronelle Debrow.)

symptoms occur in 10 to 25% of patients. A small proportion of patients with advanced disease present with an abdominal mass or exhibit symptoms from metastases. The neoplasm is asymptomatic in 10 to 15% of patients and is discovered incidentally during routine excretory urogram (18, 24).

Radiographic Studies

Excretory Urography

The classic finding seen in 30 to 70% of excretory urograms, or retrograde urograms, is a filling defect. The filling defect is normally irregular and adjacent to the wall of the collecting system. Other possible causes of a urinary filling defect, such as a kidney stone, fungus ball, blood clot, sloughed papilla, and air bubble, should be part of the differential diagnosis. The pyelograms should be examined for symmetry because a renal pelvic tumor may occupy or occlude a calyx and thus not be immediately apparent. Careful attention should be paid to the opposite renal unit because of the 1.5 to 2% incidence of synchronous bilateral renal tumors (18, 23). Renal tomography and ureteral compression should be performed as part of the excretory urogram to improve sensitivity. Up to 50% of excretory urograms will show nonfunction of the affected kidney (17).

Retrograde Urography

This study provides better visualization of the collecting system than excretory urography (Fig. 9.4), especially if there is a nonfunctioning kidney. Before performing retrograde urography, a careful cystoscopy is warranted because of the high incidence of synchronous bladder and upper tract tumors. The ureteral orifices should be examined for dilatation and protruding tumor, findings that occur in 12% of patients with upper tract tumors. A ureteral washing is obtained before retrograde urography because the high osmolality contrast may alter the cellular architecture and make cytologic interpretation difficult (35). (Ureteral washings should be interpreted cautiously in patients with suspected upper tract tumors, as will be discussed in the section on cytology.) Retrograde urography is performed by inserting a bulb-tipped catheter snugly into the ureteral orifice and gently injecting dilute (50%) contrast material. If possible, the progress of the contrast up the ureter should be observed fluoroscopically. Care is taken not to overdistend the collecting system. Such overdistention may lead to contrast extravasation, which will interfere with image interpretation. A drainage film is often helpful to rule out subtle obstruction.

Antegrade Pyelography

In general, this study is not advisable when the suspected diagnosis is transitional cell carcinoma because of the propensity of this tumor to implant in the needle or nephrostomy tract (36). Exceptions include planned endoscopic therapy and therapeutic renal decompression when other alternatives are not appropriate.

Other Imaging Techniques

Renal ultrasound is an efficient way of identifying renal masses and hydronephrosis. However, the small size of many upper tract tumors combined with the low sensitivity of ultrasound in the midureter makes this imaging modality less effective than computed tomography (CT) for tumor staging. CT imaging can be helpful in narrowing the differential diagnosis of a filling defect in the upper urinary tract. Thin CT images taken before and after the administration of contrast material may allow the differentiation of an air bubble, a radiolucent renal calculus, or a vascular impression from a transitional cell tumor. CT may be useful in distinguishing renal cell carcinoma from urothelial carcinoma in some instances. CT cannot accurately stage localized T0 to T2 carcinoma. However, it has a sensitivity of 67 to 75% and a specificity of 45% in identifying renal parenchymal or periureteric involvement (T3) (37). CT has an additional advantage in that it allows assessment of the liver for metastatic disease and assessment of the retroperitoneum for enlarged lymph nodes. However, CT cannot detect tumor in normal-sized nodes and it cannot differentiate nodal enlargement due to inflammation from tumor infiltration. Magnetic resonance imaging offers no significant advantages over CT in the imaging of urothelial tumors, except in the rare case with renal vein and inferior vena caval involvement by a tumor thrombus (38).

Cytology

A barbotage cytology specimen is usually positive in 10% of patients with grade 1 bladder tumors, in 50% of those with grade 2 tumors, and in 90% of those with grade 3 tumors (39). However, upper tract urothelial cancers present several problems with regard to cytologic examination. First, the tumor is not easily accessible for direct barbotage unless this is performed by ureteral catheterization. Second, the tumor may obstruct the ureter and thus not shed cells into the urine. Third, inflammation proximal to a urinary obstruction may make cytologic interpretation difficult. Fourth, synchronous bladder tumors may give false-positive cytology results due to cellular contamination. Fifth, clumps of normal cells that are mechanically dislodged can be misinterpreted as low-grade papillary tumors. Because of these problems, some workers have reported cytology to be of little value in the diagnosis of upper tract tumors (40). The accuracy of cytology can be improved by using a brush biopsy. In a series of 46 patients, brush biopsy was reported to have a sensitivity of 91% and a specificity of 88% in the diagnosis of upper tract transitional cell carcinoma (41).

Ureteroscopy

The recent development of small semirigid and flexible ureteroscopes enables effective examination of the upper urinary tracts with minimal morbidity. Ureteroscopy has increased the accuracy of upper tract tumor diagnosis. In a series of 43 patients, ureteroscopy increased the percentage of definitive diagnosis from 55 to 86% with a very low complication rate (42). The disadvantages of ureteroscopy include difficulty in obtaining an adequate biopsy because only very small forceps will fit through the ureteroscope working channel (this may be partially overcome by brushing the lesion under direct vision); difficulty maneuvering the flexible endoscope in the renal pelvis, especially when trying to visualize lesions in the lower pole; and the theoretical potential for tumor cell dissemination by pyelovenous backflow (43). The major advantage of ureteroscopy in the diagnosis of upper tract tumors is that it permits simultaneous, minimally invasive diagnosis and treatment of any lesions discovered. Ureteroscopic tumor treatment will be discussed in full in a subsequent section.

TREATMENT OF LOCALIZED DISEASE

Treatment options for localized upper tract tumors, from the most invasive to the least invasive, include nephroureterectomy, partial ureterectomy, endoscopic resection or ablation, and topical chemotherapy. Several generalizations can be made to clarify the decision-making process. First, high-grade (grade 3) and high-stage (T3 to T4 or greater) tumors have a poor prognosis despite aggressive treatment. Second, intermediate-grade (grade 2) tumors appear to do better with radical surgery. Third, low-grade, low-stage tumors do equally well with either conservative or aggressive therapy (Figs. 9.2 and 9.3) (44).

Important factors to ascertain before selecting a treatment plan include the clinical stage and grade of the tumor, the tumor location (tumors that are anatomically higher in the urinary tract are more likely to recur after conservative therapy), the presence or absence of a synchronous contralateral tumor, the overall and differential renal function, and the patient's general health status.

Nephroureterectomy

The en bloc removal of the kidney, ureter, and a cuff of bladder is the standard against which other therapies for upper tract tumors must be measured. The importance of removing the entire ureter is emphasized by the 25 to 30% incidence of subsequent tumor development in the ureteral stump if it is not removed at nephroureterectomy (1, 24, 45, 46). A more conservative operation should be considered only for patients with low-grade tumors, low-stage tumors, bilateral tumors, or compromised renal function.

The operation can be performed in a number of different ways. A common method is a two-incision retroperitoneal approach, using a flank incision for access to the kidney and a modified Gibson incision for access to the lower ureter. This operation has the advantage of providing excellent exposure of the kidney and distal ureter, but has the disadvantage of requiring repositioning of the patient at the midpoint of the operation. A second approach is a long midline incision that has the advantage of a single incision, but the disadvantage of slightly compromising exposure at the upper pole of the kidney. As with all transperitoneal operations, adhesions may develop, which have the potential to cause future bowel obstruction. A third approach is an extended flank incision that allows excellent access to the kidney but slightly compromises exposure of the distal ureter. The authors favor the midline approach.

No matter what the chosen route, the operation should result in complete excision of the distal ureter with a surrounding cuff of bladder. This is most easily accomplished by opening the bladder, thereby allowing an accurate excision of the ureteral orifice with a surrounding 1-cm cuff of bladder. However, endoscopic techniques have also been successfully used (47). Recently, nephroureterectomy has been performed laparoscopically. The early laparoscopic operations have had few complications but are very time-consuming. Whether the laparoscopic technique will be able to achieve adequate margins and effectively remove the lymph nodes has not yet been defined (48). The technical details of all these procedures will be detailed in other chapters in this text.

An extensive routine lymph node dissection in combination with nephroureterectomy has been recommended by some authors (49). In general, systemic dissemination has occurred by the time tumor metastases are documented in regional lymph nodes (28). Currently, the literature lacks substantial studies that support routine lymph node dissection (18).

The results of nephroureterectomy are dependent on the initial grade and stage of the tumor. Major complications occur infrequently following nephroureterectomy performed by any of the methods described previously. In one series, the complications included hemorrhage (11%), pulmonary embolism (5%), abscess (5%), ileus (5%), and pneumonia (5%) (50). Given the high incidence of subsequent tumor formation (primarily in the bladder), patients should receive follow-up care consisting of regular cystoscopy, cytology, and upper tract imaging after nephroureterectomy.

Conservative Surgery

Conservative surgery consists of partial nephrectomy, renal pelvis resection, segmental ureteral resection with primary ureteral reanastomosis, or ureteral reimplantation into the bladder with or without a psoas hitch or Boari flap. Transureteroureterostomy is contraindicated in patients with upper tract tumors because of the risk of tumor implantation in the normal contralateral ureter.

Patients selected for conservative resections should have low-grade tumors, low-stage tumors, bilateral tumors, or renal dysfunction. The possibility of tumor recurrence in the residual ureter and the potential for tumor progression are major concerns when performing conservative resection. Most series have documented that the chance of recurrence is low if conservative resection is performed for low-stage tumors, especially if the tumors are located in the distal ureter (2, 18). In a series of 49 patients with grade 1 tumors, only 1 of 15 patients who underwent a local resection had an ipsilateral recurrence. The overall results of conservative surgery in properly selected patients are identical to those of radical nephroureterectomy (1, 18, 29). Follow-up care is similar to that after nephroureterectomy, i.e., regular cystoscopy, cytology, and upper tract imaging.

Endoscopic Treatment

Endoscopic technology is advancing extremely rapidly, and more versatile instruments are constantly being developed. The introduction of excellent rigid and flexible nephroscopes and ureteroscopes has increased the potential to treat upper tract tumors endoscopically. A variety of tools are available to remove or ablate tumors, including ureteral resectoscopes, electrocautery tools, and the argon and Nd:YAG lasers. None of these methods has been shown to have any particular treatment superiority over the others.

The advantage of endoscopic treatment is decreased morbidity. After endoscopic surgery, a patient can return to normal activity in 2 to 3 days compared with the normal 6-week recovery period associated with a major operation. The drawbacks of endoscopic therapy are the inability to obtain accurate pathologic staging, the potential for tumor implantation, the potential for local recurrence, and the technical limitations of current endoscopic equipment. The same guidelines that apply to the application of conservative surgery should also apply to endoscopic surgery. These include restricting treatment to patients with low-grade and low-stage tumors or patients with bilateral tumors or renal dysfunction. Patients with a high risk of perioperative morbidity are also candidates for endoscopic surgery.

Percutaneous Ureteropyeloscopy

Conservative management of upper tract tumors by a percutaneous approach has not gained popularity in the United States because of the perceived risk of tumor cell implantation along the nephrostomy tract and of tumor dissemination by pyelovenous backflow. The increased risk of tumor implantation has been disputed by McCarron et al., who reported no cases of nephrostomy tract implantation in 33 patients in whom the collecting system was violated (51). The efficacy of percutaneous treatment of upper tract tumors is difficult to establish because few large series have been reported in the literature. In a representative report by Orihuela and Smith, who treated a series of 14 patients by percutaneous techniques, complete tumor excision was possible in 11 of 14 patients (52). Tumor recurrence was documented in 5 of these 11 patients who underwent complete resection.

Retrograde Ureteropyeloscopy

Retrograde ureteroscopic treatment of upper tract tumors is more appealing than percutaneous treatment because it avoids transgression of the urinary tract. Multiple small series have reported effective treatment of upper tract tumors by retrograde ureteropyeloscopy using a variety of modalities (53). Grossman et al. reported a series of 12 patients with upper tract tumors in whom an attempt was made to treat the tumor using rigid ureteroscopy and the Nd:YAG laser (54). Five patients could not be effectively treated for technical reasons. Of the seven patients believed to be candidates for ureteroscopic treatment, five patients had their tumors controlled by laser ablation. Follow-up care after endoscopic therapy should be by repeat ureteroscopy because recurrent lesions can be missed by retrograde urography.

Topical Chemotherapy

Thiotepa, mitomycin C, and bacille Calmette-Guérin (BCG) have all been used to treat tumors in the upper urinary tract. Problems associated with the administration of topical therapy and the increased potential for systemic absorption have limited the applicability of this therapy in the upper tract. The only true indications for topical chemotherapy are for the treatment of carcinoma in situ or recurrent superficial tumors in a solitary renal unit. Most reports on the use of topical chemotherapy are in small series of highly selected patients. Eastham and Huffman reported a series of seven patients treated with mitomycin C after endoscopic resection of upper tract transitional cell carcinoma (55). Five patients had no evidence of disease at a mean follow-up of 9 months. The treatment was well tolerated with minimal complications. Schoenberg et al. reported on nine patients with solitary functioning kidneys who were treated with endoscopic resection followed by BCG instillation (56). With an average follow-up time of 24 months, seven patients had no evidence of recurrent disease. One patient had a persistent febrile reaction requiring isoniazid therapy.

TREATMENT OF ADVANCED DISEASE

Radiation Therapy

The long-term survival of patients with high-grade (grade 3) and high-stage (T2 to T4) carcinomas of the renal pelvis and ureter is uniformly poor. Most series report a 5-year survival rate somewhere between 30 and 50%. In an attempt to improve outcome, several groups have administered postoperative radiation therapy. Randomized trials to establish the efficacy of postoperative radiation have not been performed because of the rarity of these tumors. Several case series have suggested that adjuvant radiation decreases the rate of local tumor recurrence from 70 to 15%. However, radiation therapy does not result in statistically significant prolonged survival times (57, 58).

Chemotherapy

Systemic chemotherapy is known to be effective in the treatment of metastatic bladder cancer. Currently, the most potent treatment regimen for transitional cell carcinoma is methotrex-ate, vinblastine, doxorubicin (Adriamycin), and cisplatin (MVAC). Of patients with metastatic bladder cancer, approximately 25% will have a complete response to chemotherapy. Two thirds of these patients will have a relapse within 2 years. Thus, 8% of patients will have a durable response at 3 years (59). Because of the small numbers of patients with upper tract tumors, randomized controlled studies of the effectiveness of chemotherapy are not possible. Case series of patients treated with MVAC for upper tract tumors have reported response rates similar to those seen with bladder cancer (60, 61). Multiple drug resistance mediated by P-glycoprotein expression may adversely affect chemotherapy response in patients with upper tract tumors (62).

Conclusion

Upper tract tumors are rare. Therefore, information regarding natural history and treatment is based mainly on the results of retrospective reviews of small case series. Despite the paucity of prospective data, treatment is relatively effective and is not controversial in the majority of patients. As technology improves, minimally invasive treatment of low-grade tumors is likely to increase. Effective therapy is still lacking for local advanced tumors, which have a strong propensity to metastasize and are therefore associated with poor survival.

REFERENCES

1. Huben RP, Mounzer AM, Murphy GP. Tumor grade and stage as prognostic variables in upper tract urothelial tumors. Cancer 1988;62:2016.
2. Wallace DMA, Wallace DM, Whitfield HN, et al. The late results of conservative surgery for upper tract urothelial carcinomas. Br J Urol 1981;53:537.
3. 1987 Annual cancer statistics review including trends: 1950–1985, NIH publication no. 88-2789. Bethesda, MD: U.S. Department of Health and Human Services, National Cancer Institute, 1987.
4. McLaughlin JK, Silverman DT, Hsing AW, et al. Cigarette smoking and cancers of the renal pelvis and ureter. Cancer Res 1992;52:254.
5. Jensen OM, Knudsen JB, McLaughlin JK, et al. The Copenhagen case control study of renal pelvis and ureter cancer: role of smoking and occupational exposures. Int J Cancer 1988;41:557.
6. Heuper WC, Wiley WF, Wolfe HD. Experimental production of bladder tumors in dogs by the administration of betanaphthylamine. J Industr Hyg Toxicol 1938;20:46.
7. Rehn L. Blasengeschwultse bei fuchsin-Arbeitern. Arch Clin Chir 1895;50:588.
8. Poole-Wilson DB. Occupational tumours of the renal pelvis and ureter in the dye making industry. Proceedings of the Royal Society of Medicine 1969;62:93.
9. Case RAM, Hosker ME, McDonald DM, et al. Tumours of the urinary bladder in workmen engaged in the manufacture and use of certain dye stuff intermediates in the British chemical

industry: the role of aniline, benzidine, alpha-naphthylamine, and beta-naphthylamine. Br J Industr Med 1954;11:75.

10. McCredie M, Stewart JH, Ford JM. Analgesics and cancer of the bladder and renal pelvis. J Urol 1983;130:28.

11. Jensen OM, Knudsen JB, Tomasson H, et al. The Copenhagen case control study of renal pelvis and ureter cancer: role of analgesics. Int J Cancer 1989;44:965.

12. Petersen I, Ohgaki H, Ludeke BI, et al. p53 mutations in phenactin induced urothelial cancers. Verh Dtsch Ges Pathol 1993;77:252.

13. Petrovic VJ, Bukurov NS, Djokic MR, et al. Balkan endemic nephropathy and papillary transitional cell tumors of the renal pelvis and ureters. Kidney Int Suppl 1991;34:77.

14. Brenner DW, Schellhammer PF. Upper tract urothelial malignancy after cyclophosphamide therapy: a case report and literature review. J Urol 1987;137:1226.

15. Booth CM, Cameron KM, Pugh RCB. Urothelial carcinoma of the kidney and ureter. Br J Urol 1980;52:430.

16. Grampa G. Radiation injury with particular reference to Thorotrast. Pathol Annu 1971;6:147.

17. Babaian RJ, Johnson DE. Primary carcinoma of the ureter. J Urol 1980;123:357.

18. Schwartz CB, Bekirov H, Melman A. Urothelial tumors of upper tract following treatment of primary bladder transitional cell carcinoma. Urology 1992;40:509.

19. Oldbring J, Glifberg I, Milkowlski P, et al. Carcinoma of the renal pelvis and ureter following bladder carcinoma: frequency, risk factors, and clinicopathological findings. J Urol 1989;141:1311.

20. Soloway MS, Masters BS. Urothelial susceptibility to tumor cell implantation. Cancer 1980;46:1158.

21. Sidransky D, Frost P, von Eschenbach A, et al. Clonal origin of metachronous tumors of the bladder. N Engl J Med 1992;326:737.

22. Guinan P, Vogelzhang NJ, Randazzo R, et al. Renal pelvic transitional cell carcinoma: the role of the kidney in the tumor nodes metastasis staging. Cancer 1992;62:1773.

23. Batata MA, Whitmore WF, Hilaris BS, et al. Primary carcinoma of the ureter: a prognostic study. Cancer 1975;35:1626.

24. Geiger J, Fong Q, Fay R. Transitional cell carcinoma of the renal pelvis with invasion of the renal vein and thrombosis of the subhepatic vena cava. Urology 1986;28:52.

25. Davis BW, Hough AJ, Gardner WA. Renal pelvic carcinoma: morphological correlates of metastatic behaviour. J Urol 1987;137:857.

26. Melamed MR, Reuter VE. Pathology and staging of urothelial tumors of the kidney and ureter. Urol Clin North Am 1993;20:333.

27. Mostofi FK, Sobin LH, Torloni H. Histological typing of urinary bladder tumors (international histological classification of tumors no. 10). Geneva: World Health Organization, 1973.

28. Heney NM, Nocks BN, Daly JJ, et al. Prognostic factors in carcinoma of the ureter. J Urol 1981;125:632.

29. Miyakawa A, Tachibana M, Nakashima J, et al. Flow cytometric bromodeoxyuridine deoxyribonucleic acid bivariate analysis for predicting tumor invasiveness of upper tract urothelial cancer. J Urol 1994;152:76.

30. al Abadi H, Nagel R. Transitional cell carcinoma of the renal pelvis and ureter: prognostic relevance of nuclear deoxyribonucleic acid ploidy studied by slide cytometry. an 8 year survival time study. J Urol 1992;148:31.

31. Logothetis CJ, Xu HJ, Ro JY, et al. Altered expression of retinoblastoma protein and known prognostic variables in locally advanced bladder cancer. J Natl Cancer Inst 1992;84:1256.

32. Esrig D, Elmajian D, Groshens, et al. Accumulation of nuclear p53 and tumor progression in bladder cancer. N Engl J Med 1994;331:1259.

33. Grabstald H, Whitmore WF, Melamed MR. Renal pelvic tumors. JAMA 1971;218:845.

34. Spiessl B, Beahrs OH, Hermanek P, et al. Renal pelvis and ureter. In: Spiessl B, Beahrs OH, et al., eds. UICC-TMN Atlas illustrated guide to the TMN/PTMN classification of malignant tumors. Berlin: Springer-Verlag, 1989:260.

35. Andriole GL, McClennan BL, Becich MJ, et al. Effect of low osmolar, ionic and non ionic contrast media on the cytological features of exfoliated urothelial cells. Urol Radiol 1989;11:133.

36. Sharma NK, Nicol A, Powell CS. Tract infiltration following percutaneous resection of renal pelvic carcinoma. Br J Urol 1994;73:597.

37. McCoy JG, Honda H, Reznicek M, et al. Computerized tomography for the detection and staging of localized and pathologically defined upper tract urothelial tumors. J Urol 1991;146:1500.

38. Newhouse JH. The radiological evaluation of the patient with renal cancer. Urol Clin North Am 1993;20:231.

39. Soloway MS, Morrison DA, Shelton TB. Modalities used in the diagnosis, staging and evaluation of bladder cancer. American Urological Association Update Series. 1985;4:1.

40. Nielson K, Ostri P. Primary tumors of the renal pelvis: evaluation of clinical and pathological features in a consecutive series of 10 years. J Urol 1988;140:19.

41. Sheline M, Amendola MA, Pollock HM, et al. Fluoroscopically guided retrograde brush biopsy in the diagnosis of transitional cell carcinoma of the upper urinary tract: results in 48 patients. AJR 1989;153:313.

42. Blute ML, Segura JW, Paterson DE, et al. Impact of endourology on the diagnosis and management of upper urinary tract urothelial cancer. J Urol 1989;141:1298.

43. Lim DJ, Shattuck MC, Cook WA. Pyelovenous lymphatic migration of transitional cell carcinoma following flexible ureterorenoscopy. J Urol 1993;149:109.

44. Catalona W. Urothelial tumors of the urinary tract. In: Walsh P, Retik A, Stamey T, et al., eds. Campbell's urology. 6th ed. Philadelphia: WB Saunders, 1992:1094.

45. Murphy DM, Zincke H, Furlow WL. Primary grade 1 transitional cell carcinoma of the renal pelvis and ureter. J Urol 1980;123:629.

46. Anderstrom C, Johansson SL, Pettersson S, et al. Carcinoma of the ureter: a clinicopathological study of 49 cases. J Urol 1989;142:280.

47. Ercole CJ. Endoscopic removal of the lower ureter in nephroureterectomy. Urology 1993;41:49.

48. Kerbl K, Clayman RV, McDougall EM, et al. Laparoscopic nephroureterectomy: evaluation of first clinical series. Eur Urol 1993;23:431.

49. Johansson S, Wahlqvist L. A prognostic study of urothelial renal pelvic tumors: comparison between the prognosis of

patients treated with intrafascial nephrectomy and perifascial nephroureterectomy. Cancer 1979;43:2525.

50. Vahlensieck W, Sommerkamp H. Therapy and prognosis of carcinoma of the renal pelvis. Eur Urol 1989;16:286.

51. McCarron JP, Mills C, Vaughan ED. Tumors of the renal pelvis and ureter: current concepts and management. Semin Urol 1983;1:75.

52. Orihuela E, Smith AD. Percutaneous treatment of transitional cell carcinoma of the upper tracts. Urol Clin North Am 1988;15:425.

53. Gerber GS, Lyon ES. Endourological management of upper tract urothelial tumors. J Urol 1993;150:2.

54. Grossman HB, Schwartz SI, Konnack JW. Ureteroscopic treatment of urothelial carcinoma of the ureter and renal pelvis. J Urol 1992;148:275.

55. Eastham JA, Huffman JL. Technique of mitomycin C instillation in the treatment of upper urinary tract urothelial tumors. J Urol 1993;150:324.

56. Schoenberg MP, Van Arsdalen KN, Wein AJ. The management of transitional cell carcinoma in a solitary renal unit. J Urol 1991;146:700.

57. Cozad SC, Smalley SR, Austenfeld M, et al. Adjuvant radiotherapy in high stage transitional cell carcinoma of the renal pelvis and ureter. Int J Radiat Oncol Biol Phys 1992;24:743.

58. Brookland RK, Richter MP. The postoperative irradiation of transitional cell carcinoma of the renal pelvis and ureter. J Urol 1985;133:952.

59. Steinberg GD, Trump DL, Cummings KB. Metastatic bladder cancer. Urol Clin North Am 1992;19:735.

60. Igawa M, Ueki T, Ueda M, et al. MVAC chemotherapy in advanced renal pelvic and ureteral carcinoma. Jpn J Cancer Chemother 1989;16:2577.

61. Sella A, Logothetis CJ, Dexeus FH, et al. Cisplatin based adjuvant chemotherapy in patients with invasive upper tract tumors. Proc Annu Meet Am Assoc Cancer Res. 1991;32:1106. Abstract.

62. Shinohara N, Nonomura K, Takakura F, et al. Expression of multidrug resistance gene product (P-glycoprotein) in transitional cell carcinomas of the upper urinary tract. Eur Urol 1994;26:327.

10

Radical Nephroureterectomy in Transitional Cell Carcinoma of the Renal Pelvis and Ureter

Robert E. Donohue

HISTORICAL PERSPECTIVE

Transitional cell carcinoma of the renal calyces, pelvis, and ureter is thought to arise from interaction between the transitional cell lining of those structures and carcinogens present in the urine. The reservoir function of the bladder yields prolonged mucosal contact with the carcinogens and has a high incidence of tumor formation. A diverticulum of that bladder, without smooth muscle to facilitate urine drainage, has the highest incidence of tumor formation (approaching 14%). The calyces, renal pelvis, and ureter, functioning as conduits, not reservoirs, have a much lower incidence of tumor formation.

The incidence of tumors in the bladder, renal pelvis, and ureter in the United States, Great Britain, and France is shown in Table 10.1.

About half of these tumors develop de novo. The other half are in patients with antecedent tumors of the urothelium, in those with concurrent tumors, or in those who have undergone treatment of tumors of the urinary bladder.

Upper tract tumors develop in 2% of patients with a history of bladder cancer (1–4). After cystectomy, the incidence is 2 to 4%. Patients with an associated carcinoma in situ of the urinary bladder have a higher incidence of these tumors, from 9 to 13%; patients with urethral tumors at cystectomy have a 20 to 30% incidence of upper tract neoplasms. Twenty-five percent of patients have tumor multiplicity at diagnosis (3). Recurrences are more common after papillary tumors, with renal pelvic rather than ureteral tumors, and in patients with initial multifocality (3).

The converse is also true. Patients with upper tract tumors have to be monitored closely for the development of tumors in the bladder. A total of 15 to 50% of patients with upper tract tumors have bladder tumors within 5 years (usually within 3 years) (5).

In 1841, Rayer described a patient who demonstrated the multifocal nature of the transitional cell tumor. He reported on a 58-year-old woman found at autopsy to have renal pelvic, ureteral, and bladder tumors (6). In 1902, Reynes recommended nephroureterectomy and bladder cuff removal (7).

Ideal treatment should consist of removal of the tumor and restoration of a normal urothelial lining for the remainder of the urinary tract bilaterally. The latter aim is unattainable with current treatment strategies but must be sought earnestly. Simple nephrectomy is associated with an 84% recurrence rate, partial nephroureterectomy with a 32% recurrence rate, and subtotal nephroureterectomy with a 24% recurrence rate (8).

Johansson and Wahlqvist reviewed their experience with radical nephroureterectomy (9). Their operation, a complete radical nephroureterectomy with resection of a cuff of bladder mucosa surrounding the orifice, ipsilateral adrenalectomy, and retroperitoneal node dissection, had an 84% 5 year-survival rate. Strong et al. reported a significant incidence of failure to remove the entire distal ureter and cuff of bladder mucosa with an extraperitoneal tenting technique (10). Fraley popularized instilling an antitumor agent into the bladder and then opening the bladder after draining its instilled content to gain direct access to the ureteral orifice and its surrounding mucosa and to permit dissection of the intramural ureter (11).

Currently, radical nephrectomy and total ureterectomy with a cuff of bladder mucosa surrounding the ureteral orifice are the treatment of choice for transitional cell tumors of the kidney. Ipsilateral adrenalectomy remains controversial. Node dissection, with an incidence of involvement of 16%, also remains an option.

Distal ureteral tumors are amenable to renal-sparing surgery by distal ureterectomy and ureteral reimplantation. There are several clinical situations where this treatment must be tempered, such as tumors in a solitary kidney, low-grade tumors, bilateral simultaneous tumors, tumors associated with Balkan nephropathy, tumors subsequent to analgesic abuse, and tumors in patients with renal insufficiency (12, 13).

These urothelial lining tumors reflect not a local change but a field change, and the entire urothelium must be consid-

Table 10.1. Incidence of Tumors in the Bladder, Renal Pelvis, and Ureter from the United States, Great Britain, and France

SITE	MEMORIAL (1)	BRISTOL (2)	FRANCE (3)
Bladder	3.269	2.770	7.117
Renal pelvis	89	43	264
Ureter	77	54	132

ered suspect for additional tumors and monitored accordingly with excretion urography, voided urine cytology, cystoscopy, and ureteroscopy and brush biopsy of suspicious upper tract lesions as mandated by the patient's clinical course.

SURGICAL PROCEDURE—PREPARATION AND INCISION

Preoperative evaluation should consist of total evaluation of the entire urinary tract, establishment of maximum pulmonary function, and avoidance of antiplatelet medications. A mechanical bowel preparation can be completed as an outpatient procedure, and pneumatic compression stockings should be applied before anesthesia induction.

The choice of incision is usually based on body habitus and surgeon preference. The patient may be supine on the operating table for a midline incision or rotated variably for a subcostal, costal, or intercostal approach. With the assumption of any rotation, protection of the contralateral axilla must be completed.

If a two-incision procedure is planned, the patient should be prepared for both incisions, allowing the catheter to be reached for the insertion of the sterile water and its drainage during the second part of the procedure.

LEFT RADICAL NEPHRECTOMY

The radical nephrectomy will be presented with a no-touch technique, the vessels being secured before mobilizing the remainder of the kidney.

The descending colon is mobilized in the lateral gutter to the splenic flexure. Anteriorly, Gerota's fascia should be separated from the posterior lip of the peritoneum, preferably without entering the peritoneum. The peritoneum is swept medially after separating it from Gerota's fascia. As that occurs, the renal vein usually comes into view. The left renal vein is exposed and dissected with a right-angle clamp as it goes medially until the left spermatic vein, laterally, and the lumbar vein, medially, are identified (Fig. 10.1). Both enter on the inferior surface of the renal vein. The plane outside the adventitia of the left renal vein is entered, and the vein is dissected anteriorly toward the inferior vena cava beyond the insertion of the internal spermatic vein and the lumbar vein inferiorly. A plane is developed with a right-angle clamp behind the renal vein, usually from the inferior aspect, medial to the two venous insertions identified. The renal vein has 2-0 silk ties passed around it but they are

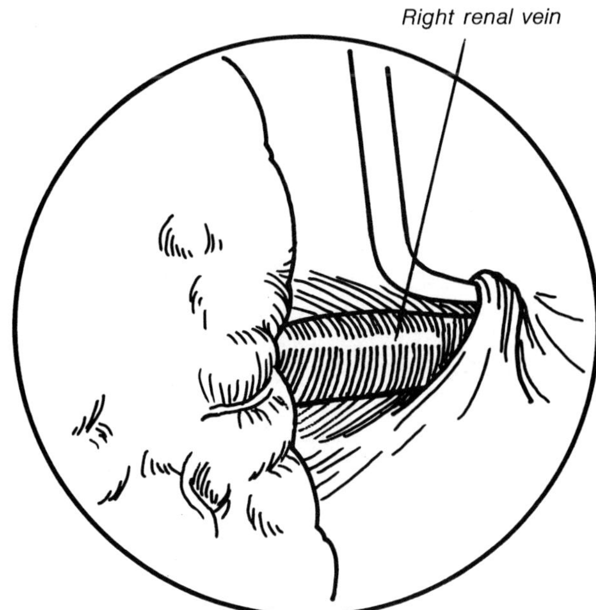

Fig. 10.1. The tissue overlying the renal vein is elevated with a right-angle clamp to allow mobilization of the vein and passage of ligatures.

not ligated. The left internal spermatic vein and the lumbar vein are ligated with 2-0 silk and divided between the ligatures.

The adrenal vein is identified entering the renal vein from above, usually medial to the point of insertion of the internal spermatic vein. Ligatures are passed around it (proximally and distally) and tied, and the vein is interrupted between the sutures (Fig. 10.2).

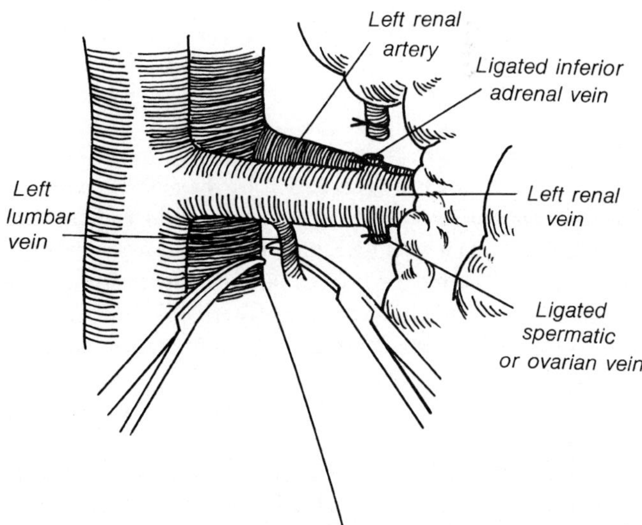

Fig. 10.2. The same technique for ligation is employed on both sides. A suture is passed around the arterial spermatic vein and lumbar vein proximally and distally after the vein has been cleaned and ligated. Sutures are passed around the main renal vein but are not tied until after the artery is ligated. The artery is identified above the vein and cleaned, isolated, and ligated, and the proximal vein can be sutured with a 5-0 cardiovascular silk suture.

Palpation above the renal vein may allow the renal artery to be identified. A right-angle clamp is passed behind this artery and then two sutures of 0 silk are passed around it and tied. The renal artery is divided between the two proximal and the third distal ligatures. If the renal artery cannot be palpated with certainty, the area above the renal vein is dissected gently parallel to the renal vein until the artery is identified. It may be necessary to retract the renal vein inferiorly with a vessel retractor to allow the area to be exposed so that the dissection for the renal artery can be completed. The artery is then isolated, doubly tied, and transected.

The renal vein ligatures are then tied, and the renal vein is divided between the ligatures. The artery and the vein can then be suture ligated with a 5-0 synthetic suture as the surgeon prefers.

The lumbodorsal fascia is entered posteriorly either bluntly or sharply. The plane inside the fascia is developed posterior to the kidney, with Gerota's fascia intact. The mobilization is continued superiorly and inferiorly around the kidney. Gerota's fascia should not be entered.

The lower pole of the left kidney is mobilized bluntly, identifying the left internal spermatic vein and the left ureter. The plane on the medial aspect of the left kidney is developed, and the renal vein is encountered.

The renal mass is then dissected bluntly from its superior attachments and the medial aspect is mobilized, identifying the left adrenal gland. This gland, with its adrenal vein ligated and cut earlier, can be dissected bluntly from its surrounding fascia.

RIGHT RADICAL NEPHRECTOMY

The ascending colon is mobilized to the hepatic flexure. The duodenum overlying the inferior vena cava is mobilized, a procedure called Kockerizing the duodenum, exposing the inferior vena cava.

The internal spermatic vein is identified as it crosses the ureter. It is followed to its insertion on the anterior aspect of the inferior vena cava. It is doubly ligated and divided. The main renal vein is cephalad to that insertion.

Dissection commences upward in the plane in the middle of the inferior vena cava. The dissection continues until the right renal vein is identified. It has no tributaries; however, 14% of patients have two right renal veins. Using a right-angle clamp, the vein is mobilized laterally for at least 1 cm, and two silk sutures are passed around it but not tied. The vein is retracted inferiorly with a vein retractor, and the renal artery is identified (Fig. 10.3). It is mobilized parallel to its path for 1 cm, and 0 silk ligatures are passed around it. The sutures are ligated and the artery is interrupted. The edge can then be suture ligated with 5-0 Prolene (Fig. 10.4). If the caliber of the vessel is smaller than the surgeon believes is proper for that kidney, a second renal artery must be searched for; 30% of patients have two renal arteries.

If the renal artery cannot be identified, the vein can be

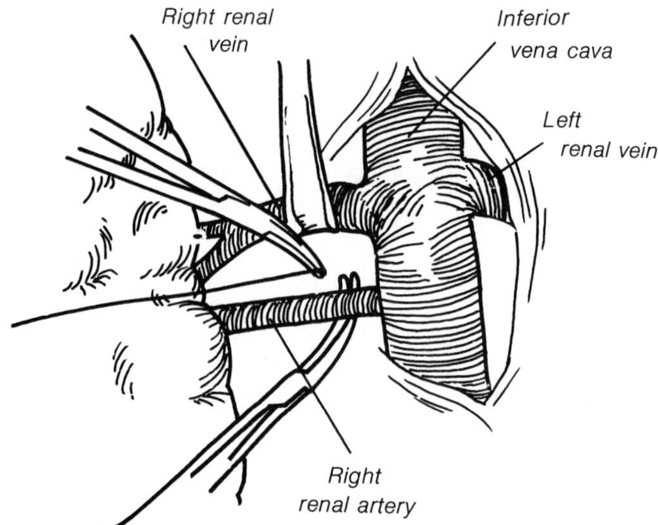

Fig. 10.3. The right renal artery is identified by palpation beneath the vein. After identification, with a right-angle clamp, the artery is cleaned in the same manner as the vein. With a right-angle clamp beneath the artery, a suture is passed on a tonsil clamp to the mouth of the right-angle clamp and the suture is passed around the artery.

retracted superiorly; the artery can often be identified in a more posterior plane. Occasionally, it is necessary to go to the other side of the inferior vena cava and identify the artery as it arises from the aorta. The left renal vein is identified and dissected from the underlying tissue as it inserts into the inferior vena cava. The right renal artery is usually identified just beneath that junction of the left renal vein and the inferior vena cava. The artery can be mobilized and doubly ligated. If adequate exposure cannot be achieved to cut the artery safely, it can be

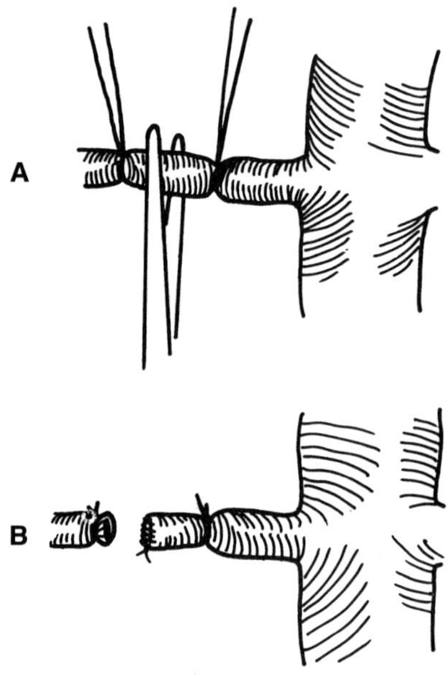

Fig. 10.4. **A.** The artery is doubly ligated, proximally and distally. **B.** Then the proximal end is oversewn with a 5-0 cardiovascular silk suture.

left doubly ligated and subsequently divided further laterally at the renal hilum.

Dissecting superiorly, the adrenal gland is identified and freed from its surrounding tissue. The medial aspect or, at times, the entire adrenal may often be located behind the inferior vena cava. The adrenal vein on the right often enters the vena cava on its posterior wall, and care must be taken to ligate that vein before removing the right adrenal gland. The adrenal artery may arise early from the right renal artery; if this occurs, the artery must be ligated if it arises proximal to the ligatures on the right renal artery. The adrenal can then be removed.

The mobilization of the superior aspect of the kidney is accomplished sharply and bluntly from the inferior surface of the liver. The ureter is not transected until it has been completely mobilized as far as the iliac vessels. The ureter can then be doubly clipped and transected; the kidney and upper ureter can be removed or the entire mass of kidney and ureter can be passed into the pelvis to be removed through a second incision.

Hemostasis is checked, and the wound is irrigated with sterile water. The flank incision is then closed in layers without a drain.

DISTAL URETERECTOMY

Sterile water is inserted into the bladder via a Foley catheter, and the catheter is clamped. A transverse incision is made above the symphysis and carried down to the bladder (Fig. 10.5). The bladder is opened longitudinally and figure-of-eight traction sutures are placed. Both ureteral orifices are identified. If there

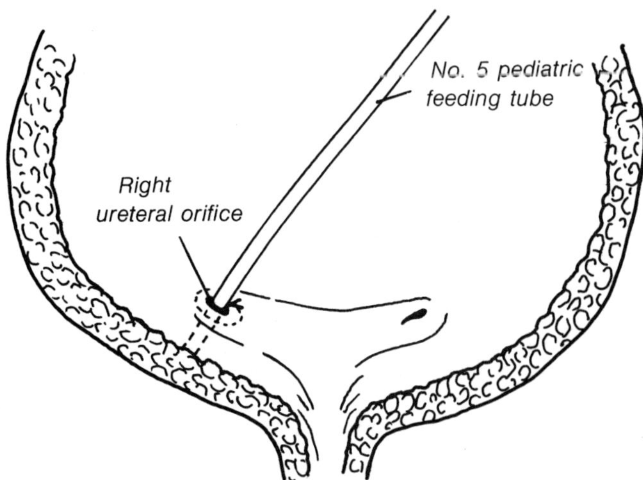

Fig. 10.6. The trigone is exposed, and a no. 5 pediatric feeding tube is passed up the orifice to be resected and sutured in place. Incision into the bladder mucosa is started in the inferomedial aspect of the bladder mucosa, allowing an appropriate cuff to be circumcised.

is difficulty with identification of either ureteral orifice, indigo carmine should be administered intravenously. A ureteral catheter or pediatric feeding tube is inserted up the remnant ureter to be removed until it meets the obstructing suture. It is sutured in place as in ureteral reimplantation surgery (Fig. 10.6).

The ureteral orifice and a circumferential piece of periureteral bladder mucosa should be removed using a needle cautery. Care must be taken to avoid the contralateral orifice. The ureteral orifice is mobilized sharply, as in ureteral reimplantation surgery, with an adequate cuff of bladder mucosa around the ureter (Fig. 10.7). The ureter is dissected sharply through the bladder wall using scissors and delivered into the retroperitoneal space (Fig. 10.8).

Attention is directed retroperitoneally at the iliac artery, which is followed from the aortic bifurcation laterally to iden-

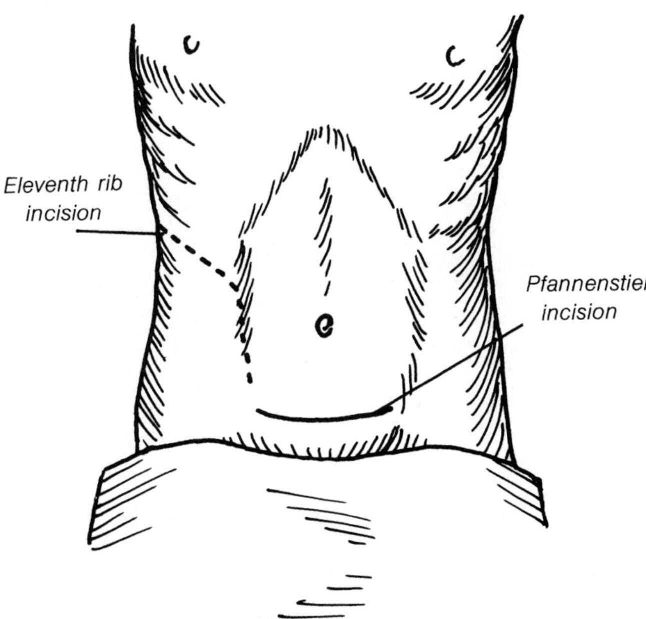

Fig. 10.5. After the patient is redraped and reprepared, a catheter is inserted, sterile water is instilled through the catheter, and the catheter is clamped. A transverse lower abdominal incision is made. The preparation and draping are done so that an extension on the ipsilateral side can be made without difficulty.

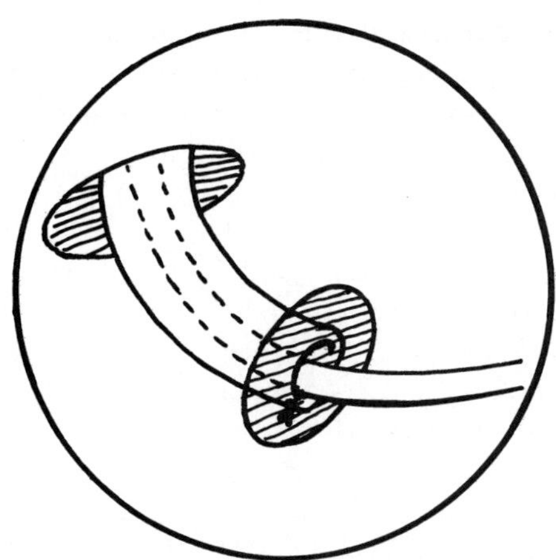

Fig. 10.7. The ureter is pulled into the bladder as mobilization progresses. This technique is the same as that used in intravesical ureteral reimplantation.

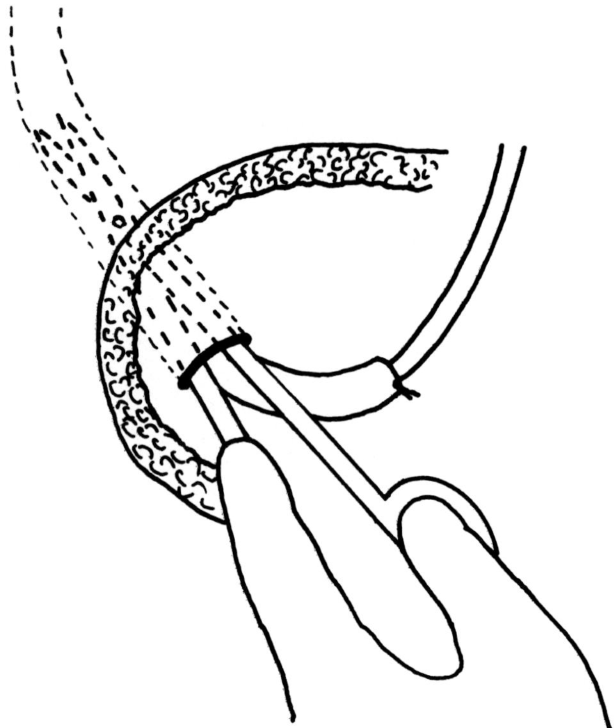

Fig. 10.8. After adequate ureteral mobilization, scissors are used to complete the tunnel to the extravesical pelvis.

tify the ipsilateral ureter. The ureter is usually located lateral to the right iliac artery bifurcation and at the bifurcation on the left side. The ureter is mobilized downward bluntly until the entire specimen is delivered from the wound.

The contralateral orifice is inspected, and clear efflux should be noted from that orifice. If difficulty in identification or concern about excretion exists, indigo carmine should be administered and efflux should be observed.

The bladder is closed in two layers. Hemostatis is achieved, and the wound is irrigated. A drain is placed in the pelvis near the site of the bladder closure.

The catheter should be filled with 240 mL of saline to demonstrate effective closure of the bladder. All leaking sites should be closed with additional sutures.

POSTOPERATIVE CARE

The external pelvic drain is usually mobilized within 3 days and removed. The suprapubic drain is likewise mobilized and removed rapidly.

Follow-up voided urine cytology and cystoscopy are recommended as in the follow-up of a bladder tumor. Excretion urography is recommended at 1 year and at 2-year intervals subsequently. A positive result on cytology or hematuria demands immediate full urinary tract evaluation.

REFERENCES

1. Batata M, Grabstald H. Upper urinary tract urothelial tumors. Urol Clin North Am 1976;3:70.
2. Williams C, Mitchell J. Carcinoma of the renal pelvis: a review of 43 cases. Br J Urol 1973;45:370.
3. Mazemann E. Tumours of the upper urinary tract calyces: renal pelvis and ureter. Eur Urol 1976;2:120.
4. Montie J. Followup after cystectomy for carcinoma of the bladder. Urol Clin North Am 1994;21:639.
5. Melamed MR, Reuter V. Pathology and staging of urothelial tumors of the kidney and ureter. Urol Clin North Am 1993; 20:333.
6. Rayer P. Traite des maladies des reins. Paris: JB Baillere, 1841;3:699.
7. Stricker O. Papillomatous tumors of the renal pelvis. Arch Klin Chir 1926;140:663.
8. Seaman E, Slawin K, Benson M. Treatment options for upper tract transitional cell carcinoma. Urol Clin North Am 1993; 20:349.
9. Johansson S, Wahlqvist T. A prognostic study of urothelial renal pelvic tumors. Cancer 1979;43:2525.
10. Strong D, et al. The ureteral stump after nephroureterectomy. J Urol 1976;115:654.
11. Fraley E. Cancer of the renal pelvis. In: Skinner DG, deKernion JB, eds. Genitourinary cancer. Philadelphia: WB Saunders, 1978.
12. Petkovic S. Conservation of the kidney in operations for tumors of the pelves and calyces: a report of 26 cases. Br J Urol 1972;44:1.
13. Zincke H, Neves R. Feasibility of conservative surgery for transitional cell cancer of the upper urinary tract. Urol Clin North Am 1984;11:717.

11

Distal Ureterectomy

Ian M. Thompson

Transitional cell carcinoma of the renal pelvis and ureter accounts for approximately 2600 newly diagnosed malignancies annually in the United States (1). Transitional cell carcinoma of the ureter constitutes only 2 to 5% of all uroepithelial tumors, perhaps due to the small total surface area of the ureter or to the short durations of exposure of the urothelium of the ureter to urinary components (2, 3). Tumors of the renal pelvis are 2.5 times more common than their counterparts in the ureter. Despite their uncommon nature, it often requires all of the urologist's diagnostic skills to establish the diagnosis of this neoplasm; the reason is their location. The more common conditions that can mimic their presence include ureteral stones, clots, sloughed papillae. With the development of improved staging techniques, improved endoscopic equipment, and techniques of local tumor biopsy or ablation, the opportunity for renal preservation has become more common for this tumor. Of all organ-preserving techniques for this tumor, distal ureterectomy provides optimal cancer control while maintaining normal urinary tract function.

PATHOGENESIS

Like the analogous epithelium of the urinary bladder, a number of agents have been implicated in the development of transitional cell carcinoma of the ureter. The most common cause in the United States has been cigarette smoking. Patients who smoke have been found to have a 2.5-fold higher risk of development of ureteral tumors (4). Although rarely seen in clinical use today, phenacetin was a common component of headache remedies of years past. Abuse of this substance was well documented to be highly associated with the development of transitional cell carcinoma of the renal pelvis and ureter (4). Other agents that have been found to be associated with the development of transitional cell carcinoma of the ureter include cyclophosphamide, chronic infection, and stone or foreign body reaction (5, 6). A rare cause of the development of this disease is Balkan nephropathy, a condition reported in the Balkan countries of Yugoslavia, Romania, and Bulgaria (7). In these patients, whose principal complications are due to renal failure, there is a hundredfold increased risk of transitional cell carcinoma of the upper tract; in 10% of these patients, the tumors are bilateral. The exact cause of this phenomenon is unknown.

PATHOLOGY

The most common type of ureter tumor is transitional cell carcinoma, which comprises more than 90% of all primary tumors (8). Other tumor types that have been reported, in order of occurrence, include adenocarcinoma, squamous cell carcinoma, small cell carcinoma, and sarcomas and metastatic lesions from the breast, colon, rectum, cervix, prostate, and bladder (1, 9–11). As previously noted, benign lesions such as stones, sloughed papillae, and blood clots can mimic ureteral tumors. Occasionally, extrinsic compression from pelvic lymphadenopathy can mimic filling defects of the distal ureter. benign polyps, although unusual, can present a diagnostic challenge (12). These latter lesions are most notable for their length and thin stalk, but histologic evaluation is necessary to establish this diagnosis. Figure 11.1 demonstrates the papillary nature of this neoplasm, with its fibrovascular core extending from the ureteral wall.

PRESENTATION

Because the majority of ureteral tumors will be low or moderate grade and associated with a papillary growth pattern at diagnosis, patients will most often present with symptoms of obstruction or bleeding. In a recent series of 108 patients with upper urinary tract tumors, hematuria was a presenting symptom in 76% and flank pain in 33% (13). These symptoms are associated with the best prognoses, whereas systemic symptoms such as weight loss, lymphadenopathy, bone or back pain, or an abdominal mass are most often associated with an advanced tumor. The importance of continued public education regarding symptom recognition is illustrated by series demonstrating delays in presentation of up to 9 years and an average delay in diagnosis of 7 months from the development of initial symptoms (14, 15).

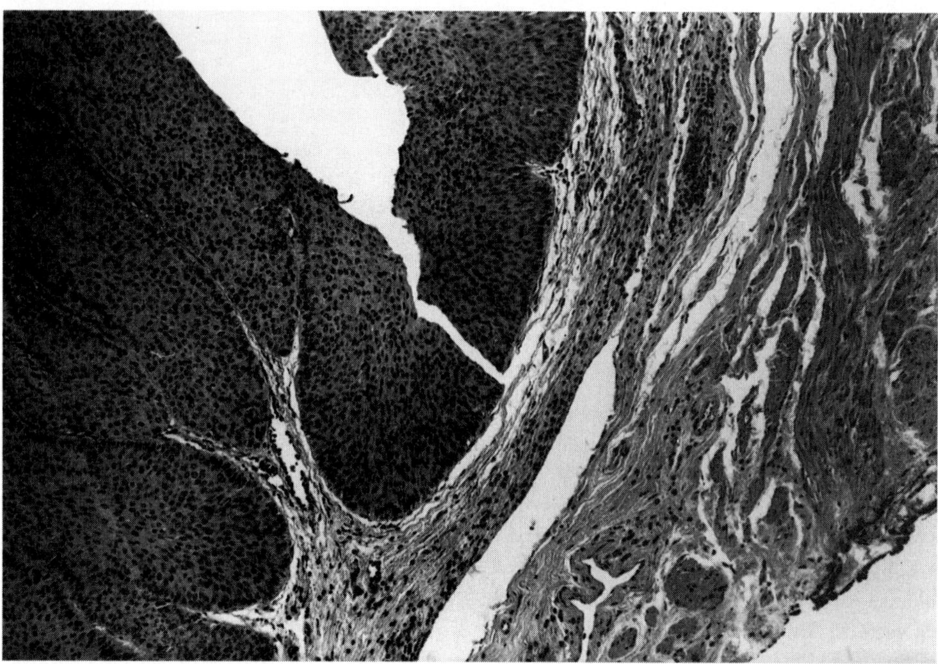

Fig. 11.1.   Papillary transitional cell carcinoma of the ureter, noninvasive.

NATURAL HISTORY AND STAGING

Many of the characteristics of ureteral tumors are similar to those of urinary bladder tumors, and it is appropriate to consider the entire urothelium—bladder, ureter, and renal pelvis—as an area at risk for coexistent disease or for recurrence. The term polychronotropism refers to this field change phenomenon, in which the entire urothelium has been exposed to agent(s) that lead to genetic instability and the risk for tumor development (Fig. 11.2). This concept meshes well with the finding that bladder tumors can be expected in 10 to 55% of patients with a history of ureteral tumors and that contralateral, metachronous ureteral tumors will develop in 2 to 10% of patients (7, 16, 17).

Early data from patients treated with bacillus Calmette-Guérin (BCG) for carcinoma in situ of the bladder showed that a significant number with distal ureteral tumors were suspicious for

pagetoid spread of transitional cell carcinoma into the distal ureter (18). More recently, a number of authors have found that the risk for subsequent upper tract transitional cell carcinoma may be most likely in patients with the highest grade and stage of disease. In 82 patients treated with BCG for recurrent superficial tumors, upper tract tumors subsequently developed in 13.4% (19). Most worrisome was the finding that 64% of these patients subsequently died of their ureteral carcinoma.

Several staging systems have been applied to ureteral tumors, the most frequent one being a modification of Jewett's system of bladder tumor staging. The TNM system that was developed by the American Joint Committee on Cancer has recently been used (20, 21). Table 11.1 lists both systems and estimates of 5-year survival by stage.

DIAGNOSIS

The first clue that a patient has a ureteral tumor will usually be provided by a radiographic study. A heightened index of suspicion should be present when a patient with a history of bladder tumors presents with hematuria or flank pain or especially when a patient is receiving BCG for high-grade bladder cancer. Intravenous pyelography (IVP) will generally demonstrate one of two findings—obstruction or some form of filling defect. If the former is noted, delayed images may outline the ureteral tumor and should always be obtained. Due to the effusive growth pattern of papillary tumors, filling defects occasionally will demonstrate contrast outline papillary fronds. Commonly, a meniscus-like cutoff of the column of ureteral contrast will have the appearance of a goblet, thus the term chalice sign. Further characterization of the extent of the lesion should be

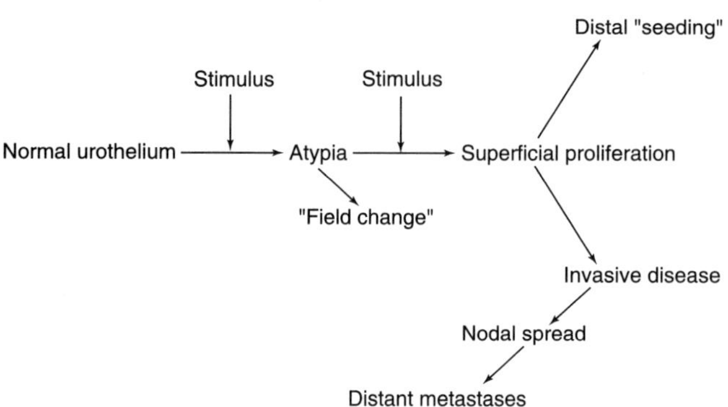

Fig. 11.2.   Theoretical pathway of tumor development and spread.

Table 11.1. Staging and Survival of Ureteral Cancer (20, 21)

MODIFIED JEWETT SYSTEM		5-YEAR SURVIVAL (%)	AJCC TNM SYSTEM	
STAGE	DESCRIPTION		STAGE	DESCRIPTION
			TX	Primary tumor cannot be assessed
			T0	No evidence of primary tumor
			TIS	Carcinoma in situ
O	Confined to mucosa	100	Ta	Papillary noninvasive carcinoma
A	Involvement through lamina propria	80–95	T1	Tumor invades subepithelial connective tissue
B	Into muscular wall	40–80	T2	Tumor invades muscularis
C	Periureteral spread	15–33	T3	Tumor invades beyond muscularis into periureteric or peripelvic fat or renal parenchyma
D	Metastatic disease	0–7	T4	Tumor invades adjacent organs or through the kidney into perinephric fat
			NX	Regional lymph nodes cannot be assessed
			N0	No regional lymph node metastasis
			N1	Metastasis in a single lymph node, 2 cm or less in greatest dimension
			N2	Metastasis in a single lymph node, more than 2 cm but not more than 5 cm in greatest dimension, or multiple lymph nodes, none more than 5 cm in greatest dimension
			N3	Metastasis in a lymph node more than 5 cm in greatest dimension
			MX	Presence of distant metastasis cannot be assessed
			M0	No distant metastasis
			M1	Distant metastasis

obtained with retrograde pyelography (Fig. 11.3). At the time of this procedure, a ureteral catheter can be passed to the level of the lesion for barbotage cytology collection or a brush can be used to obtain fragments of tissue. Such retrograde brushing of the lesion can improve the diagnostic accuracy to more than 80% (22).

With contemporary ureteroscopic equipment, small ureteroscopes can often be easily negotiated without ureteral dilation to the level of the lesion for direct visual confirmation and for biopsy (Fig. 11.4). Care must be taken to prevent ureteral perforation and potential extravasation of tumor cells. Special comment must be made concerning patients who are receiving BCG for bladder tumors. These patients have a propensity for the development of distal ureteral tumors. The development of distal ureteral stenosis in these patients must be evaluated carefully to rule out this diagnosis.

Entities that can mimic ureteral tumors include sloughed papillae, stones, and blood clots. Papillary necrosis should be suspected in those patients with characteristic calyceal findings. Radiolucent calculi should be suspected in patients who have a history of stone disease or have risk factors for uric acid stone disease (e.g., dehydration, ileostomy). In these patients, ultrasound or computed tomography (CT) scan may demonstrate the stone or an empiric trial of alkalinization may be attempted. It must be emphasized that in all patients with presumed ureteral pathologic conditions, complete evaluation of the kidney and proximal ureter is mandatory. Indeed, a frequent presentation of renal cell carcinoma may be bleeding with ureteral obstruction from clots. Thus, should the diagnosis of a clot obstructing a ureter be entertained, complete assurance that the upper tract is otherwise healthy must be obtained.

TREATMENT OPTIONS

Nephroureterectomy

Reynes has been credited as having performed the first nephroureterectomy (23). Since that time, this procedure has been described as the gold standard for urothelial tumors of the renal pelvis and ureter. Traditionally, four reasons have been given for the selection of this procedure.

1. Transitional cell carcinoma is multifocal. In many patients with upper tract transitional cell tumors, simultaneous and metachronous recurrences are common. Mufti et al. found that if tumors were multifocal, segmental upper tract resection was associated with an ipsilateral recurrence rate of 50% (24). Nephroureterectomy, by definition, eliminates this potential cause of morbidity.
2. Contralateral tumors are exceptionally rare. The risk of subsequent development of contralateral upper tract tumors is low—between 1 and 2% (15, 24). Thus, the risk of subsequent renal compromise by the treatment of a contralateral tumor is very low.
3. Ipsilateral tumor recurrence is high if the entire urothelium is not removed. Murphy et al. reported a

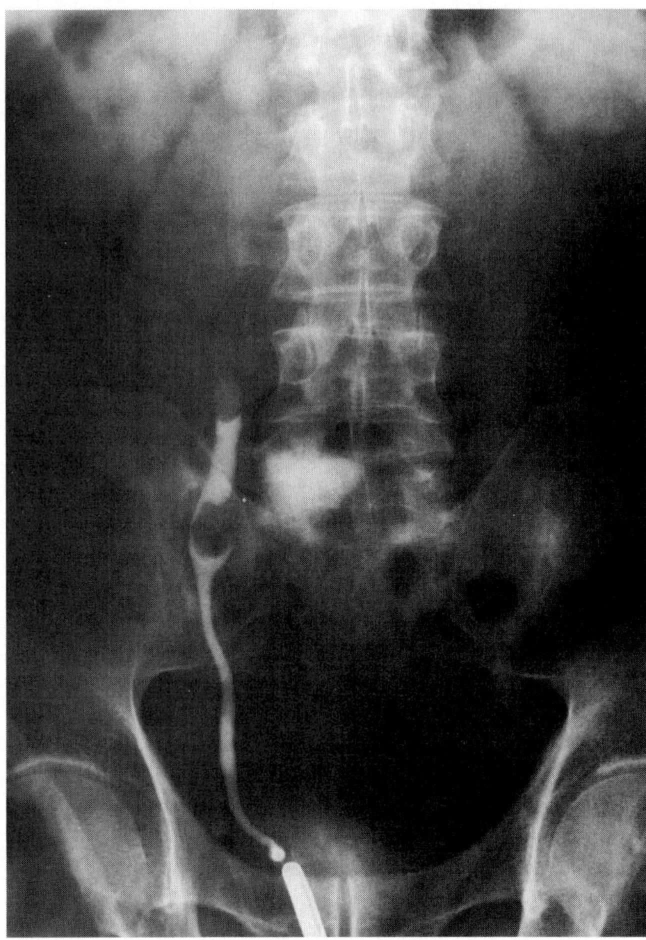

Fig. 11.3.   Retrograde pyelogram demonstrates irregular filling defect due to transitional cell carcinoma of the ureter.

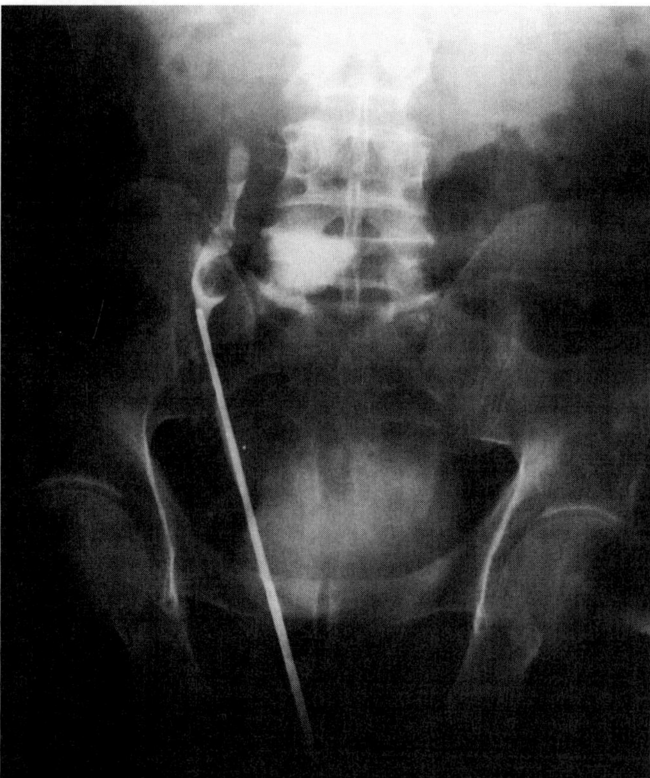

Fig. 11.4.   Ureteroscope advanced for visual confirmation and biopsy of tumor.

28% ipsilateral recurrence rate if the entire urothelium was not removed (15). Similarly, Mufti et al. found the ipsilateral recurrence rate with conservative management to be 22.4% (24).

4. Follow-up is simplified after nephroureterectomy. With recurrence rates in the 25% range if the ipsilateral urothelium is not completely removed, nephroureterectomy eliminates the need for frequent imaging of the upper tracts.

Conservative Management

Although Vest is credited with providing the first evidence that renal-preserving surgery is possible and will provide good cancer control for selected patients with upper tract transitional cell carcinoma, Robards et al. may have presented the most compelling argument for this procedure (25, 26). These authors noted that the principles of cancer control for transitional cell carcinoma of the ureter should be similar to those for the bladder. Thus, no urologist would consider performing a cystectomy for a grade 1, Ta tumor of the bladder. Similarly, perform-

ing a physiologic resection of such a tumor in the ureter (segmental or distal ureterectomy) should provide a similar opportunity for cancer control as for the same tumor in the bladder.

There are a number of opportunities for conservative management of ureteral tumors. Among them are ureteroscopic resection or fulguration, laser ablation, and segmental resection of the ureter (27, 28). Advantages of the first two techniques are the minimal risk of the procedure, rapid return of function, and minimal morbidity. Disadvantages include the relative inability to sample the adjacent urothelium, small working area, risk of extravasation of tumor cells, and, for the latter, lack of tissue for pathologic evaluation. It is perhaps for this reason that the most commonly performed conservative procedure for ureteral carcinoma is segmental ureterectomy—most commonly, distal ureterectomy. Support for the efficacy of this procedure includes the following.

1. Staging and grading of the ureteral tumor can be determined preoperatively. Using cytologic examination, grading of the ureteral tumor can determine if a low-grade lesion is present that may be amenable to distal ureterectomy. Murphy et al. found that 95% of grade 1 tumors are noninvasive on final pathologic examination (15). Clinical tumor staging can be performed using a combination of IVP, ureteroscopy, and CT imaging (as necessary). A number of characteristics of the IVP can

Table 11.2. Outcomes With Conservative Therapy for Upper Tract Transitional Cell Carcinoma (24)

	5-YEAR SURVIVAL (%)	
	NEPHROURETERECTOMY	CONSERVATIVE THERAPY
Grade I	95	100
Grade II	82	62
Grade III	54	0
pTa	90	100
pT1	95	100
pT2–3	85	70
pT4	38	12

provide a clue regarding tumor stage. Gawley et al. found that if IVP demonstrated a filling defect, the 5-year survival rate was 72% (indicating low-stage lesions) (29). Conversely, if the patient presented with nonfunction, the 5-year survival rate was only 37%.

2. Stage of the ureteral tumor, not the treatment, dictates ultimate outcome. Virtually every series that has compared nephroureterectomy with conservative therapy for ureteral transitional cell carcinoma has found that the determinant of patient survival is tumor stage (as well as grade) and is generally independent of the treatment selected. Tables 11.2 and 11.3 summarize the experience of Mufti et al. and Mills and Vaughn comparing results of conservative management with those of nephroureterectomy (24,3). As can easily be seen, minimal differences are present when the two treatments are compared at similar grades and stages.

3. Excellent cancer control can be achieved with conservative surgery in properly selected patients.

Recurrence

One compelling reason to perform nephroureterectomy is to reduce the risk of ipsilateral recurrent tumor. With proper patient selection, this development should be unusual. In a series by Wallace et al. of conservatively managed patients, they summarized 35 years of such reports (30). Data from a total of 277 patients in 13 series showed ipsilateral recurrences in 37 patients (13%). Further follow-up found that only 8 of 277 patients (2.8%) died of malignant disease during follow-

Table 11.3. Survival Following Nephroureterectomy or Conservative Therapy

	SURVIVAL (%)	
STAGE	NEPHROURETERECTOMY	DISTAL URETERECTOMY
O	100	—
A	80	100
B	50	50
C	40	0
D	14	—

up. Other authors have reported higher rates of ipsilateral recurrence, including Mufti et al.'s 22.4% and Murphy et al.'s 28% (15, 24). Conversely, Anderstrom et al., in a series of all tumor grades, found a recurrence rate of only 5% (31). Tumor grade appears to be the principal determinant of ipsilateral recurrence, with recurrence rates for grades 1, 2, 3, and 4 tumors in Zincke and Neves' series being 8%, 0%, 40%, and 100%, respectively (32).

Survival

Although it appears that the risk of ipsilateral recurrence after partial ureterectomy for transitional cell carcinoma will certainly lead to a higher ipsilateral recurrence rate than that associated with nephroureterectomy, this difference does not seem to translate into a reduction in survival time for properly selected patients. Indeed, in all series that compare these two entities, survival for grade 1 and stages Ta/T1 tumors is the same, regardless of the type of excision. It must be noted, however, that some degree of survival advantage has been suggested for some groups of patients treated with nephroureterectomy; this includes patients whose tumors are pT2 to 4 (24), T3 (3), grade 2, and grade 3 (15).

From a practical standpoint, although segmental resection of the ureter is a relatively simple procedure, the ideal patient has a tumor in a sufficiently distal location to allow distal ureterectomy and ureteral reimplantation. Fortuitously, most low-stage ureteral tumors will occur in the distal one-third of the ureter in a position to allow for this procedure (33, 34). Advantages of this procedure include a lower risk of ureteral stricture, ability to remove long distal ureteral segments (through the use of psoas hitch and Boari flap), and minimal postoperative morbidity. Additionally, the creation of a widely refluxing ureteral anastomosis high above the bladder neck will occasionally facilitate both reflux of intravesical chemotherapy and direct access for ureteroscopy.

PATIENT SELECTION AND PREOPERATIVE EVALUATION

Criteria for patient selection for distal ureterectomy include the following.

Definite Indications
• Bilateral tumors
• Solitary kidney
• Renal insufficiency
Relative Indications
• Low-grade, low-stage tumor
• Tumor in distal ureter—amenable for distal ureterectomy
Contraindications
• Multiple tumors
• Presence of carcinoma in situ
• Evidence of muscle-invasive disease

It is essential that the urologist diligently search for evidence of either multifocal tumors (through retrograde pyelography and, as necessary, ureteroscopy) or ureteral muscle invasion (usually inferred from radiographic studies and, as necessary, with CT scans). Although uncommon, the possibility of bilateral tumors should be considered, and imaging studies should assure that the contralateral collecting system is completely normal.

Preoperative medical evaluation should be tailored to the patient's medical history. Because of the advanced age of these patients (average of 65 years in many series), a meticulous review of systems (concentrating on cardiovascular and pulmonary symptoms) should be performed. All patients should undergo electrocardiography, and urinalysis results should be free of evidence of infection. Serum creatinine levels should be measured in all patients; if there is evidence of renal insufficiency, creatinine clearance should be performed. Patients who smoke should be encouraged to stop a minimum of 2 weeks preoperatively. No bowel preparation is performed, but all patients receive a single intravenous dose of a cephalosporin 1 hour preoperatively and compression stockings are placed as the patient enters the operating theater. These remain in place until the patient is ambulating postoperatively.

DISTAL URETERECTOMY

Anatomy of the Ureter

The ureter courses toward the pelvis, lying in its upper third on the anterior surface of the psoas major muscle. After crossing the iliac vessels at the level of the bifurcation of the common iliac artery, it courses laterally and posterior then medially to pass behind the bladder to enter its intramural tunnel. During its course above the pelvis, the ureter is often adherent to the posterior peritoneum and can most easily be located using this relation.

In the male, after crossing the iliac vessels, the ureter lies in proximity to the hypogastric artery and passes posterior to the vas deferens and, more distally, posterior to the superior vesical artery. After coursing retrovesically, the ureter enters its muscular hiatus at the cranial aspect of the seminal vesicle.

In the female, the ureter lies behind the round ligament and makes a steeper course into the pelvis, lying posterior to the uterine and superior vesical arteries. During this course, the ureter receives arterial tributaries from the uterine, vesical, and hypogastric arteries.

Surgical Technique

The patient is placed on the operating table in the supine position. The break in the operating table is placed cranial to the iliac crest, and the table is flexed. Either general or spinal anesthesia can be used with the understanding that, if intraoperative assessment suggests the need for nephroureterectomy, the patient with a regional block may require intubation. After preparing and draping the patient, an 18F Foley catheter with 5-mL balloon is placed in the bladder.

Any number of incisions are suitable for distal ureterectomy. We have found the lower midline incision to be ideal for this procedure. It is well understood by urologists who are almost universally facile with the technique of pelvic lymphadenectomy. If necessary, this incision can be extended superiorly to allow for nephroureterectomy. Other suitable incisions include the Gibson incision, Pfannensteil, and paramedian.

The incision is made in the midline from the umbilicus to the pubis. The fascia is divided, and the transversalis fascia is

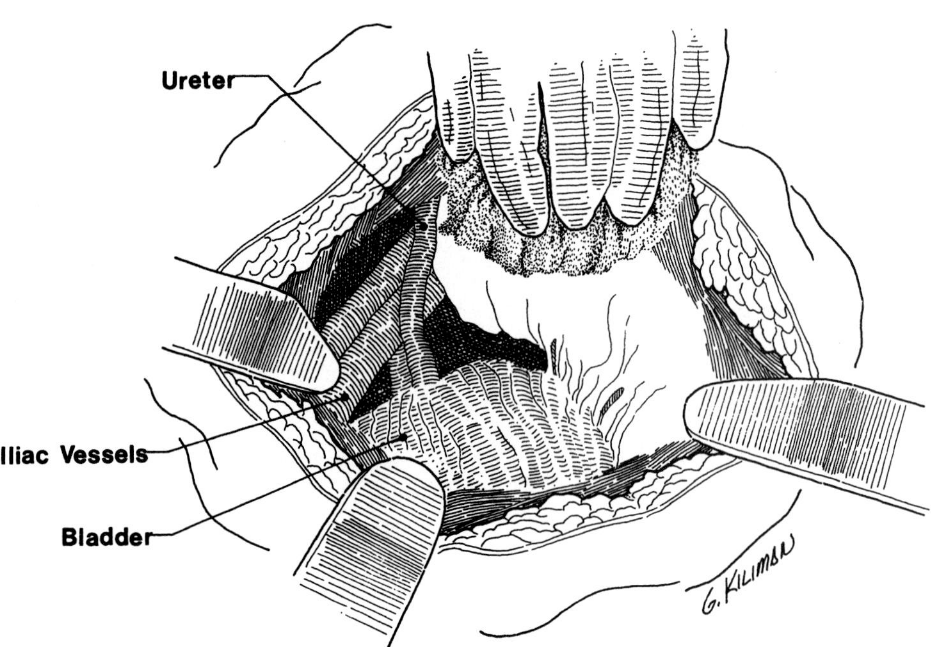

Fig. 11.5.   The incision is carried through the posterior rectus fascia. The peritoneum is swept cranially, exposing the course of the distal ureter.

consciously divided to allow access in the proper plane lateral to the bladder. As the perivesical space is dissected, attention should be directed to the placement of retractor blades. If properly placed, deep to the transversalis fascia, avulsion of the inferior epigastric vein or artery will not occur. With blunt dissection, the retroperitoneal space on the surface of the psoas muscle can be developed, and by sharply dividing lateral peritoneal attachments, the peritoneum can be swept medially and cranially. This then allows complete exposure of the course of

the ureter from well above the iliac vessels to its intramural portion. At this time, we generally place a self-retaining retractor is generally placed.

The ureter can now be identified as it crosses the iliac vessels (Fig. 11.5). It must be recalled that it is often "attached" to the posterior peritoneum and may have been reflected medially during the previous dissection. A vessel loop is placed about the ureter and it is dissected as far as possible to the intramural hiatus. Often, small ureteral vessels are encountered and should

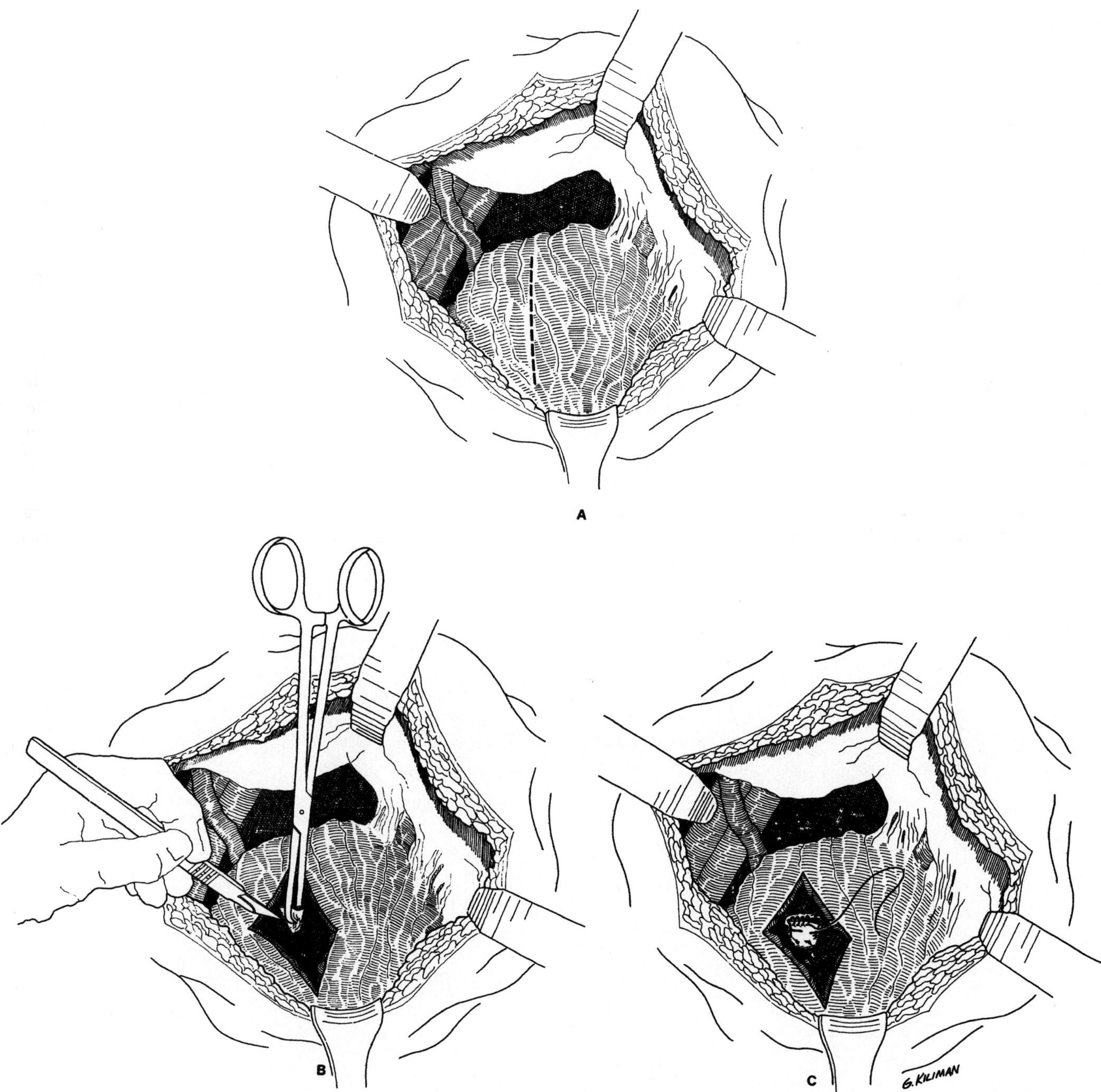

Fig. 11.6.   A. Line of incision in the bladder. **B.** The ipsilateral ureteral orifice is grasped with a long Allis clamp. The bladder mucosa about the ureteral orifice is incised. **C.** With traction on the oversewn orifice, the intramural ureter is dissected through the bladder.

be clipped with small metal clips before division to prevent troublesome bleeding during this portion of the dissection. The area of the tumor should be readily apparent by comparing radiographic studies (which must be available in the operating room) with palpation of the ureter. If there is evidence of ureteral nodularity or fibrosis or gross evidence of extramural spread, a frozen section should be considered. If pathologic inspection reveals muscular involvement, strong consideration should be given to nephroureterectomy. In general, formal pelvic lymphadenectomy is not performed but nodal regions (obturator, hypogastric, iliac) should be palpated. If abnormalities are noted, nodes should be sampled for pathologic evaluation.

After the ureter has been dissected to its entry into the intramural tunnel, a midline cystostomy is made with electrocautery (Fig. 11.6A). A malleable blade for the self-retaining retractor is then placed to retract the bladder superiorly, allowing identification of the ureteral orifice. The ureteral orifice is grasped with an Allis clamp, and a circumferential incision is made through the mucosa around the orifice with the electrocautery, a scalpel, or fine scissors (Fig. 11.6B). Following deeper dissection, the ureteral orifice is oversewn with 3-0 silk suture that is then used for traction (Fig. 11.6C). The intramural ureter is further mobilized with Metzenbaum scissors until the ureter is completely free.

The ureter is then brought out into the paravesical space, and a large clip is applied 1 cm above the ureteral tumor (Fig. 11.7). The ureter is divided above the clip and sent for frozen section to ensure that the proximal margin is free of urothelial disease. The position of the clip is noted on the pathology slip to prevent confusion on the part of the pathologist. The ureteral

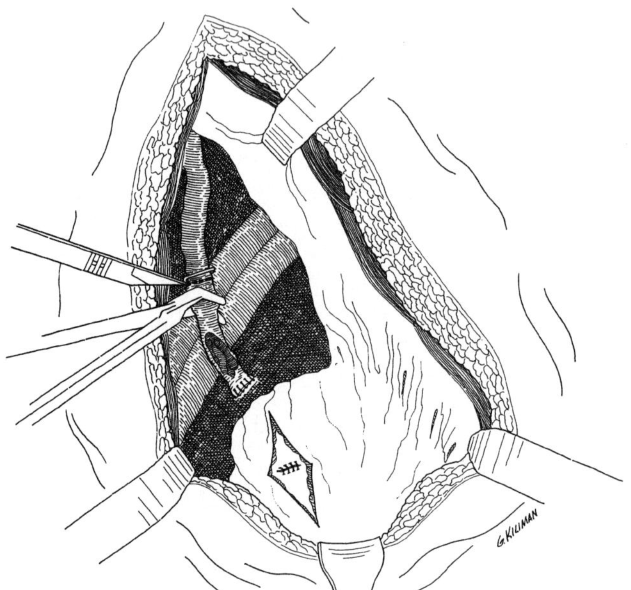

Fig. 11.7. The ureter is passed through the ureteral hiatus and dissected free of its attachments to several centimeters above the tumor. A right-angle clamp is placed 2 cm above the tumor and a clip is placed proximal to the clamp. The ureter is then divided between the two.

hiatus is closed in two layers, first closing the muscle layer with interrupted 2-0 chromic sutures followed by closure of the mucosa with interrupted 3-0 chromic sutures. If the pathologist confirms negative margins and no evidence of muscle-invasive disease, ureteral reimplantation commences. If the ureteral margin is positive for disease, a higher segment is excised. This can be performed several times until negative margins are obtained. However, if multifocal disease or muscle invasive disease is found, nephroureterectomy should be considered.

URETERAL REIMPLANTATION

Ureteroneocystostomy

Because many ureteral tumors occur so distally, direct reimplantation is often possible. To do so, adequate mobilization is necessary while preserving the periureteral blood supply (coursing in the adventitia) to prevent postoperative ischemia that can lead to stricture, obstruction, or urinary extravasation. By selecting a site for reimplantation on the superior aspect of the bladder, minimal mobilization is often necessary. A tonsil clamp is passed from within the bladder through the bladder wall (Fig. 11.8A). This maneuver can usually be performed bluntly but, on occasion, a stab incision will facilitate the clamps passage. With a spreading motion, the neohiatus is widened. A tag suture of 3-0 chromic is placed in the distal ureter, grasped with the tonsil clamp, and the ureter is gently pulled into the bladder. Using either a right-angle or long-tonsil clamp, a 2- to 3-cm submucosal tunnel is created in the direction of the bladder neck (Fig. 11.8B). A stab incision is made at the lower limit of the tunnel. A second clamp is passed retrograde through the tunnel, the ureteral tag is grasped, and the ureter is passed gently through the tunnel (Fig. 11.8C). The ureter is spatulated and anastomosed to the bladder with interrupted 5-0 chromic sutures. Two distal sutures of 4-0 chromic are placed deeply into the detrusor muscle to secure adequately the ureter and prevent retraction (Fig. 11.8D). The mucosa overlying the new ureteral hiatus is closed with interrupted 5-0 chromic sutures.

Although ureteral stenting is not required, edema commonly leads to transient obstruction. For this reason, a 6-French, double-J ureteral stent is placed. By sewing a 4-0 nylon suture to the distal stent and bringing this out the urethra, cystoscopic examination for stent removal is unnecessary. (Some stent manufacturers have stents with nylon sutures preloaded.) This stent can be removed between 10 and 20 days postoperatively. A 26-French Malecot suprapubic catheter is placed through a separate incision into the bladder and brought out medial to the wound. A large Penrose drain is placed lateral to the bladder and brought out through a separate stab incision.

Psoas Hitch

Lesions of the upper pelvic ureter usually require mobilization of the bladder and psoas hitch to achieve a tension-free anasto-

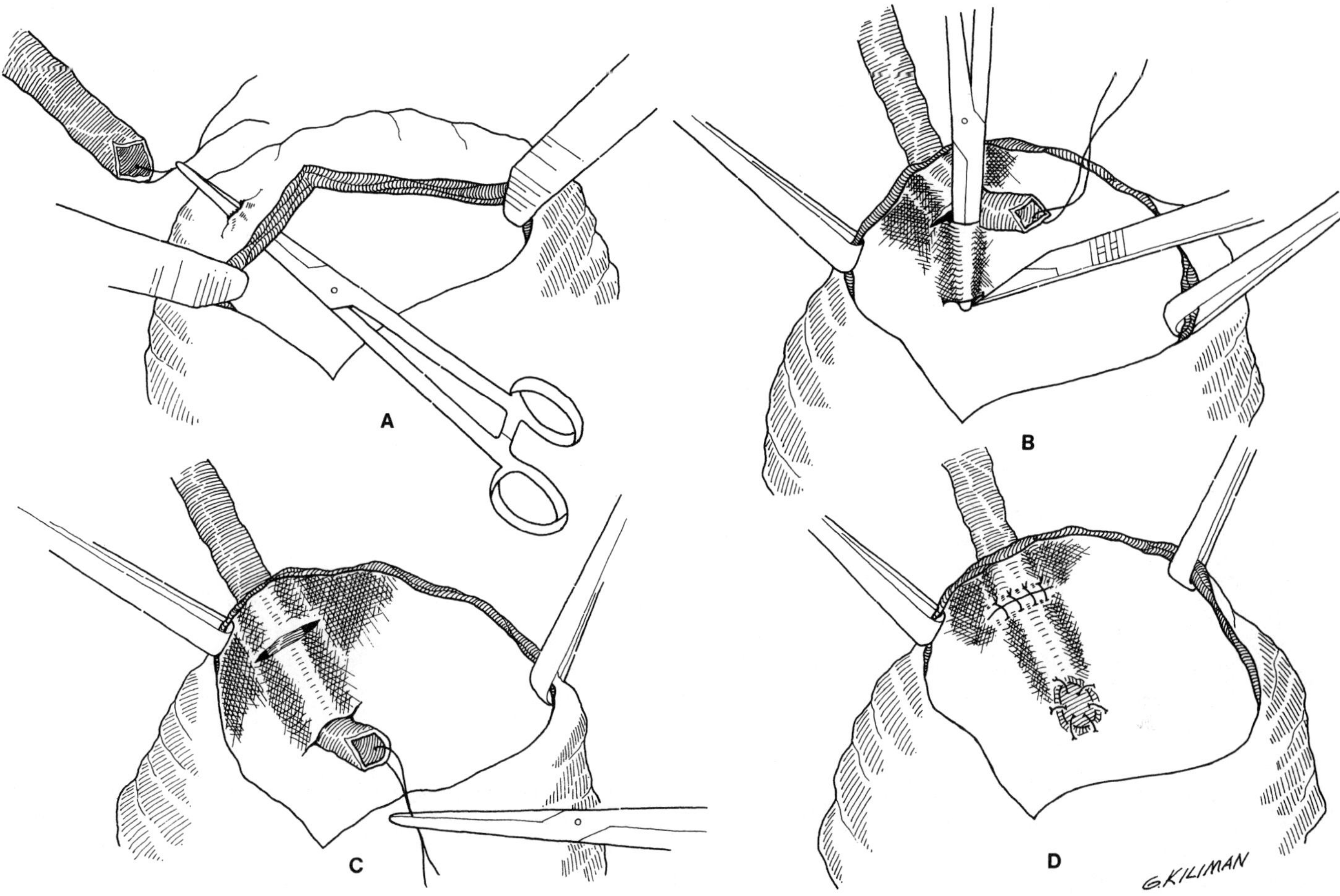

Fig. 11.8. **A.** A long tonsil clamp is passed through the bladder wall and the neohiatus widened. The ureteral traction suture is grasped and the ureter is pulled into the bladder. **B.** A submucosal tunnel has been created inferomedially from the new ureteral hiatus. **C.** With the traction suture, the ureter is gently advanced through the tunnel. **D.** The new ureteral orifice is created with interrupted sutures of 5-0 chromic catgut. Two 4-0 chromic sutures are placed distally to minimize the risk of retraction.

mosis. This maneuver will allow a minimum of 4 to 5 cm of additional length. It is often necessary to sweep the peritoneum off the dome of the bladder and to take down the superior bladder pedicle on the contralateral side to allow sufficient mobilization. The surgeon's fingers are then inserted into the bladder incision, and a horn of bladder is pulled toward the tendon of the psoas muscle and the mobilized ureteral stump (Fig. 11.9A). A row of 2-0 chromic sutures are then placed along the horn of bladder, deeply into the detrusor muscle, and then into the tendon of the psoas muscle. When performing this maneuver, it is essential to avoid incorporation of the genitofemoral nerve.

The sutures are then tied, and inspection of the hitch should reveal considerable overlap between the dissected ureter and mobilized bladder. Ureteral reimplantation is then performed as described above (Fig. 11.9B). Catheters and drains are identical. The need for an antirefluxing ureterovesical anastomosis should be discussed here. It is not clear that such an anastomosis will reduce postoperative morbidity (e.g., pyelonephritis) in adults who undergo ureteroneocystostomy. Additionally, ad-

vantages of a "fishmouth" direct ureteral anastomosis include facilitated ureteroscopic inspection of the ureter, easier retrograde pyelograms, and the theoretical advantage of reflux of intravesical agents (e.g., BCG) into the upper tract. Additional advantages of this type of anastomosis are that less ureteral length is required for the anastomosis and less ureteral manipulation is required.

Boari Flap

If the bladder will not reach the distal ureter at the time of the hitch maneuver, a Boari flap should be used to span the gap. Ideally, the surgeon should recognize the need for this procedure when the ureterectomy is performed. In general, if the distal ureteral stump lies more than 2 to 4 cm above the iliac vessels, a flap will be required. Some surgeons will routinely perform a flap for any lesion above the vessels to assure a tension-free anastomosis. Indeed, other than the additional surgical time, little additional risk is run by adding a Boari flap to the psoas hitch.

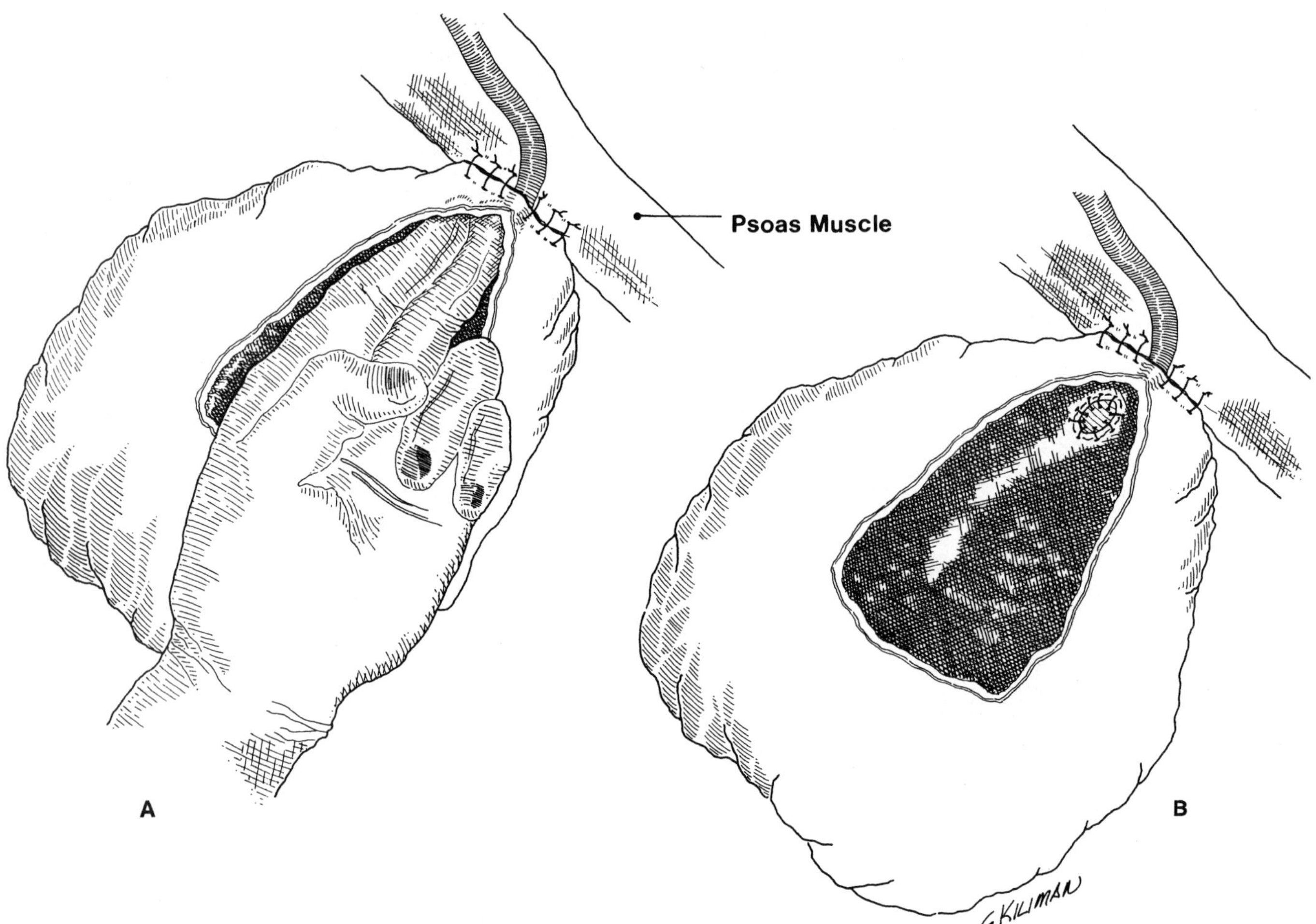

Fig. 11.9. A. The surgeon's hand is used to elevate the bladder to the ipsilateral psoas muscle. Several 2-0 chromic sutures are placed between the bladder and the psoas fascia. **B.** The ureter is brought into the submucous tunnel and anastomosed to the new site of implantation.

The peritoneum is swept off the bladder dome, and a flap with a base placed posteriorly is created. It is helpful to make the bladder flap 4 to 5 cm longer than the ureteral defect, with the flap's base being at least 4 cm wide. The apex of the flap is marked with a stay suture, and the flap is completed using electrocautery (Fig. 11.10A and B). Either a submucosal ureteroneocystostomy or a direct ureteral anastomosis is created at the apex of the flap (Fig. 11.10C and D). To prevent retraction of the flap, a psoas hitch is generally performed simultaneously. As in the ureterocystostomy above, two apical deep sutures are placed from the ureter into the detrusor muscle. Additional sutures from the bladder serosa to the ureter can be placed outside the anastomosis, but care must be taken to prevent obstruction or kinking. A ureteral stent is generally placed as is a suprapubic tube. The bladder closure is begun at the apex of the flap, tubularizing it from the ureteral anastomosis to the bladder proper. Initial interrupted sutures of 2-0 chromic at the flap's apex are replaced by a running suture of 2-0 chromic in the detrusor component of the closure.

Closure

Both the suprapubic tube and Penrose or Hemovac drain are brought out through separate stab incisions and secured with nylon sutures. The suprapubic tube is inspected to ensure that only the wings and tip of the tube are in the bladder. Allowing a long portion of the tube to rest on the trigone will often lead to severe bladder spasms, possibly causing disruption of the bladder reconstruction or tension on the ureteral anastomosis. The wound is irrigated with saline solution, and the fascia is closed. The skin is closed with staples. An elastic abdominal fishnet is often useful because it allows frequent dressing changes without the skin irritation associated with tape.

Postoperative Care

During the immediate postoperative period, urine output is recorded every 2 hours and the suprapubic catheter is checked and, if necessary, irrigated to ensure unobstructed drainage. Ambulation is begun no later than the morning of the first

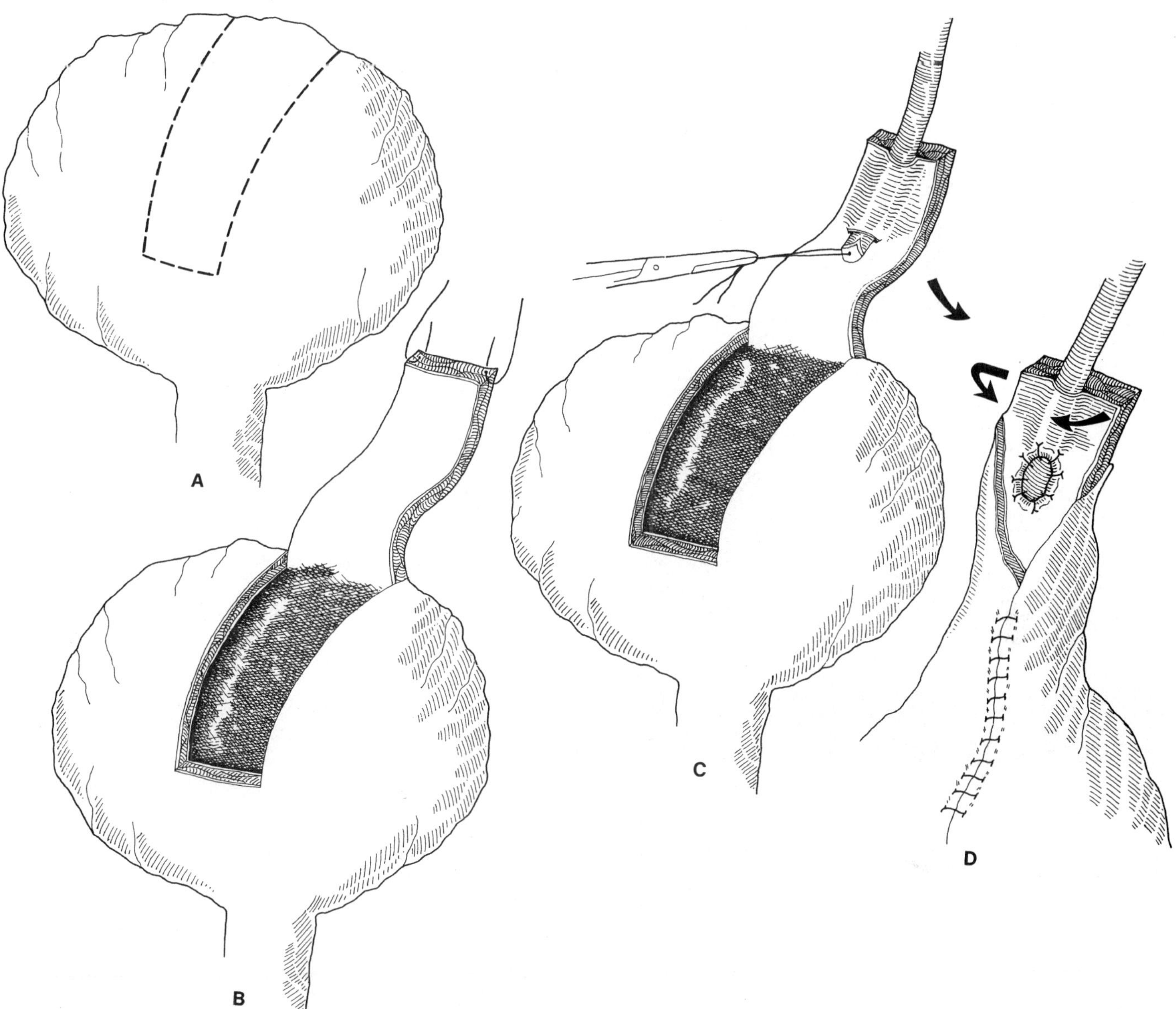

Fig. 11.10. A. A posteriorly based flap is marked to prepare the Boari flap. Although depicted here as rectangular, additional length can be obtained using an oblique or curved flap. **B.** The Boari flap has been fashioned and elevated. Traction sutures at the corners of the flap assist in manipulation during ureteral reimplantation. **C.** The ureter is brought through the submucosal tunnel in the flap. **D.** Ureteral implantation is completed. The Boari flap is closed along with the bladder using two layers of interrupted chromic catgut sutures.

postoperative day. Oral feedings are withheld until active bowel sounds are heard and the patient is passing flatus. Earlier feeding, although an extraperitoneal approach has been used, often leads to nausea or an ileus and may significantly delay hospital discharge. Serum electrolytes are monitored daily until oral intake commences. In general, complete blood counts are unnecessary because blood loss should be minimal from the procedure and postoperative bleeding is distinctly uncommon.

The suprapubic catheter is removed 5 days postoperatively and the Penrose drain is removed the following day. The double-J stent is removed 10 to 20 days postoperatively using the attached nylon string per urethra. An IVP is performed 6 weeks after surgery. Mild fullness of the collecting system and ureter is common due to residual edema. In patients who have undergone a Boari flap procedure, a persistent bladder horn will be noted on voiding cystourethrography (Fig. 11.11).

Complications

Complications are rare. Bleeding is rarely a problem, but troublesome oozing can cause clots to obstruct the suprapubic tube. Infection is also unusual if preoperative urine is sterile and perioperative antibiotics are used. The most common procedure-specific complication is obstruction at the ureterovesical

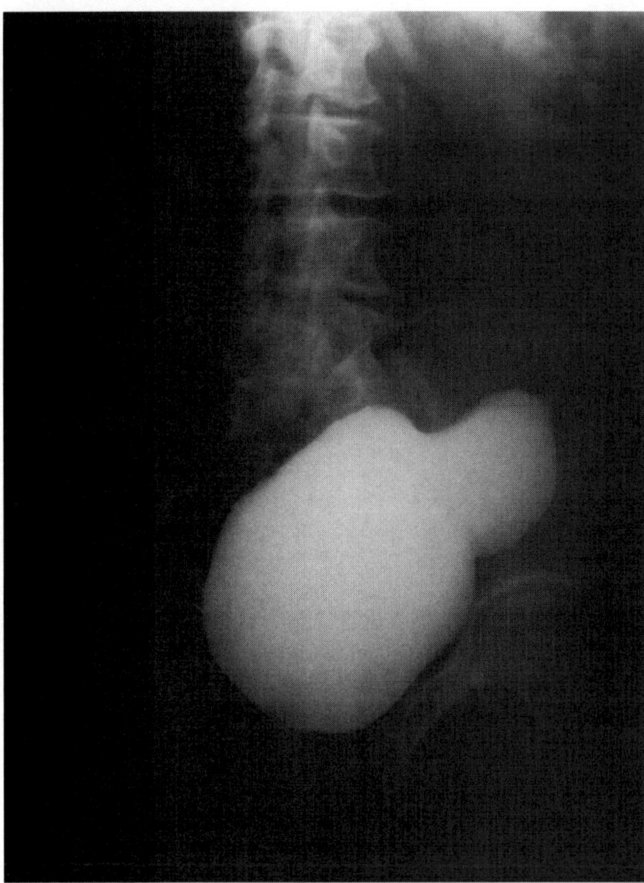

Fig. 11.11. Characteristic bladder "horn" following left Boari flap and nonrefluxing ureteroneocystostomy.

anastomosis and is usually due to overzealous ureteral skeletonization or excessive tension on the ureterovesical anastomosis. Kinking of the ureter can also cause postoperative obstruction. This can often be detected at the time of placement of the double-J stent and, if encountered, the anastomosis should be taken down and reconstructed. As previously noted, vesicoureteral reflux is not necessarily a complication but can be beneficial should reflux of chemotherapy instilled in the bladder be desired.

Follow-up

Bladder tumors can develop in between 25 and 50% of patients with a history of upper tract ureteral carcinoma (16). For this reason, surveillance cystoscopy is mandatory for all such patients. The optimal follow-up of the ipsilateral ureter is ill-defined; as a minimum, IVP or retrograde pyelography should be performed at 6 months, 1 year, and annually thereafter. (In theory, the upper tract should be followed with the same schedule as if a bladder tumor were being followed.) At the time of each surveillance cystoscopy, voided urine cytologic study should be performed.

Adjuvant Therapy

Patients with low-grade, low-stage tumors do not require adjuvant therapy because the likelihood of cure is excellent with distal ureterectomy. However, patients in whom final pathologic evaluation reveals T2 to T4 or N+ disease, the risk for local and distant recurrence is high. Methotrexate, vinblastine, doxorubicin, cisplatin (MVAC) chemotherapy has been used for upper tract tumors but its effect on these tumors in an adjuvant setting is unknown (35). Previously, a number of authors have suggested that adjuvant external beam radiation therapy will reduce local recurrence of disease (36, 37). A recent series of 26 patients with T3 to T4 N0/+ disease was reviewed to determine the effect of adjuvant radiation (38). Although local recurrence was significantly reduced by the addition of radiation therapy, no effect was noted on patient survival.

ACKNOWLEDGMENTS

The opinions expressed herein are those of the author and do not necessarily reflect those of the Departments of the Army or Defense.

REFERENCES

1. Melamed MR, Reuter VE. Pathology and staging of urothelial tumors of the kidney and ureter. Urol Clin North Am 1993; 20:333.
2. Khan AU, Farrow GM, Zincke H, et al. Primary carcinoma in situ of the ureter and renal pelvis. J Urol 1979;121:681.
3. Mills C, Vaughan ED. Carcinoma of the ureter: natural history, management and 5-year survival. J Urol 1983;129: 275.
4. McCredie M, Stewart JH, Ford JM. Analgesics and tobacco as risk factors for cancer of the ureter and renal pelvis. J Urol 1983;130:28.
5. Moloney PJ, Fenster HN, McLoughlin MC. Carcinoma in the defunctionalized urinary tract. J Urol 1981;126:260.
6. Schiff HI, Finkel M, Shapira HE. Transitional cell carcinoma of the ureter associated with cyclophosphamide therapy for benign disease. J Urol 1982;128:1023.
7. Petkovic SD. Epidemiology and treatment of renal pelvic and ureteral tumors. J Urol 1975;114:858.
8. Babaian RJ, Johnson DE. Primary carcinoma of the ureter. J Urol 1980;123:357.
9. Ray P, Lingard WF. Primary adenocarcinoma of the ureter. J Urol 1971;106:655.
10. Werner JR, Klingensmith W, Denko JV. Leiomyosarcoma of the ureter: case report and review of the literature. J Urol 1959;82:68.
11. Richie JP, Withers G, Ehrlich RM. Ureteral obstruction secondary to metastatic tumors. Surg Gynecol Obstet 1979; 148:355.
12. Fiorelli C, Durval A, DiCello V, et al. Ureteral intussusception by a fibroepithelial polyp. J Urol 1981;126:110.
13. Charbit L, Gendreau MC, Mee S, et al. Tumors of the upper urinary tract: 10 years of experience. J Urol 1991;146:1243.
14. Murphy DM, Zincke H, Furlow WL. Primary grade 1

transitional cell carcinoma of the renal pelvis and ureter. J Urol 1980;123:629.

15. Murphy DM, Zincke H, Furlow WL. Management of high grade transitional cell carcinoma of the upper urinary tract. J Urol 1981;125:25.

16. Kakizoe T, Fujita J, Murase T, et al. Transitional cell carcinoma of the bladder in patients with renal pelvic and ureteral cancer. J Urol 1980;124:17.

17. Clayman RV, Lange PH, Fraley EE. Cancer of the upper urinary tract. In: Javadpour N, ed. Principles and management of urologic cancer. 2nd ed. Baltimore: Williams & Wilkins, 1983:544.

18. Herr HW, Whitmore WF. Ureteral carcinoma in situ after successful intravesical therapy for superficial bladder tumors: incidence, possible pathogenesis and management. J Urol 1987;138:292.

19. Miller EB, Eure GR, Schellhammer PF. Upper tract transitional cell carcinoma following treatment of superficial bladder cancer with BCG. Urology 1993;42:26.

20. Batata M, Grabstald H. Upper urinary tract urothelial tumors. Urol Clin North Am 1976;3:79.

21. American Joint Committee on Cancer. Renal pelvis and ureter. In: Manual for staging of cancer. 3rd ed. Philadelphia: JB Lippincott, 1988:205.

22. Blute RD, Gittes RR, Gittes RF. Renal brush biopsy: survey of indications, techniques, and results. J Urol 1981;126:146.

23. Colston JAC. Complete nephroureterectomy. J Urol 1935;33: 110.

24. Mufti GR, Gove JRW, Badenoch DF, et al. Transitional cell carcinoma of the renal pelvis and ureter. Br J Urol 1989;63: 135.

25. Vest SA. Conservative surgery in certain benign tumors of the ureter. J Urol 1945;153:97.

26. Robards V, Thompson IM, Ross G. Primary tumors of the ureter. JAMA 1964;187:778.

27. Grossman HB, Schwartz SL, Konnak JW. Ureteroscopic treatment of urothelial carcinoma of the ureter and renal pelvis. J Urol 1992,148:275.

28. Carson CC. Endoscopic treatment of upper and lower urinary tract lesions using lasers. Semin Urol 1991;3:185.

29. Gawley WF, Harney J, Glacken P, et al. Transitional cell carcinoma of upper urinary tract: some prognostic indicators. Urology 1989;33:459.

30. Wallace DMA, Wallace DM, Whitfield HN, et al. The late results of conservative surgery for upper tract urothelial carcinoma. Br J Urol 1981;53:537.

31. Anderstrom C, Johansson SL, Pettersson S, et al. Carcinoma of the ureter: a clinicopathologic study of 49 cases. J Urol 1989; 142:280.

32. Zincke H, Neves RJ. Feasibility of conservative surgery for transitional cell cancer of the upper urinary tract. Urol Clin North Am 1984;11:717.

33. Kim KH, Leiter E, Brendler H. Primary tumors of the ureter. J Urol 1972;107:955.

34. Werth DD, Weigel JW, Mebust WK. Primary neoplasms of the ureter. J Urol 1981;125:628.

35. Scher HI, et al. Neoadjuvant MVAC (methotrexate, vinblastine, doxorubicin, and cisplatin) for extravesicular urinary tract tumors. J Urol 1988;139:475.

36. Lieber MM, Lupu AM. High grade invasive ureteral transitional cell carcinoma with a congenital solitary kidney: long-term survival after ureterectomy and radiation therapy. J Urol 1978;120:368.

37. Brookland RK, Richter MP. The postoperative irradiation of transitional cell carcinoma of the renal pelvis and ureter. J Urol 1985;133:952.

38. Cozad SC, Smalley SR, Austenfeld M, et al. Adjuvant radiotherapy in high stage transitional cell carcinoma of the renal pelvis and ureter. Int J Radiat Oncol Biol Phys 1992;24: 743.

12

Endourologic Diagnosis and Treatment of Upper Tract Urothelial Malignancies

John B. Adams, II, and Louis R. Kavoussi

Everything new is not necessarily good, but everything good was at one time new.

—Anonymous

INTRODUCTION

Urothelial malignancies effecting the upper urinary tract are relatively uncommon, accounting for 5 to 7% of all renal tumors (1–3). The standard treatment of these tumors involves nephroureterectomy, with care to remove a cuff of bladder around the ipsilateral ureteral orifice (2, 4). This technique is associated with a significant incision, notable postoperative pain, and several weeks of convalescence. To minimize the morbidity associated with open total extrication, investigators have applied endourologic methods in select patients. Advances in minimally invasive access techniques and instrumentation have made the ureteroscopic and percutaneous routes to upper tract urothelial lesions technically possible (5, 6).

The use of minimally invasive procedures to treat primary upper tract tumors is controversial for several reasons. First, with current techniques, precise staging is not always possible and this may result in inadequate treatment. Second, there is also a potential risk of tumor seeding or spillage if urothelial boundaries are violated. Third, intensive surveillance including multiple ureteroscopies may create problems associated with repeated instrumentation (i.e., strictures) and patient compliance. Fourth, minimally invasive management requires the surgeon to have expertise in a variety of endourologic techniques.

Irrespective of these concerns, there is a place for endourology in the treatment of upper tract urothelial malignancies. Endoscopic management may benefit patients with tumors in a solitary kidney; bilateral tumors; renal insufficiency; multiple low-grade, low-stage lesions; and those unable to undergo major open surgery (5). This chapter focuses on the indications, techniques, and results when using endourologic techniques to treat patients with upper tract urothelial malignancies.

CLINICOPATHOLOGIC CORRELATIONS

Regardless of the method of surgical treatment, patients with grade 1 transitional cell carcinoma (TCC) of the upper tract have a long-term survival comparable to that of age- and sex-matched control subjects (7). Survival rates range from 40 to 80% for patients with intermediate-grade tumors, whereas patients with high-grade tumors have poor 5-year survival rates in the range of 0 to 33% (8). There is a high degree of correlation between grade and stage, which can be predictive of patient prognosis (9). Patients with noninvasive or minimally invasive tumors have survival rates approaching the general population. Muscle-invasive tumors have 5-year survival rates between 30 and 80%, and patients with metastatic disease have a less than 10% 5-year survival rate (8, 10–16). Low-grade tumors tend to be superficial, and high-grade tumors usually are invasive or metastatic at presentation.

A number of other prognostic factors have also been identified. Younger patients (those younger than 60 years of age) have higher survival rates than older patients (13). Papillary tumors of all grades and stages have a 70% 5-year survival rate compared with 25% for nonpapillary tumors (13, 17). Vascular invasion correlates with decreased survival independent of tumor stage and grade (18). Metastatic disease was found to develop in 73% of patients with pathologic evidence of vascular involvement compared with 21% in those without vascular invasion. Prognostic information is also available from DNA ploidy studies (8, 19, 20–24). Low-stage tumors are predominately diploid and have a favorable prognosis. Aneuploidy is a characteristic of high-grade, high-stage tumors and is associated with poor prognosis.

TCC is a disease of the entire urothelium and comprises approximately 90% of renal pelvic tumors (16, 25, 26). However, upper tract tumors comprise less than 1% of all urothelial tumors (27). Patients have a 2 to 5% chance of tumor development in the contralateral kidney (11, 15, 28). Approximately 50% of patients with an upper tract tumor will have tumor development in the bladder at one point in the course of the disease (2, 29). Upper tract tumors are multifocal in 20 to 50% of cases (30, 31). There is also a 30 to 75% recurrence rate of TCC in the ureteral stump after nephrectomy alone (29, 32). Patients with bladder cancer and reflux do not have an increased incidence of upper tract tumors (33, 34). The exact mechanism for multifocal or recurrent disease is unknown. Some believe that spread is by intraluminal seeding, whereas others cite field changes across the entire urothelium (35, 36).

DIAGNOSIS OF TCC

Gross, painless hematuria is the most common presentation of TCC of the urothelial tract that initiates an evaluation (37–42). Flank pain, with or without hematuria, may be the presenting symptom in as many as 40% of patients with TCC localized to the upper tracts (1, 10, 25, 32, 43, 44). A small percentage may have an associated palpable flank mass or a simultaneously diagnosed renal stone (32, 45, 46).

The initial screening study for suspected upper tract lesions is an intravenous urogram with renal tomography. Radiolucent filling defects are the most common radiologic finding. The differential diagnosis includes radiolucent calculi, blood clots, benign tumors, fungus balls, inflammation, overlying bowel gas, sloughed papillae, and external compression artifact. Maneuvers that aid in distending the renal pelvis with contrast are the use of abdominal compression bands and/or placement of the patient in the prone position. A retrograde pyelogram should be performed if the collecting system or ureter is inadequately visualized.

After the filling defect has been demonstrated, further studies can be performed to verify the cause. Ultrasound can be useful to differentiate soft tissue from nonopaque renal calculi in the renal pelvis. Stones appear highly echogenic, are usually well defined, and give a characteristic back shadow not seen with tumor. However, visualization may be difficult especially if the lesion is located in the ureter.

Computed tomography can also be helpful in further characterizing filling defects in the renal pelvis and proximal ureter. A radiolucent stone will be readily differentiated from soft tissue. In the case of malignancy, enhanced and delayed views may be useful in the delineation of extrarenal spread (47, 48). However, the CT scan has limitations in preoperative local staging. McCoy et al. were not able to differentiate Ta from T2 lesions and were only fair at predicting parenchymal and fat invasion (49). The use of magnetic resonance imaging has been promising in evaluating ureteral tumors but has not been evaluated in localized renal pelvis tumors (50).

Another modality that can be helpful in the diagnosis of TCC of the renal pelvis is selective urinary cytology. High-grade lesions are more likely to have positive results on cytologic study than low-grade tumors (16). Cytologic studies of the upper tracts correlate well with the grade and stage of

tumor; a greater yield was obtained with ureteral catheterizations (51). Lavage cytology of the ureter and renal pelvis is more reliable than exfoliative urine cytology (52–54). In unclear cases, fluoroscopic and direct-vision brush or cold-cup biopsy can enhance the cytologic diagnosis and verify the location and extent of tumor (55–58).

URETEROSCOPY IN THE TREATMENT OF UPPER URINARY TRACT TUMORS

In 1929, Young inserted a pediatric endoscope into a dilated ureter and visualized the renal pelvis in a child (59). Since that time, routine techniques have been developed to safely examine the ureter and upper tracts (60–62). The therapeutic potential of ureteroscopy was first demonstrated by Das, who removed a ureteral stone in 1980 using a pediatric cystoscope (61). Over the past two decades, improvements in rigid and flexible instruments have led to the use of ureteroscopy to treat a variety of upper tract disorders, including tumors.

Ureteroscopy has been helpful in the diagnosis and treatment of upper tract malignancy. A number of investigators have used ureteropyeloscopy to establish the cause of hematuria (63–68). The entire collecting system was visualized in 23 of 29 patients (79%) by Bagley et al. when investigating a renal pelvis filling defect (63). Flexible ureteropyeloscopy was used to establish a diagnosis in all 23 patients with radiographic evidence of a filling defect. An added advantage to the ureteroscopic approach is the ability to identify and treat small discrete lesions successfully (69). Initially, flexible ureteroscopy was limited because of the restriction of the working port size and decrease in flow rate when passing instrumentation. The development of small cautery probes (less than 2 F) and thin laser fibers has increased the capability of treating small tumors (70–72). Since the development of these advances, a number of investigators have successfully treated upper tract urothelial tumors ureteroscopically (64, 73–76).

Technique of Ureteroscopy

All pertinent radiographs should be placed on the operating room viewbox for reference during the procedure. Cystoscopy is performed to inspect the bladder for any suspicious lesions.

A retrograde pyelogram performed with an 8F cone-tip catheter or Rutner occlusion catheter can help map the renal pelvis and the location of tumor. This should be done slowly, under fluoroscopic control, to avoid obscuring subtle findings with large amounts of contrast.

After sufficient imaging has been achieved, a 0.038-inch Bentson wire is passed to the renal pelvis as a safety wire. An 8F/10F coaxial dilating sheath is then used to place a 0.038 Amplatz superstiff wire as a working wire. The safety wire is sutured to the glans penis or labia majora with a 2-0 silk suture. The ureterovesical junction can be dilated by a number of methods including metallic radiopaque or beaded bougies, Amplatz fascial dilators, or high-pressure balloon dilators. We prefer using a 5-mm balloon under fluoroscopic control. Once dilated, a ureteral access sheath should be placed to allow for repeated access to the upper tract.

After adequate dilation, a rigid ureteroscope can be passed along the guide wire or a flexible scope can be passed over the guide wire to the renal pelvis. Inspection of the entire collecting system is then performed using the previously performed radiographs as a map.

A number of accessories can be used to biopsy, resect, or fulgurate the identified lesion. Brush biopsy or cup biopsy can establish a diagnosis and remove small tumors. Biopsy specimens obtained with 3F forceps pulled through the ureteroscope are small, making diagnosis difficult. Kavoussi et al. established a diagnosis in 30% of cases where three to five biopsy specimens were obtained (77). If a ureteronephroscope guide sheath could be passed to the level of the lesion, larger biopsy specimens could be obtained by pulling the entire scope out of the sheath with the biopsy forceps still protruding from the tip of the endoscope. This technique allows for larger biopsy specimens to be taken, providing an adequate diagnosis in 80% of patients (77). The presence of the guide sheath also allows for repeated atraumatic access to the lesion for additional biopsies and facilitates placement of a stent at the end of the procedure. Tumor resection can be accomplished using a rigid ureteroscopic resectoscope or the tumor may be ablated using a bugbee electrode or Nd:YAG laser fiber (Fig. 12.1). This is performed under direct vision to ensure the removal of the entire tumor. Because of the possibility of perforation, resection and cautery should be performed with care.

Postoperatively, a ureteral stent is placed until mucosal regeneration can occur and edema subsides. A double pigtail stent of adequate length should be left in place for 1 week. If a ureteric injury occurs, the stent should be left in place until radiographic evidence of healing has occurred, usually in 3 to 4 weeks.

A 3-month radiographic study should be performed to evaluate the upper tract and rule out postoperative stricture development. Cytologies should be obtained and ureteropyeloscopy and biopsies performed for suspicious findings. An intravenous pyelogram (IVP) is recommended every 3 months to monitor the upper tract for any recurrences (78). Follow-up ureteroscopy should be performed on a semiannual basis for 2 years (79). A retrograde pyelogram should be performed in patients allergic to IVP dye or if IVP results are equivocal. Close surveillance is the key to success of endourologic management of the upper tract.

PERCUTANEOUS ENDOSCOPIC MANAGEMENT OF UPPER TRACT TUMORS

Conservative management of upper tract urothelial cancers in selected patients has been reported by a number of investigators (76, 80–84). Since 1955 when the first percutaneous nephrostomy was performed, the ability to visualize and manipulate pathologic findings within the upper tracts has steadily im-

Ureteroscopic resection of renal pelvis tumor

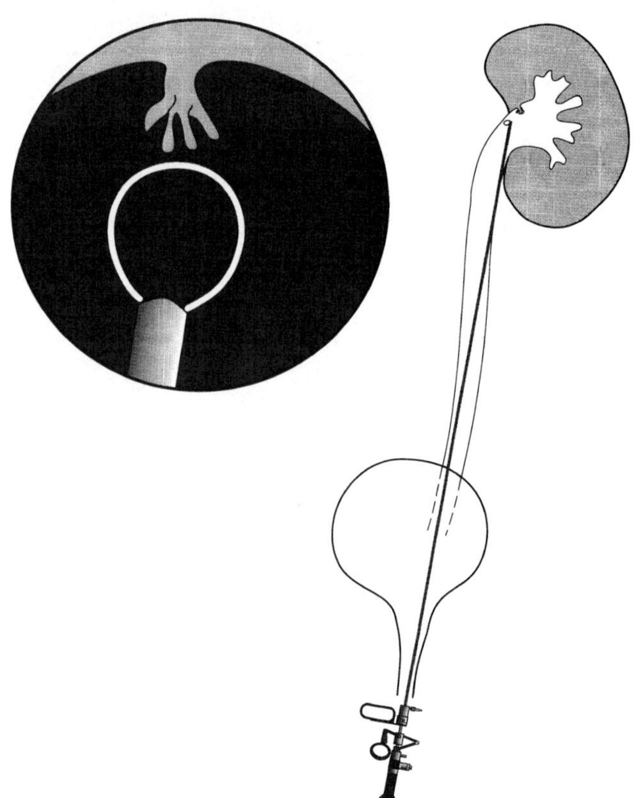

Fig. 12.1. Ureteral resectoscope for removal and fulguration of upper tract urothelial tumor. Inset: Close-up of resectoscope cutting loop with papillary tumor.

proved. Percutaneous management of upper tract tumors is a natural extension of this approach (74, 78, 85–89). Percutaneous access can be used in instances when normal access to the upper tracts is limited, such as in patients with urinary diversion. Percutaneous nephrostomy procedures can also be helpful if there is intercurrent obstruction caused by the tumor or a superimposed infection. The controversy in using primary percutaneous management of upper tract tumors arises when there is a normal contralateral kidney. It is necessary to determine in which patient population this minimally invasive technology would be appropriate.

Percutaneous Resection Technique

As with a ureteroscopic approach, appropriate imaging is first obtained. The patient is placed in the prone position, and a flexible cystoscope is used to examine the bladder. An 0.038-inch Bentson wire is advanced carefully into the renal pelvis and the cystoscope is removed. Excessive coiling of the wire in the renal pelvis may cause urothelial trauma, making visualization difficult. A 7F occlusion balloon catheter is then placed into the renal pelvis under fluoroscopic guidance to allow for visualization of the collecting system for access.

Approximately 5 mL of air or contrast agent is instilled into the calyceal system to outline the posterior calyx. The nephrostomy tract is placed so that the access sheath has a direct line with the tumor, yet enters the collecting system away from the tumor to minimize local contamination. A 16G splenic access needle is placed under fluoroscopic guidance and a 0.038 Bentson wire is passed. An 8F/10F coaxial dilator sheath is used to place a 0.038 working Amplatz wire. After securing the safety Bentson wire to the skin, the nephrostomy tract is dilated over the working wire with a 10-mm nephrostomy tract balloon, and a 30F Amplatz sheath is introduced into the renal pelvis. Flexible and rigid nephroscopes are used to visualize the entire collecting system and map the extent of tumor. Antegrade flexible ureteroscopy may be performed at this time if complete examination of the ureter has not been performed previously. Random cold-cup biopsies of the renal pelvic mucosa are taken before resection of the tumor. A standard resectoscope may be used to remove tumors, although biopsy forceps are usually adequate for small tumors (Fig. 12.2). Tumor fronds are removed with cold-cup biopsy forceps and sent for histologic analysis, after which the tumor base is biopsied and treated with cautery. Alternatively, an Nd:YAG laser set at 25 to 30 watts may be used to paint the base of the tumor.

At the conclusion of the procedure, a 7.1F single-J ureteral catheter is placed over the wire, down the ureter, and into the bladder. A 22F council-tip catheter is introduced into the renal pelvis over the stent and secured by a Tuohy-Borst side-arm

Percutaneous resection of pelvic tumor

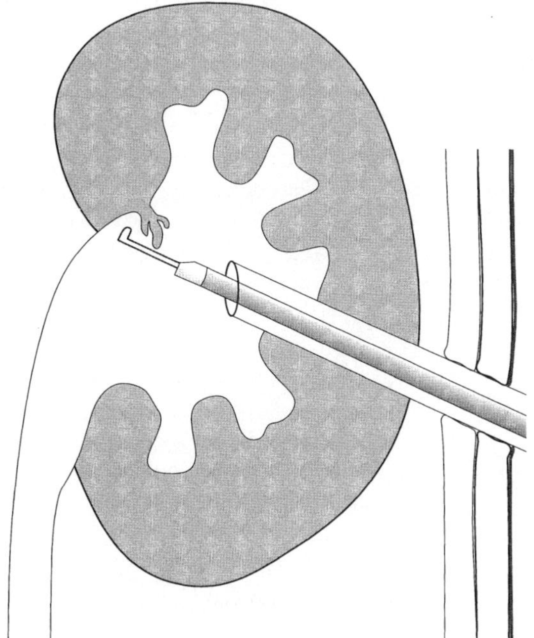

Fig. 12.2. Percutaneous access for removal of upper tract urothelial tumors.

adapter. Placement is verified fluoroscopically with contrast dye, and the tube is secured with a 2-0 silk suture. A nephrostogram is performed at 2 to 3 days postoperatively; if no extravasation is present, a second-look nephroscopy may be performed under local sedation to confirm total tumor resection. If there is no supplemental adjuvant topical therapy planned, the nephrostomy tube may be removed.

The follow-up of these patients should consist of radiographic visualization of the upper tracts every 3 months for 2 years and once a year thereafter. These examinations should be augmented with ureteroscopic visualization or biopsies if necessary.

RESULTS OF ENDOUROLOGIC MANAGEMENT OF UPPER TRACT TUMORS

The endosurgical management of upper tract urothelial tumors has results comparable to those obtained by open conservative procedures (Table 12.1). Open surgery consisting of local excision of pelvis and segmental removal of the ureter had recurrence rates of 35% and 6 to 14%, respectively (91, 92). Ureteral tumors and small renal pelvis tumors treated ureteroscopically have a recurrence rate at 2 years of 15%. Huffman et al. diagnosed upper tract tumors in 11 patients using ureteroscopy (72). Three patients had extirpative surgery because of high-grade, multifocal tumors. Of the remaining eight patients, four had no recurrences with short follow-up periods (mean, 4 months), whereas three underwent successful ureteroscopic removal of recurrent tumors. One patient was not available for surveillance.

Renal pelvic tumors were managed endoscopically by Blute et al. in 10 of 22 patients diagnosed by ureteroscopy (73). Five patients were treated with ureteroscopy alone, with two undergoing tumor fulgurations and three undergoing biopsy and fulguration. Three larger (1.5 to 4.0 cm) tumors required percutaneous management. Difficult access to a renal pelvis tumor and excision of large tumor are indications to convert to a percutaneous approach (71, 74). Ureteroscopic approaches are suitable for a small solitary tumor with minimal bleeding. When patients present with larger tumors (greater than 1 cm), a percutaneous technique is more appropriate. Multicentricity and poor accessibility are also indications for primary percutaneous access.

Woodhouse et al. reported on four patients treated by percutaneous removal of renal pelvis tumors (85). The techniques included dilation of the tract to 26F and placement of a radioactive iridium (^{192}Ir) wire in the nephrostomy tract several days postoperatively. There was evidence of local recurrence in one patient with 7- to 36-month follow-up. Tasca and Zattoni successfully managed low-grade tumors in four patients by percutaneous resection and fulguration (88). There were no recurrences at 11 to 24 months follow-up. Blute et al. recently reported a long-term follow-up on endosurgically treated upper tract tumors (78). The local recurrence rate was 39%, with renal pelvis tumors recurring after a shorter interval (7 months) than upper ureteral tumors (18 months).

Table 12.1.   Endosurgical Therapy of Upper Tract Urothelial Tumors

AUTHORS	PATIENTS	APPROACH	ADJUNCTIVE THERAPY	LOCAL RECURRENCE	OPEN ABLATION	METASTASES	FOLLOW-UP (mo)
Endosurgical							
Orihuela and Smith (5)	4 (pelvis)	Percutaneous	No	75	25	0	19
	7 (pelvis)	Percutaneous	Yes	29	29	14	22
Woodhouse, et al. (85)	15	Percutaneous	Yes	39	33	0	24
Blute et al. (78)	8 (pelvis)	Percutaneous (3)	—	0	0	0	18
	13 (ureter)	Ureteroscopy (5)	—	20	0	0	28
		Ureteroscopy (13)	—	15	0	0	21
Huffman (6)	5	Percutaneous and ureteroscopy	—	40	40	0	>12
Huffman et al. (89)	8	Ureteroscopy	Yes	38	13	0	21
Surgical							
Wallace et al. (90)	7 (pelvis)	Local excision	—	35	NA	29	9.6 yr
	7 (pelvis)	Segmental excision		14	NA	0	5.9 yr
Mazeman (91)	23 (pelvis)	Local excision	—	35	NA	—	>12
	50 (ureter)	Segmental removal		6	NA	—	>12

Adapted from Clayman RV, Kavoussi LR. Endosurgical techniques for noncalculus disease. In: Walsh PC, Retick AB, Stamey TA, et al., eds. Campbell's urology. 6th ed. Philadelphia: WB Saunders, 1992:2302.

In a series reported by Orihuela and Smith, 14 patients were initially treated with percutaneous resection (74). Complete tumor excision was performed in 11 of 14 patients; the remaining 3 underwent immediate open nephroureterectomy when invasive malignancy was discovered. A mean follow-up of 19 months showed that 3 patients were tumor free. Of the remaining 11 patients, 5 had recurrent disease, of which 3 had extirpative procedures and 2 with solitary kidneys had further conservative treatment. The technique used included dilation of the nephrostomy tract to 34F and tumor removal with a resectoscope. At 7 to 10 days postoperatively, the patients underwent additional nephroscopy to ascertain completeness of resection. Additional biopsies and cytologies were performed at that time to identify occult disease. Patients with low-grade, small, papillary tumors did well. However, local recurrences occurred in four of six patients with grade 2 or 3 TCC, indicating the need for more radical procedures in patients with medium- to high-grade lesions with normal contralateral units.

In a more recent review of 36 cases of percutaneous resection of upper tract tumors, Jarrett et al. found tumor grade to be the most important factor in predicting recurrence (92). Selected recurrence rates for grades 1, 2, and 3 tumors were 18% (2 of 11), 33% (3 of 9), and 50% (5 of 10), respectively. Cancer-related mortality was encountered in 13% (4 of 30), and all of these patients had grade 3 tumors. Thus, compared with historical experience, the percutaneous approach did not negatively affect the ultimate outcome of patients treated endosurgically.

There have been no well-documented cases of nephrostomy tract seeding in the literature. However, there have been instances of retroperitoneal recurrences after percutaneous violation of the urothelium (93). There have also been distant bladder recurrences that have not affected patient survival.

Therefore, in select patients, results imply that endourologic techniques yield tumor-free survival rates that are similar to open conservative surgery. However, longer follow-up times in larger series are necessary to make recommendations that may be applied to patients with a normal contralateral kidney.

COMPLICATIONS OF PERCUTANEOUS REMOVAL OF UPPER TRACT MALIGNANCIES

A major concern during the percutaneous removal of renal pelvis tumors is seeding of the nephrostomy tract. Intraoperative pyeloscopy was performed by Tomera et al. on 18 patients subsequently found to have TCC (93). Although all patients underwent immediate nephroureterectomy, tumor recurrence was noted locally in two patients (11%). Both patients had noninvasive, low-grade lesions, suggesting that percutaneous violation of the collecting system led to seeding of the retroperitoneum. However, several series have not noted tumor tract seeding (74, 94). In the follow-up of 14 patients undergoing percutaneous procedures, Orihuela and Smith did not report tumor implantation in the nephrostomy tract (74). There were no tumor recurrences found by McCarron et al. in the follow-up of 33 patients undergoing percutaneous procedures for removal of upper tract tumors (94). A number of measures that have been suggested to decrease the possibility of tract seeding include the use of sterile water as irrigating fluid, postoperative local irradiation to the tract with iridium wire, and establishment and resection performed in a one-stage procedure (85, 86, 95).

Another concern is systemic seeding during percutaneous resection due to pyelovenous backflow; however, no cases have been well documented to date (85). Using a large access sheath will allow irrigating fluid to easily run out around the instruments to keep intrapelvic pressure low. Also, the irrigating fluid should be kept below 40 cm above the patient to further lessen the chance of pyelovenous backflow.

A more unusual complication reported by Andrews and Segura was an explosion during fulguration of an upper tract tumor (96). Although there has been no recurrence in this case, the potential for spillage of tumor after perforation of the collecting system can be minimized by avoiding the buildup of hydrogen gas and air.

ADJUNCTIVE THERAPY

Topical therapy after percutaneous or ureteroscopic resection of upper tract malignancies has been used by a number of investigators in an attempt to decrease recurrence (74, 86, 89, 97, 98). To access the renal pelvis, a number of methods have been used. These include instillation via ureteral catheters, instillation via percutaneous catheters, or resection of the ureteral orifice with subsequent vesicoureteral reflux. Herr has reported a freely refluxing pyelovesical anastomosis created at the time of open resection in one patient (99). This patient was free of tumor at 13 months follow-up after a 6-week course of bacille Calmette-Guérin (BCG). Orihuela and Smith treated six patients at high risk for recurrence with weekly instillations of BCG through a nephrostomy tube. This procedure was well tolerated; in this small group, recurrence rates were 16% compared with 80% of those not treated with BCG (74).

Recently, Vasavada et al. treated eight patients after partial nephrectomy (two patients) or percutaneous resection (six patients) (98). Seven patients tolerated the BCG instillations without difficulty; however, one patient experienced reversible renal insufficiency. With a mean follow-up of 22 months, one patient had a local tumor recurrence and two patients had metastatic disease development. These patients had invasive TCC elsewhere in the urothelial tract at the time of upper tract treatment. These results lead to the belief that topical therapy may reduce the incidence of recurrence in patients with resected low-grade tumors of the upper tract.

LAPAROSCOPIC MANAGEMENT OF UPPER TRACT UROTHELIAL TUMORS

Clayman et al. reported the first laparoscopic nephrectomy for a solid renal mass in 1990 (100). Reservations about performing a laparoscopic radical nephrectomy have been the question of tumor spillage and the ability to remove adequately the kidney and surrounding tissues. These problems are compounded in the laparoscopic treatment of upper tract tumors because the entire ureter and bladder cuff have to be removed.

With the development of a surgical entrapment sac and early clinical results, enthusiasm for the laparoscopic removal of neoplasms has increased. The use of a stapled bladder closure without subsequent encrustation of exposed staples has solved the problem of violating the urothelial barrier (101). Kerbl et

al. reported a series of six patients undergoing laparoscopic nephroureterectomies for upper tract transitional cell cancer (102). A comparison with open nephroureterectomies revealed a longer operating room time (7.29 versus 3.37 hours), but a shorter hospital stay, quicker convalescence, and less parenteral analgesics for the laparoscopic procedure. The follow-up to address the question of adequate resection has been limited due to the relatively recent application of this procedure. Adams et al. has an intermediate follow-up of four patients undergoing nephroureterectomy for upper tract TCC (103). One patient was found to have nodal involvement at the time of laparoscopy. Two of the remaining patients had recurrences in the bladder, away from the bladder cuff. These patients have completed courses of BCG with negative follow-up of 12 to 14 months. In another series of three patients, Chandhoke et al. reported no recurrence of disease or bladder stones at the bladder staple line at 3 to 9 months follow-up (104).

The above series reporting on laparoscopic nephroureterectomy are promising but small. Further investigation and longer follow-up times are needed to demonstrate adequate tumor control.

Technique of Laparoscopic Nephroureterectomy

The laparoscopic procedure begins with the preparation of the distal ureter. With the patient in the dorsal lithotomy position, the bladder is examined, and a 7F balloon ureteral dilation catheter (5 mm, 5 cm) is inserted over a preplaced 0.035-inch Bentson guide wire into the distal ureter. The balloon is then distended with contrast. A 24F resectoscope is then introduced and is incised at the 12-o'clock position of the ureteral tunnel with an Orandi knife. The incision should extend the length of the intramural ureter to the ureterovesical junction (Fig. 12.3). The balloon is deflated and replaced with a 7F balloon occlusion catheter that is advanced into the renal pelvis. The Bentson wire is replaced with a 0.035-inch Amplatz superstiff guide wire. A 22F council-tip catheter placed over the occlusion balloon catheter is advanced into the bladder, the balloon is distended, and general traction is exerted to hold the catheter against the bladder neck. A side arm adapter is passed over the superstiff wire, fixed to the occlusion balloon catheter, and inserted into the end of the council-tip catheter. This allows for controlled drainage of the upper tract, and chemotherapeutic agents may be instilled into the renal pelvis (Fig. 12.4).

The patient is then moved into the lateral 60° flank position with an axillary roll, and all pressure points are padded. Wide cloth tape is used to secure the patient to the table. A Veress needle is placed 1 cm below the level of umbilicus, lateral to the rectus muscle, to obtain a pneumoperitoneum. The peritoneal cavity is insufflated to a pressure of 20 mm Hg, and a 1-cm horizontal incision is made 1 cm below the costal margin in the anterior axillary line. A 10- to 12-mm trocar is placed, and the peritoneal cavity is inspected. Additional trocars are placed under direct vision just lateral to the umbilicus and in the lower ipsilateral quadrant along the anterior axillary line (Fig.

Incision of distal ureteral tunnel

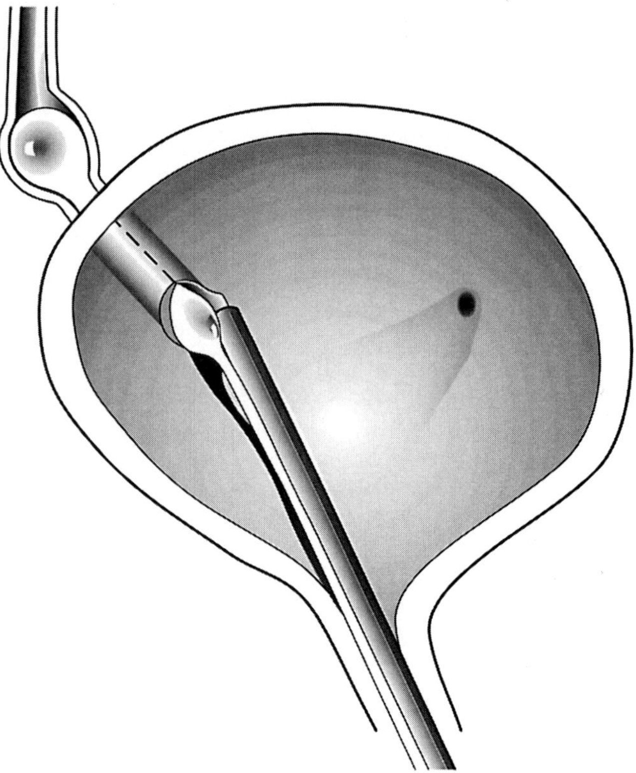

Fig. 12.3. Cystoscopic incision of intramural ureteral tunnel using an Orandi knife. This is performed over a ureteral dilation balloon.

12.5). Ports are positioned so that approximately 2 cm of sheath lie within the abdominal cavity and are secured to the skin using 2-0 polyglactin suture.

An additional 12-mm port is placed midway between the umbilicus and the pubic symphysis to provide GIA stapler access to the bladder cuff. The colon is reflected medially after incision of the peritoneum along the line of Toldt. One additional lateral trocar is placed in the posterior axillary line at the level of the umbilicus.

The peritoneal incision is extended across the iliac vessels medial to the medial umbilical ligament to expose the distal ureter. A 5-mm Babcock clamp is used to retract the ureter in a cephalad direction to aid in dissection. A combination of traction and parallel sweeping motion is used to separate the ureter from the retroperitoneal periureteral tissue. The gonadal vessels are encountered coursing from medial to lateral and are clipped and transected. Care must be taken not to avulse the ureter during retraction.

As the dissection continues toward the bladder, the vas deferens in the male or the round ligament in the female is encountered anterior to the ureter. These structures are dissected free, clipped with 9-mm occlusive clips, and transected. In addition, the medial umbilical ligament and superior vesical artery may be divided to gain access to the ureterovesical junc-

tion. A 5-cm area surrounding the point at which the ureter enters the muscle of the bladder is cleared of perivesical fat. The ureteral balloon and guide wire are removed, and a flexible cystoscope is introduced to visualize the ureteral orifice transvesically.

A 12-mm laparoscopic GIA tissue stapler is introduced through the lower midline port and positioned across the cuff of the bladder (Fig. 12.6). Retraction of the distal ureter and bladder cuff cephalad aids in positioning the stapler accurately. Cystoscopic examination confirms that the previously fulgurated cuff is incorporated. After firing the stapler, the cuff is inspected with the laparoscope for leaks and with a cystoscope for exposed staples. A Foley catheter is then placed to drain the bladder.

The camera is then moved from the umbilical port to the posterior axillary port to view the posterior portion of the kidney and associated tissues. Gerota's fascia of the upper pole is manipulated medially, and sharp dissection is used to deliver the perinephric tissues with the kidney. This gives an unobstructed view of the renal hilar vessels. On the left side, care should be taken to identify and ligate the gonadal vein, posterior lumbar vein, and adrenal vein.

After the smaller veins are secured, the main renal vein is identified and isolated. The pulsating renal artery is usually

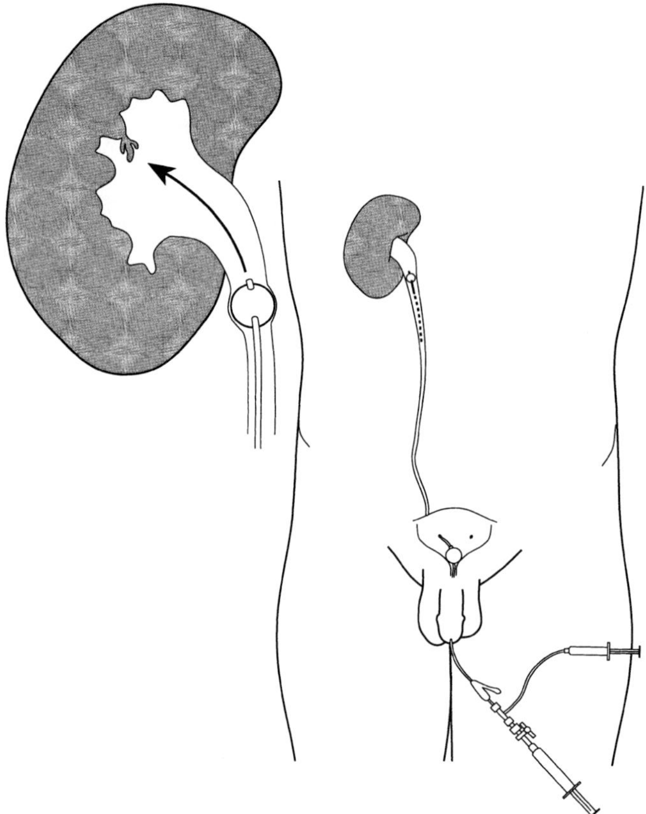

Fig. 12.4. Occlusion balloon catheter access to the upper tract through a council-tip Foley catheter. This method allows for instillation of chemotherapy into the upper tract before laparoscopic nephroureterectomy.

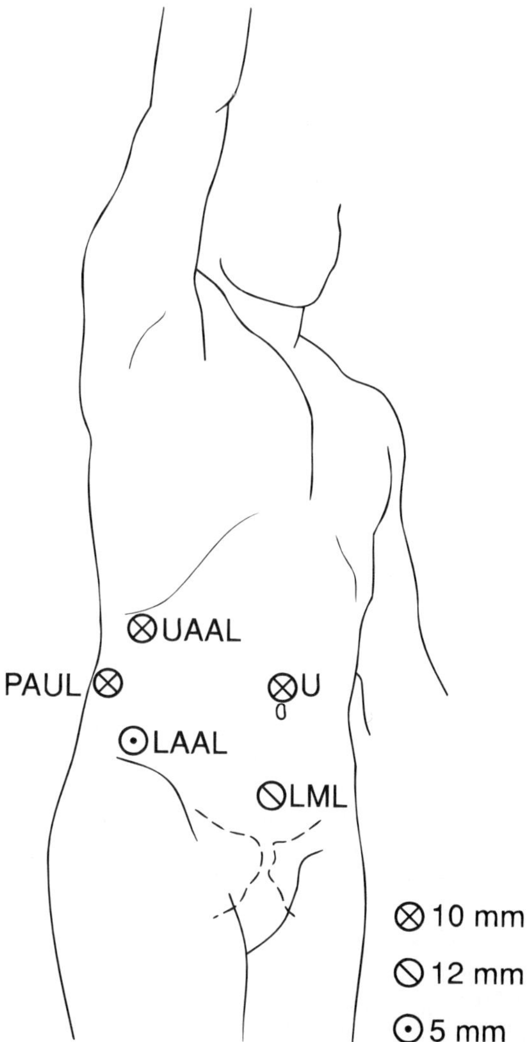

Fig. 12.5. Port placement for laparoscopic nephroureterectomy. Upper anterior axillary line (UAAL) port, posterior axillary umbilical line (PAUL) port, and umbilical (U) port are 10 mm in size. Lower midline (LML) port should be 12 mm for laparoscopic stapling of the bladder cuff. Lower anterior axillary line (LAAL) 5-mm port is optional at the surgeon's preference.

seen just posterior and isolated from the renal vein for a length of 1.5 cm. Three clips are placed on the stump of the artery, with one clip positioned on the renal side of the artery. After transection, the renal vein should decrease in size. A complete window is dissected around the renal vein, and a vascular GIA stapler is placed to include the entire vein. After firing the GIA, the renal pedicle is freed from its remaining lymphatic attachments and the kidney is free in the peritoneal cavity.

A 5- × 8-inch organ entrapment sac is placed through a 10-mm port and positioned in the pelvis. With the camera in the umbilical port, the renal hilum is grasped with a Babcock clamp through the upper anterior axillary line trocar and guided into the open lap sac. The purse strings are tightened around the hilum, and the bladder cuff and pull strings are grasped with a clamp through the umbilical port. The ureter is drawn through the port site as the trocar is removed. The

pull string is used to bring the lap sac through the opening of the port site. The ureter is then transected at the most proximal point and sent for permanent section. A high-speed morcellator or ring forceps are used to remove fragments of the kidney from the lap sac. Direct laparoscopic visualization of the lap sac during kidney removal ensures no tissue spillage or injury to viscera. Alternatively, the entire specimen may be removed through a 5-cm lower midline incision. The renal fossa is then flushed with 1 L of sterile water and suctioned with a suction irrigator.

There are a variety of methods to close trocar sites that are 10 mm or larger. Skin edges are reapproximated using a 4-0 Vicryl (Ethicon, Sommerville, NJ) subcuticular running stitch. Steri-strips are used to reapproximate the skin edges.

The nasogastric tube is removed in the recovery room. In 2 to 3 days a cystogram is performed to confirm adequate bladder closure, after which the Foley catheter is removed. If there is any evidence of extravasation, the bladder is restudied after 1 week. Clear liquids may be given on the evening of surgery, and the diet may be advanced to normal as tolerated by the patient. Postoperative analgesia is provided by parenteral morphine sulphate that is discontinued in favor of oral nonnarcotics after 24 hours. Ambulation is encouraged after postoperative day 1. Follow-up after laparoscopic nephroureterectomy is iden-

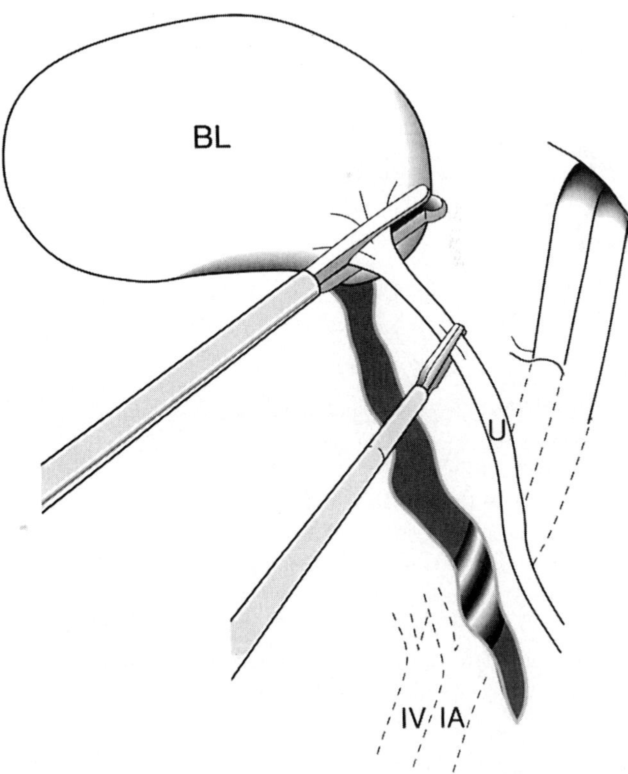

Fig. 12.6. Laparoscopic view of stapling across the bladder cuff at the ureterovesical junction. The ureter (U) is held away from the bladder (BL) using a grasper or umbilical tape to allow for stapler placement. The iliac vein (IV) and iliac artery (IA) can be used as landmarks to find the ureter as it courses from lateral to medial.

tical to the follow-up after an open procedure. This includes cystoscopic and cytologic studies every 3 months for 2 years and biannually thereafter.

CONCLUSION

Nephroureterectomy is the procedure used to treat upper tract urothelial malignancies in patients with a normal contralateral kidney. However, there is a group of patients in which parenchyma-sparing surgery may be an option. Patients with a solitary renal unit, renal insufficiency, or bilateral synchronous tumors may benefit from an endoscopic approach to upper tract lesions. Ureteroscopy can be used as a diagnostic and therapeutic tool and can be effective in treating small tumors with fulguration or laser coagulation. There is the added advantage of not violating the urothelial barrier that can potentially seed the retroperitoneum. Percutaneous techniques allow for easier access to renal pelvis tumors and make large tumor removal possible. Both techniques allow for the use of postoperative BCG or mitomycin C as supplemental therapy.

Despite the type of surgery, grade and stage of the upper tract lesion are the most important predictors of outcome. Low-grade and low-stage lesions could be successfully managed with conservative measures in certain cases. In those patients for whom nephroureterectomy is chosen, a laparoscopic approach is an alternative that is well tolerated. Preliminary studies seem promising, but longer follow-up times are needed to verify the adequacy of the dissection and removal of malignant renal lesions. Endourologic management of patients with upper tract tumors enhances the urologist's ability to adequately and effectively treat these lesions.

REFERENCES

1. Say CS, Hori JM. Transitional cell carcinoma of the renal pelvis: experience from 1940 to 1972 and literature review. J Urol 1974;112:438.
2. Catalona WJ. Urothelial tumors of the renal pelvis and ureter. In: Walsh PC, Retick AB, Stamey TA, et al., eds. Campbell's urology. 6th ed. Philadelphia: WB Saunders, 1992:1137.
3. Grabstald H, Whitmore WF, Melamed MR. Renal pelvic tumors. JAMA 1971;218:845.
4. Richie JP. Carcinoma of the renal pelvis and ureter. In: Skinner DG, Lieskovsky G, eds. Diagnosis and management of genitourinary cancer. Philadelphia: WB Saunders, 1988: 331.
5. Orihuela E, Smith AD. Percutaneous treatment of transitional cell carcinoma of the upper urinary tract. Urol Clin North Am 1988;15:425.
6. Huffman JL. Ureteroscopic management of transitional cell carcinoma of the upper urinary tract. Urol Clin North Am 1988;15:419.
7. Murphy DM, Zincke H, Furlow WL. Primary grade 1 transitional cell carcinoma of the renal pelvis and ureter. J Urol 1980;123:629.
8. Corrado F, Ferri C, Mannini D, et al. Transitional cell carcinoma of the upper urinary tract: evaluation of prognostic factors by histopathology and flow cytometric analysis. J Urol 1991;145:1159.
9. Knocks BN, Heney NM, Daly JJ, et al. Transitional cell carcinoma of the renal pelvis. Urology 1982;19:472.
10. Cummings KB, Correa RM, Gibbons RP, et al. Renal pelvic tumors. J Urol 1975;113:158.
11. Batata MA, Whitmore WF, Hilaris BS, et al. Primary carcinoma of the ureter: a prognostic study. Cancer 1975;35: 1626.
12. Mills C, Vaughn ED. Carcinoma of the ureter: natural history, management and 5-year survival. J Urol 1983;129: 275.
13. Matsuoka K, Ueda S, Yamasahita T, et al. Analysis of prognostic factors in patients with pyeloureteral carcinoma. Am J Clin Oncol 1991;14:146.
14. Heney NM, Nocks BN, Daly JJ, et al. Prognostic factors in carcinoma of the ureter. J Urol 1981;125:632.
15. Gatewood OM, Goldman SM, Marshall FF, et al. Computerized tomography in the diagnosis of transitional cell carcinoma of the kidney. J Urol 1982;127:876.
16. Nocks BN, Heney NM, Daly JJ, et al. Transitional cell carcinoma of the renal pelvis. Urology 1982;19:472.
17. Nocks BN, Heney NM, Daly JJ, et al. Prognostic factors in carcinoma of the ureter. J Urol 1981;125:632.
18. Hasui Y, Nishi S, Kitada S, et al. The prognostic significance of vascular invasion in upper tract transitional cell carcinoma. J Urol 1992;148:1783.
19. Badalament RA, O'Toole RV, Kenworthy P, et al. Prognostic factors in patients with primary transitional cell carcinoma of the upper urinary tract. J Urol 1990;144:859.
20. Blute ML, Tsushima K, Farrow GM, et al. Transitional cell carcinoma of the renal pelvis: nuclear deoxyribonucleic acid ploidy studied by flow cytometry. J Urol 1988;140:944.
21. Oldbring J, Hellsten S, Lindholm K, et al. Flow DNA analysis in the characterization of carcinoma of the renal pelvis and ureter. Cancer 1989;64:2141.
22. Al-Abadi H, Nagel R. Transitional cell carcinoma of the renal pelvis and ureter: prognostic relevance of nuclear deoxyribonucleic acid ploidy studied by slide cytometry. an 8-year survival time study. J Urol 1992;148:31.
23. Chiang PH, Huang MS, Tsai CJ, et al. Transitional cell carcinoma of the renal pelvis and ureter in Taiwan. Cancer 1993;71:3988.
24. Corrado F, Mannini D, Ferri C, et al. The prognostic significance of DNA ploidy pattern in transitional cell cancer of the renal pelvis and ureter: continuing follow-up. Eur Urol 1992;21(Suppl):48.
25. Mahadevia P, Karwa GL, Koss LG. Mapping of urothelium in carcinomas of the renal pelvis and ureter. Cancer 1983;51: 890.
26. McCarron JP, Chaski SB, Gray GF. Systematic mapping of nephroureterectomy specimens removed for urothelial cancer: pathological findings and clinical correlations. J Urol 1982; 128:243.
27. Miller A, Mitchell JP, Brown NJ. The Bristol Bladder Tumor Registry. J Urol 1969;41(Suppl):1.
28. Auld CD, Grigor KM, Fowler JW. Histopathological review

of transitional cell carcinoma of the upper urinary tract. Br J Urol 1984;56:485.

29. Kakizoe T, Fujita J, Murasc T, et al. Transitional cell carcinoma of the bladder in patients with renal pelvic and ureteral cancer. J Urol 1980;124:17.

30. Anderstrom C, Johansson SL, Pettersson S, et al. Carcinoma of the ureter: a clinicopathologic study of 49 cases. J Urol 1989;142:280.

31. Fujimoto H, Tobisu K, Mizutani T, et al. Transitional cell carcinoma of the upper urinary tract: analysis of morphology and distribution for surgical management. Jpn J Clin Oncol 1993;23:303.

32. Williams CB, Mitchell JP. Carcinoma of the ureter: a review of 54 cases. Br J Urol 1973;45:371.

33. DeTorres Mateos JA, Banus Gassol JM, Palon Redorta J, et al. Vesicoureteral reflux and upper urinary tract transitional cell carcinoma after transurethral resection of recurrent superficial bladder carcinoma. J Urol 1987;138:49.

34. Palou J, Farina LA, Villavicencio H, et al. Upper tract urothelial tumor after transurethral resection for bladder tumor. Eur Urol 1992;21:110.

35. Sidransky D, Frost P, VonEschenbach A, et al. Clonal origin of bladder cancer. N Engl J Med 1992;326:737.

36. Habuchi T, Takahashi R, Yamada H, et al. Metachronous multifocal development of urothelial cancers by intraluminal seeding. Lancet 1993;324:1087.

37. Riches EW, Griffiths IH, Thackray AC. New growths of the kidney and ureter. Br J Urol 1951;23:297.

38. Taylor WN. Tumors of the kidney pelvis. J Urol 1959;82:452.

39. Newman DM, et al. Transitional cell carcinoma of the upper urinary tract. J Urol 1967;98:322.

40. Grace DA, Taylor WW, Taylor JN, et al. Carcinoma of the renal pelvis: a 15-year review. J Urol 1968;98:566.

41. Donnelly JD, Koontz WW. Carcinoma of the renal pelvis: a 10-year review. South Med J 1975;68:943.

42. Hall L, et al. The use of the red cell surface antigen to predict the malignant potential of transitional cell carcinoma of the ureter and renal pelvis. J Urol 1982;125:23.

43. Wagle DG, Moore RH, Murphy GP. Primary carcinoma of the renal pelvis. Cancer 1974;33:1642.

44. Stragier M, et al. Primary carcinoma-in-situ of renal pelvis and ureter. Br J Urol 1980;52:401.

45. McDonald JR, Priestley JT. Carcinoma of the renal pelvis: histopathologic study of 75 cases with special reference to prognosis. J Urol 1944;51:245.

46. Leong CH, et al. Carcinoma of the renal pelvis: analysis of the diagnostic problems in 23 cases. Br J Urol 1976;63:102.

47. Baghdassarian OM, et al. Computerized tomography in the diagnosis of transitional cell carcinoma of the kidney. J Urol 1982;127:876.

48. Baron RL, et al. Computed tomography of transitional cell carcinoma of the renal pelvis and ureter. Radiology 1982;144:125.

49. McCoy JG, et al. Computerized tomography for detection and staging of localized and pathologically defined upper tract urothelial tumors. J Urol 1991;146:1500.

50. Milestone B, et al. Staging of ureteral transitional cell carcinoma by CT and MRI. Urology 1990;4:346.

51. Zincke H, et al. Significance of urinary cytology in the early detection of transitional cell cancer of the upper urinary tract. J Urol 1976;116:781.

52. Leistenschneidr W, Nagel R. Lavage cytology of the renal pelvis and ureter with special reference to tumors. J Urol 1980;124:597.

53. Eriksson O, Johansson S. Urothelial neoplasms of the upper urinary tract: a correlation between cytologic and histologic findings in 43 patients with urothelial neoplasms of the renal pelvis or ureter. Acta Cytol 1976;20:20.

54. Sarnacki CT, et al. Urinary cytology and the clinical diagnosis of urinary tract malignancy: a clinicopathologic study of 1,400 patients. J Urol 1971;106:761.

55. Sheline M, et al. Fluoroscopically guided retrograde brush biopsy in the diagnosis of transitional cell carcinoma of the upper urinary tract: results in 45 patients. AJR 1989;153:313.

56. Blute RD, et al. Renal brush biopsy: survey of indications, techniques and results. J Urol 1981;126:146.

57. Gill WB, Lu CT, Thomsen S. Retrograde brushing: a new technique for obtaining histologic and cytologic material from ureteral, renal pelvic and renal calyceal lesions. J Urol 1973;109:573.

58. Gittes, RF. Retrograde brushing and nephroscopy in the diagnosis of upper-tract urothelial cancer. Urol Clin North Am 1984;11:617.

59. Young HH, McKay RW. Congenital valvular obstruction in prostatic urethra. Surg Gynecol Obstet 1929;48:509.

60. Lyon ES, Banno JJ, Schoenberg HW. Transurethral ureteroscopy in men using juvenile cystoscopy equipment. J Urol 1979;122:152.

61. Das S. Transurethral ureteroscopy and stone manipulation under direct vision. J Urol 1981;125:112.

62. Marshall VF. Fiber optics in urology. J Urol 1964;91:110.

63. Bagley DH, Huffman JL, Lyon ES. Flexible ureteropyeloscopy: diagnosis and treatment in the upper urinary tract. J Urol 1987;138:280.

64. Bagley DH, Rivas D. Upper urinary tract filling defects: flexible ureteroscopic diagnosis. J Urol 1990;143:1196.

65. Bagley DH, McCue P, Blackstone AS. Inverted papilloma of renal pelvis: flexible ureteroscopic diagnosis and treatment. Urology 1990;32:336.

66. Street SB, et al. Ureteropyeloscopy in the evaluation of upper tract filling defects. J Urol 1986;136:383.

67. Bagley DH, Allen J. Flexible ureteroscopy in the diagnosis of benign essential hematuria. J Urol 1990;143:549.

68. Schmeller NT, Hofstetter AG. Laser treatment of ureteral tumors. J Urol 1989;141:840.

69. Kaufman RP, Carson CC. Ureteroscopic management of transitional cell carcinoma of the ureter using the neodymium: YAG laser. Lasers Surg Med 1993;13:625.

70. Carson CC. Endoscopic treatment of upper and lower urinary tract lesions using lasers. Semin Urol 1991;9:185.

71. Grossman HB, Schwartz SL, Konnak JW. Ureteroscopic treatment of urothelial carcinoma of the ureter and renal pelvis. J Urol 1992;148:275.

72. Huffman JL, et al. Endoscopic diagnosis and treatment of upper tract urothelial tumors: a preliminary report. Cancer 1985;55:1422.

73. Blute ML, et al. Impact of endourology on diagnosis and

management of upper urinary tract urothelial cancer. J Urol 1989;141:1298.

74. Orihuela E, Smith AD. Percutaneous treatment of transitional cell carcinoma of the upper urinary tract. Urol Clin North Am 1988;15:419.

75. Papadopoulos I, et al. Diagnosis and treatment of urothelial tumors by ureteropyeloscopy. J Endourol 1990;4:55.

76. Ferris DO, Daut RV. Epithelioma of the pelvis of a solitary kidney treated by electrocoagulation. J Urol 1948;59:577.

77. Kavoussi LR, Basler J, Clayman RV. Flexible fiberoptic ureteronephroscopy. 6th world congress of ESWL and Endourology, Paris, 1988. Abstract.

78. Blute ML, Segura JW, Patterson DE, et al. Impact of endourology on diagnosis and management of upper tract urothelial cancer. J Urol 1989;141:1298.

79. Grasso M. Resecting upper-tract urothelial Ca by ureteroscopy. Contemp Urol 1993;5:52.

80. Vest SA. Conservative surgery in certain benign tumors of the ureter. J Urol 1945;53:97.

81. Brown HE, Roumani GK. Conservative surgical management of transitional cell carcinoma of the upper urinary tract. J Urol 1974;112:184.

82. Gibson TE. Local excision in transitional cell tumors of the upper tract. J Urol 1967;97:619.

83. Petkovic SD. Conservation of the kidney in operations for tumors of the renal pelvis and calyces: a report of 26 cases. Br J Urol 1992;44:1.

84. Zincke H, Neves RJ. Feasibility of conservative surgery for transitional cell cancer of the upper urinary tract. Urol Clin North Am 1984;11:717.

85. Woodhouse CRJ, Kellett MJ, Bloom HJG. Percutaneous renal surgery and local radiotherapy in the management of renal pelvic transitional cell carcinoma. Br J Urol. 1986;58:245.

86. Streem SB, Pontes EJ. Percutaneous management of upper tract transitional cell carcinoma. J Urol 1986;135:773.

87. Nolan RL, Nichel JC, Froud PJ. Percutaneous endourologic approach for transitional cell carcinoma of the renal pelvis. Urol Rad 1988;9:217.

88. Tasca A, Zattoni F. The case of a percutaneous approach to transitional cell carcinoma of the renal pelvis. J Urol 1990;143:902.

89. Huffman JL, Bagley DH, Lyon EJ, et al. Endoscopic diagnosis and treatment of upper tract urothelial tumors: a preliminary report. Cancer 1985;55:1422.

90. Wallace DMA, Wallace DM, Whitfield HN, et al. The late results of conservative surgery for upper tract urothelial carcinomas. Br J Urol 1981;53:537.

91. Mazeman E. Tumors of the upper tract calyces, renal pelvis and ureter. Eur Urol 1976;2:120.

92. Jarrett TW, et al. Percutaneous management of transitional cell carcinoma of the upper urinary tract: ten year experience. J Endourol 1994;8(Suppl):125.

93. Tomera KM, Leary FJ, Zincke H. Pyeloscopy in urothelial tumors. J Urol 1982;127:1087–1088.

94. McCarron JP, Mills C, Vaughn ED Jr. Tumors of the renal pelvis and ureter: current concepts and management. Semin Urol 1983;1:75.

95. Elliot DS, Patterson DE, Segura JW, et al. Long term follow-up of endoscopically treated urinary tract transitional cell carcinoma. J Urol 1995;153:257. Abstract.

96. Andrews PE, Segura JW. Renal pelvic explosion during conservative management of upper tract urothelial cancer. J Urol 1991;146:407.

97. Inglis JA, Tolley DA. Conservative management of transitional cell carcinoma of the renal pelvis. J Endourol 1988;2:27.

98. Vasavada SP, Streem SB, Novick AC. Definitive tumor resection and percutaneous bacille Calmette-Guérin for management of renal pelvic transitional cell carcinoma in solitary kidneys. Urology 1995;45:381.

99. Herr HW. Durable response of a carcinoma in situ of the renal pelvis to topical bacille Calmette-Guérin. J Urol 1985;134:531.

100. Clayman RV, Kavoussi LR, McDougall EM, et al. Laparoscopic nephrectomy: a review of 16 cases. Surg Laparosc Endosc 1992;2:1.

101. Kerbl K, et al. Laparoscopic stapled bladder closure: laboratory and clinical experience. J Urol 1993;149:1437.

102. Kerbl K, et al. Laparoscopic nephroureterectomy: evaluation of first clinical series. Eur Urol 1993;23:431.

103. Adams JB, et al. Intermediate follow-up in patients undergoing laparoscopic removal of renal malignancy. J Urol 1995;153:255. Abstract.

104. Chandhoke PS, Clayman RV, Kerbl K, et al. Laparoscopic ureterectomy: initial clinical experience. J Urol 1993;149:992.

V

RETROPERITONEUM

13

Surgical Management of Retroperitoneal Tumors

Robert B. Smith and Samir S. Taneja

Retroperitoneal tumors comprise a diffuse group of tumors, of which metastatic carcinoma of the testicle is the most common. Primary retroperitoneal tumors are a group of rare tumors that originate from the various tissues of the retroperitoneum such as fat, muscle, vessels (arterial, lymphatic, or venous), and fibrous tissue of vestigial embryonic remnants. The retroperitoneal tumors discussed in this chapter deal with lesions arising from the various tissues mentioned in the retroperitoneum. Tumors occurring primarily from the kidney, ureter, liver, pancreas, adrenal, spleen, duodenum, or metastatic tumors with primary sites other than the retroperitoneal space will not be included. It appears that these tumors develop de novo and not by dedifferentiation from preexisting lesions.

Retroperitoneal tumors have been reported to develop after tissue injuries or after radiation injury (1, 2). Retroperitoneal sarcomas have also been reported after chemotherapy for primary testicular tumors. Sarcomatous degeneration of teratomas from the testicle has been reported as well (3). More than 80% of primary retroperitoneal tumors are malignant. With the exception of lymphomatous tumors, curability depends on completeness of resection (4) or the availability of adjuvant chemotherapeutic agents. The majority of these lesions are relatively radioresistant. From review of the literature, high percentages of these tumors have been found to be unresectable on initial exploration. A high mortality rate is also associated with the resection of such lesions (5–12).

Classification

Primary tumors are best classified according to the tissue of origin. The terminology for malignant tumors is complicated. More than 50 different types of soft tissue sarcomas have been described. All tumors are derived from mesenchymal cells or neural crest tissues. Tumors of mesodermal origin include those arising from adipose tissue (lipoma and liposarcoma), smooth muscle (leiomyoma and leiomyosarcoma), skeletal muscle (rhabdomyoma and rhabdomyosarcoma), connective tissue (fibroma and fibrosarcoma), blood vessels (hemangioma, hemangiosarcoma, hemangiopericytoma, and leiomyomas and leiomyosarcomas of venous structures), lymphatic vessels (lymphangioma or lymphangiosarcoma), and lymph nodes (lymphoma, Hodgkin's disease, and lymphosarcoma). Many portions of a single tumor may be well differentiated, whereas other portions may be completely undifferentiated. For this reason a small biopsy specimen may not give a proper assessment of the malignant potential of the entire lesion.

Tumors of neural origin include neurilemoma, schwannoma (sheath origin), ganglioneuroma, sympathicoblastoma, and neuroblastoma (sympathetic origin). Tumors of chromaffin tissue include paraganglioma, malignant paraganglioma, and pheochromocytoma. Tumors arising from embryonic remnants include urogenital ridge tumors, chordoma, and benign and malignant primary retroperitoneal teratomas.

Tumors of lymphatic origin are the most common (40%), with lymphosarcoma representing half of this group. Reticulum cell sarcoma and Hodgkin's disease account for the majority of the remaining lymphatic tumors. These tumors are treated as a systemic illness. Because surgical removal of the retroperitoneal portion of the malignancy is not the primary treatment, these tumors will not be discussed any further.

Liposarcoma (15%), leiomyosarcoma (10%), and rhabdomyosarcoma (8%) are the most common remaining tumors of the retroperitoneum. Tumors such as fibrosarcoma, extra-adrenal neuroblastoma, hemangiopericytoma, extragonadal germ cell tumors, malignant undifferentiated tumors, malignant histiocytoma, and other sarcomas are more rare.

Benign retroperitoneal tumors comprise only 15 to 20% of the total and include lipoma, leiomyoma, lymphangioma, xanthogranuloma, ganglioneuroma, neurofibroma, and extra-adrenal pheochromocytoma, in addition to rare retroperitoneal cysts arising from remnants of the urogenital ridge. It is often difficult to differentiate between a benign and malignant lipoma, leiomyoma, fibroma, or hemangiopericytoma. In addition, as mentioned previously, there is tremendous histologic variation within portions of a single tumor (13). One area may be well differentiated, making classification according to the primary cell of origin difficult when only small tissue samples are available. There is also evidence that these tumors have the potential to dedifferentiate into any other soft tissue elements.

Local recurrence is a common sequela, even with the so-called benign lesions. Complete radical resection is necessary for all the lesions because of the high probability of local recurrence and the possibility of sarcomatous degeneration of many of these "benign lesions." Previously mentioned sarcomatous degeneration may reflect only the variability in the initial lesion with the selective growth of the more undifferentiated components. Many pathologic studies of soft tissue sarcomas have indicated that there is rarely a true tumor capsule, although the tumors appear to be grossly encapsulated. The pseudocapsule consists of compressed surrounding cells that almost certainly have been violated by microscopic malignant cells (14).

Signs and Symptoms

Retroperitoneal tumors rarely produce early symptoms. They usually attain a large size before symptoms are noted. Abdominal or flank pain is the most common presenting symptom, followed by abdominal enlargement. Systemic symptoms such as weight loss, weakness, fever, nausea, vomiting, and decreased appetite are frequently associated symptoms but often occur relatively late in the course of the disease. Paraneoplastic syndromes such as hypoglycemia secondary to insulin-like factors secreted by the tumor have been observed in rare occasions with large poorly differentiated tumors. Swelling of the lower extremities, back pain, leg pain, and lower extremity paresthesia or weakness are usually signs of advanced disease.

An abdominal mass is the most consistent finding on physical examination. The mass generally does not move with respiration. On occasion, flank or abdominal tenderness may be present. Ascites may be present but is more common in patients with a lymphomatous lesion. Peripheral neuropathy involving the femoral nerve can also occur with a retroperitoneal pelvic mass. Approximately 25% of patients will experience neurologic symptoms secondary to compression of peripheral nerves

or nerve roots within the sacral or lumbar plexuses. Surprisingly, early complaints referable to the genitourinary tract are rare, despite the proximity of these tumors to the kidney, ureter, and bladder (Fig. 13.1).

Diagnosis

In the preoperative diagnostic evaluation of retroperitoneal masses, multiple tests should be considered, including an intravenous pyelogram, barium enema, upper gastrointestinal series, and computed tomography (CT) scan and/or magnetic resonance imaging (MRI). Currently, the CT scan is perhaps the most useful radiologic tool in the preoperative evaluation. CT scan is useful in assessing the size and position of the tumor and its relationship to surrounding structures. Preoperative assessment of spinal or vascular invasion may help to determine the likelihood of resectability. The improved quality of radiologic assessment made possible by CT and MRI has essentially obviated the other above-mentioned studies in most cases.

A venogram of the inferior vena cava should be performed in all cases of large retroperitoneal masses to aid in surgical planning, unless the MRI has delineated the extent of caval compression and/or invasion. An angiogram is essential in the evaluation of many retroperitoneal tumors, not only to assess the vascularity of the lesions, but also to aid in surgical planning. Hypervascular lesions such as hemangiopericytoma can be extremely dangerous to remove because of the risk of associated blood loss. Preoperative embolization can enable resection of even highly vascularized lesions. Figure 13.2 demonstrates the potential usefulness of this technique in the large hypervascular retroperitoneal hemangiopericytoma (15).

Angiosarcomas, rhabdomyosarcomas, and metastatic nonseminomatous testis tumors, in addition to hemangiopericytoma, may have a hypervascular pattern. Most retroperitoneal tumors, however, are hypovascular (Fig. 13.3). Under normal

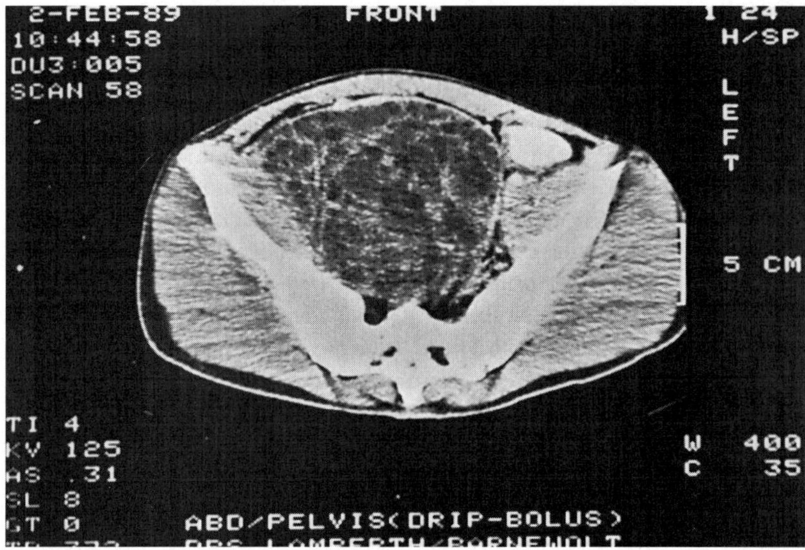

Fig. 13.1.   A huge retroperitoneal teratoma with significant distortion and displacement of the bladder. The patient denied having any voiding symptoms.

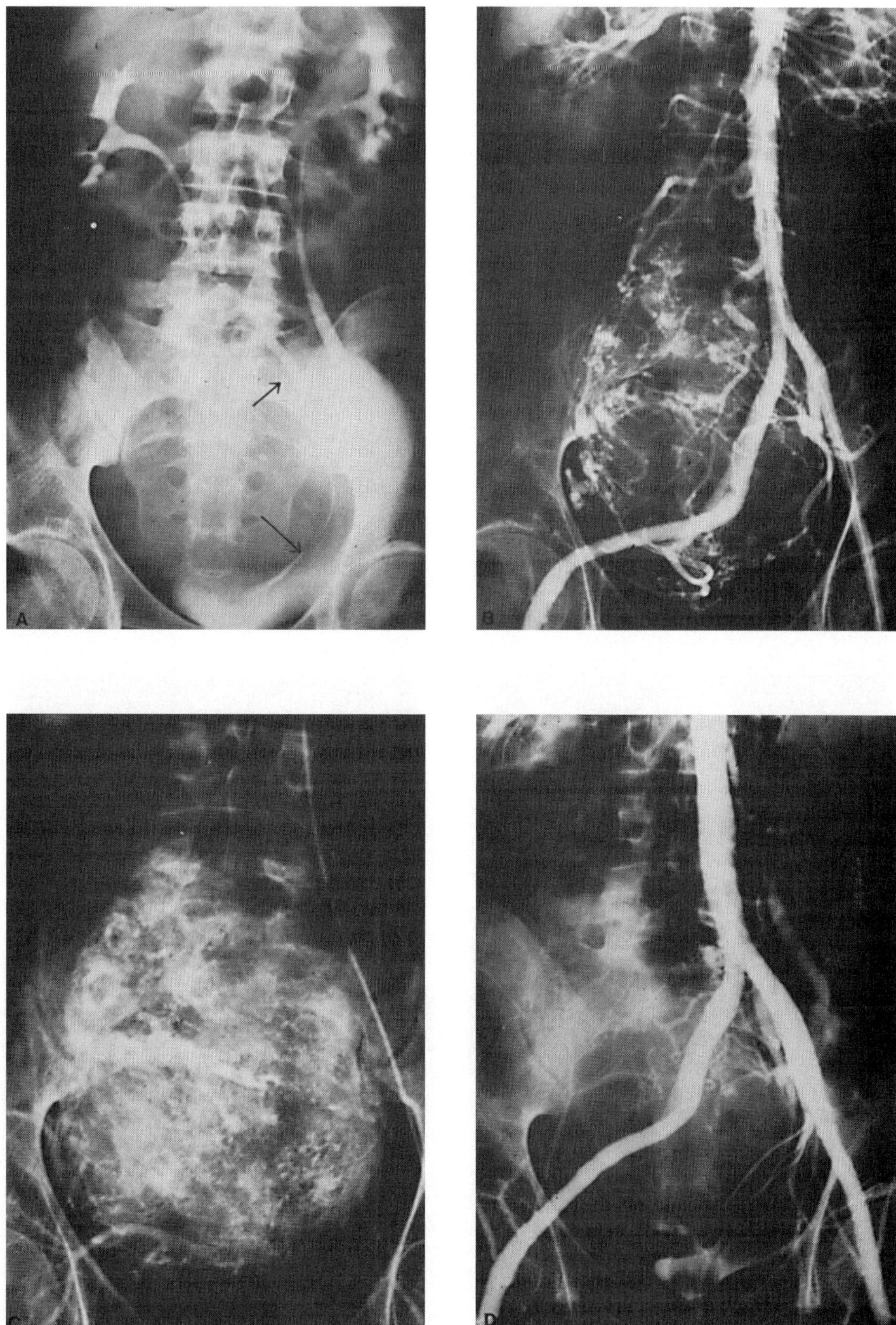

Fig. 13.2. **A.** IVP of a retroperitoneal pelvic hemangiopericytoma. Note the medial deviation of the bladder and right ureter (arrow). **B.** Angiogram. Note the hypervascularity with the blood supply from the third and fourth lumbar arteries, both hypogastric arteries, and right lateral femoral circumflex artery. **C.** The late angiogram phase showing diffuse hypervascularity of this hemangiopericytoma. **D.** Angiogram after gelatin sponge (Gelfoam) embolization (compare with B). (From Smith RB, et al. Preoperative vascular embolization as an adjunct to successful resection of a large retroperitoneal hemangiopericytoma. J Urol 1976;115:206. Copyright 1976, Williams & Wilkins, Baltimore. Reprinted by permission of publisher).

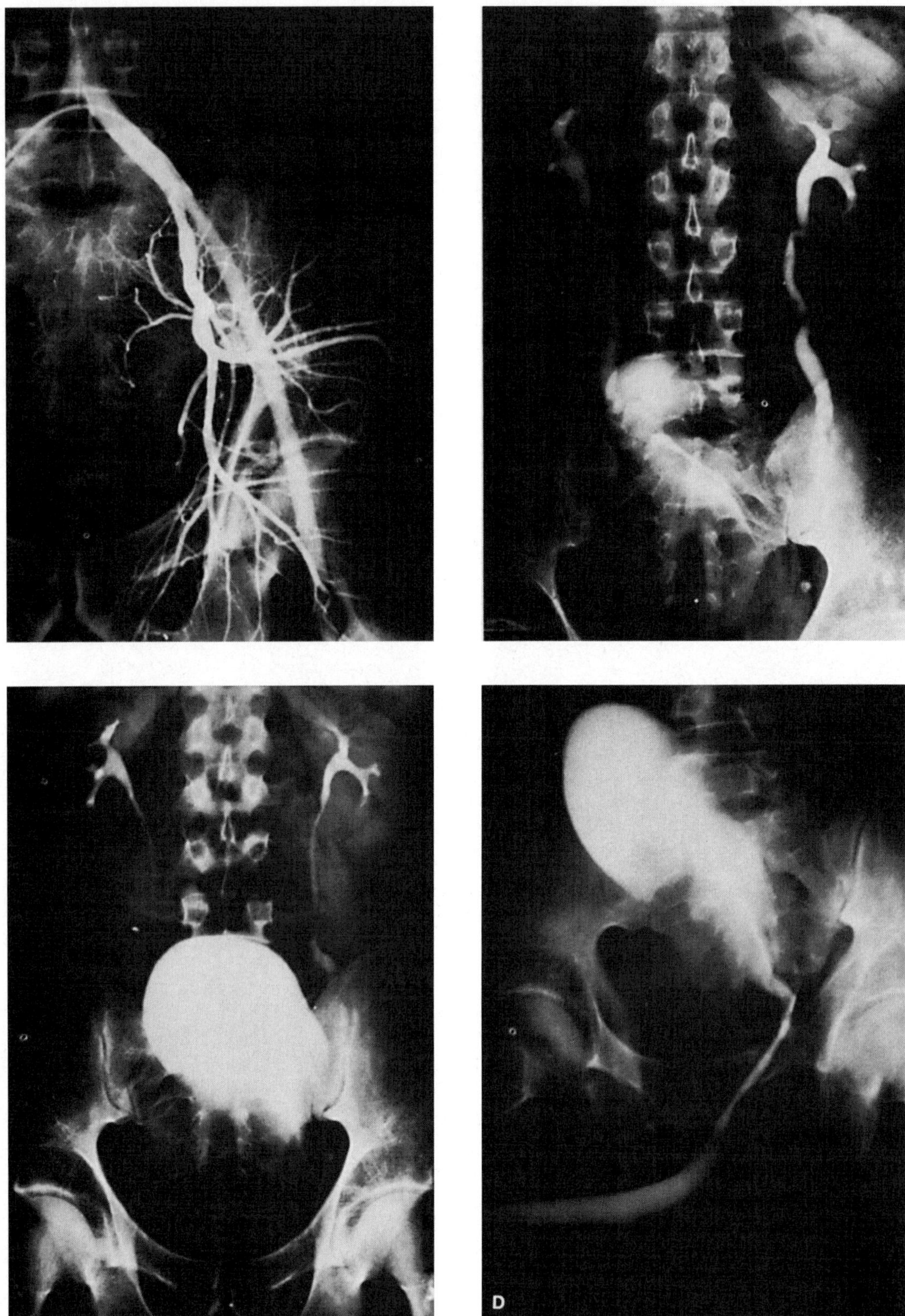

Fig. 13.3. **A.** Pelvic angiogram of a large retroperitoneal myxoliposarcoma. Note the lack of neovascularity. **B** and **C.** Intravenouse pyelogram. **D.** Voiding cystourethrogram. This lesion was excised completely, leaving the bladder, prostate, and rectum intact.

circumstances, the four-paired lumbar arteries do not contribute significant blood supply to normal retroperitoneal structures. The hypogastric artery provides the main supply to the retroperitoneum, with significant contribution from gonadal, adrenal, or renal arteries. Branches from the superior, inferior mesenteric artery and celiac axis may also contribute, in addition to the intercostal, inferior phrenic arteries. Often, hypertrophy in one of these arteries, including enlargement of a lumbar artery, may be the only indication that a retroperitoneal tumor exists (16).

A lymphangiogram or gallium scan may be indicated for evaluation of possible lymphomatous disease. In selected patients in whom the diagnosis of metastatic testicular tumor or pheochromocytoma is likely, the levels of the following substances should be measured: urinary catecholamines, vanillylmandelic acid, and the testis tumor markers beta human chorionic gonadotropin and alpha-fetoprotein. In cases suggestive of lymphoma, fine-needle aspiration biopsy may provide the diagnosis of the lesion, obviating exploratory laparotomy and biopsy.

Although fine-needle aspiration can be considered in non-lymphomatous tumor, the physician must be cognizant of the tremendous variability of the histologic pattern within a given tumor (Fig. 13.4). (13) The success of management depends on complete local excision. In addition, because many of these tumors are unresectable when the original diagnosis is made, a preoperative tissue diagnosis is essential for determining whether the lesion is radiosensitive and whether an available chemotherapy agent may be effective. Preoperative radiation therapy, with or without intra-arterial chemotherapy, may improve the chance of resecting such a lesion (7). In patients in whom a fine-needle aspiration is not successful in obtaining an adequate tissue specimen, peritoneoscopy with biopsy should be done. Whereas it is relatively safe to use fine-needle aspiration in any tumor, peritoneoscopy with direct-needle biopsy

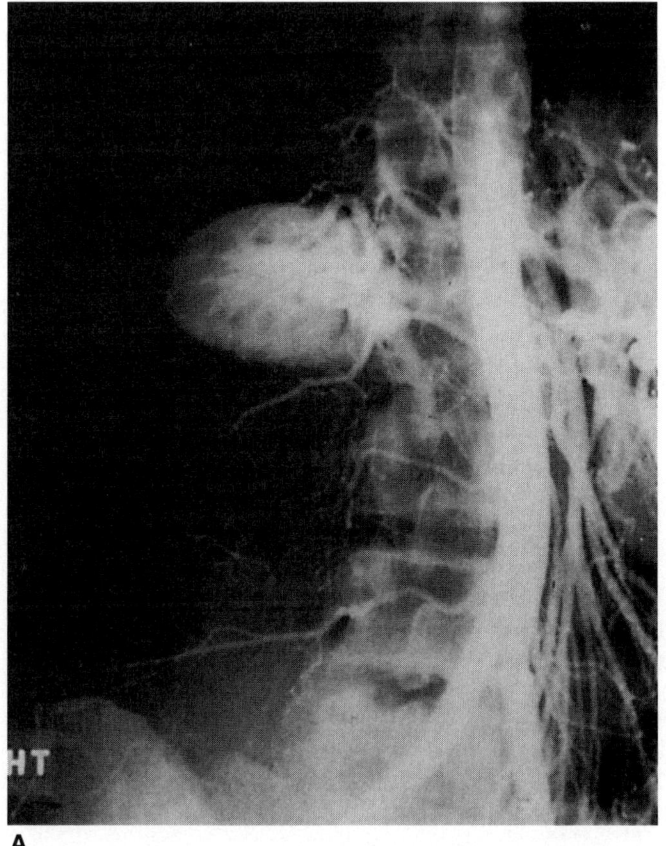
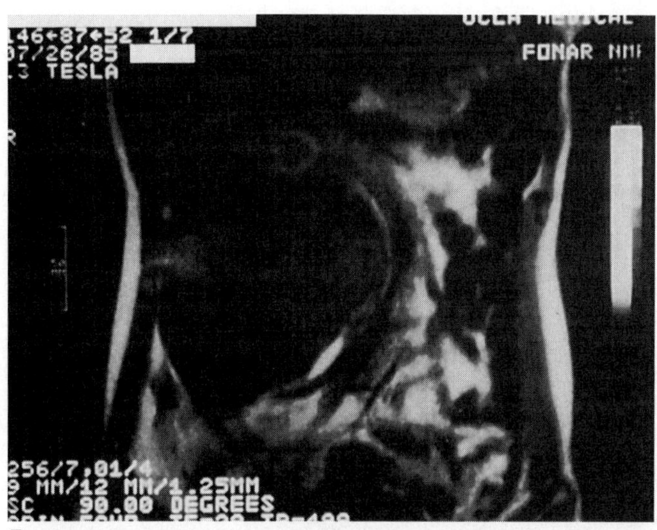
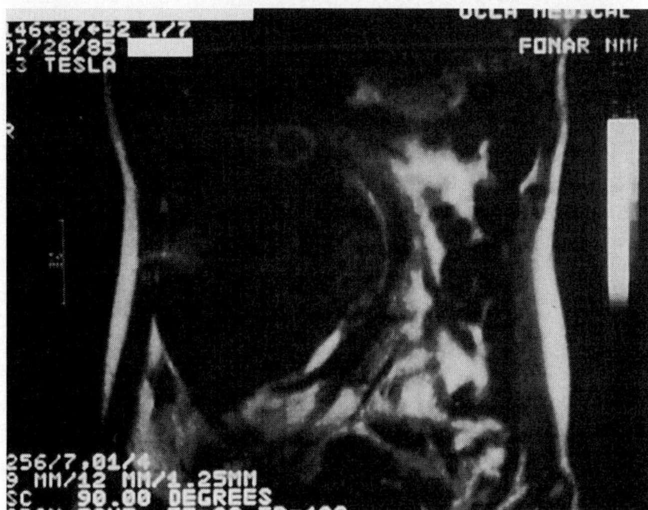

Fig. 13.4.   A large retroperitoneal liposarcoma. **A.** Angiogram demonstrating upward displacement of kidney. **B.** MRI T-1 weighted image. **C.** MRI T-2 weighted image demonstrating the great variability in the tumor.

should be used in only those patients with hypovascular lesions on angiography.

There is often a disagreement among pathologists regarding the tissue origin in some of these tumors. It appears, however, that this is much less important than the histologic grade of the tumor (the number of mitotic figures per high-power field). The American Joint Committee on Cancer has recommended a staging system where groups of patients are categorized regarding their probable therapeutic outcome (Table 13.1). Survival rate can be directly correlated to these clinical groupings (17). This system obviates exact histologic classification of the tumor.

Standard metastatic evaluation should be carried out as indicated by the nature of the primary lesion before definitive therapy is undertaken. The lung is a primary site of spread for these retroperitoneal malignant sarcomas. CT scan of the chest may be far more sensitive in the detection of small peripheral lung lesions than chest radiography alone. Liver and other visceral metastases can be detected by hepatic enzyme levels and abdominal imaging.

Table 13.1.   Stage Grouping For Soft-Tissue Sarcomas*

STAGE I
IA: G_1, T_1, N_0, M_0
      Grade-1 tumor less than 5 cm in diameter with no regional
        lymph node or distant metastases
IB: G_1, T_2, N_0, M_0
      Grade-1 tumor 5 cm or greater in diameter with no regional
        lymph node or distant metastases
STAGE II
IIA: G_2, T_1, N_0, M_0
      Grade-2 tumor less than 5 cm in diameter with no regional
        lymph node or distant metastases
IIB: G_2, T_2, N_0, M_0
      Grade-2 tumor 5 cm or greater in diameter with no regional
        lymph node or distant metastases
STAGE III
IIIA: G_3, T_1, N_0, M_0
      Grade-3 tumor less than 5 cm in diameter with no regional
        lymph node or distant metastases
IIIB: G_3, T_2, N_0, M_0
      Grade-3 tumor 5 cm or greater in diameter with no regional
        lymph node or distant metastases
IIIC: Any G, T_1, or T_2, N_1, M_0
      Tumor of any histologic grade or size (no invasion) with
        regional lymph node metastases but without distant me-
        tastases
STAGE IV
IVA: Any G, T_3, any N, M_0
      Tumor of any histologic grade or malignancy that grossly
        invades bone, major vessels, or major nerves with or with-
        out regional lymph node metastases but without distant
        metatases
IVB: Any G, any T, any N, M_1
      Tumor with distant metastases

* From American Joint Committee on Cancer. *Manual for Staging of Cancer,* 2nd edition. Edited by OH Beahrs and MH Myers. Philadelphia, JB Lippincott, 1983:111.

Treatment

The treatment of choice for these lesions is wide, local excision. It must be understood that these tumors often extend well beyond their so-called pseudocapsule. Microscopic extension tends to occur along fascial planes and may be as far as 6 to 7 cm beyond all gross disease (18, 19). Metastasis to regional lymph nodes is an uncommon event.

To maximize the possibility of a successful resection, appropriate preoperative systemic chemotherapy, radiation therapy, or infusional chemotherapy may decrease the size of primary lesions, increasing the chance of resectability. Also, some tumors may develop a dense capsule after chemotherapy, which can aid in the resection. Another advantage to preoperative therapy is the theoretical decrease in the likelihood of tumor embolization during the manipulation of the tumor at the time of resection. The surgical treatment of retroperitoneal sarcomas involves a wide resection of tumor including wide normal margins. Removal of adjacent organs or vessels may be necessary to achieve complete surgical resection. Despite some recent responses to chemotherapy and radiation therapy, a wide surgical excision is still accepted as the best means of achieving a potential long-term cure. The best results have been seen in those tumors in which a margin greater than 3 cm can be obtained. If this is not feasible, preoperative adjuvant chemotherapy or radiation therapy should be given.

Preoperative Preparation

Adequate preoperative preparation is essential. Intra-arterial lines and Swan-Ganz catheters are helpful in monitoring these potentially extensive procedures. Adequate blood should be ordered preoperatively because blood loss can be considerable. Although it is rarely necessary to type and cross for more than 6 units, the blood bank should be warned of the potential magnitude of blood loss to assure that enough units of type-specific blood are available.

Consent of the patient should be obtained to allow removal of contiguous structures that may be involved by the primary lesion. In cases involving the high retroperitoneum, en bloc resection of the kidney, vena cava, or ureter may be necessary. In cases of retroperitoneal pelvic tumors, consent should be obtained for anterior or posterior exenteration or both, along with the appropriate urinary or fecal diversion.

Complete bowel preparation (mechanical and antibiotic) is essential should bowel injury occur or should bowel resection become necessary. The patient should be well hydrated with intravenous fluids. General anesthesia, with controlled use of nitroprusside, may lessen intraoperative blood loss in high-risk patients.

SURGICAL PROCEDURE

Tumors Above the Pelvis: Thoracoabdominal Incision

It is essential that the patient be positioned properly before the incision is made. The torque flank position is ideal, with the shoulders at a 40 to 45° angle and the pelvis in as supine a position as possible. The patient should be placed as close as possible to the operating surgeon, with the table fully hyperextended (Fig. 13.5). The use of the thoracoabdominal approach for lesions above the true pelvis maximizes the chance for a complete resection. The superior exposure afforded by this approach and the access to all retroperitoneal vessels, including the ipsilateral great vessels (inferior vena cava or aorta), above the diaphragm make this the incision of choice. The thoracoabdominal incision also allows palpation of the mediastinal area and the ipsilateral lung parenchyma.

The level of the thoracoabdominal incision depends on the size and location of the tumor. Most commonly, it is made in the eighth, ninth, or tenth interspace and should extend at least to the midaxillary line posteriorly. It is our experience that resection of a rib is unnecessary to facilitate exposure but may be used at the discretion of the surgeon. The larger the mass, the higher the incision. The incision crosses over to the midline, transecting the rectus muscle in the epigastrium, which prevents denervation of the rectus muscle. The incision can then be extended inferiorly as a midline or paramedian incision toward the pubis. For large tumors, a T incision is made anteriorly or posteriorly to the main thoracoabdominal incision (Fig. 13.6).

No attempt is made to remain outside the peritoneum in operations for large retroperitoneal lesions. The peritoneum should be entered promptly to save time and to facilitate exposure. The transverse colon, descending or ascending colon,

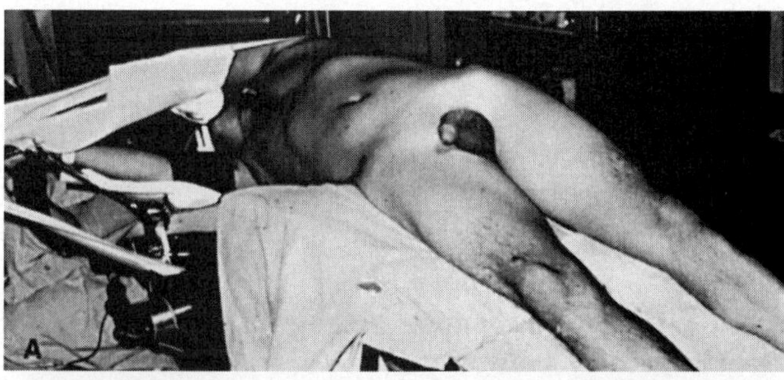

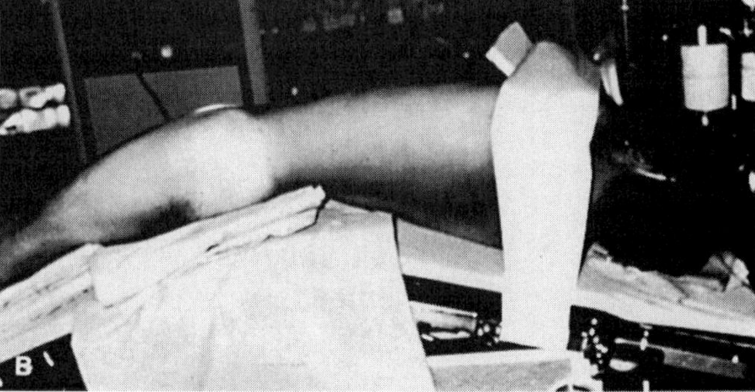

Fig. 13.5. **A.** Operative position (torque flank position). Note the shoulder angle 40 to 45° to the horizontal. The table is fully hyperextended. **B.** The pelvis is nearly in the supine position. The patient is as close as possible to the surgeon's side of the table.

small bowel, duodenum, and pancreas are completely mobilized to gain access. For left-sided tumors, the peritoneal incision is made down the left lateral peritoneal reflection from the splenic flexure around the sigmoid colon to the pelvic brim. A medial incision is also made in the colon mesentery, maintaining the integrity of the marginal artery (Fig. 13.7).

Right-sided lesions are exposed by incising the posterior peritoneum from the hepatic flexure down the ascending colon and around the cecum. The incision is then carried superiorly to the ligament of Treitz (Fig. 13.8). This allows complete mobility of the right colon, small bowel, duodenum, and pancreas on the superior mesenteric artery pedicle. Care should be taken not to occlude the superior mesenteric artery by extensive tension. All bowel contents are then placed in a Lahey bag. For left-sided tumors that are large or cross over the midline, the peritoneal incision is as shown in Figure 13.7.

If the abdominal contents have been mobilized on the superior mesenteric artery pedicle, it is important to check from time to time to make sure that the blood flow via the superior mesenteric artery has not been occluded because of a kink or excessive tension on the pedicle. Ligation of the inferior mesenteric artery aids in mobilization of the descending colon and should be performed for large, left-sided lesions. The marginal artery must remain intact, however. In older patients, diarrhea or cramping abdominal pain may result from inferior mesenteric artery ligation; this is rare in younger patients and only occasionally presents serious problems in any age group.

Although it has not occurred in our series at UCLA, ischemic damage to the colon may occur. If ischemic damage is noted, the ischemic portion of the colon should be resected primarily and the colon reanastomosed. The decision to protect the anastomosis by a proximal diverting colostomy depends on the surgeon's preference, the success of the preoperative bowel preparation, and the technical quality of the anastomosis.

After proper mobilization of the aforementioned structures, an attempt should be made to secure control of the feeding vessels as determined by a preoperative angiogram. Embolization is a valuable adjunct to the surgical procedure in lessening the amount of intraoperative blood loss. The ipsilateral great vessel (and occasionally the contralateral great vessel) should be mobilized by ligating the lumbar vessels below the level of the renal pedicle. Ischemic damage to the spinal cord should not occur; the spinal cord ends at the level of the first lumbar vertebra. Extensive experience in surgical procedures for aortic aneurysms has confirmed the safety of this maneuver (20). Reports still exist, however, of spinal ischemia following this maneuver, but these are rare (21) and are probably related to prolonged periods of hypotension associated with aneurysm resections.

There are usually four pairs of lumbar arteries found distal to the main renal artery. These arteries should be individually ligated with 3-0 or 4-0 silk ties proximally and hemostatic clips on the distal portion of the vessels. The use of hemoclips in the proximal portion is dangerous and may be a source of serious intraoperative or postoperative hemorrhage if a clip becomes dislodged. In rare cases, retroperitoneal lesions have in-

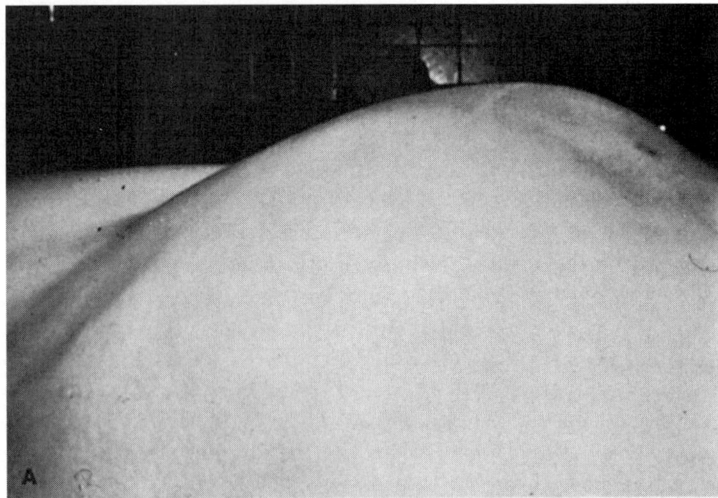

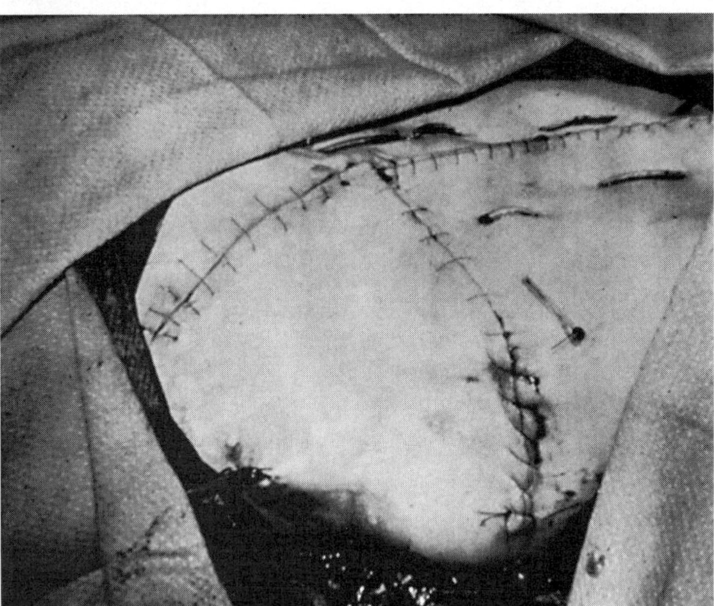

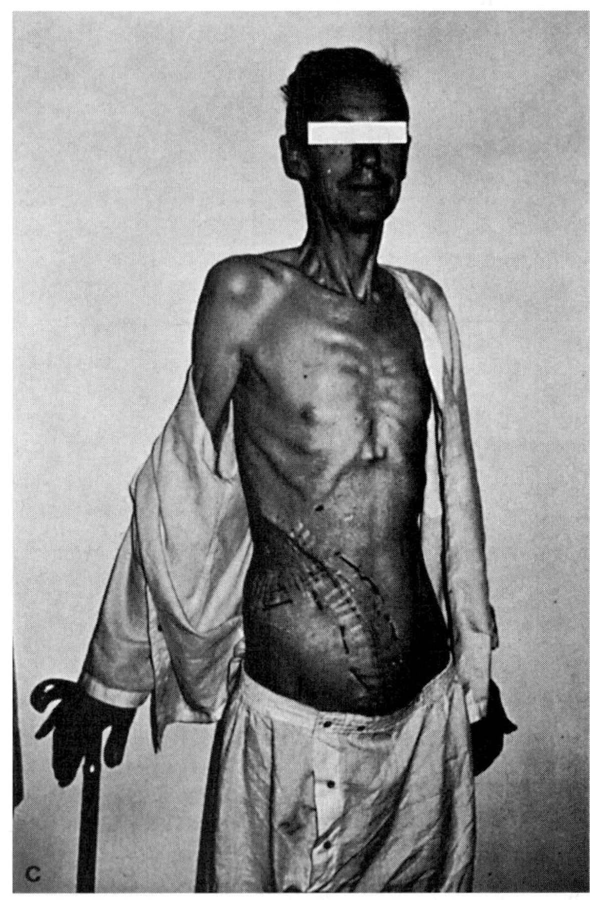

Fig. 13.6. **A.** A huge retroperitoneal tumor obvious on inspection. **B.** The thoracoabdominal incision via the 8th interspace was not sufficient to gain adequate posterior exposure. A posterior T-extension of the incision was made. **C.** Postoperative appearance of the incision.

vaded or encased the aorta or iliac artery. In these cases, the aorta or iliac artery should be resected and then replaced with a Dacron bypass graft.

Vena caval obstruction by invasion or encasement by a tumor occurs more commonly (Fig. 13.9). The vena cava can be resected en bloc with the tumors, especially if the tumors have obstructed the vena cava preoperatively. In these instances, collateral venous channels are established mainly via paraspinus venous plexus, but retroperitoneal venous collateral vessels may also be present and troublesome at the time of tumor resection. If necessary, these may be ligated to allow exposure or to ensure complete removal of the lesion.

It is dangerous to ligate the vena cava above the level of the renal veins, especially if only the right kidney remains. In these cases, all attempts should be made to maintain the integrity

of the vena cava or to perform some form of venous drainage procedure to the right renal vein via the splenic or portal vein. Even ligation of the left renal vein at its insertion in the vena cava is not without risk, despite well-documented potential collateral flow via the left adrenal, lumbar, and gonadal veins. Cases of significant morbidity with prolonged acute tubular necrosis have been reported (22) and have also been seen in our series. En bloc resection of contiguous structures invaded by direct extension should be performed if technically feasible. Resection of the posterior body wall musculature is often necessary to obtain clear margins.

Both ureters should be identified and protected. Stripping of ureteral adventitia should be avoided if possible. Major lymphatic vessels should be occluded with hemoclips to lessen the likelihood of lymphocele or chylous ascites. Care should be taken not to injure the cisterna chyli, which is in the area of the crus of the diaphragm, usually behind the right renal artery. If encountered and opened, it should be ligated or controlled with a suture or hemoclip.

If technically feasible, one or both of the sympathetic chains should be preserved to prevent ejaculatory failure. Unnecessary dissection over the anterior aspect of the lower portion of the aorta near its bifurcation could also cause ejaculatory failure. In cases of large retroperitoneal tumors, and particularly in bulky metastatic testicular tumors, it is often necessary to sacrifice both sympathetic trunks. The patient should be forewarned of this possibility and the couple encouraged to deposit semen in a sperm bank preoperatively if they wish to have children.

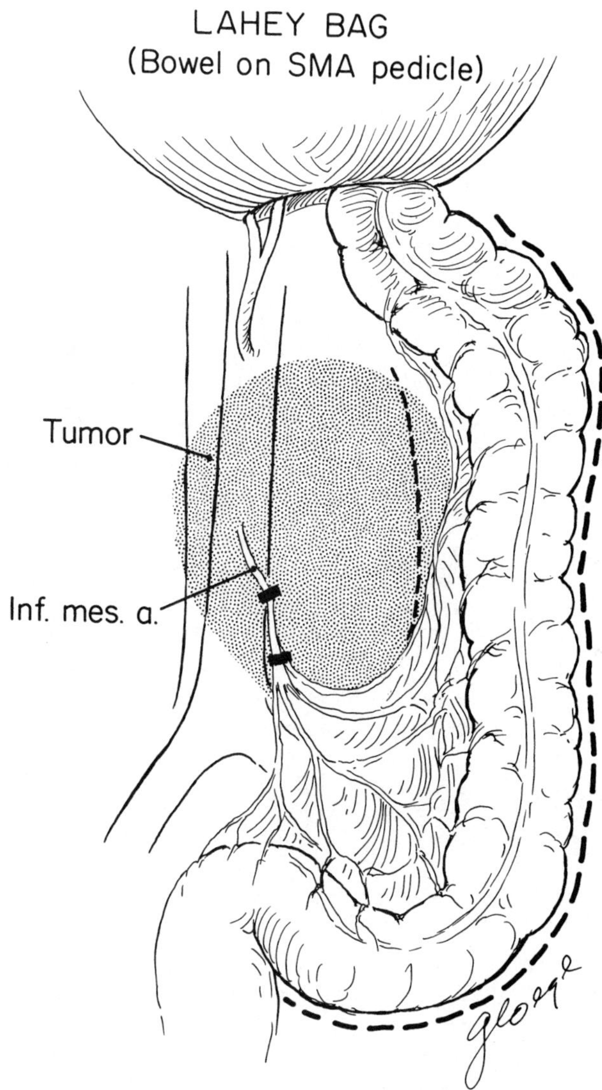

Fig. 13.7. A peritoneal incision for left-sided tumors. The incision is made down the left lateral peritoneal reflection from the splenic flexure, around the sigmoid colon, to the pelvic brim. A medial incision is also made in the colon mesentery, maintaining the integrity of the marginal artery. Ligation of the inferior mesenteric artery aids in mobilization of the ascending colon and should be performed for large left-sided lesions. This can be combined with the maneuver depicted in Figure 13.6 for large lesions.

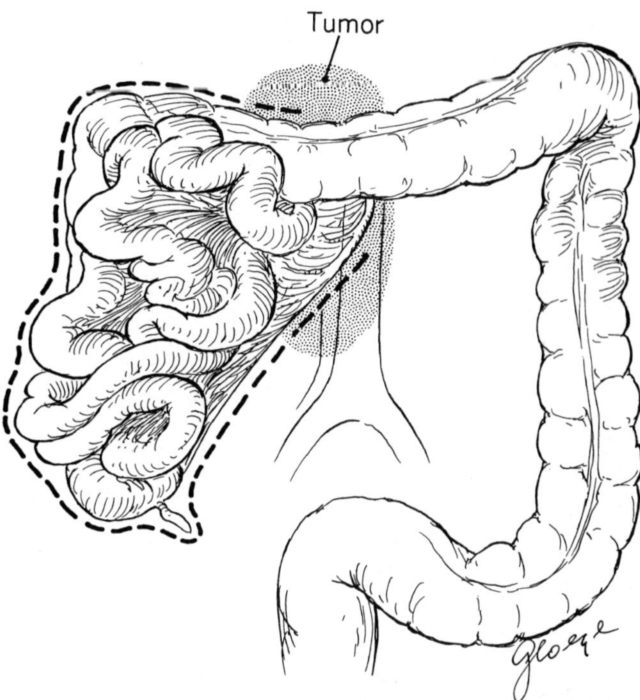

Fig. 13.8. The posterior peritoneum is incised from the hepatic flexure down the ascending colon and around the cecum. The incision is then carried superiorly to the ligament of Treitz. This allows complete mobility of the right colon, small bowel, duodenum, and pancreas on a superior mesenteric artery pedicle. Care should be taken not to occlude the superior mesenteric artery by intensive tension. All bowel contents are placed in a Lahey bag.

Reperitonealization is unnecessary but may be done. Drains are not routinely left in place unless a specific indication exists (i.e., pancreatic injury or resection). A large chest tube is left indwelling until chest drainage ceases. The thoracoabdominal incision is closed in a standard manner, taking care to resect extra rib cartilage at the costal margin; a painful postoperative wound can result if cartilage is allowed to override. Injection of bupivacaine hydrochloride (5 mL of 0.75 solution) decreases postoperative pain (23).

Tumors of the True Pelvis

A lesion in the true pelvis is best approached through a midline lower abdominal intraperitoneal or extraperitoneal incision, although a transverse or unilateral Gibson incision can be used depending on the surgeon's preference. The superior exposure afforded by the midline incision and the possibility of an intraperitoneal approach make it ideal. On occasion, the extent of pelvic retroperitoneal tumors is underestimated, especially regarding their upward extension. A low transverse or unilateral extraperitoneal incision may seriously compromise the surgeon's operative exposure. It is often possible to excise these pelvic masses without performing cystectomy or proctectomy. Figure 13.3 shows a large retroperitoneal myxoliposarcoma that

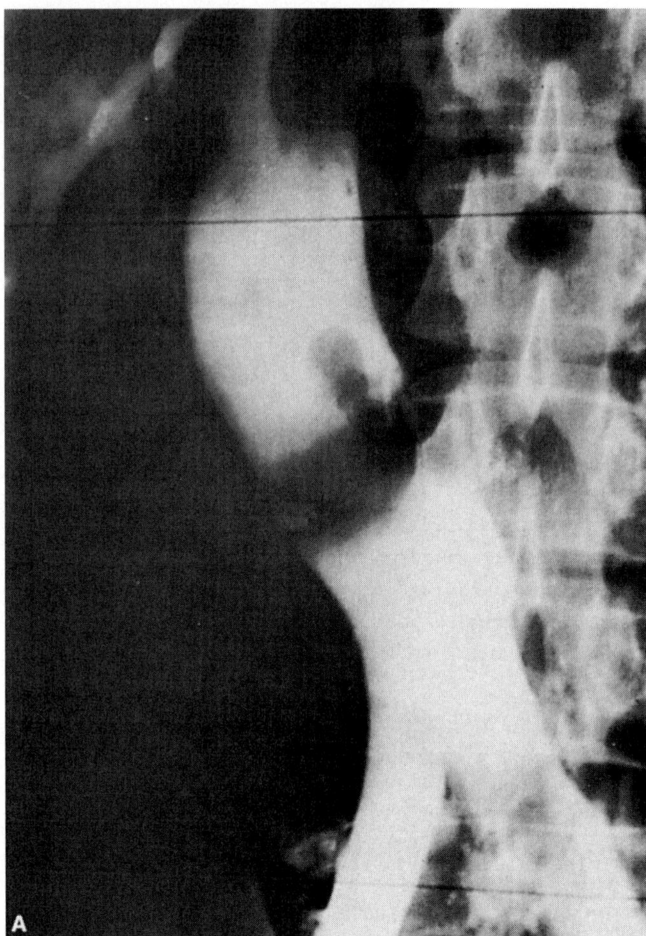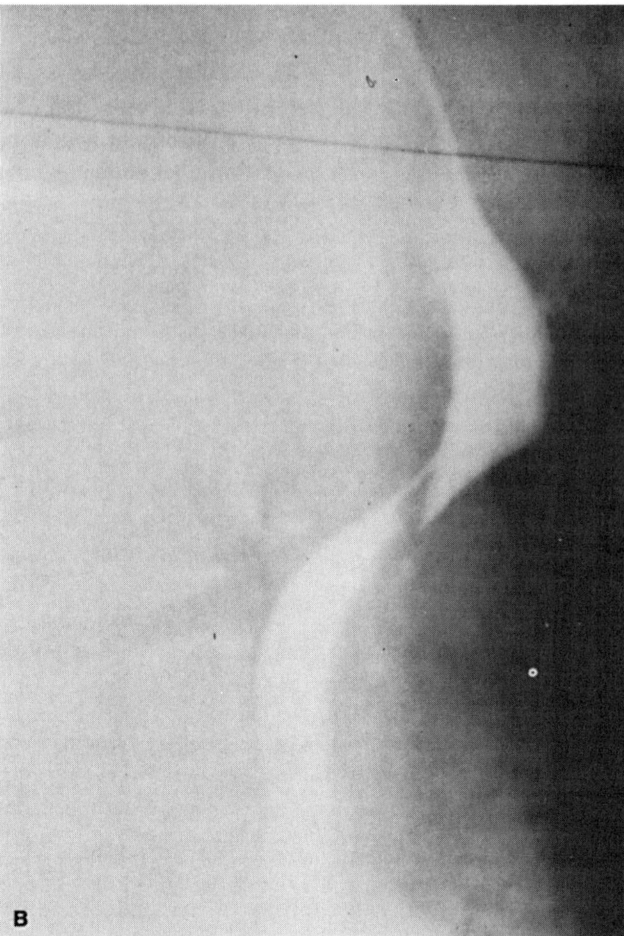

Fig. 13.9.   Inferior venacavogram. **A.** Anteroposterior view. Note the lateral deviation of the vena cava with intraluminal filling defects. **B.** Lateral view. Note the anterior displacement of the vena cava with intraluminal invasion.

was removed without removal of the bladder, prostate, or rectum. However, the surgeon must carefully prepare these patients both medically and emotionally for possible exenteration.

POSTOPERATIVE CARE AND COMPLICATIONS

Postoperative care is standard as with any major surgical procedure. A large, third-space fluid loss occurs with these procedures, and replacement of this loss with colloid is essential in the early postoperative period (usually 50 to 75 mL/hr for 36 to 48 hours). The chest tube is connected to a three-bottle suction device until significant drainage ceases. It is then usually connected to water/seal drainage for an additional 24 hours before removal to lessen the likelihood of subsequent hydrothorax or hemothorax. Nasogastric drainage is generally maintained until postoperative ileus abates. Monitoring with a Swan-Ganz catheter is used if medically indicated. We do not favor prophylactic anticoagulation in these patients because complications from this therapy, in our experience, exceeded the benefit. Pulsatile pneumatic stockings, however, have been

shown to lessen the likelihood of deep venous thrombosis in the extremities and should be used (24).

Devascularization of the spinal cord has not occurred in our series. Lymphoceles can be a problem, as can chylous ascites or chylothorax. These complications, on occasion, may require operation (25). Extraperitoneal lymphoceles can be treated with external drainage or the creation of an intraperitoneal window. Lymphoceles rarely occur when a primary intraperitoneal approach is used. Chylous ascites is almost always caused by damage to the cisterna chyli. Spontaneous resolution usually occurs unless proximal obstruction of the thoracic duct is present. Patients with significant lymphocele or chylous ascites should be maintained on a medium-chain fatty acid diet to decrease lymphatic outflow. On occasion, reoperation may be necessary to ligate the lymphatic leaks. Chylothorax usually responds to prolonged chest tube drainage and a medium-chain fatty acid diet.

Ureteral injuries, when seen, must be managed with great care because the extensive retroperitoneal mobilization necessary may devascularize a ureter. Ureteral lesions in the lower or middle third should be managed by ureteral reimplantation or implantation with a psoas hitch, a Boari flap, or a combination of these techniques. Primary reanastomosis is dangerous because of precarious blood supply, especially in the middle- or upper-third injuries to the ureter and in cases where preoperative radiation therapy or chemotherapy has been administered. Autotransplantation, ileal ureter replacement, and even nephrectomy are treatment options in upper-third injuries. Ischemic injury to the bowel should be managed by resection of the ischemic segment. Late bowel fistulas are best managed by incision and drainage and the replacement of the bowel at prolonged rest, with the institution of parenteral hyperalimentation.

On occasion, a polar renal artery can be damaged, and reanastomosis should be attempted if feasible. If this is not technically feasible, simple ligation usually suffices. In cases in which a unilateral sympathectomy has been performed, temperature difference in the lower extremity should be expected in the postoperative period.

NONSURGICAL TREATMENT MODALITIES

Radiation Therapy

Because of the high recurrence rates of retroperitoneal sarcomas after incomplete gross excision, many investigators have attempted to use radiation therapy as an adjunctive measure in effecting locoregional control or cure. The primary limitation in the use of radiation therapy for retroperitoneal tumors is the inability of surrounding viscera to tolerate high doses generally used in the extremities. This limitation results in high rates of local failure of up to 80 to 85% and survival rates of 10% following the use of radiation therapy alone (26–29). The true value of radiation therapy may be in the treatment of patients with complete resection and microscopically positive margins or even in those patients with incomplete resection at the time of primary exploration. Although no series has shown a significant improvement in survival with the use of adjuvant radiation therapy, the rate of local recurrence is affected favorably. Again, the limiting factor appears to be radiation dose.

A randomized trial of patients undergoing adjuvant radiation therapy compared radiation doses of greater or less than 5500 cGy (30). Patients receiving greater than 5500 cGy had 2-year local recurrence rates of 25% compared with 38% for those receiving lower doses. No increase in radiation-related morbidity was noted in the higher dose group due to the use of small bowel exclusion measures to reduce toxicity. The possibility that higher radiation doses will improve long-term survival remains to be confirmed in longer follow-up.

Several institutions proposed the use of intraoperative radiation therapy (IORT) in the treatment of retroperitoneal sarcomas (31, 32). Irradiation of the tumor bed intraoperatively allows an increased total radiation dose with lower levels of exposure to surrounding viscera and bowel. Updated data from these randomized trials of resection and postoperative external beam radiation therapy (EBRT) of 5000 to 5500 cGy versus resection and IORT (2000 cGy), and postoperative EBRT of 3500 to 4000 cGy reveal relatively similar survival rates among the two treated groups (33). Local recurrence was significantly less frequent in the IORT group (6 of 15 patients) than in the control group (16 of 20 patients), with a median follow-up of 8 years. Additionally, patients receiving IORT had a reduction in the incidence of radiation enteritis but an increase in the incidence of peripheral neuropathy-related complications. Although IORT does appear to allow a reduction in postoperative radiation dose, it is costly and its value in improving prognosis remains undetermined.

Interest in improving response rates to radiation has sparked an interest in the use of radiation sensitizers such as iododeoxyuridine (IdUrd). A phase I/II trial of IdUrd and preoperative EBRT delivered twice daily (125 cGy/dose) resulted in a local control rate of 45% after resection with or without postoperative EBRT at relatively short follow-up (34). Local recurrence was present in only 37.5% of patients with complete resection with or without microscopically positive margins. Although these data are based on small patient numbers and short follow-up, the concept of enhancing radiation response may represent an important trend.

Efforts to control local recurrence in patients undergoing partial resection have been less fruitful and may be very dependent on the volume of residual disease. Investigators report a drastic reduction in local recurrence rates in partial resection patients responding to adjuvant therapy with doses in the range of 6000 cGy (17% recurrence) when compared with doses of 5000 cGy (65% recurrence) (35).

Chemotherapy

Early attempts to treat soft tissue sarcomas with chemotherapy showed doxorubicin (Adriamycin) to be the only single-agent therapy with significant antitumor activity. Initial reports suggested a response rate of up to 40% (36–38), with occasional complete responses resulting in long-term, disease-free survival times of more than 5 years. Subsequent follow-up has revealed that complete responses of significant durability are rare using doxorubicin alone. The exception remains in extremity sarcomas where the use of intra-arterial infusion of doxorubicin preoperatively provides relatively low local recurrence rates and higher 5-year survival rates than those noted with retroperitoneal sarcomas (39–41). Certainly, the inability to deliver intra-arterial infusion secondary to a poorly defined arterial supply contributes to the difficulty in approaching retroperitoneal tumors.

In view of poor response rates with single-agent therapy, several combination protocols have been developed with the intent of improving the efficacy of chemotherapy as a treatment modality. Most combination therapies fail to show any improvement in survival when compared with single-agent doxorubicin. Currently, efforts are focused on the use of cytokines to enhance chemotherapeutic response rates. A phase I trial of ifosfamide, doxorubicin, and cisplatin with or without mitomycin used subcutaneously delivered recombinant granulocyte-macrophage colony-stimulating-factor (GM-CSF) with the intensive chemotherapeutic regimen (42). Five complete responses were noted among 15 patients with disseminated sarcoma of varied histologic type. Additionally, four partial responses were noted with subsequent conversion of two patients to complete response after surgical resection. It is unclear if the noted effect of GM-CSF is secondary to bone marrow stimulation or direct enhancement of antitumor immune mechanisms. Although follow-up is short, the use of GM-CSF appears to offer great promise in improving the treatment of disseminated disease.

Because adjuvant chemotherapy protocols have largely failed in controlling locoregional recurrence or affecting survival (43) investigators have attempted to use preoperative chemotherapy in combination with preoperative and intraoperative. Although most data come from extremity sarcoma protocols, such an approach does appear to have great potential in reducing local recurrence rates (44, 45). Additional attempts at extremity perfusion with various cytokines, including interferon alfa and tumor necrosis factor, also appear to offer a new adjunct in therapy for soft tissue sarcomas (46–48). Obviously, systemic side effects will limit use in the treatment of the retroperitoneal variety of tumor.

PROGNOSIS

Local recurrence remains the most common pattern of disease progression among patients undergoing resection of primary retroperitoneal sarcomas, occurring in 75% of patients with noted postoperative recurrence (49). The majority of recurrence occurs within 2 years, but can occur as late as 5 years (49). Although distant metastases will eventually develop in only 30 to 40% of these patients, local recurrence does indicate a poor prognosis and likely disease-related mortality.

In a review of 88 explorations for recurrent retroperitoneal sarcoma, complete resection was possible in 44% of patients, with additional patients benefiting from palliative resection to eliminate tumor-related symptoms. Survival on complete resection was drastically improved to a median of 48 months compared with 21 months for partial resection and 15 months for unresectable recurrences (50). Fourteen patients remained clinically free of disease at longer than 3 years follow-up. Although complete resection may not be possible, aggressive partial resection may improve survival and certainly may improve the patient's quality of life.

Despite adherence to the principles of aggressive surgical resection, survival rates for retroperitoneal sarcoma remain poor. Most series reports 10-year survival rates ranging from 14 to 33%, with lower relapse-free survival rates (50, 51). A recent review of 104 patients treated by aggressive surgical resection with or without adjuvant therapy revealed 5-year and 10-year survival rates of 36% and 14%, respectively. Respective recurrence-free rates of 28% and 9% were noted at the same intervals (52). The only predictor of improved survival was

complete surgical resection, which improved survival rates to 55% and 22% at 5 and 10 years. The use of postoperative radiation did not improve overall survival; however, those patients receiving radiation therapy of greater than 3500 cGy often saw a delay in time to progression.

A second series reaffirmed the improved survival after complete resection and identified histologic grade as an independent predictor of survival (49). Low-grade tumors resulted in an 80-month median survival time after resection compared with 20 months for high-grade tumors. Histologic type does not appear to affect survival significantly. In a third study, improved survival approaching that of complete resection was noted in patients undergoing aggressive partial resection (50).

Summary

In approaching the patient with retroperitoneal sarcoma, the surgeon must first fully stage the disease through appropriate imaging of the retroperitoneum as well as the gastrointestinal and urinary tracts. CT scan and MRI have largely replaced conventional radiologic staging methods, but angiography still may provide valuable information regarding the vascular supply of the tumor and its proximity to important vascular structures. Preoperative embolization should be reserved for select hypervascular tumors with defined arterial supply and may be extremely helpful in this subset of patients.

Aggressive surgical resection of the primary tumor, including en bloc resection of juxtaposed viscera, may provide the only chance for cure. The role for adjuvant therapies is limited by the relative ineffectiveness of chemotherapy and the inability of surrounding intra-abdominal viscera to tolerate high doses of radiation. Certainly, IORT may improve the likelihood of preventing local recurrence in complete gross resection.

Local recurrence is the most common therapeutic failure and often serves as a grim prognostic indicator. Once diagnosed, locoregional recurrences should be approached in an aggressive manner equivalent to that of the primary tumor treatment regimen.

Although recent combination chemotherapy and cytokine-based protocols carry great promise in improving overall survival, results must still be confirmed by long-term follow-up. In approaching the patient with retroperitoneal sarcoma, aggressive primary surgical therapy remains the only controllable variable in improving outcome. Combination therapy using external beam and IORT along with the previously mentioned chemotherapy protocols may further enhance the ability of the surgeon to successfully treat this biologically aggressive disease.

REFERENCES

1. Pack FT, Braund RR. The development of sarcoma in myositis ossificans. JAMA 1942;119:776.
2. Petit VD, Chamnes JT, Ackerman LV. Fibromatosis and fibrosarcoma following irradiation therapy. Cancer 1954;7:149.
3. Ulbright TM, et al. The development of non-germ cell

malignancies within germ cell tumors: a clinical pathological study of 11 cases. Cancer 1984;54:1824.

4. Kinne DW, et al. Treatment of primary and recurrent retroperitoneal liposarcomas: 25 years experience at Memorial Hospital. Cancer 1973;31:53.

5. Deweerd JH, Dockert MB. Lipomatous retroperitoneal tumors. Am J Surg 1952;84:397.

6. Bek V. Primary retroperitoneal tumors. Neoplasia 1970;17: 253.

7. Wiley AL, et al. Clinical and theoretical aspects of treatment of surgically unresectable retroperitoneal malignancies with combined intraarterial Actinomycin D and radiation therapy. Cancer 1975;36:107.

8. Rhamy RK. Retroperitoneal tumors. In: Glenn J, ed. Urologic surgery. 2nd ed. New York: Harper & Row, 1975:859.

9. McGrath PC, et al. Improved survival following complete excision of retroperitoneal sarcomas. Ann Surg 1984;200:200.

10. Bengmark S, et al. Retroperitoneal sarcoma treated by surgery. J Surg Oncol 1980;14:307.

11. Solla JA, Reed K. Primary retroperitoneal sarcomas. Am J Surg 1986;152:496.

12. Salvadori B, et al. Surgical treatment of 43 retroperitoneal sarcomas. Eur J Surg Oncol 1986;12:29.

13. Snover DC, et al. Variability of histologic pattern in recurrent soft tissue sarcomas originally diagnosed as liposarcoma. Cancer 1982;49:1005.

14. Bowden L, Booker, RJ. The principles and technique of resection of soft parts for sarcoma. Surgery 1958;44:963.

15. Smith RB, et al. Preoperative vascular embolization as an adjunct to successful resection of a large retroperitoneal hemangiopericytoma. J Urol 1976;115:206.

16. Lowman RM, et al. The angiographic patterns of the primary retroperitoneal tumors. Radiology 1972;104:259.

17. American Joint Committee on Cancer. In: Beahrs OH, Myers MH, eds. Manual for staging of cancer. 2nd ed. Philadelphia: JB Lippincott, 1983.

18. Krementz ET, Shaver JC. Behavior and treatment of soft tissue sarcomas. Ann Surg 1963;157:770.

19. Gerner RE, Moore GE. Synovial sarcoma. Ann Surg 1975; 181:22.

20. Debakey ME, et al. Aneurysms of the abdominal aorta: analysis of results of graft replacement therapy one to eleven years after operation. Ann Surg 1964;160:622.

21. Ferguson LRJ, et al. Spinal ischemia following abdominal aortic surgery. Ann Surg 1975;181:267.

22. McCullough DL, Gittes RF. Ligation of the renal vein in the solitary kidney: effects on renal function. J Urol 1975;113:295.

23. Crawford ED, et al. Intercostal nerve block with thoracoabdominal incision. J Urol 1978;121:290.

24. Coe MP, et al. Prevention of deep vein thrombosis in urologic patients: a controlled, randomized trial of low-dose heparin in external pneumatic compression boots. Surgery 1978;83:230.

25. Livingston WD, Confer DJ, Smith RB. Large lymphocele resulting from retroperitoneal lymphadenectomy. J Urol 1980; 124:543.

26. McNeer GP, et al. Effectiveness of radiation therapy in the management of sarcoma of soft somatic tissues. Cancer 1968; 22:391.

27. Gilbert HA, et al. Soft tissue sarcomas of the extremities. J Surg Oncol 1975;7:303.

28. Windeyer B, et al. The place of radiotherapy in the management of fibrosarcoma of the soft tissues. Clin Radiol 1966;17:32.

29. Harrison LB, Gutierrez E, Fischer JJ. Retroperitoneal sarcomas: the Yale experience and a review of the literature. J Surg Oncol 1986;32:159.

30. Fein DA, et al. Management of retroperitoneal sarcomas: does dose escalation impact on locoregional control? Int J Radiat Oncol Biol Phys 1995;31:129–134.

31. Sandelar WF, et al. Experimental and clinical studies of intraoperative radiotherapy. Surg Gynecol Obstet 1983;157: 205.

32. Kinsella TJ, et al. Preliminary results of a randomized study of adjuvant radiation therapy in resectable adult retroperitoneal soft tissue sarcoma. J Clin Oncol 1988;6:18.

33. Sindelar WF, et al. Intraoperative radiotherapy in retroperitoneal sarcomas: final results of a prospective, randomized, clinical trial. Arch Surg 1993;128:402–410.

34. Robertson JM, et al. Preoperative radiation therapy and iododeoxyuridine for large retroperitoneal sarcomas. Int J Radiat Oncol Biol Phys 1995;31:87–92.

35. Tepper JE, et al. Radiation therapy of retroperitoneal soft tissue sarcomas. Int J Radiat Oncol Biol Phys 1984;10: 825–830.

36. Gottleib JA, et al. Chemotherapy of sarcoma with combination of Adriamycin and dimethyltrizoneimidazolecarboxamide. Cancer 1972;30:1632.

37. Poon MC, et al. Inflammatory fibrous histious cytoma: an important variant of malignant and fibrous histious cytoma highly responsive to chemotherapy. Ann Intern Med 1982;97: 858.

38. Tan C, et al. Adriamycin: an antitumor antibiotic in the treatment of neoplastic diseases. Cancer 1973;32:9.

39. Haskell CM, et al. Adriamycin (NSC-123127) by arterial infusion: part III. Cancer Chemother Rep 1975;6:187.

40. Engel CJ, et al. Preoperative chemotherapy for soft tissue sarcomas of the extremities: the experience at the University of California, Los Angeles. In: Verweij J, Pinedo HM, Suit HD, eds. Multidisciplinary treatment of soft tissue sarcomas. Boston: Kluwer Academic, 1993:135–141.

41. Eilber FR, et al. Limb salvage for skeletal and soft tissue sarcomas: multidisciplinary preoperative chemotherapy. Cancer 1984;53:2579.

42. Edmondson JH, et al. Cytotoxic drugs plus subcutaneous granulocyte-macrophage colony stimulating factor: can molgramostim enhance antisarcoma therapy? J Natl Cancer Inst 1994;86:312–314.

43. Elias AD. Chemotherapy for soft tissue sarcomas. Clin Orthop 1993;289:94–105.

44. Gherlinzoni F, et al. A randomized trial for the treatment of high grade soft tissue sarcomas of the extremities: preliminary observations. J Clin Oncol 1986;4:552–558.

45. Edmondson JH, et al. Preliminary study of concomitant chemotherapy with preoperative irradiation for primary extremity soft tissue sarcomas. Proc Am Soc Clin Oncol 1994; 13:480.

46. Edmondson JH. Chemotherapeutic approaches to soft tissue sarcomas. Semin Surg Oncol 1994;10:357–363.

47. Eggermont AMM, et al. Limb salvage by high dose tumor necrosis factor alpha, gamma interferon, and melphalan

isolated limb perfusion in patients with irresectable soft tissue sarcomas. Proc Am Soc Clin Oncol 1992;11:412.

48. Lienard D, et al. High-dose recombinant tumor necrosis factor alpha in combination with interferon gamma and melphalan in isolation perfusion of the limbs for melanoma and sarcoma. J Clin Oncol 1992;10:52–60.

49. Potter DA, et al. Patterns of recurrence in patients with high grade soft tissue sarcomas. J Clin Oncol 1985;3:353–366.

50. Jaques DP, et al. Management of primary and soft tissue sarcoma of the retroperitoneum. Ann Surg 1990;212:51–59.

51. Shiloni E, et al. High-grade retroperitoneal sarcomas: role of an aggressive palliative approach. J Surg Oncol 1993;53:197–203.

52. Catton CN, et al. Outcome and prognosis in retroperitoneal soft tissue sarcoma. Int J Radiat Oncol Biol Phys 1994;29:1005–1010.

14

An Anatomic Approach to the Pelvis in the Male

Robert P. Myers

Consider the following:

1. Before Vesalius (1), the "pubis" (os pubis, NA) was the "pecten" (2). In the eighteenth century, "pubis" and "pecten" were used synonymously (3). In the nineteenth century, nomenclators endorsed the "pecten of the pubis" (4, 5)!
2. A reputable anatomist (6) and illustrator (7) show insertion of the deep transverse perineus and sphincter urethrae into the medial aspect of the inferior pubic rami, which is impossible.
3. "Rectourethralis" is common parlance for anterior longitudinal muscle of the rectum attached to the membranous urethra. However, this muscle inserts into the perineal body, not the urethra; the "rectourethralis" is truly misnamed.
4. The term "levator prostatae" appears widely in the anatomic literature, and an impossible medical illustration (8) purports to show a "levator prostatae." However, the only muscle capable of lifting the prostate is the puborectalis portion of the levator ani.

Pelvic anatomy is often improperly illustrated, ambiguously described, and misunderstood as the above four examples attest. Fortunately, medical illustration is becoming much more precise and accurate (9). Recently, magnetic resonance imaging (MRI) has added immensely to our understanding of the basic relationships of bone, ligaments, muscle, viscera, vessels, nerves, glands, skin, and subcutaneous tissue. Gross dissection during the first year of medical school on a formalin-fixed cadaver has its utility but never quite duplicates in-training live anatomy at the time of surgery—the lament of generations of surgeons.

The complete urologist should know the pelvis inside and out and has a duty to go beyond a strictly genitourinary frame of reference. Without a holistic approach, how can one understand complex pelvic pain or assist a team of orthopedic, vascular, colorectal, and plastic surgeons in hindquarter amputation for advanced chondrosarcoma? Obviously, coverage of all aspects of the human male pelvis is beyond the scope of this chapter.

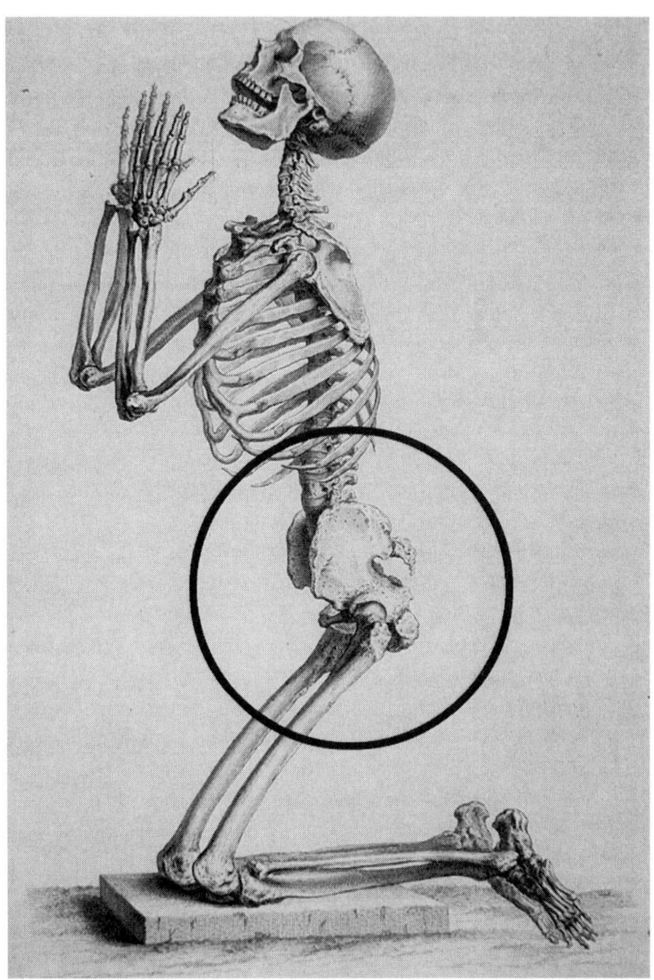

The emphasis here is on the pelvic floor and the anatomy associated with urinary continence. Readers are encouraged to consult, as needed, standard references and textbooks to fill in the gaps (such as in vasculature and neuroanatomy) and to expand their knowledge of those areas that are given only cursory attention. In logical order, bones, ligaments, and muscles are mentioned briefly to cover the outer framework; the viscera that fill the pelvic cavity follow. Incisions to enter the pelvis are described or cited, thereby setting the stage for actual pelvic surgery. Bilateral pelvic lymphadenectomy, which is a frequent precedent to cancer operations, is reviewed, followed by what is considered by this author to be most important—the relation of the fascias, prostate and membranous urethra with its external striated urethral sphincter, and the levator ani, which comprise the pelvic diaphragm.

BONES

An anatomic approach to the pelvis, male or female, begins with how soft structures (everything exclusive of bone) relate to bone, namely, the coxal bones, the sacrum, and the coccyx. Each coxal bone is formed from the fusion of ilium, ischium, and pubis with the sacrum and coccyx wedged between them to form the bony framework of the human pelvis (pelvis means basin in Latin). On the medial aspect of each coxal bone is a ridge, the arcuate line, that extends anteriorly and inferiorly, commencing at the anterior border of the auricular surface (sacroiliac junction), incorporating the iliopectineal eminence, and ending along the top of the pubis. This arcuate line, as a curvilinear ridge, gives rise to a superior pelvic aperture called the false pelvis and an inferior pelvic aperture called the true pelvis.

LIGAMENTS

Pelvic ligaments (Table 14.1) stabilize the L-5 vertebra, sacrum, coccyx, and femoral heads with each coxal bone. The inguinal ligament, extending from the anterior superior iliac spine to the pubic tubercle, provides important fascial attachment and protects medially in a lacuna vasorum the femoral vein, artery, and nerve lateral to the femoral canal. Laterally, in a lacuna musculorum, it protects the exit of the iliopsoas

Table 14.1.   Pelvic Ligaments

Anterior
  Inguinal
  Superior pubic
Posterior
  Iliolumbar
  Sacroiliac
  Sacrotuberous
  Sacrospinous
Hip
  Iliofemoral
  Ischiofemoral
  Pubofemoral
Perineum
  Anococcygeal
  Perineal body
  Transverse of the pelvis
  Arcuate of the pelvis

from the pelvis en route to insertion on the lesser trochanter. In their crisscrossing, the sacrotuberous and sacrospinous ligaments help join the sacrum to the os coxae and define each greater and lesser sciatic foramen. The hip joint capsule consisting of iliofemoral, ischiofemoral, and pubofemoral ligaments stabilizes the femoral head at the acetabulum. The anococcygeal ligament provides support for the anus, rectal sphincters, and pubococcygeus. The transverse ligament of the perineum is a thick band that bridges the inferior pubic rami, sits immediately anterior to the membranous urethra at its junction with the corpus spongiosum, and is continuous with the periosteum and the perineal membrane posteriorly. On MRI, it is a very prominent dark band (Fig. 14.1).

MUSCLES

There are 36 pairs of striated muscles directly located in the pelvis in addition to several closely associated muscles that neither originate nor insert there (Table 14.2). Operations that necessitate resection of the pubis must take into account the attachments of anterior muscles, rectus abdominis, adductor longus, and gracilis. Muscle flaps with pelvic attachment (gracilis, rectus abdominis, latissimus dorsi) all need to be understood with respect to reconstructive procedures (10). Actions of the various muscles should be studied and understood with reference to standard textbooks of anatomy such as *Gray's Anatomy* (8).

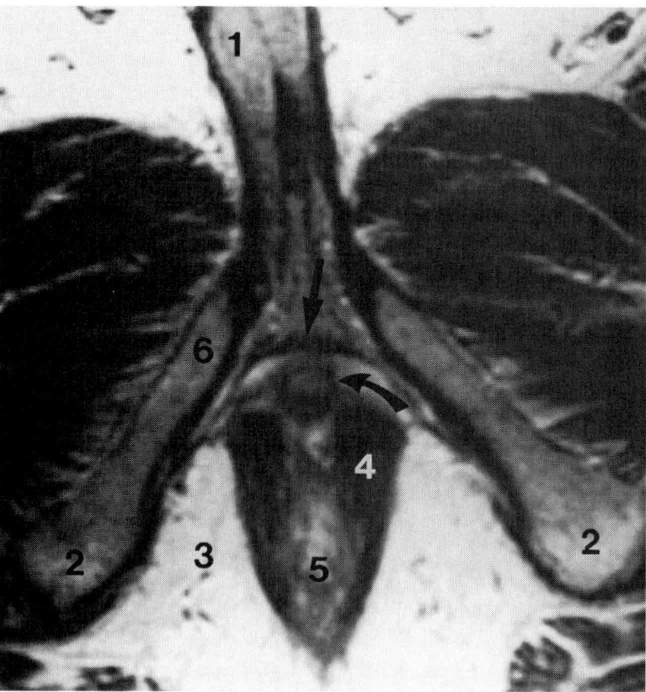

Fig. 14.1.   Transverse MRI to show perineal structural relations (56 year old). 1: Corpus cavernosum; 2: ischial tuberosity; 3: ischioanal fossa; 4: levator ani; 5: anus; 6: inferior pubic ramus; curved arrow: membranous urethra; straight arrow: transverse ligament of the perineum.

Table 14.2. Muscles With Pelvic Origin or Insertion

Exterior
  Anterior
    Pyramidalis
    Rectus abdominis
    Adductor longus
    Gracilis
    Adductor brevis
    Adductor magnus
    Pectineus
    Obturator externus
    Iliacus
    Rectus femoris
    Sartorius
  Posterolateral
    Gluteus maximus
    Gluteus medius
    Gluteus minimus
    Gemellus superior
    Obturator internus
    Gemellus inferior
    Semitendinosus
    Semimembranosus
    Biceps femoris
    Tensor fasciae latae
    Transversus abdominis
    Internal oblique
    External oblique
    Quadratus lumborum
  Posterior
    Erector spinae
    Multifidus
    Latissimus dorsi
Pelvic floor
  Piriformis
  Coccygeus
  Iliococcygeus
  Obturator internus
  Pubococcygeus
  Puborectalis
  Pubourethralis
Perineum
  Superficial transverse perineus
  Ischiocavernosus
Associated muscles that do not attach
  Anal sphincter
    Deep
    Superficial
    Subcutaneous
  Bulbospongiosus
  Sphincter urethrae
  Deep transverse perineus

The pelvic diaphragm could be considered, and has been considered, a continuous muscle with multiple insertion points. However, for the sake of understanding, it is useful to subdivide this vast sheet of muscle into component parts while still recognizing its integrity as a whole. From posterior to anterior and lateral to medial, components of the levator ani include the iliococcygeus, pubococcygeus, puborectalis, and pubourethralis. Within the true pelvis, the levator ani in continuity with the rectal sphincters provides conical investment of the bladder neck, prostate, membranous urethra, rectum, and anus. Functionally, the puborectalis brings the anus forcefully forward and upward together with the prostate. The puborectalis and some of its most distal fibers, the pubourethral muscle (11), and the bulbospongiosus constitute the three most important muscles active during ejaculation. The pubourethral muscle appears to be the modern equivalent of Krause's "levator urethrae (12)" and Wilson's muscle (13), the latter mistakenly called the sphincter urethrae in dictionaries (14, 15). To its credit, *Stedman's Medical Dictionary*'s definition, "certain fibers of the levator ani," is correct but vague.

Of particular urologic interest are the obturator muscles, especially the relatively massive obturator internus, which, joined by the gemelli after it exits the lesser sciatic foramen, inserts on the greater trochanter. After accounting for the pelvic muscles responsible for truncal stability, and the relatively few muscles necessary for hip stability and ambulation, one is still left trying to explain why there are 12 pairs of external hip rotators; that is, what possible survival function or evolutionary selective advantage could there be for so many external hip rotators? These external hip rotators are the gluteus maximus, obturator internus, obturator externus, gemellus superior, gemellus inferior, piriformis, quadratus femoris, gluteus medius (posterior part), adductor magnus (lower portion), biceps femoris (long head), iliopsoas, and sartorius.

The obturator externus, another powerful external rotator, also inserts directly on the greater trochanter. With both lower extremities relatively fixed, simultaneous contraction of the obturator internus and externus plus all of the other "external hip rotators" results in forceful forward pelvic thrust. That each obturator internus has its own nerve supply and two bursae plus the pudendal nerve and vessels beneath its fascia infers a high degree of specialization. The obturator muscles strategically flank the external genitalia; they are completely unnecessary with respect to either hip stability or ambulation. Thus, in terms of pelvic function, a procreative role of the external rotators must be considered seriously, the idea being:

1. That the muscles in question are designed as much to provide pelvic thrust as to provide external hip rotation, and

2. That their function in repetitive contraction and relaxation is more important to sexual intercourse than to locomotion.

By contrast, internal hip rotation is much weaker and is provided by an assortment of muscles, none of which appear to be primarily dedicated to internal rotation. These internal hip rotators are the tensor fasciae latae, gluteus medius (anterior part), gluteus minimus, pectineus, gracilis, adductor longus, adductor brevis, adductor magnus (upper portion), semitendinosus (with the knee flexed), and semimembranosus (with the knee flexed).

The obturator internus muscles laterally and the coccygeus and piriformis muscles posterolaterally supplement the levator ani in completing the muscular portion of the pelvic floor.

VISCERA

With its formidable array of muscles uniting trunk and lower extremities, the male pelvis as a basin harbors in retroperitoneal position the viscera and organs of pelvic exenteration: bladder, terminal ureters, prostate, seminal vesicles, vasa deferentia, membranous urethra, and rectum and anus posteriorly. As the peritoneal cul-de-sac dips to its adherent semicircular end at the base of the prostate and seminal vesicles, the pelvis also harbors considerable intraperitoneal content, including the small bowel and sigmoid colon. Intrapelvic operations usually necessitate careful packing and retracting of peritoneal contents in a cephalad direction with or without the assistance of head-down body tilt.

As the bladder distends, it pushes the intraperitoneal contents upward, but it always conforms to the surrounding viscera and organs (Fig. 14.2). In disease with detrusor hypertrophy and relative bladder wall rigidity, this conformation is less pronounced. When the bladder wall is of normal thickness or thin, one can often appreciate endoscopically loops of bowel pressing extrinsically on the posterior bladder wall near the

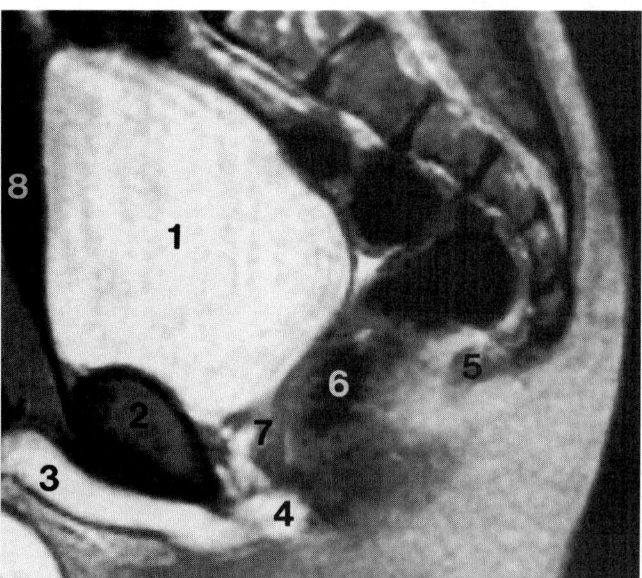

Fig. 14.2. Sagittal MRI showing how distended normal urinary bladder conforms to contiguous structures (11 year old). 1: urinary bladder filled with contrast medium; 2: pubis; 3: corpus cavernosum; 4: corpus spongiosum; 5: coccyx; 6: rectum; 7: prostate; 8: rectus abdominis.

dome before the bladder is fully distended. A complication of Nd:YAG laser ablation of bladder tumors is perforation of adjacent bowel when proper energy control is not maintained.

INCISIONS

The choice of skin incision to explore the pelvis depends on the operation to be performed (Table 14.3). What is done in accomplishing one operation should always be done with the idea that another pelvic operation may take place at a later date. Thus, the exposure for any operation should be sufficient for that operation and not so extensive as to obliterate unnecessarily the tissue planes that will be necessary at some future date.

The anterior low midline incision is the most popular source of internal pelvic exposure. If the lower end of the incision is carried too close to the penis, unnecessary external genital edema may result because of lymphatic interference. This is usually temporary, but if external beam pelvic radiation is involved as an adjunct, chronic scrotal and penile edema may ensue and is a troublesome complication.

The upper end of the midline incision is carried just short of the umbilicus for limited operations but is extended periumbilically to varying degrees for more extensive operations. With periumbilical extension, strong closure is facilitated by making the anterior rectus fascial incision paramedian cephalad to the arcuate line formed by the posterior rectus sheath.

After the rectus abdominis muscles are retracted in the midline, the glistening transversalis fascia is readily identifiable below the arcuate line. Full extraperitoneal exposure includes development of a retropubic space, followed by sweeping the bladder wall medially on both sides, and then further developing lateral spaces over the external iliac vessels and iliopsoas muscle. The posterior rectus fascia may be incised without peritoneal entry; then, with a self-retaining retractor, a generous extraperitoneal cavity is prepared as an antecedent to numerous urologic operations with or without pelvic lymphadenectomy.

The transverse incisions include the Pfannenstiel and the Cherney, the former splitting and retracting the rectus abdom-

Table 14.3. Incisions Into the Pelvic Interior

Lower abdominal
  Midline
    Extraperitoneal
    Intraperitoneal
    Extraperitoneal and intraperitoneal
  Paramedian
    Vertical
    Hockey stick
  Transverse
    Pfannenstiel
    Cherney
Perineal
Transsacral

inis in the midline, the latter transecting the rectus tendons close to their insertion on the pubis. The latter was a favorite approach by the late Ormond Culp for cystectomy and bilateral ureterosigmoidostomy (16). The rectus tendons are reattached to the anterior rectus fascia close to the pubis with horizontal mattress sutures of nonabsorbable material. The result is a very strong and cosmetically pleasing incision.

BILATERAL PELVIC LYMPHADENECTOMY

Removal of fibrofatty lymph-node–bearing tissue from within the obturator space and along the internal and external iliac vessels constitutes traditional pelvic lymphadenectomy. If the tissue can be removed en bloc, the operation is more elegant by keeping the lymphatic channels intact. Special care is necessary in isolating and ligating securely the distal ramifications of the obturator node package emanating from the femoral canal. If not properly secured, these lymphatics may drain for an interminable period or result in lymphocele formation with its resultant compression morbidity on the iliac vessels and the development of lower extremity edema. Metal clips (small, medium, and large) are a tremendous asset in securing lymphatics and extraneous vessels, especially tiny arteries emerging from the muscular back wall of the obturator space. The obturator nerve should be identified and freed carefully throughout its visible length before nodal tissue is removed. This maneuver greatly lessens the chance of inadvertent transection, the result of haste and inattention. An anatomic dissection of the appropriate nodal tissue and avoidance of significant obturator vessels are enhanced by the routine use of surgical loupe magnification ($\times$2).

The obturator lymph node group extends proximally into a V-shaped cleft beneath the external iliac vein. Lymph-node–bearing tissue at this site can be manually extracted between the tip of an index finger and thumb. From the proximal end of the obturator group, direct continuation with the common iliac lymph nodes is apparent. In extracting obturator space tissue, any use of a vein retractor against the external iliac vein must be gentle because iatrogenic intimal venous injury predisposes to phlebothrombosis with risk of pulmonary embolus from the site of retraction. In this author's experience, computed tomography of the common iliac vein proved this point in a single case and led to the abandonment of routine use of a vein retractor when performing pelvic lymphadenectomy.

Incidentally, the ischial spine can be palpated with the tip of the index finger in the floor of the obturator space after completion of the lymphadenectomy.

FASCIA

The muscular pelvic sidewalls are covered by fascia known as parietal fascia, whereas fascia covering the bladder and prostate is known as visceral fascia. Together, the parietal and visceral fascias comprise the pelvic or endopelvic fascia. All striated muscle has a fascial covering, or epimysium. Because the levator

ani and the obturator internus, for example, have a fascial surface facing the pelvic interior, their fascias then are the parietal component of the pelvic or endopelvic fascia. On the lateral sidewalls of the pelvis, there are two tendinous arches (17), one (arcus tendineus m. levatoris ani, NA) for muscular origin of the iliococcygeus and the other (arcus tendineus fasciae pelvis, NA) marking the fascial boundary between the parietal fascia where it descends off the pelvic sidewall to meet the visceral fascia in the sulcus lateral to the bladder and prostate. The tendinous fascial arch appears as a white line fascial condensation running from the pubovesical ligament to the ischial spine (see the section on pubovesical versus puboprostatic ligaments later in this chapter). The pelvic fascia should always be opened parallel and lateral to the white line to avoid bleeding from the prostatic and vesicovenous plexuses. After the pelvic fascia is opened, the adherence of pubococcygeus superiorly and puborectalis inferiorly to the anterolateral prostate and prostatourethral junction can be appreciated. The parietal fascia or epimysium of the adjacent levator adheres to the lateral surface of the prostate and urethra in one continuous sheet that passes posteriorly uninterrupted over the surface of the rectum, constituting Denonvilliers' lateral prostatic or puborectal aponeurosis (18). This aponeurosis or fascia covers veins of the prostatic plexus and the neurovascular tissue with its cavernosal nerves to the penis. Radical prostatectomy cannot be performed without incising this fascia, both at the prostatourethral junction and above or below the neurovascular bundle.

Neurovascular Preservation Versus Sacrifice

The fascial incision above and parallel to the neurovascular bundle allows the neurovascular bundle to fall laterally and remain resting on the rectal surface. In the potency-preserving nerve-sparing operation, the most efficacious point for incising the fascia to begin the process of allowing the nerve bundles to fall away is on either side of the apex, at the shoulders of the prostate if one considers the membranous urethra as the neck. Improvement with a T-shaped incision in the course of radical retropubic prostatectomy (RRP) has recently been proposed (19). This maneuver allows mobilization of the apex with dropping off of the neurovascular tissue and subsequent appropriate urethral transection without disturbing the bundles. Beneath the most superficial layer of fascia that originates from the adjacent levator ani lie veins of the prostatic venous plexus within the true multilayered visceral fascia of the prostate (20).

For wide resection that includes the neurovascular bundle with the prostate specimen in non–nerve-sparing operations, the incision in the fascia is made lateral, parallel to, and below the bundle. In this non–nerve-sparing operation, the most efficacious point for entry into the plane between the rectum and prostate lies at the base of the prostate and seminal vesicles and lateral to the neurovascular bundle, where the fascia is particularly thin and rectal injury can be minimized. Unless there is untoward inflammation, the prostate can then be separated from the rectum with the index fingers pressed against both the posterior prostate surface and the intact rectoprostatic (Denonvilliers') fascia that continues in a cephalad direction to cover both seminal vesicles. Herein the noneponymic "rectoprostatic fascia" is introduced as a replacement for the vernacular and eponymic Denonvilliers' fascia. Extension of this same fascia to cover the seminal vesicles is implicit in this new terminology.

Rectoprostatic Fascia

One of the most controversial topics among urologists is the nature of the fascia that covers the posterior surface of the prostate. The points in question are whether it is one or two layers and whether it is derived embryologically from fusion of peritoneum distal to the end of the peritoneal cul-de-sac (21–23)). From the surgical standpoint, this fascia appears to be an upward mesenchymal extension of the perineal body with which it is continuous rather than a downward extension of the peritoneum, which in the adult ends in a cul-de-sac at the base of the prostate and seminal vesicles. Semicircular adherence of the peritoneum to this fascia of the base of the prostate and seminal vesicles is constant. Although Denonvilliers called the layer "prostato-peritoneale," nothing in his description suggests two

layers, only a single layer with a texture "resembling the (scrotal) dartos."

Its laminar consistency can be confirmed histologically (24, 25), but this in no way confirms peritoneal origin. The medial portion of this fascia has been found fused to the prostate with no discrete prostate capsule at this midline point of fusion (25). MRI supports this midline predominance and documents distinct thickening of this fascia along the posterior midline (Fig. 14.3). Once the cul-de-sac peritoneum is swept away bluntly, the rectoprostatic fascia continues visibly from its prostatic portion in smooth transition over the posterior surface of the seminal vesicles and well cephalad to the most distal peritoneal attachment. Once this smooth fascial surface is established, there is nothing to suggest grossly any peritoneal origin, and it becomes counterintuitive to suggest any peritoneal origin. With painstaking scrutiny of studies to date (21–23, 26, 27) plus his own methodical sectioning, Silver could find no convincing histologic evidence that peritoneum is involved in the formation of the embryologic rectovesical septum or rectoprostatic fascia (28).

In the course of RRP, the tip of the posterior rectoprostatic fascia at the apex of the prostate must be transected from its attachment to the superior end of the perineal body. This point

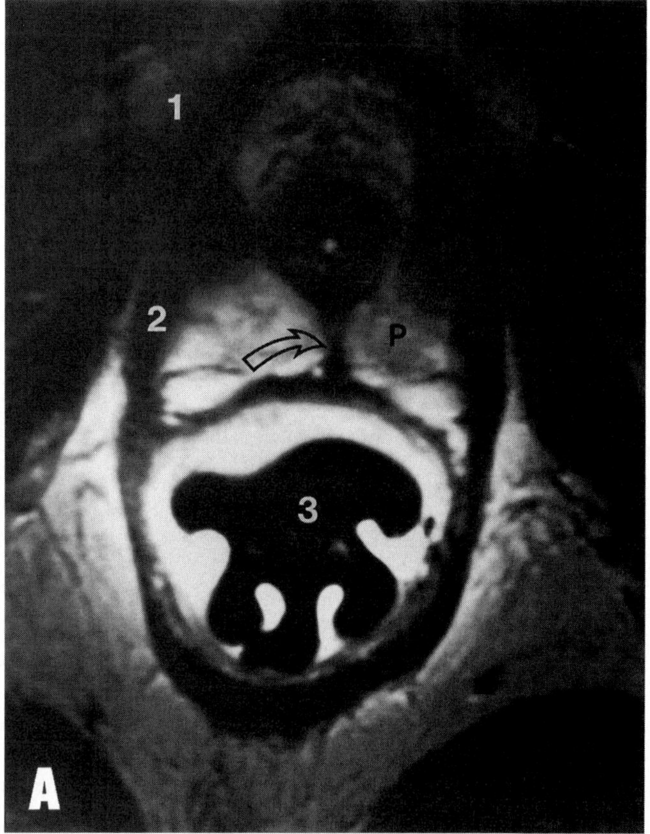
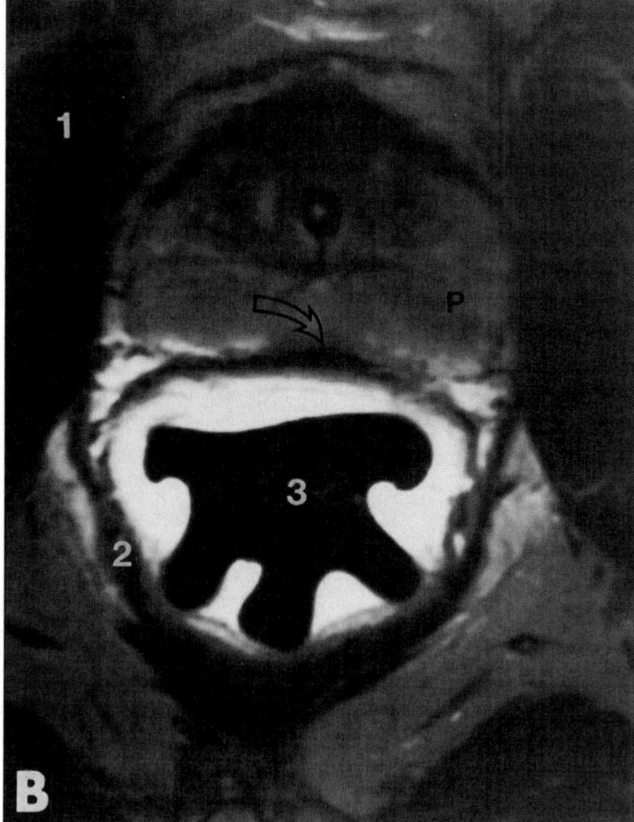

Fig. 14.3.   Transverse MRI (52 year old). **A.** Close to prostatic apex and membranous urethra with indwelling Foley catheter. 1: Inferior pubic ramus; 2: puborectalis; 3: endorectal coil; P: prostate; arrow: junction of rectourethralis. **B.** Midprostate. 1: Obturator internus; 2: pubococcygeus against rectal wall; 3: endorectal coil; P: prostate; arrow: midline thickening of rectoprostatic (Denonvilliers') fascia.

is just proximal to the attachment of the "rectourethralis" muscle to the perineal body. For the radical prostatectomist, the apical margin is the most difficult from the standpoint of complete tumor removal and is associated with the highest incidence of positive margins (29). The importance of removing the malignant prostate with its posterior surface completely covered by rectoprostatic fascia cannot be overemphasized with respect to achieving negative margins of resection. Maintaining continuity of the rectoprostatic fascia over the base of the prostate and seminal vesicles is especially important because this is a frequent site of extraprostatic spread that can be contained primarily by not violating the integrity of this important fascia (25, 30).

"RECTOURETHRALIS"

Anterior longitudinal smooth muscle fibers of the rectal wall are embedded in the superior aspect of the perineal body at a point close to the posterior apex of the prostate and the membranous urethra. From this standpoint, the attachment grossly and palpably appears to be urethral. However, histologic sections clearly demonstrate attachment to the midline perineal body (central tendon of the perineum, NA), not the urethra. Smith wrote, "In his operation for perineal prostectomy Proust cuts through the perineal body (the recto-urethral muscle) then opens this rectoprostatic space . . . " (22). Because of the interposed fibromuscular cephalad extent of the perineal body in a prerectal raphe between the urethra and the rectal smooth muscle, any urethral connection is indirect. For this reason, the term "rectourethralis" is not only imprecise but also misleading. Figures schematically showing the fibers in direct contact with the urethra (25) are incorrect. The alternative use of the term "pre-rectal muscle" (31) is more accurate from both an anatomic and histologic standpoint. Variation in the bulk and extent along the perineal body is evident, and both superior and inferior limbs are described (8). The attachment of this muscle does not have to be taken down during the course of RRP, but is of course an essential part of radical perineal prostatectomy. If the attachment is not done with care during this latter operation, inadvertent rectotomy may ensue, necessitating recognition and primary closure with or without temporary colostomy, depending on whether the rectum was prepared preoperatively.

PUBOVESICAL VERSUS PUBOPROSTATIC LIGAMENTS

In the child, male or female, the pubovesical muscle is a smooth muscle extension of the outer longitudinal detrusor muscle of the urinary bladder with attachment to the pubis. The muscle attaches on either side of the symphysis in the distal third of its posterior surface, usually in two thick bands. This muscle persists in adulthood with ligamentous cephalad continuity to the serosa of the bladder. Residual smooth muscle continuity with the detrusor over the anterior surface of the prostate, in association with these ligaments, always can be demonstrated

throughout life irrespective of the size of the prostate. What is generally not appreciated is the fact that the anterior bladder wall obscures the underlying anterior prostate in most cases. The prostate is visualized only after opening the pelvic fascia in a line parallel to and lateral to the tendinous fascial arch, and then all that can be visualized are the lateral surfaces of the prostate. The bladder covers and obscures the anterior prostate all the way to its pubovesical ligaments (Fig. 14.4). Unfortunately, illustrations abound incorrectly showing the bladder entirely superior to the prostate. With growth of the prostate and the establishment of significant adenomatous hyperplasia, the prostatic isthmus enlarges. What began as pubovesical muscle and ligaments may come to appear puboprostatic; however, these ligaments are vesical in origin, never prostatic, and should be called rightfully pubovesical ligaments (32).

The pubovesical ligaments function as a protective buffer to the underlying prostatourethral junction and striated sphincter of the membranous urethra. For satisfactory prostatourethral transection, it is often necessary to divide the pubovesical ligaments for several millimeters to provide adequate access for control of the dorsal vein complex. This maneuver should be performed judiciously to protect nerves to the striated sphincter that penetrate anteriorly (33). It has been postulated that injury to these anterior nerves may contribute to postprostatectomy incontinence. Overzealous suture placement during the control of the dorsal vein complex must be avoided, and this can be aided by conservation and minimal transection of the pubovesical ligaments.

In routine radical perineal prostatectomy when a plane of dissection is chosen beneath the anterior plexus, there is no reason to believe that it is necessary to transect the pubovesical ligaments, which lie anterior to the plexus. The only real adherence is along the midline isthmus, which demands sharp division to free the overlying plexus.

DORSAL VEIN COMPLEX; ACCESSORY PUDENDAL ARTERY

When retropubic fat is removed carefully, the pubovesical ligaments can be visualized clearly above the dorsal vein complex, which lies anterolateral to the membranous urethra. It is common to find a superficial preprostatic vein or veins exiting from the fascia into retropubic fat between the pubovesical ligaments. In about 80% of patients, this superficial vein reenters the vesicovenous plexus in the midline. Sometimes the superficial veins go directly to one or both pelvic sidewalls, and in about 10% of patients they are entirely absent (34). Unless there is significant benign prostatic hyperplasia (BPH) with a massive prostatic isthmus, the dorsal vein complex superior to the prostatourethral junction generally trifurcates to the vesicovenous plexus anteriorly and prostatovenous plexuses posterolaterally with or without lateral prostatic anastomoses to the anterior plexus (Fig. 14.4). Asymmetry is common. With increasing BPH that progressively widens the prostatic isthmus, the bladder wall is pushed cephalad, but the venous plexus

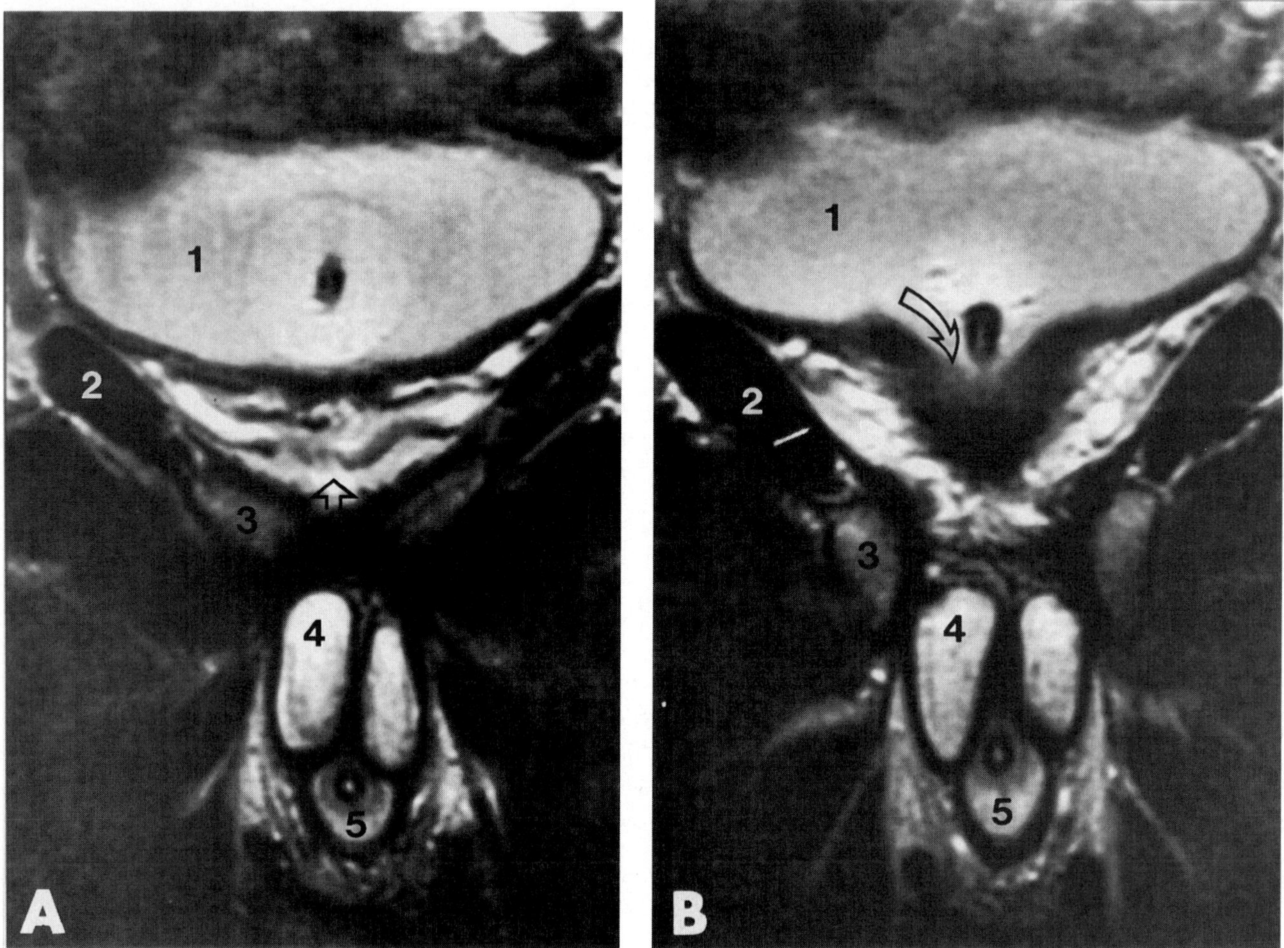

Fig. 14.4.   Coronal MRI (52 year old). Relation of venous plexus to urinary bladder and prostate at three superficial levels anterior to posterior. 1: Bladder; 2: obturator internus; 3: pubis; 4: corpus cavernosum; 5: corpus spongiosum; P: prostate. Venous plexus (arrow in A) is demonstrated to cover anterior tongue of bladder wall (arrow in B) that extends to form pubovesical ligaments flanking dorsal vein complex (arrow in C). Anterior plexus is predominantly vesicovenous.

anteriorly continues to lie above the prostatic isthmus and thus appears to be more prostatic than vesical. The continuity of the serosal surface of the bladder and the pubovesical ligaments is still maintained.

An accessory pudendal artery, unilateral or bilateral, is encountered in approximately 5% of RRP (35). Preservation may be possible during control of the dorsal vein complex; in addition, there is the risk of excessive venous bleeding while trying to keep the artery intact. The effect of preservation on potency does not appear to be significant.

With the retropubic fat removed, a pubourethral space can be appreciated (36, 37). The pubourethral space is important in transsphincteric urethroplasty (37). The tip of an index finger can be inserted into this space, which dead-ends above the penile hilum (38). Ligamentous attachment of the pubovesical ligaments continues distally with firm support of the membranous urethra against the pubis. There is good reason to believe that the very distal anterior ligamentous support of the mem-

branous urethra should not be disturbed to preserve urinary continence. RRP with pubectomy has a significantly higher degree of postoperative urinary incontinence in contrast to cases without transpubic exposure (39).

PROSTATE, PELVIC FLOOR, AND THE MEMBRANOUS URETHRA

On its anterolateral surface, the prostate is wrapped tightly in levator muscle (20, 40). However, there is no levator muscle between the prostate and rectum because of the presence of the rectoprostatic fascia. Thus, there is no levator muscle positioned to lift only the prostate exclusive of the rectum and anus. Official nomenclature recognizes a levator of the prostate (levator prostatae, NA), but Santorini's original description of the levator prostatae (3) is in accord with the modern day "puborectalis." The term "levator prostatae" should be discarded and is omitted purposely in Table 14.2.

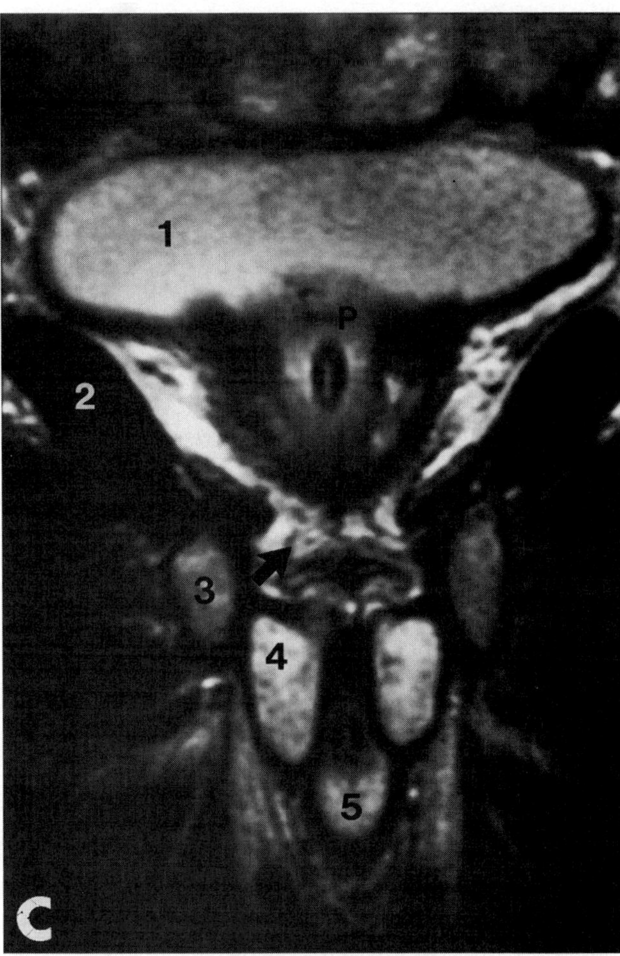

Fig. 14.4.   *(continued)*

Within the coat of levator muscle, pubococcygeus above and puborectalis below, lies a prostate that is variable in shape, in both the child and the adult. Much of this variation is related to the development of BPH, generally beginning at about 35 years of age, but distinct differences in shape can be seen well before the onset of BPH (Fig. 14.5). As the prostate grows with outbudding from the urethral lumen (beginning at approximately the ninth week of gestation), the prostatic mass progressively disrupts the integrity of the circumferential striated urethral sphincter in its upper half (41). The striated urethral sphincter (sphincter urethrae, NA) fibers end up splayed out over or absorbed into the anterior fibromuscular stroma, which forms a commissure anterior to the urethra, that is, the prostatic isthmus. The nonhyperplastic prostate has no lobar architecture. Only the hyperplastic prostate has lobar architecture, the nature of which is variable. The classic symmetrical appearance combining lateral lobes and a median lobe of BPH creates the trilobar configuration so commonly seen. Sometimes there is only lateral lobe hyperplasia, symmetrical or asymmetrical, or only median lobe hyperplasia, and rarely there is hyperplasia of anterior periurethral glands to produce an anterior

lobe. In the nonhyperplastic gland, the verumontanum (veru) or seminal colliculus often sits at the most distal posterior aspect of the prostatic urethra (20). With BPH, progressive lobar growth and distal expansion cause the prostate to overlap the membranous urethra. The veru is found usually within 1 cm from the apex, as though the process of BPH has produced superior migration of the veru. How much is congenital and how much is developmental with respect to placement of the veru is unknown. The functional striated sphincter ends where it abuts prostate stroma, but the smooth muscle sphincteric component extends proximally to the veru.

From the standpoint of urinary continence, the integrity of the smooth muscle and its nerve supply distal to the veru is most important. This is true for patients who undergo transurethral resection of the prostate (TURP) and may be equally true for patients who undergo radical prostatectomy. The striated sphincter appears to be ancillary with its passive slow twitch compression, but the integrity of the membranous urethra with both coats of smooth and striated muscle should not be broken if one seeks a continent distal sphincter mechanism. Successful radical prostatectomy and orthotopic neobladder creation depend on maintaining as much intact membranous urethral length as is considered prudent under each patient's circumstances.

The configuration of the prostatourethral junction is variable if one inspects sequential specimens taken at the time of surgery or at autopsy (Fig. 14.6). The prostatic isthmus varies in width. If narrow or minuscule, there may be an anterior apical notch and prominent posterior lip (20, 24), in which case the striated sphincter extends upward anteriorly to fill the notch.

Although drawn so often in medical illustration, the urethra coring straight through the prostate into the bladder is distinctly uncommon. A bend in the urethra of approximately 35° angled forward superior to the veru is common (42). Sometimes the urethra takes an almost right-angle bend to enter the bladder, in which case the bladder neck takes up nearly the entire anterior surface of the prostate.

Distal Urethral Continence Mechanism

How can the lessons of Turner-Warwick (43) be expanded? With respect to TURP, the veru is sacrosanct; resection must never be carried distal to the veru or there is significant risk of urinary incontinence. The reason for this is that the distal sphincter continence mechanism includes that portion of the urethra with its smooth muscle between the veru and the apex of the prostate, which together with the membranous urethra forms a functional unit that includes smooth muscle, elastic tissue, and the striated muscle of the striated sphincter (this muscle being of predominant influence distal to the apex of the prostate). If the limit of the veru is essential for postoperative urinary continence after TURP, then why should it not be essential for the same degree of continence after radical prostatectomy? It only stands to reason that if a portion of the

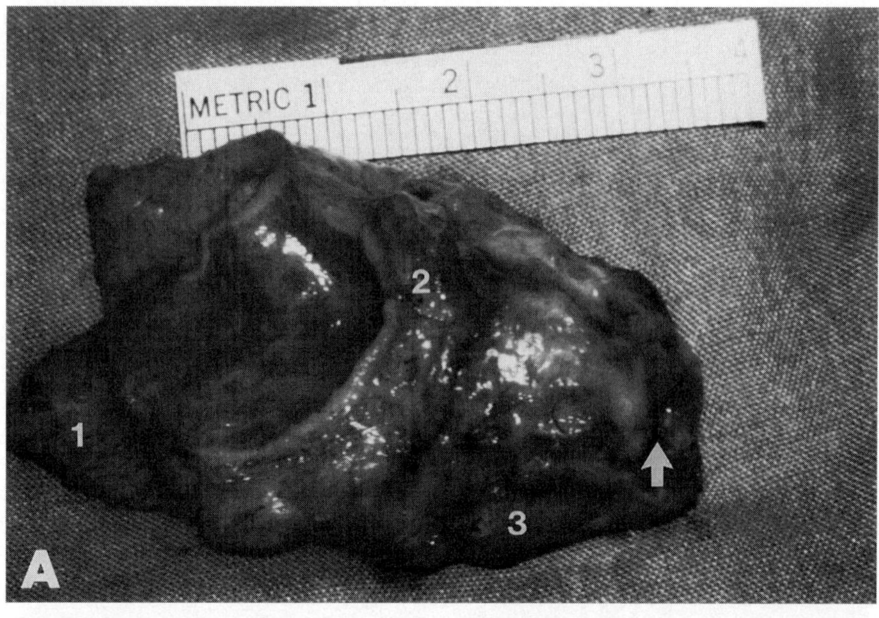

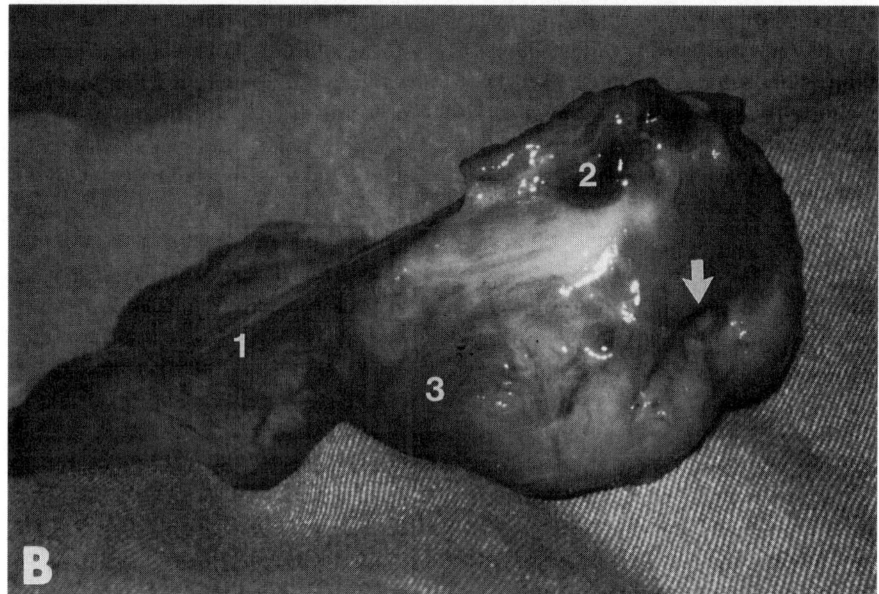

Fig. 14.5. **A** and **B**. Two prostates of remarkably different shape (each cadaveric specimen from a 16 year old). 1: Seminal vesicle; 2: wall of urinary bladder; 3: prostate; arrow: urethral opening at prostatic apex.

continence mechanism is removed as a result of radical prostatectomy, then a proportionate number of patients will be incontinent depending on how much of the continence mechanism is sacrificed.

The continence mechanism simply does not begin at the apex of the prostate—it begins at the veru! Turner-Warwick stated, "Prostatectomy by enucleation or total excision requires preservation of as much of the proximal third as possible for maximal retention of urinary continence." Furthermore, he contended that radical prostatectomy removes the proximal two thirds of the distal sphincter! When it is done properly, far less than two thirds is sacrificed, but the potential is present.

Importantly, the functional membranous urethra is more than the segment from the prostate apex to the superior surface of the corpus spongiosum. There is an intraprostatic segment distal to the veru if the veru is situated proximal to the apex. If the veru sits at the apex, there is no intraprostatic portion of the continence mechanism (20).

From an anatomic standpoint, there is little doubt that radical prostatectomy performed with urethral transection distal to the apex of the prostate threatens the establishment of satisfactory postoperative urinary continence in some cases. For the best chance of continence, measures should be taken to transect the urethra as close to the veru as possible. One method is to use

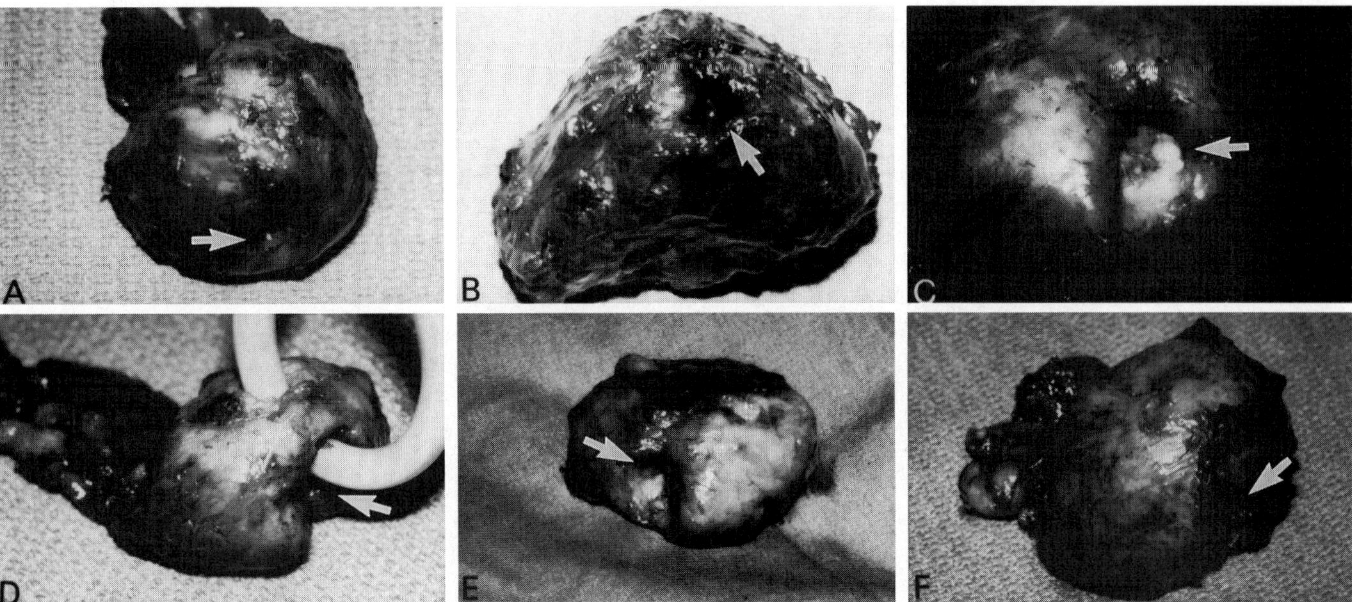

Fig. 14.6.   Variation in prostate shape. **A.** Doughnut. **B.** Conical. **C.** Anterior apical notch with posterior lip. **D.** Posterior apical notch. **E.** Asymmetric apex. **F.** Spheroid. Arrows: Urethral openings at prostatic apex. Note extreme angulation of prostatic urethra in D. (From Myers RP. Practical pelvic anatomy pertinent to radical retropubic prostatectomy. In: Ball TP Jr., ed. AUA Updated Series 1994;13(4):25. Reprinted with permission.)

a vein retractor to retract the prostatic isthmus before anterior urethral transection (39, 44). Direct urethral involvement by cancer is uncommon and occurs in about 5% of patients (1 of 20). Urethral involvement is usually associated with the more malignant, infiltrative, higher Gleason primary grades when there is apical prostatic involvement. The urethra can be transected at the inferior border of the veru without cutting into the prostate. In patients who have undergone prior TURP, the urethra may be too adherent to perform the vein retractor maneuver, and transection may be necessary flush with the apex. In this case, patients will have a shorter final membranous urethra than what might otherwise have been achieved; therefore, preoperative urethral pressure profilometry is recommended, with measurement of resting and maximum urethral pressure. Patients who are continent after TURP and have marginal maximal urethral pressures, for example, 75 cm H_2O, should be counseled about the probable high risk of postoperative incontinence. Indeed, such patients might best consider alternative treatment to radical prostatectomy.

How important the striated sphincter is to overall continence after radical prostatectomy is unclear. Striated sphincter bulk and influence appear to increase progressively from the apex of the prostate to the corpus spongiosum. Functional striated sphincter is generally not found proximal to the apex of the prostate and, if so, only to a limited and insignificant degree producing mild concavity. There is no reason to refute Clegg's contention that, "In no case is striped muscle seen to enter into close relationship with the urethra except near the apex of the gland . . ." (45). Clegg was faulted by Haines (46) because "he missed the upper part altogether," but striated sphincter embedded into prostate stroma or splayed over the anterior surface of the isthmus cannot be considered functional because it has lost its proximity to the urethra. Furthermore, Haines' material came not from adults but from two boys, aged 4 and 5 years, and his figures are consistent with prostates that have a considerable apical notch configuration allowing striated sphincter to embrace the urethra cephalad to the most posterior apical prostate (24, 41).

Schematic representations showing striated sphincter as a functional urethral sphincteric component for a significant distance within the distal prostatic urethra (43, 47) are not supported by histologic sections in the coronal plane (24, 48). As stated previously, the striated sphincter appears to have much greater influence on continence distally than proximally. This is borne out by maximal urethral pressure profilometry demonstrating the highest pressure in the most distal segment of the membranous urethra (44). This fact may provide some leeway in the point of proximal urethral transection for patients with particularly high maximal urethral pressures (e.g., 185 cm H_2O) and well-innervated pelvic floor musculature. However, in patients who do not meet these criteria and have reduced maximal urethral pressure (e.g., the patient aged 70 years with maximal urethral pressure of 125 cm H_2O), steps should be taken to preserve every millimeter of viable striated sphincter and functional membranous urethra within the bounds of satisfactory cancer surgery and achievement of negative margins of resection.

Urogenital Diaphragm or Urogenital Hiatus?

The membranous urethra passes through a hole or hiatus in the pelvic diaphragm to enter the corpus spongiosum immediately.

Oelrich (41) properly used "urogenital hiatus" to describe this aperture in the floor of the pelvis that accommodates the urethra after it leaves the apex of the prostate. Specifically, he challenged the existence of a "urogenital diaphragm" or membranous urethra within a muscle sandwich of striated sphincter and deep transversus between a superior and inferior fascia as advocated by Henle (31). That configuration, Oelrich maintained, does not exist. And there is no evidence that it does.

As maintained by others (36, 49), what Henle described as superior fascia is nothing more than the inferior fascia of the pelvic diaphragm, which he left in situ after removing the levator ani muscle exclusive of its inferior fascia. He then transected membranous urethra and striated sphincter at the level of the inferior fascia of the pelvic diaphragm. This then left the upper two thirds of the membranous urethra with its striated sphincter attached to the apex of the prostate (Fig. 14.7) and the lower one third of the membranous urethra with its striated sphincter beneath the inferior fascia of the pelvic diaphragm. He then renamed the upper two thirds of the striated sphincter the "sphincter vesicae externus" (remembering Vesalius? [Vesalius' Table 14.49 clearly shows below the prostate the male striated urethral sphincter, which he labeled "vesicae cervicis musculus," that is, "muscle of the vesical neck." "External vesical sphincter" as a label for the striated urethral sphincter appears as late as 1978 (50)]); the dismembered lower one third became part of a single muscle mass, all of which he called the deep transverse perineus. The perineal membrane served as the inferior fascia of his newly created "diaphragma urogenitale."

After careful study, one becomes acutely aware of the artifact and anatomic mischief involved—Henle dismembered the membranous urethra! With a vertically oriented striated urethral sphincter, Henle's figures of a side view of a gross specimen and another showing bladder, prostate, and membranous urethra in midline sagittal section look accurate until one realizes that the lower one third of the membranous urethra and striated sphincter is missing. Illustrations abound showing the famous and erroneous muscle sandwich with deep transversus extending bilaterally to insert into the ischia (7, 51).

Although neither MRI nor proper gross dissection supports Henle's diaphragma urogenitale, there is on any gross dissection (52) a triangular ligament (30) or urogenital trigone (30, 36) that

1. Combines perineal membrane with its thickened anterior border, the transverse ligament of the perineum,
2. Fills the gap between the inferior pubic rami and ischial rami, and
3. Provides firm fascial support for the underlying suspended corpus spongiosum.

This triangular ligament, which is primarily perineal membrane, is the end product of removing the pelvic diaphragm in its entirety, including its inferior fascia. Although this triangular ligament per se constitutes a urogenital diaphragm in one sense, it is not the muscle sandwich urogenital diaphragm as conceived by Henle that is widely and erroneously illustrated. With respect to an intact membranous urethra and striated sphincter, "urogenital hiatus" (41) is both accurate and useful (Fig. 14.8) and is finally gaining acceptance (53). It is also particularly useful, with respect to radical perineal prostatectomy, to remember Young's "triangular ligament"; the currently accepted equivalent "perineal membrane" fails to connote shape.

Deep Transverse Perineus

The variability of this muscle is such that no single description suffices (3). In this author's dissections, there appears to be no difference in the color or caliber of its fiber from those of the striated sphincter. In some preparations, the fibers are simply a part of the posterior aspect of the sphincter that sweep around and encompass the bulbourethral (Cowper's) glands. The bulbourethral glands have been described as "placed behind the membranous urethra among the fibers of the sphincter urethrae" (54). The figures of Kalischer (55) purport to show the correct and incorrect depictions of the striated sphincter, with the correct relationship showing the striated sphincter around the membranous urethra anteriorly and discrete transverse fibers heading laterally posterior to the striated sphincter. Some preparations do support Kalischer; true short transverse fibers leave a central raphe and end laterally in the fascia that surrounds the pudendal vessels running along the medial aspect of each inferior pubic ramus (Fig. 14.9). Müller used "transversus of the bulb" (56). Gil Vernet (57) wrote "the osseous inser-

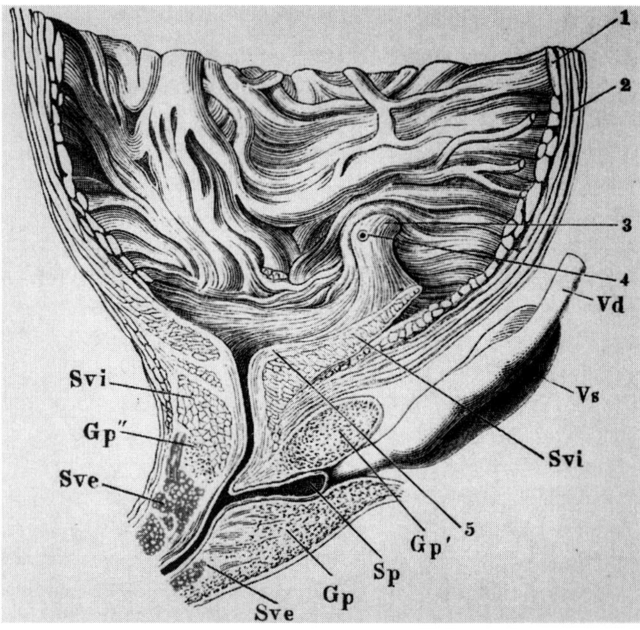

Fig. 14.7. Schematic midline sagittal section of urinary bladder, prostate, and membranous urethra with distal third of striated sphincter missing. Sve: Sphincter vesicae externus; Svi: sphincter vesicae internus; Gp, Gp', Gp": prostate; Vd: vas deferens; Vs: seminal vesicle; 1: inner layers of detrusor; 2: outer layers of detrusor; 3: ureter; 4: ureteral orifice; 5: inner longitudinal muscle of trigone. (From Henle (31)).

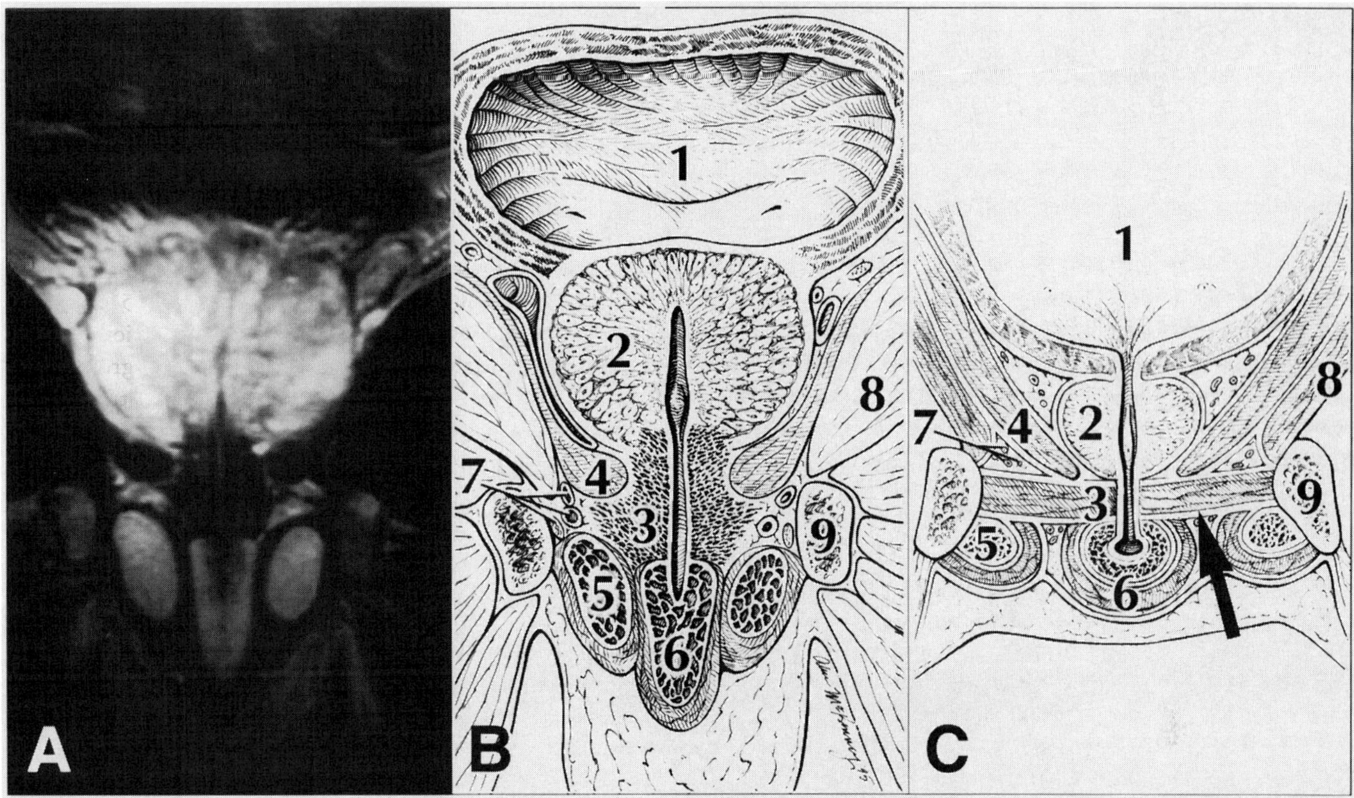

Fig. 14.8. Urogenital hiatus (correct) versus urogenital diaphragm (incorrect). **A.** Coronal MRI (T2-weighted fast-spin echo image). **B.** Artist's rendering of part A. **C.** Fictitious urogenital diaphragm (arrow) (After Netter (7)). 1: Urinary bladder; 2: prostate; 3: striated urethral sphincter; 4: puborectalis; 5: corpus cavernosum penis; 6: corpus spongiosum; 7: pudendal vessels and nerves; 8: obturator internus.

tion of this muscle is never seen . . . a physical impossibility . . . on account of . . . the fibrous tunnel that wraps the pudendal vessels and nerves." The term "lunate fascia" has been applied to the fascia surrounding the pudendal vessels within the urogenital triangle (35).

It was Gil Vernet's contention that the function of the deep transverse muscle is "to squeeze (the bulbourethral glands) during ejaculation." Histologic sections (52) showing striated sphincter with its posterior fibers construed as deep transverse perineus enveloping the bulbourethral glands tend to support Gil Vernet's view. Santorini is no doubt correct in his assessment that there is great variation, and Henle's concept of a single muscle mass may often be true, but at other times it is false.

CONCLUSION

It is easy for the urologist to have a myopic view of the pelvis, limiting knowledge only to the procedures of a urogenital nature and thereby ignoring the complex osseous, musculoskeletal, and neurovascular anatomy that surrounds intimately the structures of immediate urologic interest. Although the text of this chapter moved rapidly to a very limited discussion, the opening salvo began with an invitation to know and explore all anatomic aspects, with a Chelselden engraving (58) (pelvis circled) suggesting that despite prayer, doom may await an incomplete understanding of all the elements that comprise the human pelvis. Disaster in the form of unnecessary morbidity awaits the surgeon who is not precisely clear about the anatomy at operation and literally gets lost, thinking he or she is doing one thing but is really doing something else, something that is dangerous (for example, the unnecessary transection of the ureter during the course of radical prostatectomy in the mistaken belief that additional vascular pedicle is being "taken"; unfortunately, both the ureter and the patient are being taken).

Despite the initial plea for omniscience, this chapter in essence covered certain special highlights of male pelvic anatomy. It also questioned some widely held beliefs that obfuscate rather than clarify fundamental anatomic relationships. The ultimate goal was to provide information useful to radical prostatectomy and radical cystoprostatectomy with emphasis on preservation of the distal sphincter mechanism and thereby urinary continence. A great deal of surgical success depends on understanding the fascia with respect to proper entry points and lines of dissection. The past 25 years have seen a burst of activity toward improving pelvic operations like radical prostatectomy and orthotopic neobladder creation with preservation of not only urinary continence but also erectile function. The basis for im-

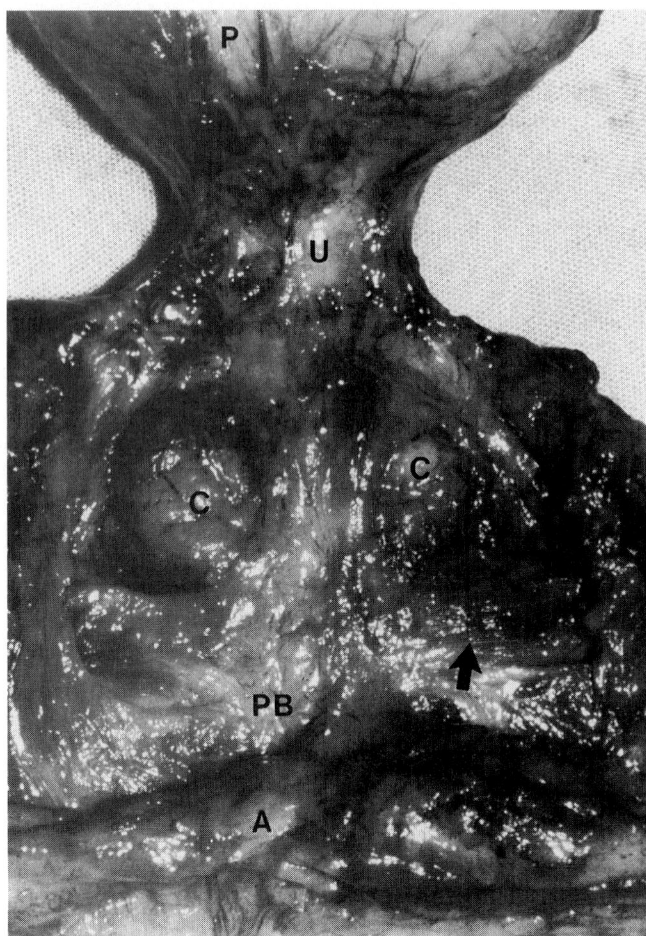

Fig. 14.9. Posterior view of prostato-urethral junction with distal perineal structures (adult cadaveric specimen). P: Prostate; U: urethra; C: bulbourethral (Cowper's) gland; PB: perineal body; A: anal wall; arrow: deep transverse perineus.

provement lies specifically in an improved understanding of pelvic anatomy.

ACKNOWLEDGMENTS

The author thanks Donald R. Cahill, PhD, Professor of Anatomy, and Chair, Department of Anatomy, Mayo Medical School, for support and advice; Bernard F. King, MD, for review of magnetic resonance images; M. Alice McKinney for medical illustration; LeAnn Stee for editorial review; and Debra Jacobson for manuscript preparation.

REFERENCES

1. Vesalius A. De humani corporis fabrica libri septem. Basel: Oporini, 1543.
2. Celsus AC. De medicina. book VIII. chapter 1. Florence: Nicolaus Laurentii, 1478.
3. Santorini GD. De virorum naturalibus. (Concerning the male genitalia.) In: Observationes anatomicae. Venetiis: Baptistam Recurti, 1724:173.
4. His W, ed. Basle nomina anatomica (BNA). Leipzig: Verlag, 1895.
5. Hyrtl J. Onomatologia anatomica. Vienna: Braumüller, 1880.
6. Hollingshead WH. The perineum. In: Textbook of anatomy. New York: Harper & Row, 1962.
7. Netter FH. Atlas of human anatomy: pelvis and perineum. Summit, NJ: Ciba-Geigy Corp, 1989. Plate 361.
8. Williams PL, Warwick R, Dyson M, et al. eds. Gray's anatomy. 37th ed. New York: Churchill Livingstone, 1989.
9. Hinman F Jr. Atlas of urosurgical anatomy. Philadelphia: WB Saunders, 1993.
10. Jordan GH. The application of tissue transfer techniques in urologic surgery. In: Webster G, Kirby R, King L, et al. eds. Reconstructive urology. Boston: Blackwell Scientific Publications, 1993:143.
11. Chilton CP. The urethra. In: Webster G, Kirby R, King L, et al. eds. Reconstructive urology. Boston: Blackwell Scientific Publications, 1993.
12. Krause W. Handbuch der menschlichen anatomie. Hannover: Hahn'sche Buchhandlung, 1879.
13. Wilson J. A description of two muscles surrounding the membranous part of the urethra. Medico-Chirurgical Transactions 1809;1:175.
14. Stedman's medical dictionary. 26th ed. Baltimore: Williams & Wilkins, 1995.
15. Dorland's illustrated medical dictionary. 27th ed. Philadelphia: WB Saunders, 1988.
16. Culp OS, DeWeerd JH. Advantages of the Cherney incision for urologic operations. J Urol 1953;445.
17. Nomina anatomica. 6th ed. New York: Churchill Livingstone, 1989.
18. Denonvilliers M. Anatomie du périnée. Bull Soc Anat de Paris, 3rd series 1836;2:105.
19. Ruckle HC, Zincke H. Potency-sparing radical retropubic prostatectomy: simplified anatomic approach. J Urol 1995;153: 1875.
20. Myers RP. Radical prostatectomy: pertinent surgical anatomy. Atlas Urol Clin North Am 1994;2:1.
21. Cunéo B, Veau V. De la signification morphologique des apnévroses périvésicales. J Anat 1899;35:235.
22. Smith GE. Studies in the anatomy of the pelvis, with special reference to the fasciae and visceral supports: part II. J Anat 1907–1908;42:252.
23. Wesson MB. The development and surgical importance of the rectourethralis muscle and Denonvilliers' fascia. J Urol 1922;8: 339.
24. Myers RP, Goellner JR, Cahill DR. Prostate shape, external striated urethral sphincter and radical prostatectomy: the apical dissection. J Urol 1987;138:543.
25. Villers A, McNeal JE, Freiha FS, et al. Invasion of Denonvilliers' fascia in radical prostatectomy specimens. J Urol 1993;149:793.
26. Tobin CE, Benjamin A. Anatomical and surgical restudy of Denonvilliers' fascia. Surg Gynecol Obstet 1945;80:373.
27. Uhlenhuth E, Wolfe WM, Smith EM, et al. Recto-genital septum. Surg Gynecol Obstet 1948;86:148.
28. Silver PHS. The role of peritoneum in the formation of the septum rectovesicale. J Anat 1956;90:538.

29. Stamey TA, Villers AA, McNeal JE, et al. Positive surgical margins at radical prostatectomy: importance of the apical dissection. J Urol 1990;143:1166.

30. Young HH. The cure of cancer of the prostate by radical perineal prostatectomy (prostatoseminal vesiculectomy): history, literature and statistics of Young's operation. J Urol 1945;53:188.

31. Henle J. Handbuch der systematischen anatomie des menschen. Eingeweidelehre. Braunschweig: F. Vieweg & Sons, 1866;2.

32. Albers DD, Faulkner KK, Cheatham WN, et al. Surgical anatomy of the pubovesical (puboprostatic) ligaments. J Urol 1973;109:388.

33. Narayan P, Konety B, Aslam K, et al. Neuroanatomy of external urethral sphincter: implications for urinary continence preservation during radical prostate surgery. J Urol 1995;153:337.

34. Myers RP. Anatomical variation of the superficial preprostatic veins with respect to radical retropubic prostatectomy. J Urol 1991;145:992.

35. Polascik TJ, Walsh PC. Radical retropubic prostatectomy: the influence of accessory pudendal arteries on the recovery of sexual function. J Urol 1995;154:150.

36. Smith GE. Studies in the anatomy of the pelvis, with special reference to the fasciae and visceral supports: Part I. J Anat 1907–1908;42:198.

37. Turner-Warwick R. The sphincter mechanisms: their relation to prostatic enlargement and its treatment. In: Hinman F Jr, ed. Benign prostatic hypertrophy. New York: Springer-Verlag, 1983:809.

38. Devine CJ, Angermeier KW. Anatomy of the penis and male perineum: part I. AUA Update Series 1994;13(2):9.

39. Golimbu M, Al-Askari S, Morales P. Transpubic approach for lower urinary tract surgery: a 15-year experience. J Urol 1990;143:72.

40. Thompson Walker JW. On the surgical anatomy of the prostate. J Anat Physiol 1906;40:189.

41. Oelrich TM. The urethral sphincter muscle in the male. Am J Anat 1980;158:229.

42. McNeal JE. Normal and pathologic anatomy of prostate. Urology 1981;17(Suppl):11.

43. Turner-Warwick R. The anatomic basis of functional reconstruction of the urethra. In: Droller MJ, ed. Surgical management of urologic disease. St. Louis: CV Mosby, 1992:770.

44. Myers RP. Male urethral sphincteric anatomy and radical prostatectomy. Urol Clin North Am 1991;18:211.

45. Clegg EJ. The musculature of the human prostatic urethra. J Anat 1957;91:345.

46. Haines RW. The striped compressor of the prostatic urethra. Br J Urol 1969;41:481.

47. McNeal JE. The prostate gland: morphology and pathobiology. Monogr Urol 1988;9:36.

48. Blacklock NJ. Surgical anatomy of the prostate. In: Williams DI, Chisholm GD, eds. Scientific foundations of urology. sect II. London: William Heinemann Medical Books, 1976:2;113.

49. Thompson P. On the arrangement of the fasciae of the pelvis and their relationship to the levator ani. J Anat Physiol 1901;35:127.

50. Lich R Jr, Howerton LW, Amin M. Anatomy and surgical approach to the urogenital tract in the male. In: Harrison JH, Gittes RF, Perlmutter AD, et al. eds. Campbell's urology. 4th ed. Philadelphia: WB Saunders, 1978:15.

51. Lich R Jr, Howerton LW, Amin M. Anatomy and surgical approach to the urogenital tract in the male. In: Harrison JH, Gittes RF, Perlmutter AD, et al. eds. Campbell's urology. 4th ed. Philadelphia: WB Saunders, 1978:17.

52. Myers RP. Practical pelvic anatomy pertinent to radical retropubic prostatectomy. AUA Update Series 1994;13:25.

53. Angemeier KW, Devine CJ. Anatomy of the penis and male perineum: part II. AUA Update Series 1994;13:17.

54. Martin CP. Urogenital system. In: Brash JC, ed. Cunningham's textbook of anatomy. 9th ed. London: Oxford University Press, 1951.

55. Kalischer O. Die urogenitalmuskulatur des dammes: mit besonderer Berücksichtigung des Harnblasen-Verschlusses. Berlin: Verlag, 1900.

56. Müller J. Über die organischen nerven der erectilen männlichen geschlectsorgane des menschen und der säugethiere. (Concerning the autonomic nerves of the male erectile genital organs of man and mammals.) Berlin: F. Dummler, 1836.

57. Gil Vernet S. L'innervation somatique et végétative des organes génito-urinaires. (Somatic and autonomic innervation of the genitourinary organs.) Acta Urol Belg 1964;32:265.

58. Cheselden W. The anatomy of the human body. London: Hitch and Dodsley, 1756.

VI

CARCINOMA PROSTATE

15

Prostate Cancer

An Overview

Robert A. Badalament, Duke K. Bahn, and Fred Lee

> *Is treatment possible in those for whom it is necessary, and necessary in those for whom it is possible?*
>
> WILLET F. WHITMORE, JR.

EPIDEMIOLOGY FACTORS

In 1995, it was projected that 244,000 new cases of prostate cancer would be diagnosed and 40,400 men would die of prostate cancer in the United States (1). Prostate cancer is the most common male malignancy, accounting for 36% of all neoplasms. Fourteen percent of the male cancer deaths are attributable to prostate cancer. It is second to lung cancer in mortality, but among men 75 years and older, prostate cancer is the most common cause of cancer death. Although frequently regarded as an indolent disease, during a 10-year period 75% of men with prostate cancer will die of this disease rather than of other causes (2). Additionally, patients dying of prostate cancer lose an average of approximately 9 years of life (3).

Epidemiologic factors associated with the development of prostate cancer include age, genetic influences, race, environmental conditions, infectious agents, hormonal status, benign prostatic hyperplasia (BPH), and prior vasectomy. The incidence and mortality increase with age (4–6). Fewer than 1% of patients with clinically detectable prostate cancer are younger than 50 years old, and approximately 75% of patients with clinically detectable prostate cancer are between 60 and 79 years of age (7). Autopsy series have demonstrated that the pathologic prevalence of prostate cancer is greater than the clinical prevalence. Sakr et al. carefully examined 152 prostate glands from young male patients 10 to 49 years old, and the histologic incidence of prostate cancer was 0%, 0%, 27%, and 34% in the second, third, fourth, and fifth decades of life, respectively (8). Cumulative data compiled by Petersen show a mean frequency of prostate cancer in the fifth, sixth, seventh, and eighth or greater decades of life to be 8%, 22%, 37%, and 53%, respectively (7).

Although the impression of many physicians is that prostate cancer in younger men has a more aggressive biologic potential than in older men, this cannot be substantiated on a stage-for-stage basis. However, younger men do have a higher incidence of metastatic disease at presentation than do older men (7). Furthermore, because longevity would otherwise be longer in younger men, an unfavorable outcome is more likely.

Prostate cancer occurs more frequently among consanguineous relatives than in the general population. Several studies have demonstrated that prostate cancer occurs 2 to 3 times more frequently among men with first-degree relatives with prostate cancer compared with those with no family history of disease (9–12). Carter et al. have described hereditary prostate cancer, which can be identified by early age onset and autosomal dominant inheritance pattern (13). It is estimated that 9% of prostate cancers result from the effects of a hereditary prostate cancer gene in the population. Because hereditary prostate cancer is an autosomal trait, women may transmit the deleterious allele to their sons. The risk of prostate cancer increases with decreasing age of prostate cancer diagnosis in the proband and increasing number of first-degree relatives (Table 15.1). Prostate cancer screening beginning at age 40 has been advocated for men with a family history of prostate cancer.

African-American men have the highest reported prostate cancer incidence; Asian men have the lowest (14, 15). African-American men tend to have higher stage disease at the time of diagnosis and shorter survival rates, even when corrected for stage (16). In a study of 112 men treated by radical prostatectomy, Badalament et al. noted that African-Americans had a higher percentage of DNA aneuploidy and a twofold higher mean prostate-specific antigen (PSA) level than whites (17).

Men who immigrate from low-risk to high-risk countries, such as those immigrating from Japan to the United States, have incidence rates between those of the country of origin and that of the United States. This observation suggests that

Table 15.1. Estimated Risk Ratios for Prostate Cancer in First-Degree Relatives of Probands by Age at Onset in Proband and Additional Affected Family Members

	RISK RATIO[a]	
AGE AT ONSET OF PROBAND (YR)	NO ADDITIONAL RELATIVES AFFECTED	1 OR MORE ADDITIONAL FIRST-DEGREE RELATIVES AFFECTED
50	1.9 (1.2–2.8)	7.1 (3.7–13.6)
60	1.4 (1.1–1.7)	5.2 (3.1–8.7)
70	1.0[b]	3.8 (2.4–6.0)

From Carter BS, Bova GS, Beaty TH, et al. J Urol 1993;150:797–802.
[a] Hazard ratio is shown with 95% confidence interval in parentheses.
[b] Reference group.

environmental factors play an etiologic role (15). Further support for an environmental role was provided in a study by Jackson et al. that compared American and Nigerian black males (18). Although the incidence of latent prostate cancer found at autopsy was similar, clinically detectable prostate cancer was sixfold higher in African-American men.

The incidence of prostate cancer is highest in industrialized countries and urban areas (19). Occupations associated with an increased risk of prostate cancer include rubber manufacturers, mechanics, newspaper workers, and plumbers. However, these reports have not been conclusively confirmed (20–24). Several studies have shown that cadmium exposure slightly increases the risk for prostate cancer (25–28). Cadmium is a trace mineral found in cigarette smoke and alkaline batteries. Welders and electroplating workers are exposed to high levels of this element. It is hypothesized that cadmium exposure may alter intraprostatic zinc or selenium concentrations, leading to malignant degeneration.

There is a strong correlation between a high-fat diet and prostate cancer (19, 29–32). Giovannucci et al. studied more than 50,000 health-care professionals and noted a significant association between fat consumption and prostate cancer (32). This association was primarily caused by animal fat, especially fat from red meat (relative risk, 2.64), rather than vegetable fat. Fat from dairy products (with the exception of butter) or fish was not related to risk. The mechanism by which dietary fat increases the risk of prostate cancer is unclear and may be related to secondary factors such as altered production of sexual hormones, fat-soluble vitamin absorption especially vitamin A, or intake of trace nutrients such as zinc (33).

The development of prostate cancer by a sexually transmitted viral agent has been postulated. An increased incidence of prostate cancer among men whose sexual partners had cervical cancer supports this theory. Epidemiologic support, however, is lacking (34). Cytomegalovirus isolated from prepubertal prostates and herpes virus isolated from prostate cancer have been shown to cause in vitro malignant transformation of human prostate cell lines and hamster cells (35, 36). Additionally, viral antibody titers have been found to be elevated in prostate cancer patients when compared with control subjects

(29, 35). RNA viruses also have been implicated. Human prostate cancers have demonstrated reverse transcriptase activity, RNA virus-like particles, and RNA tumor virus core proteins (37, 38).

Several of the previously mentioned risk factors can be mediated through endogenous hormones. The increased incidence of prostate cancer with age is possibly related to changes in the hormonal milieu. High fat ingestion may be associated with an increased testosterone level. The difference in prostate cancer incidence between Japanese and American men might be related to dietary habits. Japanese men, who eat a high-fiber, low-fat diet, have lower serum sex hormone binding globulin and higher sex hormone binding in their feces than their American counterparts who eat a high-fat, low-fiber diet (39, 40).

Further evidence supporting hormonal mediation includes the presence of prostatic steroid hormone receptors, the necessity of sex hormones for normal prostatic development, an extremely low incidence of prostate cancer among eunuchs and castrated men, a decreased occurrence of latent prostate cancer in cirrhotics who tend to have hyperestrogenism, and the favorable response in prostate cancer patients to estrogens or androgen deprivation (41–43). Additionally, Noble induced prostate cancer in experimental animals by prolonged administration of androgens (44). Several studies have demonstrated that levels of testosterone and its metabolite, dihydrotestosterone (DHT), are higher in carcinomatous than normal prostatic tissue (45–47).

Studies comparing the levels of total plasma testosterone and DHT in prostate cancer patients and control subjects are inconclusive (47–51). These studies, however, did not measure the unbound fraction, which is the biologically active portion. Serum prolactin levels have provided more consistent findings. Of seven studies, five noted higher prolactin levels in prostate cancer patients compared with patients with BPH or normal prostate (50–57); no difference was demonstrated in two studies (55, 56). Prolactin increases prostatic uptake and metabolism of testosterone. Thus, elevated prolactin levels may result in increased prostatic uptake of testosterone and accelerated conversion into DHT.

The relationship between prostatic hyperplasia and carcinoma remains undefined. The two most frequently quoted studies produced contrasting results. Greenwald et al. followed up on 838 patients with BPH and 802 age-matched control subjects for 10 years but failed to identify any difference in prostate cancer incidence between the two groups (57). Armenian et al. reported a 3.7 to 5.1 times higher age-adjusted death rate due to prostatic carcinoma among patients with BPH compared with age-matched control subjects (58). Histologic studies suggest that the etiologic factors for prostate cancer and BPH are unrelated. Studies of small-volume prostate cancers concluded that prostate cancer originates in nonhypertrophied senile tissue and compressed atrophic glands (sclerotic atrophy) outside the expanding hypertrophic nodules (57, 59).

The conflicting results from epidemiologic studies of vasectomy and its possible risk factor for prostate cancer resulted in controversy and confusion (60). Vasectomy results in antisperm antibodies, reduced prostatic secretory function, and possibly slightly increased serum testosterone. However, these effects do not provide a clear causal mechanism. Six of seven case-control studies and one of two retrospective cohort studies indicated a positive association between vasectomy and prostate cancer; these epidemiologic studies, however, contain potential sources of error, especially detection bias (61–70). Indeed, men undergoing vasectomy are arguably more likely to seek health care than those men who have not had a vasectomy.

In 1993, Giovannucci et al. reported on a prospective cohort study involving 47,855 health-care professionals (71). Men undergoing vasectomy had an age-adjusted relative risk of 1.66 compared with the nonvasectomy control subjects. Because Giovannucci's study better addressed detection bias, the National Institutes of Health (NIH) reviewed that study. The NIH concluded that the association between vasectomy and prostate cancer was weak and that detection bias still could not be excluded. Additionally, the NIH recommended that physicians could continue to perform vasectomy, that vasectomy reversal is not warranted, and that prostate cancer screening for patients who had vasectomy should not differ from those who did not.

ANATOMIC CONSIDERATIONS

Classical concepts of prostate anatomy, initially described by Lowsley (72) and later by Franks (73), were extensively modified by McNeal (74). In McNeal's model, the prostate is divided into four areas—peripheral zone, central zone, transitional zone, and periurethral gland region. In the normal prostate, these regions constitute approximately 70%, 20%, 10%, and less than 1% of the glandular prostate, respectively. The spatial orientation of these regions is illustrated in Figure 15.1.

Embryologically, the peripheral zone, transitional zone, and periurethral gland region share a common origin from the urogenital sinus and therefore are histologically similar with small, rounded, and uniform acini. The central zone has large and irregular acini, which suggests wolffian duct origin. BPH usually occurs in the transitional zone and periurethral gland region. Glandular hyperplasia predominates in the transitional zone, and stromal hyperplasia predominates in the periurethral glandular region. Approximately 70% of cancers develop in the peripheral zone, 20% in the transitional zone, and 10% in the central zone.

PROSTATIC INTRAEPITHELIAL NEOPLASIA

Prostatic intraepithelial neoplasia (PIN) refers to premalignant cytologic and architectural abnormalities (Fig. 15.2) (75, 76). The term PIN replaces synonymous terminology such as atypical hyperplasia, marked atypia, duct-acinar dysplasia, large acinar atypical hyperplasia, and intraductal dysplasia (77–79). The spectrum of dysplastic abnormalities is reflected in the three grades of PIN. These range from PIN grade 1, character-

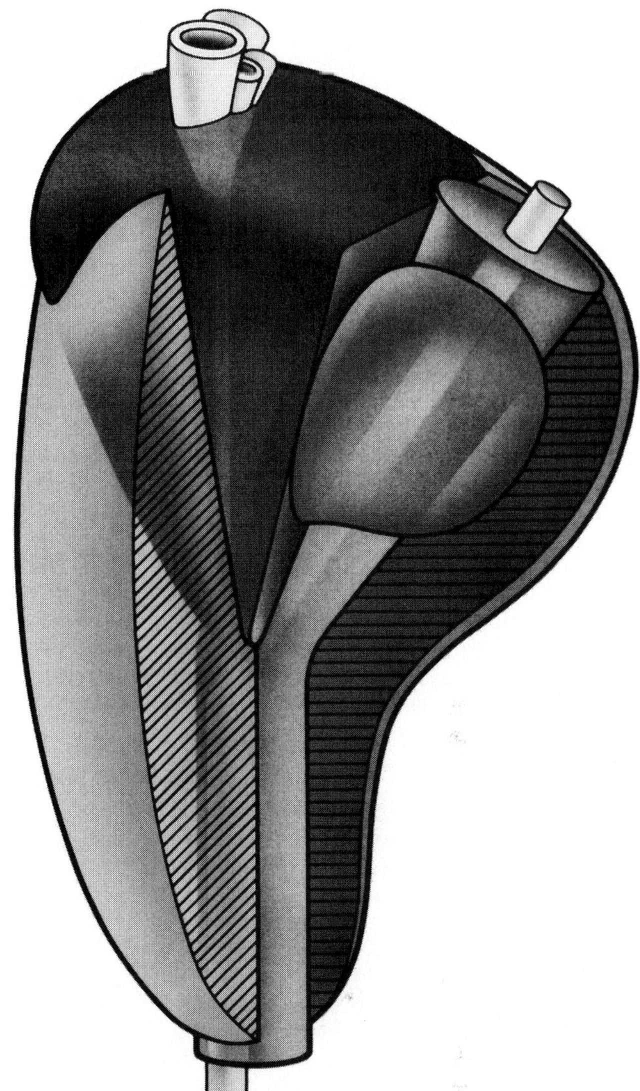

Fig. 15.1. Zonal anatomy of the prostate.

ized by variably enlarged nuclei and cell crowding, to PIN grade 3, which may be indistinguishable from carcinoma in situ.

Several observations suggest that PIN is a premalignant lesion. PIN is likely to be found about twice as often in prostates with cancer than in hyperplasia (80). The distribution of PIN within the prostate also closely parallels that for carcinoma. Foci of invasive carcinoma have been demonstrated at their points of origin from areas with high-grade PIN (81). Furthermore, immunohistochemical studies demonstrated a loss of differentiation antigens proportional to the severity of PIN. Sakr et al. identified PIN in 9%, 20%, and 44% of men during their respective third, fourth, and fifth decades of life; in these same respective groups, the incidence of actual prostate cancer was 0%, 27%, and 34% (8).

Recently, Weinstein and Epstein studied 33 men with high-grade PIN shown on needle biopsy of the prostate (82). Twenty-

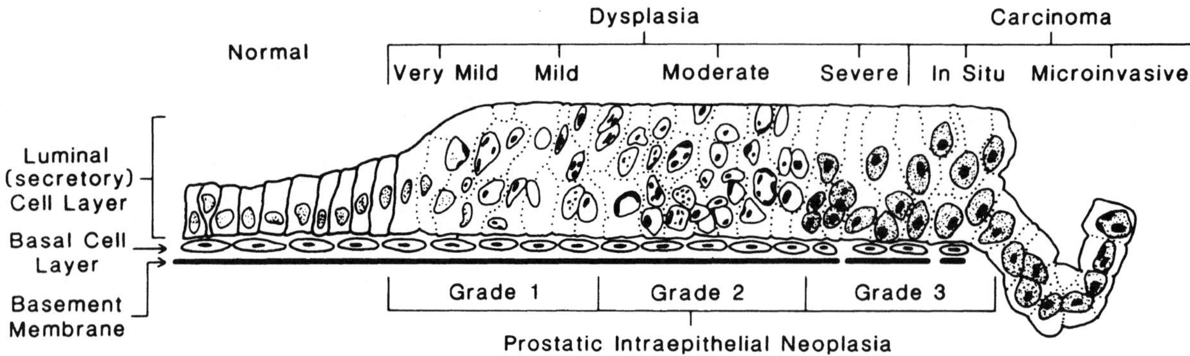

Fig. 15.2. Disease continuum of prostatic intraepithelial neoplasia (PIN). (From Bostwick DG, Brawer MK. Prostatic intra-epithelial neoplasia and early invasion of prostate cancer. Cancer 1987;59:788–794. Used with permission.)

four men (73%) had adenocarcinoma on subsequent biopsy. When PSA was greater than 4.0 ng/mL, however, 86% were subsequently proven to have adenocarcinoma. Close observation appears to be warranted for patients with high-grade PIN.

GRADING

The Gleason system is the most frequently used grading system (Fig. 15.3) (83). It is based on the degree of glandular differen-tiation and the growth pattern of the tumor in relation to the prostatic stroma; individual cellular characteristics are not considered. The pattern can vary from a well-differentiated grade 1 tumor to a poorly differentiated grade 5 tumor. The Gleason system assigns a histologic grade to both the primary and secondary patterns, and the final Gleason score represents the sum of the two. As a result, the Gleason score ranges between 2 and 10. Thus, the Gleason grading system is unique

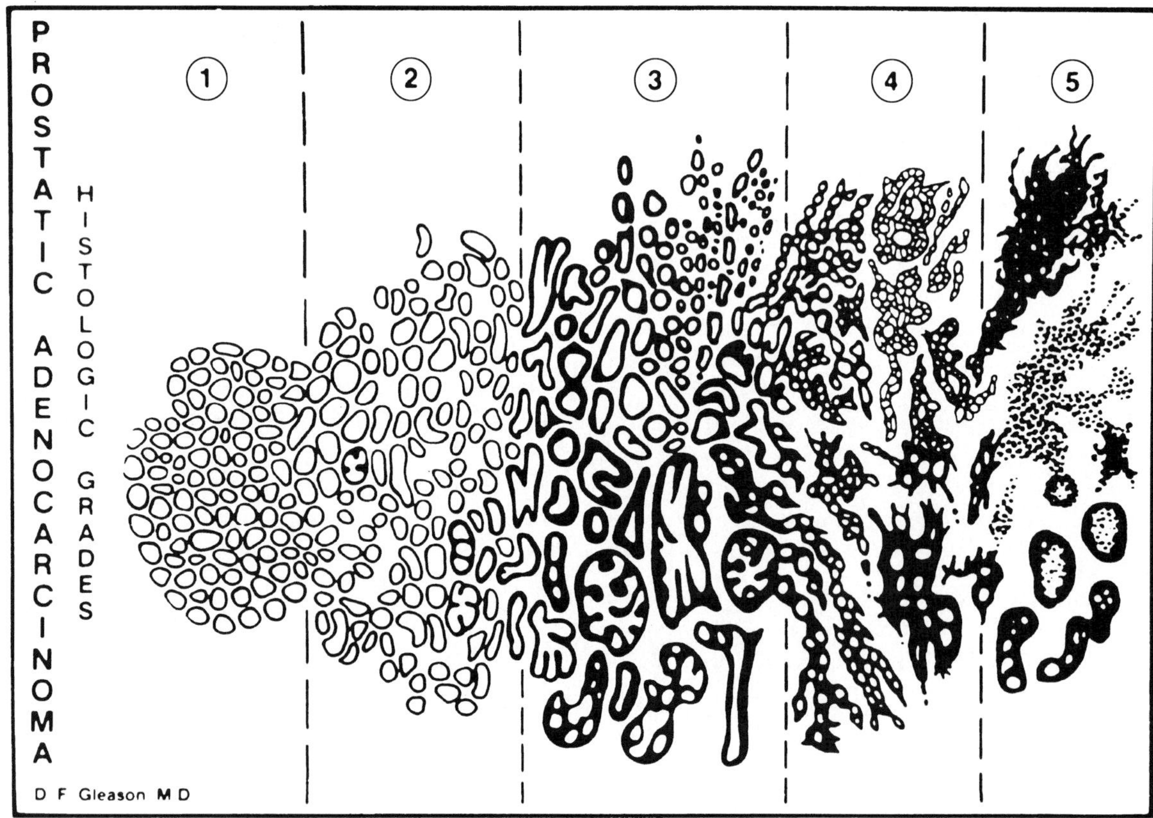

Fig. 15.3. Gleason grading system of prostatic adenocarcinoma. (From Gleason DF. The Veterans Administration Cooperative Research Group: histologic grading and clinical staging of prostatic carcinoma. In: Tannenbaum M, ed. Urologic pathology: the prostate. Philadelphia: Lea & Febiger, 1977. Used with permission.)

because the histologic grade is based on the majority of the specimen and not the most undifferentiated portion.

NATURAL HISTORY

As tumors enlarge, they become more poorly differentiated and increasingly heterogeneous (84). Tumors less than 0.5 cc are probably clinically insignificant; tumors less than 3.8 cc usually remain intraprostatic; and tumors greater than 5.0 cc are typically extraprostatic (85). It has been estimated that a tumor must undergo 30 doublings to reach a size of 1 cc (10^9 cells). Only 10 more doublings are required to achieve a volume of 1 kg (10^{12} cells) (86). The assumptions that the doubling time takes approximately 2.5 years, that a tumor must be 1 cc to be palpable, and that a 1-kg tumor causes death account for the long preclinical phase (87). Although the autopsy incidence of prostate cancer in men older than 50 years is approximately 30%, only 9.37% will be diagnosed and 0.11% will die of their disease. Prostate cancer spreads by direct extension into the seminal vesicles, bladder, membranous urethra, and pelvic sidewalls. Invasion into the rectum is relatively uncommon because of the protection afforded by Denonvilliers' fascia. Regional and distant metastases also can occur by lymphatic and hematogenous routes. Surgical staging series have demonstrated that the obturator lymph node group is the primary landing site for pelvic nodal metastases (88, 89). Subsequent lymphatic invasion involves the iliac and para-aortic lymph nodes. Lung metastases result from either further lymphatic spread via the thoracic duct or hematogenous dissemination from the prostatic venous plexus. Bone metastases most frequently involve the vertebral column, ribs, and pelvic bones (90).

CLINICAL PRESENTATION

At presentation, 58% of patients have localized disease, 15% have regional involvement, and 16% have distant metastases (1). The majority of patients are either asymptomatic or have bladder outlet obstructive symptoms. Patients can also present with severe irritative bladder symptoms in the absence of infection. Patients with metastatic disease most often complain of bone pain. Frequently, the disease is erroneously attributed to degenerative arthritis. Pathologic fracture or spinal cord compression may result from metastatic bone disease. Occasionally, palpable peripheral lymphadenopathy or lower extremity edema caused by pelvic adenopathy is the presenting symptom. Renal failure resulting from bilateral ureteral obstruction, visceral metastases, anemia, or cachexia can be the initial signs of prostate cancer. Occasionally, a patient will present with metastatic disease from an unknown primary site; in this case, PSA and prostatic acid phosphatase immunohistochemical stains of biopsy specimens are useful (91, 92).

DETECTION IN ASYMPTOMATIC MEN

Screening for prostate cancer remains controversial. It is well established that screening men older than 50 years of age in-

creases the detection rate of prostate cancers, especially early, localized tumors (93–95). Most screening protocols initially evaluate patients with digital rectal examination (DRE) and PSA. As illustrated in Table 15.2, DRE and PSA can be combined to identify the probability of prostate cancer (96). Transrectal ultrasound (TRUS) is reserved for patients with either an abnormal DRE and/or PSA.

Identified in 1979, PSA is produced almost exclusively by normal and neoplastic prostatic ductal epithelium (97). The half-life is 2.2 days, and its serum concentration is proportional to total prostate volume. Although relatively sensitive, PSA lacks the specificity to make it an ideal screening test (98–102). Despite being an imperfect tool, it is still extremely valuable. Compared with DRE, PSA detects about twice as many prostate cancers and nearly twice as many pathologically organ-confined cancers. Applications of PSA aimed at enhancing clinical use include PSA density, PSA velocity, and age-specific PSA reference ranges (103).

PSA density was introduced by Benson et al. and is the ratio of the serum PSA divided by the total prostate volume determined by TRUS (104, 105). Patients with a PSA density of greater than 0.15 can be considered at high risk for prostate cancer. Subsequent studies, however, have shown that PSA density is equal to or slightly better than PSA alone in detecting prostate cancer (106–111). Seaman et al. have shown that the major use of PSA density may be in patients with PSA values between 4.0 and 10.0 ng/mL (112).

PSA velocity was first reported by Carter et al., who established a cutoff of 0.8 ng/mL/yr to distinguish BPH from prostate cancer (113). Carter identified differences in PSA velocity 9 years before clinical diagnosis. It was believed that at least three measurements were necessary to calculate PSA velocity. In a larger study, Catalona et al. accurately confirmed these findings (94). Brawer et al. studied 710 subjects yearly for 2 years and noted that a 20% annual change identified men at significant risk for prostate cancer (114).

Oesterling et al. studied 471 men who had no evidence of cancer when evaluated by PSA, DRE, and TRUS (115). They found that "normal" reference ranges were age dependent. For men 40 to 49 years old, the reference range was 0.0 to 2.5 ng/

Table 15.2. Cancer Detection Rates Related to Levels of Serum Prostate-Specific Antigen and Digital Rectal Examination in 2634 Patients

PSA (ng/mL)	NO. OF CANCERS/NO. OF PATIENTS	
	DRE+	DRE−
≤4	46/446 (10.3%)	31/1265 (2.5%)
>4	141/438 (55.3%)	64/48 (13.2%)
4.1–10	74/194 (38.1%)	19/343 (5.5%)
>10	168/256 (65.6%)	45/144 (31.3%)

From Cooner WH. Prostate-specific antigen, digital rectal examination, and transrectal ultrasound of the prostate in prostate cancer detection. In: Stamey TA, ed. Monogr Urol 1991;12:1–13. Used with permission.
PSA, prostate-specific antigen (hybritech method); DRE, digital rectal examination.

mL; for men 50 to 59 years old, the reference range was 0.0 to 3.5 ng/mL; for men 60 to 69 years old, it was 0.0 to 4.5 ng/mL; and for men 70 to 79 years old, it was 0.0 to 5.0 ng/mL. Confirmatory studies have produced conflicting results (93, 95).

TRUS should be limited to patients with abnormal DRE and/or PSA. Lee et al. established that most early prostate cancers are hypoechoic; the degree of hypoechogenicity of prostate cancer is related to tumor morphology (116, 117). Tumors larger than 1.0 cc tend to have a positive color flow Doppler; this permits identification of subtle inner gland lesions. Contrary to the advice of some (118), Lee and Bahn do not recommend routine random sextant biopsy. The predicted PSA can be calculated by multiplying the gland volume by 0.12. The excess PSA is equal to the serum PSA minus the predicted PSA. Because each cc of prostate cancer produces about 2 ng/mL of PSA, the expected tumor volume can be estimated by dividing the excess PSA by 2. The cube root of the tumor volume provides an estimate of the average tumor dimension that should be visible on ultrasound for tumor-directed prostate biopsies. If no lesion is found in the outer gland, random sextant biopsies are generally not performed.

STAGING CLASSIFICATION SYSTEMS

Treatment selection is largely based on the extent of disease. Multiple staging systems have been proposed, and these systems are similar in designating the disease as being confined to the prostate, having local spread to either regional or distant lymph nodes, or involving bone or other parenchymal sites. The A, B, C, D system proposed by Whitmore (119) and later modified by Jewett (120) is the most commonly used system in the United States (Table 15.3).

In the Whitmore-Jewett classification, there is no universal agreement on definitions of stage A1 versus stage A2 disease. Stage A1 disease has been arbitrarily defined to be differentiated carcinoma involving three or fewer of the prostatic currettings following transurethral resection (121), or, alternatively, less than 5% of total gland volume (122). Stage A2 prostate cancer is moderate- to high-grade focal disease or diffuse cancer. Jewett noted that among stage B patients, the 15-year disease-free survival for 103 patients with 1.5-cm tumors involving less than one lobe was superior to that of 79 patients with larger tumors (27% versus 18%). Given these results, Jewett subclassified stage B tumors into stage B1 (less than one lobe) and stage B2 (one or more lobes) (120).

With the popularization of brachytherapy, Memorial Sloan-Kettering Cancer Center began to subclassify stage C tumors. Tumors with palpable invasion of one or both sulci only are designated stage C1. Tumors involving the base of one or both seminal vesicles with or without sulcal involvement are designated stage C2. Tumors with more extensive involvement of the seminal vesicles and/or involvement of adjacent structures are designated stage C3 (123). Stage D prostate cancer is divided into stage D1 (regional lymph node metastasis) and stage D2 (distant metastasis). Whitesel et al. suggested a special stage designation, stage D0, for patients who lack clinical evidence of metastasis but have elevated acid phosphatase levels (124).

The TNM system of staging prostate cancer has been adopted by the American Joint Committee for Cancer Staging and End Results Reporting (125). Except for stage T1c disease, the Whitmore-Jewett and the TNM classifications have many similarities. Patients with stage T1c disease are a unique group of men with nonpalpable and nonvisible cancer who had biopsies that were based solely on an abnormal PSA. This group is the focal point of the current controversy concerning prostate cancer screening. Many physicians fear that this group of patients has an overabundance of clinically insignificant tumors (126, 127). Ohori et al. confirm that slightly more clinically insignificant tumors are noted in stage T1c patients than in typical radical prostatectomy patients (17% versus 9%) (128). However, stage T1c patients had less advanced tumors (4% versus 29%) and more curable tumors (79% versus 62%). Other studies showed that the detection of clinically insignificant tumors has not substantially increased (94, 129, 130).

The Organ Site Coordination Center (OSCC) of the National Cancer Institute devised a classification that incorporates the Whitmore-Jewett and TNM systems (131). The advantage of the OSCC classification is that it defines the primary tumor by the more familiar A, B, C terminology and at the same time characterizes the lymph node (N) and metastatic (M) status.

Lee et al. introduced a modification of the Whitmore-Jewett classification system based on the ultrasound findings and associated staging biopsy findings (132). Strategic TRUS guided biopsy affords accurate tumor mapping and staging when modes of internal spread and escape of cancer from both outer and inner glands are known (Figs. 15.4 and 15.5). (117) For outer gland tumors, sites of tumor escape include the nearby neurovascular bundle, or the trapezoid fossa of the apex. If the tumor involves the midline, the seminal vesicles should also be sampled. For inner gland tumor, sites of escape are the apex at the junction of the anterior fibromuscular stroma with the prostate capsule and the bladder neck at the junction with the central zone.

If the lesion is less than 1.5 cm in average dimension with negative staging biopsy results (no evidence of extraprostatic invasion), it is classified as an ultrasound B1 (UB1). If the lesion is larger than 1.5 cm in dimension with negative staging biopsy results, it is classified as UB2. If the staging biopsy is positive regardless of the lesion size, it is classified as UC. Lesions not seen on ultrasound and picked up by random biopsy can be classified as UA. There is no UD because TRUS cannot image the pelvic lymph node.

CLINICAL METHODS OF STAGING

Staging of the Primary Tumor

DRE is inexpensive and easily accomplished. However, it is an imprecise method of evaluating the extent of the primary

Table 15.3. Summary of Clinical Staging Systems for Prostate Cancer

MODIFIED WHITMORE-JEWETT	TNM		OSCC		MODIFIED LEE	
A No clinical neoplasm A_1<5% total tissue A_1>5% total tissue	Tx	Primary tumor cannot be assessed	Tx	Anatomic relationship undefinable	UA	Not visible on ultrasound, detected by random biopsy
	T0	No evidence primary tumor	TA	Digitally unrecognizable neoplasm		
	T1a	≤5% of total specimen	TA1	≤5% total specimen and/or high grade		
	T1b	>5% of total specimen	TA2	>5% total specimens and/or high grade		
	T1c	Tumor identified by needle biopsy (e.g., because of elevated PSA)				
B Palpable neoplasm B_1≤1.5 cm, 1 lobe B_2>2.5 cm, >1 lobe	T2	Tumor confined within the prostate	TBx	Palpable tumor but not characterized	UB	Visible on ultrasound, negative staging biopsies (no extraprostatic invasion)
	T2a	≤half of a lobe	TB	Palpable tumor, not beyond capsule		
	T2b	>half of a lobe but not both lobes	TB1	Not more than ½ lobe		
	T2c	Both lobes	TB2	More than ½ lobe, <1 lobe	UB1	≤1.5 cm
			TB3	>1 lobe or more than 1 tumor	UB2	>5 cm
C Local invasion C_1 Invasion of one or both sulci C_2 Base of seminal vesicle C_3 More seminal vesicle involvement and/or adjacent structures	T3	Tumor extends through prostatic capsule	TCx	Extension but not characterized	UC	Visible on ultrasound, positive staging biopsies (extraprostate invasion present)
			TC1	Extension beyond margin unilaterally		
	T3a	Unilateral				
	T3b	Bilateral	TC2	Extension beyond margin with involvement of bladder base and/or rectum, and/or levator, and/or pelvic side-wall		
	T3c	Invasion of seminal vesicle(s)			UC1	≤50% prostatic involvement
	T4	Fixed tumor or invasion of adjacent structures			UC2	>50% prostatic involvement
	T4a	Bladder neck and/or external sphincter and/or rectum				
	T4b	Levator ani muscle and/or pelvic wall				
D Metastasis D_0 Elevated PAP D_1 Regional lymph node D_2 Distant metastasis	NX	Regional nodes cannot be assessed	N0	No regional node metastasis		
	N0	No nodal metastasis	N1	Microscopic lymph node metastasis		
	N1	≤2 cm single regional node	N2	Gross regional lymph node metastasis		
	N2	2–5 cm regional node(s)	N3	Extra regional lymph node metastasis		
	N3	>5 cm regional nodes	Nx	Requirements not met		
	MX	Distant metastasis cannot be assessed	M0	No evidence of metastasis		
	M0	No distant metastasis	M1	Elevated acid phosphatase		
	M1	Distant metastasis	M2	Visceral and/or bone metastasis		
	M1a	Nonregional lymph node(s)	Mx	Requirements not met		
	M1b	Bone(s)				
	M1c	Other site(s)				

tumor. In a study from The Johns Hopkins University involving 565 patients with clinical stage T2 disease, histologic examination of the radical prostatectomy specimen demonstrated extraprostatic disease in 48% (133). Further, when subdivided into clinical stages T2a, T2b, and T2c, the pathologic incidence of extraprostatic disease was 39%, 59%, and 65%, respectively. These findings suggest that the accuracy of DRE decreases with tumor volume.

Incidental prostate cancer is detected in 10% of patients undergoing prostatectomy for clinically benign disease (134).

In patients with focal low-grade (Stage A1) prostate cancer, a staging TURP has been suggested. A summary of six studies involving 281 patients with stage A1 disease demonstrated that a repeat or staging transurethral prostatectomy (TURP) identified residual cancer in 23% (135). In our practice, we favor performing ultrasound-guided biopsies rather than a staging TURP.

The relationship between serum PSA and advanced clinical stage, tumor volume, and pathologic stage is well established. For individual patients, however, PSA lacks sufficient sensitiv-

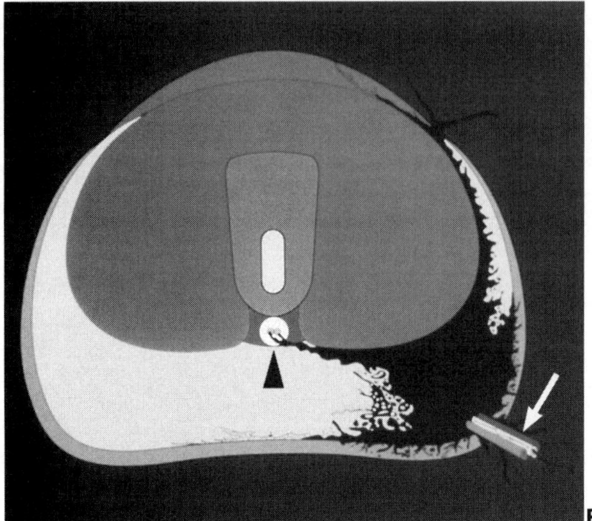
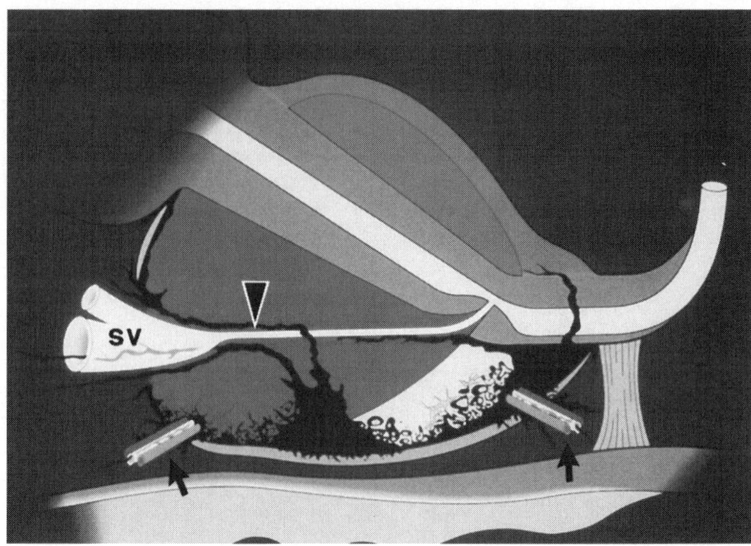

Fig. 15.4. Routes of outer gland spread. **A.** Transverse view shows extension of cancer via the neurovascular bundle (arrow) and ejaculatory duct (arrowhead). Outer gland cancers tend to remain in an ipsilateral location. **B.** Longitudinal view shows escape of cancer via the ejaculatory duct (arrowhead) and seminal vesicle (SV). Asterisk indicates the prostatic fossa (Trapezoid space). Arrow indicates neurovascular bundles. (From Lee F, Bahn DK, McHugh TA, et al. US-Guided percutaneous cryoablation of prostate cancer. Radiology 1994;192:769–776. Used with permission.)

ity to provide accurate staging information (17, 102, 111, 136). Approximately 75% of men with a PSA of less than 4.0 ng/ mL have pathologically organ-confined disease. The majority of men with a PSA of greater than 10.0 ng/mL have capsular penetration, and most men with a PSA of greater than 50 ng/ mL have positive lymph node involvement. The accuracy of PSA can be improved when used in combination with tumor grade or number of positive sextant biopsies (133, 137). Oesterling et al. indicated that among newly diagnosed, untreated patients, a bone scan is unnecessary when the PSA value is less than 10 ng/mL (138).

Magnetic resonance imaging (MRI) has great promise for staging prostate cancer. In a multicenter trial comparing body surface MRI and TRUS staging accuracies after subsequently examining the radical prostatectomy specimens, the MRI staging accuracy was found to be 69% compared with 58% for TRUS (139). Extremely high resolution has been noted when an endorectal surface coil is used. In a small study of 22 patients

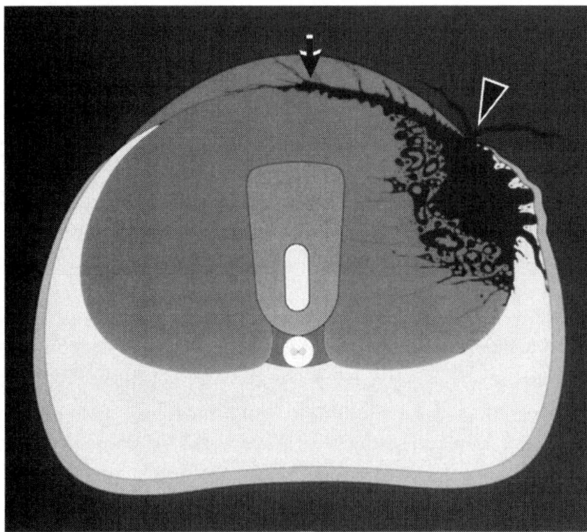
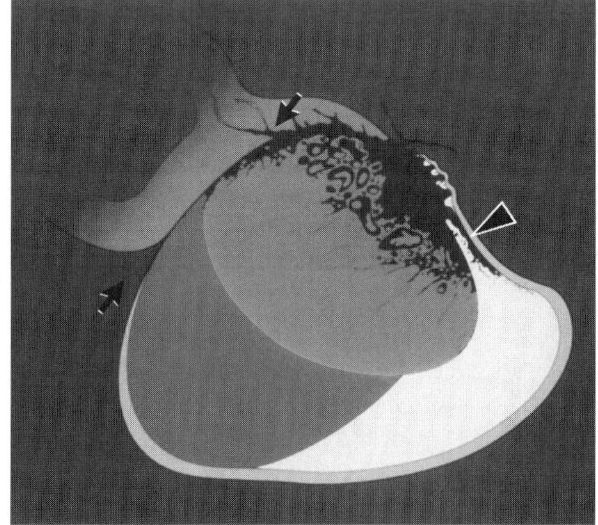

Fig. 15.5. Routes of inner gland cancer spread. **A.** Transverse view shows contralateral extension of cancer (arrow) and tumor escape at the junction of the capsule and anterior fibromuscular stroma (arrowhead). **B.** Longitudinal view shows tumor spread to the bladder neck (arrows) and into the apex of the outer gland (arrowhead). (From Lee F, Bahn DK, McHugh TA, et al. US-Guided percutaneous cryoablation of prostate cancer. Radiology 1994;192: 769–776. Used with permission.)

treated by radical prostatectomy, Schnall et al. noted an accuracy of 82% in differentiating stage B from stage C cancer (140). Recently, Chelsky et al. performed endorectal surface coil MRI in 47 patients before radical prostatectomy (141). The overall accuracy was 68%, with a 91% accuracy in detecting seminal vesical involvement. Major limitations to the use of MRI include expense, discomfort, and the inability to obtain images and perform prostatic biopsy simultaneously.

Evaluation of Regional Lymph Nodes

Lymphography, computed tomography (CT) scan, and MRI have been used in the evaluation of pelvic lymph nodal status (142–144). Lymphography is of limited value because the hypogastric and obturator lymph nodes are inconsistently visualized, resulting in false-positive rates of 10 to 17% and false-negative rates of 22 to 40%. CT scan and MRI have a reported accuracy of 80 to 90% in detecting metastatic adenopathy, but both imaging modalities are limited by their inability to identify microscopic disease. Detection of microscopic metastatic disease can be enhanced when CT is used in conjunction with fine-needle aspiration cytology to confirm a positive study (145, 146). However, a negative CT-guided aspiration cytology does not exclude metastases.

Radioimmunoscintigraphy of pelvic lymph nodes with [111]indium-labeled monoclonal antibody CYT-356 shows promise in early clinical trials (Fig. 15.6). Babaian et al. studied 19 patients with prostate cancer at high risk for metastatic lymphadenopathy and found an overall accuracy of 76%, with a sensitivity and specificity of 44% and 86% (147). The negative predictive value was 83%, and the positive predictive value was 50%. The detection threshold of this antibody scan was a cancer focus of 5 mm.

Because of the inability of imaging modalities to evaluate regional nodal status precisely, pelvic lymphadenectomy has been advocated in patients with clinically localized prostate cancer. In summarizing the literature, Donohue et al. noted that the incidence of metastatic lymphadenopathy among prostate cancer patients undergoing surgical staging varied by clinical stage. Of the patients with clinical stages A1, A2, B1, B2, and C prostate cancers, pelvic lymph node metastases were found in 2%, 23%, 18%, 35%, and 46%, respectively (148). The incidence of unsuspected pelvic lymph node metastases among radical prostatectomy patients, however, has decreased from earlier reports of 20% to contemporary studies ranging from 6.7 to 5.7% (149, 150). Using a statistical model based on clinical stage, PSA, and Gleason grade, Bluestein et al. predicted the probability of pelvic lymph node involvement (151). With this model they estimate 61% of patients with clinical stages A1 to B1 and 29% with clinical stages A1 to B2 can be spared pelvic lymphadenectomy.

The morbidity of open lymphadenectomy and low incidence of occult lymph node metastasis have led to the development of laparoscopic lymph node dissection (152–157). Compared with open excision, laparoscopy is just as accurate but less mor-

bid (154). Kerbl et al. noted that the hospital stay for a patient undergoing laparoscopic pelvic lymph node dissection for metastases was 1.7 days compared with 5.4 days for those undergoing surgical lymph node dissection (155). Additionally, laparoscopic lymphadenectomy resulted in a decrease in the return-to-work recovery time from 48 days to 7 days. Kavoussi et al. reported a 15% incidence of complications for 372 patients who underwent an intraperitoneal laparoscopic approach (156). Das and Tashima developed an extraperitoneal approach that may decrease the adverse sequelae that often accompany the intraperitoneal approach (157).

Evaluation of Distant Metastases

Physical examination, serum PSA, chest radiograph, and radionuclide bone scan are indicated to detect distant metastases. Physical examination can reveal palpable lymphadenopathy, lymphedema, exostosis, or soft tissue metastases. Although PSA and prostatic acid phosphatase, when used alone, are of limited use to stage localized prostate cancer, significantly elevated levels of either of these tumor markers are reliable indicators of metastatic disease (102). A chest radiograph diagnoses osseous metastasis in the ribs and axial skeleton. Skeletal metastases are osteoblastic because of an increase in noncalcified osteoid that replaces air spaces within the bone. This phenomenon produces a paradoxical appearance of increased bone density in areas of calcium loss.

Among newly diagnosed prostate cancer patients with a PSA less than 10 ng/mL, a radionuclide bone scan is unnecessary (138). Although a bone scan is more sensitive than a bone survey, it is also less specific (158–160). Paget's disease, degenerative arthritis, and trauma may also cause increased radionuclide uptake, thereby creating false-positive results. Radiographs, CT scans, MRI, or bone biopsy may be useful in evaluating equivocal bone scans. Diffuse symmetrical metastatic uptake (superscan) can be falsely interpreted as normal. Minimal soft tissue visualization and the absence of renal excretion of radionuclide should raise the suspicion of a falsely negative superscan (160).

TREATMENT OPTIONS: LOCALIZED DISEASE

The optimal management of men with localized prostatic carcinoma remains controversial. Treatment options include watchful waiting or expectant management, radical prostatectomy, external beam or interstitial radiation therapy, and cryotherapy. The selection of treatment is based on projected survival of the patient, quality of life issues, and patient and physician preferences.

Expectant Management

Several studies show that expectant management appears to be a reasonable option among patients with low-stage and low-grade tumors who have a life expectancy of less than 10 years.

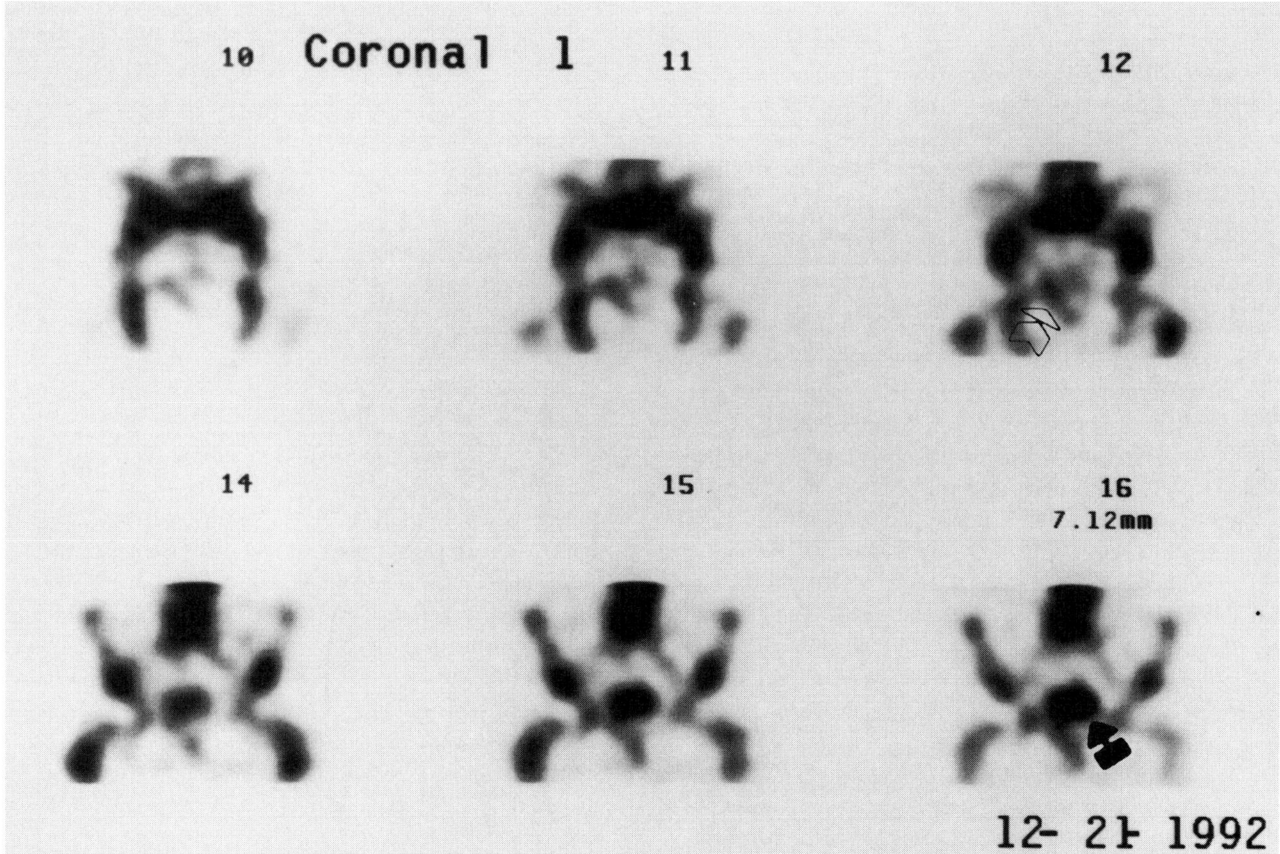

Fig. 15.6.   Coronal cuts through the pelvis of the ^{111}In CYT-356 nuclear medicine images showing the prostate tumor (closed arrow) and the lymph node involvement (open arrow). Symmetrical elongated structures represent major vessels or skeletal structures.

The details of these studies, however, should be examined before applying expectant management to all men with localized prostate cancer. Published reports concerning expectant management reflect data obtained from a highly selected group of patients (161–164). Most studies are from Sweden, where the diagnosis of cancer is usually made on cytology without biopsy confirmation. Compared with contemporary radical prostatectomy series, expectant management studies have a higher proportion of stage A1 disease, grade 1 tumors, and a lower percentage of poorly differentiated tumors. Moreover, a large proportion of patients treated expectantly eventually receive endocrine therapy.

A 10-year follow-up may not be long enough to demonstrate the true therapeutic advantage of radical prostatectomy over expectant management. Warner and Whitmore treated 75 of 4000 patients with expectant management (163). Of the patients who received follow-up care for 10 years or longer, 27% died of cancer and 82% had disease progression. Adolfsson et al. reviewed the literature since 1980 and noted that at 10 years the development of metastatic disease and death was 50% lower for men who underwent radical prostatectomy than for those treated by expectant management (165). As the men from Sweden who were treated expectantly continue to age,

the Swedish prostate cancer mortality rate, already one of the highest in the world, can be expected to rise (1).

Modeling studies that illustrate the effects of certain choices in prostate cancer treatment have contributed to the confusion about expectant management. Recently, the Prostate Patient Outcomes Research Team (PORT) published a decision analysis that promoted expectant management as a reasonable alternative to invasive treatment for many men with localized prostate cancer (166). The PORT study reported that for most patients, treatment provided less than a 1-year improvement in quality-adjusted life expectancy. However, Beck et al. (167) reanalyzed the PORT study using a different set of cure rates for intracapsular and extracapsular disease and incorporated annual metastatic rates from a meta-analysis of expectant management studies performed by Chodak et al. (168). In this study, patients with moderately or poorly differentiated tumors treated by radical prostatectomy had about 2.5 additional quality-adjusted life years compared with those who had expectant management.

Radical Prostatectomy

Since Young's report in 1905, radical prostatectomy has been considered the definitive treatment for localized prostate cancer

(169). There is no evidence that any other treatment modality produces better control of the primary lesion and lessens the chance of distant metastases than does total excision of the prostate (170). Radical prostatectomy cures a majority of men with organ-confined disease or well-differentiated to moderately well-differentiated tumors that have penetrated the prostatic capsule to the extent that it is possible to obtain a clear surgical margin (171).

Radical prostatectomy has also been used in combination with hormonal therapy in patients with extraprostatic disease. The concept of preoperative estrogen therapy to permit excision of locally advanced tumors was initially described by Scott (172). With the introduction of luteinizing hormone—releasing hormone (LH-RH) analog and the antiandrogen flutamide, this concept has been revived. Two studies involving a total of 56 patients treated with neoadjuvant hormonal therapy noted "downsizing" but not "downstaging" (173, 174).

Labrie et al. prospectively randomized 161 patients to radical prostatectomy alone or to 3 months of neoadjuvant hormonal therapy before radical prostatectomy (175). Compared with the control group, the incidence of positive margins was less (34% versus 8%) and the rate of organ-confined disease was more (49% versus 78%) in patients receiving neoadjuvant combination therapy. Long-term follow-up is needed to determine the effect on survival.

Among patients with limited lymph nodal metastasis treated by radical prostatectomy and pelvic lymph node dissection, Steinberg et al. reported 5-year and 10-year actuarial survival rates of 97% and 62% (176). Subsequent analysis of progression noted a more favorable outcome for those patients with a Gleason score of 7 or less on needle biopsy (177). Tumor volume in the lymph nodal tissue is an important prognostic factor. Lymphadenectomy among patients with a single metastatic lymph node resulted in a favorable outcome compared with those undergoing lymph node dissection with multiple metastatic lymph nodes (178–180).

At the Mayo Clinic, radical prostatectomy has been used in conjunction with early adjuvant radiation therapy or hormonal therapy. Of 1035 patients with pathologic stage C prostate cancer treated by radical prostatectomy and bilateral pelvic lymphadenectomy, 611 received no immediate adjuvant therapy, 113 received adjuvant radiation therapy, and 103 received only adjuvant orchiectomy (181). Among these three treatment groups, overall survival rates at 5, 10, and 15 years were 91%, 68%, and 46%, respectively; cause-specific survival rates were 96%, 81%, and 66%, respectively. Orchiectomy and radiation therapy demonstrated similar efficacy in controlling local recurrence. The 5-year local recurrence-free survival rate for those patients receiving adjuvant therapy was greater than 95% compared with 84% for those not receiving adjuvant therapy. Adjuvant therapy, however, did not improve the overall or cause-specific survival.

Zincke and colleagues from the Mayo Clinic reported on 370 patients with stage D1 prostate cancer undergoing radical prostatectomy, bilateral pelvic lymph node dissection, and im-

mediate adjuvant hormonal therapy (182). The overall 5-year and 10-year survival rates were 84% and 66%, which were similar to age-matched control subjects. The cause-specific survival rates at these intervals were 89% and 75%. For patients with DNA diploid tumors, overall and cause-specific survival rates were significantly better than those for patients with nondiploid tumors. The cause-specific 10-year survival rate for patients with DNA diploid tumors was 87% compared with 56% for patients with DNA aneuploid tumors.

Salvage radical prostatectomy has been performed in a small number of patients with radiorecurrent tumors (183–186). Surgery after definitive radiation therapy can be technically challenging and is associated with a higher morbidity rate. In the majority of properly selected patients, however, the tumor may be completely removed.

Table 15.4 summarizes the overall survival for men with clinically localized prostate cancer treated by radical prostatectomy (187–195). The studies in this table represent all reported cases with 15-year survival data. The clinical staging accuracy of the total group of patients was 49%. The overall survival (i.e., scoring deaths from all causes) for the total group was 82% at 5 years, 66% at 10 years, and 44% at 15 years. If, however, only the studies that originated in 1950 or later are considered, the overall survival rates at 5, 10, and 15 years were 92%, 74%, and 58%, respectively, which approximates the expected survival of an age-matched control population.

Cause-specific survival has been used to reduce the effects of age, medical condition, and other risk factors. Lepor et al. reexamined Jewett's radical prostatectomy series of 57 patients with clinical B1 prostate cancer; the 5-year, 10-year, 15-year, and 20-year cause-specific survival rates were 95%, 86%, 85%, and 82%, respectively (196). A report from the Mayo Clinic of 472 men who received follow-up care for 10 years after surgery and 166 men who received follow-up care for 15 years demonstrates 10-year and 15-year cause-specific survival rates of 90% and 82% (195).

Despite the therapeutic proven efficacy of radical prostatectomy, morbidity associated with the procedure limits its acceptance and use. The two most feared complications are urinary incontinence and erectile impotency. Before Walsh introduced improvements in the surgical technique, cumulative data from 11 series involving 1877 patients noted total incontinence in 6.1% of the patients, stress incontinence in 9.7%, and maintenance of erectile potency in only 3.9% (190–193, 197–202). Walsh's modifications to surgical technique have reduced the morbidity of radical prostatectomy (203–205). A recent study by Walsh of 600 patients treated by anatomic radical retropubic prostatectomy reports complete urinary control in 92%, complete urinary incontinence in 0%, stress incontinence in 8%, and maintenance of erectile potency in 68% (206). Similar results have been achieved by others (207–209). However, a survey performed by the American College of Surgeons of data from 2122 patients treated by radical prostatectomy in 1990 is more representative of national patterns of care (210). This survey noted urinary control in 81%, complete urinary inconti-

Table 15.4.   Overall Survival For Patients With Clinically Local Prostate Cancer Treated By Radical Prostatectomy[a]

AUTHOR	YEARS OF SURVEY	OVERALL SURVIVAL (%)		
		5-YEAR	10-YEAR	15-YEAR
Berlin et al. (187)	1935–1958	79 (113/143)	52 (63/121)	33 (22/66)
Belt and Schroeder (188)	1928–1970	69 (—)	44 (—)	22 (—)
Culp and Meyer (189)	1950–1972	— (—)	72 (83/115)	54 (50/74)
Veenema et al. (190)[b]	1951–1975	84 (—)	52 (—)	45 (—)
Hodges et al. (191)	1948–1963	80 (156/195)	55 (107/195)	27 (53/195)
Jewett (192)	1909–1951	75 (77/103)	50 (52/103)	35 (37/103)
	1951–1963	85 (49/57)	70 (40/57)	51 (29/57)
Gibbons et al. (193)[c]	1954–1982	94 (92/97)	75 (40/54)	— (—)
Gibbons et al. (194)	1954–1971	— (—)	— (—)	63 (33/52)
Zincke et al. (195)[d]	1966–1991	— (—)	75 (355/472)	60 (100/166)
Total	1909–1991	82 (487/597)	66 (740/1117)	44 (313/713)
Total	1950–1991	92 (141/154)	74 (518)	58 (202/349)
Expected Survival[e]	1970	87 —	70 —	51 —

Adapted from Badalament RA, Drago JR. Disease-a-month: prostate cancer. Chicago: Year Book, 1991;37:199–268. Used with permission.
[a] Numbers occasionally extrapolated from tables or graphic data where percentages were provided.
[b] Belt and Veenema reported on 464 and 159 patients, respectively. However, the authors did not provide information concerning number of patients followed for 5, 10, and 15 years.
[c] 15-year survival data provided in article but not presented in table because subsequent review also included this information.
[d] 26% had adjuvant hormonal therapy or radiotherapy.
[e] Based on Washington State life tables for 61-year-old men from 1969 to 1971.

nence in 4%, stress incontinence in 15%, and maintenance of erectile potency in 28% of patients.

External Beam Irradiation

Radiation therapy can be delivered by external beam irradiation, interstitial implantation, or a combination of the two methods. Although Paschkis and Tittinger first used an intraurethral source to treat prostate cancer in 1910, the modern era of radiation therapy coincides with the development of cobalt 60 radiation sources and the linear accelerator in the 1950s (211). Since that time, radiation therapy has proved to be an effective treatment option for patients with clinically localized prostate cancer. Furthermore, among patients with cancer that extends beyond the prostate but is confined to the bony pelvis (stage C), external beam irradiation provides good local control and, in some cases, has been curative (212, 213). Typically, a dose of 7000 cGy is administered to the prostate and 5000 cGy is delivered to the whole pelvis over 7 weeks.

Salvage external beam irradiation also has been offered as curative therapy in patients with positive surgical margins or rising PSA values after radical prostatectomy (214–219). External beam irradiation has proved to be an excellent form of palliative therapy for hormone-refractory patients with symptomatic osseous metastases. In these patients, 3000 cGy in 10 treatments provides complete relief of pain in 42%, partial relief in 35%, and no relief in 14% (220). Palliative external beam irradiation has proven to be efficacious among hormone-refractory patients with ureteral obstruction, spinal cord compression, and prostatic urethral bleeding (221).

Recently, Bagshaw et al. updated Stanford's experience with definitive external irradiation in 1245 patients with clinically localized prostate cancer (222). The overall survival at 5, 10, and 15 years was 64%, 50%, and 29%, respectively (Fig. 15.7). The median survival time was 10 years versus 15 years for an age-matched cohort. The cause-specific survival rates for 5, 10, and 15 years were 81%, 65%, and 50%, respectively.

Among 409 patients with clinical stage C disease treated by external beam irradiation, Bagshaw et al. reported an overall survival rate of 67% at 5 years, 40% at 10 years, and 20% at 15 years (223). The cause-specific survival rates were 71%, 49%, and 31%, respectively. del Regato et al. treated 372 patients with clinical stage C prostate cancer and noted overall survival rates at 5, 10, 15, and 20 years of 66%, 38%, 18%, and 7%, respectively (224).

Shipley et al. performed a literature review of 2611 men receiving external irradiation for clinically localized prostate cancer (225). This review documented a 0.2% incidence of treatment-related mortality, 1.9% severe complications, 0.9% incontinence, and 33 to 66% maintenance of erectile potency 5 or more years after therapy. The cause of radiation-induced impotence is not fully understood. Goldstein et al. believe that it is secondary to radiation-induced endarteritis of the branches of the internal pudendal and penile arteries (226).

Interstitial Irradiation

Interstitial radiation therapy has also been used for the treatment of organ-confined prostate cancer (227, 228). Candidates for this form of therapy are limited to patients with stage B or nonbulky stage C disease to permit seed placement. Approximately 16,000 to 18,000 cGy are delivered to the prostate over a 12-month period, resulting in a biologically equivalent dose

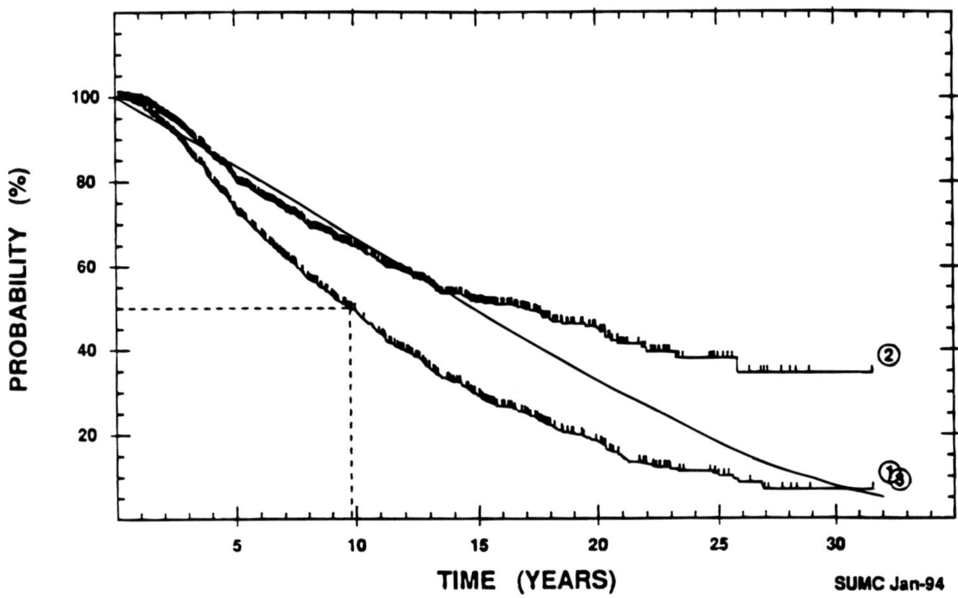

Fig. 15.7. The Stanford University experience with external beam irradiation in 1245 patients with clinically localized prostate cancer treated from October 1956 to December 1992. 1: Overall survival; 2: cause-specific survival; 3: expected survival. The median survival was 10 years. Cause-specific survival at 15 years was 50%. (From Bagshaw MA, Cox RS, Hancock SL. Control of prostate cancer with radiotherapy: long-term results. J Urol 1994;152:1781–1785. Used with permission.)

of 7000 cGy of external beam irradiation. The advantages of interstitial ^{125}I implantation include simultaneous staging of pelvic lymphadenectomy and implantation, a technically easier operation, preservation of potency in 71 to 94% of patients, and maintenance of continence in 97 to 100% of patients (227). Disadvantages include treatment failures from geographic misses, inhomogeneous distribution of seeds, and variability of radiation emitted from each seed.

Recently, Leibel et al. updated the studies at Memorial Sloan-Kettering Cancer Center (229). Among 1078 patients with clinical stage B to C disease, the overall survival rates at 10 and 15 years were 42% and 28%; the 10-year and 15-year disease-free survival rates were 26% and 12%. The most favorable group consisted of 733 patients with negative pelvic lymph node dissections. The 5-year, 10-year, and 15-year overall survival rates were 74%, 60%, and 37%, respectively; disease-free survival rates for node-negative patients were 79%, 57%, and 40%, respectively.

Currently, seed implantation is performed via a percutaneous, transperineal route under ultrasonic and/or fluoroscopic guidance (Fig. 15.8). (230, 231) Although ^{125}I is still commonly used, palladium-103 and iridium-192 are also employed. There are limited data on the efficacy of using palladium-103. Among 75 patients with stage B2 and C disease treated with iridium brachytherapy, the 18-month negative biopsy rate was 75% (232, 233).

Cryotherapy

Destruction of prostate tissue by low temperature was first clinically applied in 1966 by Gonder et al., who used a transure-

thral probe (234). Serious complications arising from an inability to monitor the freezing prevented the widespread use of the procedure. In 1993, Onik et al. revived this procedure by combining three techniques—high-resolution TRUS, percutaneous interventional radiology, and advanced cryotechnology (235).

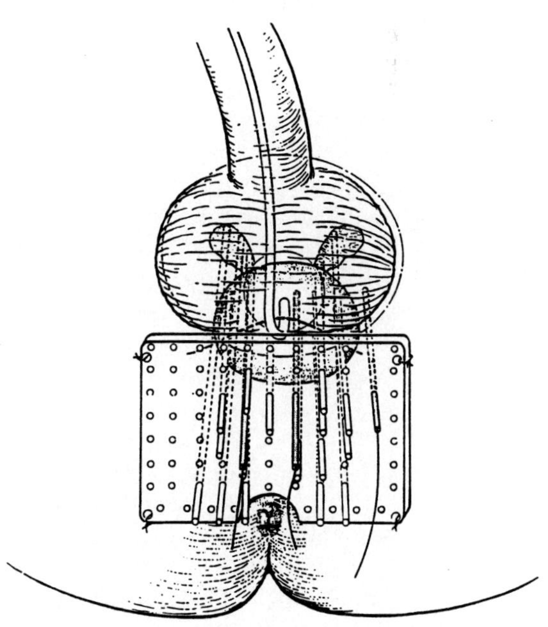

Fig. 15.8. Template-guided transperineal interstitial implantation of the prostate. (From Bagshaw MA, Kaplan ID, Cox RC. Radiation therapy for localized disease. Cancer 1993;71(Suppl):939–952. Used with permission.)

In 1994, Lee et al. reported a tailored approach to cryoablation in men with clinical stage B and C prostate tumors (Figs. 15.9 and 15.10) (236). This approach included preoperative total androgen ablation and cancer mapping based on ultrasound-guided staging biopsies. The entire prostate, and significant portions of periprostatic tissue, are frozen with five cryoprobes, each cryoprobe generating overlapping 2-cm radius ice balls. Killing temperature (less than 20°C) is monitored by properly positioned thermocouples. Patients receive two freeze and thaw cycles. A specially designed urethral warming catheter protects the urethra from freezing and subsequent sloughing. This urethral protection, however, preserves some of the periurethral tissue and thus PSA levels are often measurable after cryoablation. Patients maintain 10F size suprapubic catheters for 1 to 3 weeks or until they are able to void per urethra. This procedure is performed under general or spinal anesthesia; patients are discharged within 23 hours.

In 1995, Bahn et al. reported on 210 patients treated with cryoablation of the prostate (237). The 3-month and 6-month follow-up data were available for 130 men, and 12-month data were available for 43 patients. Positive biopsy at 3, 6, and 12 months occurred in 7.7%, 3.3%, and 2.3% of patients, respectively. Stage C patients had higher failure rates than stage B patients (21% versus 3.7%). Gleason score was related to the positive biopsy rate (5.2% among men with Gleason 4 to 6 tumors, 12% in Gleason 7 tumors, and 28.6% in Gleason 8 and 9 tumors). The mean PSA decreased from 12.6 ng/mL preoperatively to 0.35 ng/mL at 3 months, 0.54 ng/mL at 6

months, and 0.43 ng/mL at 12 months. At 3 months, a level of 1.0 ng/mL yielded a sensitivity of 70% and specificity of 88% for subsequent positive biopsy findings.

Complications were minimal; most occurred early in the study. There were no deaths, total incontinence in 2.3% (all previously irradiated), stress incontinence in 6.2%, prolonged urinary outlet obstruction in 2.9%, urethrorectal fistulas in 2.4%, pelvic pain in 1.5%, and maintenance of potency in 41%. The majority of complications occurred in previously irradiated patients, which comprised 21% of the total group. Treatment success, however, did not significantly differ between irradiated and nonirradiated patients.

Predicting and Monitoring Results of Therapy

The most sensitive indicator of tumor persistence after radical prostatectomy is a detectable PSA, which can antedate other clinical indicators of treatment failure by years (238–243). After radical prostatectomy, a detectable PSA indicates local recurrence, which could benefit from pelvic irradiation, or distant metastases requiring hormonal therapy. McCarthy et al. note that those patients most likely to benefit from pelvis irradiation at relapse initially have undetectable levels of PSA (218). Although a detectable PSA can equate persistence of tumor, Trapasso et al. point out that "the interval to clinical failure may not ultimately be clinically significant" (244).

Radioimmunoscintigraphy with [111]indium-labeled monoclonal antibody CYT-356 can identify occult extraprostatic

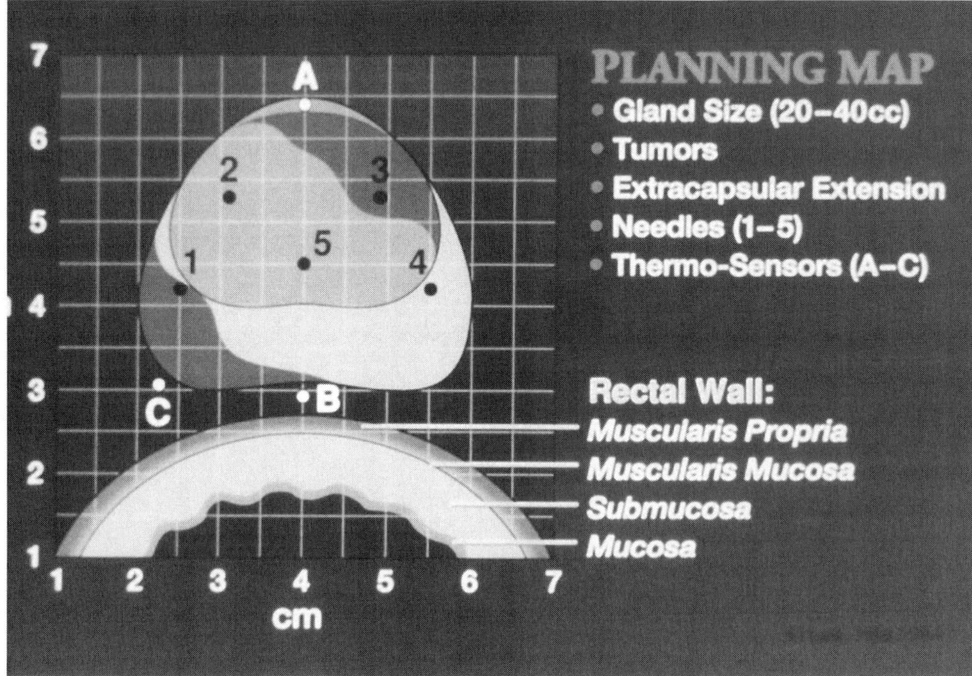

Fig. 15.9.   Planning map for cryoablation (transverse view). The shaded areas represent outer and inner gland cancers. Thermosensor A is placed in the anterior fibromuscular stroma, and other sensors (B and C) are placed adjacent to the prostatic capsule. Cryoprobes 1 and 4 are always placed so that distance y exceeds distance x. This ensures lateral extension of the ice ball for treatment of neurovascular bundle involvement without causing rectal damage. An additional probe (6) may be used when gland volume is greater than 40 mL and when extracapsular extension of the cancer is extensive.

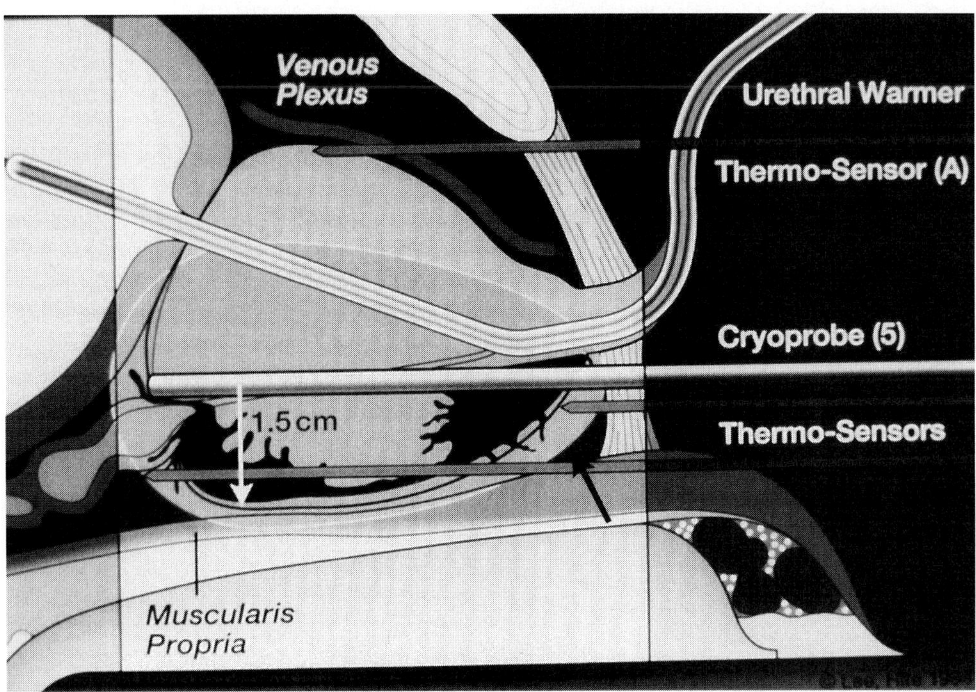

Fig. 15.10.   Midline longitudinal view of prostate with cryoprobe 5 in place (Fig. 15.9 shows transverse view). The ice ball is white. The probe is placed in the correct position for the first freeze, at least 1.5 cm from the muscularis propria (white arrow) (black arrow denotes inferior extent of ice ball with the first freeze). This is inadequate to cover the prostatic fossa (*). For the second (apical) freeze, the probe should be pulled back approximately 1 cm to treat the prostatic fossa. Thermosensor locations are for control of anterior, posterior, and apical freezes. (From Bagshaw MA, Cox RS, Hancock SL. Control of prostate cancer with radiotherapy: long-term results. J Urol 1994;152:1781–1785. Used with permission.)

fossa metastatic sites. Kahn et al. studied 27 patients with a PSA of 0.8 ng/mL or greater following radical prostatectomy; 15 had extraprostatic areas of increased radionuclide uptake identified by radioimmunoscintigraphy (245). Although biopsies were not performed on these sites to confirm metastases, these exciting preliminary data demonstrate the potential of this technique.

The role of PSA in monitoring recurrence after radiation therapy has been enhanced by Zagars (246). Among 260 patients with clinically localized prostate cancer, a nadir PSA value was typically achieved at 6 to 12 months after therapy. This value proved an important prognostic tool. Nadir values less than 1 ng/mL had only a 12% relapse rate at 5 years. Nearly two thirds of patients with nadir values of 4 ng/mL or greater had relapses at 2 years. Those patients with PSA values greater than 30 ng/mL did extremely poorly. Other researchers noted similar results (247–249).

Recently, Lee et al. used PSA as a measure of recurrence among 500 men with localized prostate cancer treated with external beam irradiation (250). Among men receiving follow-up care for more than 1 year after radiation therapy, serially increasing PSA or a PSA value of greater than 1.5 ng/mL was considered indicative of recurrence. The 5-year overall survival rate was 80%, the survival without clinical evidence of disease excluding PSA (cNED) was 72%, and the survival without clinical evidence of disease including PSA (bNED) was 51%. Additionally, these investigators noted that a pretreatment PSA

was the most important predictive factor. A pretreatment PSA of less than 15 ng/mL was associated with a 3-year bNED rate of 86%, whereas a pretreatment PSA of greater than 15ng/mL was associated with a 3-year bNED rate of 38%.

The significance of postirradiation biopsy results has been controversial (251–253). Histologic differentiation of persistent carcinoma from radiation-induced atypia is the major concern. Two studies have 10-year disease-free survival data for patients who underwent postirradiation biopsies. The 10-year disease-free survival rate for patients with negative biopsy results was 62 to 82%; for those with positive biopsy results, it was 12 to 19%. Thus, it appears that a positive postirradiation biopsy result is a powerful indicator of treatment failure.

TREATMENT OPTIONS: METASTATIC DISEASE

Hormonal Therapy

More than half a century after the concept of hormonal treatment for prostate cancer was introduced by Huggins and Hodges, androgen deprivation remains the mainstay of therapy for patients with metastatic prostate cancer (254). Prostatic neoplasms are heterogenous tumors consisting of hormone-dependent, hormone-sensitive, and hormone-independent cell populations (255). Hormone-dependent cells die when deprived of androgens. Hormone-sensitive cells grow when stim-

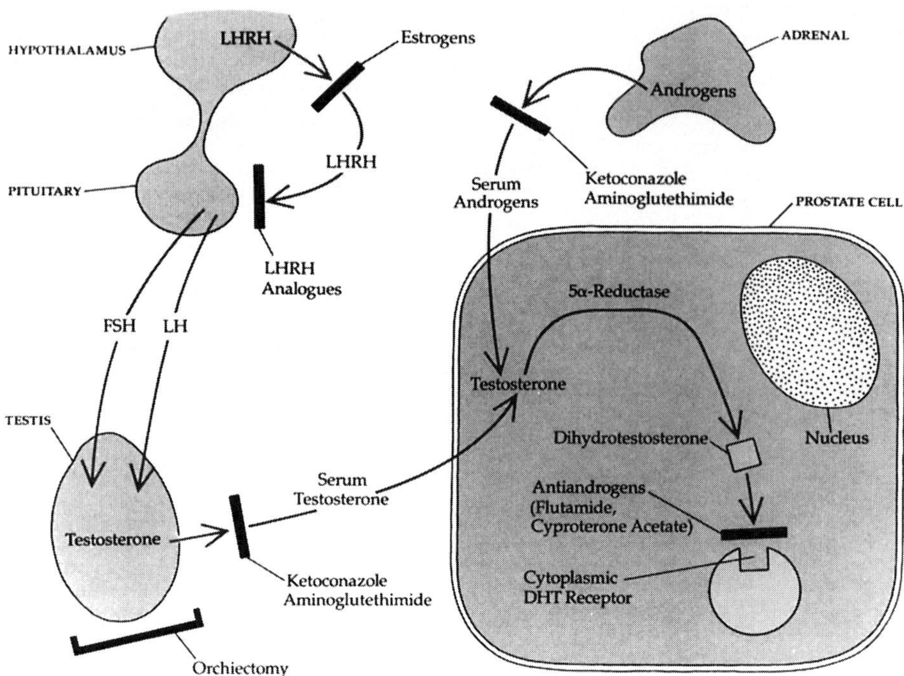

Fig. 15.11. Hypothalamic-pituitary regulation of testosterone and adrenal androgen synthesis. Sites of interruption of androgens synthesis producing androgen a deprivation are illustrated. (From Garnick MB: Urologic cancer. In: Rubenstein R, Federman DD, eds. Scientific American Medicine: selections for urologists. New York: Scientific American, 1992. Used with permission.)

ulated by androgens, but when androgens are absent, these cells enter the resting phase of the cell cycle. Hormone-independent cells grow despite androgen deprivation. The relative proportion of these three cell types determines the patient's response to androgen deprivation. Immediately after androgen deprivation, about 40% of patients exhibit objective tumor regression, 40% show disease stabilization, and 20% have tumor progression. Eventually, hormone-independent cells repopulate the tumor, and hormone-sensitive cells leave the resting phase of the cell cycle and proliferate in response to lower androgen levels than originally required. After initiation of hormonal therapy in patients with symptomatic metastatic disease, 10% die within 6 months, 50% survive 3 years, and 10% survive 10 years or longer (256).

The hypothalamus, pituitary, adrenal glands, and testis form an axis that controls androgen production (Fig. 15.11). (257, 258). The hypothalamus secretes gonadotropin-releasing hormone (GnRH) and corticotropin-releasing hormone (CRH) into the hypothalamic–pituitary venous portal system. These releasing hormones stimulate the anterior pituitary to secrete luteinizing hormone (LH) and adrenocorticotropic hormone (ACTH). LH stimulates Leydig cells in the testis to produce testosterone. ACTH stimulates adrenocortical conversion of cholesterol to androstenedione and dihydroepiandrostenedione, which are eventually metabolized to testosterone. Inhibition of testosterone secretion occurs via negative feedback on the hypothalamus, resulting in direct suppression of LH-RH and CRH and resulting in decreased secretion of LH and ACTH.

Additionally, hydrocortisone may directly inhibit adrenal androgen production at the pituitary level. In men, 90% of the testosterone is produced by the testes and the remaining 10% by the adrenal gland. About 97% of circulating testosterone is bound to plasma proteins. The remaining 3% of testosterone is unbound and available to diffuse passively into the prostate. Intracellular testosterone is converted by the enzyme alpha 5 reductase into DHT, which, in turn, binds to receptors in the nuclei, stimulating normal and neoplastic prostate cellular growth.

Orchiectomy

The goal of hormonal therapy is to interrupt the stimulation of prostatic growth by DHT. Orchiectomy is the simplest, most reliable, and most cost-efficient method (259, 260). Alternative forms of hormonal monotherapy such as estrogens (261, 262), progestational agents (262, 263), antiandrogens (264–269), and LH-RH agonists (270–273) appear to have no therapeutic advantage over orchiectomy. Castration produces a rapid symptomatic response, assures patient compliance, and is not associated with cardiovascular toxicity. Adverse effects include psychologic trauma, impotency, hot flashes, gynecomastia, and nipple tenderness.

Estrogens

The most commonly used estrogen is diethylstilbestrol (DES), although premarin and ethinyl estradiol are equally effective.

Estrogens decrease testosterone levels primarily by suppressing LH-RH release from the hypothalamus and secondarily by decreasing free testosterone by enhancing serum testosterone protein binding (274). A Veterans Administration Cooperative Research Group study using 5-mg daily dose of DES showed excessive cardiovascular and thromboembolic complications (275). Although a 3-mg daily dose of DES reliably lowered testosterone to castrate levels, cardiovascular risks were still considerable (270, 276). A 1-mg daily dose of DES did not consistently lower serum testosterone to castrate levels (277). Additional adverse reactions to administration were noted, including impotency, hot flashes, gynecomastia, nipple tenderness, and gastrointestinal disturbances. Prophylactic anticoagulation is an attractive treatment adjunct but is of unproven efficacy.

LH-RH Analogs

LH-RH analogs (leuprolide, goserelin) produce a transitory elevation in testosterone for approximately 1 or 2 weeks. Longterm administration of LH-RH analogs results in a reduction in the number of LH-RH receptors in the pituitary. This causes a decline in serum testosterone to castrate levels within 1 month. LH-RH analogs are as effective as orchiectomy or estrogen therapy (270, 278–280). The initial testosterone flare can produce temporary worsening of symptoms such as bone pain or obstructive voiding symptoms. In patients with neurologic complaints, acute spinal cord compression can ensue. Pretreatment with 2 weeks of flutamide has been shown to block the testosterone flare (281). Hot flashes and impotency are the most common adverse effects noted. LH-RH analogs produce less painful gynecomastia, gastrointestinal disturbances, edema, and thromboembolic and cardiovascular side effects than estrogens. LH-RH analogs are expensive and require monthly injections. Clinical trials of a 3-month sustained-release preparation are ongoing (282).

Antiandrogens

Antiandrogens, such as flutamide, bind to intracellular androgen receptors, thereby blocking the cellular effects of circulating testosterone and DHT (283, 284). Flutamide has been approved for clinical use in the United States in combination with leuprolide acetate. Several studies have demonstrated that when used as monotherapy in previously untreated stage D2 patients, flutamide is an effective treatment option (285–287). Furthermore, because serum androgen levels remain high, many men remain potent. The activity of flutamide, however, is greatly decreased in patients who have had relapses after conventional endocrine therapy. Flutamide may cause diarrhea and other gastrointestinal disturbances, gynecomastia, hot flashes, and hepatotoxicity, but has not been shown to be associated with cardiovascular or thromboembolic side effects (284–288).

Ketoconazole

Ketoconazole was developed as a broad-spectrum antifungal agent. Ketoconazole inhibits testicular and adrenal cytochrome P-450 dependent enzymes (289). In clinical practice it is primarily used for the acutely ill patient; castrate levels are achieved within 24 hours of a 400-mg oral dose administered every 8 hours (290). Like flutamide, ketoconazole is unlikely to produce a significant effect in patients who have had relapses after conventional hormonal therapy (291–294). Ketoconazole is associated with nausea, which may occur in up to 20% of patients and has a 1 in 8000 to 16,000 incidence of severe but reversible hepatotoxicity.

Timing of Hormonal Therapy

The proper timing for initiation of endocrine therapy remains undefined (295–298). Few physicians, if any, would dispute starting hormonal therapy in patients with debilitating symptoms from metastatic disease. In the absence of direct evidence that early hormonal therapy prolongs survival in asymptomatic patients; however, some clinicians can be reluctant to initiate hormonal therapy. Proponents of early hormonal therapy argue the following points.

1. Survival of patients with metastatic disease in the postendocrine era appears to be longer than survival in the pre-endocrine era.
2. Patients with stage C and D1 disease treated with immediate hormonal therapy live longer than those treated with delayed therapy.
3. Experimental studies using rat prostate cancer models support early androgen deprivation.
4. Reanalysis of the Veterans Administration Cooperative Research Group study showed that younger stage D patients with a Gleason score of 7 to 10 derived a survival benefit.
5. Preliminary data from a study comparing leuprolide and flutamide versus leuprolide alone suggest a survival advantage for those patients with minimal metastatic disease receiving treatment.

Those favoring delayed treatment point out the following.

1. The initiation of hormonal therapy in the asymptomatic, sexually active patient may severely alter his quality of life.
2. The adverse reactions associated with hormonal therapy may not be trivial.
3. Theoretically, altering the hormonal milieu may disrupt the clonal stability of a tumor, leading to accelerated tumor cell proliferation.

Although early initiation of hormonal therapy in asymptomatic men appears to be an attractive option, its efficacy remains unproven.

Total Androgen Ablation

The concept of total androgen ablation involves combination hormonal therapy for simultaneous suppression of testicular and adrenal androgen production. This therapeutic approach was popularized by Labrie et al., who showed prolonged survival in patients treated with total androgen ablation (299–301). A double-blind, randomized, multicenter trial involving 603 men with distant metastatic prostate cancer provided further support for this therapeutic option. Patients were given leuprolide and placebo or leuprolide and flutamide. Median survival time for the combination group was 35.6 months compared with 28.3 months for the leuprolide and placebo group; this difference in survival was statistically significant (302). The authors suggest that a subset of patients with minimal metastatic disease may respond more favorably to total androgen ablation.

Many studies, however, did not demonstrate a survival advantage from total androgen ablation (303–307). Denis et al. presented preliminary results from a meta-analysis of 5425 men with metastatic prostate cancer, half of whom were treated by conventional monotherapy and half by total androgen ablation (303). The 5-year survival rates, 16.7% for the conventional monotherapy group and 19.7% for the total androgen ablation group, were not significantly different.

Flutamide Withdrawal Syndrome

Several studies examined the effect of flutamide withdrawal in stage D_2 prostate cancer patients who had progression of disease after an initial positive response to combination therapy with the antiandrogen and LH-RH analogs (308–311). Scher and Kelly noted a significant decrease in PSA values in 10 of 25 patients and clinical improvement in a subset of patients (308). The median duration of response was about 5 months. One complete response, 3 partial responses, 26 stable responses, and 10 nonresponses were documented among 40 patients treated with flutamide withdrawal by Dupont et al. (309). Of the 30 responders, the average duration of response after flutamide withdrawal was 440 days. Other studies have documented similar findings.

The mechanism of this response is unknown. It is hypothesized that some tumor subclones become hypersensitive to androgens or a mutated androgen receptor. Conducting a trial of flutamide withdrawal should be considered with patients whose disease is progressing on total androgen ablation before more toxic treatment options are initiated.

Strontium-89

Strontium-89 is a pure beta emitter with a biologic half-life of 14 days in normal bone and 50 days in bony metastases (312). It can be injected intravenously and, following the same biochemical pathways as calcium, is incorporated into the osteoclast/osteoblast reaction around bony metastases. Ninety percent of strontium is renally excreted within 1 week. Porter and members of the TransCanada Strontium-89 Study randomized 126 patients to local field radiation therapy and either 10.8 mCi of strontium-89 or placebo (313). Compared with the patients receiving placebo, those treated with strontium-89 had a significantly favorable response in terms of consumption of analgesics, number of new painful sites, PSA levels, alkaline phosphatase levels, acid phosphatase levels, alleviation of pain, physical activity performance level, and quality of life responses to questionnaires. The most common adverse reaction was thrombocytopenia, which occurred in 70 to 80% of patients; nadir platelet counts occurred 4 to 8 weeks after injection. In about 60% of patients, a transient increase in bone pain occurred within a few days of injection. This pain flare usually responded well to a short course of steroids.

Chemotherapy

Chemotherapy can be considered after failure of hormonal therapy. First-line hormonal therapy should be continued to prevent normalization of serum testosterone levels and subsequent tumor stimulation. In general, the results of cytotoxic chemotherapy are disappointing (314–317). Eisenberger summarized the results of single-agent phase II trials in hormone-resistant prostate cancer (316). Among a total of 1162 evaluable patients, 86 (7.5%) had an objective response (complete or partial response). Commonly used single agents include cyclophosphamide (318), 5-fluorouracil (319, 320), doxorubicin (321, 322), estramustine phosphate (323, 324), methotrexate (325), and cisplatin (325, 326). Results from multiple drug regimens failed to demonstrate significant superiority over single agents in controlled phase III clinical trials (315–317, 327). Single and multiple drug regimens have not significantly prolonged survival compared with patients treated with standard palliative measures.

The combination of estramustine phosphate and vinblastine has been shown to have activity in hormone-refractory prostate cancer patients (328, 329). Both agents are microtubule inhibitors that appear to be synergistic. Among 36 hormone-refractory patients, 22 patients (61%) had a PSA decrease of at least 50% and 8 patients (23%) had a PSA decrease of at least 75%.

It is evident from the poor response of traditional chemotherapeutic regimens in patients with hormone-refractory prostate cancer that new drugs are needed. Current studies are investigating agents such as suramin (330–332), gallium nitrate (333), taxol (334), R.75251 (Liarozole) (335), interferon alfa (336, 337), and ^{90}Y-CYT-356 monoclonal antibody (338). Of these agents, suramin has been studied most intensely. Nine studies summarized by Scher and Kelly show an objective response (complete or partial) in 24% of patients and a decrease in PSA of at least 50% in 47% of patients (330). Because suramin inhibits PSA release and concomitantly administered hydrocortisone can lower PSA levels, and because many patients discontinued flutamide (possibly resulting in a flutamide withdrawal response), further studies are needed to determine the true clinical efficacy.

Quality of life, cost, and toxicity are important issues that need to be discussed with each patient before the initiation of chemotherapy. Because chemotherapy offers no survival benefit, potentially toxic regimens should be administered only to patients participating in clinical trials. The realistic goal of therapy for the individual patient with hormone-resistant prostate cancer is pain amelioration. A trial of a single agent with a low toxicity profile or the combination of estramustine phosphate and vinblastine appears to be a reasonable therapy to meet this goal.

REFERENCES

1. Wingo PA, Tong T, Bolden S. Cancer statistics. CA Cancer J Clin 1995;45:8.
2. Gann PH, Hennekens CH, Stampfer M. A prospective evaluation of plasma prostate-specific antigen for detection of prostate cancer. JAMA 1995;273:289.
3. Carter BS, Carter HB, Isaacs JT. Epidemiologic evidence regarding predisposing factors to prostate cancer. Prostate 1990;16:187.
4. Murphy GP, Natarajan N, Pontes JE, et al. The national survey of prostate cancer in the United States by the American College of Surgeons. J Urol 1982;127:928.
5. Feldman AR, Kessler L, Myers MH, et al. The prevalence of cancer: estimates based on the Connecticut Tumor Registry. N Engl J Med 1986;315:1394.
6. Satariano WAM, Swanson GM. Racial differences in cancer incidence: the significance of age-specific patterns. Cancer 1988;62:2640.
7. Petersen RO. Prostate and seminal vesicles. In: Petersen RO, ed. Urologic pathology. 2nd ed. Philadelphia: JB Lippincott, 1992:603.
8. Sakr WA, Haas GP, Cassin BF, et al. The frequency of carcinoma and intraepithelial neoplasia of the prostate in young male patients. J Urol 1993;150:379.
9. Woolf C. An investigation of the familial aspects of carcinoma of the prostate. Cancer 1960;13:738.
10. Cannon L, Bishop DT, Skolnick M, et al. Genetic epidemiology of cancer in Utah genealogies: a prelude to the molecular genetics of common cancers. J Cell Physiol Suppl 1984;3:63.
11. Spitz MR, Currier RD, Fueger JJ, et al. Familial patterns of prostate cancer: a case control analysis. J Urol 1991;146:1305.
12. Steinberg GS, Carter BS, Beaty TH, et al. Family history and the risk of prostate cancer. Prostate 1990;17:337.
13. Carter BS, Bova GS, Beaty TH, et al. Hereditary prostate cancer: epidemiologic and clinical features. (Review). J Urol 1993;150:797.
14. Paganini-Hill A, Ross RK, Henderson BE. Epidemiology of prostatic cancer. In: Skinner DG, Lieskovsky G, eds. Diagnosis and management of genitourinary cancer. Philadelphia: WB Saunders, 1988:40.
15. Haenszel W, Kurihara M. Studies of Japanese migrants: part I. mortality from cancer and other disease among Japanese in the United States. J Natl Cancer Inst 1968;40:43.
16. Baquet CR, Horm JW, Gibbs T, et al. Socioeconomic factors and cancer incidence among blacks and whites. J Natl Cancer Inst 1991;83:551.
17. Badalament RA, O'Toole RV, Young DC, et al. DNA ploidy and prostate specific antigen as prognostic factors in clinically resectable prostate cancer. Cancer 1991;67:3014.
18. Jackson MA, Kovi J, Heshmat MY, et al. Factors involved in the high incidence of prostatic carcinoma among American blacks. Prog Clin Biol Res 1981;53:111.
19. Blair A, Fraumeni JF Jr. Geographic patterns of prostate cancer in the United States. J Natl Cancer Inst 1978;61:1379.
20. Decoufle P, Stanislawczyk K, Houten L. A retrospective survey of cancer in relation to occupation: NIOSH Research Report. DHEW (NIOSH) publication no. 77-178/G. US Department of Health, Education and Welfare, 1977:77.
21. Ernster VL, Selvin S, Brown SM. Occupation and prostate cancer. J Occup Med 1979;21:175.
22. Lloyd JW, Lundin FE Jr, Redmond CK, et al. Long-term mortality study of steelworkers: part IV. mortality by work area. J Occup Med 1970;12:151.
23. Schuman LM, Mandel JS. Epidemiology of prostatic cancer in blacks. Prev Med 1980;9:630.
24. Checkoway H, DiFerdinando G, Hulka BS, et al. Medical life-style and occupational risk factors for prostate cancer. Prostate 1987;10:79.
25. Kipling MD, Waterhouse JAH. Cadmium and prostatic carcinoma. Lancet 1967;1:730.
26. Kolonel L, Winkelstein W Jr. Cadmium and prostatic carcinoma. Lancet 1977;2:566.
27. Armstrong BG, Kazantzis G. Prostatic cancer and chronic respiratory and renal disease in British cadmium workers: a case control study. Br J Ind Med 1985;42:540.
28. Elghany NA, Schumacher MC, Slattery ML, et al. Occupation, cadmium exposure, and prostate cancer. Epidemiology 1990;1:107.
29. Schuman LM, Mandel J, Blackard C, et al. Epidemiology study of prostatic cancer: preliminary report. Cancer Treat Rep 1977;61:181.
30. Slattery ML, Schumacher MC, West DW, et al. Food consumption trends between adolescent and adult years and subsequent risk of prostate cancer. Am J Clin Nutr 1990;52:752.
31. Mills PK, Beeson WL, Phillips RL, et al. Cohort study of diet, lifestyle, and prostate cancer in Adventist men. Cancer 1989;64:598.
32. Giovannucci E, Rimm EB, Colditz GA, et al. A prospective study of dietary fat and the risk of prostate cancer. J Natl Cancer Inst 1993;85:1571.
33. Pienta KJ, Esper PS. Risk factors for prostate cancer. Ann Intern Med 1993;118:793.
34. Feminella JG, Latimer JK. An apparent increase in genital carcinomas among wives of men with prostatic carcinomas: an epidemiologic survey. Pirquet Bull Clin Med 1974;20:3.
35. Sanford EJ, Geder L, Laychock A, et al. Evidence for the association of cytomegalovirus with carcinoma of the prostate. J Urol 1977;118:789.
36. Centifano YM, Kaufman HE, Zam ZS, et al. Herpesvirus particles in prostate carcinoma cells. J Virol 1973;12:1608.
37. Ohtsuki Y, Seman G, Dmochowski L, et al. Brief

communication: virus-like particles in a case of human prostate carcinoma. J Natl Cancer Inst 1977;58:1493.

38. McCombs RM. Role of oncornaviruses in carcinoma of the prostate. Cancer Treat Rep 1977;61:131.

39. Ross RK, Bernstein L, Lobo RA, et al. 5-alpha-reductase activity and risk of prostate cancer among Japanese and U.S. white and black males. Lancet 1992;339:887.

40. Ross JK, Pusateri DL, Schultz TD. Dietary and hormonal evaluation of men at different risks for prostate cancer: fiber intake, excretion, and composition, with in vitro evidence of an association between steroid hormones and specific fiber components. Am J Clin Nutr 1990;51:365.

41. Sanford EJ, Rhoner TJ, Rapp F. Virology of prostate cancer. Cancer Chemother Rep 1975;59:33.

42. Sanford EJ, Dagen JE, Geder L, et al. Lymphocyte reactivity against virally transformed cells in patients with urologic carcinoma. J Urol 1977;118:809.

43. Geder L, Sanford EJ, Rohner TJ, et al. Cytomegalovirus and cancer of the prostate: in vitro transformation of human cells. Cancer Treat Rep 1977;61:139.

44. Noble KL. The development of prostate adenocarcinoma in the Nb rat following prolonged sex hormone administration. Cancer Res 1977;37:1929.

45. Kreig M, Bartsch W, Voigt KD. Binding, metabolism and tissue level of androgens in human prostatic carcinoma, benign prostatic hyperplasia and normal prostate. Excerpta Med ICS 1980;494:102.

46. Geller J, Albert J, de la Vega Loza D, et al. Dihydrotestosterone concentration in prostate cancer tissue as a predictor of tumor differentiation and hormonal dependency. Cancer Res 1978;38:4349.

47. Habib FK, Lee IR, Stitch SR, et al. Androgen levels in the plasma and prostate tissue of patients with benign hypertrophy and carcinoma of the prostate. J Endocrinol 1976;71:99.

48. Hammond GL. Endogenous steroid levels in human prostate from birth to old age: a comparison of normal and diseased tissues. J Endocrinol 1978;78:7.

49. Ghanadian R, Puah CM, O'Donoghue EPN. Serum testosterone and dihydrotestosterone in carcinoma of the prostate. Br J Cancer 1979;39:696.

50. Bartsch W, Steins P, Becker H. Hormone blood levels in patients with prostatic carcinoma and their relation to the type of carcinoma growth differentiation. Eur Urol 1977;3:47.

51. Saroff J, Kirdani Y, Ming Chu T. Measurements of prolactin and androgens in patients with prostatic diseases. Oncology 1980;37:46.

52. Harper ME, Peeling WB, Cowley T. Plasma steroid and protein hormone concentrations in patients with prostatic carcinoma, before and after oestrogen therapy. Acta Endocrinol 1976;81:409.

53. Griffiths K, Peeling WB, Groom GU. Protein hormones and prostate cancer. Prog Cancer Res Ther 1980;144:185.

54. Rolandi E, Pescatore D, Milesi GM, et al. Evaluation of LH, FSH, TSH, Prl and GH secretion in patients suffering from prostatic neoplasms. Acta Endocrinol 1980;95:23.

55. Hammond GL, Kontturi M, Maattala P, et al. Serum FSH, LH and prolactin in normal males and patients with prostatic diseases. Clin Endocrinol 1977;7:129.

56. Jacobi GH, Rathgen GH, Altwein JE. Serum prolactin and tumors of the prostate: unchanged basal levels and lack of correlation to serum testosterone. J Endocrinol Invest 1980;3:15.

57. Greenwald P, Kirmss V, Polan AK, et al. Cancer of the prostate among men with benign prostatic hyperplasia. J Natl Cancer Inst 1974;53:335.

58. Armenian HK, Lilienfeld AM, Diamond EL, et al. Relation between benign prostatic hyperplasia and cancer of the prostate. A prospective and retrospective study. Lancet 1974;2:115.

59. Franks LM. Latent carcinoma of the prostate. J Clin Pathol 1954;68:603.

60. Guess HA, Jacobsen SJ, Oesterling JE. Seeking a link between vasectomy and prostate cancer. Contemp Urol 1994;6:52.

61. Rosenberg L, Palmer JR, Zauber AG, et al. Vasectomy and the risk of prostate cancer. Am J Epidemiol 1990;132:1051.

62. Mettlin C, Natarajan N, Huben R. Vasectomy and prostate cancer risk. Am J Epidemiol 1990;132:1056.

63. Newell GR, Fueger JJ, Spitz MR, et al. A case-control study of prostate cancer. Am J Epidemiol 1989;130:395.

64. Spitz MR, Fueger JJ, Babaian RJ, et al. Vasectomy and the risk of prostate cancer. Am J Epidemiol 1991;134:108. Letter.

65. Honda GD, Bernstein L, Ross RK, et al. Vasectomy, cigarette smoking, and age at first sexual intercourse as risk factors for prostate cancer in middle-aged men. Br J Cancer 1988;57:326.

66. Ross RK, Paganini-Hill A, Henderson BE. The etiology of prostate cancer: what does the epidemiology suggest? Prostate 1983;4:333.

67. Hayes RB, Pottern LM, Greenberg R, et al. Vasectomy and prostate cancer in US blacks and whites. Am J Epidemiol 1993;137:263.

68. Sidney S. Vasectomy and the risk of prostatic cancer and benign prostatic hypertrophy. J Urol 1987;138:795.

69. Sidney S, Quesenberry CP Jr, Sadler MC, et al. Vasectomy and the risk of prostate cancer in a cohort of multiphasic health-checkup examinees: second report. Cancer Causes Control 1991;2:113.

70. Giovannucci E, Tosteson TD, Speizer FE, et al. A retrospective cohort study of vasectomy and prostate cancer in US men. JAMA 1993;269:878.

71. Giovannucci E, Ashcerio A, Rimm EB, et al. A prospective cohort study of vasectomy and prostate cancer in US men. JAMA 1993;269:873.

72. Lowsley OS. The development of the human prostate gland with reference to the development of other structures at the neck of the bladder. Am J Anat 1912;13:299.

73. Franks LM. Benign nodular hyperplasia of the prostate: a review. Ann Roy Coll Surg 1954;14:92.

74. McNeal JE. The prostate gland: morphology and pathobiology. Monogr Urol 1988;9:36.

75. Bostwick DG, Brawer MK. Prostatic intra-epithelial neoplasia and early invasion of prostate cancer. Cancer 1987;59:788.

76. Brawer MK. Prostatic intraepithelial neoplasia: a premalignant lesion. Hum Pathol 1992;23:242.

77. Gleason DF. Atypical hyperplasia, benign hyperplasia, and

well-differentiated adenocarcinoma of the prostate. Am J Surg Pathol 1985;9(Suppl):53.

78. McNeal JE, Bostwick DG. Intraductal dysplasia: a premalignant lesion of the prostate. Hum Pathol 1986;17:64.

79. McNeal JE. Significance of duct-acinar dysplasia in prostatic carcinogenesis. Prostate 1988;13:91.

80. Troncoso P, Babaian RJ, Ro JY, et al. Prostatic intraepithelia neoplasia and invasive prostatic adenocarcinoma in cystoprostatectomy specimens. Urology 1989;34(Suppl):52.

81. McNeal JE, Villers A, Redwine EA, et al. Microcarcinoma in the prostate: its association with duct-acinar dysplasia. Hum Pathol 1991;22:644.

82. Weinstein MH, Epstein JI. Significance of high-grade prostatic intraepithelial neoplasia on needle biopsy. Hum Pathol 1993;24:624.

83. Gleason DF. Classification of prostatic carcinomas. Cancer Chemother Rep 1966;50:125.

84. Nowell PC. The clonal evolution of tumor cell populations. Science 1976;194:23.

85. McNeal JE, Bostwick DG, Kindrachuk RA, et al. Patterns of progression in prostate cancer. Lancet 1986;1:60.

86. Carter HB, Isaacs JT. Why do cells metastasize? World J Urol 1990;8:2.

87. Carter HB, Morrell CH, Pearson JD, et al. Estimation of prostatic growth using serial prostatic specific antigen measurements in men with and without prostate disease. Cancer Res 1992;52:3323.

88. Barzell W, Bean MA, Hilaris BS, et al. Prostatic adenocarcinoma: relationship of grade and local extent to the pattern of metastases. J Urol 1977;118:278.

89. McLaughlin AP, Saltzstein SL, McCullough DL, et al. Prostatic carcinoma: incidence and location of unsuspected lymphatic metastases. J Urol 1976;115:89.

90. Dodds PR, Caride VJ, Lytton B. The role of vertebral veins in the dissemination of prostatic carcinoma. J Urol 1981;126:753.

91. Feiner HD, Gonzales R. Carcinoma of the prostate with atypical immunohistologic features: clinical and histologic correlates. Am J Surg Pathol 1991;10:765.

92. Allhoff EP, Proppe KH, Chapman CM, et al. Evaluation of prostate specific acid phosphatase and prostate specific antigen in identification of prostatic cancer. J Urol 1983;129:315.

93. Richie JP, Catalona WJ, Ahmann FR, et al. Effect of patient age on early detection of prostate cancer with serum prostate-specific antigen and digital rectal examination. Urology 1993;42:365.

94. Catalona WJ, Smith DS, Ratliff TL, et al. Detection of organ-confined prostate cancer is increased through prostate-specific antigen-based screening. JAMA 1993;270:948.

95. Mettlin C, Murphy GP, Lee F, et al. Characteristics of prostate cancers detected in a multimodality early detection program. Cancer 1993;72:1701.

96. Cooner WH, Mosley BR, Rutherford CL Jr, et al. Prostate cancer detection in a clinical urological practice by ultrasonography, digital rectal examination and prostate specific antigen. J Urol 1990;143:1146.

97. Wang MC, Valenzuala LA, Murphy GP, et al. Purification of a human prostatic specific antigen. Invest Urol 1979;17:159.

98. Drago JR, Badalament RA, Wientjes MG, et al. The relative value of prostatic-specific antigen and prostatic acid phosphatase in the diagnosis and management of adenocarcinoma of the prostate: the Ohio State University experience. Urology 1989;34:187.

99. Ferro MA, Barnes I, Roberts JBM, et al. Tumour markers in prostatic carcinoma: a comparison of prostate-specific antigen with acid phosphatase. Br J Urol 1987;60:69.

100. Myrtle JF, Klimley PG, Ivor LP, et al. Clinical utility of prostate specific antigen (PSA) in the management of prostate cancer. Adv Cancer Diagn 1986;1:1.

101. Seamonds B, Yang N, Anderson K, et al. Evaluation of prostatic-specific antigen and prostatic acid phosphatase as prostate cancer markers. Urology 1986;28:472.

102. Stamey TA, Yang N, Hay AR, et al. Prostate specific antigen as a serum marker for adenocarcinoma of the prostate. N Engl J Med 1987;317:909.

103. Partin AW, Oesterling JE. The clinical usefulness of prostate specific antigen: update 1994. J Urol 1994;152:1358.

104. Benson MC, Whang IS, Pantuck A, et al. Prostate specific antigen density: a means of distinguishing benign prostatic hypertrophy and prostate cancer. J Urol 1992;147:815.

105. Benson MC, Whang IS, Olsson CA, et al. The use of prostate specific antigen density to enhance the predictive value of intermediate levels of serum prostate specific antigen. J Urol 1992;147:817.

106. Brawer MK, Aramburu EAG, Chen GL, et al. The inability of prostate specific antigen index to enhance the predictive value of prostate specific antigen in the diagnosis of prostatic carcinoma. J Urol 1993;150:369.

107. Elliss WJ, Chetner MP, Preston SD, et al. Diagnosis of prostatic carcinoma: the yield of serum prostate specific antigen, digital rectal examination and transrectal ultrasonography. J Urol 1994;152:1520.

108. Catalona WJ, Richie JP, Ahmann FR, et al. Comparison of digital rectal examination and serum prostate specific antigen in the early detection of prostate cancer: results of a multicenter clinical trial of 6,630 men. J Urol 1994;151:1283.

109. Catalona WJ, Richie JP, deKernion JB, et al. Comparison of prostate specific antigen concentration versus prostate specific antigen density in the early detection of prostate cancer: receiver operating characteristic curves. J Urol 1994;152:2031.

110. Romell FM, Agusta VE, Breslin JA, et al. The use of prostate specific antigen and prostate specific antigen density in the diagnosis of prostate cancer in a community based urology practice. J Urol 1994;151:88.

111. Blackwell KL, Bostwick DG, Myers RP, et al. Combining prostate specific antigen with cancer and gland volume to predict more reliably pathological stage: the influence of prostate specific antigen cancer density. J Urol 1994;151:1565.

112. Seaman E, Whang M, Olsson CA, et al. PSA density (PSAD): role in patient evaluation and management. Urol Clin North Am 1993;20:653.

113. Carter HB, Pearson JD, Metter EJ, et al. Longitudinal evaluation of prostate specific antigen levels in men with and without prostate disease. JAMA 1992;267:2215.

114. Brawer MK, Beatie J, Wener MH, et al. Screening for

prostatic carcinoma with prostate specific antigen: results of the second year. J Urol 1993;150:106.

115. Oesterling JE, Jacobsen SJ, Chute CG, et al. Serum prostate-specific antigen in a community-based population of healthy men: establishment of age-specific references ranges. JAMA 1993;270:860.

116. Lee F, Gray JM, McLeary RD, et al. Transrectal ultrasound in the diagnosis of prostate cancer: location, echogenicity, histopathology, and staging. Prostate 1985;7:117.

117. Lee F, Siders DB, Torp-Pedersen ST, et al. Prostate cancer: transrectal ultrasound and pathology comparison. Cancer 1991;67:1132.

118. Flanigan RC, Catalona WJ, Richie JP, et al. Accuracy of digital rectal examination and transrectal ultrasonography in localized prostate cancer. J Urol 1994;152:1506.

119. Whitmore WF Jr. Hormone therapy in prostate cancer. Am J Med 1956;21:697.

120. Jewett HJ. The present status of radical prostatectomy for stages A and B prostatic cancer. Urol Clin North Am 1975; 2:105.

121. Boxer RJ. Adenocarcinoma of the prostate gland. Urol Survey 1977;27:75.

122. Bartsch G, Dietze O, Hohlbrugger G, et al. Incidental carcinoma of the prostate: grading and tumor volume in relation to survival rate. World J Urol 1983;1:24.

123. Grossman HB, Batata M, Hilaris B, et al. Implantation of the prostate: further follow-up of first 100 cases. Urology 1982; 20:591.

124. Whitesel JA, Donahue RE, Mani JH, et al. Acid phosphatase in influence on the management of carcinoma of the prostate. J Urol 1984;131:70.

125. Schroeder FH, Hermanek P, Denis L, et al. TNM classification of prostate cancer. Prostate Suppl 1992;20:129.

126. McClennan BL. Transrectal ultrasound of the prostate: is the technology leading the science? Radiology 1988;168:571.

127. Kramer BS, Brown ML, Prorok PC, et al. Prostate cancer screening: what we know and what we need to know. Ann Intern Med 1993;119:914.

128. Ohori M, Wheeler TM, Dunn JK, et al. The pathological features and prognosis of prostate cancer detectable with current diagnostic tests. J Urol 1994;152:1714.

129. Epstein JI, Walsh PC, Brendler CB. Radical prostatectomy for impalpable prostate cancer: the Johns Hopkins experience with tumors found on transurethral resection (stages T1A and T1B) and on needle biopsy (stage T1C). J Urol 1994;152: 1721.

130. Stormont TJ, Farrow GM, Meyers RP, et al. Clinical stage B_0 or T1c prostate cancer: non-palpable disease identified by elevated serum prostate-specific antigen concentration. Urology 1993;41:3.

131. Whitmore WF Jr. Natural history of low stage prostatic cancer and the impact of early detection. Urol Clin North Am 1990;17:689.

132. Lee F, Littrup PJ, McLeary RD, et al. Needle aspiration and core biopsy of prostate cancer: comparative evaluation with biplanar transrectal US guidance. Radiology 1987;163:515.

133. Partin AW, Yoo J, Carter HB, et al. The use of prostate specific antigen, clinical stage and Gleason score to predict pathological stage in men with localized prostate cancer. J Urol 1993;150:110.

134. Sheldon CA, Williams RD, Fraley EE. Incidental carcinoma of the prostate: a review of the literature and critical reappraisal of classification. J Urol 1980;124:626.

135. Badalament RA, Drago JR. Disease-a-month: prostate cancer. Chicago: Year Book, 1991;37:199.

136. Kleer E, Larson-Keller JJ, Zincke H, et al. Ability of preoperative serum prostate specific antigen value to predict pathologic stage and DNA ploidy. Urology 1993;41:207.

137. Peller PA, Young DC, Marmaduke DP, et al. Sextant prostate biopsies: a histopathologic correlation with radical prostatectomy specimens. Cancer 1995;75:530.

138. Oesterling JE, Martin SK, Bergstralh EJ, et al. The use of prostate specific antigen in staging patients with newly diagnosed prostate cancer. JAMA 1993;269:57.

139. Rifkin MD, Zerhouni EA, Gatsonis CA, et al. Comparison of magnetic resonance imaging and ultrasonography in staging early prostate cancer: results of a multi-institutional cooperative trial. N Engl J Med 1990;323:621.

140. Schnall MD, Imai Y, Tomaszewski J, et al. Prostate cancer: local staging with endorectal surface coil MR imaging. Radiology 1991;178:707.

141. Chelsky MJ, Schnall MD, Seidmon EJ, et al. Use of endorectal surface coil magnetic resonance imaging for local staging of prostate cancer. J Urol 1993;150:391.

142. von Eschenbach AC, Jing BS, Wallace S. Lymphangiography in genitourinary cancer. Urol Clin North Am 1985;12:715.

143. Arger PH. Computed tomography of the lower urinary tract. Urol Clin North Am 1985;12:677.

144. McCarthy P, Pollack HM. Imaging of patients with stage D prostatic carcinoma. Urol Clin North Am 1991;18:35.

145. Van Poppel H, Ameye F, Oyen R, et al. Accuracy of combined computerized tomography and fine needle aspiration cytology in lymph node staging of localized prostatic carcinoma. J Urol 1994;151:1310.

146. Wolf SW Jr, Cher M, Dall'era M, et al. The use and accuracy of cross-sectional imaging and fine needle aspiration cytology for detection of pelvic lymph node metastases before radical prostatectomy. J Urol 1995;153:993.

147. Babaian RJ, Sayer J, Podoloff DA, et al. Radioimmunoscintigraphy of pelvic lymph nodes with [111]indium-labeled monoclonal antibody CYT-356. J Urol 1994;152:1952.

148. Donohue RE, Mani JH, Whitesel JA, et al. Pelvic lymph node dissection: guide to patient management in clinically locally confined adenocarcinoma of the prostate. Urology 1982;20:559.

149. Danella JF, deKernion JB, Smith RB, et al. The contemporary incidence of lymph node metastases in prostate cancer: implications for laparoscopic lymph node dissection. J Urol 1993;149:1488.

150. Petros JA, Catalona WJ. Lower incidence of unsuspected lymph node metastases in 521 consecutive patients with clinically local prostate cancer. J Urol 1992;147:1574.

151. Bluestein DL, Bostwick DG, Bergstralh EJ, et al. Eliminating the need for bilateral pelvic lymphadenectomy in select patients with prostate cancer. J Urol 1994;151:1315.

152. Levy DA, Resnick MI. Laparoscopic pelvic lymphadenectomy and radical perineal prostatectomy: a viable alternative to radical retropubic prostatectomy. J Urol 1994;151:905.

153. Guazzoni G, Montorsi F, Bergamaschi F, et al. Open surgical

revision of laparoscopic pelvic lymphadenectomy for staging of prostate cancer: the impact of laparoscopic learning curve. J Urol 1994;151:930.

154. Schuessler WW, Pharand D, Vancaillie TG. Laparoscopic standard pelvic node dissection for carcinoma of the prostate: is it accurate? J Urol 1993;150:898.

155. Kerbl K, Clayman RV, Petros JA, et al. Staging pelvic lymphadenectomy for prostate cancer: a comparison of laparoscopic and open techniques. J Urol 1993;150:396.

156. Kavoussi LR, Sosa E, Chandhoke P, et al. Complications of laparoscopic pelvic lymph node dissection. J Urol 1993;149:322.

157. Das S, Tashima M. Extraperitoneal laparoscopic staging pelvic lymph node dissection. J Urol 1994;151:1321.

158. Pollen JJ. Bone scanning in neoplastic disease. Cancer 1976;37:580.

159. O'Mara RE. Skeletal scanning in neoplastic disease. Cancer 1976;37:480.

160. Smith JA, Datz FI. Interpretation of the equivocal bone scan in patients with prostate cancer. Prob Urol 1987;1:124.

161. Johansson JE. Expectant management of early stage prostatic cancer: Swedish experience. J Urol 1994;152:1753.

162. Adolfsson J, Ronstrom L, Lowhagen T, et al. Deferred treatment of clinically localized low grade prostate cancer: experience from prospective series at Karolinska hospital. J Urol 1994;152:1757.

163. Warner J, Whitmore WF Jr. Expectant management of clinically localized prostatic cancer. J Urol 1994;152:1761.

164. George NJR. Natural history of localized prostatic cancer managed by conservative therapy alone. Lancet 1988;1:494.

165. Adolfsson J, Steineck G, Whitmore WF Jr. Recent results of management of palpable clinically localized prostate cancer. Cancer 1993;72:310.

166. Flemming C, Wasson JH, Albertsen PC, et al. A decision analysis of alternative treatment strategies for clinically localized prostate cancer. JAMA 1993;265:2650.

167. Beck JR, Kattan MW, Miles BJ. A critique of decision analysis for clinically localized prostate cancer. J Urol 1994;152:1894.

168. Chodak GW, Thiested RA, Gerber GS, et al. Outcome following conservative management of patients with clinically localized prostate cancer. N Engl J Med 1994;330:242.

169. Young HH. The early diagnosis and radical cure of carcinoma of the prostate. Bull Johns Hopkins Hosp 1905;16:395.

170. Walsh PC, Lepor H. The role of radical prostatectomy in the management of prostate cancer. Cancer 1987;60:526.

171. Walsh PC, Partin AW, Epstein JI. Cancer control and quality of life following anatomical radical retropubic prostatectomy: results at 10 years. J Urol 1994;152:1831.

172. Scott WW. An evaluation of endocrine therapy plus radical perineal prostatectomy in the treatment of advanced carcinoma of the prostate. J Urol 1964;91:97.

173. Oesterling JE, Andrews PE, Suman VJ, et al. Preoperative androgen deprivation therapy: artificial lowering of serum prostate specific antigen without downstaging the tumor. J Urol 1993;149:779.

174. Pummer K, Crawford ED, Daneshgari F, et al. Hormonal pretreatment does not affect the final pathologic stage in locally advanced prostate cancer. Urology (Symposium) 1994;44:38.

175. Labrie F, Cusan L, Gomez JL, et al. Down-staging of early stage prostate cancer before radical prostatectomy: the first randomized trial of neoadjuvant combination therapy with flutamide and a luteinizing hormone-releasing hormone agonist. Urology (Symposium) 1994;44:29.

176. Steinberg GD, Epstein JI, Piantadosi S, et al. Management of stage D1 adenocarcinoma of the prostate: the Johns Hopkins experience 1974 to 1987. J Urol 1990;144:1425.

177. Sgrignoli AR, Walsh PC, Steinberg GD, et al. Prognostic factors in men with stage D1 prostate cancer: identification of patients less likely to have prolonged survival after radical prostatectomy. J Urol 1994;152:1077.

178. Prout GR Jr, Heaney JA, Griffin PP, et al. Nodal involvement as a prognostic indicator in patients with prostatic carcinoma. J Urol 1980;124:226.

179. Zincke H, Utz DC, Taylor WF. Bilateral pelvic lymphadenectomy and radical prostatectomy for clinical stage C prostate cancer: role of adjuvant treatment for residual cancer and in disease progression. J Urol 1986;135:1199.

180. Smith JA Jr, Middleton RG. Implications of volume of nodal metastasis in patients with adenocarcinoma of the prostate. J Urol 1985;133:617.

181. Cheng CWS, Frydenberg M, Bergstralh EJ, et al. Radical prostatectomy for pathologic stage C prostate cancer: influence of pathologic variables and adjuvant treatment on disease outcome. Urology 1993;42:283.

182. Zincke H, Bergstralh EJ, Larson-Keller JJ, et al. Stage D1 prostate cancer treated by radical prostatectomy and adjuvant hormonal treatment. Cancer 1992;70(Suppl):311.

183. Mador DR, Huben RP, Wajsman Z, et al. Salvage surgery following radical radiotherapy for adenocarcinoma of the prostate. J Urol 1985;133:58.

184. Neerhut GJ, Wheeler T, Cantini M, et al. Salvage radical prostatectomy for radiorecurrent adenocarcinoma of the prostate. J Urol 1988;140:544.

185. Zincke H. Radical prostatectomy and exenterative procedures for local failure after radiotherapy with curative intent: comparison of outcomes. J Urol 1992;147:894.

186. Ahlering TE, Lieskovsky G, Skinner DG. Salvage surgery plus androgen deprivation for radioresistant prostatic adenocarcinoma. J Urol 1992;147:900.

187. Berlin BB, Cornwell PM, Connelly RR, et al. Radical perineal prostatectomy for carcinoma of the prostate: survival in 143 cases treated from 1935 to 1958. J Urol 1968;99:97.

188. Belt E, Schroeder FH. Total perineal prostatectomy for carcinoma of the prostate. J Urol 1972;107:91.

189. Culp OS, Meyer JJ. Radical prostatectomy in the treatment of prostatic cancer. Cancer 1973;32:1113.

190. Veenema JR, Gursel EO, Lattimer JK. Radical retropubic prostatectomy for cancer: a 20-year experience. J Urol 1977;117:330.

191. Hodges CV, Pearse HD, Stille L. Radical prostatectomy for carcinoma: 30-year experience and 15-year survivals. J Urol 1979;122:180.

192. Jewett HJ. The present status of radical prostatectomy for stages A and B prostatic cancer. Urol Clin North Am 1975;2:105.

193. Gibbons RP, Correa RJ Jr, Brannen GE, et al. Total prostatectomy for localized prostatic cancer. J Urol 1984;131:73.

194. Gibbons RP, Correa RJ Jr, Brannen GE, et al. Total prostatectomy for clinically localized prostatic cancer: long-term results. J Urol 1989;141:564.

195. Zincke H, Oesterling JE, Blute ML, et al. Long-term (15 years) results after radical prostatectomy for clinically localized (stage T2c or lower) prostate cancer. J Urol 1994; 152:1850.

196. Lepor H, Kimball AW, Walsh PC. Cause-specific actuarial survival analysis: a useful method for reporting survival data in men with clinically localized prostate carcinoma of the prostate. J Urol 1989;141:82.

197. Culp OS. Radical perineal prostatectomy: its past, present and possible future. J Urol 1968;98:618.

198. Alyea EP, Dees JE, Glenn JF. An aggressive approach to prostatic cancer. J Urol 1977;118:211.

199. Boxer RJ, Kaufman JJ, Goodwin WE. Radical prostatectomy for carcinoma of the prostate: 1951–1976. a review of 329 patients. J Urol 1977;117:208.

200. McDuffie RW Jr, Blundon KE. Radical retropubic prostatectomy: 59 cases. J Urol 1978;119:514.

201. Cochran JS, Kadesky MC. Private practice experience with radical surgical treatment of cancer of prostate. Urology 1981;17:547.

202. Fowler JE Jr, Clayton M, Sharifi R, et al. Early experience with Walsh technique of radical retropubic prostatectomy. J Urol 1987;29:242.

203. Reiner WG, Walsh PC. An anatomical approach to the surgical management of the dorsal vein and Santorini's plexus during radical retropubic surgery. J Urol 1979;121:190.

204. Walsh PC, Donker PJ. Impotence following radical prostatectomy: insight into etiology and prevention. J Urol 1982;128:492.

205. Peters CA, Walsh PC. Blood transfusion and anesthetic practices in radical retropubic prostatectomy. J Urol 1985; 134:81.

206. Walsh PC, Partin AW, Epstein JI. Cancer control and quality of life following anatomical radical retropubic prostatectomy: results at 10 years. J Urol 1994;152:1831.

207. Catalona WJ, Basler JW. Return of erections and urinary continence following nerve sparing radical retropubic prostatectomy. J Urol 1993;150:905.

208. Leandri P, Rossignol G, Gautier JR, et al. Radical retropubic prostatectomy: morbidity and quality of life. experience with 620 consecutive cases. J Urol 1992;147:883.

209. Surya BV, Provet J, Dalbagni G, et al. Experience with potency preservation during radical prostatectomy. Urology 1988;32:498.

210. Murphy GP, Mettlin C, Menck H, et al. National patterns of prostate cancer treatment by radical prostatectomy: results of a survey by the American College of Surgeons Commission on Cancer. J Urol 1994;152:1817.

211. Paschkis R, Tittinger W. Radiumbehandlung eines prostatasarkoms. Wiener Klinische Wochenschrift Nr, 48, 1910.

212. Hanks GE. Treatment of locally advanced prostate cancer with radiation therapy. Urology 1989;33(Suppl):37.

213. Zagars GK, von Eschenback AC, Johnson DE, et al. Stage C adenocarcinoma of the prostate: an analysis of 551 patients treated with external beam radiation. Cancer 1987;60:1489.

214. Porter AT, Forman JD. The role of radiotherapy in the management of locally advanced prostate cancer. Urology (Symposium) 1994;44:43.

215. Lange PH, Lightner DJ, Medini E, et al. The effect of radiation therapy after radical prostatectomy in patients with elevated prostate specific antigen levels. J Urol 1990;144:927.

216. Link P, Freiha FS, Stamey TA. Adjuvant radiation therapy in patients with detectable prostate specific antigen following radical prostatectomy. J Urol 1991;145:532.

217. Stein A, deKernion JB, Dorey F, et al. Adjuvant radiotherapy in patients with post radical prostatectomy with tumor extending through capsule or positive seminal vesicles. Urology 1992;39:59.

218. McCarthy JF, Catalona WJ, Hudson MA. Effect of radiation therapy on detectable serum prostate specific antigen levels following radical prostatectomy: early versus delayed treatment. J Urol 1994;151:1575.

219. Thompson IM, Paradelo JC, Crawford ED, et al. An opportunity to determine optimal treatment of pT3 prostate cancer: the window may be closing. Urology 1994;44:804.

220. Benson RC Jr, Hasan SM, Jones AG, et al. External beam radiotherapy for palliation of pain from metastatic carcinoma of the prostate. J Urol 1982;127:69.

221. Hazuka MB. Palliative irradiation for genitourinary carcinoma. In: Crawford ED, ed. Current genitourinary cancer surgery. Philadelphia: Lea & Febiger, 1990.

222. Bagshaw MA, Cox RS, Hancock SL. Control of prostate cancer with radiotherapy: long-term results. J Urol 1994;152: 1781.

223. Bagshaw MA, Kaplan ID, Cox RC. Radiation therapy for localized disease. Cancer 1993;71(Suppl):939.

224. del Regato JA, Trailins AH, Pittman DD. Twenty-year follow-up of patients with inoperable cancer of the prostate (stage C) treated by radiotherapy: report of a national cooperative study. Int J Radiat Oncol Biol Phys 1993;26:197.

225. Shipley WU, Zietman AL, Hanks GE, et al. Treatment related sequelae following external beam radiation for prostate cancer: a review with an update in patients with stages T1 and T2 tumor. J Urol 1994;152:1799.

226. Goldstein I, Feldman MI, Declose PJ, et al. Radiation-associated impotence. JAMA 1984;251:903.

227. Russell KJ, Blasko JC. Recent advances in interstitial brachytherapy for localized prostate cancer. Prob Urol 1993; 7:260.

228. Porter AT, Forman JD. Prostate brachytherapy. Cancer 1993; 71(Suppl):953.

229. Leibel SA, Fuks Z, Zelefsky MJ, et al. The effects of local and regional treatment on the metastatic outcome in prostatic carcinoma with pelvic lymph node involvement. Int J Radiat Oncol Biol Phys 1993;28:7.

230. Kaye KW, Olson DJ, Payne JT. Detailed preliminary analysis of ^{125}iodine implantation for localized prostate cancer using percutaneous approach. J Urol 1995;153:1020.

231. Nag S, Scaperoth DD, Badalament RA, et al. Transperineal palladium 103 prostate brachytherapy: analysis of morbidity and seed migration. Urology 1995;45:87.

232. Porter AT. Prostate brachytherapy. In: Mould R, ed. Brachytherapy 1990. Nucletron Int 1990;22:165.

233. Donnelly BJ, Pedersen J, Porter AT, et al. Iridium-192 brachytherapy in treatment of cancer of the prostate. Clin Urol 1991;18:483.

234. Gonder M, Soanes W, Shulman S. Cryosurgical treatment of the prostate. Invest Urol 1966;3:372.

235. Onik GM, Cohen JK, Reyes GD, et al. Transrectal ultrasound-guided percutaneous radical cryosurgical ablation of the prostate. Cancer 1993;72:1291.

236. Lee F, Bahn DK, McHugh TA, et al. US-guided percutaneous cryoablation of prostate cancer. Radiology 1994; 192:769.

237. Bahn DK, Lee F, Solomon MH, et al. Prostate cancer: US-guided percutaneous cryoablation. work in progress. Radiology 1995;194:551.

238. Goldrath DE, Messing EM. Prostate specific antigen: not detectable despite tumor progression after radical prostatectomy. J Urol 1989;142:1082.

239. Takayama TK, Krieger JN, True LD, et al. Recurrent prostate cancer despite undetectable prostate specific antigen. J Urol 1992;148:1541.

240. Stein A, deKernion JB, Dorey F. Prostatic specific antigen related to clinical status 1 to 14 years after radical retropubic prostatectomy. Br J Urol 1991;67:626.

241. Lange PH, Ercole CJ, Lightner DJ, et al. The value of serum prostate specific antigen determinations before and after radical prostatectomy. J Urol 1989;141:873.

242. Partin AW, Pound CR, Clemens JQ, et al. Serum PSA after anatomic radical prostatectomy: the Johns Hopkins experience after 10 years. Urol Clin North Am 1993;20:713.

243. Hudson MA, Bahnson RR, Catalona WJ. Clinical use of prostate specific antigen in patients with prostate cancer. J Urol 1989;142:1011.

244. Trapasso JG, deKernion JB, Smith RB, et al. Incidence and significance of detectable levels of serum prostate specific antigen after radical prostatectomy. J Urol 1994;152:1821.

245. Kahn D, Williams RD, Seldin DW, et al. Radioimmunoscintigraphy with [111]indium labeled CYT-356 for the detection of occult prostate cancer recurrence. J Urol 1994;152:1490.

246. Zagars GK. Prostate specific antigen as outcome variable for T1 and T2 prostate cancer treated by radiation therapy. Urology 1994;152:1786.

247. Willett CG, Zietman AL, Shipley WU, et al. The effect of pelvic radiation therapy on serum levels of prostate specific antigen. J Urol 1994;151:1579.

248. Schellhammer PF, El-Mahdi AM, Wright GL Jr, et al. Prostate-specific antigen to determine progression-free survival after radiation therapy for localized carcinoma of prostate. Urology 1993;42:13.

249. Zelefsky MJ, Leibel SA, Wallner KE, et al. Significance of normal serum prostate specific antigen in the follow-up period after definitive radiation therapy for prostatic cancer. J Clin Oncol 1995;13:459.

250. Lee WR, Hanks GE, Schultheiss TE, et al. Localized prostate cancer treated by external-beam radiotherapy alone: serum prostate specific antigen-driven outcome analysis. J Clin Oncol 1995;13:464.

251. Scardino PT, Wheeler TM. Local control of prostate cancer with radiotherapy: frequency and prognostic significance of positive results of post-irradiation prostate biopsy. NCI Monogr 1988;7:95.

252. Kuban DA, El-Mahdi AM, Schellhammer PF. The significance of post-irradiation prostate biopsy with long-term follow-up. Int J Radiat Oncol Biol Phys 1992;24:409.

253. Kuban DA, El-Mahdi AM, Schellhammer PF. Prognostic significance of post-irradiation prostate biopsies. Oncology 1993;7:29.

254. Huggins C, Hodges CV. The effect of castration, of estrogen and of androgen injection on serum phosphatases in metastatic carcinoma of the prostate. Cancer Res 1941;293.

255. Coffey DS, Isaacs JT. Prostate tumor biology and cell kinetics-theory. Urology 1981;17(Suppl):40.

256. Walsh PC. Physiologic basis for hormonal therapy in carcinoma of the prostate. Urol Clin North Am 1975;2:125.

257. Drago JR, Badalament RA. Biochemical mechanisms of endocrine interruption in stage D prostate cancer: part 4. Cancer of the prostate: current practice/future directions. Philadelphia: CoMed Communications, 1990.

258. McConnel JD. Physiologic basis of endocrine therapy for prostatic cancer. Urol Clin North Am 1991;18:1.

259. Grayhack JT, Keller TC, Kozlowski JM. Carcinoma of the prostate: hormonal therapy. Cancer 1987;60:589.

260. Johansson JE, Andersson SO, Holmberg L, et al. Primary orchiectomy versus estrogen therapy in advanced prostate cancer: a randomized study. results after 7 to 10 years of follow up. J Urol 1991;145:519.

261. Nesbitt RM, Baum WC. Endocrine control of prostatic carcinoma. clinical and statistical survey of 1818 cases. JAMA 1950;143:1317.

262. Blackard CE. The Veterans Administration Cooperative Urological Research Group studies of carcinoma of the prostate: a review. Cancer Chemother Rep 1975;59:225.

263. Geller J, Albert J, Yen SSC. Treatment of advanced cancer of prostate with megestrol acetate. Urology 1978;12:537.

264. Sogani PC, Whitmore WF Jr. Experience with flutamide in previously untreated patients with advanced prostatic cancer. J Urol 1979;122:640.

265. MacFarlane JR, Tolley DA. Flutamide therapy for advanced prostatic cancer: a phase II study. Br J Urol 1985;57:172.

266. Smith RB, Walsh PC, Goodwin WE. Cyproterone acetate in the treatment of advanced carcinoma of the prostate. J Urol 1973;110:106.

267. Wein AJ, Murphy JJ. Experience in the treatment of prostatic carcinoma with cyproterone acetate. J Urol 1973; 109:68.

268. Trachtenberg J. Ketoconazole therapy in advanced prostatic cancer. J Urol 1984;132:61.

269. Bamberger MH, Lowe FC. Ketoconazole in initial management and treatment of metastatic prostate cancer to spine. Urology 1988;32:301.

270. The Leuprolide Study Group. Leuprolide versus diethylstilbestrol for metastatic prostate cancer. N Engl J Med 1984;311:1281.

271. Debruyne FMJ, Denis L, Lunglmayer G, et al. Long-term therapy with a depot luteinizing hormone-releasing hormone analog (Zoladex) in patients with advanced prostatic carcinoma. J Urol 1988;140:775.

272. Presant CA, Soloway MS, Klioze SS, et al. Buserelin as primary therapy in advanced prostatic carcinoma. Cancer 1985;56:2416.

273. Schroeder FH, Lock TMTW, Chadha DR, et al. Metastatic

cancer of the prostate managed with buserelin versus buserelin plus cyproterone acetate. J Urol 1987;137:912.

274. Walsh PC. Physiologic basis for hormonal therapy in carcinoma of the prostate. Urol Clin North Am 1975;2:73.

275. The Veterans Administration Cooperative Urological Research Group. Carcinoma of the prostate: treatment comparisons. J Urol 1967;98:516.

276. Glashan RW, Robinson MRG. Cardiovascular complications in the treatment of prostatic cancer. Br J Urol 1981;53:624.

277. Kent JR, Bischoff AJ, Arduino LJ, et al. Estrogen dosage and suppression of testosterone levels in patients with prostatic carcinoma. J Urol 1973;109:858.

278. Peeling WB. Phase III studies to compare goserelin (Zoladex) with orchiectomy and with diethylstilbestrol in treatment of prostatic carcinoma. Urology 1989;33(Suppl):45.

279. Citrin DL, Resnick MI, Guinan P, et al. A comparison of Zoladex and DES in the treatment of advanced prostate cancer: results of a randomized, multicenter trial. Prostate 1991;18:139.

280. Conn PM, Crowley WF Jr. Gonadotrophin releasing hormone and its analogues. N Engl J Med 1991;324:93.

281. Labrie F, Dupont A, Belanger A, et al. Flutamide eliminates the risk of disease flare in prostatic cancer patients treated with a luteinizing hormone-releasing hormone agonist. J Urol 1987;138:804.

282. Waxman J, Sandow J, Abel P, et al. Three monthly GnRH agonist (Buseriline) for prostatic cancer. Br J Urol 1990;65:43.

283. Soloway MS, Matzkin H. Antiandrogenic agents as monotherapy in advanced prostatic carcinoma. Cancer 1993;71:1083.

284. Neri RO. Antiandrogens: preclinical and clinical studies. Urology (Symposium) 1994;44:53.

285. Sogani PC, Vagaiwala MR, Whitmore WF Jr. Experience with flutamide in patients with advanced prostatic cancer without prior endocrine therapy. Cancer 1984;54:744.

286. Prout GR Jr, Keating MA, Griffin PP, et al. Long-term experience with flutamide in patients with prostatic carcinoma. Urology 1989;34(Suppl):37.

287. Lund F, Rasmussen F. Flutamide versus stilboesterol in the management of advanced prostate cancer: a controlled prospective study. Br J Urol 1988;61:140.

288. Gomez JL, Dupont A, Cusan L, et al. Incidence of liver toxicity associated with the use of flutamide in prostate cancer patients. Am J Med 1992;92:465.

289. Sonino N. The use of ketoconazole as an inhibitor of steroid production. N Engl J Med 1987;317:812.

290. Trachtenberg J. Ketoconazole therapy in advanced prostatic cancer. J Urol 1984;132:61.

291. Trump DL, Havlin KH, Messing EM, et al. High-dose ketoconazole in advanced hormone-refractory prostate cancer: endocrinologic and clinical effects. J Clin Oncol 1989;7:1093.

292. Gerber GS, Chodak GW. Prostate specific antigen for assessing response to ketoconazole and prednisone in patients with hormone refractory metastatic prostate cancer. J Urol 1990;144:1177.

293. Jubelirer S, Hogan T. High dose ketoconazole for the treatment of hormone refractory metastatic prostatic carcinoma: 16 cases and review of the literature. J Urol 1989;142:89.

294. Eichenberger T, Trachtenberg J, Toor P, et al. Ketoconazole: a possible direct cytotoxic effect on prostate cancer cells. J Urol 1989;141:191.

295. Kozlowski JM, Ellis WJ, Grayhack JT. Advanced prostatic carcinoma: early versus late endocrine therapy. Urol Clin North Am 1991;18:15.

296. Schroeder FH. Early versus delayed endocrine treatment in metastatic prostatic cancer. In: Murphy GP, Khoury S, eds. Therapeutic progress in urological cancers. New York: Liss, 1989:253.

297. Byar DP, Code DK. Hormone therapy for prostate cancer: results of the Veterans Administration Cooperative Urological Research Group studies. NCI Monogr 1988;7:165.

298. Herr HW, Kornblith AB, Ofman U. A comparison of the quality of life of patients with metastatic prostate cancer who received or did not receive hormonal therapy. Cancer 1993;71:1143.

299. Labrie F, Dupont A, Belanger A, et al. New hormonal therapy in prostatic carcinoma: combined treatment with an LHRH agonist and an antiandrogen. J Clin Invest Med 1982;5:267.

300. Labrie F, Dupont A, Belanger A. Complete androgen blockade for the treatment of prostate cancer. In: de Vita VT, Hellman S, Rosenberg SA, eds. Important advances in oncology. Philadelphia: JB Lippincott, 1985:193.

301. Labrie F, Belanger A, Simard J, et al. Combination therapy for prostate cancer: endocrine and biologic basis of its choice as a first-line therapy. Cancer 1993;71(Suppl):1059.

302. Crawford ED, Eisenberger MA, McLeod DG, et al. A controlled trial of leuprolide with and without flutamide in prostatic carcinoma. N Engl J Med 1989;321:419.

303. Denis L, Smith PH, Carneiro De Moura JL, et al. Orchiectomy vs. Zoladex plus flutamide in patients with metastatic prostate cancer. Eur Urol 1990;18(Suppl):34.

304. Iversen P, Danish Prostatic Cancer Group. Zoladex plus flutamide vs. orchiectomy for advanced prostatic cancer. Eur Urol 1990;18(Suppl):41.

305. Fourcade RO, Cariou G, Coloby P, et al. Total androgen blockade with Zoladex plus flutamide vs. Zoladex alone in advanced prostatic carcinoma: interim report of a multicenter, double-blind, placebo-controlled study. Eur Urol 1990;18(Suppl):45.

306. Boccardo F, Decensi A, Guarneri D, et al. Zoladex with or without flutamide in the treatment of locally advanced or metastatic prostate cancer: interim analysis of an ongoing PONCAP study. Eur Urol 1990;18(Suppl):48.

307. Di Silverio F, Serio M, D'Eramo G, et al. Zoladex vs Zoladex plus cyproterone acetate in the treatment of advanced prostatic cancer: multicenter Italian study. Eur Urol 1990;18(Suppl):54.

308. Scher HI, Kelly WK. Flutamide withdrawal syndrome: its impact on clinical trials in hormone-refractory prostate cancer. J Clin Oncol 1993;11:1566.

309. Dupont A, Gomez JL, Cusan L, et al. Response to flutamide withdrawal in advanced prostate cancer in progression under combination therapy. J Urol 1993;150:908.

310. Sartor O, Cooper M, Weinberger M, et al. Surprising activity of flutamide withdrawal, when combined with aminoglutethimide, in treatment of "hormone-refractory" prostate cancer. J Natl Cancer Inst 1994;86:222.

311. Cusan L, Gomez JL, Dupont A, et al. Metastatic prostate cancer pulmonary nodules: beneficial effects of combination therapy and subsequent withdrawal of flutamide. Prostate 1994;24:257.

312. Porter AT, Vaishampayan N. Strontium-89 in metastatic prostate cancer. Urology (Symposium) 1994;44:75.

313. Porter AT, McEwan AJB, Powe JE, et al. Results of a randomized phase-III trial to evaluate the efficacy of strontium-89 adjuvant to local field external beam irradiation in the management of endocrine resistant metastatic prostate cancer. Int J Radiat Oncol Biol Phys 1993;25:805.

314. Lum BL, Torti FM. Chemotherapy of hormone-refractory prostatic carcinoma. Prob Urol 1990;4:506.

315. Yagoda A, Petrylak D. Cytotoxic chemotherapy for advanced hormone-resistant prostate cancer. Cancer 1993;71:1098.

316. Eisenberger MA. Chemotherapy for prostate carcinoma. NCI Monogr 1988;7:151.

317. Scher HI, Cordon-Cardo C. Current and future therapeutic strategies in metastatic hormonal-resistant prostate cancer: therapy based on phenotype. Prob Urol 1993;7:226.

318. Carter SK, Wasserman TH. The chemotherapy of urologic cancer. Cancer 1975;36:729.

319. Moore GE, Bross ID, Ausman R. Effects of 5 fluorouracil (NCS-19893) in 389 patients with cancer: Eastern Clinical Drug Evaluation Program. part 1. Cancer Chemother Rep 1968;52(6):641.

320. Ansfield FJ, Schroeder J, Curreri AR. Five years clinical experience with 5 fluorouracil. JAMA 1962;181:295.

321. Blum RH. An overview of studies with Adriamycin (Nsc-123127) in the United States: part 3. Cancer Chemother Rep 1975;6:247.

322. Scher H, Yagoda A, Watson RC, et al. Phase II trial of doxorubicin in bidimensionally measurable prostatic adenocarcinoma. J Urol 1984;131:1099.

323. Newling DWW, Fossa SD, Tunn UW, et al. Mitomycin C versus estramustine in the treatment of hormone resistant metastatic prostate cancer: the final analysis of the European Organization for Research and Treatment of Cancer, genitourinary group prospective randomized phase III study (30865). J Urol 1993;150:1840.

324. Janknegt RA. Estramustine phosphate and other cytotoxic drugs in the treatment of poor prognostic advanced prostate cancer. Prostate 1992;4:105.

325. Leoning SA, Beckley S, Brady MF, et al. Comparison of estramustine phosphate, methotrexate and cis-platinum in patients with advanced, hormone refractory prostate cancer. J Urol 1983;129:1001.

326. Qazi R, Khandekar J. Phase II study of cisplatin for metastatic prostate cancer: an Eastern Cooperative Oncology Group study. Am J Clin Oncol 1983;6:203.

327. Dawson NA. Treatment of progressive metastatic prostate cancer. Oncology 1993;7:17.

328. Hudes GR, Greenberg R, Krigel RL, et al. Phase II study of estramustine and vinblastine, two microtubule inhibitors, in hormone-refractory prostate cancer. J Clin Oncol 1992;10:1754.

329. Seidman AD, Scher HI, Petrylak D, et al. Estramustine and vinblastine: use of prostate specific antigen as a clinical trial end point for hormone refractory prostatic cancer. J Urol 1992;147:931.

330. Scher HI, Kelly WK. Suramin: defining the role in the clinic. Principles & Practice of Oncology Updates 1993;7:1.

331. Myers C, Cooper M, Stein C, et al. Suramin: a novel growth factor antagonist with activity in hormone-refractory metastatic prostate cancer. J Clin Oncol 1992;10:881.

332. Eisenberger MA, Reyno LM, Jodrell DI, et al. Suramin, an active drug for prostate cancer: interim observations in a phase I trial. J Natl Cancer Inst 1993;85:611.

333. Scher HI, Curley T, Geller N, et al. Gallium nitrate in prostatic cancer: evaluation of antitumor activity and effects on bone turnover. Cancer Treat Rep 1987;71:887.

334. Roth B, Yeap B, Wilding G, et al. Taxol (NSC 125973) in advanced, hormone refractory prostate cancer: an ECOG phase II trial. Proc Am Soc Clin Oncol 1992;11:196. Abstract no. 598.

335. Mahler C, Verhelst J, Denis L. Ketoconazole and liarozole in the treatment of advanced prostatic cancer. Cancer 1993;71(Suppl):1068.

336. van Haelst-Pisani C, Richardson RL, Therneau TM, et al. Phase II study of recombinant leukocyte: a human interferon roferon-A in patients with hormone-resistant prostate cancer. Proc Am Soc Clin Oncol 1990;9:150. Abstract no. 583.

337. Dreicer R, Forest P, Williams RD. A phase II study of 5FU and alpha interferon in hormone-refractory metastatic prostate cancer. Proc Am Soc Clin Oncol 1992;11:205. Abstract no. 635.

338. Axelrod HR, Gilman SC, D'Aleo CJ, et al. Preclinical results and human immunohistochemical studies with 90Y-CYT-356. J Urol 1992;147:361. Abstract no. 596.

16

Pelvic Lymphadenectomy

Sakti Das

In the field of observation, chance favors only the mind that is prepared.

LOUIS PASTEUR

The lymphatic system constitutes the initial avenue of spread from pelvic genitourinary malignancies. Metastatic spread into the pelvic lymph nodes is ominous evidence of advancing distant disease. For many years, pathologic scrutiny of surgically removed pelvic and para-aortic lymph nodes has been used for the staging and therapeutic planning of gynecologic neoplasms. During the latter half of this century, pelvic lymphadenectomy has increasingly assumed a significant role in the management of genitourinary malignancies. Pelvic lymphadenectomy is rarely a primary therapeutic procedure in the presence of minimal disease. For malignancies of bladder, prostate, urethra, and penis, pelvic lymphadenectomy is mostly considered as a staging procedure that determines the prognosis and aids in planning adjuvant therapies.

Considerable morbidities of pelvic lymphadenectomy have led to technical improvements over the years. Initial open intraperitoneal dissection was abandoned in favor of the less morbid but equally efficacious extraperitoneal approach. The geographic limits of the lymphadenectomy template have been reduced to obviate the risks of lymphedema without significantly altering the diagnostic yield of metastatic spread. The latest development of minimally invasive laparoscopic technology has encroached on this arena by popularizing laparoscopic pelvic lymph node dissection by intraperitoneal or extraperitoneal approach.

PELVIC LYMPHADENECTOMY IN PROSTATIC CANCER

Pelvic lymph node dissection in prostatic cancer may be carried out for two reasons. The first is for staging; most urologists agree that it is a staging procedure. Evidence of metastasis in the pelvic lymph nodes portends a poor prognosis with eventual more distant skeletal spread (1–4). Gervasi et al. demonstrated that local regional therapy failed in patients with small-volume nodal metastases at a rate similar to that for patients with more extensive disease (5). In a

series of patients treated with pelvic lymphadenectomy and radical perineal prostatectomy, Cline et al. found that 50% of patients with positive lymph nodes had recurrent disease within 2 years of treatment (6). More than the local stage or tumor grade, presence of lymph node metastasis is the most significant indicator of subsequent disease progression. In contrast, the absence of metastatic nodal disease after pelvic lymphadenectomy generally predicts a long-term favorable response to local therapy for carcinoma of the prostate.

The second reason is therapeutic. Despite the majority opinion that the presence of nodal disease is an indication of systemic cancer, and pelvic lymphadenectomy in such circumstances cannot be construed as a curative procedure, some authors have implied that patients with limited nodal spread can be cured with regional therapy (7). Rutishauer and Hering detected no difference in disease-free survival between node-negative patients and patients with single microscopic or macroscopic nodal invasion (8).

Several reports, mainly from the Mayo Clinic, have suggested that patients with pelvic lymph nodal metastases may gain a survival benefit from early endocrine therapy in addition to local treatment, especially in terms of time to first disease progression (9, 10). The beneficial effect of early hormonal therapy became more apparent in patients with DNA diploid carcinoma (11).

Whether pelvic lymphadenectomy has any value in radiation therapy planning remains controversial. It may be prudent to confine radiation to the prostate when lymph nodes do not harbor metastasis. The justification of extending the radiation field to the pelvic and/or periaortic nodes with the expectation of sterilizing metastatic nodal disease is questionable (12). In 90 patients with surgically proven stage D1 prostatic carcinoma treated by extended field radiation, Paulson et al. observed that the mean time to failure was 23 months (13). Radiation therapy in patients with lymph nodal metastases might delay the onset of disease progression but probably has little effect on survival.

ALTERNATIVES TO PELVIC LYMPHADENECTOMY

Imaging

In the assessment of pelvic lymph nodal status, imaging studies such as pedal lymphangiography, pelvic computed tomography scan, and magnetic resonance imaging have proven disappointing, with an unacceptably high rate of false-negative and false-positive results. Combining fine-needle aspiration of abnormal lymph nodes and computed tomography, VanPoppel et al. detected 35 true-positive and 8 true-negative histologic confirmations of 43 patients with enlarged lymph nodes out of a total 285 patients (14). The majority of these patients had locally advanced disease (stage B2 [11 patients] and stage C [18 patients]) with high expectations of lymph nodal metastases. Their 100% specificity was similar to that reported by Flanigan et al (15). The overall sensitivity of these two reports, however, was 77.8% and 50%, respectively. By decision analysis study, Wolf et al. predicted that only 2.5% of candidates for radical prostatectomy would benefit from cross-sectional imaging and necessary fine-needle aspiration (16). The aggregate benefit to the 2.5% does not outweigh the cost and inconvenience to the other 97.5%. Lymph nodal imaging may be justified when applied selectively to patients with a high probability of lymphatic metastases.

Multivariate Regression Analysis

Recently, regression analysis of available preoperative parameters has yielded promising results whereby selected patient groups may be spared surgical lymphadenectomy for lymph nodal staging. Using prostate-specific antigen (PSA) alone, Danella et al. found a sensitivity and specificity of 77% and positive predictive value of 18% when the preoperative PSA was more than 15 ng/mL (17). Using logistic regression analysis, Bluestein et al. showed that the predicted power of serum PSA could be enhanced considerably by taking into account the Gleason grade and local clinical stage (18). Analyzing these three variables with ultimate pathologic stage of 703 patients, Partin et al. created probability plots and nomograms that would allow us to compare the percentage probability of various pathologic stages to our individual patients (19). Bishoff et al. also analyzed their 481 patients and claimed that their probability curve derived from preoperative PSA, Gleason score, and clinical stage could eliminate the need for pelvic lymphadenectomy in up to 50% of patients (20). These decision analysis processes would certainly help in avoiding the unnecessary morbidities of pelvic lymphadenectomy during primary therapy for localized disease in low-risk cancer prostate patients. Patients in moderate- to high-risk categories, however, still need pathologic confirmation of distant disease before giving up hope for cure.

Lymphoscintigraphy

Radioimmunologic scanning using indium 111-labeled monoclonal antibody has been evaluated by Babaian et al. to assess pelvic lymph nodes before pelvic lymphadenectomy (21). The overall accuracy of 76% and respective sensitivity and specificity of 44% and 86% of this noninvasive technique are encouraging. Various newer technologies using fluorescence photometry and positron imaging tomography are being evaluated in other oncologic areas and may be applicable to the detection of lymph nodal spread in prostate cancer.

LYMPHATIC ANATOMY OF PELVIS

Lymphatic vessels from the pelvic viscera and pelvic parietes drain into the outlying groups of lymph nodes scattered along the iliac vessels and their branches (Fig. 16.1). The main groups of nodes include the common iliac, external iliac, and internal iliac.

The common iliac lymph nodes are arranged as medial, lateral, and intermediate or anterior chains around the common iliac artery starting below the bifurcation of the aorta. After receiving afferents from the external and internal iliac nodes, they send their efferents to the lateral aortic lymph nodes. Two to four nodes of the medial group lying in front of the L5, S1 intervertebral discs are designated as presacral or nodes of sacral promontory.

The external iliac lymph nodes are composed of the lateral, medial, and anterior or intermediate chain. The anterior or intermediate nodes are inconstant. The lateral chain receives efferents from the circumflex iliac and inferior epigastric nodes. The main route of drainage is through the medial chain lying medial to the external iliac vessels. The distal-most node of this chain lying in the femoral canal called the node of Cloquet communicates with the deep inguinal nodes. The medial chain receives afferents from the inguinal lymph nodes; infraumbilical, abdominal, and pelvic parietes; anterior pelvic viscerae; glans penis; clitoris; and part of the vagina. The efferents drain into the common iliac nodes.

The internal iliac lymph nodes surround the hypogastric artery and its branches. They receive lymphatic drainage from all the pelvic viscera, perineum, posterior thigh, and gluteal muscles and send efferents to the common iliac nodes. Important outlying members in this group include obturator lymph nodes lying in the vicinity of the obturator nerve or in the obturator canal. Several nodes along the lateral sacral arteries lying opposite the second and third sacral foramina are called the presciatic nodes.

Lymph vessels of the bladder originating from the intramural plexuses mostly drain into the external iliac nodes. Prostatic lymph vessels exiting from the posterior surface travel along with the vesical lymphatics to drain into the external iliac nodes. Lymph trunks from the anterior aspect join vessels from the membranous urethra and terminate at the internal iliac chain. The presacral and presciatic lymph nodes also have been reported to harbor metastases from prostatic carcinoma.

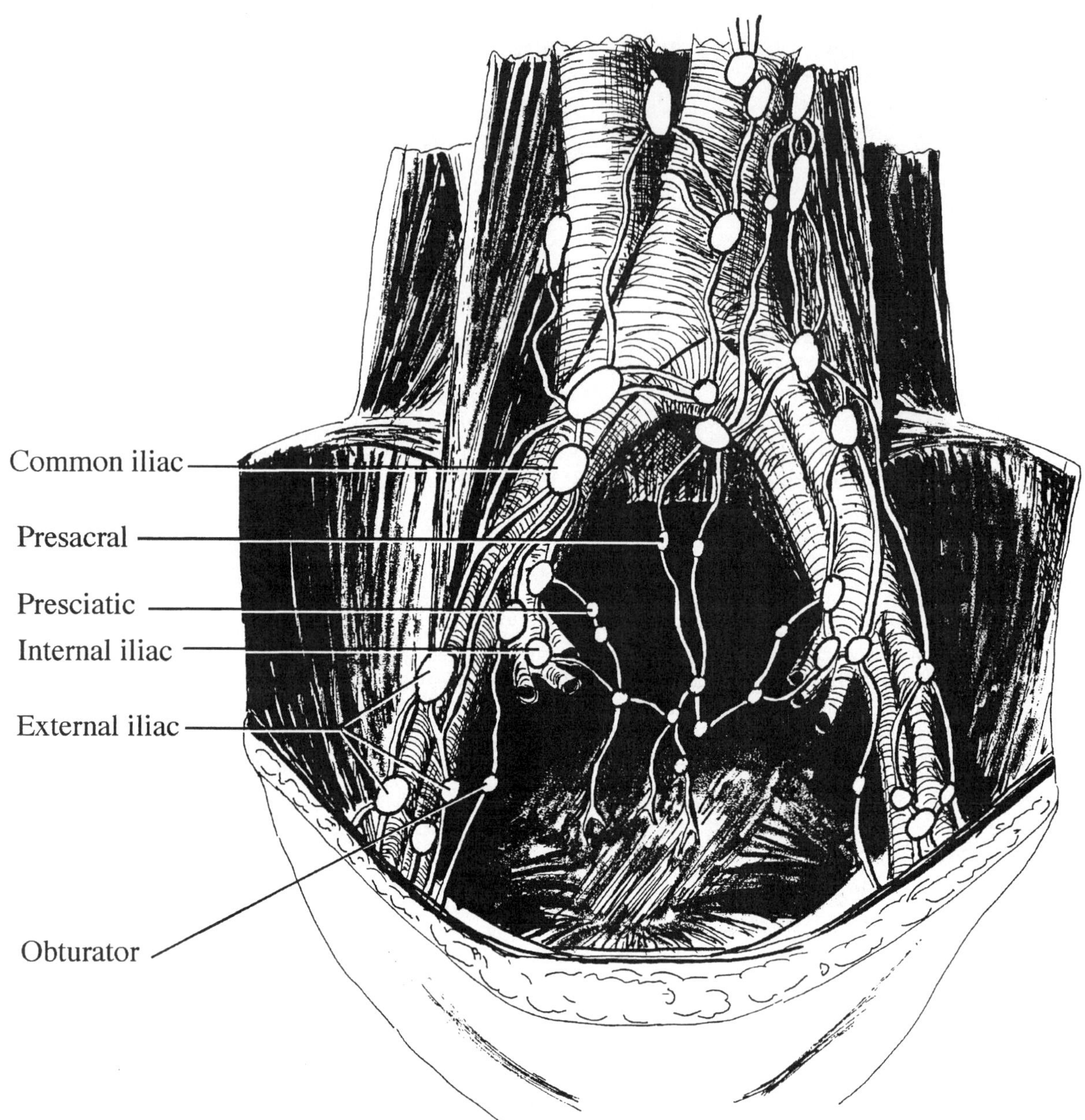

Fig. 16.1. Lymph nodal distribution in the pelvis.

THE EXTENT OF PELVIC LYMPHADENECTOMY FOR PROSTATIC CARCINOMA

The controversy about the proper extent of pelvic lymphadenectomy for prostate carcinoma remains unresolved. There is considerable evidence indicating that the obturator, hypogastric, and external iliac nodes are the initial sites of lymphatic dissemination. Raghavaiah and Jordan observed from their direct intraprostatic contrast injection study that the pattern of lymphatic drainage was one of orderly, localized, stepwise drainage to the regional pelvic lymph nodes with the obturator, hypogastric, and external iliac chain as the first echelon of draining lymph nodes (22).

Historically, the "standard" pelvic lymphadenectomy included dissection of all tissues bounded laterally by the genitofemoral nerve, distally by the superficial circumflex vessels and Cooper's ligament, medially by the bladder wall, inferiorly by the endopelvic fascia below the obturator vessels, and proximally by the bifurcation of common iliac vessels sweeping down the internal iliac arterial branches (Fig. 16.2). (23). This template included the external iliac (lateral, intermediate, and medial chain) and the internal iliac group of lymph nodes excluding the presciatic nodes and nodes at the sacral promontory. Golimbu et al. advocated extended pelvic lymphadenectomy that included removal of presacral and presciatic nodes as well (24). They observed metastases

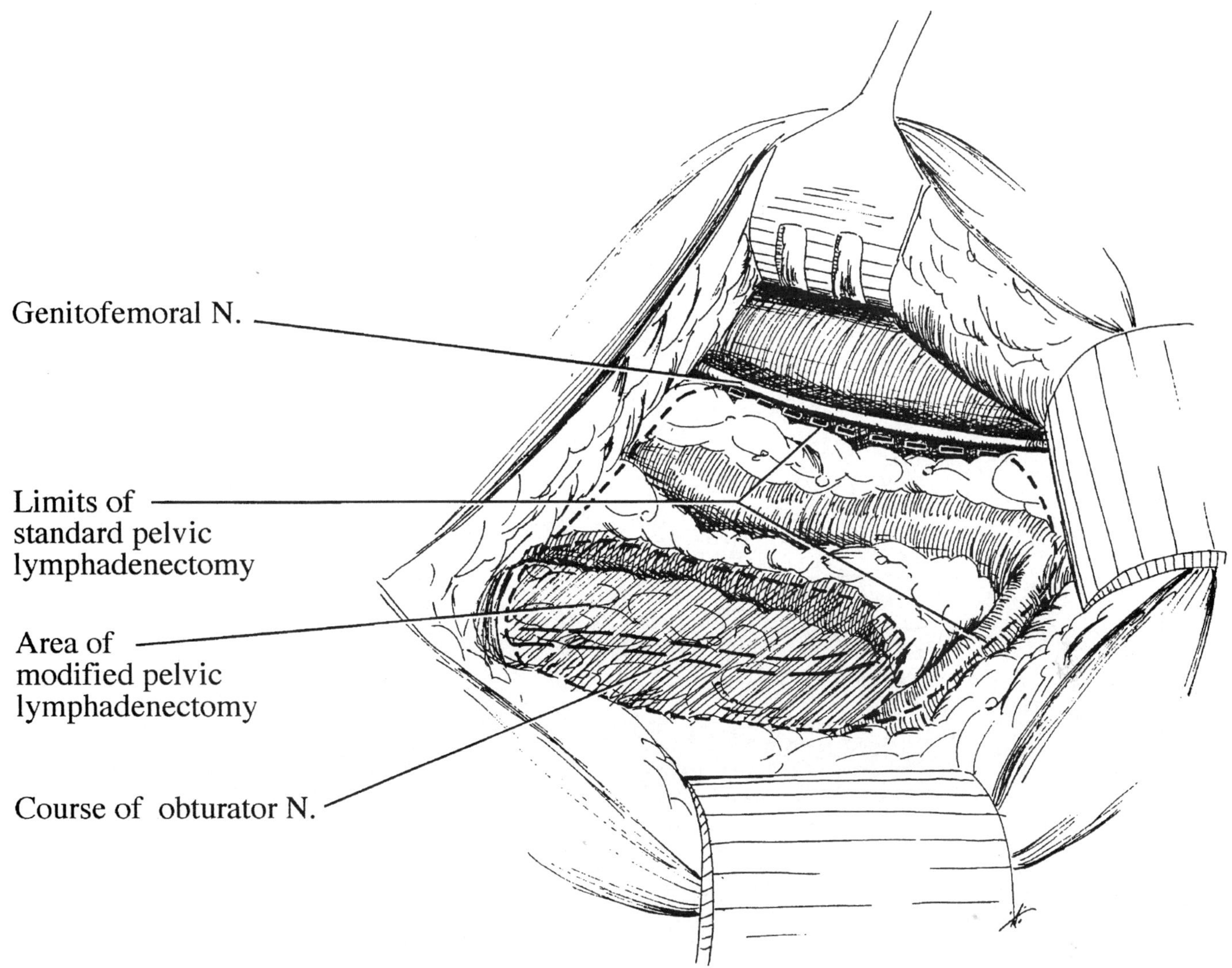

Fig. 16.2. Boundaries of standard and modified pelvic lymphadenectomy.

to the presciatic and presacral lymph nodes in 47% and 53% of cases, respectively. Isolated metastases to the presacral node were found in one patient and to the presciatic node in another patient. Extended pelvic lymphadenectomy is a technically difficult operation; unless larger clinical data validate the argument that presacral and presciatic metastases are common without involvement of the external iliac and hypogastric chain, the morbidity of such an operation may not be justified.

To reduce the morbidity associated with the standard pelvic lymphadenectomy, Whitmore proposed a more limited dissection of tissues with the lateral limit at the external iliac vein (Fig. 16.2) (25). The incidence of nodal metastases by clinical stage is claimed to be similar whether the lymphadenectomy is limited or more extensive. At a subsequent analysis, Fowler and Whitmore observed 39% solitary metastases to the lateral and intermediate chain of external iliac nodes that are excluded in the limited dissection (26). McDowell et al. emphasized more critical dissection of the hypogastric chain lying below the obturator nerve along the entire course of the hypogastric arterial branches (27). These hypogastric nodes were the only site of metastases in 29% of their patients.

The majority of urologists, however, have adopted the modified template of limited pelvic lymphadenectomy that is bounded laterally by the external iliac vein, distally by the circumflex iliac vein and Cooper's ligament, posterosuperiorly by the hypogastric artery, and inferiorly by the endopelvic fascia (28). Tissues surrounding the obturator nerve and vessels are included in the specimen. Distinct benefits include shortened operating time and lessened incidence of postoperative lymphedema. Limited pelvic lymphadenectomy has virtually eliminated genital, prepubic, groin, and lower extremity lymphedema that previously occurred in about 50% of patients after the standard lymphadenectomy.

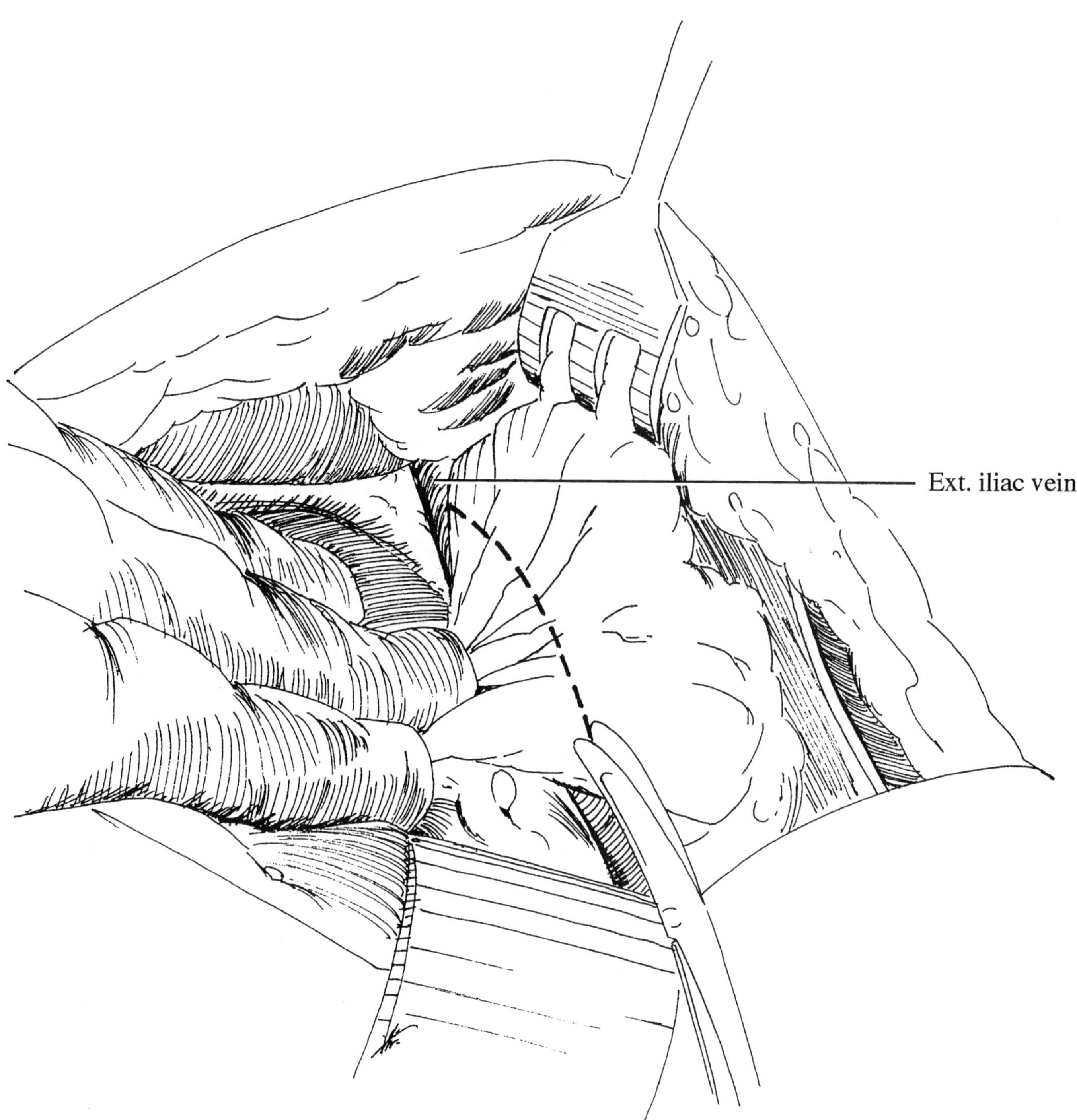

Fig. 16.3.   Commencing lymphadenectomy along the upper medial margin of the external iliac vein.

PELVIC LYMPHADENECTOMY FOR BLADDER CARCINOMA

Pelvic lymphadenectomy is usually considered a staging procedure that determines the prognosis and helps select patients for possible adjuvant chemotherapy. Lymphatic spread from bladder carcinoma has been observed mostly into the obturator and external iliac nodes with lesser involvement of the common iliac and perivesical lymph nodes. Isolated involvement of nodes proximal to the common iliac chain was not encountered without concomitant distal nodal metastases. Because of such stepwise spread, a curative effect of pelvic lymphadenectomy has been conjectured in patients with limited metastases to the primary echelon of lymph nodes. Skinner reported a 35% 5-year survival rate after meticulous pelvic lymphadenectomy and radical cystectomy in patients with nodal metastases (29).

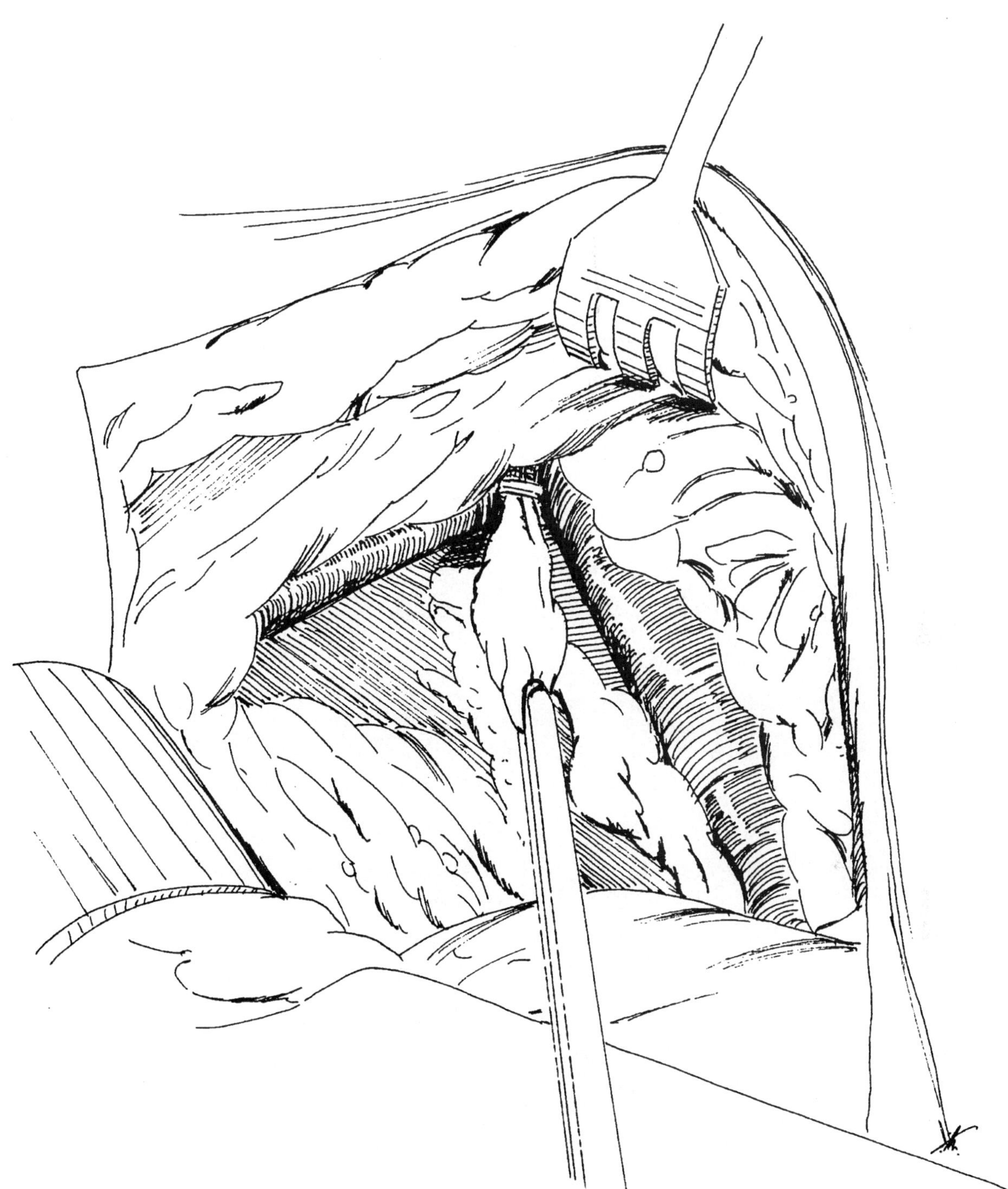

Fig. 16.4.   Dissection of the lymph node of Cloquet.

Stockle et al. reported a cure rate of 27% in 27 similar patients (30). Analyzing a large series from Memorial Sloan-Kettering, Herr suggested that pelvic lymphadenectomy adds only 1 to 2% to the 5-year survival rate of patients with bladder cancer treated with cystectomy (31). Also, in a subsequent prospective study of adjuvant chemotherapy after cystectomy, Skinner et al. had poorer results with surgery alone for node-positive disease compared with their promising earlier experience (32).

In a recent report of a controlled prospective trial of adjuvant polychemotherapy with methotrexate, vinblastine, cisplatin, and doxorubicin (M-VAC) or epirubicin (M-VEC) for non–organ-confined bladder cancer after radical cystectomy, Stockle et al. observed significant improvement in progression-free survival, especially in the subset of patients with metastatic pelvic lymph nodes (33). In accordance with similar data presented prospectively by Skinner et al. (32) and retrospectively by Fra-

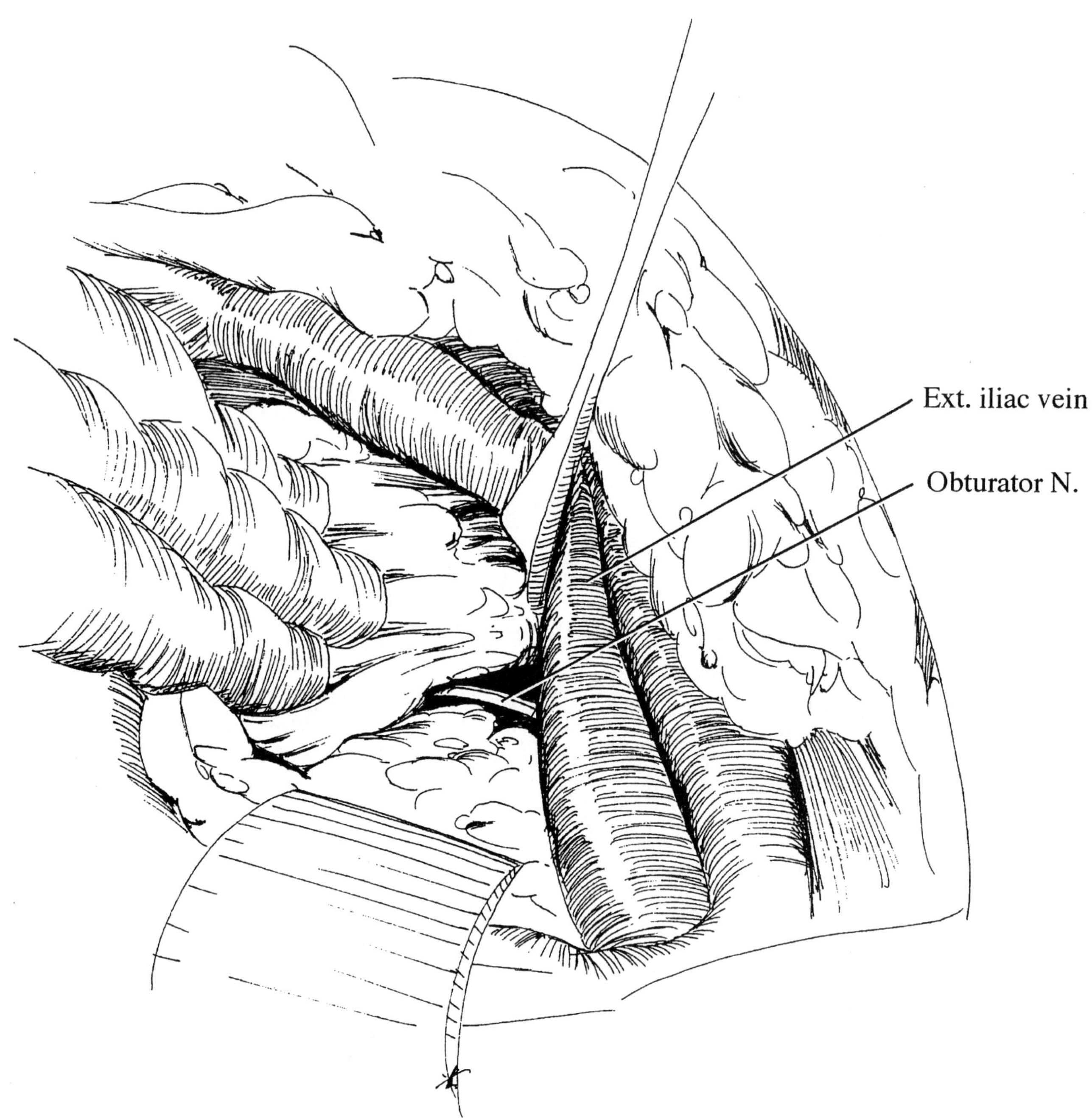

Fig. 16.5. Lymph nodal dissection around the obturator nerve.

det et al. (34), the authors found a trend that patients with limited lymph nodal metastases had greater benefit from adjuvant chemotherapy than did those with more extensive nodal disease. Despite skepticism from the critics about the validity of these studies, the need for well-designed randomized trials of adjuvant chemotherapy for node-positive bladder cancer patients calls for pelvic lymphadenectomy during radical cystectomy for the purposes of definitive staging and establishing a meticulously performed surgery alone as the control study arm (35).

The extent of pelvic lymphadenectomy in bladder carcinoma is dictated by individual philosophic belief about the utility of this procedure. Those who believe in the therapeutic curative role of pelvic lymphadenectomy pursue the standard lymphadenectomy with extension of proximal dissection up to the level of aortic bifurcation. Many, however, believe in the prognostic role of lymphadenectomy for staging that helps in selecting patients for whom adjuvant chemotherapy is suitable. Therefore, to obviate the risks of postoperative lymphedema associated with more extensive dissections, the modified limited pelvic lymphadenectomy is often recommended.

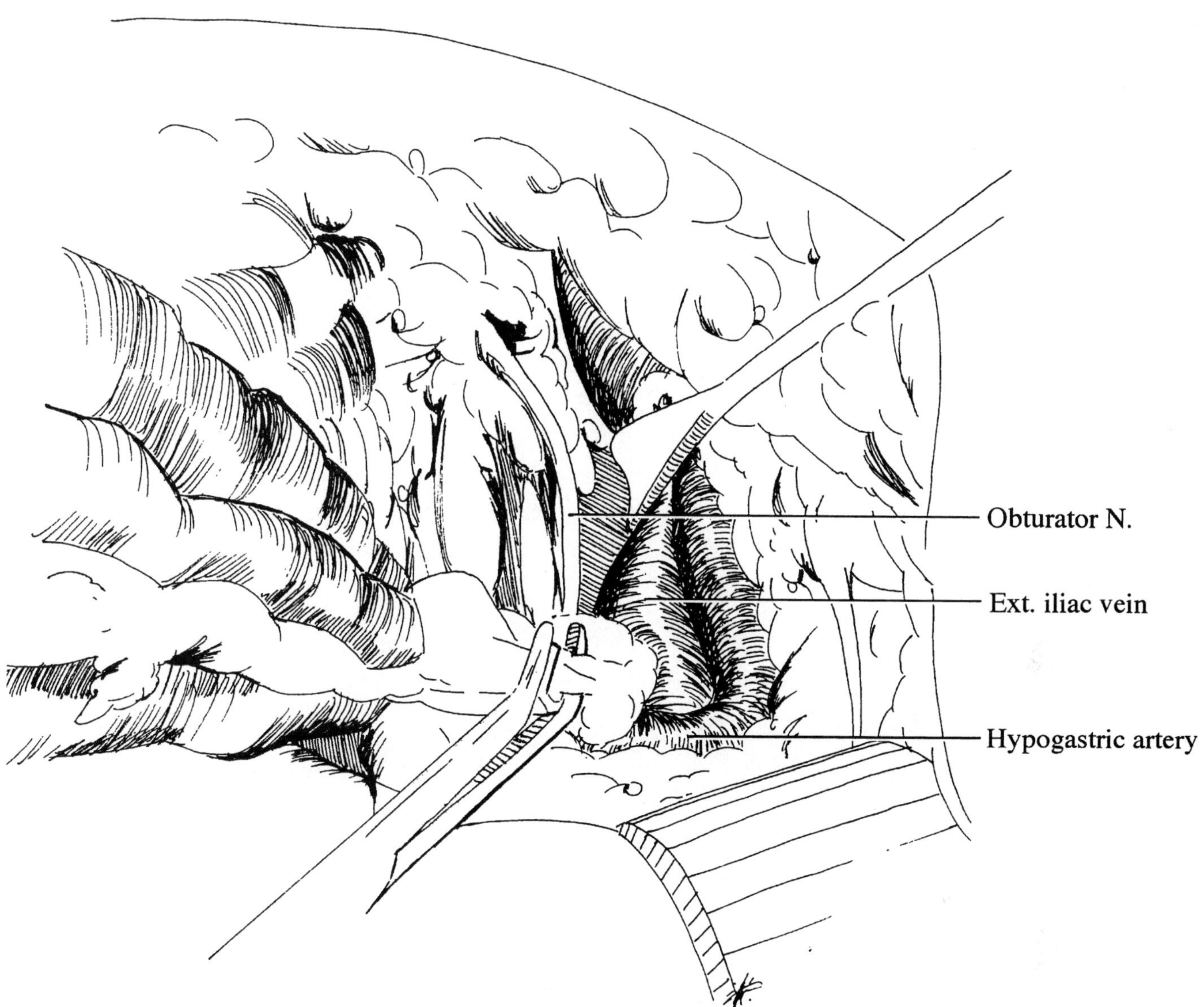

Fig. 16.6. Dissection at the hypogastric corner.

OPEN PELVIC LYMPHADENECTOMY

Preoperative Preparation

Special preparations are unnecessary for patients undergoing pelvic lymphadenectomy only for planned radiation therapy for prostate carcinoma. In the majority of instances, however, pelvic lymphadenectomy is done as part of other major extirpative surgery in the pelvis. We use mechanical and antibiotic bowel preparations to reduce the risk of sepsis during intestinal urinary diversion and inadvertent rectal injuries. In anticipation of significant blood loss during radical prostatectomy or cystectomy, we usually have the patient save 2 or 3 units of autologous blood preoperatively.

Thromboembolic disease remains a major concern for patients undergoing radical pelvic surgeries. Deep vein thrombosis rates of 1.2 to 3%, pulmonary embolism rates of 0.4 to 2.7%, and a fatal pulmonary embolism rate of 0.6% have been reported in radical retropubic prostatectomy (36, 37). In contemporary cystectomy series, comparable thromboembolic complications with pulmonary embolism rates of 1.8 to 4.1% and fatal pulmonary embolism rates as high as 2% have been reported (38). We routinely use an intermittent pneumatic compression device during surgery and continue its use until the patient is fully ambulatory. In patients with additional risk factors, we will consider added prophylaxis with subcutaneous heparin. Although increased bleeding and lymphocele formation remain valid concerns, heparin has been found to reduce the deep vein thrombosis rate from 39.4 to 9.7% (39) and the pulmonary embolism rate from 11 to 0% in prostatectomy patients (40).

We start antibiotic prophylaxis with 1 g cephalosporin intravenously 1 hour before surgery and continue it every 8 hours for three more doses.

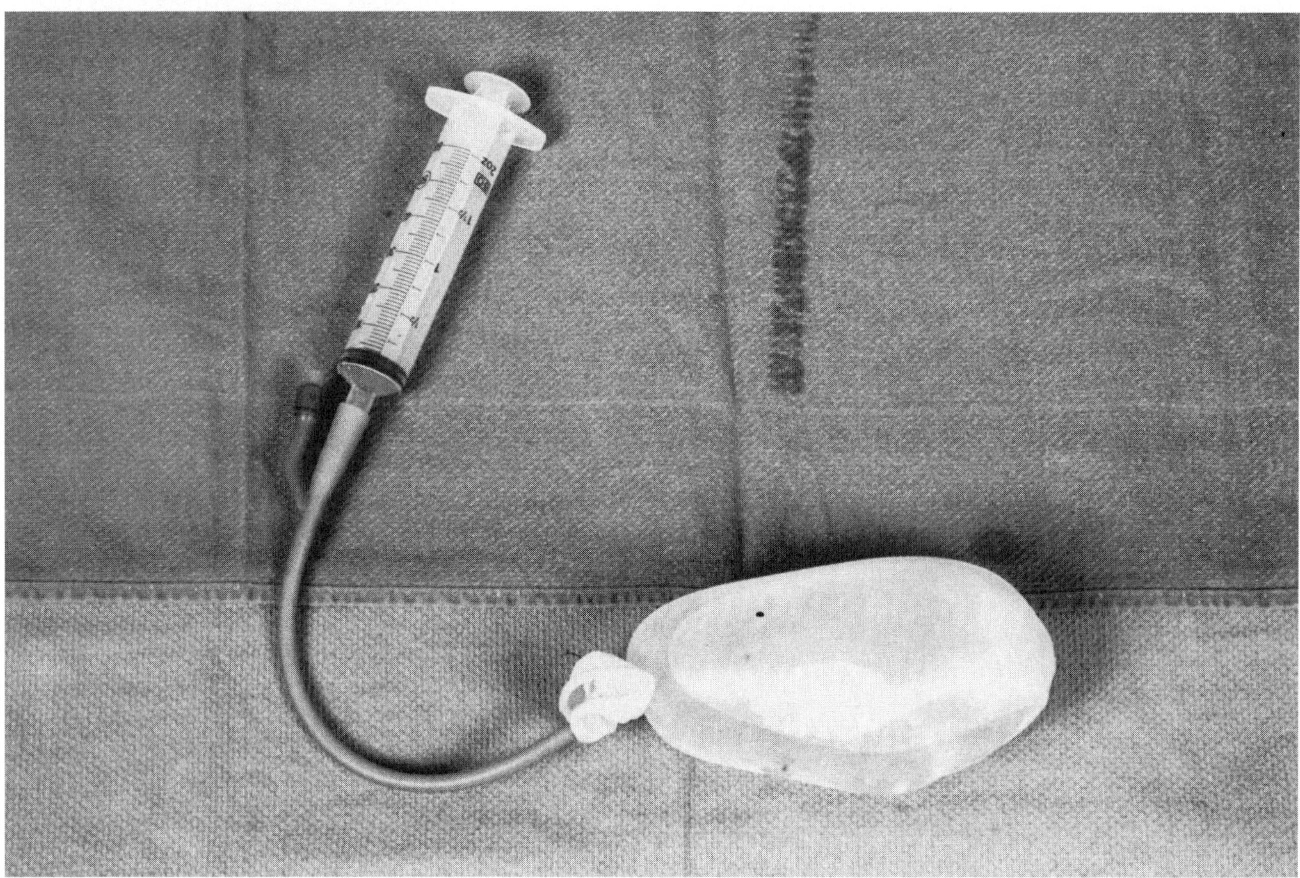

Fig. 16.7. Properitoneal balloon dissector.

Surgical Technique

The patient is placed supine, and the abdominal skin is prepared with disinfectant and draped in a sterile manner. A Foley catheter is placed per urethra and connected to continuous drainage during surgery. A midline suprapubic incision is made from the umbilicus to the symphysis pubis. The skin, subcutaneous tissue, and linea alba are incised. Rectus abdominis muscles are retracted laterally from the midline. Underlying fascia transversalis is opened to expose the retropubic space. In patients with prostate cancer, we start lymphadenectomy on the side ipsilateral to the cancer on preoperative biopsy. Laterally, the external iliac vein is exposed aided by retracting the lateral wall with a medium Richardson or Israel retractor and bluntly pushing the parietal peritoneum off the lateral pelvic wall. The spermatic cord with vas deferens is retracted above and laterally and does not have to be divided. A Deaver retractor is placed between the bladder and the hypogastric arterial location, retracting the tissues at this junction in a superior direction.

Lymphadenectomy is begun by dissecting the tissues along the superomedial margin of the external iliac vein in a subadventitial plane (Fig. 16.3). The distal limit of the dissection is the node of Cloquet that lies between the external iliac vein, Cooper's ligament, and the superior pubic ramus. Tissues containing the node at this junction are carefully dissected, placing a hemoclip at the depth to close the afferent lymphatics (Fig. 16.4). Dissecting proximally along the vein, the accessory obturator vein often comes into view and can be saved or divided between 3-0 silk ligatures. The dissected external iliac vein is now retracted laterally with the vein retractor, and the fibrofatty lymphatic tissue is dissected in continuity off the obturator internus muscle at the lateral pelvic wall. At this stage, the dissection dips down toward the endopelvic fascia, and the obturator nerve is defined by sweeping the forceps up and down in the direction of the nerve. The obturator vessels coursing posteroinferiorly may have to be divided between ligatures (Fig. 16.5). The strip of lymph nodal tissue, the so-called obturator package, is held up with Russian forceps and dissected proximally toward the angle between hypogastric artery and external iliac vein. At this corner, the modified pelvic lymphadenectomy specimen is disconnected after placing a hemoclip (Fig. 16.6). Throughout the procedure, hemoclips are used generously to control lymphatics. Unless necessitated by synchronous prostatectomy or cystectomy, a drain is not used solely for pelvic lymph node dissection. The wound is closed in layers.

Complications

Overall incidence of complications after open pelvic lymphadenectomy varies at around 22%. Wound complications such as

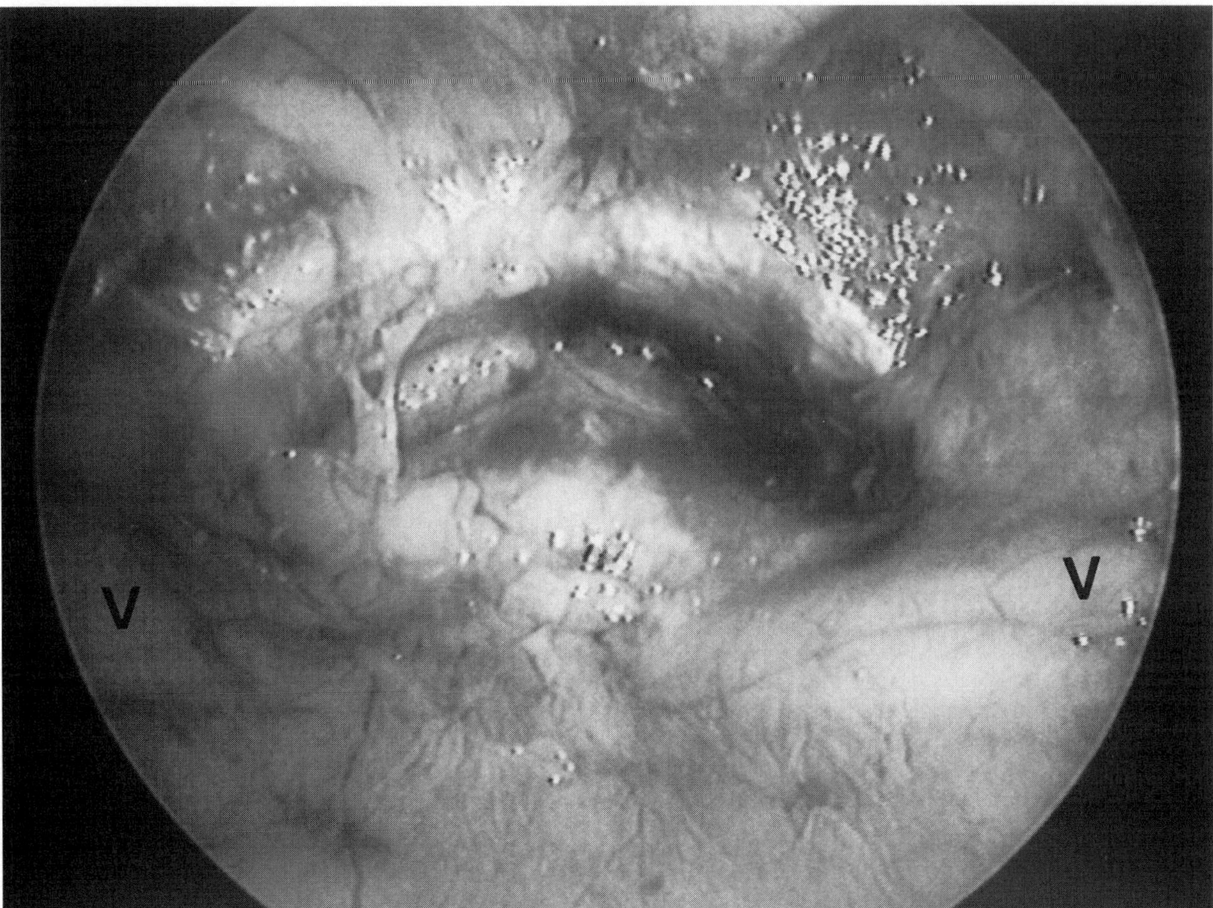

Fig. 16.8. Laparoscopic view of pelvis after balloon dissection. V: external iliac vein.

infection, hematoma, and dehiscence occurred in 3 to 26% of patients (27). Deep venous thrombosis and consequent pulmonary embolism constitute the most serious and often life-threatening complications. The use of intermittent pneumatic compression and additional prophylactic measures in susceptible patients helps reduce the risks of thromboembolic events.

Symptomatic lymphoceles have been reported in 5.5 to 8.4% of patients after extraperitoneal open pelvic lymphadenectomy (41, 42). Meticulous use of hemoclips to occlude small, potentially leaking afferent lymphatics is emphasized in prevention of lymphoceles. Prophylactic use of minidose heparin has been associated with a higher incidence of lymphoceles. Asymptomatic incidentally discovered lymphoceles should be followed conservatively with serial ultrasound studies. Symptomatic lymphoceles and those pressing on the ureters, pressing on the bladder, or causing distal edema from venous or lymphatic obstructions should be drained by percutaneous aspiration. Lymphoceles recurring after such aspiration are best managed by laparoscopic-intraperitoneal marsupialization (43). Prolonged lymph leak should be prevented by careful lymphostasis with hemoclips. Incidence of genital, prepubic, and lower extremity chronic lymphedema has been reduced to a great extent since the institution of the limited template lymphade-

nectomy preserving the lymphatic vessels over and lateral to the iliac arteries. Rare complications such as major bleeding from injury to the external iliac vessels, bladder perforations, ureteral injury, and obturator nerve injury have been reported, emphasizing the need for careful attention to surgical technique.

LAPAROSCOPIC PELVIC LYMPHADENECTOMY

As laparoscopic technology continues to make inroads into the urologic surgical arena, laparoscopic pelvic lymphadenectomy remains the most common application of laparoscopy in urology. Endoscopic lymph node dissection was pioneered by Hald and Rasmussen, who first used mediastinoscopic technique for pelvic lymph node sampling (44). Querleu et al. used the laparoscopic technique to dissect pelvic lymph nodes in patients with cervical cancer (45). Later, the laboratory work of Winfield et al. (46) and clinical report of Schuessler et al. (47) established the use of laparoscopic lymph node dissection in the staging of prostate, bladder, and penile cancer.

The primary advantage of laparoscopic pelvic lymph node dissection is in reducing patient morbidity by avoiding an open

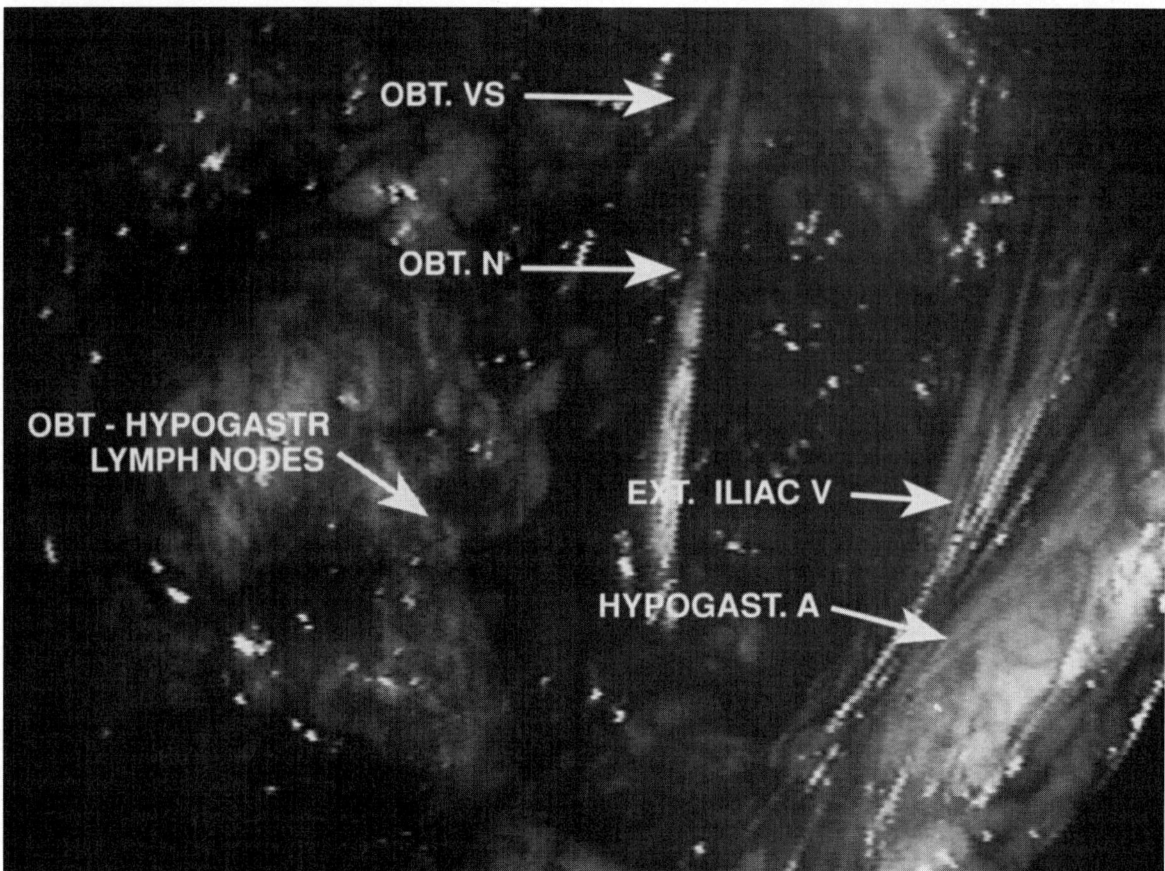

Fig. 16.9. Extraperitoneal laparoscopic lymphadenectomy on the right side.

abdominal incision. It is therefore ideally indicated for staging patients who have elected radiation therapy or perineal prostatectomy as their primary treatment (48). In patients prepared for radical retropubic prostatectomy, laparoscopic lymphadenectomy may be recommended in selected instances where there is a high probability of lymphatic metastases. Revelation of nodal metastases will preclude radical prostatectomy. Therefore, our selection criteria for staging laparoscopic lymph node dissection in prostate cancer patients include one or more of the following features: a higher grade lesion with a Gleason score of 7 or more; higher volume stage B2, C, or D0 disease; or a serum PSA level of 20 ng/mL or more.

Surgical Technique of Transperitoneal Laparoscopic Pelvic Lymphadenectomy

With the patient under general endotracheal anesthesia, a Foley catheter is placed for continuous bladder drainage. Pneumoperitoneum is established with carbon dioxide using the closed Veress needle or open Hasson cannula technique. Aside from the 11-mm camera port at the umbilicus, three other working ports are established—a 5-mm port in each iliac fossa lateral to the edge of the rectus abdominis muscle and another 11-mm port midway between the umbilicus and symphysis pubis. The patient is placed in steep Trendelenburg position to displace the intestine away from the pelvis. Using graspers and laparoscopic scissors, the parietal peritoneum is incised just lateral to the medial umbilical ligament. The vas deferens coursing laterally is electrocoagulated and divided. Lifting the lateral edge of the incised peritoneum, the external iliac vein is identified. The medial edge of the external iliac vein is stripped of all the fibrofatty tissue from the level of the common iliac artery to the femoral canal distally. The distal strip of fibrofatty tissue is disconnected from the femoral canal, and with further dissection off the lateral pelvic wall below the external iliac vein, the obturator nerve is identified. The nodal package is stripped off the obturator nerve carrying proximally toward the hypogastric artery. The proximal end of the dissection is disconnected after applying a hemoclip. The specimen is removed intact through the 11-mm suprapubic port. On the left side, the sigmoid colon needs to be released from its peritoneal bands to gain better access to the left external iliac vein. Hemostasis is checked after lowering the pneumoperitoneum insufflation pressure. Pneumoperitoneum is vented, and the port sites are closed by separately suturing the fascial layer and the skin.

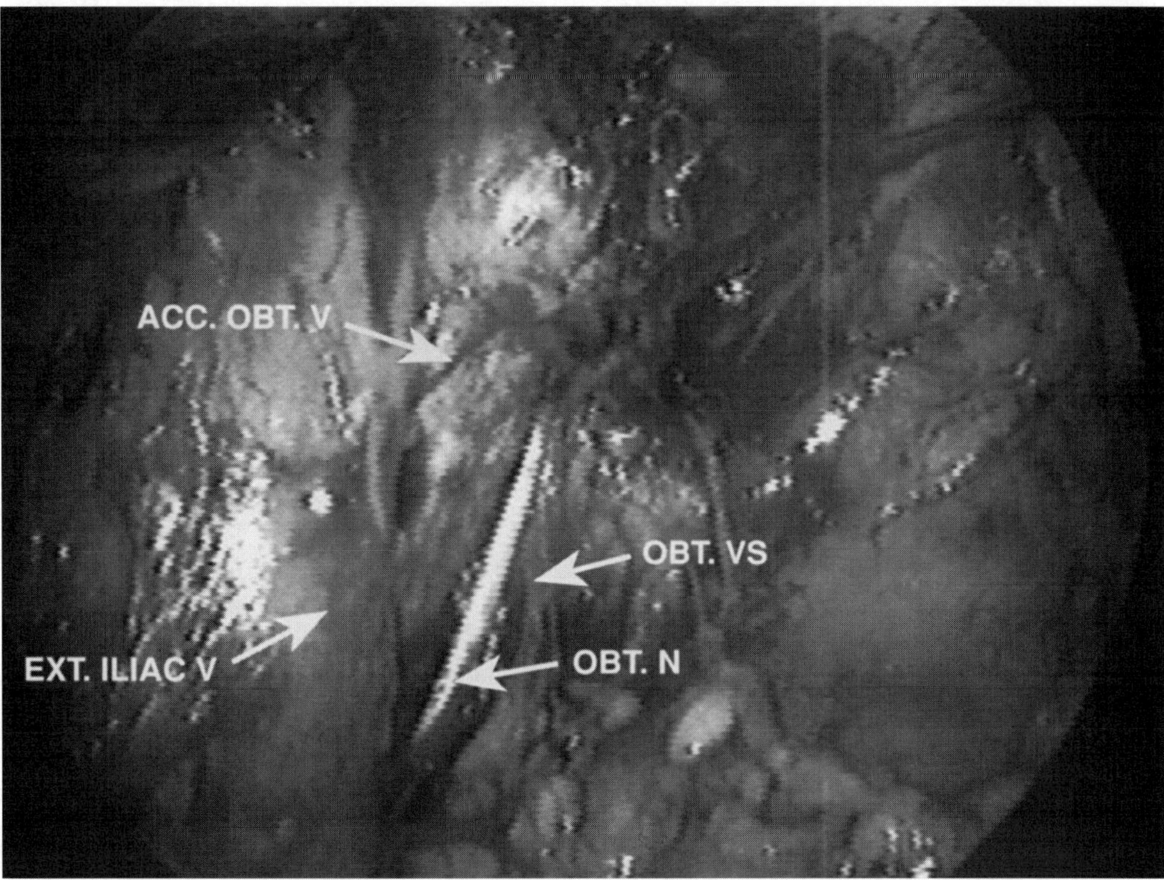

Fig. 16.10.   Extraperitoneal laparoscopic lymphadenectomy on the left side.

EXTRAPERITONEAL LAPAROSCOPIC STAGING PELVIC LYMPHADENECTOMY (49)

The advantages of the extraperitoneal over the intraperitoneal approach to staging lymphadenectomy are already evident from the comparative analysis on open pelvic lymphadenectomy patients (50). Morbidities such as ileus, intraperitoneal adhesions, or intestinal obstruction can be obviated by avoiding entry into the peritoneal cavity. Cumulative analysis by Kavoussi et al. revealed a 15% incidence of complications for 372 patients in whom intraperitoneal laparoscopic pelvic lymph node dissection was done (51). In their series of laparoscopic lymphadenectomy, Kerbl et al. reported a 13.3% incidence of major complications, most of which occurred in their initial cases, thus implying that some of these complications could be attributed to the learning of a new technique (52). However, certain risks of intraperitoneal insufflation needle and trocar insertion, such as bowel, bladder, or vascular injuries, are inherent with this approach. Our interest in developing the extraperitoneal approach to laparoscopic pelvic lymphadenectomy was generated by these reports of complications associated with the intraperitoneal approach and was further fueled by the retroperitoneoscopic balloon dissection technique reported by Gaur for laparoscopic surgeries for upper urinary organs (53).

Surgical Technique of Extraperitoneal Laparoscopic Pelvic Lymphadenectomy

The patient's position and preparation are similar to those in the transperitoneal approach described previously. Through a small midline incision below the umbilicus, the linea alba and underlying fascia transversalis are opened. The extraperitoneal retropubic space is developed by digital dissection. A distending balloon device prepared by tying a rubber glove over an 18 F catheter (Fig. 16.7) is introduced into the extraperitoneal space and distended by hand, injecting about 1200 mL of saline through the catheter. The saline is then drained and the catheter with the deflated glove is removed. The 0° laparoscopic lens in a 10-mm trocar is introduced through the incision. High- flow carbon dioxide insufflation is continued to maintain pneumoretroperitoneum of 12 to 14 mm Hg pressure. Three additional accessory ports are placed as described previously. The anatomic landmarks of the symphysis pubis, superior pubic rami, urinary bladder, and laterally the pulsations of external iliac vessels are easily discernible (Fig. 16.8).

Laparoscopic dissection is begun at the junction of the superior pubic ramus and external iliac vein. Here the node of Cloquet is grasped and dissected. Continuing laterally, the medial edge of the external iliac vein is further defined up to the common iliac artery. All the fibrofatty and lymphatic tissue medial to the vein is dissected medially and inferiorly, clearing the surface of the obturator internus muscle overlying the lateral wall of the true pelvis. Continuing inferiorly, the obturator nerve is identified and dissected carefully. The strip of lymph nodal tissue starting distally with the node of Cloquet followed by the obturator nodes is held up with laparoscopic spoon forceps, and more proximal dissection is done to include the hypogastric nodes in the package (Fig. 16.9). At this stage, the camera is often moved to the suprapubic port to obtain better visibility and a lateral perspective of the hypogastric area. Similar dissection is done on the contralateral side (Fig. 16.10). The lymphadenectomy on the left side is comparatively easier than during the transperitoneal approach because intraperitoneal dissection and mobilization of the sigmoid colon are unnecessary.

Therefore, we now recommend an extraperitoneal laparoscopic lymph node dissection for staging clinically localized prostatic carcinoma in selected patients with a high probability of lymph nodal metastases based on their clinical stage, PSA, and histologic grade. Several reports comparing the laparoscopic pelvic lymphadenectomy with standard open extraperitoneal pelvic lymphadenectomy have established that the former is minimally invasive with shorter hospital stays, shorter convalescent times, better cosmesis, and equal effectiveness in the completeness of dissection of the node-bearing area (52, 54).

The technologic advances in the fields of imaging, scintigraphy, and biochemical markers threaten the need for invasive surgical procedures for lymph nodal evaluation. Multivariate decision analysis using several parameters now aids us in selecting cases where pelvic lymphadenectomy can be omitted. The use of pelvic lymphadenectomy continues to be curtailed and its future remains uncertain.

REFERENCES

1. Paulson D, Okada K, Yoshida O, et al. Lymph node staging of potentially curable prostatic carcinoma. Prog Clin Biol Res 1990;357:167.
2. Kramer SA, Cline WA Jr, Farnham R, et al. Prognosis of patients with stage D-1 prostatic adenocarcinoma. J Urol 1981;125:817.
3. Prout GR Jr, Heaney JA, Griffin PP, et al. Nodal involvement as a prognostic indicator in patients with prostatic carcinoma. J Urol 1980;124:226.
4. Smith JA Jr, Haynes TH, Middleton RG. Impact of external irradiation on local symptoms and survival free of disease in patients with pelvic lymph node metastases from adenocarcinoma of the prostate. J Urol 1984;131:705.
5. Gervasi LA, Mata S, Easley JD, et al. Prognostic significance of lymph nodal metastasis in prostate cancer. J Urol 1989;142:332.
6. Cline WA, Kramer SA, Farnham R, et al. Impact of pelvic lymphadenectomy in patients with prostatic adenocarcinoma. Urology 1981;17:129.
7. Cheng CW, Bergstralh EJ, Zincke H. Stage D1 prostate cancer: a non-randomized comparison of conservative treatment options versus radical prostatectomy. Cancer 1993;71(Suppl):996.
8. Rutishauer G, Hering F. Lymph node staging in potentially curable prostatic carcinoma. Prog Clin Biol Res 1988;269:227.
9. Neuwirth H, deKernion JB, Stenzl A, et al. Stage D1 carcinoma of the prostate: radical prostatectomy with early endocrine therapy improves survival. 84th annual meeting of the American Urological Association, Dallas, 1989. Abstract no. 563.
10. Kramolowsky EV. The value of testosterone deprivation in stage D1 carcinoma of the prostate. J Urol 1988;139:1242.
11. Winkler HZ, Rainwater LM, Myers RP, et al. Stage D1 prostatic adenocarcinoma: significance of nuclear DNA ploidy patterns studied by flow cytometry. Mayo Clin Proc 1988;63:103.
12. Freiha FS, Bagshaw MA. Carcinoma of the prostate: results of post-irradiation biopsy. Prostate 1984;5:19.
13. Paulson DF, Cline WA, Hinshaw W. Uro-Oncology Research Group: extended field radiation therapy versus delayed hormonal therapy in node-positive prostatic adenocarcinoma. J Urol 1982;127:935.
14. VanPoppel H, Ameye F, Oyen R, et al. Accuracy of combined computerized tomography and fine needle aspiration cytology in lymph node staging of localized prostatic carcinoma. J Urol 1994;151:1310.
15. Flanigan RC, Mohler JL, King CT, et al. Pre-operative lymph node evaluation in prostatic cancer patients who are surgical candidates: the role of lymphangiography and computerized tomography scanning with directed fine needle aspiration. J Urol 1985;134:84.
16. Wolf JS, Cher M, Dall'era M, et al. The use and accuracy of cross-sectional imaging and fine needle aspiration cytology for detection of pelvic lymph node metastases before radical prostatectomy. J Urol 1995;153:993.
17. Danella JF, deKernion JB, Smith RB, et al. The contemporary incidence of lymph node metastases in prostatic cancer: implications for laparoscopic lymph node dissection. J Urol 1993;149:1488.
18. Bluestein DL, Bostwick DG, Bergstralh EJ, et al. Eliminating the need for bilateral pelvic lymphadenectomy in select patients with prostatic cancer. J Urol 1994;151:1315.
19. Partin AW, Yoo J, Carter HB, et al. The use of prostate specific antigen, clinical stage and Gleason score to predict pathological stage in men with localized prostate cancer. J Urol 1993;150:110.
20. Bishoff JT, Reyes A, Thompson IM, et al. Pelvic lymphadenectomy can be omitted in selected patients with carcinoma of the prostate: development of a system of patient selection. Urology 1995;45:270.
21. Babaian RJ, Sayer J, Podoloff DA, et al. Radioimmunoscintigraphy of pelvic lymph nodes with [111]indium-labelled monoclonal antibody CYT-356. J Urol 1994;152:1952.
22. Raghavaiah NV, Jordan WP Jr. Prostatic lymphography. J Urol 1979;121:178.
23. Fisher H, Herr H, Sogani P, et al. Modified pelvic node dissection in patients undergoing ^{125}I implantation for carcinoma of the prostate. Presented at the 67th annual

meeting of the American Urological Association, Boston, 1981. Abstract no. 299.

24. Golimbu M, Morales P, Al-Askari S, et al. Extended pelvic lymphadenectomy for prostatic cancer. J Urol 1979;121:617.

25. Herr HW. Pelvic lymphadenectomy and iodine-125 implantation. In: Johnson DE, Boilean MA, eds. Genitourinary tumors: fundamental principles and surgical techniques. Orlando: Grune & Stratton, 1982:63.

26. Fowler JE Jr, Whitmore WF Jr. The incidence and extent of pelvic lymph node metastases in apparently localized prostatic cancer. Cancer 1981;47:2941.

27. McDowell GC, Johnson JW, Tenney DM, et al. Pelvic lymphadenectomy for staging clinically localized prostate cancer: indications, complications and results in 217 cases. Urology 1990;35:476.

28. Paulson DF. Uro-Oncology Research Group: the impact of current staging procedures in assessing disease extent of prostatic adenocarcinoma. J Urol 1979;121:300.

29. Skinner DG. Management of invasive bladder cancer: a meticulous pelvic node dissection can make a difference. J Urol 1982;128:34.

30. Stockle M, Alken P, Jacobi GH, et al. Hat die pelvine lymphadenecktomie in rahmen der radikalen zystektomie eine therapeutische bedentung? Verhandl Dtsch Gesell Urol 1986; 38:39.

31. Herr HW. Bladder cancer: pelvic lymphadenectomy revisited. J Surg Oncol 1988;37:242.

32. Skinner DG, Daniels JR, Russell CA, et al. The role of adjuvant chemotherapy following cystectomy for invasive bladder cancer: a prospective comparative trial. J Urol 1991; 145:459.

33. Stockle M, Meyenburg W, Wellek S, et al. Adjuvant polychemotherapy of nonorgan-confined bladder cancer after radical cystectomy revisited: long-term results of controlled prospective study and further clinical experience. J Urol 1995; 153:47.

34. Fradet Y, Chin JL, Carrier S, et al. Adjuvant MVAC chemotherapy after radical cystectomy for invasive bladder cancer: part 2. J Urol 1992;147:446. Abstract no. 934.

35. Raghavan D. Chemotherapy for advanced bladder cancer: "Midsummer Night's Dream" or "Much Ado about Nothing"? Br J Cancer 1990;62:337.

36. Kibel AS, Loughlin KR. Pathogenesis and prophylaxis of postoperative thromboembolic disease in urologic pelvic surgery. J Urol 1995;153:1763.

37. Igel TC, Barrett DM, Segura JW, et al. Perioperative and postoperative complications from bilateral pelvic lymphadenectomy and radical retropubic prostatectomy. J Urol 1987;137:1189.

38. Thomas PJ, Nurse DE, Deliveliotis C, et al. Cystoprostatectomy and substitution cystoplasty for locally invasive bladder cancer. Br J Urol 1992;70:40.

39. Vandendris M, Kutnowski M, Futeral B, et al. Prevention of postoperative deep vein thrombosis by low-dose heparin in open prostatectomy. Urol Res 1980;8:219.

40. Bigg SW, Catalona WJ. Prophylactic mini-dose heparin in patients undergoing radical retropubic prostatectomy: a prospective trial. Urology 1992;34:309.

41. Basinger GT, Gittes RF. Lymphocyst: ultrasound diagnosis and urologic management. J Urol 1975;114:740.

42. Sogani PC, Watson RC, Whitmore WF Jr. Lymphocele after pelvic lymphadenectomy for urologic cancer. Urology 1981;17: 39.

43. Gill IS, Munch LC, Lucas BA, et al. Transperitoneal marsupialization of lymphoceles: a comparison of open and laparoscopic techniques. Presented at the 89th annual meeting of the American Urological Association, San Francisco, May 14–19, 1994. Abstract no. 1077.

44. Hald T, Rasmussen F. Extraperitoneal pelvioscope: a new aid in staging of lower urinary tract tumors. a preliminary report. J Urol 1980;124:245.

45. Querleu D, Leblanc E, Castelain B. Laparoscopic pelvic lymphadenectomy in the staging of early carcinoma of the cervix. Am J Obstet Gynecol 1991;164:579.

46. Winfield HN, Donovan JF, See WA, et al. Urological laparoscopic surgery. J Urol 1991;146:941.

47. Schuessler WW, Vancaillie TG, Reich H, et al. Transperitoneal endosurgical lymphadenectomy in patients with localized prostate cancer. J Urol 1991;145:988.

48. Thomas R, Steele R, Smith R, et al. One-stage laparoscopic pelvic lymphadenectomy and radical perineal prostatectomy. J Urol 1994;152:1174.

49. Das S, Tashima M. Extraperitoneal laparoscopic staging pelvic lymph node dissection. J Urol 1994;151:1321.

50. Freiha FS, Salzman J. Surgical staging of prostatic cancer: transperitoneal versus extraperitoneal lymphadenectomy. J Urol 1977;118:616.

51. Kavoussi LR, Sosa E, Chandhoke P, et al. Complications of laparoscopic lymph node dissection. J Urol 1993;149:322.

52. Kerbl K, Clayman RV, Petros JA, et al. Staging pelvic lymphadenectomy for prostate cancer: a comparison of laparoscopic and open techniques. J Urol 1993;150:396.

53. Gaur DD. Laparoscopic operative retroperitoneoscopy: use of a new device. J Urol 1992;148:1137.

54. Parra RO, Andrus C, Boullier J. Staging laparoscopic pelvic lymph node dissection: comparison of results with open pelvic lymphadenectomy. J Urol 1992;147:875.

17

Radical Retropubic Prostatectomy

Fuad S. Freiha

For the right patient, this is the right operation, but it needs to be done correctly.

PATRICK C. WALSH

INTRODUCTION

During the past decade, the incidence of prostate cancer in U.S. men increased by 150%—76,000 new cases in 1984 compared with 200,000 new cases in 1994 (1, 2). This steep rise is, at least, partly due to screening with prostate-specific antigen (PSA). One of the major effects of screening for prostate cancer is the migration of its stage at diagnosis. More organ-confined disease is being diagnosed now than ever before (3, 4); therefore, more patients with potentially curable disease are available for the proponents of radical prostatectomy, which is considered by many to be the most effective treatment for men with localized prostate cancer.

Radical prostatectomy is the total removal of the prostate gland, seminal vesicles, and ampulla of the vasa deferentia and is accompanied by a limited pelvic lymphadenectomy. It can be accomplished by either a retropubic or a perineal approach. The choice of the approach is a matter of training, familiarity, surgical expertise, and personal preference. This chapter deals only with radical retropubic prostatectomy.

In 1945, Millin was the first to describe the retropubic approach to the prostate gland (5). Since then, several different techniques of radical retropubic prostatectomy using this approach have been described (6–8) and modified (9–11) to make the operation more anatomical and give it definite advantages over the perineal procedure. These advantages include fewer rectal injuries, lower rates of postoperative incontinence, and a concomitant access to the pelvic lymph nodes.

Although radical prostatectomy was always considered by many to be the most effective treatment for the patient with organ-confined prostate cancer, it never gained universal acceptance because of its associated morbidity, namely impotence and incontinence, which influenced patients to choose and physicians to recommend alternate treatments such as radiation therapy. During the past decade, however, two major developments took place to make the operation more popular and more acceptable to patient and physician alike. The first is the high rate of failure of radiation therapy to sterilize local disease (12). The second is the modifications in technique introduced by Walsh et al. (13) to preserve sexual function, i.e., the nerve-sparing radical prostatectomy.

This chapter discusses some pertinent aspects of the surgical anatomy of the prostate and adjacent structures, selection criteria used to recommend the operation, the concept of nerve sparing, and a technique of radical retropubic prostatectomy.

SURGICAL ANATOMY

The extraperitoneal pelvic cavity is lined by the endopelvic fascia; the parietal leaf covers the levator ani muscles and the visceral leaf covers the lateral aspect of the prostate, seminal vesicles, and bladder. The junction of the parietal and visceral leaves is the most dependent and distal point in the pelvic cavity. An anterior condensation of fibers at this junction form the puboprostatic ligaments that insert on the distal undersurface of the symphysis pubis (Fig. 17.1). Incising the puboprostatic ligaments drops the prostate away from the symphysis pubis and exposes the dorsal vein complex.

The bulk of the prostate gland lies distal to the endopelvic fascia. Incising this fascia at the junction of its two leaves (Fig. 17.1) exposes the lateral surface of the prostate gland and anterolateral rectal wall (Fig. 17.2). Here, the prostatic capsule is covered by a very fine fascia, the lateral periprostatic fascia, which continues posteriorly over the neurovascular bundle to become the lateral rectal fascia (Fig. 17.3) and distally over the membranous urethra to become the lateral periurethral fascia. Fibers from the levator ani muscles insert on the lateral periprostatic and periurethral fascia covering the apex of the prostate and urethra.

Separating the posterior surfaces of the prostate and seminal vesicles from the anterior rectal wall is Denonvilliers' fascia, the fibers of which thicken distally to become Denonvilliers' plate, which lies between the apex of the prostate and membranous urethra anteriorly and the rectum posteriorly (Fig. 17.4).

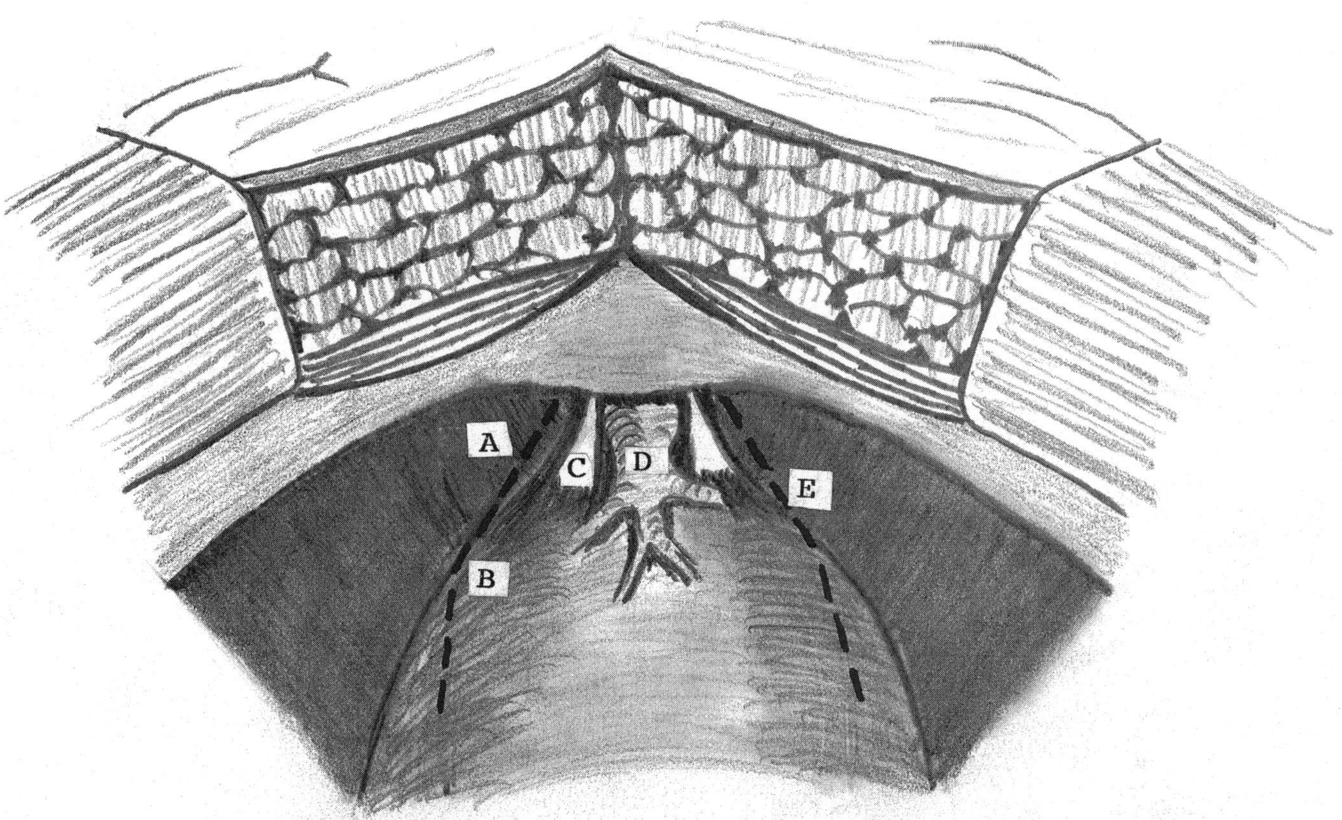

Fig. 17.1. View of the extraperitoneal pelvic cavity. A: Parietal leaf of endopelvic fascia; B: visceral leaf of endopelvic fascia; C: puboprostatic ligament; D: dorsal vein complex; E: site of incision in endopelvic fascia.

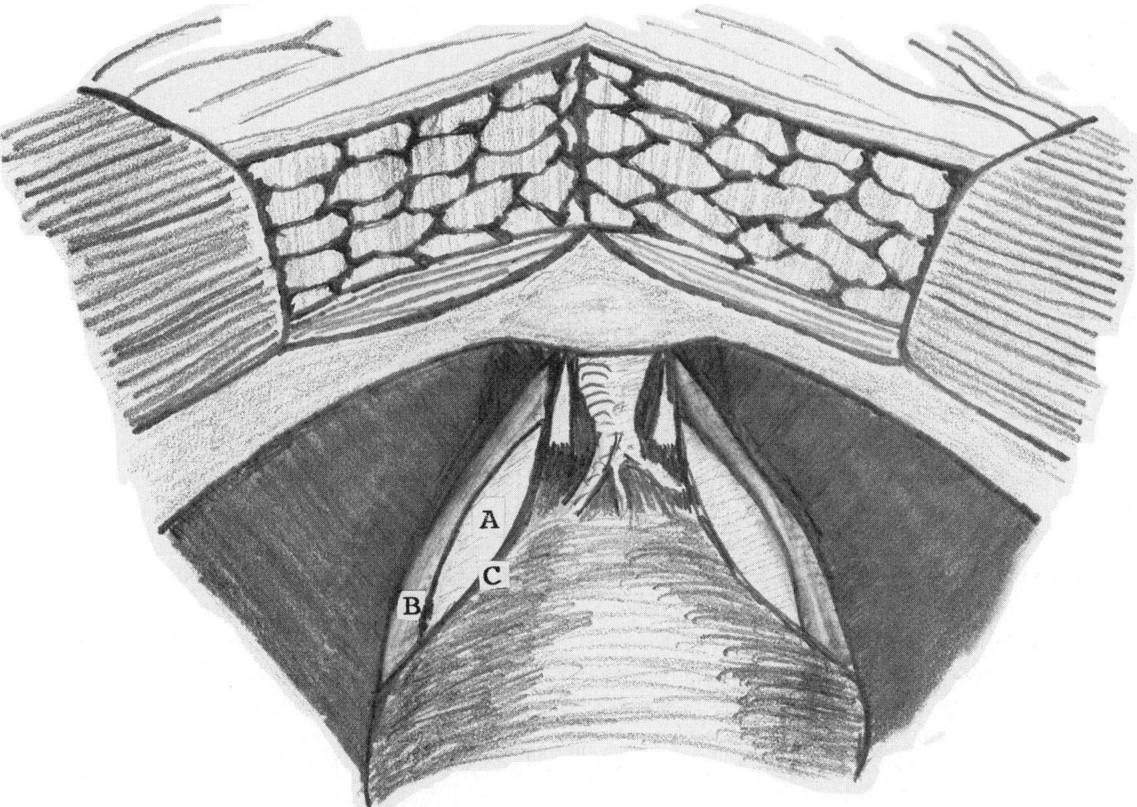

Fig. 17.2. Incised endopelvic fascia exposing the lateral aspect of the prostate gland (A) and anterolateral rectal wall (B). C: Medial cut edge of endopelvic fascia.

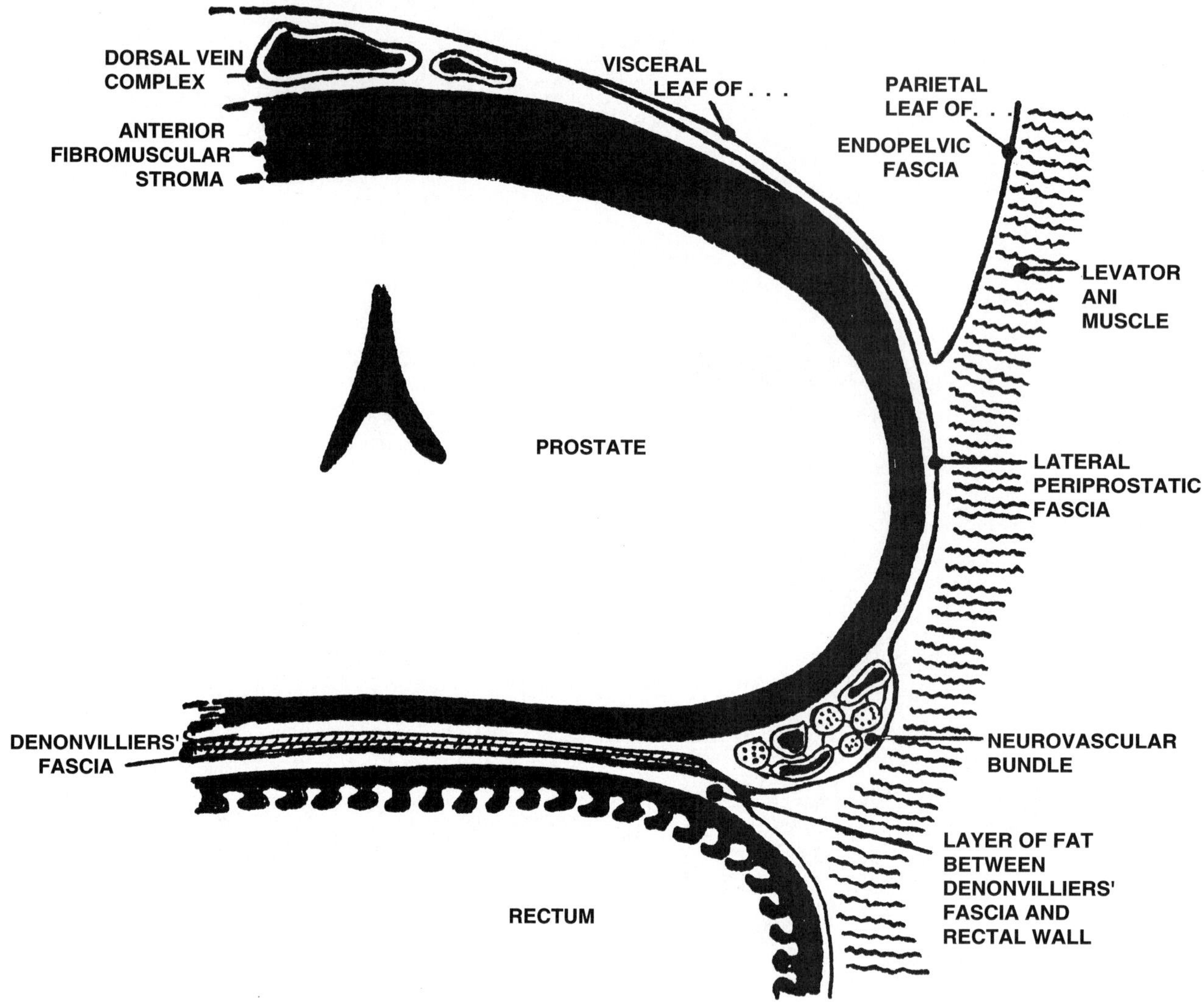

Fig. 17.3. Transverse section through the midprostate showing the different fascial layers and their relation to each other and to the prostate, neurovascular bundle, and rectum.

There is often a very thin layer of adipose tissue between Denonvilliers' fascia and the anterior rectal wall that lends ease to developing the plane between them.

Extending from the apex of the prostate distally along the membranous urethra on either side and within the lateral periurethral fascia are the prostatoischial ligaments of Mueller, often referred to as the urethral pillars. The neurovascular bundles lie just posterior to these ligaments.

There are two sets of vascular pedicles to the prostate—the superior and inferior. The superior pedicles are the largest of the two and they originate from branches of the inferior vesical vessels and penetrate the prostate posterolaterally at the prostatovesical junction. The inferior pedicles have only recently been recognized (14) and are vascular and nerve branches of the neurovascular bundle that penetrate the prostate at its apex (Fig. 17.5). They can be a source of a continuous bleeding during the operation.

The nerves in the neurovascular bundles arise from the pelvic plexus that provides autonomic innervation to the bladder, prostate, seminal vesicles, rectum, membranous urethra, and corpora cavernosa. The nerves to the corpora cavernosa control erections. It has been shown that preserving one of the neurovascular bundles may be enough to maintain erections.

The nerves from the pelvic plexus travel along the superior vascular pedicles of the prostate. Those that supply the prostate pierce the prostatic capsule with the vessels at the 5-o'clock and 7-o'clock positions. Those that supply the membranous urethra and corpora cavernosa leave the superior vascular pedicles with some vessels, curve distally, and run outside the prostatic capsule posterolaterally as the neurovascular bundles (Fig. 17.5). After giving branches that supply the prostatic apex and membranous urethra, forming what has recently been described as the inferior prostatic pedicle (14), the neurovascular bundles continue distally behind the prostatoischial ligaments of Mueller and posterolateral to the urethra until they pierce the urogenital diaphragm. From there the nerves go on to supply the corpora cavernosa.

The neurovascular bundles are closely adherent to the pros-

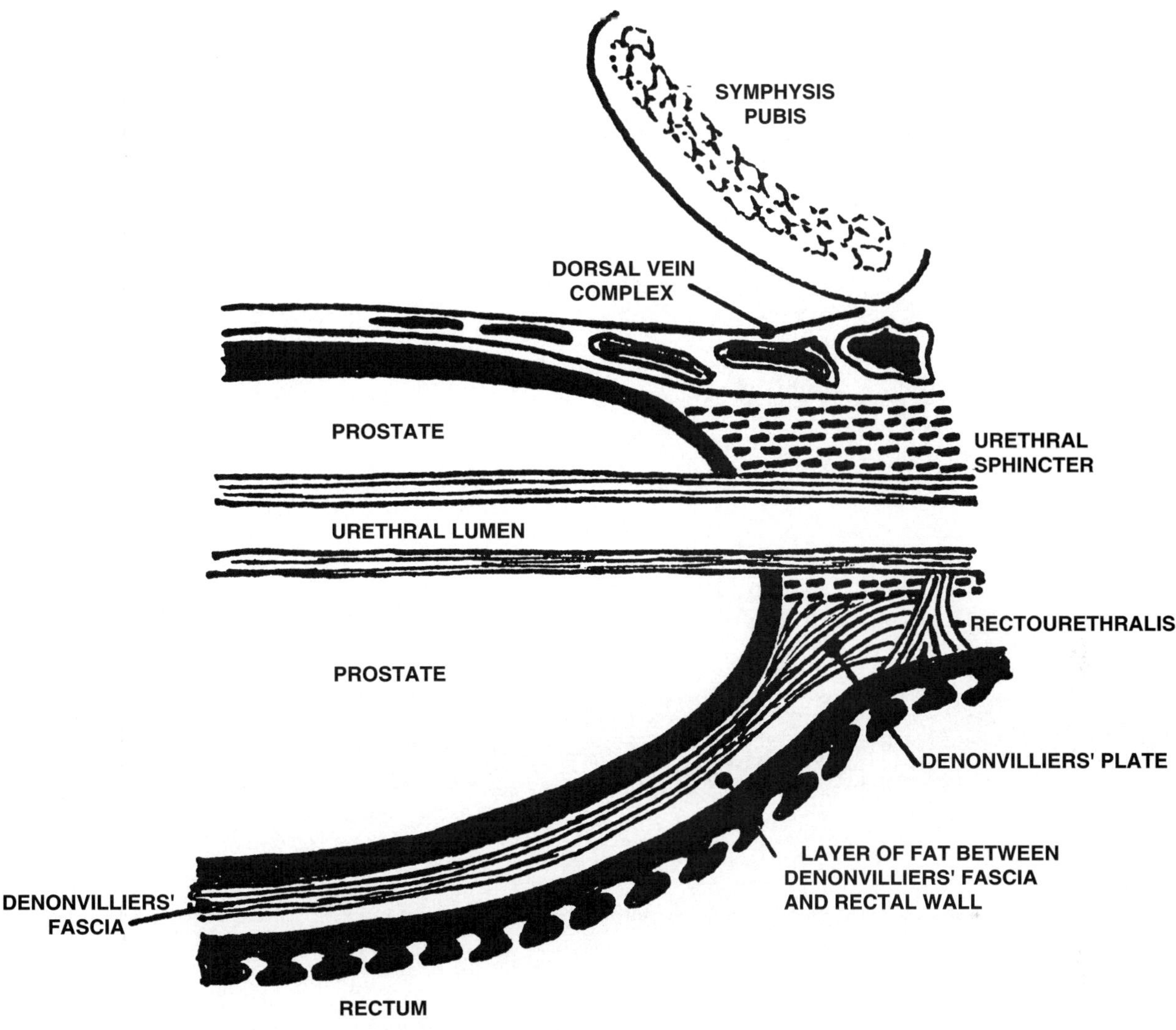

Fig. 17.4. Longitudinal section through the midprostate.

tatic capsule and often give branches that penetrate the capsule along their course. They are covered laterally by the lateral periprostatic and periurethral fascia and posteriorly by the lateral extension of Denonvilliers' fascia, which separates them from the anterior rectal wall (Fig. 17.3).

The anatomy of the dorsal vein complex and the venous plexus of Santorini is quite varied. Normally, the deep dorsal vein of the penis penetrates the urogenital diaphragm anterior to the urethra and divides into the following three major branches:

1. A superficial branch that lies between the two puboprostatic ligaments and divides into smaller branches that penetrate the anterior fibromuscular stroma, bladder neck, and bladder (Fig. 17.1), and
2. Two lateral branches that divide and form plexuses that cover most of the lateral aspect of the prostate and communicate with the obturator, pudendal, and inferior vesical veins.

The dorsal vein complex often wraps around the anterior half of the membranous urethra and may be the source of excessive blood loss during the operation.

Just behind the dorsal vein complex and beyond the apex of the prostate lies the external sphincter muscle, which encircles the anterior three fourths of the membranous urethra. It is thickest anteriorly and care must be exercised not to destroy its fibers during control of the dorsal vein complex.

PATIENT SELECTION

The ideal patient for a radical prostatectomy is a relatively young and healthy man with small-volume, organ-confined carcinoma.

Morphometric analyses of radical prostatectomy specimens studied by the step-section technique in the Department of Urology at Stanford show that the volume of cancer is the best predictor of the local extent of disease—the larger the volume,

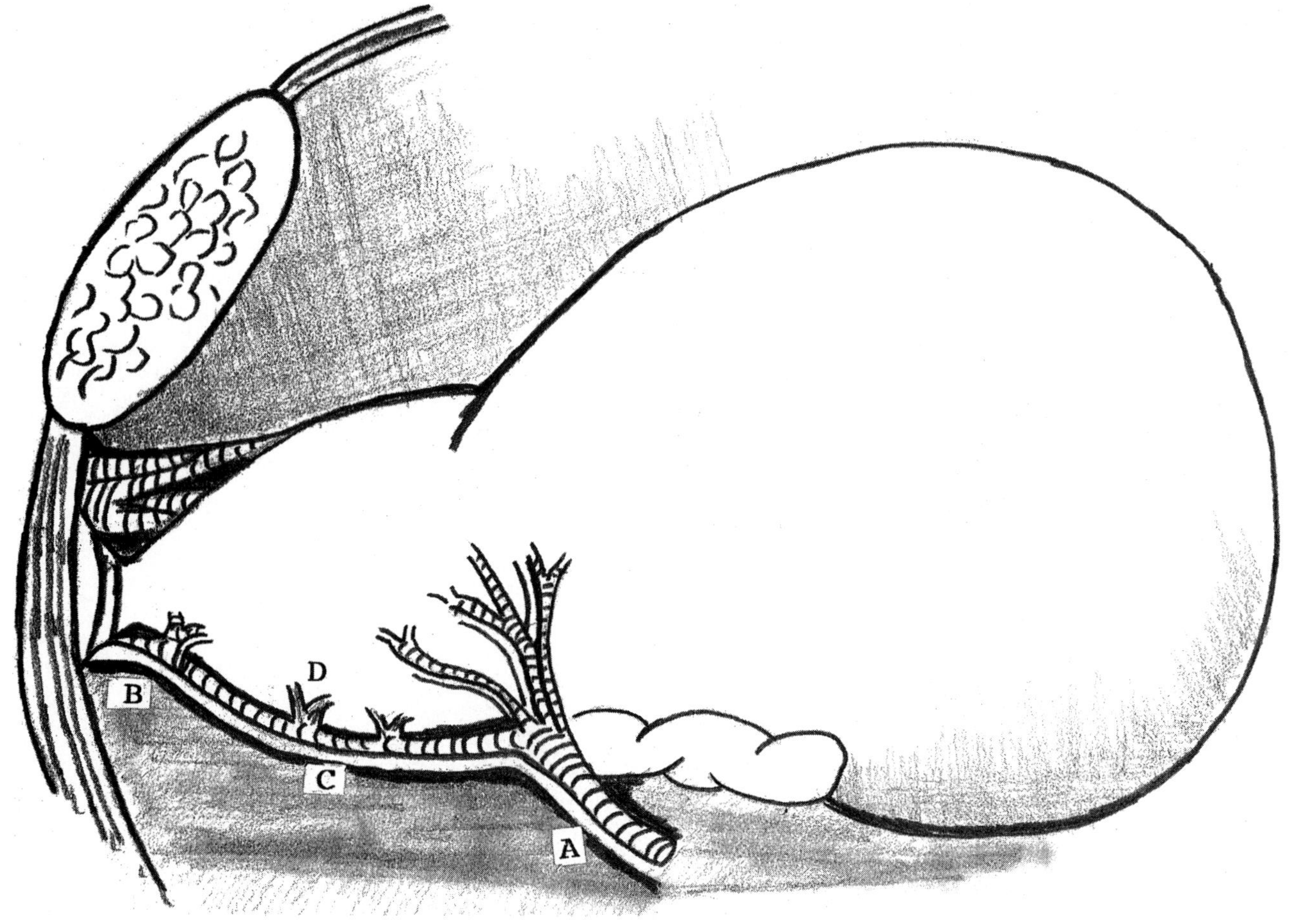

Fig. 17.5.   Lateral view of the prostate and bladder. A: Superior vascular pedicle; B: inferior vascular pedicle; C: neurovascular bundle; D: perforator veins.

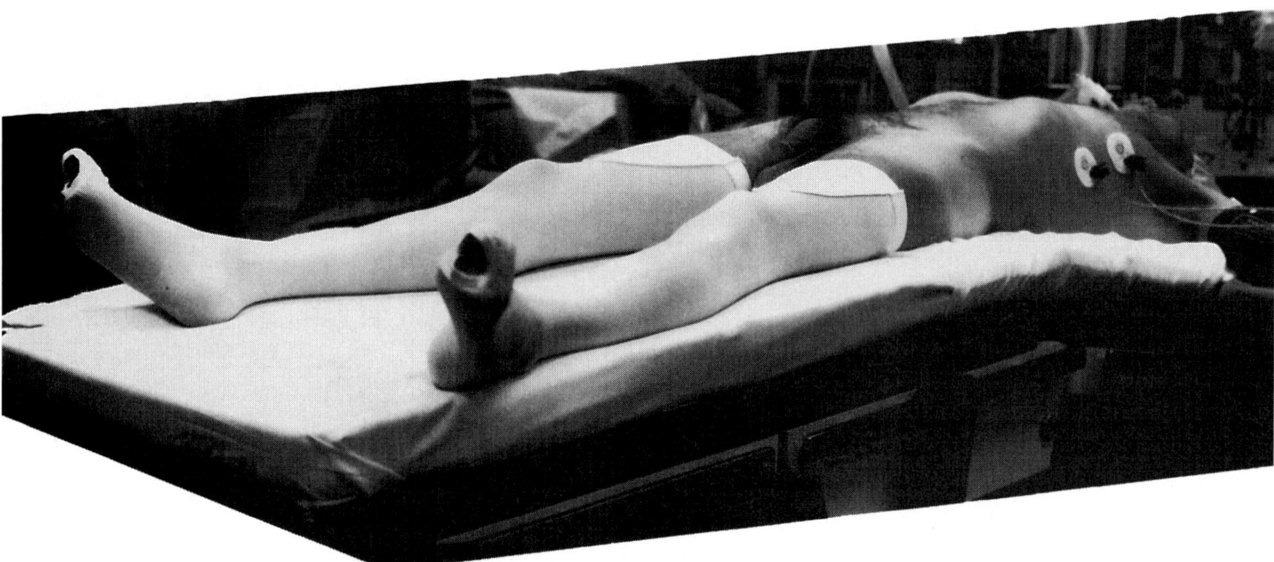

Fig. 17.6.   Position of the patient on the operating table. The legs are apart and the back is in minimal flexion.

Table 17.1.   Correlation Between Cancer Volume and Local Extent of Cancer in 376 Radical Prostatectomies

CANCER VOLUME (cc)	NO.	CAPSULAR PENETRATION (%)	SEMINAL VESICLE INVASION (%)	LYMPH NODE METASTASIS (%)
<4	201	39 (19)	6 (3)	5 (3)
4–12	132	96 (73)	21 (16)	17 (13)
>12	43	39 (91)	13 (30)	18 (42)
	—	—	—	—
Total	376	174 (46)	40 (11)	40 (11)

the higher the chance of finding capsular penetration, seminal vesicle invasion, and lymph node metastasis.

Observations in 376 consecutive radical prostatectomies performed by the author show that the great majority of cancers that are less than 4 cc in volume are totally confined to within the gland. Although some of these tumors do penetrate the capsule early in the course of the disease, they do not invade the seminal vesicles or metastasize to regional lymph nodes until they grow larger. The majority of cancers larger than 12 cc in volume are incurable by radical prostatectomy alone (Table 17.1).

Therefore, how do we estimate the volume of cancer preoperatively?

Digital Rectal Examination

Digital rectal examination (DRE) remains the best method for detecting prostate cancer. The findings at DRE are the basis for the clinical staging system now in use.

- A is impalpable cancer.
- B1 is cancer involving less than half of one lobe.
- B2 is involvement of more than half of one lobe.
- B3 is cancer in both lobes.
- C is cancer extending beyond the capsule laterally or into the seminal vesicles.

But how accurate is DRE in estimating cancer volume? In the author's experience, it is quite accurate at lower stages; 78% of patients with clinical stage B1 disease have tumors less than 4 cc in volume and only one patient has a tumor more than 12 cc. The accuracy drops as the stage advances (Table 17.2).

Table 17.2.   Correlation Between Clinical Stage and Cancer Volume in 290 Radical Prostatectomies Performed for Clinical Stage B Prostate Cancer

CLINICAL STAGE	NO.	CANCER VOLUME (cc)		
		<4	4–12	>12
B1	101	79 (78%)	21 (21%)	1 (1%)
B2	142	58 (41%)	68 (48%)	16 (11%)
B3	47	14 (30%)	15 (32%)	18 (38%)

A new TNM classification was recently developed to include those nonpalpable cancers that are discovered because of an elevated PSA and/or by transrectal ultrasound directed systematic biopsies (15).

Transrectal Ultrasound

There are great limitations to the usefulness and accuracy of transrectal ultrasound (TRUS) in volume measurements because of the lack of adequate resolution of ultrasounds and the fact that some cancers are isoechoic and that not all hypoechoic lesions are cancerous. Terris et al. compared the actual cancer volume in 110 radical prostatectomy specimens studied by the step-section technique with the cancer volume estimated by preoperative TRUS and found a significant discrepancy in 70% of cases. TRUS underestimated the cancer volume by an average of 2.4 to 3.5 cc, depending on the volume estimation method used (16).

Prostate-Specific Antigen

PSA determination has become a standard test in the evaluation and follow-up of patients with prostate cancer. It correlates well with the extent of disease. Multiple regression analysis shows that cancer volume is the main and only significant determinant of the serum levels of PSA (17). Can serum PSA levels, therefore, be used to estimate cancer volume?

Observations by the author in 356 untreated patients with clinically localized prostate cancer who were undergoing radical prostatectomy showed a strong and significant correlation between the preoperative serum level of PSA and cancer volume. The majority of patients with PSA levels of less than 10 ng/mL have tumors that are less than 3 cc in volume. As the PSA level increases, so does the tumor volume (Table 17.3).

A word of caution—because benign prostatic hypertrophy can elevate serum PSA levels, interpretation of PSA values in any patient should be coupled with the findings on DRE regarding the clinical stage of the disease, size of the prostate gland, and presence or absence of benign prostatic hypertrophy. For example, 1 of 114 patients listed in Table 17.3 under PSA levels of greater than 20 had a prostate cancer that was only 0.01 cc in volume. This patient had a serum PSA level of 28.6 ng/mL, clinical stage B1 disease, and a very large gland full of

Table 17.3.   Preoperative Prostate-Specific Antigen Levels and Cancer Volume in 356 Radical Prostatectomies

PSA (ng/ml)[a]	NO.	CANCER VOLUME (cc)			P VALUE
		AVERAGE	RANGE		
<10	140	2.91	0.1–17.7		<0.001
10–20	102	4.54	0.2–21.4		<0.001
>20	114	9.42	0.01–45.4		

[a] Yang method

benign prostatic hypertrophy that weighed 183 g. It is clear that this patient's high PSA was being driven by benign prostatic hypertrophy and not by the cancer.

In summary, the intraprostatic cancer volume determines the extent of disease, and every attempt should be made to estimate this volume before recommending treatment. Findings on DRE and the level of serum PSA should give a fairly accurate estimate of the cancer volume in the majority of patients. Using these parameters, it seems that the ideal patient for radical prostatectomy is the one who has clinical stage B1 disease and a serum PSA level of less than 10 ng/mL.

NERVE-SPARING

Penetration of prostatic carcinoma through the prostatic capsule is a phenomenon that occurs early in the course of the disease and depends a great deal on the ability of this cancer to invade and travel along perineural spaces, another early phenomenon in prostate cancer.

The nerve supply to the prostate forms a rich arborization of nerve branches that penetrate the capsule at two main sites—the superior and inferior pedicles (Fig. 17.5). From there, the nerves travel for a distance of 0.2 to 0.5 cm along the inner surface of the capsule before dividing into smaller branches that dip deep into the parenchyma. Where the nerves penetrate the capsule, they create defects that act as paths of least resistance along which cancer cells migrate and extend through the capsule into the periprostatic tissues (18). The nerve branches running along the superior pedicle arise from the neurovascular bundle at the base of the prostate and follow a fairly long course of 0.5 to 1.5 cm before penetrating the capsule. The nerves of the inferior pedicle leave the neurovascular bundle at the apex of the prostate and almost immediately penetrate the capsule. The margins of safety, therefore, may be better at the superior pedicle.

A study of 156 consecutive radical prostatectomy specimens removed for clinical stage B disease shows a 50% incidence of capsular penetration (78 of 156 specimens). In 95% of cases of capsular penetration (74 of 78 specimens), more than half of the total area of capsular penetration occurs along perineural spaces; in 50% of cases (39 of 78 specimens), extension through the prostatic capsule occurs entirely within perineural spaces. Of the 39 cases of capsule penetration along perineural spaces only, 21 are at the superior pedicle and 18 at the inferior pedicle. A positive surgical margin during nerve-sparing procedure occurred in 16 of 18 cases at the inferior pedicle and in only 7 of 21 cases at the superior pedicle. This difference is explained by the difference in length of the pedicles. The inferior pedicle is so short that it is almost impossible to preserve the neurovascular bundle at the apex of the prostate and have a safe margin (18).

The selection of patients for nerve-sparing radical prostatectomy, therefore, should be determined preoperatively based on the clinical stage of the disease and the site of cancer. Nerve-sparing procedures should be avoided on the side of the cancer, especially if the cancer is apical. Patients with clinical stage B3 disease should be advised against undergoing nerve-sparing procedures. The ideal patient for bilateral nerve-sparing is one with stage A disease where the cancer arises anteriorly and away from the course of the neurovascular bundles.

PREOPERATIVE PREPARATION

Patients are asked to donate 2 or 3 units of their own blood for autologous transfusion in case a transfusion is needed intraoperatively.

The patient is usually admitted to the hospital on the afternoon of the day before the operation. Patients with a history of or predilection for thromboembolic disease are immediately given prophylactic subcutaneous heparin at a dose of 5000 units every 12 hours, which is continued postoperatively until the patient is ambulating well. Cleansing soapsuds enemas are given until the returns are clear, followed by a neomycin enema the evening before and in the morning of the day of surgery. Prophylactic antibiotics are administered parenterally on call to the operating room and continued for two additional doses postoperatively. The choice of antibiotics is a matter of personal preference. Antiembolic stockings and sequential compression boots are routinely used.

SURGICAL TECHNIQUE

Position

Positioning the patient on the operating table is a matter of personal preference. The author places the patient in a supine position with the legs apart and minimal back extension (Fig. 17.6). Others prefer a gentle lithotomy position for easy access to the perineum in case pressure on the urethra is needed to facilitate the urethrovesical anastomosis. Access to the perineum can also be achieved by a frog-leg position or by placing the legs straight on arm boards and dropping the foot of the table.

Incision and Exposure

The retropubic space may be entered through either a midline, extraperitoneal vertical incision extending from the umbilicus to the symphysis pubis or through a Pfannenstiel's incision. The peritoneum is dissected off the pelvic wall to expose the iliac vessels from the common iliac bifurcation, proximally, to the beginning of the femoral canal, distally. Occasionally, the spermatic cord may limit the exposure. In such instances, the vas deferens is dissected free from the spermatic vessels and transected as it leaves the vessels and dips into the pelvis. The vessels are then dissected free of the posterior peritoneum and made to drop laterally. The bladder is retracted medially, further exposing the lateral wall of the pelvis in preparation for the pelvic lymphadenectomy. A 20 French Foley catheter is inserted into the bladder.

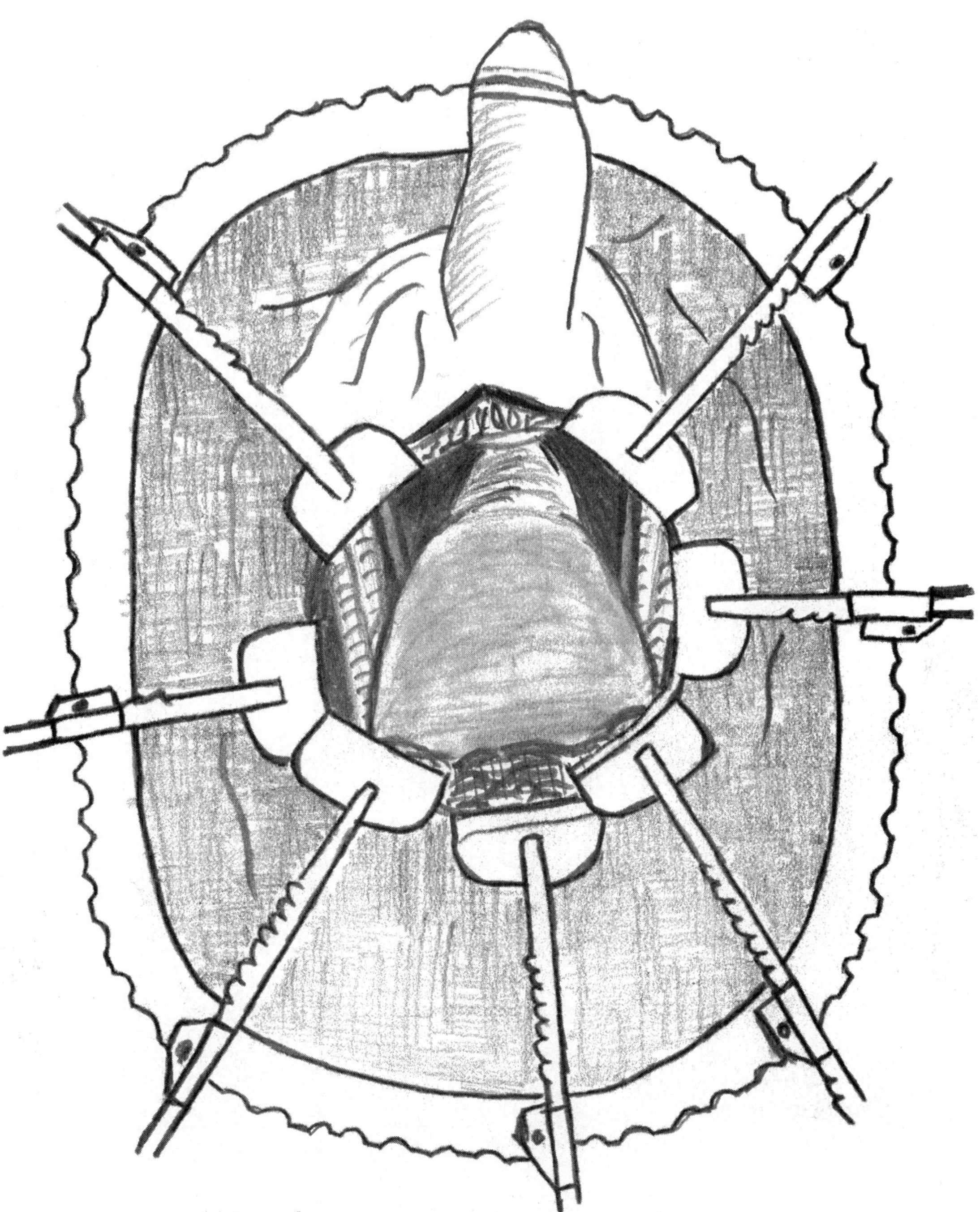

Fig. 17.7. Bookwalter retractor in place.

A retractor is placed to keep the edges of the incision and abdominal wall apart. In the author's experience, the Bookwalter ring retractor with its many versatile attachments is best suited to give an excellent exposure. It is placed as is shown in Figure 17.7.

All adipose tissue is lifted off to expose the endopelvic fascia, puboprostatic ligaments, and prostatovesical junction. The superficial branch of the dorsal vein complex is coagulated or tied and transected.

Extent of Pelvic Lymphadenectomy

When prostate cancer spreads into the lymph nodes, it does so in a systematic fashion without skip. Three echelons of nodes are involved first—the medial external iliacs, the obturator, and the hypogastric nodes. From there the cancer goes to the common iliac chain and then to the para-aortics. Because pelvic lymphadenectomy is not therapeutic, limiting the dissection to these three groups of nodes will give adequate information

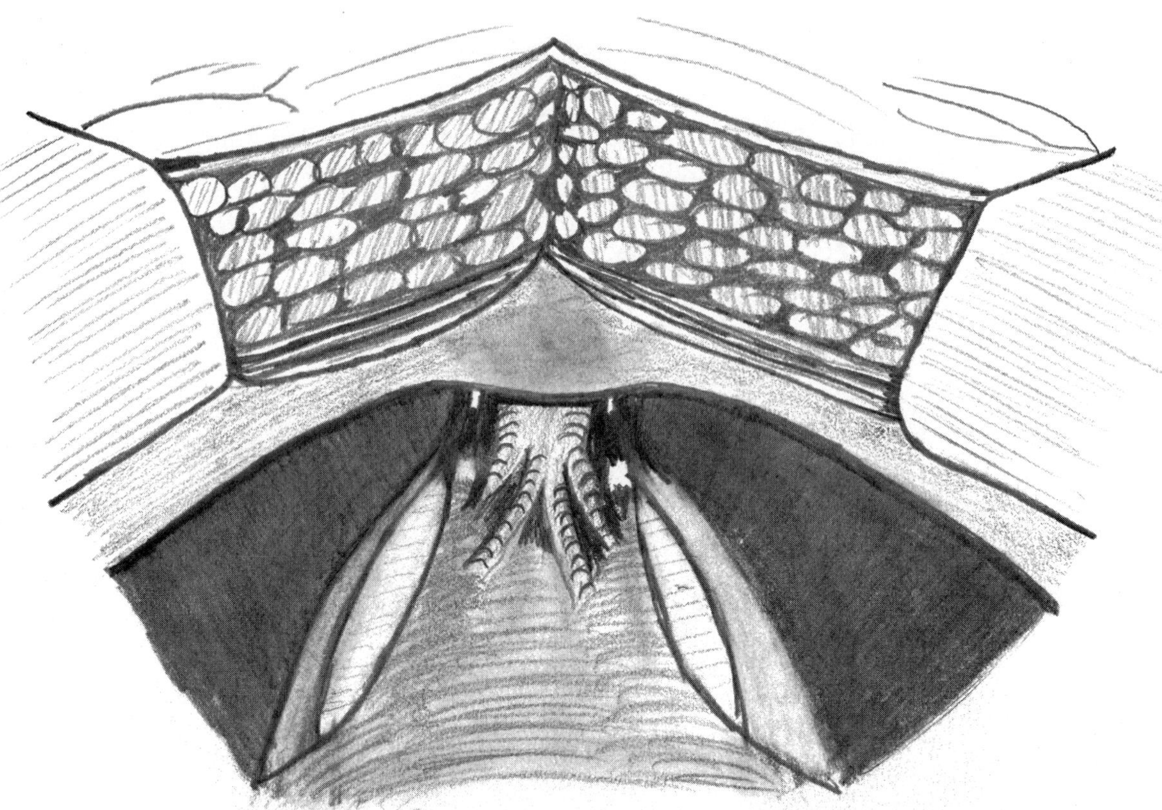

Fig. 17.8.   Transected puboprostatic ligaments exposing the dorsal vein complex.

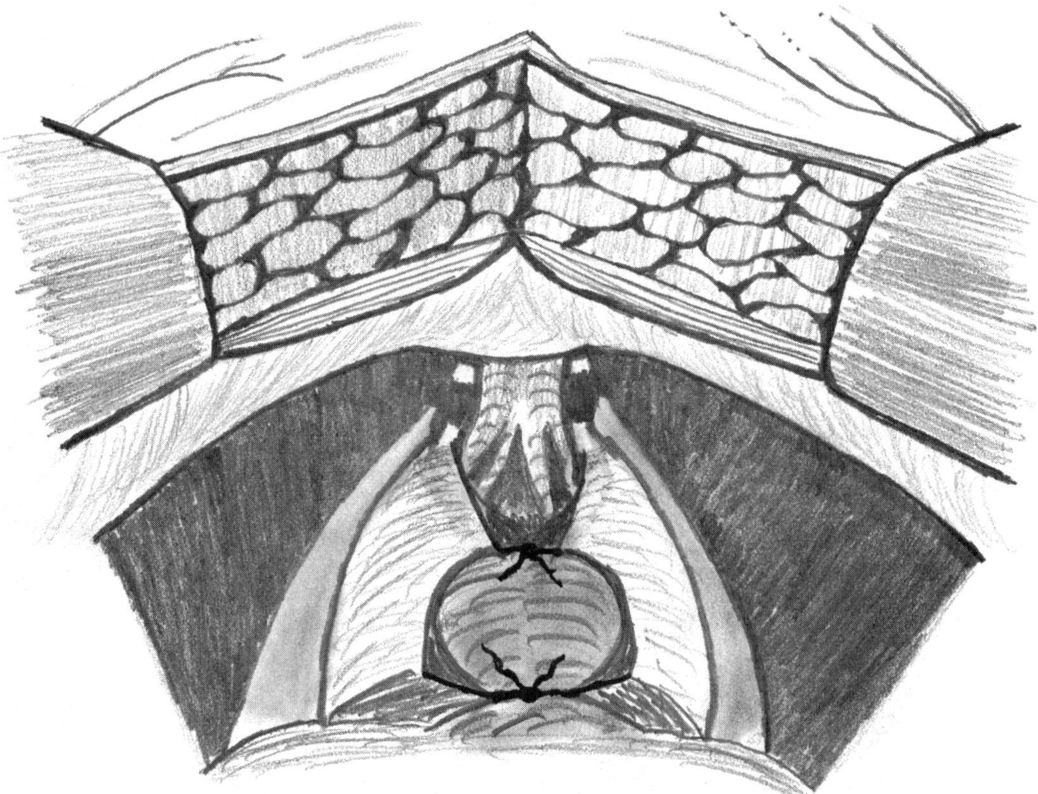

Fig. 17.9.   The medial cut edges of the endopelvic fascia are incorporated in two suture ligatures. This maneuver achieves three things: exposes the lateral surface of the prostate better, gathers the dorsal vein complex, and prevents back bleeding when the dorsal vein is transected.

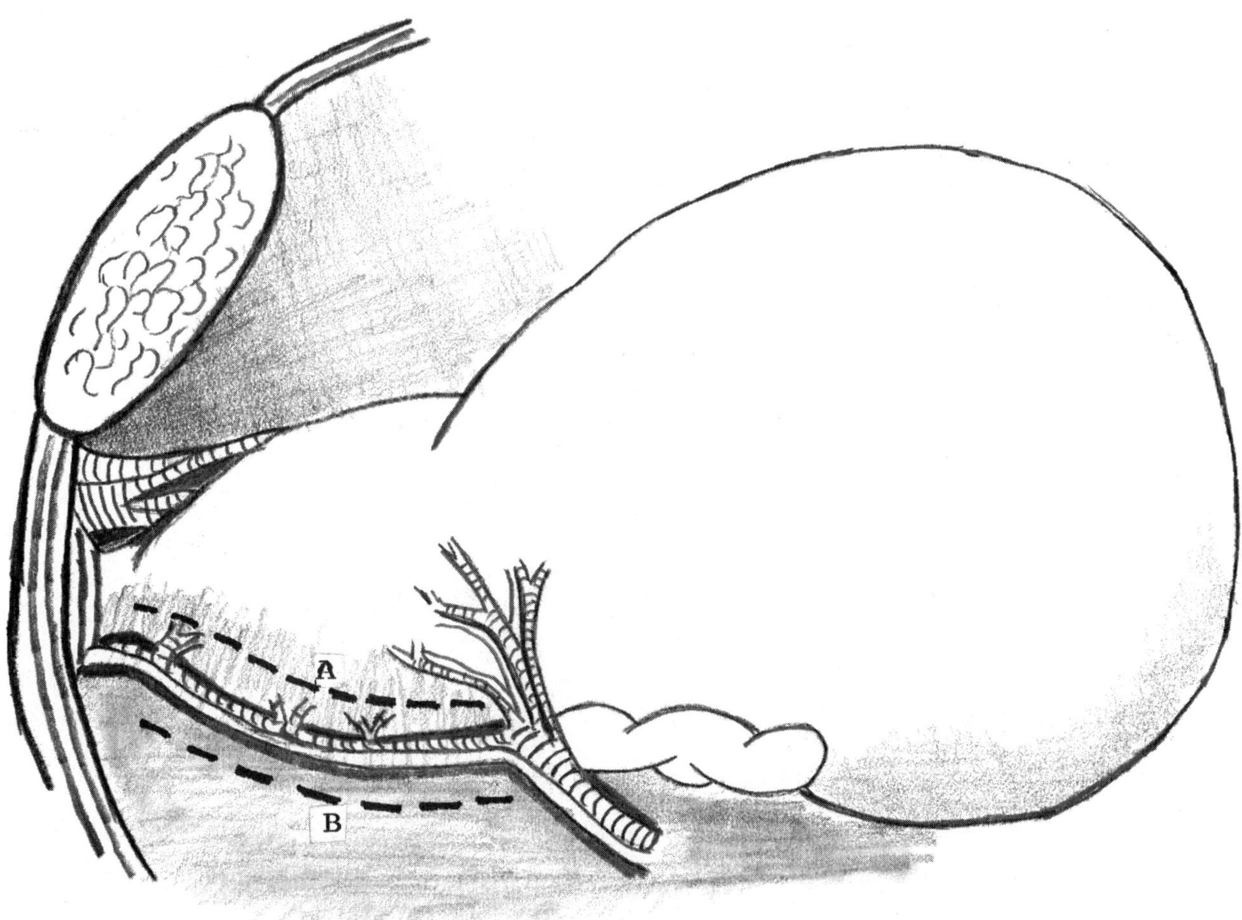

Fig. 17.10.   Lateral view showing the site of incision in the lateral periprostatic fascia (A) for nerve-sparing and the site of incision in the perirectal fascia (B) for non–nerve-sparing.

regarding the extent of disease and will limit the morbidity associated with a more radical lymphadenectomy.

A limited pelvic lymphadenectomy extends from the common iliac bifurcation along the medial aspect of the external iliac artery to the beginning of the femoral canal, where the node of Cloquet is, and along the internal iliac artery (hypogastric) medially and posteriorly to the deep pelvic vein. All lymphatic and adipose tissues within these boundaries are excised, including all tissues between the external iliac artery and vein and lateral and posterior to the obturator nerve.

The generous use of ties, hemoclips, and electrocautery is recommended during the lymphadenectomy to secure even the smallest of the lymphatics and prevent leakage of lymph fluid, which may lead to the formation of lymphoceles or excessive postoperative drainage and loss of protein.

After they are excised, the lymph nodes are carefully inspected and subjected to frozen section pathologic examination if suspicious. It is the author's practice to abandon the planned radical prostatectomy if metastasis into the lymph nodes has occurred.

Incision of Endopelvic Fascia and Division of Puboprostatic Ligaments

The endopelvic fascia is incised on either side (Fig. 17.2), with either a scalpel or electrocautery, starting at the puboprostatic ligaments anteriorly and going posteriorly along the junction of its parietal leaf covering the levator ani muscle and its visceral leaf covering the lateral aspect of the prostate, bladder, and rectum. This incision is then curved superiorly along the posterolateral aspect of the prostate until it ends at the superior vascular pedicle (Fig. 17.1). The fibers of the levator ani muscles are bluntly dissected off the prostate and membranous urethra until the Foley catheter is felt in the membranous urethra beyond the apex of the prostate.

The puboprostatic ligaments are identified and freed of all adipose tissues and of the superficial branch of the dorsal vein of the penis that runs between the two ligaments toward the bladder neck. The ligaments are transected with scissors as close to the undersurface of the symphysis pubis as is safe without impinging on the dorsal vein complex (Fig. 17.8). These cuts should be made with the tip of the scissors

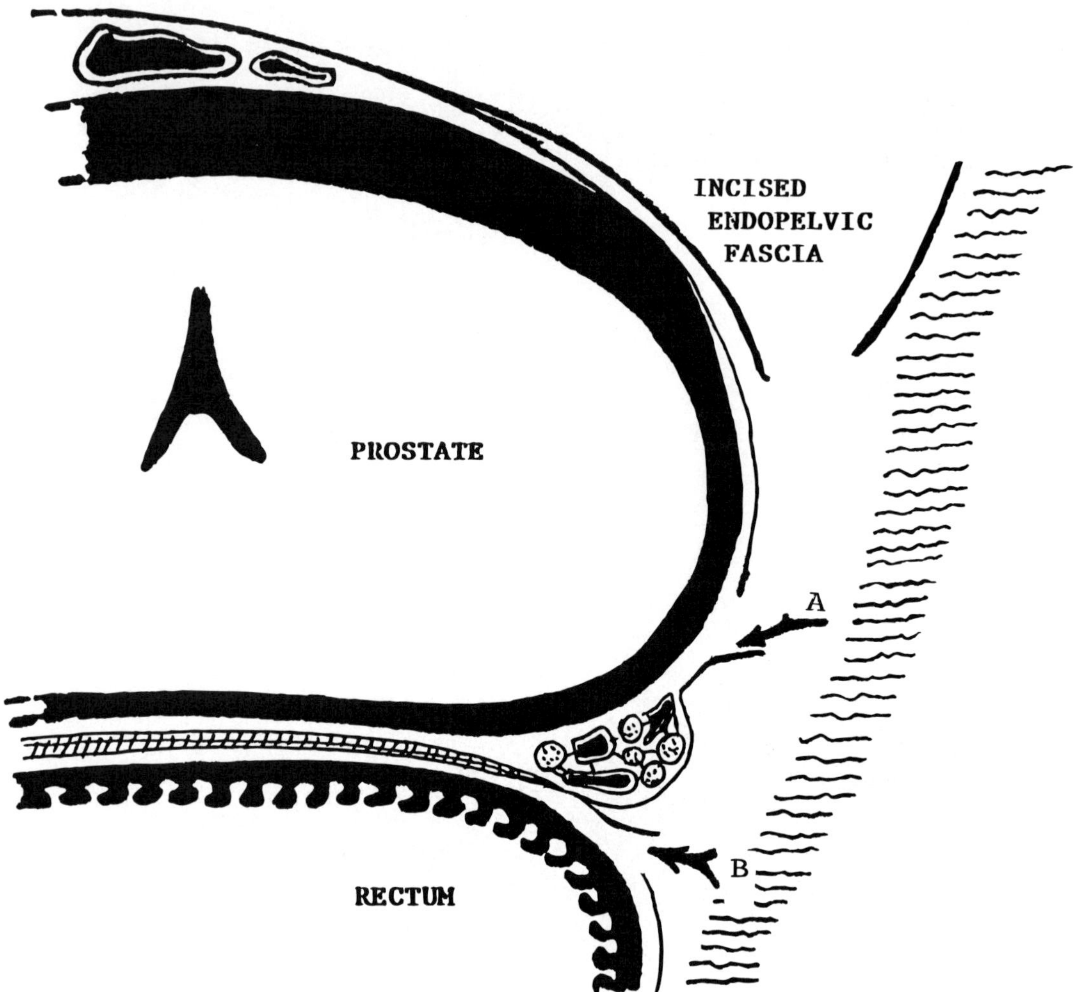

Fig. 17.11.   Cross-section through the midprostate showing the site of incision in the lateral periprostatic fascia (arrow A) in preparation for freeing the neurovascular bundle. Arrow B points to the site of incision in the perirectal fascia in non–nerve-sparing procedures and in preparation to develop the plane between Denonvilliers' fascia and the anterior rectal wall.

under direct vision. Transecting the puboprostatic ligaments allows the prostatic apex to drop posteriorly and makes access to the dorsal vein complex possible.

The medial edges of the incised endopelvic fascia (Fig. 17.2) are incorporated in a transverse suture taken deep into the anterior fibromuscular stroma of the prostate at two or three different levels between the prostatovesical junction and the apex of the prostate (Fig. 17.9). These sutures achieve three goals.

1. They expose the lateral aspect of the prostate to a better advantage in preparation for freeing the neurovascular bundle.
2. They gather the dorsal vein complex for easier control.
3. They prevent back bleeding when the dorsal vein is transected.

Nerve-Sparing

Freeing the neurovascular bundle is done at this stage and before cutting the dorsal vein complex because there is no bleeding yet to obscure the exposure and risk injury to the neurovascular bundle.

The anterior leaf of the lateral periprostatic fascia is incised along the course of the neurovascular bundle from the superior pedicle to the membranous urethra (Fig. 17.10). The plane between the neurovascular bundle and the prostatic capsule and membranous urethra is developed by sharp and blunt dissection (Fig. 17.11), teasing the bundle off these structures until it comes to lie laterally and away from the prostate and urethra (Fig. 17.12). The neurovascular bundle should be handled very gently by traction rather than by holding with a forceps to prevent crush injury to the nerves.

Use of the cautery while freeing the bundle should be avoided. If bleeding from a perforator is excessive, the vessel should be isolated and clipped with the smallest hemoclip possible.

Separating the Prostate from the Anterior Rectal Wall

Developing the plane between Denonvilliers' fascia and the anterior rectal wall to separate the prostate from the rectum can be accomplished at this stage or after the transection of

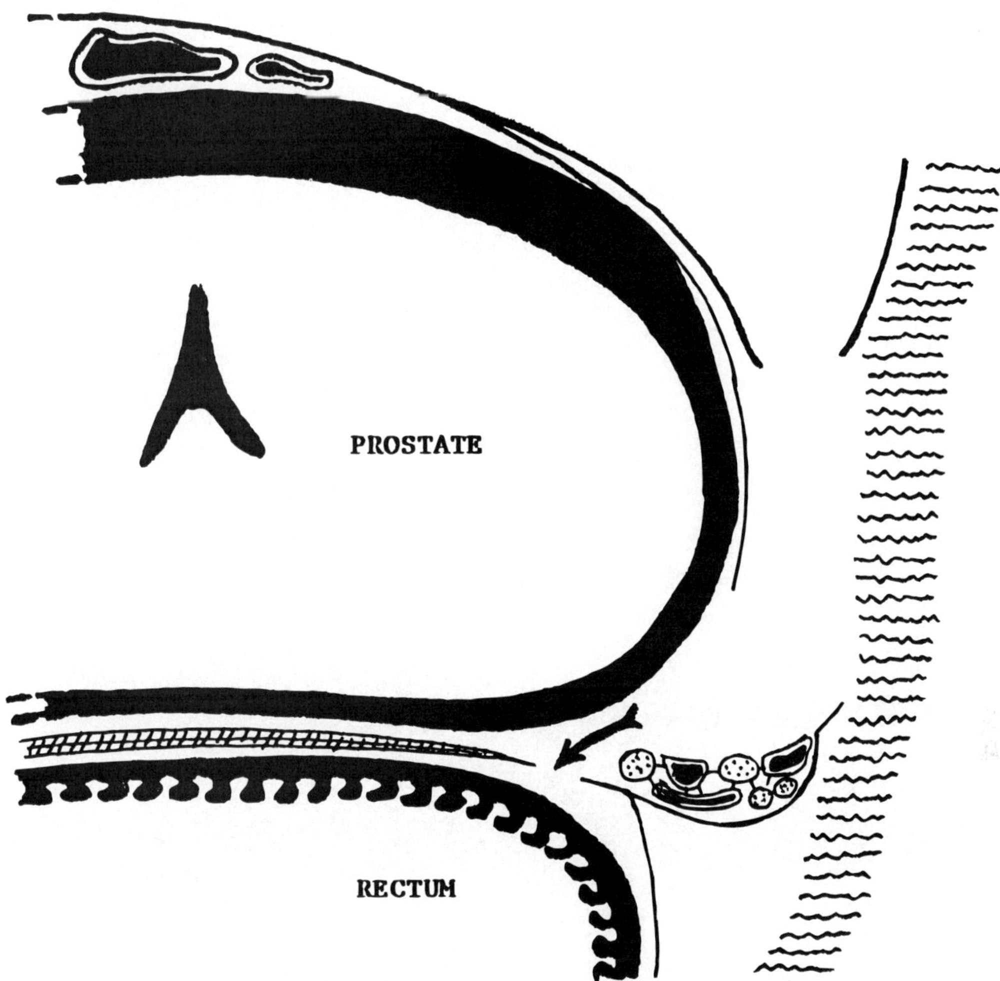

Fig. 17.12. Cross-section view showing the freed neurovascular bundle lying away from the prostate. The arrow shows the site of incision in the perirectal fascia medial to the freed neurovascular bundle in preparation to develop the plane between Denonvilliers' fascia and the anterior rectal wall.

the urethra and Denonvilliers' plate. Performing this maneuver at this stage has several advantages.

- It gives more mobility to the prostate and allows for a better apical dissection.
- It makes the superior vascular pedicles more prominent and easily amenable to transection, which also adds to the mobility of the prostate.
- It decreases bleeding.

On the non–nerve-sparing side, an incision is made in the lateral perirectal fascia lateral to the neurovascular bundle (Figs. 17.10, 17.11, and 17.13). On the nerve-sparing side, the incision is made medial to the already separated neurovascular bundle (Figs. 17.12 and 17.14). The incision in the lateral perirectal fascia should be deep enough to allow the fat layer anterior to the rectal wall to bulge through the incision (Fig. 17.15), an indication that the correct layer has been reached to allow the plane between the anterior rectal wall and Denonvilliers' fascia to be developed. The incision in the lateral perirectal fascia is enlarged to extend from the superior vascular pedicle proximally to beyond the apex of the prostate distally.

A right-angle clamp, with its tip pointing medially, is placed behind the medial cut edge of the lateral perirectal fascia just beyond the superior vascular pedicle (Fig. 17.16). Spreading the tip of the right-angle clamp will start the plane between Denonvilliers' fascia and the anterior rectal wall. With finger dissection, this plane can now be developed further distally on either side to lift the prostate and proximal urethra off the rectal wall. The superior vascular pedicles that now have become prominent are cross-clamped, transected, and tied.

Sometimes it may not be possible to develop this plane because of adhesions, especially in men who have undergone multiple biopsies. In such cases, the plane should be developed in a retrograde fashion and under direct vision after transection of the urethra and Denonvilliers' plate (see below).

Control of the Dorsal Vein Complex and Transection of the Membranous Urethra

Control of the dorsal vein complex is the most critical maneuver during radical prostatectomy because injury to the anterior fi-

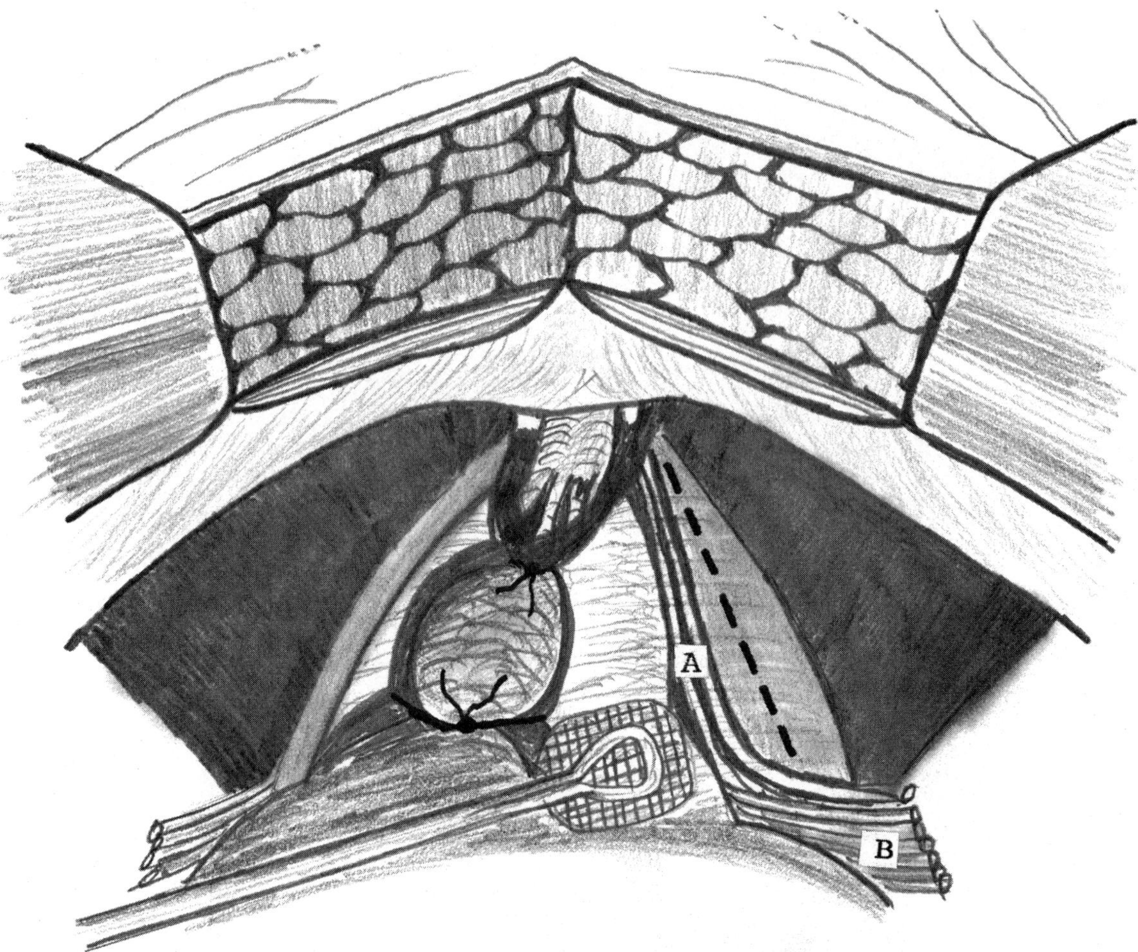

Fig. 17.13. Medial traction at the base of the prostate exposes the neurovascular bundle and more of the anterolateral rectal wall. The dotted line indicates the site of incision in the perirectal fascia in preparation to develop the plane between the Denonvilliers' fascia and the anterior rectal wall. A: Neurovascular bundle; B: superior vascular pedicle.

bers of the external sphincter and excessive blood loss are most likely to occur here.

Attempts at passing a right-angle clamp between the dorsal vein and urethra or placing a suture deep into the tissues close to the urethra are likely to incorporate some of the anterior sphincteric fibers and compromise postoperative continence. Instead, a suture of 0 chromic or any absorbable material is placed as distally and as superficially as possible, meaning close to the undersurface of the symphysis pubis rather than to the urethra, and tied (Fig. 17.17). Even if this suture does not provide complete control when the vein is cut, it is better to lose some blood rather than risk injury to the sphincter. Complete control can easily be achieved after the vein is cut.

A transverse incision is made with a scalpel across the dorsal vein complex, the prostatoischial ligaments of Mueller and anterior half of the urethra, 2 to 4 mm beyond the apex of the prostate and cephalad to the suture (Fig. 17.18). The Foley catheter is now exposed (Fig. 17.19).

If the previously placed suture in the dorsal vein complex does not completely control bleeding, a figure-of-eight suture using 0 chromic on a UR-6 needle is placed under direct vision in the lateral periurethral fascia at 3 o'clock and then across to the 9-o'clock position on the opposite side and tied. Approximating these two edges of the lateral periurethral fascia will tamponade the vein and immediately stop bleeding. While placing this suture, very little tissue should be incorporated to avoid injury to the anterior sphincteric fibers.

The Foley catheter is partially withdrawn to expose the lumen of the urethra. Full thickness sutures of 3-0 absorbable material are placed in the urethra at 3 o'clock and 9 o'clock, incorporating the lateral periurethral fascia and prostatoischial ligaments of Mueller. These sutures will later be used for the urethrovesical anastomosis.

The posterior half of the urethra is now transected, exposing Denonvilliers' plate, which is dissected off the anterior rectal wall with a right-angle clamp (Fig. 17.20). The neurovascular bundle on the side of the cancer is incorporated within this dissection, while the freed neurovascular bundle on the opposite nerve-sparing side lies laterally and away from the lateral edge of Denonvilliers' plate. Two posterior, full-thickness sutures of

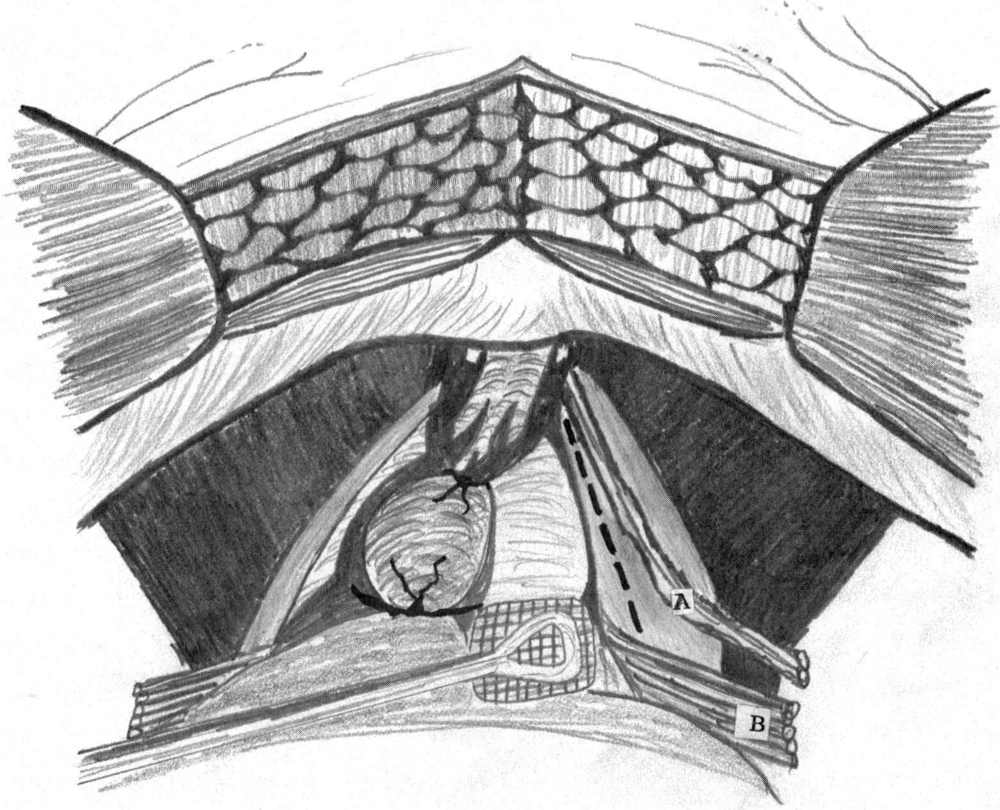

Fig. 17.14. The freed neurovascular bundle now lies laterally away from the prostate. The dotted line indicates the site of incision in the perirectal fascia, medial to the neurovascular bundle. A: Neurovascular bundle; B: superior vascular pedicle.

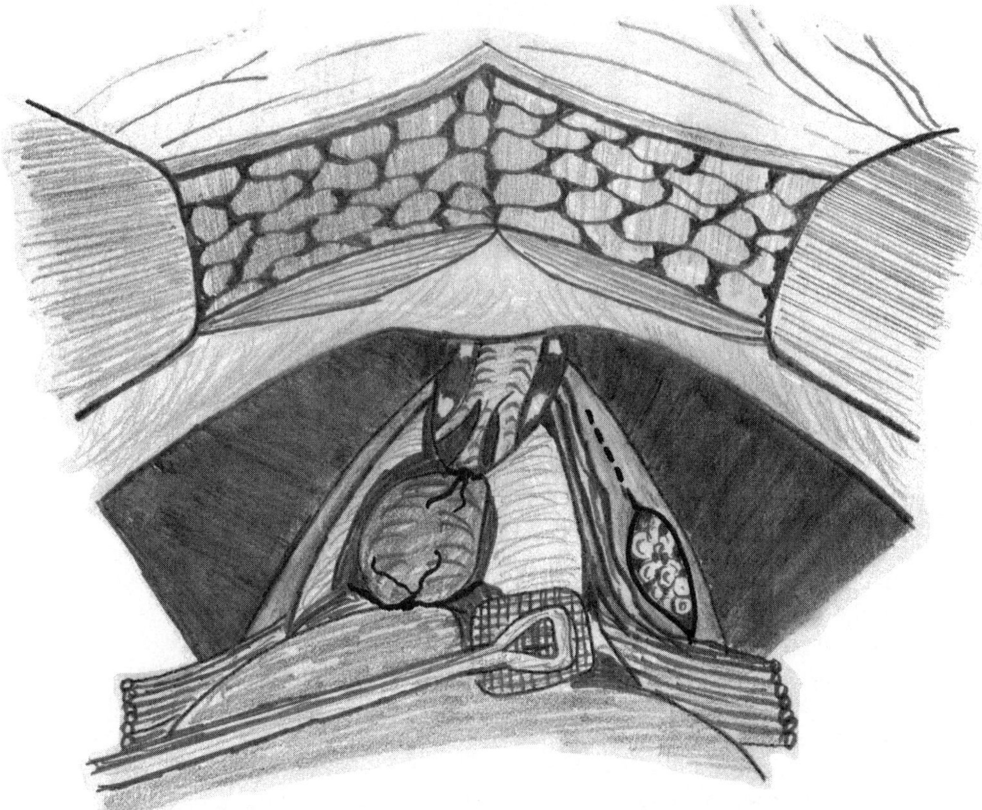

Fig. 17.15. Incision in the lateral perirectal fascia with fat bulging through the incision indicating that the proper plane between the anterior rectal wall and Denonvilliers' fascia is reached.

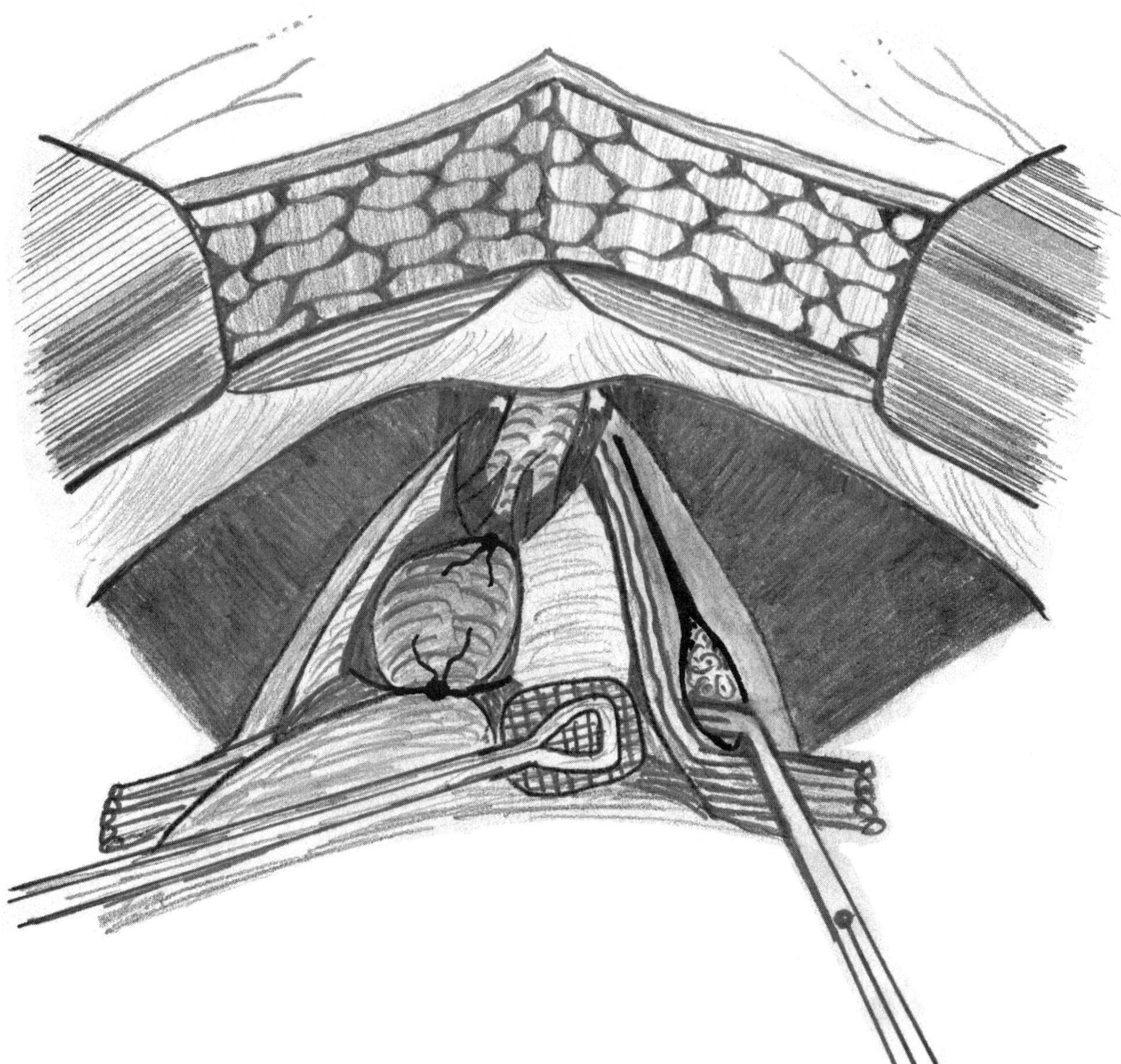

Fig. 17.16.   The right-angle clamp is placed behind the prostate to start the plane between the anterior rectal wall and Denonvilliers' fascia.

3-0 absorbable material are placed in the urethra at 5 o'clock and 7 o'clock, incorporating Denonvilliers' plate for strength. These sutures will also be used later for the urethrovesical anastomosis. Denonvilliers' plate is now incised together with the neurovascular bundle on the side of the cancer, completely separating the prostate from the urethra.

If the prostate has already been separated from the rectal wall as described previously, it can now be retracted cephalad. If it has not, the plane between Denonvilliers' fascia and the anterior rectal wall can be started by placing a right-angle clamp behind the proximal cut end of Denonvilliers' plate in the midline and spreading its tips laterally. By gently lifting the apex of the prostate and with cephalad blunt and sharp dissection under direct vision, the prostate can now be lifted off the rectal wall. A Foley catheter is now introduced into the bladder through the proximal cut end of the membranous urethra and used for traction. Continuing in the cephalad dissection, the seminal vesicles and ampullae of the vas deferens, covered by Denonvilliers' fascia, are lifted off the anterior rectal wall.

Control of the Superior Vascular Pedicles

Cephalad traction on the Foley catheter to one side of the midline or the other will lift the prostate and seminal vesicles off the rectum and expose one or the other superior vascular pedicle. With the right-angle clamp, a plane is developed between the pedicle and Denonvilliers' fascia covering the lateral aspect of the seminal vesicles. On the nerve-sparing side, this plane should be developed as close to the prostate as possible to avoid injury to the neurovascular bundle. The prior lateral dissection

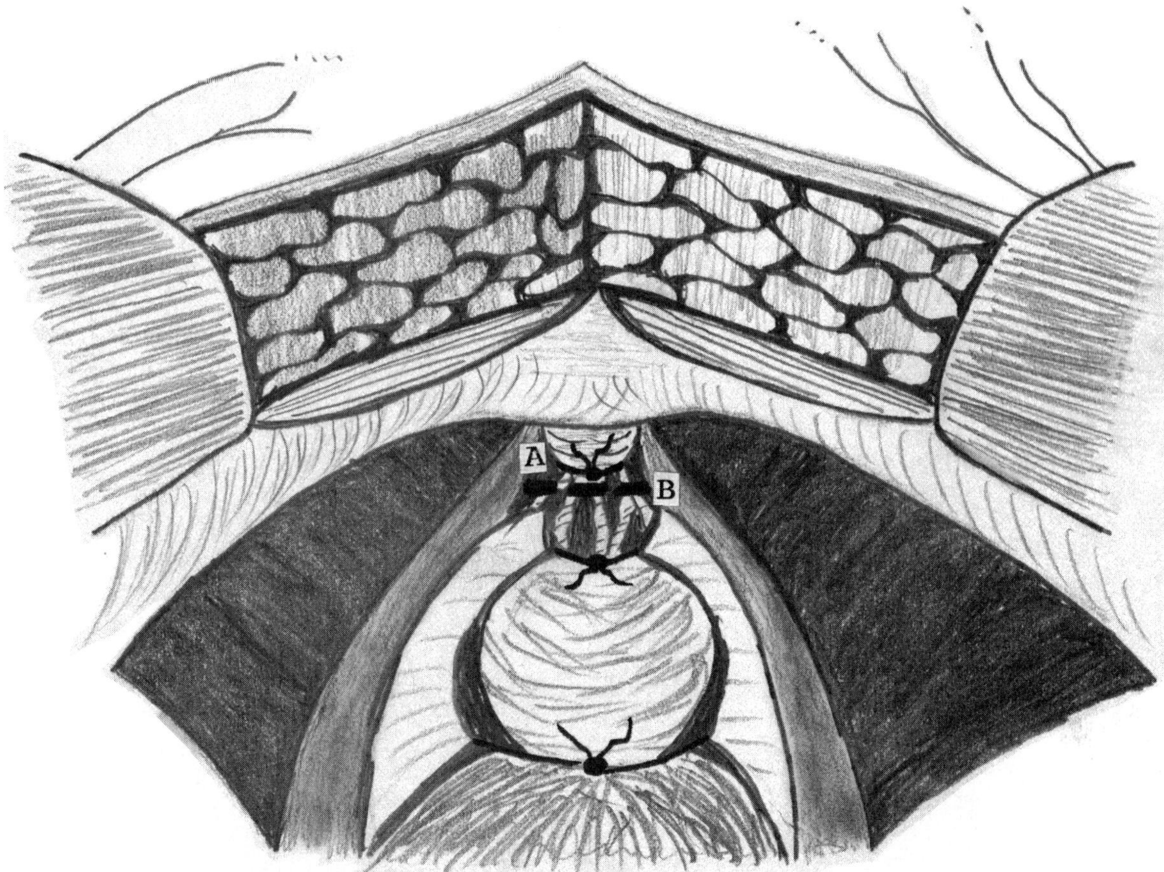

Fig. 17.17. Suture ligature around dorsal vein complex (A) and site of incision (B) in the dorsal vein complex, anterior half of urethra and prostato-ischial ligaments of Mueller beyond the apex of the prostate.

of the bundle helps keep it in sight and away from being incorporated in any ligature. On the non–nerve-sparing side, the pedicle should be clamped as posterior as possible to ensure a safe margin of resection on the side of the cancer (Fig. 17.21). The pedicles are transected between ligatures. It may take two or three ligatures on each side to completely control the pedicles.

Once the vascular pedicles have been transected, the superior edges of the seminal vesicles come into view. Blunt dissection between the bladder and superior edges of the seminal vesicles across the midline will separate these two structures and facilitate the later separation of the posterior bladder neck and trigone from the ampullae of the vas and anterior surface of the seminal vesicles.

Division of the Bladder Neck

The anterior bladder neck is incised transversely about 1 cm cephalad to the prostatovesical junction (Fig. 17.22). Cutting with the electrocautery will reduce bleeding. After the anterior half of the bladder neck is incised, the Foley balloon is deflated and the Foley catheter is withdrawn from the bladder and looped around the anterior prostate for traction (Fig. 17.23).

The ureteral orifices are identified, and incision of the posterior bladder neck is made 1 cm beyond the interureteric ridge. Incising the posterior bladder neck can be aided by placing a finger or a large right-angle clamp in the plane previously developed between the seminal vesicles and ampullae of the vas and bladder.

The bladder neck should always be widely excised, leaving about 1 cm of bladder wall on all sides of the prostate specimen. Indigo carmine can be used to facilitate the identification of the ureteral orifices.

Excision of the Seminal Vesicles

After the bladder is completely separated from the prostate by incising the bladder neck, the anterior surfaces of the ampullae of the vas and seminal vesicles, which should be covered by the anterior reflection of Denonvilliers' fascia, are bluntly separated from the trigone and posterior bladder wall (Fig. 17.24). The ampullae of the vas are transected between ligatures or hemoclips, the apex of the seminal vesicle is freed on either side, and the arteries to the seminal vesicles are clipped or tied and transected (Fig. 17.25). This completely frees the surgical spec-

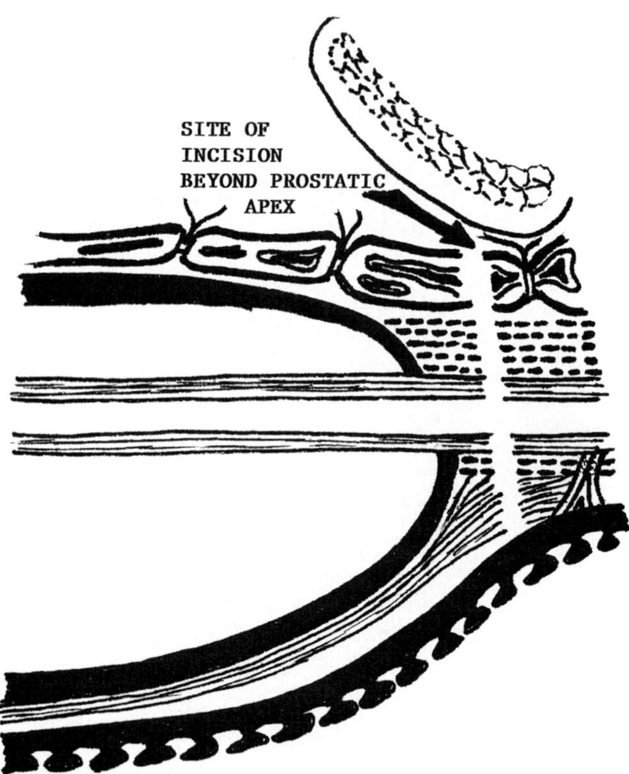

Fig. 17.18. Lateral view showing site of incision beyond the apex of the prostate.

imen that is delivered out of the incision. Hemostasis is secured with the electrocautery.

Closure of the Bladder Neck and Completion of the Urethrovesical Anastomosis

The bladder neck is partially closed either longitudinally in a tennis racket fashion (Fig. 17.26) or transversely (Fig. 17.27), leaving about a 0.5- to 1-cm opening for the urethrovesical anastomosis. The longitudinal closure starts posteriorly, carefully avoiding the ureteral orifices. Transverse closure is on either side of the midline, reducing the opening until the desired aperture is reached. Absorbable 2-0 interrupted sutures are used. The mucosa around the newly reconstructed bladder neck is everted with 3-0 or 4-0 chromic sutures to ensure a mucosal-to-mucosal urethrovesical anastomosis and prevent stricture formation.

The previously placed four urethral sutures at 3 o'clock and 9 o'clock as well as at 5 o'clock and 7 o'clock are placed in the bladder neck, full thickness, at their respective positions. A 20 French Foley catheter is inserted per urethra, across the bladder neck into the bladder. A fifth suture is placed at 12 o'clock in the bladder neck and at the same position in the anterior urethral wall, incorporating with it only the urethral mucosa and tissues from the ligated dorsal vein complex for strength. The Foley balloon is inflated to 10 cc, and gentle traction is applied

on the catheter to approximate the vesical neck to the membranous urethra. With continued traction on the Foley catheter, the sutures are gently tied starting with the 12-o'clock suture because this suture incorporates strong tissues and is the least likely to cut through the urethral wall.

Alternate methods of urethrovesical anastomoses exist. Some do not use any sutures and rely on the Foley catheter to approximate the vesical neck to the membranous urethra. Others use Vest sutures between the bladder neck and the perineum. In the author's experience, the rate of stricture formation is very significant if a mucosal-to-mucosal apposition is not achieved.

After the anastomosis is completed, traction on the Foley catheter is released and the pelvic cavity is thoroughly irrigated. A drain is left in the retropubic space and brought out through a separate stab-wound skin incision. The abdominal incision is closed.

POSTOPERATIVE CARE

Epidural or patient-controlled analgesia is used. Antibiotics are continued for only two postoperative doses. The patient should be ambulating on the evening of the day of surgery and at frequent intervals thereafter. Feeding is started only after the return of bowel function. The retropubic drain is removed when it stops draining, usually on the third postoperative day.

The average hospital stay is 5 days, including the preoperative day. The patient is discharged from the hospital when he is eating a regular diet and is having normal bowel function. The day before discharge, the patient is given a set of discharge information and instructions to read and study. On the day of discharge, the nurse or doctor will go over these instructions with the patient and will answer any questions. The patient is sent home with a leg bag, nighttime urinary drainage bag, and a copy of the following instructions:

Radical Retropubic Prostatectomy Discharge Information and Instructions

You have undergone a major urologic procedure and now comes the time for your discharge from the hospital. You will find here lots of useful information to help you know what you should or should not be doing when you are at home.

Activity

For the next 6 weeks try to walk up to 1 mile a day. You may walk a longer distance if you feel like it, but stop if you get tired. Avoid running, fast walking, walking on inclines and declines, heavy lifting (over 10 pounds), or any heavy exercise. Climb stairs slowly and carefully. These will put an extra strain on your incision, which is going to take 6 to 8 weeks to achieve complete healing. A good rule of thumb is that if anything unduly hurts your incision, then avoid it. This way you will be the best judge.

Do not ride long distances in cars. If you must, then you

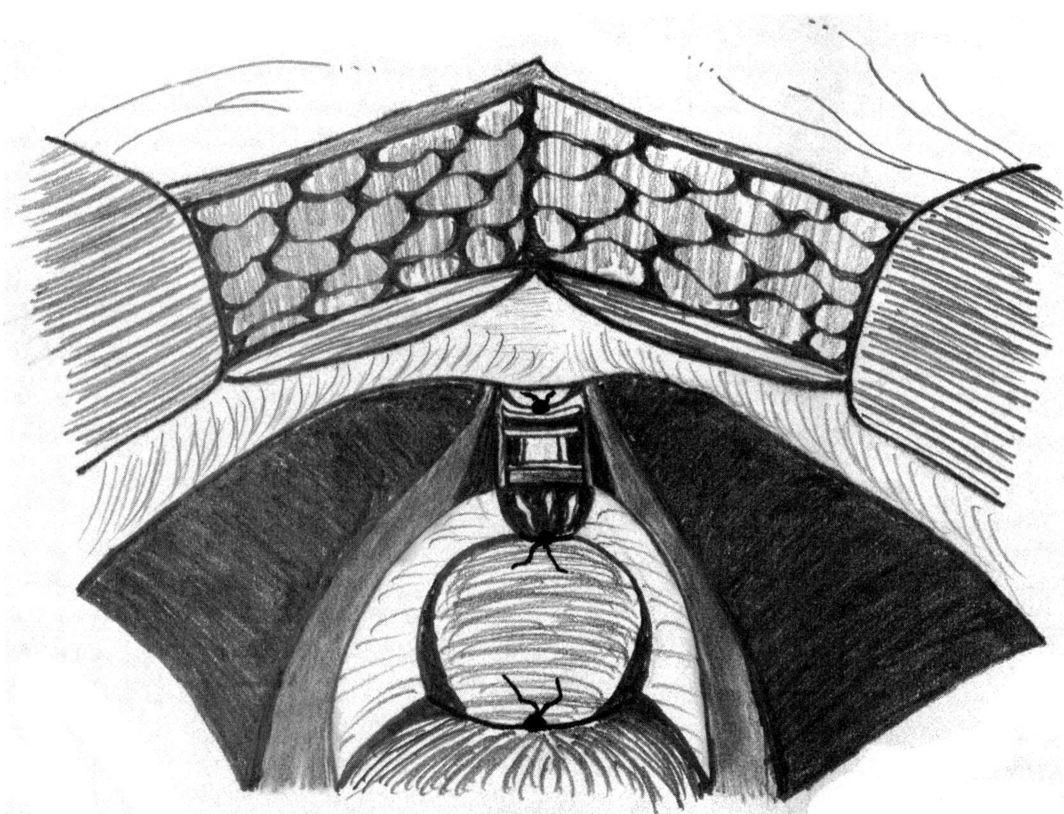

Fig. 17.19.   Incised dorsal vein complex, anterior half of the urethra and prostato-ischial ligaments of Mueller exposing the Foley catheter.

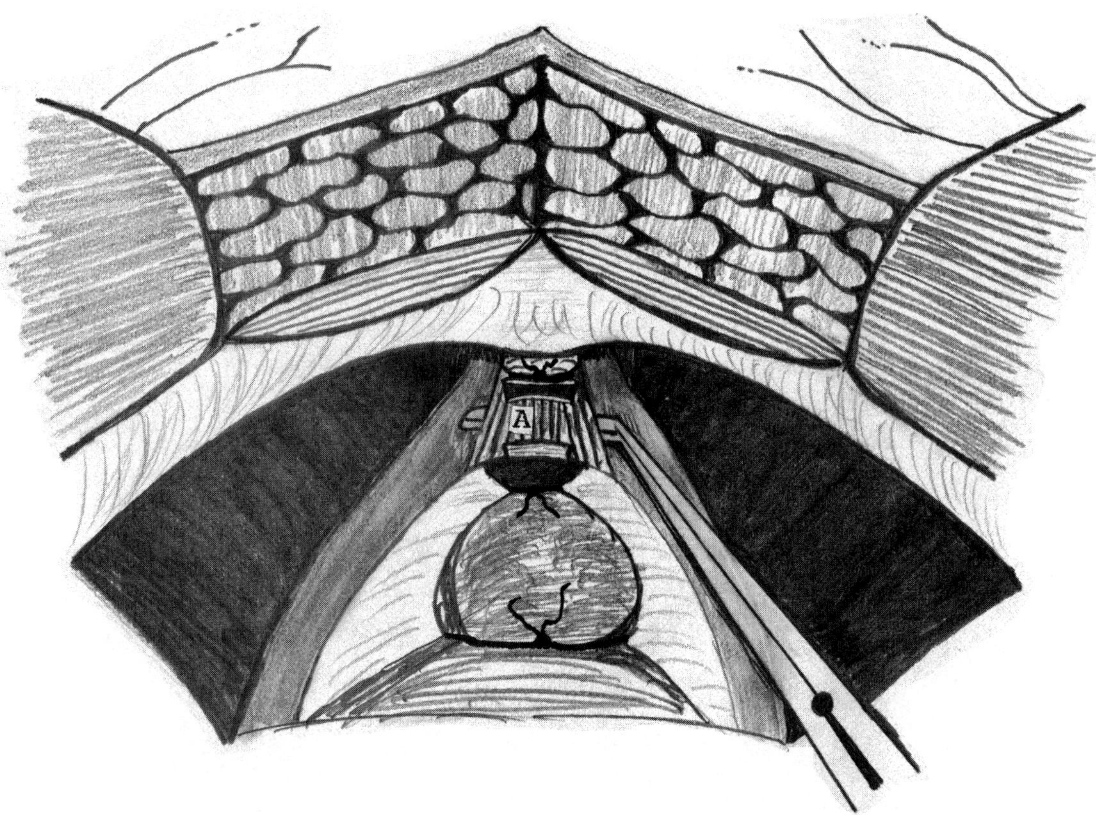

Fig. 17.20.   Denonvilliers' plate dissected off the anterior rectal wall with a right-angle clamp. A: Denonvilliers' plate.

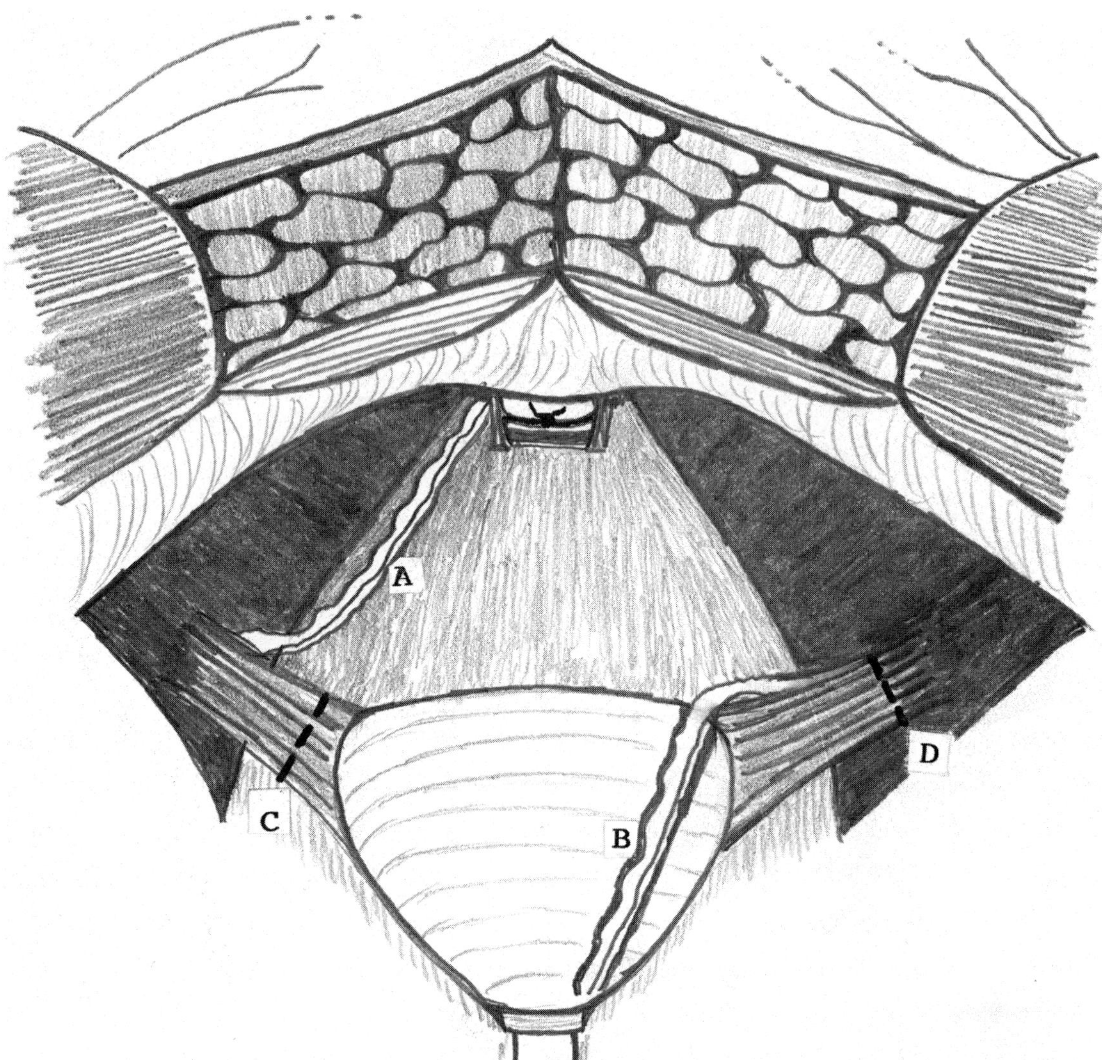

Fig. 17.21. Exposure of the superior vascular pedicles. A: Preserved neurovascular bundle; B: excised neurovascular bundle attached to the posterolateral aspect of the prostate; C: site of transection of the superior vascular pedicle on the nerve-sparing side; D: site of transection of the superior vascular pedicle on the non–nerve-sparing side.

should break your journey every half to one hour, get out of the car, stretch your legs, and walk around. It is also preferable to stretch your legs while in the car, maybe by lying on the back seat. Remember to do your calf exercises. Do not cross your legs. All these precautions will promote the venous circulation in your legs and prevent you from developing a clot.

Driving

You should not drive a car until after your catheter comes out, approximately 2 weeks after your operation. The discomfort from the catheter will make your reactions using the foot pedal suboptimal in case of emergency braking, even though you may feel you can drive. For your safety and to maximize wound healing, you should not drive during this period. After the 2 weeks you may drive, but limit this to short distances only for a further 2 weeks before you resume normal driving.

Bathing and Showers

You may shower or bathe anytime after leaving the hospital. Wash your incision with soap and water. Avoid scrubbing the incision. It is permissible for your catheter and drainage bag to get wet in the shower, but do not submerge them in water. After showering, dry the incision and the adhesive tapes by dabbing with a dry towel. Secure the firm end of the clear connecting tube to the thigh with tape. The adhesive tapes will usually fall off within the following 2 weeks.

Diet

There are no restrictions to your diet. Please note that constipation may result from taking pain medications (Vicodin) and iron tablets. This will make you strain and put extra pressure onto the area of the surgery. By eating a balanced diet with high fiber

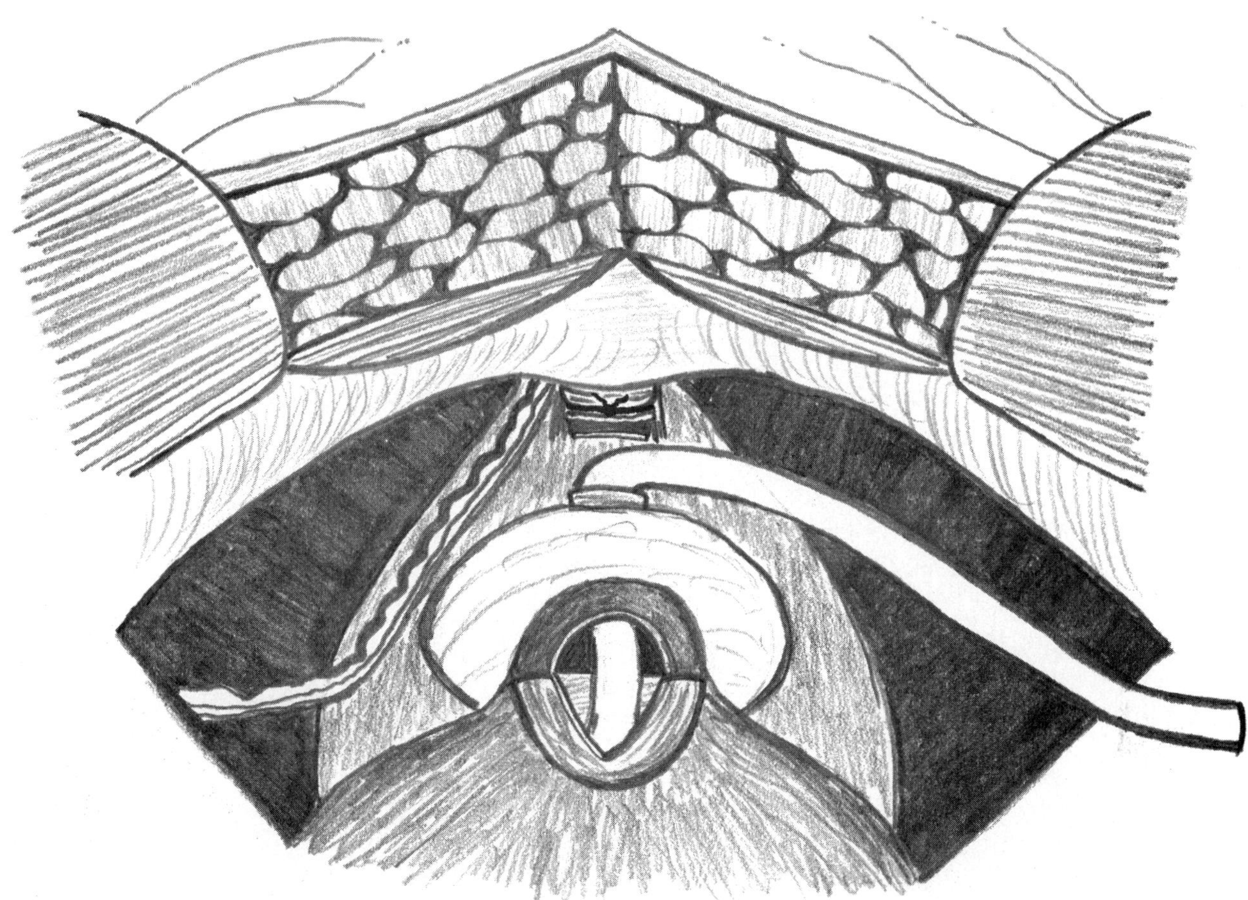

Fig. 17.22.   Incised anterior half of bladder neck.

such as fresh fruits, vegetables, whole grain, and bran, you can help avoid constipation. You will also be given stool softeners (DSS and Metamucil) to help regulate your bowels. Keep well hydrated by drinking 6 to 8 glasses of fluid each day. You may drink alcohol in moderation (1 to 2 drinks per day).

Foley Catheter

You have a catheter inside your bladder to drain the urine. This catheter will stay in for 2 weeks from the day of surgery. It prevents your bladder from storing urine and distending during the period of healing of the new connection made between your bladder and urethra. The catheter is maintained in the bladder by a water-filled balloon at its end. Make sure that the catheter is well secured to the thigh by tape and avoid traction and tension on it. Clean the catheter with soap and water where it exits from your urethra at the end of the penis and apply K-Y jelly (or polysporin cream) on a daily basis in the same way that you were shown in the hospital. Use your leg bag during the day and secure the bag by strapping it snugly but not too tightly to your thigh or calf. Tight strapping will obstruct the venous circulation and may cause swelling and a clot.

The urine may become intermittently blood-stained on walking or having a bowel movement. This is not unusual and as long as the catheter is draining well and there are no blood clots, it is of no consequence. Also, with the presence of the retaining balloon inside, the bladder gets a false feeling of fullness and you may feel the urge to urinate even though your bladder is empty. The bladder may even go into spasm and you may feel uncomfortable contractions. Blood-stained urine may leak around the catheter when your bladder spasms. Do not panic. Lie down and rest, and within a short time your bladder will readjust and the discomfort will resolve.

Occasionally, the catheter may become blocked and stop draining due to a small blood clot. Within a few hours, you will start to get the feeling of your bladder distending. Call us if this occurs and we will instruct you on what to do next.

Medications

1. Vicodin 1 to 2 tablets every 6 hours as required. This is a pain medication. With time, you may need only Tylenol for the discomfort associated with your incision.

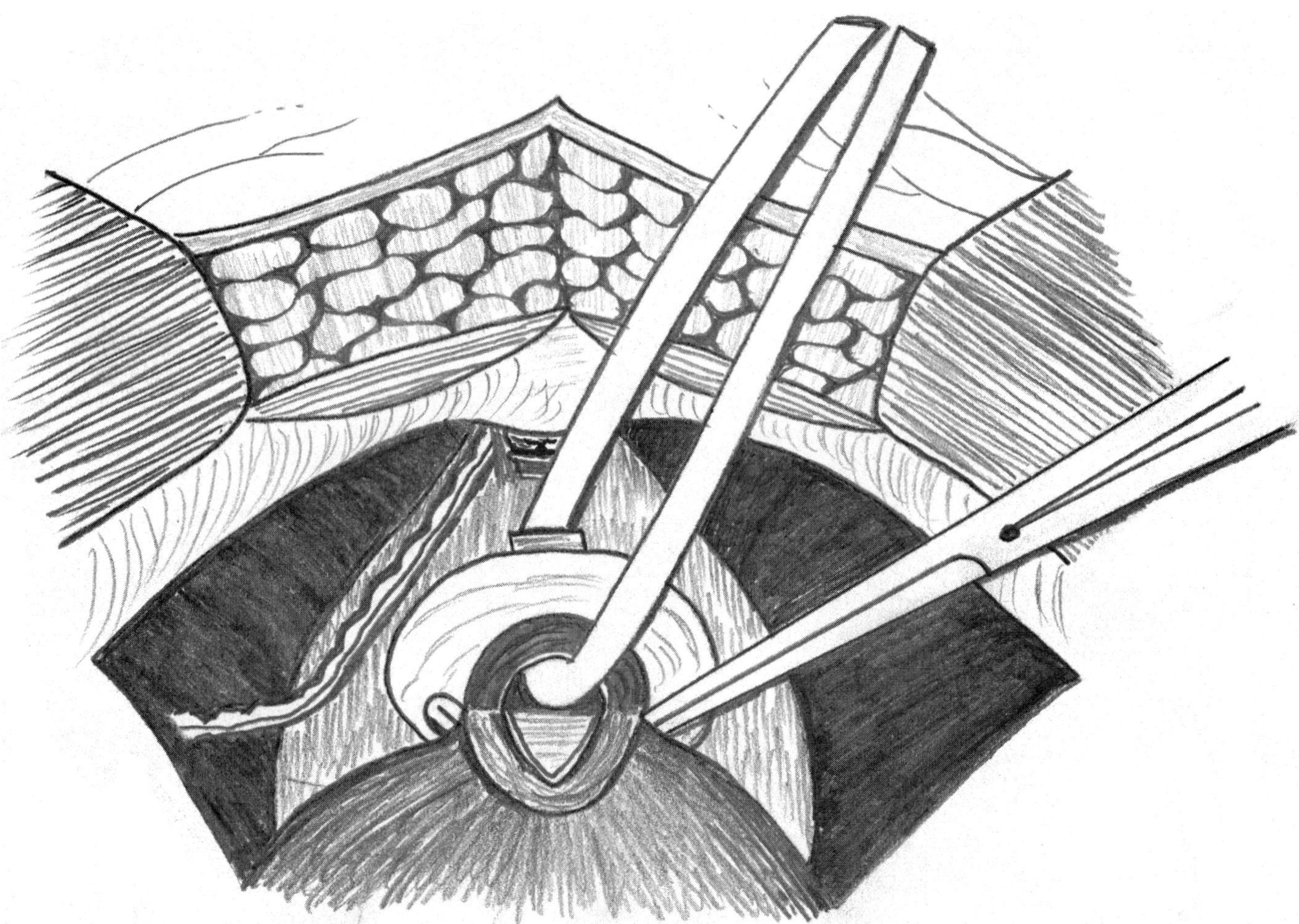

Fig. 17.23.   The Foley catheter is delivered out of the bladder and looped around the prostate for traction. A large right-angle clamp is placed behind the posterior bladder neck to facilitate its transection.

2. Ferrous gluconate 300 mg three times per day for 1 month. This is an iron tablet that helps your body in reproducing new blood cells. It can be constipating as mentioned earlier and may make your stools black. You may not need this, and your doctor will let you know.
3. DSS 240 mg twice per day. This is stool softener.
4. Metamucil 1 teaspoon twice per day. This is a stool softener.

Return to Clinic

You are scheduled to return to the urology clinic 2 weeks after your surgery.

On your return, you need to bring with you a pair of jockey shorts and some diapers made for newborn babies. These can be obtained in any supermarket in your area. These will be used during the initial period when your bladder is regaining its control.

Any Further Questions?

Try to think of any further questions that you may have while you are still in the hospital and ask us. We will be delighted to answer any and all questions you may have. Don't be afraid to ask anything that comes to mind. Remember that sometimes the simplest questions are the most important. When you are at home and any questions arise or problems are encountered, please call us. There is always a urologist available 24 hours a day, every day. In particular, call us if:

- Your incision gets red, breaks open, or drains fluid.
- The catheter is not draining urine.
- There are blood clots in the urine.
- You experience fevers, chills, and/or vomiting.

The patient returns 2 weeks after the operation for removal of the Foley catheter, serum PSA determination, and instructions regarding incontinence, activity, and perineal exercises. He is sent home that day with another set of instructions.

Radical Retropubic Prostatectomy Information and Instruction After Catheter Removal

Your Foley catheter has been removed. We have given you an antibiotic for 3 days, which should prevent any urinary infection.

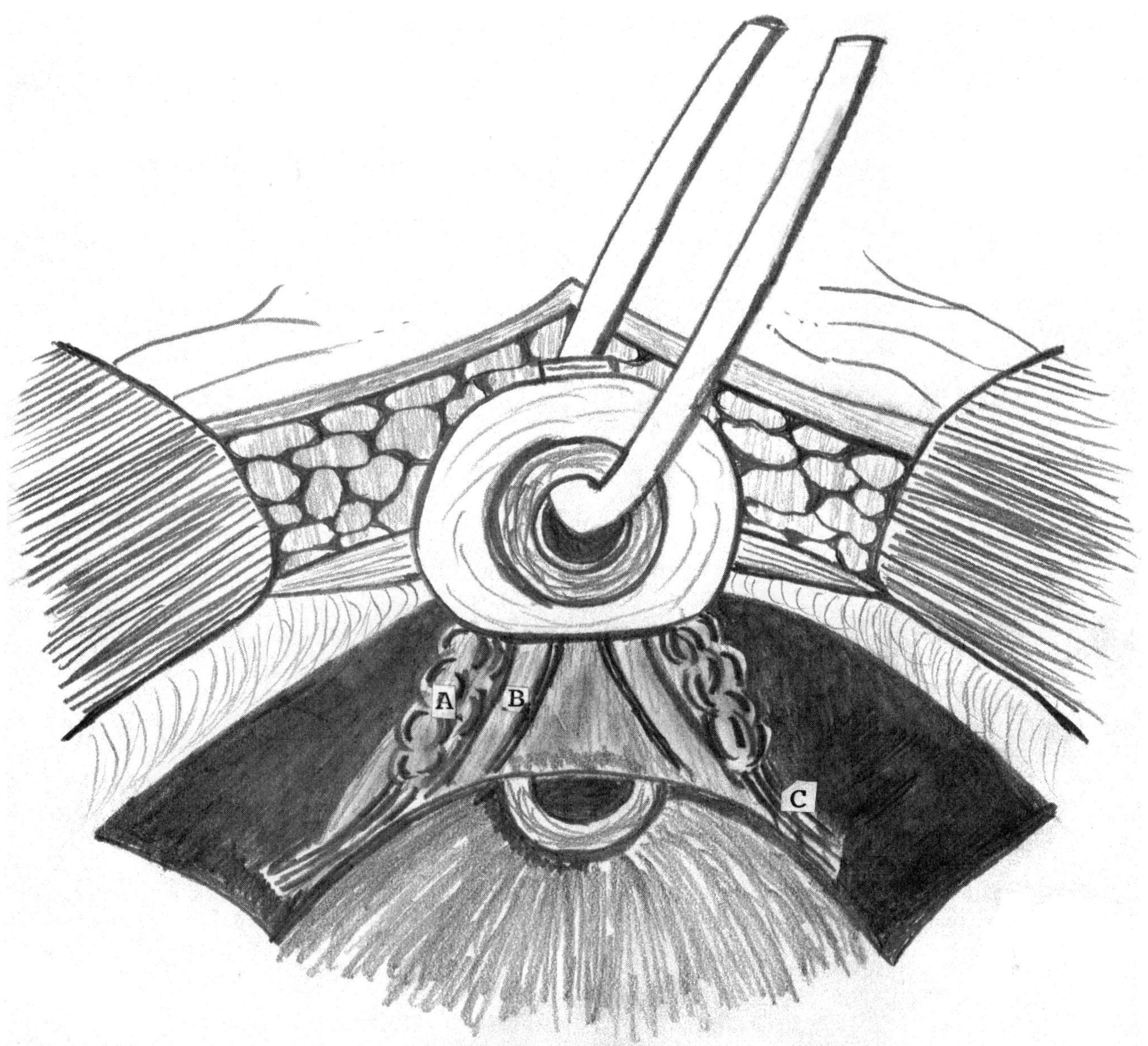

Fig. 17.24. Completely separated bladder neck, exposing the anterior surface of the seminal vesicles (A) and ampulla of the vas (B). C: Vessels to the tip of the seminal vesicles.

During the next several weeks, you will go through a period of temporary urinary incontinence. This is to be expected after radical prostatectomy, and in the majority of patients it lasts for a few months. You should start to notice a gradual and continuous improvement in your control during the first month, but in a small number of patients it may take 6 months or longer to achieve complete control. These instructions contain information to help you manage during this period and, more importantly, to help you regain your full continence.

Regaining Urinary Continence: How to Do the Exercises

The most important exercise to regain continence is stopping and restarting your stream in the middle of urination. Try to do this at least two or three times with each voiding while the stream is very strong. Try to cut it off sharply and to the last drop. Also helpful are pelvic floor exercises (Kegel exercises), which you do by tightening and relaxing your pelvic sphincter muscles. This can be done anytime during the day, and we encourage you to practice at least 200 times a day. Use the same muscle you use in stopping your urinary stream. All exercises should be done "religiously" until you regain full control.

You should become dry at night in bed within weeks. When this occurs, it is important to stop using a diaper when you go to bed. Next, you will become dry in the mornings; again, it is important to give up the morning diaper when this occurs. Your last episodes of incontinence will occur in the late afternoon or early evening, especially after an alcoholic drink. You

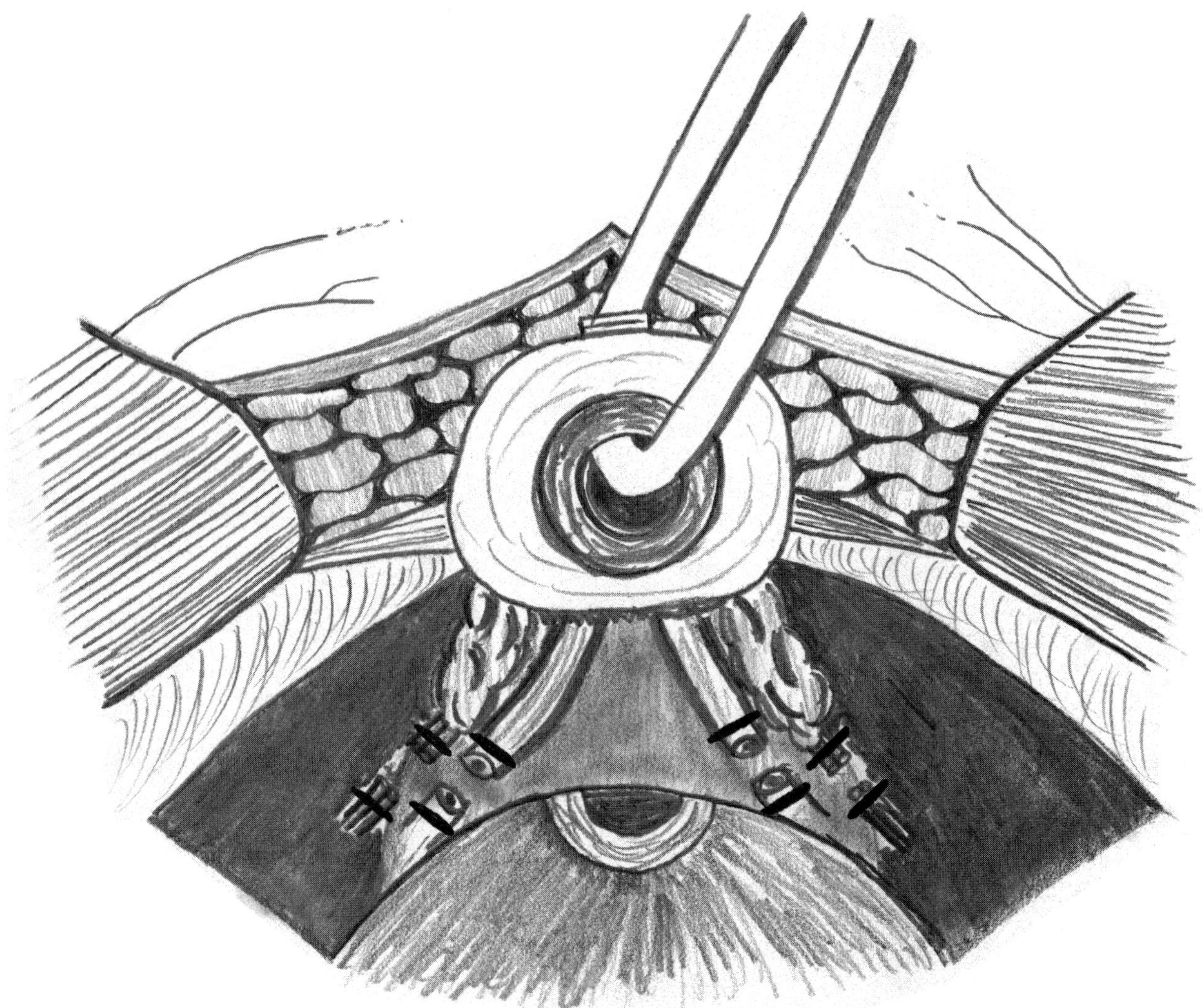

Fig. 17.25.   The ampulla of the vas and the vessels to the tip of the seminal vesicles are transected between clips.

will also need a diaper for a while during vigorous exercise, golfing, or strenuous gardening. It is important that you continue stopping and starting your urinary stream several times with each voiding until you are completely dry. If you stop exercising when you are 99% dry, you will be left with 1% incontinence, so persevere to the end.

Things to Watch For

After your prostate was removed, we reconnected your bladder to your urethra with a set of stitches. The healing process of this connection will continue over the next 3 months. In the majority of patients, this heals satisfactorily leading to a nice, wide open urinary channel. However, in a small number of patients, the healing process may lead to a much smaller channel and some degree of blockage. You need to be aware of this and to let us know if you notice the following:

- Decrease in size and force of your stream when you have a full bladder. We should be informed if the size of your stream with a full bladder is smaller than the one you had before the operation.
- Straining when you void.
- Feeling that your bladder is still full after voiding.

Future Follow-up

You will return to the urology clinic in 3 months. You will have a blood test (PSA), you will be examined, and your progress will be assessed. We will review with you at that time our final pathology report from our research laboratories, a review that will determine how often we need to see you in follow-up.

From then on, follow-up is once every 3 months for the first year and once every 6 months thereafter. With every follow-up visit, a serum PSA is determined, physical examination including DRE is performed, and the patient is interviewed regarding continence, force of the urinary stream, and sexual activity.

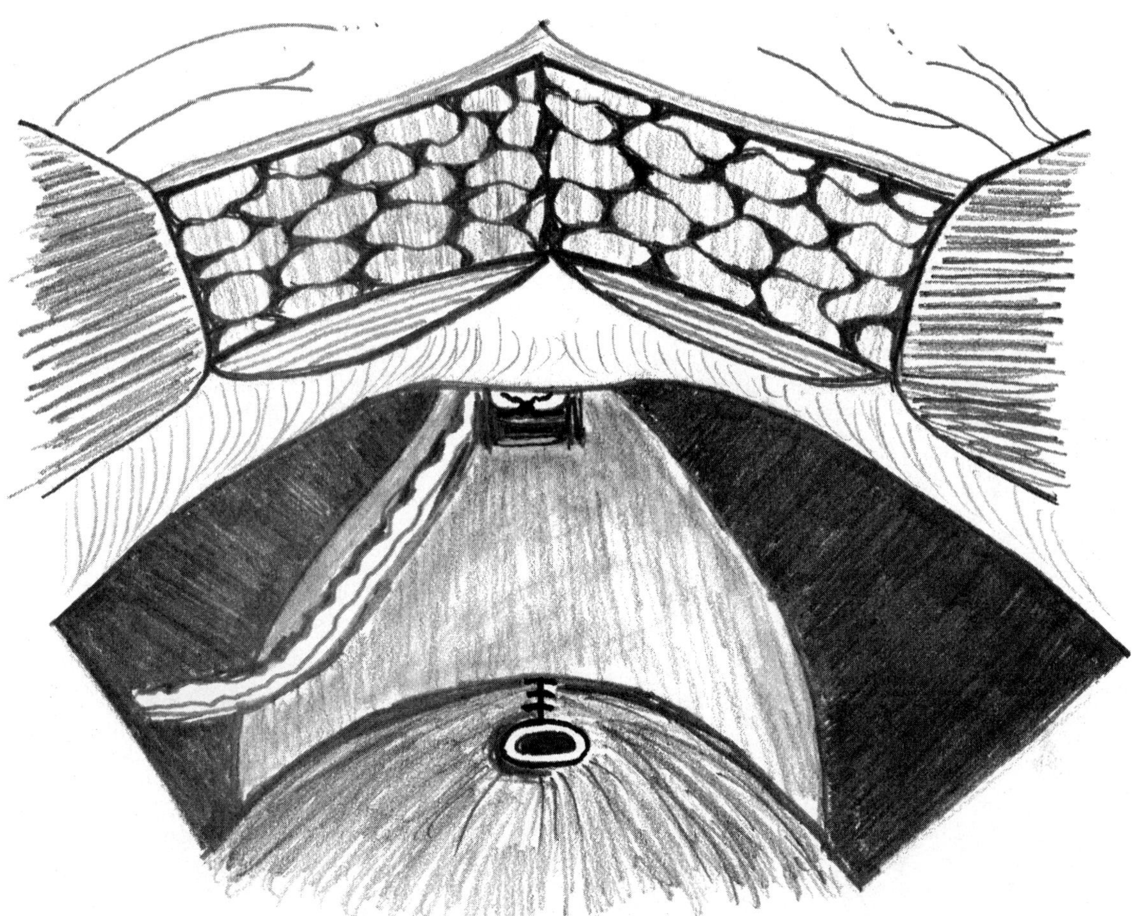

Fig. 17.26. Longitudinal closure of bladder neck (tennis racket).

COMPLICATIONS

There are two major intraoperative complications. The first is excessive blood loss, which usually occurs during control of the dorsal vein complex. The second is injury to the rectum, which occurs while dissecting the plane between Denonvilliers' fascia and the anterior rectal wall, especially if adhesions are present or infiltration by cancer has occurred.

In the author's experience, the average blood loss is 500 mL, which is usually replaced by the patient's own blood. Occasionally, the bleeding from the dorsal vein is profuse. In such cases, pressure on the vein for 10 minutes may be all that is needed to stop the bleeding. Placing deeper sutures may also be required.

Rectal injury is extremely rare. In the author's experience, it occurred 5 times in 475 consecutive radical prostatectomies. It was always recognized and closed in two layers, a continuous through-and-through layer of 3-0 absorbable material and an inverting layer of 3-0 or 2-0 absorbable sutures. We do not use nonabsorbable sutures. At the end of the operation, the anal sphincter should be dilated to release the intrarectal pressure postoperatively and avoid tension on the suture line. All five cases of rectal injury healed well without sequelae and without prolonging the hospital stay.

Late complications of radical prostatectomy are incontinence, impotence, and stricture at the urethrovesical anastomosis.

Total or severe incontinence is extremely rare, occurring in less than 2% of cases. Stress incontinence is more common and occurs in 10% of patients. It is usually minimal, occurring toward the end of the day and requiring a small pad. Severe stress incontinence occurs in 2% of cases and usually requires intervention.

Impotence after nerve-sparing radical prostatectomy is directly related to the age of the patient and the extent of disease. Older men with locally extensive disease fare less well than younger men with organ-confined disease. In general, nerve-sparing preserves potency in 50% of patients, with a range of 20 to 75% depending on the preceding factors.

Strictures are rare if a mucosa-to-mucosa anastomosis is performed. Strictures occur in less than 10% of cases and usually respond to simple dilations. Table 17.4 lists all the complications encountered by the author in 450 consecutive radical prostatectomies.

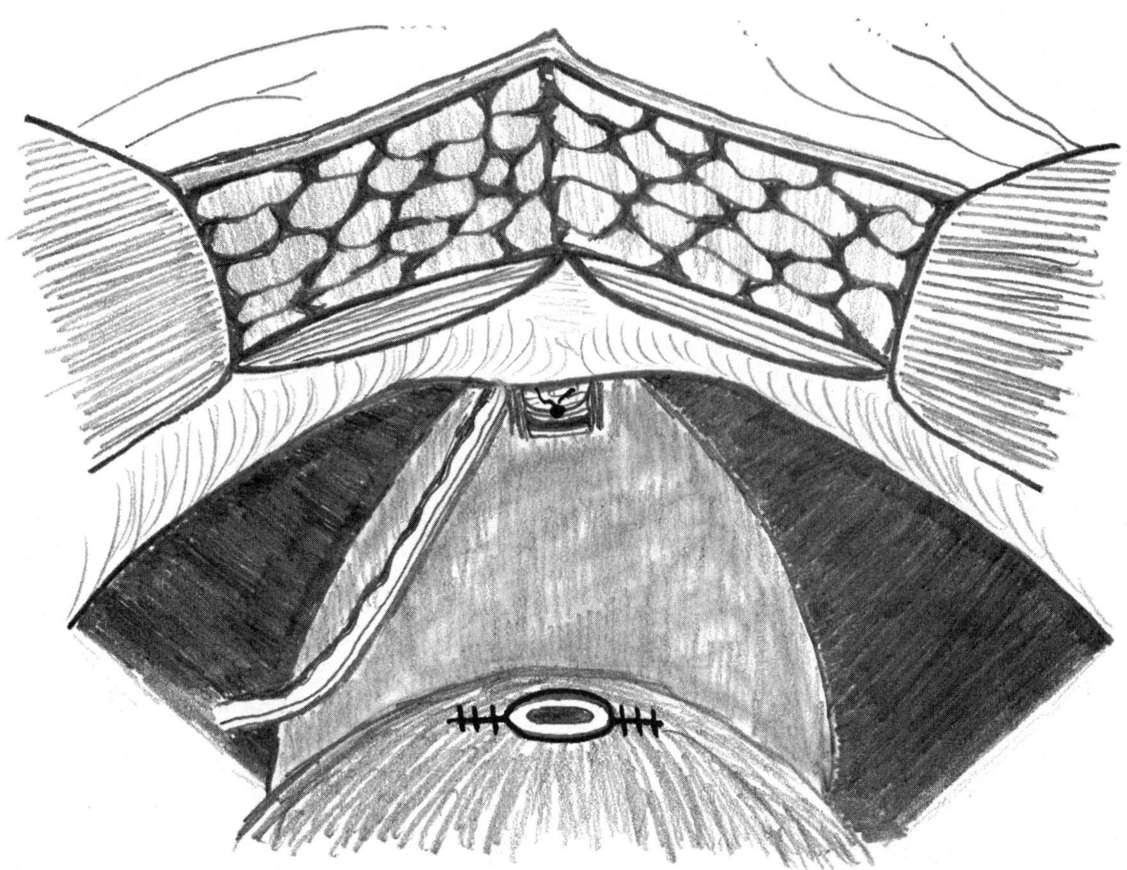

Fig. 17.27. Transverse closure of bladder neck.

Table 17.4. Complications in 475 Consecutive Radical Retropubic Prostatectomies

COMPLICATION	%
Death	0
Transfusion of more than 2 units	7
Rectal injury	1
Anastomotic stricture needing more than 1 dilation	8
Lymphocele	4
Wound infection	2
Thromboembolic disease	
Nonfatal	1
Fatal	0
Laryngeal spasm requiring tracheostomy	0.2
Incontinence	
Total	2
Significant stress	2
Minimal stress	10
Impotence	70

RESULTS

Modern radical retropubic prostatectomy is less than 10 years old, and it will be another 10 years before its results and its influence on patient survival are known.

The majority of reports on the results of radical prostatectomy for stage A prostate cancer combine the relatively few patients with stage A1 and those with stage A2 disease. The long-term disease-free survival rate is 90%, and the disease-specific mortality rate is only 1% (19). Elder et al. (20) recently reported on 25 patients with stage A2 disease who received follow-up care from 9 months to longer than 10 years after radical prostatectomy. These authors found only one instance of local recurrence and one death from other causes without evidence of prostate cancer; twenty-three patients are alive free of disease.

There are two series of radical prostatectomy for stage B disease with long-term follow-up—the Johns Hopkins Hospital Series reported by Walsh and Jewett in 1980 (21) and the Mason Clinic Series reported by Gibbons et al. in 1984 (22). Of 57 patients with stage B1 prostate cancer in the Hopkins series, 29 (51%) lived for at least 15 years without evidence of disease, 18 (32%) died of other causes within the 15-year follow-up period but had no clinical evidence of disease, and 10

(17%) died of prostate cancer. The 15-year disease-free survival rate of men with clinical stage B, excluding those with B1 disease, was 25%. Those who had disease limited to the prostate on pathologic examination of the surgical specimen had a 15-year disease-free survival rate of 50% compared with 13% for those who had disease outside the capsule or invading the seminal vesicles.

In the Mason Clinic Series of radical prostatectomy for stage B disease, the 15-year disease-free survival rate was 50%. Twenty-nine patients were at risk for 15 years. In a recent update of this series, Gibbons found a 60% observed survival in 57 men who received follow-up care for at least 15 years. This survival exceeded the life expectancy of men of the same age-group living in the same region during the same time. Of 57 patients who received follow-up care for at least 15 years, 46 (84%) are alive and free of disease or were free of disease when they died of other causes (23).

The author's series of 376 consecutive radical prostatectomies performed on previously untreated men with localized prostate cancer spans 10 years. It is worth discussing here because of certain features.

1. All 376 specimens were morphometrically studied by the step-section technique.
2. All patients received follow-up care with a serum PSA, which has the ability to detect recurrences long before the recurrences become clinically evident by DRE, computed tomography scan, or bone scan.

Of 376 patients, 40 (11%) had lymph node metastasis and 40 (11%) had seminal vesicle invasion. Although only 55 of them have had disease progression during a follow-up period of 2 to 10 years, all 80 patients are expected to have disease progression. Disease progression is defined as detectable and rising PSA anytime after the operation. One hundred seventy-four (46%) had capsular penetration, and 75% of these patients remain free of disease. Of 122 patients with organ-confined disease, 113 remain with a PSA of 0.0 ng/mL.

In summary, the radical retropubic prostatectomy described here is a well-tolerated operation with a relatively low morbidity. If performed on a select group of patients with low-volume disease, it can be curative in the majority of cases.

REFERENCES

1. Silverberg EL. Cancer statistics. CA Cancer J Clin 1984;34:3–22.
2. Boring CC, Squires TS, Tong T, et al. Cancer statistics. CA Cancer J Clin 1994;44:7.
3. Catalona W. Screening for prostate cancer: enthusiasm. Urology 1993;42:113.
4. Babaian RJ, Mettlin C, Kane R, et al. The relationship of prostate-specific antigen to digital rectal examination and transrectal ultrasonography. Cancer 1992;69:1195.
5. Millin T. Retropubic prostatectomy: new extravesical technique. report on twenty cases. Lancet 1945;2:693.
6. Millin T. Retropubic urinary surgery. Baltimore: Williams & Wilkins, 1947.
7. Memmelaar J. Total prostatovesiculectomy: retropubic approach. J Urol 1949;62:340.
8. Chute R. Radical retropubic prostatectomy for cancer. J Urol 1954;71:347.
9. Ansel JS. Radical transvesical prostatectomy: preliminary report of an approach to surgical excision of localized prostatic malignancy. J Urol 1959;82:373.
10. Campbell EW. Total prostatectomy with preliminary ligation of the vascular pedicles. J Urol 1959;81:464.
11. Mittemyer BT, Cox HD. Modified radical retropubic prostatectomy. Urology 1978;12:313.
12. Freiha FS, Bagshaw MA. Carcinoma of the prostate: results of post-irradiation biopsy. Prostate 1985;5:19.
13. Walsh PC, Lepor H, Eggleston JC. Radical prostatectomy with preservation of sexual function: anatomical and pathological considerations. Prostate 1983;4:473.
14. Villers A, McNeal JE, Redwine EA, et al. The role of perineural space invasion in the local spread of prostatic adenocarcinoma. J Urol 1989;142:763.
15. Montie JE. Staging of prostate cancer. Cancer 1994;74:1.
16. Terris MK, McNeal JE, Stamey TA. Estimation of prostate cancer volume by transrectal ultrasound imaging. J Urol 1992;147:855.
17. Stamey TA, Yang N, Hay AR, et al. Prostate specific antigen as a serum marker for adenocarcinoma of the prostate. N Engl J Med 1987;317:909.
18. Villers A, McNeal JE, Redwine EA, et al. The role of perineural space invasion in the local spread of prostatic adenocarcinoma. J Urol 1989;142:763.
19. Catalona WJ, Scott WW. Carcinoma of the prostate. In: Walsh PC, Gittes RE, Perlmutter ED, et al., eds. Campbell's urology. 5th ed. Philadelphia: WB Saunders, 1986:1463.
20. Elder JS, Gibbons RP, Correa RJ, et al. Efficacy of radical prostatectomy for stage A2 carcinoma of the prostate. Cancer 1985;56:2151.
21. Walsh PC, Jewett HJ. Radical surgery for prostatic cancer. Cancer 1980;45:1906.
22. Gibbons RP, Correa RJ, Brannen GE, et al. Total prostatectomy for localized prostatic cancer, J Urol 1984;131:73.
23. Gibbons RP. Total prostatectomy for localized prostatic cancer: long-term surgical results and current morbidity. the Virginia Mason Clinic experience. Presented at the Consensus Development Conference on Management of Localized Prostate Cancer, NIH, Bethesda, June 15–17, 1987.

18

Radical Retropubic Prostatectomy

The Anatomic Antegrade Approach

E. David Crawford

Adenocarcinoma of the prostate is the most common cancer diagnosed in U.S. males and is currently the second-leading cause of death (1). However, if current trends continue, it is likely to surpass lung cancer in the next decade as the leading cause of death. The widespread public awareness and early detection efforts for prostate cancer have resulted in the majority of patients having their conditions diagnosed at a stage when treatment with curative intent can be considered. Selection of such patients is based on clinical stage, age at diagnosis, life expectancy, grade of tumor, and personal preferences. Selection of patients for this procedure is discussed in detail in Chapter 15. Further refinements in prostate-specific antigen (PSA) assays, transrectal ultrasound, reverse transcriptase, and other methods to predict extracapsular disease are resulting in better clinical means to identify locally confined prostate cancers. Patients undergoing complete surgical extirpation of the disease now are more likely to have an organ-confined cancer than those treated a decade ago. This should result in significant improvements in cancer-specific survival rates.

Radical surgical extirpation of the cancerous prostate remains the time-honored therapy for locally confined cancer. The procedure includes the en bloc removal of the prostate, ejaculatory ducts, seminal vesicles, and investing Denonvilliers' fascia. Ideally, the procedure also involves division of the vascular and lymphatic supply before manipulation of the gland. Refinements in the technique permit preservation of urinary continence in the majority of patients. In fact, total urinary incontinence is a rare event, occurring in less than 1% of patients in our hands. The ability to maintain erectile potency sufficient for intercourse is related to a number of preoperative factors, including tumor stage, potency status, and patient age.

HISTORICAL PERSPECTIVES

The technique for radical perineal prostatectomy was described by Kuchler in 1866 (2). This report was followed in 1905 by Young's performance of the first radical prostatectomy in the United States (3). Young's selection of patients was apparently not as sophisticated as the current process because most of his patients ultimately died of metastatic disease. However, to date there have been few changes in the surgical technique that he described in 1903.

The perineal approach to radical prostatectomy remained popular until 1947, when Millin introduced the retropubic method (4). Early interest in Millin's approach stemmed from urologists' familiarity with retropubic anatomy. The addition of staging pelvic lymphadenectomy has added a new dimension to our surgical methods and serves to strengthen the use of the retropubic approach. McLaughlin et al. believe that the concept of radical prostatectomy has been extended to include an extraperitoneal pelvic lymphadenectomy (5). This conclusion is based on the fact that 35% of patients who are assumed to have clinical disease confined to the prostate will be found to have unsuspected lymph node metastases at the time of lymphadenectomy.

Our method for radical retropubic prostatectomy is a modification of the technique as first described by Ansell and later advocated by Campbell (6, 7). Dissatisfaction with Millin's classic retropubic approach prompted the development of Campbell's technique, which emphasizes dissection of the prostate from the base to the apex. Campbell reported less local contamination and manipulation during removal of the prostate, with a resultant decreased chance of disseminating cancer cells.

A successful cancer operation includes three basic principles—proper selection of patients, removal of all malignant tissues with acceptable tumor-free margins, and tissue dissection performed in the proper sequence to minimize iatrogenic lymphatic and hematogenous dissemination. This technique fulfills the latter two criteria; the first premise must be fulfilled by careful presurgical evaluation. In addition to meeting the requirements for a good cancer operation, we believe that this technique offers a number of distinct advantages over the classic perineal or retropubic approaches to prostatectomy.

This approach initially allows for a predictable anatomic dissection. Common to both the classic approach and Campbell's retropubic approach are the opportunity to perform a staging pelvic lymphadenectomy and the advantage of the urologist's knowledge of retropubic anatomy. With Campbell's approach, however, there is less time-consuming hemorrhage early in the procedure because division of the dorsal vein of the penis and periurethral venous plexus is one of the final steps. Placement of the urethral sutures under direct vision at the time of anastomosis decreases the chance of incontinence as well.

SELECTION AND EVALUATION OF PATIENTS

Radical surgical procedures performed to cure prostate cancer are based on the premise that all cancer cells reside in the tissue removed. Therefore, proper selection of patients is mandatory. The selection of patients with prostatic adenocarcinoma amenable to surgical excision has been outlined in Chapter 15. The need for total prostatic excision is based on the study by Byar and Mostofi (8). After evaluating step sections of 208 prostates removed for early carcinoma, they found that tumor was present in both posterior lobes in 80% of cases, that it was multifocal in 85%, and that it was present in one of the first two apical step sections in 75%.

The propensity for dissemination increases with the size of the neoplasm. McNeal has reported that dissemination is usually limited to tumors over 1 mL in volume (9). Therefore, patients with clinical stage T2 disease represent the ideal candidates for radical prostatectomy. We also perform radical prostatectomy in patients with stage T1 disease who have negative results from staging lymphadenectomy. We have not found that the operation performed after transurethral resection is compromised. Patients with stage T2B and T3 disease are not ideal candidates for radical prostatectomy because the propensity for extracapsular disease and lymph node involvement is high (14 to 45%) (4–10).

Because of this preoperative knowledge, many patients undergo more extensive preradical prostatectomy evaluation for pelvic lymph node involvement, including CT scanning, MRI, and laparoscopic lymph node dissection. These patients are then filtered out, and the true incidence of pelvic lymph node disease in patients undergoing radical prostatectomy significantly decreases. Thus, the current trend is a decreasing incidence of stage N+ disease. Many patients thought to have stage T2 disease are found to have pathologic stage T3 disease (10).

At this time, we do not advocate a radical surgical procedure for patients with bulky stage T3 or stage N+ disease. However, studies are in progress to assess the value of combining radical prostatectomy with some sort of hormonal manipulation. We have recently observed a group of patients who had clinical stage T3 disease who underwent laparoscopic lymph node dissection, 4 months of neoadjuvant hormonal therapy, and radical prostatectomy. Only 1 of 26 patients experienced true tumor downstaging. However, the majority experienced significant reductions in PSA and tumor volume. Extended follow-up is needed to determine whether these pathologic findings result in an improved survival rate. There are several ongoing and completed clinical trials that support or refute the value of neoadjuvant hormonal therapy before radical prostatectomy for patients with T2 or less lesions (11, 12). There may be some survival benefit conferred on this subset of patients, but further follow-up is needed.

Evaluation of the grade of the tumor is important because the higher grade tumors appear as more advanced disease (13). The candidate for radical prostatectomy should have a thorough radiologic and laboratory evaluation, in addition to a diligently performed physical examination. Tests to detect distant spread of disease include bone scan, CT scan of the pelvis, intravenous pyelogram, chest radiograph, PSA, acid phosphatase, and new molecular markers. PSA, clinical stage, and Gleason score are powerful predictors of extracapsular or disseminated disease. Bone scans and CT scans should be reserved for patients at significant risk for metastatic disease. Cystoscopic examination before the surgical procedure is indicated in patients who have symptoms suggestive of a urethral stricture or microhematuria.

The psychological aspects of the operation, including impotence, must be discussed in detail with the patient and his sexual partner during the initial and preoperative visits. Quality of life should be an important part of the decision analysis. Quality of life may be affected by any treatment, including watchful waiting. The major complications after radical retropubic prostatectomy are the risk of incontinence and impotence.

In our early series of 150 patients undergoing radical retropubic prostatectomy, 50% of patients did not engage in regular sexual activity and 50% of those who did and were impotent after radical prostatectomy desired some sort of intervention. Modification of the surgical technique can preserve potency in up to 80% of patients who undergo the procedure. In our experience, preservation of potency after the procedure is age related. It is rare for men who are 50 years old or younger to become impotent, whereas nearly 50 to 80% of those approaching 70 years of age will experience significant erectile dysfunction.

With the widespread public awareness and early detection efforts, the age at which patients undergo the operation is significantly decreasing. The majority of patients that we currently perform radical prostatectomy on are in their 50s; currently, 10% of the surgical group are younger than 50. For this group, maintenance of potency is extremely important, and extensive preoperative counseling is warranted. Patients should be made aware that their erections certainly will not be any better than they are now and probably will not be the same. However, in those in whom potency is preserved, the erections are usually adequate for intercourse and usually do not require any assistance by injections or vacuum devices.

ANATOMIC CONSIDERATIONS

Knowledge of the anatomic features of the prostate, including its blood vessels and fascia, is imperative for the success of this surgical procedure. However, urologists remain confused about the exact nature of Denonvilliers' fascia, the endopelvic fascia, and the puboprostatic ligaments.

Endopelvic Fascia

Structure

The endopelvic fascia represents a condensation of the pelvic fascia and a continuation of the transversalis fascia as it enters the pelvis. At the arcus tendineus or white line, the pelvic fascia reflects medially off the obturator internus muscle. From this white line, one leaf of the fascia sweeps medially and thickens to form a sheath covering the anterior and lateral surfaces of the prostate. This condensation is known as the endopelvic fascia. The puboprostatic ligaments represent its anterior reflection from the pubic bone, which supports the gland and blends with the prostatic capsule. These paired ligamentous structures are avascular.

The endopelvic fascia fuses with Denonvilliers' fascia at the posterolateral margin of the prostate. The anatomic importance of the endopelvic fascia lies not only in its support of the prostate, but also in the fact that it contains, beneath its lateral reflections, much of the vascular and lymphatic supply of the gland. The anterior and lateral reflections of the endopelvic fascia must be divided in the course of a radical prostatectomy. We prefer early ligation of the lateral reflections before any manipulation of the gland. Our approach is to treat these lateral reflections as anatomic pedicles and to ligate them as such.

Profuse bleeding occurring during the division of the prostatomembranous urethra is often mistakenly thought to rise from the puboprostatic ligaments. However, microscopic studies by Albers et al. show these ligaments to be mostly composed of collagen and variable amounts of smooth muscle (14). The ligaments are attached to the inferior border of the pubis, lateral to the cartilaginous symphysis, and on the prostatic side they blend with the lateral leaves of the endopelvic fascia at the prostatovesical junction. Sharp division of the puboprostatic ligaments results in their retraction because of the smooth muscle component.

Venous Drainage

A rich system of venous drainage is located in the recess between the puboprostatic ligaments and also on the lateral aspects of the prostate. Our approach to this highly vascular area involves a vertical incision in the endopelvic fascia, approximately 1 cm lateral to its reflection onto the prostatic surface (Fig. 18.1). This incision allows for development of a plane between the prostate and the rectum and also prevents inadvertent injury to the lateral prostatic venous plexus. An incision made in close proximity to the prostate risks laceration of this lateral plexus. The incision in the endopelvic fascia can be made with either electrocautery or a knife. The space is developed

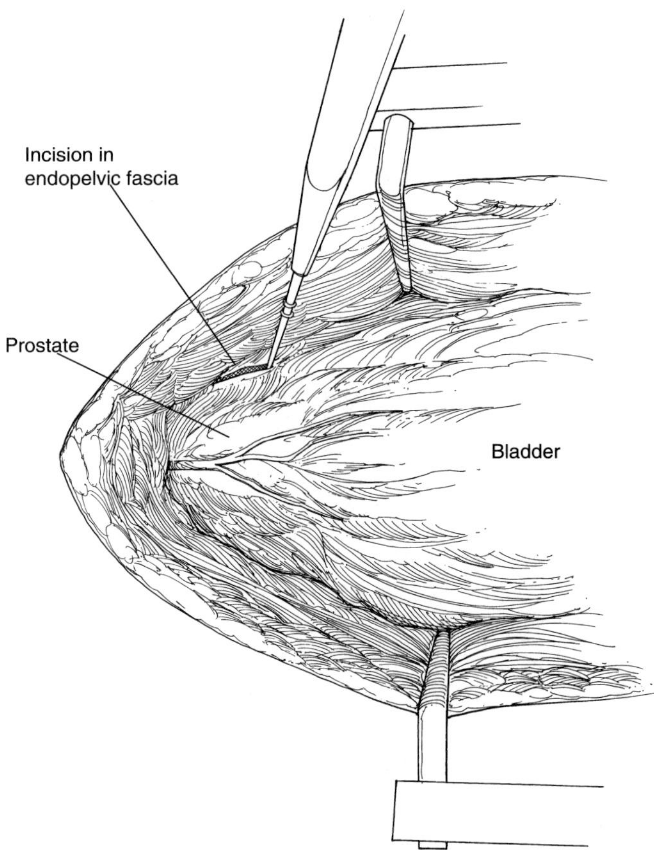

Fig. 18.1. Incision is made in the endopelvic fascia approximately 2 cm lateral to its reflection onto the prostatic surface.

posterior and lateral, and then carried cephalad toward the urethra.

The puboprostatic ligaments are divided sharply to establish a connection between the superior aspect of the previous incision in the endopelvic fascia and to expose the superficial branch of the dorsal vein in the penis (Fig. 18.2). The superficial vein trifurcates at the prostatomembranous urethral junction. In the past, we have dissected underneath the pubis to expose this trifurcation and then passed a right-angle clamp anterior to the urethra. A 0 or 2-0 chromic ligature is passed via the right angle and tied as distally as possible. The dorsal venous complex is ligated proximally with a 2-0 chromic and sharply divided between the sutures with a scissors. In the past 300 radical retropubic prostatectomies performed by our technique, a modification has been made whereby the puboprostatic ligaments are identified and sharply divided. Use of a Kitner dissector is helpful in identifying the puboprostatic ligaments before division. They frequently lie deeper than anticipated. After these are divided, cephalad and posterior traction is placed on the prostate, exposing the dorsal venous complex. With Metzenbaum scissors, it is sharply divided down to the anterior portion of the urethra. In general, very little bleeding results and it is easily controlled with suture ligatures of 2-0 chromic. It is rarely necessary to place more than two or three of these

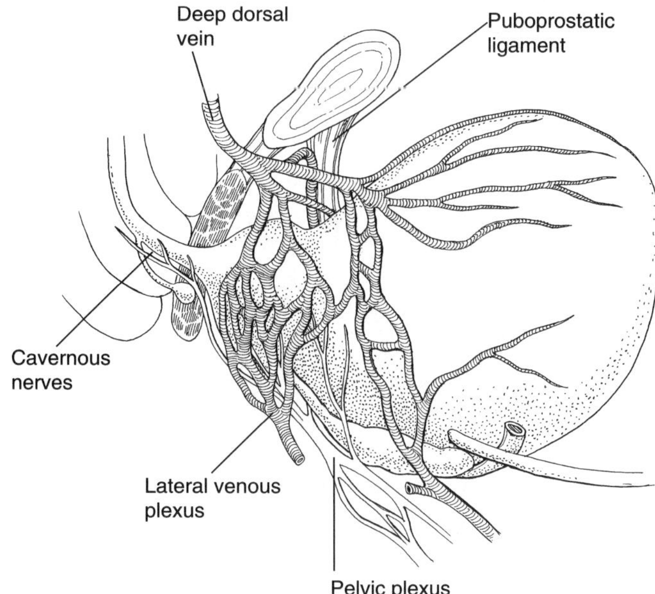

Fig. 18.2. Anatomic depiction of deep dorsal vein and its tributaries behind the symphyses pubes and the cavernous nerves coursing posterolaterally close to the prostate and the membranous urethra.

suture ligatures. Using this plus other techniques to be described has resulted in a significant reduction in transfusion rates. In the past 90 procedures performed, only 1 patient has required 1 autologous unit of blood. Blood loss is consistently within the 300 to 800 mL range.

Denonvilliers' Fascia

Anatomic descriptions of the nature and confines of Denonvilliers' fascia remain confusing. In addition, anatomists use a number of terms to describe it, including prostatoperitoneal membrane, rectal fascia, anterior and posterior layers of Denonvilliers, and pearly gates. The excellent review by Tobin contains an in-depth evaluation of Denonvilliers' fascia, its origin, and its surgical importance (15). Clinically, Denonvilliers' fascia is not only an important anatomic landmark in the surgical approach to the prostate and seminal vesicles, but it is also an effective barrier in preventing extensions of pus, extravasation of urine, and spread of malignant tumors of the prostate, seminal vesicles, and rectum.

Structure

Compressed between the posterior surface of the seminal vesicles, prostate, bladder, and the anterior rectal wall are three distinct layers. Overlying the ventral rectal surface and intermingled with the external longitudinal musculature is a layer of areolar and fatty rectal fascia known as the posterior layer of Denonvilliers' fascia. The remnant of the peritoneal cul-de-sac in the fetus is located anterior to the rectal fascia (Fig. 18.3) (15). This layer is known as the anterior layer of Denonvilliers'

fascia or the prostatoperitoneal membrane and is in the form of a V.

The apex of the V is attached to the superior layer of the urogenital diaphragm at the inferior border of the prostate (Fig. 18.4). The two limbs of the V extend dorsolaterally to cover the posterior surface of the seminal vesicles. More importantly, this fibrous membrane fuses with the prostatic capsule where the ampullae join the prostate. Therefore, an attempt to establish a plane anterior to this layer often results in the disruption of the prostatic capsule, with the resultant risk of entering the tumor or leaving an involved capsule behind.

Anterior to this layer is a framework of connective tissue that is continuous around the prostate and seminal vesicles. This framework is believed to blend with the anterior layer of Denonvilliers' fascia. There is a difference of opinion about whether this layer is a branching of the anterior layer of Denonvilliers' or a separate anatomic layer (15). Regardless of its origin, it appears that on reaching the tips of the seminal vesicles, this anterior layer splits and one leaf passes caudally over the posterior surface of the seminal vesicles, vasa, and prostatic capsule. It then extends to meet the anterior layer at the apex of the prostate.

The second leaf extends over the ventral surface of the seminal vesicles to the bladder base, where it reflects superiorly over the fundus of the bladder and then fuses with the first leaf. Between these leaves is an anatomic compartment, which is the space entered when the prostate base, seminal vesicles, and vasa are freed from the bladder and rectum.

Planes of Dissection

The clinical importance of these three layers located between the rectum and prostate is obvious. There are three potential

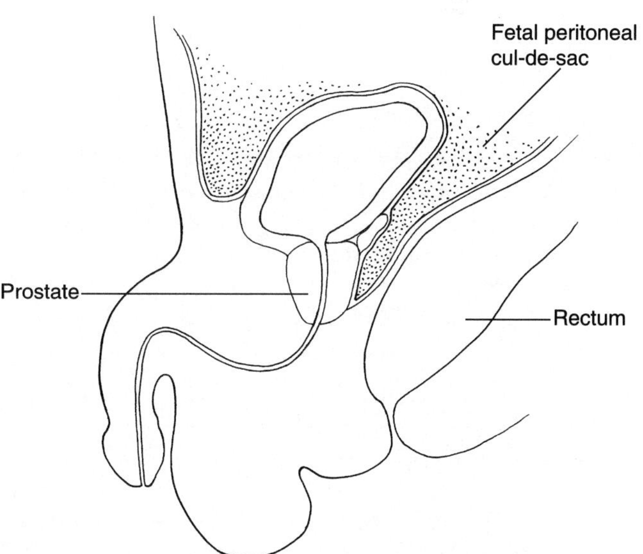

Fig. 18.3. Median view from the pelvis of a full-term fetus demonstrating the peritoneal cul-de-sac extending between the seminal vesicles, prostate, and rectum.

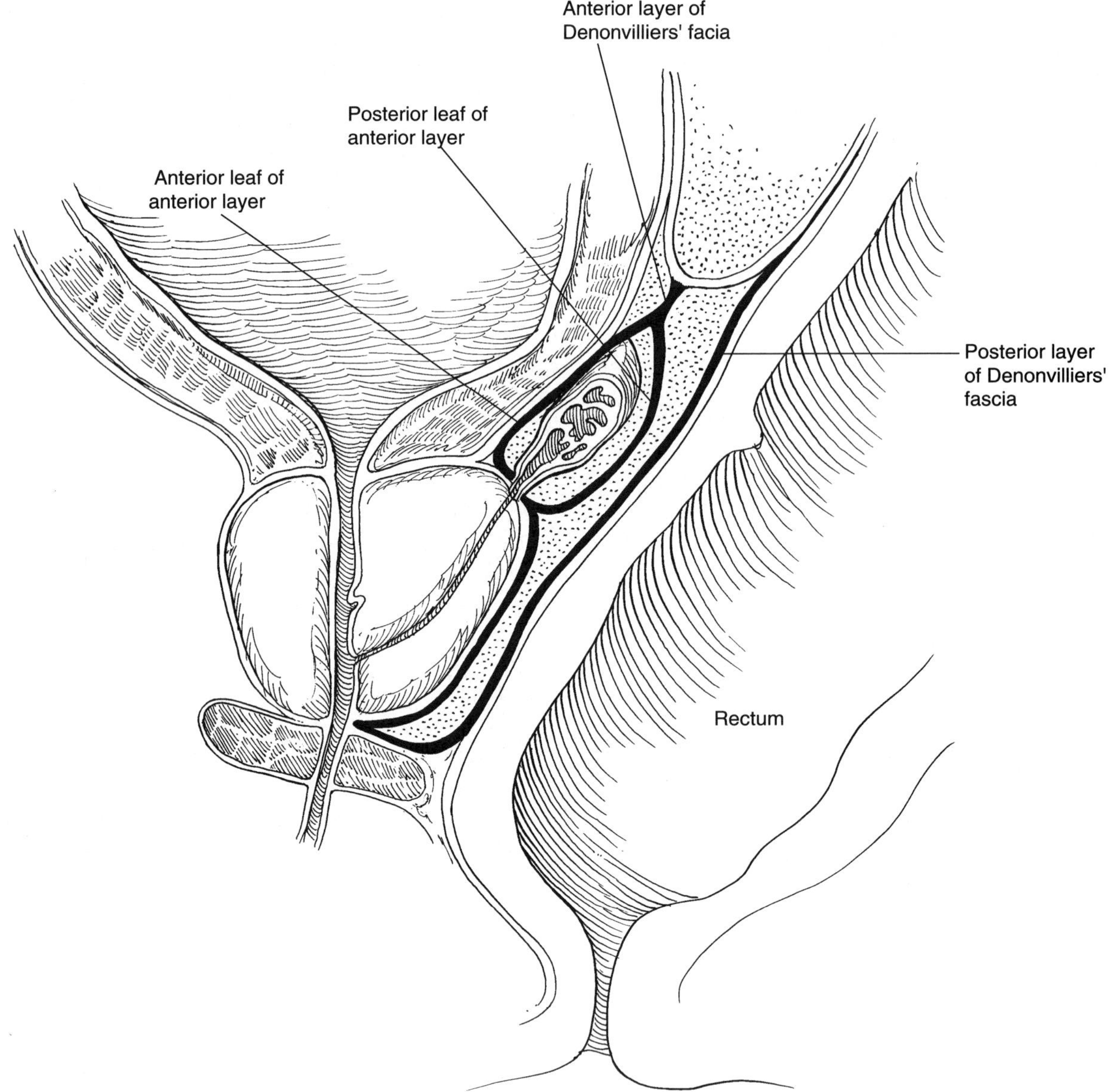

Fig. 18.4.   Midline sagittal view of the male pelvis showing the relationships among the layers of Denonvilliers' fascia, rectum, and prostate.

spaces that can be entered in an attempt to separate the prostate from the anterior rectal wall. One is between the longitudinal rectal musculature and the rectal fascia (posterior layer of Denonvilliers' fascia). The second is between the rectal fascia and the prostatoperitoneal membrane (anterior layer of Denonvilliers' fascia). The third is between the prostatoperitoneal membrane and the fibrous covering of the prostate and the seminal vesicles. The preferred plane is between the anterior and posterior layers of Denonvilliers' fascia. This plane is also referred to as the posterior compartment of Denonvilliers' fascia or the space of Proust.

SURGICAL PROCEDURE

Our preoperative preparation for patients has changed dramatically in the past 5 years. We no longer perform routine bowel preparations and do not admit patients to the hospital the evening before the procedure. They are admitted on an outpatient basis after taking nothing by mouth from midnight before the procedure. We continue to use a broad-spectrum antibiotic preoperatively and for 48 hours after the procedure.

The patient is placed in the supine position on the operating table. After adequate endotracheal anesthesia, the kidney rest is elevated under the lumbar spine area, providing slight hyperextension (Fig. 18.5). The entire abdomen, scrotum, penis, and inner thighs are prepared. The patient is draped in the usual manner with a sterile towel placed over the scrotum and under the penis. A sterile 22-French catheter is inserted and connected to a gravity drainage system. Another sterile towel is placed over the penis and preparation is made for the surgical incision.

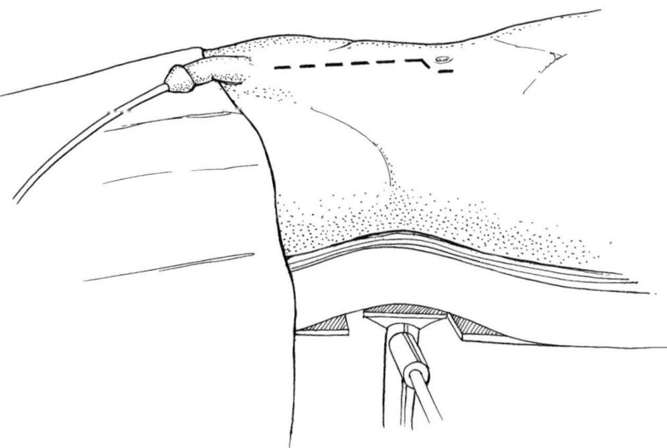

Fig. 18.5. Surgical position demonstrating elevation of the kidney rest under the lumbar spine area, placement of urethral catheter, and proposed incision site.

Incision

A midline incision is made, beginning at the symphysis pubis and extending superiorly to the lateral side of the umbilicus (Fig. 18.6). At this point, an electrocauterization unit is used for the division of the subcutaneous tissues. The rectus fascia is identified and incised, the midline is identified, and the rectus muscles are retracted laterally. The layer immediately deep to the rectus muscles is the investing fascia of the rectus abdominis muscles, which is contiguous with the transversalis fascia (Fig. 18.7). This layer is entered sharply (exposing the underlying retroperitoneal connective tissue), and dissection is carried inferiorly and laterally until the external iliac vessels

are identified. Failure to remain deep to this plane often results in inadvertent injury to the inferior epigastric vessels and also creates difficulty in approaching the prostate and pelvic vessels. The peritoneal reflection is identified with the vas and spermatic vessels coursing in its medial aspect (Fig. 18.8). The spermatic vessels are dissected free and, with sharp dissection, the reflection is freed from the psoas muscle. The vas is sharply dissected free and divided between two medium to large ligaclips (Fig. 18.9). It is not always necessary to divide the vas, and in approximately 70% of cases it may be preserved bilaterally. Some believe division of the vas may lead to an increased incidence of postoperative testicular pain and perhaps even epididymitis. The obliterated processus vaginalis will be adherent to the internal ring and requires sharp dissection to mobilize the peritoneal reflection. It is extremely important to carry the dissection laterally and cranially on each side of the colon, freeing this peritoneal reflection. This results in increased bladder mobility and a funneling effect of the bladder, permitting a subsequent urethral/bladder anastomosis that is free of any tension. This maneuver also affords excellent exposure for the pelvic lymphadenectomy and prostatectomy.

TECHNIQUE

A bilateral pelvic lymphadenectomy is done as described in Chapter 16. We currently do frozen sections only on suspicious lymph nodes.

The bladder is deflated, and slight traction is placed on the urethral catheter. The surgeon palpates the catheter balloon at the bladder neck and, with the other hand, makes a small incision with the electrocautery unit at the prostatovesicle junc-

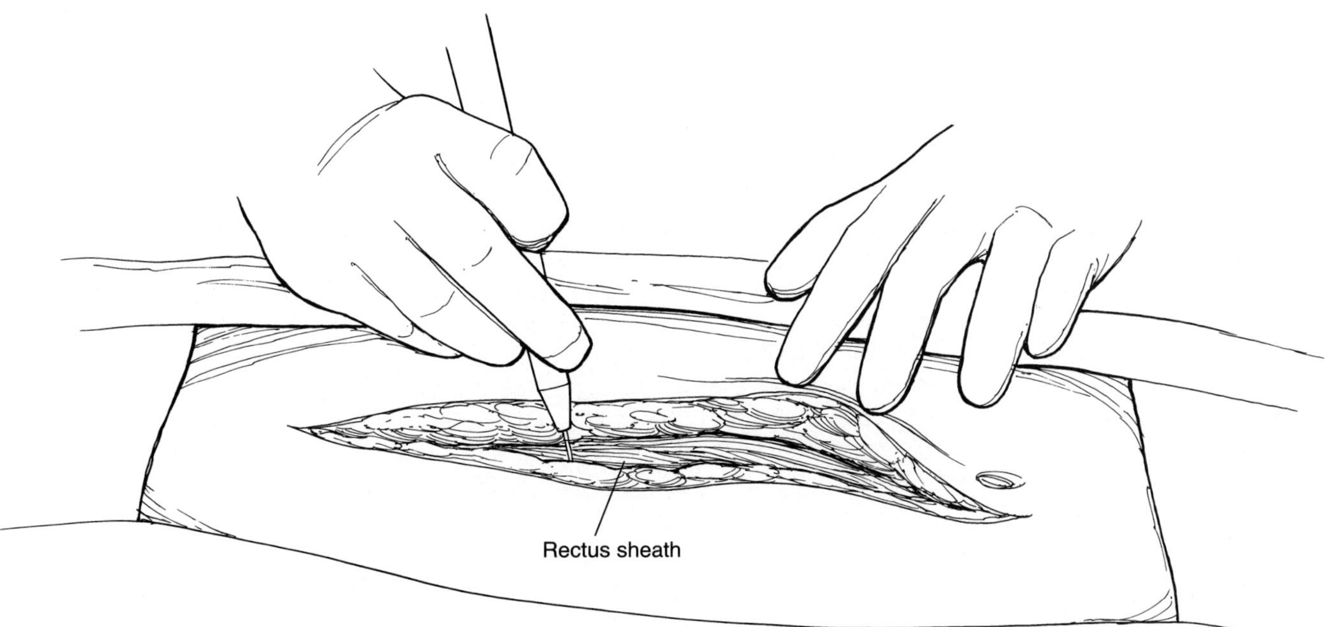

Fig. 18.6. Incision through subcutaneous tissues, exposing the rectus sheath.

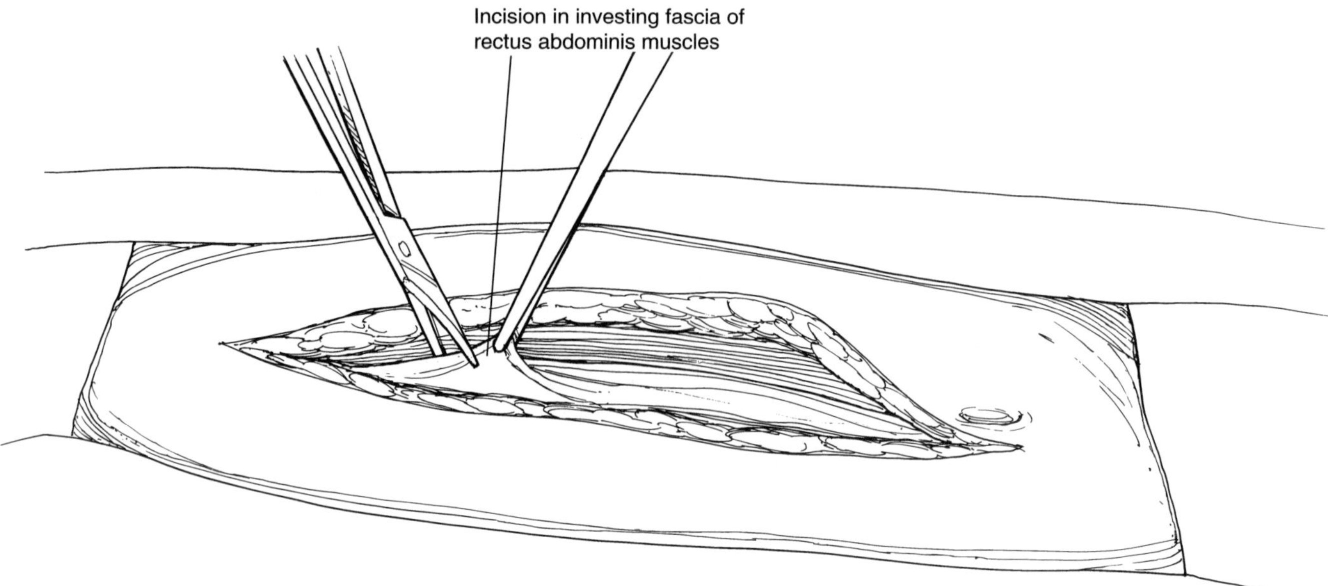

Fig. 18.7.   The incision has been carried through the rectus fascia, and the rectus muscles have been retracted laterally. An incision is being made in the investing fascia of the rectus abdominis muscles, exposing the retroperitoneal connective tissue.

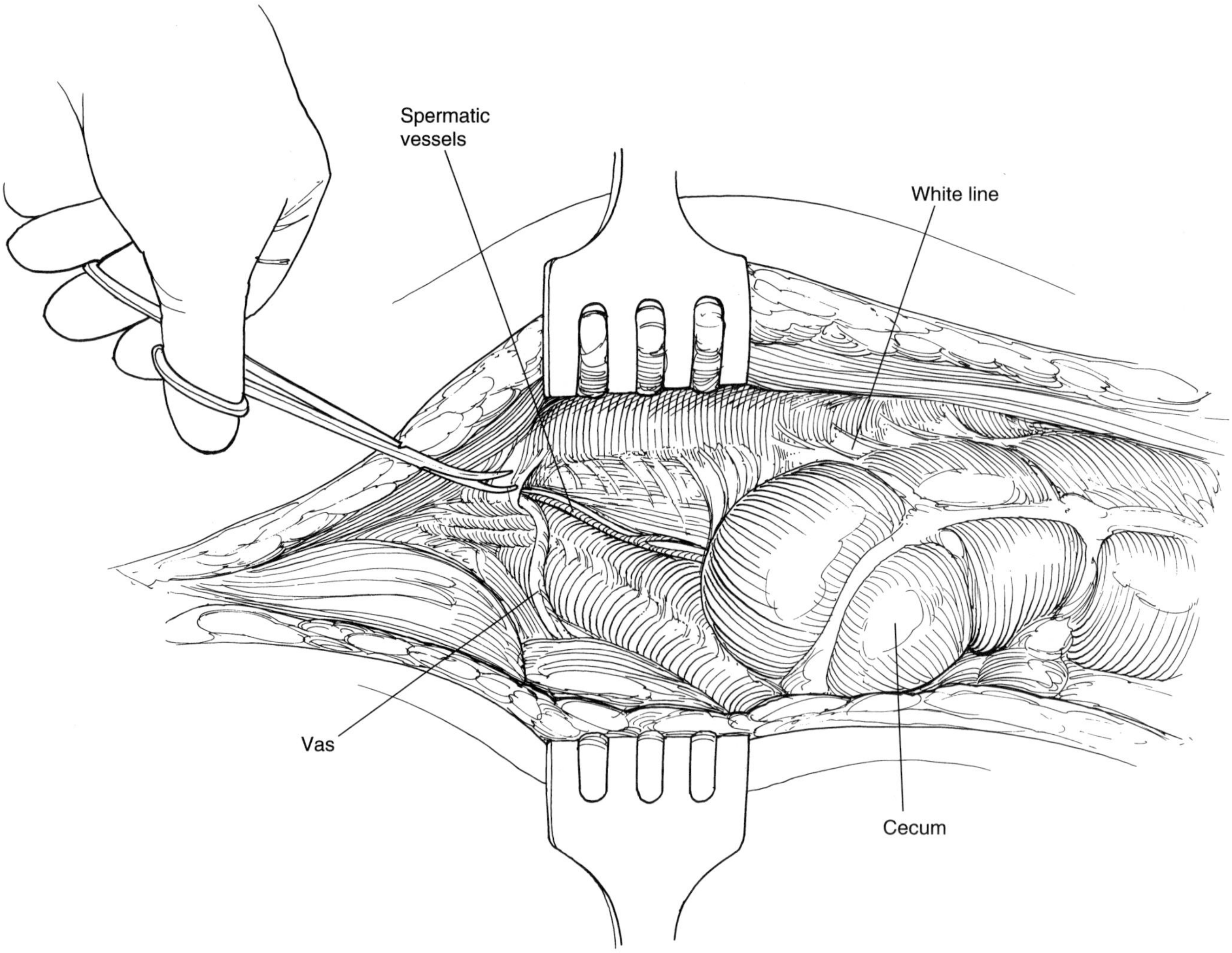

Fig. 18.8.   Peritoneal reflection with the vas and spermatic vessels identified. An incision is made at the internal ring lateral to the spermatic vessels.

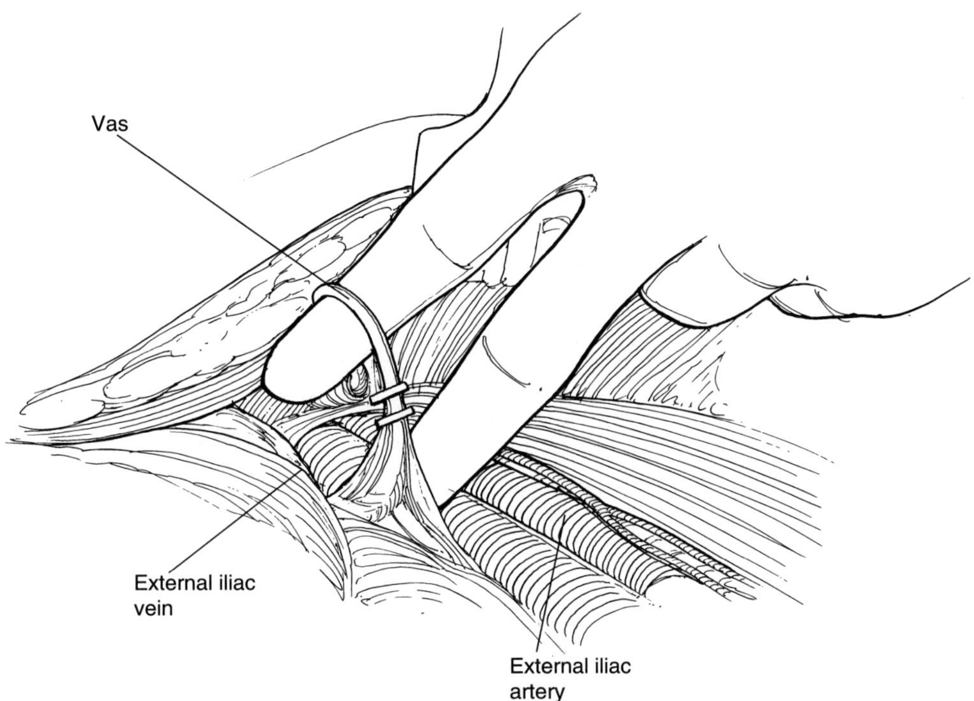

Fig. 18.9.   The vas is divided between two medium ligaclips.

tion (Fig. 18.10). The cautery current is used for the incision, and the superficial branch of the deep dorsal vein is usually encountered traversing the junction at the midline. The bladder is entered, and the incision is carried laterally between the 3-o'clock and 9-o'clock positions. The anterior bladder may be grasped with Allis forceps and elevated as the dissection is continued posteriorly. I continue to use the electrocautery unit for the entire division of the bladder neck. The catheter is removed from the bladder and advanced toward the symphysis pubis. The trigone and ureteral orifices are identified, and ureteral catheters are passed up each ureter. Indigo carmine may be injected intravenously to aid in the identification of the ureteral orifices. It is rarely necessary to use ureteral catheters or indigo carmine unless there is obvious concern for the close proximity of the trigone to the area of division.

The next step is the division of the trigonal floor from the prostate (Fig. 18.11). The first assistant places two fingers in the open bladder and provides cephalad traction. Two Allis clamps are placed on the lateral aspects of the bladder neck and are retracted laterally. This maneuver results in stretching of the junction of the trigone and prostate in a horizontal plane. Failure to execute this maneuver may result in a false plane leading into the thick posterior bladder wall and trigonal muscles. The incision should be approximately 2 cm in length and should be carried posteriorly until the ampullae of the vasa are visualized. There is little danger of injuring the rectum because the anterior compartment of Denonvilliers' fascia with the vasa and seminal vesicles is interposed between the posterior bladder wall and the rectum (Fig. 18.4).

With Metzenbaum scissors, a plane is established over the anterior surface of the seminal vesicles and vasa (Fig. 18.12). The dissection will develop a pedicle containing the tissue between the initial and trigonal incisions. This pedicle is divided with electrocautery. The posterior bladder lip is dissected from the vasa and seminal vesicles with sharp dissection. The lip may be elevated with an Allis clamp, taking care not to apply excessive cephalad traction because the bladder musculature may tear easily.

The vasa are individually mobilized and clamped with ligaclips (Fig. 18.13). The right and left ampullae of the vasa are identified. With Metzenbaum scissors, the areolar tissue is freed, both proximally and distally on the vas, and a right-angle clamp is passed under the vas. This right-angle clamp is opened and a plane developed under the vas. A medium-sized ligaclip is placed toward the bladder side of the vas, and it is divided with an electrocautery unit. We have found that the ligaclip does not usually remain on the prostate side of the vas due to manipulation. There is also evidence that tumor cells may be exfoliated in the seminal fluid and that cauterization acts to seal the vas. A similar procedure is carried out on the contralateral vas. A Babcock clamp is then placed on the distal vas (the side with the ligaclip), and gentle upward and cephalad traction is applied. This facilitates dissection over the anterior and medial surfaces of the seminal vesicle. The seminal vesicles are situated lateral to the ligated stumps. There are numerous small blood vessels entering the seminal vesicle, and the liberal use of electrocautery to control these is indicated. The dissection is carried distally on the seminal vesicles as they wrap around the lateral side of the rectum. There is little danger of entering the rectum because the posterior leaf of the anterior

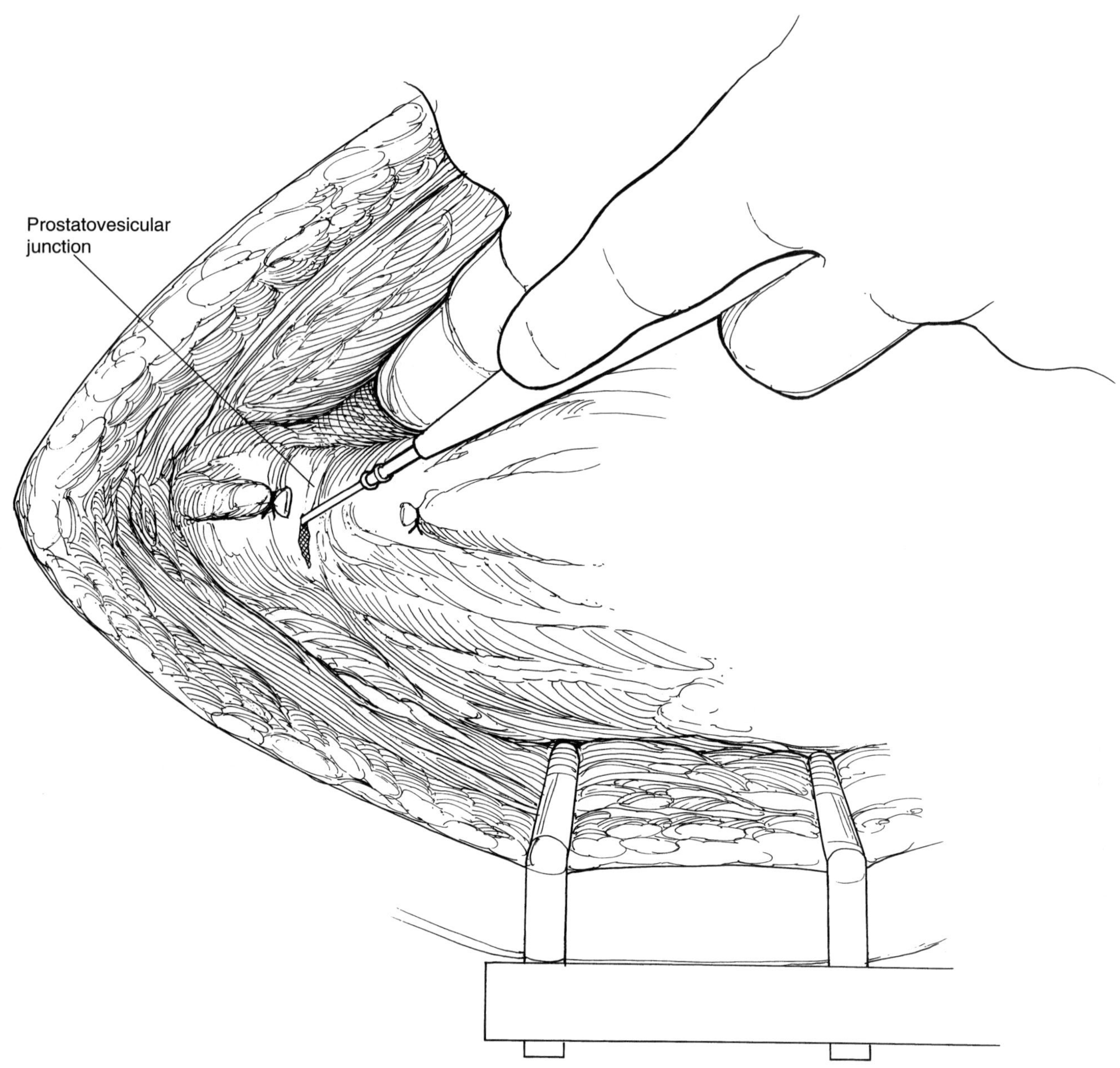

Fig. 18.10.   Incision at the prostatovesical junction made with the electrocautery unit.

layer of Denonvilliers', plus the posterior layer of Denonvilliers' fascia, are still in place.

After the tip of the seminal vesicle is identified, the blood supply is encountered. This may be controlled with a small ligaclip or with the electrocautery unit (Fig. 18.14).

The prostate is now free from the bladder and the seminal vesicles, and the vasa are free from the rectum. This maneuver has been performed within the anterior compartment of Denonvilliers' fascia. The cranial portion of the lateral pedicle is carefully divided between either ligaclips or 2-0 chromic suture ligatures (Fig. 18.15). When performing a nerve-sparing procedure, care is exercised not to extend the dissection beyond the position of the tip of the seminal vesicle. The anterior layer of Denonvilliers' fascia fuses with the prostatic capsule at the

junction of the vasa with the prostate. Therefore, any attempt to proceed bluntly through this plane often results in laceration of the prostatic capsule, with the resulting risk of tumor spill. The plane must be sharply entered proximal to the fusion with the prostatic capsule to proceed between the anterior and posterior layers of Denonvilliers' fascia. There are two ways to accomplish this.

One can sharply enter the plane proximal to the point where the anterior layer fuses with the prostatic capsule, or one can proceed in a retrograde manner, freeing the rectum from the prostate and then dividing over the dissecting finger. If there is little concern for preservation of potency, it is easier to develop the plane in the retrograde manner. To accomplish a retrograde dissection as already described, a vertical incision is

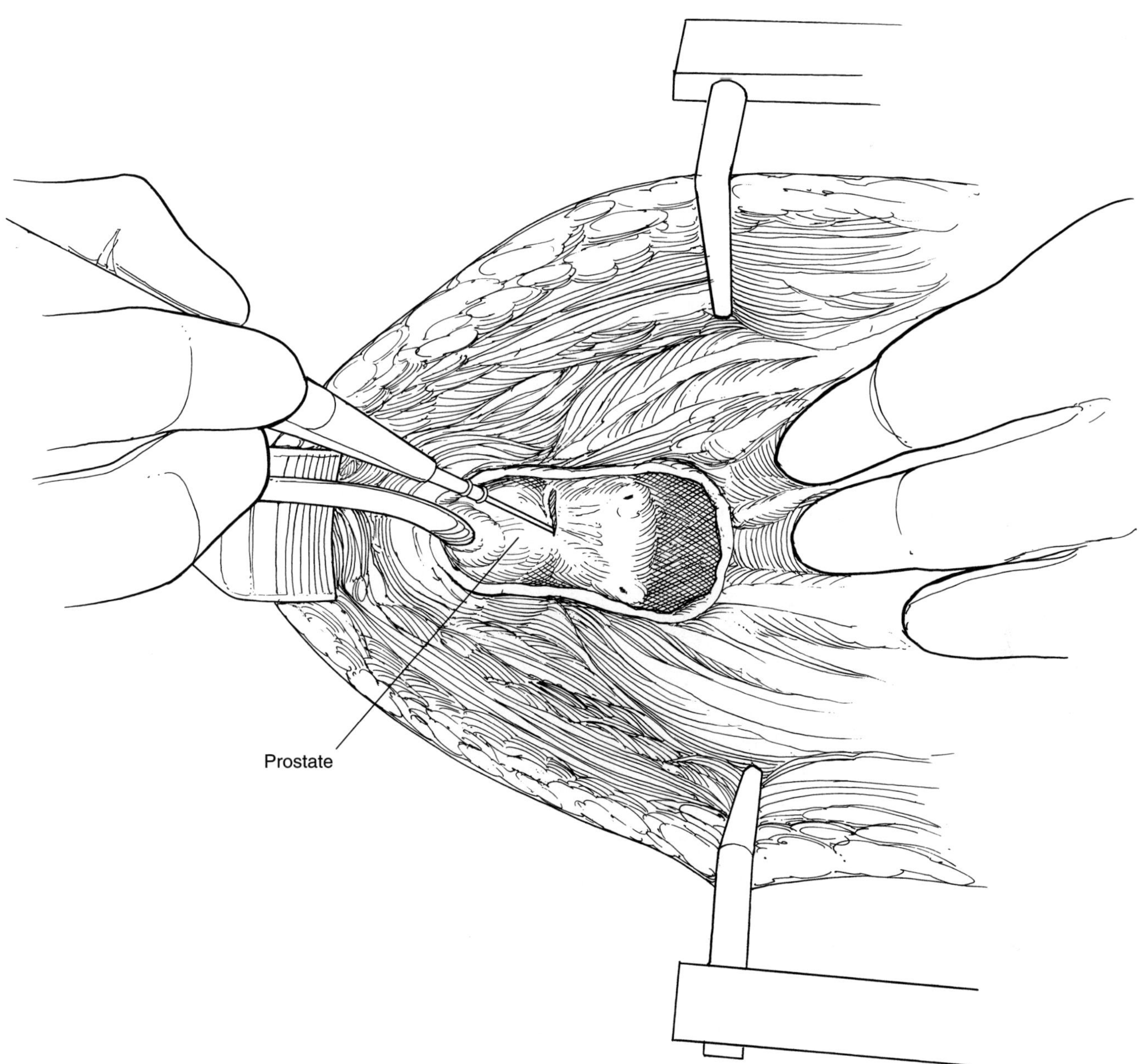

Fig. 18.11.   Ureteral catheters may be placed in both the ureteral orifices. Incision is made posteriorly in the trigone at the prostatovesical junction.

made in the endopelvic fascia approximately 1.5 cm lateral to the prostate. With blunt dissection using the index finger, a plane is established between the posterior surface of the prostate and the anterior rectal wall. To facilitate dissection, the index finger is insinuated medially until the undersurface of the urethra is palpated. Then with blunt dissection in a sweeping motion, the urethra is freed and the dissection carried posteriorally and cephalad under the prostate toward the prostate base. This blunt dissection proceeds without resistance if the proper plane between the layers of Denonvilliers' fascia is established.

With sweeping motion, the rectum is freed laterally, which results in the development of a lateral pedicle consisting mainly of the endopelvic fascia and the prostatic artery and neural complex at the base. The index finger is then brought to the prostate base just under the vasa, and an incision is made in the remaining posterior leaf of the anterior layer of Denonvilliers'. This incision is carried laterally on each side, resulting in freeing the entire posterior aspect of the prostate. At this time, the lateral pedicle can be divided between ligaclips or, as an alternative, a 0.25-in. Penrose drain is passed in a retrograde fashion from the incision in the endopelvic fascia posterior to the prostate and out the incision made at the base under the ampullae (Fig. 18.16A). Superior traction on this will result in the elevation of a pedicle, which can easily be ligaclipped. It is prudent to ensure that the rectum is dissected away by

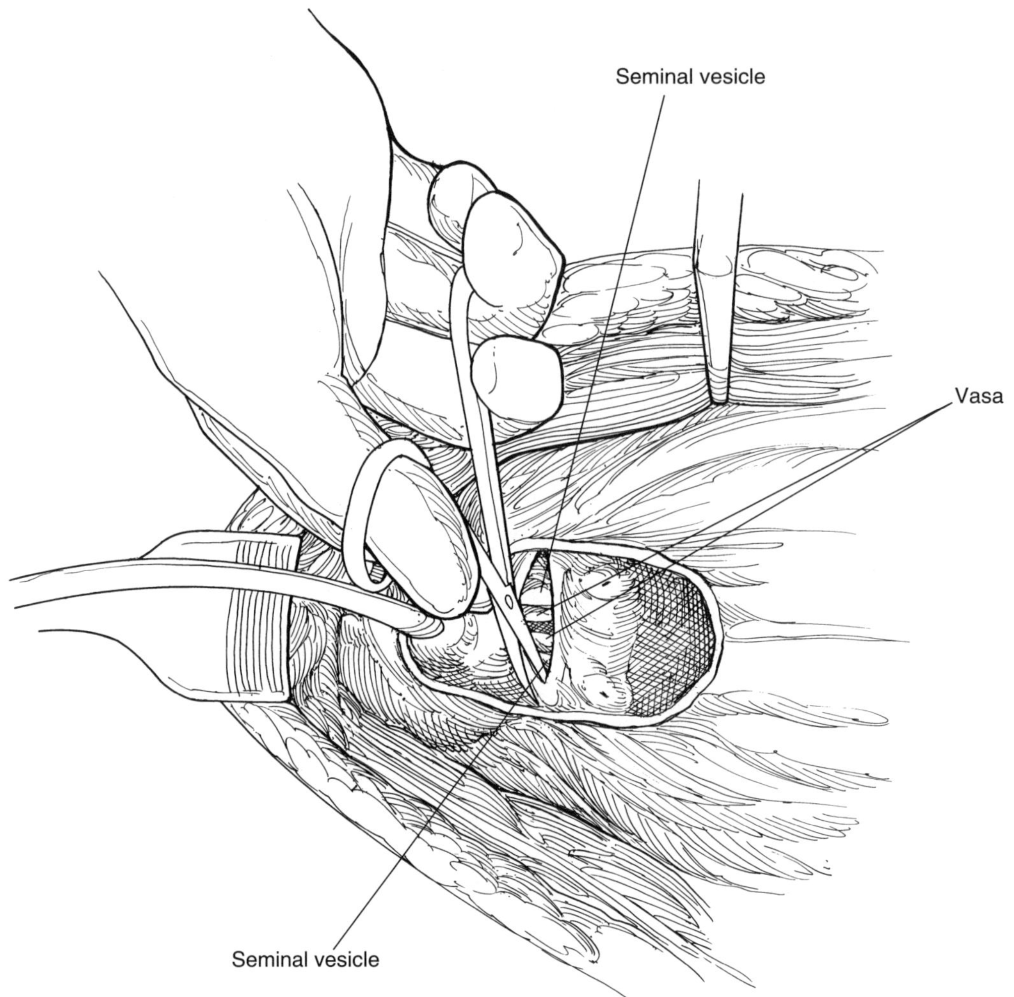

Fig. 18.12.   The incision is carried in a lateral direction, with Metzenbaum scissors establishing a plane over the anterior surface of the seminal vesicles and vasa.

sweeping finger dissection. This lateral pedicle is then divided between ligaclips; however, the vascular portion will be near the base of the prostate (Fig. 18.16B). After each of these lateral pedicles is divided, the prostate is free except for the urethra.

Nerve-Sparing Modification

If nerve sparing is intended, there are two ways to ensure this modified approach. The first involves the retrograde dissection as just described. The index finger palpates the urethra and is insinuated in a notch on each side between the urethra and the prostate apex. This contains the neurovascular structures at this point, and they are dissected from that area with blunt dissection using the index finger. The majority of time, they are easily separated and this is carried back cephalad toward the prostatic base, resulting in identification of a thin supporting structure, the endopelvic fascia. There is dense adherence at the prostatic base where the prostatic artery and neurovascular bundle are in close proximity. This needs to be sharply dissected

from the prostatic base toward the apex. The prostatic vasculature entering into the organ can either be ligaclipped or controlled with a suture. (Fig. 18.17).

The second method to preserve the neurovascular structures and to develop the lateral pedicles is by incising the posterior leaf of Denonvilliers' fascia just beneath the ampulla vas. To accomplish this, the ampulla is secured with a Babcock instrument and gently elevated. Use of a Kitner dissector will reveal the identification of the posterior leaf as it fuses with the prostatic capsule. An incision is made in this just under the prostate base, and with Metzenbaum scissors a plane is developed under the prostate. This plane will be identifiable by the presence of scant adipose tissue and loose areolar tissue. The finger is positioned in this place and should proceed to the urethra with little resistance. The usual error is to make this incision too superficial, resulting in inadvertent entering into the prostatic substance. Once this proper plane is identified, with sweeping motions the neurovascular bundles are freed from the lateral aspects of the prostate and the urethra. A similar maneuver is

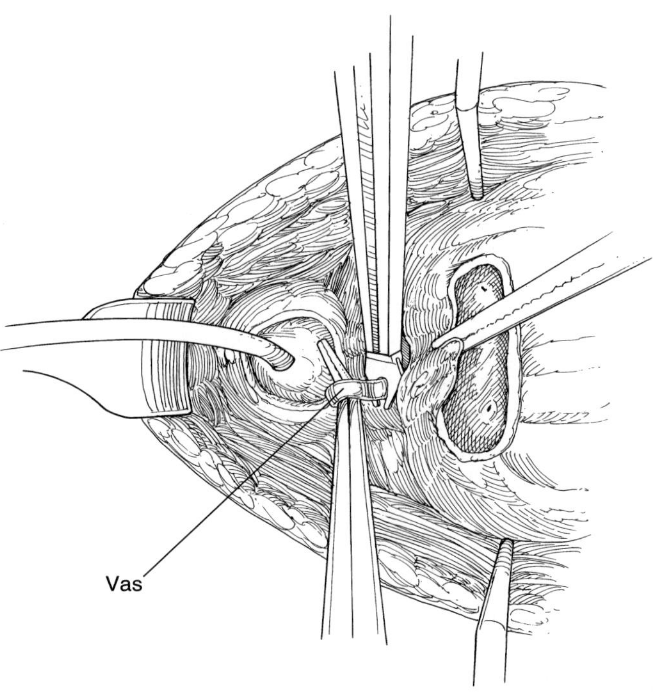

Fig. 18.13. The ampullae of the vasa are identified, dissected cranially, and divided between ligaclips. The seminal vesicles are situated lateral to the ligated stumps.

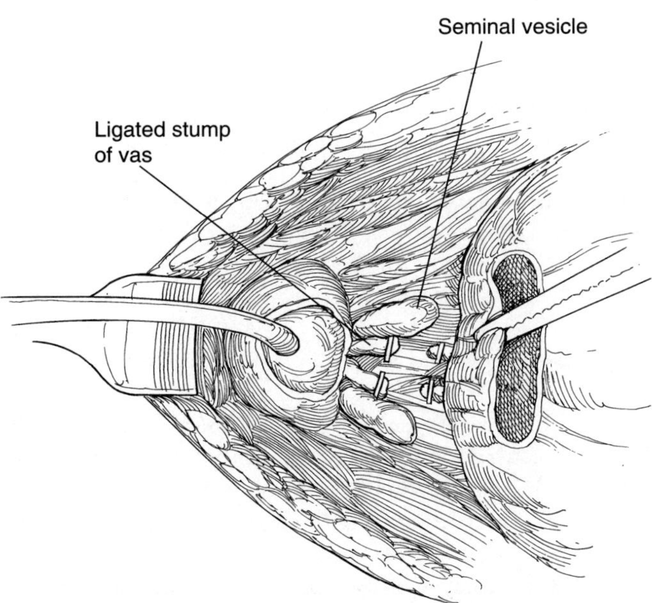

Fig. 18.14. Seminal vesicles and ampullae of the vasa have been divided. The dissection is carried dorsally, completely mobilizing the seminal vesicles and vasa from the rectum.

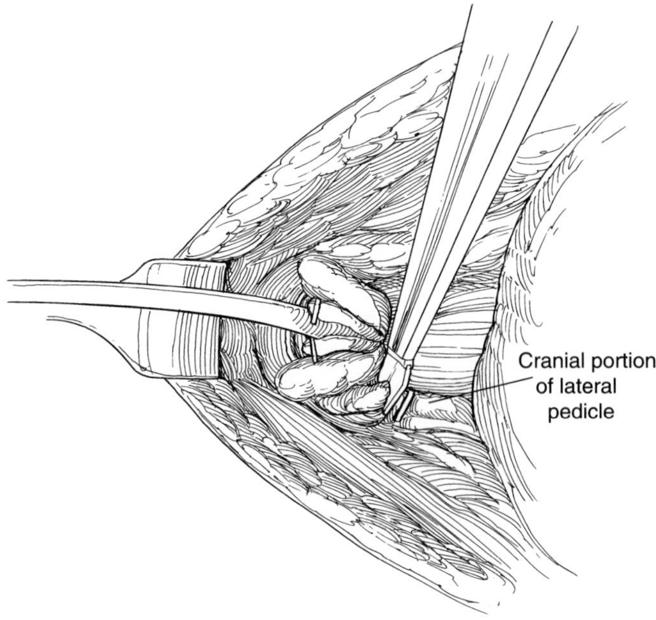

Fig. 18.15. Division of the cranial portion of the lateral pedicle of the prostate.

carried out as previously described in that the index finger is insinuated in the notch between the prostatic apex and urethra, and the neurovascular structures gently mobilized laterally. This mobilization is carried back to the prostatic base and, again, the artery and tissues are either sutured, ligated, or clipped and then sharply divided. The endopelvic fascia is thin and avascular at this point and may be divided either with cautery or Metzenbaum scissors (Fig. 18.16).

There should be minimal blood loss up to this point. Inadvertent injury to the lateral prostatic venous plexus during blunt dissection can be controlled with a laparotomy pack or a gauze sponge. The next step in the procedure is to fashion a new bladder neck in preparation for anastomosis to the urethra. The first assistant places his or her index finger in the bladder neck and elevates it superiorly (Fig. 18.18). The location of the ureteral orifices is noted, and the bladder is closed vertically from the posterior region to the anterior region with interrupted 2-0 chromic catgut sutures. Care is taken to avoid the ureteral orifices in any of these sutures. If used, the ureteral catheters are left in place for identification until the closure is complete. The bladder closure is continued anteriorly until the opening fits snugly around the average index finger. If the opening is close to the ureteral orifices, we extend the incision through the anterior bladder wall. This ensures that the anastomotic stitches will be well away from the ureteral orifices. A second layer of running 2-0 chromic sutures may be placed from the posterior to the anterior region. Again, extreme care must be exercised to avoid inadvertent suturing of a ureteral orifice. A watertight closure is attained, and the ureteral catheters are removed. The bladder mucosa of the new bladder neck is everted with 5-0 chromic sutures.

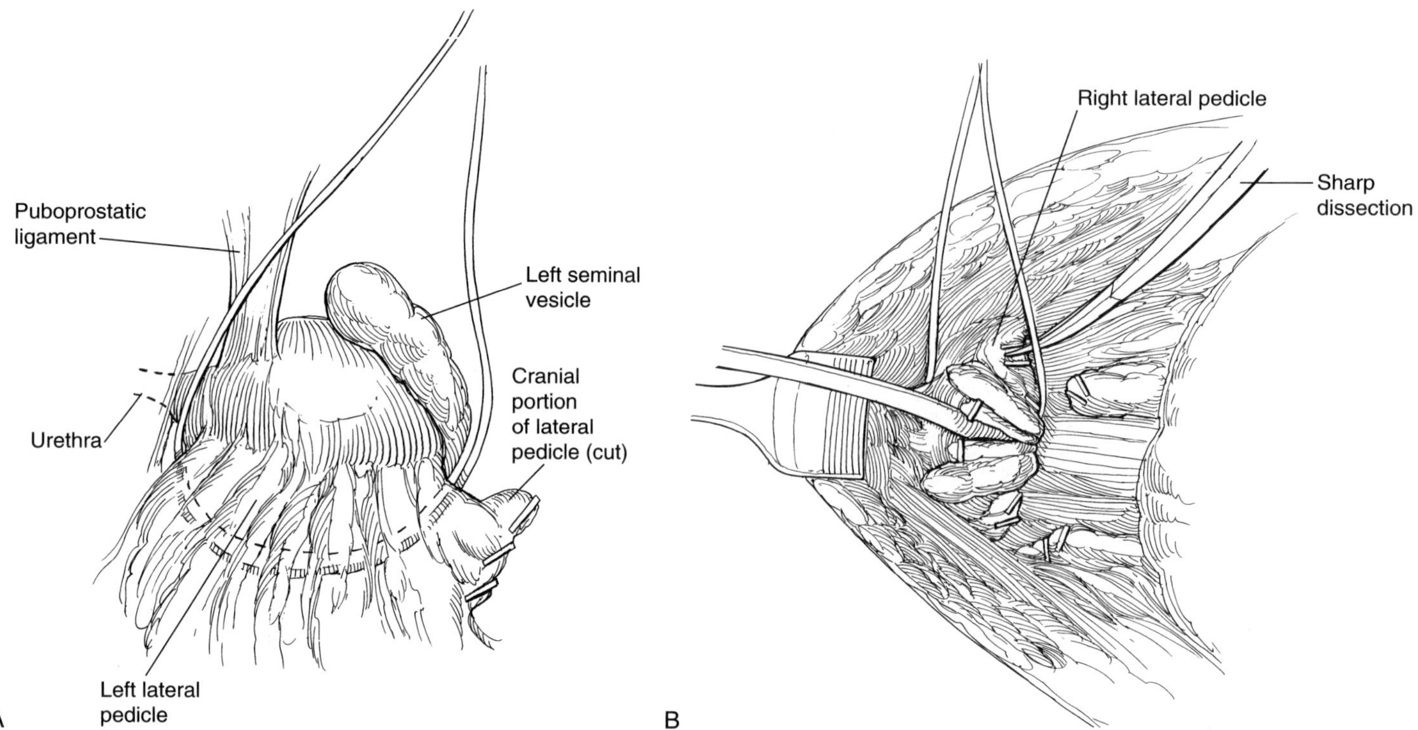

Fig. 18.16.   A. The left lateral pedicle has been isolated, and a Penrose drain is used for traction. **B.** The right lateral pedicle is divided between ligaclips (non–nerve-sparing technique).

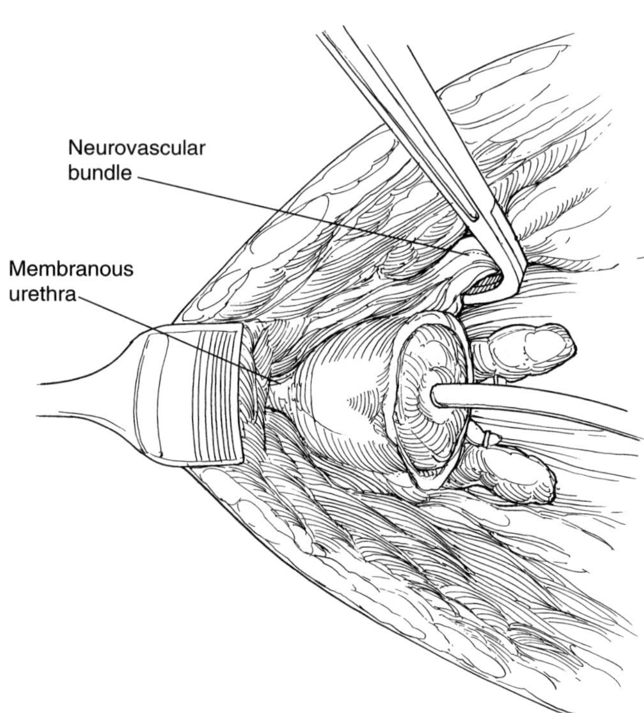

Fig. 18.17.   Nerve-sparing technique. A right-angle clamp is used to develop a plane of dissection.

The puboprostatic ligaments are divided as previously discussed. With downward traction on the prostate and a Kitner dissector, they are identified and sharply divided near the pubic bone. The dorsal vein is readily identifiable in the midline and, along with its investing tissue, is sharply divided down to the urethra (Fig. 18.19). Any bleeding is controlled with suture ligatures. Care should be taken not to place a number of sutures in the obturator internus muscle or to lacerate this muscle because it can be a formidable point of bleeding. Care should also be taken not to place these sutures so deeply as to injure the urogenital diaphragm and supporting structures.

We have not found commercially marketed dorsal venous ligators to be of any significant help in reducing this blood loss. We are also concerned about the injudicious use of right-angle clamps, which may result in inadvertent entering of the anterior prostatic tissue at the apex and subsequent positive margins.

The junction of the prostatic apex with the membranous urethra is palpated. The rectum should be completely free from the prostatic apex and membranous urethra before proceeding with division of the urethra. Any adherence may be bluntly dissected away with the index finger. Complete skeletonization of the membranous urethra should be avoided because the areolar tissues surrounding the urethra add strength to the subsequent anastomosis and reduce the risk of incontinence.

After the dorsal venous complex is controlled, attention is directed to dividing the urethra. Downward superior traction is placed on the prostate, exposing the prostatomembranous urethra. This should be clearly visualized, and a careful incision

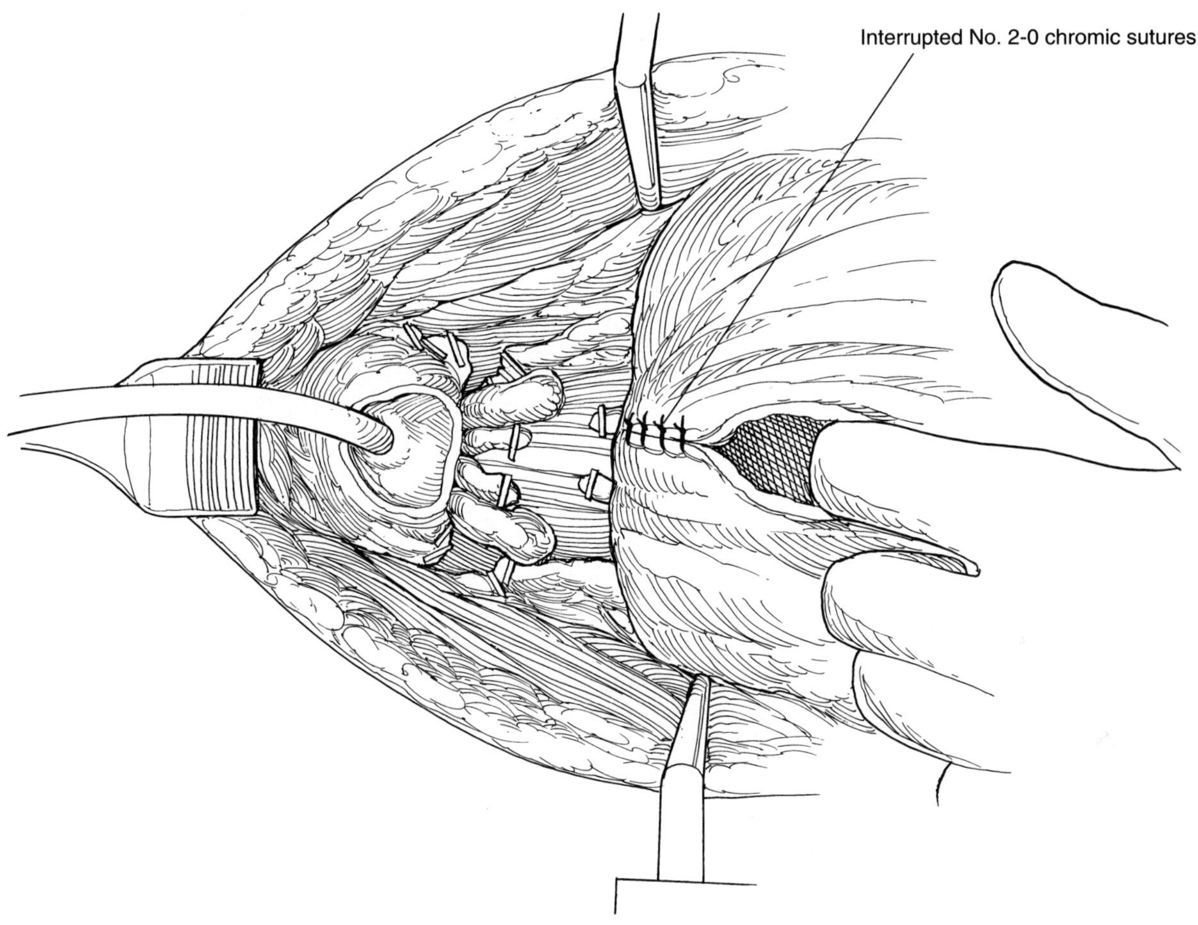

Fig. 18.18.   The bladder neck is closed with interrupted 2-0 chromic sutures so that the final opening fits snugly around the average index finger.

is made just distal to the prostatic apex, reducing the risk of any positive margin. The incision is made from 9 o'clock to 3 o'clock over the urethral catheter (Fig. 18.20). Once the urethra has been partially transected, a full-thickness section of the urethra is transfixed at the 12-o'clock position with a 2-0 chromic suture on a ⅝-inch circular needle (Fig. 18.21). This suture may be placed from inside out or from outside in. However, we find that this first stitch is most easily placed by sliding the needle along the catheter into the urethra and out again. We also find it easier to place all the stitches from inside out rather than outside in. We mark the hemostats holding the stitches with a marking pin. An alternative is to have a set of hemostats engraved with the positions frequently used, namely, 12, 2, 4, 6, 8, 10. In the event that a suture is placed from outside in, it is important to recognize this when completing the anastomosis. This may be done by using a Crile hemostat as a marker, instead of a straight one. After the urethra is further divided, sutures are placed at 2 o'clock and 10 o'clock, 4 o'clock and 8 o'clock, and finally at 6 o'clock. To place the 6 o'clock stitch, the Foley catheter is partially removed, with the tip remaining in the membranous urethra. A bridge of membranous urethra remains (Fig. 18.22), and a stitch is placed before it is divided. This membrane is then divided and any

remaining lateral attachments of the prostate are divided sharply. The specimen is then removed from the operative field.

CLOSURE

The bladder neck is placed in a position near the urethra, and the 6-o'clock suture is placed through the bladder opening. The 4-o'clock and 8-o'clock sutures are placed through the bladder neck. Those sutures that have been placed from inside out will require a tapered needle for proper placement. We find it helpful to cut the needle from each suture after it has been placed to avoid any confusion and to keep the sutures in proper order for later tying. A well-lubricated 22-French catheter with a 5-mL balloon is passed into the urethra and placed through the bladder neck. We have developed a technique for securing and easily replacing the Foley catheter if the balloon deflates. A no. 2 nylon retention suture is passed through the eye of the Foley catheter and tied over a forceps (Fig. 18.23). The needle is then passed through the eye of the Foley catheter and out, pulling the knot within the lumen of the catheter. This technique will reduce the incidence of trauma when removing the Foley catheter. The needle is then brought through either side of the bladder and out the abdominal wall.

The balloon is inflated to 10 mL and left in position. The

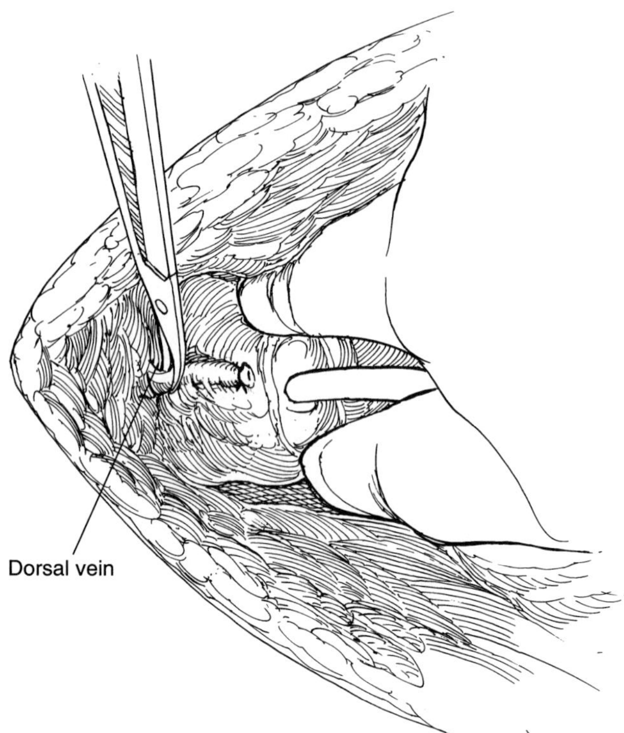

Fig. 18.19. The dorsal vein complex is divided sharply.

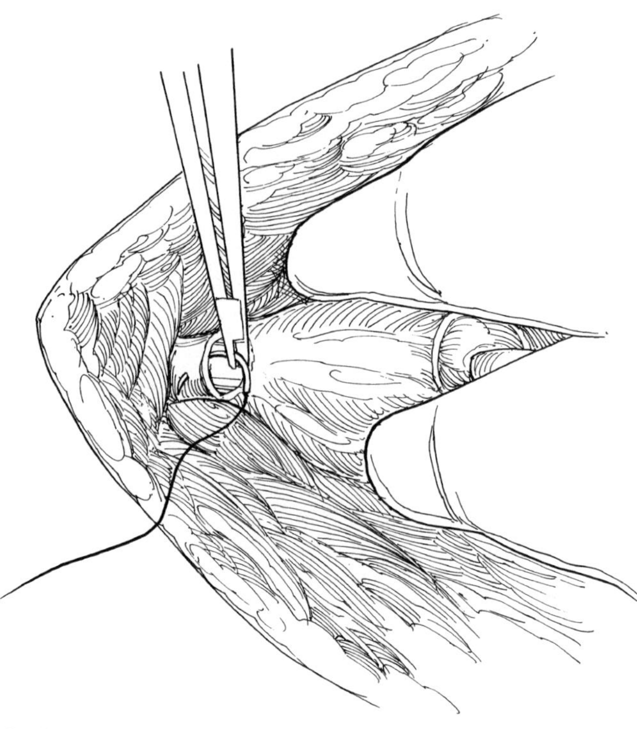

Fig. 18.21. Full section of urethra transfixed at the 12-o'clock position with a 2-0 chromic catgut suture.

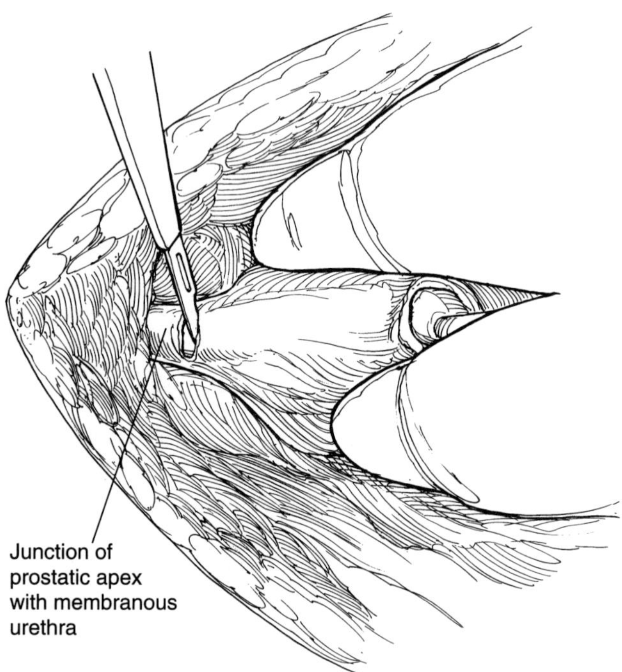

Fig. 18.20. An incision is made through the anterior circumference of the urethra lifted up by a right-angle clamp.

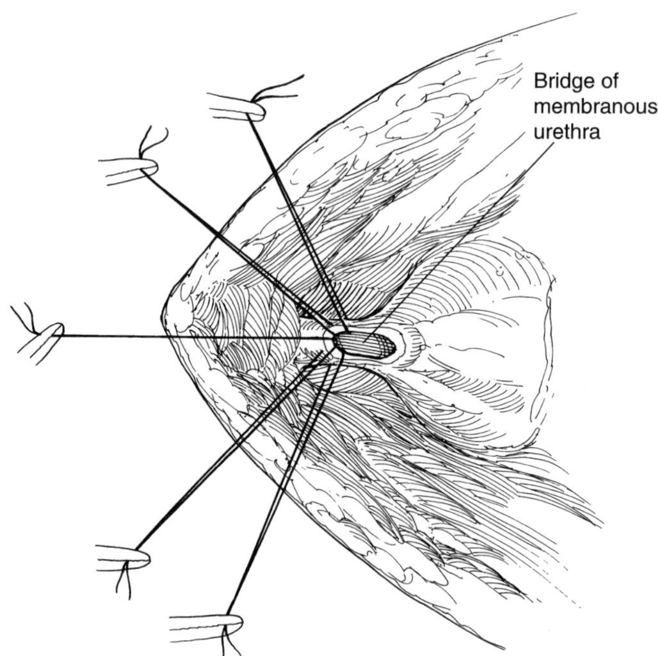

Fig. 18.22. Bridge of membranous urethra before final division and removal of the prostate.

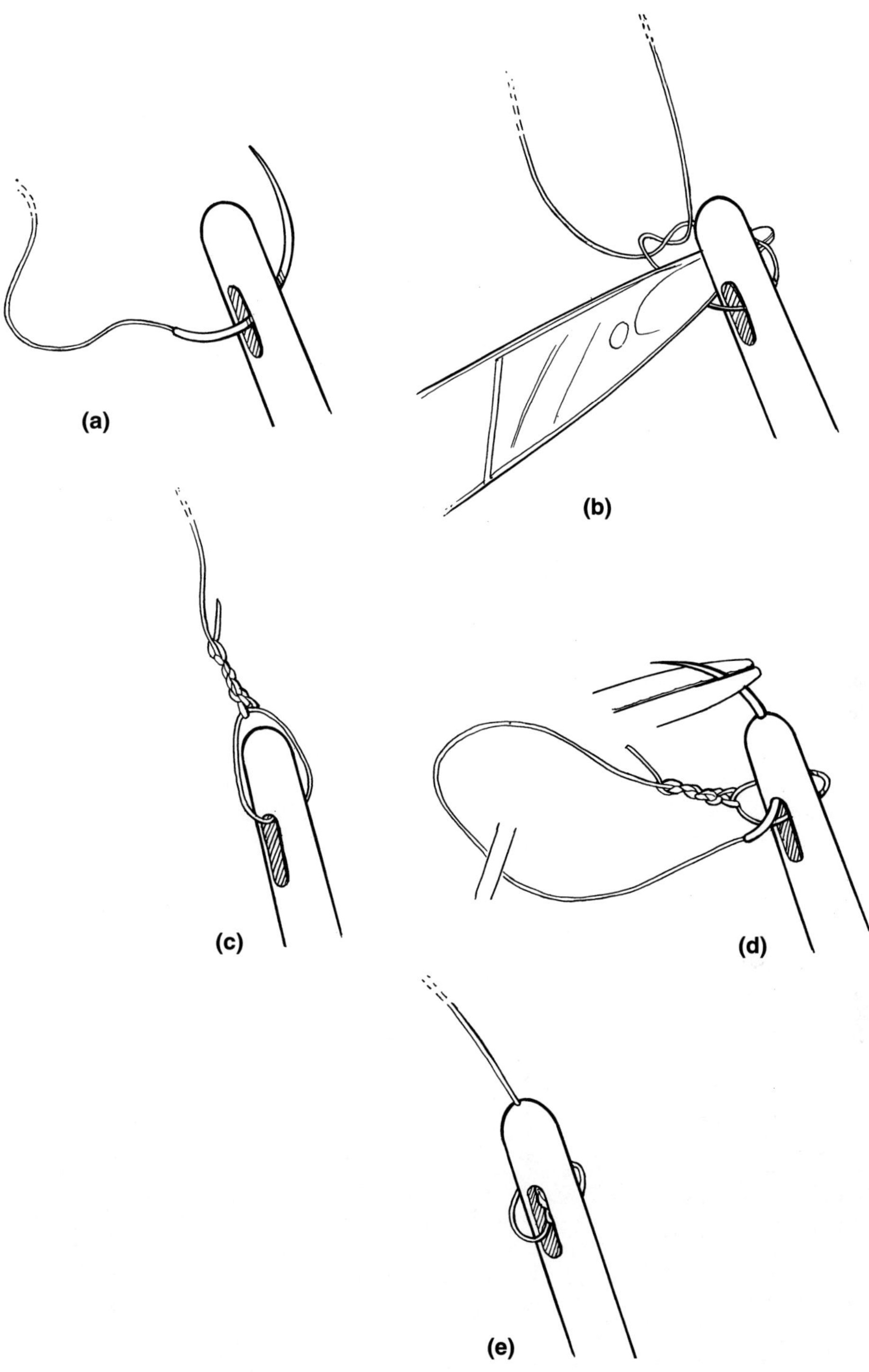

Fig. 18.23. Method for securing a Foley catheter.

remaining sutures are placed, with the 12-o'clock suture being the final one (Fig. 18.24). Gentle traction is placed on the catheter, and the bladder neck is brought down to the urethra. The sutures are tied, beginning with the 6-o'clock stitch and with lateral alternation, until the 12-o'clock stitch is tied. At this point, the bladder is irrigated until clear. We have not found it necessary to place a suprapubic tube with this procedure.

A 0.5-in Penrose or Jackson-Pratt drain is placed near the anastomotic site and brought through a separate stab wound; the surgical incision is closed (Fig. 18.25). If the rectus muscles have been divided from their tendinous insertion in the sym-

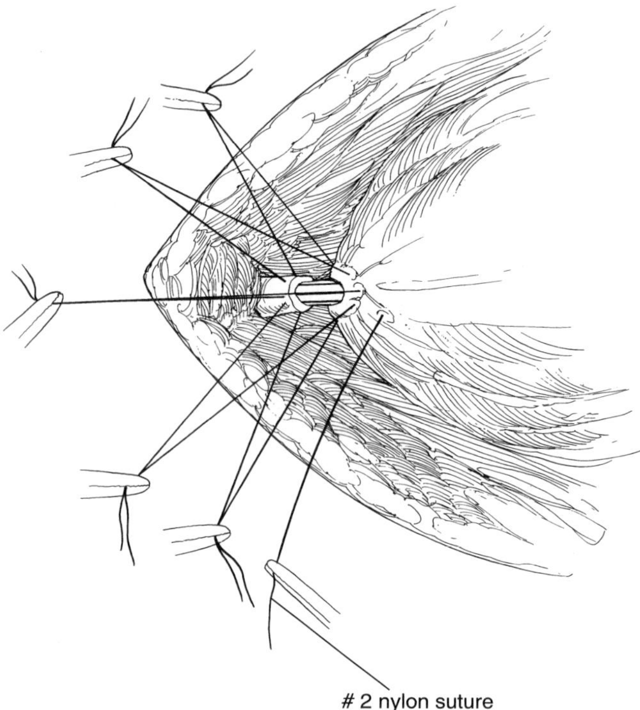

Fig. 18.24. All sutures have been placed through the bladder and are ready to tie.

physis pubis, they are approximated. The rectus fascia is closed with figure-of-eight absorbable sutures, and the subcutaneous tissues are then reapproximated. The skin is closed in the usual fashion.

In addition to hemorrhage, the two major intraoperative problems are ureteral injury and rectal perforation. Major injuries to the ureter are best treated with a formal reimplantation.

However, minor disruptions may be treated by leaving a ureteral catheter in place for 4 to 5 days postoperatively. An inadvertent rectal laceration may be closed primarily in two layers. We recommend a diverting colostomy in patients who have multiple or extensive rectal lacerations and in those who have had prior pelvic irradiation.

One major problem that can occur in the early postoperative period is rupture of the balloon, with subsequent removal of the catheter, as already discussed. We therefore place a "security stitch" as described. The catheter is brought over the anterior abdominal wall and secured to mild traction for 48 hours. Because of the secure, watertight anastomosis with this procedure, we do not use prolonged traction on the catheter.

POSTOPERATIVE MANAGEMENT

It is rare that patients need to be observed in the surgical intensive care unit. However, it is important to monitor vital signs, including urinary output, to ensure that no blood clots obstruct the catheter. In general, the urine remains free of clots and rapidly clears. Because of the pelvic lymph node dissection, a majority of patients will have some third-space fluid loss requiring 1 unit of plasma protein faction (Plasmanate). Central venous pressure lines are helpful in higher risk patients, particularly in the more elderly patients, and should be placed before the surgical procedure. We keep very mild traction on the Foley catheter by securing it to the anterior abdominal wall for 12 hours and then releasing it. A nasogastric tube, if used, is removed on the morning of postoperative day 1, and clear liquids are begun.

Patients should be ambulating on the first postoperative day and striving to increase their ambulation and eating a regular diet so that discharge can be anticipated on the second to

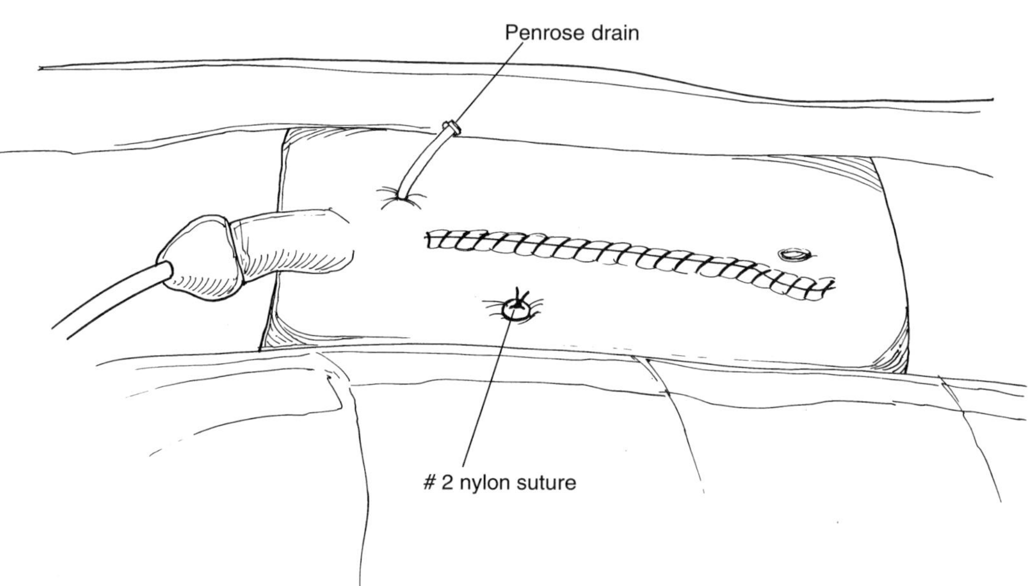

Fig. 18.25. Final wound closure.

fourth postoperative day. The catheter is left in place for 2 weeks, and the drain is advanced and usually removed by the second to third postoperative day. However, in the rare event of significant urinary leakage, it is left in place until this abates. We do not routinely obtain retrograde urethrograms before removing the catheter. Patients are provided with postoperative instructions, including information about Kegel exercises, at hospital discharge so they can begin the exercises as soon as the catheter is removed.

COMPLICATIONS

There have been several unusual complications with the procedure. In one patient, symptoms of urinary obstruction occurred several months after the procedure. On cystoscopic examination, the patient was found to have a ligaclip protruding into the urethra near the anastomosis. This clip was easily removed cystoscopically, but as a result, we have become aware of the fact that any ligaclips in and about the anastomosis should be removed before finalizing the procedure. Three patients experienced anuria 24 hours after the procedure. Evaluation revealed this to be obstructive in origin, and it was thought to be secondary to edema of the ureteral orifices. Within 24 hours, the edema subsided and the patients had normal postoperative courses. Four postoperative lymphoceles occurred.

One of the more important functional results of the operation is postoperative urinary continence. In our original series of 350 patients, 1.8% were totally incontinent. Three of these patients had undergone a salvage prostatectomy after radiation therapy. In the past 650 cases performed, the incidence of total incontinence was 1%. In more than 900 prostatectomies performed by this approach, we have had one ureteral injury. That was in a patient who had a bulky stage C lesion on a protocol of hormonal downsizing followed by radical prostatectomy. The ureteral disruption was repaired by primary reimplantation. In the same number of radical retropubic prostatectomies performed with this technique, there have been no rectal lacerations. We have had two in patients who had undergone salvage prostatectomies after radiation therapy, and none in the more than 900 patients who have had no therapy or had hormonal therapy only.

This technique for radical retropubic prostatectomy provides for predictable and careful anatomic prostatic removal. Once the anatomic planes and techniques of the procedure are understood, the operative time for the procedure, exclusive of the lymph node dissection, is between 1.5 and 2 hours. Because of its anatomic design, the procedure is readily taught to residents. Postoperative complications have been minimal, and urinary incontinence has been negligible.

REFERENCES

1. Wingo PA, Tong T, Bolden S. Cancer statistics 1995. CA Cancer J Clin 1995;45:8.
2. Kuchler H. Uber prostatavergrosserungen. Deutsch Klin 1866; 18:458.
3. Young HH. The early diagnosis and radical cure of carcinoma of the prostate: being a study of 40 cases and presentation of a radical operation which was carried out in four cases. Bull Johns Hopkins Hosp 1905;16:315.
4. Millin T. Retropubic urinary surgery. Baltimore: Williams & Wilkins, 1947.
5. McLaughlin AP, et al. Prostatic carcinoma: incidence and location of unsuspected lymphatic metastases. J Urol 1976; 115:89.
6. Ansell JS. Radical transvesical prostatectomy: preliminary report on an approach to surgical excision of localized prostatic malignancy. J Urol 1959;83:373.
7. Campbell EW. Total prostatectomy with preliminary ligation of the vascular pedicles. J Urol 1959;81:464.
8. Byar DP, Mostofi FK. Carcinoma of the prostate: prognostic evaluation of certain pathologic features in 208 radical prostatectomies. Cancer 1972;30:5.
9. McNeal JE. Origin and development of carcinoma in the prostate. Cancer 1969;23:24.
10. Partin AW, et al. The use of prostate specific antigen, clinical stage and Gleason score to predict pathological stage in men with localized prostate cancer. J Urol 1993;150:110.
11. Soloway MS, et al. Randomized comparison of radical prostatectomy alone or preceded by androgen deprivation for cT2b prostate cancer. J Urol 1995;153:391. Abstract.
12. Pedersen KV, et al. Neoadjuvant hormonal treatment with triptorelin versus no treatment prior to radical prostatectomy: a prospective randomized multicenter study. J Urol 1995;153: 391. Abstract.
13. Narayan P, et al. The role of transrectal ultrasound-guided biopsy-based staging, preoperative serum prostate specific antigen, and biopsy Gleason score in prediction of final pathologic diagnosis in prostate cancer. Urology 1995;46:205.
14. Albers DD, et al. Surgical anatomy of the pubovesical ligaments. J Urol 1973;109:388.
15. Tobin CE, Benjamin JA. Anatomical and surgical restudy of Denonvillier's fascia. Surg Gynecol Obstet 1945;80:373.

19

Radical Perineal Prostatectomy

Vernon E. Weldon

We shall not cease from exploring and at the end of our exploration we shall return to where we started and know the place for the first time.

T.S. ELIOT

INTRODUCTION

The use of serum prostate-specific antigen (PSA) levels as a tumor marker has transformed the management of localized adenocarcinoma of the prostate in at least three ways.

1. It identifies a greater number of patients with clinically significant disease at an earlier stage when the cancer is still confined and potentially curable.
2. It demonstrates the different outcomes of competing treatment modalities within 5 years, if they are not obscured by adjuvant androgen deprivation.
3. It nullifies the concept of latent prostate cancer (1) and demonstrates that untreated prostate cancer is a progressive disease, albeit with a generally slow growth rate.

Before the PSA era, two thirds of new prostate cancer cases were too advanced when detected to be curable. With PSA screening this ratio is reversed, and two thirds of newly diagnosed cases are localized and potentially curable (2). Before PSA, determination of treatment failure by evidence of clinical progression or death due to cancer often required 10 to 15 years of follow-up. With PSA, the interval required to judge treatment failure has shrunk to 5 years, with most radiation or surgical failures becoming evident by that time. Although almost all patients treated with radiation therapy have an initial decline in their serum PSA levels, up to 80% of them demonstrate failure with a rising PSA at 5 years after treatment (3, 4). Conversely, up to 80% of radical prostatectomy patients are apparently cured with undetectable PSA at a mean of 4 years after operation (5, 6). Serial PSA monitoring of untreated patients with prostate cancer demonstrates progression in 86%, but with doubling times of 2 to 4 years (7). Patients with advanced age or significant comorbidity may properly have

curative treatment for localized prostate cancer withheld based on the calculation that the decline of the host will outpace the advance of the tumor. However, if they have not died of other causes, by 10 years 42% of those with medium-grade and 74% of those with high-grade prostate cancer will have bony metastases (8). Beyond 10 years, prostate cancer is the cause of death in 56% of palliatively treated men who initially had only low-stage and low-grade cancer (9).

There also has been concern that radical prostatectomy might be misapplied to patients at the opposite extremes of the localized prostate cancer spectrum, i.e.,

1. Those with clinically insignificant, low-volume cancer, and
2. Those with high-grade cancer that, although apparently localized, may be intrinsically incurable.

With the former, recent data demonstrate that detection of clinically insignificant cancer is not a significant risk when patients are carefully selected for biopsy by including only those with a high prevalence of significant cancer (elevated PSA level or biopsy of an area of palpable abnormality) (10). With the latter, up to 43% of those with biopsy Gleason scores of 8 to 10 without lymph node metastases who undergo radical prostatectomy have undetectable PSA at 5 years (11).

The results of randomized, controlled trials assessing the influence of prostate cancer screening on cancer-related mortality (12), and the outcomes of radical prostatectomy versus observation with delayed androgen deprivation (13), will be available in another decade. Until then, the best currently available data demonstrate that the currently recommended screening criteria (abnormality on digital rectal examination or PSA level greater than 4 ng/mL) (14) detect clinically significant cancer that, when organ- or specimen-confined, has a high probability of being cured with radical prostatectomy.

With the provisional establishment of the appropriateness

and the effectiveness of radical prostatectomy, attention to reducing treatment morbidity and maximizing cost-effectiveness is necessary. In this context, the perineal approach to radical prostatectomy has a prominent role.

HISTORICAL PERSPECTIVE

Perineal access to the lower genitourinary tract was first gained by the early lithotomists. Celsus (15), in the first century AD, described a curvilinear transverse incision anterior to the anus for removing bladder stones. In 1852, Demarquay (16) described a perineal approach for removal of stones from the prostatic urethra through a semicircular incision anterior to the anus, division of the rectourethralis muscle, and blunt dissection of the rectum from the membranous urethra and the posterior surface of the prostate (identical to the modern approach). Later, the prostate was incidentally removed during the perineal excision of rectal cancer, and in 1866 Küchler (17) first described the potential use of this route for partial excision of the prostate for prostate cancer, although there is no record that he did it. Bilroth (18) applied Küchler's theory the following year. In 1883, Leisrink (19) performed the first total perineal prostatectomy for prostate cancer, with anastomosis of the bladder neck to the membranous urethra. He also removed part of the anterior rectal wall and the patient died within a few days.

Numerous blind, partial, and sometimes inadvertent attempts at removing obstructing hyperplastic prostate lobes through the perineal approach preceded Proust's description (20), in 1901, of complete perineal enucleation of the prostatic adenoma under vision, but through a vertical, midline incision that limited exposure. In 1903, Young (21) described his technique of perineal enucleation, which was similar to Proust's but used the semicircular incision of Celsus and Demarquay. This led to Young's development of his classic technique of radical perineal prostatectomy, which he first performed with Halsted's assistance in 1904 and described in 1905 (22). He reported his life's work with this operation 40 years later (23).

Young's technique of radical perineal prostatectomy is the basis of the contemporary procedure, which includes two important modifications. First, it was recognized that maintaining dissection on the ventral rectal wall allowed additional resection of the adjacent posterolateral periprostatic fascia and thereby achieved wider margins, a practice that Weyrauch attributed to Dillon in 1959 (24). Second, after Walsh and Donker (25) described preservation of the cavernous nerves and potency with radical retropubic prostatectomy, Weldon and Tavel (26) adapted these anatomical and functional conservations to radical perineal prostatectomy in 1988. They also further delineated the extended periprostatic fascial excision and wider margins that could be achieved through the perineal approach by sacrificing the ipsilateral cavernous nerve. Contemporary radical perineal prostatectomy should always selectively include one of these modifications on each side.

PATIENT SELECTION

Radical prostatectomy provides a significant advantage when it is applied to cancers that are clinically localized and likely to be confined within the available specimen in men who are likely to live long enough to benefit from it. This essentially restricts radical prostatectomy to men with tumors in clinical stages T1 to T2, N0, M0 (27) who have no other disease limiting their time at risk from their cancer to less than 10 years. A disqualifying upper age limit around 75 years is reasonable, based on data demonstrating that healthy men without any other significant disease at age 75 have a mean survival of 10.5 years, and that equally healthy men at age 80 have a mean survival of 7.5 years (28).

These generalizations are tempered by the realities of recognized adverse factors. Rates of negative specimen margins, durable undetectable PSA levels, and long-term disease-free survival are inversely related to increasing clinical stage, biopsy Gleason score, and preoperative PSA levels (5, 29, 30). Only 10% of men with clinical stage T2a disease who undergo radical perineal prostatectomy manifest PSA failure at a mean follow-up of 3 years (6). Even with stage T2b and T2c disease, although the positive-margin rates with step-section pathologic analysis are 48% and 64% respectively, the detectable PSA rate at a mean of 3 postoperative years is only 33% (6). Within the stage limitations, no Gleason score or PSA level alone unequivocally disqualifies an individual patient from radical prostatectomy, although the highest PSA level we have seen with pathologically organ-confined disease on step-section analysis was 19 ng/mL and the highest with pathologically specimen-confined disease was 26 ng/mL.

Selective refinements of clinical staging modalities help to exclude some men who are unlikely to benefit from radical prostatectomy. In patients with lymph node metastases, radical prostatectomy virtually always fails (5), and early adjuvant androgen deprivation does not prolong survival (31). Men with demonstrated lymphatic metastases should be excluded. Those with a PSA level higher than 40 ng/mL have a reasonable rate of preoperative demonstration of lymphatic metastases by computed tomographic discovery of enlarged pelvic lymph nodes and guided percutaneous fine-needle aspiration of those nodes with cytologic diagnosis. The role of recently developed radioimmunoscintigraphy in demonstrating lymphatic metastases and excluding men from operation remains to be determined.

Patients with invasion of the seminal vesicles and the perivesicular fascia also have a very high failure rate (5, 32). They may be excluded preoperatively even if the seminal vesicles are not palpably abnormal by demonstrating this invasion with transrectal sonographically guided needle biopsy of the seminal vesicles (33) when they are sonographically abnormal or when large or high-grade tumors are located at the base of the prostate. Equivocal involvement of the lateral margin is not an exclusion factor because 25% of clinical stage T3a patients are overstaged and have pathologically organ-confined disease (34). Moreover, an extended radical dissection sacrificing the posterolateral periprostatic fascia and the ipsilateral neurovascular bundle can keep many tumors with small-volume capsular penetration in those areas confined within the specimen and is associated with a durable undetectable PSA level (6). Prostate imaging beyond sonography with computed tomography or magnetic resonance imaging is not cost-effective and adds insufficiently to staging sensitivity and specificity to be useful, except after abdominal-perineal resection of the anorectum when staging by palpation and sonography are impossible.

Radical prostatectomy has a very limited role in patients with clinical stages T1a and T3 disease. With incidentally discovered, low-volume, and low-grade T1a tumors, a reasonable case for aggressive treatment of healthy men younger than age 65, who will be at risk for more than 15 years, has been made (35). However, most of them can be followed with serial PSA determinations and selected repeat transrectal sonograms with systematic biopsies to detect significant progression and the need for intervention. With clinical stage T3 disease and obvious extracapsular extension, there are some who advocate the use of radical prostatectomy, including adjuvant or neoadjuvant androgen deprivation, suggesting possible survival benefits and reduction in local complications. However, most of these patients have extensive positive margins with a high PSA failure rate that is little altered with adjuvant radiation therapy (5, 6), and only 11% of symptomatic patients with clinical stage T3 to T4 disease ever require more than a single transurethral resection and androgen deprivation for symptomatic local control (36). Radical prostatectomy or radiation therapy (3, 4, 37) provide these patients with no clear advantage beyond that of androgen deprivation alone.

ADVANTAGES AND DISADVANTAGES

Radical perineal prostatectomy, one of the oldest prototypes of a "minimal-access" surgical procedure, offers access to the prostate at its most superficial location just beneath the subcutaneous fascia, through a small perianal incision. This provides one of its major advantages—low morbidity and a short hospital stay. No muscles pull on the incision, and there is little pain. Any extravasated blood or urine drains dependently, and there is no ileus. The median total hospital stay is 3 days.

The second major advantage is the easy and direct access it provides to the apex of the prostate and the membranous urethra. This is the most troublesome area during radical retropubic prostatectomy in regard to positive margins (38) and postoperative morbidity with incontinence and anastomotic strictures. Most prostate cancers originate within the peripheral zone, and the direct perineal access to the apical and posterior aspects facilitates precise dissection and significantly reduces the number of positive margins in those areas when compared with the retropubic approach (6). Solitary positive apical margins constitute only 7% of all positive margins with the perineal approach, and solitary positive posterior and lateral margins constitute only 16% (6). In that regard, the perineal approach is superior to the retropubic approach in the treatment

of peripheral zone cancers. The single, discretionary variable providing the best chance of negative margins with an apical tumor is the perineal approach. Precise dissection of the apex also minimizes incontinence by allowing preservation of as much of the distal sphincteric mechanism as possible without compromising margins. Ready access to the membranous urethra allows vesicourethral anastomosis with precise placement of as many sutures as needed to provide a reliable, usually watertight, anastomosis with direct mucosal apposition. The anastomotic stricture rate is less than 1%.

The perineal dissection beneath Santorini's venous plexus provides its third major advantage, low blood loss, but also its major disadvantage, an increased risk of a positive anterior margin (6). Median blood loss is 600 mL and most patients receive no transfusion, with the remaining receiving 1 or 2 autologous units (26). Perioperative homologous blood is used in less than 1% of patients. However, even with a bilaterally extended dissection sacrificing the lateral prostatic fascia, a vertical strip of anterior prostatic capsule as wide as the puboprostatic ligaments (averaging 15 mm) and extending from those ligaments to the apex is exposed. The incidence of tumor penetration of the capsule anteriorly is much less than in the peripheral zone; however, when it occurs, the perineal approach is likely to result in a positive margin. In that regard, the perineal approach is inferior to the retropubic approach in the treatment of transition zone cancers. An iatrogenic increase in this problem can be eliminated by avoiding avulsion of the puboprostatic ligaments and sharply dividing them ventral to their capsular insertions. In our series, increased numbers of positive anterior margins were not evident with clinical stage T1b tumors, but they were with true clinical stage T1c tumors (no palpable or sonographically visible tumor within the peripheral zone) associated with a high PSA level (6). Particular care with the puboprostatic ligaments is necessary in those cases.

The inability to access the pelvic lymph nodes through the same incision is an inconvenience with the perineal approach. Lymph node metastases occur in only 10% of all patients currently undergoing exploration surgery for possible prostatectomy (6), but they predict virtually certain treatment failure (5) and render any advantage with radical prostatectomy very questionable. Combined preoperative clinical parameters are highly reliable in predicting negative lymph nodes in up to 58% of patients. Pelvic lymphadenectomy can be omitted in those patients with clinical stage T2b or less, biopsy Gleason score of 6 or less, and PSA of 11 ng/mL or less (node-negative predictive value of 99%) (6). With the exclusion of these very low-risk patients, the incidence of lymph node metastases in the remaining higher risk group is 22%. Noninvasive exclusion of lymphatic metastases by radioimmunoscintigraphy with [111]I-labeled monoclonal antibody CYT-356 is promising, with early reports of specificities of 86 to 90% and node-negative predictive values of 83 to 91% (39, 40). Its exact role is yet to be determined. Pelvic lymphadenectomy in the remaining patients can be accomplished within the minimal-access concept by a concurrent laparoscopic or "mini-lap" (41) approach.

The latter is quicker and less costly (no expensive disposable equipment), requires no special training, causes no more morbidity (the 6-cm incision equals the total length of the multiple laparoscopic access incisions), and does not prolong the total hospital stay (especially with ketorolac-based analgesia). Median total operative time for mini-lap bilateral pelvic lymphadenectomy and radical perineal prostatectomy, including time for repositioning, is 3.5 hours.

During nerve-sparing procedures, the perineal approach allows separation of the neurovascular bundles from the prostatic capsule under direct vision, which aids in determining whether they can be spared without risking an avoidable positive margin in equivocal circumstances. Rates of potency preservation are directly related to the number of neurovascular bundles spared and are inversely related to patient age and tumor stage. Our initial experience spared potency in 56% of patients who had a bilateral nerve-sparing modification (26).

The required exaggerated lithotomy position is occasionally prohibited by ankylosis of the spine or hips or, in the morbidly obese, by the need for excessively high ventilatory pressure that impedes cardiac filling. Most other patients with skeletal deformities can be adequately positioned; those with chronic spine and disk disease not only usually tolerate this position, but often report improvement in their symptoms afterward. The exaggerated lithotomy position provides maximal gravitational drainage of the pelvic and leg veins during radical prostatectomy. Avoidance of the initiation of thrombosis during that time may contribute to the low rate of recognized thromboembolic events afterward, occurring in only 1.5% despite concurrent pelvic lymphadenectomy and no prophylactic maneuvers other than early ambulation.

The minimal-access nature of the perineal approach with a small incision creates a difficulty with large prostates, although glands weighing up to 180 g have been removed. In those circumstances, close attention to the sequence of maneuvers that maximize specimen mobility, including early division of the vascular pedicles, is necessary. Occasionally, the seminal vesicles must be removed separately.

Prior operations including transurethral prostate resection, suprapubic transvesical simple prostatectomy, and abdominal-perineal resection of the anorectum do not create excessive problems with radical perineal prostatectomy. The first causes little trouble, particularly if radical perineal prostatectomy is deferred for 3 months until inflammation and tissue friability have completely resolved. The last is surprisingly routine once the extensive posterior scarring is passed.

SELECTED PELVIC ANATOMY

Patient outcomes and personal satisfaction with radical perineal prostatectomy and its nerve-sparing and extended radical variations are maximized by a clear understanding of the details of pelvic fascial anatomy. The pelvic fascia is derived from the mesenchyme of the adjacent pelvic organs and is continuous around and between the bladder and prostate and the rectum.

It has variable areolar and fatty constituents, related to general body habitus. Denonvilliers' membrane, the single, fibrous membrane that he called the "prostatoperitoneal membrane" (42, 43), is derived from the embryologic fusion of the most caudal portion of the peritoneal sac within the pelvis, with resorption of the serous surfaces leaving the fibrous remnants. It is interposed between the rectum and the prostate and extends caudally from the peritoneal cul-de-sac for a variable distance, but often down to the prostatic apex. Its lateral margins extend to the neurovascular bundles on each side, where the edges are often slightly everted by the branches of those bundles that penetrate the prostatic capsule. It loosely covers the dorsal surface of the seminal vesicles, but it is densely adherent to the dorsal prostatic capsule. It is separated from the rectum by the ventral rectal portion of the continuous pelvic fascia that joins the lateral rectal and lateral prostatic fascia on each side across the midline, between the prostate and the rectum and dorsal to Denonvilliers' membrane (Fig. 19.1). This ventral rectal fascia extends caudally down to the rectourethralis muscle, which blocks its further caudal extension, and terminates by blending with the fascia at the superior surface of the urogenital diaphragm.

The pelvic nerve plexuses, from which the cavernous nerves originate, are located in the lateral rectal fascia, lateral to the rectum on each side in a parasagittal plane and at the level of the tips of the seminal vesicles (44). The cavernous nerves course caudally and slightly obliquely in a ventral and medial direction as part of the neurovascular bundles, accompanied by branches of the middle rectal artery and vein. They lie within the lateral pelvic fascia at its junction with the ventral rectal fascia and over the dorsolateral aspects of the prostate and membranous urethra adjacent to the lateral margins of Denonvilliers' membrane. They penetrate the urogenital diaphragm to reach the corpora cavernosa.

Some details of rectal anatomy, particularly involving its longitudinal muscle bands, are relevant. Beneath the peritoneal reflection, the three taeniae coli, which are the bands of longitudinal muscle of the intra-abdominal colon, become concentrated on the rectum into two broad bands of longitudinal muscle located anteriorly and posteriorly. The rectourethralis muscle is formed by some muscle fascicles originating from the anterior band of longitudinal rectal muscle that insert into the posterior edge of the urogenital diaphragm near the membranous urethra (45). Caudal to the rectourethralis muscle, some fibers of the medial portion of the levator ani, the puborectalis muscle, sweep anterior to the rectum and insert onto the ventral rectal wall, while most of this muscle forms a sling around the rectum posteriorly.

Contemporary radical perineal prostatectomy uses entry within the envelope of the perirectal fascia and two different dissection planes within the pelvic fascia. When an extended radical dissection with wide excision of the posterolateral periprostatic fascia and the enclosed neurovascular bundle is planned, the dissection plane is between the rectal wall and its ventral fascia. The dissection extends laterally around the

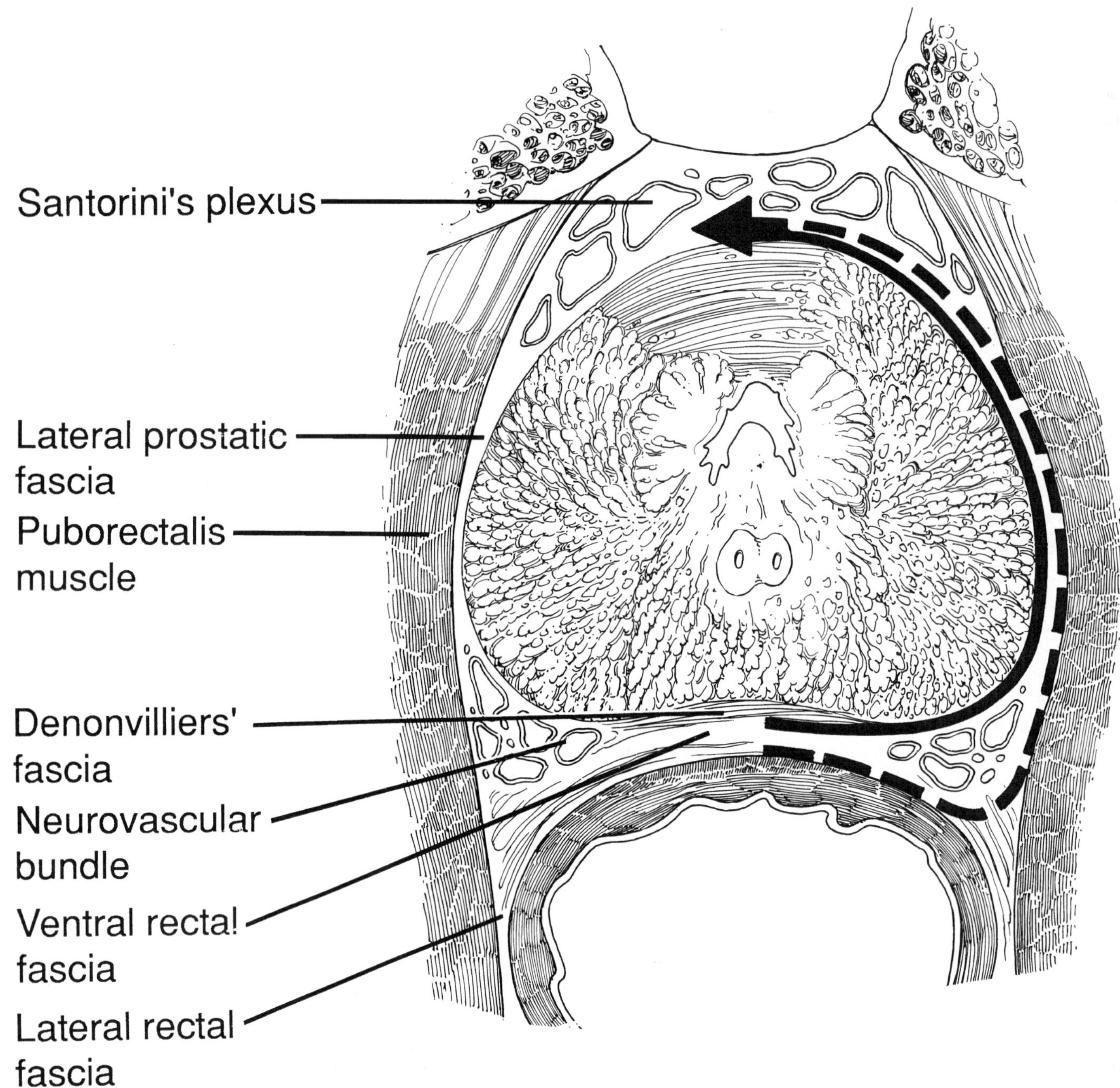

Fig. 19.1.   Transverse section through prostate at level of verumontanum. Note the continuous nature of pelvic fascia. Lateral pelvic fascia comprises lateral prostatic and lateral rectal fascia. Ventral rectal fascia is key to contemporary operative modifications. The solid line indicates the nerve-sparing dissection plane on Denonvilliers' membrane (fascia) and lateral prostatic capsule inside ventral rectal and lateral prostatic fascia. The broken line indicates the extended radical dissection plane outside these fasciae incorporating neurovascular bundle. (Reprinted with permission from Weldon VE, Tavel FR. Radical perineal prostatectomy. In: Das S, Crawford E, eds. Cancer of the prostate. New York: Marcel Dekker, 1993:225–266.)

neurovascular bundle and through the lateral rectal fascia onto the puborectalis muscle, turning ventrally on this muscle between it and the lateral prostatic fascia, and then medially onto the plane of the anterior prostatic capsule beneath Santorini's venous plexus. This removes all of the posterolateral periprostatic fascia with the specimen down to the rectal wall and the levator ani muscle. When potency sparing with preservation of the neurovascular bundle is planned, the dissection plane is between the ventral rectal fascia and Denonvilliers' membrane posteriorly and continues ventrally on the prostatic capsule inside the lateral prostatic fascia and beneath Santorini's venous plexus (Fig. 19.1). Either of these dissection planes may be used on each side during the operation, depending on the patient's potency status, the extent of tumor, and the surgeon's intent.

Confusing descriptions of pelvic fascial anatomy abound, although Tobin and Benjamin clarified it in their classic study of Denonvilliers' fascia (46). Denonvilliers described a single fascial layer that he labeled the "prostatoperitoneal membrane" (42, 43). Denonvilliers' membrane has been called the "anterior layer of Denonvilliers' fascia" and the "pearly gates." The latter acknowledges its characteristic color and its role in identifying the entry into Young's dissection plane (and the nerve-sparing dissection plane) around the prostate, with whimsical heavenly allusions. The ventral rectal fascia has been called the "posterior layer of Denonvilliers' fascia." Denonvilliers did describe a "very loose cellular tissue" posterior to his "prostatoperitoneal membrane" and between it and the rectum. However, this ventral rectal fascia is part of the circumferential pelvic fascia around the rectum above the levator ani, and, except for anatomical proximity, it is neither embryologically nor histologically related to Denonvilliers' membrane. These inaccurate clinical designations have historical interest, but they impede understanding the anatomy of the surgical dissection planes necessary for executing the contemporary modifications of radical perineal prostatectomy; they should be retired.

SELECTIVE NERVE SPARING

The contemporary era of radical prostatectomy is defined by the description of the paired neurovascular bundles and their relevance to postoperative impotence (25) and the local spread of prostate cancer (47). Sparing the cavernous nerves that lie within the neurovascular bundles can spare potency in the majority of men (26). Bilateral nerve sparing optimizes potency preservation, but unilateral nerve sparing is often adequate to preserve potency, particularly in younger men (48). However, the primary route of cancer penetration of the prostatic capsule is via the perineural spaces around the nerve branches of the neurovascular bundles that penetrate the capsule and create susceptible openings (38, 47). Additional resection of the posterolateral periprostatic fascia and the enclosed neurovascular bundle can keep tumors with capsular penetration in those areas confined within the specimen, providing negative margins and durable undetectable PSA levels in 15% of all cases (6). In contrast, patients with capsular penetration and positive margins have a 47% rate of detectable PSA levels after a mean of 3 years. Even those with only focal positive margins (3 mm or less) have a 27% rate of detectable PSA within the same time (6). Therefore, a bilateral extended dissection with additional removal of all posterolateral periprostatic fascia and the enclosed neurovascular bundles is indicated for all impotent men and for those with marginal potency who are unlikely to retain it. It is also indicated for those who do not consider potency preservation important or who, given the contingencies, are unwilling to accept any discretionary risk in the treatment of their cancer.

For potent men, optimal decisions can sometimes be difficult. However, there are reasonable strategies that minimize the risk of a related positive margin and allow selective nerve sparing. Clinical stage T1 tumors without significant peripheral zone involvement are often ideal cases for bilateral nerve sparing. A neurovascular bundle may be spared with little risk of a positive margin if it overlies a lobe with no clinically detectable tumor, particularly if the results of systematic biopsies of that lobe are negative. A neurovascular bundle may also be spared if it is adjacent to a small tumor (T2a) with a biopsy Gleason score of 6 or less and if it can be easily and cleanly dissected free. A neurovascular bundle that is adjacent to any larger or higher grade tumor, or that is unusually adherent to the capsule, should be sacrificed. With this selective approach, the risk of a positive margin related to nerve sparing was 7%, and all related positive margins were focal (3 mm or less) and associated with an undetectable PSA level at a mean follow-up of 3 years (6). Potent patients can be reassured that, even if erections are not spared, they retain the capacity for orgasm and the rhythmic, ejaculatory contractions of the perineal muscles, but not emission. When desired, erections can usually be restored by penile self-injection of prostaglandin E_1 or a vacuum-constriction device.

PREOPERATIVE PREPARATION

The contemporary modifications of radical perineal prostatectomy, particularly the extended radical modification, require more dissection on the rectal wall than the classic operation of Young. The related, low risk of an inadvertent proctotomy (1.5%) is warranted by the demonstrated benefit of an extended dissection in 15% of patients. Despite the low incidence of proctotomy, complete preoperative bowel preparation is always advisable because the potential complications are significant, including rectourethral and rectocutaneous fistulas and perineal cellulitis and abscesses. Bowel preparation permits continuation of the radical prostatectomy despite proctotomy and without a diverting colostomy, as it optimizes the chance of an uncomplicated proctotomy repair. A well-tolerated, complete cleansing can be accomplished in the outpatient setting without the inconvenience of enemas by a clear liquid diet, 45 mL of buffered oral sodium biphosphate laxative, and four bisacodyl tablets on the day before the operation as well as a bisacodyl rectal suppository on arising on the day of operation. This regimen is commercially available as a kit with patient instructions (Fleet Prep Kit no. 1; C.B. Fleet, Lynchburg, VA). Antibiotic prophylaxis appropriate for colorectal operations is provided by a single intravenous dose of cefotetan 2 g at the beginning of the operation (49).

Although blood loss during radical perineal prostatectomy is low (median, 600 mL), it is prudent to have 1 or 2 units available for transfusion (autologous whenever possible). Cystourethroscopy before radical perineal prostatectomy can be helpful. Transurethral passage of the prostatic tractor in patients in the exaggerated lithotomy position can sometimes be troublesome, and it is useful to be aware of urethral strictures, false passages, or postprostatectomy bladder neck contractures in advance. The knowledge of the presence of a significant prostatic middle lobe is advantageous during division of the posterior bladder neck. Otherwise unrecognized bladder stones or tumors may not be seen at the time of division of the bladder neck when it is done in a manner to spare most of the neck; such stones or tumors may cause postoperative complications. As a final preoperative staging procedure, the occasional, unsuspected finding of gross invasion of the bladder neck by prostate cancer, proved with biopsy, is sufficient to eliminate consideration of radical prostatectomy.

SPECIAL INSTRUMENT

Atraumatic traction and manipulation of the prostate during radical perineal prostatectomy are greatly facilitated by the prostate tractors designed by Lowsley and Young (Fig. 19.2). Lowsley's long tractor has a curved shape similar to a Van Buren male sound, which makes it much easier to pass transurethrally. After division of the membranous urethra, continued specimen traction can be provided by Young's mechanically simpler and cheaper short prostatic tractor, inserted directly through the apical prostatic urethra.

An adaptable, self-retaining retractor provides superior exposure. The table-mounted Omni-Tract Surgical "mini-crescent" retractor with accessory perineal blades and a retractor-mounted fiber-optic cable light (St. Paul, MN) is very satisfac-

tory. If this retractor is used to provide all necessary retraction, including the critical posterior (rectal) retraction, the correct angle of retraction almost always requires placement of the shaft of the posterior retractor inside the crescent ring with a modified connector (Fig. 19.3).

Other useful special instruments include Young's notched bulb retractor and lobe forceps as well as Auvard's weighted vaginal specula with long and short blades. The long Lahey right-angle gall duct forceps with longitudinal jaw serrations always holds a ligature securely at its tip and is a superior ligature carrier.

OPERATIVE PROCEDURE

Patient Position

Careful positioning of the patient in the exaggerated lithotomy position is necessary for patient safety and optimal surgical exposure. It can readily be accomplished with the following sequential steps.

While still supine, the patient is moved caudally until the sacrum is at the table break, which will become the end of the table when the foot-section is lowered completely (a removable foot-section extension is useful). The patient is in proper position if his buttocks are caudal to the table break. Foam boots with soft stirrups are placed on the feet. Stirrup poles are vertically attached to the table, with their curved stirrup attachments and table connection extensions situated at right angles to the longitudinal table axis. The legs are then flexed at the hips, and the feet are raised so that the stirrups can be attached to their poles. The table foot-section is then lowered completely. The perineum is elevated almost parallel to the floor by placing three folded cotton flannel sheets under the sacrum. During this maneuver, lifting the pelvis is easy if assistants simultaneously pull the patient's knees toward his shoulders. Adjustments to achieve the proper parallel position of the perineum can be made by rotating the stirrup poles cephalad on their table-connection brackets, but all weight should be borne by the sacral padding and not by torquing forces on the legs. The poles should be extended in length to reduce knee flexion, and they should be located sufficiently away from the end of the table to allow later attachment of a self-retaining retractor. Shoulder braces are unnecessary and may injure the brachial plexus. The arms should be abducted as little as possible to avoid the same problem. The legs and feet are inspected, and they are adjusted or padded to eliminate any focal pressure points. Broad canvas tape attached to the poles and placed over the folded sheets and the buttocks will help stabilize the position (Fig. 19.4).

After the patient is placed into position, digital opening of the anus will empty any small volume of residual liquid in the rectum from the bowel preparation. If a large volume is present, it should be drained with a rectal tube.

After antiseptic scrub of the surgical field, adequate isolation can be achieved with towels, leg drapes, and a vertical laparot-

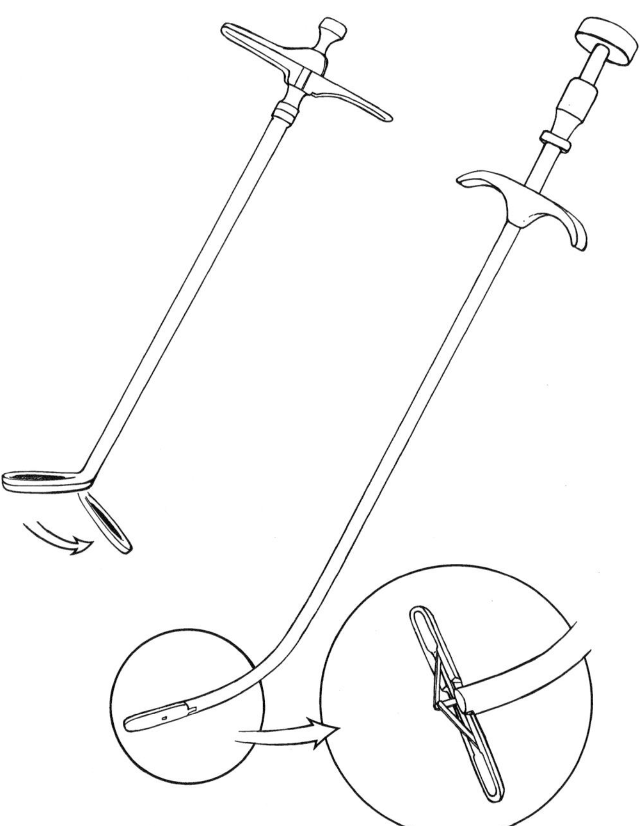

Fig. 19.2. Prostatic tractors of Young (left) and Lowsley (right), closed for transurethral passage and opened for specimen traction.

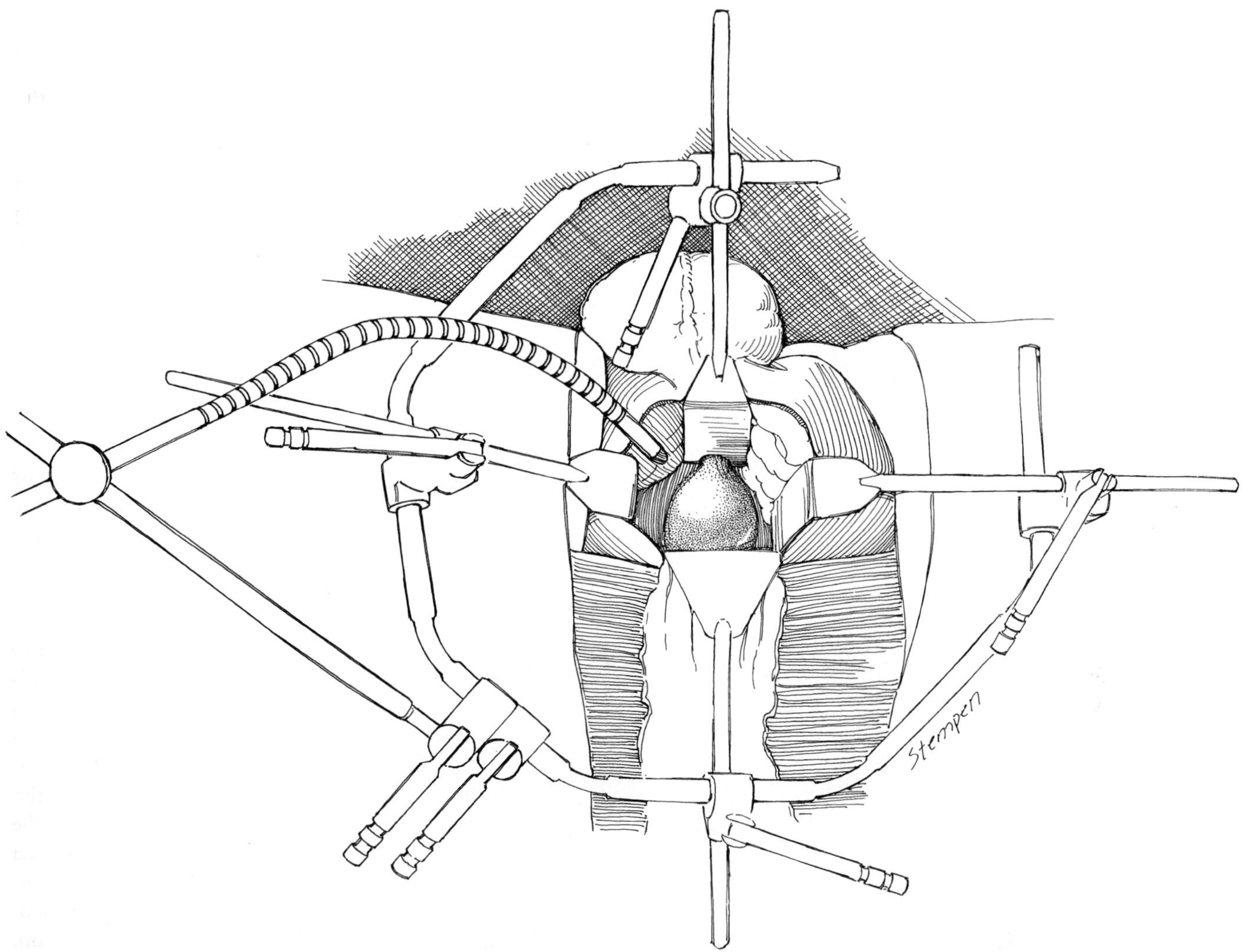

Fig. 19.3.   Table-mounted Omni-Tract Surgical mini-crescent self-retaining retractor with fiber-optic cable light. Note the location of the posterior retractor shaft mounted inside the crescent ring. (Reprinted with permission from Weldon VE, Tavel FR. Radical perineal prostatectomy. In: Das S, Crawford E, eds. Cancer of the prostate. New York: Marcel Dekker, 1993:225–266.)

omy sheet turned upside down. With an empty, prepared rectum and prophylactic antibiotics, special draping to attempt to isolate the anus is unnecessary.

Lowsley's long curved prostatic tractor can be inserted at this time. A temporary reverse Trendelenburg position, injection of water-soluble lubricant into the urethra, and preliminary passage of a 28-Ch Van Buren curved sound to assess the urethral direction are useful adjuncts. If the tractor cannot be passed easily, it should not be forced, and the Van Buren sound or a large Foley catheter is an adequate substitute.

Incision

An inverted U incision is made outside the external anal sphincter as described by Young (23). Belt's approach inside the anal sphincter can be used (50), but it has the disadvantages of a more tunneled and narrow field and it eliminates the assistance

of the functioning sphincter in maintaining an unsoiled operative field. The apex of the incision just anterior to the anal sphincter can often be located by observing the slightly rounded skin contour and increased skin pigmentation over the sphincter and by palpating the slightly softer subcutaneous tissue outside it, or by locating it 4 to 5 cm anterior to the center of the anus. The vertical arms of the incision are placed just inside the ischial tuberosities and are extended posteriorly to a point lateral to the anal center (Fig. 19.5). The skin incision is deepened 1 to 2 cm into the subcutaneous fat.

Full development of the incision requires transecting the central tendon of the perineum, opening the ischiorectal fossae, and exposing the ventral rectal wall. The central "tendon" is the vertical, midline, anterior striated muscular extension of the external anal sphincter that connects it to the transverse perineal and bulbospongiosus muscles at the perineal body. Anterior extension into those muscles should be avoided. A 2-

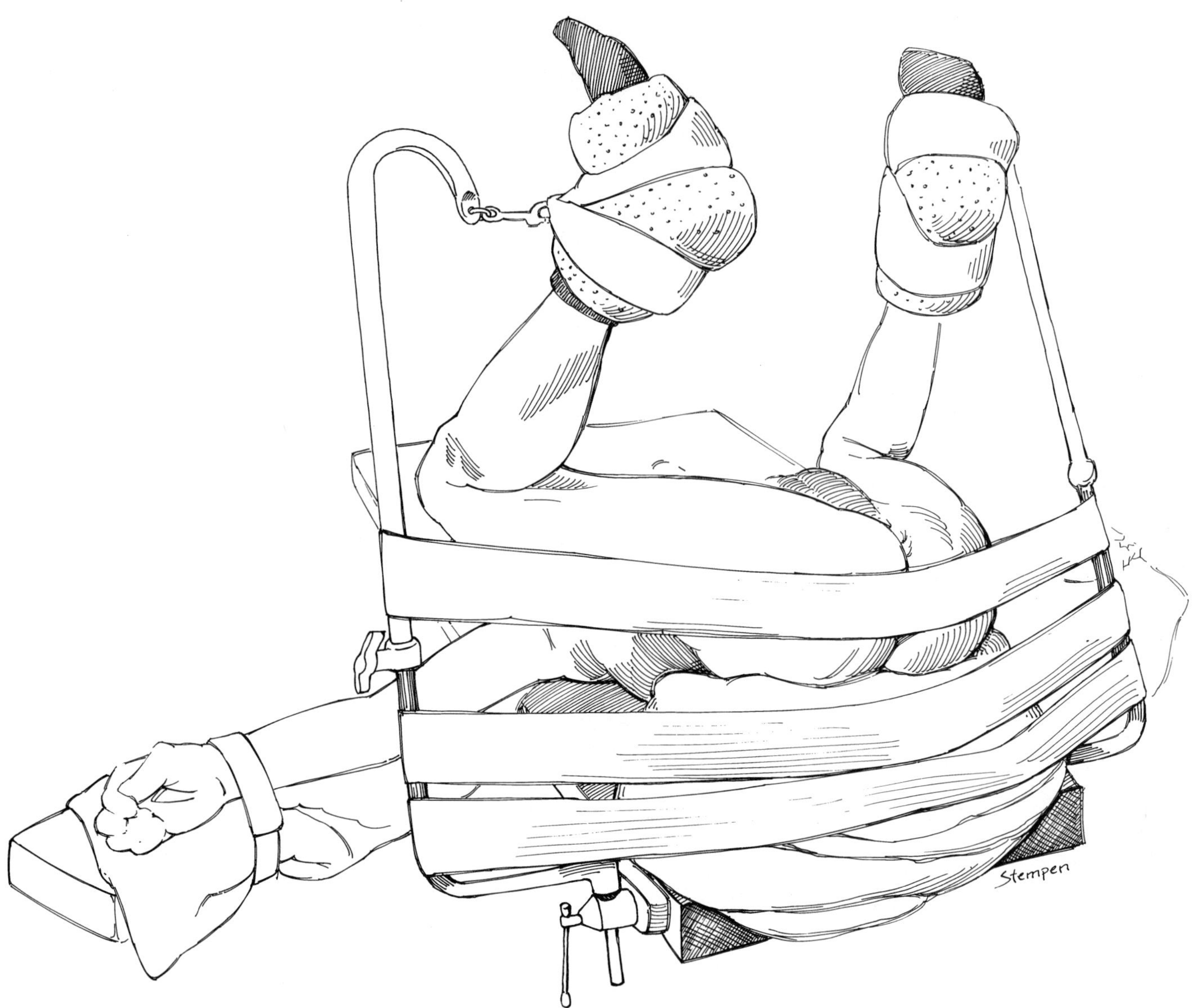

Fig. 19.4. Exaggerated lithotomy position with perineum parallel to floor. Note the folded cotton flannel sheets under the sacrum. The broad canvas tape strips between the poles and over the sheets and buttocks stabilize the patient's position. (Reprinted with permission from Weldon VE, Tavel FR. Radical perineal prostatectomy. In: Das S, Crawford E, eds. Cancer of the prostate. New York: Marcel Dekker, 1993:225–266.)

cm stab wound is made through the subcutaneous perineal fascia on each side at the posterior ends of the vertical arms of the incision and inside the ischial tuberosities, taking care not to extend posteriorly into the inferior rectal vessels and nerves located lateral to the anal center. An index finger is inserted through these stab openings on each side, outside the external anal sphincter in a cephalad and medial direction, and each ischiorectal fossa is bluntly dissected while the thick rectal wall is palpated medially. A finger is insinuated at a point of little resistance just over the rectal wall and cephalad to the anal sphincter, connecting the opened ischiorectal fossae. The central tendon is now located above this finger, and incision through all of the tissue above the finger will expose the rectum (Fig. 19.6). If a finger cannot be easily insinuated directly over

the rectal wall, it should not be forced or inadvertent proctotomy may occur. Instead, an Allis clamp applied to the subcutaneous fascia at the apex of the flap will help accentuate the central tendon by placing it on tension, and it can be transected under vision, assisted by palpation in each fossa to locate the rectum.

Rectal Mobilization

The pale color of the smooth muscle of the ventral rectal wall signals successful entry onto the correct plane of dissection. Some red, striated fibers of the medial portion of the levator ani, the puborectalis muscle, insert obliquely onto the ventral rectal wall caudal to the rectourethralis muscle. These decuss-

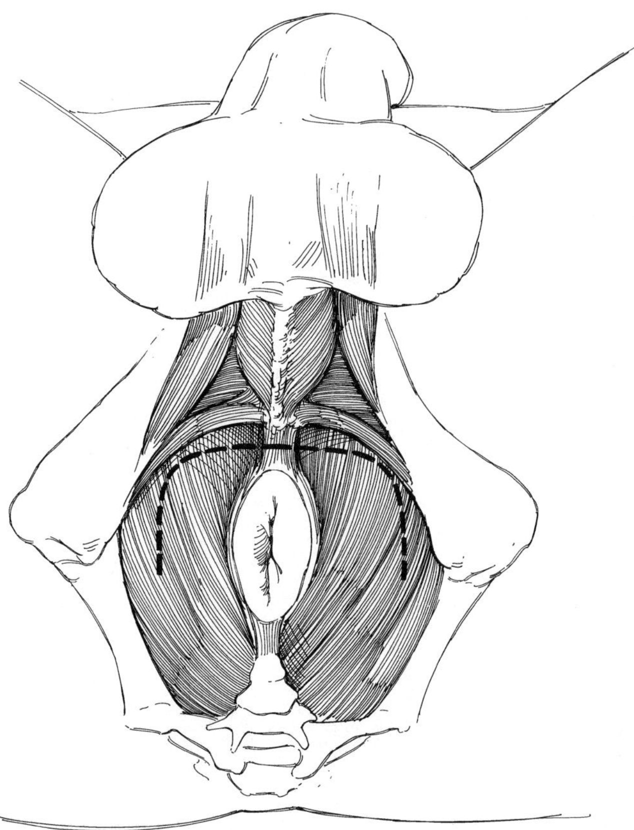

Fig. 19.5. The broken line indicates the location of inverted U skin incision relative to underlying anatomical structures. Vertical arms of incision are inside ischial tuberosities. The apex of incision crosses central "tendon" of perineum, which connects the external anal sphincter to transverse perineal and bulbospongiosus muscles at perineal body. (Reprinted with permission from Weldon VE, Tavel FR. Radical perineal prostatectomy. In: Das S, Crawford E, eds. Cancer of the prostate. New York: Marcel Dekker, 1993:225–266.)

ations are separated or incised, exposing the rectal wall more completely. Further cephalad dissection on the broad band of ventral longitudinal rectal muscle leads directly to the rectourethralis muscle, which securely attaches the rectum to the posterior urogenital diaphragm. With a prostatic tractor inserted, palpation lateral and ventral to the rectourethralis muscle will identify the underlying membranous urethra and prostatic apex.

The rectourethralis muscle must be isolated and skeletonized in preparation for its safe division. The space lateral to this muscle on each side, between it and the levator ani, is opened with scissor-spreading and digital probing. Pinching the rectourethralis muscle can further outline it. It must be visualized and isolated as a strap suspending the apex of the tent of the rectum. This is aided by placing it on tension with retraction of the posterior edge of the urogenital diaphragm with Young's notched bulb retractor (Fig. 19.7) and countertraction on the rectal wall. The latter may be accomplished by temporarily covering the nondominant hand with a second glove, inserting the index finger into the rectum, and applying

traction to the ventral rectal wall with the thumb placed over an intervening gauze sponge. Movement of the index finger will assist in identifying the suspended rectal wall. Attempted blunt disruption of the rectourethralis muscle will almost always result in an inadvertent proctotomy. It must be divided sharply and completely before the rectal wall can be safely mobilized. There are two helpful maneuvers.

1. Any isolated edge of the rectourethralis muscle, either lateral or central, can be confidently divided.
2. If the remaining muscle is broad and indefinite, it can be completely penetrated by spreading horizontally positioned scissors in the midline down to the lighter colored ventral rectal fascia.

The resulting split parallels the longitudinally oriented muscle fibers. Each remaining half is then completely incised, beginning at the newly created medial edge and extending laterally (Fig. 19.8).

Immediately after the rectourethralis muscle is completely transected, the previously tented ventral rectal wall turns at a right angle to the initial plane of dissection, parallel to the

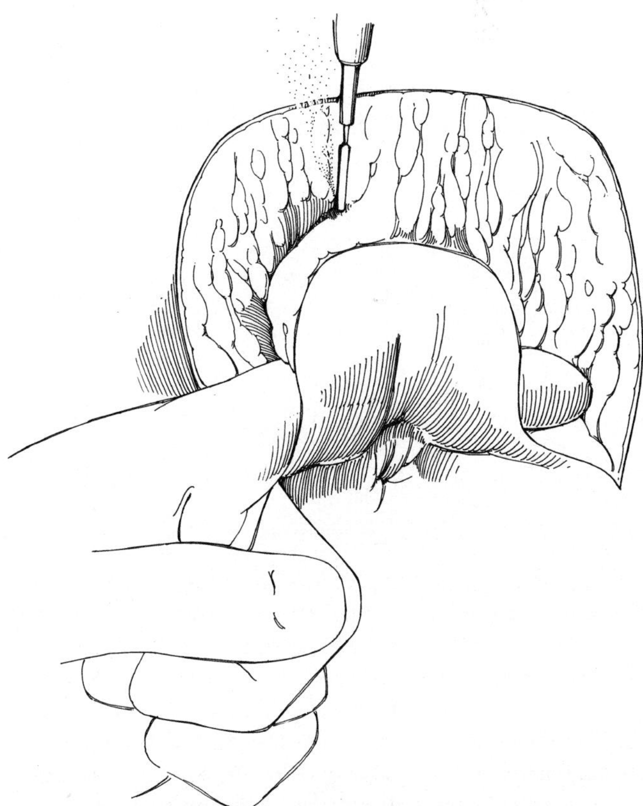

Fig. 19.6. Index finger inserted cephalad to external anal sphincter, immediately over ventral rectal wall between bluntly developed ischiorectal fossae on each side and under central tendon of perineum. The tissue divided over the finger includes central tendon. (Reprinted with permission from Weldon VE, Tavel FR. Radical perineal prostatectomy. In: Das S, Crawford E, eds. Cancer of the prostate. New York: Marcel Dekker, 1993: 225–266.)

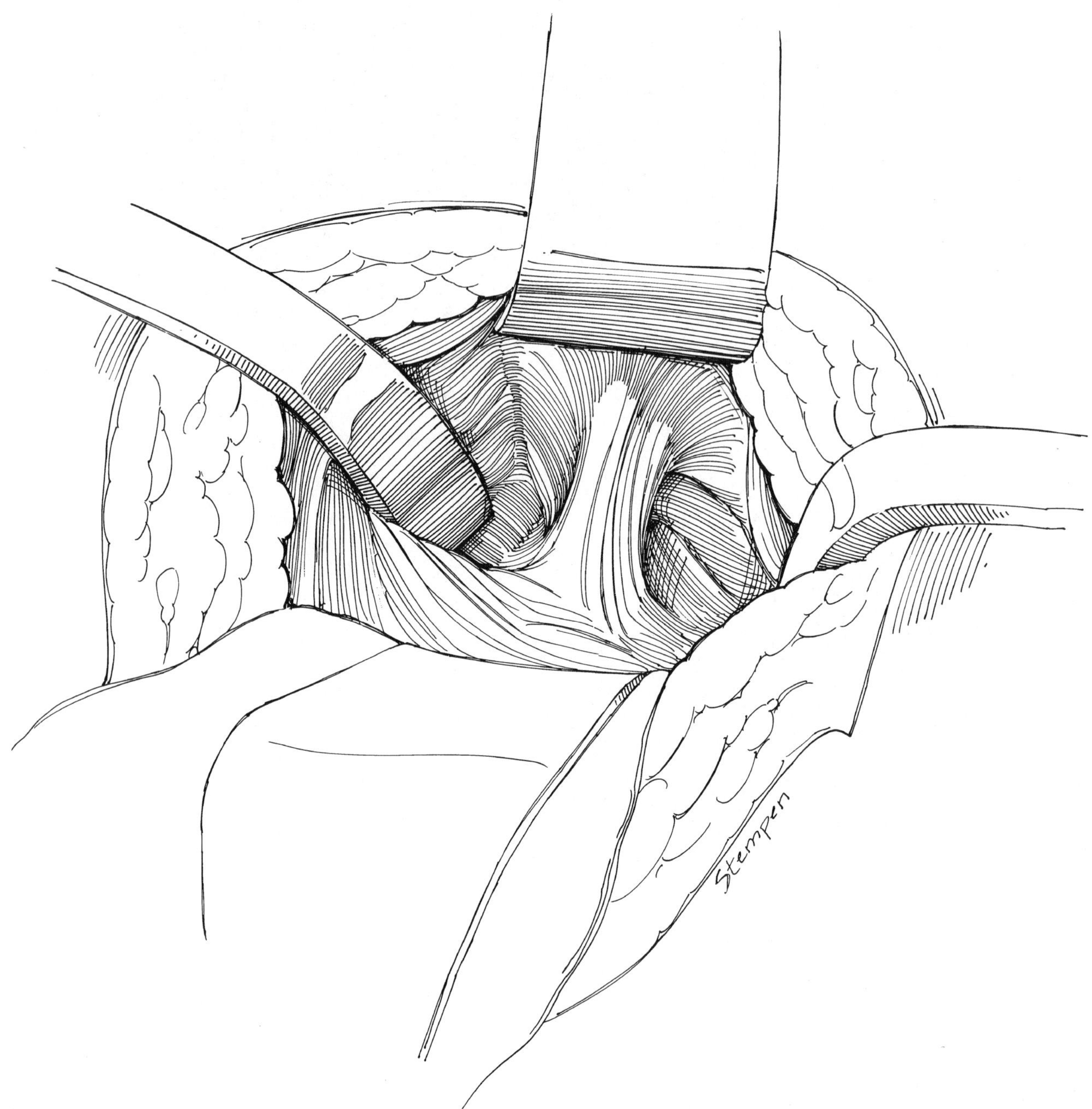

Fig. 19.7.   Rectourethralis muscle, connecting anterior band of longitudinal rectal muscle to urogenital diaphragm in midline, is placed on tension and accentuated by anterior and posterior retraction. Lateral retractors displace levator ani fibers inserting onto ventral rectal wall. (Reprinted with permission from Weldon VE, Tavel FR. Radical perineal prostatectomy. In: Das S, Crawford E, eds. Cancer of the prostate. New York: Marcel Dekker, 1993:225–266.)

dorsal surface of the prostate, and the ventral rectal fascia is encountered. The important space between it and the rectal wall is entered, and the direction of the plane of dissection turns from the horizontal to the vertical (Fig. 19.9). This space can usually be developed bluntly with careful finger dissection by keeping the fingernail against the underlying prostate while seeking the proper areas of separation with lateral and cephalad pressure and avoiding dorsal pressure on the rectal wall (Fig. 19.10). Occasionally, retraction of the rectal wall with sharp

dissection under vision may be necessary. This space must be opened down to the base of the prostate, which can be recognized by palpating the retractor blades. If a neurovascular bundle is to be sacrificed, more lateral dissection of the space on that side is needed. If a nerve-sparing dissection is anticipated, the lateral dissection should be minimized.

After this space is adequately developed, the ventral rectal fascia is exposed by retracting the ventral rectal wall. A single, opened baby laparotomy sponge is inserted with its end at the

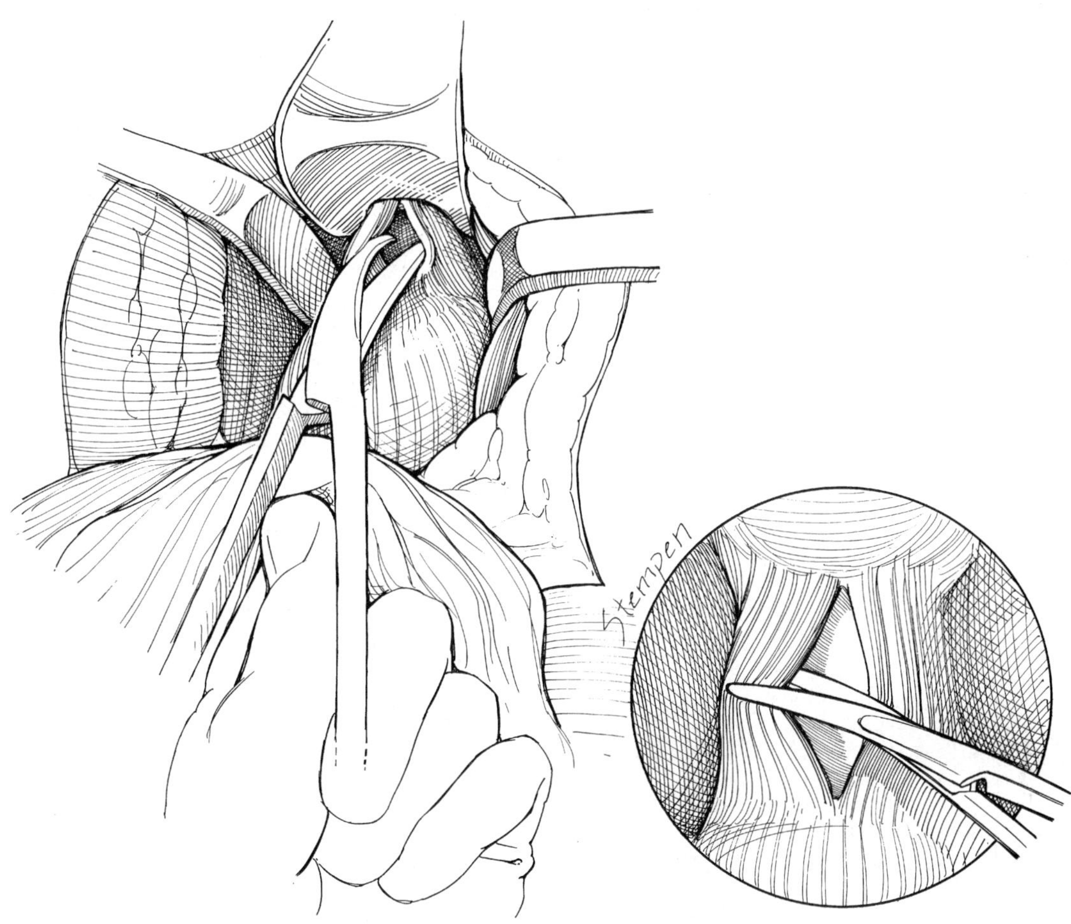

Fig. 19.8.   Division of rectourethralis muscle. After any isolated central or lateral edge is divided, any remaining broad and indefinite muscle is completely penetrated and split longitudinally by scissors-spreading in the midline. Inset: Each remaining half is then completely incised, beginning at the newly created medial edge and extending laterally.

bottom of the dissected space and a retractor is placed over it. With small prostates and a small space, a baby Deaver retractor is best. With any larger prostate, an Auvard weighted vaginal speculum with a blade of appropriate length (usually short) serves well without occupying an assistant. With the speculum, it may be necessary to stretch or divide some lateral fibers of the levator ani to insert the blade and to place a rolled wound towel under the weighted handle to obtain the proper angle of retraction.

Thus far, the operation has proceeded within the envelope of the perirectal fascia, and further progression with contemporary radical perineal prostatectomy offers two different strategies for escaping this envelope. The ventral rectal fascia is the key to the nerve sparing and extended radical modifications of radical perineal prostatectomy. The different methods of dealing with this fascia constitute the point of departure for each modification. If a nerve-sparing dissection is intended, either unilaterally or bilaterally, it is best to proceed with vertical incision of the ventral rectal fascia and mobilization of the neurovascular bundle(s) before placing the self-retaining retractor to minimize neuropathy from traction on the nerves. If an extended dissection is in-

tended, it is often convenient to proceed with division of the cephalad end of the neurovascular bundle and transverse incision of the adjacent ventral rectal fascia at the level of the prostatic base to free the rectum and more widely open the space before placing the self-retaining retractor. After the crescent ring is fixed into position, careful placement of the rectal blade, with adjustment of the angle of retraction, is important (Fig. 19.3).

Figures 19.11 to 19.24 illustrate the techniques used in a potent man with prostate cancer clinically involving more than half of the right lobe but not clinically involving the left lobe, i.e., an extended radical dissection on the right and a nerve-sparing dissection on the left.

Extended Radical Modification

This modification entails total prostatoseminal vesiculectomy with the additional excision of the ventral rectal and lateral prostatic fascia (with the enclosed neurovascular bundle). The emphasis is on maximal fascial excision rather than only on excision of the neurovascular bundle. When performed, the

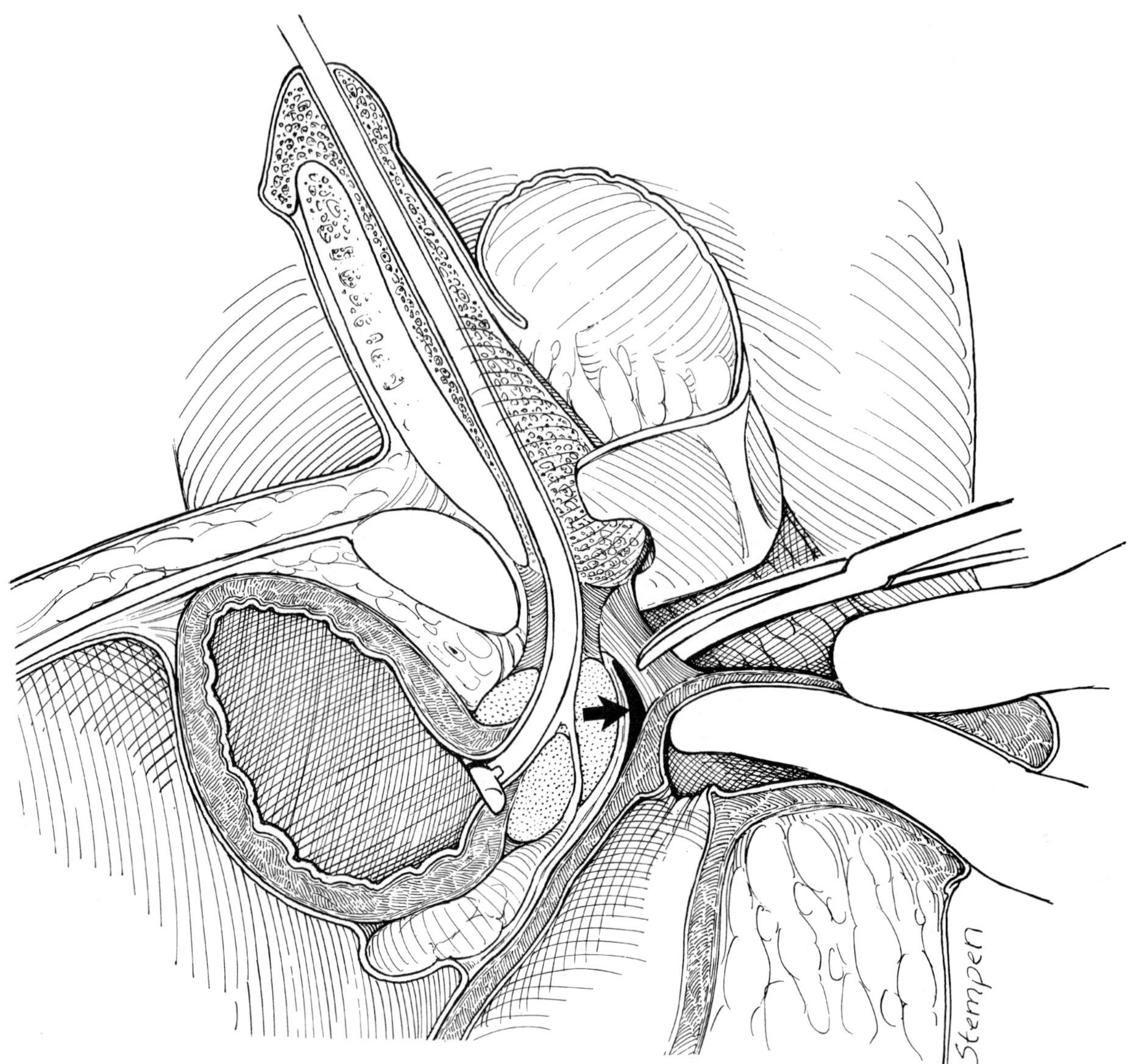

Fig. 19.9. After sharp transection of rectourethralis muscle, key space between rectal wall and its ventral rectal fascia (arrow) is entered.

widest possible posterolateral excision is achieved, with specimen margins on the ventral rectal wall and the medial aspect of the levator ani (the puborectalis muscle) (51). It may be unilateral or bilateral.

If a unilateral extended radical dissection is to be performed, dissection begins by opening the ventral rectal fascia vertically, just across the midline and medial to the neurovascular bundle to be spared, and extending from at least 1 cm over the membranous urethra to the base of the prostate (Fig. 19.11). Entry into Denonvilliers' membrane over the prostate is avoided. For a bilateral extended radical dissection, the ventral rectal fascia is maintained over the prostate. The portion to be excised is then transected transversely at the level of the membranous urethra. If it is convenient and accessible, the same portion of the ventral rectal fascia can be divided transversely at the prostatic base while avoiding the adjacent fold of the ventral rectal wall. Otherwise, this can be deferred until the prostate is more

completely mobilized. The enclosed neurovascular bundle is transected at both ends between hemostatic clips (Fig. 19.12).

Dissection then extends laterally through the thin lateral rectal fascia lateral to the neurovascular bundle onto the puborectalis muscle (Fig. 19.12). The thin lateral rectal fascia may be opened bluntly or sharply. Dissection continues ventrally in the plane between the dark red fibers of the puborectalis muscle and the white lateral prostatic fascia. This clean, avascular plane is opened with digital dissection up to the fascia containing Santorini's anterior venous complex (Fig. 19.1).

The contralateral dissection is then performed with either the same extended dissection or a nerve-sparing dissection.

Nerve-Sparing Modification

After the rectum has been mobilized and the space between the ventral rectal wall and its fascia developed, the neurovascular

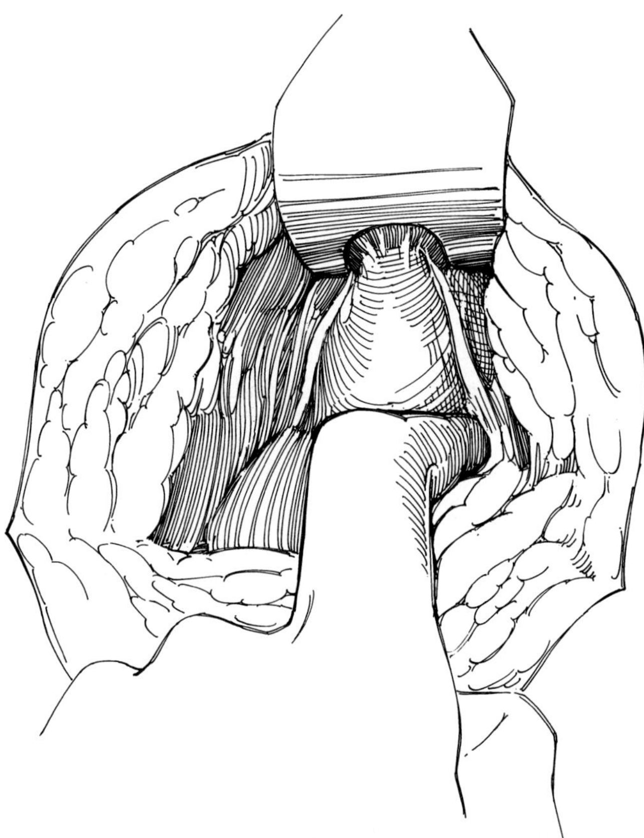

Fig. 19.10. Digital dissection at the level of the prostatic apex develops a vertical plane between the rectal wall and its ventral rectal fascia. Neurovascular bundles are within the lateral aspects of this fascia. (Reprinted with permission from Weldon VE, Tavel FR. Radical perineal prostatectomy. In: Das S, Crawford E, eds. Cancer of the prostate. New York: Marcel Dekker, 1993:225–266.)

bundles (containing the cavernous nerves) can be seen coursing vertically within the lateral aspects of the ventral rectal fascia over the posterolateral surface of the prostate and the membranous urethra. A nerve-sparing dissection begins with vertical division of the ventral rectal fascia from at least 1 cm over the membranous urethra to the base of the prostate. If a bilateral nerve-sparing dissection is anticipated, the ventral rectal fascia is opened in the midline. If the dissection is unilateral, the fascial incision is asymmetric and just medial to the neurovascular bundle to be spared. The medial edge of the divided ventral rectal fascia containing the neurovascular bundle is elevated, and it is carefully separated from the prostatic capsule to avoid inadvertent capsular disruption (Fig. 19.11). The three main areas of attachment of the neurovascular bundle to the prostatic capsule are at the superior and inferior neural pedicles, described by Villers et al. (47), and a fascial attachment at the prostatomembranous junction. Mobilization of the neurovascular bundle is facilitated by isolating these structures and separately dividing each one. The neural pedicles are divided beneath microhemostatic clips placed at their origin on the neurovascular bundle to avoid any hematoma-related neuropa-

thy (Fig. 19.13). Any unusual adherence may indicate cancer infiltration of the perineural spaces and warrants reassessment of the nerve-sparing decision.

Further lateral and ventral digital dissection around the prostate is accomplished in the avascular plane between the prostatic capsule and the lateral prostatic fascia (Figs. 19.11 and 19.12).

Injury to the neurovascular bundle is most likely during three other maneuvers.

1. Retraction, with injury by compressing with lateral blades or by stretching with excessive retraction with the notched anterior blade.
2. Division and ligation of the vascular pedicles of the prostate lateral to the seminal vesicles and adjacent to the cephalad end of the neurovascular bundles.
3. Division of the membranous urethra, and later suture of the vesicourethral anastomosis with excessive incorporation of the periurethral fascia, near the caudal end of the bundles.

Care with these maneuvers will maximize potency preservation.

Division of the Membranous Urethra and Puboprostatic Ligaments

After an extended radical or nerve-sparing dissection has removed the ventral rectal fascia over the junction of the prostatic apex with the membranous urethra, any remaining myofascial fibers are incised transversely over this junction to expose the white wall of the urethra. If an extended radical dissection has been performed, it is necessary at this time to divide the wing of lateral prostatic fascia lateral to the membranous urethra that extends to Santorini's venous plexus beneath two large hemoclips placed as ventrally as possible. The space around the urethral wall is dissected by spreading a curved forceps on the urethral wall laterally, and then encircling it with a Mixter right-angle forceps. In the proper dissection plane, passage of the Mixter forceps between the urethra and the underlying dorsal vein of the penis is unimpeded. The dorsal half of the urethral wall is incised sharply with a knife precisely at its junction with the prostatic apex (Fig. 19.14). Depressing the prostatic apex with a Küntner dissector helps visualize this junction. If a prostatic tractor is in place, the incision is deepened down to the metal shaft, the prostatic tractor is removed, and the ventral half of the urethral wall is transected with Potts' angled scissors beneath the encircling right-angle forceps. No attempt is made to dissect any urethra from within the prostatic apex because of the added risk of a positive margin with that maneuver. Belt's modification (50) of transection and preservation of the prostatic apex is antiquated; it is specifically avoided with contemporary radical perineal prostatectomy because cancer is present within 1 cm of the apical margin in 80% of radical prostatectomy specimens (34, 38).

Young's short prostatic tractor is then inserted through the transected prostatic apical urethra and rotated dorsally, allowing dissection onto the anterior prostatic capsule. If there is

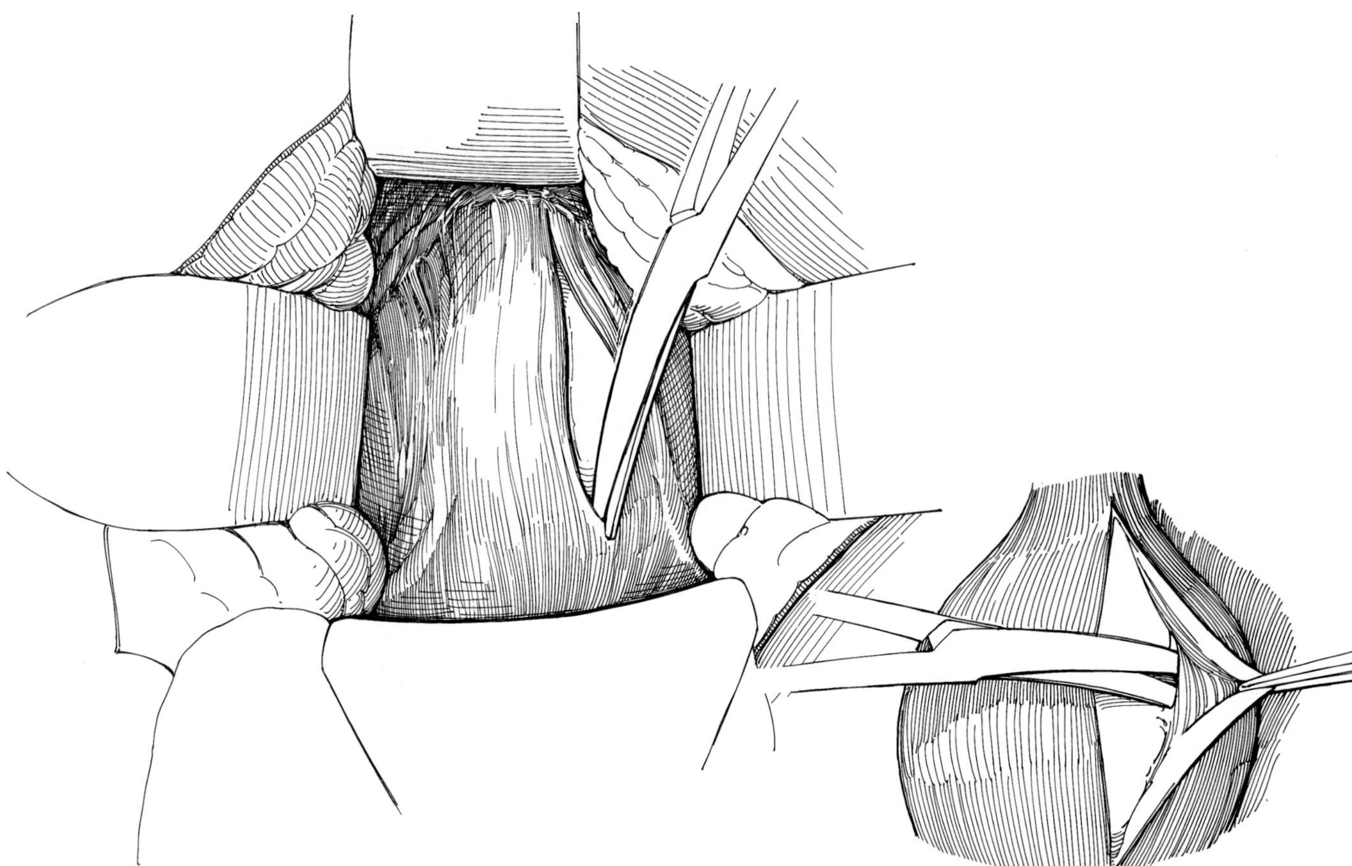

Fig. 19.11.   Vertical incision of the ventral rectal fascia medial to left neurovascular bundle, from prostate base to over membranous urethra, begins left nerve-sparing dissection. An extended radical dissection is intended on the right side. Asymmetrical incision maintains most of ventral rectal fascia with right neurovascular bundle that will be sacrificed with the prostate. Inset: Left nerve-sparing dissection with elevation of left neurovascular bundle and adjacent fascia from Denonvilliers' membrane and lateral prostatic capsule. (Reprinted with permission from Weldon VE, Tavel FR. Radical perineal prostatectomy. In: Das S, Crawford E, eds. Cancer of the prostate. New York: Marcel Dekker, 1993:225–266.)

any remaining wing of the lateral prostatic fascia extending to Santorini's plexus with an extended radical dissection, it is completely divided beneath hemoclips up to the puboprostatic ligaments.

The puboprostatic ligaments are encountered in the midline caudal to the bladder neck. Palpation lateral and cephalad to these ligaments will reveal the contour of the prostatic base and the extent of the midline structures that need to be passed. It is imperative to avoid the temptation simply to push off these structures, as that maneuver will avulse the delicate anterior prostatic capsule and, if there is an underlying transition zone tumor, create an iatrogenically positive margin (6). Those ligaments must be divided sharply, ventral to their capsular insertion (Fig. 19.15). Any soft fascia containing branches of Santorini's venous plexus that lies beneath and between those ligaments can then be pushed cephalad to expose the anterior bladder neck.

With an extended radical dissection, the wing of lateral prostatic fascia must now be transected across the bladder neck (Fig. 19.16). This is best done beneath large hemoclips near the midline because of the frequent large venous branches; more laterally, these are fewer and smaller.

If there is any troublesome bleeding from Santorini's plexus, it can be visualized with the assistance of the retractor-mounted fiber-optic light, grasped with DeBakey's vascular thumb forceps, and clipped. If this is not adequate, the area beneath Santorini's plexus is packed with an opened gauze sponge and the operation is continued. Most of the bleeding will have ceased when the pack is removed at the time of the vesicourethral anastomosis. Completing the anastomosis pulls the bladder neck ventrally and compresses the veins against the unyielding anterior endopelvic fascia and further diminishes bleeding.

Bladder Neck Division

Simple division of the vesicoprostatic junction is performed. Wide excision of the bladder neck is usually unnecessary, and it is futile when it seems necessary. In our series, bladder neck invasion occurred in only 3% of patients and was always accompanied by a positive margin at another site and by seminal vesicle invasion in 50% (6). Although bladder neck preservation does not directly enhance postoperative continence, it re-

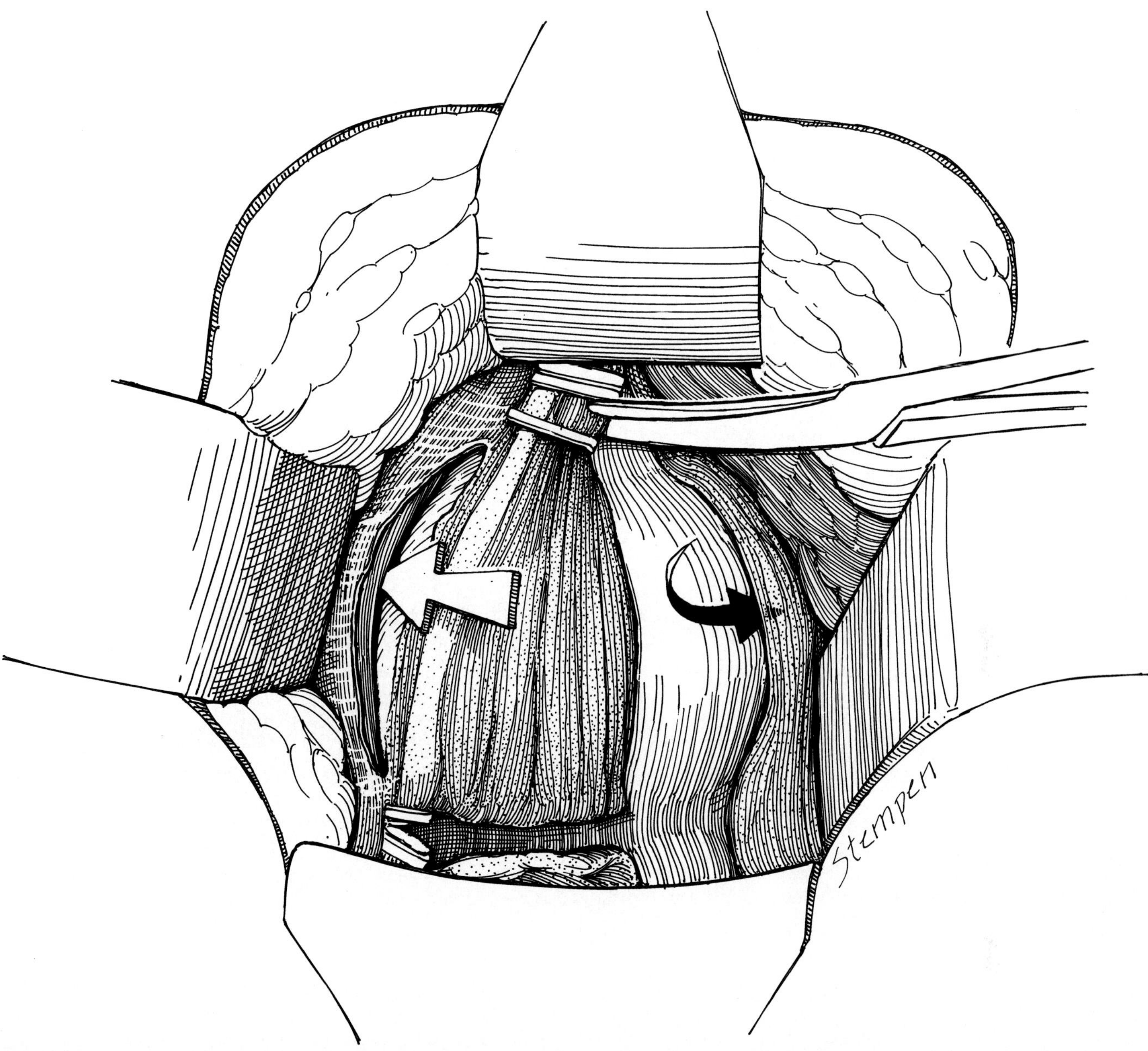

Fig. 19.12.   Right extended radical and left nerve-sparing dissections. Right ventral rectal fascia and enclosed neurovascular bundle clipped and divided transversely over membranous urethra and base of prostate. Thin right lateral rectal fascia penetrated, exposing extended radical dissection plane between levator ani and lateral prostatic fascia (white arrow). Left neurovascular bundle and ventral rectal fascia mobilized off Denonvilliers' membrane, exposing nerve-sparing dissection plane between lateral prostatic capsule and lateral prostatic fascia (black arrow). (Reprinted with permission from Weldon VE, Tavel FR. Radical perineal prostatectomy. In: Das S, Crawford E, eds. Cancer of the prostate. New York: Marcel Dekker, 1993:225–266.)

duces tension on the subsequent anastomosis. The muscle fibers of the bladder will usually separate from the prostate with digital dissection over the anterior 270° of the bladder neck circumference, especially if there is at least a moderate degree of prostatic hyperplasia. With small glands, and particularly with prior transurethral resection of the prostate, sharp scissors dissection is necessary. The correct level of transection is identified by palpating the prostatic contour and visualizing the circular bladder muscle fibers (Fig. 19.17).

After the anterior bladder neck mucosa is opened, the pros-

tatic tractor transversing the urethra impedes visualization of the posterior bladder neck and is removed. All subsequent outward traction on the specimen is achieved by pulling a 0.5-in. Penrose drain through the prostatic urethra and around the ventral prostate. After prior transurethral resection, the thin ventral prostate may fracture vertically when traction is applied on the encircling drain. In that circumstance, Young's lobe forceps may be used to grasp the entire (usually small) prostate for traction. Further sharp dissection circumcises the mucosa (Fig. 19.18). If a pedunculated middle lobe is present, it is

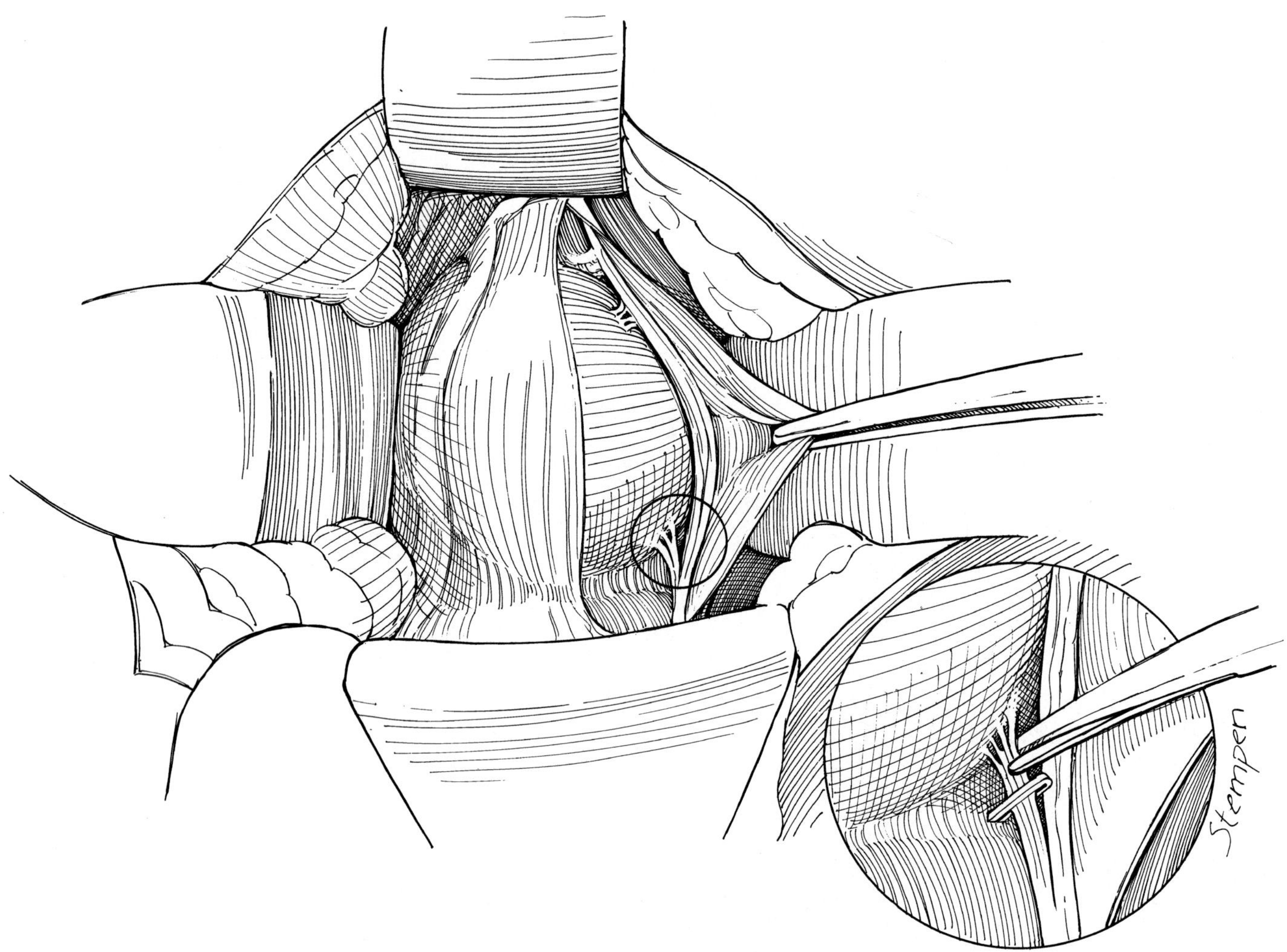

Fig. 19.13. Left nerve-sparing dissection, with mobilization of left neurovascular bundle by isolating and dividing superior and inferior neural pedicles and fascial attachment at prostatomembranous junction. Inset: Superior neural pedicle divided beneath clip.

best grasped and pulled outward with Schroeder's sharp, single-toothed uterine tenaculum forceps to facilitate incision cephalad to it across the distal trigone. The remaining, thick posterior bladder neck is transected sharply or with the electrocautery unit down to the ampullae of the vas deferentia and the seminal vesicles. The muscle in this area is often thicker than expected and, if the landmarks are not clear, completion of this division may be deferred until after the vascular pedicles are divided. The seminal vesicles and the plane between them and the posterior neck musculature are then more evident. If the ventral prostate was fractured earlier, further specimen traction can be accomplished by pulling a 0.5-in. Penrose drain between the vasal ampullae and around the entire prostate.

During division of the bladder neck, visualization of the ureteral orifices (assisted by intravenous indigo carmine) is not routinely necessary but it is very useful if the anatomy is not clear. The ureteral orifices can be seen if the bladder neck is widely open, or their location can be estimated by palpating the interureteric ridge if the bladder neck is small.

Vascular Pedicle Division

Contralateral rotation of the specimen exposes the vascular pedicle entering the base of the prostate lateral to the seminal vesicle. The cephalad extent of the prostatic base and the prominent lateral "band" formed by the vascular pedicle cephalad to the base are identified by palpation. This band, and any remaining lateral prostatic fascia associated with an extended radical dissection, are secured and divided with a "hook and clamp" technique. A closed Mixter right-angle forceps is inserted through the tissue medial to the palpable prominence of the vascular pedicle from either the dorsal or ventral direction. The insinuated right-angle forceps is then pulled in the direction of specimen traction, and an opened right-angle forceps is inserted, parallel and cephalad to the hooking forceps and around the pedicle, and closed (Fig. 19.19). If a nerve-sparing dissection has been done on that side, the laterally adjacent neurovascular bundle can be clearly seen and avoided. The hooking technique pulls the vascular

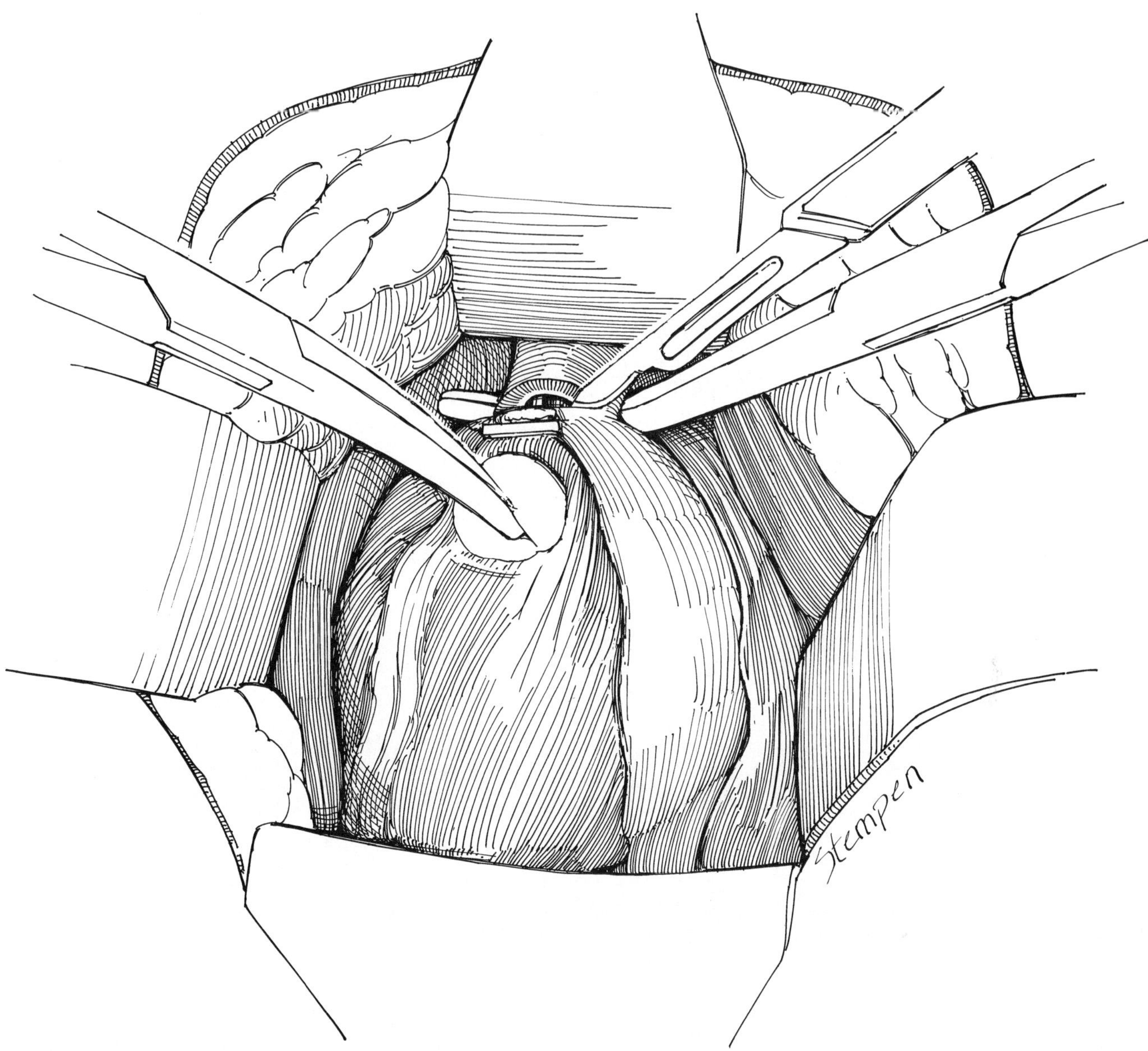

Fig. 19.14. Transection of membranous urethra at prostatic apex, with right extended radical and left nerve-sparing dissections. The knife divides the dorsal urethral wall down to the metal shaft of the long prostatic tractor. Proximal urethral wall dissected from enveloping fascia, preserving immediately adjacent left neurovascular bundle. Right-angle forceps encircle membranous urethra in unimpeded dissection plane on its wall. Right neurovascular bundle clipped and divided distally. Küntner dissector depresses prostatic apex to expose precise urethral transection. (Reprinted with permission from Weldon VE, Tavel FR. Radical perineal prostatectomy. In: Das S, Crawford E, eds. Cancer of the prostate. New York: Marcel Dekker, 1993:225–266.)

pedicle away from the neurovascular bundle and allows safe transection of the pedicle close to the prostate. The pedicle is transected caudal to the clamping forceps. There is no significant back bleeding from the stump of the pedicle on the prostate, and it is unnecessary to secure it. The proximal pedicle is secured with a single 2-0 synthetic braided absorbable ligature passed in a long Lahey right-angle gall duct forceps with longitudinal jaw serrations. Large hemostatic clips have been used on the proximal pedicles, but they have occasionally loosened during subsequent manipulation, and the ligatures are more secure. This maneuver is repeated until all of the vascular pedicle is divided and the lateral wall of the seminal vesicle is exposed. The contralateral vascular pedicle is then similarly divided.

This maneuver exposes the lateral aspects of the seminal vesicles on each side and, if the posterior bladder neck has not previously been completely transected, it provides an advantageous lateral view of the dissection plane between the seminal vesicles and the remaining bladder neck fibers. A Mixter right-angle forceps can be inserted to develop this plane and elevate the remaining bladder neck muscle for division with an electrocautery unit (Fig. 19.19).

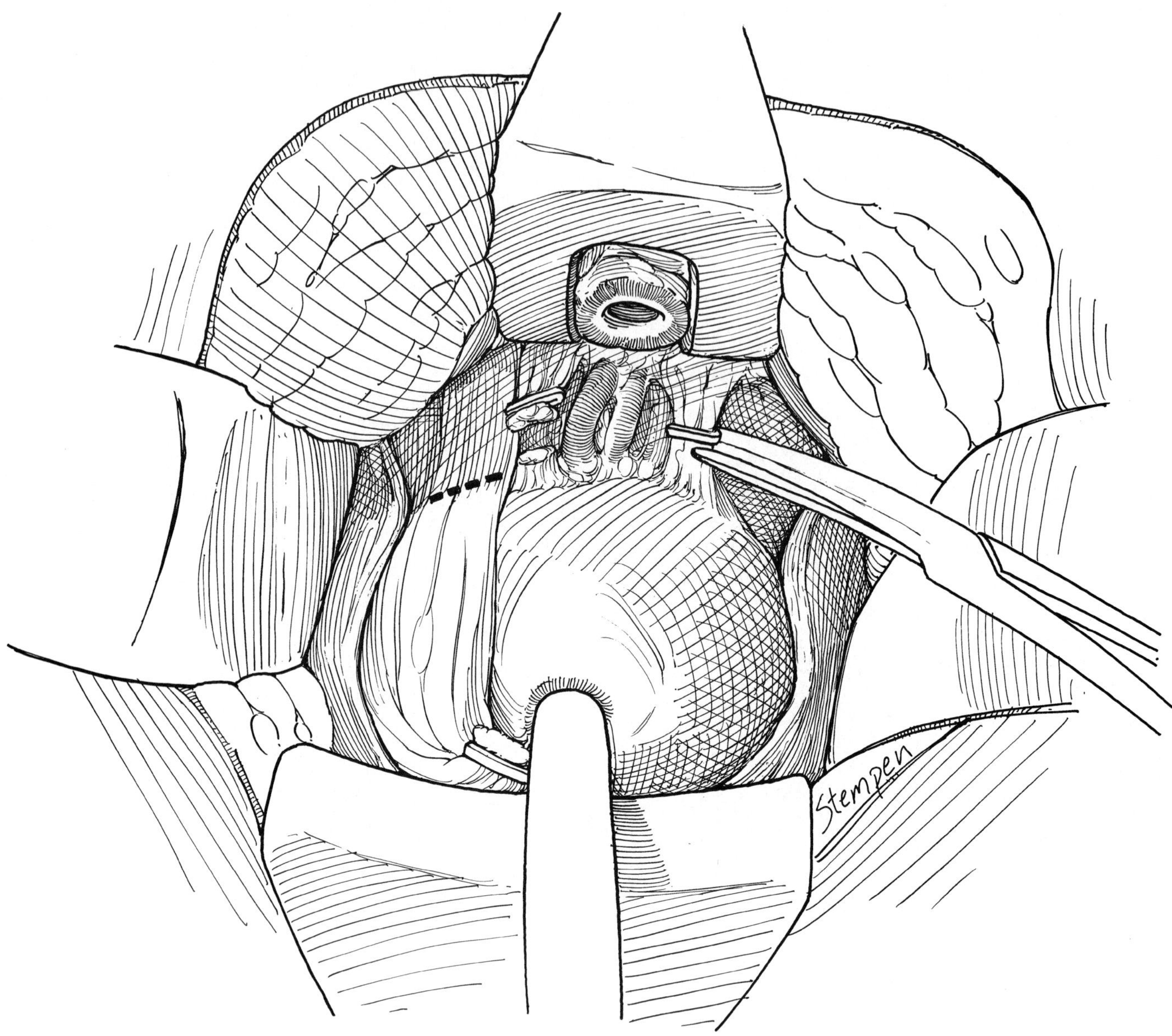

Fig. 19.15.   Sharp division of puboprostatic ligaments, with right extended radical and left nerve-sparing dissections. The short prostatic tractor entering the prostatic apex has been rotated dorsally, exposing the anterior prostatic capsule. The broken line indicates the site of division of the right lateral prostatic fascia (with an extended dissection) at the level of the bladder neck cephalad to the puboprostatic ligaments. Note the clipped right neurovascular bundle at the prostatic apex. (From Weldon VE, Tavel FR, Neuwirth H, et al. Patterns of positive specimen margins and detectable prostate-specific antigen after radical perineal prostatectomy. J Urol 1995;153:1565.)

Seminal Vesicle Dissection

After the ventral surfaces of the seminal vesicles and the ampullae of the vasa deferentia are exposed, the prostate is pulled ventrally, exposing the fascia over the dorsal aspect of these structures. If an extended radical dissection has been performed but the cephalad portion of the ventral rectal fascia at the base of the prostate has not yet been divided, it is now transected transversely. Denonvilliers' membrane is then exposed and, after the space between it and the ventral rectal fascia is developed more widely and in a cephalad direction, it is also divided

transversely over the seminal vesicles while a generous cuff is maintained with the specimen (Fig. 19.20).

Complete dissection of the seminal vesicles is performed bilaterally with the assistance of four maneuvers.

1. Scissor-spreading on the dorsal and ventral walls of the seminal vesicle.
2. Opening of the cleft between the ipsilateral vasal ampulla and the seminal vesicle, whose medial edge overlaps the ampulla dorsally (Fig. 19.21).
3. Traction and counter-traction by grasping the partially

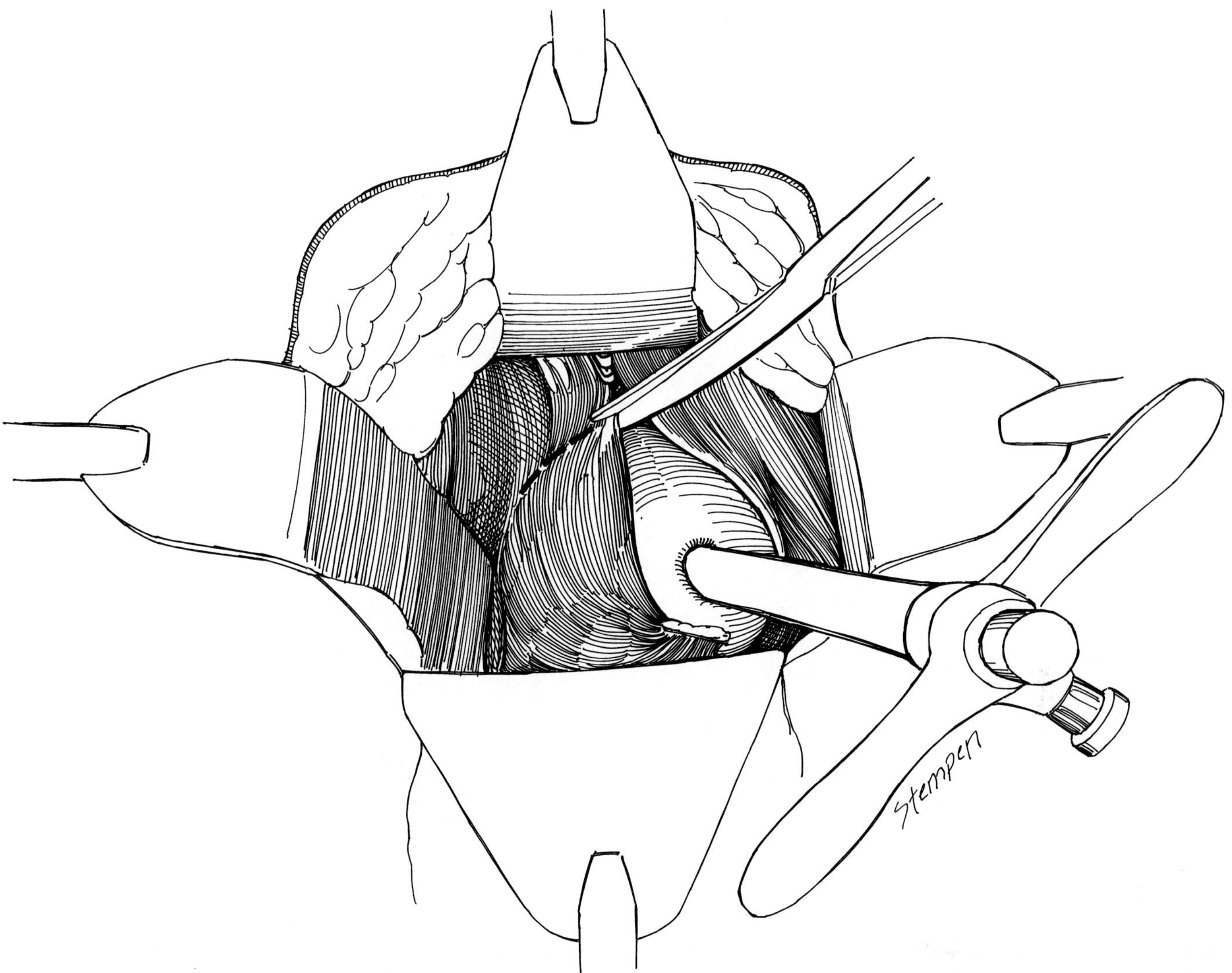

Fig. 19.16. Division of right lateral prostatic fascia across bladder neck (broken line), with right extended radical and left nerve-sparing dissections. Contralateral rotation of short prostatic tractor aids exposure. (Reprinted with permission from Weldon VE, Tavel FR. Radical perineal prostatectomy. In: Das S, Crawford E, eds. Cancer of the prostate. New York: Marcel Dekker, 1993:225–266.)

mobilized seminal vesicle with a long Russian thumb forceps and by retraction of the perivesicular fascia by an adroit assistant with a Yankauer tonsil suction tube.

4. Division of the seminal vesicle blood vessels beneath hemoclips (Fig. 19.22).

Occasionally, the seminal vesicles must be transected if intense scarring prohibits safe dissection, as after abdominal-perineal resection of the anorectum or after some transurethral prostate resections. With very large prostates that fill the small perineal field, it is often necessary to transect the seminal vesicles and remove them separately after the large prostate specimen has been removed.

After complete bilateral dissection of the seminal vesicles, the ampullae of the vasa deferentia are transected and cephalad stumps are secured with large hemoclips or ligatures, leaving 2- to 3-cm stumps with the specimen. If the vasa are transected first, traction on the specimen almost always results in inadvertent tearing of the seminal vesicles. The specimen is then removed.

Variations

In certain circumstances it may be useful and even necessary to alter the sequence of maneuvers just described. An interesting variation recommended by Belt (50) is early ligation of the vascular pedicles before dividing the membranous urethra and mobilizing the prostate. This is most easily done with small prostates situated more caudally, in which the dorsal area cephalad to the prostatic base is easily exposed. It is best executed during an extended radical dissection with transverse incision of the ventral rectal fascia at the base of the prostate and of

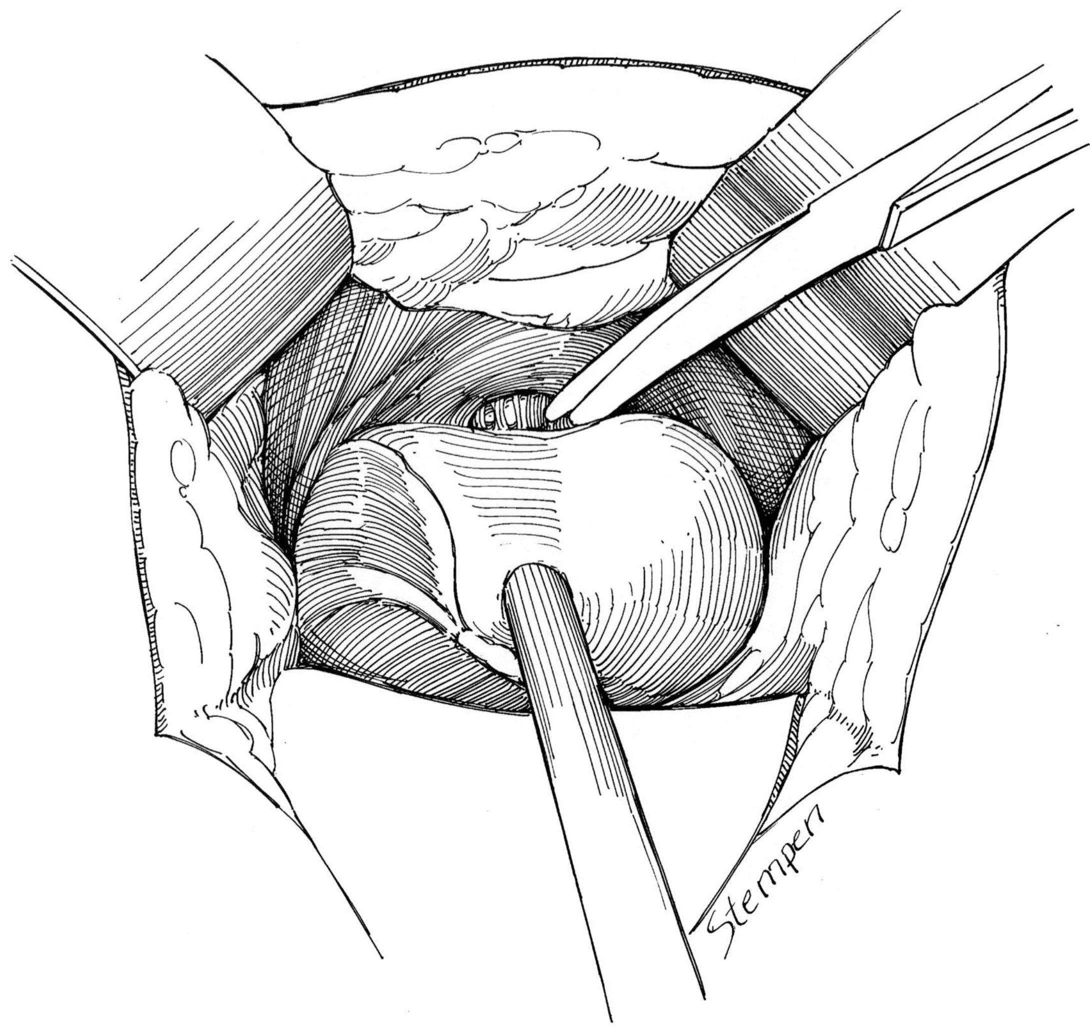

Fig. 19.17. Anterior bladder neck transection. Circular bladder neck fibers are completely separated from the prostate, exposing the mucosa, which is opened sharply. Tractor blades are beneath the mucosa. (Reprinted with permission from Weldon VE, Tavel FR. Radical perineal prostatectomy. In: Das S, Crawford E, eds. Cancer of the prostate. New York: Marcel Dekker, 1993:225–266.)

Denonvilliers' membrane over the seminal vesicles (Fig. 19.20), with the use of the hook and clamp technique to secure the vascular pedicles at the lateral prostatic base.

With very large prostates that almost fill the entire perineal wound, visualization of the posterior and cephalad portions of the dissection is hampered, and early complete mobilization of the prostate is necessary. The prostate is fixed in position by its attachments to the membranous urethra, the puboprostatic ligaments, and the vascular pedicles. When these structures are sequentially divided early in the dissection, mobility is sufficient to allow adequate visualization, even with very large prostates (52). The bladder neck and ampullae of the vas deferentia are quite mobile and do not significantly limit prostate movement. After either the nerve-sparing or extended radical modification is executed on each side, the membranous urethra, puboprostatic ligaments, and anterior bladder neck are divided as previously described (Figs. 19.14 to 19.17). It is then neces-

sary to divide the vascular pedicles entering the base of the prostate on each side, with a variation of the Belt approach to the pedicles. Outward traction on the prostate is temporarily halted, the short prostatic tractor is removed, and the prostate is returned to its bed.

It is then pulled contralaterally and ventrally with narrow ribbon retractors, exposing the vascular pedicles. Occasionally, the prostatic apex may even be rotated ventrally almost 180° and pushed into the bladder through a widely open anterior bladder neck to expose the base of the prostate and the pedicles. Both pedicles are completely divided with the hook and clamp technique. After division of these three main areas of fixation, resumption of outward traction on the prostate will now adequately expose the posterior bladder neck. With very large prostates that completely fill the wound, the seminal vesicles may need to be transected and removed separately after removal of the prostate.

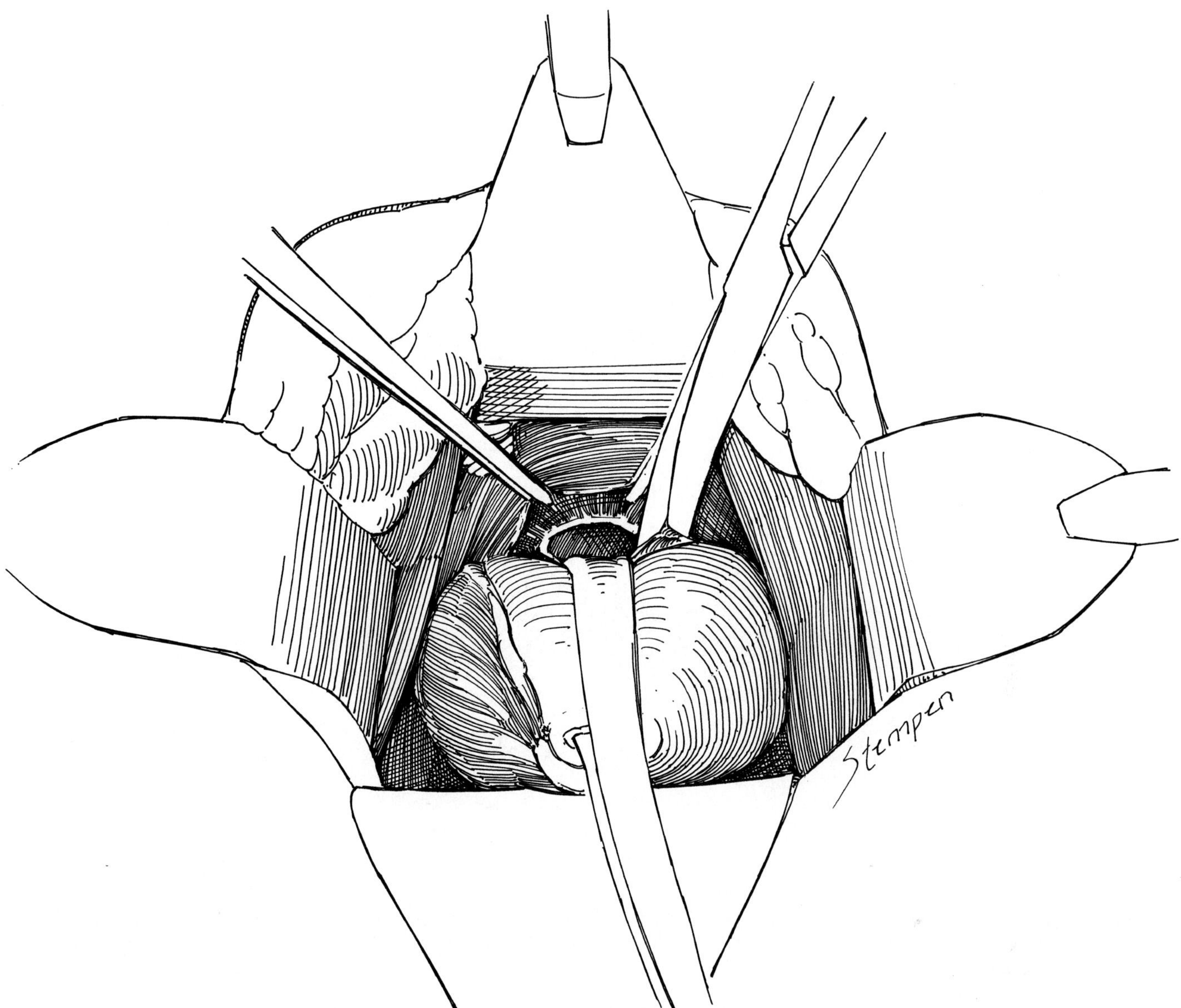

Fig. 19.18. Sharp division of posterior bladder neck. Short prostatic tractor has been removed, and specimen traction is continued with 0.5-in. Penrose drain looped through the prostatic urethra around the ventral prostate. (Reprinted with permission from Weldon VE, Tavel FR. Radical perineal prostatectomy. In: Das S, Crawford E, eds. Cancer of the prostate. New York: Marcel Dekker, 1993:225–266.)

Vesicourethral Anastomosis

The anterior bladder neck is anastomosed to the membranous urethra with interrupted 2-0 synthetic braided absorbable sutures on a 5/8 circle tapered needle. Exposure of the membranous urethra is facilitated by adjusting retraction of the notched anterior retractor blade to retract the adjacent urogenital diaphragm. A 20-Ch silicone Foley catheter with 5-mL balloon is passed through the urethra until its tip is seen at the open end of the membranous urethra. An assistant passing the catheter tip in and out through the transected urethral stump helps to identify its ventral lip. Alternatively, the catheter may be passed through the urethral stump, pulled out through the

wound, and doubled back on itself. Traction on both ends of the catheter will then usually expose the ventral lip of the membranous urethra.

Sutures are placed through-and-through, 4 to 5 mm deep, at 3-mm intervals, and outside-in beginning at the bladder neck and ending outside the urethra, taking care to include the mucosa with the muscularis on each pass. The needle is most easily passed from outside the bladder with a forehand motion of the needle carrier, and then, except for the 12-o'clock stitch, from inside the membranous urethra with a backhand motion. During suturing, the bladder neck is best grasped with a long, heavy-toothed thumb forceps, while the membranous urethra is best grasped with a long, delicate-toothed Cushing

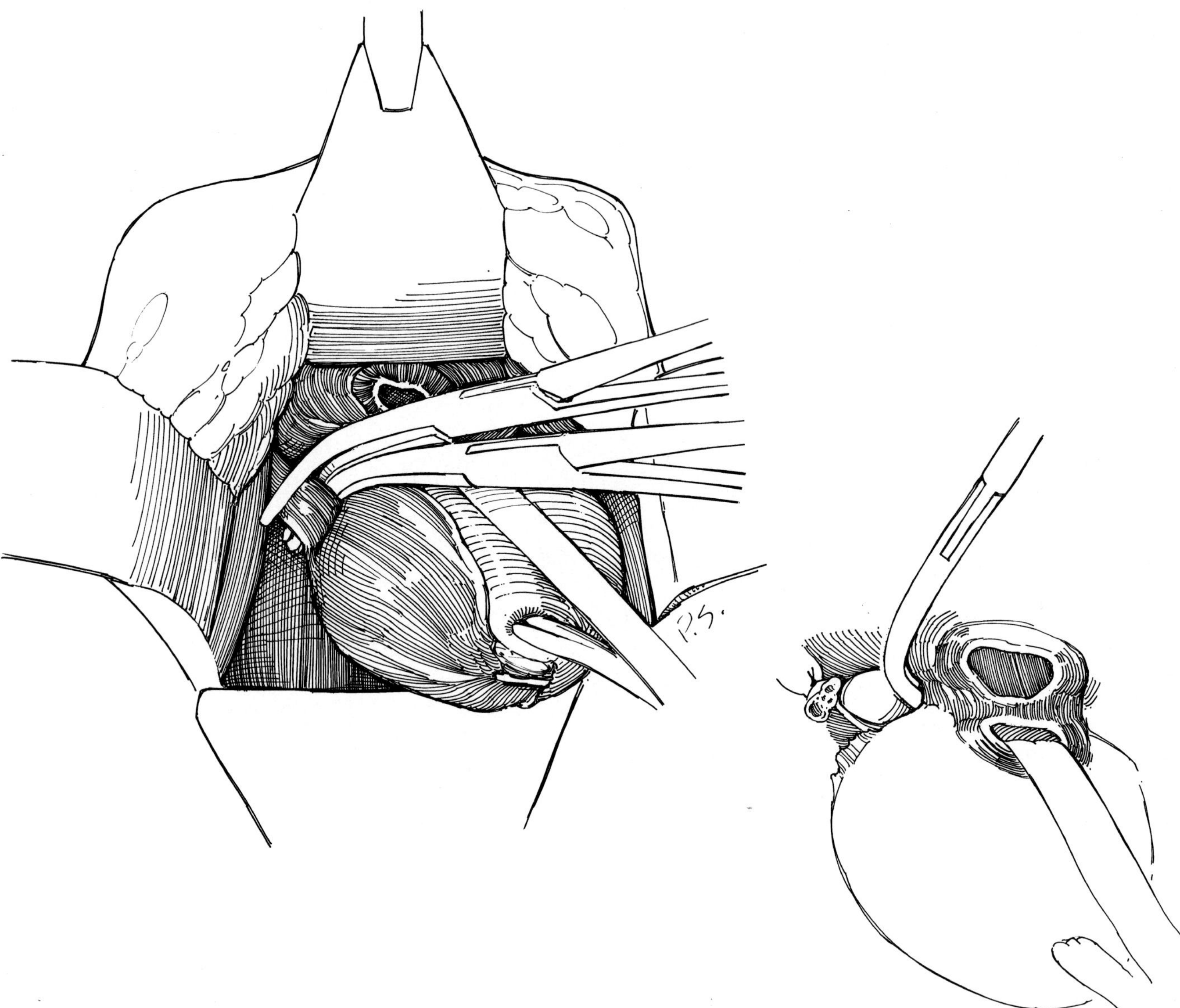

Fig. 19.19.   Vascular pedicle transection with "hook and clamp" technique. Specimen is rotated contralaterally. First, right-angle forceps are inserted medial to the pedicle to hook it and pull it down, allowing parallel passage of a second right-angle forceps above it to clamp the pedicle. Only the cephalad stump is ligated. Inset: After the vascular pedicle is completely divided and the lateral edge of the seminal vesicle is exposed, an advantageous view of the plane of transection of the posterior bladder neck is achieved. The plane between the bladder neck and the seminal vesicles is developed with right-angle forceps. (Reprinted with permission from Weldon VE, Tavel FR. Radical perineal prostatectomy. In: Das S, Crawford E, eds. Cancer of the prostate. New York: Marcel Dekker, 1993:225–266.)

thumb forceps. If the bladder neck is small, the bladder mucosa may be difficult to visualize and grasp. A medium-length thumb forceps with strong spring action inserted into the bladder neck and allowed to spring open will assist exposure. The initial three ventral sutures at 11 o'clock, 12 o'clock, and 1 o'clock are placed (Fig. 19.23), the retraction of the notched anterior retractor is eased, and these three sutures are tied. Lifting the posterior bladder neck with a heavy-toothed forceps while tying will reduce any tension. The anastomosis is then completed with little difficulty.

The tip of the catheter is inserted into the bladder, and the anterior bladder neck is progressively sutured around the circumference of the membranous urethra without "bunching." No attempt is made to tighten the bladder neck. If a nerve-sparing dissection has been done, care is taken not to include the fascia lateral to the membranous urethra in these sutures. Any bladder neck redundancy is closed as a "racquet handle" in a linear manner posteriorly (Fig. 19.24). With a small bladder neck, there may be no redundancy. Seven sutures are usually used in the anastomosis with a racquet handle closure, and eight are usually used if there is no bladder neck redundancy.

The Foley catheter balloon is then inflated to 10 mL, and

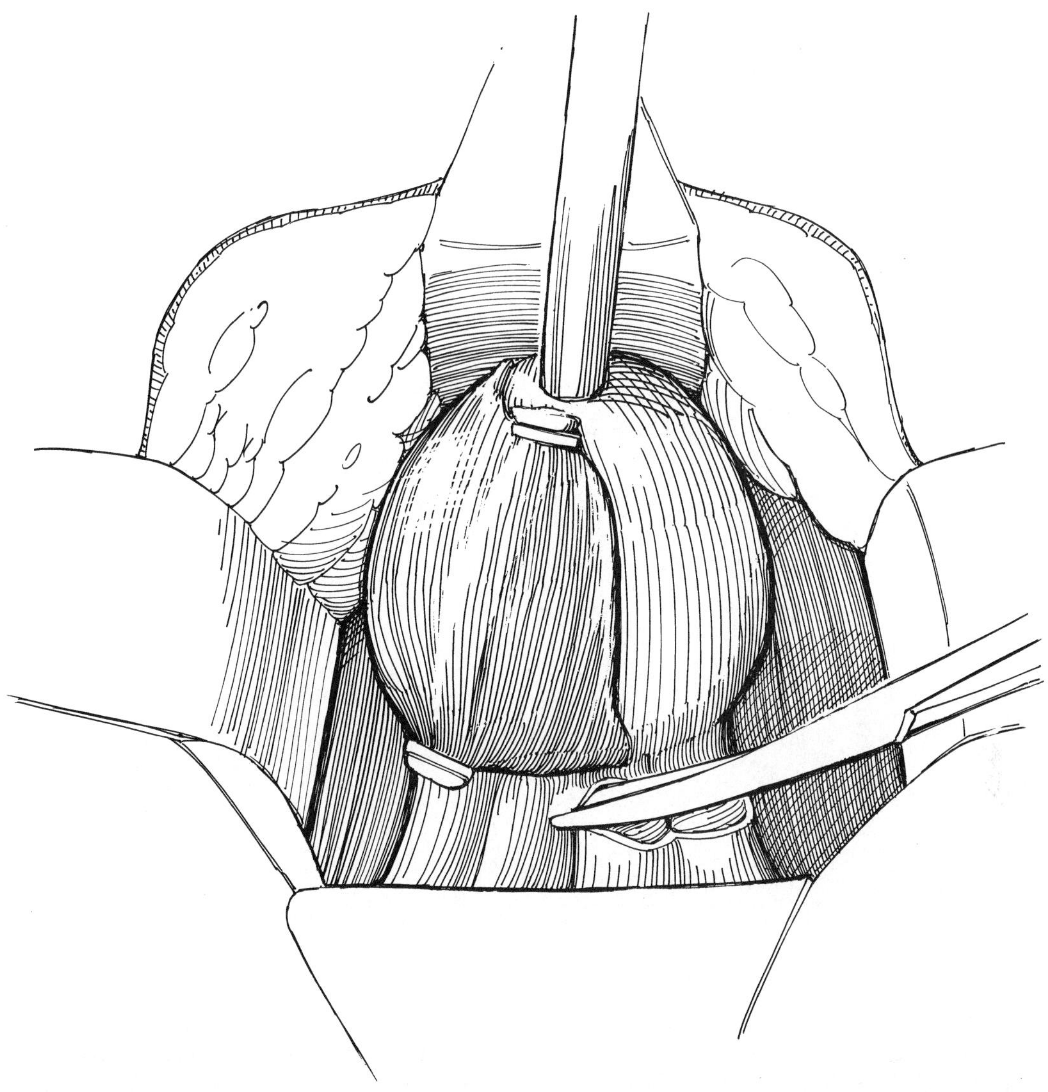

Fig. 19.20.   Dorsal seminal vesicle dissection. The prostate is rotated ventrally. Denonvilliers' membrane is incised transversely over seminal vesicles and vasal ampullae, maintaining a generous cuff of membrane with specimen. Note the clipped and divided right neurovascular bundle and ventral rectal fascia on the specimen, with right extended radical and left nerve-sparing dissections. (Reprinted with permission from Weldon VE, Tavel FR. Radical perineal prostatectomy. In: Das S, Crawford E, eds. Cancer of the prostate. New York: Marcel Dekker, 1993:225–266.)

the catheter is irrigated. The precise anastomosis is usually watertight.

CLOSURE

Before removing the self-retaining retractor, the posterior blade is removed and the rectum is inspected. An unrecognized proctotomy creates significant morbidity. It is most likely at the site of division of the rectourethralis muscle or at the transverse division of the ventral rectal fascia at the base of the prostate with an extended radical dissection. If there is any question, an index finger, temporarily covered with a second glove, is inserted into the rectum to assist complete inspection. Any proctotomy is meticulously closed in two layers—the mucosa with a continuous 4-0 synthetic braided absorbable suture and the muscularis with continuous or interrupted 4-0 synthetic absorbable monofilament suture. The broad anterior band of longitudinal rectal muscle provides a secure second layer in the midline. It may be possible to approximate some of the levator ani fibers in the midline between the vesicourethral anastomosis and the proctotomy closure with absorbable sutures. If a nerve-sparing modification has been used, the neurovascular bundles should not be included in this approximation.

A 0.25-in. Penrose drain is placed with its center looped into the depth of the wound, and each end is separately brought out the opposite corners of the wound and sutured to the skin. A drain placed in this manner will not inadvertently be pulled out with friction when the patient is sitting, unlike drains placed with an end deep in the wound. The perineal flap is closed in two layers—the subcutaneous perineal fascia with a

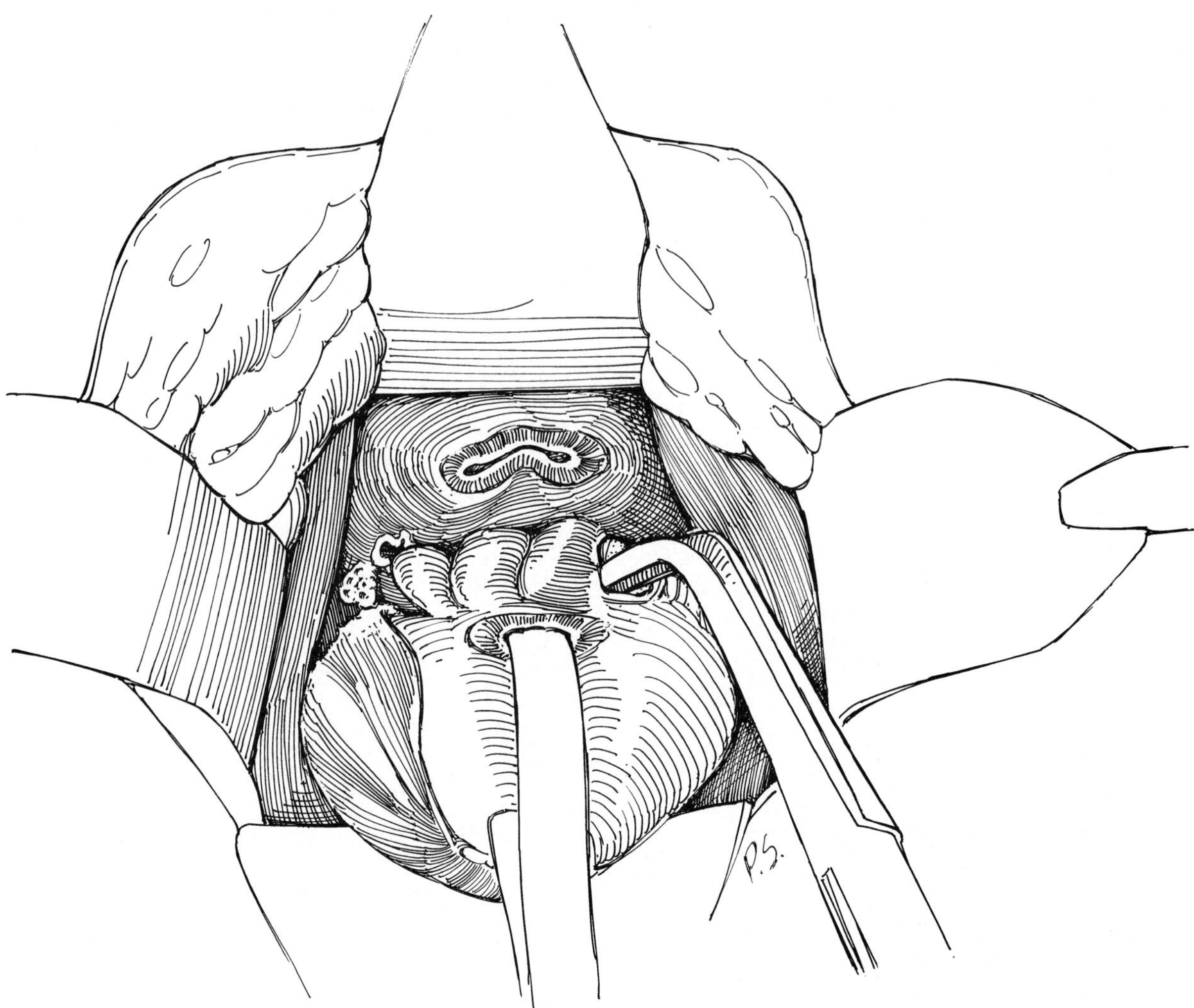

Fig. 19.21.   Ventral seminal vesicle dissection. Right-angle forceps open the cleft between the left seminal vesicle and ampulla of left vas deferens. The medial edge of the seminal vesicle extends under vasal ampulla. (Reprinted with permission from Weldon VE, Tavel FR. Radical perineal prostatectomy. In: Das S, Crawford E, eds. Cancer of the prostate. New York: Marcel Dekker, 1993:225–266.)

continuous 3-0 synthetic braided absorbable suture and the skin with a buried, continuous intradermal 4-0 synthetic braided absorbable suture. This closure will adequately resist any shearing forces on the flap that occur when the patient sits.

If a proctotomy closure has been required, the anus is dilated to accommodate three fingers to maintain low intrarectal pressure. Absorbent pads are best held in position over the wound and the drain with disposable, stretch-net pants, available in most obstetric units and adapted for use in men with a strategic anterior scissor snip. The catheter is taped to the thigh to avoid traction of the retention balloon on the anastomosis.

POSTOPERATIVE CARE

Full ambulation on the first postoperative day is encouraged. The minimal-access nature of perineal prostatectomy, with essentially extended subcutaneous access, is inherently associated with little pain, and even a concomitant mini-lap pelvic lymph-adenectomy adds little. This advantage is exploited by using ketorolac-based analgesia (absent a contraindication) administered parenterally every 6 hours for 48 hours. Additional minimal intravenous narcotics are intermittently provided by patient-controlled devices, without any continuous basal narcotic doses. Oral analgesics are usually sufficient by the second postoperative day. Minimizing narcotic use significantly reduces morbidity and enhances a rapid recovery (53). Epidural narcotics are excessive and unnecessary. This combination of perineal approach and analgesia eliminates significant ileus, and oral liquids are often tolerated within a few hours after the operation; the patient can be eating an unrestricted diet on the first or second postoperative day.

The precise anastomosis results in little extravasated urine, and the perineal drain is generally removed on the second postoperative day just before the resumption of defecation. In the unusual circumstance of prolonged urinary drainage, it may be necessary to probe the drain sites to keep them open, although

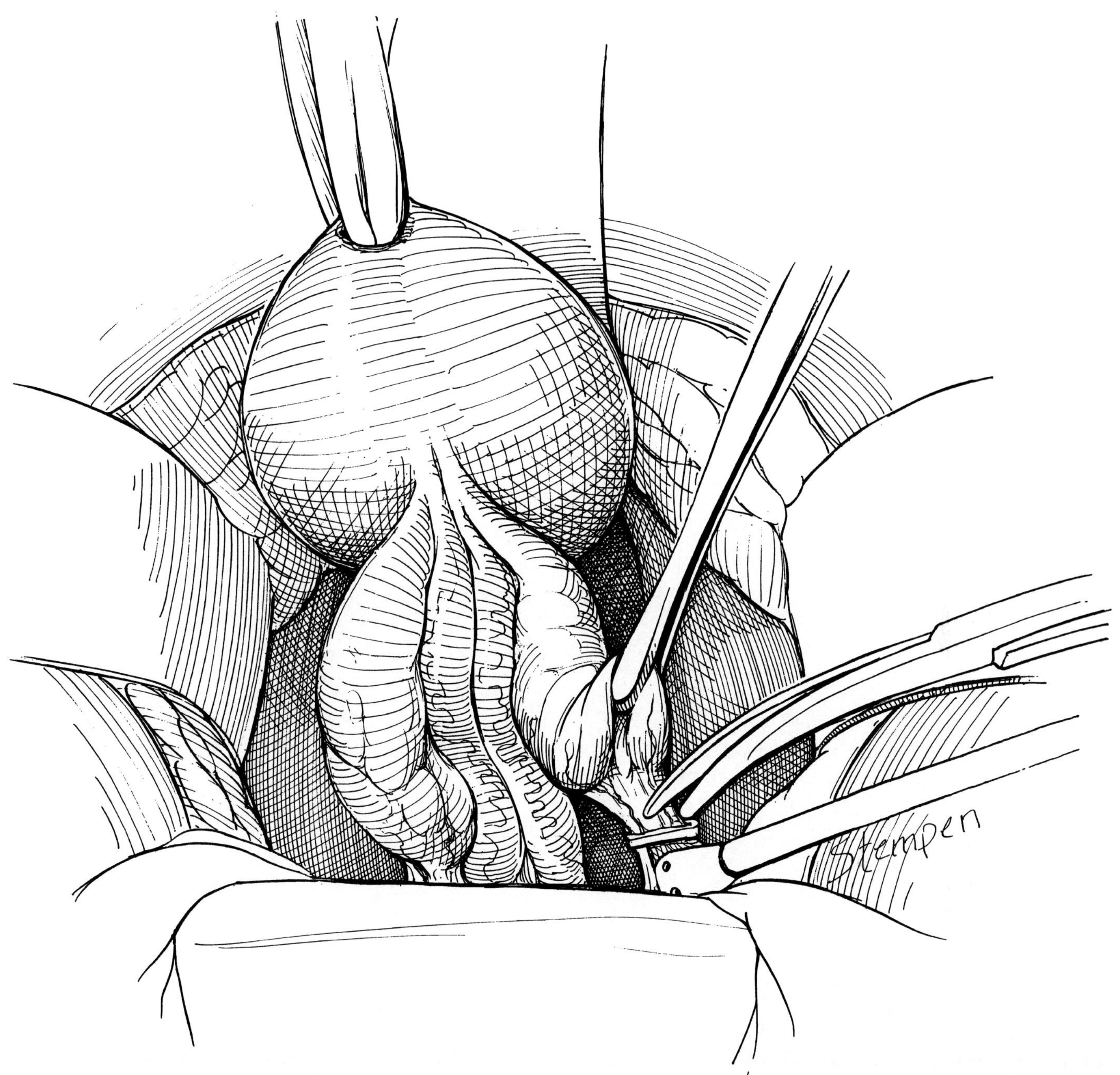

Fig. 19.22.   Dissection of cephalad area of the seminal vesicle with traction and countertraction exposing vesicular blood vessels for clipping and division.

the dependent route of drainage is usually adequate to assure egress. The complete preoperative bowel preparation, postdissection rectal wall edema, and initial liquid diet result in liquid and sometimes incontinent feces for a few days. Postdefecation sitz baths will keep the area clean. Certainly, no laxatives are indicated and nothing should be inserted into the rectum. If a proctotomy repair has been required, a liquid diet (including the palatable, commercially available, balanced nutritional supplements) is maintained for 10 days. With a proctotomy, cefotetan is continued for 48 hours.

If the urethral catheter falls out but the anastomosis has been precisely accomplished without any bladder neck tightening, another similar catheter can usually be gently reinserted without difficulty. If difficulty is encountered and urinary extravasation has ceased, the catheter may be left out. If urinary extravasation is still present and urethral catheter reinsertion is difficult, suprapubic cystostomy is preferable to aggressive urethral instrumentation.

Younger patients undergoing only radical perineal prostatectomy are often discharged from the hospital on the second

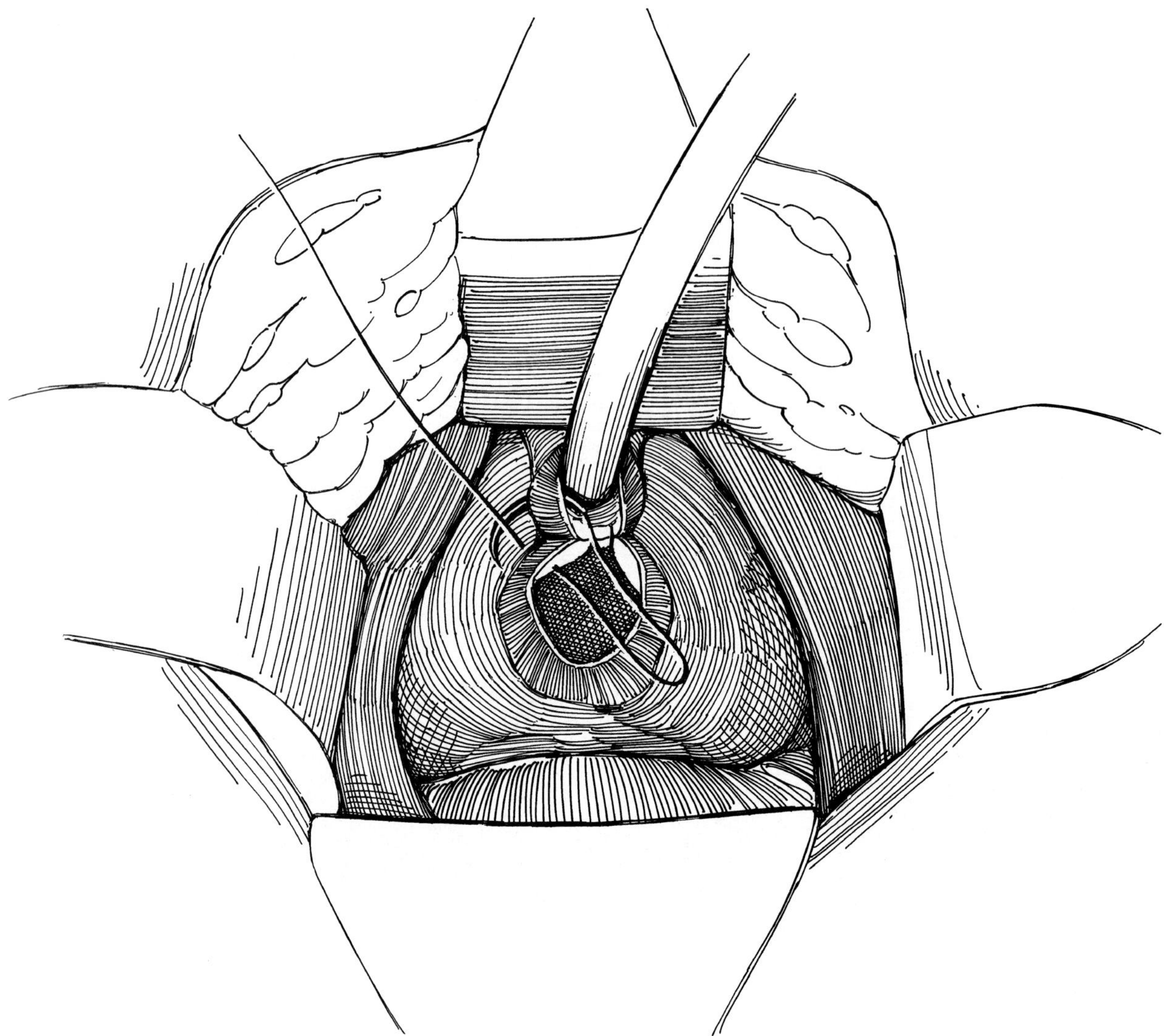

Fig. 19.23.   Initiation of vesicourethral anastomosis. Retraction of the edge of the urogenital diaphragm by anterior retractor blade aids exposure of the membranous urethra. A Foley catheter is pulled through the urethra and doubled back on itself, exposing the ventral lip of the membranous urethra. Three initial sutures at 11 o'clock, 12 o'clock, and 1 o'clock are placed and then tied after easing anterior retraction. (Reprinted with permission from Weldon VE, Tavel FR. Radical perineal prostatectomy. In: Das S, Crawford E, eds. Cancer of the prostate. New York: Marcel Dekker, 1993:225–266.)

postoperative day. Older patients, and those who also had a mini-lap pelvic lymphadenectomy, are usually discharged on the third postoperative day. The median total hospital stay is 3 days. Presuming cessation of all urinary extravasation, the catheter is removed at a convenient time after 2 postoperative weeks, with urine culture and sensitivity-specific antibiotic treatment of the usual catheter-related urinary infection. No preliminary urethrograms are needed. Although a small number of patients are immediately continent when the catheter is removed, most have a variable degree of temporary incontinence that is managed with pads. The short, remaining, functional urethral sphincter after radical prostatectomy is always marginal, but it is usually adequate with resolution of edema and absorbable sutures and return of functional elasticity. With a rare exception, complete continence can usually be expected

within 3 to 4 months. As long as the patient is warned about temporary incontinence and he can sense progress, little anguish results. Younger age and a longer membranous urethra are associated with early, complete continence.

If one or both neurovascular bundles have been spared, return of potency adequate for regular coitus requires a longer recovery period—occasionally 3 months, but 6 to 12 months is more usual; it may take up to 18 months. Again, younger age correlates with earlier and more likely return of potency.

COMPLICATIONS

Among the author's 250 consecutive patients undergoing radical perineal prostatectomy with the contemporary modifications, no perioperative deaths have occurred and none is totally

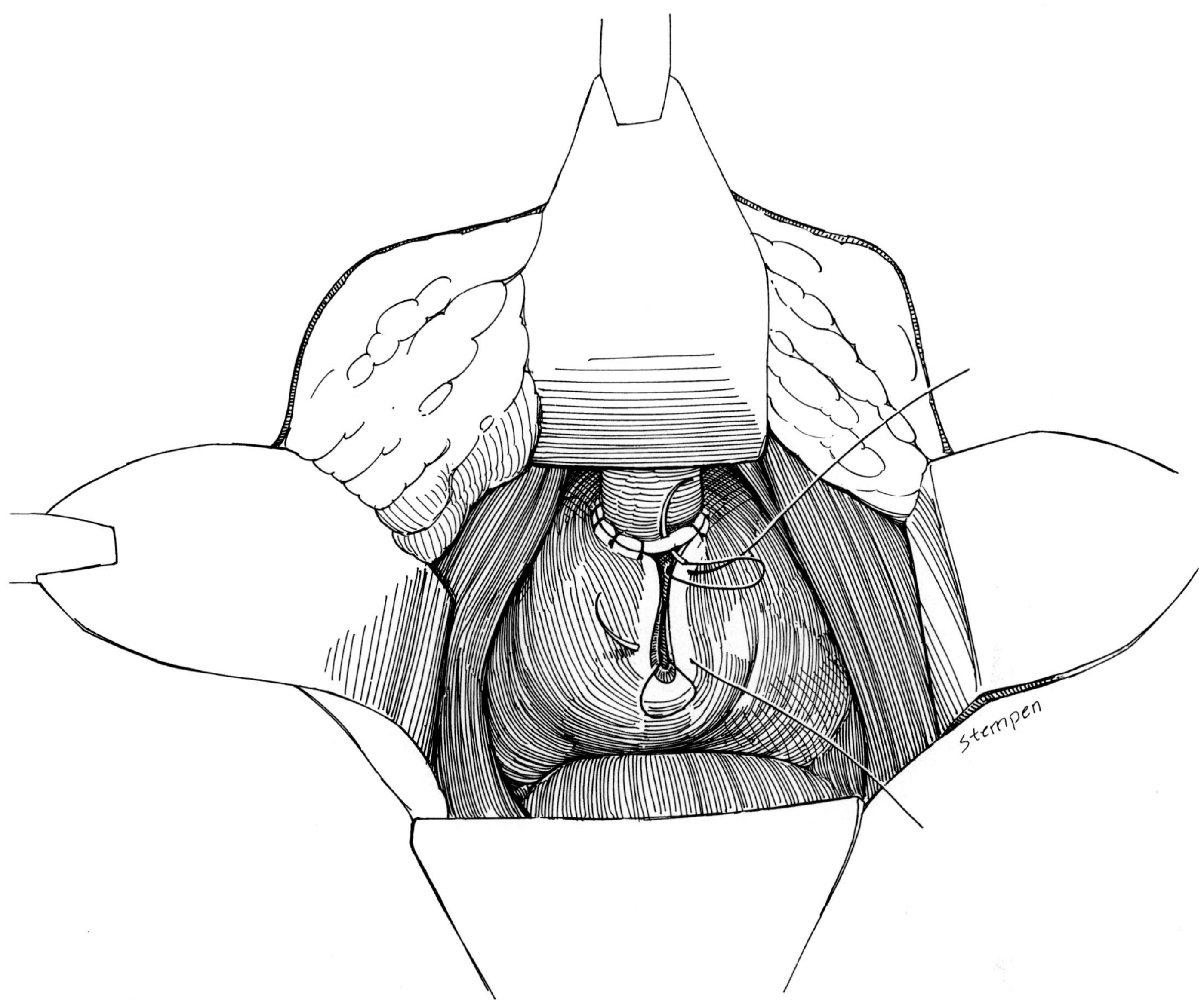

Fig. 19.24.   Completion of vesicourethral anastomosis. The anterior bladder neck is approximated around the circumference of the membranous urethral stump with interrupted sutures. The redundant bladder neck is closed posteriorly in a linear "racquet handle" manner. (Reprinted with permission from Weldon VE, Tavel FR. Radical perineal prostatectomy. In: Das S, Crawford E, eds. Cancer of the prostate. New York: Marcel Dekker, 1993:225–266.)

incontinent. No artificial sphincters have been required. Moderate stress urinary incontinence has persisted in 6%, who either wet one pad significantly or require more than one pad daily. All men who are persistently incontinent after 6 months should undergo appropriate incontinence testing; some may have an occult unstable bladder that is not suggested by history and is significantly improved by anticholinergic medication (54). Some men who complain of moderately severe incontinence have neither an objectively demonstrated unstable bladder nor any demonstrable stress incontinence when standing and coughing with a full bladder. Collagen injections just below the anastomotic area have been very helpful in some of those with residual stress incontinence, as the incontinence has always

been partial and the defect after a precise perineal dissection and anastomosis is usually an inherently deficient distal sphincteric mechanism with a supple and minimally scarred proximal membranous urethra.

Inadvertent proctotomy has occurred in 1.5% (always in the setting of complete preoperative bowel preparation). Managed by closure, anal dilation, liquid diet, and additional short-term antibiotics as described, it has caused no morbidity.

No perineal abscesses have occurred, although a few episodes of limited perineal cellulitis have required antibiotic treatment. Pulmonary complications have almost disappeared with the ketorolac—minimal narcotic regimen for postoperative pain control. Significant perioperative cardiac events including myocardial infarction and arrhythmias occurred in 1.5%. Deep venous thromboembolic events occurred in 1.5% with no prophylaxis other than early ambulation (all had a concurrent open pelvic lymphadenectomy). Transient, partial lower extremity neuropathies related to position have occurred in 2.5%. All resolved within 48 hours.

CONCLUSIONS

In an era when many more cases of localized prostate cancer are being identified, the appropriateness and effectiveness of radical prostatectomy are being more firmly established, and the high cost of medical care is causing increasing concern to society, the resurgence of interest in radical perineal prostatectomy with its contemporary modifications is timely. To allocate the limited resources properly, a focus on efficiently providing only necessary treatment, with a cost-effective analysis, will be necessary. Costs may be contained with no detriment to patients by limiting staging bone scintigrams (55), prostate imaging beyond sonography, and pelvic lymphadenectomy to those carefully defined clinical circumstances in which these modalities significantly enhance staging accuracy.

The effectiveness of radical perineal prostatectomy and the means of achieving it are described herein. Regarding costs specific to that procedure, the routine 3-day total hospital stay (with or without mini-lap pelvic lymphadenectomy) offers significant savings. These efficiencies will allow effective treatment of the increased number of men who now would benefit from it, without the same increase in proportional costs for that benefit. In this context, radical perineal prostatectomy has a promising role in the treatment of localized prostate cancer.

REFERENCES

1. Franks LM. Latent carcinoma of the prostate. J Pathol Bacteriol 1954;68:603.
2. Catalona WJ, Smith DS, Ratliff TL, et al. Detection of organ confined prostate cancer is increased through prostate-specific antigen based screening. JAMA 1993;270:948.
3. Kaplan ID, Cox RS, Bagshaw MA. Prostate-specific antigen after external beam radiotherapy for prostate cancer: followup. J Urol 1993;149:519.
4. Stamey TA, Ferrari MK, Schmid H-P. The value of serial prostate specific antigen determinations 5 years after radiotherapy: steeply increasing values characterize 80% of patients. J Urol 1993;150:1856.
5. Partin AW, Pound CR, Clemens JQ, et al. Serum PSA after anatomic radical prostatectomy: the Johns Hopkins experience after 10 years. Urol Clin North Am 1993;20:713.
6. Weldon VE, Tavel FR, Neuwirth H, et al. Patterns of positive specimen margins and detectable prostate-specific antigen after radical perineal prostatectomy. J Urol In press.
7. Schmid H-P, McNeal JE, Stamey TA. Observations on the doubling time of prostate cancer: the use of serial prostate specific antigen in patients with untreated disease as a measure of increasing cancer volume. Cancer 1993;71:2031.
8. Chodak GW, Thisted RA, Gerber GS, et al. Results of conservative management of clinically localized prostate cancer. N Engl J Med 1994;330:242.
9. Aus G, Hugosson J, Norlen L. Risk of dying of prostate cancer in different stages, grades and age at diagnosis. J Urol 1994;151(Part 2):278. Abstract.
10. Weldon VE, Tavel FR, Neuwirth H, et al. Failure of focal prostate cancer on biopsy to predict focal prostate cancer: the importance of prevalence. J Urol 1995;154:1074.
11. Partin AW, Lee BR, Carmichael M, et al. Radical prostatectomy for high grade disease: a reevaluation 1994. J Urol 1994;151:1583.
12. Gohagan JK, Prorok PC, Kramer BS, et al. Prostate cancer screening in Prostate, Lung, Colorectal and Ovarian Cancer Screening Trial of National Cancer Institute. J Urol 1994;152:1905.
13. Wilt TJ, Brawer MK. Prostate cancer intervention versus observation trial: randomized trial comparing radical prostatectomy versus expectant management for treatment of clinically localized prostate cancer. J Urol 1994;152:1910.
14. Littrup PJ, Goodman AC, Mettlin CJ, and the Investigators of the American Cancer Society-National Prostate Cancer Detection Project. The benefit and cost of prostate cancer early detection. CA Cancer J Clin 1993;43:134.
15. Celsus: De medicina (translated by C. des Estangs, 1846). Paris.
16. Demarquay JN. Calculs de l'urètre. Bull Soc Chir 1852:467.
17. Küchler H. Uber prostatavergrosserungen. Deutch Klin 1866;18:458.
18. Bilroth T. Clinical surgery (Translated by C.Dent). London: New Sydenham Society, 1881.
19. Leisrink H. Tumor prostatae: totale exstirpation der prostata. Arch Klin Chir 1883;28:578.
20. Proust R. Technique de la prostatectomie périnéale. Assoc Franc Urol 1901;5:361.
21. Young HH. Conservative perineal prostatectomy: presentation of new instruments and technique. JAMA 1903;41:999.
22. Young HH. The early diagnosis and radical cure of carcinoma of the prostate. Bull Johns Hopkins Hosp 1905;16:315.
23. Young HH. The cure of cancer of the prostate by radical perineal prostatectomy (prostato-seminal vesiculectomy): history, literature and statistics of Young's operation. J Urol 1945;53:188.
24. Weyrauch HM. Perineal prostatectomy. In: Surgery of the prostate. Philadelphia: WB Saunders, 1959:203.
25. Walsh PC, Donker PJ. Impotence following radical prostatectomy: insight into etiology and prevention. J Urol 1982;128:492.
26. Weldon VE, Tavel FR. Potency-sparing radical perineal prostatectomy: anatomy, surgical technique and initial results. J Urol 1988;140:559.
27. Schröder FH, Hermanek P, Denis L, et al. The TNM classification of prostate cancer. Prostate Suppl 1992;4:129.
28. Lew EA, Garfinkel L. Mortality at ages 75 and older in The Cancer Prevention Study. CA Cancer J Clin 1990;40:210.
29. Partin AW, Yoo J, Carter HB, et al. The use of prostate specific antigen, clinical stage and Gleason score to predict pathologic stage in men with localized prostate cancer. J Urol 1993;150:110.
30. Paulson DF, Moul JW, Walther PJ. Radical prostatectomy for

clinical stage T1–2 N0M0 prostatic adenocarcinoma: long term results. J Urol 1990;144:1180.

31. Steckel J, Dorey F, de Kernion JB. Long term follow up in men with microscopic stage D1 prostate cancer treated with and without early endocrine therapy (EET) after radical prostatectomy. J Urol 1994;151(Part 2):434. Abstract.

32. Epstein JI, Carmichael M, Walsh PC. Adenocarcinoma of the prostate invading the seminal vesicle: definition and relation of tumor volume, grade and margins of resection to prognosis. J Urol 1993;149:1040.

33. Vallancien G, Bothereau G, Wetzel O, et al. Influence of preoperative seminal vesicle biopsy on the staging of prostate cancer. J Urol 1994;152:1152.

34. Byar DP, Mostofi FK. Carcinoma of the prostate: prognostic evaluation of certain pathologic features in 208 radical prostatectomies. Cancer 1972;30:5.

35. Epstein JI, Paull G, Eggleston JC, et al. Prognosis of untreated stage A1 prostate carcinoma: a study of 94 cases with extended follow-up. J Urol 1986;136:837.

36. Gee WF, Cole JR. Symptomatic stage C carcinoma of the prostate, traditional therapy. Urology 1980;15:335.

37. Paulson DF, Hodge GB Jr, Hinshaw W. Radiation therapy versus delayed androgen deprivation for stage C carcinoma of the prostate. J Urol 1984;131:901.

38. Stamey TA, Villers AA, McNeal JE, et al. Positive margins in radical prostatectomy: importance of the apical dissection. J Urol 1990;143:1166.

39. Babaian RJ, Sayer J, Podoloff DA, et al. Radioimmunoscintigraphy of pelvic lymph nodes with [111]Indium-labeled monoclonal antibody CYT-356. J Urol 1994;152:1952.

40. Burgers JK, Hinkle G, Badalament RA, et al. Prostate cancer lymph node imaging with monoclonal antibody (CYT-356). J Urol 1994;151(Part 2):505. Abstract.

41. Steiner MS, Marshall FF. Mini-laparotomy staging pelvic lymphadenectomy (minilap): alternative to standard and laparoscopic pelvic lymphadenectomy. Urology 1993;41:201.

42. Denonvilliers CPD. Anatomie du périnée. Bull et Mém Soc Anat (Paris) 1836;11:106.

43. Denonvilliers CPD. Propositions et observations d'anatomie de physiologie et de pathologie. Thèse de l'Ecole de Médicine, Paris. 1837;185:23.

44. Lepor H, Gregerman M, Crosby R, et al. Precise localization of the autonomic nerves from the pelvic plexus to the corpora cavernosa: a detailed anatomical study of the adult male pelvis. J Urol 1985;133:207.

45. Woodburne RT. The pelvis. In: Essentials of human anatomy. New York: Oxford University Press, 1957:477.

46. Tobin CE, Benjamin JA. Anatomical and surgical restudy of Denonvilliers' fascia. Surg Gynecol Obstet 1945;80:373.

47. Villers AA, McNeal JE, Redwine EA, et al. The role of perineural space invasion in the local spread of prostatic adenocarcinoma. J Urol 1989;142:763.

48. Quinlan DM, Epstein JI, Carter BS, et al. Sexual function following radical prostatectomy: influence of preservation of neurovascular bundles. J Urol 1991;145:998.

49. Periti P, Mazzei T, Tonelli F. Single-dose cefotetan vs. multiple-dose cefoxitin: antimicrobial prophylaxis in colorectal surgery. Dis Colon Rectum 1986;32:121.

50. Belt E. Radical perineal prostatectomy in early carcinoma of the prostate. J Urol 1942;47:287.

51. Weldon VE. Extended radical perineal prostatectomy: an anatomical and surgical study. J Urol 1988;139(Part 2):488. Abstract.

52. Weldon VE. Radical perineal prostatectomy, updated. Infect Urol 1989;2:48.

53. Koch MO, Smith JA Jr, Hodge EM, et al. Prospective management of a cost-effective program for radical retropubic prostatectomy. Urology 1994;44:311.

54. Foote J, Yun SK, Leach GE. Post-prostatectomy incontinence: pathophysiology, evaluation and management. Urol Clin North Am 1991;18:229.

55. Oesterling JE. Using PSA to eliminate the staging radionuclide bone scan: significant economic implications. Urol Clin North Am 1993;20:705.

20

Brachytherapy for Prostate Carcinoma

Mark J. Noble, Stephen T. Smalley, and Eschwar Reddi

INTRODUCTION

Brachytherapy, or insertion of radioactive sources directly into or adjacent to tissues, was first suggested by Pierre Curie in 1901 and then by investigators at New York's Memorial Hospital 16 years later (1, 2). Initially, glass tubes containing radon 222 were placed in tumors for variable periods. However, this technique caused severe, localized tissue necrosis, which helped to account for its loss of popularity toward the late 1940s (2, 3). The chief reasons for this waning enthusiasm included difficulty with source availability and production, radiation safety problems, the nontrivial calculations of dosimetry, and improvements in external beam teletherapy, which was more economical and simpler to administer (3). The advent of modern computer technology, better implantation procedures, and newer radioactive sources as well as modern after loading techniques have rekindled interest in prostate brachytherapy (3).

Prostate cancer brachytherapy experiences were reported initially in 1909 (intraurethral radium) and 1915 (transperineal radium needles) (4, 5). Carlton and others reported an interstitial gold 198 seed treatment with supplemental external beam radiation therapy in 1965 (6). The Memorial Sloan-Kettering Cancer Center (MSKCC) group began implanting I-125 seeds in the prostate in 1970 (7). Both techniques required open surgical pelvic lymph node dissection and seed implantation, with the latter performed primarily by palpation of the surgically exposed prostate.

Because of concerns regarding variable seed placement, perineal templates for either temporary or permanent implants were devised that helped align needles more precisely in the prostate (8). Temporary isotopes (such as iridium 192) were also developed that allowed removal of the interstitial implants after several days (8). Recently, ultrasound guidance has gained popularity for objective, intraoperative positioning of radioactive sources, enabling such positioning without open surgical exposure of the prostate (9). Lymph nodes may be sampled laparoscopically when indicated before brachytherapy (10). This ultrasound-guided transperineal placement using either I-125 or palladium 103 promises low perioperative morbidity compared with open surgical brachytherapy or radical prostatectomy

techniques, but long-term data are not yet available regarding its efficacy or safety.

IMPLANTATION TECHNIQUE

Patient Selection

Selection criteria vary considerably among institutions using prostate brachytherapy. Nevertheless, some general patient selection guidelines can be articulated. If an open procedure is planned, patients should have good general health and be suitable surgical candidates. Operative mortality rates are extremely low, and surgical morbidity is infrequent and usually managed without difficulty. However, the indolent natural history of prostate cancer (11–16) and the availability of nonsurgical interventions, such as external beam radiation therapy or hormonal therapy, argue against subjecting patients to even a minimally increased operative risk. Operative complications with transperineal ultrasound-guided implantation have been variable (17–19), although Blasko et al. (17) and other groups have reported negligible acute operative complications. Other corroborative series and longer follow-up are needed, but it is possible that transperineal ultrasound-guided implantation will eventually prove suitable even for medically unfit patients (20–22).

Patients with known pelvic nodal metastasis should be excluded from consideration. Virtually all brachytherapy series with meaningful follow-up have documented the extremely poor prognosis of node-positive patients. The MSKCC group observed a 92% distant metastasis risk at 10 years regardless of stage, grade, probability of local control, or treatment-related parameters as well as extremely poor survival (23, 24). Gervasi et al. found that those with even one microscopically positive node have 10-year cancer outcomes that are nearly identical to those with more extensive nodal disease (20). Patients with known nodal disease should, therefore, be excluded from implantation. However, the role of a purely staging lymph node dissection (whether through an open or pelvioscopic procedure) before a closed transperineal implantation remains to be defined; the yield is likely to be low in those with favorable histologic grade and preimplantation prostate-specific antigen (PSA) levels (26). Whether the cost and minimal morbidity of such a procedure may be warranted is currently a matter of clinical judgment.

A previous transurethral resection is associated with a much higher incidence of late urinary complications, and implantation should be administered with caution and attention to techniques directed toward minimizing urethral dose (17, 27–29). Extensive corpora amylacea represent a theoretical concern because their high electron density might absorb the radiation emitted from low-energy implantation sources, which could potentially lead to underdosing of the tumor. Furthermore, extensive, large corpora amylacea may interfere with optimal placement of the radioactive seeds.

The biology of the tumor itself is extremely important. High-grade and/or large-volume tumors have been well documented to be associated with inferior local control, distant metastasis free rates, and overall survival (20, 22–24, 30–34). Tumors with these characteristics have higher local failure and/ or complication rates with implantation versus external beam radiation therapy or surgery (31–33). It must be borne in mind that most implantation techniques do not implant either the seminal vesicles or extracapsular tissue. Ergo, it is not surprising that higher grade and stage tumors with their greater propensity for extracapsular or seminal vesicle extension would diminish the effectiveness of these techniques. Therefore, tumor and patient selection factors suggest that those best suited for brachytherapy are similarly well managed by surgery or external beam therapy.

Specific Brachytherapy Approaches

There are two basic approaches—retropubic implantation and transperineal implantation—by which brachytherapy sources are placed in the prostate. There are also myriad permutations by which brachytherapy implantation can be varied such as dose, radionuclide implanted, and addition of external beam radiation therapy.

Retropubic Permanent Implantation

The technique of retropubic implantation is well known (7, 24, 30, 35). Patients are placed in a modified lithotomy position following a bimanual examination and cystoscopy. Tumors with extension beyond the verumontanum or into the bladder neck or trigone are unsuitable for implantation. An O'Connor drape is placed that facilitates rectal examination during the implant. A Foley catheter is placed, and a midline suprapubic incision is made from the umbilicus to the symphysis. An extraperitoneal pelvic lymph node dissection can be performed. The extent of lymph node dissection is variable. Omission of the external iliac artery dissection decreases postoperative edema, shortens operating time, and does not substantially alter staging accuracy (30). The endopelvic fascia is incised on both sides of the prostate to mobilize the lateral aspects of the gland,

although the puboprostatic ligaments do not require transection. The entire prostate is measured in three dimensions.

1. The lateral dimension is measured by a caliper.
2. The superior-inferior dimension is measured by a ruler.
3. The anterior-posterior dimension is obtained (when all grid needles are in place) by measuring the needles' lengths outside the gland and subtracting from total needle length (15 cm).

These measurements are then used to confirm the necessary spacing between needles and seed activity (see physics section later in this chapter).

The guide needles are inserted, usually at the superior medial margin of the prostate near the bladder base lateral to the urethra (Fig. 20.1). Then, with a finger in the rectum over an O'Connor drape, the needles are introduced in an anterior-posterior direction systematically to a depth that permits the index finger in the rectum to sense the tip of the needle before it perforates the rectal wall. The guide needles should be approximately 1 cm apart for optimal radiation overlap and dosing. After the entire gland has been covered by the guide needles, a seed applicator is attached to each individual guide needle and seeds are introduced into the prostatic tissue itself. The applicator is retracted 0.5 cm before insertion of the seeds because the seeds are approximately 0.5 cm in length and it is important not to introduce the seeds directly into the rectal wall. The applicator is then retracted a predetermined distance after the deposit of each seed into the prostate until the entire length of the needle within prostate tissue has been covered. After the removal of the guides, the patient is examined for bleeding and any seeds that may have inadvertently dropped into the pelvic space are removed. The implantation of Au-198 is easier in view of the greater depth of penetration of the radiation emitted from these sources, although this radionuclide is rarely used in the United States today.

Transperineal Brachytherapy Techniques

Several transperineal implantation techniques successfully place brachytherapy sources in a geometrically satisfactory location. One approach uses an open procedure in which placement of the radioactive sources is accomplished via clinical evaluation of the location of the needles as determined by open palpation through the lymphadenectomy incision (36–41). Patients are placed in a low lithotomy position, and an O'Connor drape is often used to avoid contamination during the interstitial implantation. A Foley catheter is placed and inflated with contrast for localization. A bilateral lymphadenectomy is performed, and the prostate is exposed. When the radioactive seeds (usually Ir-192) are to be loaded postoperatively, palpable tumor margins are marked by placement of radiopaque seeds at the lateral margin close to the base and apex of the prostate; this is done by using a simple seed implanter through the perineum that is guided by feeling the apex of the prostate with a finger in the rectum. A guide needle is then placed

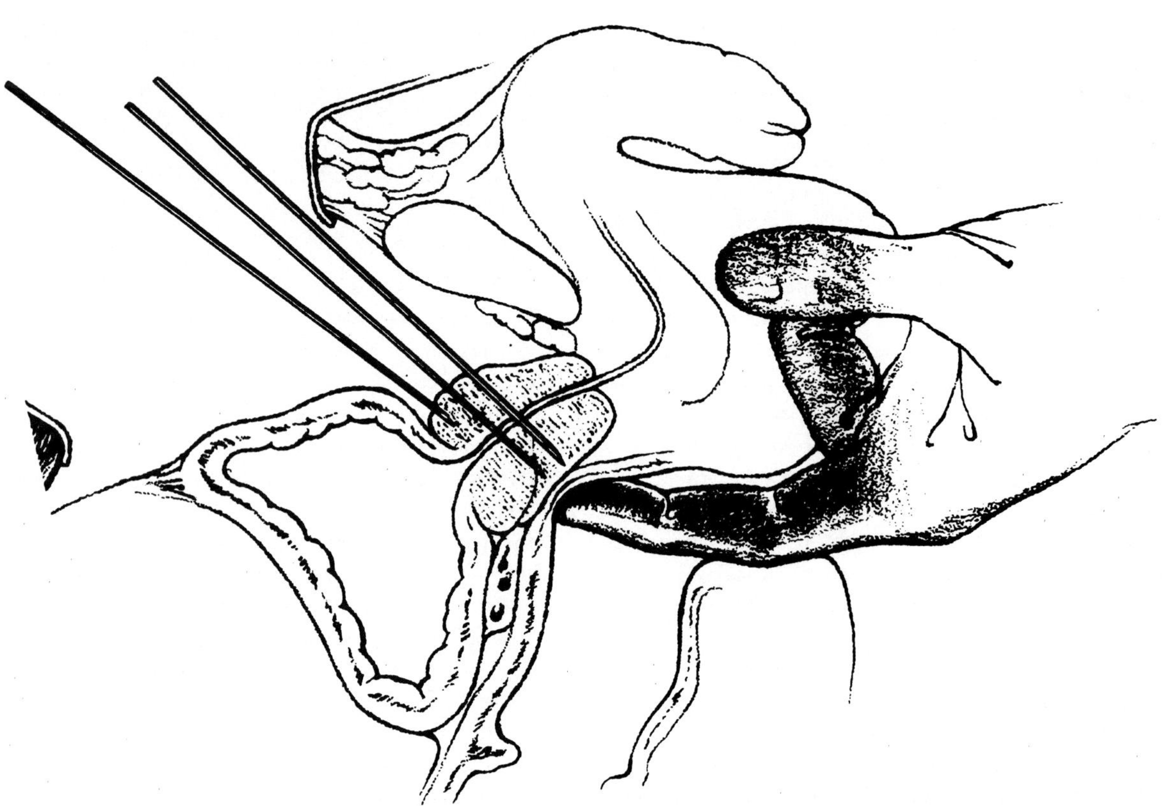

Fig. 20.1. With the patient in lithotomy position, interstitial seed placement is achieved after open surgical lymph node dissection and exposure of the prostate. A finger in the rectum enables guidance for positioning needles used to implant the seeds. (Modified from Whitmore WF Jr, Hilaris BS, Grabstald H. Retropubic implantation of Iodine-125 in the treatment of prostatic cancer. J Urol 1972;108:918. Reprinted with permission of the authors and Williams & Wilkins.)

transperineally at the inferior aspect of the pubic arch. The needle is inserted until the tip extends above the bladder neck and just under the capsule. A template of various designs can then be seated on top of this guide needle. Once the template has been secured against the perineum, the remainder of the prostate is implanted to the depth of the guide needle. Care is taken while implanting the posterior needles to avoid placing the needles in the rectal wall by palpating with the index finger in the rectum.

The seminal vesicles can be implanted if involved, although such posterior placement of needles substantially increases the risk of severe rectal complications (37, 39, 40). After needle placement, the perineal template is sutured to the perineal skin and the guide needles are fixed to the template. Patients are subsequently evaluated in the radiation oncology department, where dummy seeds are loaded within the guide needles and anterior-posterior and lateral radiographs are obtained. The dummy sources allow three-dimensional location of each radioactive seed to be determined. This facilitates computerized dosimetry in which guide needles can be differentially loaded with a variety of seed strengths to produce a relatively homogeneous dose distribution. The prostate (defined by the radiopaque markers placed at the time of surgery) is then treated to a total dose of 3000 to 3500 cGy at a dose rate of 5000 to 90 cGy/hr. The transperineal implant is then removed after a satisfactory dose has been obtained. External beam radiation is often administered 2 to 4 weeks after implant removal. External beam radiation dose varies from 3000 to 4000 cGy. The pelvic lymph nodes have been treated by some investigators with placement of a midline block over the prostate after 4000 cGy.

Other transperineal approaches do not require an open pelvis to guide needles manually. These closed procedures have been performed using fluoroscopy alone and manual clinical evaluation of the posterior extent of needle placement to ensure that the rectum is not implanted (42, 43). A computed tomography (CT) scan-based system has also been developed in which patients are scanned in the semilithotomy position with a rectal obturator attached to a planning perineal template, which is inserted flush with the perineum (44). This obturator and perineal template is then attached to an orientation and planning system device that allows parameters to be recorded so that the details of the rectal obturator and perineal template position can be accurately reproduced at the time of the implant procedure. Multiple CT scans are then obtained, with each CT scan being referenced in three-dimensional space to the location of the transperineal orientation and planning system device. The prostate gland is then reconstructed by entering the prostate volume on each slice into a computer algorithm that three-dimensionally reconstructs the prostate gland. Computerized preplanning is then performed, which determines the precise position, orientation, depth of insertion, and seed strength that will be inserted through the transperineal template at the time of the actual procedure.

The ability of transrectal ultrasound (TRUS) to define accurately the prostate volume and the adaptation of this technology to allow accurate three-dimensional placement of brachytherapy sources within the prostate have generated substantial interest. The technique and preliminary results have been published by several groups (17–18, 45–48). Transperineal ultrasound-guided implantation occurs in two steps. The initial step is a planning procedure in which the number and location of each brachytherapy seed are determined before the implantation.

The planning phase is done in the lithotomy position. Serial ultrasound images are obtained at 2- to 5-mm intervals using an axial scanner mounted in a stepping unit (Fig. 20.2). A grid is electronically superimposed on each ultrasound image. This grid corresponds to channels in a multichannel puncture guide that is attached to the ultrasound probe and will be placed adjacent to the perineum during the actual implant (Fig. 20.3). The probe is positioned so that the posterior row of dots (corresponding to the location of the needles that will be placed at the time of the actual implant) overlies the posterior aspect of the prostate in every section. These images are then recorded

on hard copy, and a three-dimensional reconstruction of the gland is performed. This allows preplanning of the three-dimensional seed distribution necessary to produce adequate dosimetry.

The implantation procedure reproduces the planning position with patients in the lithotomy position. A Foley catheter is placed, the bladder is filled, and the catheter is clamped. The ultrasound probe is introduced into the rectum and attached to the stabilization device. The perineal template is attached to the transducer in proximity to the perineum. The template holes correspond to the position of the dots seen on the electronically produced grid under ultrasound. The probe is advanced to the base of the prostate and positioned to reproduce the planning scan images. The electronic grid demonstrates the desired points for needle placement. The prostate is quite mobile, and stabilizing needles are often placed before actual seed insertion. Stabilizing needles can also delineate the location of the prostatic base under fluoroscopy (48). The needles with preloaded seeds are then advanced through their respective portals in the template. Their correct position is confirmed by ultrasound. The position of each seed can be double-checked by fluoroscopy. Kaye has reported substantial improvement in placement of the sources when fluoroscopy was added to ultrasound alone (48). In 31 patients, acceptable dosimetry was achieved in all 31 and good placement was achieved in 24 when ultrasound and fluoroscopy were combined; in 19 patients, ac-

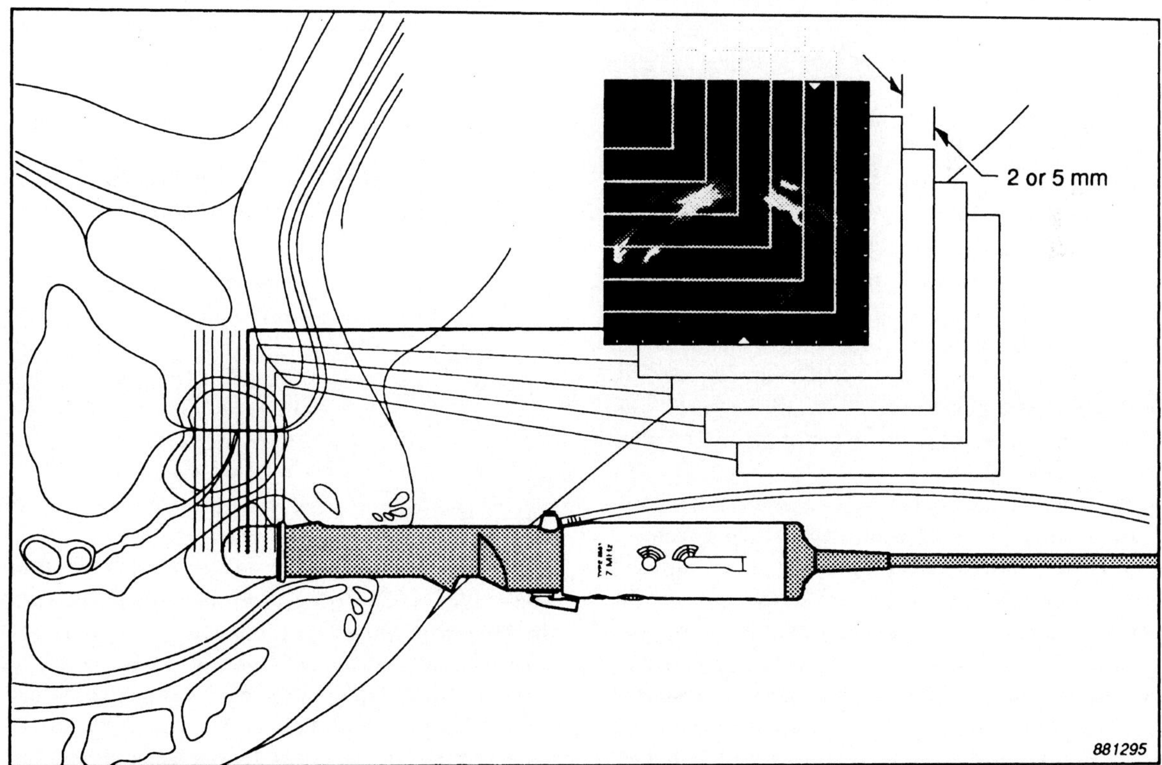

Fig. 20.2.   A transrectal ultrasound probe with a step sectioning device is used to obtain cross-sectional images of the prostate every 2 to 5 mm. (Modified from Carter SSC, Torp-Pedersen ST, Holm HH. Ultrasound-guided implantation techniques in treatment of prostate cancer. Urol Clin North Am 1989; 16:751–762. Reprinted with permission of the authors and WB Saunders Company.)

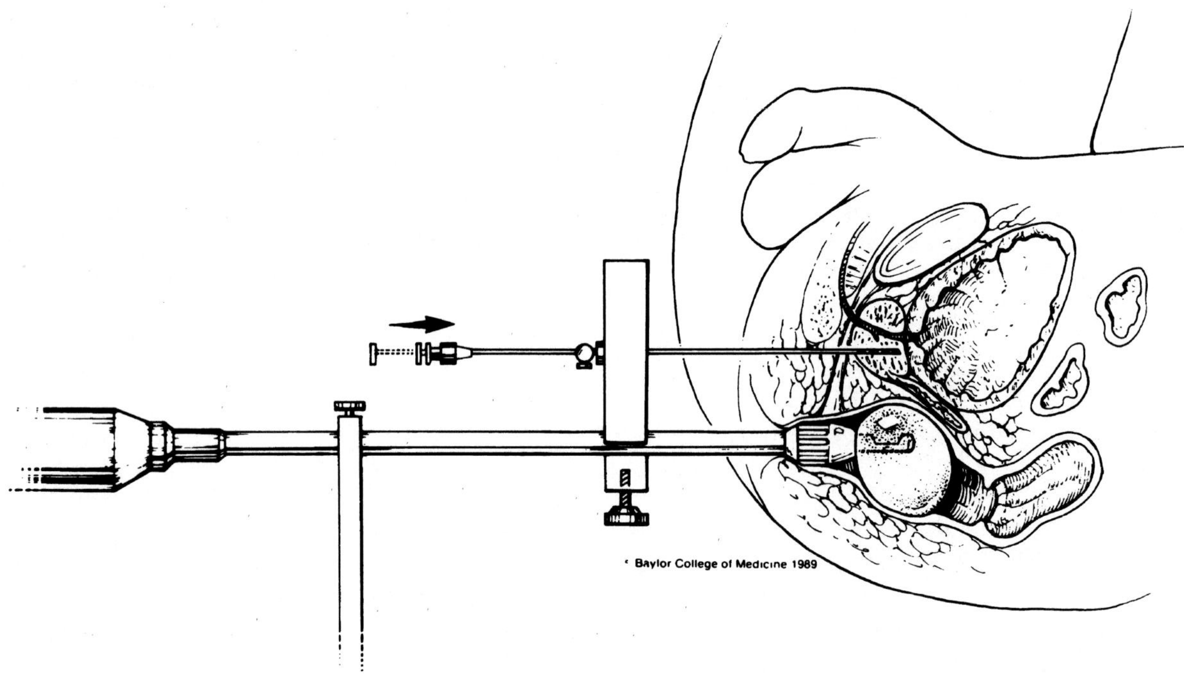

Fig. 20.3. Each seed is implanted using a needle inserted through the grid and into the prostate. Position of the needle tip is confirmed with transrectal ultrasound. (Modified from Carter SSC, Torp-Pedersen ST, Holm HH. Ultrasound-guided implantation techniques in treatment of prostate cancer. Urol Clin North Am 1989;16:751–762. Reprinted with permission of the authors and WB Saunders Company.)

ceptable dosimetry was achieved in 16 and good dosimetry was achieved in 8 when ultrasound alone was used.

During the procedure, one or two of the planned lateral puncture channels (particularly anteriorly) may be inaccessible because the bony pelvis intervenes between the template and peripheral prostate. An orthopedic drill can be used to allow the implanted needle to reach this portion of the prostate. Alternatively, the peripheral prostate may be implanted freehand by angling the needle past the margin of the pubic arch under sagittal ultrasound guidance. Finally, whereas prior transurethral resection of the prostate substantially increases complications, it is possible to use TRUS to attempt to avoid placement of seeds directly within the urethral surface itself. Nevertheless, patients need a minimum of 1 cm of prostate tissue surrounding the transurethral prostatic resection defect (17, 28, 29). Also, after implantation, a cystoscopy can be performed for removal of any seeds placed in the urethra.

Other technologic modifications of transperineal implantation have been reported. Percutaneous transperineal placement of Au-198 (45) and TRUS-guided placement of afterloading catheters followed by high–dose-rate brachytherapy with or without external beam radiation (49–52) have been described. Transperineal techniques have also been used to implant radon seeds (53). Goffinet, in a technologic tour de force, reported transperineal implantation of Ir-192 with hyperthermic probes and administered the brachytherapy concomitantly with hyperthermia (54). Reports of transurethral radiation therapy using a single Co-60 pellet (55) and an intraoperative radiation therapy technique using very high single doses (2800 to 3500 cGy)

administered after transperineal exposure of the prostate gland (56) have been described. Prostate brachytherapy will inevitably see a proliferation of technologic innovations, but it should be underscored that none of these high-technology techniques have mature results of outcome.

RADIOBIOPHYSICAL CONSIDERATIONS OF PROSTATE BRACHYTHERAPY

Study of the important radiobiophysical factors in prostate brachytherapy may sometimes appear a complex task. Although a detailed description of these factors is beyond the scope of this chapter, the basic principles are fundamental to a true understanding of the current state of the art and of future research directions.

Radioisotopes

The radioisotopes used in prostate brachytherapy are listed in Table 20.1 (57). Ir-192 is used for temporary implants. The higher energy of Ir-192 and Au-198 poseradioprotection problems. Because of the short physical half-life of Au-198, the isotope decays rapidly. Patients may be discharged from the hospital after several days, at which time the Au-198 has decayed sufficiently to no longer place the general public at risk of receiving significant doses of radiation. Because Ir-192 has such a long half-life, these seeds must be removed when a sufficient dose has been administered. Table 20.1 also illus-

Table 20.1.   Radioisotopes Used In Prostate Brachytherapy

ISOTOPE	HALF-LIFE (days)	ENERGY (keV)	INITIAL DOSE RATE (cGy/hr)[a]
Iridium 192	74.2	380 (average)[b]	60–90
Gold 198	2.7	412	64[c]
Iodine 125	60.2	28 (average)[d]	8[e]
Palladium 103	17.0	21 (average)[f]	20[g]

[a] Initial dose rate achieved with most prostate implantation techniques.
[b] Range, 136–1060 keV.
[c] Dose rate for nominally prescribed dose of 60 Gy (47).
[d] Range, 27–35.5 keV.
[e] Dose rate for 160 Gy MPD.
[f] Range, 20–23 keV.
[g] Dose rate for 120 MPD (47).

trates the substantial difference in energy between I-125 and Pd-103 versus Ir-192 and Au-198. The emissions from higher energy isotopes react with tissue almost exclusively via the Compton effect (the same interaction used by external beam radiation therapy), whereas the lower energy isotopes interact predominantly through the photoelectric process. The differences in the way these various isotopes' gamma rays interact with matter have two potentially important clinical implications.

First, although the low-energy isotopes are attenuated by tissue to a much greater extent than the higher energy isotopes (accounting for their diminished tissue penetration and much better radiation safety), the gamma rays of these low-energy isotopes are significantly affected by any high electron density substance they encounter in their path. Therefore, corpora amylacea with a high electron density will dramatically absorb and attenuate the radiation emitted from I-125 or Pd-103. Second, the lower energy gamma rays are more biologically effective, dose for dose, in killing cells than are the gamma rays emitted from the higher energy isotopes or the x rays delivered during conventional external beam treatment (58, 59). Therefore, a similar dose of radiation from either Pd-103 or I-125 would be expected to produce more tumoricidal effect than the higher energy isotopes, provided all other conditions were similar.

Dosimetry

The study of the dose distribution of radioactive implants is fraught with caveats and vagaries. There are a variety of methods used to describe the dose of absorbed radiation within a tumor. The MSKCC group has described, and many groups have adopted, the matched peripheral dose (MPD) convention, which they use to describe the dose of radiation delivered to the tumor (60, 61). The MPD is the dose of radiation absorbed at the periphery of the volume of an ellipsoid having the same dimensions as the measured, mutually perpendicular dimensions of the prostate gland. The dimensions of the prostate gland, in this case, are determined clinically at the time of a suprapubic exploration or, if a closed technique is used, by the imaging measurements used to determine the prostate gland volume. The substantially less-than-the-maximum central dose should be taken into account. Significant volumes of the prostate gland and tumor will receive larger doses than those prescribed by the MPD (62). Furthermore, the true minimal peripheral dose (the smallest dose received by the periphery of the actual tumor) will generally be lower than the MPD because the actual tumor shape will not usually conform precisely to that predicted by the ellipsoidal volume formulae (61). Because a portion of the actual tumor shape may project outside of the calculated same-volume ellipsoidal isodose contour, this portion of tumor could receive a lower dose of radiation, rendering the true minimal peripheral dose less than the MPD.

Decisions regarding the number and distribution of I-125 sources to be implanted are made on the basis of a nomogram developed by Hilaris and colleagues (62, 63). The MPD nomogram uses the average dimension method. The average dimension (D_a) is the average of the mutually perpendicular length, width, and depth $[d_a = (A + b + c) / 3]$ for the implanted volume. The required activity (A) is then derived from some equation multiplying the d_a times some factor(s) based on implanted volume.

The MPD, despite its highly theoretical description, may relate to the probability of local tumor control (24, 31, 45, 64). Hilaris reported only approximately 75% local control with MPD doses of 12,000 cGy rising to approximately 85% local control with an MPD of 16,000 cGy and to 90% local control with an MPD of 18,000 cGy (64). Morton and Peschel observed local failure in 42% of patients with MPDs less than 10,000 cGy versus local failure in only 18% of patients with MPDs greater than or equal to 10,000 cGy (31). Crusinberry et al. showed statistically significantly improved decreases in tumor volume when 15,000 cGy MPD was used versus 9000 cGy MPD when Au-198 isotopes alone were used (45). Finally, Fuks has reported that an MPD of greater than or equal to 14,000 cGy produced statistically significantly improved local control compared with MPDs of either 10,000 to 13,900 cGy or less than 10,000 cGy (24). This analysis must be interpreted with some caution in view of the fact that the relationship between dose and local control was searched for in 1000-cGy intervals from 7000 to 20,000 cGy and that the data therefore become subject to subset analysis error. Nevertheless, this is the most recent report of the MSKCC I-125 data and is noteworthy both for its long follow-up (median, 97 + months) and for the fact that local relapse occurred with a mean annual hazard of 11.2 ± 1.2% per year over the first 15 years after initial treatment. The median time to detection of local relapse was 108 months after therapy.

Unfortunately, there are many caveats to the interpretation of this dosimetry literature. One problem with the MSKCC MPD literature is that the formula on which the nomogram was based has changed with time.

1965 Memorial Protocol; $A = 5d_a$

1975 Memorial Protocol; $A = 5 d_a$ (for $d_a \leq 2.4$);
$A = 3.87 (d_a)1.293$ (for $2.4 < d_a < 3.24$);
$A = 2.76 (d_a)1.581$ (for $d_a \geq 3.24$).

1979 Memorial Protocol; $A = 5 (d_a + 1)$ (for $d_a \leq 2.4$);
$A = 3.87 (d_a + 1)1.293$ (for $2.4 < d_a < 3.24$);
$A = 2.76 (d_a + 1)1.581$ (for $d_a \geq 3.24$).

The alteration in the formulae used to determine how much activity to implant has extremely important clinical implications. First, the MPD will always be substantially greater for smaller volume tumors (65). Therefore, it is difficult to know whether a higher MPD is associated with improved local control because it, in fact, delivered a higher dose or because the tumor that was implanted was smaller and more favorable to begin with. Second, the three successive formulae will produce successive increases in MPD for most tumor volumes (65). This makes it difficult to know whether the improved local control seen with higher MPD is related to improved cancer control with higher doses or merely shorter follow-up time for those treated in more recent years when the formula would dictate a higher MPD. Third, the MPD method relies on clinical evaluation that is usually performed intraoperatively to determine prostate volume. Clinical evaluation has been observed to be substantially discrepant from ultrasound-determined prostate volume in individual patients (66). Fourth, most institutions reserve implantation only for stage A and B disease. Clinical evaluation is known to miss either paraprostatic extracapsular tumor extension or extension into the seminal vesicles in 20 to 40% or more of patients. Whereas TRUS will correlate well with measured prostate gland volume (67), it is far from an adequate tool for evaluation of either extracapsular extension or seminal vesicle involvement.

Regardless of the dosimetry convention used, it is widely acknowledged that standard I-125 (retropubic) implantation has substantial difficulty in achieving homogeneous dose distribution throughout the gland. Seeds can migrate and become lost, usually by transurethral routes, although pulmonary embolization of I-125 seeds has been reported (68). According to Sommerkamp et al., seed loss occurred in 90% of 52 patients monitored serially and averaged 8% of the total implant seed number (69). Transperineal techniques also suffer from seed loss problems. Vijverberg et al. observed seed loss in 43% of transperineal ultrasound-guided implants by 4 weeks (70). Because seed loss may occur anytime during the length of the implant (69), the total number of patients with seed loss is unknown. Poor distribution of I-125 seeds or implantation errors are variously defined but are reported to occur in 14 to 85% of implants (69, 71–73). Frequently, the superior portion of the prostate contains too few seeds (73), a problem that may not be completely resolved by the use of TRUS perineal implantation (74).

Poor distribution of seeds has been described as an important determinant of local tumor control (71, 72). The MSKCC (71) reported local failure in 7 of 29 patients (24%) with poor distribution of the 160 MPD volume versus local failure in only 4 of 83 patients (5%) with adequate distribution of the 160 MPD volume. The importance of poor seed distribution is also evident in the transperineal ultrasound-guided series. Positive postimplantation biopsy rates have been observed to significantly increase actuarially with "bad" versus "good" quality implants (70). Although it seems conceptually "intuitively" obvious that failure to place the seeds homogeneously and uniformly throughout the prostate will result in a higher failure rate, these observations have profound implications. Roy et al. (75) have documented the failure of transperineal-guided implantation to treat adequately the entire target volume in a substantial percentage of cases. For example, in the Roy series, the average MPD (the dose reported in most brachytherapy series and the dose "prescribed" by the brachytherapy team) overestimated by about 3 times the actual average minimum peripheral dose as measured by CT scans. In other words, on average, clinicians overestimate by a factor of 3 the dose that is received by the entire tumor!

For permanent implants, all the dosimetry conventions used to describe dose calculate the total absorbed dose of radiation in the tumor over the entire period of decay of the radioactive isotope. Certainly, the prostate gland and tumor do receive all of the absorbed radiation that is given off during the entire decay of the isotope. However, as the radioactivity decays, the dose rate eventually falls to extraordinarily low levels. At some point, the dose rate eventually falls to a level where it just compensates for cell proliferation. This is the so-called effective treatment time (T_{eff}). After T_{eff} has been reached, any additional radiation dose is wasted in terms of its tumoricidal effect (57, 58, 76–78). This wasted dose may amount to 3 to 30% of the total dose received by the tumor (58). Unfortunately, the T_{eff} is dependent on complex tumor cell kinetics and is impossible to predict in individuals. While we are unable to correct for this wasted dose, it seems self-evident that such a large degree of uncertainty demands that purely physical descriptions of dose distribution be interpreted with extreme caution.

Biology

The radiobiology of low–dose-rate brachytherapy is complex and incompletely characterized. Several reviews deal with the topic in general and are recommended for those wishing detailed understanding of the subject (79, 80).

The relative biologic effectiveness of the lower energy isotopes (I-125, Pd-103) is greater than that of the higher energy isotopes (Ir-192, Au-198). This is because the secondary electrons produced by the lower energy photons result in a greater density of energy deposited along the track of the radiation. This higher linear energy transfer results in more dense ionization events occurring within the tissue receiving radiation. Because radiation exerts its effect via ionization of important chemical bonds within the cells, the higher linear energy transfer of the lower energy isotopes results in greater cytotoxicity. Thus, the relative biologic effectiveness of the lower energy isotopes is greater. Therefore, a dose of radiation (expressed as either a rad or cGy) will not result in the same biologic effect if one is comparing different isotopes.

The radiation dose rate is extremely important and can significantly influence the radiobiologic effect. The dose rates produced by the various radioisotopes vary considerably (Table 20.1), and this variation occurs over a clinically important range. With external beam radiation the dose rate is about 100 to 300 cGy/min. Such a rapidly administered dose allows no time for repair of sublethal damage or repopulation of the surviving cancer cells before completion of treatment. However, much slower dose rates allow some sublethal damage repair during treatment, resulting in less damage as a result of the same radiation dose. If the dose rate falls sufficiently, cell division continues and cell population grows (albeit slowly). The dose rate at which mitotic delay begins to lengthen the cell cycle time, producing a greater dose per cell cycle, inhibition of cell division, and population shrinkage is termed the critical dose rate. Critical dose rates vary substantially among different cell lines and biologic systems.

Several investigators have attempted to predict the effect of these varying dose rates on tumor control, usually by implementation of the linear-quadratic model (57, 58, 76–78). This model requires numerous assumptions about the intrinsic radiosensitivity of the cell as well as the T_{eff} (the time until radioactivity decays to a point where the dose rate will just compensate for cell proliferation). Interestingly, both Fowler (58) and Anderson and Ling (57) have arrived at the conclusion that prostate cancers with a potential doubling time or T_p (cell cycle time multiplied by growth fraction; assuming no cell loss) of 10 days or less are more satisfactorily treated by Pd-103 with its higher initial dose rate. Those prostate cancers with a T_p of greater than 10 days are theoretically more adequately treated by I-125. The analyses have correlated with Marchese and Hall's study of I-125 radiation and potentially lethal damage repair (81), in which they suggested that I-125 may be less suitable for rapidly growing tumors with their shorter cell cycles and higher growth fractions. Unfortunately, what little data have been published regarding T_p in prostate cancer indicate that the T_p may be substantially in excess of 10 days in the usual tumor. Trott and Kummermehr, on the basis of the very long latency time to local recurrence after definitive radiation therapy, have estimated a T_p of 30 days (82). These calculations were based on a median latency time to local recurrence of only 3 years.

Recently published information suggests that the median latency time may actually be much more than 5 years after treatment (24, 33, 83). Even observation-alone series indicate that a very significant portion of untreated tumors may have median latency periods to progression in excess of 3 years (12, 15, 16, 83). Anderson and colleagues have measured average labeling indices of less than 1% and average T_p of 60 days in 38 adenocarcinomas of the prostate (84).

To summarize, although the clinical experience with I-125 has been disappointing in terms of its ability to produce local tumor control and some enthusiasm for exploration of Pd-103 as a more effective radioisotope exists, application of our best mathematical models and prostate cancer tumor kinetics to this problem fails to provide convincing evidence that Pd-103 will provide superior results. Obviously additional experience with significantly longer follow-up will be needed to reach conclusions regarding efficacy of Pd-103.

UNIVERSITY OF KANSAS MEDICAL CENTER EXPERIENCE WITH I-125 BRACHYTHERAPY

From 1976 to 1987, 115 patients at the University of Kansas Medical Center (KU) with adenocarcinoma of the prostate underwent pelvic lymphadenectomy and brachytherapy using I-125 seeds as primary treatment. Patients' ages ranged from 41 to 78 years (mean, 63.5). All patients were staged preoperatively with history, physical examination, acid phosphatase, bone scan, and pelvic CT scan. A total of 99 patients had clinically localized disease; this was defined as lack of tumor extension or fixation on rectal examination, normal serum acid phosphatase, negative bone scan, and no evidence of extension or lymphadenopathy on CT scan. Sixteen patients had nonbulky clinical stage C disease, with evidence by rectal examination and/or CT scan of extension beyond the prostate yet a negative bone scan and no pelvic lymphadenopathy. Postoperative follow-up was by rectal examination, acid phosphatase, and bone scan every 6 months and by PSA and TRUS when these latter two techniques became available. Our retropubic surgical implantation technique was modified from that of Whitmore and associates and is described earlier in this chapter in the section on retropubic implantation technique (7).

Patient follow-up ranged from 3.5 to 11.5 years (mean, 7.2), excluding one postoperative death and one patient who died in the first year of a cause unrelated to prostate cancer. Clinical stages were upgraded to D1 due to microscopically positive lymph nodes in 1 of 8 patients (13%) with stage A2, 5 of 53 patients (9%) with stage B1, 8 of 38 patients (21%) with stage B2, and 9 of 16 patients (56%) with stage C disease. Total clinical understaging for all patients was 20%. Early postoperative surgical complications are listed in Table 20.2 and comprise 9 major complications (including the 1 death in the immediate postoperative period) and 22 minor complications. Late complications (Table 20.3) include those believed to be surgical (2) and those believed to be due to radiation side effects (16).

Of 61 patients who were asked about sexual function and were potent preoperatively, only 2 claimed erectile dysfunction 12 to 18 months postoperatively. Several had transient dysfunction in the first 3 months after surgery but this resolved by 6 months. The most frequent, bothersome, long-term problem was radiation prostatitis with severe irritative voiding symp-

TABLE 20.2.—University of Kansas Experience—Early Surgical Postoperative Complications

MINOR COMPLICATION	NO.	MAJOR COMPLICATION	NO.
I-125 (115 Patients)			
Atelectasis	3	Wound dehiscence	1
Epididymitis	5	Pelvic hematoma	2
Voiding symptoms	6	Deep wound hematoma	1
Lymphocele, leg edema	2	Pulmonary embolus	1
Zoster	1	Brachial plexus injury	1
Arrhythmia	1	Enterotomy	1
Superficial wound infection	3	Iliac vein injury	1
Pneumonia	1	Myocardial infarction	1
Total	22	Total	9
Ir-192 (22 patients)			
Dysuria	4	None	
Hematuria, hematospermia	1		
Total	5	Total	0

toms (five patients); three of these patients were essentially "prostate cripples," that is, truly disabled by their frequent and painful voiding. Symptoms in the other two patients improved but did not completely resolve after transurethral resection of the prostate (including resection of many seeds) plus long-term antibiotics. Coliform organisms grew from prostate fluid in all five patients, suggesting that their I-125 seeds were colonized.

Sixteen of 115 patients died of unrelated causes 1 to 13 years postoperatively and were free of disease at death. Seven patients with surgical stage A2 disease experienced no disease recurrence (mean follow-up, 7 years). However, six of seven patients with stage A2 disease had well-differentiated carcinoma; one of seven had moderately differentiated carcinoma. Thus, nearly all stage A2 patients would have been expected to have favorable prognoses in any event based on tumor grade.

For the 48 surgical B1 patients, 41 (86%) showed no clinical evidence of disease (NCED) with a mean follow-up of 6.6 years, 2 (4%) are alive with metastases, and 5 (10%) died of metastatic disease. Metastatic disease was first detected by bone scan in

Table 20.3.   University of Kansas Experience—Late Complications[a]

RADIATION RELATED	NO.	SURGERY RELATED	NO.
Radiation proctitis	3	Hydrocele	1
Rectovesical fistula	1	Lymphocele	1
Radiation prostatitis	5		
Urethral stricture	1		
Radiation cystitis	1		
Impotence	2		
Perirectal abscess	1		
Bladder neck contraction	1		
Chronic orchalgia	1		
Total	16	Total	2

[a] All late complications were secondary to I-125 implantation. There were no late complications observed in the 22 Ir-192 patients who underwent implantation at the University of Kansas.

the seven patients at an average of 2.2 years (range, 1 to 4 years) after treatment. There were 32 well-differentiated, 14 moderately differentiated, and 2 poorly differentiated cancers.

In the 30 surgical B2 patients, 22 (73%) showed NCED with a mean follow-up of 5.2 years, 3 (10%) have metastases, and 5 (17%) have died of metastatic prostate cancer. Seventeen had well-differentiated carcinoma, 12 had moderately differentiated carcinoma, and 1 had poorly differentiated carcinoma. Positive bone scans were noted in the B2 group an average of 3.6 years after initial therapy (range, 1 to 6 years).

Of seven patients with surgical C disease, only two (29%) have NCED (mean follow-up, 7.5 years). Both of these patients had well-differentiated carcinoma, whereas the five patients with progression had moderately differentiated (four patients) or poorly differentiated (one patient) disease, as one might expect. Disease progression into bone occurred after a mean of 5 years posttreatment. Only 2 of 23 (9%) surgical D1 patients have no evidence of disease (mean follow-up, 5 years), and 7 (30%) are alive with metastases (mean, 6.7 years posttreatment). The 14 dead individuals include all three patients with high-grade tumors; the remainder had intermediate-grade pathologic conditions.

Looking at patients who had progression to bone metastases (41 of 115), we found that this occurred within a mean of 3.1 years after surgery (range, 1 to 7.5). In fact, 76% of this group had positive bone scans at 3.8 years postoperatively.

A subset of our patients was studied (after informed consent) with prostate needle biopsy between 18 and 24 months postoperatively. Tissue was studied histopathologically and placed in primary explant tissue culture for 8 weeks to see if cells would proliferate, enabling at least one subculture. Other researchers had demonstrated that it was feasible to culture prostate cells after radiation therapy; it seemed reasonable to evaluate this technique for any clinical correlation with prognosis (85, 86).

The individual performing cell culture was unaware of the pathology result(s), and those pathologists examining the histologic appearance were unaware of cell culture outcomes. Results were later compared (after long-term clinical follow-up) by two individuals not involved in either cell culture or histologic interpretation. Although the results (Figs. 20.4A and 20.4B) were preliminary, it was noted that both a negative histologic result and failure to grow cells in culture (growth arrest) were predictors of good intermediate clinical status (NCED). In addition, positive growth in cell culture was a good predictor of clinical relapse. However, an abnormal histologic result was not a reliable predictor, in that some biopsies contained radiation-altered cells that had a malignant appearance and were termed positive (yet some of these patients continued to do well clinically). Figure 20.5 shows a biopsy specimen from one of our patients demonstrating significant radiation effect and only atypical epithelial cells. Figure 20.6 shows a biopsy specimen with residual cancer present (87).

In other published reports, a positive histologic result (for cancerous cells) is seen in prostate needle biopsies at 2 years after I-125 brachytherapy in 25 to 40% of patients (88, 89);

this carries a poor prognosis after 10 years (90). It is unclear if some of the KU patients doing well (despite positive biopsy results) simply had not had sufficient time to relapse (although most relapses were within 4 years at KU), if positive or abnormal biopsies were "overcalled" by the interpreting pathologist(s), or if some other factor played a role in the results.

It is imperative that all brachytherapy-treated patients receive follow-up care as if they had undergone radical prostatectomy, with interval visits tailored to the clinical situation at hand. We ordinarily follow patients with physical examination (including digital rectal), PSA, complete blood count, serum chemistry, and urinalysis on a 3- to 6-month basis. Bone scan and TRUS examination are obtained if suspicion exists that the disease is not controlled (PSA rises or remains above the "undetectable" level, bone pain is noted, the rectal examination suggests incomplete local control, etc.). In those clinical circumstances in which a repeat biopsy is indicated 12 to 24 months after brachytherapy, TRUS is used to guide the biopsy needle because we believe it is more accurate (91) and it enables an objective comparison with the preoperative appearance of lesion(s).

RESULTS OF OTHER BRACHYTHERAPY SERIES

Local Tumor Control

Most brachytherapy series have used a purely clinical definition of local failure. That is, routine biopsy information was either not obtained or was disregarded. In addition, routine PSA and/or prostatic acid phosphatase values were not routinely used in the diagnosis of a local relapse. Table 20.4 summarizes local failure rates using a variety of brachytherapy techniques. There is a wide range of local failure ranging from 0 to 80%. The most important factors accounting for this wide range of clinical local failures are the stage and grade of tumors as well as the length of follow-up of each series.

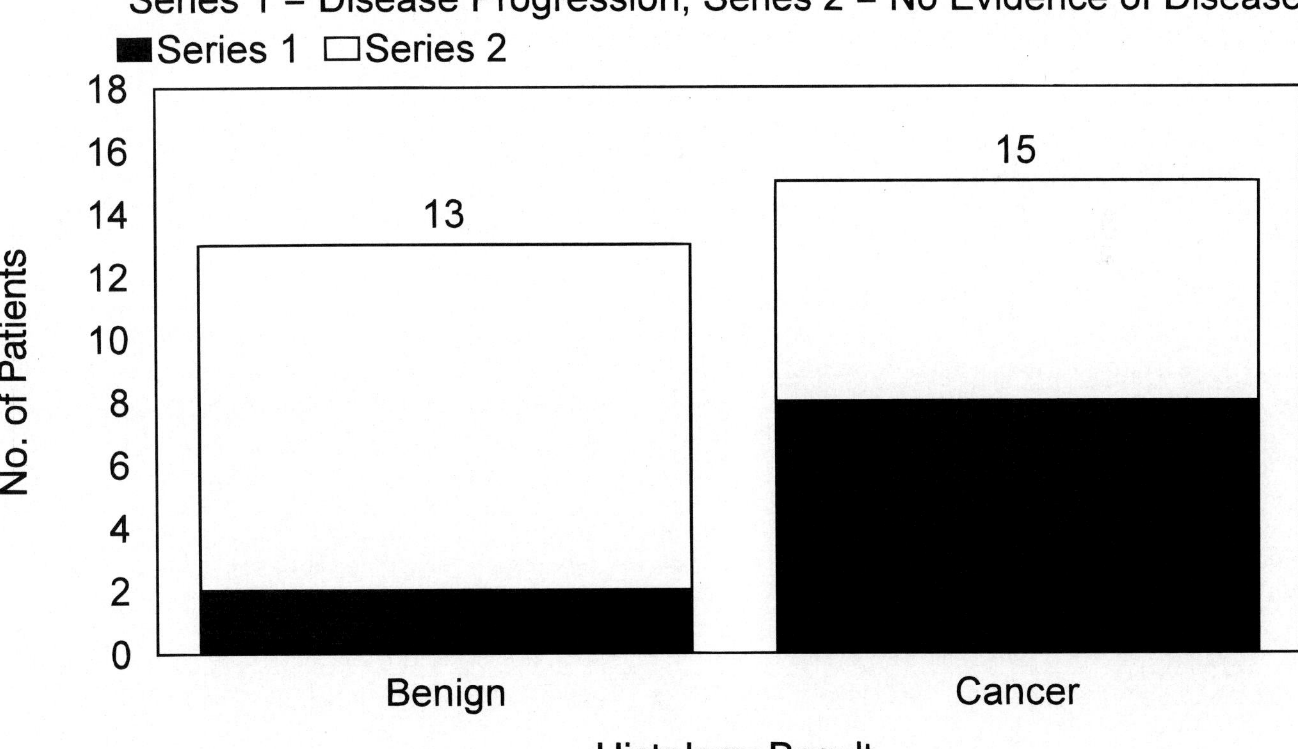

Fig. 20.4.   Clinical outcome with respect to disease progression (solid portion of bars) or no evidence of clinical disease (clear portion of bars) for patients who underwent biopsy 18 to 24 months after I-125 interstitial therapy, with outcome versus histologic result (A) and outcome versus cell culture result (B). However, 2 of 18 patients with "no growth" in cell culture were given diethylstilbestrol, making these preliminary results less precise.

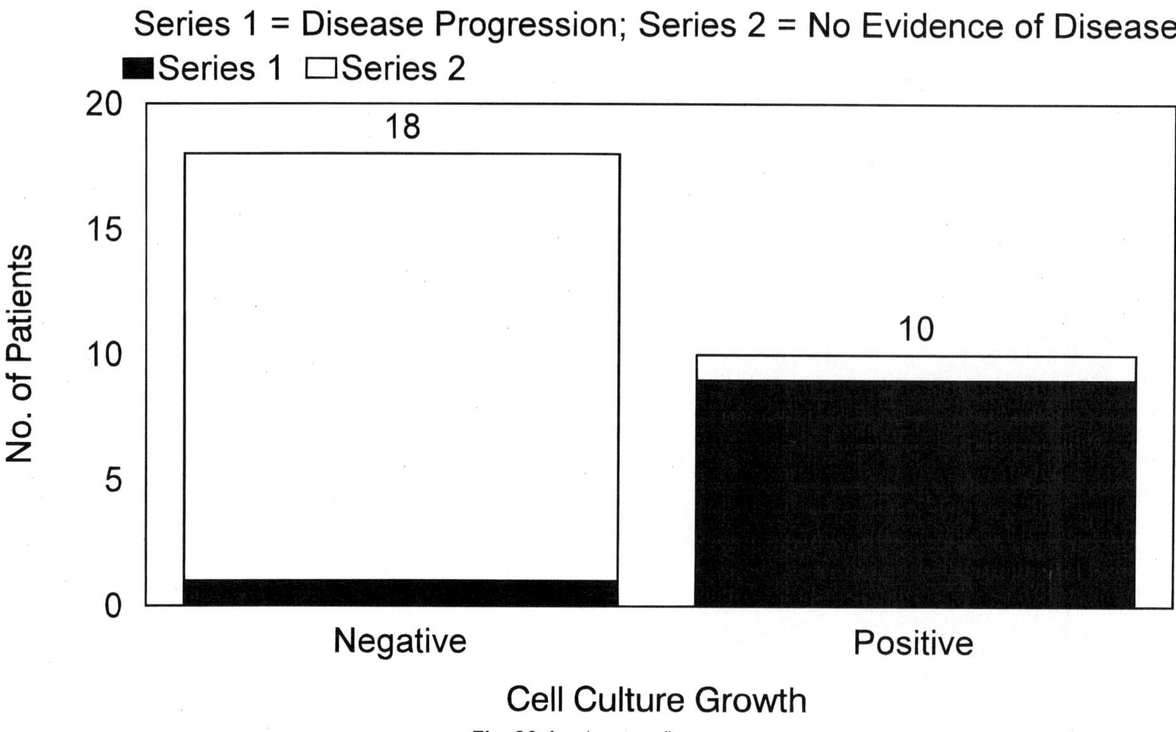

Fig. 20.4. *(continued)*

The importance of long follow-up cannot be overemphasized. The MSKCC (24) group observed an actuarial local failure rate of 79% at 15 years. The observed mean annual hazard of local relapse was $11.2 \pm 1.2\%$ yearly over the first 15 years of treatment for that series. The median time to detection of local relapse was 108 months after implantation. Kuban et al. (33) reported that only 57% of I-125 patients who ultimately experienced recurrence had manifested this clinical local failure by 5 years in contrast to externally irradiated patients who experienced 91% of their local failures by 5 years after therapy, a statistically significant difference (P = 0.002). The Baylor group also reported that, of those ultimately having local failure, at least 6 to 8 years was required before 50% of these local recurrences became manifest (83). Doornbos et al. reported that the median time to local failure was 4.5 years in those treated with surgery and brachytherapy (92). The long time to local recurrence seen in those series that have adequate follow-up time emphasizes both the indolent natural history of the disease and the uncertainty of reaching conclusions in studies lacking at least 10 to 15 years follow-up. As shown in Table 20.4, series with longer follow-up have progressively more local failure.

The negative impact of increasing tumor stage (21, 24, 31, 33, 34, 36, 95, 96) and grade (24, 33, 34, 36, 95, 96) on local tumor control is well described. This is expected as both advancing grade and stage predict a higher likelihood of extraprostatic tumor extension and seminal vesicle involvement, neither of which is easily or routinely included within the brachytherapy treatment volume. Advancing grade and stage are also known predictors of increasing tumor failure with both external beam therapy and radical prostatectomy (90, 97).

Table 20.5 summarizes several series where routine biopsies were performed after brachytherapy. These corroborate, in part, the disturbingly high clinical local failure rates seen in *mature* brachytherapy series. Unfortunately, most series reporting biopsy results exclude 40 to 75% of patients treated, which unavoidably introduces substantial bias into these reports and their interpretations. Despite this, most report positive biopsy results in 25 to 55%. The very high positive rate in the series by Lee et al. (99) may reflect inadequate therapy, selection bias, and the fact that biopsies were performed under TRUS guidance (which may increase sensitivity and specificity of post-therapy biopsies). The fact that the biopsies done by Blasko (74) were performed under TRUS guidance makes the 16% incidence of either positive or indeterminate biopsies more noteworthy. Although it seems attractive to conclude that this low positive biopsy rate is due to superior results from transper-

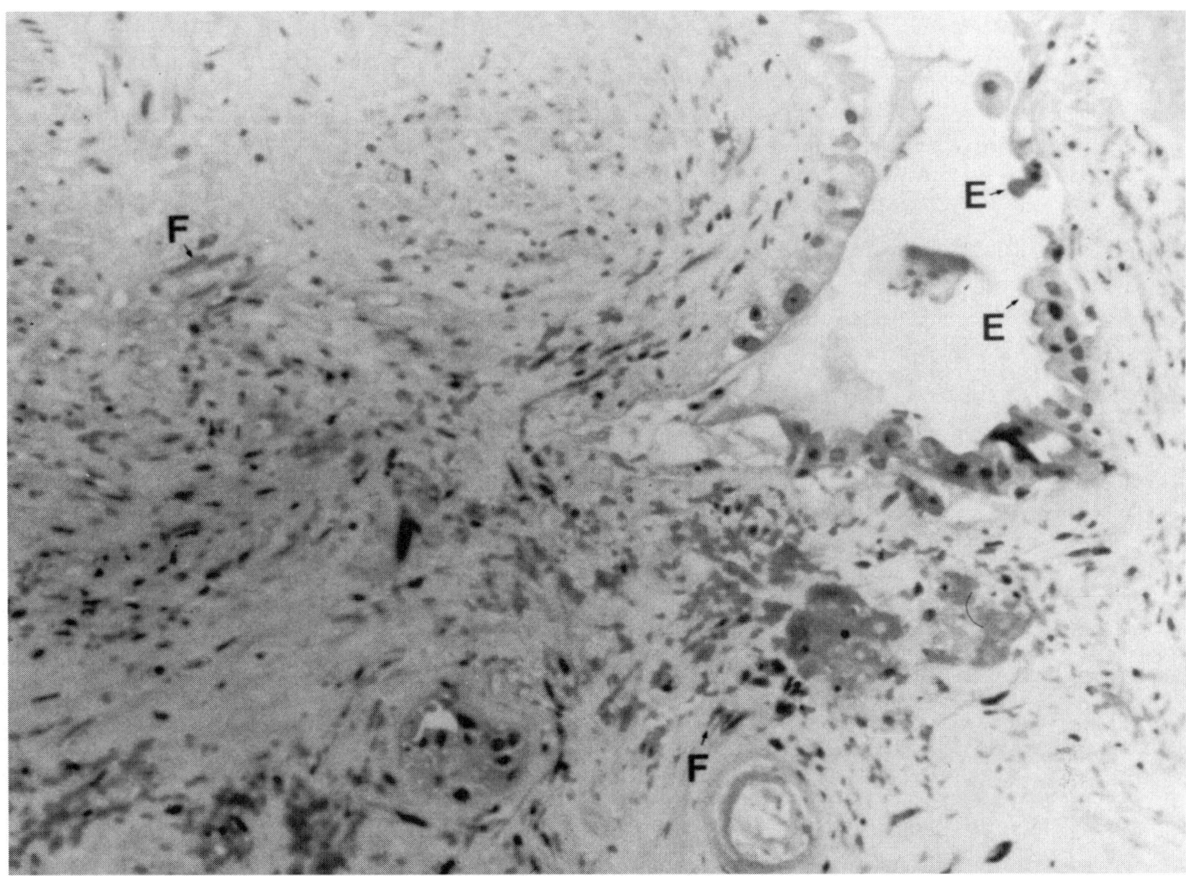

Fig. 20.5. Prostate biopsy specimen 19 months after interstitial radiation therapy with I-125. Note significant radiation changes with atypical fibroblasts (F), collections of mononuclear cells, and focally disrupted swollen epithelial cells (E) of remaining nonneoplastic glands (hematoxylin-eosin stain, ×400).

ineal ultrasound-guided implantation, Iversen et al. (19) reported a 48% incidence of positive biopsies and Carter et al. (18) reported a 25% incidence evident either clinically or by TRUS using a similar technique of transperineal implantation. Vijverberg et al. (70) observed that positive biopsies increased from only 22% at 6 months to 50% at 4 years. Although these very high rates of biopsy positivity after transperineal ultrasound-guided implantation are distressing, the biopsy positivity rate decreases in "good" quality implants, which are produced with greater frequency in groups with more experience (70). One final note regarding the Blasko et al. series—it is overwhelmingly composed of much lower grade and lower stage patients than were included in the other biopsy series. Despite this, further follow-up of this exceptional series is eagerly awaited.

Based on the reports of the high incidence of positive postradiation biopsy results, Syed et al. developed a temporary iridium-192 implant technique combined with external beam radiation to improve local control (8). This procedure is performed at the time of bilateral pelvic lymphadenectomy. The dose from the implant is approximately 3000 to 3500 cGy followed in 2 to 4 weeks by external beam radiation therapy for an additional 3000 to 3500 cGy. It is believed that a dose of 3000 to 3500 cGy given with an implant within a short time (40 to 60 hours) is radiobiologically much more effective than with protracted external beam irradiation or permanent I-125 implants.

Several years ago, Syed et al. reported an update of the results for 200 patients treated between 1977 and 1985 (93). Clinical local control was 95.5%, and the actuarial 5-year survival rate was 85%. Seventy-four patients underwent postradiation biopsies, and 13 (18%) had positive biopsy results. This incidence of positive postradiation biopsy is close to the low incidence reported by Blasko et al. The serious complication rate was 11% in the first series of 100 patients but only 4% in the second group of 100. Six patients in the first 100 required a temporary colostomy; however, modification of the source distribution to reduce the rectal dose and reduction in the total dose to the prostate in those who had prior surgery dropped the complication rate to the 4% range. No colostomies were required in the second group of 100 patients.

At the University of Kansas, our early Ir-192 results were recently reported by Reddy et al. (94), with 22 patients treated by Ir-192 implants and external radiation. The median follow-

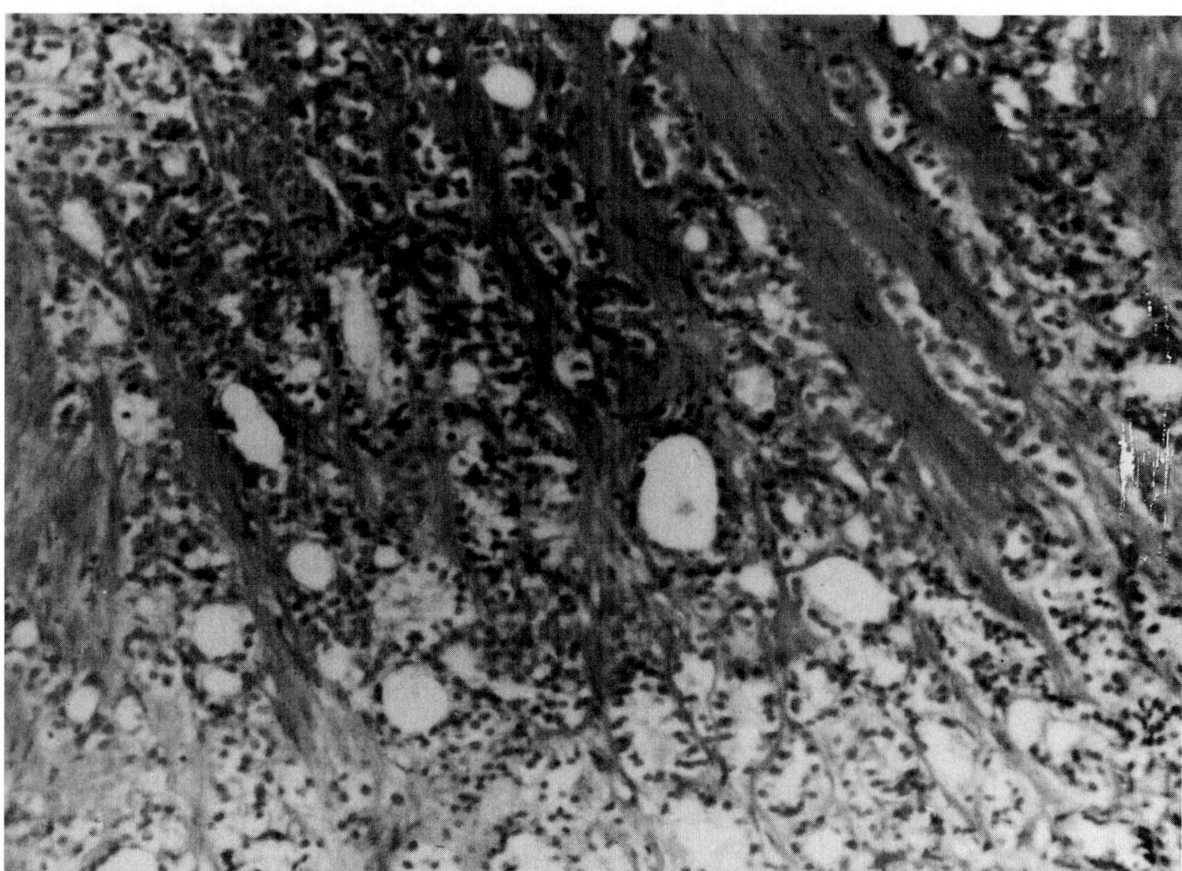

Fig. 20.6.   There is relatively mild interstitial fibrosis, and the tumor cells have cytoplasmic vacuolization and nuclear pyknosis (hematoxylin-eosin stain, ×400). This prostate biopsy specimen is positive for residual cancer 24 months following brachytherapy with I-125.

Table 20.4.   Clinical Local Failure in Prostate Brachytherapy Series[a]

AUTHOR	NO. OF PATIENTS	TECHNIQUE	F/U MEDIAN (Range) (mo)	LOCAL FAILURE (%)
Syed et al. (93)	200	Ir-192 (30 Gy); EB 40–50 Gy	84 (NS)	5.5
Reddy et al. (94)	22	Ir-192 (30–35 Gy); EB 30–35 Gy	48 (NS)	15
Blasko (74)	62	Pd-103 (90–115 Gy MPD) ± EB 45 Gy	23 (13–44)	0
Gutierrez and Merino (25)	119	Au-198 (30 Gy); EB 45 Gy	36 (12–163)	6
Giles and Brady (34)	122	I-125 180 Gy MPD	36 (3–84)	17
Kumar et al. (43)	68	I-125 160 Gy MPD	NS	15
Blasko (74)	274[b]	I-125 (120–180 Gy MPD) ± EB 45 Gy	40 (13–64)	4
Morton and Peschel (31)	141	I-125 100–170 Gy MPD	NS	23
Carey et al. (21)	67	AU-198 (30–35 Gy) + EB 40 Gy	60 (12–109)	36[c]
Kuban et al. (33)	120	I-125 160 Gy MPD	80 (36–145)	29
Lerner et al. (83)	360	Au-198 (25–30 Gy MPD) + EB 40–50	87 (14–220)	20
Fuks et al. (24)	679	I-125 100–180 Gy MPD	97	79[d]

[a] EB, external beam; NS, not stated. Series tabulated do not use PSA, PAP, or routine biopsy information to diagnose local failure.

[b] 41 of 315 (13%) treated, lost to follow-up.

[c] 7-year actuarial minimal estimate.

[d] Actuarial 15 year risk; actual local relapse observed in 52%.

Table 20.5.   Prostate Brachytherapy Biopsy Results

AUTHOR	NO. BIOPSIED	NO. TREATED	BIOPSIED (%)	POSITIVE BIOPSIES (%)
Scardino (95)	124	475[a]	26	35
Lytton (98)	29	106	27	55
Lee (99)	23	40	58[b]	91
Kandzari (72)	46	80	58	39
Klein (38)	15	35	43	27
Iverson (19)	25	33[c]	76	48
Blasko (74)	224[b]	377[c]	59	16[d]
Shellhammer (100)	71	109	65	35

[a] 803 originally treated but 328 excluded for various reasons.

[b] Biopsies done under TRUS guidance.

[c] Transperineal implantation using ultrasound.

[d] Includes indeterminate biopsy results.

up was 48 months for these patients. Clinical local control was 85%, and the overall survival rate was 95.5%. The disease-free survival rate was 85%. Four patients had dysuria, one patient had hematuria, five had diarrhea, and one experienced proctitis. There were no late serious complications. Our experience with this technique at KU shows promise, but "mature" results of outcome await additional follow-up.

A positive biopsy result 12 to 18 months or more after therapy clearly confers a much poorer prognosis, in terms of both local recurrence and increased risk of distant metastases (24, 32, 33, 87, 96, 100). For example, Scardino et al. reported 58% clinical local recurrence at 5 years and 82% at 10 years in those with positive biopsy results, whereas the 5- and 10-year recurrence risks were only 18% and 32%, respectively, in patients with negative biopsy results (95). Schellhammer et al. observed local failure in 47% of patients when biopsy results were positive versus 12% if biopsy results were negative (100). In our experience at KU (Fig. 20.4A), we similarly found a positive biopsy indicative of a poorer overall prognosis, in terms of both local recurrence and distant metastases (87, 96).

The morbidity and mortality of local failure after brachytherapy are not negligible. Kuban et al. reported that 20% of those with local failure after I-125 therapy required surgical intervention as treatment of local recurrence versus 8% of those undergoing external beam radiation therapy with local tumor recurrence (P < 0.05) (33). Although morbidity may be substantial, those who manifest relapse only with local failure may enjoy a relatively long survival. Schellhammer et al. observed an overall cancer-specific median survival of 87 months after local relapse in this select group (101).

There are reports from several groups comparing local tumor control with I-125 implants versus alternative therapy (31–33, 100, 102, 103). All found that I-125 produced either similar or inferior local control when compared with external beam and/or radical prostatectomy. Reddy et al., with a more than 9-year median follow-up, reported inferior local control rates with increasing complications for all stages if treated with I-

125 versus external beam (96). The Yale group reported inferior absolute local control rates for stages B and C when treated with I-125 implants compared with those treated in the same institution by external beam therapy (102). Schellhammer reported greater local failure in those treated with I-125 versus those treated with either external beam radiation or radical prostatectomy (97). Those treated with external beam or radical prostatectomy had similar local control rates, and the morbidity of local failure was not statistically different. Statistically significant increases in local tumor failure are observed in patients with stage B-2 and C disease as well as those with moderately or poorly differentiated histology if treated with I-125 versus external beam radiation therapy (33).

Overall, Relapse-Free, and Cause-Specific Survivals

Treatment results in prostate cancer are usually reported as overall, relapse-free, or cause-specific survival. Table 20.6 includes such results for a number of series employing brachytherapy for treatment of prostate cancer, including results for KU (although 10-year posttreatment results are not yet available). This type of table sometimes engenders a desire to compare results of brachytherapy with results of other treatment modalities for prostate cancer. This is unfortunately not possible, short of a large-scale phase III trial. All survival parameters shown in Table 20.6 are dramatically affected by patient age, tumor histology, stage, nodal status, patient comorbidity, and DNA ploidy. The effects of these variables on outcome are present in all large prostatectomy, external beam, and observation alone (11–16) reports of localized prostate cancer. These variables greatly affect the outcomes in brachytherapy series as well, and the particular mix of such variables is most likely not identical to series using other treatments.

Overall survival rates range from 70 to 90% at 5 years and from 50 to 86% at 10 years. Two brachytherapy series report 15-year survival figures ranging from 36 to 43%. Five-year survival data from observation-alone series (11, 13, 14, 106) show results within the 70 to 90% range as well. Fifteen-year overall survival results with placebo or observation alone are not as readily available, but published results are also generally within this range (11, 106). Surgical series (107–109) and external beam series (110–112) have 10- and 15-year overall survivorship that is not markedly different, given the significant variability in outcome introduced by prognostic factors. For example, the MSKCC series of 679 patients treated with I-125 had a projected actuarial local failure rate of 80% at 15 years, yet 15-year overall survival was 43% (consistent with surgery or external beam radiation therapy, given the fact that 48% had stage B2, 11% had stage B3, and 13% had stage C disease) (24). These and other data suggest that the natural history of the disease and the condition of the biologic host on survival may be the dominant factors that determine ultimate outcome.

Because of the importance of tumor and host biology, many have stressed the importance of either relapse-free or cause-specific survival results. Table 20.6 reveals that there is marked

Table 20.6.   Overall, Relapse-Free, and Cause-Specific Survival

AUTHOR	STAGE(S)	NO. OF PATIENTS	5-YR (%)	10-YR (%)	15-YR (%)
Overall survival[a]					
Gervasi (20)	T1–3; N0	359	90	62	36
Fuks (24)	T2–3; N0	679	85[b]	60[b]	43[b]
Carey (21)	T2–3; N0	41	79		
Iverson (19)	T0–2; N0	32	70		
DeLaney (102)	T1–3; N0/+	54	86	86[c]	
Boileau (104)	T1–3; N0/+	65	76		
Morton (31)	T1–3; N0/+	141	86	50	
KU (87, 96)	T1–3; N0/+	115	83		
Weyrich (105)	T2; N0/+	76	84	55	
Relapse-free survival					
Gervasi (20)	T1–3; N0	359	80	57	53
Carey (21)	T2–3; N0	41	69		
DeLaney (102)	T2–3; N0	43	86	86[c]	
Iverson (19)[d]	T0–2; N0	32	50		
Kuban (33)	T1; N0/+	11	100	90	
	T2a; N0/+	9	88	88	
	T2b; N0/+	68	77	50	
	T3; N0/+	32	50	14	
Boileau (104)	T1–3; N0/+	65	72		
Morton (31)	T1b; N0	9	88	88[c]	
	T2; N0/+	112	84	62[c]	
	T3; N0/+	20	38	30[c]	
KU (87–92, 95–98, 100, 102, 104)	T1–3; N0	92	78		
Weyrich (105)	T2; N0/+	76	66	50	
Cause-specific mortality[e]					
Lerner (83)[f]	T1b,2; N0	213	2	13	
	T3; N0	43	5	48	
Gervasi (20)[f]	T1–3; N0	359	2	17	30
Gutierrez (25)	T2; N0/+	26	0	15	
	T3; N0/+	93	32	43	
KU (87, 96)	T1–3; N0	92	11		

[a] Includes death from any cause.

[b] Refers to figures inferred from actuarial survival curve.

[c] 9-year survival.

[d] Implants performed by TRUS-directed transperineal technique.

[e] Actuarial risk of prostate cancer death.

[f] References 20 and 83 refer to the same Baylor data.

variation in relapse-free survival among different series. Relapse-free survival ranges from 38 to 100% at 5 years and from 14 to 90% at 10 years after treatment. Clearly, T stage and nodal status are highly important prognostic variables so far as relapse-free survival and cause-specific survival are concerned. Nevertheless, the numerous series with 60% or greater 10-year relapse-free survival, coupled with the Baylor series reporting 53% relapse-free survival at 15 years in all node-negative patients, clearly document the ability of brachytherapy to clinically control disease for extended periods in some patients with prostate cancer. These relapse-free survival figures seem better than those relapse-free survivals reported in observation-alone series.

Cause-specific mortality provides additional insight into potential therapeutic effects of brachytherapy. Ten-year cause-specific mortality in T1 to T2 disease is only in the range of 15%, while Gervasi et al. has reported a 30% 15-year cause-specific mortality rate (20). For patients with T3 tumors, the cause-specific mortality rate is higher, approximately 45% at 10 years. Several possible conclusions can be reached from this cause-specific mortality data.

1. Five-year cause-specific mortality grossly underestimates the true risk of cancer deaths in patients with prostate cancer. Follow-up for 10 or preferably 15 years is mandatory before drawing conclusions regarding efficacy of therapy.
2. Substantial cause-specific mortality is not observed until 10 to 15 years have elapsed since therapy. It is therefore only at this point that improved treatment efficacy could potentially be reflected in improved overall survival.

3. Whereas T3 tumors seem to be poorly treated on the basis of both the extremely high local failure rate and the nearly 50% 10-year cause-specific mortality rate, more favorable N0 tumors have only a 30% cause-specific mortality rate at 15 years. Although this is not negligible as a cause of death in node-negative patients, it appears that brachytherapy can provide many of these patients with significant delay in cancer death and clinical relapse.

Complications

Complication rates vary widely among different series. Such differences may be related to the technique of brachytherapy, the medical condition of the patients, and/or the possibility of underreporting of complications in some series (113). Patients undergoing open procedures have a greater rate of postoperative complications than those who undergo a closed transperineal implantation. The incidence of postoperative complications in those undergoing open procedures ranges from 5% to greater than 20% (21, 36, 105, 114–116). Postoperative deaths are rare (less than 1% overall). Postoperative complications related to transperineal implantation without pelvic surgery are usually 5% or less, with most complications being temporary and relatively easily managed clinically (17, 19, 49).

The overall incidence of late complications ranges from 0 (21) to 72% (36), with most late complication rates ranging from 10 to 25%. Rectal complications are generally less frequent than urinary or urethral treatment-related morbidity. Although rectal ulcerations and rectal fistulas have been frequently reported, they are relatively uncommon in most series. Several groups have reported rectal complications in less than 5% (17, 34, 41, 114), although most report mild to moderate, usually transient, rectal complications in 20 to 25% (36, 37, 49, 104, 115). Martinez et al. (37) have reported an extremely high incidence of severe rectal complications in a series of unfavorable, bulky stage C carcinomas treated by aggressive external beam plus IR-192 therapy. Others (116) have observed increased toxicity when large, bulky tumors have been implanted. Proctitis symptoms or more favorable rectal ulcers can be managed conservatively with stool softeners, analgesics, and steroid enemas. However, severe rectal ulceration should be treated by fecal diversion followed months later by evaluation of the suitability for reconstruction. If reconstruction is performed, resection of any fistulous tract(s) should precede the placement of a vascularized pedicle flap (117).

Urinary or urethral morbidity ranges from 10 to 37% (36, 105, 114–116). Blasko et al. (17), using I-125 implantation via transperineal ultrasound, have reported a significant influence of preexisting uropathy and/or transurethral resection of the prostate on subsequent urinary complications. Although incontinence occurred in 5% of patients overall, it was nonexistent in those without a prior TUR of the prostate. Urinary complications in those without preexisting uropathy and/or TUR were only 3% versus 20% in patients with preexisting problems. Additionally, they observed superficial urethral necrosis that consisted of a recurrence of severe irritative symptoms at 12 to 18 months following implant, with cystoscopic evidence of superficial mucoid necrotic debris in the proximal urethra. Although Blasko (74) reported only a 14% incidence of serious late complications using the TRUS-guided perineal technique, Iversen et al. (19) have reported a 42% incidence of serious late complications using similar technology. The MSKCC group reported rectal bleeding and/or ulceration in 47%, with some mild or greater urinary symptoms in 25 to 50% 1 year after CT-guided implantation (28). As with other implantation methods, it seems likely that increasing operator experience will produce diminished complication rates. Blasko and colleagues now attempt to avoid implantation of seeds extremely close to the urethra. Hopefully, this precaution will diminish the incidence of urethral complications (28, 29).

Although reports of sexual complications following implantation usually concentrate on impotence, a variety of other complications include ejaculatory pain, orchialgia, and hematospermia (28, 48, 72, 114, 116). Some investigators have the clinical impression that implantation results in a greater likelihood of potency when compared with external beam treatment (31). Unfortunately, several groups (36, 49, 115, 118) have reported impotency rates of 25 to 61%. The MSKCC group reported only a 7% incidence of impotency (114), which is substantially lower than the impotency rate of other treatment modalities. It is noteworthy, however, that 94% of patients who had sexual function evaluated were potent before implantation. KU rivaled MSKCC's impotency data (see previous section on KU data) with only 2 of 61 patients claiming impotency 12 to 18 months after therapy. These data compare to an expected incidence of potency of 77% in patients 50 to 70 years of age (114) and a 69% incidence of potency in the Stanford experience before external beam radiation therapy. Because quality of erection before therapy has been correlated strongly with subsequent potency (48), it is impossible to exclude selection bias as a major cause of apparently improved potency after implantation; at least two series have reported potency before implantation of 90% or more (114, 118). Furthermore, potency progressively diminishes from 1 to 3 years after implantation (115), similar to the potency profile after external beam radiation therapy (110). Thus, the initial optimistic reports of potency (MSKCC and KU) based on 15 months of follow-up may represent a select, more favorable group of patients in view of the high rate of potency before therapy. Thus, the long-term impotency rate associated with treatment may also be underestimated.

Implantation Costs

Large-scale cost comparisons that compare radical prostatectomy, brachytherapy implantation, and external beam therapy are unavailable. One small study reviewed 1984 costs for treatment of early-stage prostate cancer. Average cost was $14,400 for a radical prostatectomy, $5600 for external beam therapy using CPT-4 coding, and $12,000 for lymph node dissection and I-125 implantation. However, about 50% or more of the implantation cost was associated with the open pelvic procedure and ensuing hospital bill (119). Therefore, ultrasound-guided transperineal implantation, because it can be administered as a completely outpatient procedure (with appropriate isotope selection), may significantly diminish the cost of implantation. None of the cost analysis reports compares the longitudinal cost of therapy and morbidity management over a 1- to 2-year period after diagnosis.

SALVAGE THERAPY

Salvage prostatectomy is sometimes considered for patients who manifest a local failure as the only site of tumor recurrence after brachytherapy. Only a few series (120–122, 123) with short follow-up have reported results of salvage prostatectomy for localized brachytherapy failure. These series indicate that salvage prostatectomy, and even nerve-sparing prostatectomy, can be performed with reasonably low morbidity. Neerhut et al. (122) reported that rectal and other operative complications, although of substantial concern, decreased significantly as experience with this technique increased. Kenny and Ragde (120) reported no rectal injuries and only one urethral stricture associated with incontinence in 12 consecutive postbrachytherapy salvage prostatectomies.

It is not surprising that patients would have a greater risk of operative complications after radical radiation therapy in view of the significant fibrosis resulting from the radiation treatment. Extracapsular extension, seminal vesicle involvement, and involved surgical margins (particularly at the prostatic apex) were common in the Baylor experience (122). The greater surgical complications and the considerable incidence of pathologically involved surgical margins illustrate the importance of carefully selecting patients for this procedure. Although patients have only rarely received follow-up care for longer than 3 years, 8 of 12 patients in the Kenny and Ragde series (3 with concomitant orchiectomy) and 14 of 16 patients in the Neerhut et al. series were without evidence of tumor recurrence at the time of follow-up.

The use of prostate brachytherapy as salvage after external beam or prior brachytherapy local relapse has been reported by several groups (39, 43, 116, 124). These series uniformly show a significantly increased risk of complications, sometimes severe, when compared with brachytherapy series as a whole. Usually, follow-up is not reported or is extremely short. However, Wallner et al. (124) treated 13 patients with a second I-125 implantation after local recurrence alone. Local recurrence was noted in 6 of 13 patients, and distant metastasis was actuarially computed at 100% by 6 years. In view of both the markedly elevated toxicity of therapy and the very poor disease outcome reported thus far, brachytherapy is contraindicated as a salvage treatment.

Conclusion

There continues to be debate about the relative merits of one form of curative therapy over another (surgery versus external radiation versus brachytherapy) for localized prostate cancer. Because no prospective, randomized, controlled study has yet compared the various modalities, it is unknown which method of treatment, if any, is superior. Because some patients are simply not candidates for radical prostatectomy due to medical risk factors, at least some individuals will require radiation therapy for their disease if cure is to be one's goal (3). In the past, external beam has proven to be simpler to administer, has had lower initial risk, and may have delivered more uniform dosimetry to the entire prostate gland compared with interstitial brachytherapy. Current ultrasound-guided, transperineal placement may offer potential for improved results, although mature studies are not yet available for proper comparison. It is hoped that newer imaging modalities with greater uniformity of seed placement along with more sophisticated computer-aided calculations might ensure appropriate dosing and successful tumor cell kill using the brachytherapy technique.

REFERENCES

1. Hilaris BS. Historical review. In: Hilaris BS, ed. Handbook of interstitial brachytherapy. Acton: Publishing Sciences Group, 1975:13.
2. Janeway HH. In: Radium therapy in cancer at the Memorial Hospital New York. New York: Paul B. Hoeber, 1917.
3. Spaulding JT. Interstitial brachytherapy for prostatic carcinoma. In: Das S, Crawford D, eds. Current genitourinary cancer surgery. Philadelphia: Lea & Febiger, 1990:201.
4. Pasteau O, Degrais P. The radium treatment of cancer of the prostate. Arch Roentgen Ray (London) 1914;18:396.
5. Barringer BS. Radium in the treatment of carcinoma of the bladder and prostate. JAMA 1917;68:1227.
6. Carlton CE Jr, Dawoud F, Hudgins PT, et al. Irradiation treatment of carcinoma of the prostate: a preliminary report based on 8 years of experience. J Urol 1972;108:924.
7. Whitmore WF Jr, Hilaris BS, Grabstald H. Retropubic implantation of iodine-125 in the treatment of prostatic cancer. J Urol 1972;108:918.
8. Syed AMN, et al. Management of prostate carcinoma: combination of pelvic lymphadenectomy, temporary $^{Ir}192$ implantation, and external irradiation. Radiology 1983;149:829.
9. Ragde H, et al. Use of transrectal ultrasound in transperineal ^{125}Iodine seeding for prostate cancer methodology. J Endourol 1989;3:209.
10. Holm HH, Juul N, Pedersen JF, et al. Transperineal ^{125}Iodine seed implantation in prostatic cancer guided by transrectal ultrasonography. J Urol 1983;130:283.
11. Madsen PO, Graversen PH, Gasser TC, et al. Treatment of localized prostatic cancer; radical prostatectomy versus placebo: a 15-year follow-up. Scand J Urol Nephrol Suppl 1988;110:95.
12. Johansson JE, Andersson SO, Kraaz W, et al. Wait and see in early prostatic cancer: preliminary report of a 7-year material of 223 patients. Scand J Urol Nephrol Suppl 1988;110:77.
13. George NJR. Natural history of localised prostatic cancer managed by conservative therapy alone. Lancet 1988;1:494.

14. Barnes R, Hadley H, Axford P, et al. Conservative treatment of early carcinoma of prostate. Urology 1979;14:359.

15. Whitmore WF, Rosenberg S, Chopp R. Wait and see: experience with B1 lesions. In: Prostate cancer, part B: imaging techniques, radiotherapy, chemotherapy, and management issues. New York: Alan R. Liss, 1987:387.

16. Adolfsson J, et al. The prognostic value of modal deoxyribonucleic acid in low grade, low stage untreated prostate cancer. J Urol 1990;144:1404.

17. Blasko JC, Ragde H, Grimm PD. Transperineal ultrasound-guided implantation of the prostate: morbidity and complications. Scand J Urol Nephrol Suppl 1991;137:1.

18. Carter SSC, Torp-Pedersen ST, Holm HH. Ultrasound-guided implantation techniques in treatment of prostate cancer. Urol Clin North Am 1989;16:751.

19. Iversen P, et al. Ultrasonically guided [125]Iodine seed implantation with external radiation in management of localized prostatic carcinoma. Urology 1989;34:181.

20. Gervasi LA, et al. Prognostic significance of lymph nodal metastases in prostate cancer. J Urol 1989;142:332.

21. Carey PO, Lippert MC, Constable WC, et al. Combined gold seed implantation and external radiotherapy for stage B2 or C prostate cancer. J Urol 1988;139:989.

22. Fritjofsson A, Cederlund J, Norlen BJ, et al. Combined therapy with interstitial gold (198Au) implantation and external irradiation in the management of prostatic cancer. Scand J Urol Nephrol Suppl 1988;110:177.

23. Whitmore WF, et al. Interstitial irradiation using [125] seeds. In: Prostate cancer, part B: imaging techniques, radiotherapy, chemotherapy, and management issues. New York: Alan R. Liss, 1987:177.

24. Fuks Z, et al. The effect of local control on metastatic dissemination in carcinoma of the prostate: long-term results in patients treated with 125I implantation. Int J Radiat Oncol Biol Phys 1991;21:537.

25. Gutierrez AE, Merino OR. Adenocarcinoma of the prostate: radioactive gold seed implant plus external irradiation. Int J Radiat Oncol Biol Phys 1988;15:1317.

26. Flanigan RC, Gee WF, Patterson J, Lucas BA, et al. Complications associated with preoperative radiation therapy and iodine-125 brachytherapy for localized prostatic carcinoma. Urology 1983;22:123.

27. Green N, Treible D, Wallack H. Prostate cancer: post-irradiation incontinence. J Urol 1990;144:307.

28. Kleinberg L, Wallner K, Roy J, et al. Treatment-related symptoms during the first year following transperineal [125] prostate implantation. Int J Radiat Oncol Biol Phys 1994;28:985.

29. Mouli K, Sharifi R, Ray P, et al. Prostatorectal fistula associated with iodine-125 seed radiotherapy. J Urol 1983;129:387.

30. Whitmore WF, et al. Interstitial radiation: short-term palliation or curative therapy? Urology 1985;25(Suppl):24.

31. Morton JD, Peschel RE. Iodine-125 implants versus external beam therapy for stages A2, B, and C prostate cancer. Int J Radiat Oncol Biol Phys 1988;14:1153.

32. Schellhammer PF, et al. Morbidity and mortality of local failure after definitive therapy for prostate cancer. J Urol 1989;141:567.

33. Kuban DA, El-Mahdi AM, Schellhammer, PF. [125] interstitial implantation for prostate cancer. Cancer 1989;63:2415.

34. Giles GM, Brady LW. [125]Iodine implantation after lymphadenectomy in early carcinoma of the prostate. Int J Radiat Oncol Biol Phys 1986;12:2117.

35. Hilar BS, Whitmore WF, Batata M. Endoradiotherapy for cancer of the prostate. Proceedings of the International Endourotherapy Symposium, 1981:115.

36. Bosch PC, et al. Preliminary observations on the results of combined temporary [192]Iridium implantation and external beam irradiation for carcinoma of the prostate. J Urol 1986;135:722.

37. Martinez A, et al. Improved pathologic local control and survival for patients with bulky stage C prostate cancer treated by P.L.A. continuous R.A.-L.D.R.-[Ir]192. Mupit implant and external beam Abstract. Presented at symposium on "Prostrate Cancer: The role of interstitial implantation.", Seattle, WA, 1991.

38. Klein FA, Ali MM, Marks SE, et al. Bilateral pelvic lymphadenectomy, iridium 192 template, and external beam therapy for localized prostatic carcinoma: complications and results. South Med J 1988;1:27.

39. Brindle JS, et al. Acute toxicity and preliminary therapeutic results of pelvic lymphadenectomy combined with transperineal interstitial implantation of 192IR and external beam radiotherapy for locally advanced prostate cancer. Urology 1985;25:233.

40. Brindle JS, et al. Pelvic lymphadenectomy and transperineal interstitial implantation of [Ir]192 combined with external beam radiotherapy for bulky stage C prostatic carcinoma. Int J Radiat Oncol Biol Phys 1989;17:1063.

41. Clubb BS, Summers JL. Combined iridium-192 interstitial and external beam radiation therapy for the treatment of prostatic cancer. Cancer Treat Rep 1984;68:1027.

42. Kumar PP, et al. Transperineal [125]Iodine endocurietherapy of prostate cancer. Am J Clin Oncol 1988;11:479.

43. Kumar PP, Good RR, Bartone FF. Iodine[125] interstitial irradiation for localized prostate cancer. J Natl Med Assoc 1990;82:181.

44. Nori D, et al. Precision transperineal brachytherapy in the treatment of early prostate cancer. Endocurietherapy/Hyperthermia Oncol 1990;6:119.

45. Crusinberry RA, Kramolowsky EV, Loening SA. Percutaneous transperineal placement of gold 198 seeds for treatment of carcinoma of the prostate. Prostate 1987;11:59.

46. Greenburg S, Petersen J, Hansen-Peters I, et al. Interstitially implanted [125] for prostate cancer using transrectal ultrasound. Oncol Nurs Forum 1990;17:849.

47. Holm HH, Myschetzky P, Nielsen L, et al. An ultrasonic multipurpose/multiplane endoprobe. Acta Radiol 1990;31:630.

48. Kaye KW. Improved technique for prostate seed implantation: combined ultrasound and fluoroscopic guidance. Presented at Prostate symposium, Prostate cancer: the role of interstitial implantation, Seattle WA. 1991;6:21.

49. Bertermann H, et al. Iridium-192: five years experiences with interstitial high dose brachy and external teletherapy in locally confined prostate cancer. Presented at Prostate symposium, Prostate cancer: the role of interstitial implantation, Seattle, WA. 1991;6:21.

50. Mate TP, et al. Remote high-dose rate afterloading brachytherapy of the prostate: a preliminary report. Presented at 1991 meeting of American Urological Association in Toronto, Canada. Presented at Prostate symposium, Prostate cancer: the role of interstitial implantation, Seattle, WA. 1991;6:21. Abstract.

51. Porter AT, Scrimger JW, Pocha JS. Remote interstitial afterloading in cancer of the prostate: preliminary experience with the microselectron. Int J Radiat Oncol Biol Phys 1988; 14:571.

52. Porter AT, Scrimger JW. Remote afterloading in prostatic cancer. Prog Clin Biol Res 1989;303:219.

53. Charyulu KKN. Transperineal interstitial implantation of prostate cancer: a new method. Int J Radiat Oncol Biol Phys 1980;6:1261.

54. Goffinet DR. 192 Ir removable transperineal interstitial hyperthermia prostate implants. Presented at Prostate symposium, Prostate cancer: the role of interstitial implantation, Seattle, WA. 1991;6:21.

55. Harada T, Kigure T, Etori K, et al. Remote afterloading transurethral radiotherapy for prostatic cancer. Urol Int 1990; 45:41.

56. Takahashi M, Okada K, Shibamoto Y, et al. Int J Radiat Oncol Biol Phys 1985;11:147.

57. Anderson L, Ling C. Radiobiophysical considerations in brachytherapy: temporal and spatial aspects. Presented at Prostate symposium, Prostate cancer: the role of interstitial implantation, Seattle, WA. 91;6:21. Abstract.

58. Fowler J. The radiobiology of brachytherapy: dose rate effects of iodine palladium and iridium. Presented at Prostate symposium, Prostate cancer: The role of interstitial implantation, Seattle, WA. 1991;6:21.

59. Mitchell JB, Bedford JS, Bailey SM. Dose-rate effects on the cell cycle and survival of S3 HeLa and V79 Cells. Radiat Res 1979;79:520.

60. Anderson L, Aubery R. Computerized dosimetry for 125I prostate implants. In: Hilaris BS, Batata MA, eds. Brachytherapy oncology. New York: Memorial Sloan-Kettering Cancer Center, 1983:57.

61. Hilaris B, Nori D, Anderson L. Atlas of brachytherapy. New York: Macmillan, 1988:70.

62. Hilaris B, Batata M. Brachytherapy techniques. In: Hilaris B, Batata M, eds. Brachytherapy oncology. New York: Memorial Sloan-Kettering Cancer Center, 1983:41.

63. Anderson LL. Clinical dosimetry for [125] permanent implants. Proceedings of the 23rd annual meeting of the American Society of Therapeutic Radiologists, 1981, Miami, FL.

64. Hilaris B, et al. 125I implantation of the prostate: dose-response considerations. Front Radiat Ther Oncol 1978;12:82.

65. Rao G, Kan P, Howells R. Interstitial volume implants with [125] seeds. Int J Radiat Oncol Biol Phys 1981;7:431.

66. Hastak S, Gammelgaard J, Holm H. Transrectal ultrasonic volume determination of the prostate: a preoperative and postoperative study. J Urol 1982;127:1115.

67. Blasko J, Radge H, Schumacher D. Transperineal percutaneous iodine-125 implantation for prostatic carcinoma using transrectal ultrasound and template guidance. Endocurietherapy/Hyperthermia Oncol 1987;3:131.

68. Steinfeld A, Donahue B, Plaine L. Pulmonary embolization of iodine-125 seeds following prostate implantation. Urology 1991;37:149.

69. Sommerkamp H, Rupprecht M, Wannenmacher M. Seed loss in interstitial radiotherapy of prostatic carcinoma with [125]. Int J Radiat Oncol Biol Phys 1988;14:389, 392.

70. Vijverberg PLM, Blank LECM, Dabhoiwala NF, et al. Analysis of biopsy findings and implant quality following ultrasonically-guided [125] implantation for localised prostatic carcinoma. Br J Urol. 1993;72:470.

71. Sogani P, et al. Carcinoma of the prostate: treatment with pelvic lymphadenectomy and iodine-125 implants. Clin Bull 1979;9:24.

72. Kandzari S, Belis J, Kim J-C, et al. Clinical results of early stage prostatic cancer treated by pelvic lymphadenectomy and [125]Iodine implants. J Urol 1982;127:923.

73. Gore R, Moss A. Value of computed tomography in interstitial 125I brachytherapy of prostatic carcinoma. Radiology 1983;146:453.

74. Blasko JC. Transperineal ultrasound guided permanent implantation for prostate carcinoma: results of the Seattle series. Presented at Prostate symposium, Prostate cancer; the of interstitial implantation, Seattle, WA. 1991;6:21.

75. Roy JN, Wallner KE, Harrington PJ, et al. A CT-Based evaluation method for permanent implants: application to prostate. Int J Radiat Oncol Biol Phys 1993;26:163.

76. Dale R. The application of the linear-quadratic dose-effect equation to fractionated and protracted radiotherapy. Br J Radiol 1985;58:515.

77. Fowler J. The linear-quadratic formula and progress in fractionated radiotherapy. Br J Radiol 1989;62:679.

78. Dale R. Radiobiological assessment of permanent implants using tumour repopulation factors in the linear-quadratic model. Br J Radiol 1989;62:241.

79. Nias A. Protracted radiation. In: An introduction to radiobiology. West Sussex, England: John Wiley & Sons, 1990.

80. Hall E. Lethal, potentially lethal, and sublethal radiation damage, and the dose-rate effect. In: Radiobiology for the radiologist. Philadelphia: Harper & Row, 1978.

81. Marchese M, Hall E. Encapsulated iodine-125 in radiation oncology. Am J Clin Oncol 1984;7:613.

82. Trott KR, Kummermehr J. What is known about tumour proliferation rates to choose between accelerated fractionation or hyperfractionation. J Radiol Ther Oncol 1985;3:1.

83. Lerner S, Seale-Hawkins C, Carlton C, et al. The risk of dying of prostate cancer in patients with clinically localized disease. J Urol 1991;146:1040.

84. Anderson L. Spacing nomograph for interstitial implants of 125I seeds. Med Phys 1976;3:48.

85. Noble MJ, Lee SH, Mebust WK. Role of the matrix in modifying the growth of prostatic epithelial cells in vitro. Cleve Clin Q 1984;51:411.

86. Jones LW, Ohnuki Y, Narayan KS, et al. Growth of cultured cells following radiation for prostatic cancer. Proceedings of the AUA. 1982:132.

87. Noble MJ, Lee SH, Mebust WK, et al. Cell culture viability testing for radiation treated prostatic carcinoma. J Urol 1988; 139:191. Abstract.

88. Musselman PW, Tubbs R, Connelly RW, et al. Biological

significance of prostatic carcinoma after definitive radiation therapy. J Urol 1987;137:114. Abstract.

89. Schellhammer PF, Ladaga LE, El-Mahdi A. Histological characteristics of prostatic biopsies after [125]Iodine implantation. J Urol 1980;123:700.

90. Carlton CE, Jr. Scardino PT. Combined interstitial and external irradiation for prostatic cancer. In: Prostate cancer, part B: imaging techniques, radiotherapy, chemotherapy, and management issues. New York: Alan R. Liss, 1987:141.

91. Weaver RP, Noble MJ, Weigel JW. Correlation of ultrasound guided and digitally directed transrectal biopsies of palpable prostatic abnormalities. J Urol 1991;145:516.

92. Doornbos JF, Hussey DH, Robinson RA, et al. Results of radical perineal prostatectomy with adjuvant brachytherapy. Radiology 1992;184:333.

93. Syed AM, Puthawala A, Austin P, et al. Temporary iridium-192 implant in the management of carcinoma of the prostate. Cancer 1992;69:2515.

94. Reddy EK, Krishnan L, Mebust W, et al. Iridium-192 template therapy in localized prostate cancer. Endocurietherapy/Hyperthermia Oncol 1994;10:125.

95. Scardino PT, et al. The prognostic significance of post-irradiation biopsy results in patients with prostatic cancer. J Urol 1985;135:510.

96. Reddy EK, Mebust WK, Weigel JW, et al. Iodine-125 implantation in localized prostatic cancer. Endocurietherapy/ Hyperthermia Oncol 1990;6:239–244.

97. Schellhammer PF. Radical prostatectomy for carcinoma of the prostate and 15 year analysis of survival and local control: part 2. J Urol 1986;135:247. Abstract.

98. Lytton B, Schiff M, Shonk CR. Treatment of early stage prostatic cancer by implantation of iodine-125 seeds. Surg Clin North Am 1980;60:1215.

99. Lee F, et al. Transrectal ultrasound in the diagnosis and staging of local disease after [125]125 seed implantation for prostate cancer. Int J Radiat Oncol Biol Phys 1988;15:1453.

100. Schellhammer PF, et al. Prostate biopsy after definitive treatment by interstitial [125]Iodine implant or external beam radiation therapy. J Urol 1986;137:897.

101. Schellhammer PIF, Kuban DA, El-Mahdi AM. Treatment of clinical local failure after radiation therapy for prostate carcinoma. J Urol 1993;150:1851.

102. DeLaney TF, et al. Preoperative irradiation, lymphadenectomy, and [125]Iodine implantation for patients with localized carcinoma of the prostate. Int J Radiat Oncol Biol Phys 1986;12:1779.

103. Shipley WU, et al. Radiation therapy for localized prostate carcinoma: experience at the Massachusetts General Hospital (1973–1981). NCI Monogr 1988;7:67.

104. Boileau MA, et al. Interstitial gold and external beam irradiation for prostate cancer. J Urol 1988;139:985.

105. Weyrich TP, Kandzari SJ, Jain PR. Iodine-125 seed implants for prostatic carcinoma; five and ten year follow-up. Urology 1993;41:122.

106. Graversen PH, et al. Radical prostatectomy versus expectant primary treatment in stages I and II prostatic cancer. Urology 1990;36:493.

107. Schroeder FH, Belt E. Carcinoma of the prostate: a study of 213 patients with stage C tumors treated by total perineal prostatectomy. J Urol 1975;114:257.

108. Gibbons RP. Total prostatectomy for clinically localized prostate cancer: long-term surgical results and current morbidity. NCI Monogr 1988;7:123.

109. Lepor H, Walsh PC. Long-term results of radical prostatectomy in clinically localized prostate cancer: experience at The Johns Hopkins Hospital. NCI Monogr 1988;7:117.

110. Bagshaw MA, Cox RS, Ray GR. Status of radiation treatment of prostate cancer at Stanford University. NCI Monogr 1988; 7:47.

111. Perez CA, et al. Definitive radiation therapy in carcinoma of the prostate localized to the pelvis: experience at the MallincKrodt Institute of Radiology. NCI Monogr 1988;7: 85.

112. Zagars GK, von Eschenbach A, Johnson DE, et al. Stage C adenocarcinoma of the prostate: an analysis of 551 patients treated with external beam radiation. Cancer 1987;7:1489.

113. Parliament M, Danjoux C, Clayton T. Is cancer treatment toxicity accurately reported? Int J Radiat Oncol Biol Phys 1985;11:603.

114. Fowler JE, Barzell W, Hilaris BS, et al. Complications of [125]Iodine implantation and pelvic lymphadenectomy in the treatment of prostatic cancer. J Urol 1979;121:447.

115. Schellhammer PF, El-Mahdi AM. Pelvic complications after definitive treatment of prostate cancer by interstitial or external beam radiation. Urology 1983;21:451.

116. Cumes DM, Goffinet DR, Martinez A, et al. Complications of [125]Iodine implantation and pelvic lymphadenectomy for prostatic cancer with special reference to patients who had failed external beam therapy as their initial mode of therapy. J Urol 1981;126:620.

117. Jordan GH, et al. Major rectal complications following interstitial implantation of iodine-125 for carcinoma of the prostate. J Urol 1985;134:1212.

118. Flanigan RC, et al. Complications associated with preoperative radiation therapy and iodine-125 brachytherapy for localized prostatic carcinoma. Urology 1983;22:123.

119. Hanks GE, Dunlap KA. Comparison of the cost of various treatment methods for early cancer of the prostate. Int J Radiat Oncol Biol Phys 1986;12:1879.

120. Kenny G, Ragde H. Salvage prostatectomy. Presented at the Prostate symposium, Prostate cancer: the role of interstitial implantation, Seattle, WA. 1991;6:21. Abstract.

121. Thompson IM, Rounder JB, Spence CR, et al. Salvage radical prostatectomy for adenocarcinoma of the prostate. Cancer 1988;61:1464.

122. Neerhut GJ, Wheeler T, Cantini M, et al. Salvage radical prostatectomy for radiorecurrent adenocarcinoma of the prostate. J Urol 1988;140:544.

123. Mador DR, Huben RP, Wajsman Z, et al. Salvage surgery following radical radiotherapy for adenocarcinoma of the prostate. J Urol 1985;133:58.

124. Wallner KE, et al. [125]Iodine reimplantation for locally progressive prostatic carcinoma. J Urol 1990;144:704.

21

Cryosurgical Ablation of the Prostate

An Alternative for the Management of Localized Prostate Cancer

Jeffrey K. Cohen, Barry A. Shuman, Ralph J. Miller, Jr., and Lori Merlotti

Adenocarcinoma of the prostate is the most common malignant tumor in adult men. It is estimated that in 1995, 244,000 new cases of adenocarcinoma of the prostate will be diagnosed (1). Prevalence studies estimate that well over 50% of men surviving past the eighth decade will have histologic evidence of prostate cancer (2, 3). Improved tools for screening and detecting prostate cancer (prostate-specific antigen [PSA] and transrectal ultrasound), increased media attention, and a rapidly expanding elderly sector of the population have led to this increase in the incidence of the disease.

Treatment options abound. Patients with localized prostate cancer can elect to undergo extirpative surgery (perineal or retropubic radical prostatectomy), radiation therapy (external beam, brachytherapy, or conformational proton beam therapy), androgen ADT, or expectant management (observation until progression, at which point androgen deprivation would be instituted). Despite the variety of treatment options, there are several specific circumstances in which these patients are without respectable alternatives. It is specifically for these circumstances that investigators reexamined cryosurgical techniques for the eradication of this disease. Furthermore, the reality is that no one treatment option will be acceptable for every stage, grade, and clinical presentation. To highlight these specific patient groups, one must critically examine the standard forms of therapy for prostate cancer.

Radical prostatectomy remains the treatment of choice for clinically localized prostate cancer. Survival statistics after radical prostatectomy for organ-confined cancer are excellent and provide reproducible 10- and 15-year data (4, 5). Long-term morbidity (mainly incontinence and impotence) after this procedure has improved dramatically since introducing the anatomic approach to radical prostatectomy. Careful review of studies, however, reveals significant improvement in only the younger patient (6). Although survival statistics for the older patient after radical prostatectomy are favorable, no control population has been evaluated and long-term complications can significantly alter a patient's quality of life (7).

Recent publications have revealed several groups of patients for whom radical prostatectomy may not be beneficial. Histologic examination of radical prostatectomy specimens has revealed that capsular penetration and positive surgical margins are both closely correlated with clinical stage (T2b and T3) and cancer volume (greater than 4 cc) (8, 9). These locally extensive cancers portend an unfavorable prognosis following radical prostatectomy; this is thought to be due to our inability to remove tissue beyond the surgical resection margin (5). Additionally, radical prostatectomy (salvage) following definitive radiation therapy for prostate cancer has considerable complications. These consist of hemorrhage, positive surgical margins, and incontinence rates approaching 60% (10, 11). Because of this, salvage prostatectomy is generally reserved as a last resort. In addition, there are patients who, because of age or medical comorbidities, are not suitable candidates for radical surgery yet still have a reasonable life expectancy; hence, the need for definitive treatment.

Radiation therapy remains a standard of care in the definitive treatment of localized prostate cancer. The theoretical advantages of using radiation therapy focus on lower rates of complications (due to its noninvasiveness) and the ability to treat locally extensive disease more aggressively than could surgical resection alone. Long-term estimates, however, reveal that as little as 20% of patients are actually cured by this modality, based on PSA data (12). Retrospective series examining prostatic biopsy specimens 18 to 24 months after definitive radiation therapy reveal that 51 to 90% of patients have residual adenocarcinoma (13–16). Careful review of these reports indicates that those patients with extensive local lesions (stage C) and those with pretreatment PSA values greater than 10 ng/mL benefit only marginally from the treatment (17). Despite these shortcomings, 10-year survival statistics are statistically equal to those from radical prostatectomy (possibly a reflection of non–cancer-specific mortality) (18). Radiation therapy remains an alternative for patients who prefer a nonsurgical treatment or patients who are older with other medical comorbidities and demand or desire definitive therapy.

The use of ADT results in a systemic response. This therapy is rarely curative but will induce a remission from prostate cancer. The duration of this remission is variable, lasting for many years if treatment is instituted early. ADT is not recommended as a monotherapy for those who are younger and seeking a cure from the disease. The complications from this treatment (hot flashes, lost libido, and impotence) are often unacceptable.

Observation, or watchful waiting, has recently received increasing attention in the urologic literature. Several centers, mainly in Europe, have analyzed watchful waiting as a primary means of therapy for localized adenocarcinoma. This originated because of the constraints in their health-care delivery system and the significant discrepancy between the prevalence and perceived morbidity/mortality rates in their populations. These published series report death rates from untreated prostate cancer that are generally less than 10% (19, 20). The conclusions are weakened due to a significant percentage of patients receiving ADT, the fact that the cohorts contained a large percentage of less extensive and aggressive tumors, and the absence of a control interventional group undergoing surgery or radiation therapy. Because of the uncertainties, watchful waiting has been recommended only for patients older than 65 years of age with small (less than 1 cc), well-differentiated (Gleason's score, 2 to 4) tumors (21). Even in such circumstances, the mental stress of living with an untreated malignancy is often too great, resulting in patients subsequently opting for some form of treatment.

These inadequacies of the current therapeutic regimens prompted a reexamination of cryotherapy for the treatment of prostate cancer. Patients in whom radiation therapy has failed have no reasonable alternative but ADT. Patients with locally extensive cancers must accept high risks of treatment failure and the risks of complications with radical prostatectomy. Their chances of eradicating the cancer are low with radiation therapy. Finally, due to widespread screening, there is an increasing segment of the population believed to be too old to undergo definitive surgery, yet these patients demand treatment.

CYROSURGERY: HISTORICAL PERSPECTIVE AND MECHANISM OF ACTION

It is known that bringing tissues rapidly to subzero temperature will induce cell death and necrosis. Cell death is an effect of the ice formation and a spectrum of events secondary to hypothermia (22). Hypothermia begins the cascade of injury marked by decreased intracellular energy stores and a breakdown in the physical and physiologic functions of the cellular membrane. Rapid hypothermia leads to intracellular dehydration and cell shrinkage. When the temperature drops below $-4°C$, ice crystals form in the extracellular space and eventually cross the cell membrane gap junctions, leading to intracellular ice, membrane rupture, and cell death. On completion of the freezing process, microscopic ice crystals coalesce into sheets of ice, cre-

ating shearing forces accounting for additional destruction. Any viable cells remaining are suddenly faced with a significantly hypotonic environment (from the thawing of pure water), resulting in a sudden influx of free water by osmotic forces (membrane function remains inactivated). This causes cell swelling, rupture, and death. The freezing process causes obstruction of the small vasculature, which leads to thrombosis. This final injury causes tissue anoxia and completes the cytotoxic cascade of events from cryotherapy.

Tissue absorption after cryotherapy can take up to 3 months and is marked initially by inflammation and removal of cellular debris and later by deposition of collagen and the creation of organized scar tissue. Cryodestruction of prostatic tissue leads to increased serum levels of PSA, acid phosphatase, and creatinine phosphokinase (CPK, both MB and MM fractions). Histologically aberrant glands can be seen after cryosurgical ablation of the prostate (CSAP) and include basal cell hyperplasia, squamous cell metaplasia, and transitional cell metaplasia (23). Studies have shown that nerve and muscle cells as well as fibroblasts have the capacity to regenerate after cryodestruction. The recovery of neural function depends on the integrity of the neural sheath and may take 6 to 12 months (24).

Cryotherapeutic techniques hold several advantages over conventional surgery. They are less invasive, are associated with a shorter hospital stay, and are well tolerated by radiated tissues. They can also be applied percutaneously. All these factors may lead to a decrease in morbidity.

CSAP as it is applied today is a modification of an old concept. It is well established that bringing tissue to subzero temperatures would induce cell death and necrosis. Gondor and Soanes initially applied cryotherapeutic techniques in the 1960s to eradicate locally obstructive prostatic tissue (25). Liquid nitrogen was poured through a urethral probe, and the ice formation was monitored through digital palpation. The central gland subsequently became necrotic and sloughed, leaving behind a cavitated, nonobstructing prostate. However, complications ensued from this poorly controlled freezing process. Rectourethral fistulae resulted from transmural rectal freezing. Additionally, the prostatic urethra invariably became necrotic, allowing the necrotic prostatic parenchyma to slough into the urinary stream, frequently requiring bladder irrigation and prolonged urethral catheterization while the prostate reepithelialized.

In the 1970s, urologists at the University of Iowa examined the cryodestructive capabilities on prostate cancers (26). In attempts to improve the ability to monitor the freezing process, they performed cryosurgery through a perineal incision. After the rectum was fully mobilized, the prostate was frozen under direct vision with a paddle-shaped cryoprobe applied to the posterior surface of the prostate. The incidence of rectal injury dropped; however, cutaneous fistulae developed and sloughing continued to be a significant problem. These complications led to the demise of CSAP as a clinical alternative to either radical prostatectomy or radiation therapy. Retrospective examination of the Iowa experience, however, revealed that 10-year survival from CSAP was similar to that in contemporary surgical and radiation therapy series (27). Interest in CSAP waned due to the associated complications and not from the results as measured by survival, digital rectal examination (DRE), or acid phosphatase.

The modern era of CSAP was made possible by the advent of transrectal ultrasound. Ultrasound surveillance of cryosurgical ablation of isolated hepatic tumors revealed that the ice formation created a characteristic array of images (28). Due to the ultrasonically impenetrable nature of ice crystals, sound waves reflect off the frozen/nonfrozen interface and appear on transrectal ultrasound as an advancing hyperechoic line with an anechoic shadow behind (29). Histologic studies confirmed a precise correlation of cell death and necrosis to this ultrasonically visualized lesion (30). It is this characteristic imaging that allows the surgeon to aggressively yet safely freeze the prostate. Once the preliminary studies were complete (31), attention was then directed toward developing a technique to freeze the prostate, which would avoid the pitfalls and shortcomings of the previous attempts. The most notable issues to address included fistulization from a perineal incision and urethral sloughing.

To lessen the risks of fistulization, two separate issues arose. Initially, fistulization occurred to the rectum. This came from freezing through the rectum. With ultrasound guidance, the growth of the iceball could be stopped on reaching the anterior rectal wall. Stopping the treatment prematurely would leave a portion of the prostate (peripheral zone) susceptible to inadequate freezing. This issue was addressed by the development of a new liquid nitrogen delivery system. This new system (Accuprobe; Cryomedical Sciences, Rockville, MD) provided supercooled, pressurized liquid nitrogen for the procedure that could be delivered through thin (3-mm) probes. This new technology prevented liquid nitrogen from entering a gas phase during circulation through the probes, hence enhancing efficiency. This greater efficiency translates into much colder temperatures within the ice and a much steeper drop in temperature from the periphery to the probe in the core of the iceball. With this system, a smaller margin of normal tissue than was previously possible needs to be incorporated within the iceball to assure adequate cytotoxic temperatures within the prostate. This system eliminated the need to freeze into the rectum to achieve cytotoxic temperatures in the peripheral zone of the prostate. Cutaneous fistulae encountered in the Iowa experience were a result of the perineal incision. Percutaneous access techniques similar to the placement of a percutaneous nephrostomy were modified to allow the placement of access ports and probes transperineally directly into the prostate.

The issue of urethral sloughing was addressed by the concept of urethral warming. A catheter placed in the urethra circulates warm saline and prevents cryodestruction of the prostatic urothelium. Viable urothelium is surrounded by necrotic prostatic parenchyma that involutes, changing to scar tissue. The initial concept was tested by warm saline being delivered transurethrally via a flexible cystoscope placed at the level of the external sphincter and exiting from a suprapubic tube. This model

system, although cumbersome, prevented urethral sloughing in the first eight patients studied (32). Subsequently, several self-contained, closed-loop catheter systems have been designed to provide similar effects with less difficulty.

With the areas of previous difficulty addressed by technical modifications, a pilot study was undertaken at Allegheny General Hospital, Medical College of Pennsylvania. Beginning in June 1990, eight procedures were completed. Each procedure was well tolerated. Follow-up biopsy specimens of the treated areas revealed predominantly scar and necrosis (33). This provided the impetus to embark on a formal study of the efficacy of CSAP for the treatment of prostate cancer. The application of CSAP continues to evolve as new issues arise. The following are the indications, techniques, and results from the studies at Allegheny General Hospital.

PATIENT SELECTION AND PROTOCOL

All patients with biopsy-proven adenocarcinoma of the prostate are eligible for consideration. Contraindications to the procedure include active genitourinary infection (specifically, acute prostatitis), the presence of an uncontrollable bleeding disorder, a prostate larger than 65 g on transrectal ultrasound volumetric analysis (these patients would require downsizing by androgen deprivation before therapy), and the inability to grant informed consent.

Preoperative requirements for CSAP include a recent PSA, prostate acid phosphatase (PAP), computed tomography or magnetic resonance imaging scan of the abdomen and pelvis, and a radionucleotide bone scan. Our assessment includes review of the above studies and of the histologic slides. Each patient is examined to assess clinical stage. We do not routinely perform staging biopsies in patients with a preexisting diagnosis of prostate cancer. All patients then participate in a group discussion about the issues of prostate cancer management, the history behind cryosurgery, what to expect from the procedure, complications, and results to date. CSAP is identified as being an investigational alternative to the standards of care, surgery, and radiation. The group discussion format is used to enable patients to glean information from questions raised by others. All patients are entered into investigational protocols. As per the protocol (1990), preoperative assessment of nodal status is only recommended in patients with a PSA level greater than 10 ng/mL, no previous ADT (which would make the histologic results unreliable), and age younger than 70 years.

Postoperative surveillance consists of performing a DRE, measuring PSA levels, and performing systematic prostatic needle biopsies. All patients are instructed to have their PSA levels measured at 6 and 12 weeks, then every 3 months thereafter. Accompanying each 3-month evaluation, a DRE and a general survey for complications are done. Transrectal ultrasound-guided prostate biopsies are performed at 3 and 24 months. Biopsy between these times is optional and performed as indicated by an abnormal DRE, a rising PSA level, or any other specific concerns. Protocol biopsies involve a total of 11 cores (sextant samples from the prostate, proximal seminal and neurovascular bundle bilaterally, and the site of the entrance of the ejaculatory duct into the prostate).

If any 1 of the 11 cores contains evidence of persistent or recurrent adenocarcinoma, local treatment failure is considered to have occurred. A consistently rising PSA in the face of two consecutive sets of negative prostatic biopsy results is considered to be distant failure; thus, ADT is initiated. Any patient with local failure is offered repeat treatment with CSAP or can elect radiation therapy, surgical therapy, ADT, or watchful waiting.

METHODS

All patients are admitted through the same-day surgical unit. Preoperative preparation consists of a phospha-soda (Fleet; Lynchburg, VA) enema for rectal debulking and oral antibiotics (ciprofloxacin 500 mg by mouth twice a day for three doses and metronidazole 750 mg by mouth on arrival at the hospital). Patients are counseled about anesthesia, and either a spinal or general anesthetic is chosen.

The procedure can be performed in any operating room. Once anesthetized, the patient is placed in a relaxed dorsal lithotomy position. The lower abdomen and perineum are shaved, prepared, and draped as for a suprapubic tube placement. Cystoscopy is performed, and a suprapubic tube is placed into the dome of the bladder. We have chosen a 10.4 Fr Cook Cope Loop (Cook Urological, Spencer, IN) due to its ease of insertion, its self-retaining characteristics, and the enhanced patient comfort due to the curved tip design. On cystoscopic examination, any bladder lesions, urethral obstructive lesions, or median lobe prostatic tissue are noted; these may require further treatment postoperatively. The cystoscope is removed, and a urethral warming catheter is inserted. The catheter is perfused with body temperature saline to maintain the viability of the urethra.

Transrectal ultrasound is then performed. We recommend performing CSAP with a biplanar ultrasound probe. This is crucial to allow three-dimensional surveillance of the freezing process. Additionally, the sagittal or longitudinal scanner must be a linear array crystal (which for mechanical reasons must also be piezoelectric). The linear array sagittal transducer allows significantly more separation of the structures posterior to the prostate without the volume averaging and refractory artifacts commonly seen with mechanical sector scanning transducers. Routine volumetric analysis is performed using the formula (L × W × H) × 0.52. All hypoechoic areas are noted, and any areas of suspected capsular penetration are carefully documented.

We started using color flow Doppler (CFD) ultrasound to monitor CSAP in March 1994. CFD ultrasound graphically depicts flow through blood vessels as shades of blue or red depending on the direction of flow. Graphic analysis of the vessels can distinguish arterial and venous waveforms. The neurovascular bundle flow and location are documented as well as any aberrant vessels leading directly into the prostate. This

information is used to detect areas of increased vascularity, areas that would act as heat sinks to prevent adequate freezing. We can then modify our cryoprobe placement so that we encompass and ablate these vessels in the iceball and enhance the cytotoxic effects of the cryotherapy. The vascular supply to the prostate is variable and not in the same position for each patient.

Next, the probe access ports are placed. Each port is placed similarly and begins with a percutaneous puncture of the perineum. With a diamond-dipped needle placed in a needle guide, the transrectal ultrasound (transverse transducer) is used to guide the needle into the appropriate position in the prostate. It is then advanced under visualization by the sagittal transducer to the cephalad capsule of the prostate. A stiffened 0.038 J-tipped guide wire is placed, and the needle is removed. A modified Amplatz dilator and Teflon introducer sheath are then advanced over the wire, again using ultrasound visualization. Once in position, the dilator and wire are removed. The sheath is irrigated with saline to remove air and debris (which would interfere with freezing) and improve ultrasound visualization of the tract. All probe sites are subsequently placed.

The normal geometry of the iceball that forms at the probe tip is integral to the selection of probe sites. The iceballs generated by the Accuprobe system are symmetric and reproducible. The ice begins at the probe tip (5 mm growth past the tip in the completed iceball) and extends up the shaft for a total length of 4 cm; recently designed probes for this system are more efficient and freeze an average length of 5 cm. The maximum radius of the iceball is 2 cm, with the final iceball being egg shaped. In a multiple probe arrangement, iceballs augment the performance of any adjacent probes. Any recesses between adjacent iceballs (probes) become filled in as a result of this augmentation, so that the final contour is smooth (referred to as ice sculpting).

The typical template involves five individually controlled probes. Two probes are placed anteriorly and three posteriorly. The two anterior probes are placed between 5 and 8 mm from the anterior capsule at the midpoint between the urethra and the lateral capsule. The two posterolateral probes are placed so that the iceball growth will extend past the lateral capsule before reaching the rectum (the point of procedure termination). The posterolateral probes should also be placed as anteriorly as possible (not beyond the 2-cm radius of the iceball) to let the iceball grow out laterally to encompass the neurovascular bundles and medially to augment the performance of the other probes. A fifth probe is placed in the midline under the urethra. Additional access ports can be placed outside the prostate parallel to the neurovascular bundles to triangulate areas of extracapsular extension or seminal vesicle involvement.

After all access ports are established, the cryoprobes are placed into the sheaths. Once in place, the pre-slit Teflon sheaths are withdrawn and the machine is activated by circulating liquid nitrogen through the probes. This will create a small iceball at the tip of the probe, "sticking" the probe in place. We generally stick our probes at −70 to −100°C. The probes are suspended with rubber straps from a Bookwalter retractor ring that is suspended above the perineum.

Because objects close to the transducer cause acoustic interference, all manipulation, probe placement, and freezing are performed in an anterior to posterior sequence. After all probes are stuck in place, the system is then activated to circulate pressurized, supercooled liquid nitrogen at full flow through the probes (-180 to $-200°C$). As the tissue temperature drops below $4°C$, the tissue water changes from a liquid to a solid. This interface reflects all sound waves and is interpreted as a hyperechoic line. The lack of sound wave transmission beyond this interface is referred to as acoustic shadowing; the iceball itself is anechoic. The early freezing process is monitored with both the sagittal and transverse transducers to provide a three-dimensional image.

Once the advancing edge of the iceballs from the anterior probes has reached the posterior row of probes, the posterior probes are activated. The anterior probes continue to freeze until the iceballs reach the posterior prostatic capsule. This augments the performance of the posterior probes and assures adequate margins anteriorly. Surveillance at this point is with the sagittal transducer because it provides better delineation of the structures posterior to the prostate. A 6-cm linear array sagittal transducer allows simultaneous visualization of the entire prostate (the ice is widest at the probe tip). The contour of the rectum does not follow a straight line. At the apex and urogenital diaphragm, the rectum is anteriorly situated compared with its location at the base. A sagittal transducer will accurately show the relationship of the iceball to the entire anterior rectal wall. As the treatment continues, there is an increase in blood flow around the prostate. The signals from the neurovascular bundles increase as the iceball approaches the rectum, and portosystemic shunts through the rectum become visualized. These vascular changes are believed to be due to microvascular obstruction in the prostate. This increased peripheral flow has the potential to heat and preserve surrounding tissue. Due to this finding, we began double freezing the prostate to extinguish these signals by an encompassing iceball. The probes remain activated until the advancing edge of the iceball abuts the anterior rectal wall.

After the first freeze cycle, the prostate is allowed to thaw (passively), after which the prostate base is again frozen. This is termed a double freeze. Most prostates are longer than 4 cm, requiring a pullback of the probes to treat the apical prostate and trapezoidal area. This second freeze, termed a pullback, will encompass the apical prostate and the trapezoidal area; it is generally brought through the urogenital diaphragm. With prostates shorter than 4 cm (or 5 cm with the newer probe design), the procedure is complete following the double freeze in the initial position.

After the freezing process is completed, the probes are thawed and then removed. Manual pressure is applied to the perineum for hemostasis, and the probe insertion sites are closed with simple sutures of 3-0 chromic. The urethral warming catheter is left activated until the entire prostate has thawed, which generally takes 20 minutes. The catheter is removed, the suprapubic tube placed to straight drain, and the patient taken to the recovery room.

The usual hospital stay is 1 day. Patients are generally given a liquid diet that evening and can ambulate as tolerated. The following morning, the suprapubic tube is capped with a heparin lock, and instructions are given. Patients are discharged later that morning if eating, ambulating, and managing the suprapubic tube well. There is generally little pain postoperatively. Scrotal ecchymosis and edema (lymphedema from obstructed pelvic channels) develop within 2 to 3 days and can be dramatic; yet, it invariably resolves without treatment in 3 weeks. Patients can resume normal activities in 1 to 2 weeks, with a return to work in a similar time frame. The suprapubic tube is removed when the postvoid residuals are consistently below 100 cc. We recommend oral antibiotic therapy (ciprofloxacin) for 2 weeks after the procedure and for 1 week after suprapubic tube removal.

RESULTS

All patients undergoing CSAP are enrolled in one of several protocols, all of which have been reviewed and approved by our institutional review board. For purposes of data analysis, we have divided all patients into four categories—virgin (no prior treatment), virgin and ADT, radiation therapy failures, and radiation therapy failures on ADT. In each category, subgroups are categorized by clinical stage, histologic score, gland volume, and preoperative PSA (preoperative PSA from patients receiving ADT is the last recorded value before starting treatment). Survival is the ultimate measure of treatment efficacy in any cancer. Short-term measures following localized ablation of the prostate include serial PSA levels, DRE, and timed systematic prostatic biopsies. We have patterned our schedule of assessments to parallel those of recently published radiation therapy series to enable short-term comparison of these two locally destructive modalities.

Biopsy Results

Through January 16, 1995, 383 patients have undergone a total of 447 procedures. The mean age is 65.1 ± 6.6 years (range, 41 to 79 years). Mean and median follow-up are 17.2 ± 8.6 months and 16.3 months, respectively, with a range of 1.3 to 50.3 months. Of these, 358 (93.5%) have had at least one follow-up biopsy. At the time of initial follow-up biopsy, 54 (15.1%) were positive for residual or recurrent prostate cancer. Of those with negative biopsy results, another 132 (36.9%) have had a subsequent biopsy (either protocol biopsy or one driven by clinical suspicion), and 41 (31.1%) are positive. Combining these two groups, local treatment failure occurred in 95 patients (26.5%).

The majority of patients with biopsy-confirmed local failure have opted to undergo repeat cryosurgical ablation. In this cohort of patients undergoing more than one application of

Table 21.1. Patient Demographics by Treatment Group

	NO.	STAGE				GRADE			UNKNOWN	MEAN/MEDIAN PRE-PSA (ng/mL)
		A	B	C	D	2–4	5–7	8–10		
No prior treatment	244	67	97	56	24	90	137	16	1	12.08/8.30
ADT[a]	90	19	32	20	19	24	49	15	2	26.58/12.35
Radiation therapy	24	4	5	13	2	1	12	11	0	23.96/14.95
Radiation therapy/ADT[a]	19	1	3	8	7	1	12	4	2	29.48/15.30
RRP	6	0	0	3	3	1	4	1	0	14.16/10.05

[a] Two patients each with no preoperative Gleason assessment.

cryotherapy, the positive biopsy rate in follow-up is 28.9%. Reentry of those patients with a favorable local response after a subsequent treatment into the negative biopsy category gives a reflection of biopsy status following the last treatment. Analysis of biopsy status after the last treatment reveals 361 of 383 patients (94.3%) with a follow-up biopsy. From this cohort, 32 patients (8.9%) were positive at their initial biopsy and 35 of 136 patients (25.7%) were positive at a subsequent biopsy; this produces a total positive biopsy rate of 18.6% (67 of 383 patients) after the last cryosurgical treatment.

Patient demographics can be found in Table 21.1. The subgroups contain patients generally representative of those found in recently published series examining radical prostatectomy and radiation therapy with a trend toward decreasing histologic differentiation with increasing clinical stage. Pelvic lymphadenectomy was not routinely performed. Preoperative staging lymphadenectomy was performed in 20.6% of the study group (63 of 79 lymphadenectomies revealed benign lymph node pathologic condition).

Biopsy results for clinically localized (stages A and B) tumors of the prostate are summarized in Table 21.2. These data encompass all treatment groups. Biopsy results following the last procedure (which again incorporates those patients who had an initial positive biopsy and underwent a subsequent cryosurgical treatment) are presented in the final column of Table 21.2.

Biopsy results following CSAP for non–organ-confined prostate cancer (stages C and D) can be found in Table 21.3. Patients were labeled as having stage C disease based on DRE (revealing induration into the seminal vesicles or beyond the lateral capsule), radiographic suggestion of extracapsular tumor extension (ultrasound [38], computed tomography [1], or magnetic resonance imaging [5]), or histologic evidence of cancer beyond the capsule on any of the surveillance biopsies (25). Patients initially thought to have organ-confined disease who postoperatively were found to have extracapsular disease on their biopsy at 3 months were placed into the stage C cohort.

Biopsy results from the cohort of previously irradiated patients can be found in Table 21.4. All patients previously underwent definitive radiation therapy (external beam [35], brachytherapy [5], and both [5]) and had histologic evidence of persistent cancer at least 18 months after the completion of therapy. The mean interval from therapy to the documentation of recurrence/persistence after radiation therapy was 49.3 ± 31.4 months (range, 6.57 to 133.0 months). These patients were all treated with a single freeze with or without a pullback.

Patterns of Failure

An earlier review of these 383 consecutive patients following CSAP examined patterns of local histologic failure and isolated biochemical failure. All positive biopsy results were compared with the initial biopsy site of the carcinoma, the clinical examination, and the intraoperative ultrasound findings. The Gleason score of the postcryotherapy positive biopsies was also compared with the preoperative biopsy score.

Of 97 biopsies positive for resistant or recurrent adenocarci-

Table 21.2. Biopsy Results After Cryosurgical Ablation of the Prostate for Organ-Confined Disease

STAGE	NO.	MEDIAN PREOPERATIVE PSA (ng/mL)	INITIAL BX (%)	OVERALL POS. BX (%)	OVERALL POS. BX AFTER LAST PROCEDURE (%)
A1	34	7.7	3 (8.8)	6 (17.6)	3 (8.8)
A2	42	9.6	4 (9.5)	6 (14.3)	4 (9.5)
Unspecified A	9	6.4	0	1 (11.1)	1 (11.1)
Overall A	85	8.6	7 (8.2)	13 (15.3)	8 (9.4)
B1	45	6.7	4 (8.9)	11 (24.4)	6 (13.3)
B2	75	8.1	11 (14.7)	20 (26.7)	11 (15.1)
Unspecified B	5	5.5	0	0	0
Overall B	125	7.3	15 (12.0)	31 (24.8)	17 (13.8)

Table 21.3. Biopsy Results After Cryosurgical Ablation of the Prostate in Patients With Non–Organ-Confined Disease

STAGE	NO.	MEDIAN PREOPERATIVE PSA (ng/mL)	INITIAL BX (%)	OVERALL POS. BX (%)	OVERALL POS. BX AFTER LAST PROCEDURE (%)
C	100	10.3	22 (22.0)	38 (38)	32 (30.5)
D0	31	19.6	4 (12.9)	6 (19.4)	5 (16.1)
D1	17	30.55	6 (35.3)	7 (41.2)	5 (29.4)
Overall D	48	22.3	10 (20.8)	13 (27.1)	10 (20.8)

noma, 9.0% (6 of 67) demonstrated evidence of histologic upgrading; the scores of the remaining 91.0% were either similar or decreased. Ten biopsies (10.3%) were positive only in areas previously believed to be benign as determined by DRE, biopsy, and ultrasound. Eleven of the 97 biopsies (12.6%) were positive only in extraprostatic sites (10 seminal vesicle only and 1 seminal vesicle and neurovascular bundle only), 57 of 87 (65.6%) were positive only in intraprostatic sites, and 19 of 87 (21.8%) were positive in both intra and extraprostatic biopsies.

PSA remains a valuable biochemical marker of residual disease after cryoablation. Mean and median PSA levels at the time of a positive biopsy (4.82 and 1.96 ng/mL, respectively, for the whole cohort) were significantly greater than those without recurrent cancer at last follow-up (0.90 and 0.30 ng/mL, respectively). This trend was observed in each treatment group. Median PSA at 2 years in patients with negative biopsies was 0.5 ng/mL compared with 1.25 ng/mL in patients with positive biopsies at 2 years.

Examination of the patients with negative biopsies who were not receiving ADT revealed three trends in PSA changes.

- The first group consisted of persistently undetectable PSA values.
- The second group had PSA values that were stable yet greater than expected (0.4 ng/mL less than or equal to 4.0 ng/mL).
- The third group had PSA values that continued to rise (increase greater than 0.2 ng/mL on two consecutive samples).

This third group of 59 patients (19.7% of total) with persistently negative prostatic biopsies and rising PSA values were presumed to have micrometastatic disease and were generally then given ADT. In this subgroup with rising PSA values, 43 (72.9%) were of clinical stage B2 or higher. The remaining 16 (27.1%) were of clinical stage B1 or less.

2-Year Surveillance

Scheduled biopsies are performed initially at 3 months and then again at 2 years. We have now followed 118 patients who are eligible for 2-year biopsies. Of these patients, we have biopsy information on 76 patients (64.4%). Of these 76 patients, 13 (17%) have histologic evidence of recurrent cancer on systematic biopsy. Breakdown of this cohort by stage and grade can be found in Table 21.5. Biopsy specimens from those patients in whom failure occurred at 2 years were solely intraprostatic in seven and both intraprostatic and extraprostatic in the remaining six. Median PSA at 2 years for those with a positive biopsy result was 1.25 ng/mL; for those with a negative biopsy result, it was 0.5 ng/mL. Median PSA for the cohort of 42 patients who did not undergo biopsy at 2 years was 0.3 ng/ mL. A plot of PSA over time for this cohort followed for a minimum of 2 years is shown in Figure 21.1.

PSA Data

Serum PSA is obtained postoperatively at 6 weeks, 3 months, then every 3 months thereafter. PSA data from patients with localized disease (stages A, B, and C) who are biopsy negative are represented by Kaplan-Meier analysis in Figures 21.2, 21.3, and 21.4. Mean and median PSA of those patients followed for 2 years are 1.37 and 0.65 ng/mL, respectively (range, 0 to

Table 21.4. Biopsy Results After Cryosurgical Ablation of the Prostate in Patients Who Have Undergone Radiation Therapy

	XRT				XRT AND ADT			
STAGE	NO.	INITIAL BX (%)	OVERALL BX (%)	LAST PROCEDURE (%)	NO.	INITIAL BX (%)	OVERALL BX (%)	LAST PROCEDURE (%)
A	3	0	0	0	1	0	0	0
B	5	2 (40)	3 (60)	2 (66.7)[a]	3	1 (33)	1 (33)	1 (33)
C	14	4 (28.6)	7 (50)	6 (46.2)[b]	6	1 (16.7)	3 (50)	3 (50)
D	1	0	0	0	5	2 (40)	3 (60)	2 (50)

[a] n = 3.
[b] n = 13.

Table 21.5.   Demographics and Biopsy Results of 2-Year Biopsy Cohort

STAGE	NO.	%	NO. POS. BX (%)	GRADE	NO.	%	NO. POS. BX (%)
A	18	23.7	3 (16.7)	2–4	31	40.8	2 (6.4)
B	27	35.5	4 (14.8)	5–7	38	50.0	11 (28.9)
C	38	50.0	5 (13.2)	8–10	7	9.2	0
D	12	15.8	1 (8.3)				

10). Only one patient has had a positive biopsy with a clinically undetectable PSA.

Complications

As of January 16, 1995, we have performed CSAP a total of 447 times on 383 patients. Throughout this period, we have seen no procedure-related deaths. There has been no need to transfuse any patient. Major complications are few. Fistulization, a frequent complication in earlier attempts at CSAP, has been uncommon. Two cases of prostatorectal fistula were created in the first series of 25 patients. Both patients required formal perineal surgical repair; however, neither required a diverting colostomy. One urethrocutaneous fistula developed after perineal drainage of a prostatic abscess. This tract closed spontaneously with suprapubic tube drainage. The only other major complications include two instances of prostatic abscess (both responded to conservative drainage and antibiotics), and three cases of sepsis that all responded to intravenous antibiotics.

Other complications of concern include impotence and incontinence. As with radical prostatectomy, we have noted an age-related recovery of erectile function. From nerve regeneration studies after cryoablation, it is known that if the neural sheath is intact, electrical conduction returns over the course of 6 to 12 months (24). In men younger than 60 years of age, approximately one third will recover erections suitable for penetration of the vagina without assistance. Men older than

60 years of age have a slightly worse prognosis, with 15% of men regaining the ability to experience unassisted vaginal penetration. The majority of men will regain partial erections. All will regain ejaculatory sensation. Emission will be absent. Those men regaining partial erections are very sensitive to the intracorporeal injection of pharmacologic agents (necessitating lower doses).

Incontinence up to 6 months after CSAP is often urge related and resolves with time. Prolonged (longer than 6 months) stress urinary incontinence or gross incontinence that requires the patient to wear a pad is encountered in 3.1% (14 patients). Review of this cohort reveals that the rate of incontinence in previously irradiated patients is significantly higher at 11.8%, whereas in patients with no prior treatment it is 1.5%.

Urethral stricture disease has developed in seven patients (1.6%). Also, a contracture of the bladder neck that required intervention has developed in seven patients (1.6%). Prolonged urinary retention was seen in another seven patients (1.6%). Occasionally, a channel transurethral prostatic resection is helpful to expedite recovery to normal voiding dynamics. A complete list of complications can be found in Table 21.6.

Prostatic urethral sloughing was encountered in virtually all patients initially treated with CSAP in the 1960s and 1970s. Sloughing causes a constellation of symptoms. These begin between 3 and 5 weeks postoperatively. Mild cases may include dysuria, urgency, frequency, and the passage of white particulate matter in the urinary stream. In more severe cases, patients may express large pieces of necrotic prostatic parenchyma through the urethra. These patients may initially present with overflow incontinence and are best treated with either intermittent or indwelling urethral catheterization until the process stabilizes in 4 to 8 weeks. Patients with significant obstruction and sloughing may benefit from a channel transurethral prostatic resection (the tissue is generally avascular and necrotic). This should be reserved until conservative measures have failed. Care must be taken to avoid excessive resection, as the normal anatomic landmarks (verumontanum and surgical capsule) are generally indistinct. Of those patients with sloughing syndrome, 28 (6.3% of the total cohort) had significant retention requiring either catheter placement or surgical intervention.

The concept of urethral warming has significantly decreased the clinical appearance of this complication. The initial urethral warming device consisted of a flexible cystoscope placed at the external sphincter through which a continuous flow of warmed saline solution successfully prevented urethral necrosis. The saline exited through the suprapubic tube. In an attempt to simplify the system, the subsequent warming catheter used a dual-

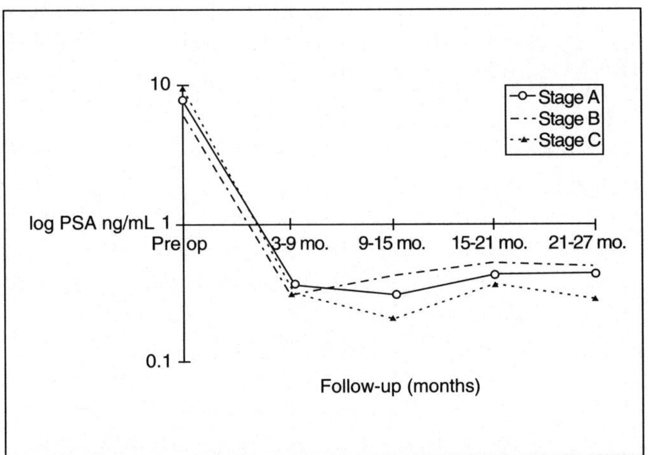

Fig. 21.1.   Logarithmic representation of serial PSA against time for cohort followed 2 years after CSAP.

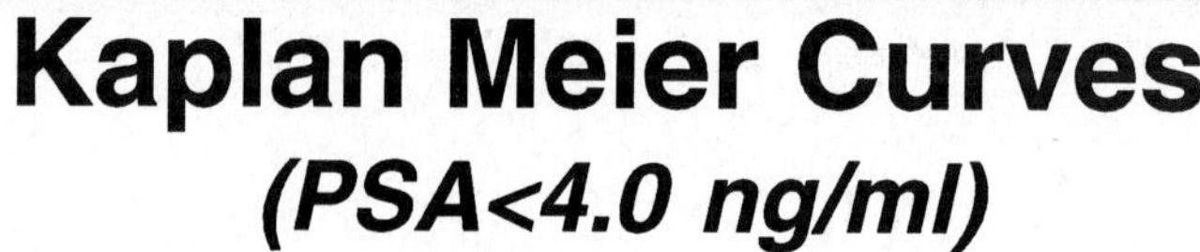

Kaplan Meier Curves
(PSA<4.0 ng/ml)

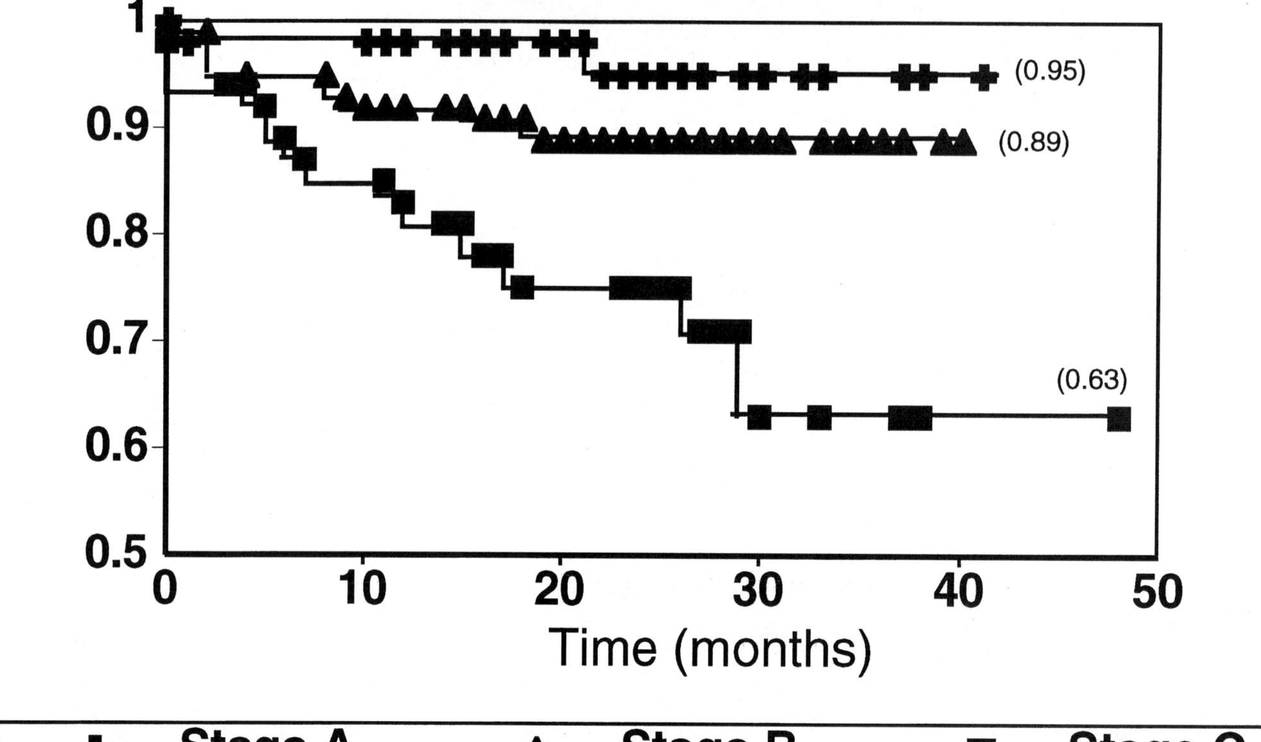

Fig. 21.2.

chamber design with a Mylar outer sheath. This closed-loop system could be passed transurethrally with ease. Sloughing with this device was 3.2%. Due to Food & Drug Administration policy, this catheter was considered a significant risk device (after being used in more than 200 patients) and mandated formal testing. A new urethral warming catheter was subsequently fashioned from stock operating room parts (34). With the newer system (used from the end of the current series to the present), the rate of clinically significant urethral sloughing is 20.4%. Review of the first 103 cases in which this system was used revealed that sloughing was much more common in virgin patients (26.5%) than in ADT patients (12.5%) or patients in whom radiation failed (6.3%). Analysis of the virgin cohort reveals that the risk of sloughing is directly proportional to gland volume. Sloughing in virgin patients with gland volumes less than 20 g occurred at a rate of 11.1%, very similar to the rate for ADT and radiation failure groups. As gland volume increased above 20 g, sloughing occurred at a rate of 35.7%. A possible explanation for this phenomenon focuses on the increased edema produced by the freezing process in larger virgin glands (higher stroma and fibrous tissue component in ADT and radiation failure glands as well). This increased edema will lead to pressure necrosis of the urethra long after the warming catheter has been removed.

DISCUSSION

Although treatment options abound for the management of clinically localized carcinoma of the prostate, there are several groups of patients for whom there is no satisfactory alternative. These groups include patients with extensive local tumors including those with significant risks of extracapsular disease (T2B, T3, T4, NxM0), patients in whom radiation therapy has failed, and those patients who deserve definitive therapy yet are older or have significant comorbid factors. High rates of treatment failure and debilitating local complications prompted the reexamination of cryosurgical ablation. The recent advent of percutaneous access techniques, transrectal ultrasound, and the concept of urethral warming/protection have led to the new era of CSAP. Complete CSAP can now be achieved with

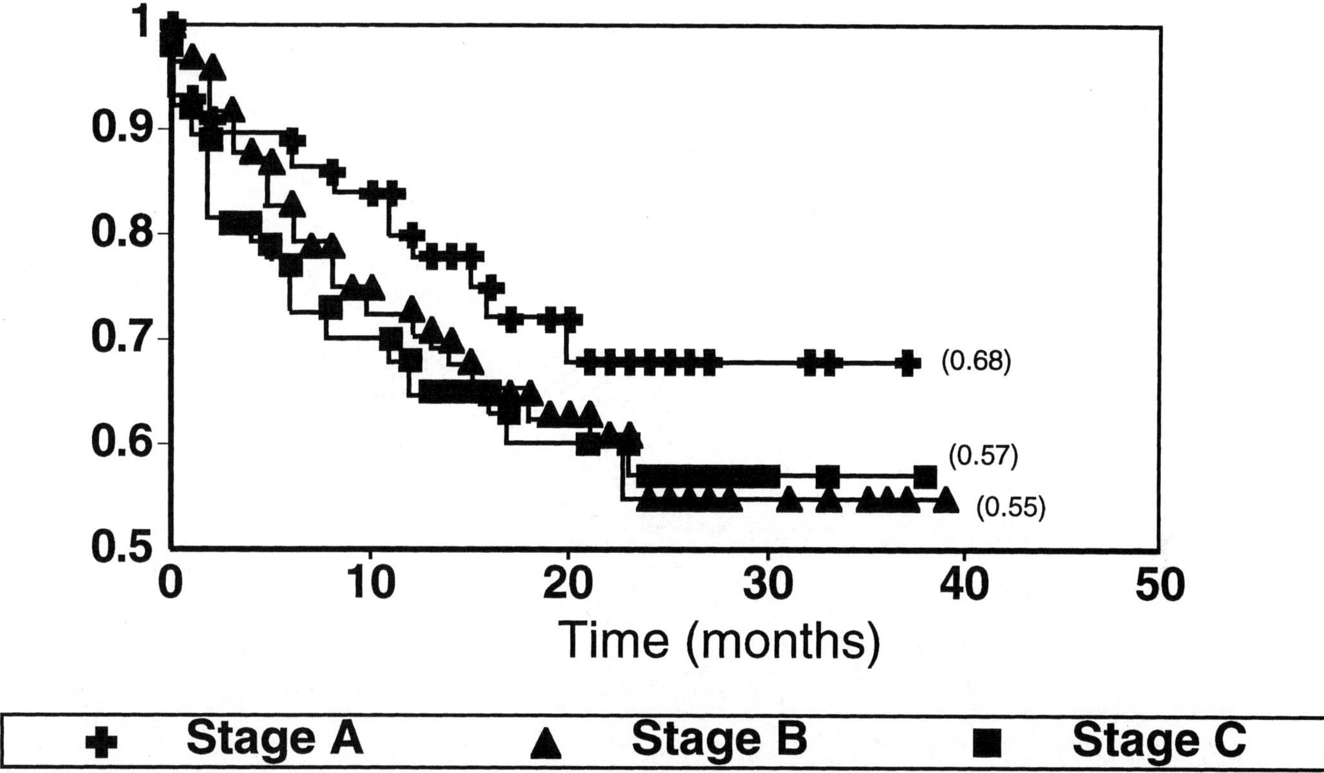

Fig. 21.3.

a minimum of surgical complications. The average hospital stay of 1 day is significantly less than that for radical prostatectomy, and the recuperative period is also much shorter.

Prostatic core biopsy and serial PSA determinations are short-term assessments of prostatic ablation. Examining the entire cohort, biopsy specimens are free of histologic evidence of carcinoma in 73.5% of patients. After repeat application of CSAP, this figure increases to 81.4%. Patients with no prior definitive therapy fare better in this regard than do those who have been previously irradiated, with negative biopsy rates of 75.9% and 55.3%, respectively, following a single application of CSAP. After we began double freezing in all patients, we have noticed a decrease in the positive biopsy results. Since the beginning of this trial, several other centers have treated large numbers of prostate cancer patients with CSAP through similar treatment protocols. Reported initial negative biopsy rates for virgin and irradiated patients range from 85 to 89.3% and from 60 to 93%, respectively (Schmidt J, Bahn D, Long J, Clark, personal communication, 1995). These figures are not significantly different from our experience, with reproducible results obtained from the use of this technique.

In the event of biopsy-proven local recurrence after CSAP, patients may choose from the same treatment options that were available to them before CSAP. In our series, 10 patients have subsequently undergone external beam radiation therapy (to date, 4 have undetectable PSA levels, 4 have decreased levels of PSA, and 2 have insufficient follow-up); 45 have undergone repeat cryosurgical treatments (an additional 6 were performed elsewhere), of which 32 (71.1%) are negative to date; 3 have had a radical prostatectomy; and 55 are currently receiving ADT.

Initial postoperative biopsy status is adversely affected by increasing clinical stage, grade, and any prior definitive radiation therapy. Because the goal of the procedure is to encompass the prostate, seminal vesicles, and local periprostatic tissues into the iceball, the exact reasons behind persistent disease (aside from suboptimal probe placement) are speculative. In vitro tissue culture studies suggest that more than 99% of cells are killed with temperatures below $-40°$ C (22). The exact relationship between temperature and cell death has not been determined in vivo. Intraoperative thermocouple studies have shown that this temperature is reached within 3 to 4 mm from

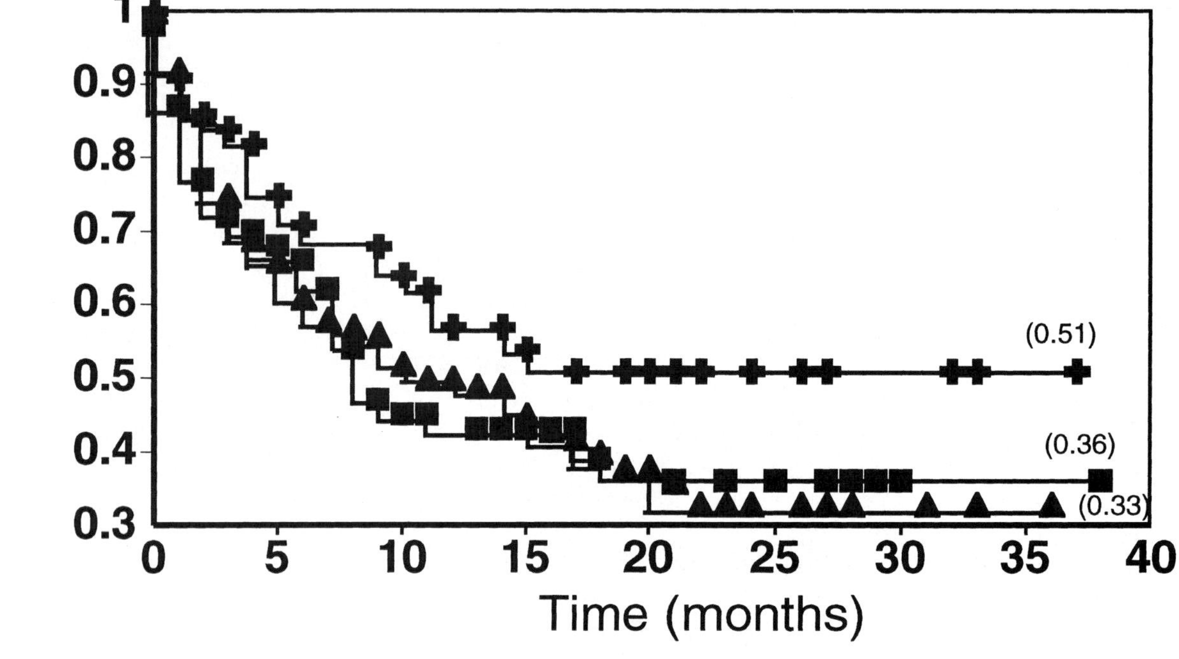

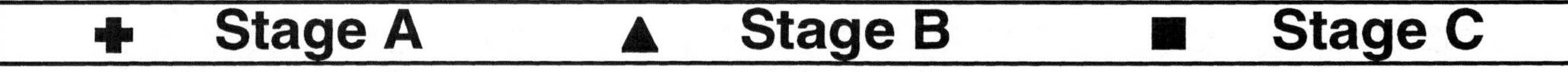

Fig. 21.4.

the edge of the iceball, and these "therapeutic" temperatures can be applied to the entire prostate including the capsule posteriorly. Intraprostatic temperature variation can be seen with increased local vascularity. Aberrant blood vessels feeding extensive tumors or in postirradiation prostates are frequently seen with CFD ultrasound. It is possible that these high flow vessels are preventing complete cryodestruction by their local warming effect. Cancer growing out the neurovascular bundles could be preserved during a single freeze cycle. Using CFD ultrasound, we have seen aberrant vessels feeding the location of residual tumors in patients failing a single freeze application of CSAP. Because of these findings, we have treated all patients with a double freeze technique since March 1994.

Examination of patients 2 years after CSAP reveals several interesting points. First, the local destructive effects of CSAP appear to be durable, as indicated by a 17% positive biopsy rate at 2 years. Second, there appears to be no significant effect of preoperative clinical stage or grade on 2-year biopsy status. Forty-two percent (32 of 76) of the patients in this cohort (patients who were treated in the early phases of the protocol)

reached and maintained undetectable levels (less than 0.4 ng/mL) of PSA. Third, to the best of our knowledge, there are no complications that present in a delayed fashion.

Serial PSA determination provides biochemical evidence of prostatic destruction. Stable serial values of PSA from those patients followed for 2 years suggest a durable response to treatment. Because the prostate undergoes treatment with subsequent necrosis and involution yet remains in situ, PSA values may not be directly comparable to those following radical prostatectomy. Reasons for persistently detectable levels of PSA include periurethral glands preserved through the use of the urethral warming catheter, persistent benign or malignant glands within the prostate, or the presence of distant micrometastases. Histologic review of prostatic biopsies following CSAP has revealed a characteristic array of changes. Most biopsy specimens reveal significant inflammation, necrosis, and fibrosis. Many biopsy specimens reveal a spectrum of benign to dysplastic glands (including basal cell hyperplasia, squamous cell metaplasia, and transitional cell metaplasia) (23). PSA stains of basal cell hyperplasia can be positive in the central portion

Table 21.6. Complications of Cryosurgical Ablation of the Prostate in 383 Patients

COMPLICATION	NO. (%)
Sloughing syndrome	39 (8.7)
Incontinence	14 (3.1)
Urethral stricture	7 (1.6)
Bladder neck contracture	7 (1.6)
Epididymitis	7 (1.6)
Urinary retention	7 (1.6)
Bleeding	6 (1.3)
UTI	5 (1.1)
Ileus	4 (0.9)
Sloughed urethral tissue	4 (0.9)
Prostatitis	4 (0.9)
Urge incontinence	3 (0.7)
Sepsis	3 (0.7)
Perineal pain	2 (0.5)
Hydrocele	2 (0.5)
Prostatic abscess	2 (0.5)
Urethrorectal fistula	2 (0.5)
Perineal necrosis	1 (0.2)
Priapism	1 (0.2)
Balanitis/phimosis	1 (0.2)
Cystitis	1 (0.2)
Numb glans penis	1 (0.2)
Stress incontinence	1 (0.2)
Thigh numbness	1 (0.2)
Hearing loss	1 (0.2)
Pleurisy	1 (0.2)
Perineal fistula	1 (0.2)
Scrotal swelling	1 (0.2)

of the gland (Masson D, personal communication, 1995). These dysplastic glands may also be a source of persistent PSA in the absence of persistent cancer.

The technique of CSAP continues to evolve. In efforts to increase rates of local tumor control, several authors have advocated preoperative androgen deprivation in all patients before CSAP (35, 36). The theoretical advantages of this approach are twofold and speculative. A smaller prostate (as a result of glandular atrophy) allows better overlapping of the iceballs and achieves lower core temperatures. Additionally, much of the prostatic microvasculature is believed to atrophy and hence eliminate much of the local heat sink effect. There have been no prospective studies examining this issue; however, these theoretical advantages do not hold true in the clinical setting. Our retrospective nonrandomized cohort does not reveal any improvement in biopsy status with preoperative androgen deprivation. Serial PSA determinations parallel those of the virgin cohort. There is no evidence suggesting a clinical outcomes advantage from preoperative ADT in the performance of CSAP (with the exception of decreasing prostatic urethral sloughing rates postoperatively).

A modification to the technique that appears superior to preoperative ADT involves double freezing of the prostate. Re-sults with patients in whom radiation therapy has failed suggest that the second freeze can significantly decrease the rates of positive biopsy. Von Eschenbach et al. initially reported a 69% negative biopsy rate that increased in a subsequent group to 92% using a double freeze (37). This was confirmed in the mixed cohort review by Shinohara and Carroll, which reported a drop in the positive biopsy rate from 43 to 5% with the initiation of double freezing (38). Intraoperative CFD ultrasonography following the initial freeze with CSAP reveals significantly increased flow through the neurovascular bundles, the portosystemic shunting through the rectum, and any other local vasculature as if the blood were shunted out of the prostate following the initial freeze. If this is true, the second freeze cycle is able to ablate more efficiently in the absence of this intraprostatic vasculature. Additionally, probe placement can be adjusted specifically to the vasculature of each patient.

Cause-specific survival is the ultimate measure of success for any treatment of adenocarcinoma of the prostate. Meaningful comparison with radical prostatectomy and radiation therapy will not be available for many years. The short-term measures of success, prostatic biopsy and serial PSA determinations, have enabled an interim comparison with these treatments.

Two recent retrospective reviews of major external beam radiation therapy series have aggressively examined their results using PSA, biopsy, and histologic data to determine success of this technique. Kavadi et al. reviewed the M.D. Anderson Cancer Center's experience in the treatment of clinically localized prostate cancer with external beam radiation therapy (17). The cohort shared similar stage, grade, and PSA demographics with our group undergoing CSAP. They determined that a 12-month nadir post–radiation-therapy PSA value of less than 1.0 ng/mL translated into a combined clinical local and distant relapse rate of 17%. For values above 1.0 ng/mL, the recurrence rates rose to more than 70%. Using a cutoff nadir PSA value of less than or equal to 1.0 ng/mL, 43% of patients attained this mark compared with 91% of virgin patients after CSAP. Examination of the radiated group by preoperative PSA demonstrated poorer results with increasing preoperative PSA levels. Preoperative PSA values between 10 and 30 ng/mL and greater than 30 ng/mL had a 15% and 4% chance, respectively, of a nadir PSA below 1.0 ng/mL compared with 95% and 60%, respectively, after CSAP.

Crook et al. reviewed their experience of routine systematic biopsies following definitive radiation therapy for clinically localized adenocarcinoma of the prostate (16). The cohort was older and with less advanced stage and grade on the average than the CSAP group. Fifty-one percent of patients had histologic evidence of viable cancer on the initial 12-month biopsy. Thirty-nine of these 115 patients eventually converted to negative biopsy status with time, for an overall positive biopsy rate of 34%. Following CSAP, the chances that a patient will have a positive biopsy after one or numerous procedures is 25% and 13%, respectively. Hence, the short-term measures of success in the treatment of prostate cancer—biopsy status and PSA levels—both appear more favorable after CSAP than after radiation therapy.

Direct comparison with historical series following radical prostatectomy is difficult due to the issues of persistent PSA after the procedure. As in radical prostatectomy, a rising PSA is generally indicative of treatment failure; however, residual, low levels of PSA after CSAP may be a reflection of several benign dysplastic changes inside the treated prostate. For clinically localized (stage B) adenocarcinoma, Epstein et al. reported a 30% rate of biochemical failure within 5 years after radical prostatectomy (39). In the current cohort following CSAP, treatment failure for clinical stages A1 to B1 (as defined by either biopsy-confirmed local recurrence or rising serial PSA values in the absence of local recurrence) occurred in 28.4% (24 of 141 [17.0%] with biopsy-confirmed local recurrence and 16 of 117 [13.6%] with rising PSA values and negative biopsy). Salvage radical prostatectomy after radiation therapy failure achieves biochemical cure in between 29.4% (11) and 47% (10) of cases. In the current series after CSAP, 3 of 10 patients (30%) (excluding those currently receiving ADT) treated for biopsy-proven recurrence after radiation therapy maintain an undetectable PSA.

CONCLUSION

CSAP incorporates modern technology and the current concepts of cancer control to apply the proven destructive abilities of cryoablation in the eradication of prostate cancer. Although long-term survival statistics are not currently available, short-term measures of success (biopsy and PSA) reveal that this technique can successfully ablate the prostatic epithelium with a minimum of treatment-related complications. Patients with extensive local tumors, high-grade tumors, and radioresistant tumors all appear to respond favorably compared with radical prostatectomy or radiation therapy. Exactly how this treatment modality will fit into the management of clinically localized adenocarcinoma of the prostate is as yet undetermined. Even at this early analysis, the short-term markers are quite favorable. Further technologic developments will advance this treatment and improve results for prostate cancer control. Further efforts using randomized prospective trials and long-term surveillance are needed to help elucidate the most efficient and appropriate treatments for localized adenocarcinoma of the prostate.

REFERENCES

1. Wingo PA, Tong T, Bolden S. Cancer statistics, 1995. CA Cancer J Clin 1995;45:8.
2. Hirst AE, Bergman RT. Carcinoma of the prostate in men 80 or more years old. Cancer 1954;7:136.
3. Rich AR. On the frequency of occurrence of occult carcinoma of prostate. J Urol 1935;33:215.
4. Gibbons RP, Correa RJ, Brannen GE, et al. Total prostatectomy for clinically localized prostatic cancer: long term results. J Urol 1989;141:564.
5. Partin AW, Pound CR, Clemens JQ, et al. Serum PSA after anatomic radical prostatectomy. Urol Clin North Am 1993;20: 47.
6. Quinlan DM, Epstein JI, Carter BS, et al. Sexual function following radical prostatectomy: influence of preservation of neurovascular bundles. J Urol 1991;145:998.
7. Fowler FJ, Barry MJ, Lu-Yao G, et al. Patient-reported complications and follow-up treatment after radical prostatectomy. Urology 1993;42:622.
8. McNeal JE, Villers AA, Redwine EA, et al. Histologic differentiation, cancer volume, and pelvic lymph node metastasis in adenocarcinoma of the prostate. Cancer 1990;66: 1225.
9. Stamey TA, McNeal JE, Freiha FS, et al. Morphometric and clinical studies on 68 consecutive radical prostatectomies. J Urol 1988;139:1235.
10. Rogers E, Ohori M, Kassabian VS, et al. Salvage radical prostatectomy: outcome measured by serum prostate specific antigen levels. J Urol 1995;153:104.
11. Pontes JE, Montie J, Klein E, et al. Salvage surgery for radiation failure in prostate cancer. Cancer 1993;71(Suppl): 976.
12. Stamey TA, Ferrari MK, Schmid HP. The value of serial prostate specific antigen determinations 5 years after radiotherapy: steeply increasing values characterize 80% of patients. J Urol 1993;150:1856.
13. Kabalin JN, Hodge KK, McNeal JE, et al. Identification of residual cancer in the prostate following radiation therapy: role of transrectal ultrasound guided biopsy and prostate specific antigen. J Urol 1989;142:326.
14. Egawa S, Wheeler TM, Greene DR, et al. Detection of residual prostate cancer after radiotherapy by sonographically guided needle biopsy. Urology 1992;34:358.
15. Freiha FS, Bagshaw MA. Carcinoma of the prostate: results of post-irradiation biopsy. Prostate 1984;5:19.
16. Crook JM, Perry GA, Robertson S, et al. Routine prostate biopsies following radiotherapy for prostate cancer. Urology 1995;45:624.
17. Kavadi VS, Zagars GK, Pollack A. Serum prostate-specific antigen after radiation therapy for clinically localized prostate cancer: prognostic implications. Int J Radiat Biol 1994;30: 279.
18. Bagshaw MA, Cox RS, Ray GR. Status of radiation treatment of prostate cancer at Stanford University. NCI Monogr 1988;7: 47.
19. Adolfsson J, Carstensen J. Natural course of clinically localized prostate adenocarcinoma in men less than 70 years old. J Urol 1991;146:96.
20. Whitmore WJ Jr, Warner JA, Thompson IM Jr. Expectant management of localized prostatic cancer. Cancer 1991;67: 1091.
21. Terris MK, McNeal JE, Stamey TA. Detection of clinically significant prostate cancer by transrectal ultrasound-guided systematic biopsies. J Urol 1992;148:829.
22. Baust JG, Chang ZH. Cryosurgery: underlying mechanisms of damage and new concepts in cryosurgical instrumentation. Proceedings from the 9th World Congress of Cryosurgery, June, 1995.
23. Masson D, Bidair M, Shabaik A, et al. Pathologic changes in

prostate biopsies following cryoablation therapy. J Urol 1995; 153:484. Abstract.

24. Trumble TE, Whalen JT. The effects of cryosurgery and cryoprotectants on peripheral nerve function. J Reconstr Microsurg 1992;8:53.

25. Gondor MJ, Soanes WA, Shulman S. Cryosurgical treatment of the prostate. Invest Urol 1966;3:372.

26. Bonney WW, Fallon B, Gerber WL, et al. Cryosurgery in prostatic cancer: elimination of the local lesion. Urology 1983; 22:8.

27. Bonney WW, Fallon B, Gerber WL, et al. Cryosurgery in prostate cancer: survival. Urology 1982;14:37.

28. Zhou XD, Zhao-You T, Ye-Qin Y, et al. Clinical evaluation of cryosurgery in the treatment of primary liver cancer: report of 60 cases. Cancer 1988;61:1888.

29. Brandt B, Hibon J, LeMaire Ph, et al. Ultrasonography and cryosurgery of the prostate. Cryosurgery 1985.

30. Littrup PJ, Mody A, Sparschu R, et al. Prostatic cryotherapy: ultrasonographic and pathologic correlation in the canine model. Urology 1994;44:175.

31. Onik G, Cobb C, Cohen J, et al. Ultrasound characteristics of frozen prostate. Radiology 1988;168:629.

32. Cohen JK, Miller RJ. Thermal protection of urethra during cryosurgery of prostate. Cryobiology 1994;31:313.

33. Onik GM, Cohen JK, Reyes GD, et al. Transrectal ultrasound-guided percutaneous radical cryosurgical ablation of the prostate. Cancer 1993;72:1291.

34. Cohen JK, Miller RJ, Shuman BA. Urethral warming catheter for use during cryoablation of the prostate. Urology 1995;45: 861.

35. Lee F, Bahn DK, McHugh TA, et al. US-guided percutaneous cryoablation of prostate cancer. Radiology 1994;192:769.

36. Lee F, Siders DB, Newby JE, et al. The role of transrectal ultrasound-guided biopsy and androgen ablation therapy prior to radical prostatectomy. Clin Invest Med 1993;16: 463.

37. von Eschenbach AC, Pisters IL, Swanson DA, et al. Results of a phase I/II study of cryoablation for recurrent carcinoma of the prostate: the University of Texas M.D. Anderson Cancer Center Experience. J Urol 1995;153:503. Abstract.

38. Shinohara K, Carroll PR. Improved results of cryosurgical ablation of the prostate. J Urol 1995;153(Suppl):385. Abstract.

39. Epstein JI, Carmichael M, Partin AW, et al. Is tumor volume an independent predictor of progression following radical prostatectomy?: a multivariate analysis of 185 clinical stage B adenocarcinomas of the prostate with 5 years of follow-up. J Urol 1993;149:1478.

22

Surveillance and Deferred Therapy for Clinically Localized Palpable Adenocarcinoma of the Prostate

Jan Adolfsson

For a difference to be a difference it must make a difference.

GERTRUDE STEIN

INTRODUCTION

Patients with low-grade clinically localized palpable prostate cancer managed with deferred treatment seem to suffer a 10 to 20% risk of dying of prostate cancer at 10-year follow-up if not dying of other disease before. Local morbidity seems low. Quality of life aspects have not been evaluated. Judging from the current literature, disease-specific survival at 10 years for deferred treatment appears somewhat lower than for radical prostatectomy and higher than for radiation therapy. However, any direct comparison of the outcome for the various managements will be biased, mainly due to varying selection and imbalances in prognostic factors. With the data available today, deferred treatment may be a treatment option for patients with a life expectancy of 10 years or less.

BACKGROUND

Deferred treatment of localized prostate cancer is usually understood as no initial antitumoral therapy at diagnosis, surveillance with regular follow-up, and treatment given if and when the tumor progress or symptoms arise. This strategy has also been called wait and watch, conservative treatment, symptom-guided treatment, and expectant management. In most cases the deferred treatment given when indicated has been endocrine therapy, but more aggressive local treatments have also been used in selected patients in some series. The initial surveillance can be regarded as first-line therapy, and the endocrine treatment as second-line therapy if and when the primary therapy fails.

In Scandinavia, particularly in Sweden and Denmark, deferred treatment of localized prostate cancer has been used since the mid-1970s. Until then, the majority of patients with newly detected prostate cancer received early endocrine therapy irre-spective of grade and stage. Gradually, however, the often deadly cardiovascular side effects of estrogen-based treatment became evident, and primary endocrine therapy in patients with early low-grade disease was questioned. Because locally aggressive therapies such as radical prostatectomy and radiation therapy were not commonly used in Scandinavia in the 1970s, a tradition of deferring therapy in patients with early prostate cancer evolved. Aside from avoiding serious side effects from endocrine treatment, the rationale for deferring treatment was that prostate cancer was usually diagnosed in elderly patients who often died of other causes; there was also an understanding that many of the early cancers had a protracted and often benign course. Deferred treatment for localized prostate cancer is still used in Scandinavian countries. However, during the past decade there has been a shift toward more aggressive local therapies, particularly radical prostatectomy. Today, deferred treatment is one of several treatment options offered to patients with clinically localized prostate cancer (1).

OUTCOME

Single Studies

Since the mid-1980s, the outcomes of several series of patients with clinically localized palpable prostate cancer managed by deferred treatment have been reported (2–13). All these studies except two (4, 13) were uncontrolled and should therefore be regraded as descriptions of the outcome in each specific patient cohort. Four of the studies (4–6, 13) were prospective, and in three (5, 6, 13) a structured long-term follow-up was performed. Like uncontrolled studies of other managements, the outcomes of these studies were dependent on selection factors that differed among the series. The contemporary reports on deferred treatment with various survival endpoints are listed in Table 22.1. Because clinically localized prostate cancer usu-

Table 22.1. Overall Survival, Progression-Free Survival, and Disease-Specific Survival Reported in the Current Literature for Deferred Treatment of Clinically Localized Palpable Prostate Cancer

AUTHOR	NO. OF EVALUABLE PATIENTS	STAGE (as reported)	OVERALL SURVIVAL (yr)			PROGRESSION-FREE SURVIVAL (yr)			DISEASE-SPECIFIC SURVIVAL (yr)		
			5	10	15	5	10	15	5	10	15
Moskovitz et al. (2)	44	T1-2	61%	34%	—	—	—	—	—	—	—
George (3)	105	Clinically localized	—	—	—	—	—	—	80%[a]	—	—
Graverson et al. (4)	50	VACURG I-II	70%	55%	32%	—	—	—	—	—	—
Johansson et al. (5)	117	T1-2	63%	40%	—	56%	43%	—	93%	85%	—
	58	T0d-2	78%	58%	—	60%	50%	—	94%[b]	87%[b]	—
Adolfsson et al. (6)	122	T1-2	—	51%	—	—	77%[c]	—	99%	84%	—
Adolfsson and Carstensen (7)	61[b]	T1-2	—	85%	—	—	—	—	98%[d]	92%[d]	—
Chisholm and Rana (8)	107	T0/T1	65%	48%	—	—	—	—	—	—	—
Egawa et al. (9)	52	A1-B	—	—	—	—	—	—	—	75%	—
Stenzl and Studer (10)	34	T0-2	67%	34%	—	—	—	—	89%	87%	—
Waaler and Stenwig (11)	28	T1-2	—	—	—	—	—	—	70%	—	—
Warner and Whitmore (12)	68	[b]	—	72%	46%[c]	—	—	—	—	—	—
Lundgren et al. (13)	88	T0-3	81%	49%	—	85%[d]	66%[c]	—	91%	74%	—

[a] 90% in Figure 22.4.

[b] Patients younger than 70 years of age.

[c] Metastasis-free survival.

[d] Subgroup of Adolfsson et al. (6).

[e] 23% at 20-year follow-up.

ally has a protracted course, 5-year follow-up is hardly appropriate when discussing survival endpoints; in the following sections, only 10-year follow-up or longer will be discussed.

Overall or crude survival rates at 10 years ranged from 34 to 72% (Table 22.1). One study reported an overall survival rate of 46% at 15 years and 23% at 20-year follow-up for patients with stage B tumors (12). In the two largest series (5, 6), the overall survival rates at 10 years were 40% and 51% (Table 22.1). In both of these series, the majority of patients who died during the first 10 years after diagnosis did so from diseases not related to prostate cancer. It is therefore not possible to rely only on overall survival in patients with early prostate cancer when comparing survival outcome of various managements because a small, or even a moderate, treatment effect may be diluted and disguised by the competing mortality.

By strict definition, disease-free survival cannot be used for series with deferred treatment because the patients still have their tumor left. Instead, progression-free survival has been used by some authors and it has been found to range from 43 to 66% at 10 years (Table 22.1). However, as endpoints, progression-free and disease-free survival are dependent on how local and distant progression are defined and assessed. This varies among the authors, and these endpoints are consequently difficult to use when comparing uncontrolled studies (14). Metastasis-free survival may be easier to assess if based on regular bone scans, and in two series (6, 13) it was reported to be 77% and 66% at 10-year follow-up (Table 22.1).

Disease-specific or cause-specific survival may theoretically be the least flawed survival endpoint for early prostate cancer when comparing uncontrolled studies. It accounts for the mortality of the studied disease only, and mortality from other causes is censored in the analysis. Thus, disease-specific survival answers the question—if a patient does not die of other disease, what is the chance of not having died of the studied disease at a specific point? Because this endpoint accounts for the mortality from the studied disease only, the accuracy of disease-specific survival greatly depends on a correct assessment of the cause of death in each case. However, the exact cause of death is difficult to define in some cases, and disease-specific survival as a survival endpoint may therefore be less robust than overall survival.

In the current literature on deferred treatment for clinically localized prostate cancer, the reported disease-specific survival rate at 10 years ranged from 74 to 87% (Table 22.1). In the two largest series (5, 6), the disease-specific survival rates at 10 years were 84% and 85% (Table 22.1). In both series, the subgroup of patients who were younger than 70 years of age at diagnosis was analyzed and the disease-specific survival rates at 10 years were 92% and 87% (Table 22.1).

The majority of studies on deferred treatment focused on survival outcomes. Only a few studies provided information on local progression or local symptoms such as bladder outlet obstruction or bleeding. In one study, with a mean follow-up time of approximately 8 years, 67% of patients had a local progression of any kind during the follow-up and 21% required a transurethral resection of the prostate because of bladder outlet obstruction (15). In another study, with a mean follow-up of 10 years, 22% of patients had tumors that progressed locally to stage T3, 16% needed a transurethral resection of the prostate or an incision of the bladder neck, and 3% experienced

Table 22.2.   Compiled 10-Year Disease-Specific Survival After Deferred Treatment of Clinically Localized Palpable Prostate Cancer Based on Data Reported in the Current Literature

	AUSTENFELD ET AL. (18) (%)	ADOLFSSON ET AL. (16)	
		WEIGHTED REPORTED MEAN (%)	CALCULATED (%)
Radical prostatectomy	89	93	93
Radiation therapy	67	74	62
Deferred treatment	87	84	83

Table 22.4.   Pooled Analysis Based on Original Patient Data from Six Series on Deferred Treatment of Clinically Localized Prostate Cancer (19)

DIFFERENTIATION	10-YR METASTASIS-FREE SURVIVAL (95% CONFIDENCE INTERVAL)	10-YR DISEASE-SPECIFIC SURVIVAL (95% CONFIDENCE INTERVAL)
Well (n = 492)	81% (75–86)	87% (81–91)
Moderate (n = 265)	58% (49–66)	87% (80–92)
Poor (n = 62)	26% (13–41)	34% (19–50)

n = Number of evaluable patients.

severe hematuria (5). Other local symptoms were rare in this study.

No study investigated how prostate cancer and deferred management affected quality of life.

Compiled Studies

Reviews

During 1993 and 1994, three reviews of the currently available literature on deferred treatment of clinically localized prostate cancer were published (16–18). The authors used more or less the same literature as a basis; in addition to a regular review, published data were compiled in various ways.

Two reviews used reported data on disease-specific survival to calculate a mean, either with the number of patients in each series as weights (16) or with a compiled variance based on the number of evaluable patients in each assessed series (18). The compiled disease-specific survival rates at 10 years in these two studies were 84% and 87% (Table 22.2). Moreover, the authors of two reviews calculated the incidence for metastasis development and the incidence of mortality from prostate cancer from the number of patients in whom metastases developed, the number of patients who died of prostate cancer, and the follow-up time reported in the evaluable series. In one of the studies (16), the yearly incidences for metastasis development and mortality from prostate cancer were 0.025 (95% confidence interval, 0.020 to 0.031) and 0.017 (95% confidence interval, 0.013 to 0.021), respectively (Table 22.3). In the other study (17), the yearly incidences for metastasis development and mortality from prostate cancer were 0.017 (95% confidence interval,

0.011 to 0.043) and 0.009 (95% confidence interval, 0.006 to 0.012), respectively (Table 22.3).

Pooled Analysis

During 1993, original data from each patient in six series of deferred treatment of clinically localized prostate cancer were pooled to a new survival analysis (19). Altogether, 819 patients were evaluable. The disease-specific survival rate at 10 years was 87% for patients with well or moderately differentiated tumors and 34% for patients with poorly differentiated tumors (Table 22.4) (Fig. 22.1). The metastasis-free survival rates at 10 years for patients with well, moderately, and poorly differentiated tumors were 81%, 58%, and 26%, respectively (Table 22.4). Although the disease-specific survival was high for patients with moderately differentiated tumors, the relatively high proportion of patients with metastatic disease among those still alive at 10 years suggests that the mortality from prostate cancer in this category of patients may increase beyond 10 years of observation time. This is, however, not yet proven. Patients with well-differentiated tumors seemed to have continuously good prognoses, whereas patients with poorly differentiated tumors had uniformly bad prognoses early in the course of the disease.

Controlled Trial

To date, there is only one published study comparing the outcome of deferred treatment for patients with clinically localized

Table 22.3.   Compiled Yearly Incidences With 95% Confidence Intervals for Metastasis Development and Prostate Cancer Mortality After Deferred Treatment of Clinically Localized Palpable Prostate Cancer Based on Data Reported in the Current Literature

	METASTASIS		MORTALITY	
	WASSON ET AL. (17)[a]	ADOLFSSON ET AL. (16)[b]	WASSON ET AL. (17)[a]	ADOLFSSON ET AL. (16)[b]
Radical prostatectomy	0.023 (0.014–0.025)	0.013 (0.010–0.015)	0.009 (0.007–0.013)	0.007 (0.005–0.009)
Radiation therapy	0.050 (0.030–0.095)	0.029 (0.025–0.033)	0.023 (0.010–0.030)	0.038 (0.023–0.059)
Deferred treatment	0.017 (0.011–0.043)	0.025 (0.020–0.031)	0.009 (0.006–0.012)	0.017 (0.013–0.021)

[a] Median annual rate.
[b] Weighted mean number of patients per person-year.

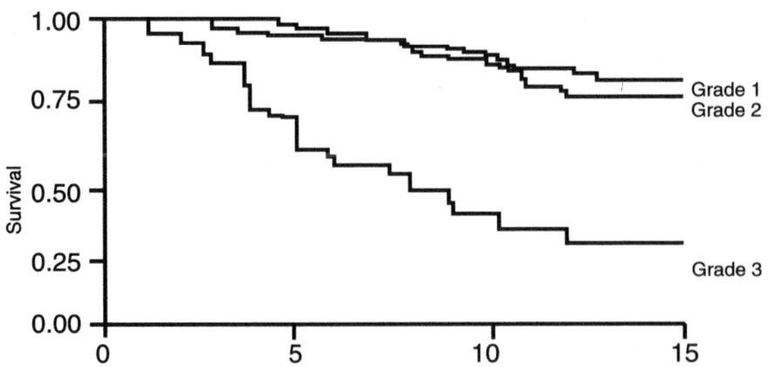

Fig. 22.1. Disease-specific survival among untreated patients with localized prostate cancer, according to tumor grade. Dates for patients who died of other causes were censored.

prostate cancer with any other treatment in a randomized study design. This study was initiated by the Veterans Administration Cooperative Urological Research Group in the late 1970s and compared deferred treatment versus radical prostatectomy. In the latest published report of this study, there was no difference between the groups with respect to overall survival at 15-year follow-up (4). The 20-year follow-up of this study has recently been presented, and there was still no difference in overall survival (Madsen PO, personal communication, 1994). However, the study has several flaws such as a low number of evaluable patients and a large number of patients lost to follow-up; the outcome must be interpreted with caution.

Summary

Judging from the various studies of deferred treatment of patients with low-grade clinically localized palpable prostate cancer diagnosed with the means available 15 to 20 years ago, the risk of dying of prostate cancer (if not having died of other disease before) up to 10 years after clinical diagnosis seems to be between 10 and 20%. For patients with high-grade tumors, the prognosis is poor.

The results in the reviews with data compilations and the pooled analysis merely mirror the outcome of the original studies (Table 22.1) because these studies provide the basis for the compiled studies. However, the similarity in the results in the reviews with various compiling techniques (Tables 22.2 and 22.3) and the narrow 95% confidence intervals in the pooled analysis (Table 22.4) suggest a certain consistency of the outcome in the various reports on deferred treatment.

The difference between overall and disease-specific survival in the individual series represents the competing mortality and up to 10 years of observation time; among all patients who died, the majority died of diseases not related to prostate cancer. There are only a few studies with observation longer than 10 years. In one with a mixed population of patients receiving early endocrine treatment or deferred treatment, the data suggest an increased mortality after 10 years (20). This was not the case in two other studies with more selected patients and follow-up times of 12.5 and 20 years (5, 12).

CONTROVERSIES

The data in the currently available series on deferred treatment of localized prostate cancer refer to patients whose conditions were diagnosed before prostate-specific antigen (PSA) was available. The patients included in these series all had conditions that were diagnosed after having abnormal results of a digital rectal examination or after transurethral resection of the prostate. Because many patients today have their conditions diagnosed after an elevated PSA is found in early detection and screening programs, the data from the currently available series on deferred treatment may appear outdated. It has been suggested that the tumors found today are smaller and with lower grades than those in the pre-PSA era (21, 22). One may consequently assume that the use of PSA today leads to a diagnosis earlier in the course of the disease than before (lead time) and it may also lead to diagnosis of tumors that would not have been diagnosed otherwise. Recently, there have been data published that suggest that the PSA might have been elevated as long as 5 to 10 years before the prostate cancer was diagnosed clinically (23, 24). This may indicate that the follow-up data from the available series on deferred treatment should be "added" with these 5 to 10 years to be comparable with the more recent treatment studies started in the PSA era. Also, with the lead time introduced by PSA detection, today's treatment studies may need 15 to 20 years of follow-up to be evaluable regarding survival.

As with all uncontrolled treatment studies, the available series on deferred treatment suffer from the selection process in various ways. One extreme is the retrospective study from the Memorial Sloan-Kettering Cancer Center series, in which the 68 evaluable patients were selected from more than 4000 patients with prostate cancer during approximately 20 years (12). The other extreme is the prospective series from Örebro in Sweden that was based on all patients with newly diagnosed prostate cancer in the catchment area during 5 years' time (5). In this series, the criteria for selection of patients to deferred treatment and the follow-up procedures were defined from the start. Although not all eligible patients were included in the surveillance protocol, all patients in the region whose conditions were diagnosed during the inclusion period were accounted for, making it possible to assess the selection of patients to the series. In this respect, this series is singular in the current literature on management of localized prostate cancer. In general, basic epidemiologic facts (such as the study base from which the evaluated patients were chosen, selection criteria, and patients lost to follow-up) are poorly described in the literature.

The two largest series on deferred treatment originate from Sweden (5, 6). The majority of patients included in these series had their conditions diagnosed with transrectal fine-needle aspiration (FNA) biopsy. All patients whose conditions were diagnosed with FNA biopsy in the two series had a palpable nodule in the prostate, and repeated biopsies confirmed the diagnosis in one of the series (6).

It has been suggested that up to 30% of patients with well-differentiated tumors diagnosed with FNA biopsy may have a false-positive diagnosis (25). The 30% was based on a study of 27 prostate specimens from radical prostatectomies in which FNA biopsies, core biopsies, and blocks were taken postoperatively and compared (26). The experience from these 27 cases must be put into relation to the much larger experience of FNA biopsies in Scandinavian countries (27, 28). In a Swedish study comparing digitally directed FNA biopsy with transrectal core biopsies directed with transrectal ultrasound, the number of patients with a clear-cut diagnosis of prostate cancer and the number of unclear findings were equal for the two techniques (29). When patients with well-differentiated tumors diagnosed with FNA or core biopsy were compared in the aforementioned pooled analysis, there was no significant difference in survival outcome (19). Consequently, the risk of a substantial number of patients with false diagnoses due to difficulties in assessing well-differentiated prostate cancer with cytology is probably much less than anticipated by some authors (25, 26).

The series on deferred treatment seemed to include a higher proportion of patients with low-grade prostate cancer compared with the series on radical prostatectomy and radiation therapy (16). In at least one of the larger series on deferred treatment, patients with poorly differentiated tumors were not included in the series (6); in another such series, patients with poorly differentiated tumors were included only during the last part of the inclusion period (5). Moreover, many patients in the deferred series (almost all patients in the Swedish series) had their conditions diagnosed by cytology after FNA biopsy. Cytologic grading has been found to undergrade prostate cancer compared with core biopsies (29–31). FNA and core biopsies have also been found to undergrade prostate cancer compared with histologic investigation of radical prostatectomy specimens (32–35). Hence, there may be a systematic undergrading in the series on deferred treatment, and at least some patients would have been upgraded if they had undergone a radical prostatectomy. The overrepresentation of patients with well-differentiated tumors in the deferred series compared with series on radical surgery and radiation may therefore be less pronounced than it may appear.

The patients in the series on deferred treatment were older than those in the series on more aggressive treatments (16). However, in two of the series (5, 7) on deferred treatment, the subgroups of patients that would have been eligible for radical surgery were analyzed separately; in these groups, the mean age was similar to that in the series on radical prostatectomy.

Differences in mean age may infer a bias in two ways when uncontrolled treatment studies are compared. First, age by itself may be a prognostic factor; e.g., younger patients have different prognoses than older patients. In this case, age acts as a confounder due to imbalances in prognostic factors if groups with different mean ages are being compared. Second, older patients are likely to experience a shorter part of the hazard rate curve for prostate cancer mortality because they have a higher risk of dying of other disease than do younger patients. If the hazard rate of dying of prostate cancer is not constant over time, various age-groups will have different risks of dying of prostate cancer. The rise in competing mortality accompanying increased age could therefore infer a difference because older patients will not live long enough to die of prostate cancer. In this case, age will also be a confounding factor but will be due to unbalanced observation periods.

Both types of confounding that may arise from varying mean ages in treatment groups are impossible to correct for in uncontrolled studies.

COMPARISONS WITH OTHER MANAGEMENT TECHNIQUES

As mentioned previously, there is to date only one published randomized trial comparing deferred treatment with any other management for localized prostate cancer (4). However, this study comparing deferred treatment versus radical prostatectomy has flaws that make it difficult to judge outcome.

The lack of reliable controlled trials in this field leaves us trying to assess the efficacy of different treatment options for localized prostate cancer from uncontrolled treatment studies. In the aforementioned three reviews of the current literature, data compilations of the outcome for various management techniques were attempted (16–18). The results of these data compilations were fairly consistent, with disease-specific survival rates at 10-year follow-up and incidences of prostate cancer mortality for radical prostatectomy that were slightly better than or equal to those for deferred treatment, although the outcome was worse for external radiation therapy (Tables 22.2 and 22.3). The incidence of metastatic disease was highest for radiation therapy, closely followed by deferred treatment; the incidence was lowest for radical prostatectomy (Table 22.3). The differences in incidences of metastatic disease may, with an extended follow-up, result in larger differences in survival between the treatment groups, but this remains to be shown.

Any comparison of outcome data generated in uncontrolled studies will be biased. Apart from bias inferred by varying inclusion criteria in the individual studies, comparisons will also be biased because of more systematic differences in the selection of patients for the different treatments. An attempt to account for these differences was made in one of the previously mentioned reviews of the current literature (16). The obvious biases were mainly due to confounding because of imbalances in prognostic factors for the various treatments. The proportion of patients with high-grade tumors was larger among patients who underwent radical prostatectomy or radiation therapy compared with those receiving deferred treatment. However, this difference may actually be less pronounced due to the varying grading procedures used, as discussed previously. There seemed to be a stage migration toward smaller local tumors in the surgical group because, in some of the surgical series, only patients with tumors that were pathologically confined to the prostate gland were included in the analysis. In the series on deferred treatment and radiation therapy, the tumors were regarded as confined after clinical investigation. Almost all patients in the surgical series and some in the radiation therapy series underwent lymph node dissection in the pelvis and most of the included patients were found to be without metastases in the regional lymph nodes; no patients in the deferred series were surgically staged. Hence, it is likely that a significant but unknown proportion of patients in the series on deferred treatment and radiation therapy had tumors that were not confined to the prostate and/or metastases in the regional lymph nodes. Some series on radiation therapy included not only patients with newly diagnosed tumors, but also patients who had their disease for some time and may have already experienced progression or other treatment failure.

With these imbalances in prognostic factors working in different directions and with various magnitudes, it is difficult, if not impossible, to judge the differences in outcome for the various management techniques. Also, differences in mean age among the groups who underwent different treatments were obvious; as previously mentioned, such differences may also infer biases in various ways.

The only way to resolve which therapy is optimal for patients with clinically localized prostate cancer is by randomized treatment studies. Two such studies, one comparing deferred treatment and radical prostatectomy (Scandinavian Prostate Cancer Group) and the other comparing deferred treatment with external radiation therapy (Umeå University), are currently being conducted in Sweden and Finland.

WHO COULD BE MANAGED WITH DEFERRED TREATMENT?

It is evident that some but not all patients with localized prostate cancer will die of their disease irrespective of primary management. Currently, there are no firm data showing a superiority for any management with respect to survival outcome up to 10 years after diagnosis. It is also evident that patients developing metastatic disease and dying of prostate cancer almost uniformly suffer from severe morbidity that is often difficult to handle.

High-grade prostate cancer will progress, and many patients will die because of it. These patients are therefore difficult to manage in a deferred way; on the other hand, it is questionable if there is any upfront therapy that is effective for the majority of these patients. There are, however, recently published data suggesting that radical prostatectomy may be effective for those whose high-grade tumor is confined to the prostate gland (36, 37).

Patients with clinically localized low-grade tumors have several treatment options and should be counseled about them all. The available data suggest that prostate cancer mortality in patients with this category of disease is affected only to a small, if any, extent by aggressive treatment during the first 10 years of follow-up in patients diagnosed with the means available 15 to 20 years ago. Whether aggressive treatment in these cases can reduce the morbidity from prostate cancer has not been investigated.

In the absence of prognostic factors that can tell us in which patients low-grade prostate cancer will progress to give symptoms and maybe eventually kill the patient, life expectancy may be the most important factor to consider when counseling the patient. With the data we have today, deferred treatment may be an option for patients with a life expectancy of 10 years or less. It must again be emphasized that these data were derived from patients whose conditions were diagnosed before PSA was available. Today (when tumors are found in a presumably earlier phase), the required time for the tumor to develop to an aggressive and advanced stage may be longer than in earlier series. Therefore, life expectancy for the patient may also be longer.

Quality-of-life issues have not been evaluated in patients with deferred treatment. As long as the patient remains untreated, functions such as urinary continence and erectile capacity remain unaffected, except for changes that are directly due to the tumor and its growth. In patients managed with a deferred strategy, the eventual problems they experience because of changes in these functions should, at least hypothetically, be less than the problems for locally aggressive treatments. If the rate of local progression with symptoms and metastatic progression is higher than for the treated groups, this will have a larger negative effect on the quality of life of the patient managed with deferred treatment; however, this remains to be shown. The knowledge of living with an untreated tumor may also have a negative effect on the quality of life, but this issue has not been studied.

MANAGEMENT

Treatment options must be thoroughly discussed at diagnosis. Only the patient can judge the pros and the cons of deferred treatment and other managements relative to his situation and preferences regarding side effects, etc. If deferred treatment is decided on, both the patient and doctor must be aware that the disease will probably progress slowly. Also, there is no guarantee that the disease will not have a more rapid course.

In the majority of clinically localized, low-grade prostate cancers, there will be a slow local progression of the tumor that initially may be difficult to assess clinically and the PSA will gradually increase with time. Usually, this process takes many years. It must be realized by both the patient and doctor that, if the tumor was truly confined from the beginning, somewhere along the course it will eventually grow to a stage where it is extending outside the capsule and by then escapes the possibility of radical cure.

A general rule is that the patient should be followed regularly, preferably by the same physician, and that the patient is kept well informed about the status of the disease during the follow-up period. Deferring therapy does not mean not taking care of the patient.

Local symptoms from an infravesical obstruction may be managed with a transurethral resection or endocrine treatment.

Symptoms from an advanced local progression or distant metastases should be treated as a progression after any other management. Anxiety because of living with the tumor or progression of the tumor must also be regarded as a symptom and treated accordingly. If the patient wants active treatment at any point during the surveillance, this should not be denied. Treatment should then be chosen with respect to the stage of the disease and the general status of the patient at that point.

Deferring treatment may give the patient many years without treatment and its side effects. The patient may not need any treatment for his prostate cancer at any point during his life.

REFERENCES

1. Jonsson PM, Danneskiold-Samsöe B, Heggestad T, et al. Management of early prostatic cancer in the Nordic countries: variations in clinical policies and physicians attitudes toward radical treatment options: a NEMT survey. Int J Tech Assess In press.
2. Moskovitz B, Nitecki S, Richter Levin D. Cancer of the prostate: is there a need for aggressive treatment? Urol Int 1987;42:49.
3. George NJR. Natural history of localised prostatic cancer managed by conservative therapy alone. Lancet 1988;5:494.
4. Graverson PH, Nielsson KT, Gasser TC, et al. Radical prostatectomy versus expectant treatment in stages I and II prostatic cancer: a fifteen-year follow-up. Urology 1990;36:493.
5. Johansson JE, Adami HO, Andersson SO, et al. High 10 year survival rate in patients with early untreated prostatic cancer. JAMA 1992;267:2191.
6. Adolfsson J, Carstensen J, Löwhagen T. Deferred treatment in clinically localized prostatic carcinoma. Br J Urol 1992;69:183.
7. Adolfsson J, Carstensen J. Natural course of clinically localized prostate adenocarcinoma in men less than 70 years old. J Urol 1991;146:96.
8. Chisholm GD, Rana A. Is the outcome of conservative management for localized prostate cancer acceptable? an overview. Eur Urol 1993;24 (Suppl):64.
9. Egawa S, Go M, Kuwao S, et al. Long-term impact of conservative management on localized prostate cancer. Urology 1993;42:520.
10. Stenzl A, Studer UE. Outcome of patients with untreated cancer of the prostate. Eur Urol 1993;24:1.
11. Waaler G, ESA. Prognosis of localized prostatic cancer managed by watch and wait policy. Br J Urol 1993;72:214.
12. Warner J, Whitmore WF Jr. Expectant management of clinically localized prostatic cancer. J Urol 1994;152:1761.
13. Lundgren R, Nordle Ö, Josefsson K, South Sweden Prostate Cancer Study Group. Immediate estrogen or estramustine phosphate therapy versus deferred endocrine treatment in non-metastatic prostate cancer: a randomized multicenter study with 15 years follow-up. J Urol In press.
14. Steineck G, Adolfsson J, Whitmore WF Jr. Local recurrence and disease free survival, doubtful parameters when comparing non-randomized studies of prostate cancer. Scand J Nephrol Urol 1991;138(Suppl):121.
15. Adolfsson J, Röström L, Löwhagen T, et al. Deferred treatment of clinically, localized low grade prostate cancer: the experience from a prospective series at the Karolinska hospital. J Urol 1994;152:1757.
16. Adolfsson J, Steineck G, Whitmore WF. Recent results of management of palpable clinically localized prostate cancer. Cancer 1993;72:310.
17. Wasson JH, Cushman CC, Bruskewitz RC, et al. Prostate Disease Outcome Research Team. A structured literature review of treatment for localized prostate cancer. Arch Fam Med 1993;2:487.
18. Austenfeld MS, Thompson IM Jr, Middleton RG for the American Urological Association Prostate Cancer Guideline Panel. Meta-analysis of the literature: guideline development for prostate cancer treatment. J Urol 1994;152:1866.
19. Chodak G, Thiested R, Gerber G, et al. Results of conservative management of clinically localized prostate cancer. N Engl J Med 1994;330:242.
20. Aus G, Hugosson J, Norlén L. Risk of dying of prostate cancer in different stages, grades and age at diagnosis. J Urol 1994;151(Suppl):278. Abstract.
21. Ohori M, Wheeler TM, Dunn K, et al. The pathological features and prognosis of prostate cancer detectable with current diagnostic tests. J Urol 1994;152:1714.
22. Smith DS, Catalona WJ. The nature of prostate cancer detected through prostate specific antigen based screening. J Urol 1994;152:1732.
23. Stenman UH, Hakama M, Knekt P, et al. Serum concentrations of prostate specific antigen and its complex with alfa-1-antichymotrypsin before diagnosis of prostate cancer. Lancet 1994;344:1594.
24. Pearson JD, Carter HB. Natural history of changes in prostate specific antigen in early stage prostate cancer. J Urol 1994;152:1743.
25. Schellhammer PF. Contemporary expectant therapy series: a viewpoint. Urology 1994;44:47.
26. Mohler JL, Erozan YS, Walsh PC, et al. Fine-needle core and aspiration biopsy; a new method for diagnosis of prostatic carcinoma. Cancer 1989;63:1846.
27. Esposti PL. Cytologic malignancy grading of prostate carcinoma by transrectal aspiration biopsy. Scand J Urol Nephrol 1971;5:199.
28. Willems JS, Löwhagen T. Transrectal fine-needle aspiration biopsy for cytologic diagnosis and grading of prostatic carcinoma. Prostate 1981;2:3281.
29. Waisman J, Adolfsson J, Löwhagen T, et al. Comparison of transrectal prostate digital aspiration and ultrasound-guided core biopsies in 99 men. Urology 1991;37:301.
30. Chodak GW, Bibbi M, Straus FH, et al. Transrectal aspiration biopsy versus transperineal core biopsy for the diagnosis of carcinoma of the prostate. J Urol 1984;132:480.
31. Carter HB, Riehle RA, Koizumi JH, et al. Fine needle aspiration of the abnormal prostate: a cytohistological correlation. J Urol 1986;135:294.
32. Catalona WJ, Stein AJ, Fair WR. Grading errors in prostatic needle biopsies: relation to the accuracy of tumor grade in predicting pelvic lymph node metastases. J Urol 1982;127:919.
33. Mills SE, Fowler JE. Gleason histologic grading of prostatic

carcinoma; correlations between biopsy and prostatectomy specimens. Cancer 1986;57:346.

34. Narayan P, Jajodia P, Stein R, et al. A comparison of fine needle aspiration and core biopsy in diagnosis and preoperative grading of prostate cancer. J Urol 1989;141:560.

35. Pontes JE, Wajsman Z, Huben RP, et al. Prognostic factors in localized prostatic carcinoma. J Urol 1985;134:1137.

36. Zincke H, Oesterling JE, Blute ML, et al. Long-term (15 years) results after radical prostatectomy for clinically localized (stage T2c or lower) prostate cancer. J Urol 1994;152: 1850.

37. Ohori M, Goad JR, Wheeler TM, et al. Can radical prostatectomy alter the progression of poorly differentiated prostate cancer? J Urol 1994;152:184.

BLADDER CARCINOMA

Carcinoma of the Bladder

An Overview

J. Brantley Thrasher

INTRODUCTION

The past decade has seen an explosion of advances in the molecular and genetic aspects of tumor biology. These advances have led to a better understanding of the mechanisms of abnormal cell proliferation, tumor invasion, and metastasis. Much of this information pertaining to changes at the genetic level and subsequent phenotypic changes is relevant to our understanding of bladder cancer.

We continue to recognize a multitude of clinical prognosticators in bladder cancer, but new molecular markers have opened up new avenues of research. Although in its infancy, the molecular biologic research of bladder cancer will lead to the most significant discoveries of the near future.

A thorough discussion of all aspects of bladder cancer or even the most recent molecular biologic research is beyond the scope of this chapter. This chapter presents an overview of the demographics and etiology of bladder cancer; pertinent molecular biologic findings and how these pertain to biologic variability noted; molecular, histologic, and clinical prognostic factors in bladder cancer; the diagnosis and staging of bladder cancer; and a contemporary overview of treatment options.

DEMOGRAPHICS

Transitional cell carcinoma of the urinary bladder is now the second most common malignancy of the genitourinary tract in the United States and is the fifth most common cause of cancer deaths among U.S. men older than 75 years of age (1). It accounts for 6.0% of all cancers diagnosed in men and 2.3% in women (1). Although the age-adjusted incidence of transitional cell carcinoma of the bladder continues to increase by 0.9% annually, cancer-specific deaths remain relatively constant at approximately 10,000 per year (7000 in men; 3600 in women) (1). Therefore, over the past three decades the 5-year cancer-specific survival rate has improved from 53% and 24% to 80% and 61% in white and black patients, respectively (1). The

noted improvement in survival accompanied by an increasing incidence is most likely attributed to early diagnosis and referral in addition to improved patient selection, surgical technique, and perioperative care.

Cancer of the bladder occurs primarily in white men. The male to female ratio is at least 3 to 1 and approaches 4 to 1 among whites. The incidence in white men is 31.5/100,000 compared with 16.2/100,000 in black men; this higher incidence rate occurs over the entire age range (2). Rates are lower among Asian and Hispanic groups than among blacks and are very low among Native Americans. Additionally, incidence and mortality rates rise with age, resulting in two thirds of cases occurring in patients 65 years or older (1).

Geographically, incidence rates are high in Western Europe and North America, with relatively low rates in Eastern Europe and Asia. The rates appear to be higher in urban areas than in rural areas both nationally and internationally (3).

ETIOLOGY

Since 1895 when Rehn first suggested a role for certain chemicals in the etiology of bladder cancer, this has been the neoplasm most strongly linked to occupational and environmental exposure to chemicals (4). Traditionally, these chemicals and other carcinogens have been hypothesized to produce carcinogenesis by the process of "initiation" and "promotion" (5, 6). Initiation is the mechanism by which stem cells that have been exposed to chemical or physical agents (mutagens) undergo an irreversible genetic change (mutation in DNA). This genetic change may be an alteration in a gene's base pairs, deletion of a component that controls cell growth, or amplification of a gene and subsequent increase in its activity (6). This resultant mutated cell must then replicate and fix the altered genome in place. Promotion is the process by which a variety of substances (promoters) react with the cell surface and/or cytoplasmic and nuclear receptors to stimulate proliferation of the initiated clone of cells. Promotion, unlike initiation, can be a reversible process and,

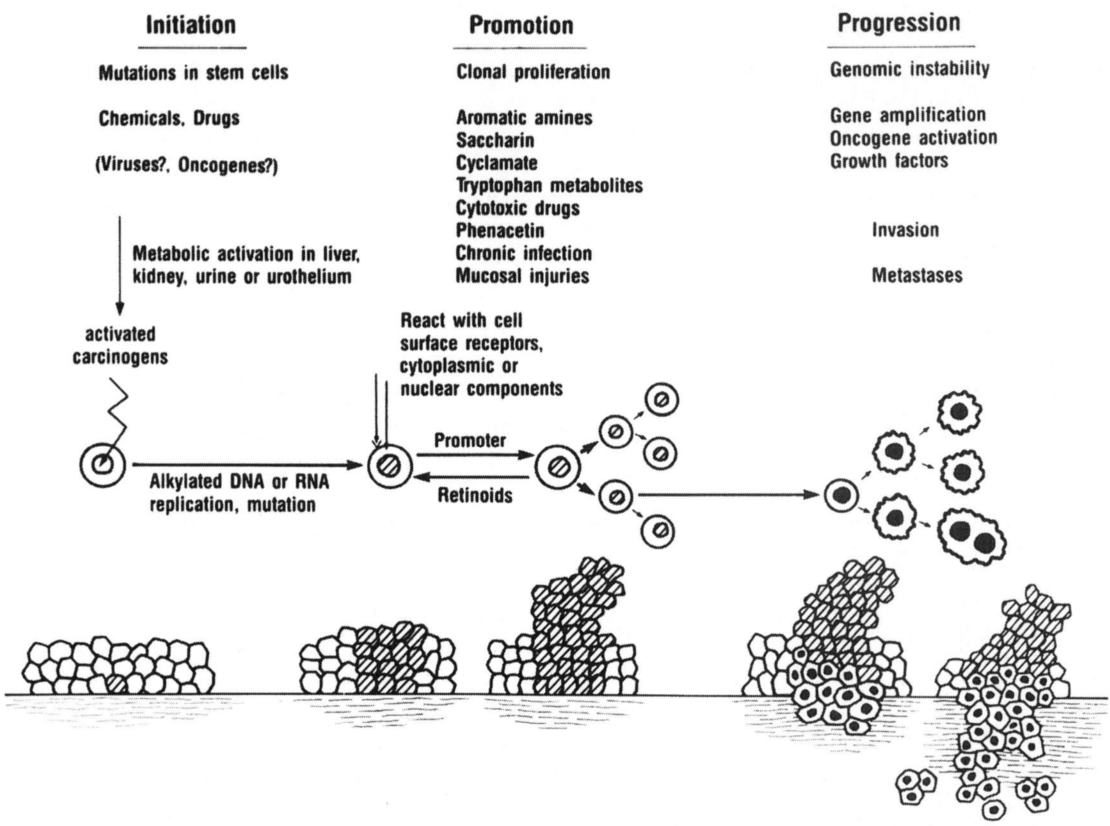

Fig. 23.1. Carcinogenesis as a multiple stage process. Initiation transforms a normal cell to a cancer cell; promotion stimulates proliferation of the initiated (mutated) cell; and progression provides for the infiltration and dissemination of cancer cells from the primary lesion. (Reprinted with permission (6).)

without initiation, will not lead to neoplastic transformation (Fig. 23.1).

A multitude of carcinogens have been implicated in the etiology of bladder cancer. Cigarette smoking has been the most commonly associated risk factor for the development of bladder cancer, with studies reporting a fourfold greater incidence of bladder cancer in cigarette smokers than in nonsmokers (7–10). As many as 40% of bladder cancers may be related to cigarette smoking, with an increase in the risk as the number of cigarettes smoked, duration of smoking, and degree of inhalation increase (11, 12). The chemical carcinogens are most likely the nitrosamines and many arylamines (2-naphthylamines, toluidines, and 4-aminobiphenyl) found in cigarette smoke. These compounds are known to function as carcinogens by inducing mutations in urothelial DNA (8).

Several occupations have long been associated with an increased risk of bladder cancer, again due to chemical carcinogens. Recent studies have estimated that between 21 and 25% of bladder cancers in whites and 27% in nonwhites are occupationally related (13). Occupations such as dye workers (14, 15), aromatic amine manufacturing workers (16, 17), rubber workers (18, 19), leather workers (20, 21), painters (14, 22, 23), truck drivers (24), aluminum workers (25), and machinists (23, 26, 27) have been shown to have an increased risk for bladder cancer development. The chemical carcinogens impli-

cated in these occupations are usually aromatic amines such as 2-naphthylamine and benzidine, both known to be especially potent human bladder carcinogens (28). The latency period for carcinoma development after exposure may be as long as 50 years but averages 18 years (29, 30).

Along these same lines, certain drugs have been implicated as etiologic factors of bladder cancer by virtue of their breakdown products. Ingestion of large quantities of the analgesic phenacetin may increase the risk for urothelial carcinoma (31). It is metabolized to paracetamol, which has a chemical structure similar to that of the aniline dyes. Therefore, this may result in the compound functioning as a carcinogen.

Similarly, cyclophosphamide, a widely used chemotherapeutic agent, is metabolized to four known breakdown products. Two of these metabolites, acrolein and phosphoamide mustard, have been shown to bind to DNA (32). Acrolein has been subsequently found to cause bladder toxicity and is believed to cause urothelial carcinomas as well as sarcomas in the bladder (33–35). 2-Mercaptoethane sodium sulfonate (Mesna), a compound that reduces cyclophosphamide-induced hemorrhagic cystitis by binding to the acrolein molecule and detoxifying the metabolite, has also been shown to reduce induction of bladder carcinoma in patients exposed to cyclophosphamide (36). This represents further evidence to support the causative association between acrolein and bladder carcinoma.

Bladder infections have also been convincingly implicated in the etiology of bladder cancer (37, 38). Whereas the majority of chemically induced bladder cancers are transitional cell carcinomas, cancers related to chronic urinary infections are generally invasive squamous cell carcinomas. Although experimental evidence has indicated that bacterial infections in the urinary tract promote bladder carcinogens in rats (39), the exact mechanisms are unclear. It is possible that bacterial enzymatic formation of nitroso compounds may play a role in the carcinogenesis. Infections with the parasite *Schistosoma haematobium* have also been associated with induction of bladder carcinoma (38). Although the schistosomal ova provide an irritative nidus by embedding in the bladder wall, secondary bacterial infection with exposure of the urothelium to nitrosamines probably plays an integral part in the formation of carcinomas in these patients (40).

Three other potential bladder carcinogens—tryptophan, sodium saccharin, and coffee—remain controversial in their association with bladder cancer. The etiologic association between tryptophan metabolites and bladder cancer has not been firmly established and requires further study. Studies have both supported and refuted this association (41, 42). Similarly, epidemiologic studies have failed to definitively document an association between ingestion of large quantities of artificial sweeteners and an increased risk of bladder cancer (43). In fact, recent epidemiologic studies and a review of the database accumulated on sodium saccharin would suggest that saccharin is not mutagenic and probably does not increase the risk for development of bladder tumors (44, 45). A similar review of case-control research on coffee drinking was recently reported, suggesting no clinically important association between the regular use of coffee and development of cancer of the lower urinary tract in men or women (46).

In summary, a multitude of etiologic factors exist for the formation of bladder cancer. The majority of these factors either are chemical carcinogens or result in the formation of chemical carcinogens that act as promoters and/or initiators in carcinogenesis. The molecular biologic changes induced by many of these agents have just recently been elucidated.

MOLECULAR BIOLOGIC CHANGES

In the mid 1970s, it became apparent that these chemical carcinogens must produce genetic damage and subsequently lead to cancer cells that carry mutant genes. During this time, Drs. Varmus and Bishop were studying animal RNA tumor viruses (retroviruses) and discovered that one of these viruses, the Rous sarcoma virus of chickens, carried a specific gene used to transform infected cells from the normal to the malignant state. This gene was termed a viral oncogene. Subsequent to this, the researchers found that the oncogene was not truly a viral gene but that it arose directly from a preexisting cellular gene that had been captured by an ancestor of the Rous sarcoma virus. This cellular gene, once captured by the virus, was used by the virus to transform cells. The kidnapped normal cellular gene was termed proto-oncogene by Stehelin, Varmus, and Bishop (47).

This work led researchers to the understanding that there were genes present in the normal cellular DNA that might serve as target genes activated by mutagenic chemicals. These proto-oncogenes might subsequently convert into oncogenes that result in the initiation of deregulated growth and cancer formation.

As our ability to perform genetic research grew, so did our ability to research the theories of oncogenes and proto-oncogenes. Studies of human tumors revealed mutations in proto-oncogenes thought to be responsible for converting them into active oncogenes. To date, approximately 20 transformed or mutated proto-oncogenes (oncogenes) have been identified in human tumors (48).

However, oncogenes appear to be only a small part of the reason cells suddenly become derailed and begin to grow out of control. Cells normally respond to external messages from neighboring cells, which leads to proliferation. A normal cell will not generally proliferate on its own. These messages may be growth inhibiting or growth stimulating and are conveyed largely by growth factors. These growth factors impinge on the surface of the cells and send messages to the interior of the cell, resulting in protein synthesis. Proto-oncogenes encode many of the proteins in this internal circuitry that enable a normal cell to respond to these external growth factors (48). Oncogenes, however, result in protein signals that activate these signaling circuits even in the absence of stimulation by growth factors (Fig. 23.2).

Another integral part of this schema, however, is the inhibition of normal cell growth. A normal cell also contains several genes that act to constrain or suppress growth. In fact, it has been suggested that normal cell growth may be regulated by a finely tuned balance achieved between the growth-promoting proto-oncogenes and the growth-constraining genes (48). Therefore, if this latter set of "antioncogenes" or "tumor suppressor genes" is mutated or disabled, cell growth may continue in an uncontrollable fashion.

The importance of many of these oncogenes as they relate to bladder cancer requires further study. However, a large body of information has now been accumulated regarding the prognostic significance of certain chromosomal changes (many of which result in loss of tumor suppressor genes) in many bladder tumors. Each chromosome has two arms that are divided into bands, with the letters p and q used to designate the short and long arms, respectively (49). Allelic loss of chromosomes 9q, 11p, and 17p have now been shown to be important genetic alterations leading to carcinogenesis in bladder cancer (50–52). Data indicating loss of chromosomal arm 9q in early stage bladder cancers suggest the presence of a tumor suppressor gene in this region whose inactivation may be important in the earlier stages of tumorigenesis (53). Additionally, chromosomal loss of 11p has been identified in approximately 30 to 40% of bladder cancers and has been associated with higher stage disease (50, 51).

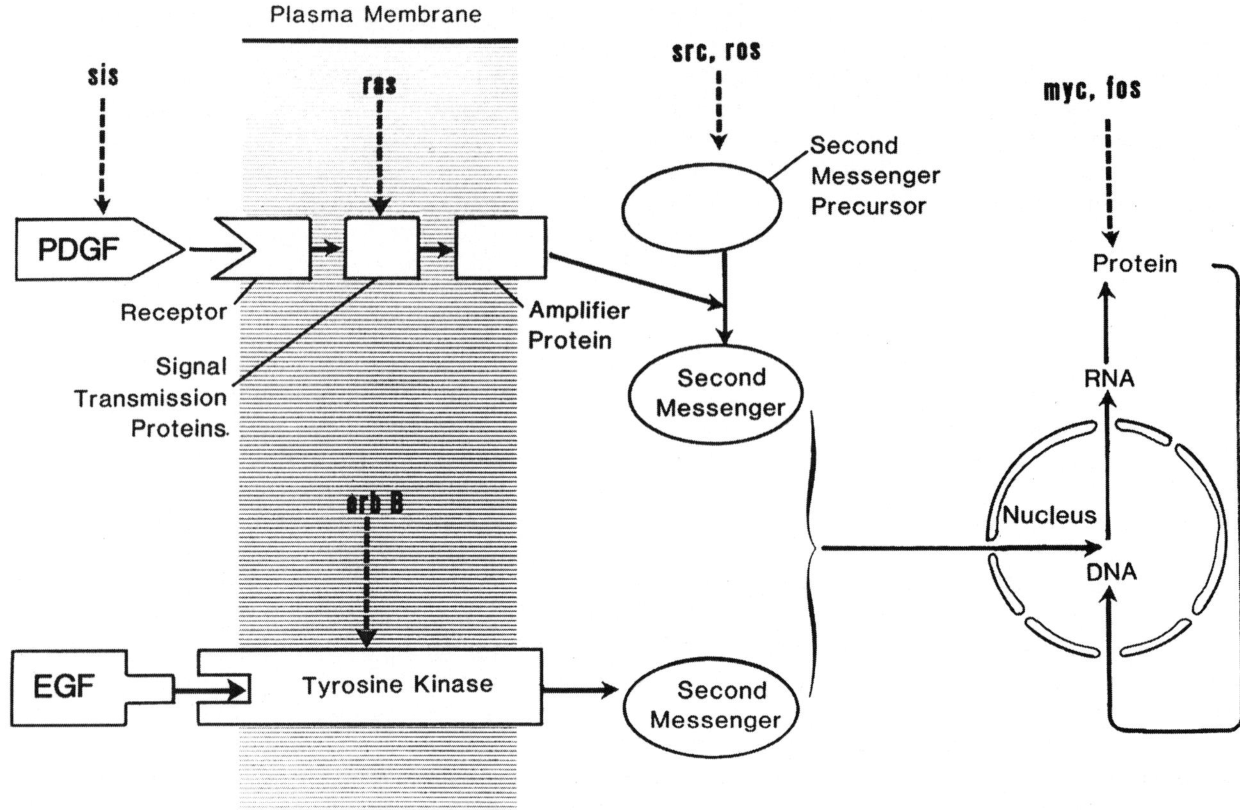

Fig. 23.2. Possible locations where oncogenes may disrupt regulation of cell growth. External signals in the form of growth factors such as platelet-derived growth factor (PDGF) or epidermal growth factor (EGF) act on plasma membrane receptors (left) and eventually act to initiate DNA transcription.

However, the most widely studied genetic alteration in bladder cancer is loss of heterozygosity at 17p where the tumor suppressor gene p53 resides. Sidransky et al. analyzed 18 primary bladder tumors and found p53 gene mutations in 61% of bladder cancers. Additionally, these mutations were usually seen in tumors of high stage and grade, with few noted in superficial tumors (54). Point mutations in the p53 gene lead to alterations within the p53 protein that inactivate the normal ("wild-type") protein (55). Additionally, in cells carrying one normal copy of the p53 gene and one mutant copy, growth may still be abnormal due to a "dominant negative" mode of action. The mutant p53 protein actually compromises the ongoing function of its normal counterpart in the cell (55). It appears that the normal role of wild-type p53 is to assure the fidelity of DNA repair and replication while loss of normal p53 results in altered cell cycle arrest and gene amplification (55).

It is now evident that tumor suppressor genes are altered in a wide variety of human tumors. Mutant versions of the p53 gene have been found in more than 50% of human tumors examined to date, making it the most common genetic alteration identified in human cancers (56). Therefore, it appears that inactivation of p53 may be a critical early step in the initiation of carcinogenesis.

The previously mentioned genetic alterations appear to cor-relate well with what is seen clinically in bladder cancer. It is possible that certain chromosomal alterations (e.g., 9q deletions) may permit uncontrolled proliferation of cells without conferring on them the ability to invade and metastasize (57). Other chromosomal alterations (e.g., 17p deletions) may not only promote cell proliferation but also confer enzymatic changes that permit the transformed cell to invade and ultimately metastasize ("progression") (Fig. 23.1) (57–59). Further studies in this regard may allow us to direct more appropriately our therapeutic approach to bladder tumors based on genetic alterations noted during clinical staging.

CLINICAL PROGNOSTICATORS IN BLADDER CANCER

Although the molecular biologic findings previously mentioned will most certainly play a key role in directing therapy for bladder cancer in the near future, further research is needed before these methods prove practically applicable for the clinician. Similarly, other molecular prognostic factors examined, such as the presence of chromosomal abnormalities (cytogenetics and flow cytometry) (60) and the presence or absence of antigen expression on tumor cells (61, 62), have been shown to relay prognostic information related to progression and risk of recurrence. Flow cytometry is probably the most objective parameter currently used to measure change in DNA. This technique uses an automated device in which individual cell nuclei are passed through a laser beam and the amount of light scatter is recorded. The device measures nuclear size and indirectly reflects the DNA content of each cell. The results are then expressed in a two-dimensional or three-dimensional graph that estimates the ploidy of the population of cells. The standard criteria for DNA changes in the bladder are as follows (63):

1. Normal—less than 11% hyperdiploid with no aneuploid line;
2. Suspicious—greater than 11%, but less than 15.9% hyperdiploid, no aneuploid line; and
3. Cancer—greater than 16% hyperdiploid or any aneuploidy.

These criteria have proved to be highly predictive for identifying early tumors up to 1 year before cytologic or cystoscopic detection (64). Also, aneuploidy has been found to be predictive of recurrence, progression, and the presence of carcinoma in situ, with 50% of these patients progressing versus 10% of those with hyperdiploid tumors (65). Nevertheless, none of these tests has proved to be sufficiently sensitive, specific, or practical to allow incorporation into general clinical use.

Conversely, clinical and histologic parameters remain the primary prognostic factors used by clinicians to determine a therapeutic course of action. Clinical indicators such as size of the initial tumor, number of tumors at initial presentation, and time to recurrence have been found to correlate with risk of recurrence and progression. Heney et al. noted that tumors greater than 5 cm had only a 25% disease-free incidence at 2 years, with a 35% progression rate compared with a 9% progression rate in those less than 5 cm (66). These authors also noted that those patients who presented with four or more tumors were at very high risk for recurrence when compared with those presenting with less than four tumors (66). Fitzpatrick et al. confirmed these findings by reporting a recurrence rate of 69% for those patients with multiple tumors at presentation versus 46% for the entire group (67). Fitzpatrick et al. also found that patients who had recurrence within 3 months of their initial resection had further recurrences 90% of the time versus those without recurrences at 3 months, in which the risk for recurrence was 21% (67).

Histologic parameters are equally important for providing prognostic information. Tumor stage, tumor grade, and the status of the surrounding urothelium have all been shown to be useful prognostic factors. It has long been recognized that the histologic stage of transitional cell carcinoma of the bladder is predictive of recurrence, progression, and survival. Most urologists and oncologists have now begun to use the TNM staging system (Table 23.1) (68) and in doing so, it has become evident that those tumors confined to the mucosa (Ta) have a different biologic potential than those that have invaded lamina propria (T1) or the muscularis propria (T2 and T3a). It is probably best to describe stage T1 tumors as minimally invasive because their risk for progression more closely parallels stage T2 tumors

Table 23.1.   TNM Classification for Bladder Cancer

TIS	Carcinoma in situ
TA	Papillary noninvasive carcinoma (confined to mucosa)
T1	Papillary tumor—lamina propria invasion
T2	Superficial muscle invasion
T3A	Deep muscle invasion
T3B	Invasion of perivesical fat
T4	Invasion of contiguous viscera
N1	Solitary pelvic nodal metastasis <2 cm
N2	One or more pelvic nodes >2 cm and <5 cm
N3	Fixed pelvic mass or >5 cm pelvic node
M1	Distant metastasis or nodes positive above the aortic bifurcation

Reprinted with permission from Thrasher JB, Crawford ED. Management of invasive and metastatic bladder cancer. In: Lipshultz LI, ed. Current problems in urology. Chicago: Mosby-Year Book, 1992;2:35.

than Ta tumors (69). Heney et al. noted that 4% of patients who initially had stage Ta tumors demonstrated subsequent progression, whereas 30% of patients with stage T1 tumors had progression (66). In the same study, the incidence of recurrence among Ta tumors was 45% versus 67% for T1 tumors. Additional evidence for the potentially ominous nature of T1 disease is the reports indicating muscle-invasive recurrences in 40 to 50% of T1 patients (70) and an incidence of involved lymph nodes of 17% in those who eventually undergo cystectomy (71).

Muscle-infiltrating carcinoma (stage T2 and T3a) has an even more grave prognosis, with 50% of patients who present with the disease having relapse at distant sites and usually dying of the disease within 2 years (72). Recent evidence indicating that patients with T2 disease found to have no tumor after pathologic examination of the cystectomy specimen (pT0) have survival statistics no different from those with invasive tumor found in the cystectomy specimen (pT2) would suggest that these patients are dying because of micrometastases that were not identified at the time of the operation (73). This implies that the process of metastasis may have occurred very early in the development of these aggressive tumors, indicating a different biologic potential from most Ta or T1 tumors.

Tumor grade usually correlates very closely with tumor stage. Generally, grade 3 cells are rarely seen in mucosally confined tumors (67). Most grade 3 tumors present with at least superficial invasion (66). In contrast, less than 10% of grade 1 tumors and approximately 40 to 50% of grade 2 tumors are invasive at presentation (74). Additionally, grade 1 tumors are associated with approximately 80 to 95% 5-year survival rates, whereas grade 3 tumors are associated with a 40 to 50% 5-year survival rate (75, 76).

The status of the adjacent urothelium in patients with bladder carcinoma appears to be an important prognostic factor. Approximately 85% of papillary tumors associated with carcinoma in situ will present with an invasive recurrence within 2 years (61). Additionally, the incidence of recurrence is significantly greater if there is adjacent moderate to severe dysplasia compared with patients with normal adjacent mucosa. Moreover, findings of moderate to severe dysplasia increase the risk of progression from 8 to 33% (66).

These data suggest that these clinical parameters are late phenotypic indications of probable genotypic changes that predestine some tumors to act aggressively and metastasize early while others remain confined to the bladder urothelium. The molecular parameters described in a previous section are much more sensitive because the clinical and histologic parameters are merely a reflection of prior changes at the molecular level. Unfortunately, however, the molecular parameters are not clinically applicable at this time but will become an integral part of our diagnostic and therapeutic methodology in the near future.

DIAGNOSIS AND PREOPERATIVE STAGING

Patients with bladder carcinoma usually present with gross or microscopic hematuria and/or irritative voiding symptoms (77). After first excluding urinary infection, voided urine is obtained for cytologic studies and an excretory urogram is performed to exclude upper tract lesions. This test is followed by cystoscopy to evaluate the lower urinary tract. The advantage of performing the excretory urogram before cystoscopy is that if the upper urinary tracts were not visualized adequately, retrograde ureteropyelograms can be performed at cystoscopy. Exfoliative cytology is an important adjunct because the identification of a low-grade lesion or no cystoscopic evidence of a lesion in conjunction with a positive cytologic result would lead the clinician to search for either carcinoma in situ or an unidentified lesion elsewhere in the urinary tract.

The cystoscopic demonstration of bladder cancer or a report of a positive cytologic result with radiographically normal upper tracts prompts the scheduling of transurethral resection of the bladder tumor and/or multiple biopsies with the patient under anesthesia. Preoperative evaluation includes an electrocardiogram, chest radiograph, serum creatinine, and liver function tests. Patients with an elevated alkaline phosphatase level undergo a ^{99m}technetium bone scan.

Further radiographic modes of staging remain controversial. Recently, intravesical ultrasound has been investigated for staging bladder tumors (78). Although this method has been reported to correctly determine stage in greater than 90% of patients with muscle-invasive tumors, it cannot differentiate between superficial stages (Ta versus T1) nor can it reliably diagnose extravesical extension or pelvic lymph node metastases. Both magnetic resonance imaging (MRI) and computed tomography (CT) scan can more completely stage these patients, and recent studies comparing CT with MRI report that MRI is the most accurate modality (79, 80). With the recent additions of gadolinium-labeled DTPA, pulse sequence optimization, and endorectal surface coils, MRI appears to be more accurate than CT scanning in the determination of local tumor extension and in the detection of bone marrow metastases (79). Both methods appear to perform equally well in detecting

lymph node involvement. The primary disadvantages of MRI lie in its inaccuracy after transurethral resection or radiation therapy (79, 81). CT scanning suffers from the same inaccuracies, requiring scanning with either modality before transurethral resection. MRI or CT scanning will determine bladder wall thickening and involvement of adjacent structures. Both methods will identify pelvic and abdominal adenopathy and provide a baseline for later comparisons. The two modalities have similar staging characteristics, but recent developments in MRI have led to the increased use of this modality for staging bladder cancer.

After the patient is anesthetized, either vaginoabdominally in the female patient or rectoabdominally in the male patient, bimanual examination is performed to determine the mobility of the bladder and extent of the tumor. A palpable mass noted at this time indicates a high likelihood of local and/or distant metastatic disease. When a bladder tumor is discovered, a biopsy is performed and as much of the tumor as can be safely resected is removed. Adequate staging requires that the resection be deep enough to include the muscularis propria. All suspicious lesions should be biopsied in a similar fashion, making note of the number, site, and configuration of all lesions. It is our policy to perform cold-cup biopsies of the tumor margin, dome, posterior wall, right and left lateral walls, trigone, and prostatic urethra to aid in determining the status of the remaining urothelium. As mentioned previously, this information is important in predicting risk of recurrence and progression and may also change the therapeutic approach to the tumor (i.e., segmental resection versus cystectomy with or without urethrectomy). Additionally, a bladder diagram is created to document the location of tumors or atypical findings. After thorough cystoscopic evaluation, transurethral resection and/or biopsies, laboratory studies, radiologic evaluations, and bimanual examination, the patient's disease can be clinically staged. As previously noted, many urologists and oncologists in the United States are currently moving to the tumor, nodes, and metastasis staging system developed by the International Union Against Cancer (Table 23.1) (68).

TREATMENT

Superficial Transitional Cell Carcinoma

Approximately 75 to 85% of patients will present with transitional cell carcinoma of the bladder confined to the mucosa. Although the risk of recurrence in these patients is 70 to 75%, only 10 to 15% will have progression to muscle-invasive disease (82). Therefore, these tumors present little mortal threat to the patient and are more of a nuisance, requiring repeated transurethral resections. Transurethral resection is generally curative, and the approach can be repeated due to the low likelihood of progression in most of these patients. Similarly, the Nd:YAG laser has been used to create a coagulation necrosis of superficial transitional cell carcinomas. The laser appears to be as effective as electrocautery at eliminating superficial cancers. The question of which method results in fewer recurrences requires further study. It is evident, however, that laser therapy for these lesions results in a very small risk of bleeding, which is a clear advantage over electrocautery. The obvious disadvantage is lack of tissue for pathologic assessment (83).

A small subset of these patients have tumors that exhibit a more aggressive behavior with early progression and poor responsiveness to transurethral therapies. As previously discussed, these tumors are typically of high grade (66), associated with carcinoma in situ (61,84–86), and multiple at the time of diagnosis (66, 67). These patients generally require a more aggressive approach than simple transurethral resection.

Intravesical chemotherapy as an adjunct to transurethral resection has been shown to prevent recurrences of these tumors. However, intravesical immunotherapy with bacille Calmette-Guérin (BCG) has proved to be the most effective intravesical agent tested to date for treatment of carcinoma in situ and the high-risk superficial tumor described previously (87–89). Randomized trials have reported a reduction in both recurrence rates and progression to muscle invasion in patients with superficial bladder cancer who are treated with BCG (90, 91). The evidence to support a reduction in the rate of progression to muscle invasion has been the most important contribution of intravesical BCG therapy.

Despite the excellent response rates of these difficult superficial cancers to intravesical agents, a few will remain recalcitrant to repeated transurethral resections and intravesical therapies. In these patients, a second course of induction treatment or an induction course of a new agent is a reasonable approach. However, recurrence or stage/grade progression of the tumor at this juncture should result in immediate radical cystectomy and bilateral pelvic lymph node dissection because the biologic potential of this tumor has become obvious (92, 93).

Minimally Invasive (T1) Transitional Cell Carcinoma

Contemporary treatment options for stage T1 bladder carcinoma include transurethral resection, radiation therapy, transurethral resection and intravesical therapy, and cystectomy. Transurethral resection alone will cure some of these patients, but progression rates average 29% overall and 40% in those patients with grade 3, T1 tumors (94). Similarly, radiation therapy will result in more than 50% of these patients achieving progression-free (but not recurrence-free) survival at 3 to 5 years. Both transurethral resection alone and radiation therapy produce progression and survival rates inferior to those noted with transurethral resection followed by intravesical therapy or cystectomy.

The introduction of BCG has changed the way many urologists now treat stage T1 bladder carcinomas. The overall progression rate of patients treated with transurethral resection followed by BCG has been shown to be 14% versus 29% for those treated with transurethral resection alone (94). However, many continue to recommend immediate cystectomy, espe-cially in grade 3 stage T1 lesions, owing to the aggressive nature of these tumors, high risk of progression, and excellent survival rates reported with cystectomy. Contemporary cystectomy series report 5-year cancer-specific survival rates for pT1 tumors of 78 to 90% (92–94).

Although both therapeutic options can be defended (it is the author's preference to err on the side of early cystectomy), a reasonable compromise is transurethral resection followed by an induction course of BCG. Those patients who respond may undergo a second course of BCG with close follow-up surveillance. In this scenario, nonresponders would wait approximately 3 months for definitive therapy, with the risk of progression to muscle invasion calculated to be 3% during this period (94). However, because recent evidence has shown that 41% of patients who have pT1 tumors after the preceding treatment develop muscle-invasive tumors within 24 months (median, 9 months) (70), immediate cystectomy should be recommended for nonresponders.

Muscle-Invasive and Metastatic Transitional Cell Carcinoma

A thorough review of the treatment of muscle-invasive and metastatic transitional cell carcinoma of the bladder is beyond the scope of this chapter. The interested reader is referred to reviews covering the subject matter (82, 95). Radical cystectomy remains the standard approach to the treatment of muscle-invasive bladder cancer. Contemporary surgical series report 5-year survival rates of 62 to 88% for stage P2 disease, 57 to 74% for stage P3A, and 29 to 57% for stage P3B (82). Additionally, refinements in surgical techniques have led to an operative mortality rate of less than 5%, and a risk of pelvic recurrence after radical cystectomy of 5 to 10% (82). Other therapeutic options such as transurethral resection alone, partial cystectomy, Nd:YAG laser therapy, and radiation therapy lead to high recurrence rates and poor survival rates and should be considered in those patients who are medically unable to undergo radical cystectomy (82).

Although radical cystectomy remains the best option for cure of muscle-invasive bladder cancer, 50% of patients who are treated locally for invasive bladder cancer will have a relapse at distant sites and usually die of the disease within 2 years postoperatively (72), presumably because of microscopic metastases that were present at diagnosis. This led to the development of combination chemotherapy regimens to treat this metastatic disease. The most effective combinations tested to date are cisplatin, methotrexate, and vinblastine (CMV) (96) and methotrexate, vinblastine, doxorubicin, and cisplatin (M-VAC) (97). Overall response rates have varied from 57 to 71% in published reports, with 10 to 15% of patients experiencing durable complete response rates (95). In addition, those patients with low-volume disease and nodal involvement only exhibit a greater response only when compared with those with advanced metastatic disease; those with TIS and nontransitional cell or mixed histology tumors respond poorly (95).

The promising results reported with these chemotherapeutic agents have led to investigations of neoadjuvant (before definitive therapy) and adjuvant (after definitive therapy) chemotherapy, including integrated chemoradiation therapy protocols. Although many of the reported studies appear promising—especially those involving chemoradiation therapy (98) and adjuvant chemotherapy (99–101)—the true efficacy of neoadjuvant and adjuvant chemotherapy awaits the results of prospective randomized trials with larger patient populations and adequate maturation of the data. Currently, these approaches remain investigative and do not represent a substitute for definitive surgery.

CONCLUSION

Our understanding of the pathogenesis of bladder cancer remains in its infancy. Further research into the genetic alterations that subsequently result in the phenotypic changes seen clinically will most certainly direct therapy in the future. In the meantime, we rely on histologic and clinical parameters to give us an indication (albeit late) about the risk of recurrence and progression for each patient.

Recently, intravesical immunotherapy has changed our approach to the high-risk superficial bladder cancer patient and those with minimally invasive (stage T1) disease. The use of BCG has reduced both recurrence and progression rates in these patients. The treatment of muscle-invasive bladder cancer continues to rely on radical cystectomy and bilateral pelvic lymph node dissection as the standard of care. The discovery of effective combination chemotherapy regimens has led to new hope for those patients with advanced bladder cancer. Investigation continues into integrated chemoradiation therapy approaches that may eliminate the need for radical cystectomy in certain subsets of patients. Additionally, chemotherapy in the neoadjuvant and adjuvant settings may lead to better cure rates as prospective information becomes available. Ultimately, however, it is hoped that the identification of the early genetic changes will allow clinicians to identify those patients with potentially aggressive carcinomas and intervene before the late stages.

REFERENCES

1. Boring CC, Squires TS, Tong T, et al. Cancer statistics. CA Cancer J Clin 1994;44:7.
2. Cancer statistics review 1973–1986. Rockville MD: U.S. Department of Health and Human Services, NIM.
3. Muir C, Waterhouse J, Mack T, et al., eds. Cancer incidence in five continents. IARC 1987;5:
4. Rehn L. Blasengeschwulste bei Fuchsin-Arbeitern. Arch Klin Chir 1985;50:588.
5. Cohen SM, Ellwein LB. Cell proliferation in carcinogenesis. Science 1990;249:1007.
6. Pode D, Fair WR. The development of bladder cancer. AUA Update Series 1988;7:314.
7. Burch JD, Rohan TE, Howe GR, et al. Risk of bladder cancer by source and type of tobacco exposure: a case-control study. Int J Cancer 1989;44:622.
8. Morrison AS, Buring JE, Verhoek WG, et al. An international study of smoking and bladder cancer. J Urol 1984;131:650.
9. Salminen E, Pukkala E, Teppo L. Bladder cancer and the risk of smoking-related cancers during follow-up. J Urol 1994; 152:1420.
10. Hartge P, Silverman DT, Schairer C, et al. Smoking and bladder cancer risk in blacks and whites in the United States. Cancer Causes Control 1993;4:391.
11. Anton-Culver H, Lee-Feldstein A, Taylor TH. The association of bladder cancer risk with ethnicity, gender, and smoking. Ann Epidemiol 1993;3:429.
12. Burns PB, Swanson GM. Risk of urinary bladder cancer among blacks and whites: the role of cigarette use and occupation. Cancer Causes Control 1991;2:371.
13. Silverman D, Levin L, Hoover R. Occupational risks of bladder cancer in the United States: part II. nonwhite men. J Natl Cancer Inst 1989;81:1480.
14. Morrison AS, Ahlbom A, Verhoek WG, et al. Occupation and bladder cancer in Boston, USA, Manchester, UK, and Nagoya, Japan. J Epidemiol Commun Health 1985;39:294.
15. Risch HA, Burch JD, Miller AB, et al. Occupational factors and the incidence of cancer of the bladder in Canada. Br J Ind Med 1988;45:361.
16. International Agency for Research on Cancer. Overall evaluations of carcinogenicity: an updating of IARC monographs. IARC Sci Publ 1987;(Suppl17):1.
17. Schulte PA, Ringen K, Hemstreet GP, et al. Risk factors for bladder cancer in a cohort exposed to aromatic amines. Cancer 1986;58:2156.
18. Checkoway H, Smith AH, McMichael AJ, et al. A case-control study of bladder cancer in the United States rubber and tire industry. Br J Ind Med 1981;38:240.
19. Delzell E, Monson RR. Mortality among rubber workers: part III. cause-specific mortality, 1940–1978. J Occup Med 1981; 23:677.
20. Decoufle P. Cancer risks associated with employment in the leather and leather products industry. Arch Environ Health 1979;34:33.
21. Marrett LD, Hartge P, Meigs JW. Bladder cancer and occupational exposure to leather. Br J Ind Med 1986;43:96.
22. Myslak ZW, Bolt HM, Brockmann W. Tumors of the urinary bladder in painters: a case-control study. Am J Ind Med 1991;19:705.
23. Silverman DT, Levin LI, Hoover RN, et al. Occupational risks of bladder cancer in the United States: part I. white men. J Natl Cancer Inst 1989;81:1472.
24. Silverman DT, Hoover RN, Mason TJ, et al. Motor exhaust-related occupations and bladder cancer. Cancer Res 1986;46: 2113.
25. Rockette HE, Arena VC. Mortality studies of aluminum reduction plant workers: potroom and carbon department. J Occup Med 1983;25:549.
26. Anton-Culver H, Lee-Feldstein A, Taylor TH. Occupation and bladder cancer risk. Am J Epidemiol 1992;136:89.
27. Brooks DR, Geller AC, Chang J, et al. Occupation, smoking, and the risk of high-grade invasive bladder cancer in Missouri. Am J Ind Med 1992;21:699.

28. Case RAM, Hosker ME, McDonald DB, et al. Tumors of the urinary bladder in workmen engaged in the British chemical industry: role of aniline benzidine, alpha-naphthylamine, and beta-naphthylamine. Br J Ind Med 1954;11:75.

29. Cole P, Hoover R, Friedell GH. Occupation and cancer of the lower urinary tract. Cancer 1972;29:1250.

30. Lower GM Jr. Chemically induced human urinary bladder cancer. Cancer 1982;49:1056.

31. McCredie M, et al. Phenacetin-containing analgesics and cancer of the bladder or renal pelvis in women. Br J Urol 1983;55:220.

32. Calabresi P, Parks RE Jr. Alkylating agents, antimetabolites, hormones, and other antiproliferative agents. In: Goodman LS, Gilman AZ, eds. The pharmacological basis of therapeutics. 5th ed. New York: Macmillan, 1975:1254.

33. Durkee C, Benson R Jr. Bladder cancer following administration of cyclophosphamide. Urology 1980;16:145.

34. Cox PJ. Cyclophosphamide cystitis and bladder cancer: a hypothesis. Eur J Cancer 1979;15:1071.

35. Thrasher JB, Miller GJ, Wettlaufer JN. Bladder leiomyosarcoma following cyclophosphamide therapy for lupus nephritis. J Urol 1990;143:119.

36. Schmähl D, Habs MR. Prevention of cyclophosphamide-induced carcinogenesis in the urinary bladder of rats by administration of mensa. Cancer Treat Rev 1983;10(Suppl):57.

37. Kantor AF, Hartge P, Hoover RN, et al. Urinary tract infection and risk of bladder cancer. Am J Epidemiol 1984;119:510.

38. Brand KG. Schistosomiasis-cancer: etiological considerations, a review. Acta Trop (Basel) 1979;36:203.

39. Yamamoto M, Wu HH, Momose H, et al. Marked enhancement of rat urinary bladder carcinogenesis by heat-killed Escherichia coli. Cancer Res 1992;52:5329.

40. El-Menzabani MM, El-Aaser AA, Zackary NI. A study of the aetiological factors of bilharzial bladder cancer in Egypt: part I. nitrosamines and their precursors in urine. Eur J Cancer Clin Oncol 1979;15:287.

41. Cohen SM, Arai M, Jacobs JB, et al. Promoting effect of saccharin and D,L-tryptophan in urinary bladder carcinogenesis. Cancer Res 1979;39:1207.

42. Renwick AG, Thakrar A, Lawrie CA, et al. Microbial amino acid metabolites and bladder cancer: no evidence of promoting activity in man. Hum Toxicol 1988;7:267.

43. Morrison AS, Buring JE. Artificial sweeteners and cancer of the lower urinary tract. N Engl J Med 1980;302:537.

44. Chappel CI. A review and biological risk assessment of sodium saccharin. Regul Toxicol Pharmacol 1992;15:253.

45. Renwick AG. A data-derived safety (uncertainty) factor for the intense sweetener, saccharin. Food Addit Contam 1993;10:337.

46. Viscoli CM, Lachs MS, Horwitz RI. Bladder cancer and coffee drinking: a summary of case-control research. Lancet 1993;341:1432.

47. Stehelin D, Varmus HE, Bishop JM, et al. DNA related to the transforming gene (S) of avian sarcoma viruses is present in normal avian DNA. Nature 1976;260:170.

48. Weinberg RA. Oncogenes and tumor suppressor genes. CA Cancer J Clin 1994;44:160.

49. DeWolf WC. Malignancy: underlying concepts of etiology, natural history, and treatment. In: Gillenwater JY, Grayhack JT, Howards SS, Duckett JW, eds. Adult and pediatric urology. 2nd ed. St. Louis: Mosby-Year Book, 1991:373.

50. Fearon ER, Feinberg AP, Hamilton SH, et al. Loss of genes on the short arm of chromosome 11 in bladder cancer. Nature 1985;318:377.

51. Olumi AF, Tsai YC, Nichols PW, et al. Allelic loss of chromosome 17p distinguishes high grade from low grade transitional cell carcinoma of the bladder. Cancer Res 1990;50:7081.

52. Tsai YC, Nichols PW, Hiti AL, et al. Allelic losses of chromosomes 9, 11, and 17 in human bladder cancer. Cancer Res 1990;50:44.

53. Sidransky D, Messing E. Molecular genetics and biochemical mechanisms in bladder cancer: oncogenes, tumor suppressor genes, and growth factors. Urol Clin North Am 1992;19:629.

54. Sidransky D, von Eschenbach A, Tsai YC, et al. Identification of p53 gene mutations in bladder cancers and urine samples. Science 1991;252:706.

55. Levine AJ, Momand J, Finlay CA. The p53 tumor suppressor gene. Nature 1991;351;453.

56. Hollstein M, Sidransky D, Vogelstein B, et al. p53 mutations in human cancer. Science 1991;253:49.

57. Droller MJ. Bladder cancer: part I. Monogr Urol 1993;14:39.

58. Moch H, Sauter G, Moore D, et al. p53 and erb B-2 protein overexpression are associated with early invasion and metastasis in bladder cancer. Virchows Archiv A Pathol Anat Histopathol 1993;423:329.

59. Liu BCS, Liotta LA. Biochemistry of bladder cancer invasion and metastasis: clinical implications. Urol Clin North Am 1992;19:621.

60. Pauwels R, Smeets W. Cytogenetic studies in bladder cancer. Probl Urol 1988;2:297.

61. Graham SD Jr. Predictive markers in recurrence and invasion of transitional cell carcinoma. Probl Urol 1988;2:320.

62. Aprikian AG, Sarkis AS, Reuter VE, et al. Biological markers of prognosis in transitional cell carcinoma of the bladder: current concepts. Semin Urol 1993;11:137.

63. Hermansen DK, Badalament RA, Fair WR. Flow cytometry in urology. AUA Update Series 1988;7:210.

64. Devonec M, Darzynkiewicz Z, Whitmore WF Jr, et al. Flow cytometry for follow-up examinations of conservatively treated low stage bladder tumors. J Urol 1981;126:166.

65. Gustafson H, Tribukait B, Esposti PL. DNA profile and tumour progression in patients with superficial bladder tumours. Urol Res 1982;10:13.

66. Heney NM, Ahmed S, Flanagan MJ, et al. Superficial bladder cancer: progression and recurrence. J Urol 1983;130:1083.

67. Fitzpatrick JM, West AB, Butler MR, et al. Superficial bladder tumors (stage pTa, grades 1 and 2): the importance of recurrence patterns following initial resection. J Urol 1986;135:920.

68. Wallace DM, Chisholm GD, Henry WF. TNM classification for urological tumors (UICC)–1974. Br J Urol 1975;47:1.

69. Thrasher JB, Crawford ED. Minimally invasive transitional cell carcinoma (T (1) and T (2)). In: Resnick MI, Kursh E, eds. Current therapy in genitourinary surgery. 2nd ed. St. Louis: BC Decker, 1992:74.

70. Herr HW. Progression of stage T (1) bladder tumors after intravesical bacillus Calmette-Guérin. J Urol 1991;145:40.

71. Skinner DG, Tift JP, Kaufman JJ. High dose, short course preoperative radiation therapy and immediate single stage radical cystectomy with pelvic node dissection in the management of bladder cancer. J Urol 1982;127:671.

72. Skinner DG, Lieskovsky G. Management of invasive and high-grade bladder cancer. In: Diagnosis and management of genitourinary cancer. Philadelphia: WB Saunders, 1988;1: 295.

73. Thrasher JB, Frazier HA, Robertson JE, et al. Does a stage pTO cystectomy specimen confer a survival advantage in patients with minimally invasive bladder cancer? J Urol 1994;152:393.

74. Webb JN. The histopathology of bladder cancer. In: Zingg EJ, Wallace DMA, eds. Bladder Cancer. Berlin: Springer-Verlag, 1985:23.

75. Gilbert HA, Logan JL, Kagan AR, et al. The natural history of papillary transitional cell carcinoma of the bladder and its treatment in an unselected population on the basis of grading. J Urol 1978;119:488.

76. Lutzeyer W, Rubben H, Dahm H. Prognostic parameters in superficial bladder cancer: an analysis of 315 cases. J Urol 1982;127:250.

77. Thrasher JB, Frazier HA, Robertson JE, et al. Clinical variables which serve as predictors of cancer-specific survival among patients treated with radical cystectomy for transitional cell carcinoma of the bladder and prostate. Cancer 1994;73:1708.

78. Salo JO. Intravesical ultrasound for staging bladder tumours. Scand J Urol Nephrol 1987;21:203.

79. Barentsz JO, Ruijs SHJ, van Erning LJTO. Magnetic resonance imaging of urinary bladder cancer: an overview and new developments. Magn Reson Q 1993;9:235.

80. Tanimoto A, Yuasa Y, Imai Y, et al. Bladder tumor staging: comparison of conventional and gadolinium-enhanced dynamic MR imaging and CT. Radiology 1992;185:741.

81. Hawnaur JM, Johnson RJ, Read G, et al. Magnetic resonance imaging with gadolinium-DTPA for assessment of bladder carcinoma and its response to treatment. Clin Radiol 1993; 47:307.

82. Thrasher JB, Crawford ED. Current management of invasive and metastatic transitional cell carcinoma of the bladder. J Urol 1993;149:957.

83. Smith JA Jr. Laser surgery for transitional-cell carcinoma: technique, advantages, and limitations. Urol Clin N Am 1992;19:473.

84. Althausen AF, Prout GR Jr, Daly JJ. Noninvasive papillary carcinoma of the bladder associated with carcinoma in situ. J Urol 1976;116:575.

85. Prout GR Jr, Griffin PP, Daly JJ, et al. Carcinoma in situ of the urinary bladder with and without associated vesical neoplasms. Cancer 1983;52:524.

86. Solsona E, Iborra I, Ricos JV, et al. Carcinoma in situ associated with superficial bladder tumor. Eur Urol 1991;19: 93.

87. Brosman SA. Experience with bacillus Calmette-Guérin in patients with superficial bladder cancer. J Urol 1982;128:27.

88. Lamm DL, Blumenstein BA, Crawford ED, et al. A randomized trial of intravesical doxorubicin and immunotherapy with bacille Calmette-Guérin for transitional cell carcinoma of the bladder. N Engl J Med. 1991;325: 1205.

89. Lamm DL, Crawford ED, Blumenstein B, et al. SWOG 8795: a randomized comparison of bacillus Calmette-Guérin and mitomycin C prophylaxis in stage T (A) and T (1) transitional cell carcinoma of the bladder. J Urol 1993;149: 282. Abstract no. 275.

90. Herr HW, Laudone VP, Badalament RA, et al. Bacillus Calmette Guérin therapy alters the progression of superficial bladder cancer. J Clin Oncol 1988;6:1450.

91. Pagano F, Bassi P, Milani C, et al. A low dose bacillus Calmette-Guérin regimen in superficial bladder cancer therapy: is it effective? J Urol 1991;146:32.

92. Amling CL, Thrasher JB, Frazier HA, et al. Radical cystectomy for stages T (A), TIS and T (1) transitional cell carcinoma of the bladder. J Urol 1994;151:31.

93. Malkowicz SB, Nichols P, Lieskovsky G, et al. The role of radical cystectomy in the management of high grade superficial bladder cancer (PA, P1, PIS and P2). J Urol 1990; 144:641.

94. Herr H, Jakse G. pT (1) bladder cancer. Eur Urol 1991;20:1.

95. Thrasher JB, Crawford ED. Chemotherapy for advanced bladder cancer. AUA Update Series 1994;13:182.

96. Harker WG, Meyers FJ, Freiha FS, et al. Cisplatin, methotrexate, and vinblastine (CMV): an effective chemotherapy regimen for metastatic transitional cell carcinoma of the urinary tract, a Northern California Oncology Group study. J Clin Oncol 1985;3:1463.

97. Sternberg CN, Yagoda A, Scher HI, et al. Methotrexate, vinblastine, doxorubicin, and cisplatin for advanced transitional cell carcinoma of the urothelium: efficacy and patterns of response and relapse. Cancer 1989;64:2448.

98. Kaufman DS, Shipley WU, Heney NM, et al. Treatment of invasive bladder carcinoma with transurethral surgery, radiotherapy, and chemotherapy with potential bladder sparing. Probl Urol 1992;6:518.

99. Skinner DG, Daniels JR, Russell CA, et al. The role of adjuvant chemotherapy following cystectomy for invasive bladder cancer: a prospective comparative trial. J Urol 1991; 145:459.

100. Stockle M, Meyenburg W, Wellek S, et al. Advanced bladder cancer (stages pT (3b), pT (4a), pN (1), and pN (2)): improved survival after radical cystectomy and 3 adjuvant cycles of chemotherapy: results of a controlled prospective study. J Urol 1992;148:302.

101. Stockle M, Meyenburg W, Wellek S, et al. Adjuvant polychemotherapy for nonorgan-confined bladder cancer after radical cystectomy revisited: long-term results of a controlled prospective study and further clinical experience. J Urol 1995;153:47.

24

Transurethral Resection of Bladder Tumors

Marc Beaghler, H. Roger Hadley, and Herbert C. Ruckle

INTRODUCTION

Bladder cancer represents the fourth most common noncutaneous malignancy in the United States (1). It is estimated that more than 50,000 cases of transitional cell carcinoma (TCC) will be diagnosed annually, making it the fourth most prevalent noncutaneous malignancy. The majority of these cases (75%) will have cancer confined to the superficial urothelium; complete transurethral resection provides the first line of treatment for the majority of these bladder tumors. However, despite complete resection of these superficial malignancies, up to 75% will recur eventually (1–3). The urologist must be aware, therefore, of the clinical implications, treatment options, and natural history of this disease to properly manage this important clinical entity.

This chapter details the natural history of bladder cancer, preoperative considerations, anesthetic requirements, operative techniques for resection of both superficial and invasive lesions, and management of intraoperative and postoperative complications.

Historical Perspective

Endoscopic surgery has progressed from the reflection of candlelight through a hollow tube to today's flexible endoscopes with fiberoptic technology and video monitor capabilities. Although there were very primitive uses of reflected light throughout the centuries to inspect body cavities, it was not until the invention of the incandescent lightbulb that truly practical cystoscopes were in service. These developments later gave rise to modern endoscopy and their widespread use in laparoscopy, arthroscopy, gastroscopy, colonoscopy, and bronchoscopy (4).

The natural evolution to diagnostic endoscopy occurred as a result of therapeutic procedures performed through endoscopes. Early attempts at transurethral endoscopic surgery progressed with the development of electrocautery devices that could be implemented transurethrally. In 1910, Beers began treating intravesical tumors transurethrally with a monopolar cautery device. Stevens and Bugbee further refined fulguration of bladder tumors with a coagulating electrode. In 1926, Stern devised one of the first resectoscopes that was subsequently modified by McCarthy. The Stern-McCarthy resectoscope was a major advance that made transurethral operative procedures practical and safe (5).

Roger Barnes was one of the great innovators involved in transurethral surgery. He wrote the first textbook on transurethral surgery in 1938, outlining several important principles that continue to have great importance today. He was one of the first advocates of bladder-sparing surgery. In 1967, he stated that although many bladder tumors recurred, 80% of cancers could be controlled by adequate endoscopic surgery (2). Barnes believed that, in many patients, an adequate resection consisted of removing the bladder tumor, including a portion of the bladder mucosa 1 cm beyond the tumor, and that with systematic endoscopic follow-up, many bladders could be preserved safely. Barnes has influenced many urologists, and his teachings are accepted by proponents of bladder preservation and minimally invasive surgery (5, 6).

Evaluation of the Patient Suspected to Have Bladder Cancer

The majority of patients whose conditions were diagnosed as bladder cancer were noted to have hematuria that subsequently led to the discovery of their malignancy. The hematuria may be microscopic or gross and typically painless and intermittent. In general, patients that have unexplained hematuria with greater than 3 erythrocytes per high-power field should be evaluated with a complete examination of the upper and lower urinary tracts that includes upper tract imaging (intravenous pyelogram), cystoscopy, and possibly urinary cytology (7).

An intravenous pyelogram is generally the study of choice to examine the upper urinary tract. If the patient has an allergy to radiographic contrast, ultrasound imaging of the kidneys and bladder and retrograde pyelography should be performed. Urine cytologies may be helpful, especially in patients with irritative voiding symptoms that may be due to carcinoma in situ (8). Cystoscopy, which is most commonly performed in the urologist's office, should systematically evaluate all areas of the bladder including the trigone, ureteral orifices, lateral sidewalls, dome, and bladder neck. The ureteral orifices should be examined and observed for bloody effluent. Using rigid cystoscopy, both the 30° and 70° lens must be used. If the anterior bladder neck is not adequately inspected, a 120° lens or flexible cystoscope should be used to evaluate this area. In males, flexible cystourethroscopy can be performed with less patient discomfort than rigid endoscopy. With the use of a topical intraurethral anesthetic (lidocaine 2%), men report the discomfort of flexible cystoscopy to be similar to urethral catheterization. Flexible cystoscopy can be performed in a variety of patient positions including prone, dorsal lithotomy, and, most commonly, the supine position. An advantage of flexible cystoscopy is its ability to see the anterior bladder neck clearly by retroflexing the endoscope onto itself. This portion of the examination is critical and should be the final step in flexible endoscopy of the lower urinary tract (9–11).

With the development of innovative accessories, small papillary lesions, erythematous patches, or other suspicious areas of the bladder may be biopsied or fulgurated in the urologist's office. Small biopsy and fulguration instruments may be implemented through a standard rigid cystoscope. A 1.8F biopsy forceps that will pass through the 5F working channel of the flexible cystoscope is now available for the simultaneous cautery and biopsy of bladder lesions (12–14). These minimally invasive procedures are successfully performed in selected patients in the office and obviate a hospital stay or outpatient procedures that require a general anesthetic. If resection of a bladder tumor is required, however, patients are best examined in the operating room under an anesthetic.

Indications for Transurethral Resection of Bladder Tumors (TURBT)

Transurethral resection of a bladder lesion suspected to be cancer is indicated for both diagnosis and treatment of that lesion. Further management is dependent on the histologic type and stage (level of invasion) of the bladder lesion resected. Although the majority of bladder lesions are TCC, other types include squamous cell carcinoma, adenocarcinoma, and rhabdomyosarcoma. Because these less-common lesions often require further treatment and generally are not cured by transurethral surgery, our discussion will be primarily of TCC.

Preoperative Considerations

The patient scheduled for TURBT will have had the bladder tumor noted during a prior cystoscopy. Typically, a preoperative cystoscopy will have been performed because of hematuria, routine surveillance cystoscopy for a history of bladder cancers, or other reasons such as a bladder mass noted on imaging studies or physical examination.

Preoperative evaluation of patients found to have bladder tumors should include a CBC, serum electrolytes, and (if appropriate) coagulation studies. If a large bladder tumor is to be resected, packed red blood cells should be available if a transfusion is necessary (15). A chest radiograph and electrocardiogram may be required depending on the patient's age and medical history. If at the time of cystoscopy a large sessile bladder tumor is noted, liver function studies should be considered to help stage the lesion.

Aspirin and nonsteroidal anti-inflammatory agents should be discontinued 1 week before the operation. Patients taking Coumadin may have to undergo anticoagulation with heparin if the Coumadin cannot be safely discontinued. Although some authors have suggested that prophylactic antibiotics are unnecessary in the presence of sterile urine, it is our practice to administer 1 g of cephazolin or ampicillin parenterally 30 minutes before the procedure. If it is thought that the patient may be at increased risk of urinary tract infection, an aminoglycoside may be added (16).

Anesthetic Considerations

Regional anesthesia, such as a spinal block, is safe and effective for transurethral surgery. Spinal anesthesia has many advantages over a general anesthetic in that the patient does not require endotracheal intubation, sedation is minimal, and emergence from the anesthetic is less likely to be accompanied by wide variations of blood pressure. In addition, regional anesthesia permits continuous observation of mental status, which may be altered by excessive absorption of irrigant fluid. General anesthesia, however, is preferable in certain situations, such as for spinal disorders (15).

Transurethral resection of small papillary lesions can be performed using local anesthesia. Engberg et al. described resection of small papillary tumors by administering a local anesthetic through a specially designed needle that fits through the working element of a 20F cystoscope. In the majority of patients, little or no pain was experienced using this technique (17). Biopsies and treatment of small papillary lesions may also be performed using the flexible cystoscope and topical anesthesia alone. Use of the flexible cystoscope and small-caliber laser fibers has been described for the treatment of bladder tumors (12–14).

Instrumentation

Standard and continuous flow resectoscopes come in two varieties—the Iglesias type and the Stern-McCarthy resectoscope. The difference in the two resectoscopes is the action mechanism that moves the resectoscope loop. In the Iglesias type of resectoscope, the loop extends forward by pressure of the thumb against a grip held by the fingers and retracts by a spring-like mechanism. The Stern-McCarthy resectoscope depends on a ratchet-like motion on a rack and pinion to extend and retract the cautery loop. Some surgeons prefer the Stern-McCarthy mechanism because they feel that they have added control when resecting either bladder tumors or prostatic tissue. Selection of a resectoscope depends most on the surgeon's experience and preference.

During the 1980s, the endoscope manufacturers developed a continuous-flow resectoscope. The continuous flow instrument allows for uninterrupted resection and provides a mechanism to maintain the bladder at a desired capacity during resection of bladder tumors. The continuous-flow resectoscope can be used with low-pressure suction placed on the outflow port or the effluent can be allowed to simply drain from the exit port (18). In addition, the continuous-flow resectoscope's ability to maintain the bladder at a given fixed volume will keep bladder wall thickness constant, which lessens the likelihood of bladder perforation (19).

Performing the operation using a video screen for visualization is becoming increasingly popular. Although video monitoring of transurethral surgery was used to aid in instruction, there are several other benefits that make it an attractive means to perform endoscopic surgery (18, 20). Using a camera allows the operating room staff to participate more actively in the performance of the procedure. For example, if the irrigant is not flowing, the staff will appreciate the impaired visualization of the operating field and the necessity of quickly reacting to the situation. In a time when surgeons face an occupational risk of human immunodeficiency virus exposure from blood and urine, there is less risk of unwanted contact if a video monitor is used to visualize the operation and the surgeon is able to stand at arm's length from the patient. Also, the resectoscope can be maneuvered to maximum angulation without placing the surgeon in an awkward position or forcing the surgeon to use his or her nondominant eye.

If video monitoring is used for teaching, the instructing surgeon can direct the procedure from the monitor image. It is our experience that residents learn transurethral surgery much more quickly if instant feedback can be given, which is only possible with video monitoring (18, 20).

Resection of Bladder Tumors

All instruments and video equipment should be inspected and tested before the operation. To provide for clean amputation of the resected tissue, the cutting loop must be adjusted to a position so that when retracted, it gently grazes the insulated sheath. The cutting and coagulation currents of the electrocautery unit are set at the appropriate levels, which will vary with the type of electrocautery unit used. The most efficacious settings may differ from the suggested base settings and should be adjusted based on experience and visible effects noted during resection (15).

After the administration of anesthesia, the patient is placed in the dorsal lithotomy position, washed with germicidal soap, and draped in a sterile fashion. A bimanual examination with the bladder empty is performed. Palpation of the bladder allows the surgeon to assess the presence of a bladder mass. Fixation of the bladder to the pelvic sidewall or adjacent structures is noted. In the male patient, it is important to note any evidence of synchronous prostate malignancy or prostatic induration that may signal invasion of the bladder tumor into the prostate.

Even if the diagnosis of bladder cancer was made in the office, it is important to again visualize the entire bladder to assure that all tumors have been identified. The bladder is mapped noting the size, location, and appearance of all tumors. In addition to the 30° and 70° lenses, it may be necessary to use the 120° lens or a flexible cystoscope to inspect the entire bladder neck.

Sterile water or an isotonic solution such as sorbitol is used as an irrigant. Water has the advantage over other solutions in that it lyses red blood cells and provides the best visualization during resection. The use of sterile water is safe provided the bladder has not been perforated. In the event that the bladder is perforated and significant amounts of water are absorbed into the general circulation, intravascular hemolysis and resultant renal tubular necrosis may occur. It is our practice, therefore, to change from water to sorbitol if there is suspicion of bladder perforation (21).

We prefer to use a 28F resectoscope sheath because the tissue can be removed most efficiently through the larger sheath. However, if it is determined that the patient's urethral size is not sufficient for the 28F resectoscope, we will use an appropriately smaller resectoscope. After calibrating the urethra with Van Buren sounds, the resectoscope is inserted into the bladder with the aid of the Timberlake obturator. An alternative is to use an optical dilator. This instrument is a tapered tube that is 20F at the distal end and 30F at the proximal end. Using a 0° lens and the optical dilator, the urethra can be calibrated under direct vision (18). If urethral or bladder neck strictures preclude insertion of the resectoscope, the surgeon must be prepared to dilate or incise these obstructions. In some instances it is necessary to resect hyperplastic prostatic tissue to access the bladder tumor adequately. This can be performed without increasing the probability of bladder recurrence in the prostatic urethra (22).

The majority of bladder tumors are low grade and have a papillary architecture. A bladder lesion with a sessile configuration usually indicates a higher grade and stage tumor compared with a papillary lesion. It should be noted, however, that even papillary tumors may be high grade. If the tumor is located on the posterior wall, it can be resected using the extended resectoscope loop and a rocking motion, which will amputate the tumor at the base (Fig. 24.1). Attention must be paid to the bladder capacity at all times so as not to distend the bladder and increase the risk of bladder perforation (Fig. 24.2).

Cutting current should be used to cleanly amputate the tissue. Just before beginning the cut, the water should be turned on to wash away bubbles generated by the electrocautery. The cutting current should be turned on just before the loop is advanced into the tissue to allow for less tissue distortion as the cut is initiated. If the patient has many small papillary lesions, we generally obtain tissue for diagnosis and then simply fulgurate the remaining lesions. Small lesions may be biopsied and fulgurated with a single device designed for this purpose (14).

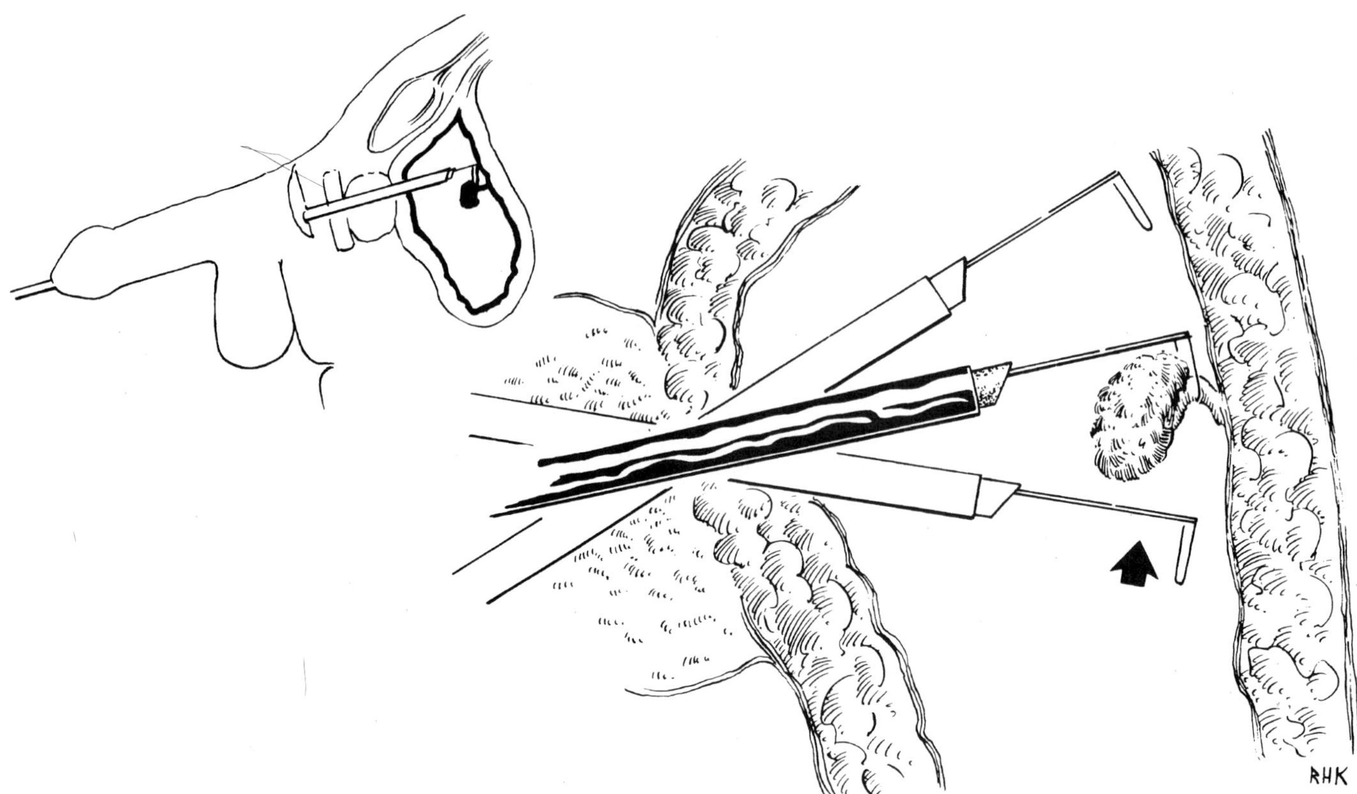

Fig. 24.1.   Resection of bladder tumor located on the posterior bladder wall. The loop of the resectoscope is extended and the tumor is amputated using a rocking motion.

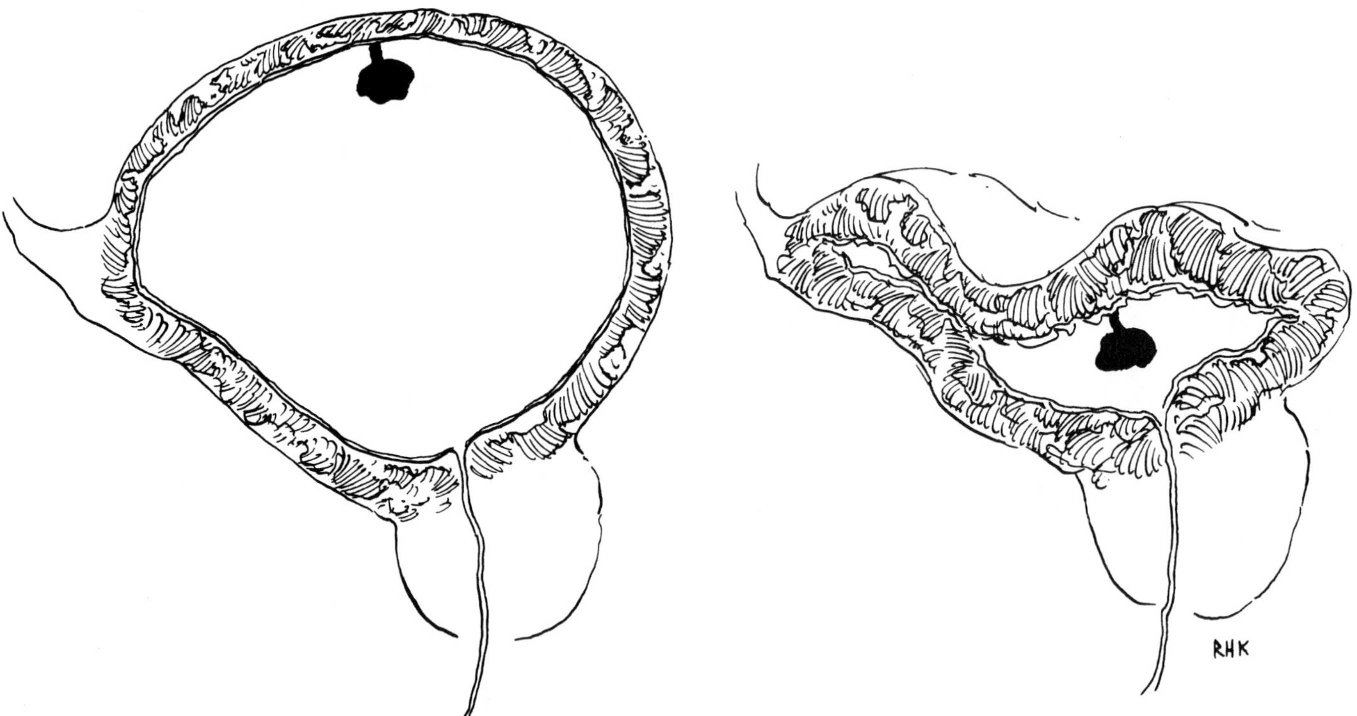

Fig. 24.2.   A full bladder has a much thinner wall than an empty bladder. To prevent bladder perforation, attention must be paid to bladder capacity at all times.

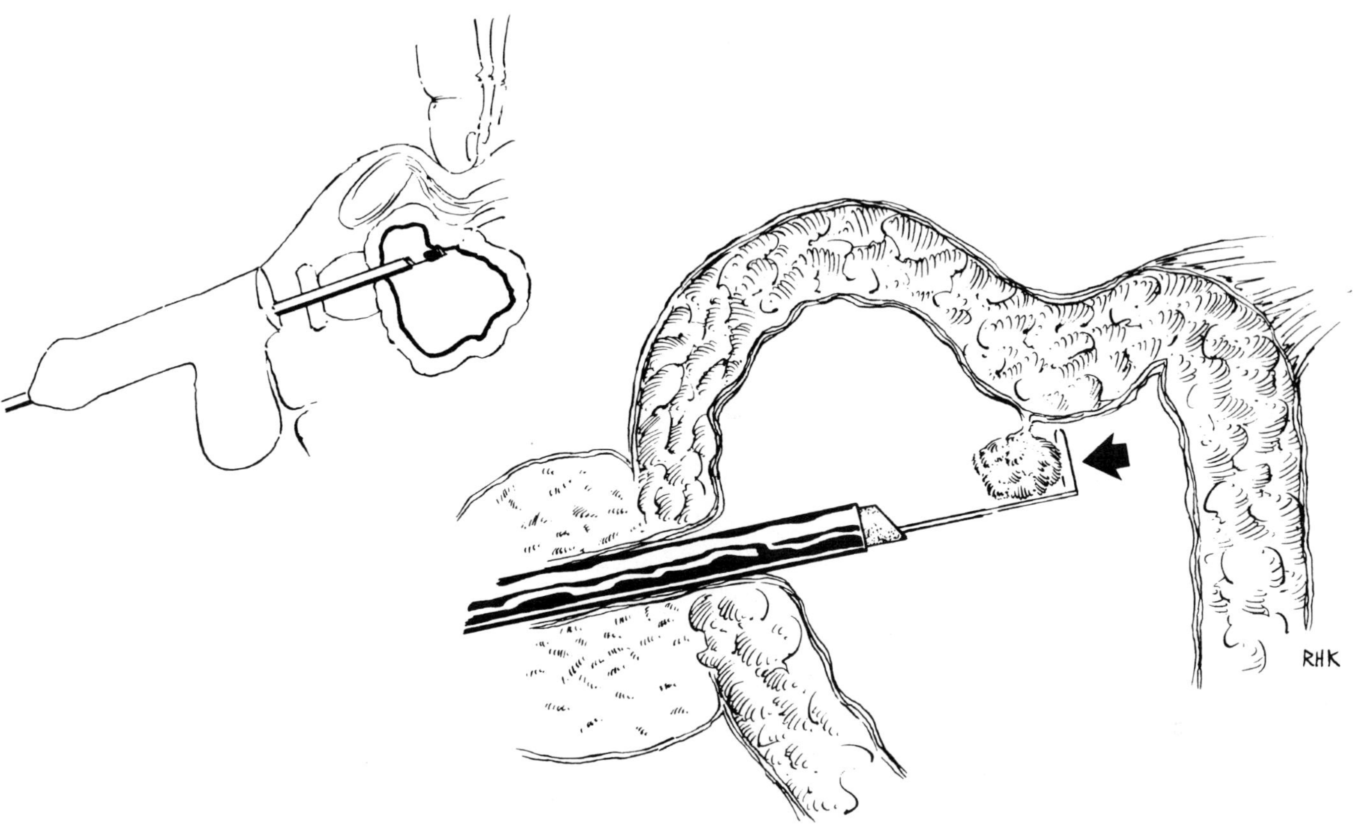

Fig. 24.3. Resection of tumors located at the dome of the bladder can be facilitated by the application of suprapubic pressure. An assistant's help in this endeavor is invaluable.

Resection of tumors in the dome of the bladder may be facilitated by the application of suprapubic pressure to improve resectoscope angle to the tumor (Fig. 24.3). An assistant's help in this endeavor can be invaluable. Resection of tumors in the base of the bladder can be aided by digital transrectal or transvaginal manipulation of the bladder base. Drapes that allow for access to the rectum while keeping a clean field are commercially available.

Tumors located at or near the ureteral orifice are treated like lesions located in other regions of the bladder. The difference is that after the tumor is completely resected, care must be taken not to coagulate the ureteral orifice directly. To remove the bladder cancer adequately, however, it may be necessary to resect the ureteral orifice. We generally place a ureteral stent if extensive coagulation is required for tumors involving the ureteral orifice (15).

If tumors are resected from the anterior lateral walls of the bladder, the obturator nerve may be stimulated, resulting in sudden and violent adduction of the ipsilateral leg. This sudden movement may cause bladder perforation. Several techniques can be used to decrease the obturator reflex, including lowering the power of the cutting current or injecting the obturator nerve with a local anesthetic. Occasionally, the patient will require administration of a general anesthetic in combination with a systemic paralytic agent to prevent the reflex (15, 18, 23).

Regardless of the location, complete resection of the bladder tumor is axiomatic to the prevention of tumor recurrences. In addition to resection of the primary visible tumor, we prefer to include a deep resection into the detrusor muscle (Fig. 24.4). The deep specimen is used to help determine the depth of invasion of the bladder cancer. We also resect a 1-cm area around the base of the tumor and vigorously cauterize the bed of the cancer. The deep specimen is sent to the pathologist separately.

A thorough transurethral resection of muscle-invasive transitional cell bladder cancers may have a curative therapeutic effect. Barnes et al. noted that patients with stage B (T2 to T3a) disease treated by transurethral resection alone had a 31% 5-year survival rate. They believed that many invasive bladder tumors subjected to an aggressive deep and wide resection could be controlled by transurethral resection alone (24). Herr and others have also found that in patients with T2 and T3a lesions, aggressive TURBT results in 5-year survival rates similar to those achieved with more radical treatment modalities (25–27).

Complications

Bladder perforation and hemorrhage are the two most common complications associated with TURBT (28). Other intraopera-

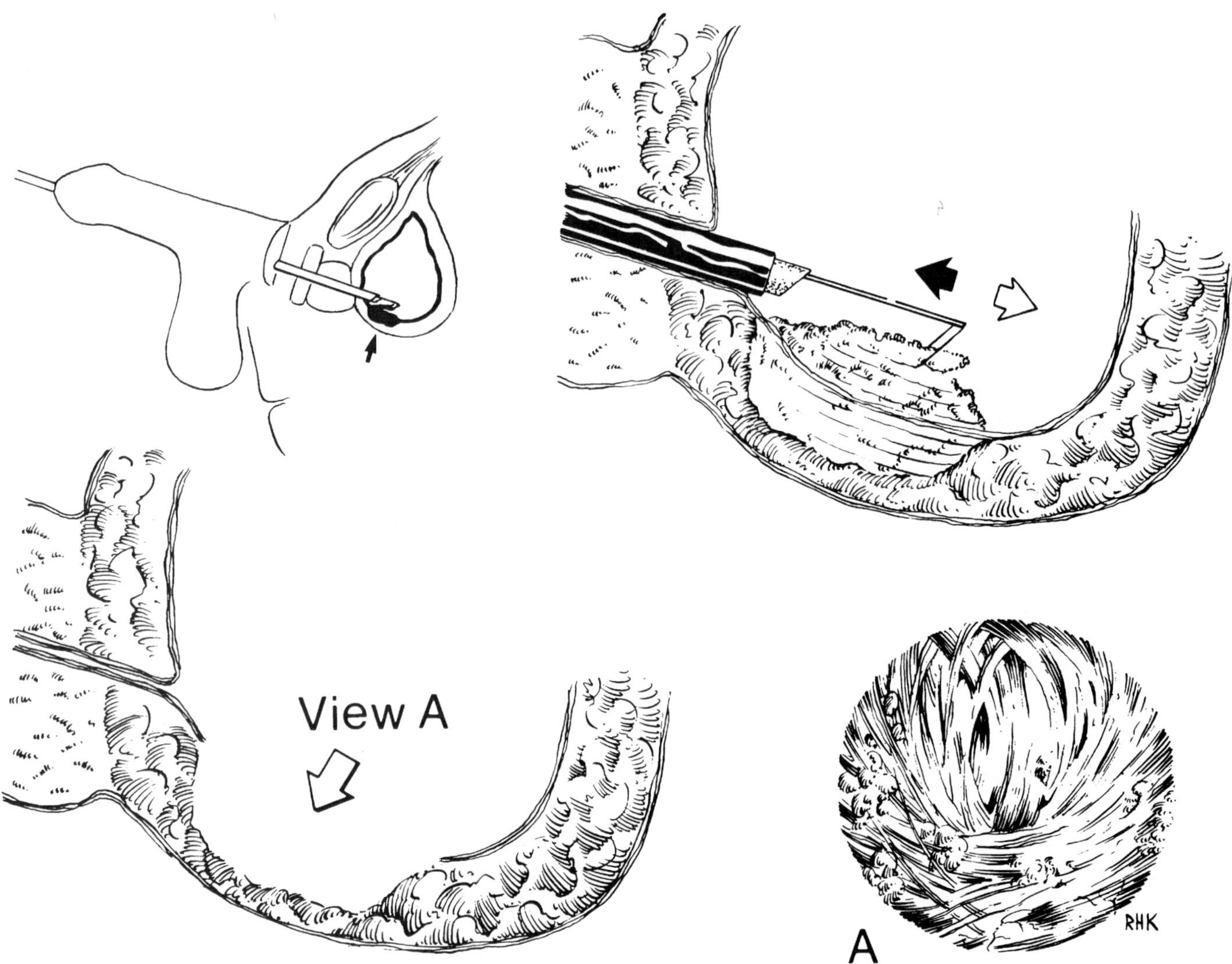

Fig. 24.4. Resection of a sessile bladder tumor is performed in a systematic fashion. We resect into the detrusor muscle and send a separate deep specimen to the pathologist.

tive complications include damage to the ureteral orifices, urethra, and glans penis. Postoperative complications include hyponatremia, hypovolemia, and hemolysis. Late complications include urethral stricture formation, vesicoureteral reflux, and bladder neck contracture (15, 21).

Perforation of the bladder is one of the most significant complications of TURBT. Perforation should be suspected if fat is visualized in the base of the resection. Other findings include abdominal pain and distention. If the volume of irrigant inflow is less than that of outflow, a bladder perforation must be considered. If a significant bladder perforation is noted, the surgeon should change the irrigant to an isotonic solution, achieve hemostasis, and terminate the procedure. A cystogram will help define the extent of the bladder injury and differentiate between intraperitoneal and extraperitoneal perforations. Intraperitoneal perforations result in extravasation of contrast that outlines the loops of the intestine. An extraperitoneal bladder perforation produces a sunburst pattern of contrast in the retroperitoneum (15, 21).

Large intraperitoneal perforations generally require exploration, débridement, and primary closure. Small intraperitoneal perforations can be managed by placing an intraperitoneal drain and a large urethral catheter for several days. Parenteral antibiotics are continued in the postoperative period.

In cases of extraperitoneal perforation, patients may be managed with continuous bladder drainage without operative suprapubic drainage. Postoperative antibiotics are administered. Generally, 7 to 10 days is sufficient to allow extraperitoneal perforations to heal.

The following steps may help prevent bladder perforation during TURBT.

1. Avoid overdistention of the bladder during resection. The bladder wall is thickest while the bladder is nearly empty (Fig. 24.2).

2. Resect bladder lesions in a systematic fashion. Meticulous hemostasis and clear visualization are prerequisites to safe resection.
3. Tumors located along the lateral sidewalls may cause stimulation of the obturator reflex. The lowering of cutting current and avoiding overdistention of the bladder will lessen the likelihood of stimulation of this reflex. If these measures fail, a general anesthetic with the use of a paralytic agent may be required to proceed with safe tumor resection (15, 21, 28).

Invasive hypervascular tumors can produce troublesome bleeding. A systematic resection of the bladder tumor, with attention to achieving meticulous hemostasis during the procedure, will generally prevent massive bleeding. A roller ball electrode can be used to cauterize the base of the resected tumor and aid in achieving hemostasis. Distention of the bladder or a low blood pressure may give the surgeon a false sense of confidence that hemostasis has been achieved. Final inspection of the resected site for hemostasis, therefore, should be done with the bladder empty and the patient's blood pressure near the preanesthetic level. A large-caliber urethral catheter placed at the completion of the operation is useful should overhead or hand irrigation be required.

Postoperative Care

After resection is completed, the bladder is emptied of resected tissue. This may be accomplished by placing the beak of the resectoscope at the base of the bladder and allowing the fragments to drain or siphon through the sheath. The bladder is filled and this procedure is repeated. Any remaining fragments can be removed under direct vision by trapping the resected fragments with the loop of the resectoscope. Alternatively, a Toomey syringe or Ellik evacuator can be used to remove tissue fragments.

A 22F or 24F catheter is placed into the bladder and connected to gravity drainage. Rather than continuous bladder irrigation, we prefer "as needed" intermittent hand irrigation while the catheter is in place.

Small papillary tumors may be resected by an outpatient procedure with catheter drainage only during the postanesthetic recovery time. Overnight catheter drainage should be used, however, if the resection traversed a significant portion of the bladder wall.

We prefer to continue intravenous antibiotics for 24 hours in simple bladder tumor resection, with a subsequent change to an oral antibiotic administered for 3 to 5 days. If a bladder perforation occurred during resection, we generally continue parenteral antibiotics for 5 to 7 days.

Patients who have bladder spasms may be helped with an anticholinergic medication while the catheter is in place. A stool softener during the postoperative period will prevent impaction that may cause postoperative bleeding.

Periodic follow-up is essential in the treatment of bladder tumors. Our standard protocol is that patients undergo cystoscopy and urine cytology at 3-month intervals for the first 2 years. If no recurrences are noted, the interval of follow-up cystoscopy and cytology is increased to 6 months. If after an additional 2 years no recurrent bladder lesions are seen, the patient undergoes annual cystoscopy and cytology. Solitary, well-differentiated papillomas require less aggressive follow-up.

Upper tract imaging should also be obtained at frequent intervals. TCC of the bladder can recur in the upper urinary tract; therefore, it is important to image the upper urinary tract. It is our practice to obtain a yearly intravenous pyelogram for the first 2 years after resection, then every other year thereafter if there is no recurrence (29).

Intravesical Chemotherapy

Intravesical instillation of chemotherapeutic or immunologic agents is used for either prophylactic or therapeutic treatment of TCC of the bladder (30). The three most commonly used agents are bacille Calmette-Guérin (BCG), thiotepa, and mitomycin C. Prospective randomized comparisons among these three agents have demonstrated BCG to be superior in terms of prevention of tumor recurrence (31, 32).

Intravesical therapy is recommended for patients at high risk for tumor recurrence or disease progression after transurethral resection. Patients with a single papillary low-grade lesion are at low risk (less than 5%) for recurrence and progression (33). However, patients who have multiple primary tumors, multiple tumor recurrences, carcinoma in situ, or high-grade superficial tumors are at high risk for recurrence and should be considered for intravesical therapy. Intravesical therapy is used in a therapeutic role, as a prophylactic agent, or as an adjuvant to transurethral resection (1, 3, 33). Therapeutic uses include tumors that are too numerous or large to be resected, inaccessible lesions, and carcinoma in situ. Intravesical therapy is used in a prophylactic role after a transurethral resection in patients with recurrent bladder tumors or patients who are at high risk for tumor recurrence (Table 24.1).

Therapeutic use of intravesical chemotherapeutic or immunologic agents is indicated in cases of established disease that have been incompletely treated by transurethral resection. Herr reviewed a large number of clinical trials using thiotepa, Adriamycin, mitomycin, and BCG for therapeutic intravesical therapy. He defined a complete response to therapy as no evidence

Table 24.1.   Indications for Intravesical Therapy

Therapeutic uses
    Large or inaccessible tumors
    Carcinoma in situ
Prophylactic uses
    Multiple tumor recurrences
    High-grade superficial tumors
    Tumor recurrence at 3 months
    Multiple tumors

of disease by cystoscopic, biopsy, or cytologic means. BCG had a complete response rate of 71%, which is significantly better than that achieved by the other forms of therapy (30).

Intravesical therapy used for prophylaxis has similarly been reviewed. In this role, BCG has also been determined to be superior to the other available chemotherapeutic agents. In a recent study by Nadler et al., a 54% tumor-free rate was achieved using one to two 6-week courses of BCG (34). However, they concluded that the potential for tumor recurrence remains and that patients treated with BCG need long-term follow-up with cystoscopic and cytologic examination performed at least biannually for 2 to 5 years and then yearly for the rest of their lives. These recommendations are based on the three patterns of recurrence noted in this study. Early recurrences tended to be more aggressive. Recurrences occurring between 2 and 5 years were variable, and late recurrences (after 5 years) were almost always of low stage or grade.

The optimal schedule for BCG intravesical therapy has not been established. Most authors agree that patients should receive a once-weekly instillation of BCG for 6 weeks. The agent is suspended in a solution of normal saline and instilled into the bladder. Patients are asked to retain the suspension in their bladders for 2 hours. After 3 months, repeat cytology and cystoscopy are performed. Lamm has recently suggested that the overall efficacy of intravesical BCG could be improved by maintenance therapy (35). If recurrent carcinoma is noted, the physician has several options. A second course of BCG may be administered, a different intravesical agent can be given, or further surgical therapy may be necessary. Treatment may need to be individualized and will depend on the pattern and type of recurrence (36).

Side Effects of BCG

BCG produces both local and systemic reactions. In the bladder, BCG produces an intense inflammatory reaction. Patients may experience dysuria, frequency, urgency, and hematuria, and they may pass tissue in their urine. These symptoms usually resolve after 24 hours and rarely require treatment. Rare systemic complications include fever, pneumonitis, hepatitis, arthralgia, skin rash, ureteral obstruction, epididymo-orchitis, and hypotension.

Patients suspected of having systemic complications of BCG may require treatment with antituberculosis medications. Relative contraindications for intravesical BCG include active tuberculosis and serious immunosuppression (35, 37).

Laser Resection and New Techniques

The efficacy and feasibility of treating superficial bladder tumors using lasers are well established (38). Nd:YAG lasers and, more recently, the Holmium laser have been used to treat superficial bladder tumors and, in selected cases, invasive bladder tumors (39). Laser treatment has several advantages over standard electrocautery resection. Laser therapy can be per-

formed with essentially no blood loss, laser fibers can be placed through flexible cystoscopes, and laser therapy produces little discomfort. Disadvantages include difficulty in adequately staging superficial lesions and possible small bowel perforations from the forward scatter of laser energy.

A new grooved bar electrode has been developed for the treatment of benign prostatic hypertrophy and uses cutting current to vaporize prostatic tissue (40). This device is used in place of a standard electrocautery loop. We have used this instrument to treat superficial bladder tumors and it appears to produce results similar to laser therapy and standard electrocautery resection, with minimal blood loss.

Conclusion

TURBT represents one of the first successful forms of minimally invasive surgery. Most patients present with superficial TCC of the bladder that can be cured with adequate transurethral resection. The role of transurethral surgery in the diagnosis and treatment of this important clinical entity is paramount. Meticulous attention to detail, a thorough understanding of the indications for transurethral surgery, and techniques to avoid and treat complications are essential for success with these operations.

Video endoscopy, laser technology, and further modifications in chemotherapeutic therapies will continue to affect the management of bladder cancer. However, for the majority of superficial lesions, transurethral surgery will still be the method of choice for diagnosis and treatment.

REFERENCES

1. Lamm DL, Griffith G, Pettit LL, et al. Current perspectives on diagnosis and treatment of superficial bladder cancer. Urology 1992;39:301.
2. Barnes RW, Bergman T, Hadley HL, et al. Control of bladder tumors by endoscopic surgery. J Urol 1967;97:864.
3. Soloway MS. Managing superficial bladder cancer: an overview. Urology 1992;40:5.
4. Gomella LG, Strup SE. History of laparoscopy: urology's perspective. J Endourol 1993;7:1.
5. Collins CW. History: endoscopic prostatic surgery. In: Barnes RW, ed. St. Louis: CV Mosby, 1943:17.
6. Hadley HL, Roger W. Barnes: pioneer resectionist and teacher of endoscopic surgery. J Urol 1991;145:276. Abstract.
7. Mariani AJ. The evaluation of adult hematuria. AUA Update Series 1989:178.
8. Lamm DL. Carcinoma in situ. Urol Clin North Am 1992;19:499.
9. Synder JA, Smith AD. Supine flexible cystoscopy. J Urol 1986;135:251.
10. Bagley DH. Flexible endoscopy in the urinary tract. Semin Urol 1986;4:198.
11. Babayan RK. Flexible cystoscopy for office procedures. Contemp Urol 1990:3.
12. Herr HW. Outpatient flexible cystoscopy and fulguration of recurrent superficial bladder tumors. J Urol 1990;144:1365.

13. Grasso M, Beaghler MA, Bagley DH, et al. Actively deflectable flexible cystoscopes: no longer solely a diagnostic instrument. J Endourol 1993;7:527.

14. Beaghler MA, Grasso M. Flexible cystoscopic bladder biopsies: a technique for outpatient evaluation of the lower urinary tract urothelium. Urology 1994;44:756.

15. Schmidt JD, Anwar H. Transurethral resection of vesical neoplasms. In: Greene LF, Segura JW, eds. Transurethral surgery. Philadelphia: WB Saunders, 1979:255.

16. Chodak GW, Plaut ME. Systemic antibiotics for a prophylaxis in urologic surgery: a critical review. J Urol 1979;121:695.

17. Engberg A, Spangberg A, Urenes T. Transurethral resection of bladder tumors under local anesthesia. Urology 1983;12:385.

18. Soloway MS, Patel J. Surgical techniques for endoscopic resection of bladder cancer. Urol Clin North Am 1992;19:467.

19. Iglesias JJ, Sporen A, Gellman AC, et al. New Iglesias resectoscope with continuous suction and low intravesical pressure. J Urol 1975;114:929.

20. Widran, J. Video transurethral resection using controlled continuous flow resectoscope. Urology 1988;31:382.

21. Michaels EK. Cystourethroscopy and transurethral resection of the prostate and bladder. In: Fowler JE, ed. Urologic Surgery. Boston: Little, Brown & Co., 1992:641.

22. Laor E, Gravstad H, Whitmore WL. The influence of simultaneous resection of bladder tumors and prostate on the recurrence of prostatic urethral tumors. J Urol 1981;126:171.

23. Augspurg R, Donohue RE. Prevention of obturator nerve stimulation during transurethral surgery. J Urol 1980;123:170.

24. Barnes RW, Dick AL, Hadley HL, et al. Survival following transurethral resection of bladder carcinoma. Cancer Res 1977;37:2895.

25. Herr HW. Transurethral resection in regionally advanced bladder cancer. Urol Clin North Am 1992;19:695.

26. Solsona E, Iborra I, Ricos JV, et al. Feasibility of transurethral resection for muscle infiltrating carcinoma of the bladder: prospective study. J Urol 1992;147:1513.

27. Droller MJ. Treatment of regionally advanced bladder cancer: an overview. Urol Clin North Am 1992;19:685.

28. Dick A, Barnes R, Hadley HL, et al. Complication of transurethral resection of bladder tumors: prevention, recognition and treatment. J Urol 1980;124:810.

29. Smith H, Weaver D, Barejenbruch O, et al. Routine excretory urography in follow-up of superficial transitional cell carcinoma of bladder. Urology 1989;34:193.

30. Herr HW. Intravesical therapy for superficial bladder cancer. AUA Update Series 1989:90.

31. Soloway MS, Perito PE. Superficial bladder cancer: diagnosis, surveillance and treatment. J Cell Biochem Suppl 1992;161:120.

32. Prout GR, Bart BA, Griffin PP, et al. Treated history of noninvasive grade I transitional cell carcinoma. J Urol 1992;148:1413.

33. Herr HR, Laudone VP, Whitmore WE. An overview of intravesical therapy for superficial bladder tumors. J Urol 1987;138:1363.

34. Nadler RB, Catalona WJ, Hudson MA, et al. Durability of the tumor-free response for intravesical bacillus Calmette-Guérin therapy. J Urol 1992;152:367.

35. Lamm DL, Stodgill VD, Stodgill BJ, et al. Complications of BCG in 1278 patients with bladder cancer. J Urol 1985;135:272.

36. Soloway MS. Intravesical therapy for bladder cancer. J Urol 1994;152:379. Editorial.

37. Orihuela E, Herr HW, Pinsky CM, et al. Toxicity of intravesical BCG and its management in patients with superficial bladder tumors. Cancer 1987;60:326.

38. Smith JA. Laser surgery for transitional-cell carcinoma: technique, advantages and limitations. Urol Clin North Am 1992;19:473.

39. Watson G, Shroff S, Thomas R, et al. The Holmium laser for multifunctional use in urology. Lasers Urol 1974;2129:116.

40. Stewart S, Benjamin D, Ruckle H, et al. Transurethral electrovaporization of the prostate: a new technique for treatment of symptomatic BPH. J Endourol 1994;8(Suppl):145.

25

Laser Surgery for Carcinoma of the Bladder

Joseph A. Smith, Jr.

The usefulness of surgical lasers is predicated by the unique tissue effects observed with thermal transformation of light energy. Lasers can be used to coagulate, incise, or vaporize tissue and can, under certain circumstances, provide a combination of the above. Selective absorption of laser energy by the target tissue is possible, thereby increasing the efficiency of therapy and decreasing the risk of side effects. The transmission of laser energy by small, flexible, optical fibers facilitates energy delivery either directly in a hand-held mode or through an endoscope. Adaptations allowing side fiber emission of laser energy have further expanded the therapeutic capabilities for surgical lasers.

Since they were first introduced into clinical practice almost 15 years ago, lasers have been used for ablation of transitional cell carcinoma of the bladder. Justification for the use of lasers as an alternative to standard methods of electrocautery resection has been based on theoretical therapeutic advantages and an observed decrease in treatment-related morbidity. The development of new laser wavelengths and instrumentation has facilitated and expanded the use of lasers in a number of areas of urologic surgery, including treatment of bladder cancer.

BASIC LASER PHYSICS

To safely and effectively apply laser energy as a surgical tool, the surgeon must have a basic understanding of the physics and tissue effects of lasers. The tissue-destructive properties of a laser beam can be therapeutically beneficial if properly used but can also produce unique complications if misdirected or applied with inadequate knowledge or experience.

The word laser is an acronym for light amplification by stimulated emission of radiation. White light from an incandescent bulb is a divergent mix of multiple wavelengths. In contrast, laser light consists of nearly a single wavelength (monochromatic) that travels in a unidirectional manner (columated) and can be deflected for projection onto tissue surfaces. In theory, the beam is nondivergent, although the angle of divergence from surgical laser fibers is at least 5° and often much greater.

Surgical lasers are powered by electricity, which is used to ignite a flashlamp. Atoms of the active medium in the laser resonator are energized from the ground state to an excited state by photons produced by the flashlamp. When the atoms spontaneously decay to the ground state, a photon of a specific wavelength is emitted. Spontaneously emitted photons interact with excited state atoms and stimulate them to decay and emit monochromatic photons. Because the original incident photon is also released, stimulated emission of radiation involves a factor of two energy gain with each atomic interaction. Photons are deflected from a totally reflecting mirror at one end of the laser cavity and a partially reflecting mirror at the other. Photon reflection through the laser resonator significantly increases laser output because photons have greater opportunity to stimulate excited state atoms to decay. Photons exit as a nearly nondivergent beam through the partially reflecting mirror at one end of the resonator. The beam may pass directly from the laser or be coupled to a flexible fused silica glass optical fiber.

The active medium, i.e., the source from which the photons are emitted, determines the wavelength of a particular laser. It may be a gas (carbon dioxide, argon), a liquid (rhodamine-B, coumarin green), or solid state (neodymium, potassium titanyl phosphate [KTP]).

TISSUE EFFECTS OF LASER ENERGY

The tissue effects and, thereby, the surgical potential of a laser result from transformation of light energy into heat (1). Cellular destruction generally is not evident when temperatures less than 60°C are maintained for only a few seconds. Above 60°C, protein denaturation ensues, although minimum volatilization and tissue vaporization occur below 100°C. Above 100°C, cellular water evaporates and charring and tissue vaporization are observed.

Several important factors influence the extent of thermal destruction that occurs when a laser beam is projected onto tissue surfaces. The most obvious factor and the one most easily controlled is the wavelength of the laser. Body tissues contain chromophores, such as hemoglobin, which selectively absorb different wavelengths of light. The absorption characteristics of a particular laser wavelength depend on the relative tissue absorption and can vary significantly from one wavelength to another.

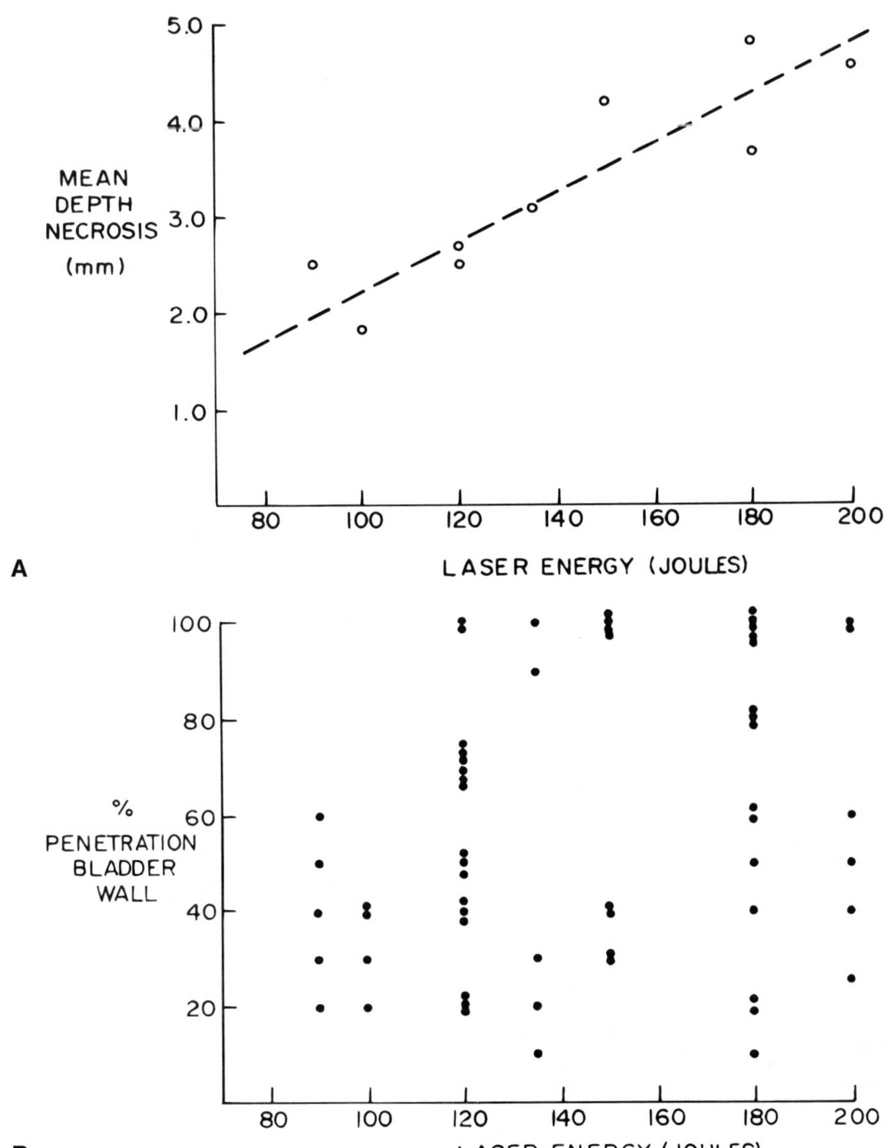

Fig. 25.1. **A.** Mean depth of bladder wall necrosis as a function of laser energy. Note the linear correlation. **B.** Percent bladder wall penetration by Nd:YAG laser as a function of laser energy. Each experiment is represented by a separate dot. Variability in bladder penetration is due to spot size, fiber variability, tangential laser application, duration of treatment, and differences in tissue characteristics.

Energy Density

In addition to wavelength, there are other parameters that can be used to predict and, to some extent, control the tissue effects and depth of penetration of a particular laser. Stated simply, energy density is the amount of energy delivered to a given area of tissue. It is determined by the formula: power (watts) $\times$ duration (seconds)/area^2 (cm^2). The power output of a particular laser is controlled from the instrument panel. Duration can be modified by controlling the time length of a particular pulse or by varying the speed with which the beam is moved across the tissue surface.

An influential component of the formula for energy density is the size of the treatment area, which is a function of offset distance and divergence angle. Surgical laser fibers with a wide angle of divergence produce a lower energy density than nondi-

vergent fibers by treating a larger surface area with the same amount of energy. The distance between the fiber tip and the tissue surface also influences the energy density by significantly changing the treated surface area (Fig. 25.1). Contact techniques increase energy density by limiting the treatment surface area.

The angle of divergence from the fiber tip is unique to each device. The end-fire probes used during the past decade typically have an angle of divergence of only 5° to 15°. Tissue injury from short-duration (2 to 3 sec), high-energy density exposure may extend for several centimeters due to thermal transport. Widely divergent beams (up to 90°) produce a much lower energy density. Long-duration (60 to 90 sec), low-power (40 to 60 W) exposure with these fibers can coagulate a large volume of tissue with coagulation depths of more than 1 cm.

Coagulation

When tissues are heated to less than 60°C for only a few seconds, tissue warming without irreversible damage is observed. Between 60 and 100°C, protein denaturation occurs, causing tissue coagulation. Although coagulation is irreversible and destructive, immediate tissue removal does not occur. The thermally injured tissue either sloughs or resorbs secondarily (Fig. 25.2). Laser-treated tissue sloughed from the urinary tract is amorphous and does not cause urinary retention. Hemostasis during and after treatment is usually excellent as the coagulation process extends to blood vessels within the volume of treated tissue. Poorly absorbed wavelengths, such as Nd:YAG, cause primarily tissue coagulation. Coagulation rather than vaporization may be favored by lowering the energy density. In general, low-power, long-duration laser exposure increases the amount of coagulation and the depth of tissue injury compared with higher power used for a short duration.

Vaporization

When high tissue temperatures (generally exceeding 100°C) are achieved, immediate tissue vaporization ensues. Surface carbonization may be observed and a smoke plume generated. Some degree of coagulation accompanies carbonization, so hemostasis is usually good although less than that observed with pure coagulation techniques. Vaporization is more difficult to achieve underwater than in an air environment. This is particularly pertinent for urologic endoscopic use as the irrigating fluid causes surface cooling. Excessive charring of the tissue surface results in increased tissue surface absorption and limits

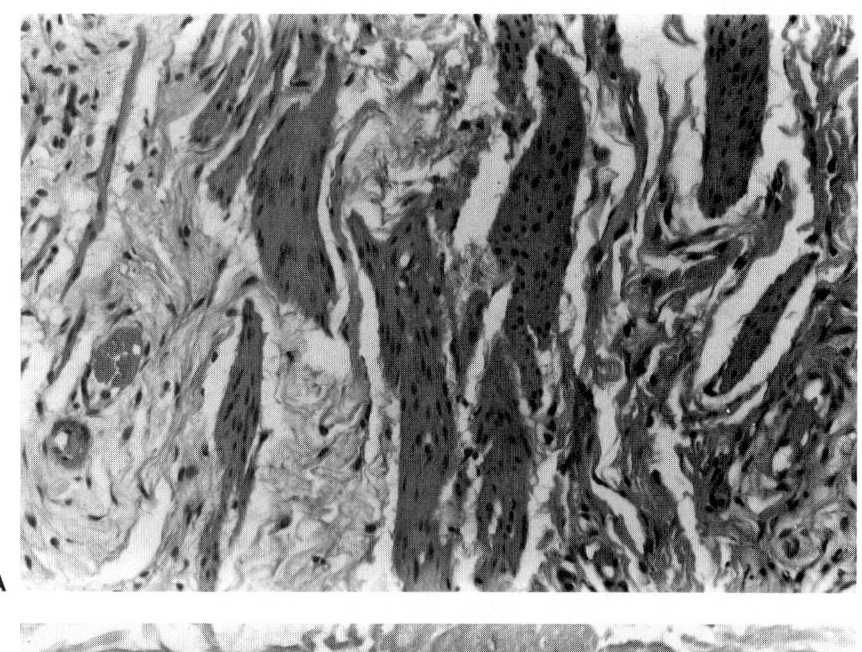

A

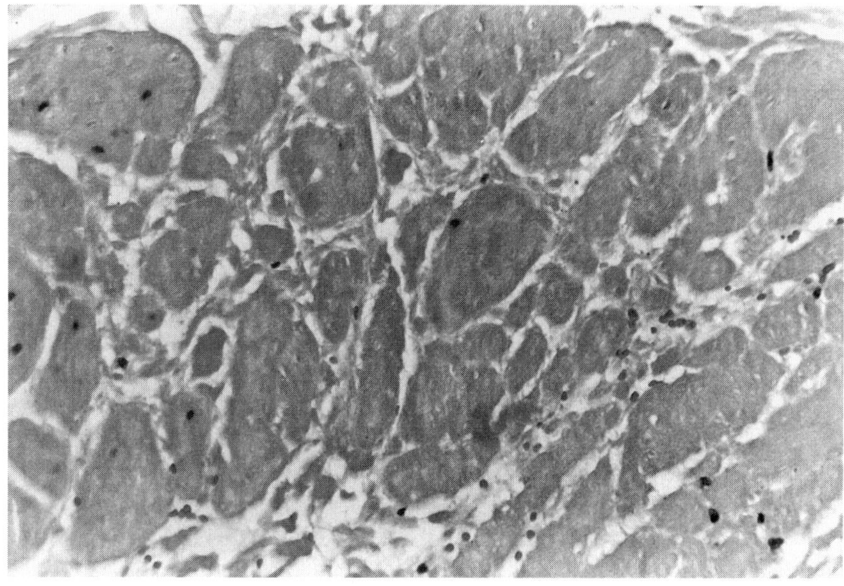

B

Fig. 25.2. **A.** Normal bladder wall. **B.** Bladder wall 5 days after Nd:YAG laser treatment. Note absence of smooth muscle nuclei but preservation of the cytoskeleton.

further penetration of laser energy deep into the tissue. Vaporization is increased by using highly absorbed wavelengths, using a high laser power output, or decreasing the treated surface area (as with contact tips).

CHOICE OF LASER WAVELENGTH

Laser instruments differ primarily in the wavelength of the emitted light. Wavelength is a function of the active medium that may be a solid, liquid, or gas as described previously. In addition, frequency doubling crystals may be used to modify the wavelength of existing laser light.

Nd:YAG Laser

Since its introduction into clinical practice in 1979, the Nd:YAG laser has been and remains the most frequently used laser in urologic surgery. The active medium consists of neodymium atoms contained within an yttrium aluminum garnet lattice. The Nd:YAG laser emits invisible infrared 1064-nm wavelength light. Light at this wavelength is poorly absorbed by water and body pigments. Due to poor absorption, the light penetrates deeply into the tissue.

In a fluid environment, the poor absorption of the laser energy results in thermal coagulation of surface and subsurface tissue. However, the tissue maintains its structural and architectural integrity. A certain percentage of the energy is transmitted through the target organ. Thus, the thermal effects may extend to adjacent organs. After noncontact Nd:YAG laser treatment, hemostasis is usually total. The coagulated tissue takes on a white, fluffy appearance. The tissue sloughs secondarily over a several-week period, although complete healing may take up to 3 months.

KTP Laser

A KTP laser uses a potassium titanyl phosphate crystal to double the frequency of an Nd:YAG laser, thereby producing 532-nm wavelength green light. Interaction of Nd:YAG light with the KTP crystal causes substantial energy loss. For that reason, the energy output of a dual wavelength laser in KTP mode is only approximately half that of the same laser in Nd:YAG mode. The 532-nm wavelength provides an intermediate level of vaporization and coagulation. The energy can be transmitted by the same standard optical fiber used for Nd:YAG treatment. Tissue effects are similar to those achieved with an argon laser, although greater power can be produced than with most surgical argon lasers.

KTP lasers have been used for treatment of superficial bladder cancer. In some circumstances, the KTP laser provides an increased safety margin compared with an Nd:YAG laser because of limited coagulation depth. However, treatment is slower than with an Nd:YAG laser and treatment for large tumors may be more difficult. KTP lasers have also been used for treatment of external genital, urethral, and ureteral lesions.

Combined techniques for treatment of benign prostatic hypertrophy using coagulating energy followed by vaporization of prostate tissue with a KTP laser have been described.

Argon Laser

Argon has several potential lasing lines between 488 and 514 nm. Light at this wavelength is poorly absorbed by water but strongly absorbed by body pigments such as melanin and hemoglobin. Consequently, tissue absorption is between that of an Nd:YAG and a carbon dioxide laser. The selective absorption of argon energy by hemoglobin has led to its use for treatment of hemangioma. Argon lasers have also been used for treatment of superficial transitional cell carcinoma of the bladder. Commercially available surgical argon lasers, however, have a relatively limited power output and generally can be used only for small (less than 1 cm) tumors. Overall, Nd:YAG or KTP lasers have proven preferable because of higher energy outputs and deeper tissue coagulations.

Carbon Dioxide Laser

The 10,600-nm wavelength of a carbon dioxide laser is strongly absorbed by water. Thus, the energy is rapidly absorbed at the tissue surface, creating high temperatures. The depth of penetration is limited, usually less than 1 mm. Vaporization is observed along with carbonization. A smoke plume is produced, and a dedicated smoke evacuator should be used if infectious material is being treated.

The relatively long wavelength of the carbon dioxide laser creates problems for transmission via flexible fibers. Far infrared wavelengths such as this are absorbed by optical glass. Attempts have been made to develop cystoscopes using a series of reflecting mirrors. So far, however, a practical carbon dioxide laser cystoscope has not been developed. Carbon dioxide lasers have proven useful for treatment of various lesions of the external genitalia and with open surgical applications. The beam is delivered to tissue via a series of articulating arms and reflecting mirrors. A lens may be used to focus or defocus the beam to vary the spot size.

Holmium:YAG Laser

The holmium:YAG laser emits light in the mid infrared region of the electromagnetic spectrum (2100 nm). Unlike the continuous wave lasers described previously, energy emission occurs in a rapid pulse over a few milliseconds. The light is readily transmitted by a flexible optical fiber. Holmium:YAG laser light is highly absorbed by water and produces explosive vaporization and cutting. Because there is more vaporization, the hemostatic abilities are less than those of a continuous wave Nd:YAG laser. The holmium:YAG laser has been used for urinary tract stone fragmentation in addition to coagulation of soft tissue lesions.

Argon Dye Laser

Dye lasers can be used to produce coherent monochromatic laser light over a wide range of wavelengths. The argon pumped dye laser uses an argon laser instead of a flashlamp to power a dye laser. By selecting the proper wavelength (choosing the proper dye), one can selectively excite a tissue chromophore. Hematoporphyrin derivative has been used in several studies due to selective uptake by carcinoma in situ in the bladder (2–4). Hematoporphyrin derivative is activated by wavelength-specific (630-nm) argon pumped dye laser light. The use of an inefficient laser to pump another inefficient laser causes tremendous energy loss. For this reason, energy output of the argon pumped dye laser is limited to 5 to 10 W.

PATIENT SELECTION

Although some investigators still believe that the tumor recurrence rate is decreased after laser treatment compared with electrocautery resection (5), laser therapy of superficial bladder cancer is performed most often because of the observed decrease in morbidity and duration of hospital stay. Commonly, patients with superficial bladder cancer undergoing laser treatment have a history of recurrent low-grade papillary transitional cell carcinoma that has been biopsied previously. When papillary tumors are seen on a routine surveillance cystoscopy, laser treatment can be an effective, low-morbidity method for eradication of these recurrent lesions.

Laser vaporization or coagulation results in tumor destruction that does not allow retrieval of tissue for adequate histologic examination. Preoperative cold-cup biopsies can partially address this issue and allow pathologic examination to determine tumor grade and give some staging information. Nevertheless, sessile-appearing tumors in which invasion cannot be excluded reasonably by visual inspection should generally be treated by electrocautery resection with biopsies of the underlying muscle tissue of the bladder wall. Some investigators have also believed that first-time tumors should be treated by electrocautery resection rather than laser treatment so that adequate histologic material is available (6).

Tumor size is another consideration. Lesions greater than 1 to 2 cm are difficult to treat with laser treatment alone and may require a debulking electrocautery resection before a laser treatment of the tumor base. This may, however, obviate many of the practical advantages of laser treatment if electrocautery resection is required anyway.

Tumor location is a relatively minor issue. Virtually all parts of the bladder are accessible for laser treatment. Extra caution is appropriate for tumors on the bladder dome where loops of small bowel may be adjacent. Treatment of tumors overlying the ureteral orifice appears to be associated with a very low risk of stricture and obstruction of the ureter.

TREATMENT TECHNIQUE

A number of treatment techniques have been described for laser destruction of bladder tumors. Additionally, differences exist depending on the laser wavelength. Finally, the amount and manner of energy delivery depend on the preoperative assessment of tumor stage.

Superficial Tumors

Laser treatment of superficial transitional cell carcinoma of the bladder (stages Ta to T1) is usually performed on an outpatient or ambulatory surgery basis. When treatment is performed without anesthesia, the patient is able to perceive the laser energy and often describes it as a burning type of discomfort. However, this treatment seems to be tolerated better than electrocautery resection. The exact reason for this is uncertain. However, laser energy probably results in rapid heating and destruction of nerve fibers in a well-defined volume of tissue. Electrocautery resection is associated with more irregular propagation of the energy along nerve and muscle bundles. The decision to perform laser therapy with general or regional anesthesia is based primarily on the surgeon's experience, patient's personality, and size, number, and location of tumors.

When a rigid cystoscope is used, the patient is placed in a standard lithotomy position. Most cystoscope instrument companies have a laser insert that adapts to the standard cystoscope with either a 19F or 21F sheath. The laser insert allows stabilization of the fiber tip and a watertight entry port. The laser fiber is inserted through the channel, and the tip of the laser fiber is positioned just beyond the end of the visualizing telescope. When using a noncontact approach with a standard 400- or 600-μm end-fire optical fiber, the fiber tip is positioned 3 to 5 mm from the tumor surface. With an Nd:YAG laser, 30 to 40 W of energy are usually sufficient for complete tumor coagulation. The duration of the treatment usually is controlled by the speed with which the aiming beam is moved across the tumor surface. The laser can be operated in a continuous mode whereby energy is emitted whenever the foot pedal is depressed. An aiming beam, from either a flashlamp or a helium neon laser, marks the point of impact since the Nd:YAG laser beam is invisible to the human eye. Sterile water, normal saline, or amino acid solutions can be used for irrigation. A continuous-flow system is not required because the irrigant can be turned off during treatment since bleeding is usually nonexistent.

Laser treatment is best performed as a dynamic process rather than a series of adjacent static impulses. The beam is slowly moved across the surface of the tumor in a "painting" fashion. The tumor undergoes a white discoloration indicative of adequate thermal coagulation (Fig. 25.3). Care should be taken to avoid excessive laser energy application in any given area. Usually 2 to 3 sec are required in a given area for complete thermal coagulation to be evident. Techniques have been described wherein a ring of coagulated tissue is created around the tumor base to seal blood and lymphatic vessels. Practically, this is unnecessary because bleeding does not occur even if the energy is applied initially to the center of the exophytic portion of the tumor.

It is unnecessary to treat the tumor base initially, but it is

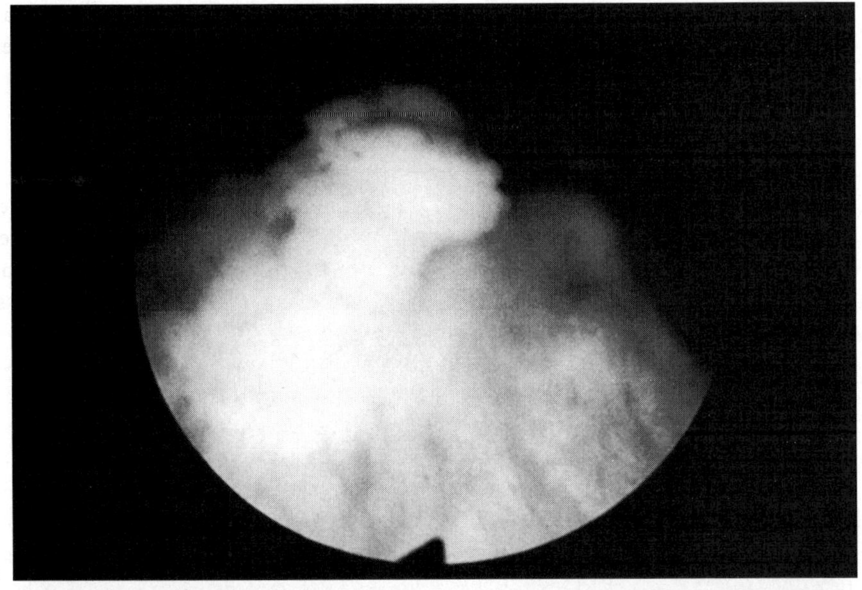

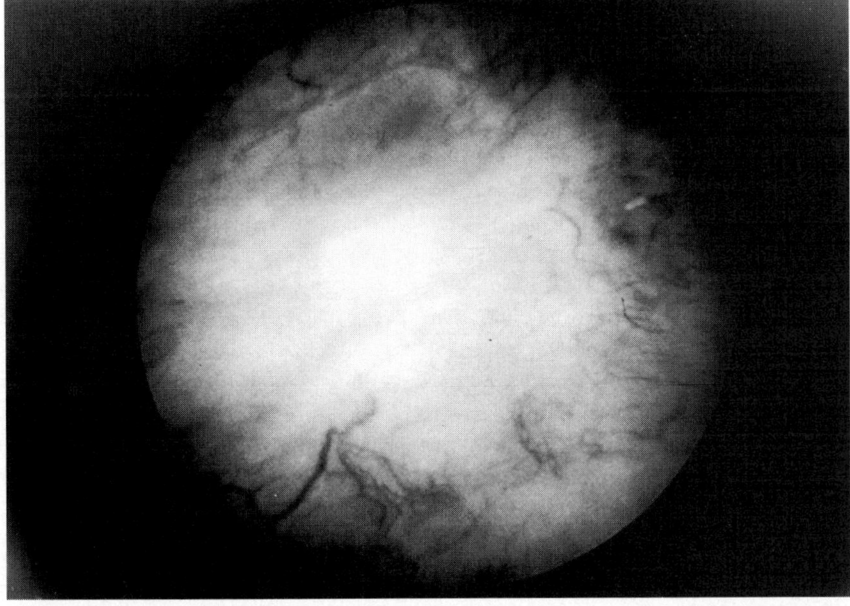

Fig. 25.3.   A. Papillary transitional cell carcinoma after Nd:YAG laser irradiation. The white discoloration is evidence of adequate thermal necrosis. **B.** Six weeks later, tumor slough has occurred. A pale white scar is evident on the bladder wall.

important to make certain that all aspects of the lesion have been thermally coagulated. After the papillary frondular tissue is coagulated, it usually can be dislodged with the tip of the fiber or the cystoscope to expose deeper portions and the tumor base. Treatment is best performed with the bladder in as collapsed a state as possible to avoid excessive thinning of the bladder wall. This allows an added margin of safety for adjacent organs. If the tumor is located in the air bubble, either the air can be evacuated or the patient can be tilted to remove the tumor from the air bubble. If this proves to be difficult, treatment can be performed through the air bubble itself, but there is usually some surface carbonization and smoke production. The temperature of the irrigating fluid does not seem to be a major factor in determining tissue or treatment effect.

Subsurface boiling may be observed during treatment, producing a popcorn-like effect. These microexplosions, although sometimes dramatic, carry no particular significance. If the fiber tip inadvertently touches the bladder wall, there usually is some superficial carbonization and a cratering effect. The foot pedal is simply released and the fiber withdrawn from the tissue surface. If there is any tissue adherent to the fiber tip, it should be wiped away with a moist sponge before proceeding with therapy. If necessary, cleavage of the fiber tip will restore the fiber to its original condition.

The depth of coagulation cannot be monitored satisfactorily intraoperatively. In general, coagulation depth is predicted preoperatively based on known characteristics of the wavelength, power, duration of laser output, and spot size. Under most circumstances, 3 to 5 mm of complete tissue coagulation can be anticipated.

If a small amount of bleeding occurs, especially after a cold-cup biopsy, hemostasis usually is accomplished in the course of laser treatment. However, even a relatively small amount of blood undergoes rapid carbonization and can both obscure and prevent effective energy delivery to the tumor surface.

Superficial tumors in bladder diverticula can be treated satisfactorily with a laser. Although, by definition, there is no muscular backing to a diverticulum, actual free perforation of the diverticulum and bladder wall is uncommon. Usually, there is some shrivelling of the mucosa of the diverticulum as the coagulation process occurs. The iliac blood vessels and obturator nerve are often adjacent to diverticula but, if appropriate energy densities are used, direct injury is unlikely. The obturator nerve is not stimulated by laser energy. Obturator spasm and a leg jerk, as may be observed with electrocautery, do not occur.

Treatment of tumors directly overlying the ureteral orifices is performed in the same manner as if the tumor were located elsewhere in the bladder. Stents should be removed from the ureteral orifice before treatment is performed because the laser energy may melt the stent. Metal guide wires can be used alternatively. After an extensive treatment overlying the ureteral orifice, postoperative management with a stent may be advisable because of temporary edema. However, the long-term risk of ureteral stenosis appears to be quite low.

A postoperative Foley catheter is usually unnecessary because of the lack of bleeding. The thermally coagulated tissue either sloughs as imperceptible particles or is resorbed. If the treatment was believed to be adequate, follow-up cystoscopy can be performed as per the routine for a particular patient depending on tumor grade, stage, and prior history.

Intravesical drugs can be used after laser treatment, and the indications for their use should be the same as those after electrocautery resection. However, since raw surfaces of the bladder wall are not exposed after laser treatment, intravesical drugs such as bacille Calmette-Guérin or chemotherapy can be introduced more rapidly after treatment with an apparent decreased risk of systemic absorption (7).

Invasive Tumors

The ability of an Nd:YAG laser to produce transmural coagulation without perforation has allowed laser treatment of some invasive bladder cancers. Even in a controlled setting, however, the treatment depth is variable (8). However, application of energy to both the inner and outer bladder wall through both a cystoscope and a laparoscope allows overlapping zones of thermal necrosis and complete transmural coagulation (9). When treated with this technique, the bladder wall maintains structural integrity due to rapid fibroblast infiltration and collagen deposition. The location of most invasive bladder tumors near the trigone makes laparoscopic visualization and energy application somewhat difficult.

Patients being considered for laser treatment of invasive bladder cancer should first undergo a standard transurethral electrocautery resection. This accomplishes two things. First, it allows accurate histologic examination for tumor staging. Second, resection debulks the surface of the tumor. Logically, if laser therapy is considered a method for extending the margin of resection, the electrocautery resection should extend deeply into the bladder muscle.

Under most circumstances, it is best to delay laser treatment for at least 3 to 5 days after an electrocautery resection. This allows any bleeding to cease and an overlying clot to lyse. Active bleeding or blood clot interferes with delivery of energy. General or regional anesthesia usually is required because relatively large amounts of laser energy are needed. The irregular appearance of the resection crater does not allow visual determination of treatment adequacy. Therefore, systematic application of laser energy to the entire resection crater and an adequate surrounding margin should be performed (Fig. 25.4).

Because the goal of treatment is transmural necrosis, energy output up to 45 or 50 W may be appropriate. When an end-fire fiber with a 5° to 15° angle of divergence is used, the energy is maintained in a given area for 2 to 3 seconds. If a laparoscope has been inserted, the small bowel can be displaced from the treatment area. After adequate energy has been applied through the cystoscope, the Nd:YAG laser fiber can be inserted through the laparoscope and energy applied to the intraperitoneal surface of the bladder in the same region if visualization is adequate. Steaming or subtle coagulation of the intraperitoneal bladder surface behind the tumor can often be seen laparoscopically during cystoscopic Nd:YAG laser therapy. Otherwise, the intended treatment site may be difficult to determine.

The most appropriate patients for laser treatment of invasive bladder cancer are those with minimally invasive lesions (10, 11). Lasers have been used to treat bulky, invasive bladder cancers. However, the surface effect that is obtained in this circumstance usually offers no demonstrable benefit compared with electrocautery debulking and cauterization of the tumor surface.

A catheter is not required postoperatively but may be used depending on the amount of the bladder surface area requiring treatment. Follow-up cystoscopy is performed after 1 month to assess healing and to detect any obvious residual tumor. Reepithelialization of the bladder surface overlying residual cancer is feasible but, most often, there is no residual tumor present when complete reepithelialization occurs within 2 to 3 months of treatment.

COMPLICATIONS

Laser treatment of bladder cancer is used most often because of the observed decrease in patient morbidity and treatment-related complications. Usually, there is minimal discomfort after treatment. A distinct advantage is the almost complete lack of bleeding that occurs with coagulative procedures. Bleeding that may be present from a preoperative biopsy usually is coagulated adequately during the course of energy application.

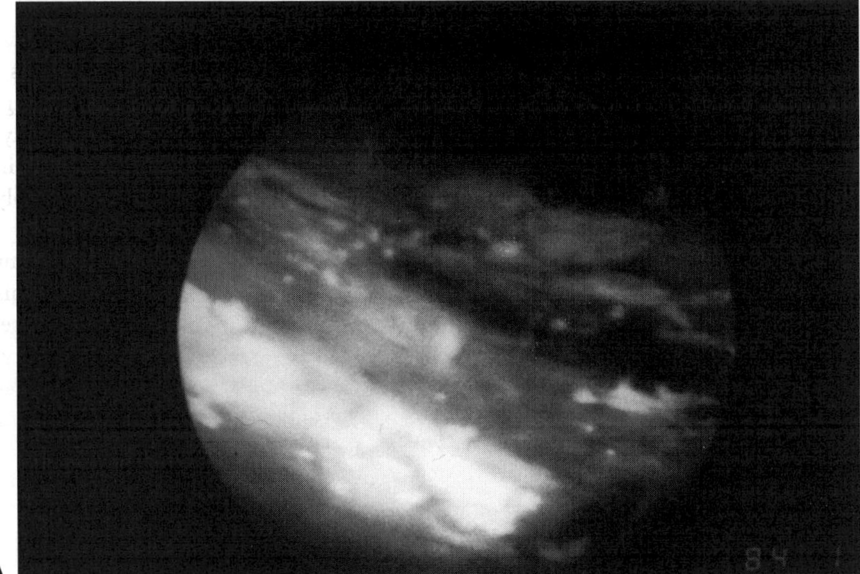

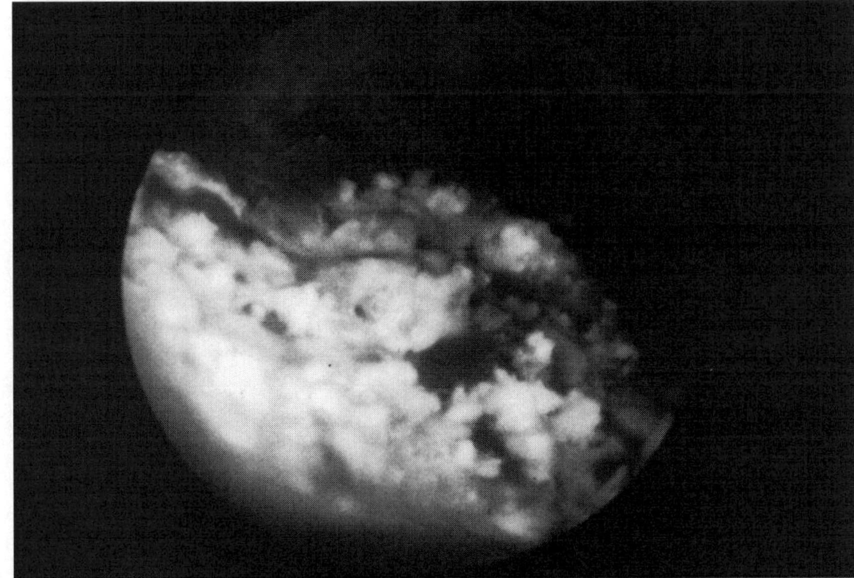

Fig. 25.4. A. Endoscopic appearance of invasive bladder carcinoma site after aggressive transurethral resection. **B.** Same site after treatment with the Nd: YAG laser.

The coagulation that occurs from the laser energy itself causes virtually no bleeding as either an immediate or delayed phenomenon.

The most feared complication of laser treatment of bladder cancer is perforation of an adjacent viscus. The small bowel or colon may lie in direct approximation with the peritoneal surface of the bladder. Thus, the risk for bowel perforation is greatest with laser treatment on the posterior bladder wall or dome.

Most patients with bowel perforation present with signs and symptoms within 8 to 24 hours of treatment, but symptomatic presentation has been delayed for as long as 2 weeks. Abdominal pain, physical examination findings consistent with an acute abdomen, and free intraperitoneal air are all associated with bowel perforation from laser therapy. It is important to recognize that bowel perforation may occur in the absence of any

evident bladder perforation. Results of a cystogram may be normal. The thicker muscle wall of the bladder makes it less prone to perforation, and forward scatter of the energy places the bowel at risk.

Immediate laparotomy is indicated if small bowel or colon perforation is suspected. The site of laser energy is identified. The zone of tissue injury may be far greater than is visibly evident, so resection of the affected site is indicated most often.

Hofstetter et al. treated more than 500 tumors and reported only two incidences of small bowel perforation, at least one of which was related to the inadvertent use of excessive energy levels (12). Smith has had no cases of small bowel perforation in more than 150 laser treatments of superficial bladder tumors (6).

RESULTS

Initially, laser treatment of superficial bladder cancer was promoted as a means to decrease the recurrence rate (13, 14). Anecdotal clinical observation and some experimental data support the contention that some recurrences of superficial bladder cancer occur because of implantation of viable tumor cells dislodged at the time of resection. Because of this, the thermal, noncontact coagulation achieved with the laser has the potential to favorably affect the recurrence rate from implantation.

Generally, both prospective and retrospective clinical series have failed to support a favorable effect of laser treatment on the recurrence rate of bladder cancer (15, 16). In most retrospective series, the patient population under study is one of the most influential factors in determining recurrence rate. This complicates comparisons of laser-treated patients with historical series of those undergoing electrocautery resection. Prospective studies have shown no apparent salutary effect of laser treatment on the overall recurrence of superficial bladder cancer.

However, there is good evidence attesting to the effectiveness of laser therapy in eradicating existing and visible superficial bladder tumors. Multiple series have shown a local recurrence rate of approximately 5 to 10%, a figure that compares favorably with electrocautery resection. In a randomized prospective study, Beisland and Seland found a local recurrence rate of 43% for stage T1 transitional cell carcinoma treated with electrocautery resection alone compared with only 7% for Nd:YAG laser treatment (15).

There are no studies comparing various laser fibers, wavelengths, or contact versus noncontact treatment of superficial bladder tumors. There has been only a single published report on holmium:YAG treatment of bladder tumors (16). If adequate vaporization or coagulation of the lesion occurs, good results can be anticipated in terms of local eradication of visible tumors with any of the laser wavelengths. Overall, the Nd:YAG laser has proven to be the most versatile and allows treatment of larger tumors. There is no evidence that other laser treatment techniques offer an increased margin of safety.

Laser therapy is firmly established as an effective treatment for superficial bladder cancer. The ability to eradicate existing, visible tumors is comparable or, perhaps, superior to results obtained with electrocautery resection. Overall, there is no demonstrable favorable effect on tumor recurrence. Therefore, the indications for adjuvant intravesical treatment with either bacille Calmette-Guérin or cytotoxic drugs are unchanged after laser therapy compared with standard treatment recommendations.

Laser treatment of superficial bladder cancer has been associated with an observed decrease in treatment-related morbidity. Bleeding is almost nonexistent, and catheter drainage of the bladder is not required. Treatment can be performed more readily on an ambulatory basis. A complication unique to laser therapy, perforation of an adjacent viscus, is unusual if appropriate treatment parameters are used. There are a number of laser wavelengths and fibers that have been used successfully to treat superficial bladder cancer. None has been proven to be inherently superior to another, although an Nd:YAG laser used in a noncontact manner produces the optimum coagulation. The primary limitations of laser treatment of superficial bladder cancer are the lack of tissue available for histologic examination and the difficulty in treating tumors that exceed 2 cm with laser treatment alone. Laser treatment of invasive bladder cancer is limited by difficulties and inaccuracies with clinical staging of invasive transitional cell carcinoma and by the inability to predict and control the depth of coagulation.

REFERENCES

1. Stein BS. Laser physics and tissue interaction. In: Smith JA Jr, ed. Lasers in urologic surgery. Chicago: Mosby Year Book Medical Publishers, 1994:10.
2. Benson RC Jr. Endoscopic management of bladder cancer with hematoporphyrin derivative phototherapy. Urol Clin North Am 1984;11:637.
3. Hisazumi H, Misahi T, Myoshi N. Photoradiation of bladder tumors. J Urol 1983;130:685.
4. Prout GR Jr, Linn CW, Benson RC Jr, et al. Photodynamic therapy with hematoporphyrin derivative in the treatment of superficial transitional cell carcinoma of the bladder. N Engl J Med 1987;317:251.
5. Hofstetter A, Frank K, Keiditsch E. Laser treatment of the bladder: experimental and clinical results. In: Smith JA Jr, ed. Lasers in urologic surgery. St. Louis: CV Mosby, 1985:63.
6. Smith JA Jr. Endoscopic applications of laser energy. Urol Clin North Am 1986;13:405.
7. Cho YH, Chi SH, Hernandez AD, et al. Adriamycin absorption after Nd:YAG laser coagulation compared to electrosurgical resection of the bladder wall. J Urol 1992;147:1139.
8. Smith JA, Landau S. Neodymium: YAG laser specifications for safe intravesical use. J Urol 1989;141:1238.
9. Scaletscky R, Milam DF, Smith JA. Combined laparoscopic and cystoscopic Nd:YAG laser photocoagulation of the porcine bladder wall. J Urol 1993;149:411. Abstract.
10. Smith JA Jr. Treatment of invasive bladder cancer with a neodymium: YAG laser. J Urol 1986;135:55.
11. Beisland HO, Sander S. Neodymium:YAG laser irradiation of stage T2 muscle-invasive bladder cancer: long-term results. Br J Urol 1990;65:24.
12. Hofstetter A, Kriegmair M, Baumgartner R. Evaluation of laser treatment of bladder cancer. In: Smith JA Jr, ed. Lasers in urologic surgery. Chicago: Mosby Year Book Medical Publishers, 1994:114.
13. Hofstetter A. Treatment of urological tumors by neodymium YAG laser. Eur Urol 1986;12(Suppl):21.
14. Malloy TR, Wein AJ, Shanberg A. Superficial transitional cell carcinoma of the bladder treated with neodymium:YAG laser: a study of the recurrence rate within the first year. J Urol 1984;131:251. Abstract.
15. Beisland HO, Seland O. A prospective randomized study on neodymium:YAG laser irradiation versus TUR in the treatment of urinary bladder cancer. Scand J Urol Nephrol 1986;20:209.
16. Johnson DE. Use of the holmium:YAG laser for treatment of superficial bladder carcinoma. Lasers Surg Med 1994;14:213.

26

The Technique of Radical Cystectomy

A Standard Anatomic Approach

Donald A. Elmajian and Donald G. Skinner

The successful management of carcinoma of the bladder depends on the proper and timely selection of treatment from a wide range of therapeutic methods. Superficial disease, i.e., disease confined to the mucosa and submucosa, can most frequently be managed without removing the bladder. Cystectomy is indicated in the 15 to 25% of patients who present with disease invasive into or beyond the bladder musculature or in the 10 to 15% of patients with superficial disease in whom invasive or metastatic disease subsequently develops. Furthermore, the majority of patients who present initially with a high-grade superficial transitional cell carcinoma do not respond completely to transurethral resection or intravesical pharmacotherapy; therefore, successful management in these cases also usually requires aggressive therapy.

Radical cystectomy generally implies the en bloc removal of the anterior pelvic organs—the prostate, seminal vesicles, and bladder with its visceral peritoneum and perivesical fat in men and the urethra, bladder, cervix, vaginal cuff, uterus, ovaries, and pelvic peritoneum in women. Recent studies of pelvic anatomy and a review of prior cystectomy specimens suggest that the urethra and anterior vaginal wall can be preserved in up to 75% of women, thus allowing lower urinary tract reconstruction in the majority of both women and men. A pelvic-iliac lymph node dissection, of varying extent, is usually included but should be denoted together with the term "radical cystectomy" to clarify whether a meticulous dissection was performed. Particularly in women, the operation is sometimes called an anterior pelvic exenteration with bilateral pelvic lymph node dissection. This is the optimal ablative surgical procedure for the treatment of invasive carcinoma of the bladder in the properly selected patient who has an appropriate surgical risk.

After the diagnosis of a high-grade or muscle-invading tumor has been established, efforts should be made to rule out metastatic disease. History, physical examination, biochemistry profile, and chest radiograph should be obtained. An elevated alkaline phosphatase should raise suspicion of occult bone metastasis, and bone scan should be performed. Elevated liver function tests should raise the possibility of hepatic involvement and warrant a computed tomography (CT) scan to evaluate the liver. The sensitivity of CT scan and magnetic resonance imaging (MRI) in the evaluation of pelvic nodal disease is poor; therefore, routine CT or MRI in all potential cystectomy patients is not warranted.

PREOPERATIVE PREPARATION

Patients normally are admitted to the hospital by 10:00 AM the day before surgery. They can have a regular breakfast but then are maintained on a clear liquid diet until midnight before the operation. Our mechanical preparation of the bowel begins with 120 mL orally of Neoloid (Kenwood Laboratories, Fairfield, NJ), a palatable emulsion of castor oil, at 10:00 AM. Patients then receive 1 g by mouth of neomycin at 10:00 AM, 11:00 AM, 12:00 noon, 1:00 PM, 4:00 PM, 8:00 PM, and 12 midnight. They also receive 1 g by mouth of erythromycin base at 12:00 noon, 4:00 PM, 8:00 PM, and 12 midnight. Slow-responding patients receive 1 bottle orally of magnesium citrate at 4:00 PM. This regimen is of short duration, exceedingly effective in decompressing and cleansing the small and large bowel, prevents dehydration associated with prolonged catharsis, renders enemas unnecessary, and maintains good nutritional support. Preoperative intravenous hydration with 5% dextrose and 0.5 normal saline solution at 125 mL/hr is instituted at 4:00 PM the day before surgery.

One of the most important aspects of preoperative preparation in patients undergoing cutaneous urinary diversion is determination of the stoma site. This is jointly done by the surgeon and enterostomal therapist, examining the patient in the supine, sitting, and standing positions. Optimal stoma placement is essential to postoperative management, patient acceptance of the procedure, and patient ability to care for the ileostomy effectively. In patients who choose a continent catheterizable reservoir, the ileostomy site may be chosen lower (well caudal to the belt or underwear line) and closer to the pubis for concealment because skin folds and creases are unimportant in patients who do not require an external appliance. Alternatively, placement higher on the abdominal wall may facilitate intermittent catheterization if concealment is of little concern to the patient. Patients are marked by scratching the skin with a needle tip and then swabbing the skin with a methylene blue soaked cotton applicator.

SURGICAL TECHNIQUE

Position

The patient is placed in the hyperextended supine position with the iliac crest located at the break in the operating table (Fig. 26.1). Female patients, in addition, are placed in a slight frog-leg position with their feet and ankles well padded and secured to the table with tape, particularly if lower urinary tract reconstruction is contemplated, to allow access to the vagina. Care is taken to provide adequate support of the legs laterally with appropriate-sized bumps. The vagina is prepared into the field. A 20F Foley catheter is placed after the patient is draped.

Incision

The incision extends in the midline from the pubic symphysis to the upper epigastrium, directing the incision away from the stoma site around the umbilicus. The anterior rectus sheath is incised along the linea alba, the rectus abdominus muscles retracted laterally, and the transversalis fascia and peritoneum incised superiorly in the incision. As the incision is extended caudally, the urachal remnant is identified and circumscribed, fanning laterally as one moves toward the bladder, so that it can be removed en bloc with the specimen. Care is taken to remain medial to the inferior epigastric vessels running along the undersurface of the rectus abdominus muscles. If the patient

has previously had a segmental cystectomy or cystotomy through a vertical incision, then this incisional tract too should be similarly circumscribed, full thickness, and removed en bloc with the bladder. The medial insertion of the rectus muscles onto the pubic symphysis is incised for a distance of 1 to 2 to facilitate subsequent pelvic exposure.

A systematic generalized abdominal examination should be performed once the peritoneal cavity has been opened in an effort to detect possible intrahepatic metastatic disease or concomitant unrelated disease as well as to assess the extent of intercurrent disease. Any adhesions present should be incised and freed at this time.

Retroperitoneal Dissection

A large Richardson retractor is used to elevate the right abdominal wall; the cecum and ascending colon are reflected medially, allowing the surgeon to incise the peritoneum along the avascular line of Toldt. The dissection continues by incising the peritoneal attachments around the cecum and extending this incision cephalad along the root of the small bowel mesentery up to the point where the duodenum crosses the midline, further defining the central retroperitoneum. The hallmark of this dissection is a filmsy, avascular fibroareolar plane that allows for combined sharp and blunt dissection. The described peritoneal attachments can be visualized as a triangle whose apex is in the ileocecal area, whose base is represented by the third and fourth portions of the duodenum, and whose right and left walls are defined by the right avascular line of Toldt and medial portion of the sigmoid mesentery (Fig. 26.2). This mobilization is an important part of setting up the surgical field to perform a cystectomy and is necessary for proper subsequent packing of the intraabdominal contents.

The left colon and sigmoid mesentery are then mobilized medially out of the retroperitoneum by incising in the left paracolic gutter along the avascular line of Toldt to the lower pole of the left kidney. The base of the sigmoid mesentery is

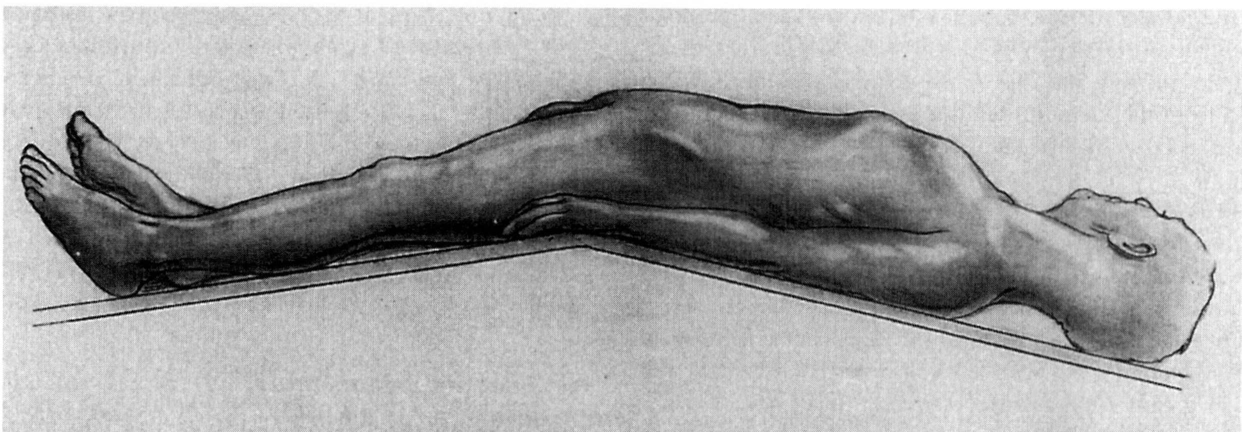

Fig. 26.1.   Hyperextended supine position with iliac crest located at the break in the operating table. (From Skinner D, Lieskovsky G, eds. Diagnosis and management of genitourinary cancer. Philadelphia: WB Saunders, 1988:608. Reproduced by permission of WB Saunders, Co.)

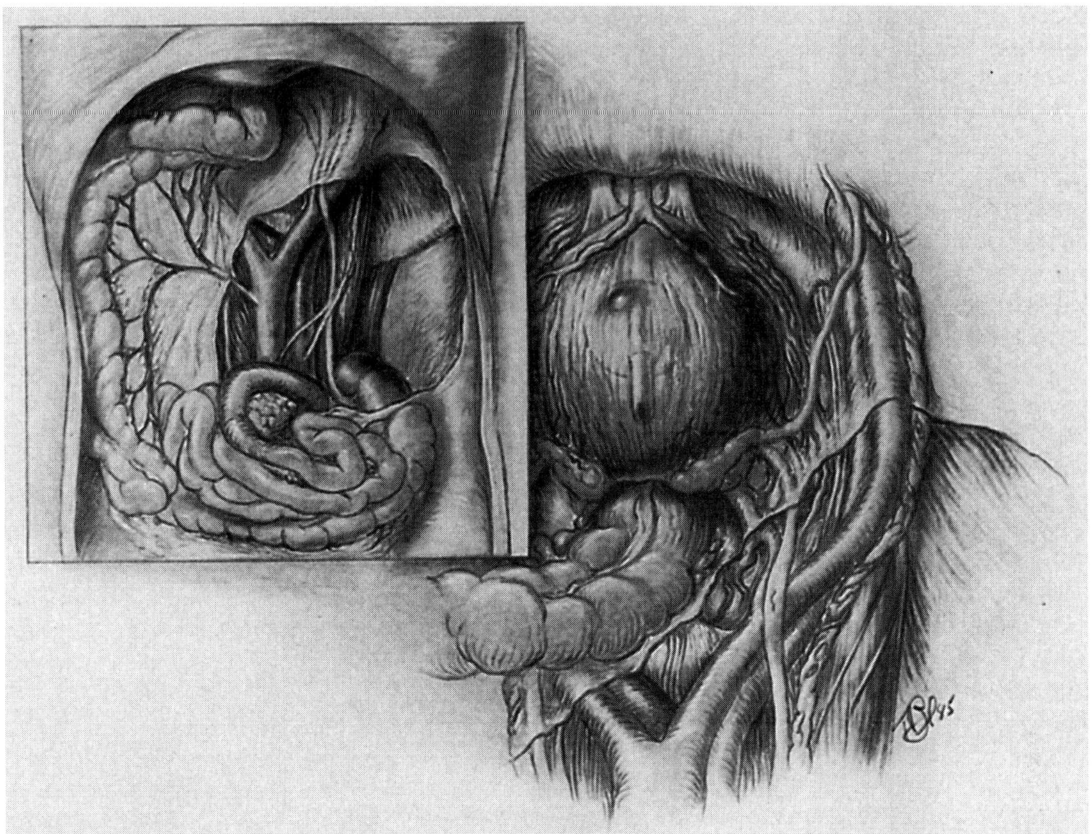

Fig. 26.2.   A view from the head of the operating table demonstrating mobilization of the ascending colon and small bowel mesentery to the level of the duodenum. (From Skinner D, Lieskovsky G, eds. Diagnosis and management of genitourinary cancer. Philadelphia: WB Saunders, 1988:609. Reproduced by permission of WB Saunders, Co.)

reflected off the aorta and sacral promontory by dividing multiple adherent bands. This maneuver creates a long window from the pelvis to the origin of the inferior mesenteric artery through which the left ureter can be passed without angulation or tension for subsequent anastomosis to the urinary diversion (Fig. 26.3). Great care should be exercised to preserve the mesenteric blood supply by dissecting along the base rather than into the colonic mesentery.

A self-retaining Finochietto retractor is positioned, and attention is directed toward packing the bowel. The right colon and small intestine are packed in the epigastrium with three moist laparotomy pads and a moist towel rolled to the width of the abdomen. No attempt is made to pack the descending colon, which should be left as mobile as possible. Successful packing is an art that greatly facilitates the operation. In general, the left hand should be used to position the intestine. Open, moist laparotomy pads can be swept along the palm of the left hand using the right hand to tuck the pad under the viscera to be packed. First the right and then the left gutters should be packed, followed by packing the remaining small intestine with the third laparotomy pad. The rolled moist towel can then be positioned to finish the packing; it should lie horizontally above the level of the aortic bifurcation. Occasionally, a large Deaver retractor on the rolled towel facilitates the cepha-

lad exposure, but usually the region above the aortic bifurcation is readily visible without retraction.

At this time, the ureters are identified and dissected into the deep pelvis several centimeters beyond the point where they cross the common iliac vessels. The ureter is ligated between two large hemoclips positioned 1.5 to 2.0 cm apart and then divided just proximal to the distal clip. A small piece of ureter, representing the ureteral margin, distal to the proximal clip, is excised and sent for frozen section. The remaining ureter is further mobilized cephalad, wrapped in a sponge, and tucked under Gerota's fascia out of harm's way. Ligation of the ureter allows for passive dilation during the remainder of the cystectomy portion of the procedure and facilitates subsequent ureteral anastomosis to the urinary diversion. Frequently, a medial vessel must be clipped and divided to accomplish adequate mobilization, but the ureter should remain attached to the gonadal vessels, an important source of additional blood supply.

Pelvic Lymph Node Dissection

The proximal extent of the lymph node dissection is initiated 1 to 2 cm above the aortic bifurcation. The fibroareolar and lymphatic tissue is dissected overlying the distal aorta and vena cava extending laterally to the genitofemoral nerve, which rep-

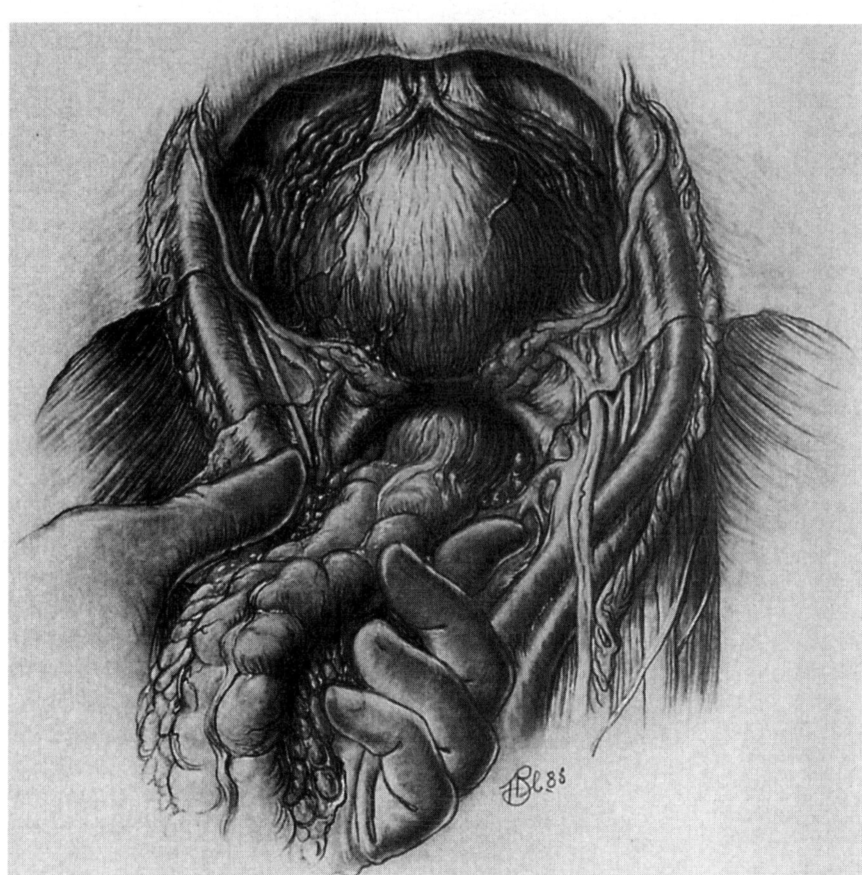

Fig. 26.3.   The descending colon and its mesentery have been mobilized medially and reflected off the aorta and sacral promontory. A window at the base of the sigmoid mesentery has been created to allow the ureter to pass without angulation. (From Skinner D, Lieskovsky G, eds. Diagnosis and management of genitourinary cancer. Philadelphia: WB Saunders, 1988:610. Reproduced by permission of WB Saunders, Co.)

resents the lateral limits of the dissection. The proximal limits of dissection are clipped to prevent lymphatic leak, but the distal limits are left unclipped unless a vessel is encountered as this tissue is removed with the specimen. In a man, the dissection is medial to the spermatic cord; in a woman, the infundibulopelvic ligament is ligated and divided as it courses over the common iliac vessels into the pelvis.

The dissection is carried off the distal aorta and vena cava onto the common iliac vessels over the sacral promontory and into the deep pelvis. The common iliac arteries are mobilized, ligating small arterial and venous branches running on the sacral promontory. In this location, the adherent fibroareolar tissue to the vertebral body can be cauterized and a sponge can be used to sweep the tissue off the sacral promontory along the sweep of the sacrum into the deep pelvis.

After the proximal portion of the lymph node dissection is complete, a finger can be passed—from proximal to distal—under the pelvic peritoneum, over the external iliac vessels, to the femoral canal. The opposite hand can be used to sweep the peritoneum from the undersurface of the transversalis fascia, anterolateral to the bladder, to connect with the right hand dissection at the femoral canal. This maneuver elevates the peritoneum into the surgeon's hand, defining the limits of

lateral peritoneum to be incised. The peritoneum is divided medial to the spermatic cord in men and lateral to the infundibulopelvic ligament in women. The only structure of consequence encountered is the vas deferens in men and the round ligament in women, which is clipped and divided.

A large right-angle rake retractor is used to elevate the lower abdominal wall and to retract the spermatic cord in men and the distal round ligament in women. To facilitate exposure, tension on this retractor should be directed vertically toward the ceiling rather than horizontally, parallel to the floor.

All fibroareolar and lymphatic tissue is dissected circumferentially from the distal external iliac artery and vein. Medium hemoclips are meticulously applied on the distal tissue to prevent lymphatic leakage. The distal limits of dissection along the artery are represented by the deep circumflex iliac vein, the lateral limits by the genitofemoral nerve and psoas muscle, and the medial distal limit by the pectineal (Cooper's) ligament. The lymph node of Cloquet (or Rosenmuller) represents the distal medial limit of dissection along the external iliac vein in the femoral canal, and afferent lymphatics into this large lymph node should be clipped. The distal vessels should now be circumferentially skeletonized. Care should be taken to identify, ligate, and divide an accessory obturator vein draining posteriorly into the backwall of the common iliac vein 40% of the time in this location.

After the distal limits of the dissection are completed, the proximal portion of the external iliac artery and vein is skeletonized. The surgeon should be aware of a small arterial and venous psoas muscular branch found along the proximal portion of these vessels, otherwise no major vascular branches are typically encountered. The fibroareolar and psoas fascia medial to the genitofemoral nerve can be incised to facilitate dissection. On the left side, the genitofemoral nerve often pursues a more medial course and may be related intimately to the vessels; if so, it is excised.

Attention is now turned to the external iliac vessels that are retracted medially, and a sponge is used to bluntly sweep all fibroareolar and lymphatic tissue from the lateral wall of the pelvis posteriorly into the obturator fossa (Fig. 26.4). The vessels are then retracted laterally, and this tissue can be swept medially out of the obturator fossa with left-handed traction. Great care must be exercised not to tear the hypogastric vein and to identify and protect the obturator nerve. The nerve is carefully dissected and retracted laterally so that the index finger of the left hand can be passed medial to the obturator nerve parallel to the endopelvic fascia at the obturator canal. The middle finger (third finger) of the left hand is then passed along the endopelvic fascia medial to this region, which effectively isolates the obturator vessels between the two fingers as they exit the pelvis in the obturator canal, medial to the obturator nerve. These vessels should be ligated and divided, allowing the obturator group of nodes to be swept medially with the specimen.

Lateral Dissection

The following portion of the dissection, development of the lateral pedicle, is perhaps the most important step in the performance of a radical cystectomy. Using countertraction with the left hand, the left index finger is gently swept medial to the hypogastric artery in the deep pelvis, parallel to the sweep of the sacrum, extending all the way to the endopelvic fascia. This maneuver defines two pedicles, the first (the lateral pedicle)

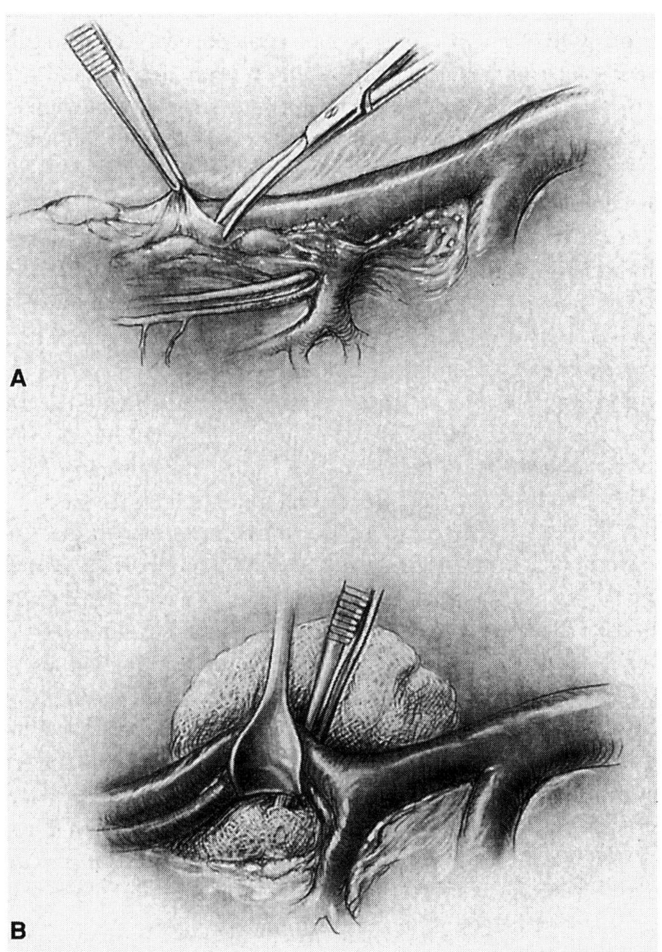

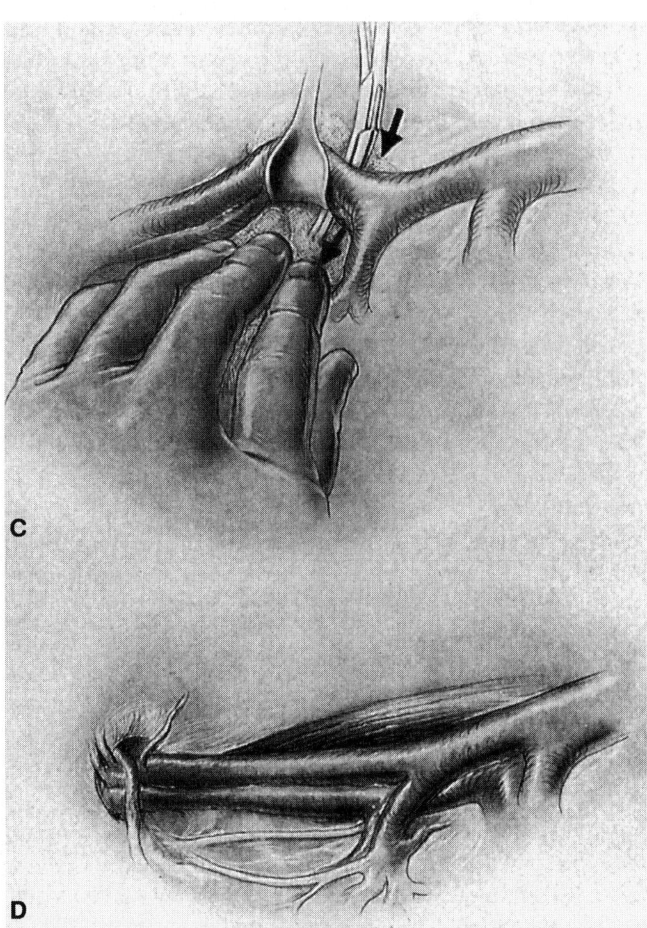

Fig. 26.4.   The external iliac vessels are skeletonized (**A**) and a gauze sponge is used to sweep all fibroareolar and lymphatic tissue along the pelvic sidewall (**B and C**) and out of the obturator fossa, en bloc, toward the specimen (**D**). (From Skinner D, Lieskovsky G, eds. Diagnosis and management of genitourinary cancer. Philadelphia: WB Saunders, 1988:612. Reproduced by permission of WB Saunders, Co.)

extending from the anterior pelvic organs to the hypogastric vessels and the second (the posterior pedicle) extending from the anterior pelvic organs to the rectum. Again, using the left hand for countertraction with the medial fingers posterior to the lateral pedicle, the hypogastric artery is further skeletonized. The first branch from the posterior portion of the hypogastric artery, the superior gluteal artery, should be identified and preserved if possible. The anterior division of the hypogastric artery, distal to the superior gluteal artery, is doubly ligated with large hemoclips and divided. Occasionally, because of the extent of disease or because of anatomic variation, it becomes necessary to ligate the hypogastric artery proximal to the takeoff of the superior gluteal artery. Some patients in whom this is done complain of buttock claudication with exercise postoperatively; thus, this artery should be preserved if possible.

The lateral pedicle is then ligated and divided all the way to the endopelvic fascia or as far as is technically feasible (Fig. 26.5). Blunt dissection with the fingers posterior to the lateral pedicle facilitates development of the plane and protects the rectum. Large right-angle hemoclip appliers are ideally suited for this maneuver; it is important to position a dual set of clips so that at least 0.5 to 1.0 cm of tissue projects beyond each

clip as the pedicle is divided to prevent the clips from being dislodged, which leads to troublesome bleeding in this location.

Posterior Dissection

Attention now is drawn toward the posterior pedicle. A double-hook thyroid tenaculum can be placed on the fundus of the uterus in women and a large clamp can be placed on the urachal remnant in men to give anterior retraction for visualization of the pouch of Douglas. The peritoneum lateral to the rectum is incised, extending that incision anteriorly into the cul-de-sac to join the incision from the other side (Fig. 26.6). One should recall that the anterior and posterior reflections of the peritoneum fuse caudally to the urogenital diaphragm, an extremely important anatomic boundary in men, lying between the posterior surface of the prostate and seminal vesicles, and the anterior surface of the rectum. The peritoneal incision in the cul-de-sac should be made on the rectal side rather than on the bladder side so that the plane behind the posterior leaf of Denonvilliers' fascia and the anterior rectal wall is entered and developed (Fig. 26.7).

This defines and allows entry into Denonvilliers' space. In this plane, the rectum can easily be swept from the posterior

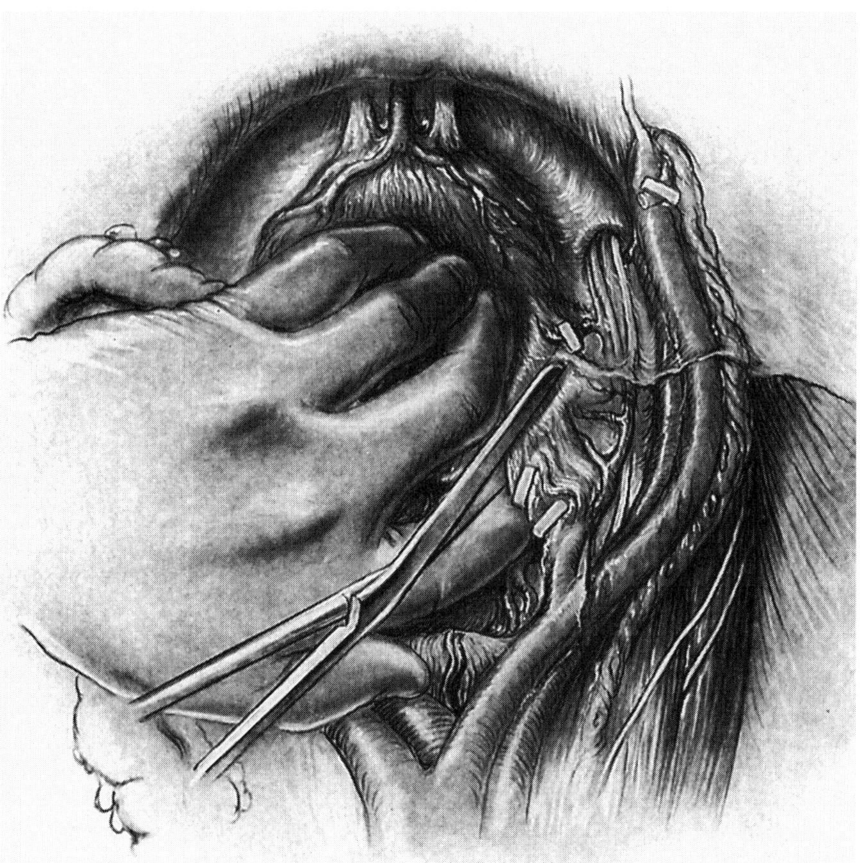

Fig. 26.5.   The lateral pedicle, extending from the anterior pelvic organs to the hypogastric vessels, is demonstrated with the left hand. This pedicle can be ligated and divided to the endopelvic fossa. The rectum is protected by the fingers posterior to the pedicle. (From Skinner D, Lieskovsky G, eds. Diagnosis and management of genitourinary cancer. Philadelphia: WB Saunders, 1988:614. Reproduced by permission of WB Saunders, Co.)

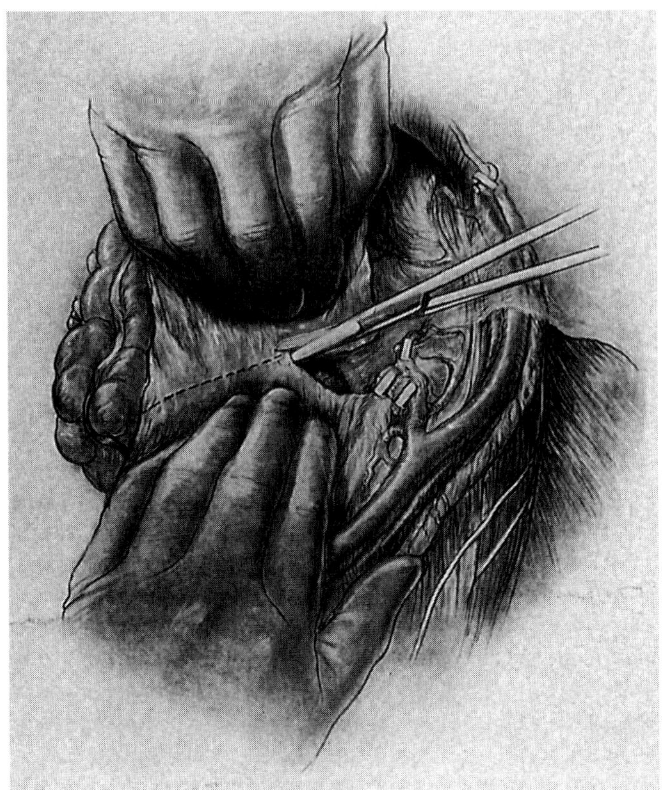

Fig. 26.6.   The peritoneum lateral to the rectum is incised into the cul-de-sac to join the incision from the other side. The incision should be made just on the rectal side to allow entry into Denonvilliers' space. (From Skinner D, Lieskovsky G, eds. Diagnosis and management of genitourinary cancer. Philadelphia: WB Saunders, 1988:615. Reproduced by permission of WB Saunders, Co.)

vaginal wall in women and from the bladder, seminal vesicles, and prostate in men. If the incision in the cul-de-sac is made anteriorly, entry may occur between the two layers of Denonvilliers' fascia or even anterior to that fascial plane, making dissection off the rectum difficult with increased risk of incidental rectal injury. Occasionally, this plane may be obliterated secondary to carcinoma or previous high-dose radiation therapy, making dissection in this area difficult. In instances in which patients have received previous cumulative high-dose radiation (greater than 6000 cGy), dissection of this plane can be greatly facilitated by an initial perineal dissection.

The surgeon's right hand, palm up, should be used to finish the dissection in this plane with a posterior sweeping motion of the fingers on the prostate, separating the rectum from the posterior leaf of Denonvilliers' fascia, thereby defining a left and a right posterior pedicle. This motion thins and develops the posterior pedicle (which now appears like a collar around the lateral sides of the rectum), facilitates use of hemoclips, and protects the rectum from injury during division of the posterior pedicles. Once defined, the pedicles are clipped and divided all the way to the endopelvic fascia in men, which is also incised on each side and swept away from the posterolateral sidewall of the prostate (Fig. 26.8).

In women, the posterior pedicles (including the cardinal ligaments) are similarly developed, clipped, and divided but only for approximately 4 to 5 cm beyond the cervix. At this point, the posterior vaginal wall is opened and the vagina circumscribed anteriorly, leaving the cervix with the specimen. The anterior vaginal wall is dissected from the posterior bladder wall down to the region of the urethra. This maneuver defines two distal posterior pedicles extending like a collar from the bladder to the lateral surface of the vagina on either side. These pedicles are clipped and divided, freeing the bladder from its posterior attachments except for the urethra. In some patients with large, posteriorly based, deeply penetrating tumors or in women with bladder neck or urethral involvement, it is advantageous to leave the anterior vaginal wall attached to the bladder; the lateral vaginal wall is then incised down to the location of the urethral meatus.

A comment should be made about the position of the surgeon. Typically, for a right-handed surgeon, the right pelvic lymph node dissection and dissection of the right lateral pedicle are performed with the surgeon on the left side of the patient. The surgeon then changes sides to perform the left pelvic lymph node dissection and development and division of the left lateral pedicle. The remainder of the dissection is then best accomplished with the surgeon on the left side of the table.

Anterior Dissection

For the first time attention is turned anteriorly. In men, the fibroareolar tissue is swept laterally from the anterior surface of the prostate. The puboprostatic ligaments are identified and sharply divided close to the pubis (Fig. 26.9A). Under direct vision, a blunt-tipped right-angle clamp should be passed anterior to the urethra and posterior to the dorsal vein complex (Fig. 26.9B). This thick complex should be ligated with 00 absorbable suture material and divided as close to the apex of the prostate as possible. Bleeding from the divided stump frequently can be easily controlled with 00 absorbable sutures. In patients who have undergone a previous segmental resection or open prostatectomy, this plane can be difficult to develop. In such situations, this portion of the operation can be facilitated by incising the periosteum of the pubis with electrocautery. A periosteal elevator can be used to easily develop this subperiosteal plane down to the region of the urethra. Anterior dissection in a woman is similar except that the dorsal vein anlage is generally less prominent and more easily controlled.

Urethral Preparation

In both men and women undergoing cutaneous forms of urinary diversion, urethral preparation is relatively straightforward. In men, having divided the dorsal venous complex, the membranous urethra comes into view and can be stretched with traction several centimeters above the urogenital diaphragm. A large curved Kocher clamp is placed on the urethra distal to the apex of the prostate. Care must be taken in placing this clamp to

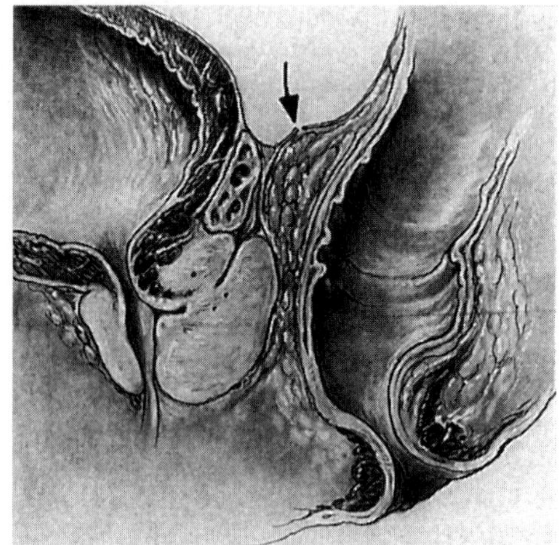

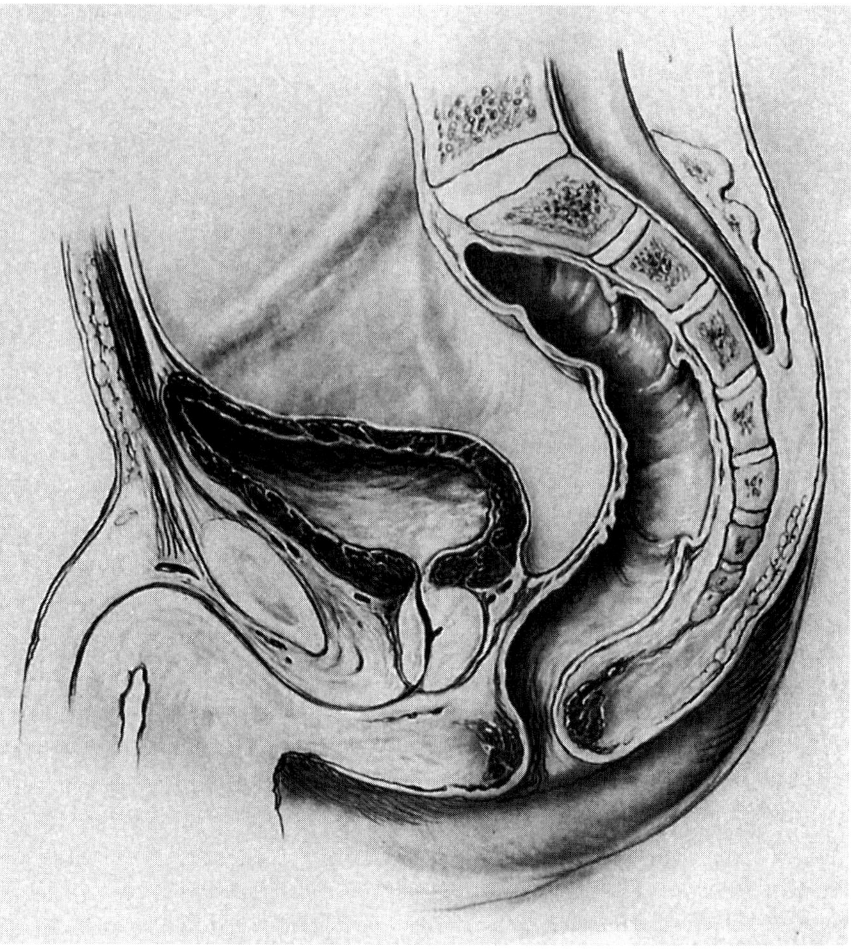

Fig. 26.7.   Denonvilliers' fascia. This represents the caudal fusion of peritoneum to the urogenital diaphragm during embryologic development. Entrance into Denonvilliers' space (the space between the posterior peritoneum and the rectum) is gained by incision close to the peritoneal fusion in the cul-de-sac at the anterior rectal wall. (From Skinner D, Lieskovsky G, eds. Diagnosis and management of genitourinary cancer. Philadelphia: WB Saunders, 1988: 616. Reproduced by permission of WB Saunders, Co.)

avoid rectal injury. The index finger of the left hand is placed beyond the clamp protecting the rectum, and the urethra (with the catheter in situ) is divided distal to the clamp, thus avoiding spillage of vesical contents. The specimen is removed en bloc (Fig. 26.9C).

In women, after the urethropubic ligaments have been divided, a large, curved Kocher clamp is placed on the urethra, the anterior vaginal wall is opened distally and incised circumferentially around the urethral meatus, and the specimen is removed. The vaginal cuff is closed with running absorbable 0 sutures. Preservation of the anterior vaginal wall, when feasible, results in a functional vagina when the cuff is closed transversely. When the anterior vaginal wall is removed, because of the local extent of the primary tumor, closure (usually longitudinally) results in a small, largely obliterated vagina. It is important to suspend the closed vagina on one side to the pectineal (Cooper's) ligament to prevent prolapse or development of an enterocele.

Most men, and now most women, with bladder cancer can undergo continent lower urinary tract reconstruction to the divided urethra (orthotopic urinary diversion) without compromising survival. This has obvious lifestyle advantages for both sexes. Urethral preparation in this instance is of critical importance.

In women, to preserve the continence mechanism, the distal urethra and pelvic floor must not be disturbed. The anterior vaginal wall is carefully dissected off the posterior bladder wall to the urethrovesical junction. Anteriorly, a right-angle clamp is used to carefully dissect the dorsal venous complex off the anterior bladder surface at the urethrovesical junction. This may be accomplished in several steps, ligating each of several major venous complexes with absorbable 00 suture material. Alternatively, the anterior urethra and venous complex can be sharply divided, thus preventing significant dissection in this area. Individual sutures incorporating the urethra and venous complex can control any significant bleeding encountered from this area.

The urethrovesical junction is further skeletonized laterally

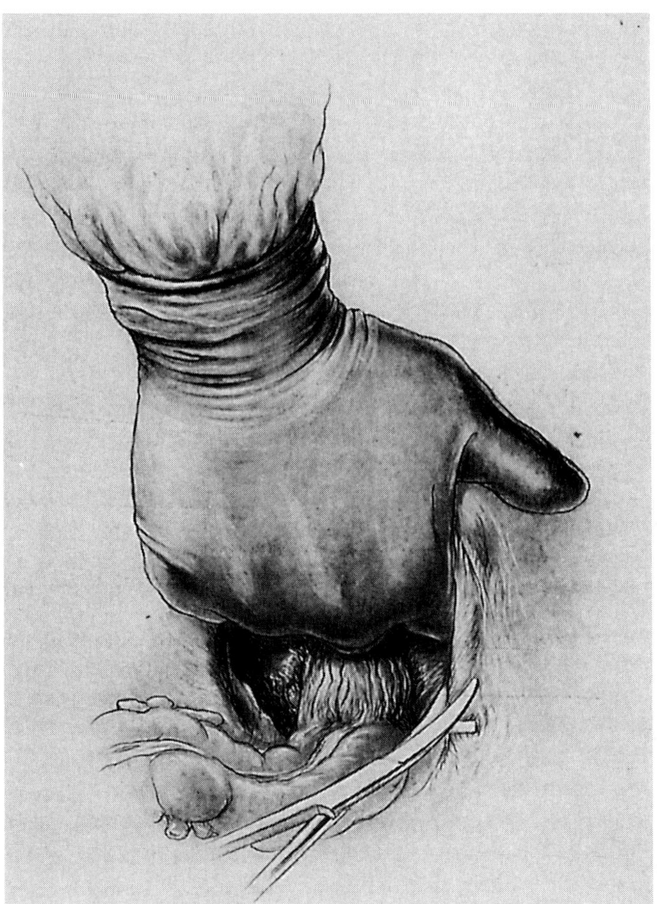

Fig. 26.8. The posterior pedicles extending from the anterior pelvic organs to the lateral surface of the rectum can be divided under direct vision after developing Denonvilliers' space. (From Skinner D, Lieskovsky G, eds. Diagnosis and management of genitourinary cancer. Philadelphia: WB Saunders, 1988:616. Reproduced by permission of WB Saunders, Co.)

with sharp dissection. Importantly, all dissection is proximal to the urethropubic ligaments. At this time, the specimen is tethered to the patient only by the urethra. A curved Satinsky clamp is placed on the urethra at or just distal to the bladder neck, and the anterior urethra is opened in a 270° fashion just distal to the clamp in the proximal third of the urethra. Six or often eight absorbable 00 sutures are placed, equally spaced, into the open urethra; the catheter is divided distally; and two or more additional sutures are then placed in the posterior urethra. The posterior urethra is divided, and the specimen is removed en bloc. The urethral margin from the specimen is excised and sent for frozen section. The vagina is closed transversely with running absorbable 0 sutures in two layers; one end will later be suspended to the pectineal (Cooper's) ligament.

In men, after ligation and division of the dorsal vein complex, traction can be placed on the apex of the prostate to elongate the membranous urethra above the urogenital diaphragm. The urethra can be skeletonized laterally by sharply dividing the so-called lateral pillars that are extensions of the rhabdosphincter and posteriorly by division of the rectoure-

thralis muscle or caudal extent of Denonvilliers' fascia. The anterior urethra is divided 270° circumferentially, as in women, so that the specimen is attached to the urethra posteriorly. Six 00 absorbable sutures are placed, equally spaced, around the open urethra using straight or curved clamps to orient future placement into the neobladder neck. The rhabdosphincter and dorsal venous complex are included in these sutures whenever possible. The catheter is clamped and divided, after which two additional sutures are placed in the posterior urethra that should include the rectourethralis muscle or distal Denonvilliers' fascia. The posterior urethra is then divided, and the specimen is removed. The urethral margin is excised from the specimen and sent for frozen section.

The pelvis is irrigated with warm water, and careful hemostasis is confirmed. The anterior rectal wall is examined to assure it has not been violated. The nodal tissue present in the presciatic notch, anterior to the sciatic nerve, is collected and sent separate from the specimen for histologic analysis because this is a frequent area of local recurrence. The presacral nodal package that was swept off the inferior vena cava, aorta, and common iliac vessels, off the sacral promontory, and down the sweep of the sacrum into the deep pelvis, is collected and also sent separately for evaluation.

On completion of the cystectomy and urinary diversion, we routinely place a 22F gastrostomy tube into the body of the stomach to enhance patient comfort in the postoperative period. The tube is removed on postoperative day 7 or later if complete bowel function is delayed. We also routinely administer sodium warfarin for postoperative prophylactic anticoagulation. Fifteen milligrams is given via the gastrostomy tube in the recovery room and then given orally on a daily basis using the prothrombin time as a guide for each dose. We aim for a prothrombin time of 18 seconds or 1.5 times control, which we believe substantially reduces our incidence of pulmonary embolism in this group of high-risk patients.

URINARY DIVERSION

Great strides have been made in the area of continent urinary diversion. In 1982, we began performing continent urinary diversion according to the method described by Kock in the *Journal of Urology*. Over the years, several important modifications have been made. Our current experience involves more than 1200 patients. The advantages in terms of lifestyle, self-esteem, relationships, sexuality, and independence are overwhelming. Multiple forms of continent cutaneous diversion have since evolved and are now commonplace worldwide.

In 1986, we began to offer select male patients continent diversion to the urethra rather than to the skin (orthotopic diversion) in an effort to more closely approximate normal bladder function. We have performed this procedure in 400 men and have achieved low complication rates, excellent continence, and high patient satisfaction. Once again, multiple other forms of orthotopic diversion have evolved, and clearly this has be-

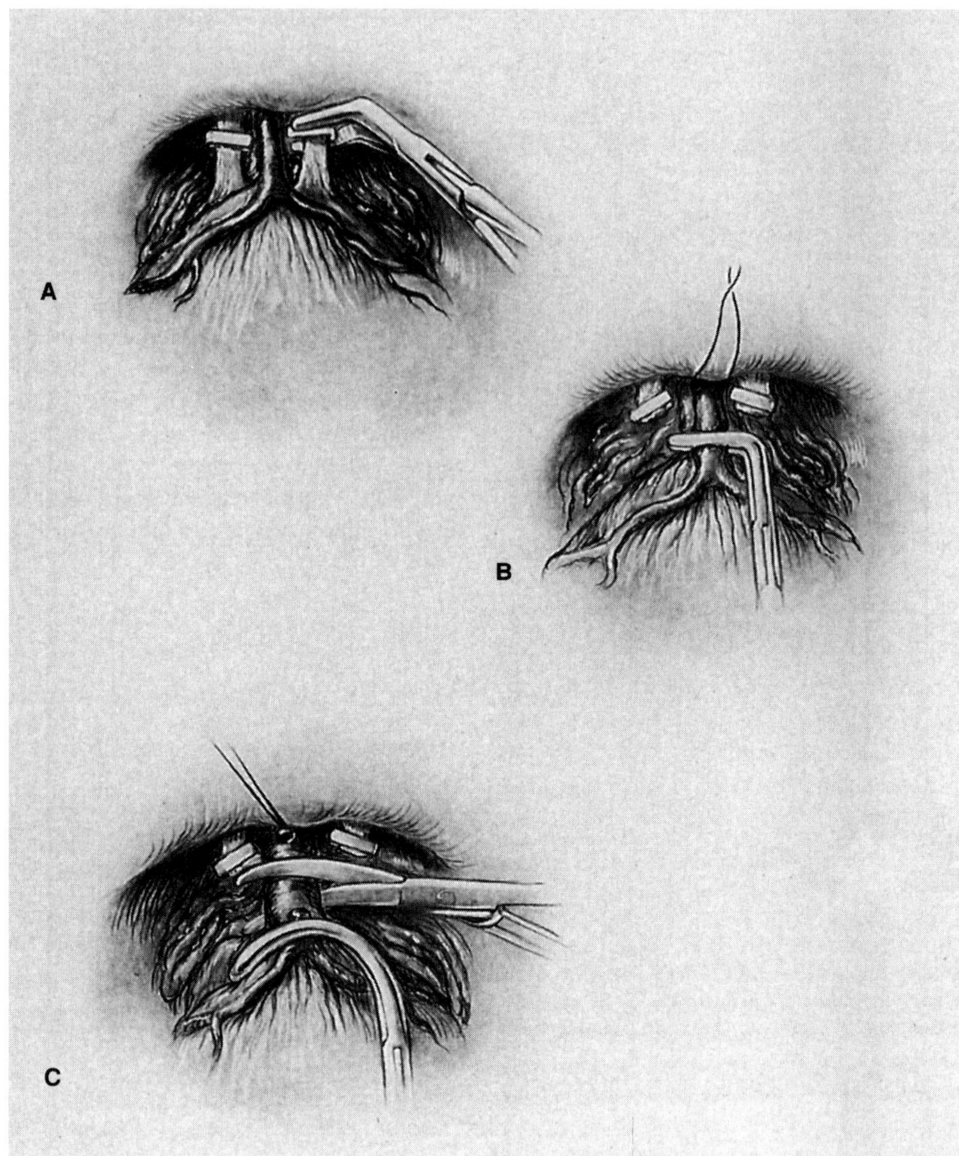

Fig. 26.9. **A.** The puboprostatic ligaments can clearly be visualized in a man. **B.** A right-angle clamp can be passed posterior to the dorsal vein complex and anterior to the urethra, allowing ligation and division of Santorini's plexus. **C.** The urethra can be transected and the specimen removed. Urethral sutures should be placed before complete urethral transection in patients undergoing orthotopic diversion. (From Skinner D, Lieskovsky G, eds. Diagnosis and management of genitourinary cancer. Philadelphia: WB Saunders, 1988:617. Reproduced by permission of WB Saunders, Co.)

come the optimal form of diversion in the vast majority of men when feasible.

Recently, we evaluated the first 266 men undergoing radical cystectomy, bilateral ileoinguinal lymphadenectomy, and a Kock orthotopic ileal neobladder from May 1986 to June 1993. There were 19 early (7.1%) and 25 late (9.4%) complications related to the reservoir itself. Overall, there were seven bleeding episodes, only one of which was directly related to overdosing of sodium warfarin. We had three patients in whom pulmonary embolus developed, one of which was fatal. There were no complications referable to the gastrostomy tube. There were three operative mortalities (1.1%). In addition to the pulmonary embolism in one patient, a fatal intraoperative arrhythmia devel-

oped in one patient. Another patient received an inadvertent potassium chloride bolus while in the intensive care unit.

Traditionally, en bloc urethrectomy has been performed in women undergoing radical cystectomy because the continence mechanism was poorly understood and the incidence of urethral recurrence was believed to be prohibitively high. Recent neuroanatomic studies from Innsbruck, Austria, of the female pelvis and urethra have led to a better understanding of the female continence mechanism. The female urethra consists of both smooth muscle and skeletal muscle with a gradual transition from smooth muscle at the bladder neck and proximal third of the urethra to skeletal muscle at the distal third of the urethra. The smooth musculature of the proximal urethra is innervated by branches from the pelvic plexus coursing along the lateral aspect of the rectum, uterus, vagina, and bladder neck. Anterior exenteration effectively denervates this proximal urethral sphincter mechanism. The striated musculature of the distal third of the urethra, the so-called rhabdosphincter, is innervated from branches of the pudendal nerve that run along the pelvic floor under the levator ani muscles. Preservation of the distal two thirds of the urethra, together with its nerve supply, is crucial for urinary continence in women. These anatomic studies support transection of the radical cystectomy specimen just distal to the urethrovesical junction at the proximal urethra with subsequent orthotopic diversion to the retained urethra with preservation of continence based on the rhabdosphincter mechanism. This is technically possible and was described earlier in this chapter.

With this information, we performed a histologic review of 67 consecutive female cystectomy specimens removed for primary bladder cancer from July 1982 through July 1990. Seventeen women (25%) had overt tumor or carcinoma in situ of their bladder neck (urethrovesical junction). Nine of these 17 patients (13%) had carcinoma or carcinoma in situ of the urethra. Additionally, 4 of these 67 patients (6%) had deeply penetrating, posteriorly based tumors involving the anterior vaginal wall, and 2 of these 4 patients had urethral involvement with tumor. However, in no instance was there histologic evidence of tumor or atypia of the urethra or vaginal wall when the bladder neck was histologically uninvolved. Therefore, we believe that in the approximately 75% of women with transitional cell carcinoma of the bladder undergoing radical cystectomy who have biopsy-proven histologically normal bladder necks, orthotopic diversion can and should be considered.

Beginning in June 1990 and extending through November 1993, we performed radical cystectomy and orthotopic urinary diversion (Kock ileal reservoir) in 14 women who met the above criteria and were considered appropriate surgical candidates. In all instances, frozen section analysis of the urethrovesical junction revealed no significant histologic abnormality. There were two early (prolonged ileus) and one late (urethroileal stenosis) complication. All patients report complete diurnal continence without the need for protection. Of the 14 patients, 12 (86%) are able to void to completion by means of increasing intra-abdominal pressure (Valsalva) and relaxing their external sphincter. Two patients are unable to void and require intermittent catheterization to empty; both represent our early experience in which Burch suspension procedures were performed in an effort to guarantee continence. These findings were objectively confirmed by fluorourodynamic evaluation that revealed high-volume, low-pressure reservoirs with excellent rhabdosphincter function. In fact, all subjective and objective data in these patients were superior to the results of orthotopic diversion in men. This initial experience has been encouraging and represents a major step forward in the management of women undergoing cystectomy. Prospective evaluation and careful follow-up will be required to define the true risk of urethral and vaginal wall recurrence.

MANAGEMENT OF THE URETHRA

Contraindications to orthotopic diversion in men are carcinoma in situ or overt carcinoma in the urethral margin sent for frozen section, or the presence of prostatic stromal invasion on a preoperative deep transurethral biopsy of the prostatic urethra. When known preoperatively, en bloc urethrectomy is performed at the time of cystectomy in these rare patients. In this instance, the patient is positioned initially in the hyperextended frog-leg position, with the perineum prepared and draped into the operative field. An associate initiates the urethrectomy at the same time the cystectomy is started from above. This two-team approach eliminates the added time associated with cystourethrectomy performed by one surgeon, and in our hands, the urethrectomy portion of the procedure is completed at about the same time the bladder is ready to be removed. Alternatively, the operation can be performed by a single surgeon. In this instance, the procedure is initiated with the patient in the exaggerated lithotomy position with the perineum horizontal in relation to the floor. This position is similar to that used to perform perineal prostatectomy.

In either situation, the entire urethra and corpus spongiosum are mobilized out to the glans by inverting the penis according to the method of Whitmore. In women, orthotopic diversion is contraindicated when disease is present at or beyond the bladder neck, when the anterior vaginal wall is involved with tumor, or when the urethral margin is positive on frozen section analysis. Therefore, in the 25% of patients in whom this applies, urethrectomy is routinely performed with cystectomy as described.

The incidence of anterior urethral recurrence in patients undergoing cutaneous diversion historically has been approximately 10%. Patients at high risk for recurrence, and who therefore require secondary urethrectomy, are those who have histologic evidence of carcinoma in situ or overt transitional cell carcinoma of the prostatic urethra or prostatic stroma. In patients with multifocal carcinoma in situ of the bladder, secondary urethrectomy is performed only when saline urethral washings, performed at routine follow-up intervals, reveal malignant cells.

Recently, we have shown that the overall probability of an anterior urethral recurrence developing at 5 years in patients undergoing Kock continent orthotopic urinary diversion is 5%. Furthermore, the probability of recurrence developing in the retained urethra at 5 years in patients whose pathologic specimen reveals carcinoma in situ or involvement of the prostatic stroma is 4% and 0%, respectively. Therefore, we now believe that patients undergoing Kock continent orthotopic diversion who are found to have carcinoma in situ of the prostatic urethra or invasive transitional cell carcinoma into the prostate and who previously would require secondary urethrectomy, may safely be followed by physical examination and urethral cytology, with delayed urethrectomy reserved for instances of recurrence. Patients with cutaneous diversions and high-risk pathologic conditions should continue to undergo prophylactic urethrectomy.

The technique described in this chapter has remained standard during the past 25 years. In 1984, we reported a 1.5% perioperative mortality rate and an overall 17% complication rate in 197 consecutive patients undergoing radical cystectomy with bilateral pelvic lymph node dissection from August 1971 through August 1982. One hundred of these patients received high-dose preoperative radiation therapy (1600 cGy), which resulted in an increased rate of wound infection (6% versus 1%) and prolonged ileus (7% versus 4%) relative to those patients undergoing surgery alone. In 266 men who underwent radical cystectomy, bilateral pelvic-iliac lymphadenectomy, and Kock orthotopic ileal neobladder, there was a 1.1% operative mortality rate, a 12.4% early complication rate, and a 5.6% late complication rate attributable to the radical cystectomy exclusive of the urinary diversion (Table 26.1). The similarity in the two series is striking and emphasizes that strict adherence to a well-established anatomic surgical technique, such as that outlined, will consistently optimize patient outcome.

In summary, a single-stage radical cystectomy with bilateral pelvic iliac lymph node dissection can be performed with an acceptably low surgical mortality and morbidity. Attention to preoperative preparation, surgical technique, and postoperative detail minimizes the adverse outcomes that may result from procedures of this magnitude. The operation remains the optimal procedure for the management of multifocal or invasive bladder cancer. A continent form of urinary diversion is now considered preferable in these patients, with orthotopic diversion in the majority of men and select women providing the best functional result.

SUGGESTED READINGS

Boyd SD, Lieskovsky G, Skinner DG. Kock pouch bladder replacement. Urol Clin North Am 1991;18:641.

Colleseli K, Strosser H, Moriggl B, et al. Hemi-Kock to the female urethra: part 2. anatomical approach to the continence mechanism of the female urethra. J Urol 1994;151:1089. Abstract.

Crawford ED, Skinner DG. Salvage cystectomy after irradiation failure. J Urol 1980;123:32.

Dretler SP, Ragsdale BD, Leadbetter WF. The value of pelvic lymphadenectomy in the surgical treatment of bladder cancer. J Urol 1973;109:414.

Elmajian DA, Esrig D, Freeman JA, et al. Orthotopic lower urinary tract reconstruction utilizing the Kock ileal reservoir: updated experience in 266 patients. American Urologic Association, April 1995. Abstract.

Kock NG, Nilson AE, Nilson LO, et al. Urinary diversion via a continent ileal reservoir: clinical results in 12 patients. J Urol 1982;128:469.

Nichols RL, Broido P, Condon RE, et al. Effect of pre-operative neomycin-erthromycin intestinal preparation on the incidence of infectious complications following colon surgery. Ann Surg 1973;178:453.

Skinner DG. Management of invasive bladder cancer: a meticulous pelvic node dissection can make a difference. J Urol 1982;128:34.

Skinner DG, Boyd SD, Lieskovsky G, et al. Lower urinary tract reconstruction following cystectomy: experience and results in 126 patients using the Kock ileal reservoir with bilateral ureteroileal urethrostomy. J Urol 1991;146:756.

Skinner DG, Lieskovsky G. Contemporary cystectomy with pelvic node dissection compared to preoperative radiation therapy plus cystectomy in management of invasive bladder cancer. J Urol 1984;131:1069.

Stein JP, Stenzl A, Esrig D, et al. Lower urinary tract reconstruction following cystectomy in women using the Kock ileal reservoir with bilateral ureteroileal urethrostomy: initial clinical experience. J Urol 1994;152:1404.

Tarter TH, Freeman JA, Chen S, et al. Urethral recurrence in patients with ileal neobladders. Proceedings of the American Urologic Association, April 1995. Abstract.

Whitmore WF Jr, Mount BM. A technique of urethrectomy in the male. Surg Gynecol Obstet 1970;131:303.

Table 26.1.   Complications of Radical Cystectomy and Bilateral Ileoinguinal Lymph Node Dissection in 266 Men

COMPLICATIONS	EARLY (%)[a]	LATE (%)[b]
Bleeding	6 (2.3)	0
Small bowel obstruction	7 (2.6)	1 (0.4)
Sepsis	1 (0.4)	0
Myocardial infarction	1 (0.4)	3 (1.1)
Rectotomy	1 (0.4)	0
Pneumonia	1 (0.4)	0
Thrombophlebitis	1 (0.4)	0
Drug reaction	1 (0.4)	0
Pulmonary embolus[c]	3 (1.1)	0
Deep venous thrombosis	4 (1.5)	1 (0.4)
Air embolus	2 (0.8)	0
CVA	2 (0.8)	0
Pancreatitis	1 (0.4)	0
Potassium chloride bolus[c]	1 (0.4)	0
Colonic leak	1 (0.4)	0
Anterior urethral stricture	0	2 (0.8)
Incisional hernia	0	2 (0.8)
Psoas abscess	0	1 (0.4)
Chronic renal failure	0	1 (0.4)
Lower extremity edema	0	1 (0.4)
Pelvic lymphocele	0	1 (0.4)
Intractable diarrhea	0	1 (0.4)
Distal ureteral stricture	0	1 (0.4)
Total	33 (12.4)	15 (5.6)

[a] Within 3 months of surgery.
[b] Longer than 3 months after surgery.
[c] Perioperative mortality.

27

Salvage Cystectomy and Perineal Cystoprostatectomy

E. David Crawford and Marc Wolach

In the United States, radical cystectomy is the standard treatment for invasive bladder cancer. Radiation therapy is offered to those who will not or cannot undergo cystectomy. An unknown percentage of those who experience treatment failures will become candidates for salvage cystectomy. For many years, British urologists have advocated radiation therapy, with cystectomy reserved for those patients in whom response is not achieved or those who experience relapse. Jenkins et al. recently published a review of 182 patients treated in this manner. Their overall, corrected 5-year survival rate was 40%. Fifty-eight percent of patients had persistence or recurrence of their cancer, and thus were potential candidates for salvage cystectomy or perineal cystoprostatectomy (1).

HISTORICAL PERSPECTIVES

The first attempt to remove a bladder tumor surgically was made during the 1700s by LeCat, who removed the tumor with forceps introduced through the female urethra (2). Little progress was made in the surgical ablation of bladder tumors, until Thompson described the perineal-digital approach in the late 1800s (3). This was followed by Billroth's description of the open suprapubic method (4). The current surgical technique of cystectomy had its beginning in 1887 when Bardenheuer described removal of the bladder and implantation of the ureters into the bowel (5). Unfortunately, he was unable to implant the ureter, and the patient died in the early postoperative period. Cystectomy did not gain great popularity until the 1940s, with the development of satisfactory methods of diversion, better anesthesia, fluid therapy, and effective antibiotics. Although these advances sparked interest in cystectomy, the goal of long-term survival remained elusive.

Radiation therapy for bladder cancer began in 1906 (6). At that time, it was believed to be an unsatisfactory method of treatment (7). Even with the development of newer methods of radiation, the survival rates have remained dismal when radiation therapy alone is used. In an effort to improve local control and survival, several groups are reporting the use of concomitant radiation therapy and chemotherapy. These studies include radiation therapy and misonidazole (8) radiation therapy and concomitant 5-fluorouracil, upfront methotrexate, cisplatin, and vincristine (MCV) followed by radiation therapy plus cisplatin. Follow-up times are short, and it remains to be seen if the higher local response rates reported will translate to higher 5-year survival rates.

SELECTION OF PATIENTS

Patients selected for salvage cystectomy are those who have biopsy-proven tumor recurrence or those who have crippling invasive bladder symptoms after definitive radiation therapy. Patients undergoing this procedure should have a thorough metastatic evaluation (including a chest radiograph), bone scan with spot films and/or biopsy of suspicious areas, liver profile and computed tomography (CT) scan if functional test results are abnormal. Bimanual examination under anesthesia and palpation of lymph node areas are generally unrewarding because of radiation-produced fibrosis. CT scans have not been proven to be universally useful because it is not always possible to distinguish between radiation-induced fibrosis and tumor. However, we continue to obtain a CT scan of the entire retroperitoneum and pelvis.

SURGICAL PROCEDURE

The 5-year survival rate for patients undergoing salvage cystectomy is 37 to 51.5%. Operative deaths range from 0 to 14%. In a review of 37 patients undergoing salvage cystectomy, Crawford and Skinner showed that the selective use of an initial perineal approach in most patients, and the use of staged cystectomy after preliminary urinary diversion in high-risk patients, resulted in decreased morbidity and mortality rates (Table 27.1). Should a rectal laceration occur during cystectomy, a diverting colostomy should be performed at the time of repair. Primary closure alone is associated with a higher morbidity and mortality (Table 27.2).

Table 27.1.   Relationship of Staged and/or Perineal Approach to Early Complications

	NO. OF PATIENTS	NO. OF COMPLICATIONS (%)
Staged procedure		
With perineal approach	7	—
Without perineal approach	6	1 (16)
Single-stage procedure		
With perineal approach	8	2 (25)
Without perineal approach	16	5 (31)
Total	37	8 (24)

From Crawford ED, Skinner DG. Salvage cystectomy after irradiation failure. J Urol 1980;123:2. Copyright 1980, The Williams & Wilkins Co., Baltimore.

The classic radical cystectomy is generally not feasible because skeletonization of the pelvic vessels and removal of the lymph nodes are generally not possible because of the fibrosis produced by higher doses of radiation. Therefore, a total cystectomy that consists of surgical removal of the pelvic peritoneum, bladder, prostate, and seminal vesicles in male patients and anterior exenteration in female patients is performed. We have found that, in male patients, there is often a dense desmoplastic radiation fibrosis in the pelvis that makes it difficult to separate the prostate from the rectum. With the initial perineal approach, the rectum can be separated from the prostate under direct vision, rather than by performing the dissection deep in the pelvis through the abdominal incision. Patients undergoing this procedure often have concomitant medical problems that increase the operative and perioperative risk (perhaps thus justifying radiation as the primary therapy).

Proper position of the patient is extremely important when the early perineal approach is performed. The patient is placed in the exaggerated lithotomy position, with sandbags beneath the sacrum, bringing the perineum parallel to the table (Fig. 27.1). The perineal area is prepared and draped, and a sterile towel is sutured anterior to the anal opening to isolate it from the operative field.

A Lowsley retractor is passed through the urethra into the bladder. A curved skin incision is made 1.5 cm anterior to the anus and carried posterior and lateral to the medial aspect of

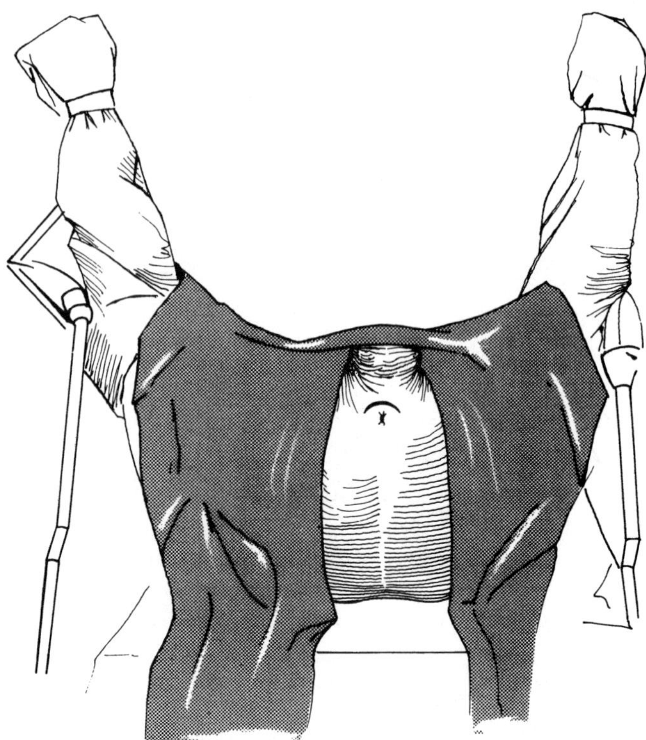

Fig. 27.1.   Exaggerated lithotomy position. Lowsley retractor is passed per the urethra into the bladder. A sterile towel (not shown) is sutured anterior to the anus.

the ischial tuberosities. The superficial perineal fascia is then divided sharply, and with blunt dissection, the ischiorectal fossae are developed lateral and anterior to the rectal wall (Fig. 27.2). The central tendon of the perineum is isolated and sharply divided. The rectal sphincter is identified posteriorly, and a bifid retractor is placed in the wound. The rectal fascia is identified and, with a sharp and blunt dissection, a plane is established anterior to the rectal wall. The rectourethralis muscle is encountered in the midline and divided sharply (Fig. 27.3). The anterior layer of Denonvillier's fascia fuses with the prostatic capsule and may be entered sharply to continue the dissection cranially around the seminal vesicles (Fig. 27.4). It is also feasible to proceed deep to this layer. The lateral

Table 27.2.   Results of Treatment of Rectal Laceration

AUTHOR	RECTAL LACERATIONS	TREATMENT (No. of patients)	OUTCOME (No. of patients)
Crawford and Skinner (9)	1	Colostomy	Successful
Smith and Whitmore (10)	2	Colostomy (1)	Death
		Delayed colostomy (1)	Death
Swanson et al. (11)	2	Colostomy	Successful
Freiha and Faysal (12)	3	Primary closure (2)	Pelvic abscess (2)
		Primary closure with colostomy (1)	Successful
Konnak and Grossman (13)	3	Primary closure	Death (1)
			Leak (1)
			Requiring colostomy

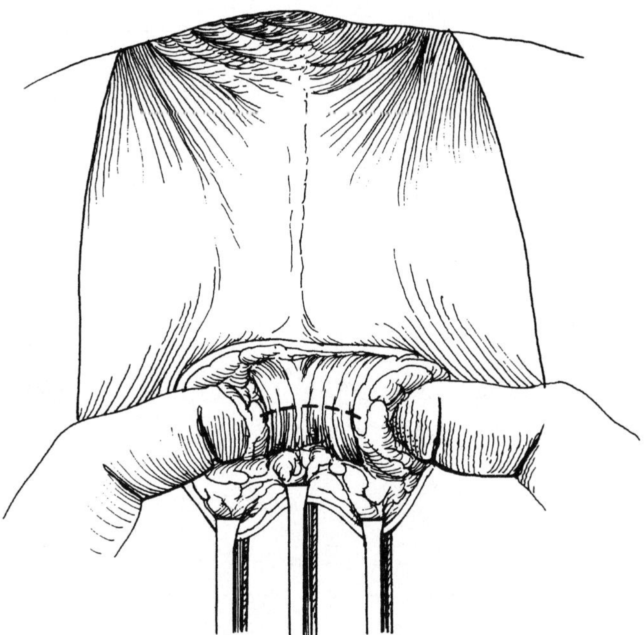

Fig. 27.2. Development of the ischiorectal fossae and isolation of the central tendon of the perineum.

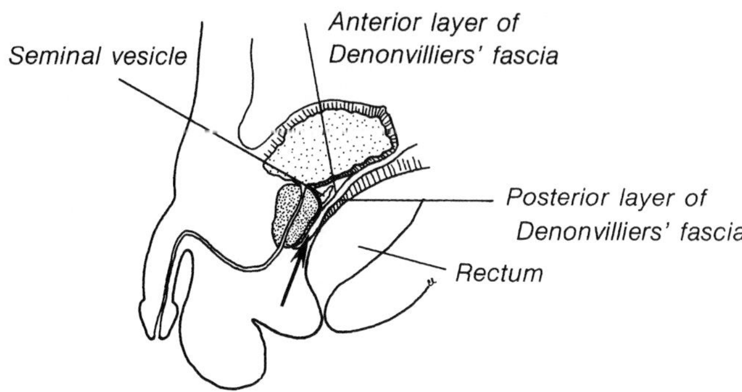

Fig. 27.4. The arrow indicates the plane of dissection. The anterior layer of Denonvilliers' fascia must be incised to mobilize the seminal vesicles.

aspects of the incision are developed, and the procedure is completed.

We do not divide the urethra at this time because this would constitute a premature commitment to cystectomy. The rectum is inspected for any lacerations, and the incision is closed in two layers. A Penrose drain is left in place for 48 hours or until most of the drainage subsides. Cystectomy is then done as described in Chapter 26. The initial perineal approach requires approximately 30 minutes of operative time. This initial investment results in time saved when the abdominal portion of the cystectomy is performed. More importantly, the risk of rectal laceration in a heavily irradiated field is reduced.

PERINEAL CYSTOPROSTATECTOMY

Based on our experience with initial perineal dissection for salvage cystectomy, we have now developed the procedure of perineal cystoprostatectomy whereby the bladder and prostate are dissected and removed entirely through a perineal approach. Perineal cystoprostatectomy has been performed in high-risk male patients who require a perineal approach to free the prostate from the rectum.

Our first patient had a prior urinary diversion and required only the cystoprostatectomy. The five others undergoing the operation all had failure of radiation therapy and/or partial cystectomy (Table 27.3). After the perineal cystoprostatectomy, an ileoconduit was performed through a lower midline incision in the majority of cases.

Procedure

The usual preoperative preparation for patients undergoing a standard cystectomy is performed, including autologous blood donation, full bowel preparation (including neomycin cleansing enemas), antiembolic and sequential compression boots. The patient is placed in the exaggerated lithotomy position on the table with a 6-in "jelly roll" beneath his sacroiliac joints. As in a perineal prostatectomy, proper patient position is essential. The patient is prepared and draped with an O'Connor-Sullivan drape for digital rectal examination.

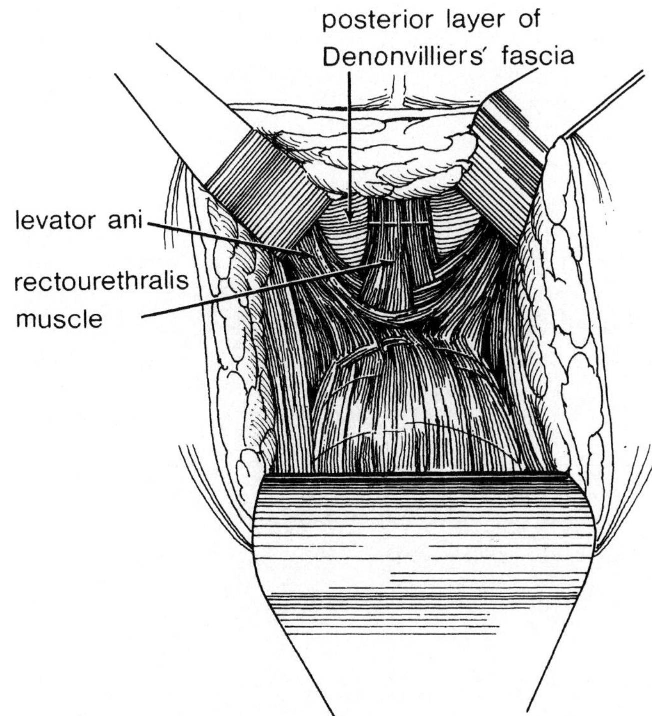

Fig. 27.3. Rectourethralis muscle is encountered in the midline and divided.

Table 27.3.   Perineal Cystoprostatectomy

PATIENT AGE (yr)	DIAGNOSIS	PRIOR THERAPY	COMPLICATIONS	EBL (ml)	TIME
35	CaProstate	Radiation therapy, conduit	—	400	120
68	CaBladder	Radiation therapy, chemotherapy	—	800	160
63	Squamous cell carcinoma	Internal urethrotomy	Ileus	500	160
67	CaBladder	Radiation therapy	Rectal laceration	1400	240
78	CaBladder	Radiation therapy, TURBT	—	500	120

An inverted U incision, as described earlier in this chapter, is made outside the anal sphincter and carried deep, isolating and dividing the central tendon. We have found the best way to accomplish this is by developing the ischiorectal fossae and then the space between the rectal wall. The white color of the rectal wall is identified, which is the landmark for the correct plane to proceed to the rectourethralis and prostatic apex. The prostate apex is divided, and the prostate dissected free as in a standard perineal prostatectomy (Fig. 27.5).

After successful mobilization of the prostate, the rectum is freed posteriorly from the bladder base. This is accomplished bluntly with a long sponge stick. Any dense adhesions can be divided sharply with scissors. The goal of this maneuver is to reach the cul-de-sac and position the rectum posteriorly so that it is not injured.

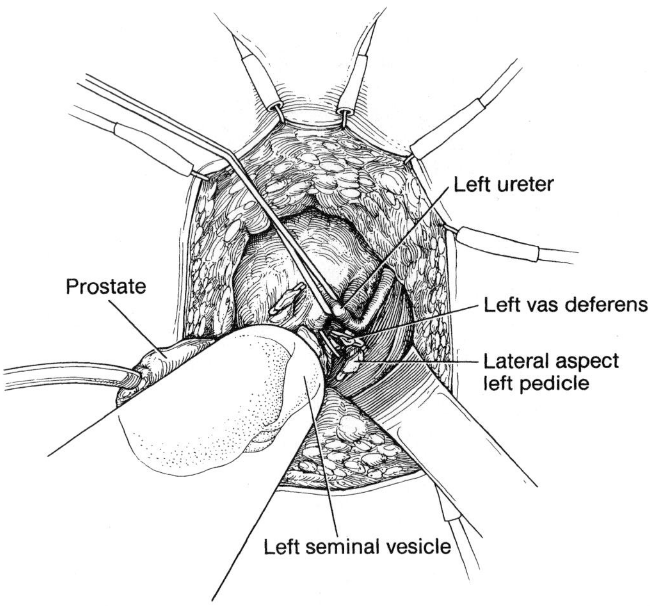

Fig. 27.6.   The left ureter is identified and will be ligated and divided. One third of the left lateral pedicle has already been divided.

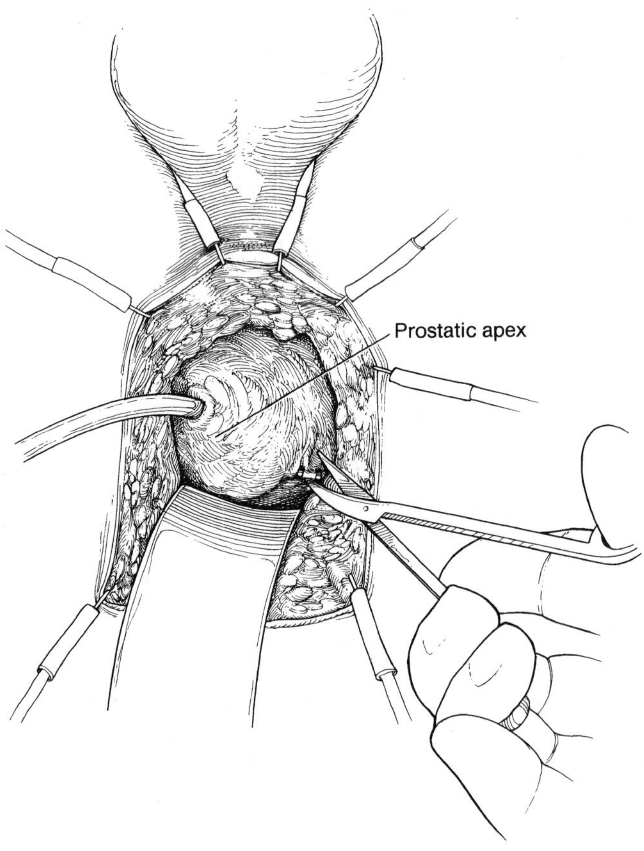

Fig. 27.5.   The prostate has been mobilized, and the left lateral pedicle is being developed.

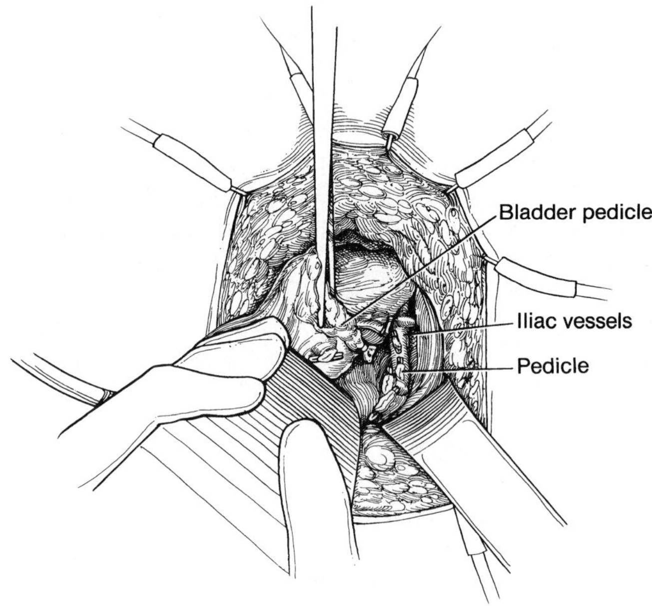

Fig. 27.7.   The complete left lateral pedicle has been divided, resulting in lateral mobility of the specimen. The contralateral pedicle is divided (not shown).

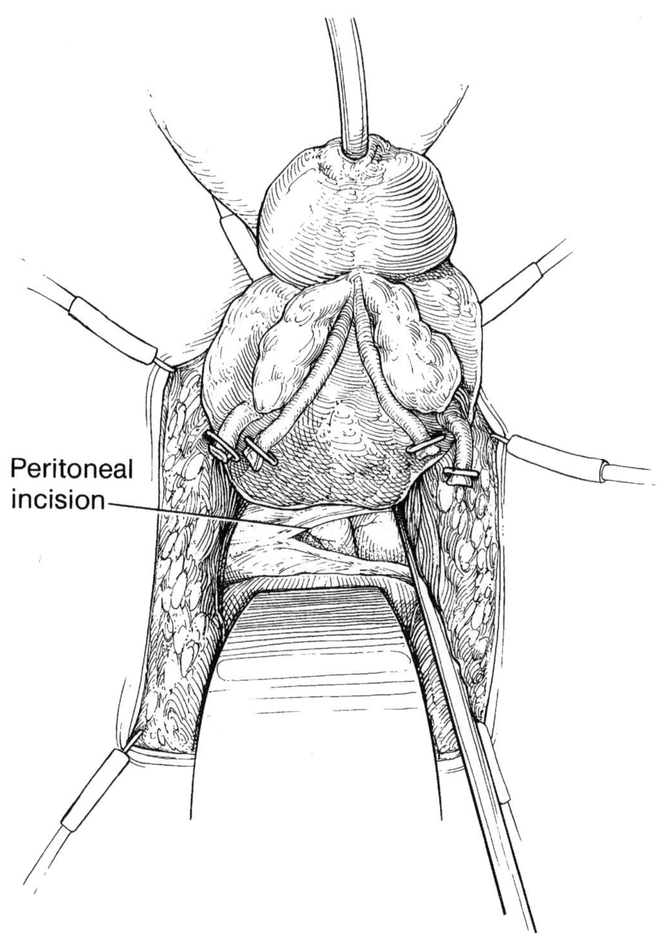

Fig. 27.8. An incision is made in the peritoneal cul-de-sac to mobilize the posterior and lateral aspects of the bladder.

We have found that an Omni-Tract surgical retractor with perineal blades or a Bookwalter retractor provides adequate exposure during the initial portions of the operation.

After the maneuvers to mobilize the prostate have been accomplished, attention is directed to developing the lateral pedicles of the bladder (Fig. 27.4). These are readily defined by both finger dissection and with the aid of a sponge stick. We have found that the pedicles are more apparent from this approach than from the standard abdominal route. These pedicles are divided between ligaclips. It is important to have an assortment of ligaclip applicators available, including both straight and right-angle clips. After one third of the pedicle is divided, the ipsilateral ureter is visualized and divided (Fig. 27.6). It is helpful to have ureteral catheters in place to aid in this identification because the course of the ureters are more lateral than one would expect.

The remainder of the lateral pedicle is divided, which should result in increased bladder mobility (Fig. 27.7).

The internal and external iliac vessels can be visualized through the incision. We have not yet attempted to remove any lymph nodes via this approach. The majority of our patients have had radiation failures, which resulted in a dense des-

moplastic reaction around the vessels. The contralateral pedicle and ureter are divided in a similar manner.

Further mobilization of the lateral and inferior aspects of the bladder is accomplished by both blunt and sharp dissection. The specimen is gradually advanced through the incision by gentle traction applied to the prostate with a tenaculum clamp. The urachus and peritoneum remain as the only remaining attachments of the bladder. The umbilicus will invert and there will be a noticeable resistance to further mobilization of the bladder secondary to the urachal attachments.

It is possible to remove the bladder by remaining extraperitoneal. The peritoneal surface of the bladder can be dissected off by blunt dissection with a sponge stick and the urachus divided sharply. This is a dissection that is accomplished quite a distance into the incision, requires long instruments, and is tedious. Another maneuver to complete the operation is to incise the peritoneum at the level of the cul-de-sac or lateral to the urachus (Fig. 27.8) and carry the incision in a circumferential manner. The final step is sharp division of the urachus between ligaclips (Fig. 27.9). After this is completed, the specimen is delivered through the wound (Fig. 27.10).

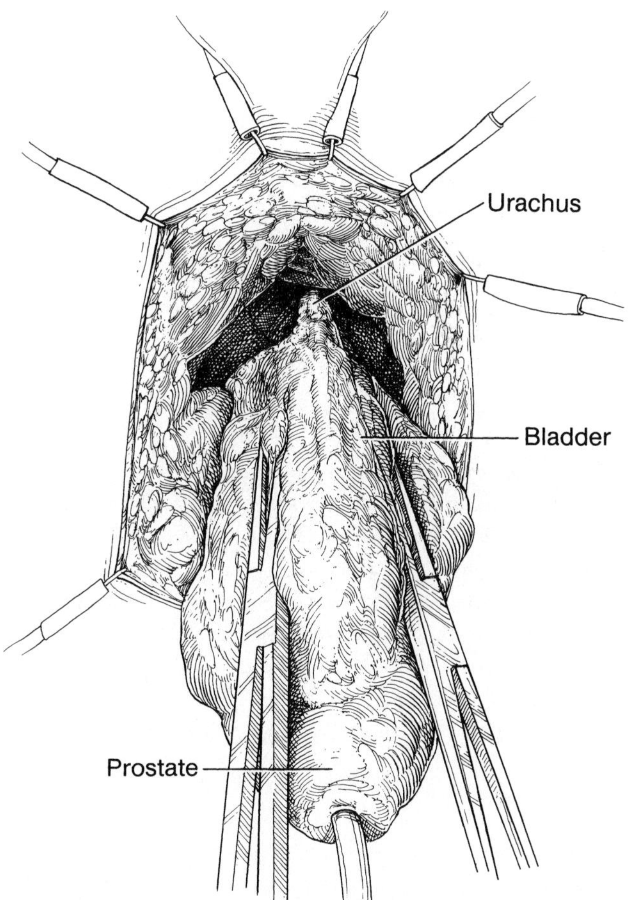

Fig. 27.9. The urachus is identified and divided.

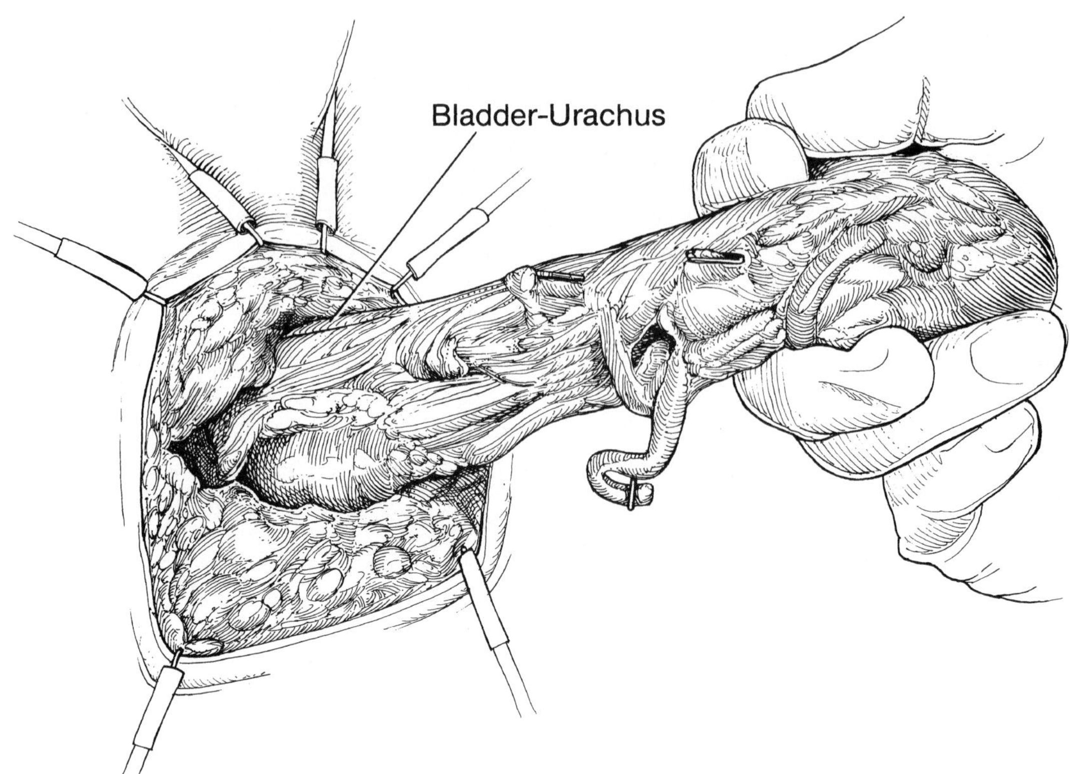

Fig. 27.10. The specimen is being removed from the operative site.

Mean operative time is 2.5 hours, and mean blood loss has been 500 mL. To date, the six patients that have undergone this procedure had either radiation and/or chemotherapy and surgery failures. It is anticipated that the surgical procedure would be less difficult in the untreated patient who requires a cystoprostatectomy. This procedure is termed a simple cystoprostatectomy unless a bilateral pelvic lymph node dissection accompanies it. We have had one major complication, which was a rectal injury occurring when mobilizing the prostate at the level of the rectourethralis muscle. This was closed primarily without further sequelae.

This procedure can be classified as minimally invasive and is technically easier and less time-consuming than attempts to remove the organ laparoscopically. The challenge remains the urinary diversion. This could be in the form of a ureterosigmoidostomy in patients who have not had prior radiation therapy. Another option would be a laparoscopic-assisted procedure. We are currently developing both of these options. The procedure has not been performed in the female patient, but should not be more difficult.

REFERENCES

1. Jenkins BJ, et al. Reappraisal of the role of radical radiotherapy and salvage cystectomy in the treatment of invasive (T2/T3) bladder cancer. Br J Urol 1988;62:343.

2. Murphy LJT. From the Renaissance to the nineteenth century. In: Murphy LJT, ed. The history of urology. Springfield, IL: Charles CJ Thomas, 1972.

3. Thompson H. Tumours of the bladder. London: J & A Churchill, 1884.

4. Billroth T. Extirpation eines Harnblasenmyoms nach vorausgehenden tiefen und hohen Blasenschnitt (C. Gussenbauer). Arch Klin Chir 1875;18:411.

5. Bardenheuer B. Der Extraperitonealer Explorativschnitt. Stuttgart: Enke, 1887.

6. Gray AL. The roentgen ray treatment of malignant disease of the bladder through a suprapubic incision: report of a case. Am J Surg 1906;20:307.

7. Riches E. Surgery and radiotherapy in urology: the bladder. J Urol 1963;90:339.

8. Abratt RP, et al. Radical irradiation and misonidazole for T2-grade 3 and T3 bladder cancer: 2 year follow up. Int J Radiat Oncol Biol Phys 1984;10:1719.

9. Crawford ED, Skinner DE. Salvage cystectomy after irradiation failure. J Urol 1980;123:32.

10. Smith JA Jr, Whitmore WF Jr. Salvage cystectomy for bladder cancer after failure of definitive irradiation. J Urol 1981;125: 643.

11. Swanson DA, et al. Salvage cystectomy for bladder carcinoma. Cancer 1981;47:2275.

12. Freiha FS, Faysal MH. Salvage cystectomy. Urology 1983;23: 496.

13. Konnak JW, Grossman HB. Salvage cystectomy following failed definitive radiation therapy for transitional cell carcinoma of bladder. Urology 1985;26:550.

SUGGESTED READINGS

Boccon Gibod L, Leleu C, Steg A. Salvage cystectomy: the case for a combined abdominoperineal approach. Eur Urol 1984;10: 370.

Jakse G, Grommhold H. Combined radiation and chemotherapy for locally advanced bladder cancer. In: Progress and controversies in oncological urology. New York: Alan R. Liss, 1984:365.

Johnson DE, Lamy S, Bracken RB. Salvage cystectomy after radiation failure in patients with bladder carcinoma. South Med J 1977;70:1279.

Marks LB, et al. Invasive bladder carcinoma: preliminary report of selective bladder conservation by transurethral surgery, upfront MCV (methotrexate, cisplatin, and vinblastine) chemotherapy, and pelvic irradiation plus cisplatin. Int J Radiat Oncol Biol Phys 1988;15:877.

Rotman M, et al. Treatment of advanced bladder carcinoma with irradiation and concomitant 5-fluorouracil infusion. Cancer 1987; 59:710.

Sauer R, et al. Preliminary results of treatment of invasive bladder carcinoma with radiotherapy and cisplatin. Int J Radiat Oncol Biol Phys 1988;15:871.

Shipley WU, et al. Cisplatin and full dose irradiation for patients with invasive bladder carcinoma: a preliminary report of tolerance and local response. J Urol 1984;132:899.

Shipley WU, et al. Treatment of invasive bladder cancer by cisplatin and radiation in patients unsuited for surgery. JAMA 1987;258:931.

28

Partial Cystectomy

Inderbir S. Gill, David P. Wood, and Rodney J. Taylor

The primary aim of surgical treatment for muscle-invasive bladder cancer is to maximize patient survival; quality of life issues such as bladder preservation are secondary concerns. Accordingly, the current gold standard treatment for muscle-invasive bladder cancer in medically fit patients is radical cystectomy.

Bladder-sparing therapeutic strategies like "radical" transurethral resection, partial cystectomy, systemic platinum-based chemotherapy, and radiation therapy have recently gained attention. However, unselective use of bladder-preservation procedures such as partial cystectomy may result in inferior survival compared with radical cystectomy. In the management of bladder cancer, partial cystectomy has limited indications due to three legitimate reasons.

1. High rate of local tumor recurrence in the remaining bladder.
2. Lower locoregional recurrence rate after radical cystectomy for muscle-invasive transitional cell carcinoma.
3. High success rate of transurethral treatment of superficial transitional cell carcinoma.

Further, the historically high patient morbidity associated with radical cystectomy has been significantly decreased with recent advances in pelvic surgical techniques, e.g., nerve-sparing radical cystoprostatectomy, continent urinary diversion, neobladder construction, and effective treatment of postsurgical impotence. The above arguments lend further support to the current bias toward radical cystectomy in the management of muscle-invasive cancer.

The Fourth International Consensus Meeting on Bladder Cancer in Antwerp, Belgium, in March 1993 found that "only a small proportion of carefully selected patients may be cured by transurethral surgery alone or by partial cystectomy alone" (1). Thus, partial cystectomy constitutes a viable therapeutic option in only a select subset of patients with muscle-invasive bladder cancer. However, the availability of newer cisplatin-based chemotherapeutic regimens may renew interest in bladder-sparing procedures in selected patients.

This chapter examines the current place of partial cystec-tomy in the treatment of carcinoma of the urinary bladder. Pros and cons of partial cystectomy (Table 28.1), patient selection, preoperative evaluation, and patient preparation are presented. Operative technique is discussed as it pertains to the location of the bladder segment to be excised. Postoperative management, complications, and data on local recurrence rates and overall patient survival are outlined. We conclude with a brief review of laparoscopic partial cystectomy.

PATIENT SELECTION

Bladder Cancer

Overall, only a small percentage (5 to 18%) of patients with bladder cancer are potential candidates for partial cystectomy (2, 3). Because of the high risk of tumor recurrence in the bladder remnant (38 to 78%) (4, 5), the criteria for patient selection are necessarily rigid. Minimal criteria include a solitary, primary tumor located at the dome of a bladder of adequate capacity without any concomitant carcinoma in situ or history of bladder tumors (1). Patients with a solitary, high-grade (grade 2 to 3), invasive (T1 or T2) primary bladder tumor located at a distance from the trigone (so as to allow a circumferential 2-cm margin of resection) are candidates for partial cystectomy. The tumor should be truly unifocal, and there should be no history of bladder tumors. The bladder and prostatic urethra should be extensively biopsied to rule out coexisting tumors, carcinoma in situ, or even advanced dysplasia. The preoperative bladder capacity should be approximately 300 mL or greater (6). There is some evidence that T3a (B2) tumors may be preferentially treated with radical cystectomy. In nonrandomized, retrospective studies, 5-year survival rates for patients with T3a disease were 48% (range, 26 to 73%) after radical cystectomy (7–9) compared with 37% (range, 18 to 45%) after partial cystectomy (2, 10, 11).

Other indications for partial cystectomy for cancer may include superficial disease that is inaccessible for transurethral resection, and (rarely) symptomatic palliation in a poor-risk patient with bladder cancer. Partial cystectomy may be the

Table 28.1. Partial Cystectomy: Advantages and Disadvantages

Advantages
  Maintains physiologic voiding
  Maintains erections
  Avoids bowel in the urinary tract
  Less radical surgery with decreased patient morbidity
  Improved quality of life, thus high patient acceptance
Disadvantages
  High local tumor recurrence rate (40–70%)
  Tumor spillage or seeding intraoperatively

treatment of choice for tumors located in a bladder diverticulum.

Urachal Cancer

Primary adenocarcinoma of the bladder comprises 1 to 2% of all bladder tumors. Adenocarcinomas may be vesical (70%) or urachal (30%) in origin (12). Urachal lesions tend to progress through the bladder wall toward the umbilicus and usually present at a late stage as a palpable, infraumbilical, midline mass (13, 14). Resectable urachal tumors are best treated with an extensive, en bloc partial cystectomy. Nevertheless, local recurrence rates are high (70 to 80%) and 5-year survival rates are poor (6 to 15%) (15).

Cancer in a Diverticulum

Tumors arising in diverticulae comprise 1.5 to 10% of all bladder tumors (16). As a general rule, cancers located in a diverticulum are of higher grade and have higher recurrence, metastatic, and mortality rates than those of similar histologic type located in the rest of the bladder. Because the diverticular wall is thin and lacks a muscular layer, these tumors should be thought of as T4 tumors. In general, disease failure occurs systemically rather than locally (17, 18).

PREOPERATIVE STUDIES

Systematic staging of invasive bladder tumors is critical. Radiologic staging should include an intravenous pyelogram. To aid in assessing the local stage of the tumor, bimanual examination under anesthesia should be performed. Random bladder biopsies are performed at multiple sites to rule out concomitant carcinoma in situ. We prefer to biopsy the bladder neck and prostatic urethra with a resectoscope loop to obtain a generous specimen. Transurethral resection of the bladder tumor with fulguration of the base is performed as completely as possible. This not only allows staging of the bladder tumor but also minimizes the risk of tumor spillage during subsequent partial cystectomy.

On confirmation of unifocal invasive bladder cancer, routine metastatic and preoperative evaluations are initiated. Liver function tests, if abnormal, may indicate hepatic involvement. Abdominopelvic computed tomography is performed to rule out intra-abdominal visceral metastases or gross pelvic lymphadenopathy. A bone scan is obtained only in the presence of an elevated serum alkaline phosphatase level or bone pain.

PREOPERATIVE PATIENT PREPARATION

Urine should be sterile, and any urinary tract infection is treated with appropriate antibiotics before surgery. Some centers recommend preoperative radiation therapy (1000 to 1500 cGy of external beam radiation over 3 to 4 days) before partial cystectomy in an effort to reduce the risk of tumor seeding (19).

The patient ingests only clear liquids 24 hours before the operation, and mechanical bowel preparation is performed as per the surgeon's preference. Bowel preparation is necessary because the patient and surgeon should be prepared for a radical cystectomy in the event that negative margins cannot be obtained intraoperatively, too much bladder needs to be excised, or if locoregional spread is present.

OPERATIVE TECHNIQUE

The patient is positioned supine, and the operating table is flexed at the sacrum. Care should be taken not to hyperextend the patient excessively because this may result in postoperative femoral neuropathy. The external genitalia are draped into the operative field. A Foley catheter is placed intraoperatively, and the bladder is filled with 100 mL of a tumoricidal agent (thiotepa, silver nitrate, sterile water) as per the surgeon's preference.

The surgical technique of partial cystectomy varies with the location of the bladder tumor. In general, tumors located on the anterior wall or dome of the bladder can be approached by an entirely extraperitoneal technique. Tumors on the posterior wall are approached transperitoneally; however, posteriorly located tumors are rarely treated by partial cystectomy. Lateral wall tumors are approached by either an extraperitoneal or transperitoneal approach, depending on location and ease of bladder mobilization.

Anterior Tumor

Through a low midline incision, the rectus muscles are separated, and the transversalis fascia is incised in the midline to enter the prevesical space. Care is taken not to dissect the perivesical tissue off the tumor-bearing bladder segment. The bladder is mobilized from the pelvic side wall bilaterally. A self-retaining ring retractor is positioned. Bilateral pelvic lymph node dissection is performed.

Sponges are positioned around the bladder to isolate it from the abdominal cavity. The bladder tumor is identified by gentle palpation through the intact bladder wall; alternatively, intraoperative flexible cystoscopy can be performed to locate the tumor precisely. Allis clamps are placed widely to tent up the surrounding bladder wall; the Foley catheter is unclamped.

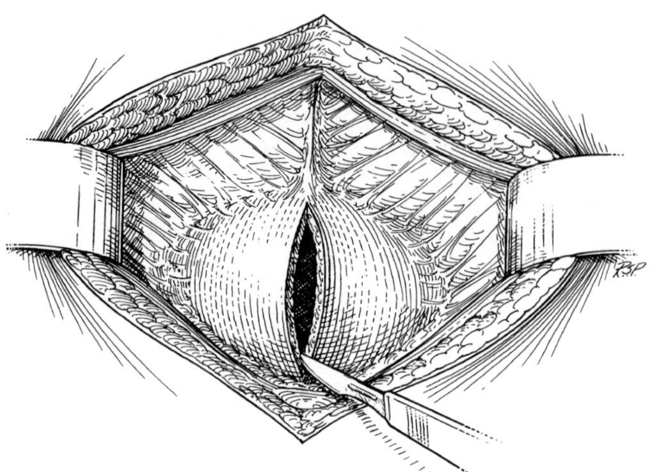

Fig. 28.1. Anterior cystotomy incision.

After confirming an empty bladder, an anterior cystotomy is made (Fig. 28.1), and the interior of the bladder is examined (Fig. 28.2). A circumferential 2-cm margin around the bladder tumor is excised with electrocautery (Fig. 28.3), and the specimen, including overlying perivesical fat, is sent for permanent section. An additional 0.5- to 1-cm wide, full-thickness strip of bladder mucosa and muscle is then excised with sharp scissors (Fig. 28.4); electrocautery is not used in this step to eliminate cautery artifact for purposes of histopathologic examination.

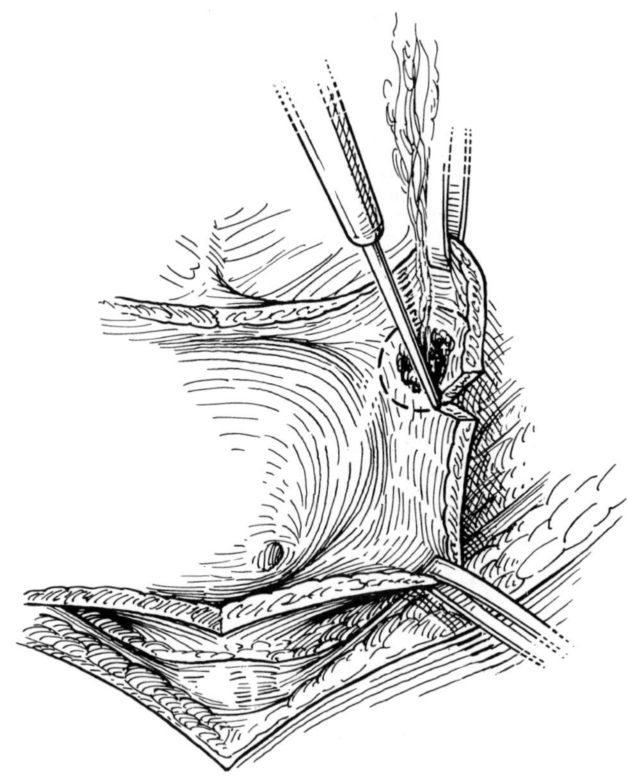

Fig. 28.3. Electrocautery knife is used to excise the tumor with a 2-cm margin circumferentially.

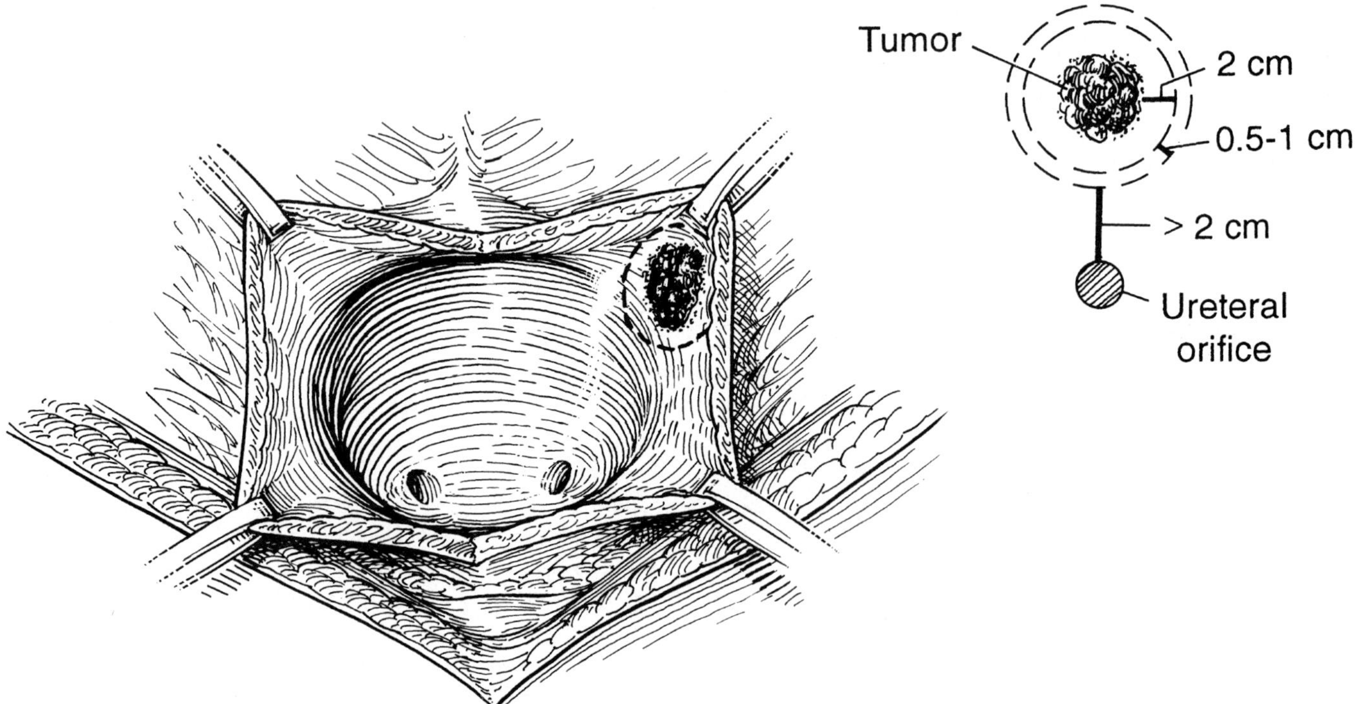

Fig. 28.2. Location of tumor in relation to the ureteral orifices. The broken line outlines the 2-cm circumferential margin of resection. Inset: First, the tumor along with a 2-cm margin is excised and sent for permanent section. Next, a 0.5- to 1.0-cm wide strip of bladder wall is excised and sent for frozen section. Ideally, the distance between the margin of resection and the ureteral orifice should be greater than 2 cm.

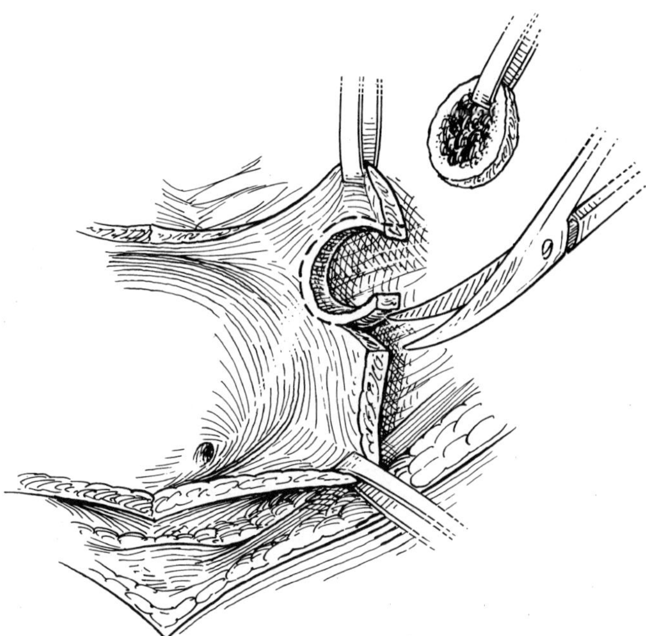

Fig. 28.4. An additional 0.5- to 1.0-cm wide strip of bladder wall is excised. This step should be performed with scissors.

The outer margin of this 0.5- to 1.0-cm strip constitutes the true surgical margin; after orienting the bladder strip with a stay suture, it is sent for frozen section to rule out tumor or mucosal dysplasia. In the event that the frozen section result indicates tumor at the surgical margin, a wider resection is performed, if possible. If not, a radical cystectomy may be required.

Hemostasis is obtained with electrocautery. A 22F or 24F Foley catheter is placed. A meticulous two- or three-layered bladder closure is performed (Fig. 28.5). The repair is tested for watertightness by instilling sterile water through the Foley catheter. At the surgeon's discretion, a Jackson-Pratt drain may

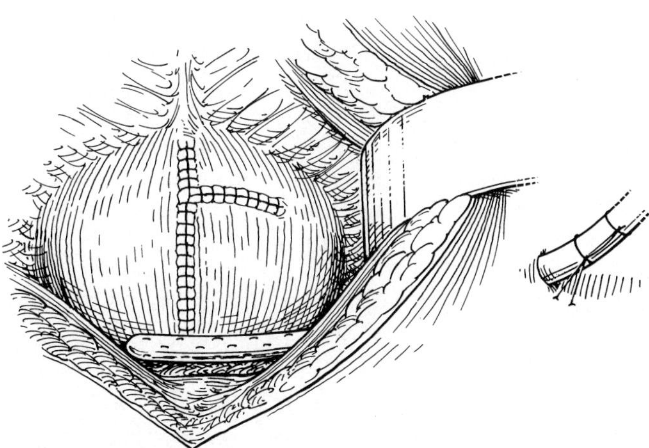

Fig. 28.5. Bladder closure is performed in three layers. A Jackson-Pratt drain may be placed in the space of Retzius. Suprapubic cystostomy should be avoided to minimize tumor seeding.

be placed in the space of Retzius, taking care that the drain is located at some distance from the cystotomy incision.

Alternatively, an anterior tumor can be excised by a closed technique. A large vascular clamp is placed around the mobilized tumor-bearing segment of the bladder. Partial cystectomy is performed, and frozen section of the margins is obtained. Bladder closure is performed in two or three layers. This technique has the significant advantage of theoretically eliminating the chances of local tumor spillage (20).

Lateral Tumor

Although the technique of partial cystectomy for a tumor located low on the lateral wall of the bladder is similar to that mentioned in the previous section, two points bear emphasis.

1. The ipsilateral aspect of the bladder must be mobilized.
2. The tumor may involve the ureter.

The ipsilateral aspect of the bladder is mobilized in a manner akin to radical cystectomy, albeit limiting the dissection to one side only. It is the authors' opinion that if the bladder tumor involves the ureter, thereby requiring a distal ureterectomy and ureteral reimplantation, attempts at partial cystectomy should be discontinued and a radical cystectomy should be performed.

Urachal Tumor

The surgical procedure involves a wide en bloc resection of the dome of the bladder, urachus, bilateral medial umbilical ligaments, rectus fascia, overlying peritoneum, perivesical fat, and the surrounding anterior abdominal wall, including the umbilicus (13).

POSTOPERATIVE MANAGEMENT

Prophylaxis against deep vein thrombosis (sequential compression devices or miniheparinization) and atelectasis (incentive spirometry) is routine. The patient is encouraged to ambulate the night of surgery, and diet is advanced as tolerated. A cystogram is performed at 1 week, and the Foley catheter is removed if no leak is identified. The Jackson-Pratt drain is removed 24 hours later, after confirming absence of urinary leakage.

FOLLOW-UP

Close, life-long surveillance is mandatory after partial cystectomy for cancer. Periodic chest radiographs and urine cytologies are performed. An abdominopelvic CT scan is obtained 6 months postoperatively. Any suspicious area on follow-up cystoscopy is biopsied and treated appropriately. Management of recurrent disease depends on its grade, stage, and location (local or systemic). Treatment options, singly or in combination, include intravesical chemotherapy, transurethral resection, salvage cystectomy and urinary diversion to the abdominal wall or urethra, systemic chemotherapy, or radiation therapy.

COMPLICATIONS

Improvements in surgical technique have decreased the morbidity and mortality after partial cystectomy. Earlier studies reported a 10% perioperative mortality rate (21). However, several recent authors have noted no mortality associated with partial cystectomy (10, 22). Currently, the overall complication rate of partial cystectomy ranges from 11 to 29%, with the majority of these complications being minor (11, 23). This section addresses only those complications that are specific to a partial cystectomy.

Urinary leakage is usually a technical complication of partial cystectomy (6). Predisposing factors for development of a urinary fistula include history of radiation therapy or bladder surgery. Causes of urine leakage include incomplete bladder closure, leakage from the ureteral reimplantation site, or unrecognized injury to the ureter or bladder. Timing of occurrence of urinary leakage can help in identifying its cause. Immediate postoperative leakage occurs due to inadequate closure; delayed leakage (4 to 6 days) is usually secondary to ischemic necrosis. Late leakage (longer than 1 month) is often due to malignant seeding of the incision site. Diagnosis is established by a gravity cystogram with a postdrainage film. The key to managing a urine leak is establishing adequate drainage. The existing Foley catheter is irrigated, and if suboptimal, replaced. Occasionally, the balloon of a standard Foley catheter occupies the base of the bladder, thus elevating the eye of the catheter; this leads to inadequate drainage of the floor of the bladder. Insertion of a large-bore straight catheter, without a balloon, ensures maximal drainage of the bladder. If a postoperative ultrasound or CT scan identifies a perivesical fluid collection, it can be drained percutaneously.

Tumor implantation of the wound (0 to 18%) is a serious complication that can lead to patient mortality (3, 10, 23–25). Tumor seeding may present as a subcutaneous nodule, pelvic mass, or formation of a fistula—vesicocutaneous, vesicovaginal, rectovesical, or colovesical. It is important to be aware of this problem and take steps to minimize its occurrence (Table 28.2).

Bladder capacity after partial cystectomy is an important issue that can affect the patient's lifestyle. Significant postoperative reduction of bladder volume has been reported in 13 to 39% of patients, resulting in debilitating irritative symptoms in 4 to 8% and subsequent urinary diversion in 3% (10, 25). Predisposing risk factors for postoperative bladder contraction include a history of radiation therapy or bladder surgery. Although it has been suggested that a bladder remnant (intraoperatively big enough to accommodate only a Foley catheter) will gradually reexpand to an adequate functional capacity (26), contrary opinion holds that no more than 50% of the bladder can be safely removed during the course of a partial cystectomy (27).

LOCAL RECURRENCE

Because of the "field change" concept of transitional cell carcinoma, radical cystectomy has rightfully remained the mainstay

Table 28.2. Steps to Minimize the Risk of Tumor Spillage

Consider external beam radiation therapy (1000–1600 cGy) for 2–4 days preoperatively (19)

Preoperative transurethral resection of the bladder tumor with extensive fulguration of the tumor base

At the start of the partial cystectomy, irrigate the bladder thoroughly with sterile water through a Foley catheter; consider instilling a tumoricidal agent (thiotepa, mitomycin, or silver nitrate) in the bladder

Before making the cystotomy, pack the bladder away from the abdominal organs with sponges

Do not cut into the tumor

Do not traumatize adjacent bladder mucosa (e.g., by placing self-retaining retractor inside the bladder) to minimize mucosal denudation and tumor implantation

If the patient has an enlarged prostate, do not perform an open prostatectomy during the same operative session

Avoid placing a suprapubic tube

Irrigate the wound copiously with sterile water before closing

of treatment for muscle-invasive disease, with partial cystectomy being reserved for a highly select group of patients. The main advantage of partial cystectomy, i.e., bladder sparing, is also its main disadvantage. By leaving behind intact, globally at-risk bladder urothelium, which continues to be susceptible to field changes, the potential for disease recurrence and progression remains. Reported tumor recurrence rates vary from 38 to 78% (4, 5), with 75% of such recurrences occurring within 2 years (11). The two most important predictors of tumor recurrence are the number of tumors present and history of tumor recurrence (10); however, this should not be a problem if—as mentioned previously—patients are selected properly. After partial cystectomy, higher-stage tumors recur more rapidly than lower-stage tumors (5, 11).

PATIENT SURVIVAL

The overall 5-year and 10-year survival rates after partial cystectomy are 49% and 24% (Table 28.3) (2, 4, 5, 10, 11, 21–24, 28–30). Clearly, grade and stage of the primary tumor affect patient survival (31). Sweeney et al. reviewed the literature to compare 5-year survival rates after partial and radical cystectomy according to the stage of bladder tumor (32). Five-year survival rates after partial cystectomy for T2 tumors (29 to 80%), T3a tumors (14 to 62%), and T3b tumors (0 to 33%) were comparable to radical cystectomy for T2 (50 to 88%), T3a (26 to 60%), and T3b (6 to 46%) tumors (32). Thus, in properly selected patients with muscle-invasive cancer, partial cystectomy (while offering a lower morbidity) results in 5-year survival rates comparable to those for radical cystectomy. However, strict patient selection is paramount. In general, adverse patient outcomes after partial cystectomy correlate with the following characteristics.

Table 28.3. Partial Cystectomy: Patient Survival According to Stage and Grade

	5-YR SURVIVAL (%)	10-YR SURVIVAL (%)
Grade		
1	85	42
2	59	36
3	36	10
Stage		
TA	83	21
T1	71	50
T2	49	25
T3A	38	5
T3B	17	—
T4	2	0
Overall	49	24

These statistics are compiled from a review of the literature (2, 4, 5, 10, 11, 21–24, 28–30).

A. History of tumor recurrence (10).
B. Multiple tumors (33).
C. Higher grade and stage of primary tumor (31, 33).
D. Large tumor size (23, 31).
E. Tumor location (posterior wall tumors have a better prognosis than tumors at the bladder neck) (2, 21).
F. History of bladder surgery (10).

Whether adjuvant therapies (systemic cisplatin-based chemotherapy, radiation therapy) confer a survival advantage in patients undergoing partial cystectomy remains to be substantiated. It appears that patients opting for bladder-sparing alternatives survive longer with combination therapy (i.e., partial cystectomy with neoadjuvant systemic chemotherapy and/or radiation therapy) than with monotherapy (partial cystectomy alone) (1). Preoperative radiation therapy has been proposed to decrease wound seeding (19). However, the beneficial effect of radiation therapy remains unproven for two reasons.

1. Comparably minimal wound implantation rates have been achieved without adjuvant radiation therapy.
2. Adjuvant radiation therapy has not been shown to enhance 5-year survival rates in patients undergoing radical cystectomy (32).

Systemic chemotherapy, both adjuvant and neoadjuvant, has been used in combination with partial cystectomy. In a series of 111 patients treated with neoadjuvant methotrexate, vinblastine, Adriamycin, and cisplatin (MVAC) chemotherapy and transurethral resection, 32 patients subsequently underwent partial cystectomy. At a median follow-up of 1.5 years, 75% of patients undergoing partial cystectomy had a functional bladder and were disease free (34). In another series of 30 patients undergoing neoadjuvant MVAC chemotherapy, 14 patients (47%) had a complete response and another 14 patients (47%) had a partial response. Of the 14 partial responders, 9 underwent partial cystectomy; the 3-year disease-free sur-

vival rate in this group was 78% (7 of 9 patients) (35). These studies indicate that combination therapy has the potential to improve the success rate of bladder-preservation therapeutic strategies. Nonetheless, prospective randomized trials are required to address this issue definitively by eliminating selection bias.

LAPAROSCOPIC PARTIAL CYSTECTOMY

Recently, laparoscopic techniques have been reported for performing partial cystectomy for cancer (36) and for a patent urachus (37). In the patient with cancer, a high-grade, invasive transitional cell carcinoma located on the anterior wall of the bladder was treated with laparoscopic partial cystectomy. After preoperative cystoscopic photoirradiation of the tumor, transperitoneal laparoscopic pelvic lymph node dissection was performed. Using an endoscopic GIA stapler and a contact tip laser, the tumor-bearing bladder segment was excised and placed in a plastic bag for intact retrieval from the abdomen. The bladder rent was sutured laparoscopically. The patient was discharged from the hospital on the third postoperative day (36). A patent urachal fistula was excised by a comparable transperitoneal laparoscopic approach. The urachal tract was dissected in its entirety from the undersurface of the anterior abdominal wall and excised. Extracorporeally tied catgut endoligatures were placed to occlude the bladder rent. The patient was discharged on the third postoperative day with complete resolution of symptoms (37). No long-term follow-up data are available.

In a similar fashion, bladder diverticulectomy has been performed laparoscopically (38, 39). Both the extraperitoneal and transperitoneal laparoscopic approaches have been used. Division of the diverticular neck can be performed either with an Endo-GIA stapler or with electrosurgical scissors. Bladder reconstruction can be performed by laparoscopic suturing or stapling techniques. The above reports represent the preliminary application of laparoscopy in this field. Proper patient selection and adequate laparoscopic expertise are essential before considering the minimally invasive approach. The laparoscopic approach must currently be considered investigational, especially because of the uncertain status of partial cystectomy in the management of invasive bladder cancer.

CONCLUSION

Bladder preservation maintains continence, potency, and physiologic voiding. However, these advantages must be weighed against the high tumor recurrence rate in the bladder remnant following partial cystectomy and the risk of local contamination. As a general guideline for the majority of patients with muscle-invasive bladder cancer, partial cystectomy is not an appropriate alternative to radical cystectomy. However, for carefully selected patients with a unifocal, primary bladder cancer in a favorable location, partial cystectomy may afford a 5-year survival rate comparable to radical cystectomy, especially in combination with other therapies. Further work is required in this field to determine which combinations of bladder-sparing strategies are most likely to afford patient survival equivalent to radical cystectomy.

REFERENCES

1. Koiso K, Shipley W, Keuppens F, et al. The status of bladder preserving therapeutic strategies in the management of patients with muscle-invasive bladder cancer. Int J Urol 1995; 2:49.
2. Utz DC, Schmitz SE, Fugelso PD, et al. A clinicopathologic evaluation of partial cystectomy for carcinoma of the urinary bladder. Cancer 1973;32:1075.
3. Jardin A, Vallencien G. Partial cystectomy for bladder tumors. In: Kuss R, Khoury S, Denis LJ, et al eds. Bladder cancer, part A: pathology, diagnosis, and surgery. New York: Alan R. Liss, 1984:375.
4. Kaneti J. Partial cystectomy in the management of bladder carcinoma. Eur Urol 1986;12:249.
5. Faysal MH, Frieha FS. Evaluation of partial cystectomy for bladder cancer. Urology 1979;14:352.
6. Wood DP, Fair WR. Complications of cystectomy. In: Marshall FF, ed. Urologic complications: medical and surgical, adult and pediatric, 2nd ed. Chicago: Year Book Medical Publishers, 1990;17:274.
7. Whitmore WF Jr, et al. Radical cystectomy with or without prior irradiation in the treatment of bladder cancer. J Urol 1977;118:184.
8. Pearse HD, Reed RR, Hodges CV. Radical cystectomy for bladder cancer. J Urol 1978;119:216.
9. Montie JR, Straffon RA, Stewart BH. Radical cystectomy without radiation therapy for carcinoma of the bladder. J Urol 1984;131:477.
10. Cummings KB, Mason JT, Correa RJ, et al. Segmental resection in the management of bladder carcinoma. J Urol 1978;119:56.
11. Resnick MI, O'Conor VJ. Segmental resection for carcinoma of the bladder: review of 102 patients. J Urol 1973;109:1007.
12. Nocks BN, Heney NM, Daly JJ. Primary adenocarcinoma of urinary bladder. Urology 1983;21:26.
13. Loening SA, Jacobo E, Hawtery CE, et al. Adenocarcinoma of the urachus. J Urol 1978;119:68.
14. Sheldon CA, Clayman RV, Gonzalez R, et al. Malignant urachal lesions. J Urol 1984;131:1.
15. Pode D, Fair WR. Urachal tumors. AUA Update Series 1991; 10:33.
16. Micic S, Ilic V. Incidence of neoplasm in vesical diverticula. J Urol 1983;129:734.
17. Wesselhoeft CW Jr, Perlmutter AD, Berg S, et al. Pathogenesis and surgical treatment of diverticulum of the urinary bladder. Surg Gynecol Obstet 1963;116:719.
18. Faysal MH, Frieha FS. Primary neoplasm in vesical diverticula : a report of 12 cases. Br J Urol 1981;53:141.
19. Werf-Messing B van der. Carcinoma of the bladder treated by suprapubic radium implants. Eur J Cancer 1969;5:277.
20. Haddad FS. Partial cystectomy for bladder cancer: a new technique. Urology 1991;38:458.
21. Magri J. Partial cystectomy: a review of 104 cases. Br J Urol 1962;34:74.
22. Evans RA, Texter JH. Partial cystectomy in the treatment of bladder cancer. J Urol 1975;114:391.
23. Lindahl F, Jorgensen D, Egvad K. Partial cystectomy for transitional cell carcinoma of the bladder. Scand J Nephrol 1984;18:125.
24. Novick AC, Steward BH. Partial cystectomy in the treatment of primary and secondary carcinoma of the bladder. J Urol 1976;116:570.
25. Ojeda L, Johnson DE. Partial cystectomy: can it be incorporated into integrated therapy program? Urology 1983; 22:115.
26. Baker R, Kelley T, Tehan T, et al. Subtotal cystectomy and total bladder regeneration in treatment of bladder cancer. JAMA 1958;168:1178.
27. Merrell RW, Brown HE, Rose JF. Bladder carcinoma treated by partial cystectomy: a review of 54 cases. J Urol 1979;122: 471.
28. Schoberg TW, Sapolsky JL, Lewis CW. Carcinoma of the bladder treated by segmental resection. J Urol 1979;122:473.
29. Brannan E, Ochsner MG, Fuselier HA, et al. Partial cystectomy in the treatment of transitional cell carcinoma of the bladder. J Urol 1978;119:213.
30. Long RTL, Grummon RA, Spratt JS, et al. Carcinoma of the urinary bladder: comparison with radical, simple, and partial cystectomy and intravesical formalin. Cancer 1972;29:98.
31. Kaubisch S, Lum BL, Reese J, et al. Stage T1 bladder cancer: grade is the primary determinant for risk of muscle invasion. J Urol 1991;146:28.
32. Sweeney P, Kursh ED, Resnick MI. Partial cystectomy. Urol Clin North Am 1992;19:701.
33. Lutzeyer W, Rubben H, Dahm H. Prognostic parameters in superficial bladder cancer: an analysis of 315 cases. J Urol 1982;127:250.
34. Herr HW, Scher HI. Neoadjuvant chemotherapy in partial cystectomy for invasive bladder cancer. In: Lepor H, Lawson RK, eds. Therapy for genitourinary cancer. New York: Kluer Academic, 1992:99.
35. Simon SD, Srougi M. Neoadjuvant M-VAC chemotherapy in partial cystectomy for the treatment of locally invasive transitional cell carcinoma of the bladder. In: Splinter AW, Scher HI, eds. Neoadjuvant chemotherapy in invasive bladder cancer. New York: Wiley Liss, 1990:169.
36. Lowe BA, Novy MJ, Strang E. Laparoscopic segmental cystectomy. J Urol 1992;147:408. Abstract.
37. Newfang T, Ludtke FE, Lepsien G. Laparoscopic excision of an urachal fistula: a new therapy for a rare disorder. Minim Invas Ther 1992;1:245.
38. Parra RO, Jones JP, Andrus CH, et al. Laparoscopic diverticulectomy: preliminary report of a new approach for the treatment of bladder diverticulum. J Urol 1992;148:869.
39. Das S. Laparoscopic removal of bladder diverticulum. J Urol 1992;148:1837.

29

Continent Urinary Diversion

A Review

Sakti Das

Historically, the modern evolution of continent urinary diversion actually represents a renascence of the original urinary diversion with ureterosigmoidostomy attempted by Simon in 1852 on a patient with ectopia vesicae (1). Despite its prohibitive surgical mortality, ureterosigmoidostomy remained a popular choice because of its relative simplicity of technique. Progressive understanding of the metabolic side effects and renal deterioration coupled with major psychological upheaval from anal incontinence prompted the search for innovative alternatives in urinary diversion. Reports of continent cutaneous diversion using cecum as the reservoir by Gilchrist et al. in 1950 (2) and bladder substitution by Couvelaire in 1951 (3) did not gain wide acceptance because their claim of achieving true continence was viewed with skepticism. Therefore, around the same time, external cutaneous urinary diversion via ileal loop popularized by Eugene Bricker became the surgical standard of diversion by virtue of its simplicity and relatively few early complications (4). Because of the inordinate surgical mortality and morbidity associated with extirpative cancer surgery in those early days, most patients were resigned to the changes in body image caused by the external urinary diversion. Patients were content to survive the onslaught of cancer and its extirpation.

With advancements in surgical techniques and outcomes aided by improved supportive care, various aspects of quality of life after cancer surgeries have become more important. The modern patient's discontent with incontinence, whether "external stomal" or "sphincteric," has a more significant social, psychological, and somatic effect than previously acknowledged. Moreover, progressive understanding of the morbidities of ureterosigmoidostomy and some disillusionment with the long-term results and complications of ileal conduit diversion have added incentives for a more intensive quest. In the 1980s, dedi-cated research by urologists in different parts of the world led to the development of a number of continent urinary diversions and bladder substitutions that are clinically feasible for the surgeon and psychologically and socially acceptable for the patient (5–12).

PRINCIPLES OF CONTINENT URINARY DIVERSION

Continent urinary diversion implies the diversion or substitution of the lower urinary tract, after which the patient has reasonable control of elimination. Certain requisite principles must be prudently observed to safeguard patients from potential harm. As cautioned by Bricker nearly half a century ago, one must remember that "urinary continence must not be achieved to the detriment of renal function." Improvement in quality of life should be constantly gauged against potential detriment to life. Continent urinary diversion should critically consider the following criteria.

The Reservoir Fashioned to Substitute for the Lower Urinary Tract Should Collect and Store Urine Under Low Pressure

Hinman has elegantly analyzed the principles involved in the construction of a urinary reservoir from intestinal segments (13). The important factors in consideration are the configuration, accommodation, viscoelasticity (compliance), and contractility. The concepts of geometric capacity prove that simple longitudinal opening of a tube and folding it back on itself as a pouch virtually doubles the volume capacity compared with the same length of unopened tube. Because of its larger radius, the reservoir or pouch thus created also accommodates a larger volume at physiologic pressure (Laplace's law). The larger radius with greater mural tension is more compliant and has larger capacity at low pressure. Longitudinal opening of the bowel prevents synchronized circular contractions with their resultant rise in pressure. Hinman concludes that only surgical techniques incorporating detubularization will benefit from the consequent alterations in geometry, accommodation, compliance, and contractility that reduce harmful contractions and at the same time yield the largest capacity from the shortest segment of bowel.

Damage to the Upper Urinary Tract Should be Prevented by Avoiding High Reservoir Pressure and Obstruction at Any Point in the Onward Egress of Urine

Principles of creating a low-pressure reservoir with detubularization are now universally accepted. However, one must be aware of the need for abdominal pressure or need to empty the detubularized neobladder connected to the urethra. Patients with such conditions should be monitored for high residual urine, necessitating intermittent catheterization to avoid upper tract distention from functional obstruction (14).

Stenosis of the ureteral implantation into the reservoir has been observed in 3 to 5% of patients (15). All ureteral anastomoses should be stented for a variable period postoperatively.

Controversy of Reflux Into the Upper Urinary Tract

A number of antireflux techniques, namely the submucosal tunnel, mucosal trough, split cuff nipple, and intussuscepted ileal nipple, have been used successfully for ureteral implantation into the reservoir. Recently, however, the need for prevention of reflux from a capacious low-pressure system has been questioned (16). Studer et al. have popularized a neobladder fashioned from detubularized ileum with an intact proximal segment into which the ureters are directly anastomosed (12). Patients do not have reflux while voiding because the intra-abdominal pressure is equally transmitted to the neobladder and to the afferent proximal segment; thereby, no differential pressures are created. Even on radiographic cystograms, reflux observed at cystometric capacity shows complete emptying of the renal pelvis on the postvoiding films. Therefore, in these low-pressure systems, reflux is probably of no clinical significance in the absence of outlet obstruction. According to Studer, "Too high a complication rate from the various antireflux valves described with other low pressure reservoirs would not be admissible and their particular advantages of preventing reflux should not be outweighed by the complications."

Upper Urinary Tract Infections Should be Minimized

Although technical improvements in ureterosigmoidostomy have reduced the incidences of lethal sepsis, symptomatic upper urinary tract infections with radiologic deterioration of the kidneys are still seen in approximately 50% of patients. Bacteriuria after ileal conduit diversion occurs in 14 to 100% of patients and has been studied in more detail over the years (17). In contrast, there is a paucity of information about urinary infection after continent diversion. Urinary infection is rare in patients with orthotopic bladder substitution who void per urethra. Cher and Roehrborn found sterile urine in 12 of 13 patients with intermittent self-catheterization of ileocecal or Kock pouch who were not receiving suppressive antibiotics (18). Nevertheless, Mansson et al. reported significant bacteriuria with *Escherichia coli*, *Klebsiella pneumoniae*, *Pseudomonas aeruginosa*, and *Proteus morganii* in 22 of 35 patients with a right colon continent reservoir (19).

McDougal surmises that the increased incidence of infection in patients with urinary intestinal diversion is most likely the result of the decreased bacteriostatic activity of the urine, a reservoir of bacteria whose survival is not significantly impaired by the intestinal mucosal cell, translocation of bacteria from the bowel lumen into the blood when the bowel segment is distended, and in certain diversions unimpeded access to the renal parenchyma (20). It is encouraging, however, that despite bacteriuria, clinical signs of infections are rare unless associated with obstruction. Mansson et al. believe that continuous production of immunoglobulin, especially secretory immunoglobulin A, and mucins is important in preventing bacterial adherence to the mucosa (21). Long-term suppressive antibiotic therapy is usually not effective in sterilizing the urine in these instances, and antibiotics should be used judiciously only in patients with symptomatic infection.

Postoperative Fluid—Electrolyte and Acid-Base Imbalances Should be Minimized

The mechanism and effects of electrolyte and anion exchanges between urine and serum across the intestinal mucosa have been the subjects of academic curiosity since Boyd reported chronic acidosis in 1931 (22) and Ferris and Odel observed hyperchloremic acidosis after ureterosigmoidostomy in 1950 (23). Recently, McDougal has comprehensively reviewed the metabolic consequences of urinary intestinal diversion (20).

In both the ileum and colon, the fluid and electrolyte transfer occurs as an active process of absorption and secretion. Bicarbonate absorption depends on the rates of cation and anion exchanges. Because of selective hyperabsorption of chlorides more than the sodium ions, a net loss of bicarbonate ions in the lumen results in acidosis. Potassium flux in the bowel, however, is a passive process to maintain electrical neutrality when sodium is absorbed. Additional potassium loss can occur from chronic diarrhea and diuresis secondary to water absorption.

When stomach is used for the construction of a urinary reservoir, hypokalemic, hypochloremic metabolic alkalosis can occur (20). Hydrogen ion obtained from intracellular carbonic acid is secreted into the lumen in exchange for potassium. This secretion of hydrogen ion results in bicarbonate release into the systemic circulation with resultant alkalosis.

Minor degrees of hyperchloremic acidosis have been observed after enterourethrostomies and in catheterizing continent reservoirs. Up to 80% of patients who undergo ureterosigmoidostomy will demonstrate hyperchloremic metabolic acidosis (23). In other types of continent diversion using ileum or colon, the incidence varied between 10 and 65% (24). It is likely that a more careful metabolic study and arterial blood gas analysis will yield a higher incidence of these alterations, as evidenced in a recent study of patients with continent diversion in which all patients had mild systemic acidosis and a defect for urinary acidification (25). The factors influencing the occurrence and degree of metabolic alterations include the following.

1. The absorptive and secretory characteristics of the intestinal segment interposed in the urinary tract.
2. The duration of urinary contact with intestinal mucosa.
3. The total surface area of intestinal mucosa as modified by the length and configuration of the intestinal segment.
4. The baseline renal function and its capacity to withstand additional electrolytic changes.
5. The histologic and functional alterations of the mucosal villi, the extent of which depends on the time elapsed since the surgical procedure.

The activity of transport processes has been suggested to diminish with time.

Deleterious electrolyte derangements have been less common in patients with continent reservoir and intestinal orthotopic bladder substitution compared with those after ureterosigmoidostomy. However, periodic postoperative monitoring of electrolyte and acid-base status is essential so that corrective therapy with hydration, alkalizing medications such as sodium citrate or sodium-potassium bicitrate, and blockers of chloride transport such as chlorpromazine and nicotinic acid can be instituted appropriately in the event of any metabolic acidosis.

Malabsorptive Nutritional Disorders Should be Minimized

Removal of long segments of intestines for urinary reconstruction can lead to nutritional deficiencies from alteration of absorption processes. Use of large segments of the stomach may impair vitamin B_{12} absorption by decreased secretion of necessary intrinsic factor into the intestinal lumen. Vitamin B_{12} is absorbed from terminal ileum, and its deficiency is also expected when terminal ileum is used in urinary reservoir construction. Indeed, 25% of patients with an ileocolonic neobladder reported by Steiner et al. had low serum vitamin B_{12} levels (26). Resection of the distal ileum and ileocecal valve may result in decreased bile salt absorption, fat malabsorption, steatorrhea, and a consequent decrease in the absorption of fat-soluble vitamins. Increased transport of bile acids to the right colon may result in troublesome diarrhea that can be prevented with oral cholestyramine therapy (27). The loss of the ileocecal valve can lead to an excess of colonic bacteria in the ileum, thereby interfering with the absorptive processes and causing diarrhea. The overall incidence of postoperative diarrhea is uncommon and if present usually subsides in 3 to 4 months. Vitamin B_{12} deficiency should be assessed for years because the body reserve may become depleted. Loss of segments of large bowel is well tolerated and usually not associated with significant nutritional problems.

Carcinogenesis Factor

Clinically in 6 to 29% of patients with ureterosigmoidostomy and experimentally in the laboratory, it has been proved that a close apposition of urothelium and colonic mucosa in the presence of urine and feces leads to development of adenocarcinoma of colonic origin at the ureterointestinal anastomotic site (28, 29). The cause of this carcinogenesis is unclear. It is conjectured that urinary nitrates may be converted to active carcinogen nitrosamine by the fecal bacteria (30). Colonic epithelium further alters nitrosamine into a more actively carcinogenic hydroxylated form. Other possible etiologic factors include superoxide radicals and epidermal growth factor receptor proliferation induced by the urothelial colonic juxtaposition with feces and urine (31). Because modern continent urinary diversions are excluded from fecal stream, chances of carcinogenesis may be minimized. Moreover, in experimental animals, ileal epithelium proved to be immune to carcinogenesis (32). Therefore, a continent urinary reservoir constructed from small intestine may have the least propensity toward malignant transformation. The issue of carcinogenesis under similar circumstances of urinary diversion is riddled with ignorance and conjectures. Whether chronic bacterial colonies in a continent reservoir are also capable of converting carcinogens in the long run will be determined by further research and clinical vigilance.

Continence Should be Maintained So That Patients Can Control Urinary Elimination at Socially Acceptable and Convenient Intervals

Continence depends on the characteristics of the reservoir and its outlet. Technical considerations of creating a low-pressure commodious reservoir have been discussed previously. Essentially, detubularization and reconfiguration of the bowel segment create a urinary reservoir of generous capacity and low pressure, the two necessary elements for continence. Lower pressure in the reservoir also allows for the achievement of a better degree of resistance across the continence zone, resulting in dryness.

The outlet characteristics of the continent cutaneous diversions are constantly evolving. In 1950, Gilchrist et al. believed that continence can be dependent on the antiperistaltic function of the terminal ileum supplemented by the functional ileocecal valve (2). Other authors working on intact cecal reservoir found that Gilchrist's principles were unreliable. Since then, a variety of valve mechanisms have evolved that can provide reliable continence. The features of these continent catheterizable conduits include ileal spout valve, flutter valve, ink-well valve, intussuscepted ileum, and intussusception through ileocecal valve.

Other techniques based on the principle of enhancing the wall tension of the catheterizing conduit use plication of ileum or narrowing of the lumen by excising and resuturing ileum with reinforcing invagination sutures of the ileocecal valves when necessary. Whenever feasible, appendix can be used in the Mitrofanoff principle, carrying its base to the skin as a catheterizable stoma and implanting the tip of the appendix in a tunneled fashion into the reservoir (33). Bissada et al. (34) have shown that the appendix tip can be brought at the umbilicus as catheterizing stoma, making the procedure even simpler (see Chapter 32). Ultimately, the choice of continent mechanism to be constructed is settled by individual preference, taking into consideration the technical ease for the surgeon and the ease of catheterization by the patient.

Two prerequisites need to be fulfilled to achieve continence with orthotopic neobladder construction.

1. A detubularized, low-pressure reservoir of good capacity.
2. An intact urethra and its distal sphincteric mechanism.

The urethra should be carefully prepared as in radical prostatectomy, with special attention to maintaining the innervation of the urogenital diaphragm (35). The smooth muscle component of the distal urethral sphincter is innervated by predominantly sympathetic noradrenergic fibers and some parasympathetic cholinergic fibers. The striated sphincter muscle consists of fast twitch (for rapid contractions) and slow twitch (for prolonged enhanced tone and contraction) fibers that receive triple innervation—the pelvic nerves, pudendal nerve, and a combination of somatic and autonomic nerves. Anastomosis between the urethra and the intestinal neobladder should be accomplished with multiple interrupted sutures approximating the mucosae of the bowel and urethra.

Although daytime continence after bladder substitution is achieved and shows progressive improvement in a large percentage of patients, nocturnal incontinence remains a troublesome quality-of-life issue in a number of patients and continues longer than diurnal incontinence. Factors contributing to nocturnal incontinence include relaxation of the pelvic floor muscles and external sphincter during sleep; loss of the physiologic urethral sphincter recruitment reflex in response to contractions of the neobladder, probably due to damage to the pelvic nerves associated with radical cystectomy; and increased urinary output due to fluid shift into the hypertonic acidic urine of the intestinal neobladders.

CONTRAINDICATIONS TO CONTINENT URINARY DIVERSION

All individuals considered for cystectomy should be potential candidates for continent urinary diversion. The additional surgical trauma from continent diversion as an alternative to conduit diversion should not be prohibitive. It is important, however, to carefully discuss intermittent self-catheterization and therefore assess and ascertain the motivation and compliance of the patient. A noncompliant, uninterested patient or one with mental or physical disability that may hinder the capability of self-catheterization should not undergo continent urinary diversion. Compromised renal function with serum creatinine level greater than 2 mg is a relative contraindication. Often, the deteriorated renal function secondary to ureteral obstruction can be improved with percutaneous nephrostomy drainage. Obstruction due to the bladder cancer is expected to improve after cystectomy. Chronic inflammatory bowel diseases such as ulcerative colitis and Crohn's disease are contraindications.

Contraindications to orthotopic neobladder construction with enterourethral anastomosis include transitional cell carcinoma (TCC) of the prostate, TCC invading the prostatic stroma, multifocal urethral TCC, or carcinoma in situ. Urethrocystoscopic evaluation with necessary biopsy of any suspicious areas should be performed before surgery. All orthotopic neobladder patients run the risk of urethral recurrence of 3 to 18% and must be carefully followed with periodic cystoscopic and cytologic studies (36). Patients with recurrent urethral strictures are probably better served with cutaneous continent diversion. Similarly, a history of pelvic irradiation and intraoperative rectal injury during cystectomy should preclude a neobladder construction. Advanced age is not necessarily a contraindication. Although better continence rates have been reported in patients younger than 70 years, one should take physiologic age rather than chronologic age into the consideration of lower urinary tract reconstructions.

TYPES OF CONTINENT DIVERSION

The evolution of techniques of continent urinary diversion has continued steadily since the original attempt at ureterosigmoidostomy by Simon in 1852. During the past several decades, many ingenious technical innovations based on our better understanding of the reservoir and continence mechanism have established the validity, feasibility, and wider acceptance of continent diversion. The major milestones in this journey toward the ideal continent diversion can be classified as follows.

1. Continent urinary reservoir attached to an intact urinary sphincter mechanism (ureteroenterourethrostomy, neobladder, orthotopic bladder substitution) using detubularized ileum, ileocecal segment, sigmoid colon, or stomach (see Chapter 33).
2. Continent urinary reservoir using a surrogate sphincter mechanism.
   A. Using the anal sphincter:
      1. Ureterosigmoidostomy with its various modifications;
      2. Rectal bladder with abdominal terminal colostomy;
      3. Rectal bladder with juxta-anal fecal colostomy.

B. Artificial urinary sphincters:
1. Primary—around an incontinent outlet conduit;
2. Secondary—around an incontinent urethra.
3. Continent urinary reservoir with abdominal stoma for inter-mittent catheterization. In addition to low-pressure com-modious reservoir, continence is maintained by:
A. Various ileal valve mechanisms—intussuscepted nip-ple, spout valve, flutter valve, or ink-well valve;
B. Intussuscepted ileocecal valve;
C. Continence dependent on intact ileocecal valve and en-hanced wall tension of ileum by plication or tapering;
D. Continence based on intact appendix as outlet (see Chap-ter 32);
E. Mitrofanoff principle—using the appendix with its base as stoma and the tip tunneled into the reservoir.

URETEROENTEROURETHROSTOMY OR ORTHOTOPIC BLADDER SUBSTITUTION

In these procedures, a low-pressure, commodious reservoir or neobladder is created from intestinal segments such as detubu-larized ileum, ileocecal segment, sigmoid colon, or stomach for the purpose of collection and storage of urine. Emptying of this reservoir is achieved by spontaneous urethral voiding or by intermittent urethral catheterization. Because of the inherent necessity of preserving a competent outlet sphincter mechanism and the urethral conduit, it is essential to adhere to strict selec-tion criteria before these operations are undertaken.

In the past, women were excluded from bladder substitution procedures because of the higher risk of incontinence antici-pated with the short female urethra and relative weakness of the pelvic outlet muscles. However, recent surgical reports ad-hering to strict surgical principles of preserving the neuromus-cular integrity of the female continence mechanism have proven the feasibility of bladder substitution in female patients (37, 38). Other contraindications due to neoplastic involvement of the urethra have been discussed previously. Camey and LeDuc initially reported that in approximately 15% of patients, it was difficult to bring the ileum up to the urethra because of the short ileal mesentery (5). Such difficulties are not encountered in the newer ileal, ileocolonic, or sigmoid reservoir. The differ-ent techniques of bladder substitution procedures are elabo-rated in Chapter 33.

URETEROSIGMOIDOSTOMY

For nearly a century, ureterosigmoidostomy remained the pop-ular choice of urinary diversion until Bricker established the ileal conduit diversion in 1950 (4). With increasing experience, follow-up, and understanding of metabolic alterations, a num-ber of serious complications of ureterosigmoidostomy have be-come evident. The early complications relate to obstruction or leakage of the ureterocolonic anastomosis. Subsequently recur-rent pyelonephritis occurs in at least 50% of patients even after successful nonrefluxing ureteral implantation. Bissada et al.

(34) recently reported renal unit deterioration in 23% of pa-tients. Incidence of renal calculi and ureteral anastomotic ob-struction increases with time. For the management of hyper-chloremic acidosis, patients are invariably condemned to ingest potassium and alkali for life, which might become hazardous to elderly individuals with cardiac diseases. Reports of adeno-carcinoma developing commonly at the ureteral implantation site have been a subject of major concern, especially for younger patients. The need for frequent bowel evacuation during the night with occasional fecal soiling is a major impediment to quality of life.

Despite these prohibitive morbidities, interest in external appliance-free diversion has led to ingenious modifications of ureterosigmoidostomy. Kock et al. incorporated the following three concepts into ureterosigmoidostomy.

1. The rectum is functionally isolated by an isoperistolic intussuscepted nipple valve at the sigmoidorectal junction.
2. Ureters are implanted into the rectum using an antirefluxing technique.
3. The capacity of the rectal reservoir is augmented and intraluminal pressure decreased by adding a detubularized and folded ileal patch to the anterior wall of open rectum (39).

Early follow-up shows promising results regarding continence and urographic evidence of improvement or stabilization of the upper urinary tract. The question of long-term complications remains unanswered.

With a clear understanding of the potential side effects, alterations in quality of life, and need for lifelong follow-up, ureterosigmoidostomy remains a surgical alternative for pa-tients who are not candidates for orthotopic bladder substitu-tion or continent diversion.

RECTAL BLADDER WITH ABDOMINAL COLOSTOMY

To obviate the problem of fecal contamination and electrolytic imbalances in ureterosigmoidostomy, the sigmoid colon can be disconnected and brought out as a terminal colostomy. The remaining rectum with implanted ureter works as a continent urinary reservoir (40). The colostomy is managed with daily colonic enemas and usually does not require elaborate external appliances. Postoperative electrolyte imbalances are virtually absent. Recurrent pyelonephritis, however, continues to be a problem in approximately 30% of patients. Although the iso-lated rectal bladder offers some advantages, it is a noncompliant reservoir with significant occurrence of enuresis. In addition, any advantages gained over ureterosigmoidostomy are at the expense of the presence of a colostomy.

RECTAL BLADDER WITH JUXTA-ANAL COLOSTOMY

In this ingenious procedure, a rectal bladder is constructed. The transected proximal sigmoid colon is then brought down through the anal sphincter and sutured to the perineum in the form of a neoanus for fecal elimination. The intact anal sphincter is supposed to provide continence for both urine and feces (41). Various modifications of this surgical concept have met with sporadic success. In general, urologists have not been enthusiastic about this technically difficult procedure with inconsistent outcome.

NEOBLADDER WITH ARTIFICIAL SPHINCTER FOR CONTINENCE

Artificial urinary sphincters have been used successfully to achieve continence after substituting the bladder with an ileocolonic pouch (42). In patients with an absent or predictably damaged sphincter mechanism, the prosthesis has been implanted as a primary procedure at the time of neobladder creation. In the majority of instances, however, the device is used as a secondary procedure to rectify postoperative incontinence.

CONTINENT URINARY RESERVOIR WITH ABDOMINAL STOMA

The evolution of continent abdominal stoma dates back to 1899 when Watsuji described intussuscepted nipple construction for gastrostomy (43). For many years, urologists and enteric surgeons strived for the creation of the ideal continent internal reservoir. The idea of a continent, catheterizable reservoir rapidly progressed after Gilchrist et al. reported the ileocolonic reservoir with the end of the ileum brought out as the stoma (2). In recent years, innovations based on the sound understanding of reservoir hydraulics and ease of catheterization have resulted in several gratifying choices. Authors in subsequent chapters have elaborated on the available popular procedures.

CONCLUSION

In 1950, Eugene Bricker, the pioneer of modern urinary diversion, stated that "the concept of radical and amputative surgery could be carried to such a stage that what was left with the patient became a consideration of equal importance to that which was removed." Our continued quest into these considerations of the biologic alterations and complications of urinary diversion has widened our understanding and has helped us in the prevention and management of these postoperative morbidities. Modern urologists have widened these considerations to include maintaining self-image and improving overall quality of life as major concerns.

In the absence of effective systemic therapy, cystectomy remains the therapeutic choice for patients with invasive bladder cancer. Cystectomy itself profoundly affects the mental and emotional attitudes, personal and sexual relationships, working abilities, and leisure activities of the modern patient. The most obviously disruptive effect on the patient's lifestyle, however, results from any external urinary diversion. Avoiding the use of an external appliance becomes the major concern for the patient and relates directly to body image and social conve-

nience. To that end, numerous surgical techniques continue to evolve modifying the inlet, the reservoir, and the outlet to achieve the most suitable continent diversion. Almost all our patients are candidates for continent diversion after cystectomy. Whether a catheterizable reservoir or the more anatomic bladder substitution will be suitable needs to be judged and selected on an individual basis.

There can be no therapeutic panacea in a situation of such variance. When selecting alternative types of treatment we should remember that the surgical procedure that causes least alterations, provided cure is not vitiated, will afford the greatest quality of life. The physician must evaluate each individual's situation in relation to what is technically feasible and what is personally acceptable to the patient.

REFERENCES

1. Simon J. Ectopia vesicae (absence of the anterior walls of the bladder and pubic abdominal parietes); operation for directing the orifices of the ureters into the rectum; temporary success; subsequent death; autopsy. Lancet 1852;2:568.
2. Gilchrist RK, Merricks JW, Hamlin MH, et al. Construction of a substitute bladder and urethra. Surg Gynecol Obstet 1950;90:752.
3. Couvelaire R. Le reservoire ileal de substitution apres la cystectomy total chez l'homme. J d'Urol Nephrol 1951;57: 408.
4. Bricker EM. Bladder substitution after pelvic evisceration. Surg Clin North Am 1950;30:1511.
5. Camey M, LeDuc A. L'enterocystoplastie avec cystoprostatectomie totale pour cancer de la vessie. Ann Urol 1979;13:114.
6. Kock NG, Nilson AE, Nilsen LO, et al. Urinary diversion via a continent ileal reservoir: clinical results in 12 patients. J Urol 1982;128:469.
7. Ashken MH. An appliance-free ileocecal urinary diversion: preliminary communication. Br J Urol 1974;46:631.
8. Benchekroun A. Continent cecal bladder. Br J Urol 1982;54: 505.
9. Mansson W. The continent cecal reservoir for urine. Scand J Urol Nephrol 1984;85:8.
10. Hautmann RE, Egghart G, Frohneberg D, et al. The ileal neobladder. J Urol 1988;149:39.
11. Thuroff JW, Alken P, Riedmiller H, et al. The Mainz pouch (mixed augmentation ileum and cecum) for bladder augmentation and continent diversion. J Urol 1986;136:17.
12. Studer UE, Ackerman G, Casanova GA, et al. Three years' experience with an ileal low-pressure bladder substitute. Br J Urol 1989;63:43.
13. Hinman F Jr. Selection of intestinal segments for bladder substitution: physical and physiological characteristics. J Urol 1988;139:519.
14. Cheng C, Hendry WF, Kirby RS, et al. Detubularization in cystoplasty: clinical review. Br J Urol 1991;67:303.
15. LeDuc A. Mucosal groove antireflux uretero-ileal implantation. In: Hohenfellner R, Wammack R, eds. Societe internationale d'urologie reports: continent urinary diversion. Edinburgh: Churchill Livingstone, 1992:103.

16. Rogers E, Scardino PT. A simple ileal substitute bladder after radical cystectomy: experience with a modification of the Studer pouch. J Urol 1995;153:1432.

17. Stewart WW, Cass AW, Matsen JM. Bacteriuria with intestinal loop urinary diversion in children. J Urol 1979;122:528.

18. Cher ML, Roehrborn CG. Incorporation of intestinal segments into the urinary tract. In: Hohenfellner R, Wammack R, eds. Societe internationale d'urologie reports: continent urinary diversion. Edinburgh: Churchill Livingstone, 1992:3–47.

19. Mansson W, Colleen S, Mardh PA. Urine from continent caecal reservoirs: studies on chemical composition and bacterial growth. Eur Urol 1989;16:18.

20. McDougal WS. Metabolic complications of urinary intestinal diversion. J Urol 1992;1199:147.

21. Mansson W, Colleen S, Low K, et al. Immunoglobulins in urine from patients with ileal and colonic conduits and reservoirs. J Urol 1985;133:713.

22. Boyd JD. Chronic acidosis secondary to ureteral transplantation. Am J Dis Child 1931;42:366.

23. Ferris DO, Odel HM. Electrolyte pattern of the blood after bilateral ureterosigmoidostomy. JAMA 1950;142:634.

24. Boyd SD, Schiff WM, Skinner DG, et al. Prospective study of metabolic abnormalities in patients with continent Kock pouch urinary diversion. Urology 1989;33:85.

25. Koch MO, McDougal WS, Reddy PK, et al. Metabolic alterations following continent urinary diversion through colonic segments. J Urol 1991;145:270.

26. Steiner MS, Morton RA, Marshall FF. Vitamin B_{12} deficiency in patients with ileocolic neobladders. J Urol 1993;149:255.

27. Einarsson K. Metabolic effects caused by exclusion of intestinal segments. Scand J Urol Nephrol Suppl 1992;142:21.

28. Schipper H, Decter A. Carcinoma of the colon arising at ureteral implant sites despite early external diversion: pathogenetic and clinical implications. Cancer 1981;47:2062.

29. Starling JR, Uehrling DT, Gilchrist KW. Value of colonoscopy after ureterosigmoidostomy. Surgery 1984;96:784.

30. Stewart M, Hill JM, Pugh RCB, et al. The role of N-nitrosamine in carcinogenesis at the ureterocolic anastomosis. Br J Urol 1981;53:115.

31. Husmann DA, Spence AM. Current status of tumor of the bowel following ureterosigmoidostomy: a review. J Urol 1990;144:607.

32. Gittes RF. Carcinogenesis in ureterosigmoidostomy. Urol Clin North Am 1986;13:201.

33. Mitrofanoff P. Cystostomie continente trans-appendiculaire dans le traitment des vessies neurologiques. Chirurgie Pediatrique 1980;21:297.

34. Bissada NK, Morcos RR, Morgan WM, et al. Ureterosigmoidostomy: is it a viable procedure in the age of continent urinary diversion and bladder substitution? J Urol 1995;153:1429.

35. Walsh PC, Quinlan CM, Morton RA, et al. Radical retropubic prostatectomy: improved anastomosis and urinary continence. Urol Clin North Am 1990;17:679.

36. Alken P. The risk of urethral reconstruction after radical cystectomy. Scand J Urol Nephrol Suppl 1992;142:95.

37. Light JK. Total vesicourethral replacement in the female. In: Webster G, Kirby R, King L, et al., eds. Reconstructive urology. 2nd ed. Boston: Blackwell Scientific Publications, 1993:495–500.

38. Colleselli K, Strasser H, Moriggl B, et al. Hemi-Kock to the female urethra: part 2. anatomical approach to the continence mechanism of the female urethra. J Urol 1994;151:500. Abstract no. 1089.

39. Kock NG, Ghoneim MA, Lycke KG, et al. Urinary diversion to the augmented and valved rectum: preliminary results with a novelle surgical procedure. J Urol 1988;140:1375.

40. Ghoneim MA, Shehab El-Din AB, Ashamallah A, et al. Evolution of the rectal bladder as a method of urinary diversion. J Urol 1981;126:737.

41. Tacciuoli M, Laurenti C, Racheli T. Sixteen years' experience with the Heitz Boyer-Hovelacque procedure for exstrophy of the bladder. Br J Urol 1977;49:385.

42. Light JK, Scott FB. Total reconstruction of the lower urinary tract using bowel and the artificial urinary sphincter. J Urol 1984;131:953.

43. Watsuji J. (Cited by Skinner DG, Boyd SD, Lieskovsky G. Clinical experience with the Kock continent ileal reservoir for urinary diversion. J Urol 1984;132:1101).

30

Ileal and Colonic Conduit Urinary Diversion

Jerome P. Richie

Everything should be made as simple as possible, but not simpler.

ALBERT EINSTEIN

The challenge of devising a practical and effective alternative means of elimination of urine when the bladder could no longer function properly dates back to 1851, when John Simon diverted the flow of urine into the bowel (1). The first crude attempts involved crushing clamps or placement of foreign bodies to establish a fistula between the ureter and rectum, and most patients died of peritonitis or uremia. Tizzoni and Poggi, in 1888, were the first to transplant ureters into an isolated loop of ileum interposed between the ureters and the urethra (2).

The close proximity of the sigmoid colon and the attractive advantage of an intact sphincter mechanism made implantation of the ureters into the intact sigmoid colon a logical alternative for urinary diversion. As early as the 1880s, numerous investigators were attempting to solve the problems of ureterointestinal anastomoses into the intact sigmoid colon. Ureterosigmoidostomy was the procedure of choice for urinary diversion from 1880 until 1950. The techniques developed for use with ureterosigmoidostomy are worthy of review because much of our current knowledge about urinary diversion rests on these techniques.

The problem of reflux, especially of fecally contaminated material, was recognized as a potential problem with this form of urinary diversion. Coffey, in 1911, heralded the modern era of ureterointestinal diversion (3). He was studying the problem of prevention of reflux in the biliary system and in ureterosigmoidostomy and devised a flap valve or "tunneled" technique (Coffey I). With this technique, the slit end of the ureter was introduced into the bowel and attached by a transfixing suture, with the muscular coat of bowel and peritoneum sutured over the ureter in a submucosal gutter. Charles Mayo was the first to use this technique clinically, and the technique became known as the Coffey-Mayo operation. Subsequent work with intubated ureteral stents led to the description of the Coffey II operation in 1927.

Numerous investigators described techniques for implantation of ureters into the colon. There was, however, general dissatisfaction because of high mortality and morbidity. All these techniques relied on scarring and slough of the distal end of the ureter and resulted in varying and unpredictable amounts of obstruction at the ureterointestinal anastomosis. In 1949, Nesbit provided a major breakthrough with the creation of a direct elliptical spatulated anastomosis with suture approximation of ureteral mucosa to bowel mucosa (4). This technique, however, did not solve the problem of reflux.

Leadbetter and Clarke, with a far-sighted accomplishment, combined the tunneled technique of Coffey and the elliptical mucosa to mucosa anastomosis of Nesbit, thereby describing the "combined" technique in 1950 (5). This technique has withstood the test of time and remains the preferred technique for ureterocolonic anastomoses for colonic conduits. An equally effective and innovative technique, the open transcolonic implantation, was provided by Goodwin et al. in 1953 (6). This technique, similar to a Leadbetter-Politano ureteral reimplant in the bladder, allows creation of a submucosal tunnel from within the lumen of the sigmoid colon.

The results of ureterosigmoidostomy were far from ideal, but other reasonable options for urinary diversion were limited. The known complications could be attributed to obstruction, reflux, and pyelonephritis. Hydronephrosis was reported in 32% of patients, pyelonephritis in 57% of patients, and electrolyte abnormalities in 46% of patients, even with nonrefluxing anastomoses (7). Ureterosigmoidostomy was a contributing factor in the demise of many of these patients. The major alternatives included colostomy with rectal bladder or rectal pouch and colostomy through the rectal sphincter. None of these procedures produced satisfactory long-term results.

The end of the ureterosigmoidostomy era was heralded by several factors. Ferris and Odel, in a classic paper, explained the method of hyperchloremic acidosis as the troubling electrolyte abnormality. They related this problem to the increased absorption of urinary contents, especially chloride, resulting from prolonged contact of urine with bowel mucosa (8). Furthermore, the incidence of colon carcinoma has been reported in up to 11% of patients (9). At the same time, Bricker popularized the creation of a cutaneous conduit, initially from the colon at the time of pelvic exenteration and subsequently from the distal ileum (10). The conduit form of diversion had the advantage of shortened contact time of mucosa with urine and lessened the likelihood of hyperchloremic acidosis, a significant change from the previous systems of ureterosigmoidostomy. Surgeons, disappointed with the short-term and long-term results of ureterosigmoidostomy, easily accepted this new form of diversion; it rapidly became the procedure of choice after radical cystectomy. In 1954, Bill et al. described ileal conduit procedures for children, and many people with benign bladder dysfunction (such as neurogenic bladder or myelodysplasia) underwent urinary diversion for social reasons (11). The short-term follow-up was quite impressive, and hyperchloremic acidosis and pyelonephritis were much less of a problem than with ureterosigmoidostomy. However, as long-term data became available, ileal conduits were discovered to be far from an ideal form of urinary diversion.

Stomal stenosis was noted in up to 25% of patients, many of whom required several revisions of the ileal conduit stoma. Pyelonephritis and calculi formation were noted in 10% and 15% of patients. Most importantly, in patients with normal pyelographic appearance of the kidney before diversion, 8% had shown signs of deterioration within 3.5 years after diversion (12). Follow-up studies up to 10 years after diversion confirmed this high rate of deterioration of the kidneys. Although stenosis or technical problems could be defined as the cause of deterioration in some patients, there remained a number who had renal damage for no apparent cause. Reflux, especially of infected urine, had to be considered a contributing factor as it had been in patients with ureterosigmoidostomy.

Dissatisfaction with the ileal conduit led to the third era of urinary diversion, the addition of antireflux technique in colonic conduits. In 1966, Mogg popularized the colon conduit (13). The conduit form prevented the problems of electrolyte absorption, and the antireflux tunnel, borrowed from the developments in the ureterosigmoidostomy era, diminished the problems of reflux and renal deterioration. Strong laboratory evidence supported the superiority of nonrefluxing colonic conduits over ileal conduits; pyelonephritis after 3 months of diversion in an animal preparation was reduced from 83% in ileal conduits to 13% with colon conduits (14). Clinical experience has attested to the long-term superiority of colonic conduits.

The fourth era of urinary diversion is the continent cutaneous diversion or orthotopic bladder. Although many complex procedures had been described previously, difficulties with infection, the need for catheterization, and the complexity of the procedures in general had precluded widespread acceptance. Medical advances, especially the acceptance of the use of intermittent self-catheterization, have changed the premise for construction of continent supravesical diversion procedures. Experience with continent diversions after proctocolectomy led Kock to adapt this technique to continent ileal reservoirs for urinary diversion (15). Vast clinical experience has been gained and recorded with the use of a long segment of ileum with nipples to prevent reflux and provide continence (16). A variety of techniques have been described for use of a long segment of ileum or the ileocecal segment and entire right colon, with a variety of techniques to prevent reflux and provide continence. The continent cutaneous diversions and orthotopic bladder are discussed in detail in Chapters 31–33.

The ideal bladder substitute has yet to be described. Conduits are currently the procedure of choice for urinary diversion, but many problems remain. The construction of the conduit requires exact and meticulous attention to detail; complications may rapidly lead to mortality and increased morbidity. This section will deal with one option for urinary diversion in patients with benign and malignant disease and will include technical preparation as well as certain "tricks of the trade."

INDICATIONS

The majority of urinary diversion procedures are performed after radical cystectomy for carcinoma of the bladder. In such patients, several factors must be taken into consideration.

1. One must be cognizant of the multifocal nature of urothelial tumors and be certain that the remaining urothelial system is free of carcinoma before urinary diversion. Frozen sections of the distal ureteral margins should suffice to exclude carcinoma in situ of the ureter.
2. In selecting the proper conduit, the amount of prior therapy—especially radiation therapy—must be considered. Large fields and high doses of radiation therapy, especially in a patient with prior abdominal surgery, may render the distal ileum and distal ureter dangerous because of the likelihood of improper healing. Careful observation of the bowel at the time of initial exploration and before excessive manipulation is essential to avoid using bowel that has been damaged by radiation.
3. One must consider the age of the patient and the overall prognosis. With only a 60 to 70% 5-year survival rate, the potential problems of reflux and renal deterioration (especially in the fully developed adult kidney) may not outweigh the risks inherent in creation of antireflux anastomosis. Indeed, one may use the freely refluxing anastomosis to obtain retrograde studies of the ureters and renal pelvis for follow-up of the patient after radical cystectomy and Bricker urinary diversion.
4. In creation of a sigmoid conduit, the surgeon relies on anastomoses between the middle and superior hemorrhoidal arteries for adequate blood supply to the distal colonic segment. Because the hypogastric artery is ligated during cystectomy, the blood supply to the distal colon may be tenuous.

For the above reasons, a reasonable choice after cystectomy is the distal ileal conduit. In patients with increased amounts of radiation therapy, a jejunal or transverse colonic conduit may be selected, preferably without an antireflux mechanism. In many patients, continent cutaneous diversion or orthotopic bladder may be considered. These techniques are time consuming and may place the patient at increased risk if there are substantial medical problems. Patient motivation is an important factor, because many newer procedures can carry a higher morbidity and reoperation rate than the standard ileal conduit urinary diversion. Nonetheless, in selected patients, these alternatives are reasonable to consider, especially when one considers quality of life.

In patients who undergo total exenteration, the colonic conduit is clearly the procedure of choice. This technique obviates an ileo-ileal anastomosis, and the distal colonic blood supply to the rectosigmoid is of no concern. We reserve the nonrefluxing conduit predominantly for children with benign disease or for patients with neurogenic bladder who require diversion. Preservation of the remaining renal function is a significant concern for long-term survival of these patients.

PREOPERATIVE PREPARATION

Bowel preparation for the patient who will undergo ileal conduit diversion need not be as stringent as for the patient in whom a colonic segment will be used. Nonetheless, the routine preparation in all patients should consist of both mechanical and antibiotic measures to lessen potential complications of wound infection and sepsis. Although longer-term mechanical cleansing and a clear liquid diet was the preparation of choice, in the current time of reduced hospital stays, patients are generally admitted to the hospital on the day of surgery. In such circumstances, Colyte (Reed and Carnrick, Piscataway, NJ) can be used orally for effective mechanical bowel cleansing (17). Neomycin, 1 g orally every hour for 4 doses and then every 4 hours, and erythromycin base, 1 g orally 4 times daily, are begun one day preoperatively (18). This regimen effectively inhibits growth of anaerobic bacteria.

The patient should be well hydrated preoperatively. A central venous catheter may be placed and its position verified by radiograph.

Selection of the stomal site is a critical and important preoperative step. The preferred placement is midway between the umbilicus and the anterior superior iliac spine, in the right lower quadrant for a right-handed patient (Fig. 30.1A). The stoma should be just medial to the lateral border of the rectus muscle. The selected site should avoid bony protuberances, previous surgical scars, or areas of unevenness in the subcutaneous tissues. The aid of an experienced enterostomal therapist preoperatively is invaluable, both for the selection of the stomal site and for effective preoperative instruction of the patient and family. The site should be evaluated with the patient in supine, sitting, and standing positions, and if any question exists, the patient can wear an appliance filled with saline for several hours to verify proper positioning.

ILEAL CONDUIT

The patient is placed in the supine position with the table slightly extended, thereby widening the distance between the

costal cartilage and the true pelvis. A left paramedian incision is preferred, with extension to the symphysis pubis if cystectomy is to be performed in conjunction with the ileal conduit diversion (Fig. 30.1A). Fascial layers are divided in line with the incision, and the peritoneal cavity is entered. At the time of initial exploration, careful attention must be paid to the condition of the distal ileum. Radiation enteritis is manifest by pale discoloration of the bowel or numerous hyperemic vessels on the surface of the bowel serosa.

Preparation of Ureters

Posterior peritoneotomies are performed where the ureters cross the common iliac arteries, and a right-angled clamp and then moistened umbilical tape are passed underneath the ureter. Dissection should allow most of the periureteral adventitia to remain with the ureter to prevent ischemia. The ureters should be mobilized distally to well below the iliac vessels and then divided between chromic ligatures or large hemoclips. This will allow the proximal ureter to dilate, thereby facilitating the ureteroenteric anastomoses. If in conjunction with the cystectomy, sections of the proximal ureter should be analyzed for presence of frank carcinoma or carcinoma in situ. The ureters are mobilized craniad to the level of the lower pole of the kidney (Fig. 30.1B). Stay sutures of 4-0 chromic are placed at the cut end of the ureter to facilitate mobilization and to reduce damage to the ureter by excessive use of forceps.

A tunnel must be created posterior to the colonic mesentery and anterior to the great vessels to allow the left ureter to be brought to the right side. This tunnel should allow the left ureter to swing across in a gentle arc with absolutely no tension. The effective craniad limit of the tunnel is the inferior mesenteric artery. Blunt and sharp dissection can be used to free the area, and hemostasis can be obtained with small hemoclips. The left ureter is then drawn through the tunnel to lie in close proximity to the right ureter near the psoas muscle (Fig. 30.1B).

Preparation of Ileal Segment

In the absence of radiation changes, the preferred segment is the distal ileum, approximately 10 to 15 cm proximal to the ileocecal valve. The anatomy is relatively constant and permits dissection of the mesentery just medial to the ileocolic artery, basing the selected segment on the last branch of the superior mesenteric artery before the bifurcation (Fig. 30.2). A segment approximately 25 cm in length should be selected, with longer segments chosen for more obese patients or those in whom the segment must be placed in an unusual position. The mesenteric incision should be much longer for the distal segment, as it will be necessary to provide length to reach the cutaneous surface. The proximal mesenteric incision should be short to protect the blood supply to the isolated segment (Fig. 30.2). If any question exists regarding the blood supply to the isolated segment, cross-table illumination will reveal the mesenteric

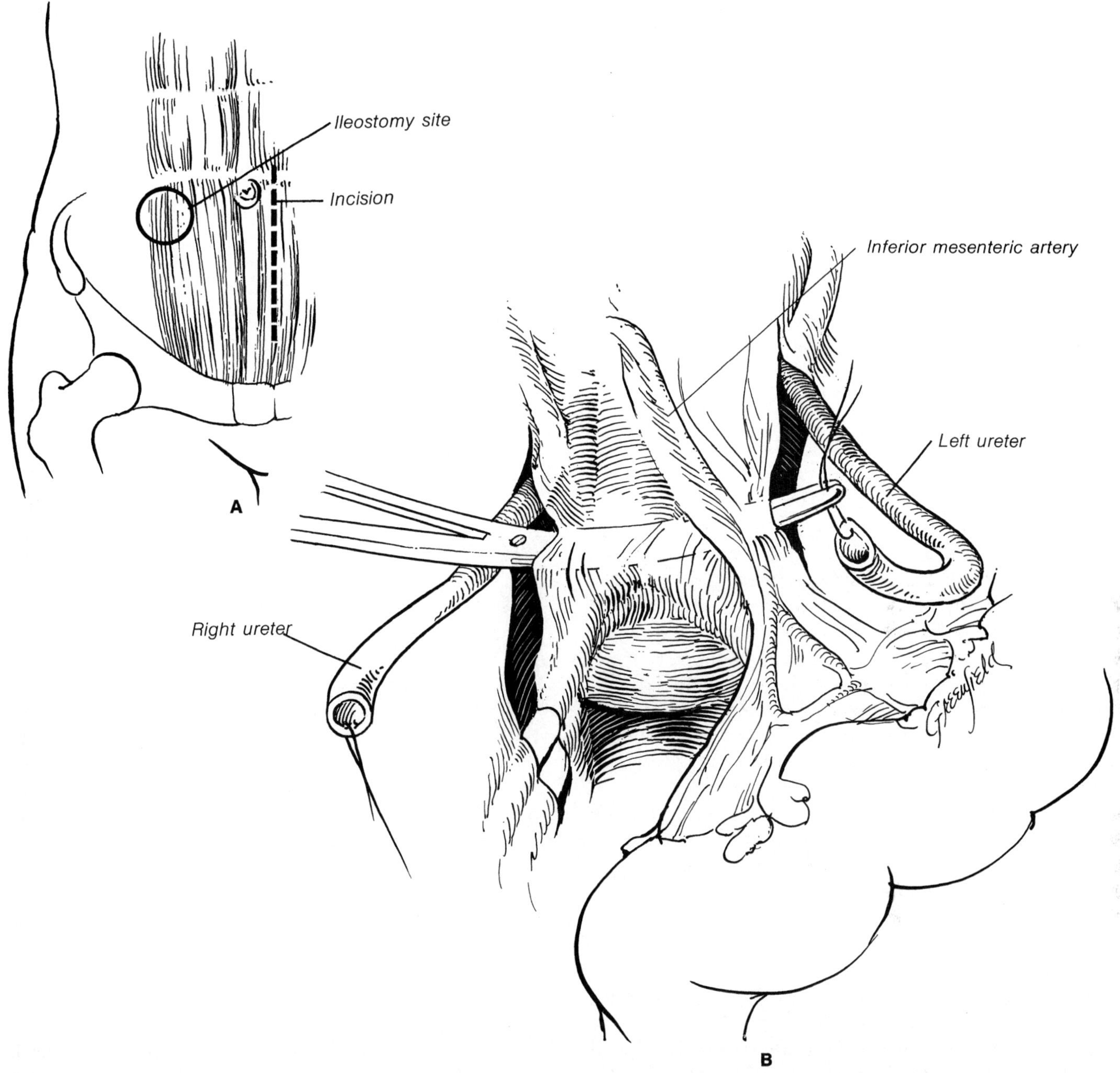

Fig. 30.1.   A. Ideal placement for the stoma in the right lower quadrant. The stoma should lie at the lateral border of the rectus muscle, halfway between the umbilicus and the anterior superior iliac spine. A left paramedian incision is preferred. **B.** A tunnel has been created underneath the sigmoid mesentery, and the left ureter is being pulled through the newly created tunnel. Stay sutures of 4-0 chromic catgut minimize manipulation of the ureteral mucosa.

arcades. A 0.25-in Penrose drain is placed at the proximal and distal ends of the proposed mesenteric incisions, and the peritoneal reflection is divided. Small vessels in line with the mesenteric incisions are doubly clamped, divided, and ligated with 4-0 silk ligatures. The mesentery is cleared from the bowel surface for a distance of 2 to 3 cm, and bowel clamps are applied. The clamps are placed in a 45° angle away from the antimesenteric surface on the intact bowel side and straight across at a 90° angle on the conduit side (Fig. 30.2). This maneuver avoids ischemia of the antimesenteric side of the proximal and distal bowel segments to be anastomosed by enteroenterostomy.

Incision of the proximal bowel segment is performed first, and the conduit end immediately closed with a running Parker-Kerr suture of 3-0 chromic. A running layer of vertical mattress sutures is placed to close the butt end of the loop and reinforced by a second running layer of seromuscular mattress sutures, creating a double inverting seromuscular closure (Fig. 30.3A). Additional reinforcement is provided by interrupted Lembert

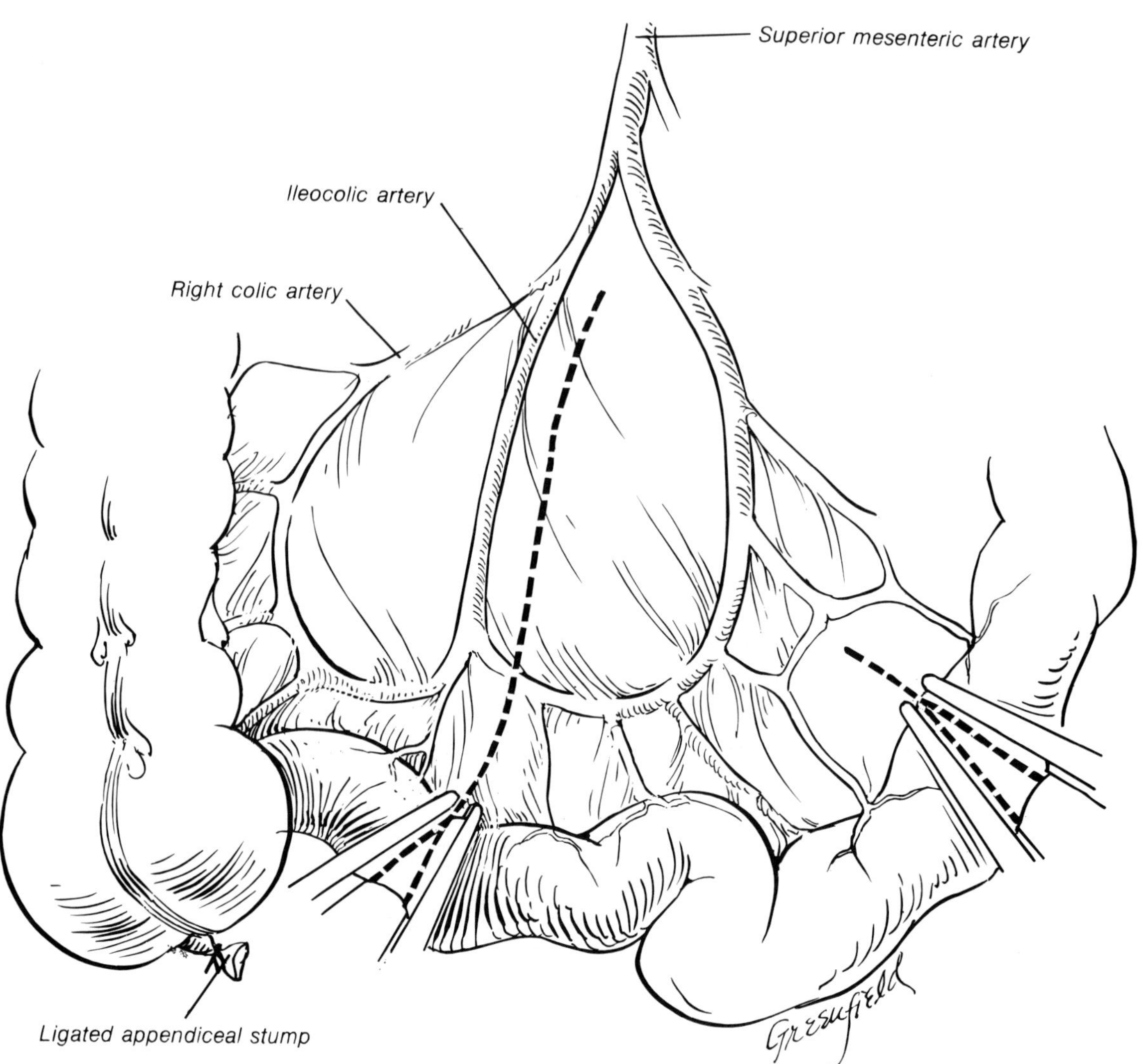

Fig. 30.2. Mesenteric incision for the creation of an isolated ileal conduit. A short proximal incision and a longer distal mesenteric incision ensure adequate mobility without compromise of blood supply. Clamps are placed at a 45° angle on the intact bowel side to prevent ischemia.

sutures of 4-0 silk in the seromuscular portion of the bowel only (Fig. 30.3). Prompt closure of the proximal end of the loop ensures an isoperistaltic segment. The distal end of the conduit is divided between clamps and the segment allowed to drop caudad (Fig. 30.3B). A standard enteroenterostomy is performed. We prefer a two-layer closure with interrupted 4-0 silk sutures for each layer (Fig. 30.4). The mesenteric window is closed with interrupted 4-0 silk sutures with care taken not to compromise the blood supply to the enteroenterostomy. TA-55 and GIA staplers can be used as an alternative. Permanent staples should not be placed in the butt end of the ileal conduit.

Ureteroileal Anastomosis

The bowel is packed out of the way, and the closed end of the loop is placed near the psoas muscle to estimate the appropriate length for the ureters. The left ureter is then divided and spatulated on its medial border, and a stay suture is placed to mini-mize trauma (Fig. 30.5A). Care must be taken to ensure that the ureter has not been twisted or angulated. A small ellipse of serosa and mucosa is removed sharply approximately 2 cm from the closed end of the loop. Forceps placed into the lumen of the ureter allow exact placement of sutures of 5-0 coated Vicryl (Ethicon, Sommerville, NJ) (cutting needle) without trauma to the ureteral mucosa. The apical suture is placed first, approximated to the ileum by incorporating a small amount of mucosa and a larger amount of serosa, and tied with the knots on the outside (Fig. 30.5B). This technique allows the ureter to extend into the enterotomy and obviates tension of the anastomosis. The stay suture is used to manipulate the ureter from side to side, allowing precise placement of alternating interrupted sutures until the anastomosis is secure. Five to six sutures will usually suffice, and stents are not routinely used. The last two or three sutures are placed and tagged, and a fine right-angle ensures the patency of the ureter and the ileal opening before the final closure. A similar procedure is

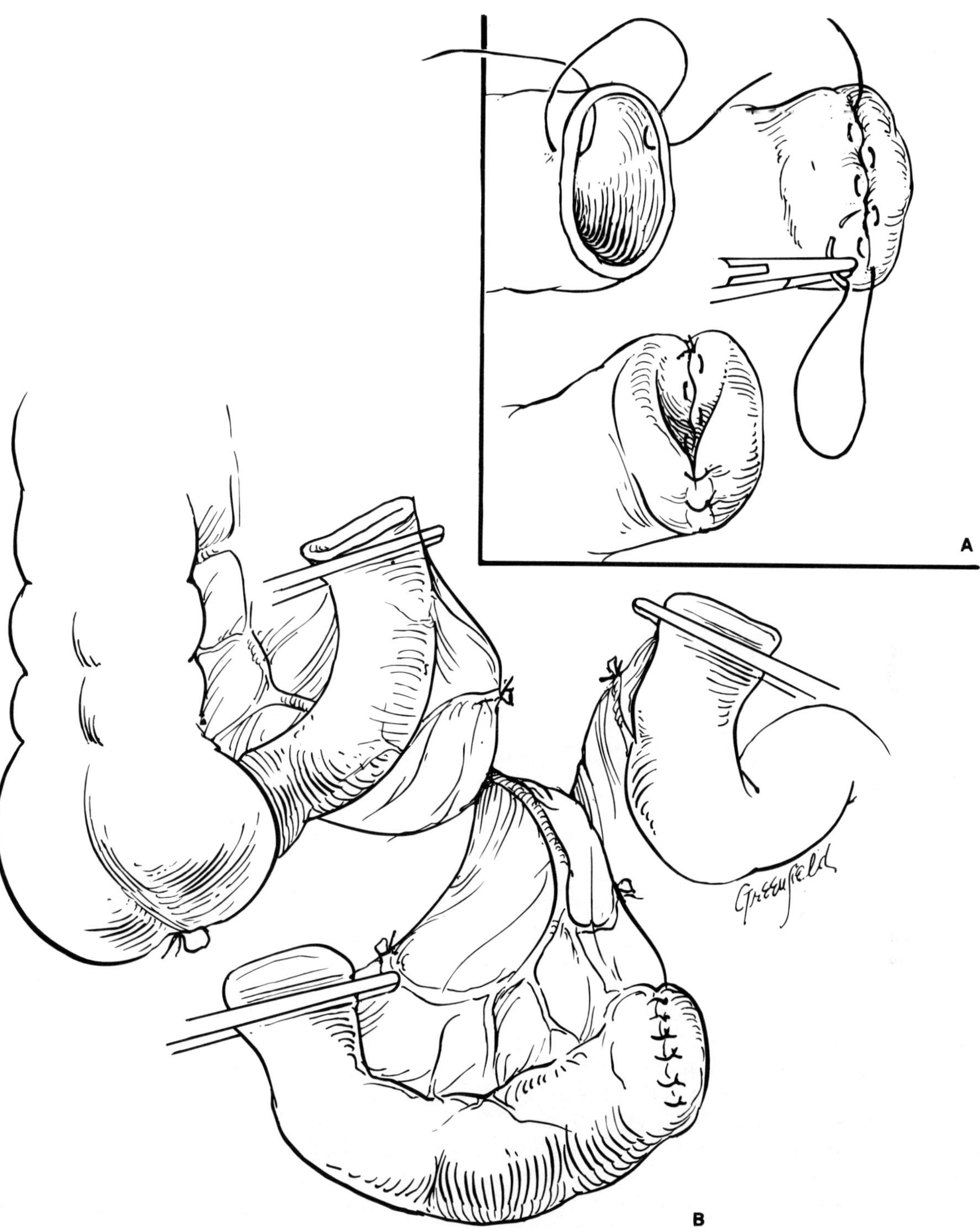

Fig. 30.3. **A.** Inset: Closure of the butt end of the ileal conduit is accomplished by double-layered running inverted sutures (Parker-Kerr) and is reinforced by a separate layer of interrupted 4-0 silk sutures. **B.** The isolated ileal conduit is positioned caudad in preparation for enteroenterostomy.

performed for the right ureter, with placement on the right side of the loop approximately 1 cm more distal from the closed end of the loop (Fig. 30.5C).

After the anastomoses are completed, the closed end of the ileal conduit may be sutured to the psoas muscle or sacral promontory with one or two seromuscular sutures of 4-0 silk.

Great care must be taken to prevent angulation of the ureters during this step. No attempt is made to place the anastomoses into the retroperitoneal space because radical cystectomy, performed concomitantly in many cases, makes this impossible. The small trap that is left between the sigmoid mesentery and the base of the ileal loop should be closed carefully with inter-

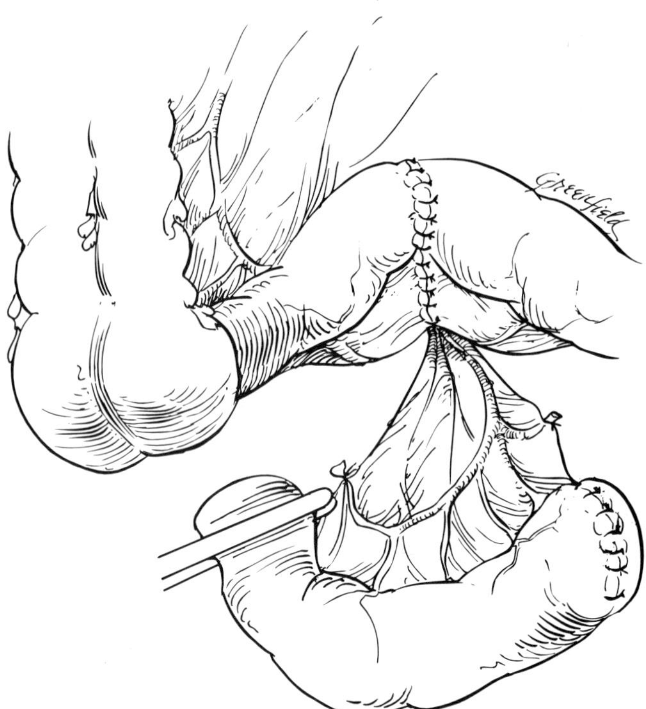

Fig. 30.4. Enteroenterostomy has been completed, and the mobile isolated segment is ready to receive the ureters.

rupted 4-0 silk sutures to prevent internal small bowel herniation and possible obstruction.

Stomal Preparation

The muscular layers of the abdominal wall are grasped with heavy Kocher clamps, and the subcutaneous tissue is grasped with towel clips and held at the approximate level of closure before construction of the ileal stoma. This technique will avoid shifting or shuttering of the muscular layers during wound closure with subsequent obstruction of the ileal conduit. At the preselected site (marked by a scratch or tattoo before skin preparation), an ellipse of skin and subcutaneous tissue approximately the size of a quarter is excised with the orientation along Langer's line (Fig. 30.6A). A plug of subcutaneous fat is removed with care not to undermine the cutaneous edges of the incision, and the anterior rectus fascia is exposed at the lateral border of the rectus muscle. Army-Navy retractors or lateral perineal retractors are helpful in providing the exposure in obese patients. A cruciate incision is made in the anterior rectus fascia, creating an opening large enough to admit two fingers (Figs. 30.6B and 30.6C). The rectus muscle may be separated by blunt dissection with Kelly clamps, with care taken to avoid the inferior epigastric vessel (Fig. 30.6D). A cruciate incision is made in the posterior rectus fascia and peritoneum, with care taken to avoid injury to the underlying bowel (Fig. 30.6E). The opening should easily permit two fingers to pass without tension. Slight angulation from the skin

surface through the various layers will create a cone-shaped opening and prevent any problem with dead space (Fig. 30.6F).

Before delivery of the loop through the stomal site, four quadrant sutures of 3-0 chromic catgut are placed through the anterior rectus fascia and the posterior rectus fascia and are temporarily clamped. This technique excludes the rectus muscle and allows a firm anchoring of the ileal loop to both the anterior and posterior rectus fascia, thereby preventing herniation. The ileal segment is then brought through the opening and should protrude at least 3 to 4 cm above the skin level (Fig. 30.7A). If this can be accomplished without tension, the tagged anterior and posterior rectus fascia sutures are placed through the seromuscular layer of the emerging ileum and are tied (Fig. 30.7A). Additional sutures may be placed between the anterior rectus fascia and the seromuscular layer of the ileum to close any additional gaps and prevent herniation. Eversion of the stoma is created by a modified Brooke technique. It is imperative that a protruding or "bud" stoma be created rather than a flat or level stoma because of subsequent problems of application of the appliance and leakage. Quadrant sutures of 4-0 Dexon are placed through the subcuticular tissue just at the cutaneous margin, through the seromuscular layer of the ileum, approximately 1 cm above the fascial fixation, and through the full thickness of the bowel at its distal edge (Fig.

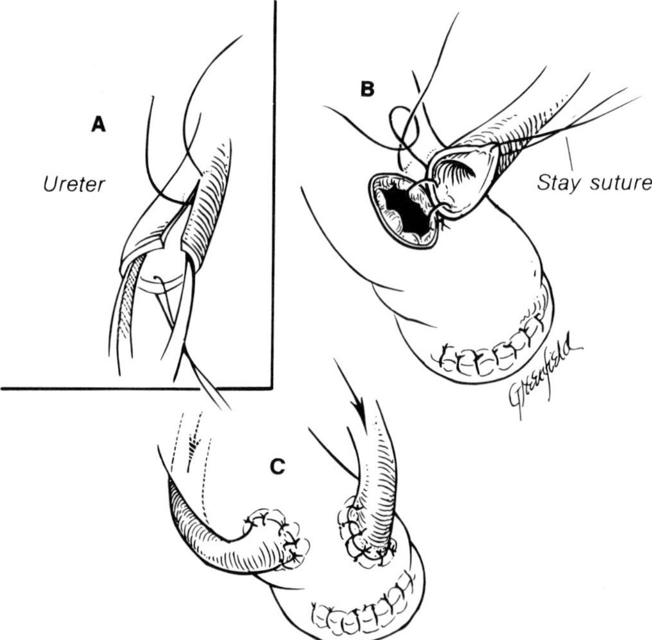

Fig. 30.5. **A.** Elliptical spatulation of the ureter is performed, and the apical suture is placed. Note the use of forceps to spread the ureter and to prevent handling of the mucosa. Note also the stay suture placed at the 12-o'clock position to aid in completion of the anastomosis. **B.** The apical suture of the ureteroileal anastomosis has been completed, and additional sutures are being placed in staggered fashion. The stay suture on the 12-o'clock position of the ureter aids in manipulation of the ureter from side to side for better visualization. **C.** Both ureteral anastomoses have been completed. The right ureteroileal anastomosis is 1 cm distal to the left anastomosis, preventing ischemia between the two anastomoses.

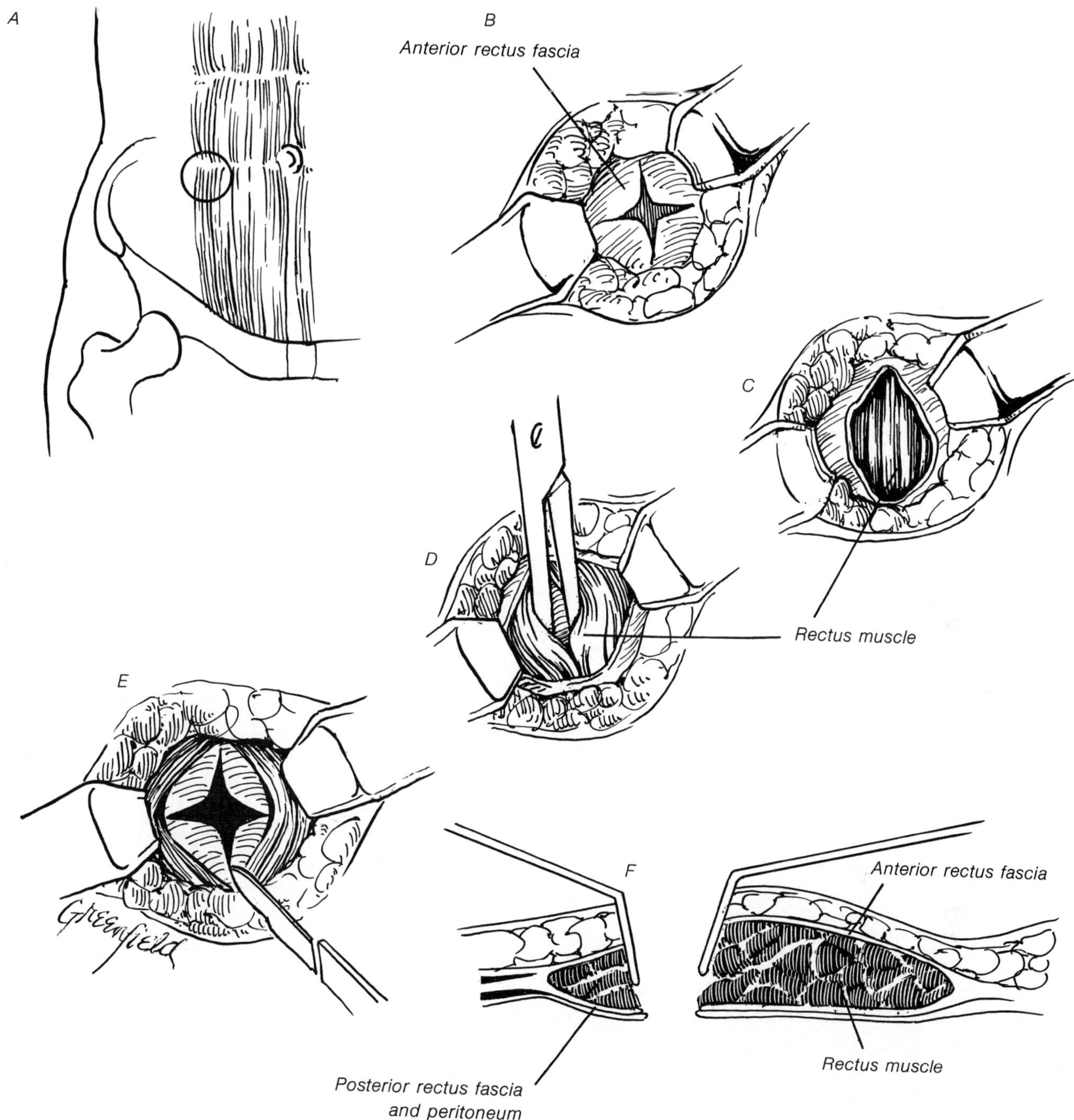

Fig. 30.6. **A.** An ellipse of skin and subcutaneous tissue is excised at the predetermined stomal site. **B and C.** A cruciate incision is made in the anterior rectus fascia, exposing the rectus muscle. **D.** The rectus muscle is separated in line with the incision. **E.** A cruciate incision is made in the posterior rectus fascia and peritoneum. **F.** Lateral view of the stomal creation. Note the cone-shaped appearance preventing undermining of the skin edge.

30.7B). Placement of four quadrant sutures in this fashion will allow turning of the stoma on itself, much like the French cuff of a sleeve, and allow fixation with a good protruding stoma (Fig. 30.7C). Additional sutures may be placed between the subcuticular tissue and the mucosa of the everted stoma. Care must be taken in the area of the mesentery at 12-o'clock to 1-o'clock to prevent strangulation or compromise the blood supply. Protrusion of the stoma at least 1 cm above the skin level allows effective diversion of efflux into the external collecting system and should prevent ileostomy dysfunction in well over 90% of patients (19). The completed ileal conduit is shown in Figure 30.8. Stents are not routinely used unless the patient has undergone radiation therapy or there is concern about the healing potential of the patient. Other authors, however, prefer to use stents routinely (20).

In patients with severe pulmonary problems or neurogenic

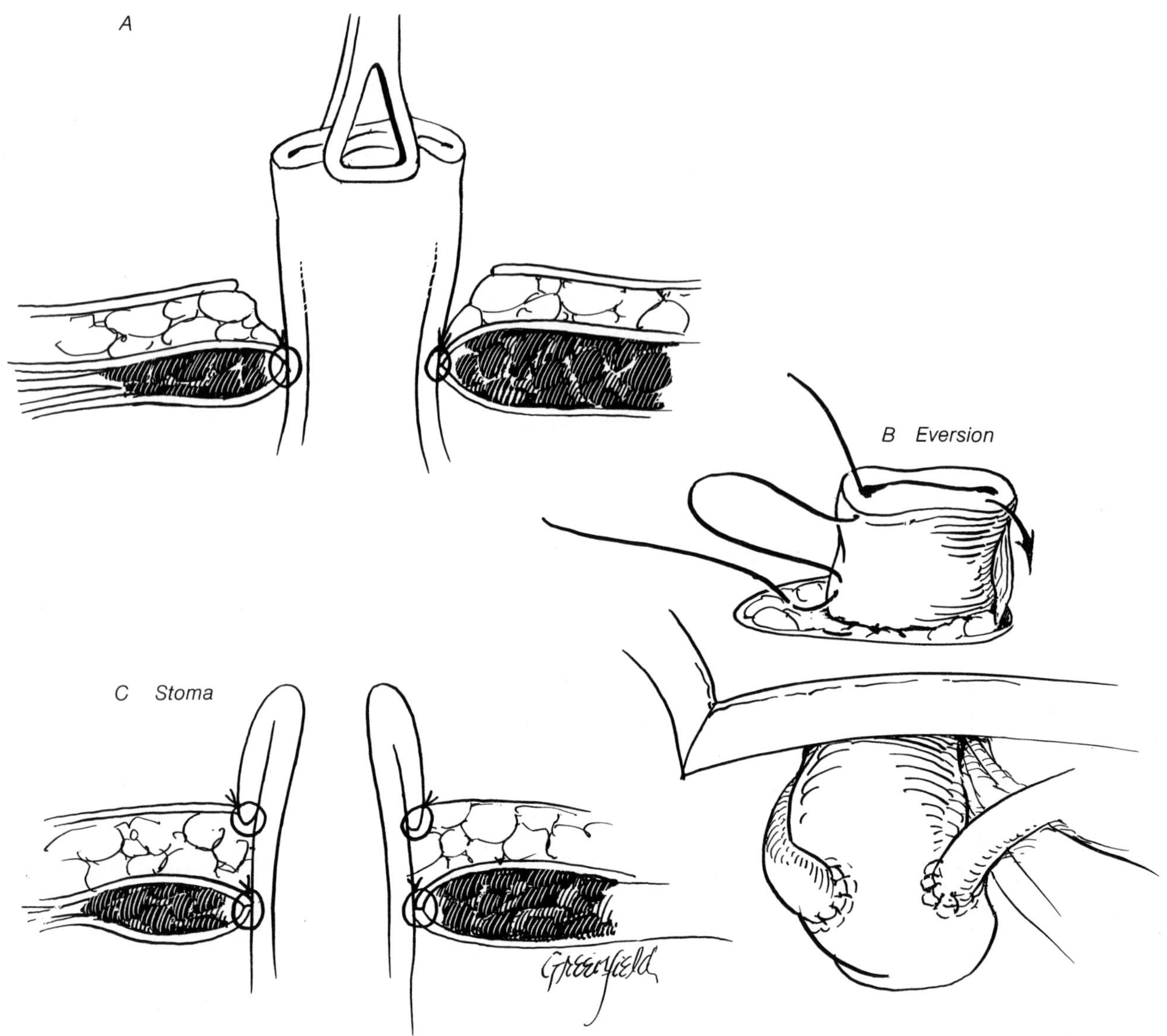

Fig. 30.7. **A.** The stoma, grasped with a noncrushing clamp, has been delivered to well above the skin level. Fixation sutures of 3-0 chromic incorporate anterior rectus fascia, posterior rectus fascia, and seromuscular portion of the emerging ileal loop. This effectively excludes the rectus muscle. **B.** Maturation of the stoma is accomplished by interrupted sutures in the subcuticular layer, emerging ileum, and full-thickness ileum. Four quadrant sutures are placed. **C.** Tying the four quadrant sutures results in a French cuff with a double layer of ileum, creating a bud or protruding stoma.

bladder, in whom prolonged ileus may be anticipated, a gastrostomy tube may be placed. Otherwise, a nasogastric tube is left for several days until active bowel sounds are present. A no. 10 closed-suction drain (Jackson-Pratt) is routinely used. A 16F red rubber catheter is sewn into the loop to prevent obstruction from edema.

Postoperative Care

Nasogastric drainage is established by low intermittent suction for 3 to 4 days until bowel function is adequate as manifested by bowel sounds and passage of flatus. Adequate hydration in the postoperative period is important, and the use of volume expanders is necessary in conjunction with radical cystectomy.

Instructions by an enterostomal therapist are important for the care of the ileostomy and for the fitting of the permanent appliance.

A postoperative urinary pouch is applied in the operating room. The author's preference is one of the vinyl pouches cut to fit the diameter of the stoma with an additional $\frac{1}{16}$-in clearance between the stoma and the opening in the face plate. Karaya washers are to be avoided because they react with the urine and produce a gelatinous mass with swelling. Attendance by an enterostomal therapist in the postoperative period will help familiarize the patients with the stoma and the proper techniques for applying the collecting device.

Permanent equipment of plastic pouches with various mounting rings, belts, and valves for emptying the urine is

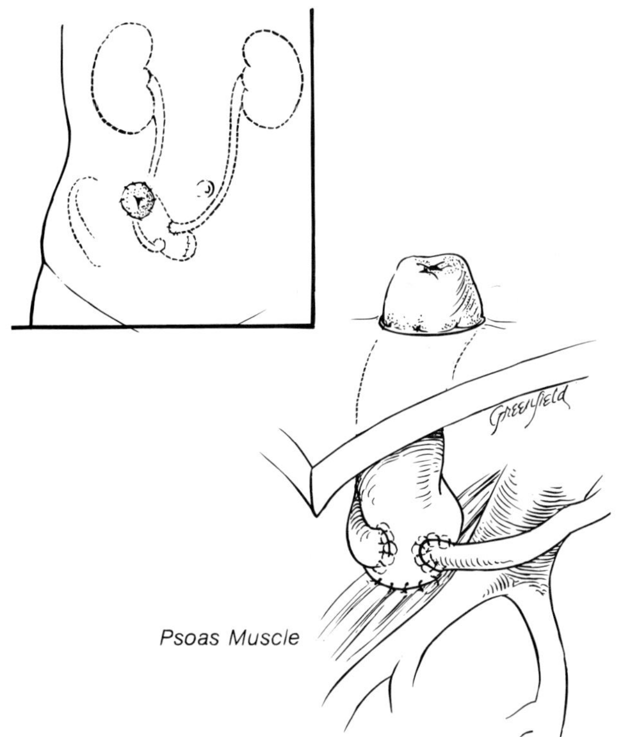

Fig. 30.8. Completed ileal loop. The ileal conduit has been anchored to the psoas muscle, and the ureters lie without tension or angulation. A protruding bud stoma has been created.

available and can be fitted in the postoperative period. However, shrinkage of the stoma will occur over the first several weeks and may necessitate ordering a smaller size face plate with time. The ileostomy should be recalibrated for shrinkage approximately 3 to 4 weeks postoperatively and again 6 weeks later. A maximum distance of $\frac{1}{16}$ in should exist between the stoma and face plate; otherwise, skin reaction with urine will occur.

Periodic follow-up visits with the enterostomal therapist are important at 3 months, 6 months, and 1 year postoperatively to ensure adequate manipulation of the stomal appliance. Loop cultures and residual urine should be measured at each visit. An intravenous pyelogram should be obtained early in the postoperative period and again at 6 months to 1 year postoperatively.

Long-Term Complications

The two most common complications following ileal conduit urinary diversion are stomal stenosis and ureteral ileal strictures. Stomal stenosis can be obviated by careful construction of the stoma using an everting technique to have a bud or protruding stoma. In patients with a retracted stoma, the enterostomal therapist can be helpful in using different face plates or other techniques to prevent problems. If severe stricturing around the stomal site occurs, revision of the ileal conduit may be necessary.

Ureteral ileal anastomotic strictures most commonly occur as a later phenomenon representing some component of ischemia. The classic treatment is open surgical revision, although endourologic procedures with percutaneous nephrostomy and balloon dilation along with indwelling stents have allowed correction of the problem without open surgical repair (21). In elderly patients or patients with poor prognosis, a permanent indwelling stent may be used (22).

Summary

The ileal conduit urinary diversion has withstood the test of time. Although reflux may be associated with some progressive renal deterioration in isolated patients, the ease of operation—coupled with relatively stable long-term effects—has allowed ileal conduit urinary diversion to achieve a place of prominence in patients who require urinary diversion. The potential for complications exists; therefore, meticulous attention to detail must be incorporated into the construction of an isolated ileal conduit urinary diversion.

COLONIC CONDUIT

The advantage of the colonic conduit is the ability to create antireflux mechanisms. This form of urinary diversion, popularized by Mogg in 1966, has the theoretical advantage of preventing reflux and therefore reducing pyelonephritis or renal deterioration. Although colonic conduit seems to be superior in the long run, this superiority depends on preventing reflux and not increasing the incidence of obstruction at the ureterocolonic anastomoses. The experience gained from ureterosigmoidostomy has been used and applied to the isolated colonic conduit.

Although the sigmoid conduit may be used, this segment should not be incorporated in conjunction with a radical cystectomy because of the tenuous blood supply to the distal colon. The most common indication in 1995 for colonic conduits is the transverse colon conduit in patients who have received large amounts of radiation.

Thorough knowledge of the anatomy of the colon and its segmental blood supply is mandatory. Transverse colon conduits will be based on the middle colic artery, whereas sigmoid conduits will be based on the inferior mesenteric artery. As a suitable length of the colon is selected, it should be made longer than anticipated because it will tend to contract once divided. Generally, a segment approximately 20 to 25 cm in length is used. Distal and proximal mesenteric incisions are made as described for ileal conduit urinary diversion. The colon is closed with a careful end-to-end bowel anastomosis using interrupted silk sutures or staples. The ureters are mobilized as for ileal conduit urinary diversion.

The advantage of the colonic conduit is the ability to create antirefluxing tunnels. Tunnels are created with staggered, 3-cm linear incisions in the taenia, near the proximal end of the conduit. It is helpful to inject several milliliters of 1 to 100,000 solution of epinephrine and saline beneath the muscularis to reduce bleeding and allow development of the submucosal plane. Circular muscle fibers are divided until the mucosa can be visualized. Once the mucosal plane has been developed, a spatulated mucosal-to-mucosal ureteral colonic anastomosis can be performed. The tunnel can then be closed with fine Vicryl or Dexon sutures. The tunnel should be 3 to 4 cm long and sufficiently developed to provide ample room for the ureter. Good muscular backing is important to prevent reflux.

The stomal creation is similar to that described for ileal conduit diversion. The opening in the skin should be no more than 1.5 inches in diameter; colonic stomas do have a tendency to be more redundant than ileal stomas. The colon should be secured to the anterior and posterior fascia with interrupted 3-0 chromic sutures and an everting nipple formed with 3-0 Vicryl sutures. Loop stomas or myotomies are unnecessary because the long-term complications from colonic stomas are unusual.

Ravi et al. reported on 30 patients who underwent transverse colon conduit as a primary urinary diversion between 1986 and 1992. Many of these patients underwent refluxing ureteral colonic anastomoses; all patients had been treated with high-dose pelvic irradiation. There was no operative mortality, but there was a complication rate of 37% and a reoperation rate of 20%. Eighty-three percent of patients showed normal or improved serum creatinine levels postoperatively. This form of diversion can be considered in high-risk patients (23).

REFERENCES

1. Simon J. Ectopic vesical (absence of the anterior walls of the bladder pubic abdominal parietes); operation for diverting the orifices of ureters into the rectum: temporary success: subsequent death: autopsy. Lancet 1852;2:568.
2. Tizzoni G, Poggi A. Die wiederherstelung der Harnblase: experimentelle untersuchungen. Zbl Shir 1911;15:921.
3. Coffey RC. Physiologic implantation of the severed ureter or common bile duct into the intestine. JAMA 1911;56:397.
4. Nesbit RM. Ureterosigmoid anastomosis by direct elliptical connection: a preliminary report. J Urol 1949;61:728.
5. Leadbetter WF, Clarke BG. Five years' experience with ureteroenterostomy by the combined technique. J Urol 1954;73:67.
6. Goodwin WE, et al. Open, transcolonic uretero-intestinal anastomosis. Surg Gynecol Obstet 1953;97:1.
7. Wear JB Jr, Barquin OP. Ureterosigmoidostomy: long-term results. Urology 1973;1:192.
8. Ferris DO, Odel HM. Electrolyte pattern of the blood after bilateral ureterosigmoidostomy. JAMA 1950;142:634.
9. Zabbo A, Kay R. Ureterosigmoidostomy and bladder exstrophy: a long-term followup. J Urol 1986;136:396.
10. Bricker EM. Bladder substitution after pelvic evisceration. Surg Clin North Am 1950;30:1511.
11. Bill AH Jr, et al. Urinary and fecal incontinence due to congenital abnormalities in children: Management by implantation of the ureters into an isolated ileostomy. Surg Gynecol Obstet 1954;98:565.
12. Richie JP. Intestinal loop urinary diversion in children. J Urol 1974;111:687.
13. Mogg RA. The treatment of neurogenic urinary incontinence using the colonic conduit. Br J Urol 1965;37:681.
14. Richie JP, Skinner DG, Waisman J. The effect of reflux in the development of pyelonephritis in urinary diversion: an experimental study. J Surg Res 1974;16:256.
15. Kock NG, et al. Urinary diversion via a continent ileal reservoir: clinical results in 12 patients. J Urol 1982;128:469.
16. Skinner DG, Boyd SD, Lieskovsky G. Clinical experience with the Kock continent ileal reservoir for urinary diversion. J Urol 1984;132:1101.
17. Wishnow KI, et al. Effective outpatient use of polyethylene glycolelectrolyte bowel preparation for radical cystectomy and ileal conduit urinary diversion. Urology 1988;31:7.
18. Nichols RL, et al. Effect of preoperative neomycinerythromycin intestinal preparation on the incidence of infectious complications following colon surgery. Ann Surg 1973;178:453.
19. Artz CP, Hardy JD. Management of surgical complications. 3rd ed. Philadelphia: WB Saunders, 1975.
20. Regan JB, Barrett DM. Stented versus nonstented ureteroileal anastomoses: is there a difference with regard to leak and stricture? J Urol 1985;134:1101.
21. Vandenbroucke F, Van Poppel H, Vandeursen H, et al. Surgical versus endoscopic treatment of non-malignant uretero-ileal anastomotic strictures. Br J Urol 1993;71:408.
22. Sanders R, Bissada NK, Bielsky S. Ureteroenteric anastomotic strictures: treatment with Palmaz permanent indwelling stents. J Urol 1993;150:469.
23. Ravi R, Dewan AK, Pandey KK. Transverse colon conduit urinary diversion in patients treated with very high dose pelvic irradiation. Br J Urol 1994;73:51.

31

Continent Cutaneous Diversion

Kock Pouch

Stuart D. Boyd, Gary Lieskovsky, and Donald G. Skinner

The continent cutaneous urinary diversions owe their success to surgical pioneers such as Kock and Gilcrist, whose work in this area began more than 30 years ago (1, 2). Kock's continent ileal reservoir for urinary diversion is a modification of the continent ileostomy that he developed in the 1960s for patients undergoing proctocolectomy for ulcerative colitis. The main feature of his urinary diversion is the creation of a reservoir that has extremely low internal pressures, with afferent and efferent intussuscepted valves that prevent reflux and provide continence. Kock and his associates have shown how detubularized, double-folded ileal reservoirs demonstrate pressure characteristics and absorptive capacities unique among the various intestinal segments (3–7). These reservoirs can maintain a much lower internal pressure compared with the tubularized reservoirs. This low pressure is found to be critical for the long-term viability of the diversion. The Kock reservoir has also proven to be extremely reliable in preventing reflux due to a durable antireflux valve that requires minimal revision. With the presence of chronic bacteriuria in the reservoir secondary to intermittent catheterization, prevention of reflux is vital for maintaining renal function.

Our series of continent cutaneous ileal reservoirs for urinary diversion now exceeds 700 patients. A number of technical modifications and adjustments to Kock's original description have been made at our institution. These are aimed at reducing the incidence of late complications and the need for reoperation (8–10). In the past 10 years, the reservoir has also been modified for use in lower urinary tract reconstruction (bladder substitution) with primary anastomosis to the urethra. This form of neobladder diversion is becoming increasingly popular and has nearly replaced cutaneous diversions in most instances. Our experience has demonstrated that the continent diversions are not too difficult to perform or maintain. In fact, continent diversions, whether to the skin or to the urethra, should be able to replace conduit diversion in most instances. Patients will continue to demand to be informed about these types of diversions and about the associated quality-of-life issues.

SELECTION AND EVALUATION OF PATIENTS

Any patient who is a candidate for a urinary diversion is potentially suitable for a cutaneous Kock reservoir, as long as adequate bowel is available and life expectancy is reasonable. The patients should have the intelligence, maturity, and manual dexterity to care for their own diversion. The presence of prior radiation therapy does not preclude the procedure. We have performed continent diversions on a number of patients who have received up to 6500 cGy of pelvic radiation. In these cases, one has to be more careful in selecting the bowel segment, and patients who have had other abdominal operations before their radiation therapy will have an increased risk of complication. Radiated bowel will have a decreased compliance, and the resulting reservoir will take longer to get up to its maximum capacity.

During the past 10 years, bladder substitution procedures have become increasingly popular among male and female patients (Fig. 31.1) (11). The ability to void per urethra after cystectomy has a tremendous effect on a patient's quality of life. Bladder substitution, however, cannot be used in patients without a viable urethra, in men with bladder tumors involving the prostatic apex or anterior urethra, or in women with tumor at the bladder back. These now appear to be the practical indications for cutaneous diversion. Obesity does not appear to be an overriding factor in any patient. Unlike Camey, we have not had to abort any procedure for fear that a thick ileal mesentery would not allow the reservoir to reach to the skin or to the urethra (12).

If conversion of an ileal conduit to a continent Kock diversion is being contemplated, it is important to radiographically examine the ureteroileal anastomoses before surgery. If there is free reflux up the ureters on a loop-o-gram and no evidence of ureteral obstruction on intravenous urogram, the base of the old conduit with its implanted ureters may be preserved. At surgery, this portion of the conduit may be anastomosed directly to an appropriately shortened afferent limb of the Kock pouch.

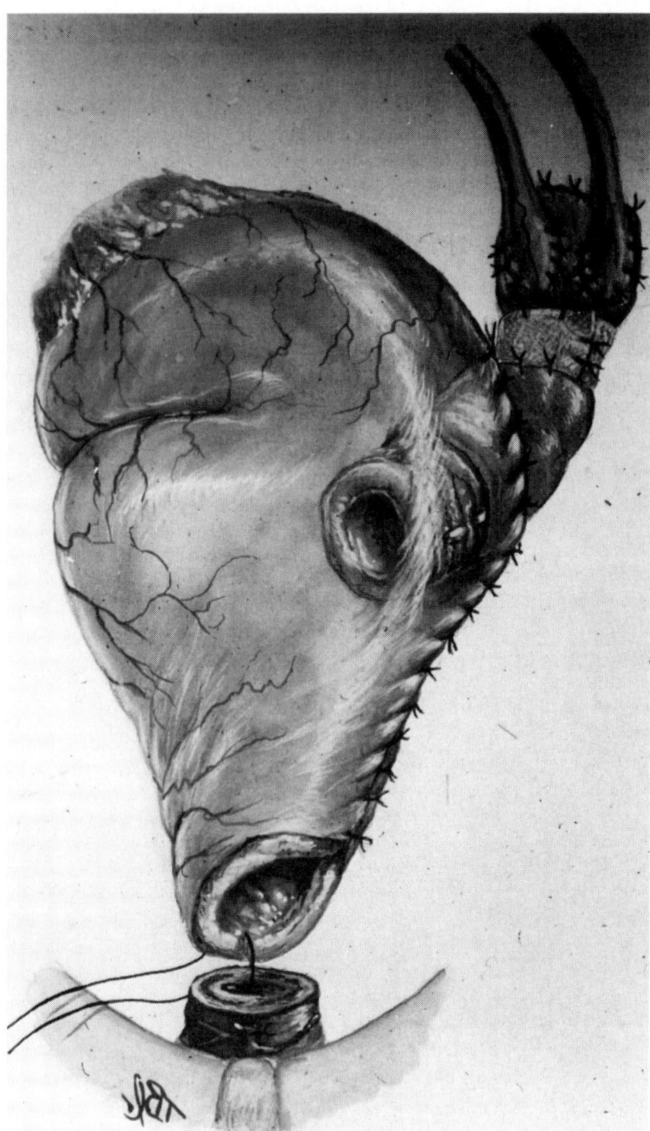

Fig. 31.1. The Kock reservoir adapted for bladder substitution with direct anastomosis to the urethra for internal urinary diversion. The procedure is not applicable in men with bladder cancer in whom the tumor extends into the prostatic urethra.

PREOPERATIVE PREPARATION

Patients are usually admitted to the hospital 1 day before surgery and ingest a clear liquid diet. A laxative is administered the morning of the preoperative day, and oral neomycin and erythromycin base are given on that afternoon and evening. Good hydration is maintained by initiating intravenous fluids that night. Routine preoperative parenteral nutrition is not used unless the patient's serum albumin/total protein levels are low.

The enterostomal therapist is invaluable in preparing cutaneous diversion patients before surgery. Detailed patient instruction by a dedicated therapist before and after surgery makes the postoperative transition and the catheterization ex-

perience much smoother and easier. The enterostomal therapist also provides necessary input in predetermining the general location of the cutaneous stoma. The stoma site can usually be low on the abdominal wall because avoidance of skin folds for ostomy bag placement is not a factor.

SURGICAL PROCEDURE

The patient is placed in a hyperextended supine position to widen the distance between the ribs and pelvis. A midline abdominal incision is made, curving to the left of the umbilicus and extending to the pubis if a cystectomy is to be performed in conjunction with the diversion. When a simultaneous cystectomy is being performed, that portion of the procedure should be completed first. In patients being converted from a previous ileal conduit diversion, a similar amount of time as that needed for the cystectomy will probably be spent delineating the old conduit and mobilizing the intestine. At this time, if preoperative radiologic evaluations of the ileal conduit reveal that the ureteroileal anastomoses are still in good condition, the base of the old conduit—with its implanted ureters—should be delineated and saved. We have had one case in which the ileal conduit was found to be greater than 80 cm in length and the entire continent diversion was created out of the old ileal conduit. The more likely scenario, however, is that just the base of the conduit will be saved for anastomosis end-to-end to an appropriately shortened afferent limb of the pouch.

In the patient without prior diversion, the ureters should be mobilized early, well below the iliac vessels, and divided between large ligaclips. This will allow the proximal ureter to dilate during the procedure and facilitate the ureteroileal anastomoses. A tunnel should be created beneath the mesentery of the descending colon and anterior to the aorta to allow the left ureter to smoothly swing over to the midline. This tunnel should be just below the inferior mesenteric artery.

Selection of the Ileal Segment

The segment of ileum to be used for the diversion must first be delineated (Fig. 31.2). If there has not been a prior bowel anastomosis, and in the absence of radiation-induced changes, the distal ileal division (efferent end) should be made approximately 15 to 20 cm from the cecum. This will allow for a long mesenteric division in the avascular plane between the terminal branch of the superior mesenteric artery and the ileocolic artery. This division can be made back to the base of the mesentery and will provide the necessary length and mobility for the diversion to reach the skin easily. If there is an existing ileal conduit, the prior small bowel anastomosis should be identified and excised. The prior mesenteric division should be opened for its full extent, and the efferent end of the pouch begun at this point.

Silk sutures are used to mark the individual segments of the reservoir—17 cm for the efferent (distal) limb, 22 cm for each of the two arms of the reservoir, and 17 cm for the afferent

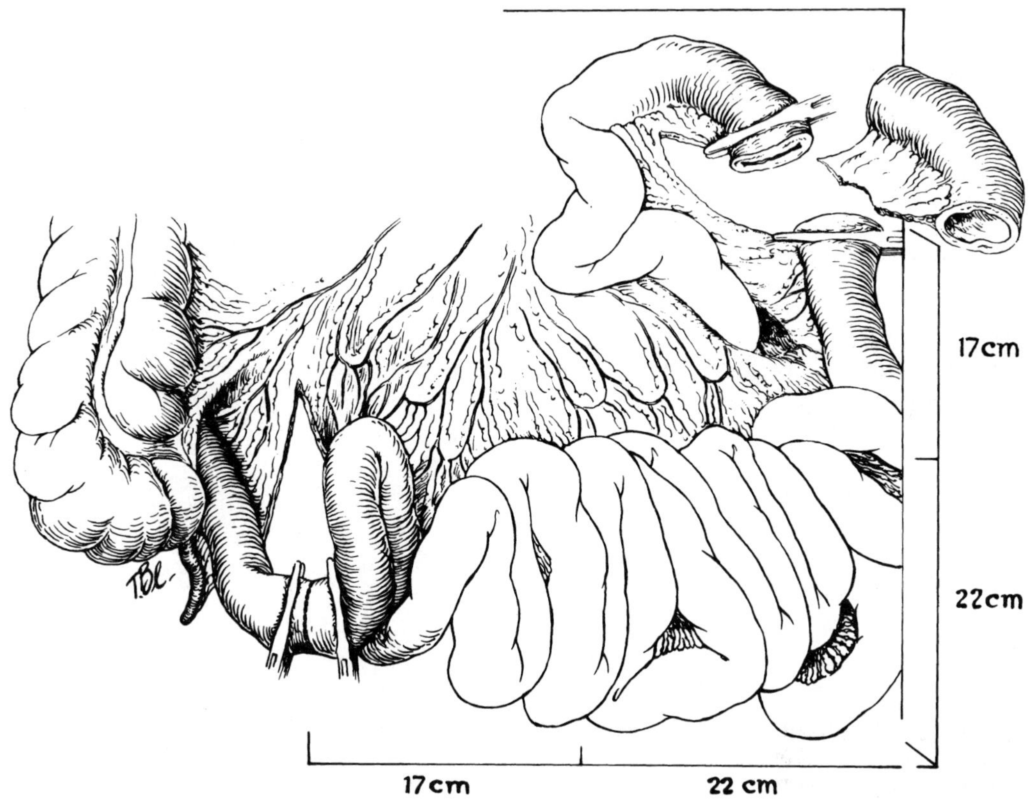

Fig. 31.2. Ileum delineated for the Kock pouch—17 cm for the efferent limb, 22 cm for each of the two segments of the reservoir, and 17 cm for the afferent limb. A 5-cm wedge of ileum and mesentery is resected proximal to the afferent limb to provide better mobility. (From Skinner DG, Boyd SD, Lieskovsky G. Creation of the continent Kock ileal reservoir as an alternative to cutaneous urinary diversion. In: Skinner DG, Lieskovsky G, eds. Genitourinary cancer. Philadelphia: WB Saunders, 1988.)

(proximal) limb. Approximately 5 cm of ileum proximal to the afferent end is discarded, along with a small triangular wedge of mesentery. This provides improved mobility to the pouch and to the small bowel anastomosis; because this mesentery division will be quite short, an excellent blood supply to the pouch is ensured. The small bowel continuity is reestablished with a standard, sutured or stapled enteroenterostomy, depending on the surgeon's preference. The mesenteric defect is closed with running absorbable sutures, with care taken not to impinge on the mesentery to the reservoir or to compromise the blood supply to the enteroenterostomy. The end of the afferent limb is oversewn. If stapling is used, we recommend that this end still be oversewn with 3-0 PGA suture so that the staple line is definitely excluded from the urine.

Construction of the Reservoir

The two 22-cm ileal segments for the reservoir are directed caudally in a U shape (Fig. 31.3). Before opening the reservoir, the segments are apposed with a running 3-0 PGA suture placed in the serosa just above the mesentery on each side. The reservoir is then opened with a cautery knife by incising the ileal segments just above the apposing suture line (Fig. 31.4). This incision should be extended for 2 to 3 cm up the afferent

and efferent limbs, along their antimesentery border, so that when the nipple valves are constructed, they will be well separated. This aids both in the closure of the pouch and in subsequent endoscopic evaluation of the mature pouch. The back wall of the reservoir is closed with two layer running 3-0 PGA suture (Fig. 31.5).

This back wall closure extends just for the length of the reservoir segments and does not extend up into the opening in the afferent and efferent limbs.

Construction of Valves

The antireflux and continence valves are created from the afferent and efferent limbs by intussuscepting the bowel. The intussusception is made easier and more secure by first dividing the mesentery beneath the portion of the limb to be intussuscepted (Fig. 31.6). The cautery knife is used to create the mesentery opening for 8 cm along the bowel's serosal surface. The windows of Deaver in the mesentery are incised, and the individual vessels are picked up with forceps and cauterized. If the mesentery is not stripped away, it may serve as the leading edge for later slippage or extussusception of the valve.

An additional opening in the mesentery is made one vascular arcade distal to the 8-cm opening just created. A 2-cm strip ples to apply three rows of parallel staples as shown. The TA-55 stapler uses a pin that leaves a pinhole that needs to be separately sutured at the base of each staple line. This pinhole has been noted to be the occasional site of a valve fistula. We have now switched to a custom GIA stapler that places a double row of 3.5-mm staples without a knife and does not create a pinhole. We have also found that it is necessary to place only two double rows of staples rather than three rows. This creates a well-vascularized but still well-secured valve. The staple rows should be placed in the anterior half of the valve, leaving the posterior side free so that another row of staples can subsequently fix the nipple to the back wall of the pouch. Do not be alarmed if the tip of the nipple valve appears slightly dusky or congested. The overall length of the valve, after it has healed, should always be much longer than the needed functional length of 2.5 cm. The staples at the base of the valves are the most important for preventing valve slippage, and these staples bury themselves well beneath the mucosa. Because the staples at the tip of the nipple valves really do not contribute to the maintenance of the valve and because they are more likely to remain exposed and become a potential site for stone formation,

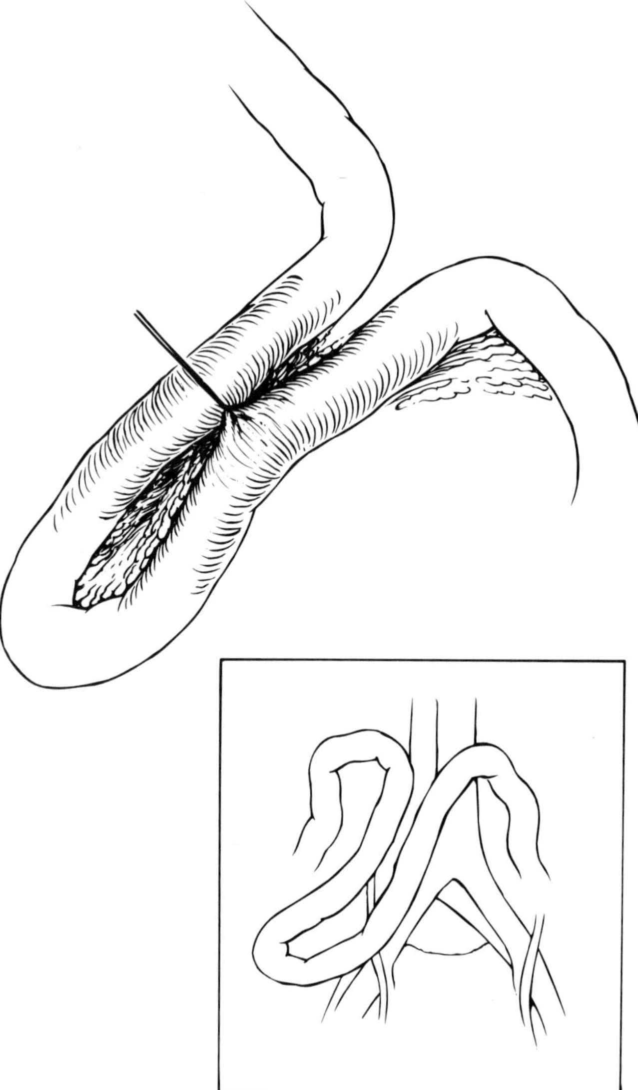

Fig. 31.3.   The reservoir segments are directed caudally in a U shape. (From Skinner DG, Boyd SD, Lieskovsky G. Creation of the continent Kock ileal reservoir as an alternative to cutaneous urinary diversion. In: Skinner DG, Lieskovsky G, eds. Genitourinary cancer. Philadelphia: WB Saunders, 1988.)

of PGA mesh is passed through this additional opening to serve as an anchoring collar for the base of the nipple valves. Marlex mesh was originally used for this purpose, but Marlex tends to be erosive and can become a source of infection and stone formation. We abandoned using Marlex mesh as an anchoring collar after our initial 150 cases.

The intussusception of the nipple valves is accomplished by passing two Allis forcep clamps just over halfway up the open limb to the anchoring collar, grasping the mucosa, and inverting the ileum into the pouch (Fig. 31.7). A valve at least 5 cm long will be created, still leaving a 1-cm lip of pouch at the opening for subsequent reservoir closure.

Noncrushing staples are used to secure the valves (Fig. 31.8); we originally used a standard TA-55 stapler with 4.8-mm sta-

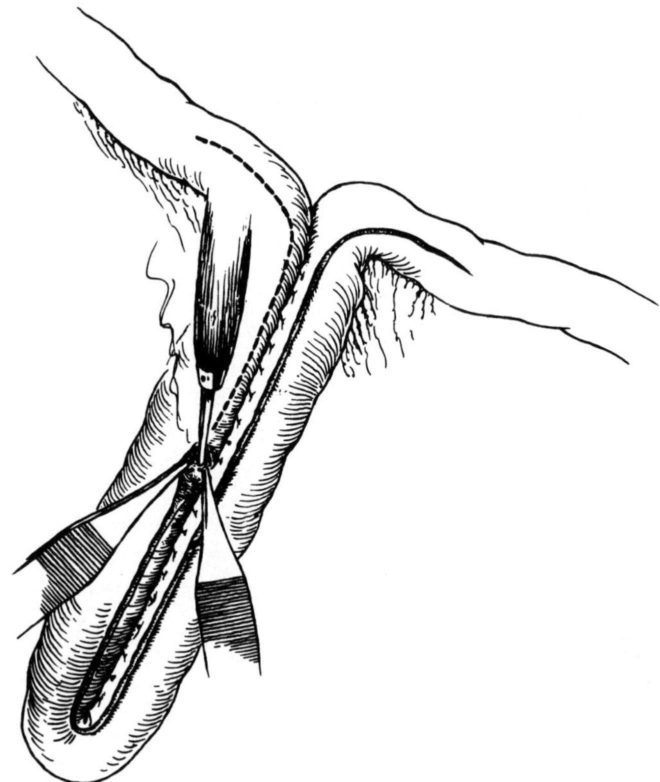

Fig. 31.4.   The inner walls of the reservoir segments are apposed with running 3-0 PGA sutures and opened with the cautery knife. The incision is extended for 2 to 3 cm up the afferent and efferent limbs along their antimesenteric border. (From Skinner DG, Boyd SD, Lieskovsky G. Creation of the continent Kock ileal reservoir as an alternative to cutaneous urinary diversion. In: Skinner DG, Lieskovsky G, eds. Genitourinary cancer. Philadelphia: WB Saunders, 1988.)

the distal six staples are removed from the corresponding end of the staple cartridge before stapling.

The effectiveness of the nipple valves are further ensured by fixing them to the back wall of the reservoir. This can be accomplished by either of two methods (Fig. 31.9). We prefer to slip the outer arm of the stapler between the two leaves of the valve, with the other arm remaining outside the reservoir, and staple the valve to the back wall just next to the mesentery. This places only two layers of tissue in the stapler, one wall of the nipple valve and the wall of the pouch, while fixing the valve in a secure fashion. A standard, full-length staple cartridge is used. A second technique is demonstrated in Figure 31.9. This requires making a small opening in the back wall of the pouch near the tip of the valve. The outer arm of the stapler is passed through this opening from the outside and advanced up the inside of the valve. When stapled, this fixes the full thickness of the valve to the back wall just lateral to the mesentery. The small opening in the reservoir is closed with 3-0 PGA sutures.

With either technique, additional 3-0 PGA sutures are used to further secure the tip of each valve to the pouch wall (Fig. 31.10). The secure fixation of the nipple valve to the pouch wall not only helps prevent long-term valve slippage but also

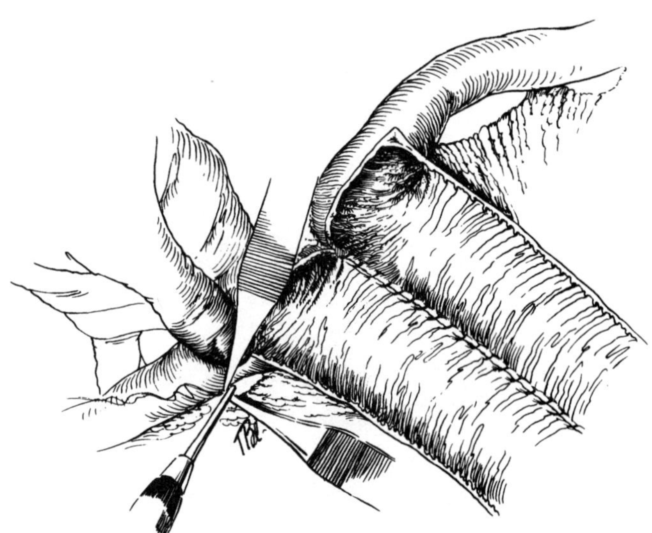

Fig. 31.6. An 8-cm mesenteric window is opened with the cautery knife beneath the portion of each limb to be intussuscepted. The window should begin 1 cm back from the opening of the limb into the reservoir. A second 1-cm window in the mesentery is made one vascular arcade beyond to accommodate each anchoring collar. (From Skinner DG, Boyd SD, Lieskovsky G. Creation of the continent Kock ileal reservoir as an alternative to cutaneous urinary diversion. In: Skinner DG, Lieskovsky G, eds. Genitourinary cancer. Philadelphia: WB Saunders, 1988.)

increases the efficiency of the antireflux and continence mechanisms as the reservoir fills and stretches. The PGA mesh is anchored to the base of the valves and the ileal limb with sutures of 3-0 PGA (Fig. 31.10). One should not include the mesentery in these sutures. The collar further stabilizes the valves and also serves as an anchoring point for fixing the efferent valve and limb to the abdominal wall. A 30F catheter can be passed up the nipple valve and through the mesh site while the mesh is being sutured. This will allow the mesh to be affixed snugly without being too tight. The redundant mesh can be excised.

Reservoir Closure

The reservoir is completed by folding the ileum in the opposite direction to which it was opened and suturing it closed (Fig. 31.11). The closure is accomplished with a two-layer, running 3-0 PGA suture, which is meticulously placed to ensure watertightness. The principle of opening, folding, and closing is important because it causes the motor activities of the different ileal segments of the pouch to counteract themselves, thus creating an extremely low-pressure reservoir. This helps assure the long-term viability of the diversion.

Ureteroileal Anastomoses

The bowel is packed out of the way, and the proximal closed end of the afferent limb is secured to the tissue overlying the sacral promontory with 3-0 PGA suture (Fig. 31.12). Each ureter is carefully trimmed to an appropriate length, spatulated,

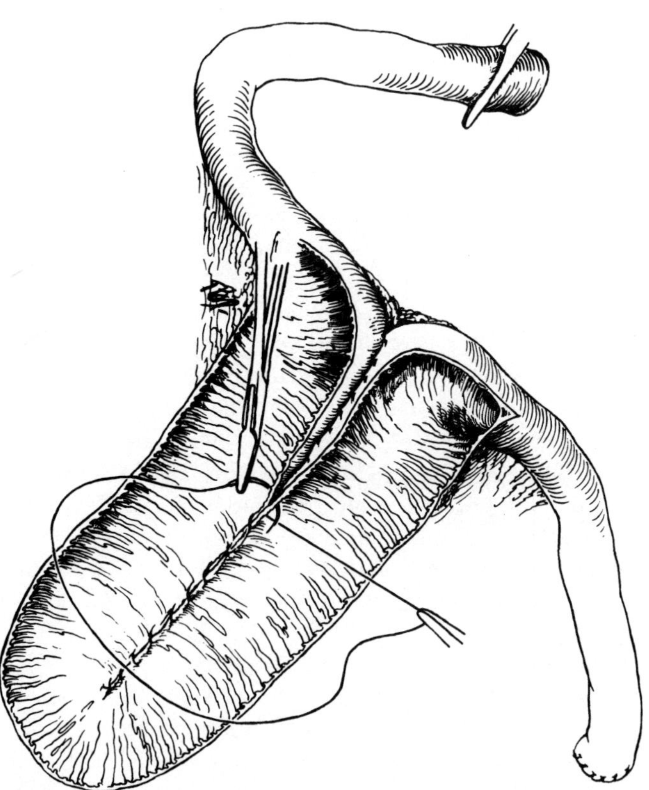

Fig. 31.5. The reservoir segments are opened and the back wall of the reservoir is closed in a watertight manner with two layers of running 3-0 PGA sutures. (From Skinner DG, Boyd SD, Lieskovsky G. Creation of the continent Kock ileal reservoir as an alternative to cutaneous urinary diversion. In: Skinner DG, Lieskovsky G, eds. Genitourinary cancer. Philadelphia: WB Saunders, 1988.)

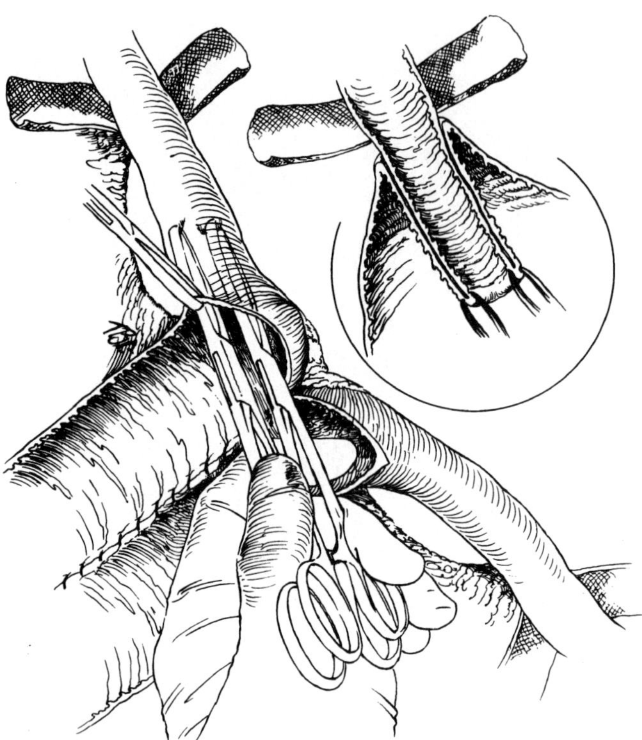

Fig. 31.7. One-centimeter anchoring collars of PGA mesh are positioned in their mesenteric openings. Two Allis forcep clamps are passed up each limb just over halfway to the anchoring collar, the mucosa is grasped, and the ileum intussuscepted, creating a nipple valve at least 5 cm long. (From Skinner DG, Boyd SD, Lieskovsky G. Creation of the continent Kock ileal reservoir as an alternative to cutaneous urinary diversion. In: Skinner DG, Lieskovsky G, eds. Genitourinary cancer. Philadelphia: WB Saunders, 1988.)

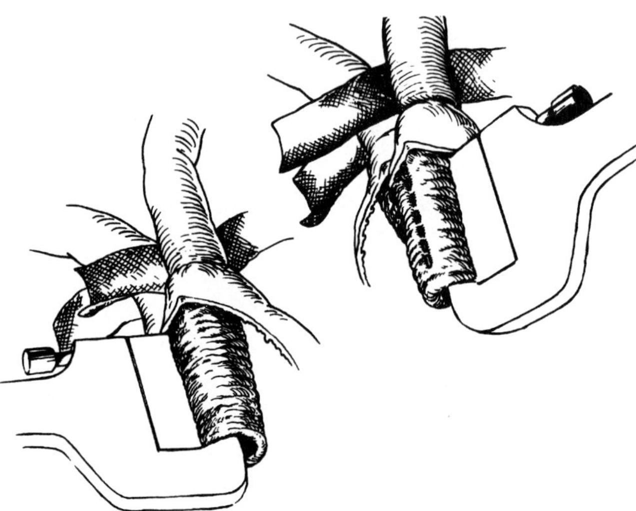

Fig. 31.8. The nipple valves are first stabilized by stapling two with special pinless TA-55 or knifeless GIA staplers. Note that the distal six staples are preremoved from the staplers. (From Skinner DG, Boyd SD, Lieskovsky G. Creation of the continent Kock ileal reservoir as an alternative to cutaneous urinary diversion. In: Skinner DG, Lieskovsky G, eds. Genitourinary cancer. Philadelphia: WB Saunders, 1988.)

and anastomosed to a small opening created on each side of the afferent limb. The anastomoses are accomplished in a standard end-to-side fashion using interrupted 4-0 PGA suture (13). Approximately eight sutures are usually required. After each anastomosis is half completed, the ureters are stented with 8F infant feeding tubes that are perforated with extra holes and fed up through the afferent limb and valve to remain indwelling in the pouch. These stents may be fixed to the end of the cutaneous catheter through a small opening in the pouch or left free in the pouch and removed endoscopically in approximately 3 weeks.

Stoma Preparation and Pouch Fixation

The stoma can usually be located low on the right side of the abdomen, overlying the rectus muscle. An approximate site for the stoma can be made preoperatively by the enterostomal therapist, but the exact site should be selected after the pouch is created so that the efferent limb can reach the skin as perpendicular to the pouch as possible. This is especially important in the obese patient.

After the stoma site is determined, a 2-cm plug of skin is removed. The subcutaneous fat is opened directly beneath the stoma with the cautery knife, and the anterior rectus fascia is exposed. A 3-cm vertical incision is made through the rectus fascia, and the muscle and peritoneum are split just widely enough to accommodate the tips of two fingers. Two horizontal mattress sutures of 1 PGA are then passed through each side of the anterior rectus fascial opening and positioned correspondingly through each side of the efferent anchoring collar and the base of the valve (Fig. 31.12). These sutures should be color-coded to avoid any confusion and to maintain the alignment when the efferent limb is brought up through the stoma site.

Before the sutures are tied, an additional 1-cm strip of Marlex mesh is anchored with no. 1 nylon suture to the posterior rectus fascia, just cephalad and lateral to the abdominal wall opening for the stoma. This Marlex strut is brought through the window of Deaver in the mesentery adjacent to the PGA mesh (Fig. 31.12). An Allis clamp is used to carefully bring the efferent limb up through the stomal opening, while being certain not to cross the mattress sutures. The mattress sutures are securely tied, thus fixing the base of the efferent valve to the rectus fascia. When the sutures are properly placed and tied, the efferent limb should exit the pouch without angulation. The Marlex strut is then further sutured to the posterior rectus fascia medial to the mesentery with another no. 1 nylon suture (Fig. 31.12). The Marlex serves to secure the mesentery side of the limb, without risk of erosion, and prevents parastomal hernias and concomitant catheterization difficulties. The redundant efferent limb above the skin line is excised. A flush or slightly recessed stoma is completed by suturing the ileum circumferentially to the skin with interrupted 3-0 PGA. A slightly recessed stoma will usually allow the stoma site to

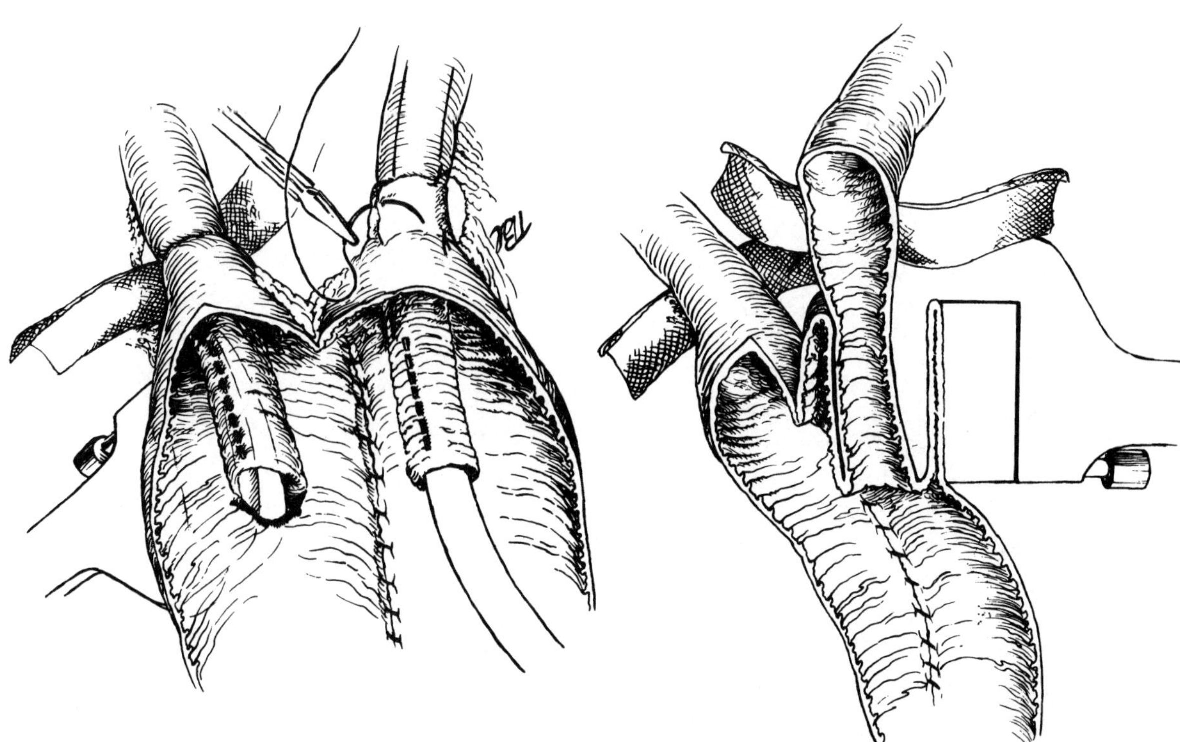

Fig. 31.9.   The nipple valves are further fixed to the back wall of the reservoir using either of two methods. The preferred technique is demonstrated on the right. The arm of the stapler is inserted from the outside, next to the mesentery, between the two leaves of the valve. The stapler is fired, fixing one leaf of the valve to the back wall. A second method is shown on the left. A hole is made in the back wall of the reservoir opposite the tip of the valve. The arm of the stapler is passed through the hole, up the inside of the valve, and fired. The hole in the back wall is closed with 3-0 PGA suture. The PGA mesh anchoring collar is firmly sutured to the base of each valve and limb. (From Skinner DG, Boyd SD, Lieskovsky G. Creation of the continent Kock ileal reservoir as an alternative to cutaneous urinary diversion. In: Skinner DG, Lieskovsky G, eds. Genitourinary cancer. Philadelphia: WB Saunders, 1988.)

constrict down to the size of the catheter over the first few months and give an even better cosmetic appearance to the stoma.

A 24 to 26F catheter is placed through the stoma site and positioned centrally in the pouch. Normal saline is instilled through the catheter to make certain that the pouch can be easily irrigated postoperatively and to check the watertightness of the suture lines. After being properly positioned, the catheter is secured at the stoma site with two no. 1 nylon sutures. A 1-in. Penrose drain is placed through a separate stab incision in the abdominal wall and positioned below the pouch. The abdomen is then closed.

POSTOPERATIVE CARE

The general care of these patients in the immediate postoperative period will be the same as for patients undergoing cystectomy and ileal conduit diversion. Gastric drainage, either by a nasogastric tube or gastrostomy tube, is maintained until bowel function is adequate, usually in 4 to 5 days. Hydration is maintained initially by intravenous fluids. Patients are encouraged to resume eating a normal diet as soon as possible and to begin early ambulation.

The one unique care feature of the continent diversion is the need to periodically irrigate the reservoir with normal saline to make certain that it stays clear of mucus. Typically, the catheter is rinsed every 4 hours with 30 to 60 mL of normal saline. By the third postoperative day, patients are instructed in self-irrigation techniques. Once patients are self-reliant, they can be discharged to home health care, usually within 8 to 10 days of the operation. It is extremely important that patients keep themselves well hydrated and continue the catheter irrigation at home. Discharge medication should include an oral antibiotic.

The catheter remains indwelling in the reservoir for 3 weeks. At the end of 3 weeks, the patients are readmitted for a 1-day stay. A Kockogram (cystogram of the pouch) is performed. If the system is well healed, the catheter is removed and the patient is instructed in self-catheterization techniques. The ureteral stents are removed at this time. Catheterization is begun at 2- or 3-hour intervals. If no difficulties are encountered during the 24-hour stay, the Penrose drain can be removed and the patient is discharged from the hospital.

The ideal catheters for home use are 20F Coudé tip, reusable catheters. Each patient usually maintains a supply of two or three catheters. Catheters can be kept in a plastic-

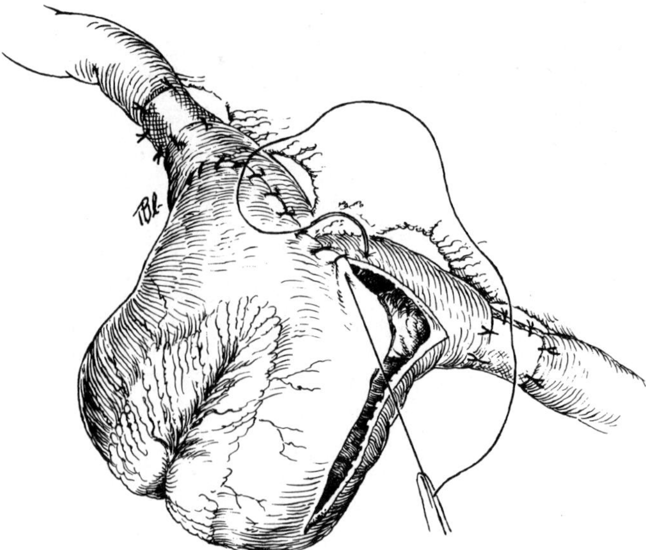

Fig. 31.11.   The reservoir is completed by folding the ileum back on itself and suturing with two-layer, running 3-0 PGA. (From Skinner DG, Boyd SD, Lieskovsky G. Creation of the continent Kock ileal reservoir as an alternative to cutaneous urinary diversion. In: Skinner DG, Lieskovsky G, eds. Genitourinary cancer. Philadelphia: WB Saunders, 1988.)

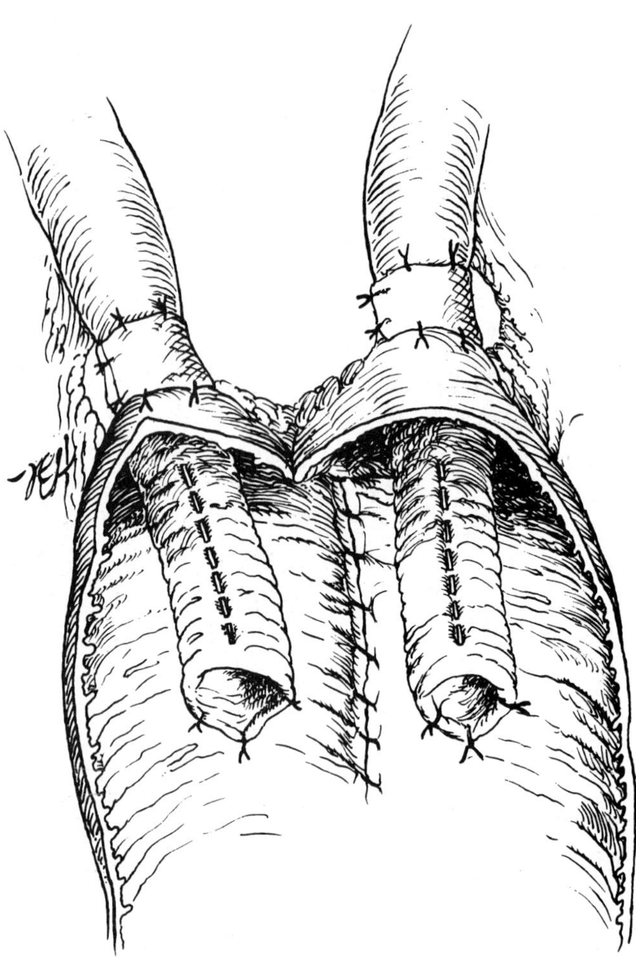

Fig. 31.10.   The fixation of the valves is completed by suturing the tips of the valves to the reservoir wall with 3-0 PGA sutures. (From Skinner DG, Boyd SD, Lieskovsky G. Creation of the continent Kock ileal reservoir as an alternative to cutaneous urinary diversion. In: Skinner DG, Lieskovsky G, eds. Genitourinary cancer. Philadelphia: WB Saunders, 1988.)

lined bag and easily carried in a purse for women or in a tobacco pouch for men. The catheterization interval is usually increased by 1 hour each week while at home. The goal after 4 to 6 weeks is to have patients catheterize themselves every 6 hours during the day and be able to sleep through the night. Patients should be instructed to be independent and to feel free to travel. Oral antibiotics are usually maintained until the catheterization schedule has stabilized. All patients wear a small absorbency pad over their stoma to prevent mucous spotting of their clothing. The pads are removed for swimming or bathing.

RESULTS

The overall early and late complication rates for patients undergoing cystectomy and continent diversion should not differ significantly from what we see in patients undergoing cystectomy and ileal conduit urinary diversion. The late complications unique to continent cutaneous diversions usually involve continence problems. Leakage of urine from the stoma sufficient to warrant reoperation occurred in 10 to 15% of our patients in the early part of our series. The problem was usually totally correctable at surgery by resecuring or replacing the continence valve (14). The newer methods of nipple fixation, the use of the Marlex strut, and the pinless stapler have reduced this rate to 5%. Problems with catheterization in the cutaneous Kock diversion occur in only 1% of patients if the method of stabilization of the efferent limb is used. The antireflux mechanism of the Kock diversion has a 98% reliability, which is difficult to obtain by any other method. The incidence of ureteroileal stenosis is 3%, similar to that seen in a standard ileal conduit. Electrolyte problems are rare; so far, vitamin B_{12} deficiency has not been noted in significant numbers although vitamin B_{12} replacement theoretically may be necessary after 5 to 10 years.

Patient satisfaction with the continent Kock diversion is excellent. Only 1% of our patients have requested conversion of their continent diversion to a conduit type diversion. There is no question that in the areas of self-confidence, self-image, interpersonal relations, and sexual desires, a significant difference exists between continent diversion and ileal conduit —continent diversion is favored (15). The most vocal advocates of continent diversion remain those patients who previously have had a noncontinent urinary diversion and subsequently were converted. In the future, orthotopic diversion will be made available to most male and female bladder cancer patients. When the diversion to the urethra is not appropriate, however, continent cutaneous diversion is still an excellent option.

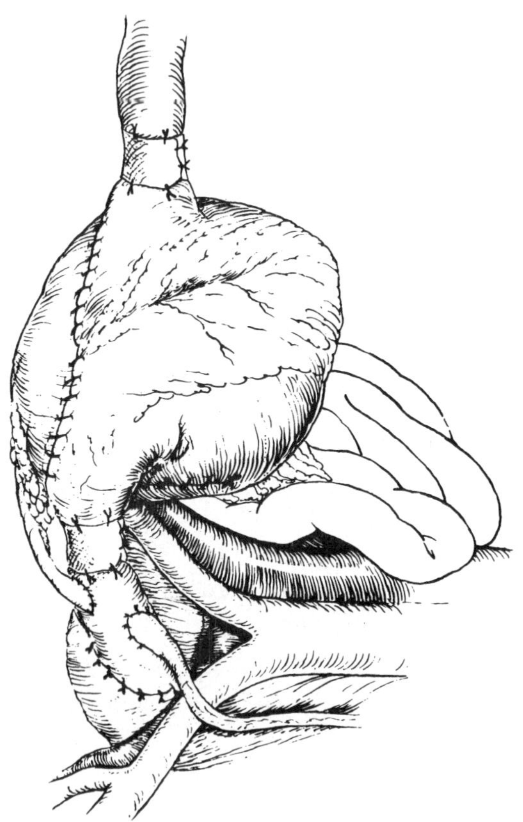
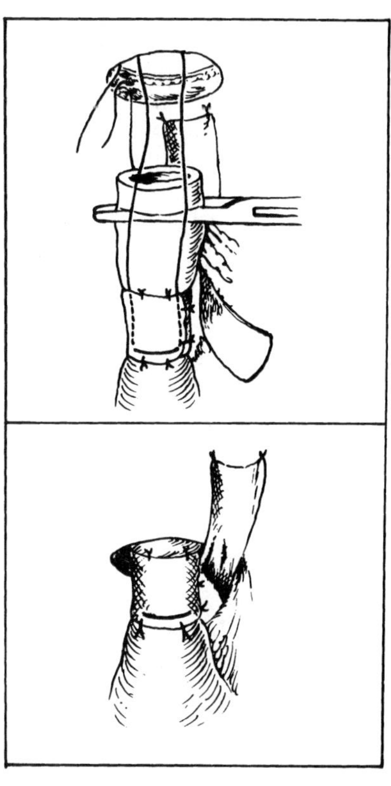

Fig. 31.12.   The end of the afferent limb is fixed over the sacrum, and a standard ureteroileal end-to-side anastomosis is performed. After the stoma site is selected and a 2-cm skin plug is removed, two horizontal mattress sutures of I PGA are fixed to the anterior rectus fascia and correspondingly on each side of the anchoring collar and the base of the efferent valve. A I-cm strut of Marlex mesh is passed through the mesenteric opening for the anchoring collar and is sutured to the posterior fascia laterally with no. I nylon. The efferent limb is pulled up through the stoma, the mattress sutures are tied, and the Marlex strut is sutured medially to the posterior fascia. (From Skinner DG, Boyd SD, Lieskovsky G. Creation of the continent Kock ileal reservoir as an alternative to cutaneous urinary diversion. In: Skinner DG, Lieskovsky G, eds. Genitourinary cancer. Philadelphia: WB Saunders, 1988.)

REFERENCES

1. Kock NG, et al. Urinary diversion via a continent ileal reservoir: clinical results in 12 patients. J Urol 1982;128:469.

2. Gilcrist RK, et al. Construction of substitute bladder and urethra. Surg Gynecol Obstet 1950;90:752.

3. Kock NG. Ileostomy without external appliances: a survey of 25 patients provided with intra-abdominal intestinal reservoir. Ann Surg 1971;173:545.

4. Kock NG, et al. Changes in renal parenchyma and the upper urinary tracts following urinary diversion via a continent ileum reservoir: an experimental study in dogs. Scand J Urol Nephrol Suppl 1978;49:11.

5. Kock NG, et al. Urinary diversion via a continent ileum reservoir: clinical experience. Scand J Urol Nephrol Suppl 1978;49:23.

6. Kock NG. Continent ileostomy: historical perspective. In: Dozois R, ed. Alternatives to conventional ileostomy. Chicago: Year Book, 1985:133.

7. Berglund B, Kock NG, Myrvold HE. Volume capacity and pressure characteristics of the continent cecal reservoir. Surg Gynecol Obstet 1986;163:42.

8. Skinner DG, Boyd SD, Lieskovsky G. Clinical experience with the Kock continent ileal reservoir for urinary diversion. J Urol 1984;132:1101.

9. Skinner DG, Lieskovsky G, Boyd SD. Technique of creation of a continent internal ileal reservoir (Kock pouch) for urinary diversion. Urol Clin North Am 1984;11:741.

10. Skinner DG, Lieskovsky G, Boyd SD. Continuing experience with the continent ileal reservoir (Kock pouch) as an alternative to cutaneous urinary diversion: an update after 250 cases. J Urol 1987;137:1140.

11. Boyd SD, et al. Continent and orthotopic urinary diversion following radical cystectomy: should these reconstructive procedures now be considered standard of care? Surg Oncol Clin North Am 1995;4:277.

12. Camey M. Bladder replacement by ileocystoplasty following radical cystectomy. Semin Urol 1987;5:8.

13. Ritchie JP. Techniques of ureterointestinal anastomoses and conduit construction. In: Crawford ED, Borden TA, eds. Genitourinary cancer surgery. Philadelphia: Lea & Febiger, 1982:227.

14. Lieskovsky G, Skinner DG, Boyd SD. Complications of the Kock pouch. Urol Clin North Am 1988;15:195.

15. Boyd SD, et al. Quality of life survey of urinary diversion patients: comparison of ileal conduits versus continent Kock ileal reservoirs. J Urol 1987;138:1386.

32

Continent Cutaneous Diversion Using the Ileocecal Bowel Segment

Nabil K. Bissada

Cutaneous and urethral continent urinary diversions have become the most popular procedures in most patients who need supravesical urinary diversion. In current continent urinary diversion procedures, a detubularized bowel segment is used to make a low-pressure, high-compliance reservoir of adequate capacity. This can be accomplished by using small bowel, sigmoid colon, ascending colon, or ileocolonic segments. Complete detubularization of the bowel segment is essential. Different techniques were successful in preventing reflux. The most demanding task in continent urinary diversion is construction of an adequate continence mechanism (1–6). This chapter reviews the development of cutaneous continent urinary diversion using the ileocecal bowel segment and describes the currently popular techniques in this category.

Continence in patients undergoing ileocecal continent cutaneous diversions relies on using either the appendix or the terminal ileum and ileocecal valve.

USE OF THE APPENDIX AS A CATHETERIZABLE CONTINENCE MECHANISM

The appendix and an ileocecal reservoir were reported as early as 1908 by Verhoogen (7). The use of the appendix in the urinary tract was popularized by Mitrofanoff (8). Currently, the appendix provides continence in patients having right colon or ileocolic reservoirs by one of three techniques.

1. The Charleston pouch technique relies on the use of the in situ appendix with minimal augmentation of the appendicocolic junction (9–13). Leak point pressure studies in cadavers and in vivo indicate that the in situ appendix without surgical manipulation can provide an adequate antileakage mechanism in some patients undergoing continent urinary pouches as constructed today (14, 15). Patients with low or borderline appendiceal leak pressure require minimal reinforcement to raise the leak pressure significantly (16). We have previously demonstrated that dilating a narrow appendix

is safe, effective, and compatible with providing an adequate continence mechanism (11).

As a readily available native continence mechanism, the in situ appendix has many advantages. The most obvious advantage is that the painstaking efforts needed to create a continence mechanism de novo would be unnecessary. Therefore, the technical difficulty, surgical time, and potential for complications are reduced. As a single-lumen, smooth tubular structure, the appendix is simple to catheterize; fistula or false passage formation is less likely. The lack of manipulation of the appendix results in a longer and more mobile tube that can traverse even the obese abdominal wall with ease. The proximal appendix remains intraabdominal so that intraabdominal pressure peaks (Valsalva, cough) are transmitted to the appendix and the pouch, thereby reducing stress incontinence. Sutures and staples are eliminated, thereby reducing tissue necrosis, erosion, and the nidus for stone formation.

2. The second technique is based on the Mitrofanoff principle, in which the appendix with its mesenteric blood supply is isolated together with a button of cecum and the distal tip is tunneled into the urinary reservoir to provide the continence mechanism (8, 17).
3. The modified Mainz pouch technique leaves the appendix attached to the cecum and buries the appendix after rolling it back on itself (18).

The Charleston Pouch Continent Urinary Diversion

The Charleston pouch relies on constructing an ileocolonic reservoir using detubularized and reoriented terminal ileum and ascending colon. The ureters are reimplanted in the colonic part with a simple antireflux technique. Whenever present, the in situ appendix is used to provide a continent catheterizable stoma. Leak pressure measurements are performed intraoperatively and when necessary, the appendicocolic junction is reinforced (16). The open end of the appendix is brought out of the abdomen at the umbilical site (19).

Preoperative Preparation

Patients are evaluated for general medical condition, psychological fitness, renal function, and to exclude colonic pathologic conditions. Stools are tested for occult blood. In patients older than 40 years of age, evaluation by colonoscopy or an air-contrast barium enema is desirable. Bowel preparation by the surgeon's preferred technique is ordered. We use mechanical bowel preparation and order parenteral antibiotics including metronidazole 1.5 g on call to the operating room.

Surgical Technique of Charleston Pouch

A midline abdominal incision is used, which extends from approximately 1 inch below the xiphoid process, makes a semicircle on the left side of the umbilicus, and then continues in the midline to the symphysis pubis. After abdominal exploration and other required procedures such as a cystectomy, the terminal ileum, cecum, ascending colon, and appendix are examined.

The right colon is mobilized to the hepatic flexure. The mesentery is visualized by transillumination, and the mesenteric vessels are examined to determine the blood supply to the pouch. Bowel segments consisting of the terminal 15 cm to 20 cm of ileum, cecum, appendix, and ascending colon are isolated with their appropriate blood supply (Fig. 32.1). The

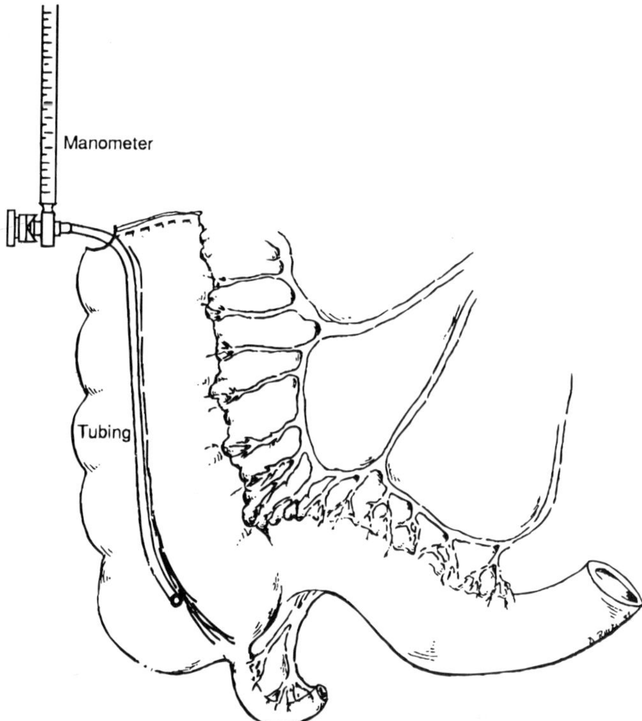

Fig. 32.2. Appendiceal leak point measurement. An arterial line tubing is inserted via the open end of the colon and the tip is advanced to the cecum. The butt end of arterial line tube is fitted with simple standing column manometer. The colon is then filled with normal saline, and the opening in the colon is occluded by the fingers. The open end of the ileum is also occluded by an intestinal clamp. Gentle pressure on the filled colon is applied, and the intracolonic pressure is noted. Leakage via the open end of the appendix is watched. The pressure at which leakage starts is the appendiceal leak point pressure.

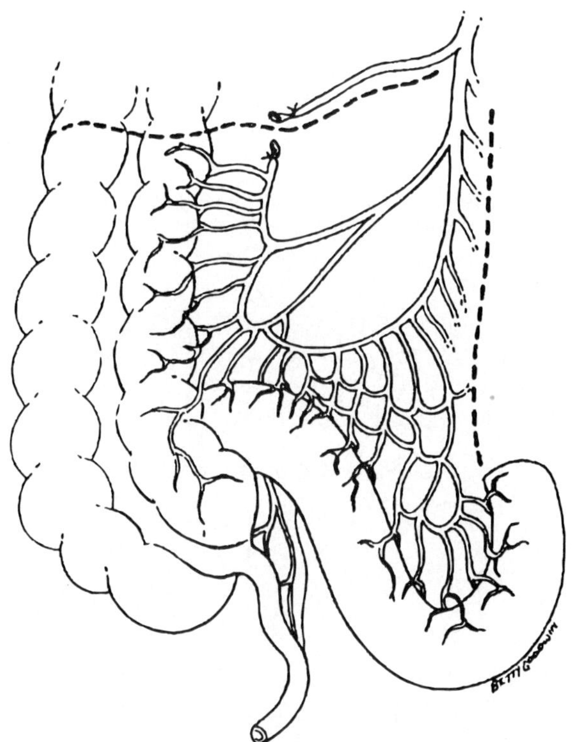

Fig. 32.1. Charleston pouch. Cecum, appendix, ascending colon, and appropriate length of terminal ileum are isolated with their blood supply.

mesenteric windows are developed. The bowel is divided at the desired sites using gastrointestinal anastomosis staple cartridges (GIA). Bowel continuity is then accomplished. Our preference is a side-to-side stapled anastomosis using the stapling device. Part of the existing staple line in the ileum and colon near the antimesenteric border is excised. This allows the two blades of the stapling device to be inserted into the lumens of the ileum and the colon. The antimesenteric borders of the ileum and the colon are brought together, and the stapling device is engaged and closed. The position of the stapling device inside the lumens is checked to ensure that it is at the antimesenteric borders. The GIA device is then activated. The device is removed and the anastomosis is inspected. The openings in the ileum and colon used for the insertion of the device are then closed by another application of the GIA device. One or two 3-0 silk sutures are used to enforce the approximation of the ileum and colon just at the end of the stapled anastomosis.

The staple lines of the isolated segment used to form the urinary reservoir are excised, and the segment is irrigated. The distal end of the appendix is excised, and the lumen is calibrated. If the lumen is narrow, it is gently dilated to 12 or 14F. The colon is filled with normal saline. Appendicular leak point pressure (intracolonic pressure at which fluid escapes via

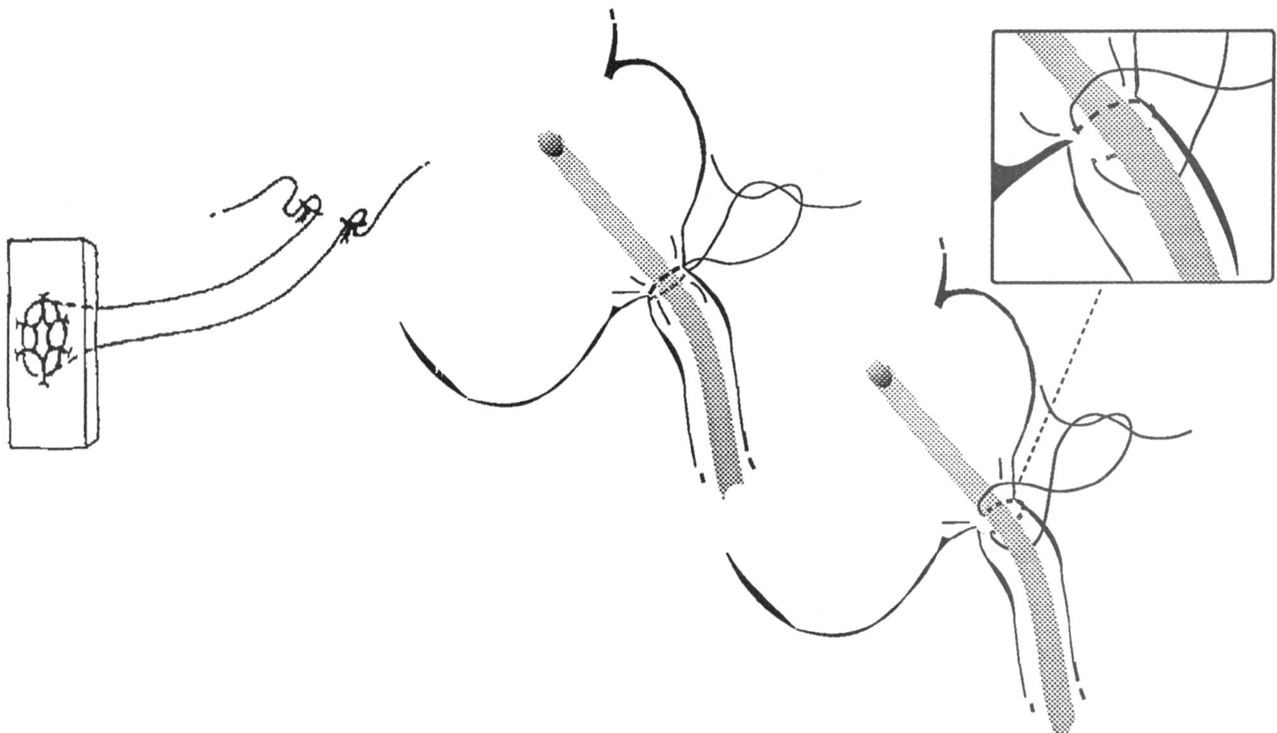

Fig. 32.3.   Maneuvers to augment the appendicocolic mechanism. Left: Invaginating 1 cm of appendix into the cecum and maintaining the invagination with two or three nonabsorbable sutures (2-0 silk or 2-0 Prolene). Middle: Purse-string suture at the appendicocolic junction is tied over 10 or 12F catheter. Right and insert: Imbricating suture in the cecum exactly at the origin of the appendix. This is the most common technique used in the past few years. A 2-0 Prolene suture is used.

the distal end of the appendix) is then measured to determine the need for any reinforcement of the appendicocolic junction, which is performed at this time. For pressure measurements, we use a simple standing column manometer and arterial line tubing (Fig. 32.2). In most patients, the leak point pressure is less than 75 cm water. In this case, two or three sutures of 2-0 silk or Prolene are used to invaginate about 1 cm of appendix into the cecum (Fig. 32.3, left).

Recently, a purse-string or an imbricating Lambert suture placed in the colon exactly at the appendicocolic junction is tied snugly over a 10 or 12F catheter in the appendix. Leak point pressure measurement is then repeated. This is almost always in excess of 75 cm water pressure. The ileum and colon are then completely detubularized by incising along the anti-mesenteric border (Fig. 32.4). Each is formed into an inverted U-shaped patch. The ileal and colonic patches are then approximated with continuous absorbable suture (Fig. 32.5). A polyglycolic acid absorbable stapling device is available and can be used for this approximation. However, its use may result in delay or failure to achieve adequate reservoir capacity; we no longer use it. Instead, we use 3-0 polyglycolic acid suture on a straight Keith needle. This allows fast approximation with appreciable reduction in operative time.

Ureteral reimplantation is done next. The mobilized ureters are reimplanted into the ascending colon. Each ureter is passed through an adequate hiatus in the colon. An incision is made

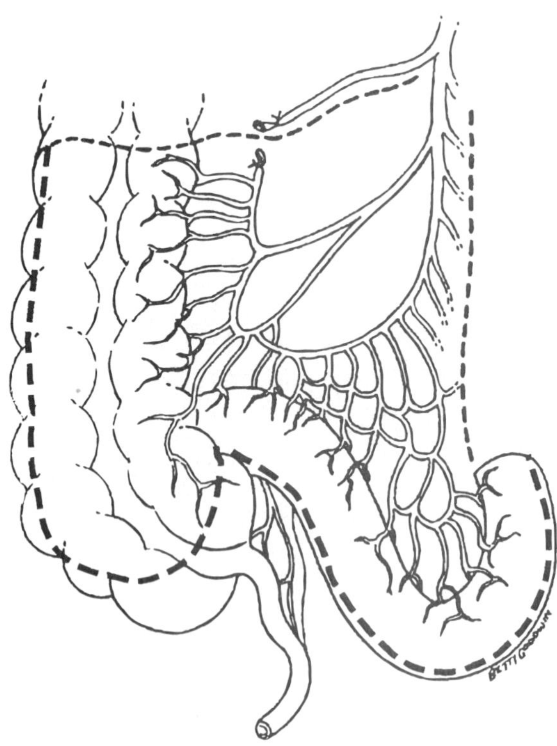

Fig. 32.4.   Ileum and colon are completely opened along the antimesenteric border.

in the mucosa to create a sulcus about 2.5 cm between the hiatus (ureteral entrance into the colon) and the site for anastomosis to the colonic mucosa. Two mucosal flaps are created by gentle scissors dissection. The ureter is then spatulated and anastomosed to the colonic mucosa at the end of the sulcus with five interrupted sutures using 5-0 polydioxanone sutures. The mucosa is loosely approximated over the ureter with one or two sutures. A single J ureteric stent is then passed up the ureter to drain the kidney during the postoperative period. It is secured to the colonic mucosa close to the anastomosis with a 4-0 chromic suture. A 24F Malecot catheter is left indwelling in the pouch (cecostomy tube). The two intestinal patches are then approximated with continuous suture of 3-0 polyglycolic acid suture to create a large globular pouch (Fig. 32.6).

The stoma site is prepared by making a triangular skin flap with its base on the right side and with its tip at the umbilicus. A 1.5-cm core is then removed from the umbilical scar, including the skin and down to the peritoneum. The appendix is then passed through this opening. It is spatulated for about 1.2 cm, and the tip of the triangular skin flap is anastomosed to the spatulated borders. The remaining circumference of the open end of the appendix is anastomosed to the surrounding skin. The pouch is filled with saline via the Malecot catheter and then is catheterized via the appendix to ensure that catheterization is easy. Occasionally, the position of the cecal part of the reservoir near the appendicocolic junction has to be adjusted to ensure easy cathe-

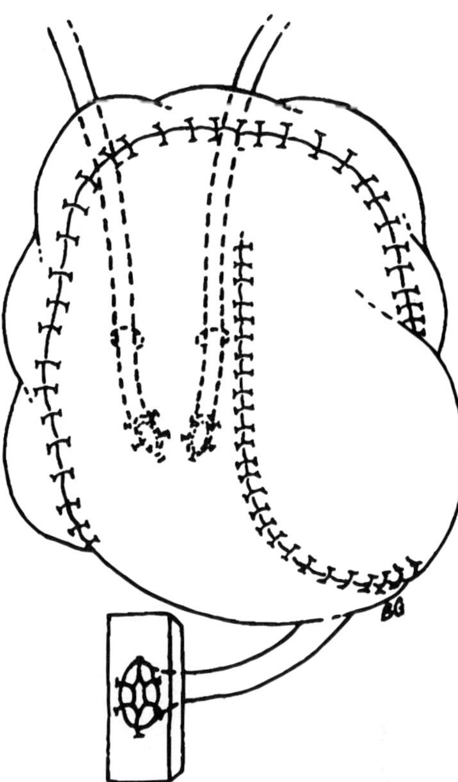

Fig. 32.6. The ileal and colonic patches approximated anteriorly to close the pouch.

terization. In this case, a 3-0 polyglycolic acid suture is used to fix that area of the reservoir in the desired position. A 10 to 12F red rubber catheter (one size smaller than the appendicular lumen) is left as a stent in the appendicular stoma.

Postoperative Care

Gastric decompression is achieved by means of either a nasogastric tube or by gastrostomy. We have used a gastrostomy tube in more than half the patients. For this we use a Stamey suprapubic cystostomy tube that is punched through a stab wound in the abdominal wall. The stomach is inflated with 250 mL of air through the nasogastric tube by the anesthetist. The Stamey tube is then punched through the stomach wall and placed inside the stomach. Three absorbable sutures are used to attach the stomach to the anterior abdominal wall next to the gastrostomy tube entrance. The nasogastric tube is removed the next morning, and the gastrostomy tube is connected to straight drainage. This is continued until the patient is passing flatus.

The ureteral stents are maintained for approximately 10 to 11 days and are then removed on two consecutive days. The following day, the Penrose drain is shortened and is removed in 2 to 3 days. As an alternative to Penrose drains, Jackson-Pratt drains that are converted to straight drainage may be used for 24 to 48 hours postoperatively. Irrigation of the cecostomy tube is started in the immediate postoperative period and continued 2 to 3 times daily to ensure removal of the mucus

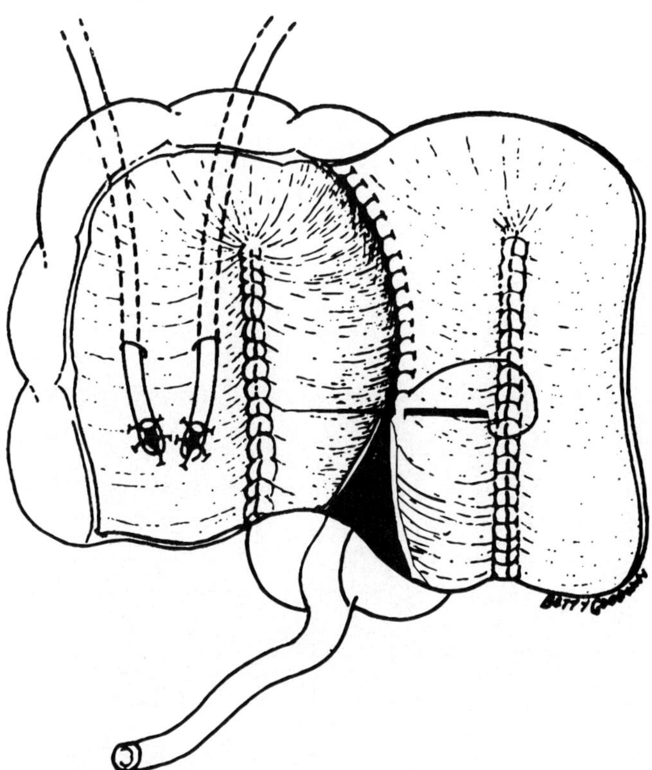

Fig. 32.5. The ileum was folded into an inverted U-shaped patch using 3-0 polyglycolic acid continuous suture on a straight Keith needle. The colon was also folded in a similar manner. The ileal and colonic patches are being approximated. Ureters are implanted in the colonic patch.

from the reservoir and avoid blockage of the cecostomy and the stenting appendiceal catheters. The patient is usually discharged from the hospital 2 weeks postoperatively. The patient is instructed about the care of the catheters and the need to continue to irrigate the catheters, usually twice daily, depending on the amount of mucus present.

The patient returns to the office 3 to 4 weeks later (approximately 5 to 6 weeks postoperatively). A gravity pouchogram and an upper tract study (intravenous pyelogram or renal scan) are performed to ensure absence of extravasation and reflux (on the pouchogram) and good visualization and absence of significant dilation (on the upper tract study). In addition, urine culture is usually performed 3 days before the return appointment so that appropriate antibiotics can be prescribed during the visit.

If the results of the imaging studies outlined above are satisfactory, the patient is instructed about intermittent catheterization technique. We do this as an outpatient procedure in the office. The stenting catheter is removed. The patient is then instructed about the technique of clean intermittent catheterization (CIC). The reservoir is filled with saline through the cecostomy tube, and the patient repeats CIC several times to ensure that he or she masters this technique and is able to empty the urinary reservoir adequately. The cecostomy tube is then removed, and a dressing is applied on its site. The patient is instructed to continue CIC every 2 hours for 1 week, every 3 hours for 6 more weeks, and then every 4 hours. Pouch irriga-

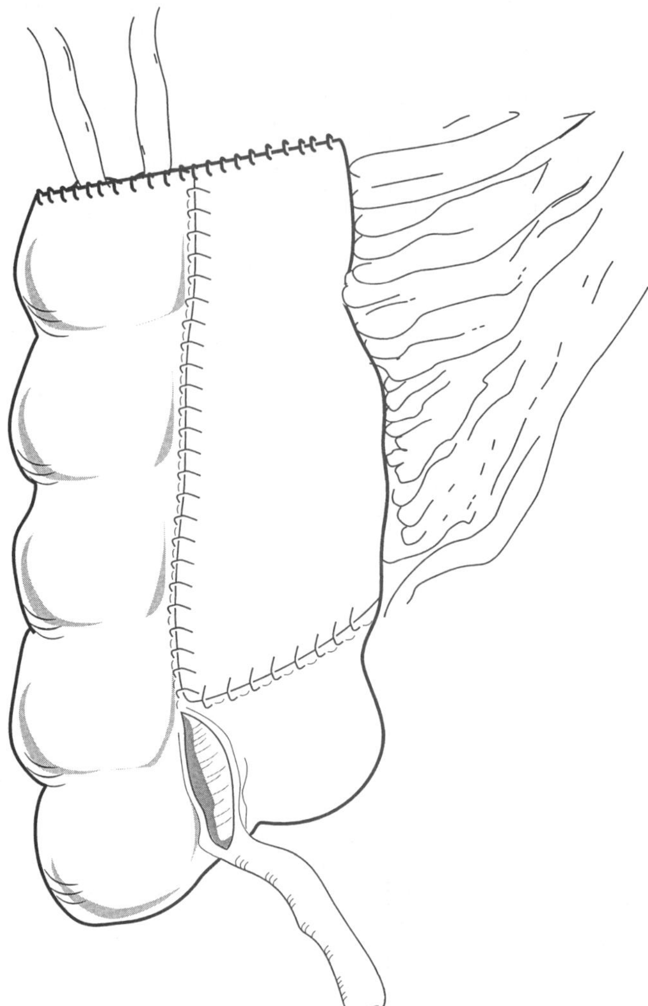

Fig. 32.8. Reservoir is closed by approximating the remaining ileal and colonic edges.

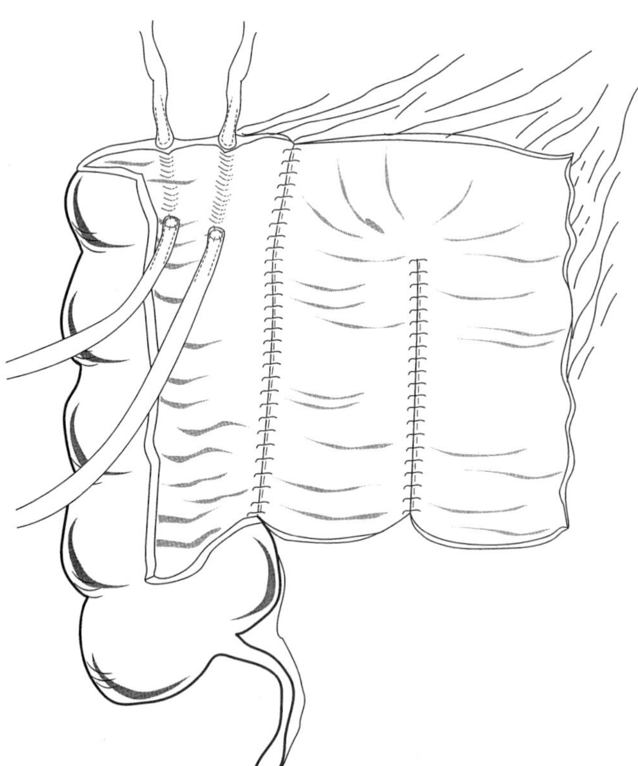

Fig. 32.7. Appendiceal Mainz pouch. A small bowel plate is formed and approximated to the adjacent border of the opened part of the colon. Ureters are implanted in the colon.

tion is performed once or twice daily depending on the amount of mucus.

Patients are also instructed about the manifestations of possible complications and how to recognize and report them appropriately. At the 3-month postoperative visit, urinalysis, urine culture, serum creatinine, and electrolytes are obtained. Patients are usually instructed to perform 4-hourly catheterizations and often can be allowed to skip one catheterization at night to allow adequate sleep. They keep a urinary diary for 2 to 3 days before each outpatient visit. Most patients do not need to cover the umbilical stoma, although a few may prefer to use an adhesive bandage or occasionally a piece of gauze. Follow-up continues indefinitely, although at less frequent intervals.

After 2 years, a physical examination and laboratory evaluation (including the measurement of vitamin B_{12} levels) are performed every 6 months and a radiologic evaluation is performed on a yearly basis. We also administer intramuscular vitamin B_{12} supplementation, 100 μg, every 2 to 3 months.

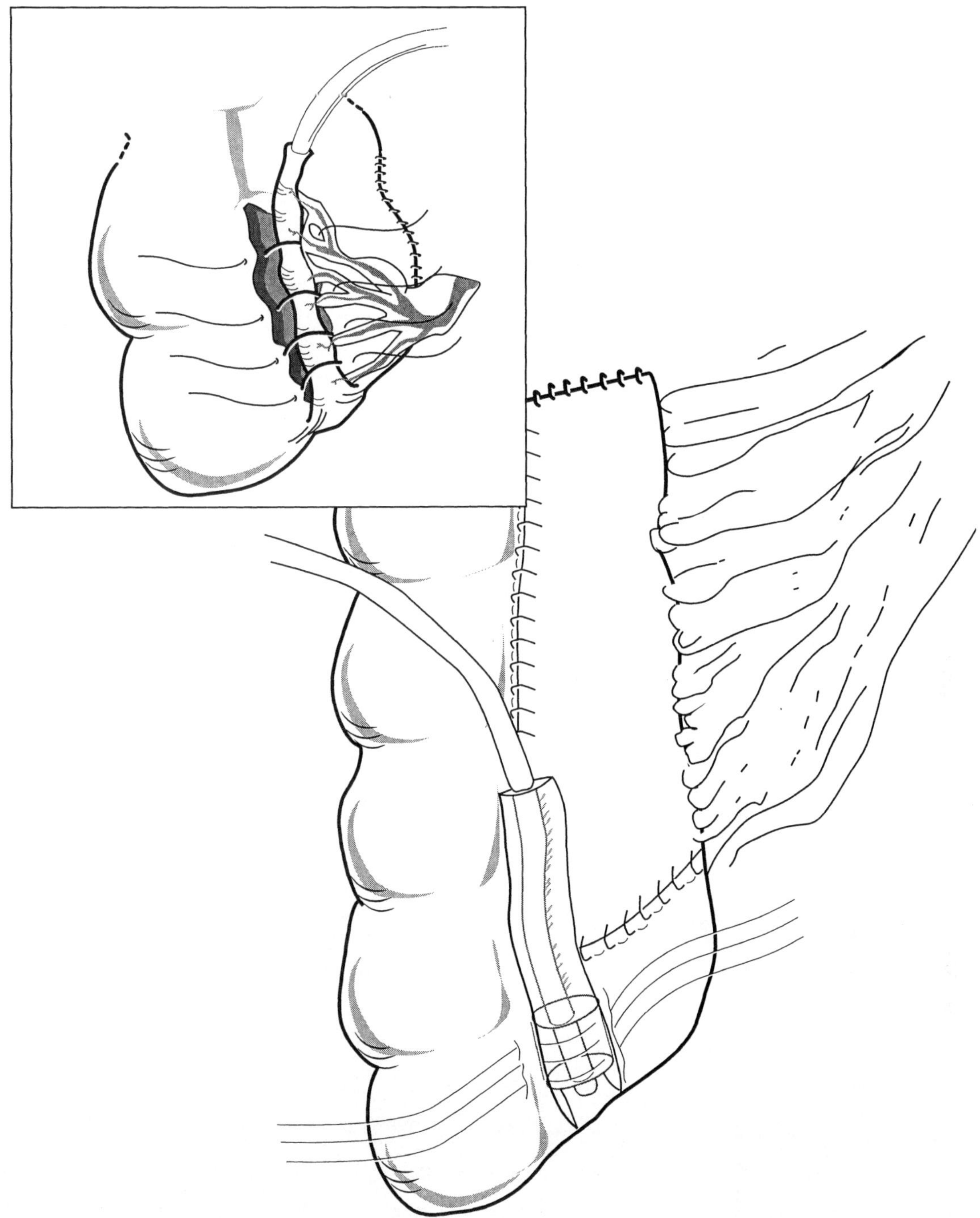

Fig. 32.9. Seromuscular incision is made in the tenia of the intact cecal wall to expose the mucosa. Submucosal bed is created by dissecting the seromuscular tissue. The appendix is folded over and its proximal 4 cm lie in the colonic mucosa. The seromuscular layer is approximated over the appendix. Insert: The seromuscular layer over the appendix should be closed with care to preserve the appendicular blood supply.

Technique of Charleston Pouch in Patients With Prior Appendectomy

In the absence of an appendix, a short segment (5 to 6 cm) of tapered terminal ileum (neoappendix) is used for the continence mechanism. Usually, a slightly longer segment of ileum than in the standard Charleston pouch is isolated. The most distal 5 to 6 cm are used for continence. The more proximal part of the isolated ileal segment (approximately 12 to 18 cm) is incorporated into the reservoir. The distal segment that is used for continence is tapered by placing a 12F red rubber catheter through the open end and into the cecum. A GIA stapling device is then used to place staples on the new tapered segment while removing two thirds of the ileal circumference at the

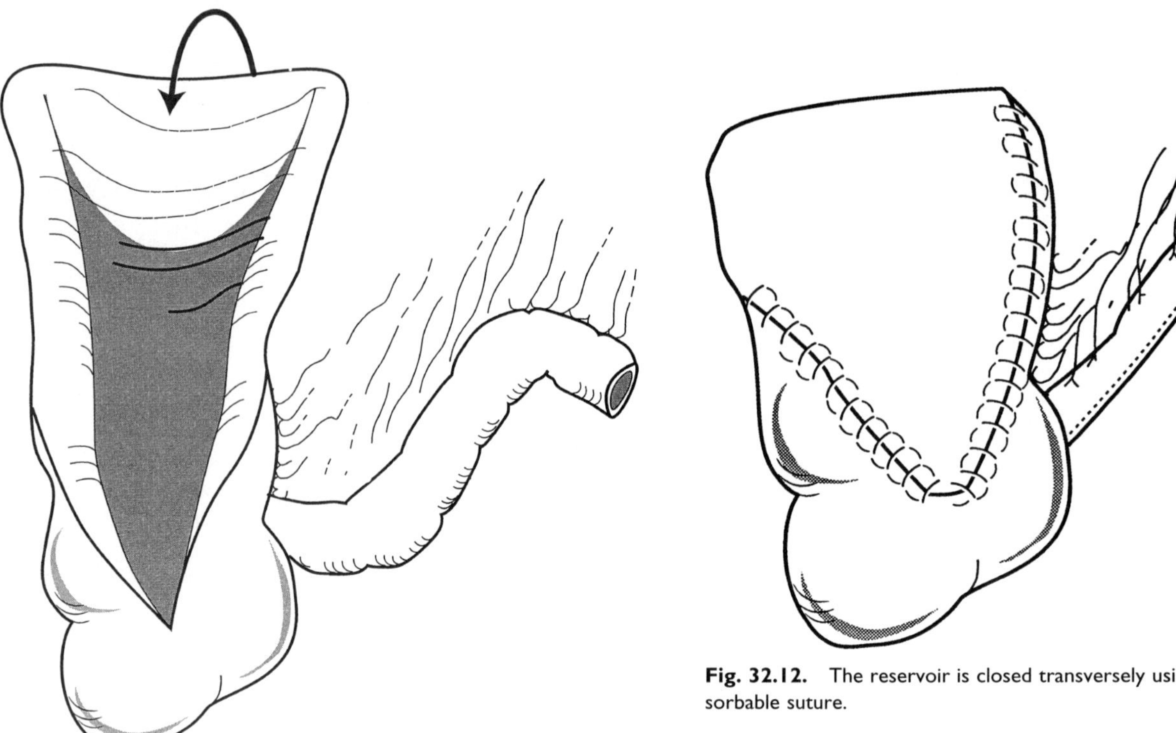

Fig. 32.10. Indiana pouch. An 8- to 10-cm segment of terminal ileum and a 25-cm segment of cecum and ascending colon are isolated. The colonic segment is opened along the antimesenteric border along the entire length of the colon, sparing only 1 to 2 cm of cecal cap.

Fig. 32.12. The reservoir is closed transversely using a running 3-0 absorbable suture.

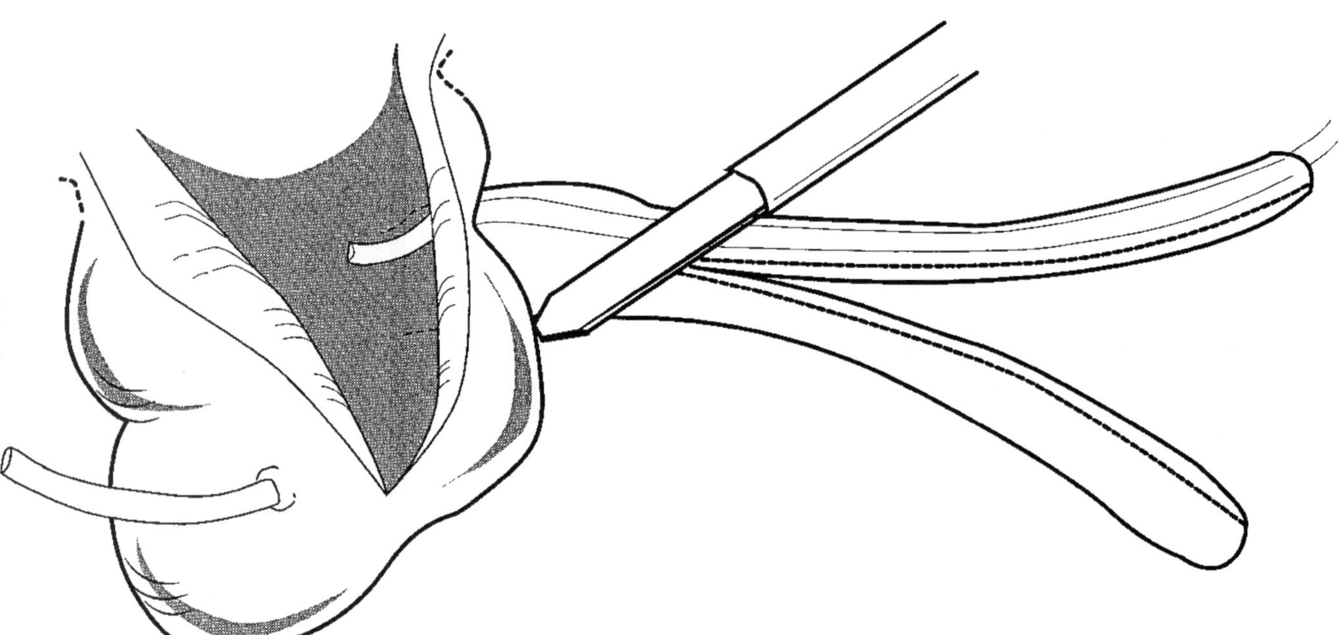

Fig. 32.11. The terminal ileum is tapered over a 12F catheter using metal GIA staples. Three-zero silk sutures will be used to plicate the area of the ileocecal valve.

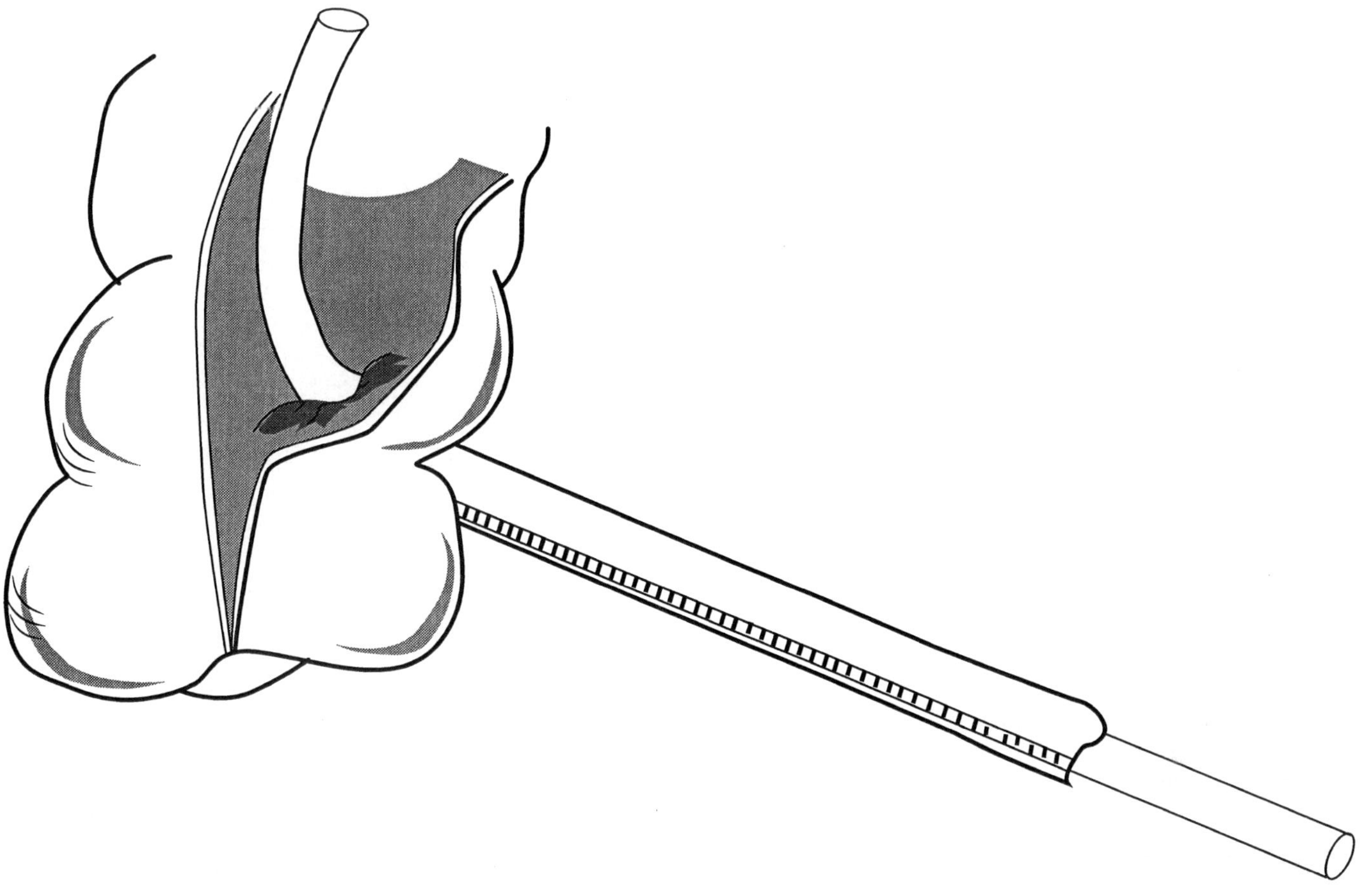

Fig. 32.13. Miami pouch. The ileal segment is tapered over 14F catheter using metal staples. The distal-most part of the tapered ileum will be reinforced with three purse-string sutures tied snugly over the 14F catheter.

antimesenteric border. This results in a narrow, well-vascularized segment that resembles the appendix.

The continence mechanism is accomplished by placing two imbricating or purse-string sutures, which are tied snugly over a 12F catheter in the tapered ileum near the ileocolic junction. Leak pressure is then measured to determine the adequacy of the continence mechanism. Usually, two to four sutures 8 mm apart from each other starting at the ileocolic junction are required. Once the continence mechanism is considered satisfactory with a leak point pressure of greater than 80 cm water, the colonic and the ileal segment to be used for the reservoir are completely detubularized and formed into inverted U-shaped patches. The remainder of the procedure is identical to that described before for appendiceal Charleston pouch procedure.

The Modified Mainz Pouch Technique

The appendiceal Mainz pouch uses an ileocolic urinary reservoir, and the appendix is used for continence (18). It requires the presence of a normal appendix of 9 to 10 cm in length, a diameter of 0.6 to 0.8 cm at the base, and the absence of inflammatory changes. For creation of the reservoir, 12 cm of cecum and ascending colon and about 2 feet of ileum are used.

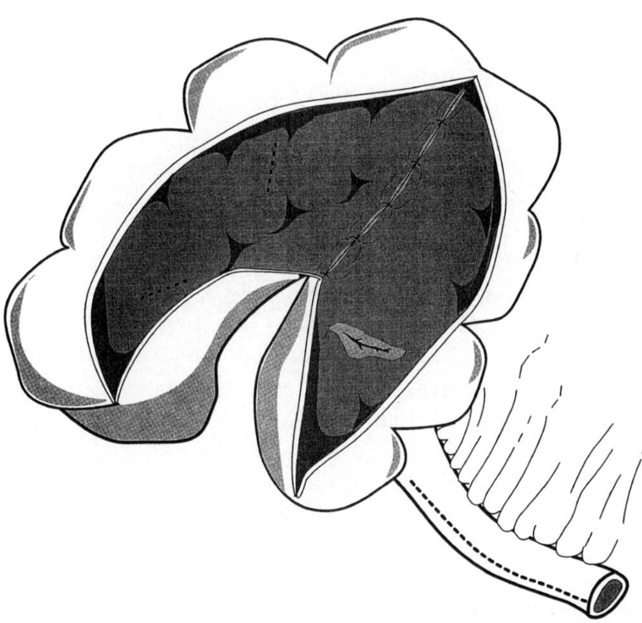

Fig. 32.14. The colon is completely opened, folded in a U shape, and the adjacent edges are sutured to each other. The ureters are implanted.

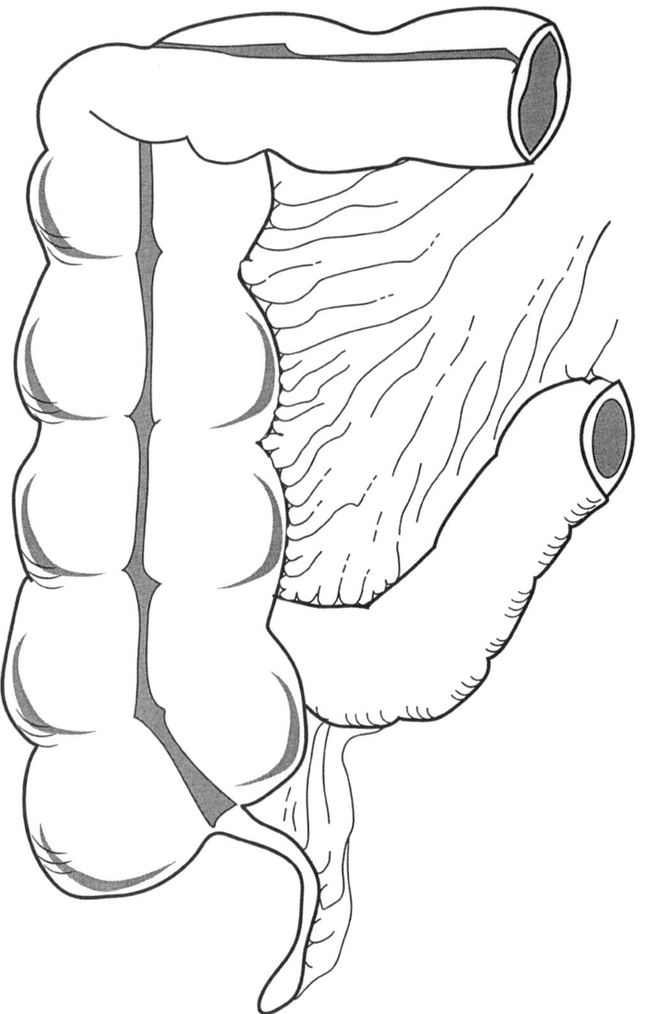

Fig. 32.15. Florida pouch. An extended right colonic segment and a terminal segment of ileum are isolated based on the right colic and ileocolic vessels.

After the appropriate bowel segment is isolated, an antimesenteric incision is made in the ileum and the upper three fourths of the colon, keeping the caudal 4 to 5 cm of the cecum intact. A small bowel plate is made. This is approximated to the adjacent border of the colon (Fig. 32.7). Ureteral reimplantation is performed, and the reservoir is closed by approximating the remaining ileal and colonic edges (Fig. 32.8). A seromuscular incision is then made in the tenia of the intact cecal wall to expose the mucosa (Fig. 32.8). Extended dissection of the seromuscular tissue creates a broad submucosal bed for the appendix. The appendicular mesentery is freed of excessive fatty tissue. The seromuscular layer is closed over the embedded appendix (Fig. 32.9), with care taken to preserve the blood supply to the appendix (Fig. 32.9 inset). This creates a tunnel length of about 4 cm and leaves a free mobile part of the appendix to bring to the skin. The appendicocutaneous stoma is accomplished in the right lower quadrant or can be placed at the umbilicus. A cecostomy and an appendicular stent are

used. Postoperative care is similar to that after Charleston pouch techniques.

USE OF THE TERMINAL ILEUM AND ILEOCECAL VALVE FOR CONTINENCE

The unaltered ileocecal valve is inadequate to maintain continence. Several authors introduced techniques to improve continence in patients having right colonic or ileocolonic urinary reservoirs. These techniques rely on either the augmented ileocecal valve with tapered terminal ileum for providing continence or the use of intussuscepted ileal or ileocecal nipple. The main concern with intussuscepted ileal or ileocecal nipple valve is the tendency to slide. This is the basis for devising complicated maneuvers to stabilize the intussusception. Most of these techniques rely on metal staples to stabilize the intussusception. We do not believe that these techniques offer any advantage over those using tapered terminal ileum and simple augmentation of the ileocecal valve and/or the terminal ileum.

The Indiana, Florida, and Miami pouches and their modifications are current notable procedures that are commonly done and that use tapered ileum and augmented terminal ileum or ileocecal valve (20–23). These relatively simple techniques rely on imbrication or plication of the ileocecal valve along with tapering of the adjoining ileal segment. They provide a reliable continence mechanism. As previously described, we have used a short segment of tapered terminal ileum (neoappendix) for continence with similar outcome (24).

The Indiana Continent Urinary Reservoir

The initial experience at Indiana University relied on a minor modification of the pioneering technique described by Gilchrist (25). In this technique, the cecum and ascending colon were used to create a reservoir. The ureters were tunneled with an antireflux technique. The terminal ileum was used as the efferent limb, relying on the ileocecal valve to provide continence. A series of modifications were necessary to improve continence. The reservoir was initially detubularized by the addition of an ileal patch. Later, a longer segment of cecum and ascending colon was used (20). The continence mechanism in the Indiana pouch relied on a plicated, 10- to 12-cm segment of terminal ileum. Lambert sutures were used to plicate the efferent limb, and a second layer of running sutures was used to reinforce the Lambert suture line. Subsequently, the terminal ileum was tapered by stapling technique as described in the Miami pouch technique (22).

In the most recent experience, an 8- to 10-cm segment of terminal ileum and a 25- to 30-cm segment of cecum and ascending colon are isolated (21). This segment is based on the ileocecal and right colic vessels. An ileocolostomy is performed to establish continuity of the alimentary tract. The colonic segment is detubularized by incising the antimesenteric border of the colon along the entire length of the colon, sparing only

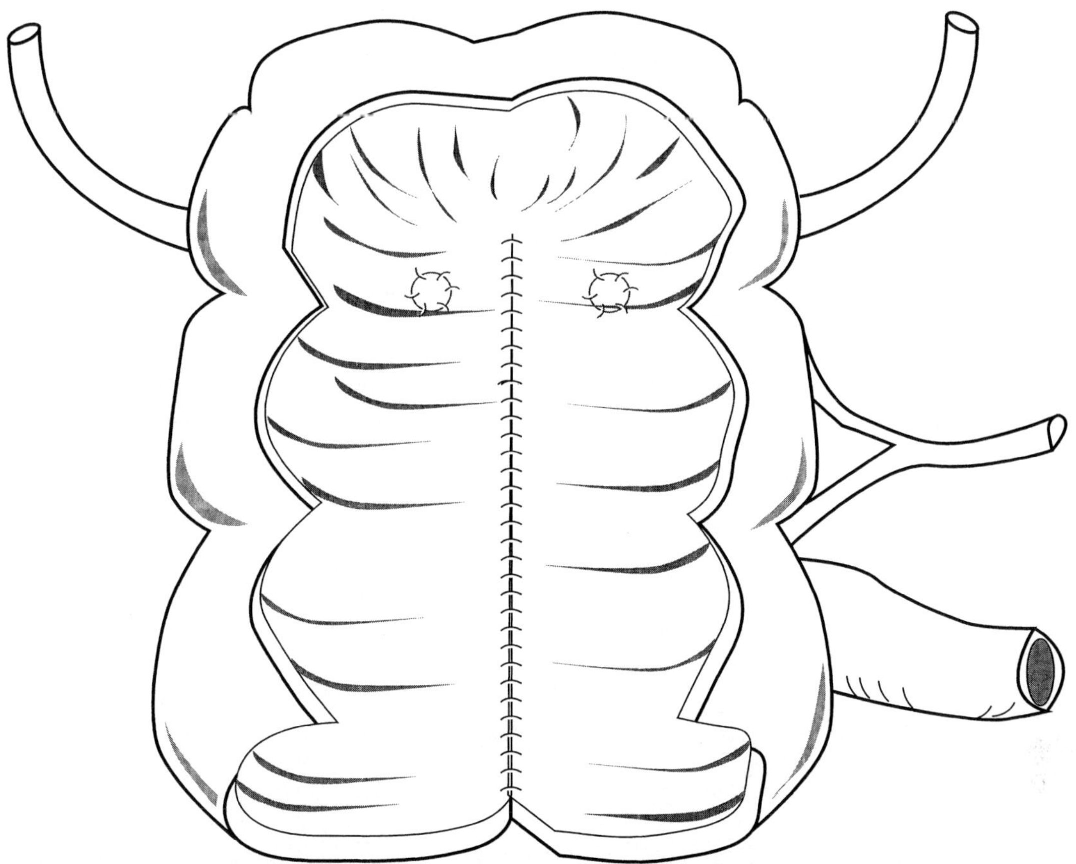

Fig. 32.16.   The colon is opened completely, folded into two limbs, and the adjacent edges are approximated. The ureters are implanted without tunneling.

1 to 2 cm of the cecal cap (Fig. 32.10). If the appendix is present, an appendectomy is performed.

The terminal ileum is tapered using metal GIA staples (Fig. 32.11). This tapering is performed over a 12F catheter. Three-zero silk Lambert sutures are used to plicate the area of the ileocecal valve. A lubricated 18F catheter is passed through the tapered ileum and imbricated ileocecal valve area. It should pass easily through the tapered ileum. Resistance should be felt when the catheter passes through the imbricated area. If no resistance is felt, additional Lambert sutures are placed further along the adjacent ileum until some resistance is noted on catheter passage. However, if the catheter cannot be passed, sutures are removed from the ileal portion of the plication until the catheter passes with some resistance.

A large Malecot catheter is placed through the cap of the cecum to drain the reservoir postoperatively. The reservoir is then closed by folding the cephalad end of the segment down to the bottom of the antimesenteric incision (Fig. 32.12). The reservoir is closed transversely using a single layer of running 3-0 absorbable suture. After the reservoir is closed, it is placed in the right lower quadrant and the ureteral implantation is performed.

The left ureter is passed through the left colon mesentery. The ureters are implanted using a tunneled antirefluxing tech-

nique. Care must be taken during this part of the procedure so that the implanted ureters are not affected by the folding over of the ascending colon.

The Florida and Miami Pouch Techniques

As stated previously, the current technique of Indiana continent urinary diversion shares similarities to the Miami and Florida continent urinary diversion. They all use a right colon reservoir. In the technique described by Bejany and Politano (22), the distal ileum is tapered by stapling (Fig. 32.13), and then the distal-most part of the tapered ileum is reinforced with three purse-string sutures tied snugly over a 14F red rubber catheter. The reservoir itself is formed by the cecum and ascending colon. The colon is completely detubularized, folded in a U shape, and the adjacent edges are sutured to each other (Fig. 32.14). The ureters are implanted in a nontunneled fashion after passing them through a large hiatus to avoid obstruction. The distal ends of the ureters are spatulated. The mucosa of the colon is incised to create a mucosal sulcus 1.5 to 2 cm in length. The ureter is laid into the sulcus and its spatulated distal end is sutured to the colon with 4-0 Vicryl (Ethicon, Sommerville, NJ) sutures. The adventitia of the ureter is lightly fixed to the colonic mucosa with 4-0 Vicryl. The reservoir is then closed

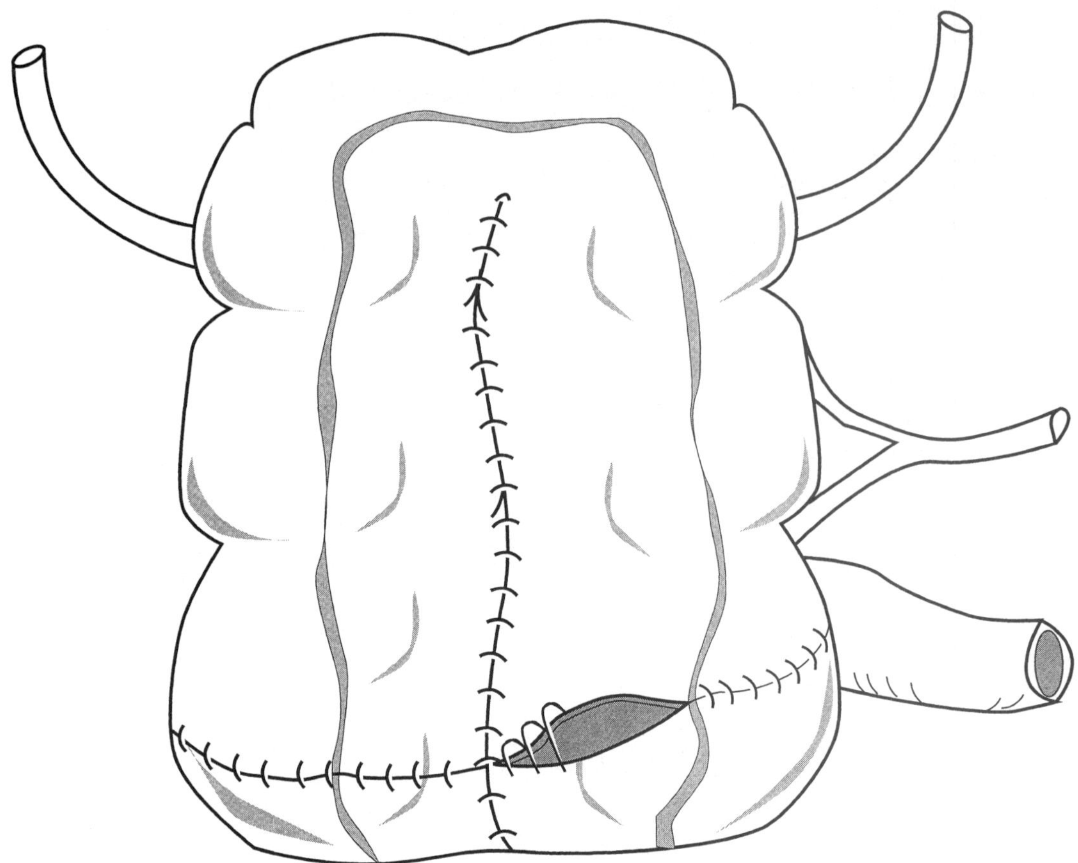

Fig. 32.17. Colonic closure completed.

by approximating the remaining edges of the colon. The end of the tapered ileal segment is brought to the skin level.

In the Florida pouch technique described by Lockhart et al., an extended right colonic segment (Fig. 32.15) is isolated based on the right colic and ileocolic vessels (23). The colon is folded and the two limbs are approximated (Fig. 32.16). Absorbable staples were recently used for this approximation. The ureters are implanted without tunneling to avoid obstruction (26). Colonic closure is completed (Fig. 32.17). The terminal ileum is used as the efferent continence mechanism. It is plicated with two parallel rows of silk sutures over a 12Fr Robinson catheter. More recently, a tapered ileal segment similar to the Miami technique was also used. Plicating sutures are extended through the ileocecal valve and cecum to augment the continence mechanism.

COMMENT

Cutaneous and urethral continent urinary diversions are now the most popular procedures for most patients who need supravesical urinary diversion. Several forms of continent cutaneous urinary diversions that use the right colon or ileocolic bowel segment have been presented. Our preference has been the appendiceal Charleston pouch whenever the appendix is present. Although we and several other authors have successfully used other forms, the classic Charleston pouch has many advantages. It is simple and can be adopted by most modern urologists. It provides excellent continence and ease of catheterization. It avoids using excessive length of small bowel with subsequent metabolic consequences. It is also cosmetically pleasing; the stoma site has been unnoticeable in the majority of our patients.

REFERENCES

1. Bissada NK. Current status of supravesical urinary diversion and bladder substitution. In: Rous SN, ed. Urology Annual. New York: WW Norton, 1993:69.
2. Lieskovsky G, Boyd SD, Skinner DG. Management of late complications of the Koch pouch form of urinary diversion. J Urol 1987;137:1146.
3. Quinlan DM, Leonard MP, Brendler CB, et al. Use of the Benchekroun hydraulic valve as a catheterizable continence mechanism. J Urol 1991;145:1155.
4. Scheidler DM, Klee LW, Rowland RG, et al. Update on the Indiana continent urinary reservoir. J Urol 1989;141:302. Abstract.
5. Thuroff JW, Alken P, Riedmiller H, et al. The Mainz pouch (mixed augmentation ileum cecum) for bladder augmentation and continent urinary diversion. World J Urol 1985;3:179.

6. Wilson TG, Moreno JG, Weinberg A, et al. Late complications of the modified Indiana pouch. J Urol 1994; 151:331.

7. Verhoogen J. Neostomie uretero-cécale. Assoc Franc di Urol 1908;12:352.

8. Mitrofanoff P. Trans-appendicular continent cystostomy in the management of neurogenic bladder. Chir Pediatr 1980;21:297.

9. Bissada NK, Marshall IY. Toward construction of an ideal continent urinary reservoir: the Charleston pouch with an in-situ appendix. Scand J Urol Nephrol 1992;142(Suppl):150.

10. Bissada NK. A new continent ileocolonic urinary reservoir: the Charleston pouch with minimally altered in-situ appendix stoma. Urology 1993;41:524.

11. Bissada NK. Characteristics and utility of the in-situ appendix as a continent catheterizable stoma for continent urinary diversion in adults. J Urol 1993;150:151.

12. Bissada NK. Experience with the in-situ appendix as a catheterizable stoma for continent urinary diversion: the Charleston pouch. J Urol 1993;149:325. Abstract.

13. Bissada NK. Experience with ileocecal continent urinary diversion: the Charleston pouch. Contemp Urol 1995;7:47.

14. Marshall IY, Bissada NK. Study of the unaltered in-situ appendix as a native continence mechanism: cadaveric and clinical correlation. J Invest Surg 1995;8:147.

15. Marshall I, Bissada NK. Studies on the use of in-situ appendix as a native continence mechanism. J Urol 1992;147:391. Abstract.

16. Bissada NK, Marshall IY. Intra-operative adjustment of the continence mechanism in patients undergoing continent urinary diversion. J Urol 1994;151:241. Abstract.

17. Duckett JW, Snyder HM III. Continent urinary diversion: variations on the Mitrofanoff principle. J Urol 1989;63:58.

18. Riedmiller H, Burger R, Muller S, et al. Continent appendix stoma; a modification of the Mainz pouch technique. J Urol 1990;143:1115.

19. Bissada NK. The case for choosing the umbilical site for continent urinary diversion stoma. Submitted for publication.

20. Rowland RG, Mitchell ME, Bihrle R, et al. Indiana continent urinary reservoir. J Urol 1987;137:1136.

21. Rowland RG, Kropp BP. Evolution of the Indiana continent urinary reservoir. J Urol 1994;152:2247.

22. Bejany DE, Politano VA. Stapled and non-stapled tapered distal ileum for construction of a colonic continent urinary reservoir. J Urol 1988;140:491.

23. Lockhart JL, Pow-Sang JM, Persky L, et al. A continent colonic urinary reservoir: the Florida pouch. J Urol 1990;144:864.

24. Bissada NK. Satisfactory experience with the Charleston pouches for continent urinary diversion. Proceedings of XXVIII world congress of the International College of Surgeons, Bologna: Italy, 1992.

25. Gilchrist RK, Merricks JW, Hamlin HH, et al. Construction of a substitute bladder and urethra. Surg Gynecol Obstet 1950;90:752.

26. Helal M, Pow-Sang J, Sanford E, et al. Direct (nontunneled) ureterocolonic reimplantation in association with continent reservoirs. J Urol 1993;150:835.

33

Continent Diversion to the Urethra

Perinchery Narayan and Viswanathan Gajendran

Life is short and the art long, occasion instant, experiment perilous.

HIPPOCRATES

Cystectomy is the most effective form of treatment for deep muscle invasive bladder cancer. This procedure, however, has not been acceptable to many patients because of the need for urostomy, with its social and personal inconveniences. Attempts at avoiding urostomy have resulted in the use of bowel segments as continent bladder substitutes. The past 10 years have witnessed significant advances in the technique of bladder substitution procedures. This has made cystectomy a more widely acceptable procedure.

Ideally, a bladder substitute should function as a low-pressure reservoir, with antirefluxing, nonobstructing ureteric anastomoses; have the ability to empty completely; and be continent with either an abdominal stoma or anastomosis to the urethra. The choice of bowel segment is influenced by the physical characteristics of bowel, technical simplicity of pouch construction, and extent of metabolic sequelae. Ultimately, the choice is based on results of long-term success with various substitutes.

Tizzoni and Poggi are credited with designing the first bladder substitution procedure in 1888, which was performed in a dog (1). Many of the present-day advances should be credited to Camey. He first performed an enterocystoplasty in 1958 and refined the technique during the ensuing years (2).

In this chapter, we describe and illustrate several of the common continent diversions to the urethra and discuss their advantages and disadvantages. The suture materials, stents, catheters, and drains mentioned in the text are standard but may easily be substituted, depending on the surgeon's preferences.

GENERAL CONSIDERATIONS

Bowel Selection

Hinman has outlined several principles to guide the urologist in selecting bowel for bladder substitution (3). The first consideration is geometric configuration—volume rises by the square of the radius. The second consideration is accommodation—at any physiologic pressure, the reservoir with the larger radius will hold a greater volume. The third is compliance. However, little difference in viscoelastic properties of bowel segments persists after 6 months. The fourth consideration is contractility—disruption of normal tubular structure will dampen the intraluminal pressure spikes.

Patient Selection

The selection of patients for continent diversion to the urethra has to be carefully planned. The factors that influence the selection criteria are both patient and disease related.

Patient Factors

Continent diversion has been restricted to male patients until recently. This is because of certain technical problems and inadequate understanding of the urinary continence mechanism in women. However, recent studies have elucidated the functional anatomy responsible for continence and innervation of the urethra in women (4–7). With encouraging results in a small group of 13 women from UCLA and gratifying European experience, it appears that continent diversion to the urethra can be applied in select women undergoing cystectomy (5, 6). However, the disturbing report of 60% hypercontinence requiring clean intermittent catheterization (CIC) in women undergoing the procedure emphasizes that the procedure has to be applied with caution in women (8). It is simpler and more convenient to have an abdominal stoma for CIC in a woman rather than a failed continent diversion to the urethra.

Age is an important factor because abdominal muscle strength is required to bear down to empty the bladder. Because older age is associated with poor abdominal muscle tone, the ideal candidates are usually relatively young patients who are physically fit and have good abdominal muscle strength.

Manual dexterity, motivation and desire to work through initial problems, and adequate intelligence to do so are some of the other requirements. Although ideally continent reservoirs to the urethra will eliminate the need for self-catheterization, several situations may necessitate CIC. These include an occasional failure to empty the bladder and conversion to abdominal stoma for technical reasons; further CIC is often required during initial weeks after the procedure. Patients having intestine as urinary reservoirs need to have lifelong follow-up care to detect metabolic complications. In addition, recurrent disease and complications related to the procedure need to be detected at an early stage to institute appropriate management. Hence, the patients selected for these procedures must be intelligent to understand the consequences of the procedure and the need for rigorous compliance. They must be well-motivated to get involved in the program for a successful outcome.

Disease Factors

The ideal bladder substitute should allow the patient to maintain body image and void normally. However, this goal should not result in compromise of principles of cancer surgery. A relatively young male, who does not need urethrectomy as part of his treatment and who has not had prior high-dose radiation to the bladder, is an ideal candidate for continent diversion to the urethra. The incidence of concurrent urethral and bladder transitional cell cancer is approximately 7% (9). We do not routinely perform urethrectomy unless preoperative evaluation reveals prostatic urethral involvement or frozen section shows cancer at the urethral margins. However, 8 to 12% of patients with bladder cancer have a recurrence in the urethra as it continues to be exposed to potential carcinogens (10). Therefore, urethrocystoscopy and urinary cytology are recommended in such patients annually after continent diversion.

There is a significant incidence of concurrent prostate cancer in patients undergoing cystectomy for bladder cancer (11, 12). When adequately excised, concomitant prostate cancer may not be an additional risk factor in these patients, as evidenced by the findings of Androulakakis et al. (13). These authors, in a 12-year follow-up, demonstrated that prognosis was dependent only on the stage and grade of bladder cancer.

Carcinoma in situ or an invasive tumor at the bladder neck is a relative contraindication, as is the presence of metastases. Preexisting bowel conditions are relative contraindications; choice of bowel segments have to be carefully made, based on the assessment of the bowel problems.

Ileitis, short bowel syndrome, chronic diarrhea, and malabsorption syndromes preclude the use of small bowel for reservoir construction. Colon cancers and premalignant conditions of the colon rule out the use of large bowel for reservoir construction. The use of stomach is limited by hyperacidity. However, in patients with existing metabolic acidosis, stomach will provide an alternative source for construction of urinary reservoir. Patients who already have artificial sphincters for incontinence or prosthesis for impotence are not ideal candidates for continent diversion to the urethra.

Patient Preparation

All bladder substitution patients receive an oral mechanical bowel preparation (Colyte, a colon electrolyte lavage preparation; Reed and Carnrick, Piscataway, NJ) while ingesting a clear liquid diet for 48 hours. A parenteral first-generation cephalosporin is used in the perioperative period, and each patient receives prophylaxis with either pneumatic compression stockings or sodium warfarin to prevent deep vein thrombosis.

Bladder Substitution Using Small Bowel Segments

Camey or similar procedures have been the most performed urinary reservoirs using the urethra as the outlet. In 1979, Camey and LeDuc reported their positive experience with patients who underwent construction of an ileal bladder substitute after radical cystoprostatectomy (2). The long-term results revealed 90% continence rate in patients if they adhered to a voiding interval of 2 to 3 hours (14). Nighttime incontinence was a major problem. Short or fatty mesentery in 15% of patients led to abandoning the procedure. The operative mortality rate was 5%. The intraluminal pressure of the pouch reached 80 cm water, even in patients with significant daytime continence. Camey has subsequently modified his technique with detubularization (see below).

Camey I Technique (Fig. 33.1)

A major component of the original Camey procedure is careful dissection of the urethra from the apex of the prostate. Camey preserved the apex of the prostate gland to ensure continence, but this is acceptable only in young patients with benign bladder disease. The indication for bladder substitution in patients with benign disease is rare since alternative bladder-preserving techniques are possible.

A 35- to 40-cm segment of ileum is chosen so that its midportion can reach the urethra without tension. The segment with its mesentery is isolated, and continuity of the bowel is reestablished with an ileoileostomy. An opening of 1 cm in diameter is created in the antimesenteric border of the ileal segment 3 to 4 cm to the right of midpoint. This makes the left limb longer because it has to travel over the rectosigmoid to meet the left ureter above the iliac vessels. This opening is then sutured to the membranous urethra with six to ten absorbable sutures over a 20Fr, 6-hole Foley catheter.

The 6-hole Foley catheter is advanced into the right limb so that it will lie in the direction of peristalsis rather than against it (Fig. 33.1A). The ureters are brought into the lumen of the ileum at each end through a stab incision. A strip of mucosa about 1 cm wide is excised, creating a 3-cm trough (Fig. 33.1B). The ureter is laid in the trough and fixed with interrupted 4-0 chromic catgut sutures placed on both sides between the edges of the trough and side walls of the ureter (Fig. 33.1C). Excess ureter is cut, the cut end splayed open and fixed to the ileal mucosa.

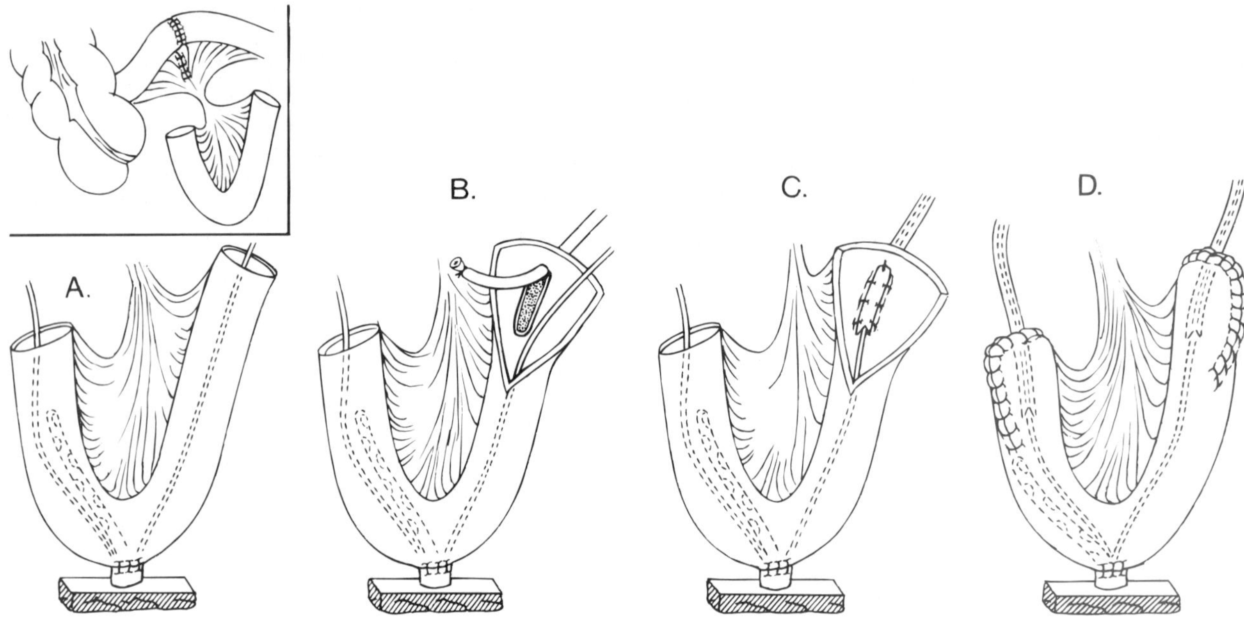

Fig. 33.1.   The Camey enterocystoplasty.

Polyethylene feeding tubes (8Fr size) are used to stent the ureters. The tubes are brought out through a stab wound in the ileum and abdominal wall. The open ends of the ileal segment are closed with a running through-and-through 3-0 chromic catgut suture and an inverting layer of interrupted 3-0 silk sutures (Fig. 33.1D). Each limb of the ileal segment is fixed to the psoas muscle, lateral to the common iliac artery, with two or three sutures of 2-0 chromic catgut. The ureteral stents are removed after 5 to 7 days. Stents are removed one at a time to permit differential pouch and ureteric urine collection. The patient receives pouch irrigations with sterile saline every 6 to 8 hours. Pericatheterograms are done at 10 days and repeated every week if leaks occur. The urethral catheter is removed after 3 weeks.

Detubularized Procedures

Urodynamic and metabolic factors dictate that the bladder substitute should be spherical to achieve higher capacity and compliance with minimal absorption of solutes when the ileum is used (15). This is achieved with detubularization. The advantages of a detubularized reservoir are as follows.

1. The volume is maximized; hence, maximum capacity is obtained from any given length of bowel.
2. Detubularization results in antimesenteric disruption of circular smooth musculature. Further cross-folding of the bowel to make a pouch results in contractions becoming incoordinate and asynchronous in the reservoir wall. This minimizes development of high-pressure peaks. There is also a compressor chamber effect, which causes the pressure peaks from contraction of one section of the bowel to be dampened by the other sections.

3. A spherical reservoir has maximum radius that minimizes end-filling pressure (Laplace's law).
4. Because of maximal radius at a given pressure, wall tension is maximized (tension α pressure α radius); thus, a sensation of fullness is more likely.
5. When constructing a spherical reservoir for a given volume, the length of the bowel resection and area available for reabsorption for the reservoir are minimized.

Several techniques have been described using various configurations, such as an M, W, S, or U, to construct detubularized bladder substitutes. As long as the reservoir is made from cross-folded ileal segments, configuration is relatively unimportant.

The Modified Camey Procedure (Fig. 33.2)

Camey modified his original operation with detubularization to overcome the high intraluminal pressures resulting from using intact ileum (14). The ileal segment is opened at its antimesenteric border and is folded into a U-shaped configuration (Fig. 33.2A). The adjacent limbs of the U are joined together with continuous sutures of 3-0 polyglycolic acid (PGA), thus creating a patch of opened ileum (Fig. 33.2B). The ureters are brought to the luminal side as before and are fixed. The patch is folded up, and the edges are sutured with 3-0 PGA to conform into a pouch (Fig. 33.2C), leaving a 1-cm defect at the most dependent part for urethroileal anastomoses. Closure of the reservoir is then completed, and urethroileal anastomoses performed with 2-0 chromic catgut sutures (Fig. 33.2D).

Vesica Ileal Padovanna Pouch (Fig. 33.3)

The Italian Group described a procedure similar to the Camey II technique, except that the spatulated ileum was rolled on

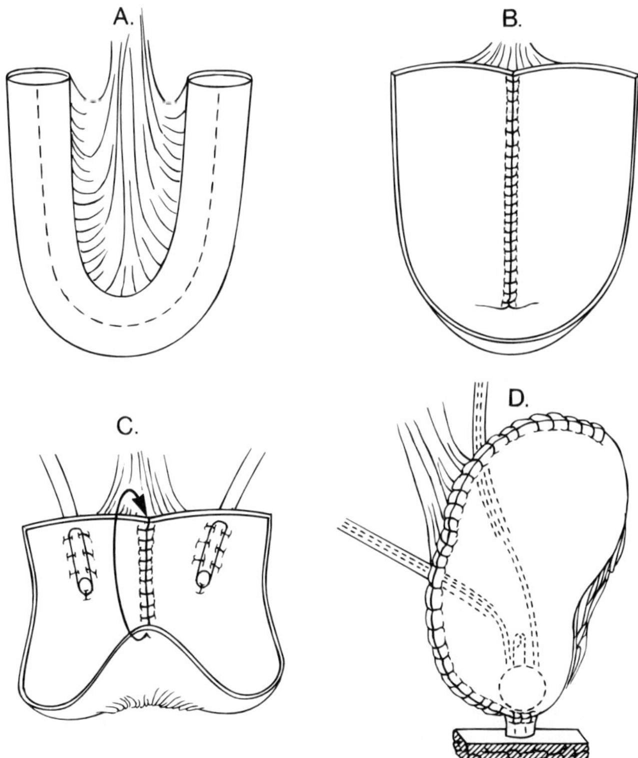

Fig. 33.2. The modified Camey enterocystoplasty with detubularization of the ileal segment.

itself (as in a jelly roll) to produce a posterior plate that is then closed anteriorly (16). This group reported 92% daytime continence and 87% nocturnal continence.

Hemi-Kock Urethral Pouch (Fig. 33.4)

Kock described a technique in 1982 for constructing a continent urinary reservoir with a cutaneous stoma (17). The reservoir has an afferent ileal limb in which ureters are implanted; the efferent limb is used for catheterization. The ileal limbs are intussuscepted to prevent reflux and for continence. The Hemi-Kock procedure consists of anastomosis of the reservoir to the urethra and eliminates the need for an efferent ileal limb

(18). The pouch offers the advantage of adequate urine storage with acceptable low intraluminal pressures at maximal filling.

Several modifications of the procedure have been attempted to improve results. The essential features of the procedure are as follows.

A 45-cm segment of ileum is isolated 30 to 40 cm proximal to the ileocecal valve (Fig. 33.4A); a distal 30-cm segment is detubularized on the antimesenteric border, folded, and sewn together on one side to create a U-shaped intestinal plate that is then folded transversely, creating the reservoir (Fig. 33.4B). The proximal 15 cm are used for intussusception into the open ileum for a distance of 5 cm and are held in place by three to four rows of staples (using the TA-55 automatic stapler) and by several 3-0 silk seromuscular sutures placed at the outer base of the nipple (Fig. 33.4C). The ureters are joined to this segment of ileum either separately end-to-side or together with the common lumen anastomosed to ileum end-to-end. The urethra is anastomosed to an opening left in the most dependent portion of the suture line, uniting the edges of the reconfigured pouch (Fig. 33.4D).

Hemi-Kock urethral pouch is technically simple to perform. The intussusception is an effective means of preventing reflux. The ureteroileal anastomoses are easy to perform and are less often associated with stenosis. Smaller lengths of ureter can be used for anastomoses, allowing for adequate safety margins, using the longer proximal ileal segment that can reach higher. Use of staples predisposes to stone formation, which appears to be the main disadvantage with this procedure. Stenosis of the afferent valve is a rare complication that can be endoscopically dilated (19). If repeated dilations are required, such patients will need open surgical revision.

Modified Camey Procedure (Narayan) (Fig. 33.5)

The principal author has been performing a modified Camey-type procedure, which is his preference for bladder reconstruction. A 45-cm length of ileum is isolated and the bowel continuity restored using end-to-end ileoileal anastomosis (Fig. 33.5A). The isolated ileal segment is placed in W configuration. The segment is opened incising the antimesenteric border, leaving 4 to 6 cm at each end. The adjacent medial borders

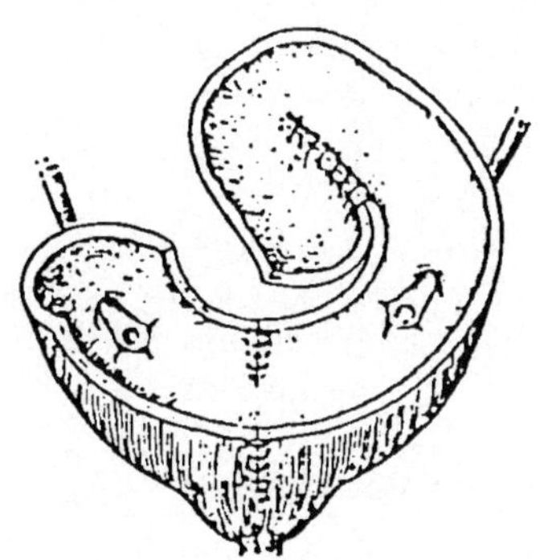
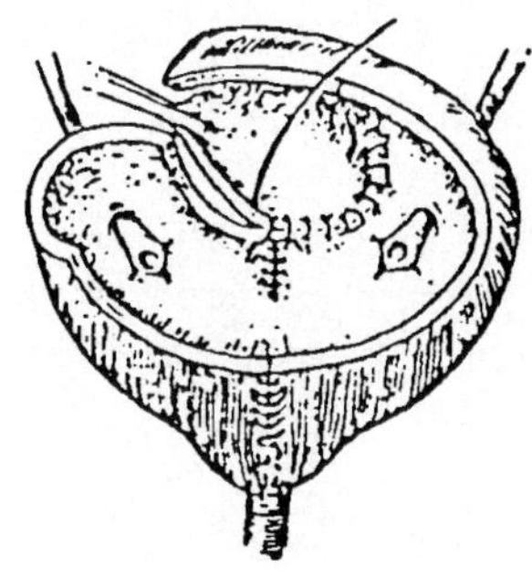

Fig. 33.3. Vesical ileal Padovanna pouch.

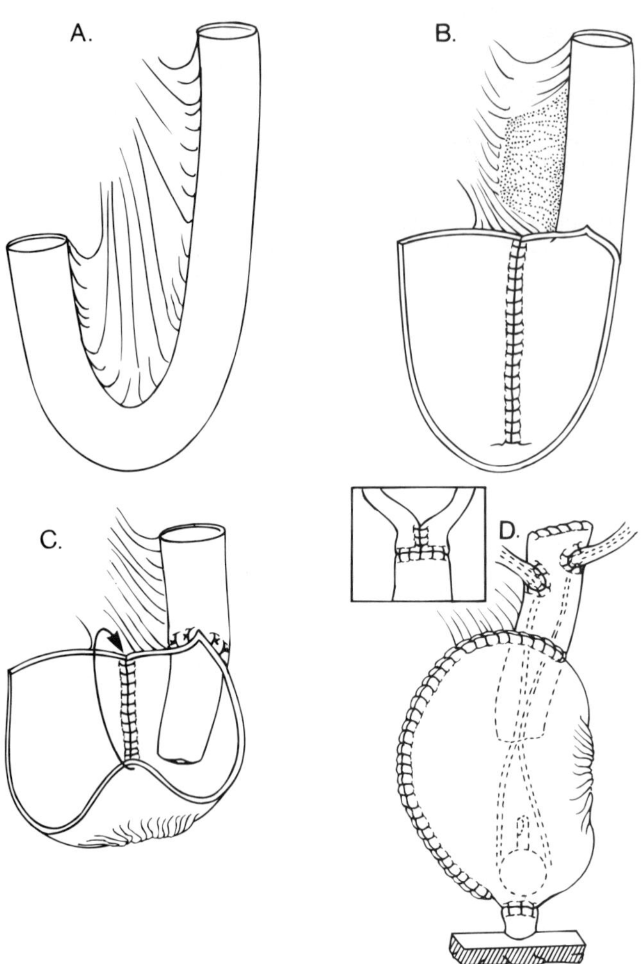

Fig. 33.4.   The Hemi-Kock operation.

win et al. in 1959 (Fig. 33.6) (20). Antireflux mechanisms consist of modified extraluminal intussuscepted ileum ("triple nipple"), ureters reimplanted with the split-cuff technique into a tubular afferent ileal limb, or the attachment to an isoperistaltic limb of 20 cm (Fig. 33.7) (21). The split-cuff technique reduces the length of ileum required for the pouch formation to 50 cm.

In a recent editorial, Studer cautioned that the role of antireflux techniques should not be overrated and that increased renal damage due to complications from strictures, stenoses, or malfunctions of antireflux techniques should be avoided (15). It is unclear whether an antireflux technique is required in a bladder substitute system with sterile urine. Although reflux will occur when the pressure exceeds that in the ureter, unlike normal bladder, there is no coordinated contraction producing an increased intravesical pressure in an orthotopic bladder substitute. The emptying is under its passive end-fill pressure mainly by outlet relaxation and then, if necessary, by abdominal straining. The end-fill pressure is low in a compliant system because the intraabdominal pressure acts equally on the reservoir and the ureters and no reflux occurs during straining. This has been confirmed manometrically (20). The only way reflux can occur is when the reservoir gets filled beyond the patient's normal voiding volume, producing a differential increase of pressure in the reservoir. This could be easily avoided by timed voiding. Absolute or relative indications for antireflux techniques may depend on basal and/or end-filling pressures, amplitude of pressure spikes, leak-point pressure of the outlet mechanism (which if low may serve as a safety valve), and presence or absence of chronically infected urine.

Modified Studer's Pouch (Fig. 33.8)

At Stanford, Freiha has circumferentially imbricated the proximal ileum at three or four different levels to enhance the antireflux mechanism.

Schreiter's Pouch (Fig. 33.9)

Schreiter described a technique to construct an S pouch using small intestine (22). The S pouch has been used in gastrointestinal surgery for ileoanal anastomosis after proctocolectomy. Seventy centimeters of terminal ileum are detached 25 to 30 cm proximal to the ileocecal valve. The isolated segment is detubularized at the antimesenteric border and formed into an S-shaped plate. The distal ileal portion is left tubular for 3 cm, tapered, and anastomosed to the urethra. The pouch is formed by folding this plate along its longitudinal axis. The antireflux mechanism consists of intussuscepted tubular proximal ileal limb, into which ureters are implanted.

deKernion et al. observed a high incontinence rate due to peristalsis of the distal short tubular, intact ileal segment that was used to anastomose with the urethra (10). They also included this segment into the S plate and anastomosed the ure-

are sutured together, resulting in a plate (Fig. 33.5B). The ureters are anastomosed to tubular portions of the bowel at either end using an end-to-side anastomosis over a single J urinary diversion stent (Fig. 33.5C). The left limb is left a little longer to accommodate the fact that the pouch is a little more to the right than to the left in its intra-abdominal location. The left ureter is not tunneled under the mesentery but anastomosed to the ileum intraperitoneally. Omentum is wrapped around the ureter as necessary if a length of it is exposed intraperitoneally between the retroperitoneum and anastomosis. The plate is constructed into a pouch by cross-folding and suturing the lower and upper edges together. A 1-cm opening is made at the most dependent portion of the pouch for anastomosis with the membranous urethra over a 20F Foley catheter using interrupted 3-0 chromic catgut or PGA sutures. This procedure is simple to perform and comprehensively includes all recent technical advances of bladder reconstruction using bowel segments.

Studer Procedure

Studer et al. have modified the orthotopic ileal bladder replacement similar to the cup patch technique as described by Good-

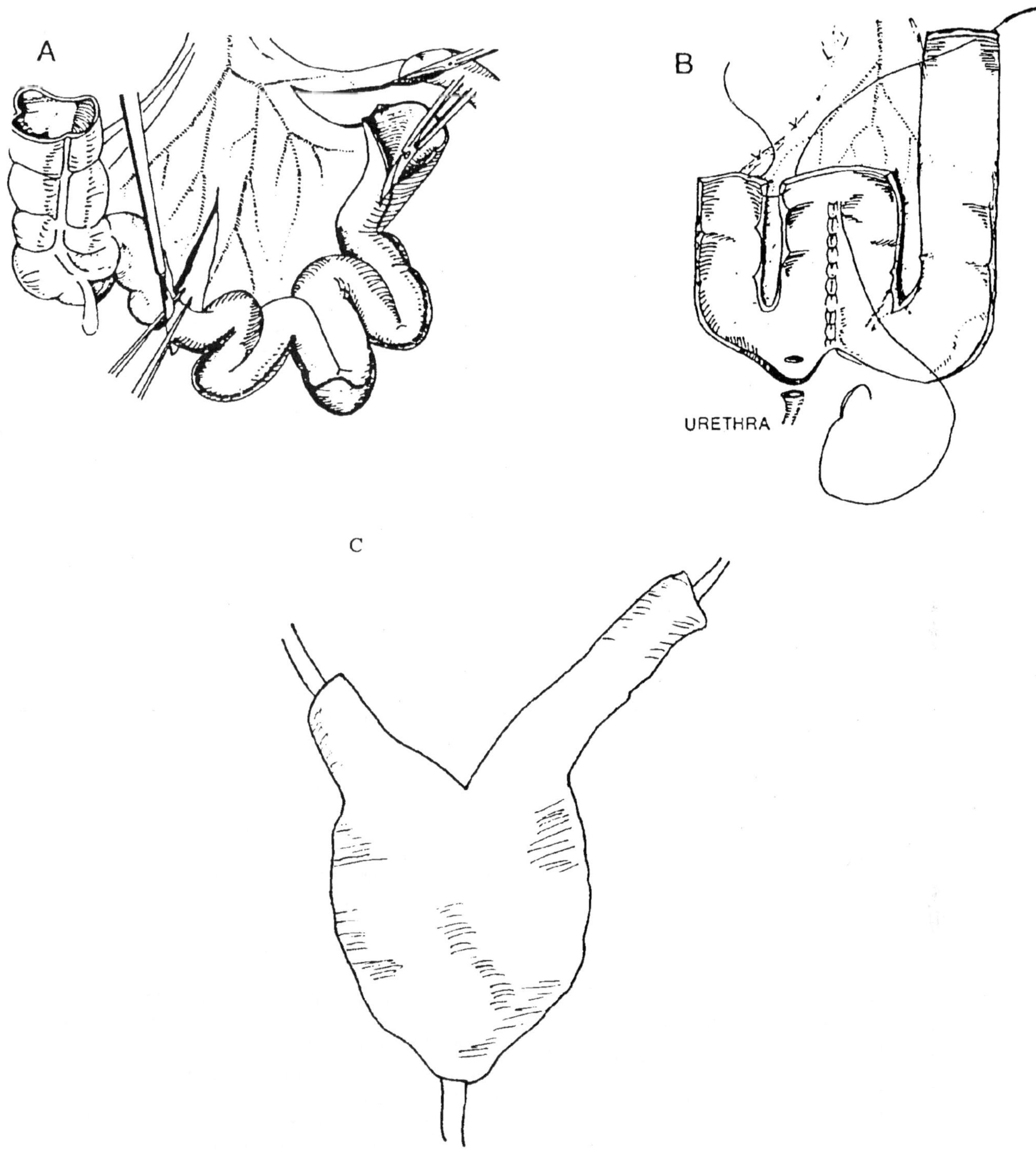

Fig. 33.5.   Narayan's detubularized ileocystoplasty.

thra to an opening made in the bowel wall at the anticipated lowest point of the pouch.

M Pouch (23)

To further increase the volume of the ileal neobladder, an M-shaped configuration was designed by Hautmann et al. (23). The other features of this technique are as follows.

1. The ureters are implanted directly into the pouch using LeDuc antireflux technique.
2. The urethra is connected to a separate opening in the small U-shaped flap created by displacing the antimesenteric detubularizing incision anteriorly over 5 cm of ileum.

In an experience with 100 patients, satisfactory results have

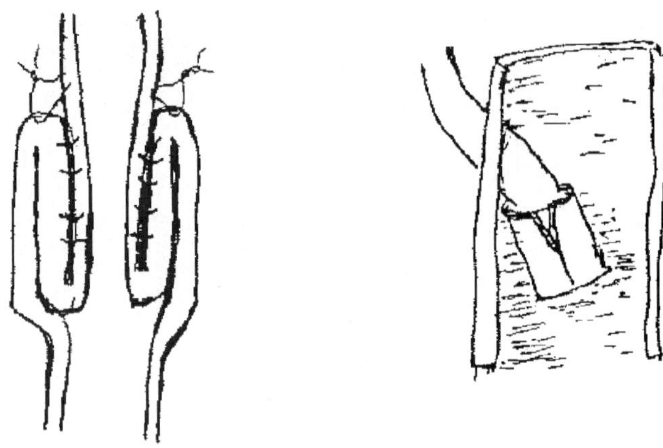

Fig. 33.6. Methods to create antireflux mechanism for ureteroileal anastomosis (Studer). Left: Triple nipple valve. Right: Split-cuff technique.

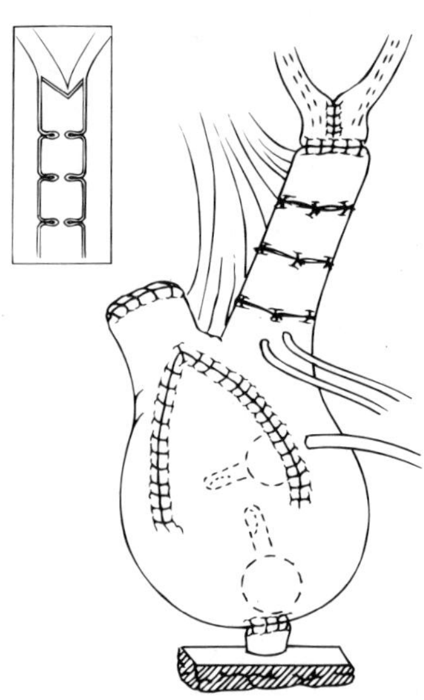

Fig. 33.8. Modification of the ileal reservoir (Freiha) to prevent reflux by circumferentially imbricating the proximal segment.

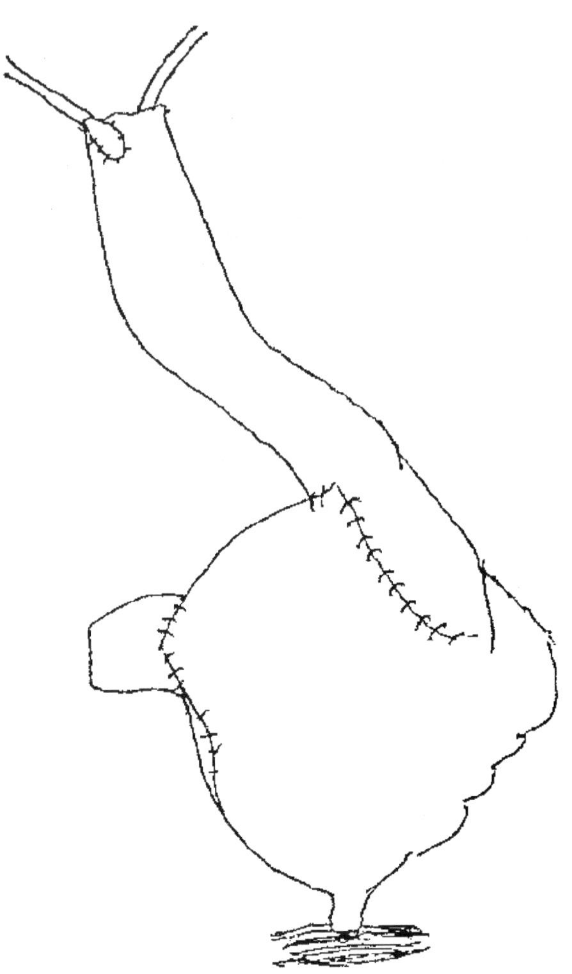

Fig. 33.7. Use of 15-cm isoperistable segment of ileum.

been reported. The average maximum capacity was 821 mL, with a mean resting pressure at amplitudes of 30 cm water, and total day and night continence in more than 90% of patients. However, late complications included urethral stricture (57%), slight acidosis (37%), and slight deterioration of upper urinary tracts (12%).

Ileocolic Bladder Substitutes

An ileocecal segment has been used in various configurations to form a neobladder. The Mainz pouch and Le Bag offer the advantage of a larger volume using a shorter segment of bowel than necessary for an ileal orthotopic reservoir (24, 25).

Tubularized Ileocecal Bladder (Fig. 33.10)

Gil-Vernet popularized the use of ileocecal segments in urologic surgery in 1965 (26). The ileocecal valves are used for antireflux requirements. A segment of terminal ileum, cecum, and ascending colon are isolated. The continuity of bowel is restored by an ileocolonic anastomosis. Appendectomy is done. The proximal end of the ileum is closed. The ileocecal valve is reinforced with several seromuscular interrupted sutures of 3-0 silk. The open end of the ascending colon is partially closed to reduce the lumen to a diameter of 1 cm for urethrocolonic anastomosis. The reservoir is turned counterclockwise to 180°, and the urethra is anastomosed to the reduced lumen of the ascending colon over a balloon catheter using interrupted su-

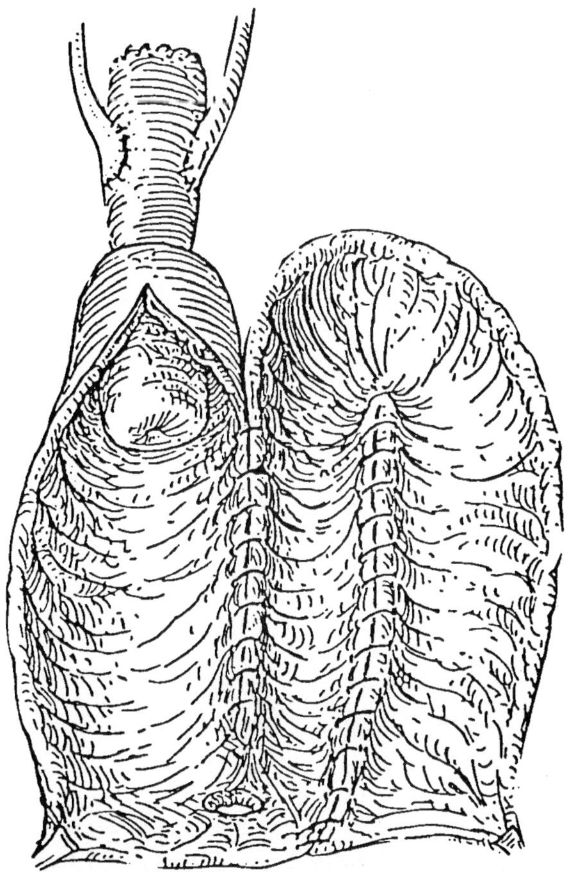

Fig. 33.9. Schreiter's pouch.

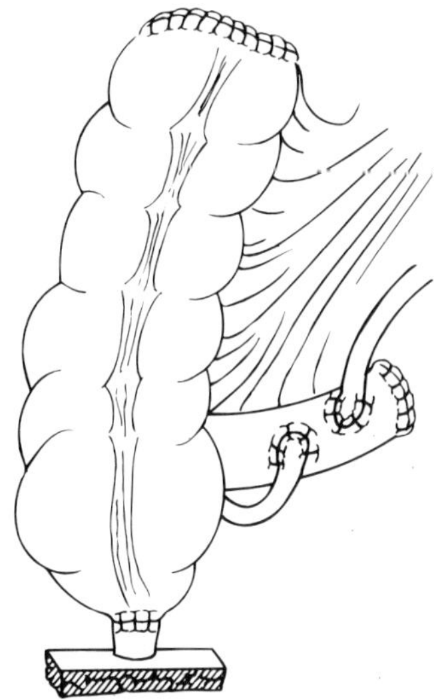

Fig. 33.11. The ileocecal bladder as described by Khafagy M, et al. (27).

tures of 2-0 or 0 chromic catgut. The ureters are reimplanted in the wall of terminal ileum.

Khafagy et al. used a similar technique but rather than rotating the reservoir, anastomosed the urethra to a dependent opening in the cecum (27) (Fig. 33.11).

Detubularized Ileocecal Bladder Substitutes: Le Bag

Light and Engleman described the detubularized ileocolonic pouch, Le Bag, for total bladder replacement (25). The cecum and 15 cm of terminal ileum are isolated and opened along the antimesenteric border, except for the most proximal 2 to 3 cm of the ileal segment. The medial edges are approximated with continuous 3-0 PGA sutures. The pouch is rotated 180° counterclockwise, and the proximal ileum is anastomosed to the urethra over a balloon catheter. The ureters are implanted into the cecum using standard antireflux submucosal tunnel. Closure of the pouch is completed.

The major disadvantage of this procedure is urgency and incontinence resulting from the interposition of the tubular segment between the reservoir and the urethra. The operation can be modified to eliminate the tubular segment, avoid rotation of the cecum, and anastomose the most dependent part of the cecum to the urethra (Fig. 33.12). The Mainz procedure described in the following section has essentially all the above modifications.

Mainz Pouch (Fig. 33.13)

Scharfe et al. first reported the use of Mainz pouch in 1988 for continent supravesical substitution (24).

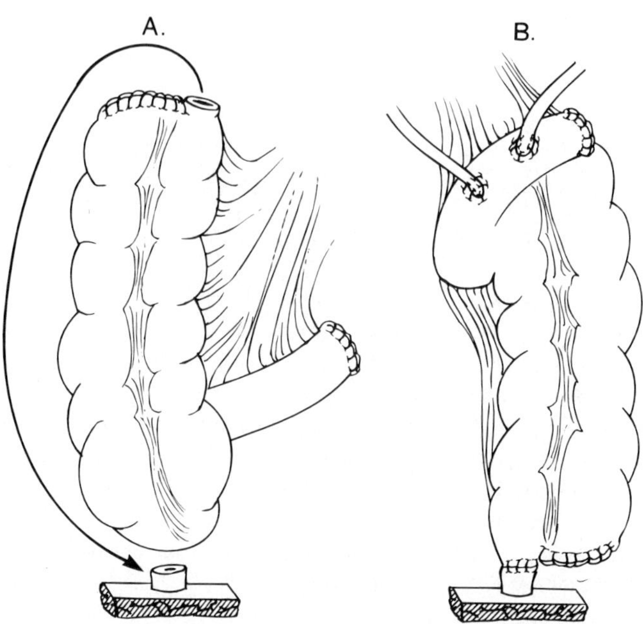

Fig. 33.10. The Gil-Vernet ileocecal cystoplasty.

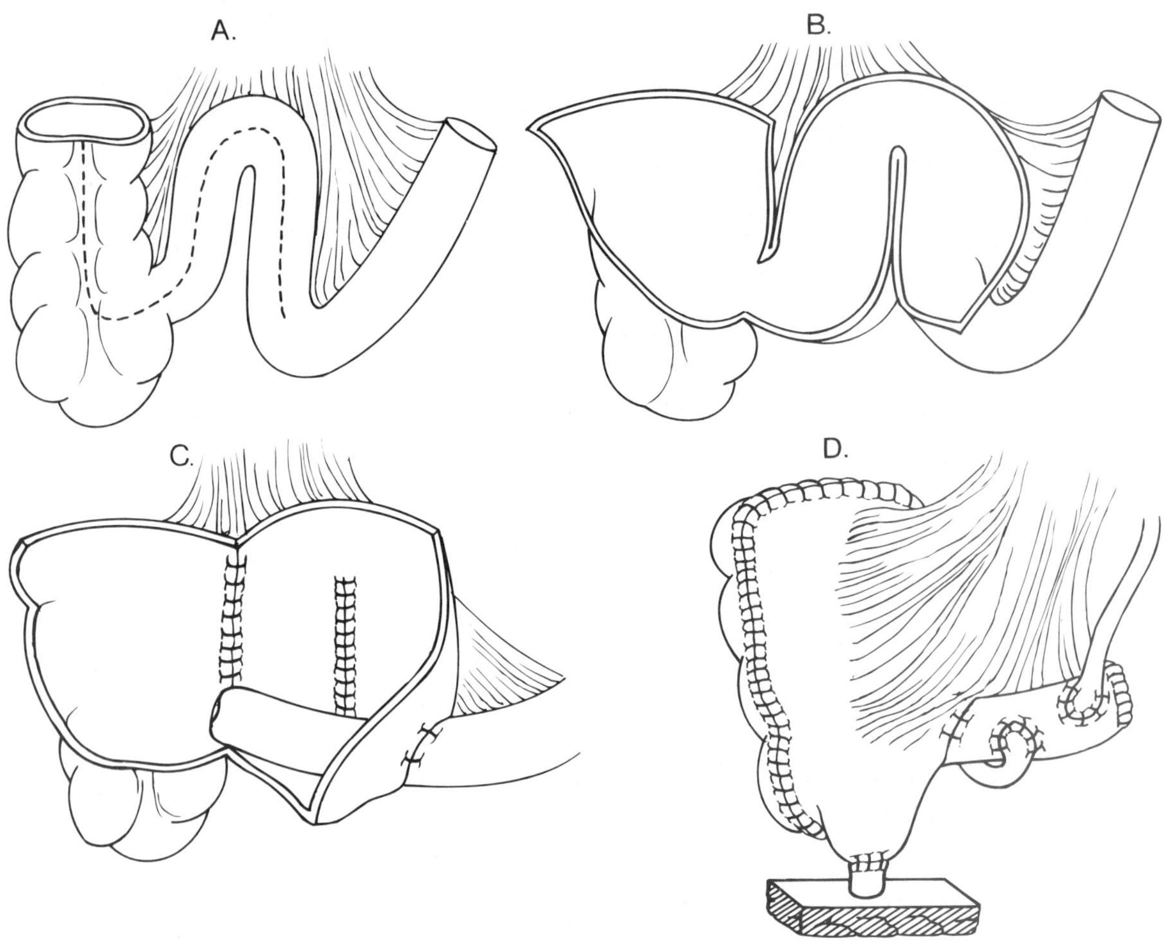

Fig. 33.12.   Le Bag.

The patient is placed in a modified lithotomy position, allowing a surgical assistant to apply perineal pressure when necessary during fixation of the enterourethral anastomoses. The pouch is constructed from 10 to 15 cm of cecum and ascending colon and two contiguous 10 to 15 cm segments of terminal ileum (Figs. 33.13A, 13B). The essential features are detubularization and reconfiguration of the bowel by incision and reanastomosis along the antimesenteric borders using continuous 3-0 PGA sutures (Fig. 33.13C). The ureters are implanted into the cecum by submucosal tunnels and stented with 90 cm 7F silastic stents (Fig. 33.13D). The pouch is drained by two 20F catheters—one suprapubic and one urethral. Penrose drains are placed adjacent to the pouch (Fig. 33.13E).

Ureteric stents are removed after the patient has been eating a normal diet for a minimum of 2 to 3 days. Stents are removed one at a time to permit differential pouch and culture urine collection. Pouch irrigation is done every 6 to 8 hours as long as the suprapubic tubes remain. Pericatheterograms are obtained at 10 days and repeated weekly if extravasation has occurred. Urethral catheters are removed 2 to 3 weeks postoperatively. The suprapubic tubes are removed after the patient voids satisfactorily. Patients are maintained on once-daily suppressive antibiotics for 4 to 6 weeks postoperatively. Intermittent catheterization is taught to patients as a safeguard against obstruction by mucus.

Results

In our initial experience with pouch construction (28), reestablishment of bowel continuity and creation of ureteroureterostomy added a mean of 2.5 hours (range, 2 to 3 hours) to the standard radical cystectomy. The enterourethral anastomosis healed in 2 to 3 weeks in 90% of patients. Five percent of patients required 4 to 6 weeks for complete healing. Sixty percent of patients voided well and are dry at night with voiding at 6-hour intervals. Patients often need to be seated and perform Valsalva or Credé's maneuver for voiding. Metabolically, there was clear evidence of sodium, potassium, and chloride absorption from pouch urine with a consequent mean decrease in urine osmolality to 321. Mild hyperchloremia (60% of patients) and hypocarbia (30% of patients) were noted. Although all patients had low vitamin B_{12} levels, megaloblastic anemia did not develop in any patient.

Urodynamically, patients maintained an average of 83% of

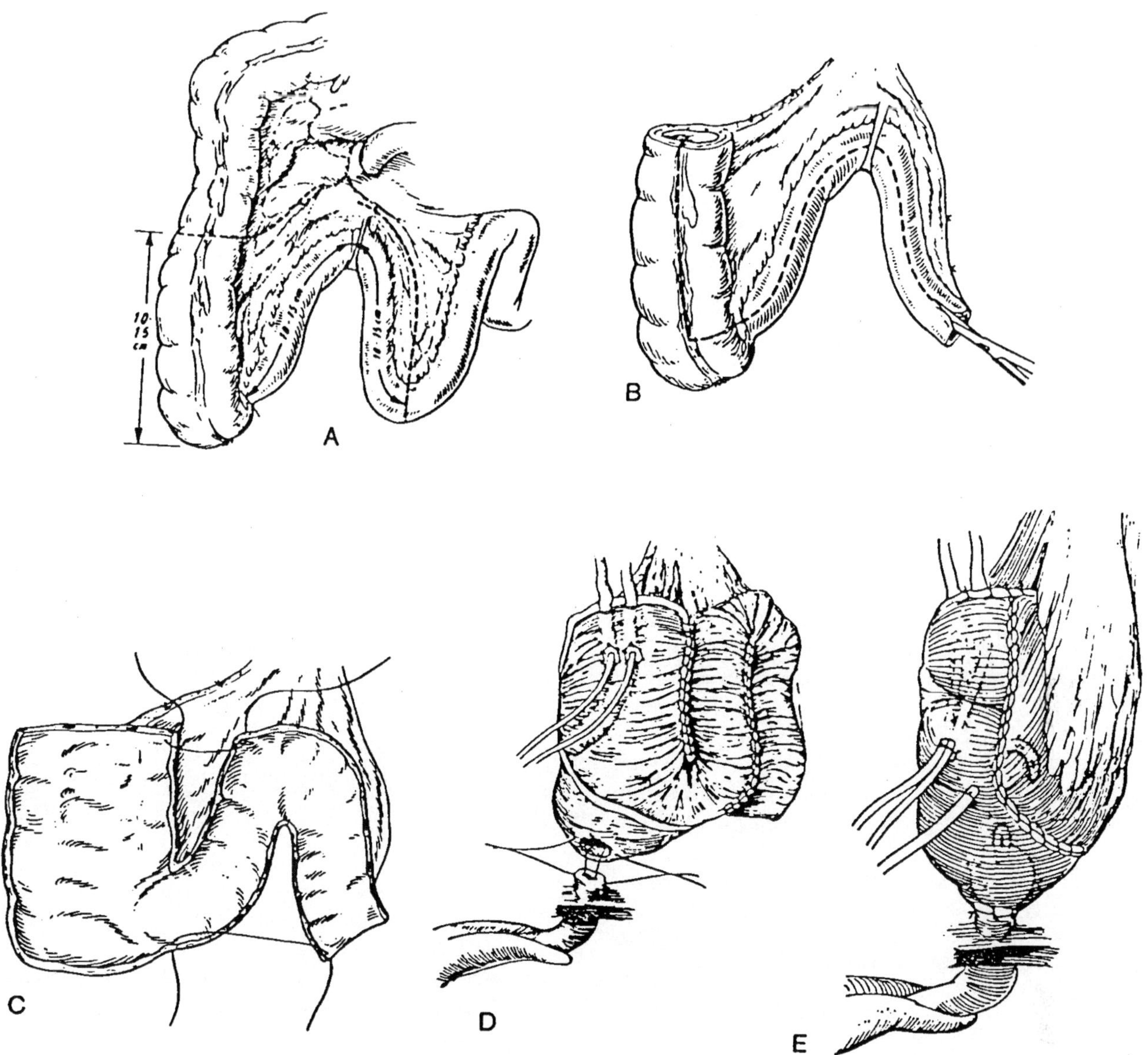

Fig. 33.13. The Mainz pouch.

their preoperative peak urethral pressure. The mean reservoir capacity was 830 mL at 6 months. Peristaltic pressure waves were noted even at 12 to 18 months although they tended to decrease when capacity increased. Continence was maintained during mean pressure waves by phasic increases in external sphincter tone that exceeded the amplitude of the pouch pressure. Resting pouch pressure at full capacity ranged from 10 to 16 cm of water. Nocturnal incontinence was related to urethral sphincter relaxation associated with sleep.

Strictures at the enterourethral anastomosis developed in 3% of patients; two were successfully managed by visual urethrotomies.

The choice of Mainz pouch in our patients originally was based on the following criteria.

1. The location of the cecum, which allows easy enterourethral anastomosis.

2. The relative surgical simplicity of both pouch reconstruction and antireflux ureteric reimplantation.
3. The use of a shorter bowel, which is theoretically less likely to cause metabolic problems from absorption of electrolytes.

More recently, we exclusively use ileum for urethral anastomosis and use a modified ileocolonic pouch for reservoirs with abdominal stoma. Modifications have included use of a shorter segment of cecum (10 cm) and longer segments of ileum (30 cm) to ensure adequate pouch volume.

SUBSTITUTION USING COLON

Partially Detubularized Right Colon (Fig. 33.14)

In 1986, Goldwasser et al. described the use of right colon for bladder replacement (29). In this procedure, the cecum,

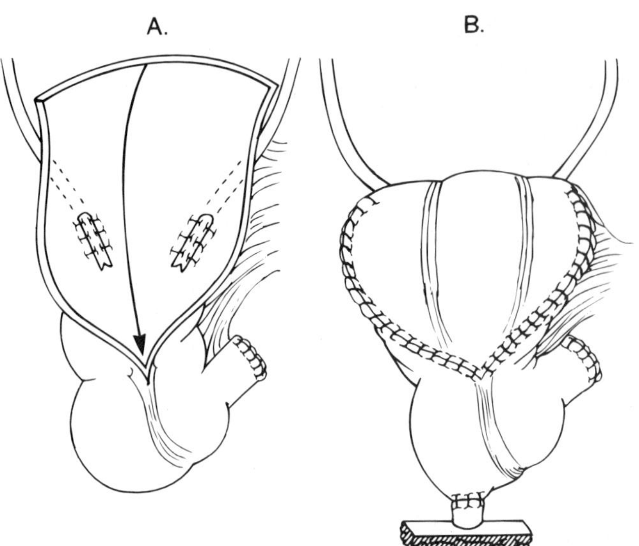

Fig. 33.14.   The partially detubularized right colic reservoir.

ascending colon, and hepatic flexure are isolated and opened along the antimesenteric taenia down to the cecum (Fig. 33.14A). The terminal ileum is closed, and an appendectomy is performed. The ureters are implanted into the back wall of cecum using an antireflux tunnel for mucosal anastomosis. The most dependent part of the cecum is anastomosed to the urethra over a Foley catheter. The opened ascending colon and hepatic flexure are folded down and sutured to the edges of the cecum using 3-0 PGA (Fig. 33.14B).

Significant bacteriuria was encountered in all patients and persisted until all tubes were removed. Stricture of urethra developed in two patients and was successfully treated in both. No significant metabolic derangement was detected in any patient. Two thirds of the patients were continent during the night if they voided every 2 to 3 hours. Urodynamic evaluations revealed acceptable capacity, residual volume, filling, and peak pressures. Pouch contractions of low amplitude (less than 40 cm water) occurred in 70% of patients. The maximal urethral closing pressure in patients ranged between 35 and 60 cm water.

The Mansson pouch is a variant of the Goldwasser pouch in which the entire colon is spatulated (30). This seems to offer advantages over the Goldwasser technique. All patients were continent during the day and night with lower basal filling pressures of less than 22 cm water.

The Sigmoid Pouch (Fig. 33.15)

The sigmoid colon may also be used for bladder replacement. Theoretically, this is the easiest segment for surgical reconstruction. If it is long and redundant, it is easy to obtain a large segment with a long vascular pedicle. The splenic flexure and descending colon need not be mobilized to obtain an end-to-end tension-free anastomosis. The sigmoid colon can be simply

reconstructed into a detubularized reservoir, and ureteral implantation is easy to perform using any of the antireflux techniques. Its removal is not associated with diarrhea, malabsorption, or bacterial overgrowth. A disadvantage is that the colon may be prone to develop cancers when in long-term contact with urine; this needs to be studied further. It is imperative that the patient should undergo colonoscopy before surgery to rule out precancerous and cancerous lesions.

The procedure involves isolation of sigmoid segment and detubularization of the segment by opening along the antimesenteric tenia and suturing together the adjacent medial edges (Fig. 33.15B). Anastomosis to the urethra is performed at the dependent part. The ureters are implanted end-to-side into the side wall of the sigmoid colon (Fig. 33.15C). Closure of the pouch is done at a right angle to the longitudinal axis of the colon.

This procedure was conceived, refined, and popularized by surgeons from the University of Minnesota (31). Satisfactory mean bladder capacity of 760 mL and pouch filling pressure of less than 20 cm water have been reported from this center.

Recent Advances: Orthotopic Continent Urinary Diversion in Women

Although continent diversion with urethral voiding would provide similar advantages in women as it does in men, it has not been attempted in women until recently. This is because cystectomy in women usually includes anterior exenteration with urethrectomy, and preservation of urethra has always posed oncologic and functional problems. Careful selection of patients with unifocal vesical neoplasms that do not involve the bladder floor must be made, reducing the already low risk of urethral relapse. Multiple bladder biopsies should be performed to exclude the presence of carcinoma in situ. Sparing the urethra and its complex sphincteric mechanisms will facilitate construction of an orthotopic urinary reservoir.

Continence in women is maintained by urethral support and suspension system in addition to the intrinsic anatomy of the urethra (5). The urethral support and suspension system are composed of functionally complementary and interdependent entities aimed at sustaining the urethra and maintaining the vesicourethral junction and the proximal urethra in an intra-abdominal position as well as to guarantee a constant vesicourethral angle. This support system is composed of musculofascial structures that include intrapelvic fascia from which urethral fascia derives medial bundles of levator ani muscle and pubococcygeal muscles (pelvic diaphragm), connective support bundles of the anterior vaginal wall that surround the proximal urethra in a sling-like fashion, and the urogenital diaphragm. The suspension system is composed of anterior and posterior pubourethral ligaments.

The anatomical and functional integrity of bladder neck and smooth and striated sphincteric muscles contribute to the closing pressure of the urethra and maintain continence in association with the support and suspension system. Rhabdosphinc-

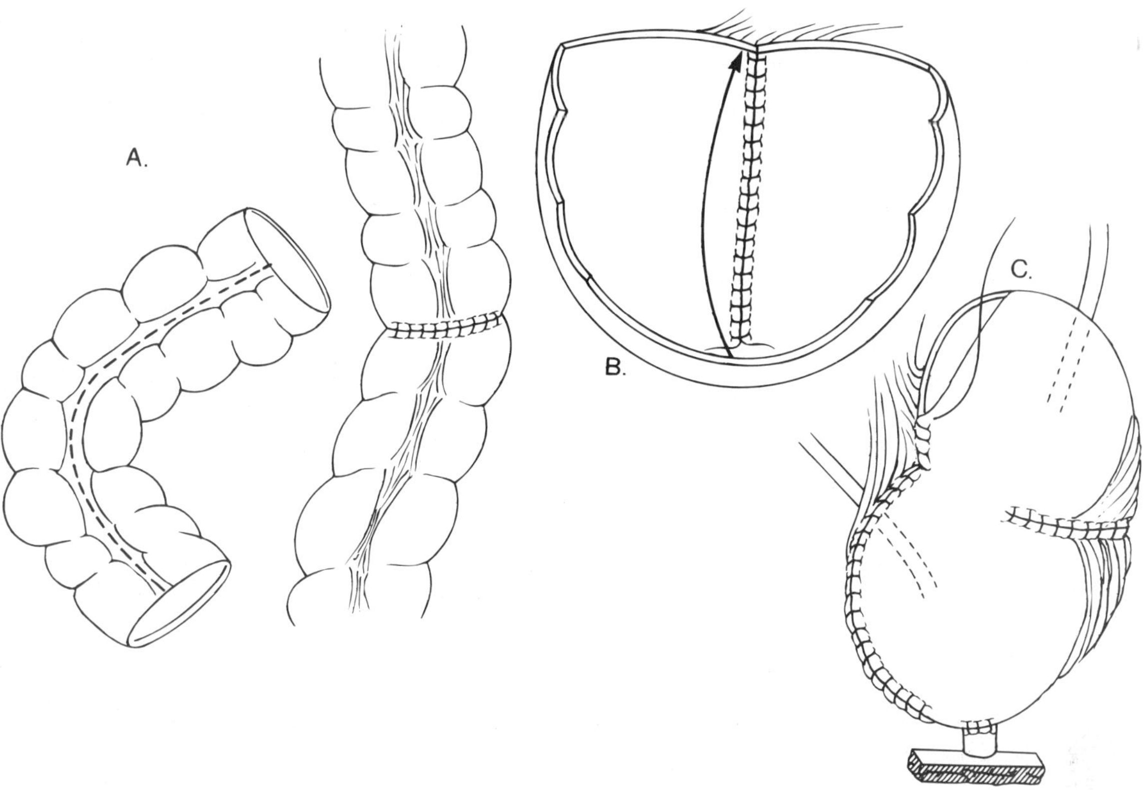

Fig. 33.15. The sigmoid pouch.

ter has been identified in the lower third of the urethra, mostly in the anterior part of the urethra. The middle third demonstrates gradual transition to smooth muscle. Nerve fibers of the pudendal nerve have been traced to the lower urethra, and those of the pelvic plexus enter the proximal third of the urethra. Experimental data have confirmed the need for integrity of this innervation for maintaining continence (4). It is possible to preserve these nerve fibers that run along the pelvic viscera toward the vagina and the urethra by nerve-sparing cystectomy; thus, orthotopic urinary diversion is a feasible option in selected women undergoing radical cystectomy.

The surgical technique should preserve the continence mechanism without compromising oncologic radicality. In particular, isolating the urethra from the vaginal wall and sectioning below the bladder neck, sparing as much urethra as possible, is an important step. The pubovesical ligaments should be sectioned close to the bladder. The pelvic fascia and the periurethral neurovascular plexus that run lateral to the bladder in the paravaginal tissue should be carefully preserved.

Suspension procedures anchoring the vaginal fornices to Cooper's ligament during the procedure or periurethral collagen injection at a later date can also be done to achieve continence, if required. The little available data demonstrate encouraging results. A special problem of hypercontinence has been reported in 40% of patient's requiring CIC (8). The mechanism is unclear, although it seems to be related to the length of the urethra and perhaps to the overenthusiastic suspension proce-

dures. The technique is still evolving, and better results may be anticipated as more centers offer the procedure to women undergoing cystectomy.

Gastrocystoplasty (Fig. 33.16)

As an alternative to intestines, gastric tissue has been used to reconstruct the lower urinary tract (32). Stomach has excellent fibroelastic properties that result in a capacious and compliant reservoir. Also, there is a rich blood supply and a significant muscularis to provide antireflux mechanism for ureteric implantation. In patients with metabolic acidosis, hydrogen and chloride secretion by the stomach is a distinct advantage to counter the metabolic problem. The mucus produced is less precipitable and causes less problems than small or large bowel mucus. Stomach may especially be useful in patients with deficient bowel or existing bowel problems or in patients who have had prior abdominal radiation.

Usually, a right gastroepiploic artery-based flap is chosen because this artery tends to be larger and more common than the left gastroepiploic artery. The omentum is incised parallel to the gastroepiploic artery 2 cm or more from the vessels. A pyramid-shaped gastric wedge is outlined with the apex close to the lesser curve (Fig. 33.16A). The length of the wedge along the greater curve may be around 15 cm. Usually one third to one half the stomach is required. The vascular pedicle of the flap formed from the root of the gastroepiploic artery to

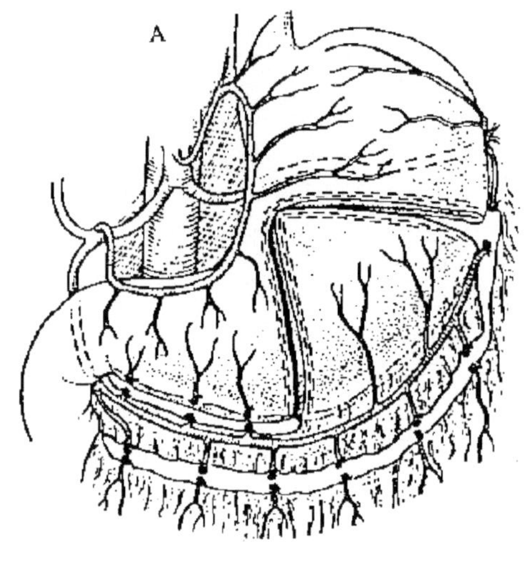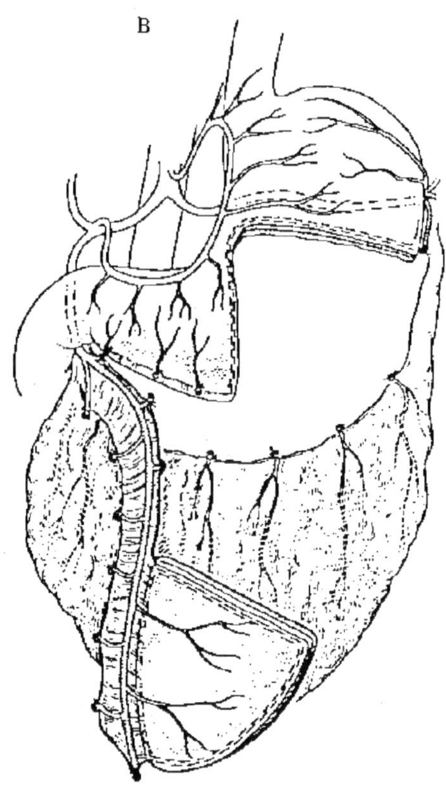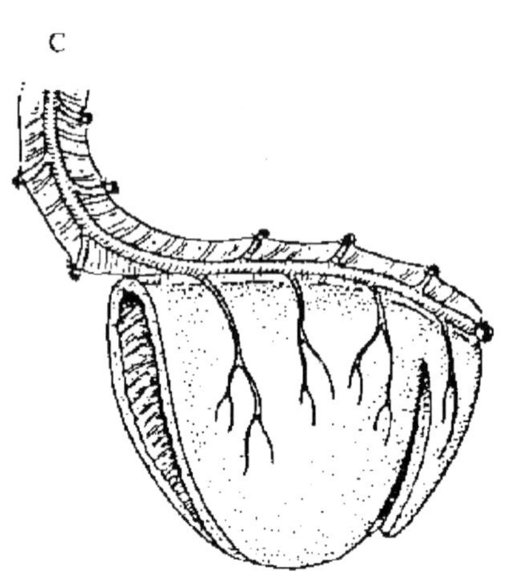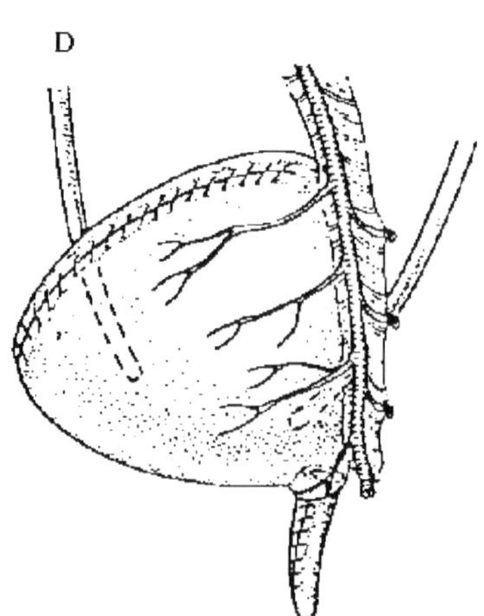

Fig. 33.16.   Gastrocystoplasty.

the right base of the wedge should be long enough to reach the pelvis. The short vessels between the right gastroepiploic artery and the stomach are suture ligated and divided, leaving the vessels supplying the flap intact. The ligatures should be well away from the artery; a loose ligature with an expanding hematoma may compromise the vascularity of the flap. The

stomach wedge is resected using a 90-mm gastrointestinal anastomosis stapler (Fig. 33.16B). This minimizes blood loss and avoids spillage of gastric juice. The stomach is then closed using 3-0 running interlocking PGA through-and-through sutures followed by 3-0 silk interrupted seromuscular sutures.

The wedge flap is brought through the mesocolon and the

mesentery of small bowel without twisting or tension so that the pedicle is in the retroperitoneum. The wedge is rotated 180° so that the apex now reaches the membranous urethra. The posterior apex is directly sutured to the membranous urethra using interrupted 4-0 chromic catgut sutures. It can also be tubularized to obtain further length of urethra to enhance continence (Fig. 33.16C). The ureters are reimplanted using a submucosal tunnel onto the posterior leaflet (Fig. 33.16D). The pouch is closed leaving a Malecot catheter. The anterior wall of the reservoir is anchored to the abdominal wall at the site of the suprapubic tube.

Irrigation of the pouch with 30 to 60 mL of normal saline is done frequently. H_2 receptor antagonists are administered for 1 month; they are continued for longer if dysuria-hematuria syndrome develops. The cause of this syndrome is unknown. It is known to occur in patients with renal impairment with oliguria, acid urine, and intact urethral sensation. However, it can also occur in patients with alkaline urine. Resistant cases are treated with omeprazole 20 mg/day orally or with phosphate-buffered saline bladder irrigation.

Patients who have undergone gastrocystoplasty should be warned that persistent secretion of chloride and hydrogen ions from the gastric mucosa will lead to severe dehydration and metabolic alkalosis if a viral infection that causes diarrhea and vomiting develops. These patients should take salt supplements and may require intravenous salt replacement.

Gastrocystoplasty is a recently conceived technique. The short-term results are satisfactory. The stomach stretches and attains good capacity with time. The end-filling pressure becomes acceptable with increase in capacity. Metabolic acidosis improves with significant recovery of renal impairment. The fibroelastic properties seem to provide excellent muscle backing for effective ureteric reimplantation and bladder neck continence procedures.

In an experience with 21 patients with renal impairment, Nguyen and Mitchell reported satisfactory results; renal function improved in all but five patients (33). Thus far, the procedure has mainly been performed in the pediatric population. However, it promises to be a good alternative in adults with compromised renal function.

Composite Flaps

The use of combination of segments from stomach and small or large bowel is another evolving technique. This may be especially useful in patients who have undergone pelvic irradiation.

Complications

Complications of the bladder substitution procedures are similar to any intraabdominal surgery that involves the gastrointestinal and urinary tracts. These may include pulmonary atelectasis and infection, wound infection and dehiscence, intestinal obstruction, anastomotic leakages, intraperitoneal abscess, anastomotic obstruction, and fistulae. Complications that are unique to these procedures are metabolic and electrolyte disorders and voiding dysfunctions.

Metabolic and Electrolyte Disorders

The variables that determine the degree of metabolic derangement seem to be the total intestinal surface area exposed to urine, type of bowel used, and renal function. Other than stomach, it appears that the differences in absorption between different bowel segments are minor and the amount of absorption is unlikely to be significant in the presence of good renal function (15). The well-known potential complication of hyperchloremic acidosis is mainly due to reabsorption of ammonium ions from the urine but is also, in part, due to reabsorption of hydrogen ions together with chloride ions (34). The secretion of bicarbonate ions from the intestinal mucosa is considered not to add significantly to the acidosis. Recently, it has been demonstrated that colonic absorption of chloride ions is greater; hence, ileum may be preferable to colon for constructing urinary reservoirs, especially in patients with renal impairment (35). With proper patient selection, the metabolic disorders are uncommon and most often mild. If troublesome, they may be treated easily with oral supplementation of bicarbonate, citrate salts, and dietary restriction of chloride.

Resection of up to 60 cm of ileum in patients who retain terminal ileum and ileocecal valve is generally well tolerated (15). A resection between 60 and 100 cm may reduce bile acid reabsorption, but increased hepatic production maintains the overall bile acid pool. Minor disturbances in lipid metabolism and osmotic diarrhea due to cathartic effect on the colon of the excess bile acid load can occur. If more than 100 cm of ileum are resected, lipid malabsorption is inevitable. Unabsorbed fat is lost into the colon, resulting in steatorrhea. There are also fat-soluble vitamin A, D, E, and K deficiencies. Increased oxalate absorption leading to oxalate renal stones and altered bile acid metabolism leading to decreased solubility of cholesterol (resulting in cholesterol biliary stones) may occur. Cholestyramine can bind malabsorption bile acid and may be used to treat diarrhea, but chronic use of this drug should be avoided.

Vitamin B_{12} deficiency is known to occur after small bowel resection and can be avoided by preserving at least 15 cm of terminal ileum (36). Other patients will require monitoring to detect early B_{12} deficiency and provide injections of vitamin B_{12} every 4 to 6 months.

Voiding Difficulties

Voiding efficiency depends on the balance between effective voiding pressure and bladder outlet resistance. The bowel substitutes cannot contract voluntarily and need good abdominal muscle power for effective voiding. Stricture at the urethral anastomotic site, although rare, can cause obstructed flow. This can be managed by visual urethrotomy. Hypercontinence in women may be a significant problem. This problem is being investigated, and further studies are ongoing.

Urinary Continence

A complication that significantly affects quality of life in patients with orthotopic bladders is urinary incontinence. Continence requires a low pressure in the bladder substitute and a high pressure in the outlet mechanism during filling. The size and shape of the reservoir may therefore affect continence, but other factors may also be important.

Care must be taken to preserve the distal sphincter mechanism at cystectomy and maintain maximal urethral length without compromising cancer margins. Results from major centers suggest that continence is better and achieved faster in patients who have undergone nerve-sparing cystectomy (36). It is uncertain whether this relates to the preservation of branches of the pelvic nerves that are thought to innervate the distal sphincter mechanism, the preservation of maximal functional length of urethra, or careful dissection of the urethra (4, 37). Younger patients seem to gain continence more rapidly than older ones (38).

In contrast to radical prostatectomy, after cystectomy there is no reflex rise in outlet pressure of the membranous urethra during filling because there is no longer any afferent side of this reflex. This loss of reflex urethral pressure can cause incontinence and may be a particular problem at night, compounded by an increased nocturnal urine output and relaxed distal sphincter (39). Mass peristalsis by colon may also be a contributory factor. Timed voiding prevents nocturnal incontinence.

Postmicturition dribble is sometimes noted by patients. This is due to urine remaining in the bulbar urethra; the normal milking of the urethra after voiding may not occur with bladder substitutes. This is remedied by milking the urethra empty after voiding.

Delayed Surgical Complications

The incidence of strictures at ureterointestinal anastomosis has been variably reported as 6 to 10% (40, 41). Good vascularity of the ureteral stump and tension-free anastomosis largely overcome these complications. Because the ureteral obstruction may be asymptomatic leading to autonephrectomy, periodic evaluation is essential (36).

Strictures at the urethrointestinal anastomotic site may occur and are amenable to visual urethrotomy.

Vesicoureteric reflux has been dealt with in detail previously. Stenosis of the afferent nipple valve has been reported and successfully corrected endoscopically (19).

Follow-up

As has been stressed previously, it is essential that patients who undergo continent urinary diversion understand the importance of regular follow-up. Close follow-up is required for early detection of disease recurrence, metabolic abnormalities, and complications associated with the diversion procedure. The recommended protocol consists of metabolic evaluation at 3-month intervals and imaging studies and cytology at 6- to 12-month intervals to detect disease recurrence and complications. These recommendations can be modified to suit individual patients based on symptomatology and findings at follow-up. The use of static and dynamic Gd-DTPA contrast medium magnetic resonance imaging in evaluation of orthotopic continent diversion, as reported by Tempany et al., appears to be a promising test (42). This test may provide information contained in multiple different studies. This will also be useful in the presence of azotemia or contrast allergy.

Conclusions

Continent orthotopic bladder substitution is an attractive procedure after cystectomy. It leaves the body image intact but has to be carefully and selectively applied using the following important principles that will determine the long-term success and acceptability of the procedure.

1. Proper patient selection is the foremost requirement.
2. Selection of bowel segment has to be made carefully based on patient and disease factors.
3. Detubularization and reconfiguration of the bowel results in satisfactory low pressure reservoir while using the shortest possible length of bowel.
4. Anastomoses have to be tension free.
5. Although the role of reflux in these reservoirs is controversial, some form of antireflux technique is currently recommended.
6. Urethra should not be anastomosed to a tubular bowel segment.
7. Patients should be instructed to urinate at defined intervals because of decreased sensation of pouch filling.
8. Patients should comply strictly with follow-up requirements.
9. The technique may be selectively applied to women.

The attractions for the patient to have an orthotopic diversion are obviously compelling. From the viewpoint of urologists, the evolving technical simplicity, reasonable continence, preservation of upper tracts, lack of bacteremia, and ease of conversion to a cutaneous stoma if required have recently made these procedures more applicable.

REFERENCES

1. Tizzoni G, Poggi A. Die Wiederhestellung der Harnblase. Experimentalle untersuchungen. Zentralbl Chir 1888;15:921.
2. Camey M, LeDuc A. L'enterocystoplastie apres cystoprostatectomie total pour cancer de vessie. Ann Urol (Paris) 1979;13:114.
3. Hinman F Jr. Functional classification of conduits for continent diversion. J Urol 1990;144:27.

4. Hubner WA, Trigo-Rocha F, Plas EG, et al. Urethral function after cystectomy: a canine in vivo experiment. Urol Res 1993; 21:45.

5. Cancrini A, DeCarli P, Fattahi H, et al. Orthotopic ileal neobladder in female patients after radical cystectomy: 2 year experience. J Urol 1995;153:956.

6. Grossfeld GD, Stein JP, Bennett EJ, et al. Lower urinary tract reconstruction in the female using the Kock ileal reservoir with bilateral ureteroileal urethrostomy: update of continence: results and fluorourodynamic findings. J Urol 1995;153:242. Abstract.

7. Colleselli K, Strasser H, Poisel S, et al. Continence after anterior exenteration (female, male) and radical prostatectomy: anatomical approach. J Urol 1995;153:305. Abstract.

8. Hautmann R, Paiss J, Kleinschmidt K, et al. The ileal neobladder in the female: why it works or not. J Urol 1995; 153:243. Abstract.

9. Schellhammer PF, Whitmore WF Jr. Transitional cell carcinoma of the urethra in men having cystectomy for bladder cancer. J Urol 1976;115:56.

10. deKernion JB, Stenzel A, Mukamel E. Urinary diversion and continent reservoir. In: Gillenwater JY, Grayhack JT, Howards SS, Duckett JW, eds. Adult and pediatric urology. 2nd ed. St. Louis: CV Mosby, 1991:1185.

11. Mahadevia PS, Koss LS, Tarr JJ. Prostatic involvement in bladder cancer. Cancer 1986;58:2096.

12. Winfield HN, Reddy PK, Lange PH. Coexisting adenocarcinoma of the prostate in patients undergoing cystoprostatectomy for bladder cancer. Urology 1987;30:100.

13. Androulakakis PA, Schneider HM, Jacobi GH, et al. Coincident vesical transitional cell carcinoma and prostatic carcinoma. Br J Urol 1986;58:153.

14. Camey M. Radical cystectomy with ileocystoplasty: 30 year experience. Eur Urol 1988;14(Suppl):27.

15. Studer EU, Turner W. The ileal orthotopic bladder. Urology 1995;45:185.

16. Pagano F, Artibani W, Ligato P, et al. Vesica ileale padovanna: a technique for total bladder replacement. Eur Urol 1990;17: 149.

17. Kock NG, Nilson AE, Nilson LO, et al. Urinary diversion via a continent ileal reservoir: clinical results in 12 patients. J Urol 1982;128:469.

18. Ghoneim M, et al. Cystectomy and diversion for carcinoma of the bilharzial bladder. In: Smith PH, Pavone-Macaluso M, eds. Management of advanced cancer of prostate and bladder. New York: Alan R. Liss, 1988:315.

19. Stein JP, Huffman TL, Freeman JA, et al. Stenosis of afferent reflux valve in the Kock pouch continent urinary diversion: diagnosis and management. J Urol 1994;151:338.

20. Studer EV, Casanova G, Zingg F. Bladder substitution with an ileal low-pressure reservoir. Eur Urol 1988;14(Suppl):36.

21. Studer EV, Spiegel T, Casanova GA, et al. Ileal bladder substitute: antireflux nipple or afferent tubular segment? Eur Urol 1991;20:315.

22. Schreiter F. The S bladder: a complete continent antireflux functional replacement of the bladder sphincter muscle function. Urologe 1987;26:201.

23. Hautmann RE, Egghart G, Frohneberg D, et al. The ileal neobladder. J Urol 1988;139:39.

24. Scharfe T, et al. Mainz pouch for augmentation, bladder substitution or continent urinary diversion. Eur Urol 1988; 14(Suppl):32.

25. Light J, Engleman U. Le Bag: total replacement of the bladder using an ileocolonic pouch. J Urol 1986;136:27.

26. Gil-Vernet J. The ileocolic segment in urologic surgery. J Urol 1965;94:418.

27. Khafagy M, et al. Radical cystectomy and ileocecal bladder reconstruction for carcinoma of the urinary bladder. A study of 130 patients. Br J Urol 1987;60:60.

28. Narayan P, Broderick GA, Tanagho EA. Bladder substitution with ileocecal (Mainz) pouch—clinical performance over 2 years. Br J Urol 1991;68:588.

29. Goldwasser B, Barrett D, Benson R. Bladder replacement with use of detubularized right colonic segment: preliminary report of a new technique. Mayo Clin Proc 1986;61:615.

30. Mansson W, Colleen S. Experience with a detubularized right colonic segment for bladder replacement. Scand J Urol Nephrol 1990;24:53.

31. Reddy PK. Detubularized sigmoid reservoir for bladder replacement after cystoprostatectomy: preliminary report of new configuration. Urology 1987;29:625.

32. Adams MC, Mitchell ME, Rink RC. Gastrocystoplasty: an alternative solution to the problem of urological reconstruction in the severely compromised patient. J Urol 1988;140:1152.

33. Nguyen DH, Mitchell ME. Gastrocystoplasty. In: Whitfield HN, ed. Smith's operative surgery: genitourinary surgery. Newton, MA: Butterworth-Heineman, 1993;1:252.

34. Kock MO, McDougal WS. The paraphysiology of hyperchloremic metabolic acidosis after urinary diversion through intestinal segments. Surgery 1985;98:561.

35. Davidson S, Akerlund E, Forsell-Aronson E, et al. Absorption of sodium and chloride in continent reservoirs for urine: comparison of ileal and colonic reservoirs. J Urol 1994;15:335.

36. Lockhart JG. Reconstruction and diversion. J Urol 1995;153: 1439. Editorial.

37. Dixon J, Gosling J. Structure and innervation in the human. In: Torrens M, Morrison JFB, eds. The physiology of the lower urinary tract. Berlin: Springer-Verlag, 1987:3.

38. Hautmann RE, Miller K, Steiner V, et al. The ileal neobladder: 6 year experience with more than 200 patients. J Urol 1993;150:40.

39. Presti JC Jr, Schmidt RA, Narayan P, et al. Pathophysiology of urinary continence after radical prostatectomy. J Urol 1990; 143:975.

40. Helal M, Pow-Sang J, Sanford E, et al. Direct (nontunnelled) ureterocolonic reimplantation in association with continent reservoirs. J Urol 1993;150:835.

41. Mansson W. The continent cecal urinary reservoir: In: King LR, Stone AR, Webster GD, eds. Bladder reconstruction and continent urinary diversion. Chicago: Year Book, 1986:209.

42. Tempany CMC, Masoudi FA, Marshall FF. The use of dynamic magnetic resonance imaging to evaluate orthotopic continent urinary diversion. Urology 1995;45:886.

VIII

TESTES

34

Testicular Cancer

An Overview

Joseph C. Presti Jr.

INTRODUCTION

Testicular cancer is rare, with approximately two to three new cases per 100,000 males being reported in the United States each year. It is the most common solid tumor malignancy of men between the ages of 20 and 34. In 1994, approximately 6800 new cases were diagnosed in the United States (1). At diagnosis, approximately 65% of cases are localized, whereas 20% have regional spread and 15% have distant metastases. Due to the development of platinum-based chemotherapy regimens, the overall cure rate exceeds 90%. Overall 5-year survival rates have increased from 78% in 1974–1976 to 91% in 1980–1985 (P < 0.05). Because of the increasing success rates in patient survival, enthusiasm about developing treatment regimens that reduce treatment-related morbidity without increasing disease-related mortality has increased.

EPIDEMIOLOGY AND RISK FACTORS

Ninety to 95% of all primary testicular tumors are germ cell tumors (seminoma and nonseminoma); the remainder are nongerminal neoplasms (Leydig cell, Sertoli cell, gonadoblastoma). This chapter will focus on germ cell tumors only.

The incidence of testicular cancer shows significant geographic, socioeconomic, and racial variations. The incidence is highest in Scandinavia, Switzerland, and Germany, is intermediate in the United States and Great Britain, and is lowest in Africa and Asia. Scandinavian countries report up to 6.7 new cases per 100,000 males annually compared with 0.8 per 100,000 males in Japan. The incidence of testicular cancer in African Americans is approximately one fourth of the incidence in white American men. Within a given race, individuals in the highest socioeconomic classes have an incidence that is approximately double those in the lowest classes.

Testicular cancer is slightly more common on the right than on the left, which parallels the increased incidence of cryptorchidism on the right side. One to 2% of primary testicular tumors are bilateral, and up to 50% of men with these tumors have a history of unilateral or bilateral cryptorchidism. Although primary bilateral testicular tumors may occur synchronously or metachronously, they tend to be of the same histologic type. Seminoma is the most common histologic type in bilateral primary testicular tumors, whereas malignant lymphoma is the most common bilateral testicular tumor.

Although the cause of testicular cancer is unknown, both congenital and acquired factors have been associated with tumor development. A history of cryptorchidism is the strongest risk factor for testicular cancer development. Approximately 6% of testis tumors develop in patients with histories of cryptorchidism, with seminoma being the most common (2). However, 5 to 10% of these tumors occur in the contralateral, normally descended testis. The relative risk of malignancy development appears related to the level of descent of the testis and is highest for the intra-abdominal testis (1 in 20) and lowest for the inguinal testis (1 in 80). Although orchiopexy facilitates examination of the testis, it does not alter the malignant potential of the testis.

Exogenous estrogen administration during pregnancy has been associated with an increased relative risk for testis tumors, ranging from 2.8 to 5.3 (3, 4). Other acquired factors such as trauma and infection-related testicular atrophy (mumps orchitis) have been associated with testicular tumors; however, a causal relationship in humans has not been firmly established.

PATHOLOGY

Model for Germ Cell Tumor Development

The current model for germ cell tumor development resulted from the work of Dixon and Moore (5), Teilum (6), and Mostofi (7) (Fig. 34.1). During development, totipotential germ cells can travel down normal differentiation pathways and become spermatocytes. However, if these totipotential germ cells follow abnormal developmental pathways, seminoma or embryonal

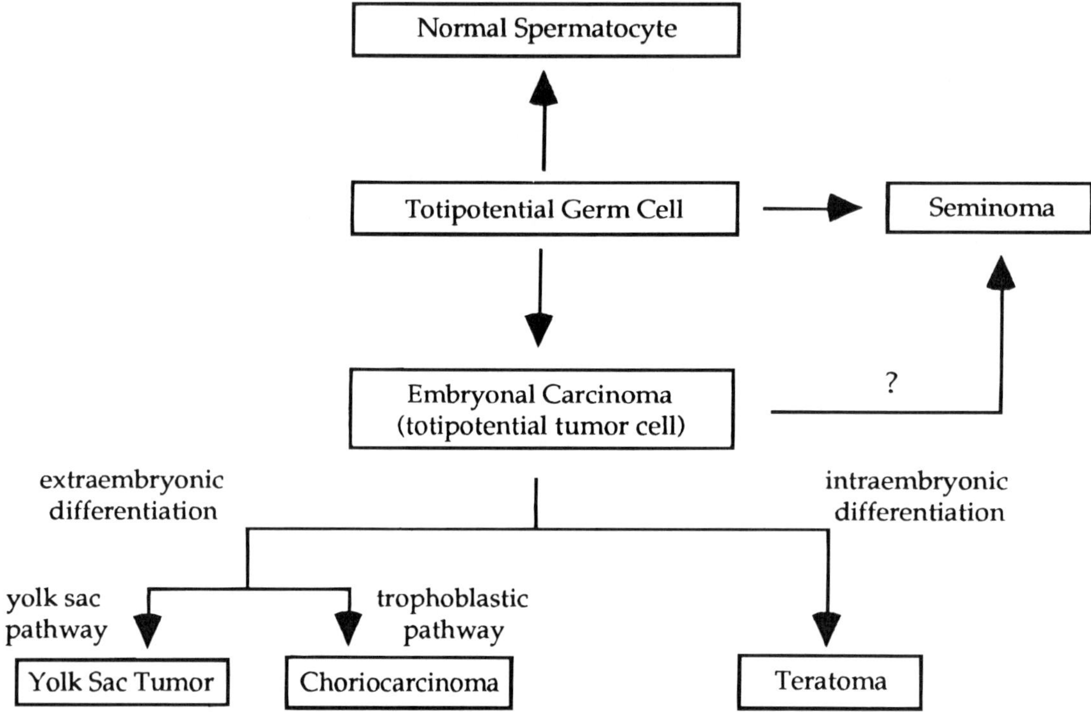

Fig. 34.1.   Model for germ cell tumor development of the testis.

carcinoma (totipotential tumor cell) develops. Embryonal cells may undergo further differentiation along intraembryonic pathways, resulting in teratomas. Alternatively, embryonal cells may follow extraembryonic pathways of differentiation, resulting in either choriocarcinoma or yolk sac tumors. This model helps to explain the specificity of certain tumor markers to select histologic subtypes. Yolk sac tumors produce alpha-fetoprotein (AFP), mimicking the production of AFP by the yolk sac in normal embryogenesis. Likewise, choriocarcinomas produce human chorionic gonadotropin (hCG), mimicking the production of hCG by the normal placenta.

HISTOLOGIC TYPE

The classification of germ cell tumors of the testis by histologic type proves to be the most useful with respect to treatment and prognosis. The two major divisions are seminoma and non-seminomatous germ cell tumors (NSGCT), which include embryonal, teratocarcinoma, teratoma, choriocarcinoma, and mixed tumors. The distribution of the histologic subtypes is shown in Table 34.1.

Seminoma

Seminomas may be classified into one of three histologic subtypes. Classic seminoma accounts for 85% of all seminomas and is most common in the fourth decade of life. Gross examination demonstrates coalescing, gray nodules. Microscopically, monotonous sheets of large cells with clear cytoplasm and densely staining nuclei are seen. Lymphocytic infiltrates are seen in up to 20% of cases. Syncytiotrophoblastic elements are seen in approximately 10 to 15% of cases; this approximately corresponds to the incidence of hCG production in seminomas.

Anaplastic seminoma accounts for 5 to 10% of all seminomas. Diagnosis requires the presence of three or more mitoses per high-power field, and cells demonstrate a higher degree of nuclear pleomorphism and cellular atypia than the classic type. Anaplastic seminoma more commonly presents at a higher stage than the classic seminoma; however, when stage is taken into consideration, this histologic subtype does not alter prognosis.

Spermatocytic seminoma accounts for 5 to 10% of all seminomas. More than half the patients with spermatocytic seminoma are older than 50 years of age. Microscopically, cells vary in size and are characterized by densely staining cytoplasm and round nuclei that contain condensed, filamentous chromatin.

Table 34.1.   Distribution of Histologic Subtypes of Testicular Germ Cell Tumors

CELL TYPE	INCIDENCE (%)	INCIDENCE (%)[a]
Seminoma	40	30
Teratocarcinoma	25–30	25
Embryonal carcinoma	20–25	30
Teratoma	5–10	10
Choriocarcinoma	1	<1
Mixed	—	15

[a] Mixed tumors considered as a separate category.

The metastatic potential of spermatocytic seminoma is low. They are not associated with cryptorchidism or other nonseminomatous elements. Orchiectomy alone in the face of a negative metastatic workup is adequate treatment.

Embryonal Cell Carcinoma

Two variants of embryonal cell carcinoma are commonly seen—the adult type and the infantile type or yolk sac tumor (also called endodermal sinus tumor). Gross examination often demonstrates extensive hemorrhage and necrosis. The adult variant histologically demonstrates significant pleomorphism and indistinct cellular borders. Mitotic figures and giant cells are common. Cells may be arranged in sheets, cords, glands, or papillary structures. Embryoid bodies are commonly seen and resemble 1- to 2-week-old embryos consisting of a cavity surrounded by syncytiotrophoblasts and cytotrophoblasts.

The infantile variant or yolk sac tumor is the most common testis tumor of infants and children. When seen in adults, it usually occurs in mixed histologic types and is possibly responsible for AFP production in these tumors. Microscopically, cells demonstrate vacuolated cytoplasm secondary to fat and glycogen deposition and are arranged in a loose network with large intervening cystic spaces. Pathognomonic for yolk sac tumors are Schiller-Duval bodies, which are glomeruloid-like structures consisting of a flattened parietal layer of cells and a central tuft of cuboidal cells surrounding a central fibrovascular core.

Teratoma

Teratomas occur in both children and adults. By definition, they contain more than one germ cell layer in various stages of maturation and differentiation. Grossly, the tumors appear lobulated and contain variable-sized cysts filled with gelatinous or mucinous material. Mature teratomas may have elements resembling benign structures derived from ectoderm, mesoderm, and endoderm; immature teratomas consist of undifferentiated primitive tissue. Unlike ovarian teratomas, which occasionally demonstrate hair or tooth formation, mature teratomas of the testis do not attain such high degrees of differentiation. Microscopically, ectoderm may be represented by squamous epithelium or neural tissue; endoderm may be represented by intestinal, pancreatic, or respiratory tissue; and mesoderm may be represented by smooth or skeletal muscle, cartilage, or bone. The metastatic potential of mature teratoma in the adult remains controversial.

Choriocarcinoma

Pure choriocarcinoma is rare. Lesions tend to be small within the testis and usually demonstrate central hemorrhage on gross inspection. Regression of the primary tumor may result in only a hemosiderin-laden scar within the testis. Microscopically, syncytiotrophoblasts and cytotrophoblasts must be visualized. Syncytiotrophoblastic elements tend to surround central aggregates of cytotrophoblasts. The syncytial elements are typically large, multinucleated cells with vacuolated, eosinophilic cytoplasm. Nuclei are large, hyperchromatic, and irregular. Cytotrophoblasts are uniform cells with distinct cell borders, clear cytoplasm, and a single nucleus.

Clinically, choriocarcinomas behave in an aggressive fashion characterized by early hematogenous spread. Small intratesticular lesions may be associated with widespread metastatic disease.

CARCINOMA IN SITU

In a series of 250 patients with unilateral testicular cancer, Berthelson et al. demonstrated the presence of carcinoma in situ in 13 contralateral testes (5.2%) (8). This is approximately twice the overall incidence of bilateral testicular cancer. Although the natural history of this entity is incompletely defined, it should be noted that 5 of these 13 patients have received follow-up care for 3 years and that invasive disease developed in 2 of these 5 patients. Currently, the optimal treatment of carcinoma in situ of the testis remains controversial.

PATTERNS OF SPREAD

With the exception of choriocarcinoma, which demonstrates early hematogenous spread, germ cell tumors of the testis typically spread via lymphatics in a stepwise fashion. Lymph nodes of the testis extend from T1 to L4 but are concentrated at the level of the renal hilum due to their common embryologic origin with the kidney. The primary landing site for the right testis is the interaortocaval area at the level of the right renal hilum. Stepwise spread, in order, is to the precaval, preaortic, paracaval, right common iliac, and right external iliac lymph nodes. The primary landing site for the left testis is the periaortic area at the level of the left renal hilum. Stepwise spread, in order, is to the preaortic, left common iliac, and left external iliac lymph nodes. In the absence of disease on the left side, no crossover metastases to the right side have ever been identified. However, right-to-left crossover metastases are common (9, 10). These observations have resulted in modified surgical dissections to preserve ejaculation in select patients.

Certain factors may alter the primary drainage of a testis neoplasm. Invasion of the epididymis or spermatic cord may allow spread to the distal external iliac and obturator lymph nodes. Scrotal violation or invasion of the tunica albuginea may result in inguinal metastases.

The retroperitoneum is the most commonly involved site in metastatic disease; however, visceral metastases may be seen in advanced disease. The sites involved, in decreasing frequency, include lung, liver, brain, bone, kidney, adrenal, gastrointestinal tract, and spleen (11).

As mentioned previously, choriocarcinoma is the exception to the rule and is characterized by early hematogenous spread, especially to the lung. Choriocarcinoma also has a predilection for unusual sites of metastasis such as the spleen.

Table 34.2. Comparison of Clinical Staging Systems for Testicular Cancer

BODEN/GIBB	MSKCC	MD ANDERSON
A (confined to testis)	A	I
B (spread to regional nodes)	B1 (<5 cm)	IIa (<10 cm)
	B2 (5–10 cm)	IIb (>10 cm)
	B3 (>10 cm)	
C (spread beyond retroperitoneum)	C	III

CLINICAL STAGING

Many clinical staging systems have been proposed for testicular cancer; however, most are variations of the original system proposed by Boden and Gibb (12). In this system, a stage A lesion was confined to the testis, stage B demonstrated regional lymph node spread, and stage C was spread beyond retroperitoneal lymph nodes. In the United States, the Memorial Sloan-Kettering Cancer Center (MSKCC) system is commonly used for NSGCT; the M.D. Anderson System is often used for seminoma (Table 34.2) (13). The TNM classification of the American Joint Committee has attempted to standardize clinical staging of testis cancer and is shown in Table 34.3 (14).

CLINICAL PRESENTATION

History and Physical Examination

Painless enlargement of the testis is the most common symptom of testicular cancer. Enlargement is usually gradual, and delays in the patient seeking medical attention are common. Typical intervals from initial recognition of the lesion by the patient to definitive therapy (orchiectomy) range from 3 to 6

Table 34.3. TNM Classification for Testicular Cancer

T—Primary tumor
- Tx Cannot be assessed
- T0 No evidence of primary tumor
- Tis Intratubular cancer (CIS)
- T1 Limited to testis
- T2 Invades beyond tunica albuginea or into epididymis
- T3 Invades spermatic cord
- T4 Invades scrotum

N—Regional lymph nodes
- Nx Cannot be assessed
- N0 No regional lymph node metastasis
- N1 Metastasis in a single lymph node 2 cm or less
- N2 Metastasis in a single lymph node >2 cm and <5 cm or multiple nodes none >5 cm
- N3 Metastasis in lymph node >5 cm

M—Distant metastasis
- Mx Cannot be assessed
- M0 No distant metastasis
- M1 Distant metastasis present

months. The length of delay correlates with the incidence of metastases (15). Patient education and instruction for self-examination are critical. Acute testicular pain is seen in approximately 10% of cases and may be the result of intratesticular hemorrhage or infarction.

Approximately 10% of patients present with symptoms related to metastatic disease. Back pain (retroperitoneal metastases irritating nerve roots) is the most common symptom. Other symptoms include cough, hemoptysis, or dyspnea (pulmonary metastases); nausea or vomiting (retroduodenal metastases); and lower extremity swelling (vena caval obstruction). Approximately 10% of patients are asymptomatic at presentation, and the tumor may be detected incidentally following trauma or may be detected by the patient's sexual partner.

On physical examination, a testicular mass or diffuse enlargement is found in the majority of cases. The mass is typically firm and nontender, and the epididymis should be easily separable from it. A hydrocele is associated with testicular tumors in up to 5 to 10% of cases, and transillumination of the scrotum may aid in evaluation. Aspiration of the hydrocele should be avoided; positive cytologies have been reported in hydroceles associated with testicular tumors (16). Palpation of the abdomen may reveal bulky retroperitoneal disease, and assessment of supraclavicular, scalene, and inguinal nodes should be performed. Gynecomastia is present in 5% of all germ cell tumors but may be present in 30 to 50% of Sertoli and Leydig cell tumors. Its etiology seems to be related to complex hormonal interactions involving testosterone, estrone, estradiol, prolactin, and hCG (17).

An incorrect diagnosis is made at the initial examination in up to 25% of patients with testicular tumors. This may result in delay in treatment or a suboptimal surgical approach (scrotal incision) for exploration. Epididymitis or epididymo-orchitis is the most common misdiagnosis in patients with testicular cancer. Hydrocele is the second most common misdiagnosis. Other diagnoses to be considered include spermatocele, granulomatous orchitis, and varicocele. Although most intratesticular masses are malignant, one benign lesion—an epidermoid cyst—may rarely be seen. These are usually very small benign nodules located just underneath the tunica albuginea; however, they can occasionally be large. Frozen sections are often difficult to distinguish from teratoma.

TUMOR MARKERS

Several biochemical markers—AFP, hCG, and lactic acid dehydrogenase (LDH)—are important in the diagnosis and management of testicular carcinoma. AFP is a glycoprotein with a molecular weight of 70,000 d and a half-life of 4 to 6 days. Although present in fetal serum in high levels, beyond the age of 1 year it is present in only trace amounts. Although present to varying degrees in many NSGCT (Table 34.4), it is never found in seminomas. If preorchiectomy serum AFP levels are elevated, the patient must have a component of NSGCT and should be treated accordingly.

Table 34.4. Incidence of Elevated Tumor Markers by Histology in Testicular Cancer

	hCG (%)	AFP (%)
Seminoma	7	0
Teratoma	25	38
Teratocarcinoma	57	64
Embryonal Carcinoma	60	70
Choriocarcinoma	100	0

hCG is a glycoprotein with a molecular weight of 38,000 d and a half-life of 24 hours. It is composed of two subunits—alpha and beta. The alpha subunit is similar to the alpha subunits of luteinizing hormone, follicle-stimulating hormone, and thyroid-stimulating hormone. The beta subunit conveys the activity to each of these hormones and allows for a highly sensitive and specific radioimmunoassay in the determination of hCG levels. The normal male should not have significant levels of beta-hCG. Although more commonly elevated in NSGCT, hCG levels may be elevated in up to 7% of seminomas. The magnitude of hCG elevations in seminoma is typically lower than that seen in NSGCT.

LDH is a cellular enzyme with a molecular weight of 134,000 d that has five isoenzymes normally found in muscle (smooth, cardiac, skeletal), liver, kidney, and brain. Elevation of total serum LDH and, in particular, isoenzyme-I was shown to correlate with tumor burden in NSGCT (18). LDH may also be elevated in seminoma (19).

Other markers have been described for testicular cancer including placental alkaline phosphatase and gamma-glutamyl transpeptidase. However, these have not contributed as significantly to patient management as those mentioned above.

IMAGING

Scrotal ultrasonography can readily distinguish between intratesticular and extratesticular masses. It also facilitates testicular examination when adequate physical examination is precluded by the presence of a large hydrocele or following trauma.

After the diagnosis of testicular cancer has been established by inguinal orchiectomy, careful clinical staging is mandatory. Chest radiographs (posteroanterior and lateral) and computed tomography (CT) scan of the abdomen and pelvis will assess the two most common sites of metastatic spread—the lungs and retroperitoneum. The role of CT scanning of the chest remains controversial because of its decreased specificity. Routine chest radiographs will detect 85 to 90% of pulmonary metastases. In the face of a negative abdominal CT scan, a routine chest radiograph appears adequate (20). Pedal lymphangiography (LAG) can add 10 to 15% to the sensitivity of CT scanning in detecting retroperitoneal nodal involvement, yet it is rarely used due to its invasiveness and low specificity. Lymphangiography may be warranted in patients undergoing a surveillance protocol.

TREATMENT AND PROGNOSIS

Serum tumor markers (AFP, hCG, LDH) should be obtained before surgical intervention. Inguinal exploration with cross-clamping of the spermatic cord vasculature and delivery of the testis into the field is the procedure of choice for a possible testicular tumor. If cancer cannot be excluded by examination of the testis, then radical orchiectomy is warranted. Scrotal approaches and open testicular biopsies should be avoided because they may result in scrotal recurrences or disruption of the normal lymphatic drainage. Further therapy is dependent on the histologic type of the tumor and clinical stage.

Low-stage Seminoma (I, II-A)

Seminoma is exquisitely radiation sensitive. Radical orchiectomy followed by retroperitoneal irradiation (usually 2500 to 3000 cGy) cures 95 to 98% of clinical stage I seminomas. This dose of radiation is usually well tolerated with minimal, if any, gastrointestinal side effects.

Low-volume retroperitoneal disease (IIa, less than 10 cm in diameter) can also be treated effectively with retroperitoneal irradiation, with an average 5-year survival rate approaching 90%. Prophylactic mediastinal irradiation in clinical stage IIa has been abandoned because this may cause significant myelosuppression and thus compromise the patient's ability to receive chemotherapy in the future. Chemotherapy should be used as salvage therapy for patients who experience relapse after irradiation.

High-stage Seminoma (II-B, III)

Patients with bulky seminoma should receive primary chemotherapy. Seminomas are also sensitive to platinum-based regimens as are their NSGCT counterparts. Some of the successful regimens include cisplatin, etoposide, bleomycin (PEB); vinblastine, cyclophosphamide, dactinomycin, bleomycin, and cisplatin (VAB-6); cisplatin and etoposide (EP). At MSKCC, all seminomas receive good-risk chemotherapy regimens (EP).

Ninety percent of patients with stage III disease will experience a complete response with chemotherapy. Residual retroperitoneal masses following chemotherapy are often fibrosis (90%). The only indication to perform surgical resection of a residual mass following chemotherapy for seminoma is if the mass is well circumscribed and larger than 3 cm. Under these circumstances, approximately 40% of cases will harbor residual seminoma (21).

High-stage disease treated by orchiectomy and primary chemotherapy has a 5-year disease-free survival rate of 32 to 75%, yet the lower value comes from older series where more crude chemotherapy regimens were used.

Low-stage NSGCT

Standard treatment for stage A disease in the United States has included retroperitoneal lymph node dissection (RPLND).

However, because 75% of patients with clinical stage A disease will be cured by orchiectomy alone and RPLND is associated with morbidity, alternatives have been explored. These options include surveillance, modified RPLND, and nerve-sparing RPLND.

Surveillance in stage A NSGCT was proposed because, as mentioned previously, 75% of patients with clinical stage A disease have pathologic stage A disease. In addition, infertility related to disruption of sympathetic nerve fibers is common after complete RPLND. Clinical staging has been significantly improved in the presence of CT scanning and LAG. In addition, effective chemotherapy regimens are available if patients have relapses. Patients are considered candidates for surveillance if the tumor is an NSGCT confined within the tunica albuginea (T1), the tumor does not demonstrate vascular invasion, tumor markers normalize after orchiectomy, radiographic imaging shows no evidence of disease (chest radiograph (CXR), CT, and LAG in select patients), and the patient is considered reliable.

Surveillance is an active process on the part of both the physician and patient. Patients are followed monthly for the first 2 years and bimonthly in the third year. Tumor markers are obtained at each visit, and CXR and CT scans are obtained every 3 to 4 months. Plain films of the abdomen are used to monitor the initial LAG (if performed). Follow-up continues beyond the initial 3 years; however, the majority of relapses will occur within the first 8 to 10 months. Sites of relapse during surveillance, in decreasing frequency, are retroperitoneum alone, chest alone, and both chest and retroperitoneum (22). With rare exceptions, patients who experience relapse can be cured by chemotherapy and/or surgery.

RPLND had been the preferred treatment of low-stage NSGCT in the United States. A thoracoabdominal or midline transabdominal approach may be used, and all nodal tissue between the ureters from the renal vessels to the bifurcation of the common iliac vessels is removed.

Although effective in surgically staging and potentially curing a subset of patients, RPLND is associated with significant morbidity, especially with respect to fertility in this young age-group. With a standard RPLND, sympathetic nerve fibers are disrupted, resulting in loss of seminal emission. A modified RPLND has been developed that preserves ejaculation in up to 90% of patients. By modifying the dissection below the level of the inferior mesenteric artery to include only the nodal tissue ipsilateral to the tumor, contralateral sympathetic fibers are preserved; thus, ejaculation is maintained (23, 24). In addition to the use of templates, sympathetic nerves can also be directly visualized and preserved at the time of surgery in more extensive dissections, resulting in preservation of ejaculation (25). This technique is especially appealing if, during a planned modified RPLND, cancer is found on frozen section. Under such circumstances a complete bilateral dissection is recommended, yet a nerve-sparing approach may be used.

Patients with negative nodes or N1 disease do not require adjuvant therapy, whereas those with N2 disease are recommended to receive two cycles of adjuvant chemotherapy as their relapse rate approaches 50% (26, 27).

The management of "marker-only" patients (negative staging workup yet tumor markers remain elevated after orchiectomy) remains controversial. As a result of small numbers of such patients, no large trials have been able to determine the optimal mode of therapy. A recent report advocates two cycles of chemotherapy in these patients (28).

Survival in patients with NSGCT treated by orchiectomy and RPLND ranges from 90 to 100%.

High-stage NSGCT

Patients with bulky retroperitoneal disease (nodes greater than 3 cm or three or more 1-cm cuts on CT scan) or metastatic NSGCT are treated with primary platinum-based combination chemotherapy following orchiectomy. If tumor markers normalize and a residual mass in excess of 3 cm is apparent on imaging studies, resection of that mass is mandatory—20% of the time it will harbor residual cancer, 40% of the time it will be teratoma, and 40% of the time it will be fibrosis (Figs. 34.2 and 34.3). (29) Typically, patients with residual masses following chemotherapy undergo complete bilateral RPLND; however, select patients may benefit from more limited resections (30). Even if patients attain a complete response after chemotherapy (normal tumor markers, no mass on CT scan or CXR), a recent report suggests that RPLND is indicated because viable germ cell tumor may be seen in up to 10% of cases (31). One group has reported excellent results in preserving ejaculation in a high percentage of patients undergoing complete RPLND following chemotherapy when meticulous attention is paid to the preservation of sympathetic lumbar roots (32). In patients who have residual masses in both the retroperitoneum and chest, resection of all masses is warranted; discordant histology between chest and retroperitoneum occurs in 35% of patients (33).

In those patients with residual cancer in the resected tissue, the histologic type is usually embryonal cell carcinoma; however, malignant teratoma is seen in less than 5% of cases. Patients with carcinoma in the resected specimen receive an additional two cycles of chemotherapy. Malignant teratoma is unresponsive to chemotherapy, and only 15% of patients will survive after surgical resection. If tumor markers fail to normalize after primary chemotherapy, then salvage chemotherapy is required (cisplatin, etoposide, bleomycin, ifosfamide).

Occasionally, a patient's condition is diagnosed as advanced NSGCT on the basis of a needle biopsy performed on a metastatic site rather than by orchiectomy. Such patients will receive chemotherapy and may require an RPLND. However, a delayed orchiectomy must be performed because viable cancer is often demonstrated in the testis (34).

Although the above-mentioned treatment plan cures up to 70% of patients with high-volume disease, there are still cases in which the disease does not respond. In addition, we would like to lessen the possible morbidity of chemotherapy including

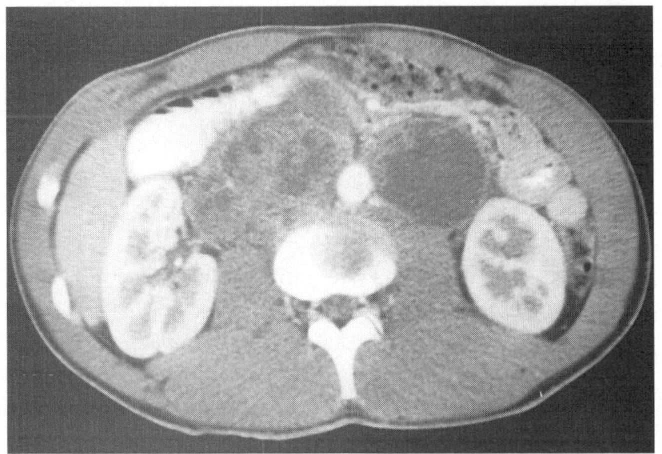 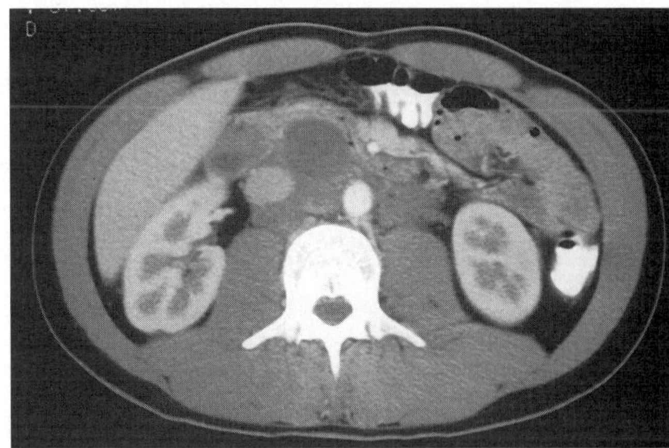

Fig. 34.2. **A.** CT scan of a patient with bulky retroperitoneal mass after radical orchiectomy for NSGCT. **B.** CT scan performed after four cycles of chemotherapy demonstrating a residual mass that was resected and found to be necrosis.

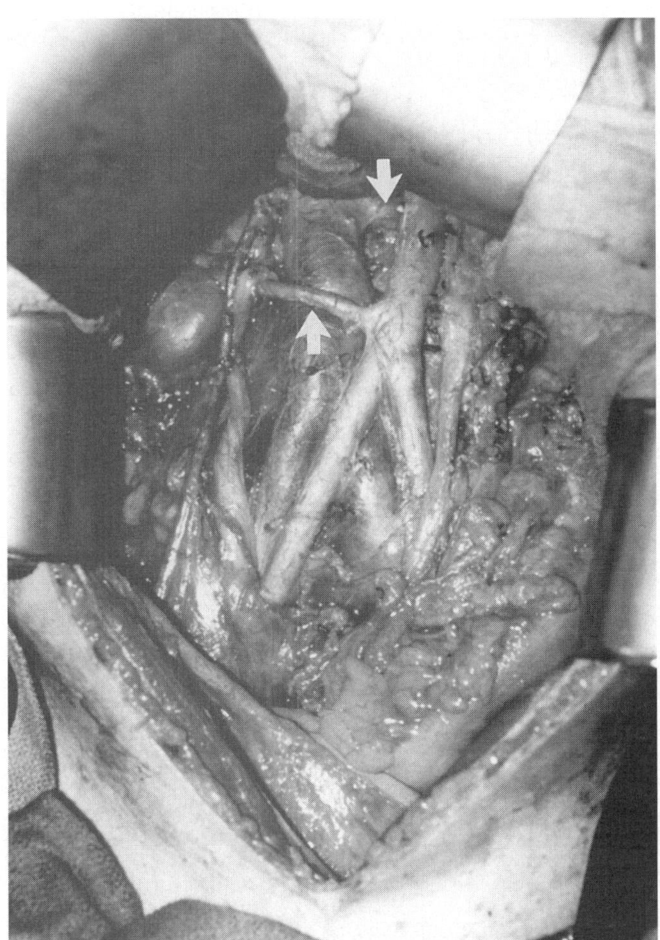

Fig. 34.3. Intraoperative picture after a complete bilateral RPLND for a residual mass after chemotherapy. Note anomalous right renal artery (up arrow) and retroaortic left renal vein (down arrow).

sepsis, neuropathy, renal toxicity, infertility, and death in patients whose conditions are likely to respond. The utility of being able to discriminate between patients whose conditions are likely to respond to standard chemotherapy (good risk) and those who may require more aggressive regimens (poor risk) is apparent.

At MSKCC, a mathematical model is used to predict the likelihood of attaining a complete response to standard chemotherapy (35). In a multivariate analysis only three parameters achieved statistical significance, namely serum lactate dehydrogenase, serum hCG, and total number of metastatic sites. At MSKCC, patients considered to be good risk will receive four cycles of cisplatin and etoposide; poor-risk patients will receive more aggressive regimens (VAB-6, high-dose regimens with autologous bone marrow transplantation).

More recently, the rate of decline of serum tumor markers during chemotherapy has been used to predict response in patients with advanced disease (36). Indiana University stratifies patients into three categories of extent of disease—minimal, moderate, and advanced (Table 34.5). Patients with minimal or moderate extent of disease receive good-risk regimens (three cycles of PEB); patients with advanced extent of disease receive more intensive regimens.

EXTRAGONADAL GERM CELL TUMORS

Epidemiology and Pathology

Extragonadal germ cell tumors are rare and account for approximately 3 to 5% of all germ cell tumors. Debate continues about whether these lesions originate from "burned-out" testicular primaries or whether they originate de novo. Some have suggested that all retroperitoneal tumors have their origin from a testicular primary, whereas mediastinal germ cell tumors are truly ectopic. Two theories exist about their origin as primary extragonadal lesions.

Table 34.5. Indiana University Staging System for Testicular Cancer

Minimal extent
  Elevated markers only
  Cervical nodes ($\pm$ nonpalpable retroperitoneal nodes)
  Unresectable nonpalpable retroperitoneal disease
  Less than 5 pulmonary metastases per lung field, all <2 cm
    ($\pm$ nonpalpable retroperitoneal nodes)
Moderate extent
  Palpable abdominal mass only (no supradiaphragmatic disease)
  Moderate pulmonary metastases; 5–10 per lung field, none larger
    than 3 cm, or a solitary pulmonary metastasis of any size > 2
    cm ($\pm$ nonpalpable retroperitoneal nodes)
Advanced extent
  Advanced pulmonary metastases: >10 pulmonary metastases per
    lung field or multiple pulmonary metastases with largest >3 cm
    or primary mediastinal germ cell tumor ($\pm$ nonpalpable retroperi-
    toneal nodes)
  Palpable abdominal mass plus supradiaphragmatic disease
  Liver, bone, or CNS metastases

1. During embryonic migration, primitive germ cells are displaced from their normal pathway and attain ectopic positions.
2. Pluripotential cells are displaced early in embryogenesis and become sequestered in ectopic sites.

The most common sites of origin, in decreasing order, are mediastinum, retroperitoneum, sacrococcygeal area, and pineal gland. All germ cell types can be observed. More than half of the retroperitoneal and mediastinal tumors are seminomas.

Clinical Presentation

Clinical presentation varies according to the site and volume of disease. Mediastinal lesions may present with pulmonary complaints. Retroperitoneal lesions may present with abdominal or back pain and a palpable mass. Sacrococcygeal tumors are most commonly seen in neonates and may present with a palpable mass and bowel or urinary obstruction. Pineal tumors may present with headache, visual or auditory complaints, or hypopituitarism.

The metastatic workup is similar to that of testicular germ cell tumors. Common sites of spread include regional lymph nodes, lung, liver, bone, and brain. A careful testicular examination is mandatory along with ultrasonography to exclude an occult testicular primary.

Treatment and Prognosis

Treatment of extragonadal germ cell tumors parallels that of testicular tumors. Low-volume seminoma can be managed with radiation therapy. High-volume seminoma should receive primary chemotherapy. Prognosis parallels that of testicular seminoma. Primary chemotherapy should be used for nonseminoma-

tous elements with surgical excision of residual masses; however, prognosis remains poor for these patients.

FUTURE DIRECTIONS

The multidisciplinary approach to testicular cancer has resulted in excellent survival data even in advanced stages. Ongoing refinements in both surgical technique and chemotherapeutic regimens are aimed at minimizing morbidity while maintaining comparable survival data. Particular areas of interest include marker-only patients and chemorefractory patients. Further clinical trials are needed in risk assessment, cost analysis, and outcome analysis to better optimize patient care.

REFERENCES

1. Boring CC, Squires TS, Tong T, et al. Cancer statistics, 1994. CA Cancer J Clin 1994;44:7.
2. Batata MA, Chu FCH, Hilaris BS, et al. Testicular cancer in cryptorchids. Cancer 1982;49:1023.
3. Henderson BE, Ross RK, Pike MC. Epidemiology of testicular cancer. In: Skinner DG, Lieskovsky G, eds. Diagnosis and management of genitourinary cancer. Philadelphia: WB Saunders, 1988.
4. Schottenfeld D, Warshauer ME, Sherlock S, et al. The epidemiology of testicular cancer in young adults. Am J Epidemiol 1980;112:232.
5. Dixon FH, Moore RA. Tumors of the male sex organs. In: Atlas of tumor pathology. Washington, DC: AFIP, 1952.
6. Teilum G. Special tumors of the ovary and testis and related extragonadal lesions. In: Comparative pathology and histological identification. 2nd ed. Philadelphia: JB Lippincott, 1976.
7. Mostofi FK. Testicular tumors: epidemiologic, etiologic and pathologic features. Cancer 1973;32:1186.
8. Berthelson JG, Skakkebaek NE, Sorensen BC, et al. Screening for carcinoma in situ of the contralateral testis in patients with germinal testicular cancer. Br Med J 1982;285:1683.
9. Donahue JP, Zachary JM, Magnard BR. Distribution of nodal metastases in nonseminomatous testis cancer. J Urol 1982;128:315.
10. Ray B, Hajdu SI, Whitmore WF Jr. Distribution of retroperitoneal lymph node metastases in testicular germinal tumors. Cancer 1974;33:340.
11. Bredael JJ, Vugrin D, Whitmore WF Jr. Autopsy findings in 154 patients with germ cell tumors of the testis. Cancer 1982;50:548.
12. Boden G, Gibb R. Radiotherapy and testicular neoplasms. Lancet 1951;2:1195.
13. Doornbos JF, Hussey DH, Johnson DE. Radiotherapy for pure seminoma of the testis. Radiology 1975;116:410.
14. Spiessl B, Beahrs OH, Hermanek P, eds. Testicular carcinoma. In: TNM Atlas. 3rd ed. Berlin: Springer-Verlag, 1992.
15. Oliver RT. Factors contributing to delay in diagnosis of testicular tumors. Br Med J 1985;290:356.
16. Orecklin JR. Testicular tumor occurring with hydrocele and positive cytologic fluid. Urology 1974;3:232.
17. Stepanas A, Samaan NA, Schultz PN, et al. Endocrine studies

in testicular tumor patients with and without gynecomastia: a report of 45 cases. Cancer 1978;41:369.

18. Liu F, Fritsche HA, Trujillo JM, et al. Serum lactate dehydrogenase isoenzyme 1 in patients with advanced testicular cancer. Am J Clin Pathol 1982;78:178.

19. Stanton GF, Bosl GJ, Whitmore WF Jr, et al. VAB-6 as initial treatment of patients with advanced seminoma. J Clin Oncol 1985;3:336.

20. See WA, Hoxie L. Chest staging in testis cancer patients: imaging modality selection based upon risk assessment as determined by abdominal computerized tomography scan results. J Urol 1993;150:874.

21. Motzer R, Bosl G, Heelan R, et al. Residual mass: an indication for further therapy in patients with advanced seminoma following systemic chemotherapy. J Clin Oncol 1987;5:1064.

22. Sogani PC, Fair WR. Surveillance alone in the treatment of clinical stage I nonseminomatous germ cell tumor of the testis (NSGCT). Semin Urol 1988;6:53.

23. Lange PH, Narayan P, Fraley EE. Fertility issues following therapy for testicular cancer. Semin Urol 1984;4:264.

24. Pizzocaro G, Salvioni R, Zanoni F. Unilateral lymphadenectomy in intraoperative stage I nonseminomatous germinal testis cancer. J Urol 1985;134:485.

25. Donohue JP, Foster RS, Rowland RG, et al. Nerve-sparing retroperitoneal lymphadenectomy with preservation of ejaculation. J Urol 1990;144:287.

26. Williams SD, Stablain DM, Einhorn LH. Immediate adjuvant chemotherapy versus observation with treatment at relapse in pathologic stage II testicular cancer. N Engl J Med 1987;317:1433.

27. Richie JP, Kantoff P. Is adjuvant chemotherapy necessary for patients with stage B1 testicular cancer? J Clin Oncol 1991;9:1393.

28. Davis BE, Herr HW, Fair WR, et al. The management of patients with nonseminomatous germ cell tumors of the testis with serologic disease only after orchiectomy. J Urol 1994;152:111.

29. Donohue JP, Rowland RG. The role of surgery in advanced testicular cancer. Cancer 1984;54:2716.

30. Wood DP Jr, Herr HW, Heller G, et al. Distribution of retroperitoneal metastases after chemotherapy in patients with nonseminomatous germ cell tumors. J Urol 1992;148:1816.

31. Toner GC, Panicek DM, Heelan RT, et al. Adjunctive surgery after chemotherapy for nonseminomatous germ cell tumors: recommendations for patient selection. J Clin Oncol 1990;8:1683.

32. Wahle GR, Foster RS, Bihrle R, et al. Nerve-sparing retroperitoneal lymphadenectomy after primary chemotherapy for metastatic testicular carcinoma. J Urol 1994;152:428.

33. Tiffany P, Morse MJ, Bosl G, et al. Sequential excision of residual thoracic and retroperitoneal masses after chemotherapy for stage III germ cell tumors. Cancer 1986;57:978.

34. Calvo F, Hodson N, Barrett A, et al. Chemotherapy of primary (in-situ) testicular tumours: response in advanced metastatic disease. Br J Urol 1983;55:560.

35. Bosl GJ, Geller NL, Cirrincione C, et al. Multivariate analysis of prognostic variables in patients with metastatic testicular cancer. Cancer Res 1983;43:3403.

36. Toner GC, Geller NL, Tan C, et al. Serum tumor marker half-life during chemotherapy allows early prediction of complete response and survival in nonseminomatous germ cell tumors. Cancer Res 1990;50:5904.

35

Radical Inguinal Orchiectomy

Michael J. Schutz

The application of surgical oncologic principles to the diagnosis and treatment of the primary site in testis cancer is best achieved with radical inguinal orchiectomy. These principles include early vascular and lymphatic control of the tumor, minimal handling of the testis, and preservation of the tissue layers surrounding the testis. These measures reduce the possibility of tumor spread during orchiectomy. The inguinal approach also allows the removal of the spermatic cord up to and proximal to the internal inguinal ring, reducing the possibility of recurrences in the inguinal canal from retained vascular and lymphatic structures of the spermatic cord.

In contrast, transcrotal orchiectomy does not allow removal of the spermatic cord up to the internal inguinal ring, and one can violate the fascial layers around the testicle with tumor spillage and the possibility of scrotal or inguinal lymph node metastases. A 24% incidence of scrotal or inguinal lymphatic cancer recurrence has been seen in the transcrotal approach (1). Later series, however, have shown no survival differences with close follow-up and aggressive adjuvant treatment (2). An initial inguinal approach may have avoided the potential morbidity of adjuvant therapy. Transcrotal needle biopsy or fine-needle aspiration also violates the scrotal lymphatics and the fascial layers overlying the testis and should be discouraged (3).

INDICATIONS

Radical inguinal orchiectomy is indicated whenever there is suspicion of a testis tumor or a tumor of the paratesticular structures. The history may include complaints of an ache or heaviness in the testicle, epididymitis that does not improve with antibiotic therapy, scrotal mass, or new onset or change in a hydrocele (4). Physical examination may reveal a testicular mass or hydrocele that does not allow complete examination of the testicle. Scrotal ultrasound may be helpful in cases where the physical examination is difficult or inconclusive. Surgical exploration is necessary if testicular neoplasm is suspected.

Baseline serum human chorionic gonadotropin, alpha-fetoprotein (AFP), and lactate dehydrogenase levels should be obtained before surgery. When present, these testicular tumor markers are very useful in the treatment and follow-up of testis cancer. Many testicular tumors do not produce elevated tumor markers. Normal or nondetectable serum tumor markers should not influence or deter the decision to proceed with surgical exploration in patients in whom testicular tumor is suspected.

PROCEDURE

Radical inguinal orchiectomy is performed with the patient in the supine position. The patient is prepared from the upper thigh to the umbilicus, including the external genitalia. The scrotum is draped into the field (Fig. 35.1). No perioperative antibiotics are necessary.

INCISION

The proper skin incision allows easy access to the inguinal canal and its contents. The internal inguinal ring lies midway between the anterior superior iliac spine and the pubic tubercle. An 8- to 10-cm incision is made beginning at the pubic tubercle and extending toward the anterior superior iliac spine (Fig. 35.2). The incision may be slightly more oblique or horizontal, depending on the tension lines in the skin (5).

The subcutaneous fat and Scarpa's fascia are sharply dissected. Branches of the superficial inferior epigastric vein and the superficial circumflex iliac vein may be encountered and should be ligated or cauterized and divided (5).

The external oblique aponeurosis and the external inguinal ring are identified and exposed. The external oblique aponeurosis is sharply incised in the direction of its fibers, and the ilioinguinal nerve underneath is identified (Fig. 35.3). The nerve is dissected free from the cremaster muscle and isolated away from the surgical field with hemostats on the external oblique aponeurosis. The fascial incision is extended through the external inguinal ring distally and over the internal inguinal ring proximally.

DISSECTION

After the external oblique aponeurosis is incised, it is elevated and dissected from the underlying cremasteric fascia and the

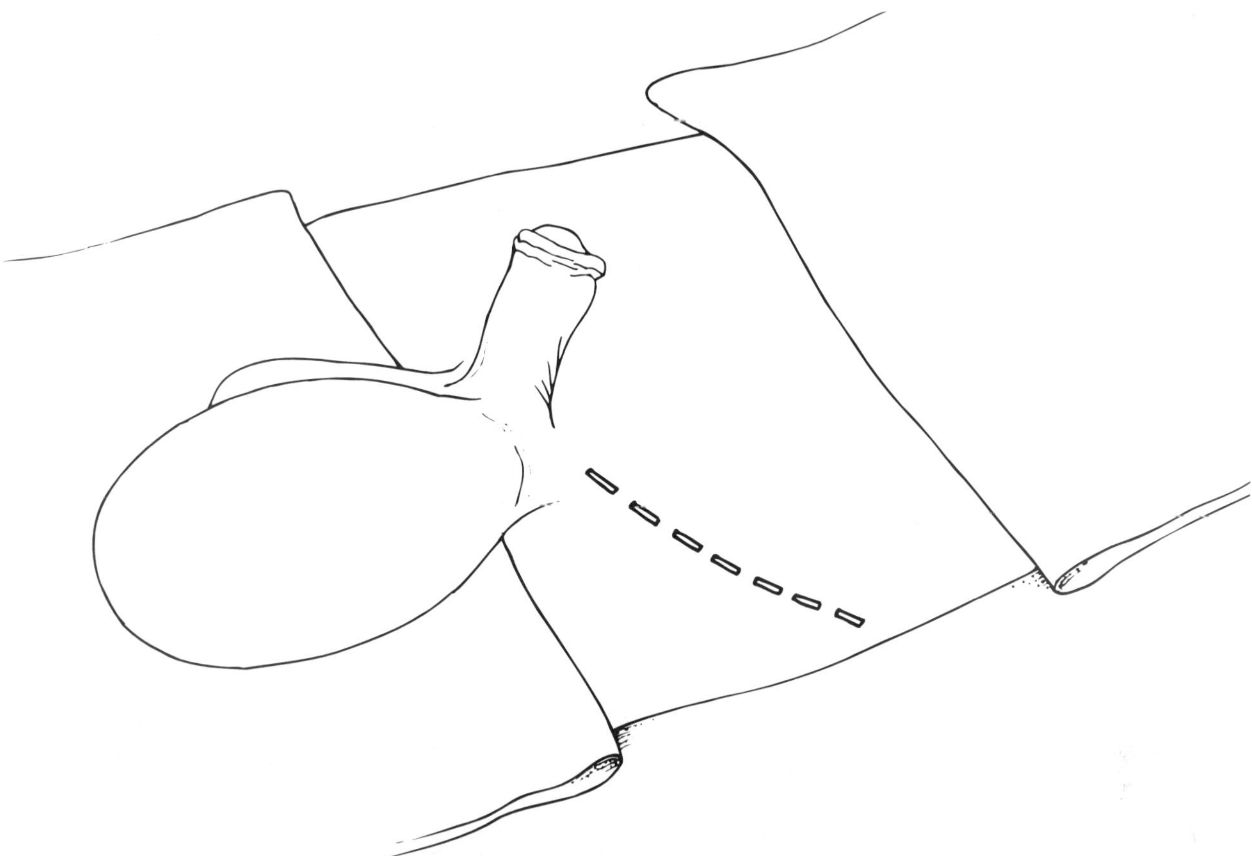

Fig. 35.1. Patient draped for left inguinal orchiectomy. Dotted line marks proposed incision.

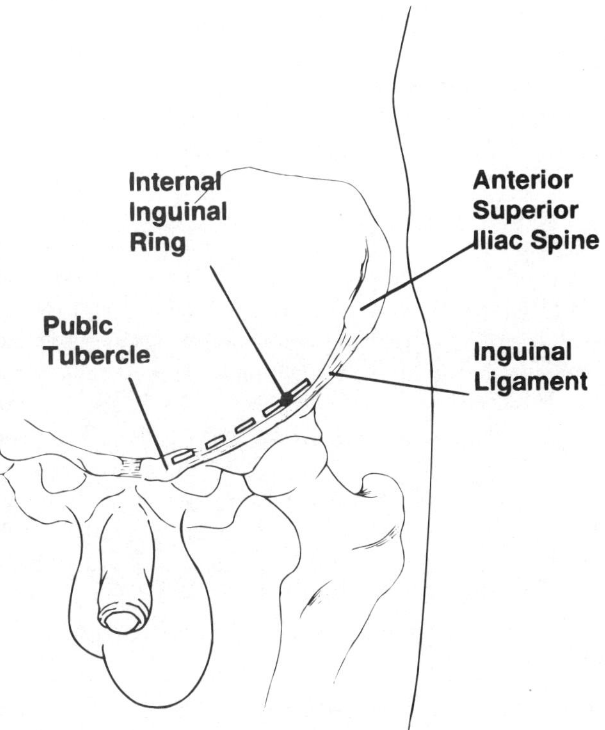

Fig. 35.2.   Anatomic landmarks and proposed incision for radical inguinal orchiectomy.

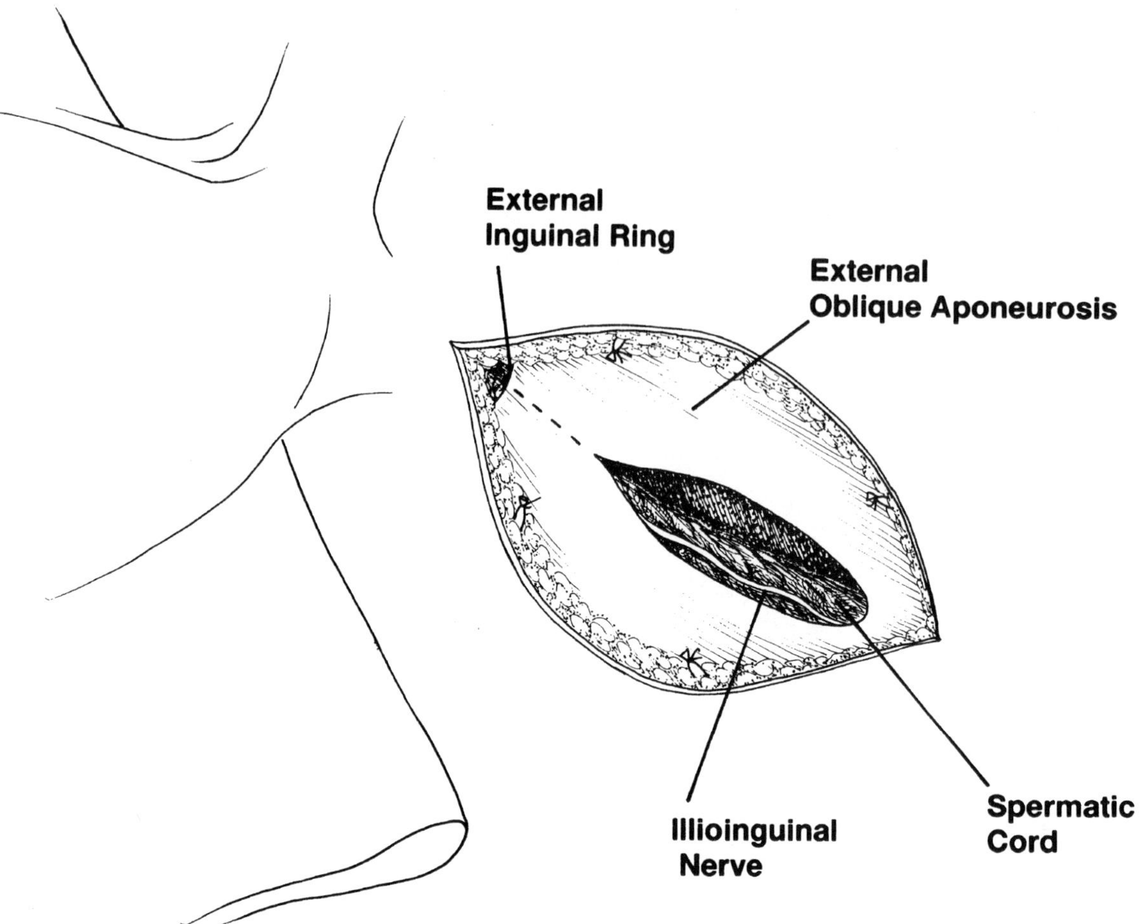

Fig. 35.3. The external oblique aponeurosis is opened, and the ilioinguinal nerve is identified. The external inguinal ring is seen at the distal limit of the incision.

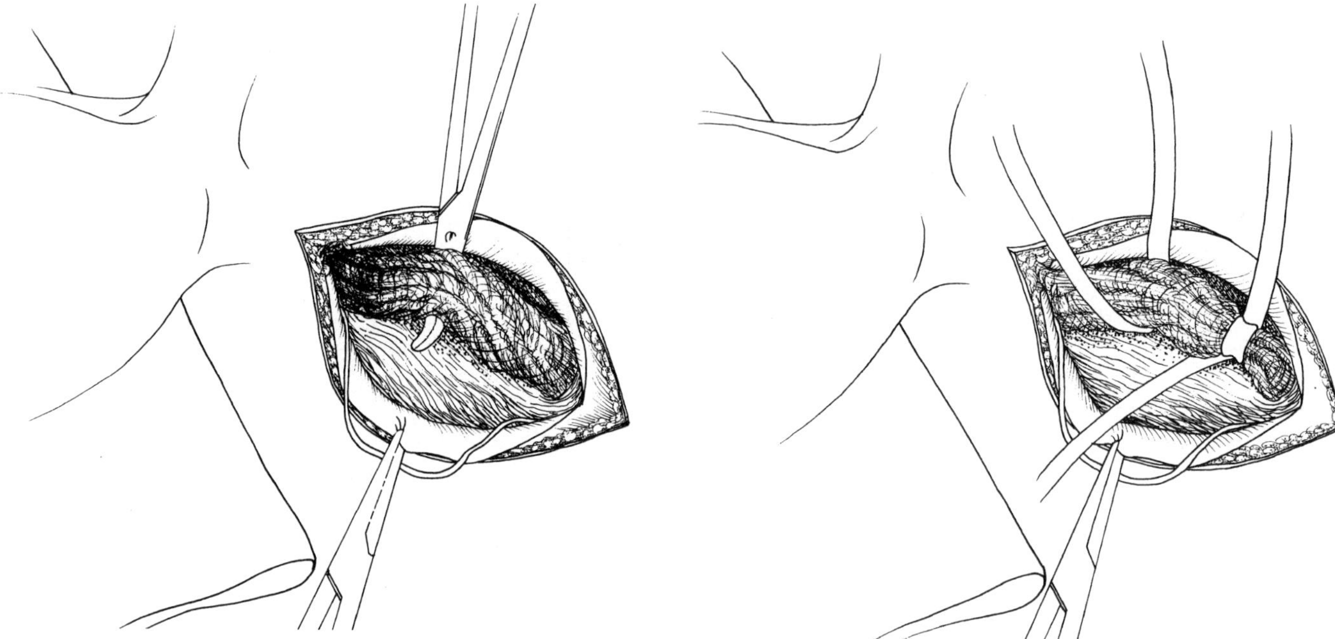

Fig. 35.4. The ilioinguinal nerve is isolated from the area of dissection by a hemostat, and a clamp is passed beneath the spermatic cord at the pubic tubercle.

Fig. 35.5. A Penrose drain is doubly looped around the spermatic cord just distal to the internal inguinal ring. A second drain is used for traction.

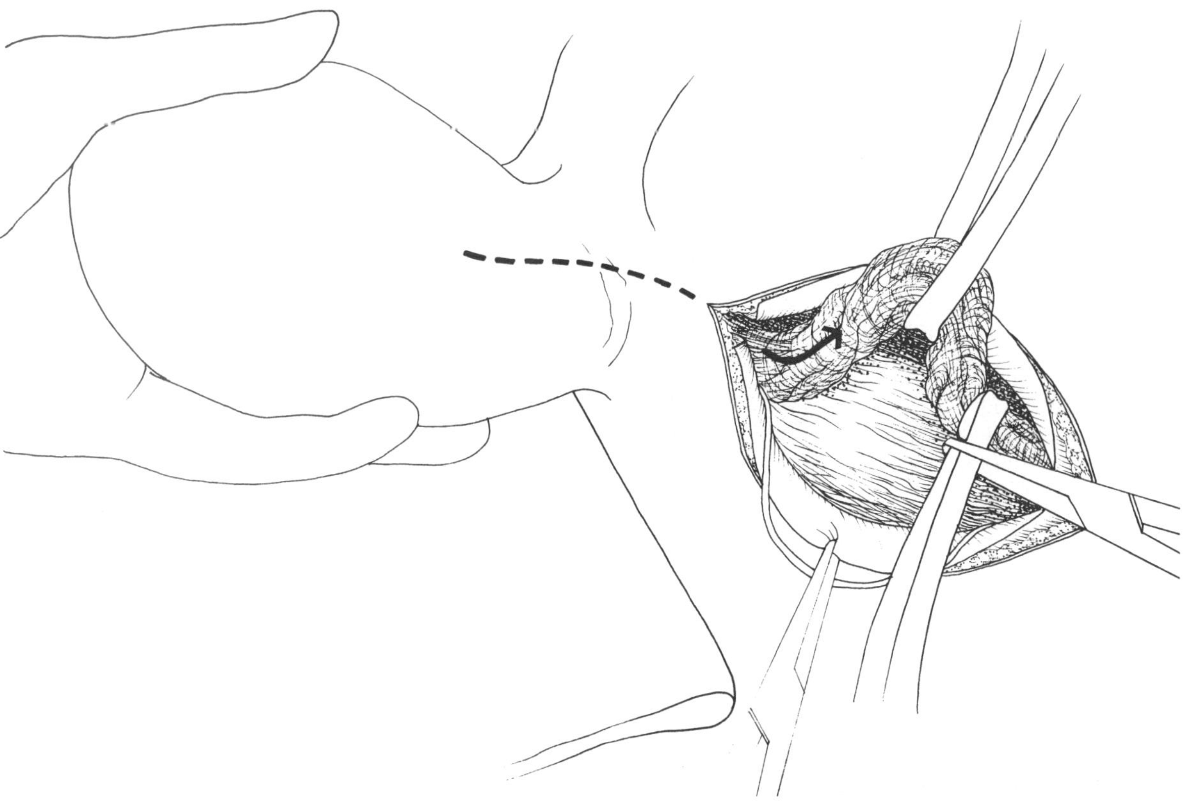

Fig. 35.6. Gentle external pressure is placed on the testicle as it is delivered from the scrotum into the wound.

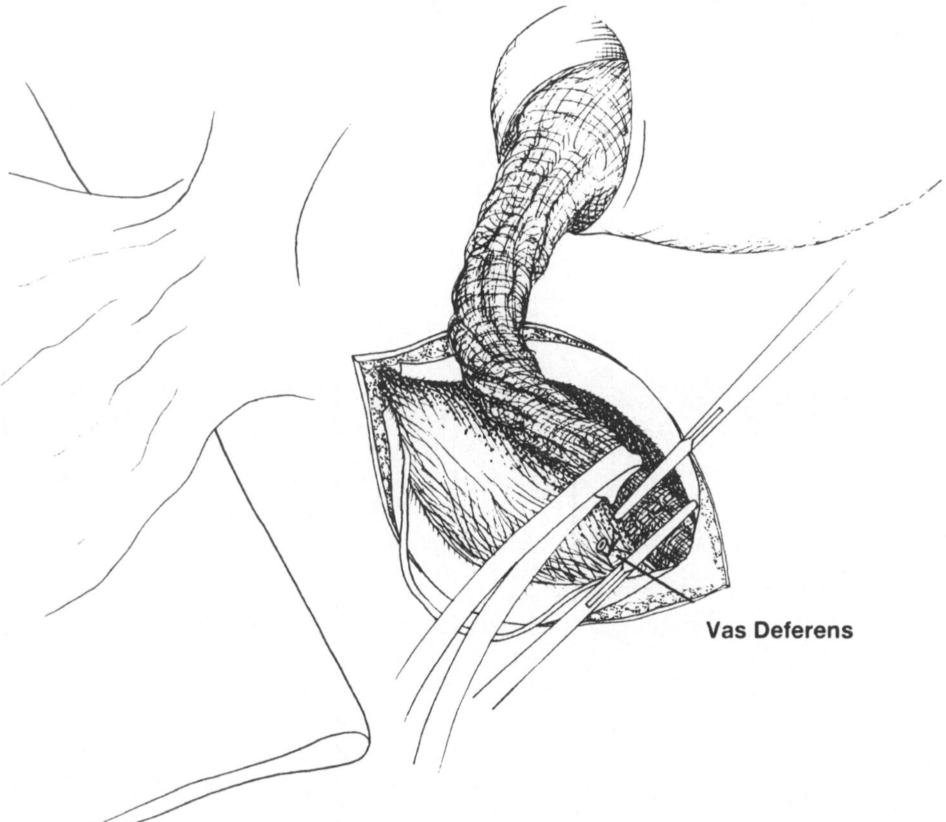

Fig. 35.7. The testicle is isolated in a towel. The spermatic cord is clamped and the vas deferens has been ligated and divided.

spermatic cord. The pubic tubercle is identified where the spermatic cord passes over it. The spermatic cord and cremaster muscle are bluntly dissected from the pubic tubercle until an instrument can be passed beneath the spermatic cord (Fig. 35.4). The spermatic cord is then doubly looped with a 0.5-in Penrose drain that is tightened and clamped to prevent blood flow.

The spermatic cord and cremaster muscle are dissected free from the floor of the inguinal canal using the Penrose drain for traction. Perforating external spermatic veins may be identified and should be ligated or cauterized. The spermatic cord should be mobilized from the internal inguinal ring distally to the external inguinal ring (Fig. 35.5).

The testicle is now brought up from the scrotum through the incision with gentle external pressure on the scrotum. Incision of Scarpa's fascia may be necessary to deliver the testicle into the incision. Large tumors may require extension of the incision into the upper scrotum to allow removal of the testicle (Fig. 35.6). Care must be taken not to violate the fascial coverage of the testicle. As the testicle is brought superiorly through the incision, the gubernaculum is identified. The gubernaculum is divided, taking care not to violate the testicle or the tunica vaginalis. Blood vessels can be divided and ligated with absorbable suture, and other attachments can be divided with electrocautery. The scrotal skin should not be excised unless there is tumor extension into the scrotum. If such tumor extension exists, the involved scrotal skin should be excised with an adequate margin. After the testicle is freed from the scrotum, the testicle is draped and isolated from the incision. If there is a question about diagnosis, a biopsy and frozen section examination can be performed without contaminating the wound.

The testicle and spermatic cord are now attached only by the spermatic vessels and vas deferens at the internal inguinal ring. Any hernia sac, which should be found at the anteromedial aspect of the spermatic cord, should be dissected from the spermatic cord to the internal inguinal ring and closed. The spermatic cord and vas are dissected deep to the internal inguinal ring. The vas and the spermatic vessels are separated, clamped, and divided. The testicle is removed from the field. The vas and spermatic vessels are ligated with a large, nonabsorbable suture such as 0 silk (Fig. 35.7). This allows identification of the end of the spermatic cord if the patient needs a retroperitoneal lymphadenectomy at a later time.

Closure

The wound is inspected for hemostasis and irrigated with saline. The scrotal skin can be invaginated, and the inside of the scrotum can be inspected. The floor of the inguinal canal is inspected and if a direct inguinal hernia is found, a hernia repair is performed. The ilioinguinal nerve is returned to the inguinal canal. The external oblique aponeurosis is approximated with a 2-0 Vicryl (Ethicon, Sommerville, NJ) suture. The subcutaneous tissue is approximated with 2-0 or 3-0 chromic suture. The skin is closed with skin clips or with a subcuticular 4-0 Vicryl suture. No drains are placed in the scrotum or inguinal canal.

Postoperative Care

Radical inguinal orchiectomy can be done on an outpatient basis. After the patient tolerates clear liquids and voids, he is discharged and oral pain medication is prescribed. The patient returns in 1 week for removal of the skin staples and further evaluation and treatment of the testicular cancer. The morbidity and mortality of the radical inguinal orchiectomy should be low, similar to that of an inguinal herniorrhaphy.

Pathology

Specific information is needed from the pathologic examination of the testicle and spermatic cord. The specific histologic type of testis cancer should be stated. Any elevation of preoperative AFP levels should alert one to the presence of nonseminomatous elements. If the pathologist reports a pure seminoma and the AFP level is elevated, the surgeon should ask the pathologist to reexamine the testicle for nonseminomatous elements. The coverings of the testicle, paratesticular structures, and spermatic cord should be examined for direct extension as well as vascular and lymphatic involvement. These findings will influence recommendations for further therapy.

REFERENCES

1. Dean AL, Jr. The treatment of teratoid tumors of the testes with radium and x-ray. J Urol 1925;13:149.
2. Giguere JK, et al. The clinical significance of unconventional orchiectomy approaches in testicular cancer: a report from the testicular cancer intergroup study. J Urol 1988;139:1225.
3. Markland C, et al. Inadequate orchiectomy for patients with testicular tumors. JAMA 1973;224:1025.
4. Dowd JB. Surgery of testicular tumors. Surg Clin North Am 1962;42:779.
5. Redman JF. Applied anatomy of the groin: part 2. AUA Update Series 1989;8:74.

Thoracoabdominal Retroperitoneal Lymphadenectomy

Seth P. Lerner and Peter T. Scardino

INTRODUCTION

Near the turn of this century, descriptions of the histologic classification of testicular neoplasms and the lymphatic drainage of the testis provided the impetus for surgeons to develop a rational surgical approach for the cure of testis cancer. Radical orchiectomy was recognized as the treatment of choice for primary tumor, and refining of the technique and timing of the retroperitoneal lymph node dissection (RPLND) yielded significant improvements in long-term survival over radical orchiectomy alone. Together with the improvements in diagnosis and staging, the development of effective platinum-based chemotherapy in the 1970s has rendered testis cancer a "conquered disease" and, in some cases, has obviated the need for lymphadenectomy.

Retroperitoneal lymphadenectomy remains a cornerstone of the management of patients with nonseminomatous germ cell tumors (NSGCT) for three major reasons. First, although the operation is formidable, it can be done safely. Major surgical morbidity is rare in low-stage disease. Loss of ejaculation can be avoided by limiting the dissection to areas of high probability of metastases and by preserving the postganglionic sympathetic nerves. Second, the procedure accurately stages the pathologic extent of the disease and provides the best indication for prognosis, thereby defining which patients will benefit from adjuvant chemotherapy. Third, a thorough, meticulous lymphadenectomy can remove all retroperitoneal node-bearing tissue that has a significant risk of harboring metastases, virtually eliminating the risk of local retroperitoneal recurrence.

This chapter reviews the historical origins of retroperitoneal lymphadenectomy, presents the rationale for the procedure, describes the operative technique for a thoracoabdominal extraperitoneal approach, and indicates the complications of this procedure. Finally, the merits and results of lymphadenectomy with or without adjuvant chemotherapy are briefly reviewed, and a plan of periodic postoperative evaluations is mentioned. Our focus is on patients with early stage (A, B1, and B2),

nonseminomatous tumors. Patients with advanced disease (B3 or C) are not treated initially with retroperitoneal dissection but rather with intensive combination chemotherapy.

HISTORICAL PERSPECTIVES

Modern systematic and accurate accumulation of information about the lymphatic drainage of the testes began with the studies published by Most in 1898 of the metastatic deposits of testicular tumors in the retroperitoneum (1). Cuneo and Marcille identified four to eight lymphatic channels from each testis that pass out of the mediastinum, traveling with the spermatic cord, to drain into the periaortic lymph nodes near the renal hilum, the embryologic origin of the testis (2). On the right side, one lymphatic channel drained to the external iliac nodes just below the bifurcation of the common iliac artery. These observations clearly demonstrated the distinct drainage of the testis, separate from the scrotum, which drains to the inguinal and distal iliac nodes.

Jamieson and Dobson mapped the lumbar nodes to determine the extent of a "truly radical operation" in their classic description of the primary lymphatic drainage of the testis (3). After injecting the testes of 10 stillborn fetuses with Prussian blue, they reported that the dye from the right side drained to the infrarenal interaortocaval, precaval, and preaortic nodes. Left-sided drainage was primarily to the left para-aortic and preaortic nodes. They further noted secondary drainage to the contralateral nodes as well as the nodes above the renal vein and common iliac nodes.

Kinmonth et al. developed the technique of pedal lymphangiography in the 1950s (4). Injecting dye into the lymphatics of the foot, however, did not routinely opacify the lumbar nodes, whereas direct injection of the testis confirmed Jamieson and Dobson's original work (5–7). Direct injection of contrast media into the lymphatics of the spermatic cord demonstrated constant crossover from right to left (left-to-right crossover occurred much less frequently) and retrograde filling of the left supraclavicular lymph node via the thoracic duct (5–7). After inguinal or scrotal surgery, opacification of the iliac or inguinal nodes occurred via collateral lymphatic drainage that included the surgical scar (5).

Before these elegant studies demonstrating the lymphatic drainage of the testes, orchiectomy was the sole treatment of testicular cancer. In 1899, Kober reported an 80% mortality rate at 3 years for 114 patients treated with orchiectomy alone (8). In 1907, Howard reported his experience with 36 evaluable patients treated by orchiectomy alone (9). Recurrent disease developed in 27 patients, and 18 of these patients had massive retroperitoneal metastases. Only 8 patients (22%) that received follow-up care survived long term. Chevassu reported an 81% death rate for 100 patients after orchiectomy alone (10).

The detailed descriptions of the lymphatic drainage of the testis and the knowledge of the generally poor survival after simple orchiectomy for testis cancer prompted surgeons to extend the field of resection. In 1897, Stinson described the use of radical orchiectomy including dissection of the inguinal lymph nodes as the proper procedure for control of primary tumor (11). Primary ligation of the spermatic cord was described as essential to prevent metastases from tumor manipulation (12).

Kocher was the first to operate transperitoneally on the lumbar lymphatics in 1882, but found unresectable metastases (12). The first successful transperitoneal resection of large nodal metastases was performed by Roberts in 1902 (13). The patient died postoperatively, however, from a bowel obstruction and peritonitis. Gregoire performed the first truly retroperitoneal approach for advanced retroperitoneal nodal metastases, but Cuneo was the first to successfully resect all of the retroperitoneal node-bearing tissue in a patient with positive nodes (12). Chevassu modified Cuneo's lateral extraperitoneal approach, yet he and others reported limited success despite improvements of this method (14–17). Surgical extirpation of the retroperitoneal nodes, however, became the cornerstone of therapy in 1948 when Lewis, using the Hinman operation, reported 192 operations without a single mortality. His 5-year survival rate for 28 patients with nonseminomatous tumors treated by orchiectomy, retroperitoneal lymphadenectomy, and radiation therapy was 46% (17).

The rationale and results were thus established and attention was turned to refining the procedure to remove all the retroperitoneal node-bearing tissue safely and completely. The limits of the area of resection were expanded until the dissection included all nodal tissue from the suprarenal regions bilaterally, to the bifurcation of the aorta, from ureter to ureter, in addition to the ipsilateral common iliac nodes.

The Thoracoabdominal Approach

Marshall described the transdiaphragmatic approach to treat combined kidney, chest, and abdominal trauma in 1946 (18). Wylie et al. extended the incision through the abdominal musculature to treat combined thoracoabdominal trauma (19). In cancer surgery, Sweet described the thoracic approach for carci-

noma of the esophagus just proximal to the gastroesophageal junction, and others used the thoracoabdominal incision for splenorenal anastomosis and splenectomy (20–21). Chute et al. and Mortensen adapted this approach for greater exposure in removing renal tumors (21, 22). Cooper et al. modified the approach to allow for wide exposure of the primary lymphatic drainage of the testis near the renal vessels (23).

Although suitable for large renal tumors and unilateral retroperitoneal lymphadenectomy, extension of the dissection to the contralateral side was difficult using the thoracoabdominal approach described by Cooper et al. This technique produced satisfactory results; however, anatomic studies and clinical experience pointed to the need for a bilateral (ureter-to-ureter) dissection should involvement of the contralateral nodes be found at the time of surgery. With their report in 1959, Mallis and Patton established the transperitoneal infrahilar bilateral dissection with no operative deaths and minimal complications (24). This was soon followed by accounts of Staubitz et al. and Whitmore confirming the efficacy of this approach (25, 26).

In 1971, Skinner and Leadbetter reported their series of 58 patients with an average hospital stay of 8 to 10 days, only one major operative complication, and no operative mortalities (27). The survival rate was 90% if the nodes were uninvolved and 52% if the nodes were involved. Skinner modified and extended the thoracoabdominal incision to facilitate a complete bilateral dissection that included the ipsilateral suprahilar and contralateral hilar region. This modification is particularly suited for resection of large retroperitoneal masses. However, the wide exposure allows the surgeon to perform a completely extraperitoneal dissection in the case of early stage testicular cancer (28).

Donohue recognized that the suprahilar lymph nodes were involved in up to 25% of patients with infrahilar lymph node metastases, even when the infrahilar nodes were grossly normal. After demonstrating the feasibility of a midline transperitoneal approach to the retroperitoneum with cadaver dissections, Donohue developed an extended bilateral transperitoneal approach to include mobilization of the pancreas and bilateral para-aortic suprahilar resection (29). The initial results were excellent; 93% of patients had no nodal involvement, and 67% with involved nodes remained alive and free of disease after 2 years (30). Skinner reported a disease-free survival rate of 95% for patients with no nodal involvement and 71% for patients with involved nodes who did not receive chemotherapy or who received single-agent adjuvant chemotherapy (31). The transperitoneal infrahilar dissection remains the most popular procedure used today, but the thoracoabdominal and transperitoneal suprahilar procedures have attracted increasing numbers of adherents, in view of the data indicating a substantial incidence of suprahilar metastases, especially in the presence of grossly involved nodes (32).

Modified Templates and Nerve-Sparing RPLND

The detailed mapping studies of Ray et al. and Donohue et al. permitted consideration of modified templates that allowed the contralateral nodes to be left intact for patients with grossly negative lymph nodes or minimal gross involvement at the time of retroperitoneal lymphadenectomy (Fig. 36.1) (33, 34). Contralateral metastases were never observed in patients with solitary ipsilateral metastases (33). Ray et al. further hypothesized that the modified template dissection may reduce the incidence of ejaculatory dysfunction (33). Whitelaw and Smithwick had previously demonstrated that antegrade ejaculation could be maintained in 100% of patients with unilateral preservation of the L1 to L3 nerves and in 46% of patients with unilateral preservation of the L3 nerve (35). The clinical studies of Narayan et al. and the cadaver dissections by Colleselli and colleagues describing the postganglionic sympathetic efferent nerves of the thoracolumbar outflow provide the current anatomic basis for preservation of emission and antegrade ejaculation (36, 37).

Numerous investigators reported preservation of antegrade ejaculation in 80% or more of patients after unilateral lymphadenectomy for low-stage disease (Table 36.1) (38–42). Emphasis was placed on limiting the contralateral dissection inferiorly to the inferior mesenteric artery and preserving the hypogastric plexus at the bifurcation of the aorta and between the common iliac arteries. This continues to be the most common form of nerve-sparing RPLND used today.

These attempts to spare the nerves focused on modifications of the extent of lymphadenectomy. Jewett et al. subsequently described a modified bilateral RPLND to preserve the postgan-

Table 36.1. Modified Retroperitoneal Lymphadenectomy: Preservation of Antegrade Ejaculation

| | | PRIMARY TUMOR | | |
AUTHOR	NO. OF PATIENTS	RIGHT (%)	LEFT (%)	TOTAL (%)
Fossa et al. (38)	36	100	67	81
Fritz and Weissbach (39)	37	NS	NS	78
Pizzocaro et al. (40)	61	86	88	87
Richie (41)	52	NS	NS	88
Donohue et al. (42)	77	NS	NS	75

NS, not stated.

glionic sympathetic nerves for patients with stage I and II nonseminomatous germ cell tumors that resulted in 18 of 20 patients recovering antegrade ejaculation (43). Donohue et al. reported similar results with preservation of antegrade ejaculation in 100% of 75 patients (44). In a recent update, Donohue et al. reported that 98% of 167 patients maintained postoperative antegrade ejaculation (42).

RATIONALE FOR SURGICAL TREATMENT

The retroperitoneal lymph nodes are the first site of metastases in up to 90% of patients with nonseminomatous germ cell tumors (45). The clinical understaging rate with computed tomography is 20 to 30% for stage A tumors, and the false-positive rate is 15 to 23% (42, 45, 46). Retroperitoneal lymphadenectomy provides accurate pathologic staging for patients with clinical stage A or B NSGCT and determines the need for adjuvant chemotherapy. Patients with pathologically proven negative lymph nodes have a 6 to 8% risk of metastatic relapse, usually in the lungs, and require careful surveillance with no further therapy (46). Patients with pathologically proven nodal metastases benefit from adjuvant chemotherapy. Treatment with two courses of cisplatin-based chemotherapy reduces the risk of relapse from 49% to 0 to 6% (46, 47). With this treatment, long-term disease-free survival rates approach 100% for patients who had pathologic stage A cancers and 95 to 98% for patients who had pathologic stage B1 or B2 tumors (30, 31, 41, 46, 47).

Many authors in a variety of medical centers have reported series of retroperitoneal lymphadenectomy with low morbidity and virtually no mortality (Table 36.2) (25–27, 31, 32, 48–50). Antegrade ejaculation can be preserved in the majority of patients, even those with small-volume grossly positive nodes (51). The issue of loss of ejaculation, if a bilateral RPLND is necessary, should no longer be the determining factor when deciding on a course of therapy for a testicular tumor, due to the advent and clinical use of rectal probe electroejaculation (52).

Patients presenting with large-volume retroperitoneal nodal metastases from nonseminomatous testis cancer should undergo

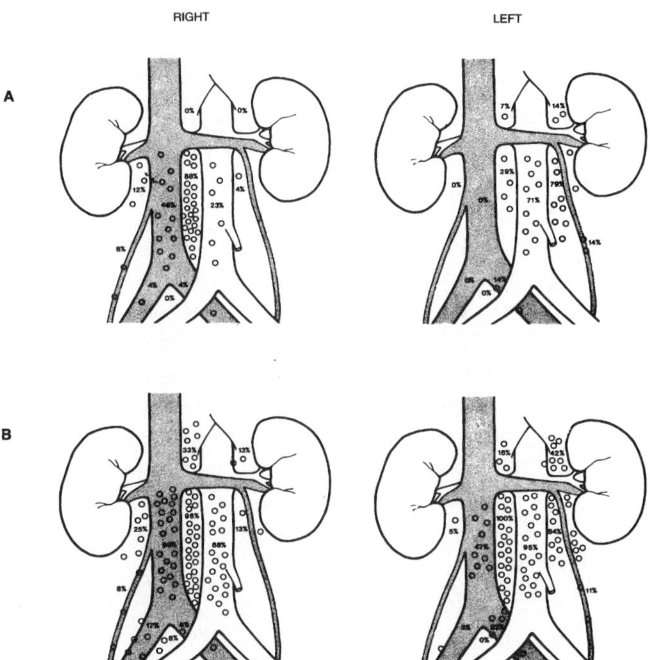

Fig. 36.1. Distribution of retroperitoneal lymph node metastases in early stage, nonseminomatous testicular cancer based on the appearance of the nodes during operation. **A.** Grossly negative (stage B1). **B.** Grossly positive (stage B2). (Reprinted with permission from Donohue JP, Zachary JM, Maynard BR. Distribution of nodal metastases in nonseminomatous testis cancer. J Urol 1982;128:315–320.)

Table 36.2. Morbidity and Mortality After Thoracoabdominal Retroperitoneal Dissection for Nonseminomatous Testicular Carcinoma (49)

PATHOLOGIC STAGE	NO. OF PATIENTS	NO. OF COMPLICATIONS		NO. OF DEATHS
		MAJOR	MINOR	
A	56	3	3	0
B1	12	0	0	0
B2	29	0	0	0
B3	12	2	0	1
C	40	7	3	1

initial chemotherapy. We generally continue chemotherapy for two cycles after normalization of serum tumor markers, with a minimum course of therapy of three cycles. We perform a postchemotherapy retroperitoneal lymphadenectomy when there is a residual mass in the retroperitoneum or teratoma in the primary testis tumor because of the high incidence of residual teratoma or malignant elements in the retroperitoneum (53–55). The need for lymphadenectomy when a patient has a complete clinical response to chemotherapy is controversial (54, 56, 57). We generally offer surveillance when we are assured that the patient is capable of adhering to a rigorous follow-up schedule.

The current debate concerns the role of retroperitoneal lymphadenectomy in the management of patients with clinical stage A NSGCT. Surveillance is associated with a 30% progression rate, with the majority of metastases occurring in the retroperitoneum (58). Surveillance requires a rigorous follow-up schedule and a highly motivated patient to identify patients with occult metastatic disease early in the course of disease progression. Recurrence often consists of bulky retroperitoneal metastases requiring chemotherapy and surgery to achieve a complete response (58). Distant metastases usually occur within the first year, whereas retroperitoneal metastases may occur 5 or more years after orchiectomy (59). Among patients whose disease progresses and requires chemotherapy, most will become infertile; those who require RPLND are more likely to lose ejaculation because the margins of dissection will be wider (57, 58).

Risk factors for progression include a high percentage of embryonal carcinoma, lymphatic or vascular invasion, and tumor extending beyond the tunica albuginea (T2 to 4) (60). Moul et al. determined that the percentage of embryonal carcinoma was the strongest predictor of occult metastatic disease in patients with stage A NSGCT (61). In addition, de Riese et al. demonstrated that patients with 100% embryonal carcinoma in the primary tumor were at high risk for retroperitoneal metastasis (62). In those patients with less than 100% embryonal carcinoma in the primary tumor, the percentage of aneuploid tumor cells in S phase (as determined by flow cytometry) was most predictive of pathologic stage.

Since 1983, we have offered surveillance to selected patients with clinical stage A NSGCT, minor components of embryonal

carcinoma, and no lymphovascular invasion (63). We recommend RPLND for patients with one or more high-risk pathologic features (75% or more embryonal carcinoma, lymphatic and/or vascular invasion, and/or T2 to 4 primary tumors). The probability of occult retroperitoneal metastases in these high-risk patients is 50 to 60%. Chemotherapy is reserved for patients with pathologically proven metastatic disease. Other investigators, however, have suggested that high-risk patients may best be treated with adjuvant chemotherapy (64). Although overall cure rates are comparable to patients treated with RPLND, chemotherapy has a significant potential for both short-term and long-term toxicity. Long-term recurrence and survival rates after chemotherapy are unknown.

MARGINS OF DISSECTION

A thorough knowledge of the lymphatic drainage of the testicle and the pattern of metastatic spread from left-sided and right-sided tumors is essential for the urologic surgeon to plan the margin of retroperitoneal dissection in each stage of disease. Patients with a partial response to chemotherapy and a residual mass, or large-volume (greater than 2 cm) adenopathy at the time of a primary lymph node dissection, should undergo a complete bilateral retroperitoneal lymphadenectomy from ureter to ureter, suprahilar to aortic bifurcation, including the ipsilateral common iliac lymph nodes. Patients with grossly negative lymph nodes at the time of surgery should undergo a dissection designed to remove all lymph nodes that are at risk of harboring metastases while preserving the contralateral sympathetic chain and associated postganglionic sympathetic nerves and the hypogastric plexus (Fig. 36.2). Dissection of the ipsilateral postganglionic sympathetic nerves can be achieved in the majority of cases without compromising the completeness of the lymphadenectomy but preserving antegrade ejaculation in more than 95% of patients (42, 43).

Although similar results can be achieved by either the transabdominal or thoracoabdominal approach, we prefer the latter. The major advantages of a transabdominal approach are the ease of the incision and the access it provides to both suprahilar regions (29). The advantages of the thoracoabdominal incision are the wide exposure of the operative field, access to the ipsilateral lung and mediastinum for palpation and excisional biopsy of suspicious lesions, and a completely extraperitoneal dissection, which decreases the risks of ileus, pancreatitis, and bowel obstruction secondary to adhesions (65).

PREOPERATIVE PREPARATION

As soon as the tissue diagnosis is established and the appropriate staging studies are completed, one may proceed with retroperitoneal lymphadenectomy. Autologous blood donation (2 units) is offered but not routinely recommended for the patient with a clinical stage A or B1 tumor because the volume of intraoperative blood loss rarely necessitates homologous blood transfusion. We generally do not offer autologous blood donation for patients undergoing postchemotherapy node dissec-

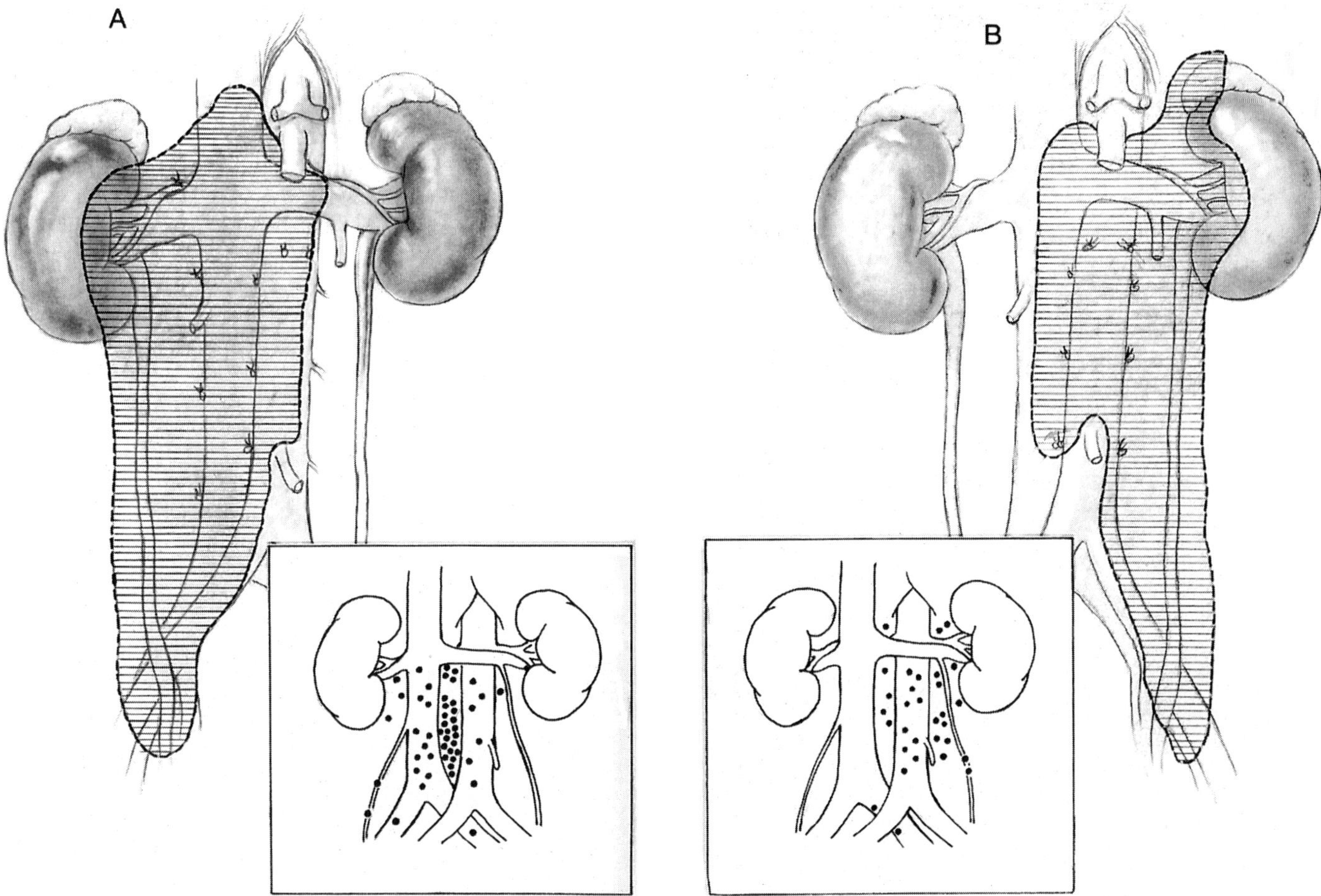

Fig. 36.2. Limits of modified nerve-sparing RPLND on the right side (**A**) and left side (**B**) for patients with grossly negative nodes. The dissection is complete within the anatomic area defined and is designed to remove all nodes likely to contain metastases (Fig. 36.1) yet preserve the contralateral sympathetic chain and hypogastric plexus. The postganglionic sympathetic nerves (L1 to 3) can be identified prospectively and preserved within the field of dissection. Insets: Margins of dissection overlaid on distribution of nodes in stage B1.

tions. Routine preoperative studies are performed in the outpatient clinic before the surgery date and include a complete blood count, electrolytes, blood urea nitrogen and creatinine determinations, and a chest radiograph. An enema may be administered for evacuation of the large bowel. Pulmonary function tests with carbon monoxide diffusion capacity and arterial blood gas determination are obtained for patients who have received bleomycin.

Patients are admitted to the hospital the morning of surgery and are hydrated before placement of an epidural catheter and induction of general anesthesia. This hydration, together with an intravenous mannitol infusion begun before manipulation of the kidney and dissection of the renal hilum, maximizes renal blood flow and minimizes the risk of arterial thrombosis or renal ischemic injury from vasospasm.

SURGICAL PROCEDURE

Anesthesia

General endotracheal anesthesia is recommended and can be safely maintained with a variety of agents. Consultation with the anesthesiologist should be considered well in advance of the planned surgery for the patient who has received bleomycin chemotherapy. The inspired fraction of oxygen should be kept at the minimum level to maintain safe oxygen saturation to prevent adult respiratory distress syndrome. We routinely use room-air oxygen without difficulty. Careful attention should be given to intraoperative intravenous fluid delivery because excess fluids may increase the risk of pulmonary complications in these patients. The use of a controlled hypotensive anesthetic technique may reduce intraoperative blood loss and the blood transfusion rate, particularly for patients with more advanced retroperitoneal disease (66). Placement of an epidural catheter for administration of a local anesthetic agent and narcotics facilitates this technique and provides excellent postoperative analgesia; it also facilitates early ambulation and a decreased risk of thromboembolic events (67).

Position

The following text and illustrations describe a left thoracoabdominal extraperitoneal approach. The patient is positioned supine so that the soft tissue of the flank, the area between the 12th rib and the iliac crest, lies directly over the break in the table (Fig. 36.3). The torso of the patient is positioned flush with the left side of the table. The right arm is extended on an arm board, and the left arm is placed in a generously padded

Kraus arm support, rotating the chest 20 to 30° to the opposite side. A rolled sheet is placed under the patient's left side between the scapula and anterior superior iliac spine, and a second roll is placed against the right flank. These maneuvers elevate the shoulder without placing tension on the brachial plexus

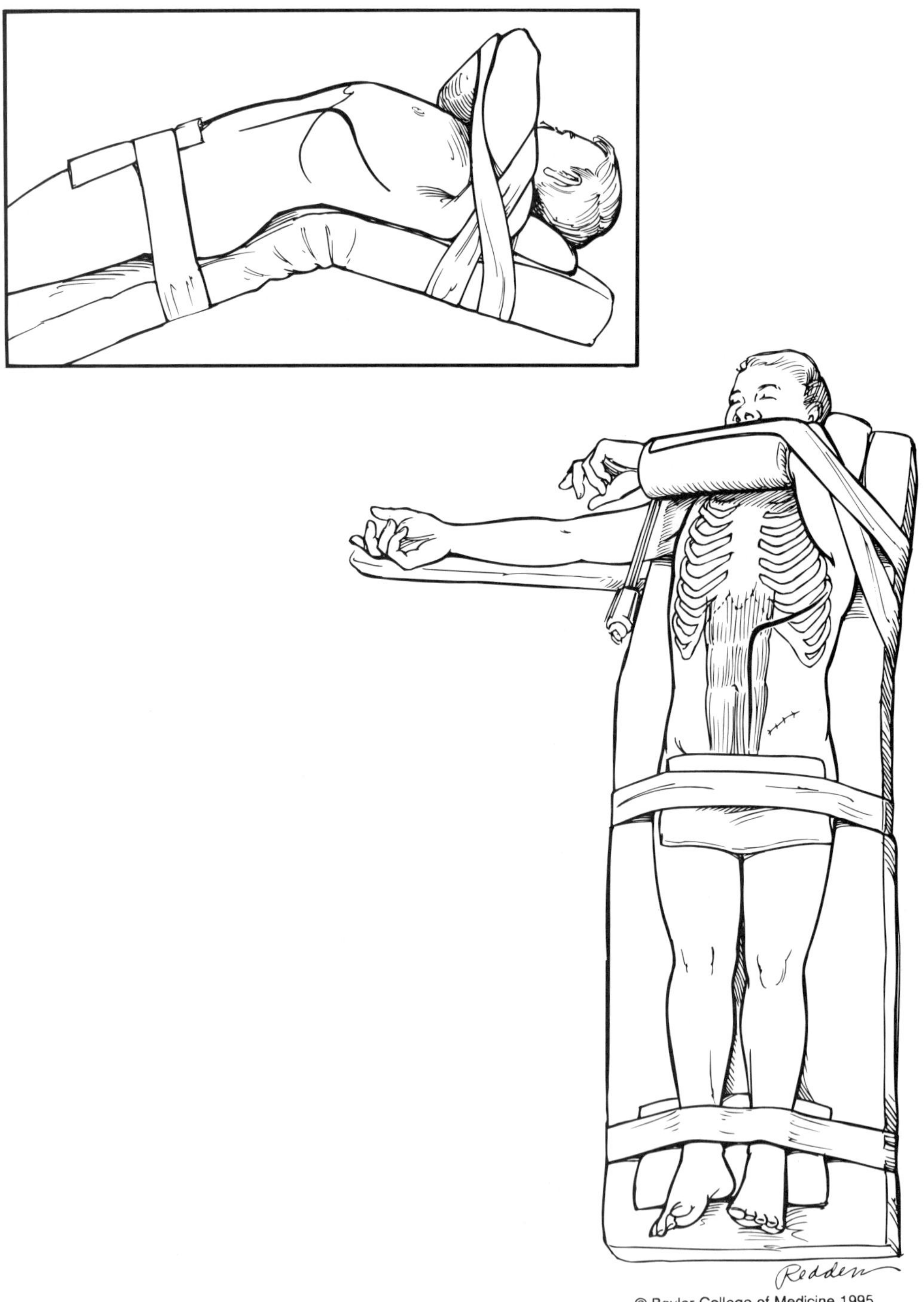

Fig. 36.3.   Left thoracoabdominal position and incision. The patient is placed supine with the left side flush with the edge of the operating table. The upper torso is rotated 20 to 30° anterior to elevate the posterior axillary line. The left arm is secured in a generously padded Kraus support. The table is maximally flexed over the flank, and the abdomen is parallel to the floor. The incision begins at the posterior axillary line over the eighth or ninth rib and is extended medially across the costal margin to a point high in the midepigastrium and extended inferiorly as a paramedian incision.

and elevate the posterior axillary line. The pelvis is kept flat; we no longer flex the contralateral leg at the hip and knee, but rather place the legs in the extended position. All pressure points are padded, and the patient is secured to the table in this position with wide adhesive tape.

Incision

The skin incision begins at the posterior axillary line over the eighth or ninth rib and is extended medially across the costal margin to a point high in the midepigastrium and extended inferiorly as a paramedian incision to the symphysis pubis (Fig. 36.3). The latissimus dorsi and external oblique muscles are incised over the rib with the electrocautery, exposing the periosteum and the intercostal muscles (Fig. 36.4). A subperiosteal resection of the rib is performed as described in Figure 36.4.

The anterior rectus sheath is incised, and the rectus muscle is reflected laterally to preserve its innervation. It is divided in the cephalad portion of the incision with electrocautery. Care should be taken to control the superior epigastric vessels that lie on the posterior surface of the muscle. The key to developing the retroperitoneal plane of dissection is to insinuate the Mayo scissors between the fibers of the transversus abdominis and spread underneath the costal margin (Fig. 36.5). The peritoneum is then gently mobilized from the posterior surface of the transversus abdominis medially, and the costal margin is divided with heavy scissors.

Mobilization of the Peritoneum

The parietal pleura is incised through the periosteum of the resected rib, exposing the diaphragm and lung (Figs. 36.6 and 36.7). The ipsilateral lung may be palpated for nodules; any suspicious areas should be excised. The diaphragm is elevated by retraction on the divided costal margin, and the peritoneum is retracted caudally with the left hand over a sponge or laparotomy pad. Sharp dissection is particularly helpful to initiate the plane between the peritoneum and the diaphragmatic muscle fibers. If the dissection is too close to the peritoneum, it will shred; if it is too close to the diaphragm, troublesome bleeding results. The peritoneum is then mobilized off the diaphragm by gently sweeping the peritoneum posteriorly with the aid of a sponge stick. The diaphragm is divided in the direction of its fibers, taking care not to disturb the terminal fibers of the phrenic nerve. The dissection is carried cephalad and lateral until exposure of the white fibers of the central tendon is obtained (Fig. 36.8).

Establishing the plane of dissection of the peritoneal envelope cephalad and lateral provides exposure for the remainder of the peritoneal mobilization. With a delicate sweeping motion, palm facing upward, the surgeon separates the peritoneum from the transversus abdominis lateral to medial (Fig. 36.8). Sharp dissection is usually necessary to free the peritoneum from the lateral margin of the posterior rectus sheath. The peritoneum is then bluntly mobilized to the linea alba, incising the posterior rectus sheath as the mobilization is completed.

A folded laparotomy pad moistened on the end is placed over the divided costal margin. A Finochietto retractor is placed so that the divided costal margin interdigitates with the opening of the blade. Towel clips placed through the opening of the blade and incorporating the skin and chest wall muscles are helpful to secure the retractor in place (Fig. 36.9).

Before mobilizing the kidney and dissecting the renal hilum, we begin a mannitol drip (100 g/500 mL normal saline) to run over 3 to 4 hours. Posteriorly, the pararenal fat and Gerota's fascia are dissected off the quadratus lumborum and psoas muscles to the level of the aorta. The kidney is then balloted to demonstrate the reflection of the peritoneal envelope laterally. There is a thin fascial layer between the peritoneum and Gerota's fascia that is incised (Fig. 36.9). The peritoneum is then dissected off the anterior layer of Gerota's fascia across the midline to the contralateral ureter. Finally, the pancreas and duodenum are elevated to identify the junction of the left renal vein and the inferior vena cava, the superior mesenteric artery, the aorta and the origins of both renal arteries, and the entire retroperitoneum. Care must be taken to clip the large retroperitoneal lymphatics that often join the lacteals draining the intestinal tract at this level.

Superior Margin of Dissection

The dissection is begun by incising the fibroareolar tissue over the left renal vein that is mobilized circumferentially. Care must be taken to identify a lumbar vein that may insert posteriorly. The spermatic and adrenal veins are ligated and divided (Fig. 36.10). The superior mesenteric artery passes anteriorly over the left renal vein and forms the upper limit of dissection of the tissue anterior to the aorta. The lymphatics overlying the root of the superior mesenteric artery are elevated with a fine right-angle clamp, ligated with clips, and divided. Large lacteals running parallel with the superior mesenteric artery can be a source of significant postoperative lymph collection if they are not securely ligated. The tissue is dissected off the lateral aorta above the left renal artery to the left crus of the diaphragm (Fig. 36.10). Inferior traction of the kidney places tension on the tissue between the adrenal gland and the aorta over the left crus. The celiac ganglion is contained within this tissue and may be mistaken for cancerous tissue due to its gritty texture. This tissue is dissected off the left crus and is clipped and divided, allowing mobilization of the upper pole of the kidney. The origin of the left renal artery is easily identified at this point and is dissected 1 to 2 cm from the aorta. The dissection at the base of the superior mesenteric artery is also carried out to the right, over the aorta and inferior vena cava, to the origin of the right renal vein. This completes the superior margin of dissection.

Exposure of the Great Vessels

The tissue overlying the aorta is divided longitudinally to the bifurcation of the aorta. The dissection of this tissue is facili-

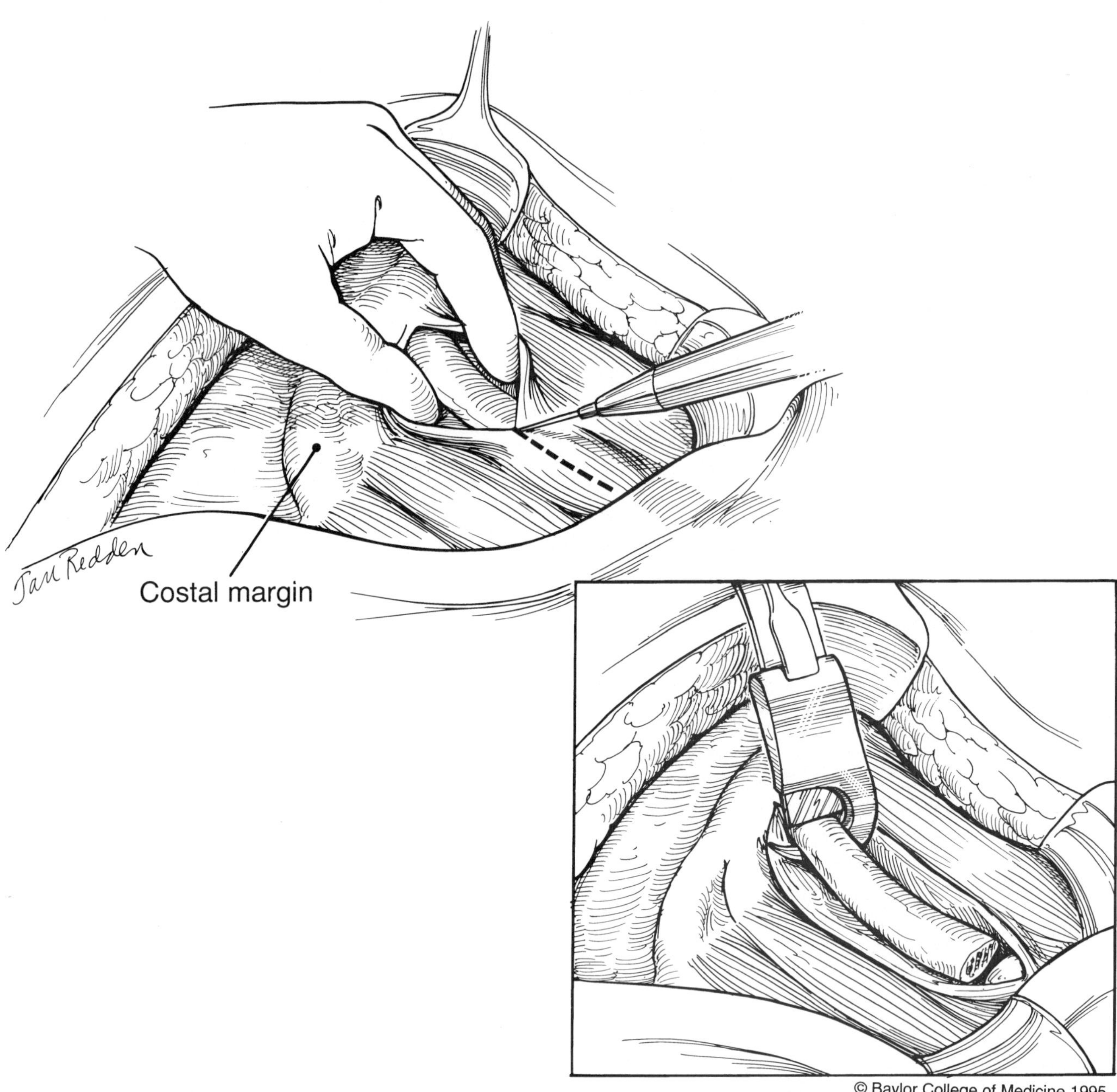

Fig. 36.4.   A subperiosteal resection of the rib is performed after division of the external oblique and latissimus dorsi muscles with the electrocautery tool. Inset: The guillotine is used to divide the rib proximally and distally.

tated by inserting a finger between the adventitia of the aorta and the thick envelope of fibroareolar lymphatic tissue (Fig. 36.11). If the lymph nodes appear grossly negative, the right lateral margin of the dissection is the lateral border of the inferior vena cava above the inferior mesenteric artery (Fig. 36.12). The lateral margin below the inferior mesenteric artery is the anterior surface of the aorta and the midportion of the common iliac artery. This leaves the interaortocaval tissue below the inferior mesenteric artery undisturbed and avoids damage to the sympathetic nerves responsible for emission and antegrade ejaculation.

Kaswick et al. demonstrated, in cadaver dissections, that complete mobilization of the great vessels by ligation and division of the infrarenal lumbar vessels is required to remove all retroaortic and retrocaval tissue (68). The aorta is retracted with a vein retractor to identify the origin of the lumbar vessels, which are doubly ligated with 3-0 silk ties and small hemoclips and divided (Fig. 36.11).

Attention is turned to the renal hilar dissection. Dissection and removal of Gerota's fascia facilitate the hilar dissection and ensure complete removal of all lymph-node–bearing adipose tissue (Fig. 36.13). On the left side, the adrenal gland is usually

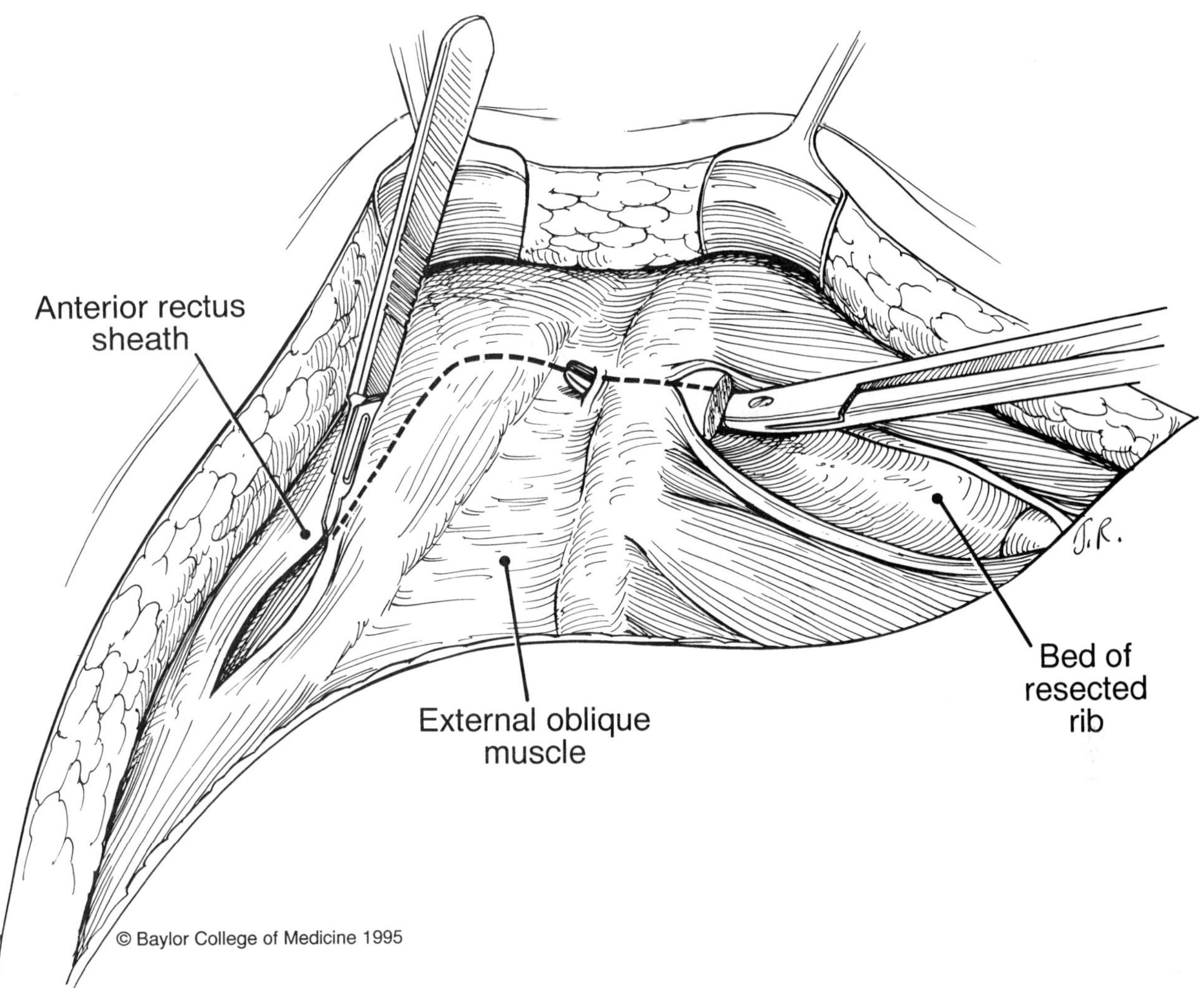

Fig. 36.5.   The anterior rectus sheath is divided, exposing the rectus muscle, and the incision is carried laterally to the bed of the resected rib. The Mayo scissors are inserted beneath the costal margin, and the peritoneum is gently dissected away from the transversus abdominis. The costal margin is divided with heavy scissors.

removed because of its intimacy with the lymph nodes in the left suprahilar area. This is unnecessary for a right-sided dissection because the right suprahilar lymph nodes lie between the inferior vena cava and aorta superior to the left renal vein. With the kidney completely mobilized anteriorly and posteriorly, the hilar lymphatic tissue is dissected away from the renal artery, vein, and pelvis. With these structures in clear view, the tissue is split anteriorly over the vessels and swept posteriorly. The para-aortic lymph nodes inferior to the left renal vein and artery and medial to the renal pelvis are the most frequent sites of metastases from left-sided tumors and must be completely removed.

Dissection Between the Great Vessels

Attention is turned medially, and the tissue over the vena cava is divided to the level of the inferior mesenteric artery (Fig. 36.12). The inferior vena cava is retracted to the right, and the

left lumbar veins are doubly ligated with 4-0 silk ties and small hemoclips and then divided. The right lumbar veins are exposed, and the interaortocaval tissue clipped just medial to the right lumbar veins. A prospective nerve-sparing dissection can be performed when adenopathy is absent or minimal. The postganglionic nerves emerge proximal to the right-sided lumbar veins and can be traced into the interaortocaval region where they can be dissected from the lymph-node–bearing tissue. Encircling the nerves with vessel loops prevents damage during dissection.

The cephalad limit of dissection on the right side is the right renal artery. The cisterna chyli lies posterior to the right renal artery on top of the right crus of the diaphragm and must be carefully ligated with hemoclips to prevent a lymph leak. The left renal vein is retracted, and the tissue over the right renal artery is split longitudinally. This packet of tissue is dissected off the crus, retracted inferiorly, clipped, and divided (Fig. 36.12). The posterior margin of dissection is the white

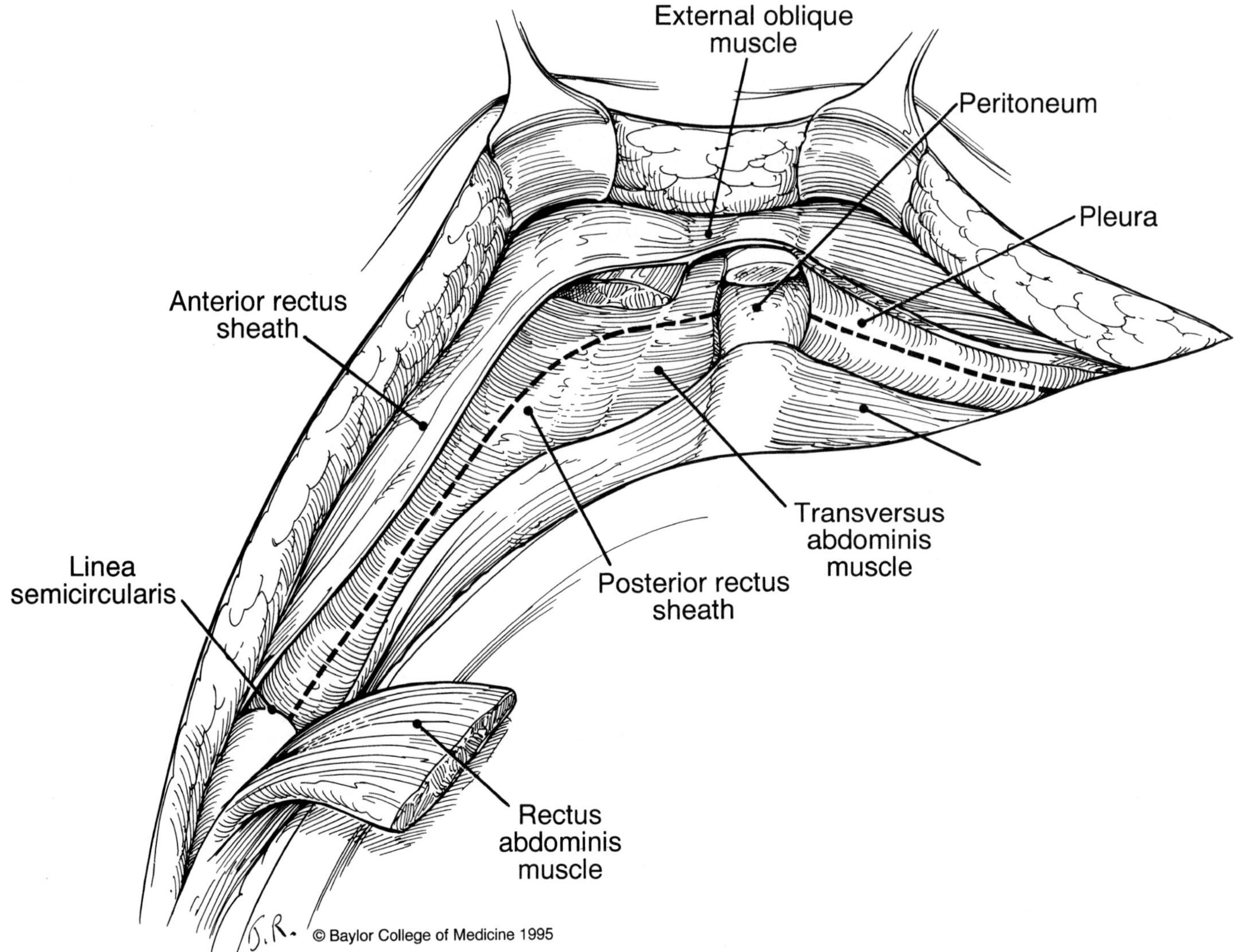

Fig. 36.6.   The rectus muscle is reflected laterally to preserve its innervation and divided in the cephalad portion of the incision. The peritoneum bulges through the defect in the costal margin, and the parietal pleura is divided in the bed of the resected rib. The transversus abdominis and posterior rectus sheath are incised after dissection of the peritoneal envelope.

fascial fibers of the prevertebral ligament. The interaortocaval lymph nodes are dissected off this fascia and swept to the left side underneath the previously mobilized aorta.

Completion of Lymphadenectomy

The distal limit of dissection is the bifurcation of the left common iliac artery. Care is taken not to dissect medial to the artery to preserve the hypogastric nerves distal to the aortic bifurcation overlying the left common iliac vein (Fig. 36.12). The tissue over the artery is clipped, divided, and swept to the left with the remainder of the specimen. The lateral margin is the genitofemoral nerve. The ureter is bluntly dissected from the specimen and retracted laterally. The left sympathetic chain can be spared if there is no gross evidence of lymph node metastases. The lumbar vessels pass posteriorly in the groove between

the psoas and paravertebral muscles and should be clipped. The spermatic vessels are traced to the internal inguinal ring, and are removed below the ligature remaining after radical orchiectomy.

The wound is irrigated with warm water. Careful survey of the entire field of dissection is undertaken to assure adequate perfusion of the kidneys, meticulous hemostasis, and secure ligation of all lymphatics, particularly at the superior and inferior margins of the dissection (Fig. 36.14).

Closure

Closure is facilitated if the flexion is taken out of the table. The costal margin is approximated to take tension off the diaphragm, which is then closed securely in two layers with a running 0 polyglycolic acid suture. A watertight closure of the

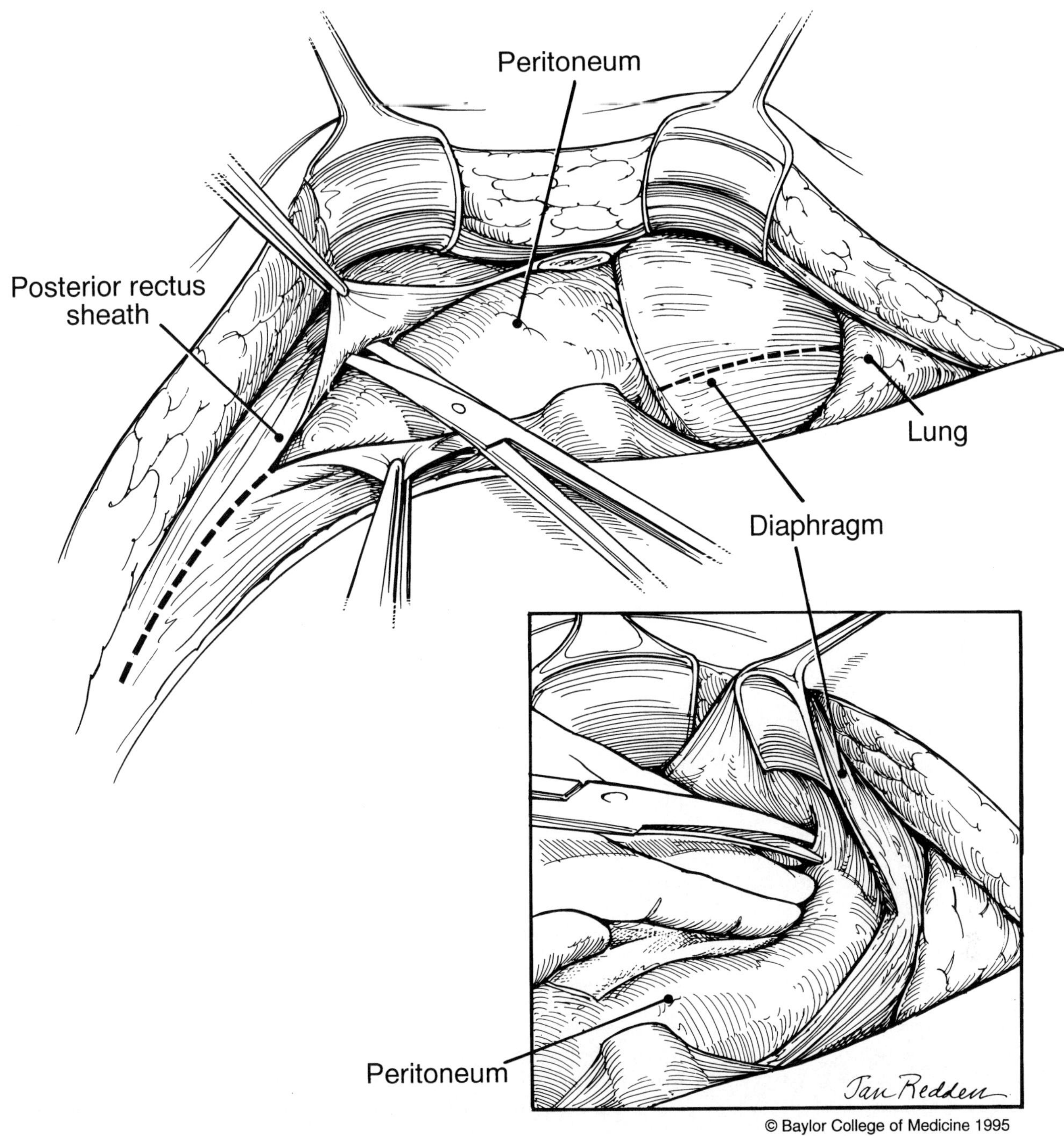

Fig. 36.7. The diaphragm and lung are exposed after division of the pleura. The peritoneum is most adherent along the lateral margin of the posterior rectus sheath, and careful sharp dissection is required to maintain the integrity of the peritoneum. The diaphragm is divided parallel to its fibers. Inset: A sponge is used to retract the peritoneum inferiorly, and the diaphragm is elevated with a Richardson retractor. After the diaphragmatic fibers are sharply divided at their insertion onto the peritoneum, much of the mobilization of the peritoneum from the diaphragm can be accomplished with blunt dissection and a sponge stick.

diaphragm is essential to prevent prolonged serous drainage from the thoracostomy tube. A no. 20 thoracostomy tube is placed one interspace above the incision and positioned with its tip oriented posteriorly in the apex of the chest cavity.

The thoracic portion of the incision is closed with buried no. 1 nylon or Prolene interrupted figure-of-eight sutures that incorporate all muscular layers. All sutures are individually placed before any are tied. The medial sutures must incorporate the diaphragm to separate the pleural cavity from the retroperitoneal space. The external oblique aponeurosis and rectus fascia

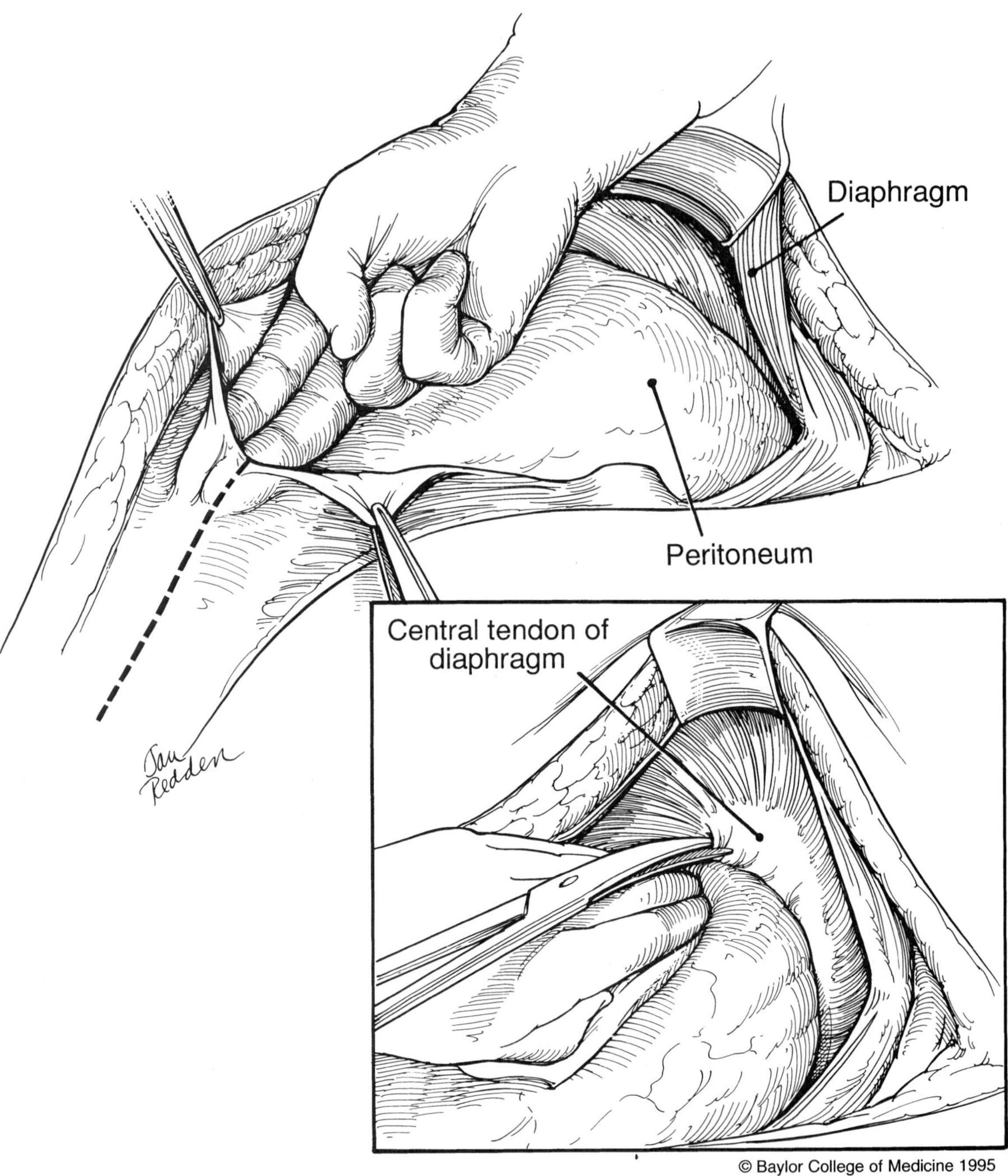

Fig. 36.8.   The posterior sheath is divided only after the peritoneal envelope is mobilized to the midline. Inset: The cephalad dissection of the peritoneal envelope is carried to the level of the central tendon of the diaphragm.

medial to the costal margin are closed in a similar fashion with interrupted buried no. 1 nylon or Prolene figure-of-eight sutures. The transudate from the denuded portion of the retroperitoneum is reabsorbed in a matter of days; therefore, drains to this area are discouraged.

POSTOPERATIVE CARE

Because no intraperitoneal dissection is required, the postoperative ileus resolves rapidly and the nasogastric tube is usually removed by the second or third postoperative day. There is, however, a large denuded surface of the retroperitoneum due to the extensive dissection, which results in third-space fluid loss comparable to that seen with severe pancreatitis or a large third-degree burn. To maintain normal intravascular volume, these patients require massive infusions of albumin solution and saline. A typical patient will receive between 3000 and 4000 mL of saline and 1000 to 1500 mL of 5% albumin (but no blood products) during the operation. Postoperatively the

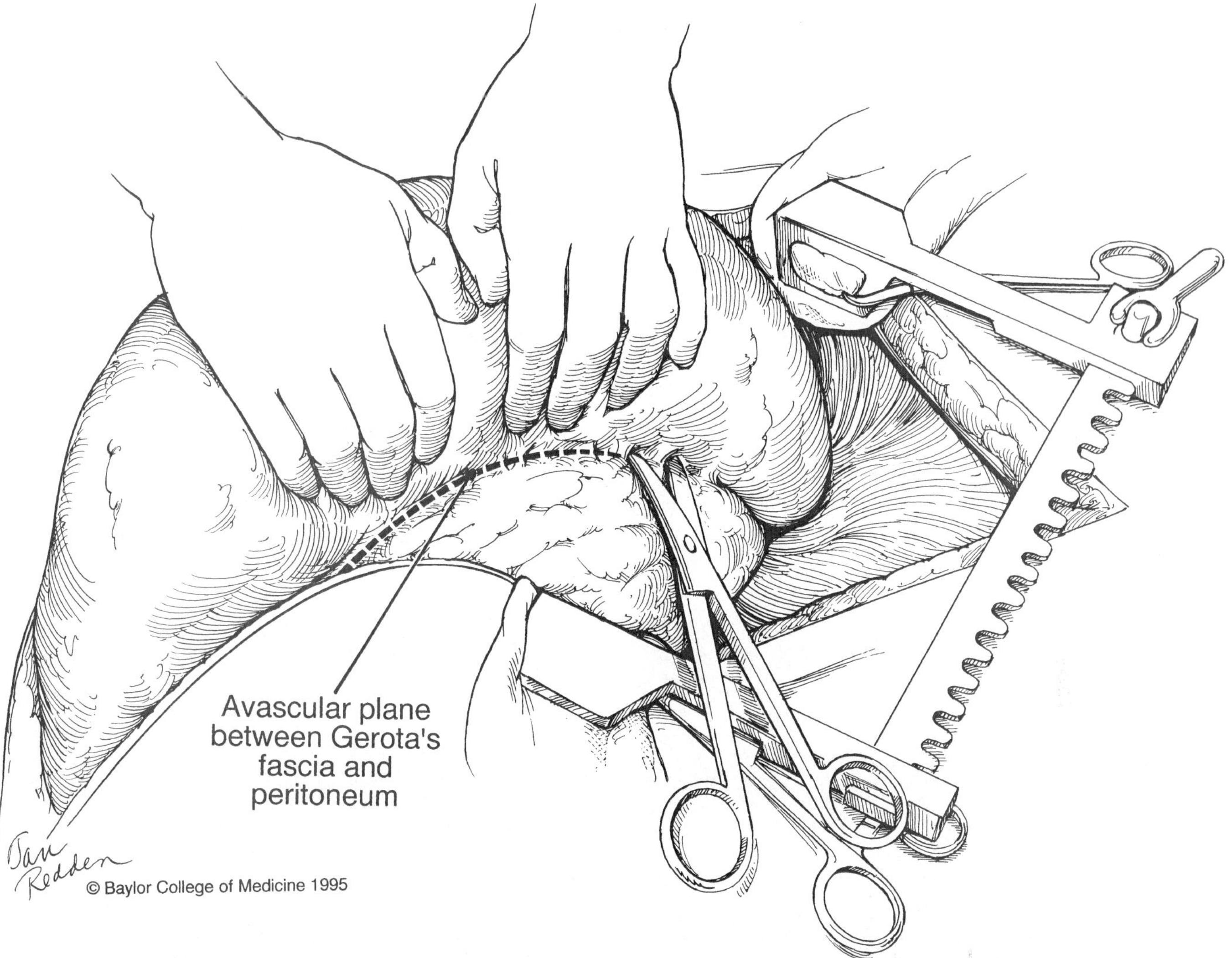

Fig. 36.9.   A moistened laparotomy pad is placed over the divided costal margin, and a Finochietto retractor is secured with towel clips. Gerota's fascia is elevated off the posterior musculature to the level of the aorta. This maneuver facilitates identification of the avascular plane between the posterior peritoneum and Gerota's fascia, which is incised. The peritoneal envelope is then dissected off the anterior layer of Gerota's fascia to the contralateral ureter.

5% dextrose and saline infusion is continued at the rate of 150 mL/hr, and 5% albumin is infused at 50 mL/hr for day 1, 25 mL/hr for day 2, and then discontinued.

Volume status is monitored adequately by measurements of hematocrit, vital signs, and urine output. By the third postoperative day the urine output will increase significantly, signaling the reabsorption of the large third-space fluid load. Parenteral fluids are therefore curtailed. Central venous and arterial lines are helpful adjuncts in patients with massive abdominal disease, but are not mandatory in young, generally healthy patients with minimal disease.

The tube thoracostomy is connected to a closed, vented suction at 15 to 20 cm negative water pressure. A single-view chest radiograph is obtained in the recovery room to assure proper placement of the tube and full expansion of the lung.

We routinely remove the chest tube the following morning. Hospital stay is generally 5 to 7 days for uncomplicated cases.

COMPLICATIONS

The thoracoabdominal extraperitoneal approach to RPLND has been used in patients ranging in age from 15 to 65 years, with a surprisingly low complication rate. The most frequent intraoperative complication, although rare, has been injury to the renal vessels. This can almost always be repaired, thus avoiding a nephrectomy. Stripping away Gerota's fascia and meticulous dissection of the tissue around the renal hilum minimize the risk of vascular injury and facilitate identification of small polar vessels. Renal artery vasospasm is a frequent occurrence that may lead to parenchymal ischemia. To prevent or reverse

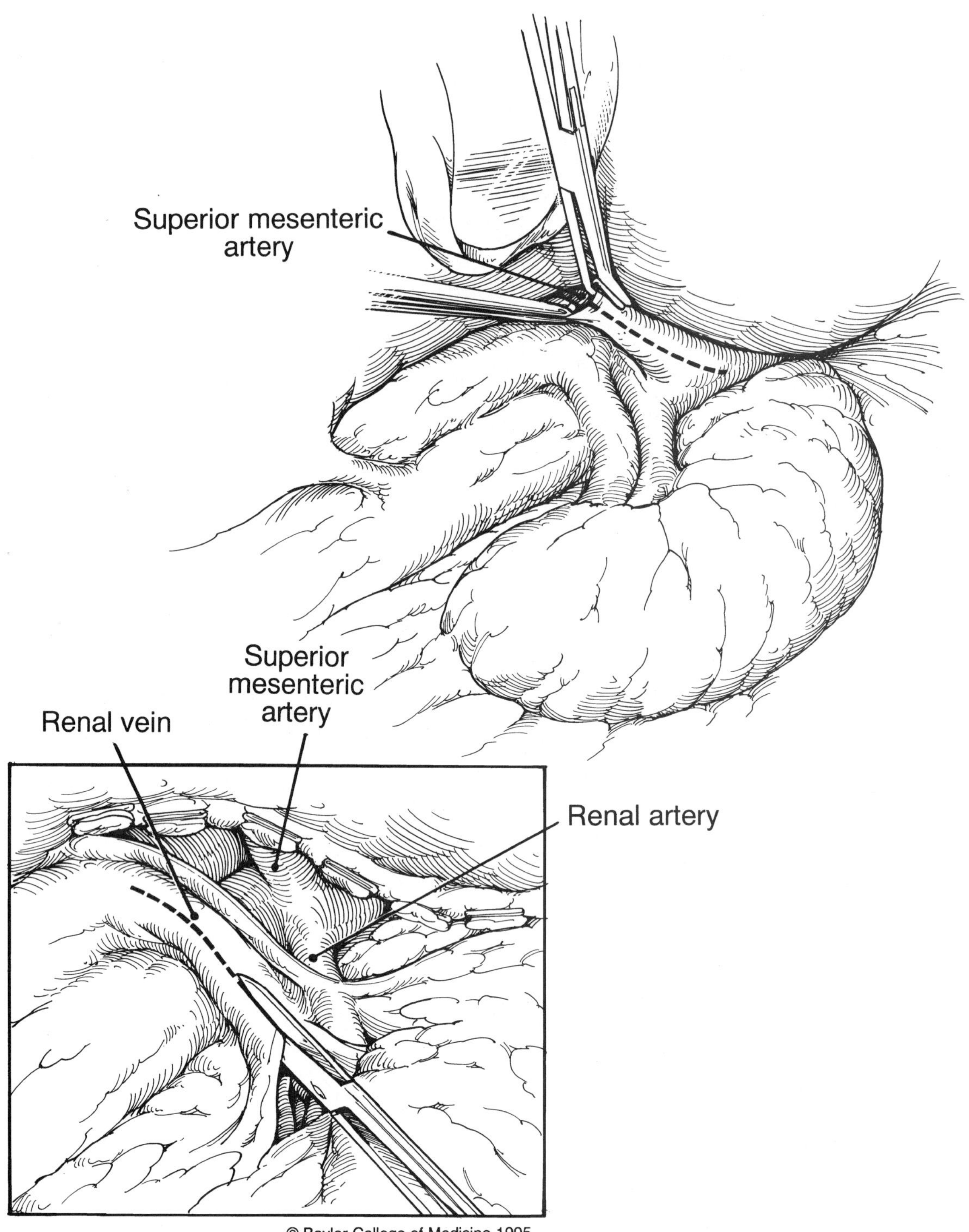

Fig. 36.10.   Identification of the left renal vein leads the surgeon to the aorta and left renal artery posteriorly and to the superior mesenteric artery superiorly. The dissection is begun at the base of the superior mesenteric artery, where numerous small lymphatics are clipped and divided to expose the adventitia of the artery. The dissection is continued over the aorta to the left crus of the diaphragm. Inset: The superior margin of this dissection must be carefully controlled with hemoclips to prevent lymphatic leakage. The tissue over the left renal vein is incised, and the dissection is continued to the midportion of the inferior vena cava.

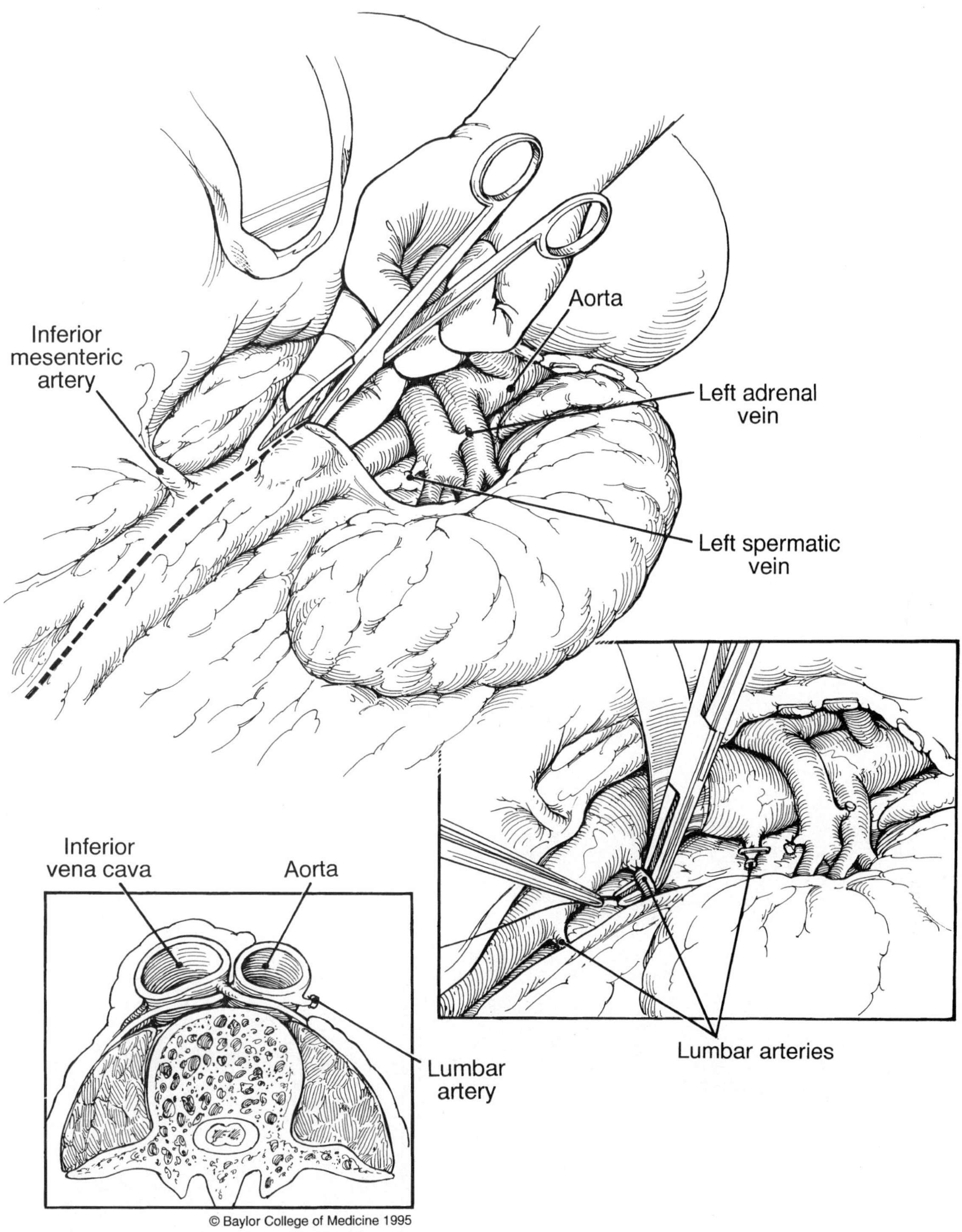

Fig. 36.11. Exposure of the great vessels. The left renal vein is completely mobilized after ligating and dividing the left adrenal and spermatic veins. The vein is then retracted, and the origin of the left renal artery is identified and carefully dissected over 1 to 2 cm. The node-bearing tissue is then divided over the infrarenal aorta to the level of the inferior mesenteric artery. Care must be taken not to disturb the plexus of nerves at the base of the inferior mesenteric artery. The line of incision is then carried inferiorly over the midportion of the left common iliac artery to its bifurcation. Right inset: The node-bearing tissue is dissected off the anterolateral aorta, exposing the ipsilateral lumbar arteries that are doubly ligated with 3-0 silk ties and hemoclips and divided. Left inset: Cross-sectional view below the renal hilum illustrates the dissection.

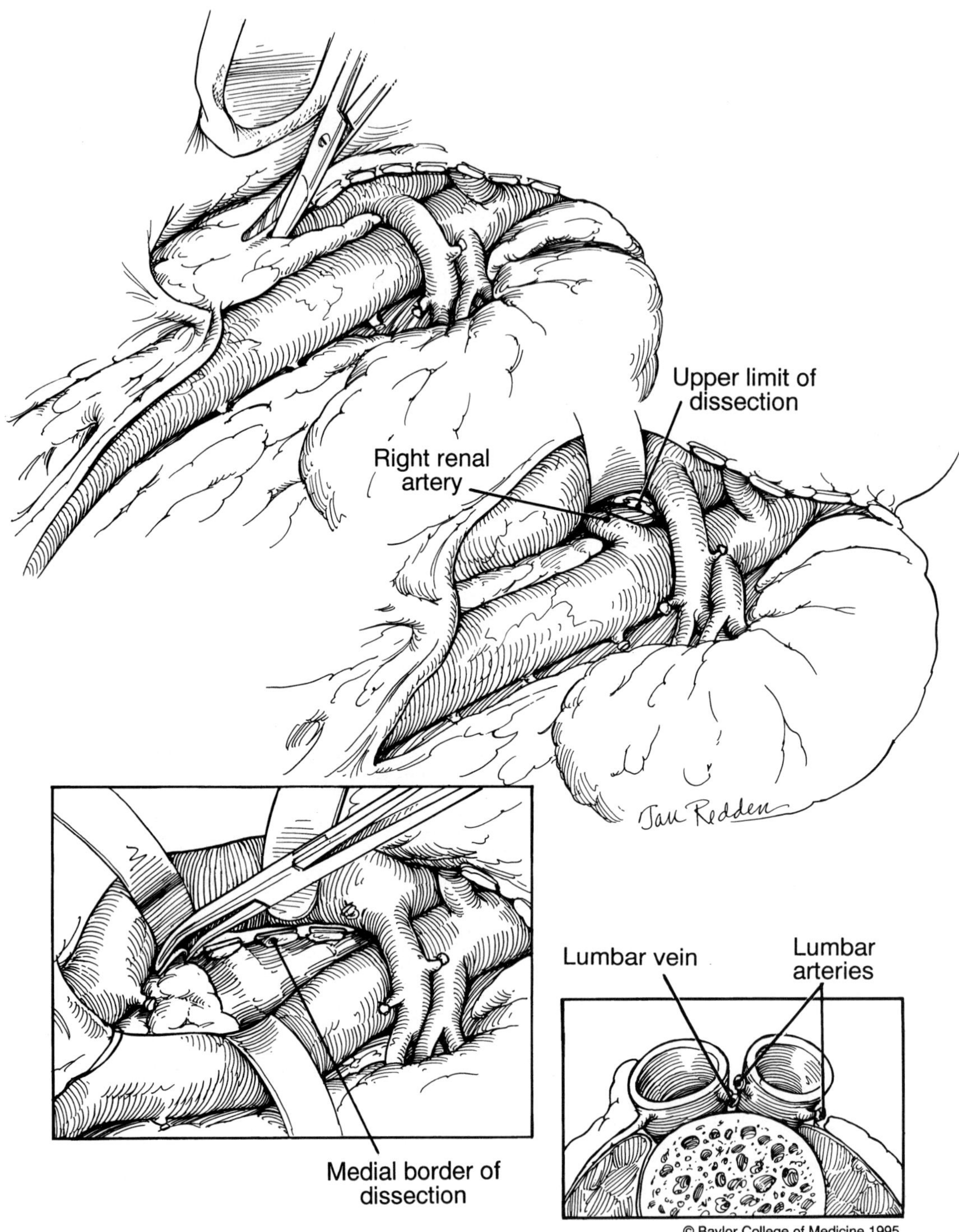

Fig. 36.12.   The interaortocaval dissection. The tissue along the midportion of the inferior vena cava is clipped laterally and divided inferiorly to the level of the inferior mesenteric artery. The vena cava and the left renal vein are retracted superiorly to expose the origin of the right renal artery, which is carefully dissected over 1 to 2 cm. The tissue cephalad to the renal artery is carefully mobilized, clipped, divided, and swept inferiorly along the prevertebral fascia. Care must be taken to ligate the cisterna chyli, which lies over the right crus of the diaphragm posterior to the right renal artery. Left inset: The medial lumbar veins between the renal artery and inferior mesenteric artery are doubly ligated with silk ties and hemoclips. The posterolateral margin of dissection is controlled with hemoclips behind the inferior vena cava. During a prospective nerve-sparing procedure, care must be taken to identify the postganglionic sympathetic nerves at their origin adjacent to the lumbar veins. Right inset: After ligating and dividing the medial lumbar arteries between the renal artery and the inferior mesenteric artery, the tissue can be swept off the prevertebral fascia and under the aorta toward the left side.

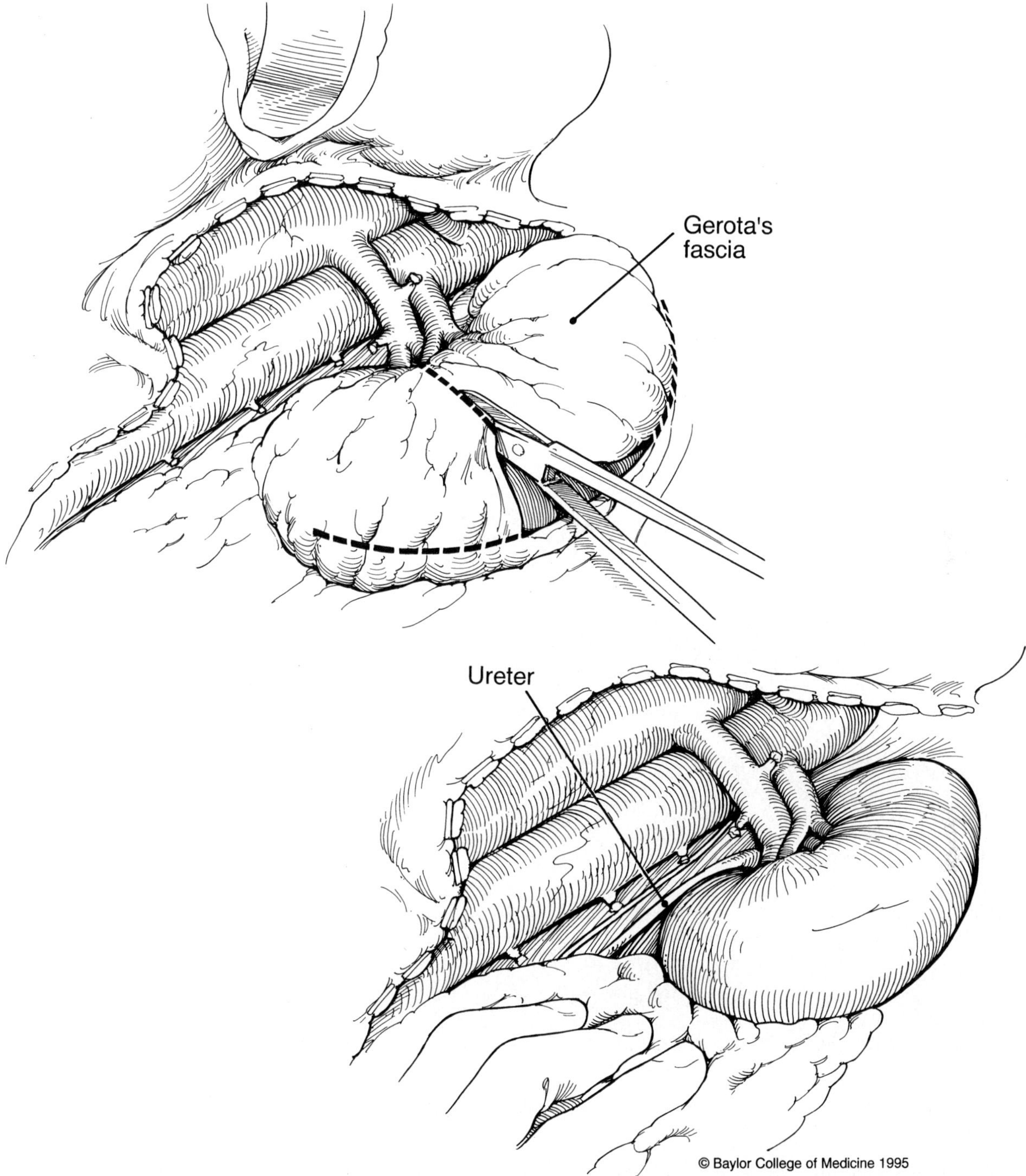

Fig. 36.13.   The lymph node tissue is now completely mobilized from the aorta and vena cava. Gerota's fascia is mobilized off the kidney to facilitate exposure of the renal hilum. The branches of the renal vessels are easily identified with this approach, and the lymph-node–bearing tissue is then dissected from the vessels. The left adrenal gland is usually removed with Gerota's fascia, and the lymphadenectomy specimen is swept inferiorly off the posterior musculature. Small perforating vessels along the left paravertebral groove should be clipped (not shown). The ureter is carefully dissected from the retroperitoneal tissue to the level of the common iliac artery.

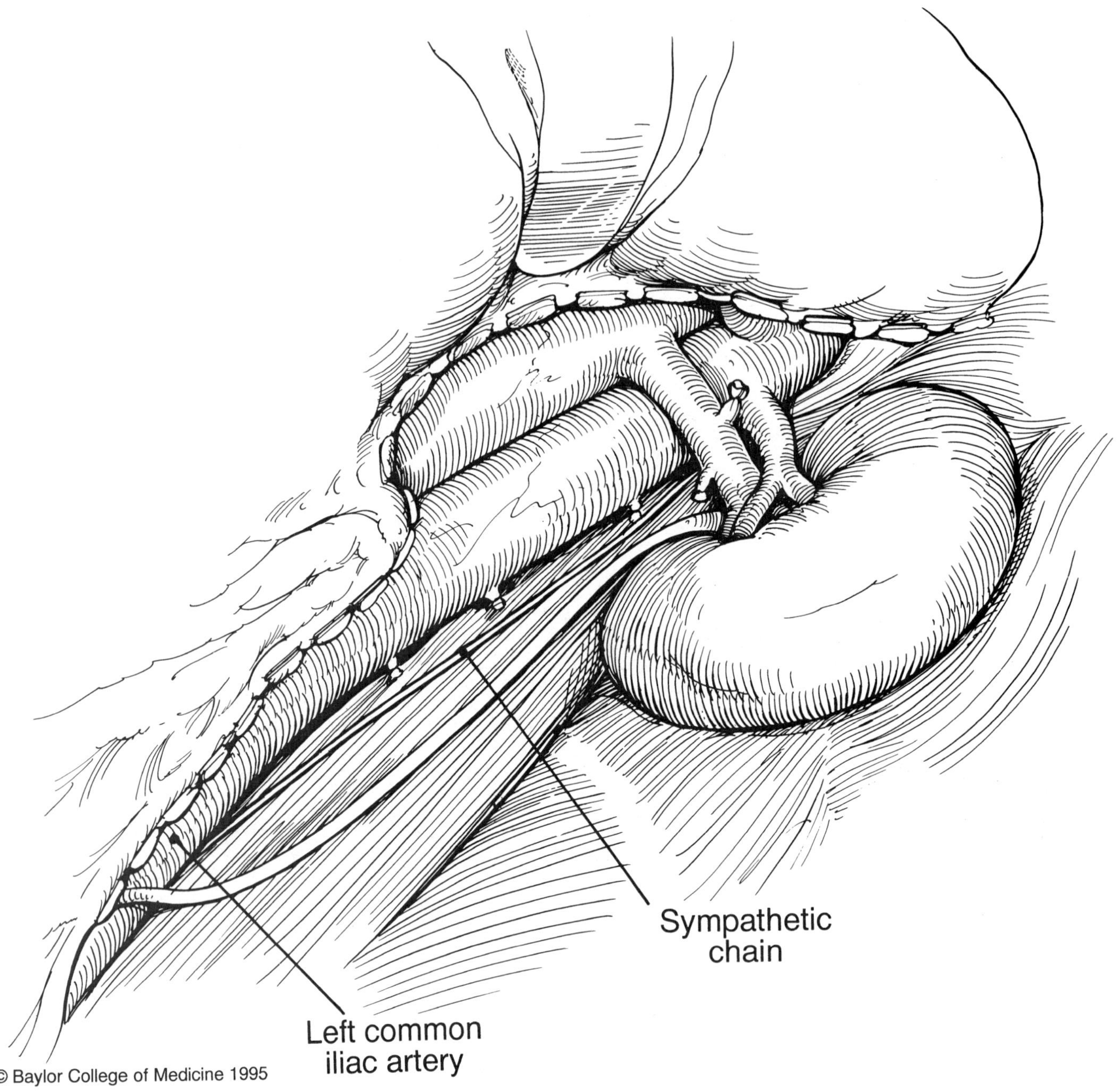

Fig. 36.14. The completed node dissection. The medial inferior limit of dissection is established at the bifurcation of the common iliac artery, preserving all the tissue inferior to the inferior mesenteric artery and medial to the common iliac artery. The sympathetic chain may be preserved in the absence of gross nodal metastases.

the vasospasm, a mannitol drip can be administered and intravascular volume can be maintained with crystalloid and albumin. These can be supplemented with direct irrigation of the artery with lidocaine or papaverine. Renal artery thrombosis should be recognized intraoperatively and repaired if possible.

Major injury to the renal vein can usually be repaired, and nephrectomy is seldom necessary. Bleeding from an avulsed lumbar vessel may occur but can be avoided by individual ligation of each pair caudad to the renal vessels. Vascular Allis forcep clamps control bleeding and allow repair of major vascular structures or ligation of small vessels with 5-0 polypropylene (Prolene) suture.

Ischemic injury to the spinal cord should not occur as long as lumbar arteries are not ligated above the renal artery (28). The spinal cord ends at the first lumbar vertebrae, and its collateral blood supply is provided by the arteria radicularis magna (artery of Adamkiewicz) that originates from the thoracic aorta in 50% of patients and from the lumbar artery in the other 50% (69–71). When the artery originates from the lumbar artery, a collateral artery to the spinal cord originates from the thoracic aorta (69, 70).

Postoperative complications, including wound infection, prolonged atelectasis or pneumonia, and prolonged ileus, have been reported in 6 to 12% of patients (25, 46, 49, 72). Chylous ascites has been reported in 1% of patients, the majority having vena caval obstruction. Most patients respond to conservative measures or total parenteral nutrition (73). Delayed bleeding, lymphoceles, thrombophlebitis, and pulmonary emboli have been rare. In more than 900 reported cases, there has been only one operative death. This was caused by a pulmonary embolus 3 weeks after the procedure (74).

ADJUVANT CHEMOTHERAPY AND FOLLOW-UP

There is no evidence that adjuvant chemotherapy, particularly low-dose chemotherapy, will substitute for an incompletely performed retroperitoneal lymphadenectomy in which tumor-bearing lymph nodes have been left behind. For patients in whom the lymph nodes are negative after a complete retroperitoneal dissection, the reported recurrence rate is 6% and virtually all recurrences are in the lungs (30).

For patients with positive lymph nodes, we recommend two courses of cisplatin and etoposide. The Intergroup Study, sponsored by the National Cancer Institute, demonstrated that the relapse rate in such patients can be reduced from 47% to 3% with short-course chemotherapy (cisplatin, bleomycin, and vinblastine) (47).

Whether adjuvant chemotherapy should be given to these patients is a matter of judgment. The advantages include a reduced recurrence rate and low morbidity compared with intensive rescue chemotherapy regimens. Mortality is comparable whether adjuvant or rescue chemotherapy is used. The major disadvantage is the exposure of all patients to chemotherapy agents that will benefit only some patients. It has not been determined that the use of short-course adjuvant chemotherapy diminishes the response rate to intensive combination chemotherapy for the small fraction of patients who experience recurrence.

After definitive treatment of early stage tumors, patients must be monitored carefully and regularly. We perform a physical examination, with special attention to the supraclavicular nodes, breasts, abdomen, and contralateral testis, every 2 months for the first year, every 3 months for the second year, every 4 months for the third year, every 6 months for the fourth and fifth years, and annually thereafter. Serum levels of beta human chorionic gonadotropin, alpha-fetoprotein, and lactate dehydrogenase are assayed and a chest radiograph is obtained at each of these office visits. Routine computed tomography of the abdomen is unnecessary in the asymptomatic patient because the risk of recurrence in the retroperitoneum is less than 1%. Other studies are performed as indicated. All patients are instructed to perform self-examination of the testis at monthly intervals up to age 50.

ACKNOWLEDGMENT

The authors thank Carolyn Schum and Irene Albright for editorial assistance.

REFERENCES

1. Most I. Ueber maligne Hodengeschwulste und ihre Metastaten. Arch Pathol Anat Klin Med 1898;154:138.
2. Cuneo B, Marcille M. Topographie des ganglions ilio-pelviens. Bull Soc Anat (Paris) 1901;6(Suppl):653.
3. Jamieson JK, Dobson JF. The lymphatics of the testicle. Lancet 1910;2:493.
4. Kinmonth JB, Taylor GW, Harper RK. Lymphangiography. Br Med J 1955;1:940.
5. Busch FM, Sayegh ES, Cheanult OW Jr. Some uses of lymphangiography in the management of testicular tumors. J Urol 1965;93:490.
6. Chiappa S, Uslenghi C, Bonadonna G, et al. Combined testicular and foot lymphography in testicular carcinomas. Surg Gynecol Obstet 1966;123:10.
7. Wahlqvist L, Hulten L, Rosencrantz M. Normal lymphatic drainage of the testis studied by funicular lymphography. Acta Chir Scand 1966;132:454.
8. Kober GM. Sarcoma of the testicle: conclusions based upon 114 cases. Am J Med Sci 1899;67:535.
9. Howard RJ. Malignant disease of the testis. Practitioner 1907;79:794.
10. Chevassu M. Le diagnostic clinique des cancers du testicule. Presse Med 1910;18:363.
11. Stinson JC. A new operation for malignant disease of the testicle: the necessity of a more extensive operation than castration for carcinoma, sarcoma, etc. of the testicle. Med Rec 1897;52:623.
12. Dew HR. Malignant disease of the testicle: its pathology, diagnosis, and treatment. New York: Paul B. Hoeber, 1926.
13. Roberts JB. Excision of the lumbar lymphatic nodes and spermatic vein in malignant disease of the testicle. Ann Surg 1902;36:539.
14. Hinman F. The operative treatment of tumor of the testicle. JAMA 1914;63:2009.
15. Young HH. Neoplasms of the urogenital tract. In: Young HH, Davis DM, eds. Young's practice of urology. Philadelphia: WB Saunders, 1926.
16. Hinman F, Johnson CM, Carr JL. The clinicopathologic classification of tumors of the testis in relation to prognosis. Trans Am Assoc Genitourin Surg 1941;34:211.
17. Lewis LG. Radical orchiectomy for tumors of the testis. JAMA 1948;137:828.
18. Marshall DF. Urogenital wounds in an evacuation hospital. J Urol 1946;55:119.
19. Wylie RH, Hoffman HL, Williams DB, et al. The thoracoabdominal casualty. Ann Surg 1946;124:463.
20. Sweet RH. Transthoracic gastrectomy and esophagectomy for carcinoma of the stomach and esophagus. Clinics 1945;3:1288.
21. Chute R, Soutter L, Kerr WSJ. Value of thoracoabdominal

incision in removal of kidney tumors. N Engl J Med 1949;
241:951.

22. Mortensen H. Transthoracic nephrectomy. J Urol 1948;60:855.

23. Cooper JF, Leadbetter WF, Chute R. The thoracoabdominal approach for retroperitoneal gland dissection: its application to testis tumors. Surg Gynecol Obstet 1950;90:486.

24. Mallis N, Patton JF. Transperitoneal bilateral lymphadenectomy in testis tumor. J Urol 1959;80:501.

25. Staubitz WJ, Early KS, Magoss IV, et al. Surgical management of testis tumors. J Urol 1974;111:205.

26. Whitmore WFJ. Surgical management of adult germinal testis tumors. Semin Oncol 1979;6:55.

27. Skinner DG, Leadbetter WF. The surgical management of testis tumors. J Urol 1971;106:84.

28. Skinner DG. Considerations for management of large retroperitoneal tumors: use of the modified thoracoabdominal approach. J Urol 1977;117:605.

29. Donohue JP. Retroperitoneal lymphadenectomy: the anterior approach including bilateral supra-hilar dissection. Urol Clin North Am 1977;4:509.

30. Donohue JP, Einhorn LH, Williams SD. Is adjuvant chemotherapy following retroperitoneal lymph node dissection for nonseminomatous testis cancer necessary? Urol Clin North Am 1980;7:747.

31. Skinner DG, Scardino PT. Relevance of biochemical tumor markers and lymphadenectomy in management of non-seminomatous testis tumors: current perspective. J Urol 1980; 123:378.

32. Donohue JP. Surgical management of testicular cancer. In: Einhorn LH, ed. Testicular tumors: management and treatment. New York: Masson Publishing USA, 1980.

33. Ray B, Hadju SI, Whitmore WF Jr. Distribution of retroperitoneal lymph node metastases in testicular germinal tumors. Cancer 1974;33:340.

34. Donohue JP, Zachary JM, Maynard BR. Distribution of nodal metastases in nonseminomatous testis cancer. J Urol 1982;128: 315.

35. Whitelaw GP, Smithwick RH. Some secondary effects of sympathectomy with particular reference to disturbance of sexual function. N Engl J Med 1951;245:121.

36. Narayan P, Lange PH, Fraley EE. Ejaculation and fertility after extended retroperitoneal lymph node dissection for testicular cancer. J Urol 1982;127:685.

37. Colleselli K, Poisel S, Schachtner W, et al. Nerve-preserving bilateral retroperitoneal lymphadenectomy: anatomical study and operative approach. J Urol 1990;144:293.

38. Fossa SD, Klepp O, Ous S, et al. Unilateral retroperitoneal lymph node dissection in patients with nonseminomatous testicular tumor in clinical stage I. Eur Urol 1984;10:17.

39. Fritz K, Weissbach L. Sperm parameters and ejaculation before and after operative treatment of patients with germ cell testicular cancer. Fertil Steril 1985;43:451.

40. Pizzocaro G, Salvione R, Sanoni F. Unilateral lymphadenectomy in intraoperative stage I nonseminomatous germinal testis cancer. J Urol 1985;134:485.

41. Richie JP. Modified retroperitoneal lymphadenectomy for patients with clinical stage I testicular cancer. Semin Urol 1988;6:216.

42. Donohue JP, Thornhill JA, Foster RS, et al. Retroperitoneal lymphadenectomy for clinical stage A testis cancer (1965–1989): modifications of technique and impact on ejaculation. J Urol 1993;149:237.

43. Jewett MA, Kong Y-SP, Goldberg SD, et al. Retroperitoneal lymphadenectomy for testis tumor with nerve-sparing for ejaculation. J Urol 1988;139:1220.

44. Donohue JP, Foster RS, Rowland RG, et al. Nerve-sparing retroperitoneal lymphadenectomy with preservation of ejaculation. J Urol 1990;144:287.

45. Wise PG, Scardino PT. Thoracoabdominal retroperitoneal lymphadenectomy for testicular cancer. In: Skinner DG, Lieskovsky G, eds. Diagnosis and management of genitourinary cancer. Philadelphia: WB Saunders, 1987:779.

46. Donohue JP, Thornhill JA, Foster RS, et al. The role of retroperitoneal lymphadenectomy in clinical stage B testis cancer: the Indiana University experience (1965 to 1989). J Urol 1995;153:85.

47. Williams SD, Stablein DM, Einhorn LH, et al. Immediate adjuvant chemotherapy versus observation with treatment at relapse in pathological stage II testicular cancer. N Engl J Med. 1987;317:1433.

48. Johnson DE, Bracken RB, Blight EM. Prognosis for pathologic stage I nonseminomatous germ cell tumors of the testis managed by retroperitoneal lymphadenectomy. J Urol 1976; 116:68.

49. Skinner DG, Melamud A, Lieskovsky G. Complications of thoracoabdominal retroperitoneal lymph node dissection. J Urol 1982;127:1107.

50. Baniel J, Foster RS, Rowland RG, et al. Complications of primary retroperitoneal lymph node dissection. J Urol 1994; 152:424.

51. Jewett MAS, Wesley-James T, Sturgeon JFG, et al. Retroperitoneal lymphadenectomy with nerve-sparing for advanced stage testis tumor after chemotherapy. J Urol 1989; 141:301. Abstract no. 525.

52. Shaban SF, Seager SWJ, Lipshultz LI. Clinical electroejaculation. Med Instrum 1988;22:77.

53. Donohue JP, Roth LM, Zachary JM, et al. Cytoreductive surgery for metastatic testis cancer: tissue analysis of retroperitoneal masses after chemotherapy. J Urol 1982;127: 1111.

54. Donohue JP, Rowland RG, Kopecky K, et al. Correlation of computerized tomographic changes and histological findings in 80 patients having radical retroperitoneal lymph node dissection after chemotherapy for testis cancer. J Urol 1987; 137:1176.

55. Hendry WF. Abdominal surgery postchemotherapy in metastatic non-seminoma. In: Horwich A, ed. Testicular cancer: investigation and management. Baltimore: Williams & Wilkins, 1991;265.

56. Fossa SD, Ous S, Lien HH, et al. Post-chemotherapy lymph node histology in radiologically normal patients with metastatic nonseminomatous testicular cancer. J Urol 1989; 141:557.

57. Toner GC, Panicek DM, Heelan RT, et al. Adjunctive surgery after chemotherapy for nonseminomatous germ cell tumors: recommendations for patient selection. J Clin Oncol 1990;8: 1683.

58. Pizzocaro G, Zanoni F, Salvioni R, et al. Difficulties of a surveillance study omitting retroperitoneal lymphadenectomy

in clinical stage I nonseminomatous germ cell tumors of the testis. J Urol 1987;138:1393.

59. Rorth M, Jacobsen GK, van der Maase H, et al. Surveillance alone versus radiotherapy for clinical stage I nonseminomatous testicular cancer. J Clin Oncol 1991;9:1543.

60. Peckham MJ, Barrett A, Horwich A, et al. Orchiectomy alone for stage I testicular nonseminoma. Br J Urol 1983;55:754.

61. Moul JW, Foley JP, Hitchcock CL, et al. Flow cytometric and quantitative histological parameters to predict occult disease in clinical stage I nonseminomatous testicular germ cell tumors. J Urol 1993;150;879.

62. de Riese WT, Albers P, Walker EB, et al. Predictive parameters of biologic behavior of early stage nonseminomatous testicular germ cell tumors. Cancer 1994;74:1335.

63. Lerner S, Winkel E, Scardino PT. Management of stage A non-seminomatous germ cell tumors: results of a selective surveillance protocol from a single institution. J Urol 1993;149:456. Abstract no. 972.

64. Oliver RTD, Raja MA, Ong J, et al. Pilot study to evaluate impact of a policy of adjuvant chemotherapy for high risk stage 1 malignant teratoma on overall relapse rate of stage 1 cancer patients. J Urol 1992;148:1453.

65. Wise PG, Scardino PT. Thoracoabdominal retroperitoneal lymphadenectomy for non-seminomatous testicular cancer. Urol Clin North Am 1983;10:371.

66. Stirt JA, Korn EL, Reynolds RC. Sodium nitroprusside-induced hypotension in thoraco-abdominal radical retroperitoneal lymph node dissection. Br J Anaesth 1980;52:1045.

67. Hendolin MA, Mattila K, Poikolainen E. The effect of lumbar epidural analgesia on the development of deep vein thrombosis of the legs after open prostatectomy. Acta Chir Scand 1981;147:425.

68. Kaswick JA, Bloomberg SD, Skinner DG. Radical retroperitoneal lymph node dissection: how effective in removal of all retroperitoneal nodes? J Urol 1976;115:70.

69. Adams HD, van Geertruyden HH. Neurologic complications of aortic surgery. Ann Surg 1956;144:574.

70. Coupland GA, Reeve TS. Paraplegia: a complication of excision of abdominal aortic aneurysm. Surgery 1968;64:878.

71. Ferguson LRJ, Bergan JJ, Conn JJ, et al. Spinal ischemia following abdominal aortic surgery. Ann Surg 1975;181:267.

72. Einhorn LH, Williams SD. The management of disseminated testicular cancer. In: Einhorn LH, ed. Testicular tumors: management and treatment. New York: Masson Publishing USA, 1980.

73. Baniel J, Foster RS, Rowland RG, et al. Management of chylous ascites after retroperitoneal lymph node dissection for testicular cancer. J Urol 1993;150:1422.

74. Scardino PT. Thoracoabdominal retroperitoneal lymphadenectomy for testicular cancer. In: Crawford ED, Borden TA, eds. Genitourinary cancer surgery. Philadelphia: Lea & Febiger, 1982;271.

37

Anterior Transabdominal Approach for Radical Retroperitoneal Lymphadenectomy

Anatomy and Nerve-Sparing Technique

Michael A.S. Jewett

Although first described in the nineteenth century, retroperitoneal lymphadenectomy (RPL) was not standardized until the military experience during World War II (1). The surgical approach was transabdominal or thoracoabdominal, but the former has become the more commonly performed procedure today. No substantial improvements were made until the 1970s when several significant advances occurred. The tumor markers alpha-fetoprotein (AFP) and the β-subunit of human chorionic gonadotropin (β-hCG) were sensitively measured with immunoassay. Computed tomography (CT) scanning was described and applied to the retroperitoneum. The geographic patterns of lymph node metastases were mapped from operative experience. Finally, platinum-based chemotherapy was developed with dramatically improved results and frequent cure. These were unprecedented advances in the treatment of testis cancer, and the mortality rate decreased rapidly. More recently, the implications of infertility due to loss of antegrade ejaculation have been defined and nerve-sparing techniques have been described to reduce morbidity. These developments have rationalized the procedure so that we can now fine tune its indications.

History of RPL

The first report of removing a large malignant teratoma from the retroperitoneum appeared in 1882 (1). In 1902, three years after the testicular lymphatic drainage was described, the first systematic RPL was reported. This patient died, but in 1906 the first successful procedure was reported. At that time, mortality from testis tumor was 85% and treatment was essentially orchidectomy only. The huge experience from the Walter Reed Army Hospital during World War II was reported by Lewis, who performed a unilateral dissection on 169 patients, 34% with metastatic disease. A multidisciplinary approach and the first staging system were developed with an established histo-

logic classification. Anesthesia improvements with positive pressure ventilation allowed Chute to develop the thoracoabdominal exposure in 1949 and apply it to the management of testis tumors. Leadbetter championed this approach, including resection of contralateral retroperitoneal disease. Travel described a transperitoneal approach with mobilization of the posterior peritoneum by incising from the cecum to the ligament of Treitz. Bowel was mobilized to expose the renal pedicles as well as aorta and vena cava. Mallis and Paton extended the skin incision from xiphoid to pubis and mobilized colon onto the chest to enhance visualization of the retroperitoneum.

Primary RPL was therefore adopted in North America for patients with early stage nonseminoma testicular cancer. Some were found to be inoperable, but the cure rate in those who did undergo the procedure was high. We now know that patients with positive nodes are cured more than 50% of the time (2). Patients undergoing RPL with negative nodes had accurate pathologic staging established to determine prognosis and had avoided further treatment. The Europeans were more oriented toward radiation therapy because of the perceived morbidity of surgery and the general availability of radiation resources. However, mortality is almost unknown with RPL and morbidity is minimal. Therefore, the two surgical approaches—one transperitoneal through a midline abdominal incision and the other retroperitoneal through a thoracoabdominal incision—were popularized. The transabdominal approach is the more widely practiced and will be described in this chapter with a discussion of the indications and the role of adjuvant treatment.

Clinical Staging

The systems for clinical staging have been modified from the Walter Reed Hospital in the United States or the Royal Marsden Hospital in the United Kingdom. The TNM system is not yet widely used. Stage I or A refers to no evidence of metastases after orchidectomy. For stage II or B, there are several staging systems in use that subdivide the extent of retroperitoneal nodal disease by the size and number of nodes. We use stage IIA when referring to disease up to 5 cm in diameter, although others divide the extent of disease at 2 or 3 cm and the number of involved nodes. Stage IIb is greater than 5 cm with no evidence of pulmonary or visceral metastases. Marker levels are not used in staging except when there is no evidence of metastases on imaging. Detectable marker levels indicate occult metastases. To establish stage, patients need to undergo CT of the abdomen, pelvis, and chest plus a chest radiograph in addition to markers.

Improvements in clinical staging have been critical for the improved treatment results with testis tumors. The advances have been in the use of tumor markers and in imaging. The radioimmunoassay for β-hCG was 1000 times more sensitive and was measurable in up to 50% of patients. AFP was detected initially in animals, then in humans with hepatomas, and in men with germ cell tumors in the 1960s. Staging accuracy was immensely improved, and previously undetectable metastases or recurrences could be detected and treated earlier. The sensitivity of detection of retroperitoneal metastases for one or both of these markers is 70% based on surgical series in which pathologic staging was obtained (3). In our experience, the specificity of a persistently elevated marker level is high for metastatic disease after orchidectomy; however, occult disease outside the retroperitoneum cannot be excluded, particularly with high levels. Low but elevated levels, in the range of 5 to 15 ng/mL, should be followed serially and regarded with suspicion as a possible false-positive result.

Patients who have elevated markers as the only evidence of metastatic disease, i.e., those for whom all imaging study results are normal, pose a particular problem. Although most patients have predictable lymphatic pattern metastases to the retroperitoneum as the first site of spread, some may have hematogenous spread. Another possibility is small-volume metastases in nodes that cannot be imaged. The natural history of these patients is not well defined, and we do not really know what proportion need systemic therapy for cure. These patients are generally treated with chemotherapy initially although there may be a role for RPL.

Clinical staging accuracy also improved with CT scanning, a major improvement over the intravenous urogram for assessment of the retroperitoneum. The accuracy of abdominal imaging remains approximately 60%, with false-positive rates of 20% and false-negative rates of 20 to 30% (3). This presents several problems.

First, this may result in overtreatment of the retroperitoneum with surgery or chemotherapy in false-positive results. This is of particular concern if chemotherapy is used as a primary modality. Second, the extent of disease may be underestimated and an RPL that is unlikely to be curative without adjuvant chemotherapy may be performed. This is particularly

possible when there are multiple smaller nodal metastases that, in our experience, appear to be associated with a higher risk of occult systemic metastases that will require later chemotherapy for relapse.

The pattern of retroperitoneal metastases has been well documented so that imaging can be interpreted with greater accuracy by the informed practitioner (4, 5). This knowledge should reduce false-positive results due to vascular anomalies and bowel loops as well as heighten suspicion of smaller nodes that may be significant due to their location. In the early period with surveillance of clinical stage I patients, we believed that our inexperience with interpretation of retroperitoneal imaging contributed to a higher relapse rate (6). Presumably, similar systematic errors can occur in clinical series reporting results with more advanced disease, which might bias results of treatment; this is particularly true if surgical confirmation is not regularly obtained. Platinum-based chemotherapy provides effective curative therapy but may be overprescribed for false-positive stage II patients. Bipedal lymphangiography has been generally abandoned in the past few years because of its invasiveness, risks, and lack of additional useful information in most patients (7).

Ultrasonography is a sensitive test for the diagnosis of primary testis tumor, especially in nonpalpable disease. However, it is not used as widely as CT in defining retroperitoneal metastatic disease.

Pattern of Retroperitoneal Metastases

The careful mappings of the pattern of retroperitoneal metastases by Ray et al., Donohue et al., and Weissbach et al. were equally important to surgeons (4, 5, 8). For the first time, the extent of the lymphadenectomy could be defined on the basis of expected sites of disease. Right-sided tumors may metastasize to the left paraaortic nodes at the level of the renal hilum. Left-sided tumors do not cross the midline in the absence of gross disease. Both sides may spread to the interaortocaval nodes and along the spermatic vessels to the respective drainage areas or landing sites in the renal hilum on the left and along the inferior vena cava (IVC) on the right, where the testicular vein drains into the IVC. This information has also been useful to the radiation therapist treating seminoma because there is no reason to expect differences in the patterns of spread to the retroperitoneal nodes. Image interpretation is now more precise because the zones of higher risk can be defined for individual patients.

Other Treatment Modalities

Radiation therapy for nonseminoma was preferred over lymphadenectomy until World War II in some centers in North America. Radiation therapy continued to be the treatment of choice for patients with suspected retroperitoneal metastases in Britain until the era of chemotherapy. Comparison of survival after radiation and surgery was difficult to determine due to the lack of accurate clinical staging at the time. Combination platinum-based chemotherapy (developed in the 1970s) rapidly ended the use of radiation therapy, which was less effective and compromised the patients' ability to receive full doses of chemotherapy.

Modern chemotherapy began when MacKenzie reported results with actinomycin D alone (with a 50% overall response rate), as did the Indiana group from 1965 to 1972 (9). Single-agent chemotherapy failed to produce complete responses beyond 1 year. Based on the success of triple therapy for tuberculosis, a triple chemotherapy regimen of actinomycin D, chlorambucil, and methotrexate was advocated for advanced testis tumor in the early 1960s. In 1970 the EORTC reported a study of 237 patients treated with bleomycin, of whom 6 had testicular cancer and 3 had choriocarcinoma. Samuels et al. reported 83 patients with metastatic testis tumors who received high-dose bleomycin with vinblastine or bleomycin plus cyclophosphamide, vincristine, methotrexate, and 5-fluorouracil 5 years later (10).

Platinum-based chemotherapy was first described for testis cancer by Einhorn and Donohue in 1972. In a preliminary series in 1975 and 1977, these authors reported a comparison of Adriamycin, high-dose bleomycin and vincristine with cisplatin, vinblastine and high-dose bleomycin; the latter protocol was superior (9). The previously attained complete response rates of up to 30% rose to more than 70% overall for patients with metastatic disease. Einhorn and Donohue deserve credit for these advances, which have been the most significant ones in the evolution of treatment of testis tumors. Patients with clinical stage I and completely resected stage II disease can now be followed without further treatment. The "safety net" of chemotherapy has led to considerable worldwide experience with surveillance rather than prophylactic RPL or radiation therapy for stage I nonseminoma, with a 30% progression rate. Therefore, up to 70% of patients can avoid therapy but at the price of laborious follow-up with repeated CT scanning of the abdomen. Defining primary tumor risk factor has identified patients who may be better managed by surgery than observation (11).

Fertility Issues in the Treatment of Testis Tumors

The last stage in the developments to rationalize RPL was a better understanding of fertility in testis cancer patients and the potential for iatrogenic infertility. There is no issue of erectile impotence other than due to psychological factors or androgen deprivation after bilateral orchidectomy (for bilateral tumors). The major morbidity of RPL is dry ejaculation with subsequent infertility. This is due to damage to the retroperitoneal sympathetic nerves that normally induce seminal emission by contraction of the seminal vesicles and closure of the bladder neck before ejaculation (12). When this complication was understood, attempts were made to limit the boundaries of dissection to preserve these sympathetic nerves. Mapping of the location of retroperitoneal metastases at surgery demonstrated the most likely sites of nodal disease, so that the dissection was limited

to the primary regional lymphatics with preservation of contralateral sympathetic nerves and ganglia. There is some theoretical risk of leaving residual disease with these limited approaches. Most protocols included postoperative chemotherapy in an adjuvant setting or for relapse, which potentially masked the real incidence.

Bilateral RPL for more extensive tumor rarely preserves antegrade ejaculation, and recovery of ejaculation is rare even with prolonged follow-up care. We have modified the technique of RPL to allow bilateral thorough dissection with identification and preservation of some or all of the sympathetic nerves and their ganglia before beginning the lymphadenectomy (13). Not only has this nerve-sparing technique eliminated the major morbidity of previous RPL techniques, it can preserve ejaculation in selected patients requiring bilateral lymphadenectomy for bulky disease. Other investigators, most notably the Indiana group, have also developed good nerve-sparing techniques that achieve the same objectives (14–16). The technique used can be either complete bilateral dissection with nerve identification and sparing or some type of template dissection that matches the surgical field to the likely sites of occult metastases (e.g., a left-sided tumor does not usually metastasize to the right, so removal of nodes in the left paraaortic region may be sufficient). Increasingly, nerves are being identified even if templates are being used. The rates for preservation of seminal emission and therefore antegrade ejaculation are 90% or more. The nerves can be electrostimulated intraoperatively to aid in the identification of dominant fibers (17).

The other modalities of therapy, chemotherapy and radiation therapy, can also affect future semen quality. Newer combinations of drugs may be less cytotoxic to the seminiferous epithelium, particularly with the elimination of the alkylating agents. Radiation is rarely used with nonseminomas, and scrotal shielding is commonly used.

Approximately 75% of patients will ultimately recover normal semen quality. Concern that the planned therapy not affect fertility is very important. The value of pretreatment sperm banking is controversial, but patients at least need to know that treatment can affect ultimate semen quality. The decision to bank semen before treatment can be left to the patient.

Indications for and Effectiveness of RPL

The indications for and the effectiveness of RPL for germ cell tumors have been controversial. Staubitz (18) prospectively studied 65 patients at Roswell Park Memorial Institute. The patients underwent bilateral RPL through a transperitoneal incision. No adjuvant chemotherapy or radiation therapy was given. The 5-year survival rates were 86% and 60% for pathologic stage I and II disease, respectively, although some patients were excluded because of inoperable disease. Others reported on the role of lymphadenectomy alone for retroperitoneal metastases. Finally, the Testis Tumor Group conducted a randomized controlled trial of the role for adjuvant chemotherapy (2). A total of 195 patients with positive retroperitoneal lymphadenopathy were randomly assigned to immediate postoperative cisplatin-based chemotherapy or observation. Ninety-eight patients were observed; 49% had recurrence, and 3 of these patients died of testis cancer. Six patients who received chemotherapy had a relapse, but five did not receive a full course of chemotherapy. The high cure rate with surgery alone (51%) was significant. The international authors of this study found no prognostic factors for relapse but they did not have serial tumor markers documented before RPL nor clearly stratified the bulk of gross disease at the time of RPL. There is no question that RPL can cure patients with retroperitoneal metastases.

Given the demonstrated successes with surgery and the improvements in combination chemotherapy, the focus has changed to minimizing the overall morbidity of treatment. Clinical staging of the retroperitoneum by imaging and markers in the presence of small-volume metastases is not as accurate as we would desire because of a significant false-positive rate. Patients are at risk of overtreatment whichever primary modality is used.

RPL is indicated in three stages of disease—selected clinical stage I, small volume stage II, and after chemotherapy for residual retroperitoneal masses.

In stage I patients, the description of the results of observation or surveillance after orchidectomy has helped to define a more appropriate algorithm of treatment that rationalizes the use of RPL (15, 16, 19). Seventy percent of patients have no metastases and will have negative nodes. Most of the 60% who have metastases somewhere will have positive nodes, and the majority will be cured by RPL alone (20). Failure analysis of the approximately 30% of clinical stage I patients who experience disease progression when initially managed by surveillance after orchidectomy has provided a more accurate definition of risk factors for metastases. Therefore, it has helped to define the patients who need treatment. The definition of high risk for future relapse is based on the pathologic features of the primary tumor and probably can be applied to 25 to 40% of all clinical stage I patients. However, up to 50% of those so defined have not experienced a relapse at the current time. Therefore, their management remains controversial. Further observation and treatment at the time of progression will spare up to 50% of patients further therapy and result in similar overall survival.

There is increasing experience with the use of laparoscopy in the staging of the retroperitoneum in men with possible nodal metastases (21, 22). The procedure can be done with minimal morbidity in experienced hands and may have a role to play in the management of early stage patients with stage I and low-volume stage II disease. It is too early to predict if the procedure will have a therapeutic role. Prophylactic or staging RPL in stage I confirms the stage of disease and will be therapeutic in those with small-volume nodal metastases (20). However, 70% will undergo unnecessary surgery.

The greatest experience in the management of stage II disease is with RPL. However, the early reports were based on patients who were staged surgically and some inoperable patients were excluded. Before the mid-1970s, CT scans were not in general use and imaging was limited to IVP and lymphangiography. In addition, markers were not routinely done until

this time. It is very difficult to extrapolate from this experience except to recognize that surgery alone was capable of curing some patients (1). Excellent results are obtained with RPL alone without adjuvant chemotherapy in cases of small-volume disease consisting of 2- to 3-cm masses seen on CT (23–26).

Combination platinum-based chemotherapy provided both a safety net for patients who had disease progression after surgery and a useful adjuvant to surgery. Patients thought to be at risk of progression were then given adjuvant chemotherapy before clear identification and measurement of risk factors such as size of nodes and marker levels. We still do not have good information on the risk of progression after RPL based on the size of nodes or preoperative marker levels. The relation of marker levels to the extent of metastases is not documented, although in the Danish study high preorchiectomy levels heralded a 50 to 60% relapse (27).

Our unpublished experience is that patients with normal or low marker levels have a lower incidence of systemic metastases. Therefore, we currently prefer to treat patients with one or more marker levels greater than 100 ng/mL with initial chemotherapy even if the imaging reveals limited disease in the retroperitoneum only.

Adjuvant chemotherapy given at reduced dosage compared with standard therapy for metastatic disease may have a role to play, although optimal dosages, drug combinations, and long-term follow-up are yet to be defined. We have been performing nerve-sparing procedures for more than 10 years and have not routinely used adjuvant chemotherapy in patients who are carefully selected after orchidectomy and are found on imaging to have retroperitoneal nodal disease without supradiaphragmatic or visceral metastases.

Tumor marker levels, histologic type of the primary, and size, extent, and location of metastases may be useful in selecting initial therapy. It is generally agreed that masses larger than 3 to 5 cm are best managed by initial chemotherapy (we have used 5 cm as our upper limit). One important issue is how size is reported. Bidimensional diameters on CT will sometimes understate true size if the mass is cigar shaped or ovoid rather than more spherical. The difference in volume will vary exponentially, leading to a gross underestimate of tumor volume and therefore cell number. In addition, there may be a number of nodal masses rather than one or two masses, and we do not have a consistent system for reporting total volume. Although it is reasonable to assume that the risk of progression after RPL is related to true total tumor burden in the retroperitoneum, we do not have clear evidence of this. Measurement inconsistencies may be one reason that the data are unavailable.

Clinical staging is now included in reports by surgeons to allow comparison of results with those achieved with other modalities (16, 20).

The role of initial or primary RPL as opposed to primary chemotherapy for clinical stage II nonseminomatous testicular tumors remains controversial (16, 28). The acute morbidity of both approaches is known, and RPL is better tolerated than three to four courses of chemotherapy. The long-term morbidity of RPL is well defined and is very small, whereas long-term morbidity (particularly the risk of second malignancy) appears to be greater for combination chemotherapy (29–31). There is also a small but persistent mortality rate with chemotherapy that is not reported with surgery. The presence of teratoma in the primary testicular tumor increases the likelihood of residual retroperitoneal masses after chemotherapy and the presence of teratoma in those masses (32). It may, therefore, be advisable to recommend initial RPL rather than chemotherapy for these patients if they have a small volume of retroperitoneal disease as they will have a high risk of requiring surgery as a second treatment after chemotherapy. Individual case series of the alternative approaches appear to be equivalent in terms of survival, and differences will be measured in quality of life and cost-effectiveness.

The role of surgery after chemotherapy is now well established. However, there is a need to define in a better manner those patients who benefit from resection of residual abdominal masses (33). To date, full bilateral RPL including excision of the mass(es) as practiced in some centers has not been compared with a modified procedure with excision of the mass only. Those with necrosis/fibrosis without active tumor elements remain free of disease and may not require full bilateral RPL if intraoperative biopsy does not reveal tumor (34). At this time, no parameters such as tumor response to therapy are sufficiently reliable to avoid excision of a residual mass. Complete resection of all masses visible on CT or ultrasound is required to avoid leaving carcinoma in 20% or more of patients and teratoma in up to 50% of patients that may subsequently metastasize or enlarge. Adjuvant chemotherapy appears to benefit those with residual active carcinoma.

Technique of RPL

Our technique of nerve identification and preservation while performing a full bilateral lymphadenectomy has been described (13, 35). We continue to do a full dissection so that we are confident that we have cleared all areas. When nodes are grossly negative, it is reasonable to consider reducing the extent of dissection to the areas of greatest risk, especially if stage I patients are undergoing primary surgery.

We discovered that the nerves are predictably situated and that dissection of nodal disease can be complete with nerve preservation even in patients with advanced disease. The anatomic limits of dissection are the ureters laterally, 1 to 2 cm above the renal arteries superiorly, and to the bifurcation of the common iliac arteries (including the aortic bifurcation) inferiorly (Fig. 37.1). Posteriorly, the anterior spinal ligament and psoas muscles are skeletonized. Attempts to preserve some of the lumbar arteries and the inferior mesenteric artery should be made.

A vertical incision is made from the xiphisternum to a point midway between the umbilicus and the pubis to enter the peritoneal cavity. The small bowel and right hemicolon are mobilized into a bowel bag by incising the retroperitoneum across

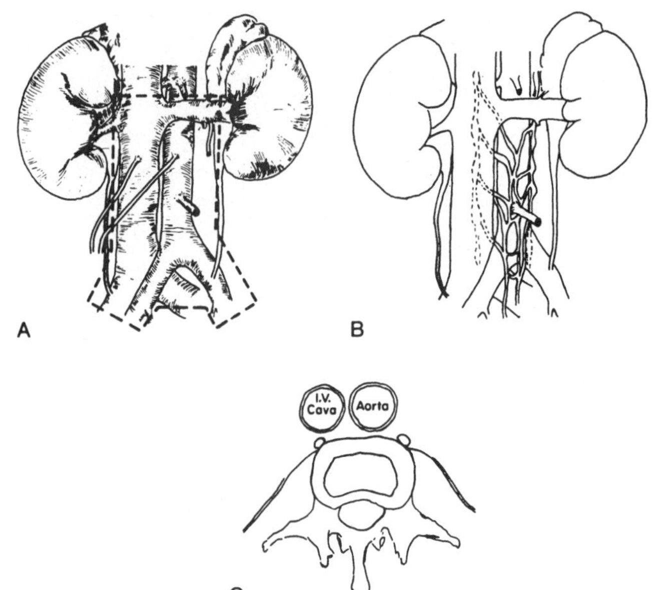

Fig. 37.1. **(A)** Surgical boundaries of bilateral retroperitoneal lymphadenectomy. **(B)** Lumbar sympathetic chain and postganglionic fibers forming the superior hypogastric plexus. **(C)** Cross-section of the sympathetic trunks in relation to the psoas muscles, vertebral bodies, and great vessels.

the root of the mesentery and around the cecum (Fig. 37.2). The inferior mesenteric vein may be divided, and the bowel bag is placed on the patient's chest. This exposes the retroperineum without the volume of the small bowel in the way.

Dissection is then begun by incising the retroperitoneal tissue in the midline anterior to the IVC. The left side of the cava is exposed, including the distal left renal vein to its origin up to the left common iliac vein, by peeling the adipose and lymphatic tissue medially (Fig. 37.3A). Care should be taken to cauterize or ligate small vessels. The IVC is carefully rolled to the right with ligation and division of the left lumbar veins as required (Fig. 37.3B). The right sympathetic chain lies posterior to the midline of the cava immediately to the right of the ligated left lumbar veins, which serve as markers for the ganglia. From the fusiform ganglia, fine nerve fibers can be seen coursing anteromedially and inferiorly to the right side of the aorta on the surface of the nodal tissue. These fibers are the lumbar splanchnic nerves and can be individually skeletonized from the underlying interaortocaval lymphatic tissue, which is ultimately mobilized posteriorly from the anterior spinal ligament and withdrawn inferiorly leaving the web of sympathetic nerves.

Before proceeding further, the left ureter is visualized by creating a plane across the midline anterior to the retroperitoneal lymphatic tissue but behind the inferior mesenteric artery, mesocolic fat, and other soft tissues. This dissection may require division of the inferior mesenteric artery, but it should be 1 or more cm distal to its origin to avoid nerve injury. The left ureter can be exposed up to the perinephric tissue, visualizing the left psoas muscle and leaving the left paraaortic retroperito-

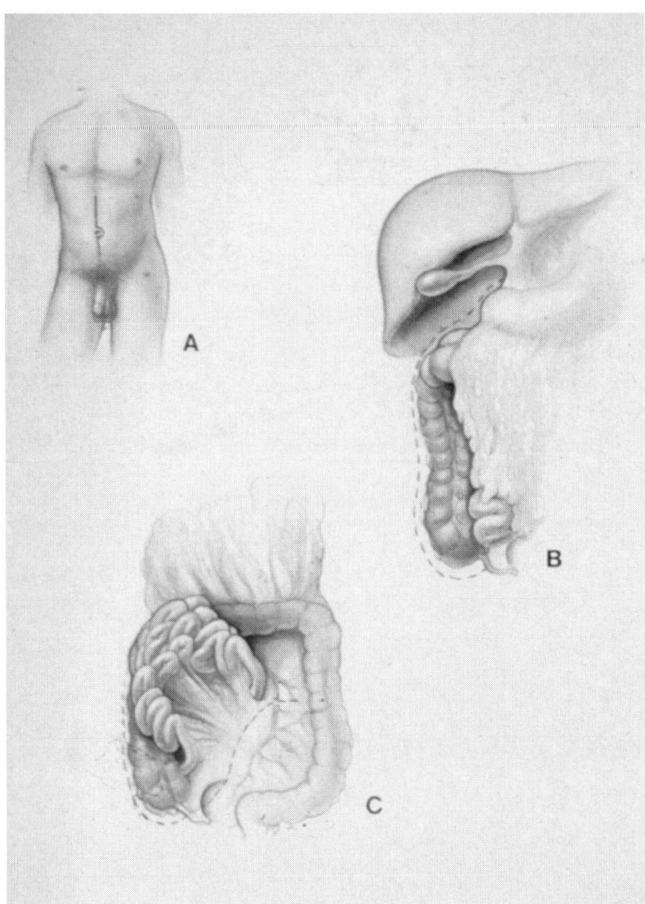

Fig. 37.2. **(A)** Retroperitoneal lymphadenectomy is performed through a midline abdominal incision from xiphoid process to midlower abdomen. **(B)** The hepatic flexure is taken down, followed by incision of the posterior peritoneum along the right colic gutter to the cecum. **(C)** The right colon is mobilized and the rest of the small bowel mesentery incised cephalad to the ligament of Treitz.

neal adipose tissue containing the lymph nodes intact. This bulk of tissue is carefully reflected medially on the anterior surface of the psoas to expose the left sympathetic chain (Fig. 37.3C). The lumbar vessels on the left are identified with this dissection as they pass medial to the sympathetic chain. Again, as with the right-sided vessels, they occasionally are lateral or bifurcate around the chain. These vessels can be sacrificed as needed. The lumbar splanchnic nerves are identified originating from the sympathetic ganglia coursing medially and anteriorly onto the side of the aorta. Superiorly, there may be a branch anterior to the renal artery coming from a higher ganglia but this is difficult to preserve.

At this point the surgeon has a sense of the patient's sympathetic anatomy, which is variable. It is useful to electrostimulate the nerves and observe their role by flexible cystoscopic observation of the bladder neck and seminal emission, by abdominal ultrasonography to visualize the vesicles contract, or by measuring the bladder neck contract urodynamically.

The aorta can now be exposed in the midline by fully mobi-lizing the left renal vein and by splitting the soft tissue over it. Dissection is carried close to the aorta. The individual sympathetic nerve branches, having been identified on both right and left sides from preceding dissection, are seen on the anterior and lateral surfaces of the aorta. They are further skeletonized, taking care to preserve those branches that form variable plexuses on the anterior aorta (Fig. 37.4). This allows withdrawal of the interaortocaval lymphatic tissue and the left paraaortic tissue from between the anterior spinal ligament posteriorly and the nerves anteriorly. The plexus at and below the level of the inferior mesenteric artery condenses to form the two hypogastric nerves that pass over the aorta and proceed inferiorly into the pelvis. Identification and preservation of these two nerves allow all lymphatic tissue over the aortic bifurcation and common iliac veins down to the sacral promontory to be removed without sacrificing ejaculation (Fig. 37.5). Inferiorly, it is our practice to limit the dissection to the bifurcation of the common iliac arteries.

The remnant of the spermatic cord is removed ipsilaterally with as much of the vas deferens as is easily removable. This is important, especially in postchemotherapy cases where metastases may be present along the cord at the pelvic brim.

Frequently, nodal metastases or tumor masses are immediately adjacent to or involve nerves. It is unnecessary to preserve all postganglionic nerves to ensure ejaculation. Therefore, the surgeon should not hesitate to sacrifice nerves unilaterally or even in a limited manner bilaterally to ensure complete removal of disease. The use of intraoperative electrostimulation is helpful (17).

RPL Complications and Their Management

There is potential for a number of serious complications with RPL. Fortunately, most are preventable with attention to detail and experience. The complications have been well described (36–38). The major complications include vascular injury to the renal vessels and lacerations of the great vessels, particularly during surgery for residual masses after chemotherapy that may require prosthetic replacement of the vessels. Intraoperative topical application of papaverine to the renal arteries and care with retraction prevents severe spasm and intimal injury with thrombosis. The right renal artery is at risk during dissection between the great vessels, particularly with lower pole accessory vessels or lower level takeoff of the main artery. Intraoperative recognition and prompt repair are necessary if injury does occur. Preservation of renal function is advisable because nephrotoxic chemotherapy or excretion of chemotherapeutic agents may be necessary.

Small bowel obstruction can be minimized by reapproximating the retroperitoneum intraoperatively. Ureteral injury should not occur, but they are the lateral limits of dissection and the right ureter may be tented up during the mobilization of the right hemicolon during the exposure.

Incisional hernia seems to be more likely to occur with long incisions in young men who have active lifestyles if great care

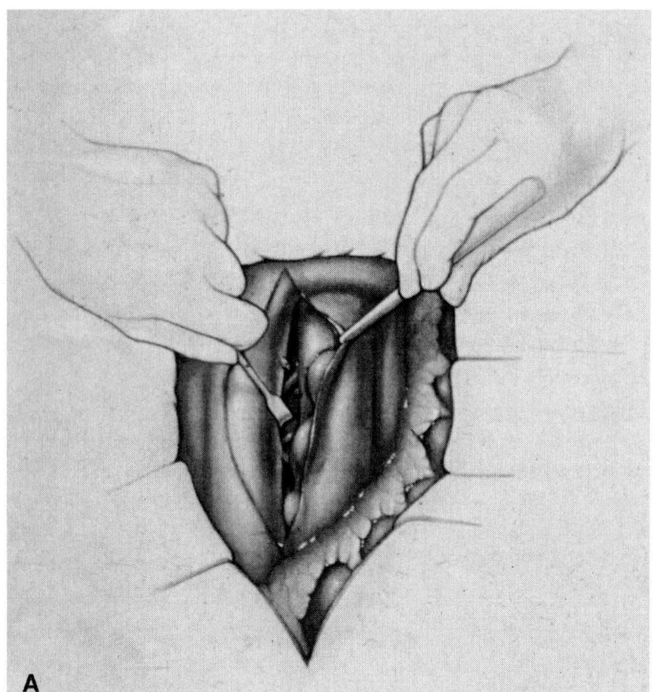

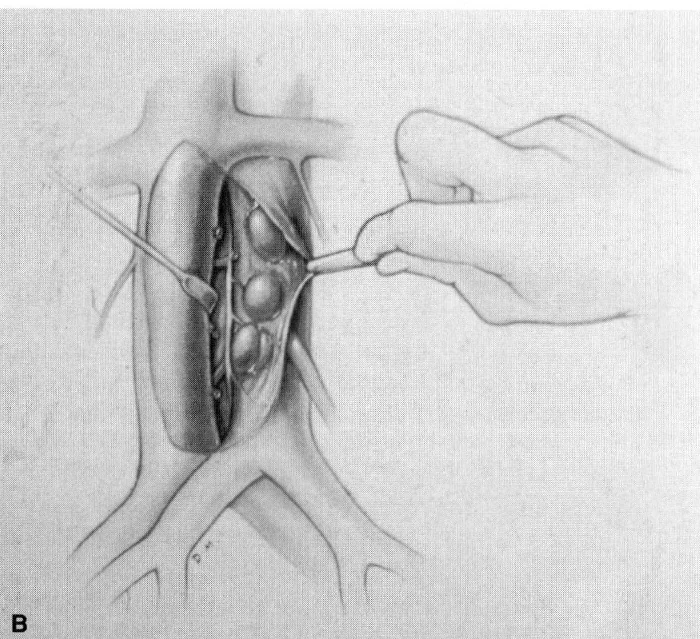

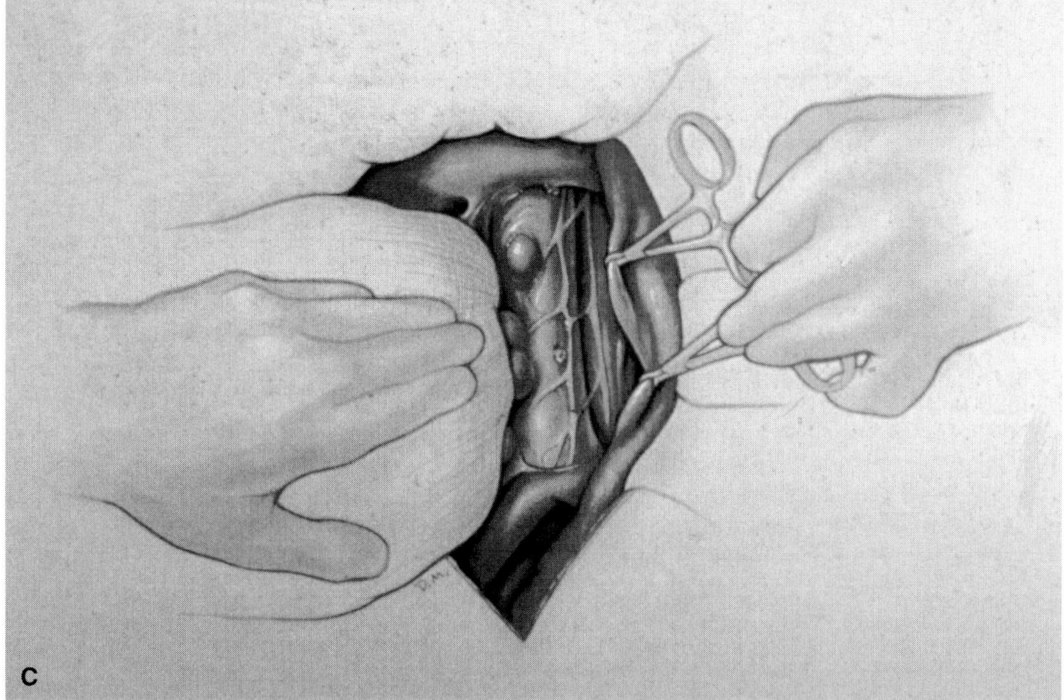

Fig. 37.3. **(A)** Dissection is begun by incising the retroperitoneal tissue in the midline anterior to the inferior vena cava. **(B)** The inferior vena cava is rolled laterally with ligation and division of the left lumbar veins as required. **(C)** A plane is created across the midline anterior to the retroperitoneal lymphatic tissue but behind the inferior mesenteric artery and associated soft tissue. The left ureter is exposed to reveal the left psoas muscle. The left paraaortic retroperitoneal tissue is then reflected medially to expose the left sympathetic chain.

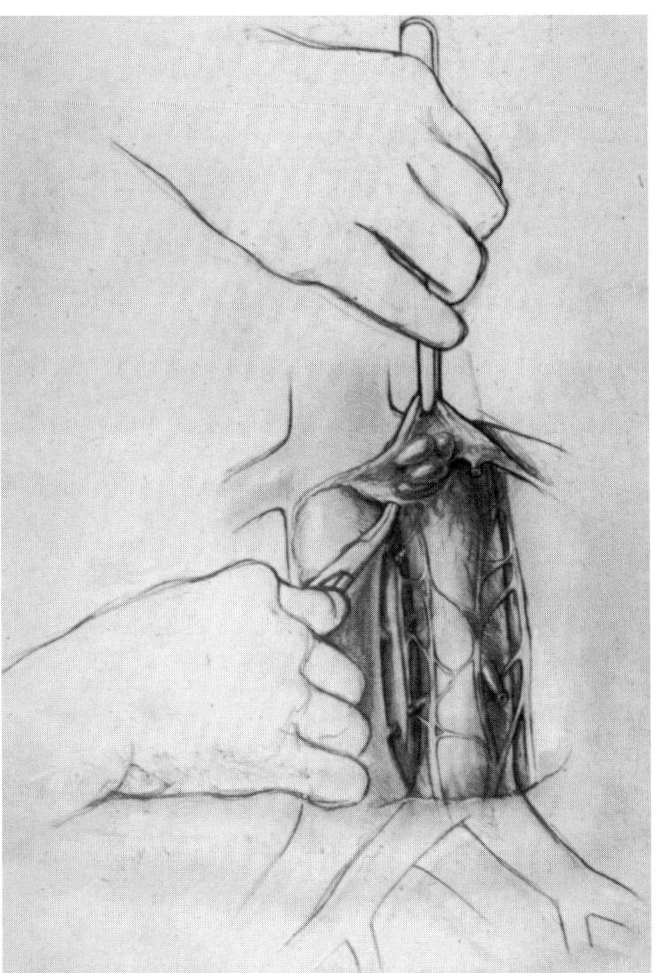

Fig. 37.4. After exposure of the sympathetic chains and the origin of the postganglionic fibers, the aorta is exposed in the midline at the level of the left renal vein.

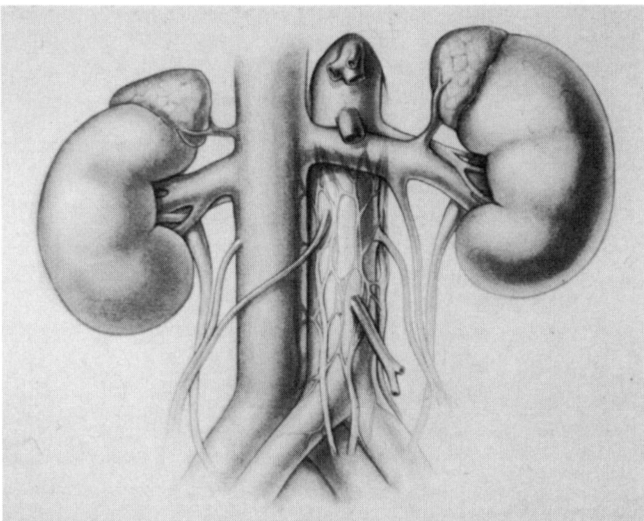

Fig. 37.5. After removal of the interaortocaval, left paraaortic, and pre-aortic lymphatic and adipose tissue, the retroperitoneum is clear, with the postganglionic sympathetic nerve completely skeletonized.

is not taken in closure. The usual acute problems of wound infection, hematoma, prolonged ileus, and atelectasis may be seen. Wounds are not usually drained. A nasogastric tube is left in, especially when the bowel has been isolated in a bowel bag for several hours.

The complication rates have not been clearly increased by increased stage of disease, except for the potential for bleomycin-associated lung toxicity (fibrosis and diffusion defects) in patients pretreated with chemotherapy. These patients are closely managed intraoperatively with lower fluid volume replacement and oxygen concentrations. Postoperatively, oxygen above room air concentrations should be avoided, and fluid replacement should keep patients slightly dry.

Mortality with RPL is now extremely rare and limited to patients who have been heavily pretreated.

REFERENCES

1. Heritz DM, Jewett MAS. The evolving role for retroperitoneal lymphadenectomy. Prob Urol 1994;8:118.
2. Williams SD, Stablein DM, Einhorn LH, et al. Immediate adjuvant chemotherapy versus observation with treatment at relapse in pathological stage II testicular cancer. N Engl J Med 1987;317:1433.
3. Sternberg CN. Role of primary chemotherapy in stage I and low-volume stage II nonseminomatous germ-cell testis tumors. Urol Clin North Am 1993;20:93.
4. Ray B, Hajdu SI, Whitmore WFJ. Lymph node metastases in testicular germinal tumors. Cancer 1974;33:340.
5. Donohue JP, Maynard B, Zachary M. The distribution of nodal metastases in the retroperitoneum from nonseminomatous testis cancer. J Urol 1982;128:315.
6. Sturgeon JF, Jewett MA, Alison RE, et al. Surveillance after orchidectomy for patients with clinical stage I nonseminomatous testis tumors. J Clin Oncol 1992;10:564.
7. Wischnow KI, Johnson DE, Tenney D. Are lymphangiograms necessary before placing patients with non-seminomatous testicular tumors on surveillance? J Urol 1984;141:1133.
8. Weissbach L, Boedefeld EA. Localization of solitary and multiple metastases in stage II nonseminomatous testis tumor as basis for a modified staging lymph node dissection in stage I. J Urol 1987;138:77.
9. Einhorn LH, Donohue JP. Improved chemotherapy in disseminated testicular cancer. J Urol 1977;117:65.
10. Samuels ML, Holoye PY, Johnson DE. Bleomycin combination chemotherapy in the management of testicular neoplasia. Cancer 1975;36:318.
11. Read G, Stenning SP, Cullen MH, et al. Medical Research Council prospective study of surveillance for stage I testicular teratoma. J Clin Oncol 1992;10:1762.
12. Lange PH, Chang WY, Fraley EE. Fertility issues in the therapy of nonseminomatous testicular tumors. Urol Clin North Am 1987;14:731.
13. Jewett MA, Kong YS, Goldberg SD, et al. Retroperitoneal lymphadenectomy for testis tumor with nerve-sparing for ejaculation. J Urol 1988;139:1220.
14. Colleselli K, Poisel S, Schachtner W, et al. Nerve-preserving

bilateral retroperitoneal lymphadenectomy: anatomical study and operative approach. J Urol 1990;144:293.

15. Donohue JP, Thornhill JA, Foster RS, et al. Retroperitoneal lymphadenectomy for clinical stage A testis cancer (1965–1989): modifications of technique and impact on ejaculation. J Urol 1993;149:237.

16. Donohue JP, Thornhill JA, Foster RS, et al. The role of retroperitoneal lymphadenectomy in clinical stage B testis cancer: the Indiana University experience (1965–1989). J Urol 1995;153:85.

17. Dieckmann KP, Huland H, Gross AJ. A test for the identification of relevant sympathetic nerve fibers during nerve-sparing retroperitoneal lymphadenectomy. J Urol 1992; 148:1450.

18. Staubitz WJ, Early KS, Magoss IV, et al. Surgical management of testis tumors. J Urol 1976;111:205.

19. Peckham MJ, Barrett A, Husband JE, et al. Orchidectomy alone in testicular stage I nonseminomatous germ cell tumours. Lancet 1982;2:678.

20. Donohue JP, Thornhill JA, Foster RA, et al. Primary retroperitoneal lymph node dissection in clinical stage A nonseminomatous germ cell testis cancer. Br J Urol 1993;71:326.

21. Klotz L. Laparoscopic retroperitoneal lymphadenectomy for high-risk stage 1 nonseminomatous germ cell tumor: report of four cases. Urology 1994;43:752.

22. Gerber GS, Bissada NK, Hulbert JC, et al. Laparoscopic retroperitoneal lymphadenectomy: multi-institutional analysis. J Urol 1994;152:1188. Discussion 1191.

23. Hartlapp JH, Weissbach L, Bussar-Maatz R. Adjuvant chemotherapy in nonseminomatous testicular tumour stage II. Int J Androl 1987;10:277.

24. Pizzocaro G, Monfardini S. No adjuvant chemotherapy in selected patients with pathologic stage II nonseminomatous germ cell tumors of the testis. J Urol 1984;131:677.

25. Richie JP, Kantoff PW. Is adjuvant chemotherapy necessary for patients with stage B1 testicular cancer? J Clin Oncol 1991;9:1393.

26. Motzer RJ. Adjuvant chemotherapy for stage II nonseminomatous testis cancer; what is its role. Semin Urol Oncol. In press.

27. Rorth M, Jacobsen GK, von der Maase H, et al. Surveillance alone versus radiotherapy after orchiectomy for clinical stage I nonseminomatous testicular cancer. Danish Testicular Cancer Study Group. J Clin Oncol 1991;9:1543.

28. Horwich A, Norman A, Fisher C, et al. Primary chemotherapy for stage II nonseminomatous germ cell tumors of the testis. J Urol 1994;151:72. Discussion 77.

29. Baniel J, Foster RS, Gonin R, et al. Late relapse of testicular cancer. J Clin Oncol 1995;13:1170.

30. Bokemeyer C, Schmoll HJ. Treatment of testicular cancer and the development of secondary malignancies. J Clin Oncol 1995;13:283.

31. Travis LB, Curtis RE, Hankey BF. Second malignancies after testicular cancer. J Clin Oncol 1995;13:533. Letter.

32. Toner GC, Panicek DM, Heelan RT, et al. Adjunctive surgery after chemotherapy for nonseminomatous germ cell tumors: recommendations for patient selection. J Clin Oncol 1990;8: 1683.

33. Steyerberg EW, Keizer HJ, Fossa SD, et al. Prediction of residual retroperitoneal mass histology after chemotherapy for metastatic nonseminomatous germ cell tumor: multivariate analysis of individual patient data from six study groups. J Clin Oncol 1995;13:1177.

34. Herr HW, Toner GC, Geller NL, et al. Patient selection for retroperitoneal lymph node dissection after chemotherapy for nonseminomatous germ cell tumors. Eur Urol 1991;19:1.

35. Jewett MA. Nerve-sparing technique for retroperitoneal lymphadenectomy in testis cancer. Urol Clin North Am 1990; 17:449.

36. Baniel J, Foster RS, Rowland RG, et al. Complications of primary retroperitoneal lymph-node dissection for low-stage testicular cancer. World J Urol 1994;12:139.

37. Jewett MAS, Wesley-James T. Early and late complications of retroperitoneal lymphadenectomy. Can J Surg 1991;34:368.

38. Donohue JP, Rowland RG. Complications of retroperitoneal lymph node dissection. J Urol 1981;13:338.

PENIS AND URETHRA

Penile and Urethral Carcinoma

An Overview

Byron D. Joyner and W. Scott McDougal

PENILE CARCINOMA

History

Nearly 2 millennia ago, Celsus reported a case of amputation of the penis followed by cautery of the penile stump. This is clearly one of the earliest references to the management of penile cancer (1). The Egyptians, Hebrews, Persians, and Indians were also familiar with this disease entity, as they mentioned it in their writings (2). In 1761, the anatomist Morgagni described, in amusing detail, a partial penectomy performed by Valsalva (3). Thiersch, in 1875, is credited with the first radical extirpative cure of carcinoma of the penis (4). The concept of removing the lymph nodes for malignancy was given impetus in 1886 by Sir William MacCormack who reported on five cases whereby total penectomy was performed with bilateral inguinal lymphadenectomy (5). This concept was further championed by Curtis (1898) who performed similar en bloc operations as those performed by MacCormack (6). Fourteen years later, in 1912, Gibson improved on this technique by providing the patient control of his urinary stream through manipulation of the scrotum (7).

In 1924, Barringer and Dean described an innovative, tissue-sparing technique of partial amputation of the penis, 1.5 cm proximal to the lesion, followed by radiation therapy to the groin (8). This allowed the patient to stand while voiding and afforded him a better body image. In 1907, Hugh Hampton Young began performing partial penectomy in association with unilateral groin dissection, a procedure he formally reported in 1931 (9). He included femoral nodes in addition to the inguinal nodes in this en bloc dissection.

In 1948, Daseler et al. described in detail the anatomical lymph node drainage of the penis based on 450 cadaveric dissections (10). Boronofsky, 5 years later, described the technique of a sartorius muscle flap to cover the femoral vessels that are exposed during ilioinguinal lymphadenectomy (11).

In 1977, Cabanas capitalized on Daseler's work by describing the "sentinel lymph node," located superomedial to the junction of the epigastric and saphenous veins (12). The hypothesis suggested that this node was the first echelon of metastatic disease of invasive penile cancer. If this node was sampled and if the results were negative, then a complete node dissection could be avoided. This new idea challenged the old school of thought and hoped to minimize the well-known morbidity in ilioinguinal lymphadenectomies. Cabanas's hypothesis was controversial then and still remains so, as do many aspects of the management of penile cancer.

Epidemiology

Cancer of the penis is rare. It constitutes less than 1% of all male malignancies in the United States. It occurs most commonly in the sixth and seventh decades of life, with an age range of 20 to 90 years (13, 14). One report that combines several large series of penile cancer cites a mean age of 58 years at presentation (15). Children have been known to have carcinoma of the penis but this is vanishingly rare (16).

Circumcision is the only known prophylaxis against carcinoma of the penis. This fact only comes from indirect observations. For example, in the Jewish population in which ritualistic neonatal circumcision is performed, carcinoma of the penis is virtually unknown. Carcinoma of the penis in the Jewish population is so rare that any occurrence warrants skepticism (17). There are only 10 documented cases of carcinoma of the penis in men who have been circumcised as infants.

Although circumcision at birth is protective against penile carcinoma, circumcision at a later time has less protective advantage. As an example, the Muslims who practice prepubertal circumcision have a slightly higher incidence of carcinoma of the penis when compared with the Jewish population. However, the incidence of carcinoma of the penis in Muslims does not approach that of uncircumcised age-matched controls. Relative to men circumcised at birth, the risk of penile cancer was 3.2 times greater among men who were never circumcised and 3.0 times greater among men who were circumcised after the neonatal period (18). Some period of exposure to smegma, however brief, may account for the decreased protective effect of postnatal circumcision (19).

Circumcision is not practiced as widely in Asia and Africa where the incidence of carcinoma of the penis is between 10 and 20% of all male malignancies (20). One example of the prophylactic effects of circumcision is that reported by Dodge and Linsell of two African tribes in Uganda (21). The Gisu tribe, which practices circumcision, has a dramatically lower incidence of penile carcinoma than that of its neighboring tribe that does not perform ritualistic circumcision.

Schrek and Lenowitz demonstrated that penile cancer has no racial predisposition. They concluded that there were probably more uncircumcised black males compared with their white counterparts (22).

It is thought, but not proven, that smegma (the by-product of the action of *Mycobacterium smegmatis* on desquamated cells) causes chronic irritation within the preputial sac (23). Perhaps it is this chronic irritation that leads to a degeneration of normal cells into cancer cells. The incidence of penile carcinoma in situ degenerating into invasive carcinoma is unknown. It is no wonder then that the most common location of carcinoma of the penis is on the glans (48%) and preputial skin (21%) (24).

Sexually transmitted diseases have long been incriminated as a causative agent in penile cancer. However, there have been several confounding factors such as low socioeconomic status, low circumcision rates, and poor hygiene (25). Recently, viral etiologies have been reported in the literature linking the venereal human papilloma viruses indirectly with squamous cell carcinoma of the penis. More recent direct studies using polymerase chain reaction have yielded strong support for an etiologic role of human papilloma virus 16 in squamous cell carcinoma of the penis (26, 27). Herpes simplex virus has been associated with penile carcinoma and cervical carcinoma. There is a three- to eight-fold increase in the incidence of cervical carcinoma among the sexual partners of males with penile carcinomas (28).

Anatomy

The penis is composed of three bodies of cavernous tissue that are bound together by the fascia penis. The glans penis is an extension of the corpus spongiosum and is covered by the preputial envelope, an extension of the phallic skin.

Arterial blood supply to the penis is derived from the internal pudendal artery, a terminal branch of the hypogastric artery. When the internal pudendal artery passes through the urogenital diaphragm it becomes the penile artery, which subsequently divides into three branches—the bulbourethral artery, cavernosal artery, and dorsal penile artery.

Aboseif et al. identified three separate drainage systems of the penis—superficial, intermediate, and deep veins (29). The superficial dorsal vein drains the skin of the dorsal penis and preputial skin, but not the glans. The intermediate drainage system is composed of the circumflex veins and the deep dorsal veins. The deep venous system provides the primary run-off for the corpora cavernosa.

Lymphatic Drainage

The fact that the primary lymphatic drainage of the penis is via the superficial inguinal nodes has been known since 1886, when MacCormack described five cases of epithelioma of the penis (5). In 1901, Brezna described the lymphatic drainage of the penis. But, it was Rouviere's review of 38 years of work that was most comprehensive (30).

Rouviere divided the lymphatic drainage of the penis into two main nodal systems—superficial and deep. The superficial system drains the cutaneous envelope while the deep system drains the glans and the erectile bodies. The deep nodal system, in turn, drains into the deep pelvic nodes. Rouviere simplified the lymphatic drainage of the penis, but, in reality, the lymphatic drainage is quite unpredictable with multiple and complex cross-communications.

In 1948, 10 years after Rouviere's review, Daseler described the inguinal and iliac inguinal nodes based on detailed dissection of 450 cadaveric groin dissections (10). He described a quadrilateral area that defined the boundaries of the superficial inguinal nodes. He further divided this quadrilateral area into five zones—the superolateral, superomedial, inferomedial, inferolateral, and central zones. Penile lymphatics drain primarily to the central and the two medial zones.

Even with all these attempts to define the lymphatic drainage of the penis, it is still not a static system and the drainage from each of the areas of the penis varies in number, location, intercommunication, and pathway. For example, between 4 and 10 lymphatic vessels travel from the prepuce to the penile root, in conjunction with dorsal lymphatics, and from there the lymphatics from the penile skin variably bifurcate to the left and right. The unpredictable lymphatic drainage is the primary reason for the false-negative rate observed in Cabanas's controversial sentinel node theory. There is no definitive pattern to the lymphatic drainage of the penis.

Premalignant Cutaneous Lesions

Verrucous carcinoma

Verrucous carcinoma of the penis, also referred to as giant condyloma of Buschke-Lowenstein, is an unusual and rare cancer, accounting for approximately 8 to 16% of all penile cancers (31). In 1948, Akerman (32) first described this entity in the oral cavity and larynx. Its first appearance in the literature with regard to the penis is debatable. The lesion, a slowly evolving tumor that has relentless expanding potential, occurs primarily on the glans and prepuce of the penis. Although it is often known as a variant of squamous cell carcinoma, it has a low metastatic potential of 10%, which some reports have ascribed to tumor hybrids. These are minute foci of invasive squamous cell carcinoma coexisting within the larger verrucous carcinoma (33, 34). These foci apparently give the verrucous carcinoma its metastatic potential.

Therapy for verrucous carcinoma of the distal penis is partial penectomy. If the lesion involves the base or shaft, so that partial penectomy would not allow for a penile length adequate to allow the patient to stand to direct his urine stream, then total penectomy with perineal urethrostomy should be performed. Conservative treatments such as cryosurgery, laser surgery, Mohs' surgery, and topical chemotherapeutic agents tend to be controversial but might be appropriate. The rarity of metastasis from verrucous carcinoma of the penis argues against prophylactic ilioinguinal lymphadenectomy or sentinel lymph node biopsy. However, any clinically suspicious nodes would warrant excisional biopsy.

Carcinoma in situ

Bowen's disease. Bowen's disease was initially described as extrapenile lesions in 1912 (35). It is characterized by slightly elevated and papular lesions with a firm consistency and a dull red color. If found on the shaft or at the base of the penis, then the lesion is referred to as Bowen's disease. Because the lesion typically involves hair follicles, topical local therapy is not recommended. The standard form of therapy is surgical excision or Mohs' operation.

Erythroplasia of queyrat. Described by Queyrat in 1911 (35), erythroplasia of Queyrat is a variant of carcinoma in situ and often confused with Bowen's disease. The two lesions are histologically identical. However, erythroplasia of Queyrat occurs on the preputial envelope and the glans penis, and Bowen's disease occurs on the penile shaft. Unlike Bowen's disease, erythroplasia of Queyrat might be managed with topical 5-fluorouracil, which has a long-term efficacy in preventing recurrences (36). For glandular lesions that do not respond to topical 5-fluorouracil, Mohs' operation might be helpful. Laser surgery also has proven efficacy (37). In all cases of erythroplasia of Queyrat, circumcision should be performed to remove the preputial sac and the smegma factor.

Balanitis Xerotica Obliterans

Balanitis xerotica obliterans (BXO) is a localized form of lichen sclerosis et atrophicus. Once thought to be a rare entity, it was found to occur routinely in the preputial skin of men circumcised for phimosis (38). It is characterized by a white cicatricial patch on the prepuce extending to and around the urethral meatus, often resulting in meatal stenosis. The lesion occurs in both circumcised and uncircumcised men but occurs more commonly in the latter (39). Diagnosis is confirmed by biopsy that demonstrates atrophic epidermis with loss of rete pegs, a homogenization of the collagen on the upper third of the dermis, and a zone of lymphocytic and histiocytic infiltration. Rare reports have associated BXO with squamous cell carcinoma (40, 41).

Treatment consists of topical steroid cream. If this initial treatment fails, then local excision is recommended. In all cases where foreskin is present, circumcision should be performed. Meatotomy or meatoplasty might be required for cases of meatal stenosis. Close follow-up is suggested.

Leukoplakia

Leukoplakia is similar in appearance to BXO, lichen planus, and candidiasis. It forms in white patches, usually around the glans or involving the meatus. Histologic examination reveals hyperkeratosis, parakeratosis, and lymphocytic infiltration. Treatment consists of circumcision in uncircumcised men. Bleomycin has been efficacious for large lesions (42).

Kaposi's Sarcoma

Approximately 18% of patients with acquired immunodeficiency syndrome with Kaposi's sarcoma will manifest this lesion on the penis or genitalia. Grossly, the appearance is that of a violaceous induration for which conservative therapy is recommended, including radiation and laser therapies (43).

Staging

The most commonly used staging system for penile cancer is that proposed by Jackson (44), which is largely a clinical staging system (Table 38.1). It does not take into account the characteristics of the presenting penile lesion or the description of the nodal burden. The second most commonly used staging system for penile cancer is the TNM system. It is an improvement on Jackson's system in that it provides a better idea of the depth of invasion (Table 38.2). However, the TNM staging system does not address differentiation of the primary lesion nor does it provide a useful classification for determining the necessity of regional therapy. Staging biases have developed although neither of the staging systems is perfect. As a result, early investigators have used the systems indiscriminately without universal agreement. Consequently, many of the studies

Table 38.1. Jackson Staging System for Penile Cancer (44)

Stage I	Tumor limited to glans and prepuce
Stage II	Invasion into penile shaft or corpora
Stage III	Proven operable regional (inguinal) lymph node metastasis
Stage IV	Tumor invading adjacent structures, inoperable regional lymph node metastasis, or distant metastasis

Table 38.2.   American Joint Committee Staging System for Penile Cancer

T0	No primary tumor
Tis	Carcinoma in situ
Ta	Noninvasive verrucous carcinoma
T1	Tumor invades subepithelial connective tissue
T2	Tumor invades corpus spongiosum or cavernosum
T3	Tumor invades urethra or prostate
T4	Tumor invades other adjacent structures
N0	No nodal metastasis
N1	Metastasis in a single, superficial inguinal node
N2	Metastases in multiple superficial inguinal nodes
N3	Metastasis in deep inguinal or pelvic lymph node(s)
M0	No distant metastasis
M1	Distant metastasis

From Beahrs OH, Henson DE, Hutter RVP, et al. Manual for staging of cancer. 3rd ed. Philadelphia: JB Lippincott, 1988.

are flawed; for example, they have neglected to distinguish between superficial and invasive primary penile cancer (45, 46).

Therefore, we have modified the Jackson staging system to reflect current therapy (47). The modified system appropriately provides the ability to predict, with reasonable certainty, the likelihood of positive regional lymph nodes. Therefore, it offers a more rational approach to management of squamous cell carcinoma of the penis. The modified staging system is outlined in Table 38.3.

Survival

Inguinal metastasis influences the prognosis of carcinoma of the penis more than any other factor, including tumor grade, gross appearance, or morphologic and microscopic tumor burden. With this in mind, it is important to be able to predict which patient will have regionally metastatic disease. Survival and the likelihood of regional spread are correlated with the degree of differentiation of the primary tumor and depth of invasion. The prognosis for patients with carcinoma of the penis is significantly worsened by the presence of inguinal metastases, which is, in turn, directly related to the differentiation of the

Table 38.3.   Modified Staging System for Penile Carcinoma (47)

Stage I	Superficial, does not extend into the subcutaneous tissue; well differentiated
Stage IIA	Locally invasive without involvement of the corpora spongiosum or corpora cavernosum; well or moderately differentiated
Stage IIB	Invasion to the corpus spongiosum and/or poorly differentiated
Stage III	Palpable inguinal nodes that persist after 6 weeks of antibiotics
Stage IV	Inoperable groin nodes, iliac node involvement, distant metastases

tumor, i.e., well, moderately, or poorly differentiated. The prognostic significance of differentiation is evident by the reported progression rates to regional lymphatic involvement of 82% in poorly differentiated, 46% in moderately differentiated, and 24% in well-differentiated primary lesions (48).

Management

Cancer of the penis is a surgically curable disease. The gold standard for invasive squamous cell carcinoma of the penis is partial or total penectomy. There is no controversy about whether the primary squamous cell carcinoma of the penis should be excised.

The Primary Tumor

A biopsy of the penile lesion is the cornerstone of making the diagnosis of penile cancer. This histologically confirms the diagnosis and assesses the grade and stage of the tumor. A 1-cm, elliptical, wedge-shaped biopsy specimen is removed and should include normal tissue to check for invasion. Approximation of the wound is performed using 3-0 chromic suture.

Therapeutic Options

There are various therapeutic options after the diagnosis of penile cancer has been confirmed. These include topical chemotherapy, radiation therapy, laser (carbon dioxide or Nd:YAG) therapy, and cryosurgery. Mohs' micrographic surgery (MMS), introduced in 1941 by Frederic Mohs, is a technique of excising neoplasm microscopically and examining the underside of the tissue layer by layer to determine the extent of tumor. This technique controls silent, unpredictable "extensions" of penile cancer and assures eradication of the neoplasm while maximally sparing adjacent normal tissue. Respectable 5-year cure rates of 74% have been achieved by Mohs et al. (49). These results are comparable to the more radical surgical techniques (50).

Systemic chemotherapy with cisplatin, bleomycin, vincristine, and methotrexate as single-agent therapies have modest antitumor activity. Pizzocaro and Diva (51) reported preliminary data that multiagent chemotherapy may play a role in metastatic squamous cell carcinoma of the penis and urethra. Adjuvant chemotherapy in the management of metastatic penile and urethral carcinomas has yet to be defined.

These therapeutic options offer less-mutilating therapies. However, if the lesion is invasive, complete excision of the primary tumor with adequate surgical margins free of tumor gives the best chance of cure with the least likelihood of local recurrence.

Regional Lymphadenectomy

Very few would argue for a regional lymphadenectomy in patients with stage I disease. Indeed, local excision alone carries a 95 to 100% cure rate. Conversely, few would also argue with the necessity for a regional lymphadenectomy in stage III disease. The 5-year survival rate without lymphadenectomy in this group approaches 0% (52), with lymphadenectomy, it ranges between 30 and 66% (53).

Even when metastatic to regional lymph nodes, cancer of the penis is one of the few diseases that can be cured by regional lymphadenectomy. The cure rate for inguinal lymphadenectomy, when nodes are positive for malignancy, may be as high as 80%. A cure rate of this magnitude with surgery in the face of regional nodal metastases parallels the experience with testicular carcinoma, in which surgical monotherapy results in a cure in a significant number of node-positive patients. This is not true with other genitourinary malignancies (e.g., the bladder, prostate, or kidney, in which node-positive patients have a dismal cure rate). Why then is there any discussion concerning ilioinguinal lymph node dissection for treatment of penile cancer when the potential for a cure is extraordinarily substantial?

The problem arises from the significant morbidity of the inguinal node dissection in contrast to the limited morbidity of retroperitoneal and pelvic lymphadenectomy for the other genitourinary tumors, namely testicular and prostate.

The controversy exists in patients with an invasive primary lesion who have palpably negative regional lymph nodes (stage II). Should the practitioner proceed with a regional lymphadenectomy immediately or carefully follow the patient and, if nodes appear, perform a ("delayed") lymphadenectomy at that time? In those patients in whom a delayed lymphadenectomy is performed, 8 to 42% survive 5 years (52, 54). If a regional lymphadenectomy is performed immediately in a patient with nonpalpable nodes and microscopic metastases are found pathologically, 84% will survive 5 years. Thus, the cure rate is much better if regional disease is removed when microscopic rather than palpable (52).

Therefore, we strongly advise performing an immediate regional lymphadenectomy in patients with stage IIB disease (47). In this group, the likelihood of pathologically positive nodes is high and offsets the morbidity to those who would undergo the procedure for no benefit, i.e., those with negative nodes. Moreover, complications of groin dissection are much less common in those undergoing a lymphadenectomy for microscopic disease versus delayed dissection for nodes that are palpably positive at a later date (55).

For patients with stage III disease in whom nodes are palpably positive, 70% will have pathologically positive nodes (54). Thus, the morbidity of lymphadenectomy is well justified in patients with palpable adenopathy that persists after excision of the primary lesion and a subsequent course of 6 weeks of antibiotic therapy. Because there is also such a high probability of regional spread in stage IIB disease (in excess of 60%), it is advised to perform bilateral regional lymphadenectomy in all patients with stages IIB and III disease. If the nodes are positive, an iliac lymphadenectomy is also performed on the ipsilateral side, realizing that if positive this will result in only an occasional 5-year survival.

Extent of Regional Lymphadenectomy

As previously described, there is considerable crossover of lymphatics. For this reason, if one groin is involved, there is a 60% chance of metastasis to the opposite groin (56). The iliac nodes are unlikely to be involved if the groin nodes are negative (53). Recurrences after a groin dissection portend a poor prognosis and are very difficult to manage.

With these facts in mind, it has been our practice to perform a regional lymphadenectomy bilaterally. We do not limit it to the superficial nodes, but include both superficial and deep nodes. This reduces the risk of local groin recurrence from that which would occur if only a superficial dissection were performed. If the groin is positive, then an iliac node dissection is performed on the side of positivity.

URETHRAL CARCINOMA

History

The first documented case of urethral carcinoma was apparently that of a young man who had a small lesion of the urethra. This case was reported by Thiaudierre (57) in 1834 and challenged in 1932 by Kirwin (58), who doubted that such a patient could have been cured by local excision and cautery. Consequently, Hutchinson in 1861 is credited with the first verified case of carcinoma of the urethra; Wasserman in 1895 is credited with the first series of 20 men with urethral cancer (59). That same year, Wasserman reported a series of 20 women with urethral cancer (60).

In 1939, Kreutzmann and Colloff (61) divided primary urethral carcinoma into two categories—anterior (penile) and posterior (bulbous and prostatic) urethral. These categories were based on the significant differences in survival from each of the urethral segments—54% anterior and 13% posterior. In the same year, Young detailed a new surgical procedure that would spare the penis and testicles while radically excising a small posterior urethral tumor.

Since 1939, several reports on improving surgical technique for urethral carcinoma have been described (62–65). Several investigators (66–68) have also reported on the relatively high incidence of urethral recurrence after definitive treatment of bladder cancer. In 1977, a staging system was devised by Ray et al. (69).

Epidemiology

Cancer of the urethra, like that of cancer of the penis, is rare. In fact, approximately 1500 cases of primary urethral cancer in females and less than than 400 cases in males have been reported in the world literature (70). Urethral cancer is the only genitourinary neoplasm with a predilection for women, with the ratio being 4:1. It arises generally between the sixth and seventh decades of life but has been reported in boys as young as 13 years old and men in their nineties. Although the mean age for men is typically older than 50, the peak incidence is 58 years old, similar to that for penile carcinoma (71).

Etiologic factors for urethral carcinoma in the male have not been conclusively identified; however, chronic inflammation is significantly common to most urethral carcinomas. Inflammation might be in the form of venereal disease, prostatitis, urethritis, or urethral stricture disease. The incidence of urethral stricture in men is approximately 24 to 76%, occurring most commonly in the bulbomembranous urethra; incidentally, this correlates with the most common site of urethral carcinoma (50 to 75%).

A history of smoking and exposure to carcinogens in the work area have been indirectly linked to urethral carcinoma but no conclusive data exist.

In women, urethral cancers account for 0.02% of all neoplasms and 0.01% of all urologic malignancies (72). Urethral cancers tend to occur more commonly in white women (88%) than in black women (12%), except for cancers of urethral diverticulum, which are more common in black women (73). Again, as in male urethral carcinoma, inflammatory diseases have been implicated as the causative process in female urethral carcinoma. Chronic irritation, caruncles, fibrosis, coitus, certain viral infections, and urethral diverticular disease have all been implicated but not substantiated (74–78).

Benign inflammatory disease processes are common and often delay the diagnosis of urethral carcinoma. Therefore, the prompt diagnosis of all urethral cancers demands a high index of suspicion.

Anatomy

Male Urethra

The male urethra is approximately 21 cm in length and is divided functionally into two segments—posterior and anterior. The posterior urethra is subdivided into the membranous and prostatic urethral segments. The anterior urethra is subdivided into the bulbar and pendulous urethra. Many authors describe "bulbomembranous" lesions, implying that the bulbar region is "posterior"; this terminology continues because of the similarity to lesions of the membranous urethra with respect to clinical presentation, management, and prognosis (79).

The prostatic urethra is approximately 3 cm long and is surrounded by the prostate. The prostatic urethra is lined by transitional cell epithelium and contains the ejaculatory ducts and the prostatic utricle. The verumontanum is the landmark dividing the prostatic and membranous urethra.

The membranous urethra is the smallest segment of the urethra, averaging 1.8 to 2.0 cm in length. It is contiguous with the urogenital diaphragm and acts as part of the external sphincter mechanism. Cowper's glands are housed in this area while the ducts course distally to empty into the bulbar urethra.

The bulbar urethra is the expanded proximal portion of the anterior urethra. Like the membranous urethra, the bulbar urethra is lined with stratified or pseudostratified columnar epithelium.

The pendulous urethra is contained within the corpus spongiosum and is the longest segment of the male urethra. It is lined with pseudostratified columnar epithelium, except at its most distal portion where it expands into the fossa navicularis, which is lined with stratified squamous epithelium.

The histopathology of the urethra, like its epithelial lining, varies through its length. The most common neoplasms to occur in the prostatic urethra are transitional cell carcinomas. Adenocarcinomas and squamous cell carcinomas occur most commonly in the membranous and bulbar urethra. Squamous cell carcinoma is typically found in the pendulous urethra.

There is ample blood supply to the urethra. The internal pudendal artery, a branch of the internal iliac artery, gives rise to two arteries that supply the anterior urethra—the bulbar and urethral arteries. The bulbar artery supplies the bulbar urethra and bulbospongiosus muscle; the urethral artery supplies the corpus spongiosum. The deep dorsal artery courses distally to supply the glans penis. The prostatic and membranous urethra are supplied by branches of the inferior vesical and internal pudendal arteries.

Female Urethra

The female urethra is approximately 4 to 5 cm in length, extending from the bladder neck to the external urethral meatus. Like the male urethra, it is somewhat arbitrarily divided into anterior and posterior segments. The posterior segment accounts for the proximal two thirds of the urethra, which is lined with transitional cell epithelium. The anterior segment constitutes the distal one third and is lined with stratified squamous epithelium.

In women, as in men, the most common urethral cancers are squamous cell carcinoma (approximately 70%) (80, 81). Transitional cell carcinomas account for approximately 15%; adenocarcinomas account for approximately 10 to 13%. Primary melanomas occur but are exceedingly rare.

Clinically, 45% of urethral tumors in women are located in the anterior urethra, 7% in the posterior urethra, and 48% extend the entire urethral length. Benign lesions of the female urethra (e.g., urethral caruncle, cysts, condyloma acuminata, urethral prolapse, and periurethral abscess) are more common than malignant tumors. Nevertheless, any lesion that persists after conservative therapy should be biopsied.

Lymphatic Drainage

Male Urethra

The lymphatic drainage of the male urethra can be divided into two anatomical regions. Lesions in the anterior urethra contained within Buck's fascia drain to the deep inguinal and external iliac nodes. Penetration of Buck's fascia results in drainage of these lesions to the superficial inguinal nodes. Lesions in the anatomical posterior urethra drain to three areas—the deep inguinal nodes along the dorsal vein, the obturator nodes along the pudendal vessels, and the dorsal aspect of the presacral nodes (82).

Female Urethra

Urethral cancers spread initially by local extension and lymphatic metastasis. In the female, the lymphatic drainage of the distal urethra is to the superficial and deep inguinal nodes. The lymphatics of the proximal urethra drain preferentially into the deep pelvic nodes (external and internal iliac, obturator, and presacral nodes). Lymph node metastases are clinically recognized in 20 to 50% of females at the time of presentation (83).

Unlike carcinoma of the penis—in which nearly half of the patients will present with palpable lymphadenopathy, of which only half of these will harbor tumor metastasis—if a patient with urethral carcinoma presents with palpable inguinal adenopathy, nearly all of these patients will have positive nodes at lymphadenectomy. Therefore, patients with palpable lymphadenopathy should be managed aggressively.

Staging

Male Urethral Carcinoma

There have been several modifications of the staging system for urethral carcinoma proposed by Ray et al. in 1977 (69, 83) (Table 38.4).

This staging system is different from the International Union Against Cancer (UICC) system, which is listed in Table 38.5.

Female Urethral Carcinoma

The most important prognostic factor in female urethral carcinoma is tumor location (84). The histologic subtype is less significant and does not seem to influence treatment or patient survival.

There are two staging systems for female urethral cancer. Grabstald et al. (85) developed a staging system in 1966 (Table 38.6). Stages 0 and A are identical to Ray et al's system (69). Grabstald's stage B, however, is infiltration of periurethral muscle; stage C is (1) infiltration of the muscular wall of the

Table 38.5. The International Union Against Cancer Staging System for Male Urethral Cancer

T	Primary (clinical)
TpT	Primary (pathologic)
TX	No evidence of primary tumor
Tis	Carcinoma in situ
Ta	Noninvasive papillary, polypoid, or verrucous carcinoma
T1	Invades subepithelial connective tissue
T2	Invades corpus spongiosum, prostate, or periurethral muscle
T3	Invades corpus cavernosum or beyond prostatic capsule, anterior vagina, or bladder neck
T4	Invades adjacent organs

From Spiessl B, Beahrs OH, Hermanek P, et al. UICC TNM classification: illustrated guide to the TNM/pTNM classification of malignant tumors. Heidelberg: Springer-Verlag, 1989:264–271.

vagina; (2) infiltration of the muscular wall of the vagina with penetration of the mucosa; and (3) infiltration of other adjacent structures, such as the bladder, labia, and clitoris. Stage D is involvement of the inguinal lymph nodes, pelvic lymph nodes below the bifurcation of the aorta, or lymph nodes above the bifurcation of the aorta or distant metastasis (86). The staging system of Grabstald was modified by Prempree et al. in 1984 (87) (Table 38.7).

Management

Male Urethral Carcinoma

Certain authors have successfully treated early stages of urethral carcinoma with local excision and primary anastomosis (88, 89). Others have recently used a combination of transurethral resection and topical chemotherapy (90). Staging of small posterior urethral lesions is fraught with inaccuracy; these lesions tend to be extremely aggressive, and inadequate treatment of

Table 38.6. Urethral Cancer Staging (Grabstald) for Women

Stage 0	Cis (tumor limited to mucosa)
Stage A	Submucosal (tumor extending to but restricted to submucosa)
Stage B	Muscular (tumor infiltrating periurethral musculature)
Stage C	Periurethral
Stage C1	Infiltration of vaginal wall musculature
Stage C2	Infiltration of muscular wall of vagina with invasion of vaginal mucosa
Stage C3	Infiltration of adjacent organs such as the bladder, labia, and clitoris
Stage D	Metastasis
Stage D1	To inguinal lymph nodes
Stage D2	To pelvic nodes below the aortic bifurcation
Stage D3	To lymph nodes above the aortic bifurcation
Stage D4	Distant

Table 38.4. Staging System for Male Urethral Cancer (69)

Stage 0	Confined to mucosa, carcinoma in situ
Stage A	Into but not beyond lamina propria
Stage B	Into but not beyond corpus spongiosum or prostate
Stage C	Beyond corpus spongiosum or prostate capsule
Stage D1	Inguinal or pelvic lymph node metastasis
Stage D2	Distant metastasis

Table 38.7. Prempree Modification of Taggart Staging System for Female Urethral Cancer (87)

Stage I	Limited to the distal half of the urethra
Stage II	Involving the entire urethra, with extension to the periurethral tissues but not involving the vulva or bladder neck
Stage III	
a	Involving the urethra and vulva
b	Invading the vaginal mucosa
c	Involving the urethra and bladder neck
Stage IV	
a	Invading parametrium or paracolpium
b	Metastases
	Inguinal nodes
	Pelvic nodes
	Paraaortic nodes
	Distant

early lesions could have lethal consequences. Therefore, local transurethral resection with chemotherapy is not a recommended therapy for early stages of urethral cancer.

The patient with urethral cancer who is the ideal candidate for radical surgery has stage 0, A, or B disease that does not extend proximal to the midbulb. It should be emphasized that patients with locally advanced disease of the urethra are best treated with en bloc excision of the penis, scrotum, and anterior pubis and cystoprostatectomy (91). In certain patients with more advanced proximal urethral lesions, anterior exenteration plus emasculation is necessary to effect a cure. These procedures can involve an extensive soft tissue loss and generally require transfer flaps for closure.

In 1989, McDougal and Koch described a technique of primary phallic reconstruction during exenterative surgery for invasive bulbomembranous urethral carcinoma (65). In this technique, the testes and spermatic cord are transferred into the natural penile skin and glans penis tube to provide bulk and prevent contraction. The cosmetic results are excellent, and the psychological trauma of mutilating emasculation is substantially reduced.

Radiation, hormonal, and chemotherapies have had only limited use in the management of urethral carcinoma and should be used only as an adjunct to surgical therapy.

Female Urethral Carcinoma

Low-stage, small external urethral tumors limited to the mucosa can be treated effectively by local excision or laser surgery. Both the carbon dioxide and Nd:YAG lasers have proven efficacy in these lesions (92, 93). Stage 0, A, and B lesions in the distal one third of the urethra have been treated with partial urethrectomy (73). There are also adequate data to suggest that irradiation using radium-226 or iridium-192 needles or wires applied interstitially will treat low-stage urethral cancers in women (94–98). Intracavitary and external beam radiation can

be used as supplemental therapies to interstitial radiation (99). However, Bracken et al. have reported significant complications (80).

In selected patients, stages B and C urethral cancers can be treated with total urethrectomy, preserving the bladder. Patients with advanced disease involving the entire urethra with extension into the bladder and vagina require an anterior exenteration, including removal of the entire urethra, uterus and appendages, bladder, anterior and lateral vaginal walls, and pelvic lymph nodes, and en bloc resection of the pubic symphysis and inferior pubic ramus.

Operative Technique

Penectomy

Partial penectomy is the generally accepted operation for squamous cell carcinoma of the penis if there is a 1.5- to 2-cm tumor-free margin distal to the level of the amputation. A total penectomy and perineal urethrostomy should be performed for all penile cancers that are at the base of the penis or for lesions that will not allow at least a 2-cm tumor-free margin so that the patient may direct his urine stream while standing. Because the extent of the primary lesion is often underestimated, the patient should give informed consent for both procedures. The patient should be placed in a dorsal lithotomy position, in case a total penectomy and perineal urethrostomy should be required.

Iliac Inguinal Lymphadenectomy

The classic iliac inguinal lymphadenectomy includes the removal of the superficial and deep inguinal nodes in continuity with the iliac nodes. It should be borne in mind that the iliac nodes are removed only if the groin nodes are positive.

Certain patients with metastatic penile carcinoma present with extremely challenging problems. For example, patients with recurrent tumor burden in a previously dissected groin or local tissue necrosis due to extensive tumor involvement or irradiation still require groin dissections. Under these circumstances, a more extensive dissection is required in which large portions of skin, muscle, fascia, nerve, and/or vessels must be removed. Groin and abdominal wall skin with the inguinal fascia may be sacrificed if necessary. Dissections of this nature are often so extensive that it is not possible to achieve wound closure with the local tissues. Appropriate transfer of skin, fascia, and muscle may be necessary and may be accomplished with a vertical rectus abdominis myocutaneous flap.

Conclusion

Carcinoma of the penis is a rare disease occurring predominantly in elderly, uncircumcised men. It is thought that the primary cause of carcinoma of the penis is a chronic irritation within the preputial sac. This irritation can be removed by surgery, which serves as both prophylaxis against (neonatal circumcision) and potential cure from (partial or total penectomy) this disease. Controversial issues surrounding the management of carcinoma of the penis primarily reflect the complex cross-communications of the lymphatic drainage and the frustrating inability to stage this cancer accurately.

Carcinoma of the urethra, which is also rare, is the only genitourinary cancer that is more common in females than in males. Despite squamous cell carcinoma being the most common type of urethral cancer, the diverse histopathology of the urethra reflects the changes in its epithelial lining along its length. The challenge of management of carcinoma of the urethra, like that of carcinoma of the penis, is to balance a complete excision of the entire tumor with an acceptable aesthetic result.

The most important aspect in management, common to all cancers, is to effect a cure. However, the disfiguring consequences that can leave the patient psychologically devastated are often overlooked in treatment attempts. Yet, with adequate planning, attention to detail, and counseling, satisfactory results can be achieved.

REFERENCES

1. Celsus C (Translated by Spencer WG). Celsus de Medina. Cambridge: Harvard University Press, 1935;2:276.
2. Lenowitz H, Graham AP. Carcinoma of the penis. J Urol 1946;56:458.
3. Morgagni GB. The seats and causes of diseases, book IV, letter L, article 50, 1761.
4. Lewis LG. Young's radical operation for the cure of cancer of the penis: a report of 34 cases. J Urol 1931;26:295.
5. MacCormack W. Five cases of amputation of the penis for epithelioma. Br Med J 1886;1:343.
6. Curtis BF. American textbook of diseases of the skin. Philadelphia: WB Saunders, 1898:76.
7. Gibson CL. Cancer of the penis. Ann Surg 1912;56:471.
8. Barringer BS, Dean AL Jr. Epithelioma of the penis. J Urol 1924;11:497.
9. Young HH. A radical operation for the cure of cancer of the penis. J Urol 1931;26:285.
10. Daseler EH, Anson BJ, Reimann AF. Radical excision of the inguinal and iliac lymph glands. Surg Gynecol Obstet 1948; 87:679.
11. Boronofsky IA. Technique of inguinal node dissection. Surgery 1953;33:886.
12. Cabanas RM. An approach for the treatment of penile carcinoma. Cancer 1977;39:456.
13. Dean AL Jr. Epithelioma of the penis. J Urol 1935;33:252.
14. Persky L. Epidemiology of cancer of the penis: recent results. Cancer Res 1977;60:97.
15. Hoppmann HJ, Fraley EE. Squamous cell carcinoma of the penis. J Urol 1978;120:393.
16. Kini MG. Cancer of the penis in a child, aged 2 years. Indian Med Gazette 1944;79:66.
17. Licklider S. Jewish penile carcinoma. J Urol 1961;86:98.
18. Maden C, et al. History of circumcision, medical conditions and sexual activity and risk of penile cancer. J Natl Cancer Inst 1993;85:1251.
19. Schellhammer PF, Jordan GH, Schlossberg SM. Tumors of the Penis. In: Walsh PC, Retik AB, Stamey TA, et al., eds. Campbell's urology. Philadelphia: WB Saunders, 1992:1271.
20. Macaluso JN Jr, Sullivan JW, Tomberlin S. Glomus tumor of glans penis. Urology 1985;25:409.
21. Dodge OG, Linsell CA. Carcinoma of the penis in Uganda and Kenya Africans. Cancer 1963;16:1255.
22. Schrek R, Lenowitz H. Etiologic facts in carcinoma of the penis. Cancer Res 1947;7:180.
23. Pratt-Thomas HR, Heins HC, Lathame E, et al. The carcinogenic effect of human smegma; an experimental study: preliminary report. Cancer 1956;9:671.
24. Burgers JK, Badalament RA, Drago JR. Penile cancer. Urol Clin North Am 1992;2:247.
25. Riveros M, Lebron RF. Geographical pathology of cancer of the penis. Cancer 1963;16:798.
26. Varma VA, Sanchez-Lanier M. Unger ER, et al. Association of human papilloma virus with penile carcinoma: a study using polymerase chain reaction and in situ hybridization. Hum Pathol 1991;22:908.
27. Sarkar FH, Miles BJ, Plieth DH, et al. Detection of human papilloma virus in squamous neoplasm of the penis. J Urol 1992;147:389.
28. Goldberg HM, Pell-Ilderton R, Daw E, et al. Concurrent squamous cell carcinoma of the cervix and penis in a married couple. Br J Obstet Gynecol 1979;86:585.
29. Aboseif S, Breza J, Lue T, et al. Penile venous drainage in erectile dysfunction: anatomical, radiographical, and functional considerations. Br J Urol 1989;64:183.
30. Rouviere H (Translated by Tobias MJ). Anatomy of the human lymphatic systemic. Ann Arbor, MI: Edwards Bros., 1938.
31. Lowe D, McKee PH. Verrucous carcinoma of the penis (Buschke-Lowenstein tumour): a clinico-pathological study. Br J Urol 1983;55:427.
32. Akerman LV. Verrucous carcinoma of the oral cavity. Surgery 1948;23:670.
33. Youngsberg GA, Thornthwaite JT, Inoshita T, et al. Cytologically malignant squamous cell carcinoma arising in a verrucous carcinoma of the penis. J Dermatol Surg Oncol 1983;9:474.
34. Medina JE, Dichtel W, Luna MA. Verrucous-squamous cell carcinoma of the oral cavity: a clinico-pathological study of 104 cases. Arch. Otolaryngol In press.
35. Bowen JT. Precancerous dermatoses: a study of two cases of chronic atypical epithelial proliferation. J Cutan Dis 1912;30:241.
36. Goette DK, Elgar M, DeVillez RL. Erythroplasia of Queyrat: treatment with topically applied fluorouracil. JAMA 1975;232:934.
37. Boon TA. Sapphire probe laser surgery for localized carcinoma of the penis. Eur J Surg Oncol 1988;14:193.
38. Ledwig PA, Weigand DA. Late circumcision and lichen sclerosus et atrophicus of the penis. J Am Acad Dermatol 1989;20:221.
39. Bainbridge DR, Whitaker RH, Shepherd BGF. Balanitis xerotica obliterans and urinary obstruction. Br J Urol 1971;43:487.
40. Bart RS, Kopf AW. Tumor conference number 18: squamous cell carcinoma arising in balanitis xerotica obliterans. J Dermatol Surg Oncol 1978;4:556.

41. Dore B, Irani J, Aubert J. Carcinoma of the penis in lichen sclerosus atrophicus: a case report. Eur Urol 1990;18:153.

42. Sakoda R, Oka M, Nakashima K. Leukoplakia of the penis: bleomycin treatment. Br J Urol 1978;50:355.

43. Wishnow KI, Johnson DE. Effective outpatient treatment of Kaposi's sarcoma of the urethral meatus using neodymium: YAG laser. Lasers Surg Med 1988;8:428.

44. Jackson SM. The treatment of carcinoma of the penis. Br J Surg 1966;53:33.

45. deKernion JB, Tynberg P, Persky L, et al. Carcinoma of the penis. Cancer 1973;32:1256.

46. Skinner DG, Leadbetter WF, Kelly SB. The surgical management of squamous cell carcinoma of the penis. J Urol 1972;107:273.

47. McDougal WS. Carcinoma of the penis: improved survival by early regional lymphadenectomy based on the histological grade and depth of invasion of the primary lesion. J Urol 1995;154:1364.

48. Horenblas S, VanTinteren H, Delemarre JFM, et al. Squamous cell carcinoma of the penis: part III. treatment of regional nodes. J Urol 1993;149:492.

49. Mohs FE, Snow SN, Larson PO. Mohs micrographic surgery for penile tumors. In: Crawford DE, Das S, eds. Penile, urethral, and scrotal cancer. Urol Clin North Am 1992;19:291.

50. Schellhammer PF, Jordan FH, Schlossberg SM. Tumors of the penis. In: Walsh PC, Retik AB, Stamey TA, et al., eds. Campbell's urology. 6th ed. Philadelphia: WB Saunders, 1992:1264.

51. Pizzocaro G, Diva L. Adjuvant and neoadjuvant therapy with vincristine, bleomycin, methotrexate for resected or unresectable inguinal metastasis of carcinoma of the penis. Proceedings of the Eur Conf Clin Radiol Madrid, Spain. 1987. Abstract.

52. McDougal WS, Kirchner FK Jr, Edwards RH, et al. Treatment of carcinoma of the penis: the case for primary lymphadenectomy. J Urol 1986;38:136.

53. Horenblas S, VanTinteren H. Squamous cell carcinoma of the penis: part 4. prognostic factors of survival: analysis of tumor, nodes and metastasis classification system. J Urol 1994;151:1239.

54. Ornellas AA, Seixas ALC, Marota A, et al. Surgical treatment of invasive squamous cell carcinoma of the penis: retrospective analysis of 350 cases. J Urol 1994;151:1244.

55. Fraley EE, Zhang G, Manivel C, et al. The role of ilioinguinal lymphadenectomy and significance of histological differentiation in treatment of carcinoma of the penis. J Urol 1989;142:1478.

56. Ayyappan K, Ananthakrishnan N, Sankaran V. Can regional lymph node involvement be predicted in patients with carcinoma of the penis? Br J Urol 1994;73:549.

57. Thiaudierre PD. Nouvelle espece de retrecissment de l'uretre; nouveau procede operatoire. Bull Gen De Therap 1834:210.

58. Kirwin TJ. Primary epithelioma of the urethra. J Urol 1932;27:539.

59. Young HH. A new radical operation for carcinoma of the bulbous urethra: new use for penis. Surg Gynecol Obstet 1939;68:77.

60. Wasserman. Epithelioma primitif de L'urethre. (Quoted by McCrea LE, Furlong JH Jr. Primary carcinoma of the male urethra. Urol Surv 1951;1:30.)

61. Kreutzman HAR, Colloff B. Primary carcinoma of the male urethra. Arch Surg 1939;39:513.

62. Kaufman JJ, Goodwin WE. Carcinoma of the male urethra: one stage surgical treatment by radical perineal excision and rectal transplantation of the divided trigone. Surg Gynecol Obstet 1953;97:627.

63. Marshall VF. Radical excision of locally extensive carcinoma of the deep male urethra. J Urol 1957;78:252.

64. Uhle CAW, Holfelner ED. Treatment of carcinoma of the male urethra by radical surgical infrapubic removal: a case report. J Urol 1952;68:302.

65. McDougal WS, Koch MO. Phallic reconstruction during exenterative surgery for invasive urethral carcinoma. J Urol 1989;141:1201.

66. Ashworth A. Papillomatosis of the urethra. Br J Urol 1956;28:313.

67. Cordonnier JJ, Spjut HJ. Urethral occurrence of bladder carcinoma following cystectomy. J Urol 1962;87:398.

68. Ahlering TE, Lieskovsky G, Skinner DG. Indications for urethrectomy in men undergoing single stage radical cystectomy for bladder cancer. J Urol 1984;131:657.

69. Ray B, Canto AR, Whitmore WF Jr. Experience with primary carcinoma of the male urethra. J Urol 1977;117:591.

70. Levine RL. Urethral cancer. Cancer 1980;45:1965.

71. Grabstald H. Tumors of the urethra in men and women. Cancer 1973;32:1236.

72. Sailer SL, Shilpley VU, Wang CC. Carcinoma of the female urethra: a review of result with radiation therapy. J Urol 1988;140:1.

73. Narayan P, Konety B. Surgical treatment of female urethral carcinoma. In: Crawford ED, Das S, eds. Penile, urethral, and scrotal cancer. Urol Clin North Am 1992;19:373.

74. Fagan FE, Hertig AT. Carcinoma of the female urethra: review of the literature. J Urol 1981;126:124.

75. Marshall FC, Uson AC, Melicow MM. Neoplasms and caruncles of the female urethra. Surg Gynecol Obstet 1960;110:723.

76. Mevorach RA, Cos LR, DiSant'Agnese PA, et al. Human papillomavirus type 6 in grade I transitional cell carcinoma of the urethra. J Urol 1990;143:126.

77. Monaco AP, Murphy GB, Dowling W. Primary cancer of the female urethra. Cancer 1958;11:1215.

78. Clayton M, Siami P, Guinan P. Urethral diverticular carcinoma. Cancer 1992;70:665.

79. Carroll PR, Dixon CM. Surgical anatomy of the male and female urethra. In: Crawford DE, Das S, eds. Penile, urethral, and scrotal cancer. Urol Clin North Am 1992;19:339.

80. Bracken RB, Johnson DE, Miller LS, et al. Primary carcinoma of the female urethra. J Urol 1976;116:188.

81. Carroll PR. Surgical management of urethral carcinoma. In: Crawford DE, Das S, eds. Current genitourinary cancer surgery. Philadelphia: Lea & Febiger, 1990:380.

82. Skinner DG, Lieskovsky G, eds. Diagnosis and management of genitourinary cancer. Philadelphia: WB Saunders, 1988:622.

83. Ray B, Guinan BD. Primary carcinoma of the urethra. In: Javopour N, ed. Principles and management of urologic cancer. Baltimore: Williams & Wilkins, 1979:445.

84. Forman JD, Lichter AS. The role of radiation therapy in the

management of carcinoma of the male and female urethra. In: Crawford ED, Das S, eds. Penile, urethral, and scrotal cancer. Urol Clin North Am 1992;19:383.

85. Grabstald, H, Hilaris B, Henschke U, et al. Cancer of the female urethra. JAMA 1966;197:835.

86. Mostofi FK, Davis CJ Jr, Sesterhenn IA. Carcinoma of the male and female urethra. In: Crawford ED, Das S, eds. Penile, urethral, and scrotal carcinoma. Urol Clin North Am 1992;19:347.

87. Prempree T, Amornmarn R, Patanaphan V. Radiation therapy in primary carcinoma of the female urethra. Cancer 1984;54:729.

88. Hopkins SC, Nag SK, Soloway MS. Primary carcinoma of the male urethra. Urology 1994;23:128.

89. Konnak JW. Conservative management of low grade neoplasms of the male urethra: a preliminary report. J Urol 1980;123:175.

90. Hilliyard RW, Ladaga L, Schellhammer PR. Superficial transitional cell carcinoma of the bladder associated with mucosal involvement of the prostatic urethra: results of treatment with intravesical bacillus Calmette-Guerin. J Urol 1988;139:290.

91. Zeirdman EJ, Desmond P, Thompson IM. Surgical treatment of carcinoma of the male urethra. In: Crawford ED, Das S, eds. Penile, urethral, and scrotal carcinoma. Urol Clin North Am 1992;19:359.

92. Stoehler G, Chausey C, Jocham D, et al. The use of neodymium: YAG lasers in urology: indications, techniques and critical assessment. J Urol 1985;134:1155.

93. Schaefter AJ. Use of CO2 laser in urology. Urol Clin North Am 1986;13:393.

94. Antoniades J. Radiotherapy in carcinoma of the female urethra. Cancer 1969;24:70.

95. Delclos L, Wharton JT, Rutledge FN. Tumors of the vagina and female urethra. In: Fletcher GH, ed. Textbook of radiotherapy. 3rd ed. Philadelphia: Lea & Febiger, 1980:812.

96. Johnson DE, O'Connell JR. Primary carcinoma of the female urethra. Urology 1983;21:42.

97. Taggart CG, Castro JR, Rutledge FN. Carcinoma of the female urethra. Am J Roentgenol 1972;114:145.

98. Weghaupt K, Gerstner GJ, Kucera H. Radiation therapy for primary carcinoma of the female urethra: a survey of over 25 years. Gynecol Oncol 1984;17:58.

99. Sullivan J, Grabstald H. Management of carcinoma of the urethra. In: Skinner DG, deKernion JB, eds. Genitourinary cancer. Philadelphia: WB Saunders, 1978:419.

39

Carcinoma of the Penis

Management of the Primary

Jagdeesh N. Kulkarni

Management of the primary malignant lesion of the penis requires following the standard oncologic surgical principles such as wide excision of the tumor with adequate healthy margins tridimensionally to achieve relapse-free survival. In most cases, this may necessitate extirpation of the male phallus, producing lasting morbidity and psychosexual problems. Over the years, various attempts at conservative treatment have been made to achieve an effective, functional, and near-normal phallus with the help of careful anatomical considerations and technical nuances in surgical and radiation therapy techniques. However, the adequacy and safety of these conservative treatments still remain uncertain. Moreover, various collective reviews are plagued by personal biases, small numbers of patients, inherent ambiguities of staging criteria, and paucity of adequate information about pathologic grade and stage of the tumor. The treatment problem becomes compounded because of extremely slow or negligible progress made in reconstruction of the penis in terms of erectile functional restoration. However, should the surgical margin be compromised, there is a danger of relapse. Nonsurgical treatments may result in a cicatrized, nonerectile, and dilapidated phallus.

HISTORICAL ASPECTS

Celsus (1) may be credited with the first report of excision of a presumed cancerous lesion of the penis. Although Valsalva (reported by Morgagni in 1761) (2) performed the first partial amputation of the penis, the first detailed description of curative surgery came from Thiersch in 1875 (3). Subsequently, MacCormack (4) and Curtis (5) suggested bilateral inguinal lymphadenectomy adjunctive to total amputation of penis. In 1907, Young (6) advocated en bloc groin adenectomy with excision of the primary tumor. Classical radical ileoinguinal node dissection became an established surgical procedure after detailed anatomical description of lymphatic drainage by Daseler et al. in 1948 (7). This was modified by Baronofsky (8) with transposition of sartorius muscle to cover femoral vessels.

Radical ileoinguinal lymphadenectomy improved cancer-free survival rates, but the lasting morbidity became a menacing problem to physicians and patients. In 1977, Cabanas (9) reported the concept of sentinel node biopsy (at the level of epigastric saphenous vein junction), with the hope of finding the first echelon of spread and avoiding formal node dissection if pathologic study results were negative. Other authors (10, 11) have reported failures with this approach and doubted its safety.

Currently, the limited node dissection (saphenous-sparing groin node dissection) reported by Catalona (12) is under careful scrutiny. Simultaneously, radiation therapy techniques have been evolving, from the earliest reports of using external beam radiation therapy to the latest brachytherapy with iridium-192 wires (13).

PATHOLOGY

In practice, the clinician may encounter three distinct pathologic conditions—skin lesions, carcinoma in situ, and overt or frank tumors.

Skin Lesions

These lesions may contain either squamous carcinoma cells or may progress to frank malignancy. Therefore, they require treatment and careful follow-up.

Cutaneous Horns

Overgrowth and cornification of the epithelium can lead to many projections that, on microscopic study, show extreme hyperkeratosis, dyskeratosis, and acanthosis and may contain squamous carcinoma at the base (14).

Condyloma Acuminatum

These are typically soft, friable, reddish papillary lesions that hang from preputial skin or meatus and are known to progress to squamous carcinoma (15).

Leukoplakia

This cutaneous lesion may present as plaque with irritative symptoms and may coexist with or precede carcinoma (16).

Balanitis Xerotica Obliterans

As the name suggests, these lesions are seen around the meatus and extend onto the glans. These lesions require close follow-up because of reported malignant degeneration (17).

Buschke-Lowenstein Tumor (Verrucous carcinoma, giant condyloma acuminatum (Fig. 39.1)

This lesion generally starts as a small papillary swelling that grows into large, exophytic lesions. These large lesions eventually destroy the glans penis and urethra. Lymph node metastases are rare with these tumors (16).

Carcinoma In Situ

Histologically, three different conditions are included under the category of carcinoma in situ—erythroplasia of Queyrat (18), Bowen's disease (19), and Bowenoid papillosis (20).

Both erythroplasia of Queyrat and Bowen's disease present clinically with erythematous, plaque-like lesions in an uncircumcised male. Occasionally, Bowen's disease may show ulcerative lesions. On microscopic study, both show noninvasive cellular changes of carcinoma in situ. Moreover, 20 to 50% may progress to invasive lesions (21). Bowenoid papillosis presents with multiple papules on the penile shaft in young men between 20 and 40 years of age. On microscopic study, there is invasion of dermis. This condition should be treated like carcinoma.

Overt or Frank Tumors

These tumors may present as nonhealing ulcers or discharging sinus from a phimotic preputial sac. There may sometimes be papillary or cauliflower-like overgrowths. Advanced lesions show fungating, foul-smelling masses or ulcerations with everted edges with induration of the shaft. Occasionally, there may be destructive lesions involving the whole penis, which leads to autoamputation.

On microscopic study, these tumors reveal the features of squamous cell carcinoma with varying degrees of acanthosis

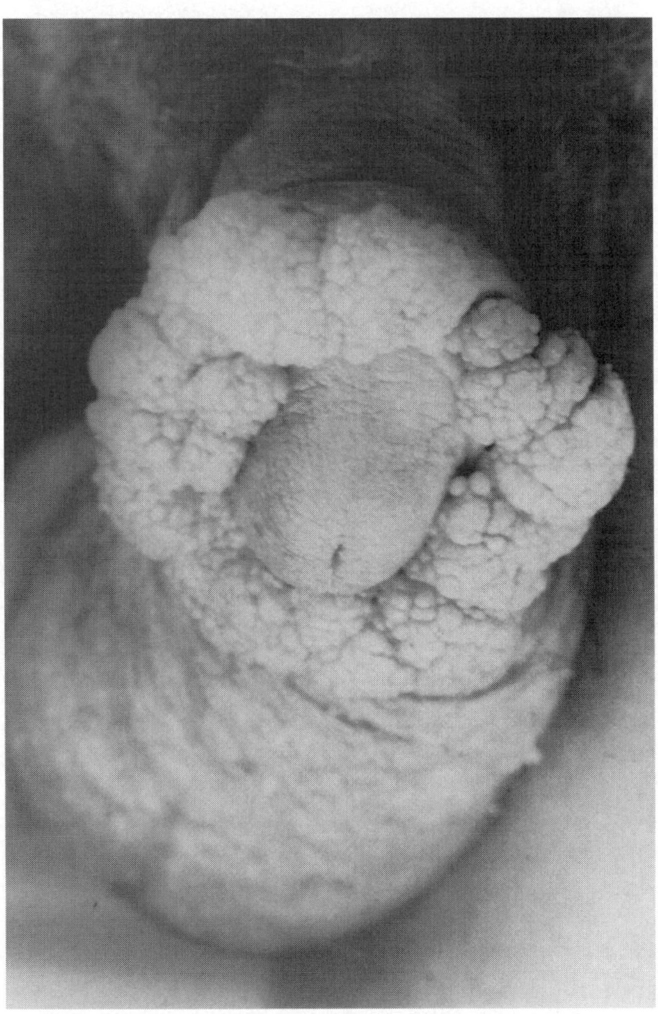

Fig. 39.1.   Giant condyloma acuminatum.

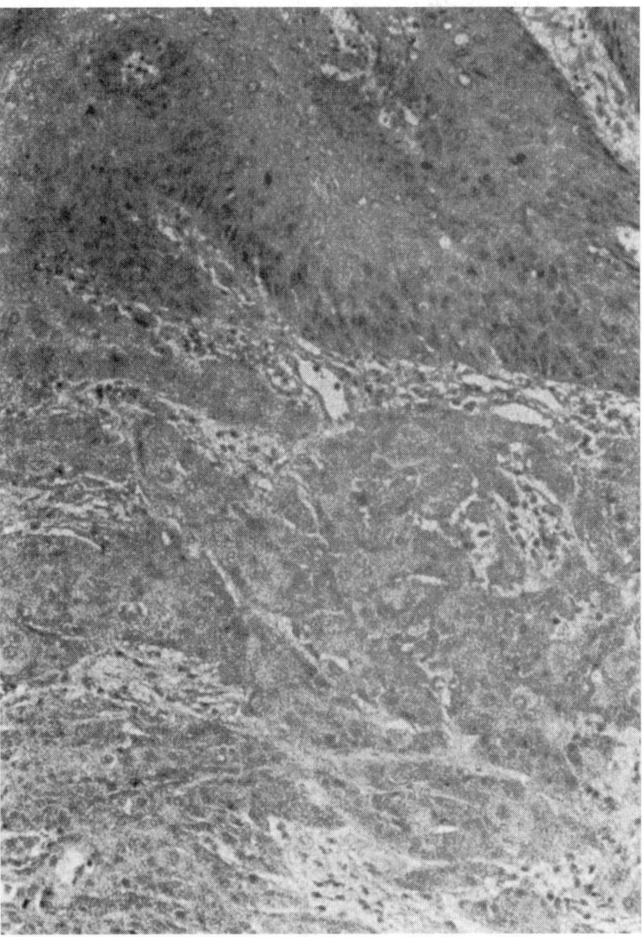

Fig. 39.2.   Photomicrograph of squamous carcinoma of the penis (hematoxylin-eosin stain, ×400).

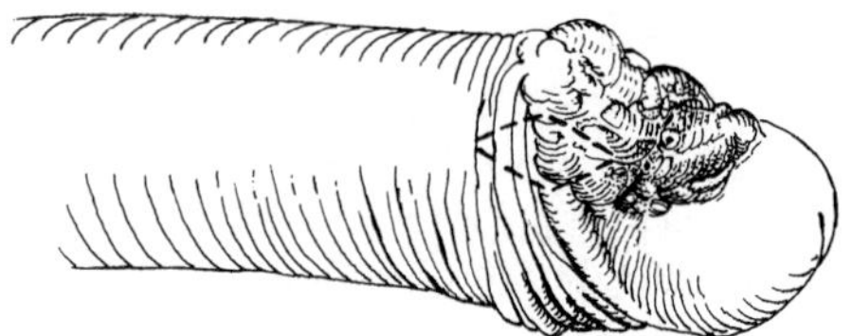

Fig. 39.3. Wedge biopsy.

and hyperkeratosis. Malignant features include a disorganized cellular pattern and cells showing pleomorphic nuclei, loss of polarity, and mitotic figures (Fig. 39.2). Spread to the inguino-iliac nodes is most common. Despite rich vascularity and venous system possessed by the penis, hematogenous spread is rare.

MANAGEMENT

Biopsy

Before planning definitive treatment, histologic confirmation of the lesion in terms of type, grade, and invasion is mandatory. Lesions that are small and involve only penile skin or prepuce can be diagnosed safely after circumcision or wide excision (after achieving a 2-cm healthy margin all around). However, lesions involving glans necessitate incisional biopsy (Fig. 39.3), including a 1-cm wedge of normal tissues and tumor segment followed by 3-0 chromic catgut suture to arrest oozing.

Treatment

Management decisions are often categorized by the type, size, extent, and location of the tumor (Fig. 39.4). Broad therapeutic approaches for the management of the primary tumor are surgical and nonsurgical.

Surgical Treatment

The aim of surgery is to achieve at least 2 to 3 cm of healthy margin with maximum organ preservation. Nonamputational surgeries, such as circumcision or wide excision, are adequate for lesions that are less than 3 cm in size and/or are noninvasive and involve the foreskin or prepuce without involving glans. Selected cases of noninvasive carcinomas involving the skin of the shaft and some dermatologic lesion can be treated by degloving or complete excision of the penile shaft skin (Figs. 39.5–39.7), followed by coverage with split thickness skin graft or scrotal skin. Inadequate surgical margins may lead to recurrence (22, 23).

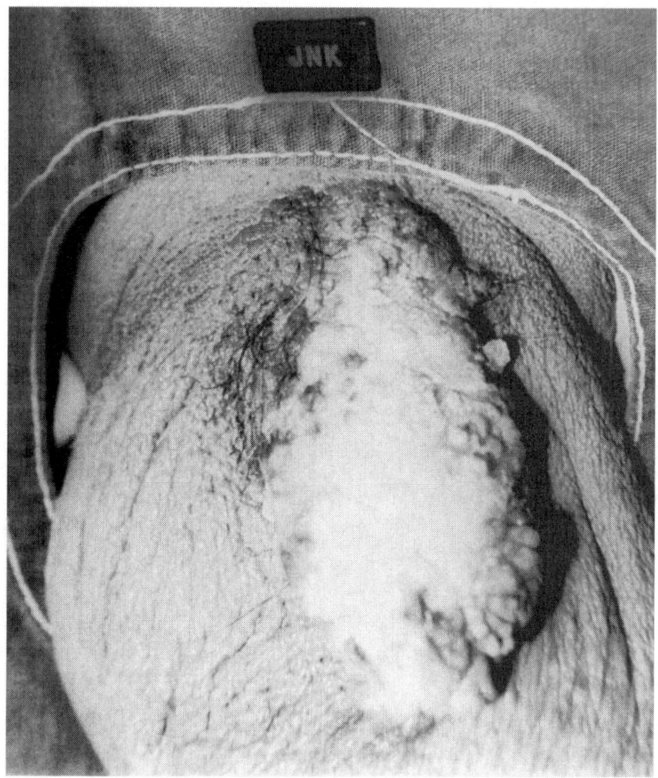

Fig. 39.5. Severe leukoplakia with papillary tumors of the shaft and prepuce.

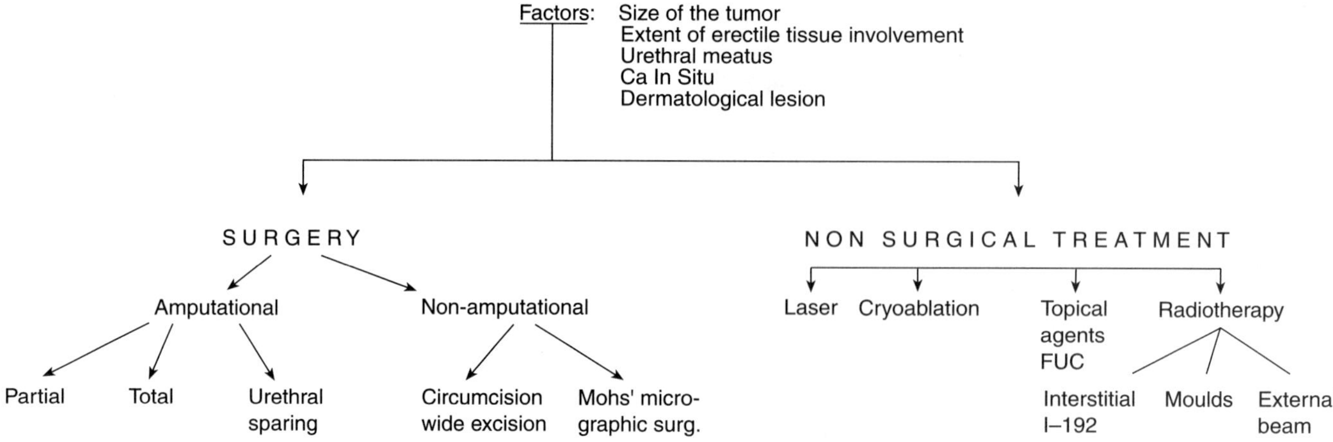

Fig. 39.4. Flow sheet showing management strategies.

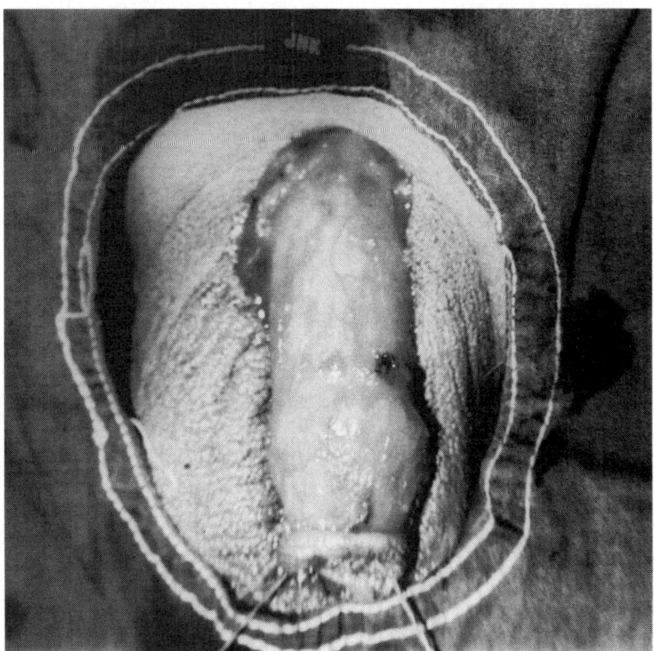

Fig. 39.6. Degloving of the penile skin.

Mohs' Micrographic Surgery (24)

The basis of this type of surgery is excision of the neoplastic tissue layer-by-layer and examination of the undersurface tissue using frozen section under a microscope. This technique helps in eradicating the neoplastic tissue and its outgrowth, which are invisible to the naked eye, and simultaneously maximally sparing the normal tissue. Generally, this technique can be

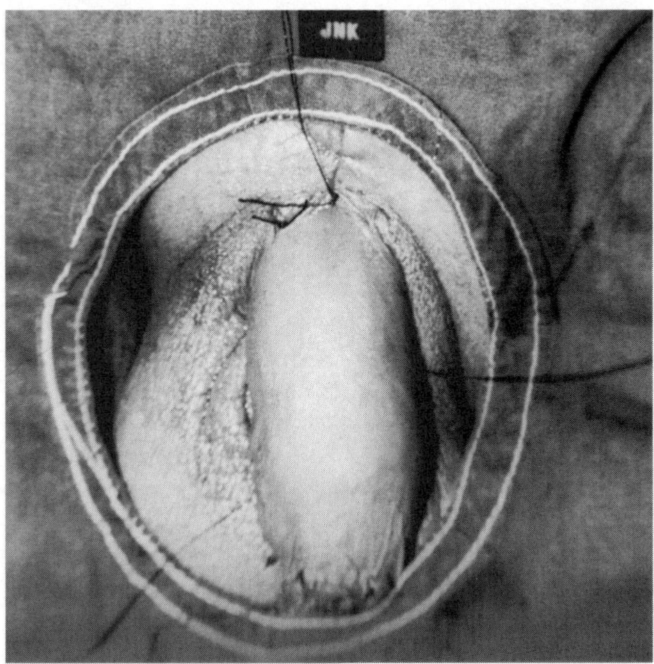

Fig. 39.7. Split skin graft tube covering whole penis.

applied to the lesions involving glans without involvement of the urethral meatus.

There are two types of techniques by which adequate microscopic control of the excision can be performed—fixed tissue technique and fresh tissue technique. The technique chosen depends on the size of the lesion and invasion of erectile tissue. If the tumor is small and noninvasive, with minimal erectile tissue involvement, the fresh tissue technique can be used (which saves time). Larger and invasive lesions require the fixed tissue technique to obviate bleeding. Although the author has seen excellent results with micrographic surgery, wide acceptance has not yet occurred due to lack of feasibility and an inadequate number of cases reported.

Amputational Surgery

Tumors involving the glans and shaft require partial or total amputation of the penis. Partial amputation is adequate if 2 to 3 cm of stump of the shaft can be left behind to achieve projectile micturition in the standing position. Sometimes, penile length can be enhanced by incising the suspensory ligaments and mobilizing lateral skin flaps to the prepubic area. d'souza has advocated subtotal penis amputation with transpo-

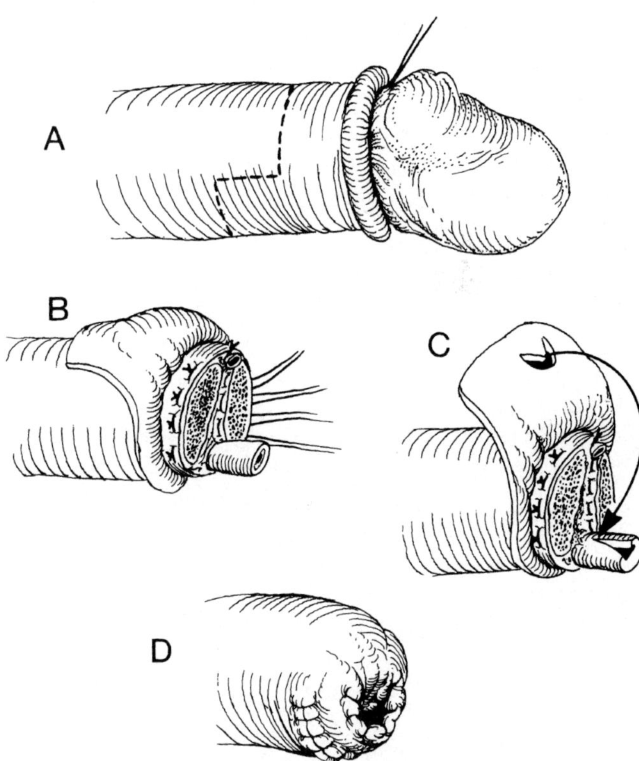

Fig. 39.8. Steps of partial amputation. **A.** The skin incision is outlined. **B.** Corporal bodies are transected and closed in the horizontal mattress sutures. Urethral stump is dissected to project 1 cm beyond the corporal stump. **C.** A crescentic buttonhole in the dorsal skin flap is made for anastomosis of the spatulated urethra. **D.** Urethrocutaneous anastomosis and reapproximation of skin flaps.

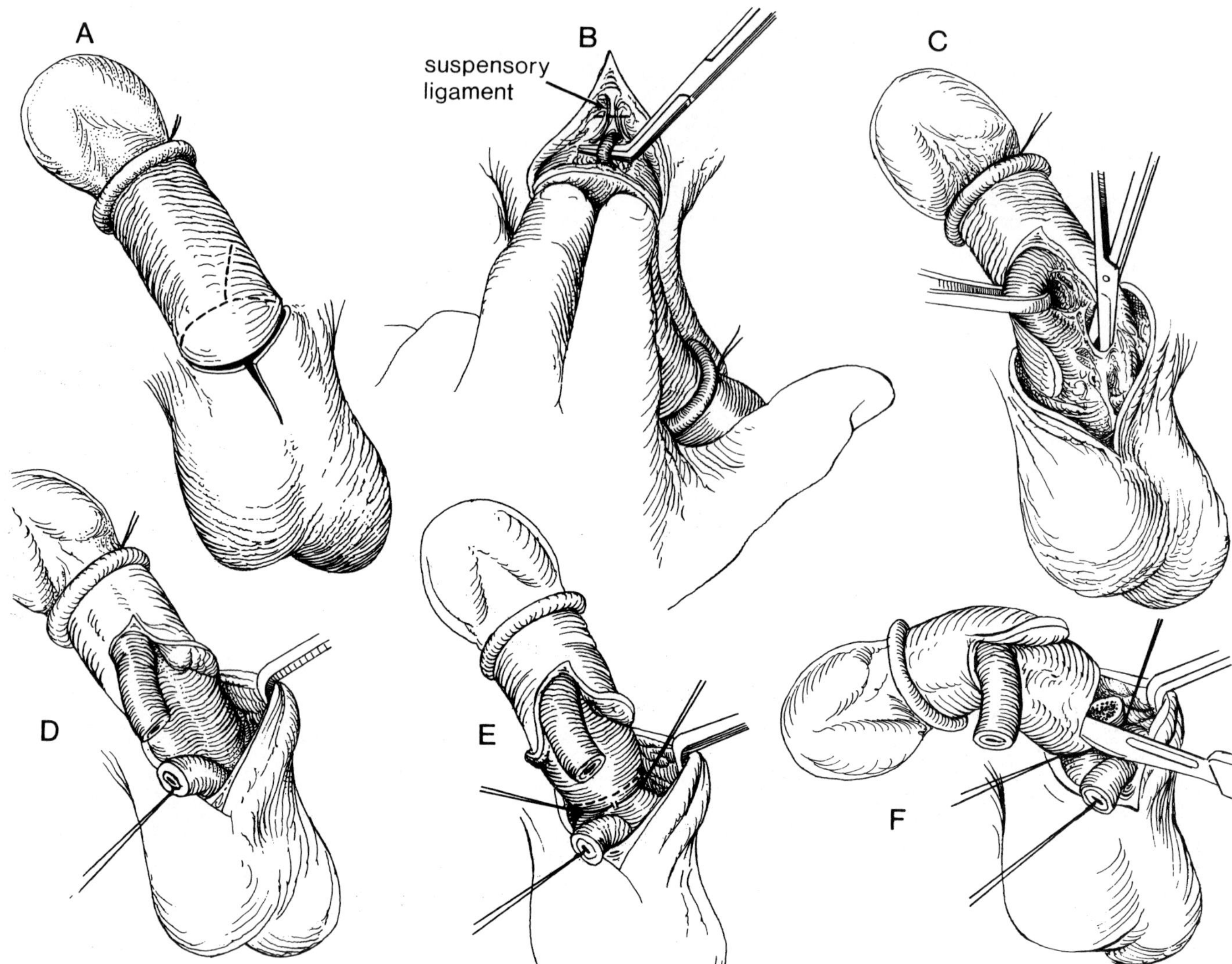

Fig. 39.9. Steps of total amputation. **A.** Skin incision at the root of the penis. **B.** Suspensory ligament and dorsal vein are isolated and divided. **C.** Urethra is dissected off the corpora. **D.** Urethra is transected. **E.** Corpora cavernosa are ligated at the level of pubic arch. **F.** Corpora are divided.

sition of the urethra in the middle of the scrotum after bivalving the scrotum (25). Large invasive tumors involving the whole shaft of the penis require total amputation of the penis with perineal urethrostomy, which allows micturition in a sitting position. Bissada (26) reported urethra-sparing total or subtotal amputation in selected patients with invasive tumors of the penis involving only dorsum, with cavernosa and spongiosum being free. This procedure can be followed by phallic reconstruction if there is no relapse at 1 year.

Partial Amputation

These patients generally have saprophytic infections, and our policy is to institute proper antibiotics for 3 days preoperatively. Preoperative shower and wash with Betadine solution and a thorough scrubbing with cetrimide precede the isolation of the primary lesion with either glove finger or condom. At the previously decided site, a circular incision is made all around the shaft of the penis. The incision is deepened, and subcutaneous veins are isolated with fine catgut sutures. After the Buck's fascia is incised, the deep dorsal vein and arteries are secured with 3-0 catgut sutures. The urethra is dissected off the corpora cavernosa and transected 1 cm distal to the proposed level of cavernosal incision. Corpora cavernosa are divided between two clamps to prevent bleeding. With 2-0 chromic catgut, cavernosal ends are sutured horizontally to form the stump. The urethra is spatulated and sutured to the skin with 4-0 chromic catgut or Vicryl (Ethicon, Sommerville, NJ) at the center of the incision. The rest of the skin is closed with 3-0 chromic catgut sutures (Fig. 39.8). An indwelling 16F Foley catheter is inserted through the neourethrostomy and removed after 48 hours.

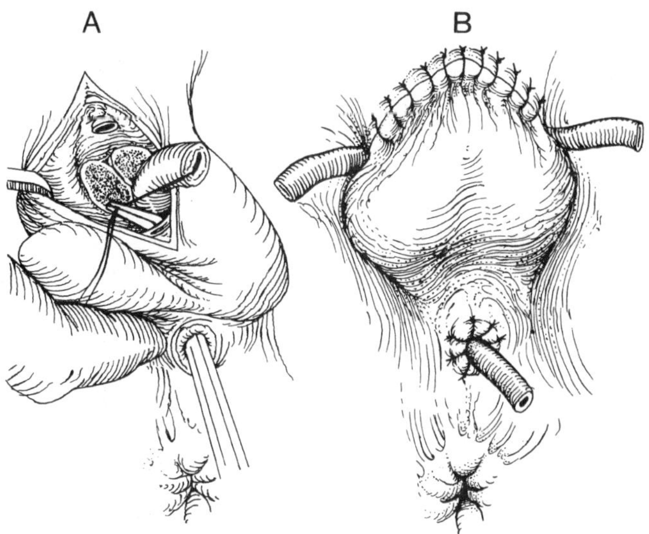

Fig. 39.10.   **A.** Proposed site of perineal urethrostomy. **B.** Perineal urethrostomy is completed, and transverse closure of skin is done.

TOTAL AMPUTATION OF THE PENIS

A circular incision is made around the root of the penis. The incision is deepened dorsally to cut the suspensory ligament. The dorsal vein and artery are isolated and divided between 3-0 chromic catgut sutures. This allows complete mobilization of corpora cavernosa off the pubic arch. Ventrally, corpus spongiosum containing urethra is isolated from the corporal bodies and transected distal to the bulbar portion. Corporal bodies are further mobilized and divided between 0 chromic sutures to prevent bleeding (Fig. 39.9). It is unnecessary to dissect corpora completely off the pubic ramus unless the primary lesion is extensive or proximal. The urethra is dissected off the surrounding structures up to the level of the urogenital diaphragm. At the midpoint between the scrotum and anal verge, 1 cm circular disk of the perineal skin and subcutaneous tissue is excised. Proximal urethral cut end is brought out at this urethrostomy site. Care is taken to avoid angulation by straightening the urethra and, if necessary, by further dividing the tissues around. Cutaneourethrostomy is completed with interrupted 4-0 chromic catgut or Vicryl sutures after the urethra is spatulated

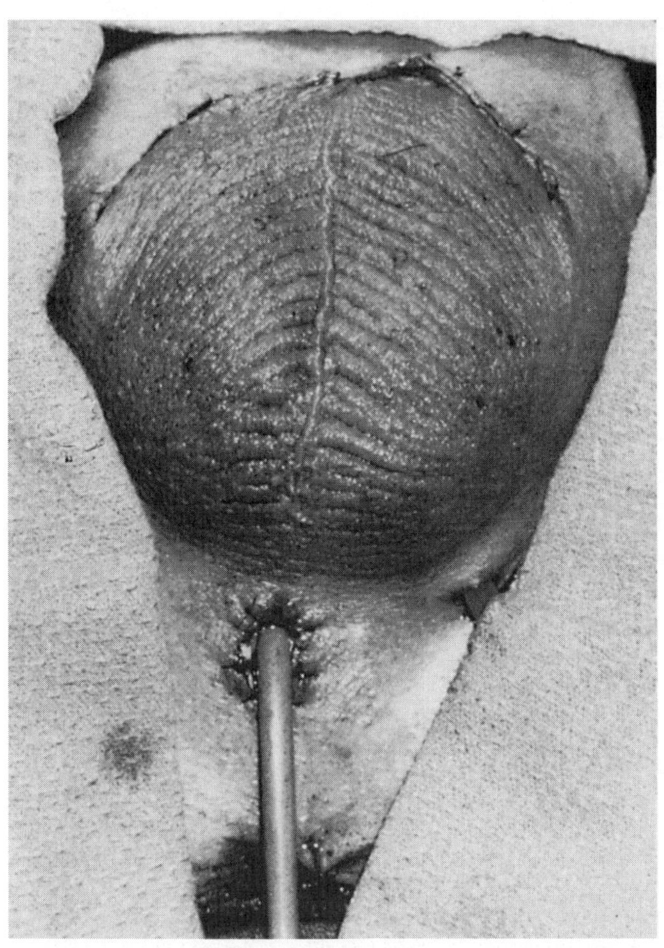

Fig. 39.11.   Perineal urethrostomy after total amputation of the penis.

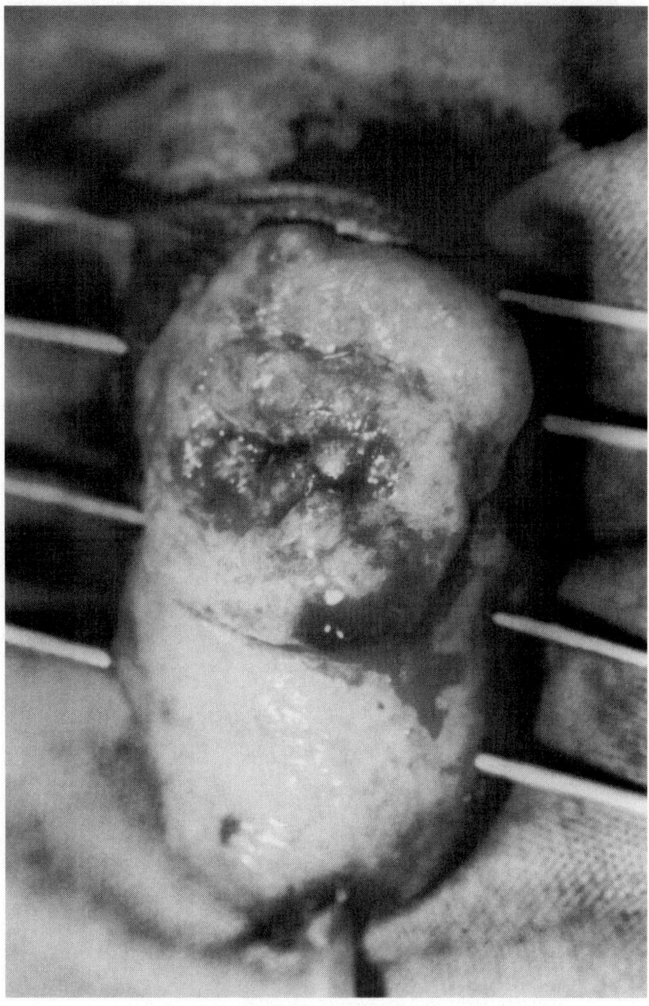

Fig. 39.12.   Brachytherapy template in position.

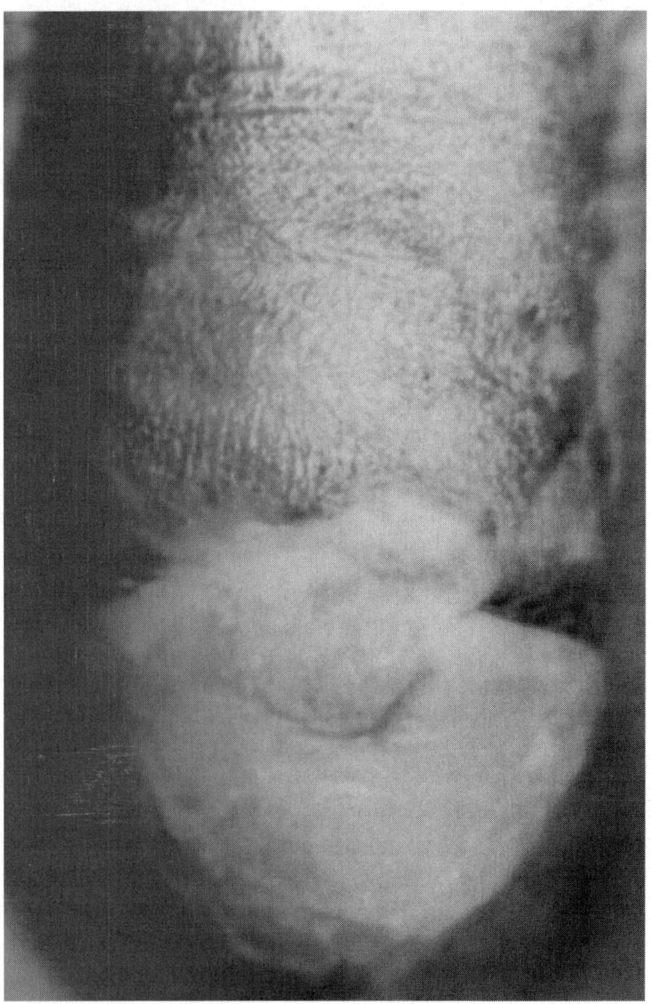

Fig. 39.13. Follow-up showing near total regression at 6 weeks.

ventrally. The skin incision is closed in layers horizontally to lift the scrotum (Fig. 39.10). An indwelling 16F Foley catheter drains the bladder for 4 days (Fig. 39.11).

NONSURGICAL TREATMENT

Various nonsurgical treatments have been in vogue for several years as alternatives to amputational surgery. Early skin lesions or carcinoma in situ can be treated effectively with topical 5-fluorouracil cream (27). Other nonamputative treatments (28) such as cryosurgery for verrucous carcinoma and surface lasers—Nd:YAG (29) or carbon dioxide (30)—have been used successfully in selected cases of in situ or noninvasive tumors. Viable cells in the posttreatment biopsy specimens necessitate surgical excision.

The role of radiation therapy in treating penile carcinoma has been constantly evolving. The earliest successful results of external beam therapy have been replaced by the latest techniques using interstitial brachytherapy (13). Despite its obvious cosmetic and psychological advantage in organ preserva-tion, the lack of uniformity in dose delivery systems, prolonged time to regression, and positive posttherapy biopsy results are causes for concern. Currently, interstitial brachytherapy with the use of iridium-192 (31, 32) wires is popular.

At our institute (32), interstitial brachytherapy is offered to selected young patients with lesions less than 3 cm that are noninvasive, do not involve the meatus, and have no groin adenopathy. Larger lesions after debulking surgery were treated with this approach but resulted in relapse and required salvage surgery. Under general anesthesia, circumcision or debulking of tumor is done. A 16F Foley catheter is introduced. At 1-cm distances, needles are inserted through the tumor and glans (Fig. 39.12). With an afterloading technique, the patient receives radiation therapy with iridium-192 wires as per previously calculated dose. Patients undergo careful follow-up to look for relapse (Fig. 39.13). The other form of interstitial brachytherapy—contact or plesiobrachytherapy—is used for noninvasive tumors of the glans by using surface molds containing radioactive substances.

Systemic chemotherapy for primary tumors in penile carcinomas was reported by Ichikawa et al. (33) using bleomycin. However, the collective experience with chemotherapy (34) has been far from satisfactory and is generally reserved for palliation in advanced disease.

REFERENCES

1. Celsus C (Translated by Spencer WG). Celsus de medicina. Loeb Classical Library Service. Cambridge: Harvard University Press, 1935;2:276.
2. Morgagni GB. The seats and causes of disease, book IV, letter L, 1761:50.
3. Lewis LG. Young's radical operation for the cure of cancer of the penis: a report of 34 cases. J Urol 1931;26:295.
4. MacCormack W. Five cases of amputation of penis for epithelioma. Br Med J 1886;1:343.
5. Curtis BF. American textbook of diseases of the skin. Philadelphia: WB Saunders, 1898:76.
6. Young HH. A radical operation for the cure of cancer of the penis. J Urol 1931;26:285.
7. Daseler EH, Anson BJ, Reimann AF. Radical excision of the inguinal and iliac lymph glands. Surg Gynecol Obstet 1948; 87:679.
8. Baronofsky IA. Technique of inguinal node dissection. Surgery 1953;33:886.
9. Cabanas RM. An approach for the treatment of penile carcinoma. Cancer 1977;39:456.
10. Perinetti E, Crane DB, Catalona WJ. Unreliability of sentinel node biopsy for staging penile carcinoma. J Urol 1980;124:734.
11. deKernion JB. Ilio-inguinal lymphadenectomy. In: Crawford ED, Borden T, eds. Genito-urinary cancer surgery. Philadelphia: Lea and Febiger, 1982:318.
12. Catalona WJ. Modified inguinal lymphadenectomy for carcinoma of penis with preservation of saphenous veins: technique and preliminary results. J Urol 1988;140:306
13. Gerbaulet AA, Lambin P. Radiation therapy of the cancer of

the penis: indications, advantages and pitfalls. Urol Clin North Am 1992;19:325.

14. Hassan AA, Orteza AM, Milan DF. Penile horn: review of literature with 3 case reports. J Urol 1967;97:315.

15. Pareira-Bringel PJ, de Andrade Arruda R. 5 fluoro uracil cream 5% in treatment of intra-urethral condylomata. Br J Urol 1982;54:295.

16. Hanash KA, Furlow WL, Utz DCF, et al. Carcinoma of the penis: clinicopathological study. J Urol 1970;104:284.

17. Rheinschild GW, Olsen BS. Balanitis xerotica obliterans. J Urol 1974;104:860.

18. Queyrat L. Erythroplasia du gland. Soc Franc Dermotol Syphiloe 1911;22:378.

19. Bowen J. Precancerous dermatoses: a review of two cases of chronic atypical epithelial proliferation. J Cutan Dis 1952;30:241.

20. Kopf AW, Bart RS. Tumor conference, part 2: multiple bowenoid papules of the penis. a new entity? J Dermatol Surg Oncol 1977;3:265.

21. Mikhail GR. Cancers, precancerous and pseudocancers on the male genitalia. J Dermatol Surg Oncol 1980;6:1027.

22. Gursel EO, Georgountzos C, Uson AC, et al. Penile cancer. Urology 1973;1:569.

23. Narayana AS, Olney LE, Loening SA, et al. Carcinoma of the penis: analysis of 219 cases. Cancer 1985;49:2185.

24. Mohs FE, Snow SN, Larson PO. Mohs' micrographic surgery for penile tumors. Urol Clin North Am 1992;19:21.

25. d'souza LJ. Subtotal amputation for carcinoma of the penis with reconstruction of penile stump. Ann R Coll Surg Engl 1976;58:398.

26. Bissada N. Conservative extirpative treatment of cancer of the penis. Urol Clin North Am 1992;19:283.

27. Tolia BM, Castro VL, Mouded IM, et al. Bowen's disease of the shaft of penis: successful treatment with 5 fluorouracil. Urology 1976;7:617.

28. Hughes PSH. Cryosurgery for verrucous carcinoma of the penis. Cutis 1979;24:43.

29. Rothenberger K, et al. The neodymium YAG laser in the treatment of penis carcinoma. Proceedings of 4th congress of the International Society of Laser Surgery. Tokyo, 1981.

30. Rosenberg SK, Fuller TA. Carbon dioxide rapid super-pulsed laser treatment of erythroplasia of Queyrat. Urology 1980;16:181.

31. El-Demiry MIM, Oliver RTD, Hopestone NF, et al. Re-appraisal of role of radiotherapy and surgery in the management of carcinoma of the penis. Br J Urol 1984;56:724.

32. Chaudhary AJ, Bhavalat RL, Kulkarni JN, et al. Interstitial brachytherapy in Ca penis: a preliminary report. Prog Urol 1991;1:1028.

33. Ichikawa T, Nakano I, Hirokawa I. Bleomycin treatment of the tumors of penis and scrotum. J Urol 1969;102:699.

34. Blum RH, Carter SK, Agre K. A clinical review of bleomycin: a new antineoplastic agent. Cancer 1973;31:903.

40

Carcinoma of the Penis

Management of the Regional Lymphatic Drainage

R. Lee Cox and E. David Crawford

INTRODUCTION

In 1886, MacCormack described the concept of regional lymphadenectomy for treatment of carcinoma of the penis (1). Surgical treatment of this disease without lymphadenectomy dates back to the time of Celsus. Valsalva performed a partial penectomy in 1761 (2). In 1931, Lewis reported on 34 patients treated between 1907 and 1931 by Young, who performed an en bloc partial penectomy and bilateral lymphadenectomy through a curvilinear lower abdominal incision. They were pleased with their results and believed this represented the standard of care for patients without evidence of distant metastatic disease (3, 4). In 1948, Daseler provided an extensive review of the anatomy of the iliac and inguinal lymphatics based on 450 cadaver dissections (5).

Carcinoma of the penis remains a disease that is amenable to surgical cure of both the primary lesion and regional metastatic disease. Although the value of lymphadenectomy in the treatment of penile carcinoma is indisputable, it is associated with significant morbidity. This morbidity gives rise to many of the controversies in the literature regarding surgical management of the regional nodes in carcinoma of the penis (6).

STAGING

Currently, there are two staging systems that are used to categorize patients with penile carcinoma. The Jackson system (7) (Table 40.1) and the TNM system (8) (Table 40.2) are both useful in their own ways, but the TNM system is becoming more popular in the current literature.

CATEGORIES

Patients with penile carcinoma fall into definable categories that help the urologic surgeon decide whether a regional lymphadenectomy should be performed. The correlation between clinical suspicion and pathologic findings with regard to regional nodes is summarized in Table 40.3.

The first category is composed of patients with TIS (14) (carcinoma in situ), Ta (15) (verrucous carcinoma), or T1 disease (16). These patients roughly correspond to patients with a Jackson stage 1 disease. They have a very low potential for the development of metastases and should be managed with local treatment of the primary tumor and serial examinations of the penis and inguinal nodes. If adenopathy is clinically apparent at diagnosis, then they should be treated with antibiotics and reevaluated. If adenopathy persists after 4 to 6 weeks of therapy, then the residual nodes should be biopsied or lymphadenectomy performed. In the case of verrucous carcinoma, the potential for metastases is so low that lymph node biopsy is favored and lymphadenectomy deferred unless the biopsy result is positive (15). The literature is less clear in the case of TIS and T1 tumors. Moderately and poorly differentiated T1 tumors have metastatic potential and perhaps should be placed in category 2 (16).

The second and most controversial category to manage is composed of patients with invasive cancer (T2 to 4) with no evidence of distant metastatic disease (M0) and clinically negative groin examinations after treatment of the local tumor and 4 weeks of antibiotic therapy. Options for management include the following.

1. Close clinical observation and ileoinguinal lymphadenectomy of the affected side or sides if adenopathy develops (9, 10, 17).
2. Imaging (computed tomography, magnetic resonance imaging, and/or lymphangiography) and close clinical observation if negative (18).
3. Fine-needle aspiration cytology of nodes opacified by lymphangiography and close observation if negative (19, 20).

Table 40.1. Jackson's Staging System

Stage I	Tumors confined to the glans and/or prepuce
Stage II	Tumors extending onto the shaft of the penis
Stage III	Operable, metastatic, inguinal adenopathy
Stage IV	Primary tumor extending off the shaft of the penis or inoperable metastatic, inguinal adenopathy or distant metastatic disease

4. Sentinel node biopsy (removal of the node at the junction of the superficial epigastric and greater saphenous veins) and close observation if negative (21).
5. Formal lymphadenectomy (bilateral) within 4 to 6 weeks of treatment of the primary tumor (early lymphadenectomy) (13, 22–24).

Because significant morbidity is attributed to regional lymphadenectomy for carcinoma of the penis, policies of watch and wait are attractive, but there is an approximately 10 to 20% chance of metastases development while observation is carried out in clinically negative patients (9, 12, 13,). Imaging studies are useful in detecting distant metastatic disease and large pelvic nodes, but add little to the evaluation of a patient who has clinically negative examination (18). While sentinel node biopsies and fine needle aspiration cytologies are both very helpful if positive, false-negative results do occur (9, 20, 25).

Data from multiple institutions agree that patients undergoing early lymphadenectomy have a better 5-year survival rate than those undergoing delayed lymphadenectomy—88% versus 38% (13), 57% versus 13% (22), and 62% versus 8% (24). This argues strongly for early lymphadenectomy despite the

Table 40.2. TNM Staging System of Carcinoma of the Penis

Primary Tumor (T)	
TX	Primary tumor cannot be assessed
T0	No evidence of the primary tumor
TIS	Carcinoma in situ
Ta	Noninvasive (verrucous) carcinoma
T1	Tumor invades subepithelial connective tissue
T2	Tumor invades corpus cavernosa or spongiosum
T3	Tumor invades urethra or prostate
T4	Tumor invades other adjacent structures
Regional lymph nodes (N)	
NX	Regional lymph nodes cannot be assessed
N0	No regional lymph node metastasis
N1	Metastasis in a single, superficial, inguinal node
N2	Metastasis in multiple or bilateral, superficial, inguinal nodes
N3	Metastasis in deep inguinal or pelvic lymph node(s), may be unilateral or bilateral
Distant Metastases (M)	
MX	Presence of distant metastasis cannot be determined
M0	No distant metastases
M1	Distant metastases are present

Table 40.3. Clinical Suspicion Versus Pathologic Findings at Lymphadenectomy

	NO. OF PATIENTS	REFERENCE
Clinically negative/pathologically positive (%)		
13.7	116	9
16.0	113	10
18.0	38	11
16.6	12	12
66.6	9	13
Clinically positive/pathologically positive (%)		
92.4	106	10
86.0	76	11
55.5	9	12

substantial morbidity associated with the procedure. Therefore, we advocate bilateral lymphadenectomy in these patients after treatment of the local cancer and 4 to 6 weeks of antibiotics.

Several other points should be made. They include the following.

1. Tumors involving the proximal shaft have a higher incidence of nodal metastases than those involving the glans, distal, or midshaft (23).
2. Moderately and poorly differentiated tumors have a higher incidence of metastases than well-differentiated tumors (16, 26).
3. It is controversial if pelvic lymphadenectomy is necessary in conjunction with inguinal lymphadenectomy (especially if the inguinal nodes are negative) (11, 27–29).

It has been our policy to perform a bilateral pelvic lymphadenectomy through a midline abdominal incision before inguinal node dissection. The pelvic lymphadenectomy does not add to the morbidity of the inguinal dissection (30). More recently, we have performed this procedure laparoscopically. If there is extensive pelvic nodal disease, then the operation is palliative at best and the surgeon may abort the planned inguinal node dissection and spare the patient the associated morbidity or, in certain cases, proceed for palliation. If there is only microscopic pelvic adenopathy, then the operation may have therapeutic value (9, 11, 27).

The third category of patients are those with invasive carcinoma and palpable adenopathy after treatment of the primary tumor and 4 to 6 weeks of antibiotics. These patients have an approximately 50% incidence of proven metastases (12). They should all undergo a bilateral ilioinguinal lymphadenectomy. Again, we prefer to perform the pelvic lymphadenectomy first for the same reasons. These patients should have imaging studies for evidence of metastases and possible percutaneous biopsy of suspicious pelvic nodes to help when counseling the patient about disease status. This might potentially spare the patient the morbidity of a node dissection. Large (greater than 4 cm) inguinal nodes are often associated with perinodal infiltration and a high likelihood of positive pelvic nodes (10). Ayyappan et al.'s data suggest that patients with clinically palpable pelvic nodes (55% positive), inguinal nodes greater than 2 cm, and fixed or ulcerated inguinal nodes also have an increased risk of positive iliac nodal disease (23). Patients with these risk factors might be appropriate candidates for laparoscopic pelvic lymphadenectomy before inguinal node dissection if computed tomography scanning does not demonstrate adenopathy that is amenable to percutaneous biopsy (fine-needle aspiration cytology).

The fourth category is composed of patients who present with an unresectable primary tumor, unresectable inguinal adenopathy, extensive pelvic nodal disease, or distant metastases. These patients are not candidates for therapeutic lymphadenectomy and should be offered systemic chemotherapy.

Those patients who are observed and in whom unilateral inguinal adenopathy later develops should be treated initially with unilateral ileoinguinal lymphadenectomy (10). At least 88% of patients in whom adenopathy develops during followup will have proven metastases (24).

The following sections discuss the anatomy and surgical techniques relevant to the performance of a full, bilateral ileoinguinal lymphadenectomy.

ANATOMICAL CONSIDERATIONS FOR ILEOINGUINAL LYMPHADENECTOMY

The surgery of ileoinguinal lymph node dissection is fraught with morbid complications that are often directly related to the technique of surgical dissection. A proper conception of the lymphatic distribution, the vascular supply, and the extent or limits of necessary dissection, is imperative for a therapeutic lymphadenectomy with minimal morbidity.

Lymphatic Drainage of the Penis

Penile lymphatics are essentially divided into two sets. Those draining the prepuce and penile skin converge and coalesce into larger lymphatic trunks in the dorsum of the penis. These channels course toward the root of the penis, then pass laterally to terminate into the superficial inguinal nodes on both sides. A more extensive network of lymphatics draining the glans penis courses along the corona to the dorsum and merge to form larger vessels that follow the dorsal vein of the penis to the symphyseal area to ultimately drain into the superficial and deep inguinal nodes. Corporal lymphatics essentially follow the same pathway as that of the glans penis. Further efferent drainage of inguinal lymphatics occurs through lymph channels located in the femoral canal into external iliac and pelvic nodes.

Regional Anatomy

The superficial fascia of the lower abdomen and thigh is composed of two layers; the superficial fatty layer (Camper's fascia) and the deeper fibroelastic layer (Scarpa's fascia). The deep fascia enveloping the muscles of the thigh and gluteal region is called the fascia lata. It is attached superiorly to the posterior surface of the iliac crest, sacrum, sacrotuberous ligaments, ischium, pubic arch, symphysis pubes, pubic crest, and inguinal ligament. Distally, it is attached at the knee to the condyles of the femur and tibia and to the head of the fibula. Fascia lata is thinnest on the medial side and thickest on the lateral aspect of the thigh.

The superficial fatty layer of the superficial fascia of the abdomen continues uninterrupted into the lower extremity. The deeper fibroelastic layer, however, fuses with the fascia lata about 2 cm below the inguinal ligament.

The skin and subcutaneous tissue of the groin are supplied by the superficial external pudendal, superficial circumflex iliac, and superficial epigastric arteries. These vessels course in the superficial fatty layer of the superficial fascia and run parallel to the inguinal ligament. Because of this transverse or horizontal disposition of the blood vessels in the superficial fascia of the groin, a transverse incision is more likely to preserve adequate blood supply to the margins of the incision.

The femoral triangle is an anatomic area on the anterior thigh. It is bounded superiorly by the inguinal ligament as its base, laterally by the sartorius, and medially by the adductor longus. The adductor canal at the confluence of sartorius and adductor longus forms its apex. Its floor is formed by the fascia covering the iliopsoas and pectineus muscles. Its roof is formed by the fascia lata. The deep group of inguinal lymph nodes is located in the femoral triangle in the vicinity of the femoral vessels.

The greater saphenous vein, originating from the foot, ascends to the anteromedial aspect of the thigh. Coursing all along in the superficial fascia of the lower extremity, it ultimately passes through the fossa ovalis, an opening in the fascia lata 3 to 4 cm below the medial aspect of the inguinal ligament. The greater saphenous vein pierces the loose cribriform fascia covering the fossa ovalis and terminates into the femoral vein. At this site, the femoral vein and artery are encased in the femoral sheath, a funnel-like projection of the transversalis fascia (anteriorly) and the iliacus fascia (posteriorly). These blend to the adventitia of the femoral vessels at about a 4-cm distance from the inguinal ligament. The femoral sheath contains three distinct compartments, the most medial being the femoral canal, which contains the lymphatics and the lymph nodes. The middle compartment is occupied by the femoral vein, and the lateral compartment contains the femoral artery. The femoral nerve courses lateral to the femoral artery in a plane deep to the iliacus fascia (Fig. 40.1).

Inguino-femoral Lymph Node Distribution

The lymph nodes in this area are divided into both superficial and deep groups. The superficial inguinal nodes, along with the greater saphenous vein and its tributaries, are located within the membranous layer of the superficial fascia (Scarpa's fascia) of the femoral triangle, sandwiched between the superficial fatty layer (Camper's fascia) and the fascia lata. Daseler catego-

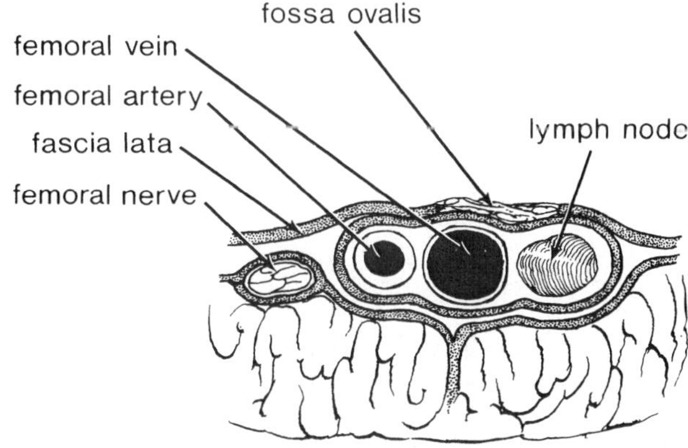

Fig. 40.1.   Femoral sheath.

rized the superficial inguinal nodes into different zones. Four quadrant zones were outlined by horizontal and vertical lines drawn at the saphenofemoral junction. Daseler's fifth quadrant was the saphenofemoral junction (Fig. 40.2) Quadrant: 1 lymph nodes are located around the superficial circumflex iliac vein. Quadrant 2, located in the superior medial area, contains lymph nodes around the superficial epigastric and superficial external pudendal vein. Of particular importance in Daseler's dissection was the fact that lymph nodes were often detected 1 cm above the inguinal ligament. Quadrant 3 is inferomedial in position and contains nodes around the greater saphenous vein. The inferolateral quadrant 4 contains lymph nodes clustered around the lateral accessory saphenous vein and termination of the superficial circumflex iliac vein. Each quadrant may contain several lymph nodes or may be completely void of them. The superficial nodes send their efferents to the glands of deeper

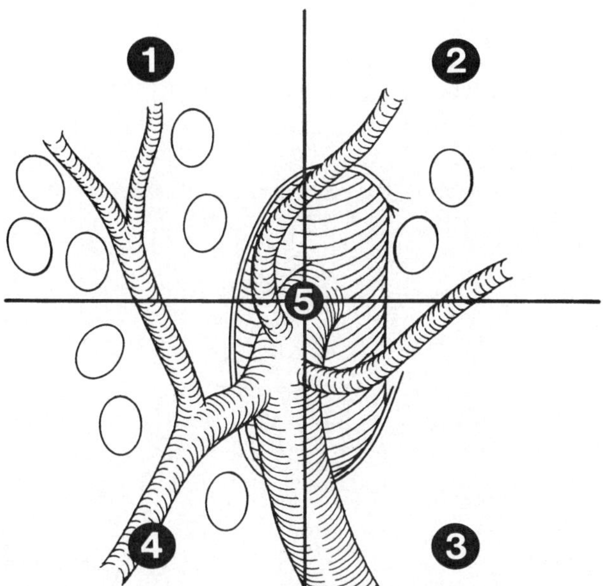

Fig. 40.2.   Zonal division of superfical inguinal nodes according to Daseler.

location situated along the femoral vessels (deep inguinal nodes) and then into the retroperitoneal iliac chain in the pelvis.

The deep inguinal nodes are situated beneath the fascia lata in the femoral triangle. They form a small chain of nodes in the adipose tissue surrounding the femoral vessels within the femoral sheath. Distally, they may extend into the adductor canal and proximally, they continue underneath the inguinal ligament to merge with the external iliac chain. The most consistent member of the deep inguinal group is the node of Cloquet or Rosenmuller, located in the femoral canal medial to the femoral vein.

ILEOINGUINAL LYMPHADENECTOMY

Oral antibiotic therapy during the 6-week period following treatment of the primary lesion of the penis helps in reducing infectious inflammation of the inguinal lymph nodes. A low residual diet on the day before surgery and a cleansing enema on the night before surgery minimize the risk of bowel movements and wound contamination in the immediate postoperative period. Parenteral broad-spectrum antibiotics are started just prior to surgery. Intermittent compressive stockings are applied to the lower extremities.

Although a variety of incisions and approaches have been proposed by individual advocates, we prefer to start with a midline suprapubic incision for bilateral pelvic lymphadenectomy, followed by curvilinear groin incisions for inguinal dissection (Fig. 40.3A). In patients with clinically or histologically positive inguinal adenopathy, or with invasive and extensive primary lesions, we recommend bilateral groin dissection. However, when an initially negative groin develops adenopathy during follow-up, unilateral dissection only of the involved side is recommended. The patient is positioned supine with a roll under the sacrum. The ipsilateral thigh is abducted, externally rotated, and flexed at the knee (Fig. 40.3B). A urethral catheter is left indwelling. The entire abdomen and thighs are prepared and draped.

PELVIC LYMPHADENECTOMY

A midline incision is made from the umbilicus to the symphyses pubes. Extraperitoneal pelvic lymphadenectomy is carried out on the ipsilateral or more involved side, taking down node-bearing adipose connective tissue around the distal common iliac artery, external iliac vessels, internal iliac artery, and the obturator fossa. If gross nodal metastases are evident and proven on frozen section analysis, then an inguinal lymphadenectomy is not warranted. If the nodes are negative, contralateral pelvic lymph node dissection is carried out with frozen section examination. In contrast to pelvic lymphadenectomy for prostatic carcinoma, the lymph node dissection is carried beyond the circumflex iliac vessels further distally, down to and behind the inguinal ligament, with special attention to dissecting nodal tissue from the femoral canal (Fig. 40.4). The dissected pelvic lymph nodal mass is removed separately at the level of

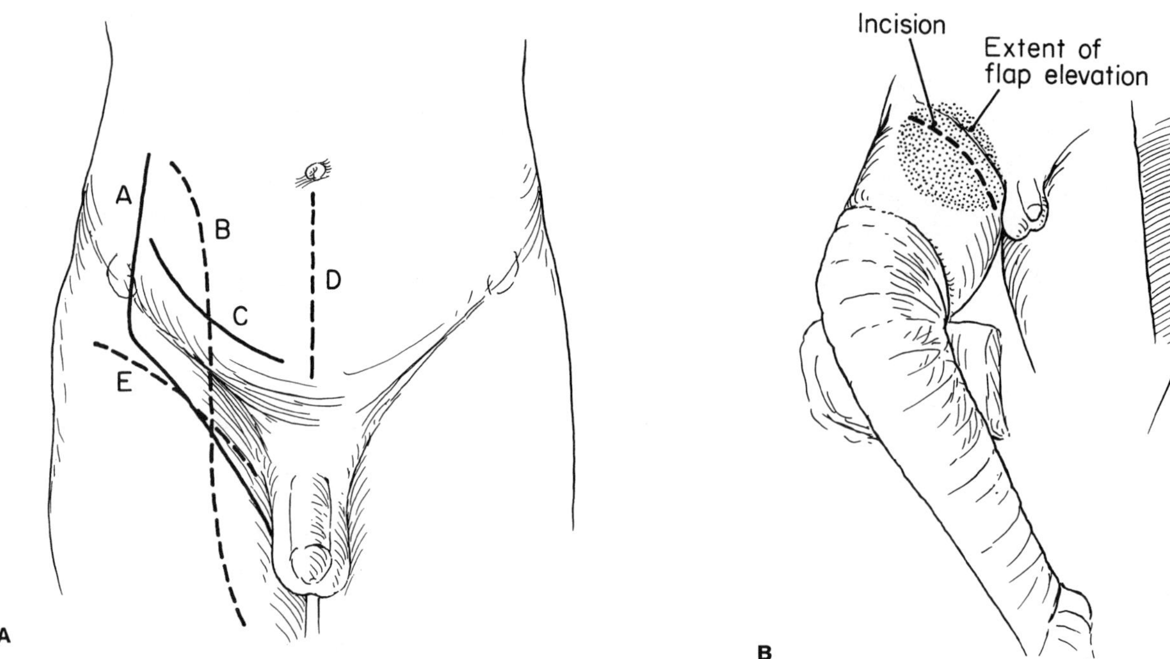

Fig. 40.3. *A,* Incisions employed for ileoinguinal lymphadenectomy. The skin-bridge technique is depicted in *C* and *E.* My current recommendation is a suprapubic midline incision coupled with a curvilinear thigh incision *(D* and *E). B,* Patient position for right ilioinguinal lymphadenectomy. The leg is abducted at the thigh, flexed at the knee, and externally rotated. An indwelling urethral catheter is inserted and the scrotum draped out of the operative field.

the inguinal ligament. We believe that any attempt at en bloc removal of pelvic and inguinal nodes, without actual division of the inguinal ligament, is an exercise in futility. The wound is closed in layers without a drain.

INGUINAL LYMPHADENECTOMY

A curvilinear incision is made in the upper thigh, starting below the anterior superior iliac spine, running 5 to 10 cm

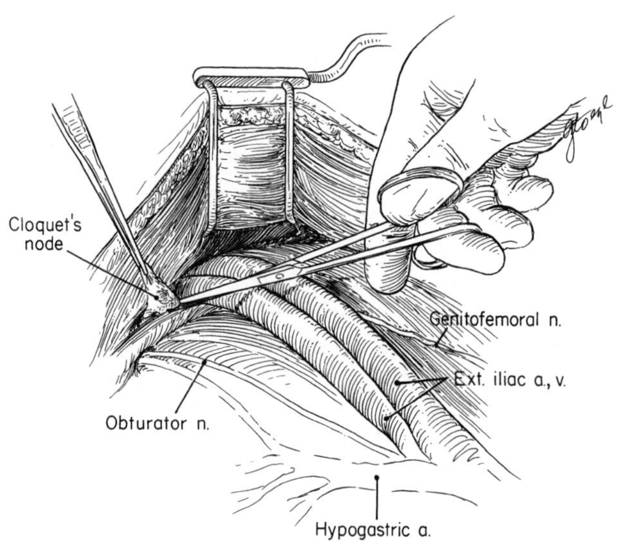

Fig. 40.4. The completed pelvic lymphadenectomy. Attention is given to the meticulous removal of the contents of the femoral canal.

distal and parallel to the inguinal ligament, and ending medially up to the prominent adductor longus tendon. The goal of the dissection is to clear the superficial and deep inguinal lymph nodes located in the femoral triangle.

Meticulous attention is devoted to developing viable skin flaps. The skin flaps should include the superficial fatty layer of the subcutaneous adipose tissue leaving only a thin layer of membranous Scarpa's fascia containing the superficial lymph nodes. Initially, skin edges are carefully handled with skin hooks, then grasped manually to finally be lifted up with Deaver retractors. We prefer to develop the skin flaps up to the margins of the femoral triangle, except proximally, as this flap is carried up to about 2 cm above the inguinal ligament (Fig. 40.5).

Starting superiorly, the fibrofatty tissue of the Scarpa's fascia is sharply divided down to the external oblique aponeurosis and then dissected towards the inguinal ligament (Fig. 40.5). Subcutaneous vessels are carefully electrocoagulated or divided between fine catgut ligatures throughout the dissection to ensure hemostasis and to minimize lymph leakage. Medially, the node-bearing tissues are stripped from the adductor longus muscle and dissection is continued to clear the femoral canal. The femoral vein and artery, enclosed in femoral sheath, lie immediately lateral. The fascial sheath overlying the vessels is stripped to expose the vein and the artery (Fig. 40.6). Lateral to the femoral artery, the femoral nerve is noted shining underneath the fascia covering the iliacus muscle. We do not dissect the nerve and its branches because no significant nodal tissue exists in this area. Dissecting laterally, the origin of the sarto-

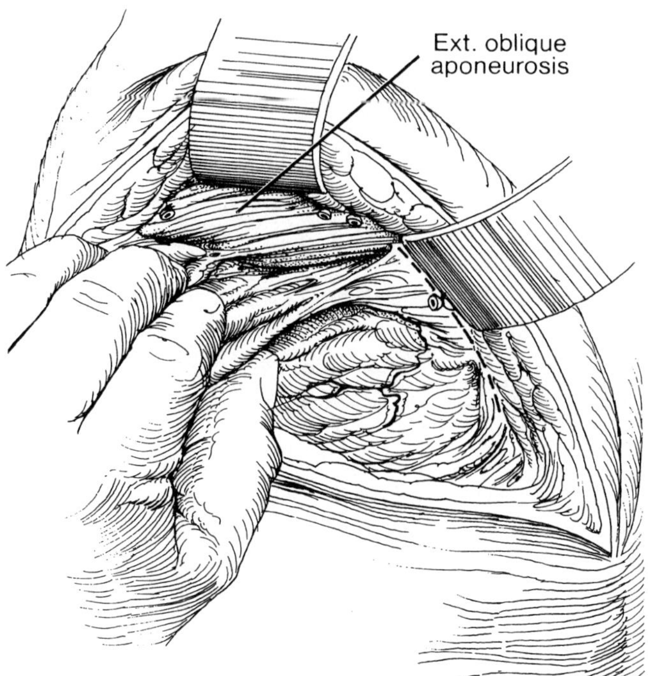

Fig. 40.5. Proximal skin flap is developed. Fibrofatty superficial fascia is dissected down to external oblique aponeurosis.

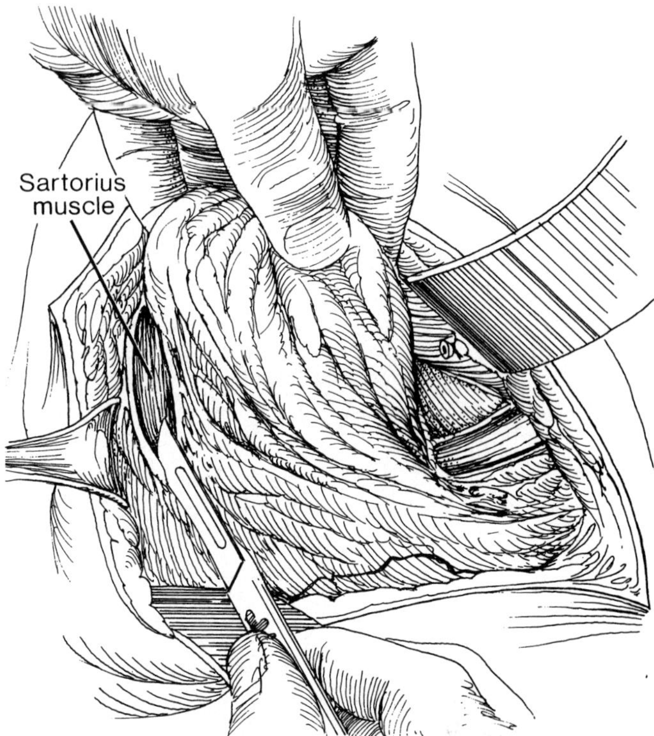

Fig. 40.7. Outer limit of dissection at the lateral margin of the femoral triangle.

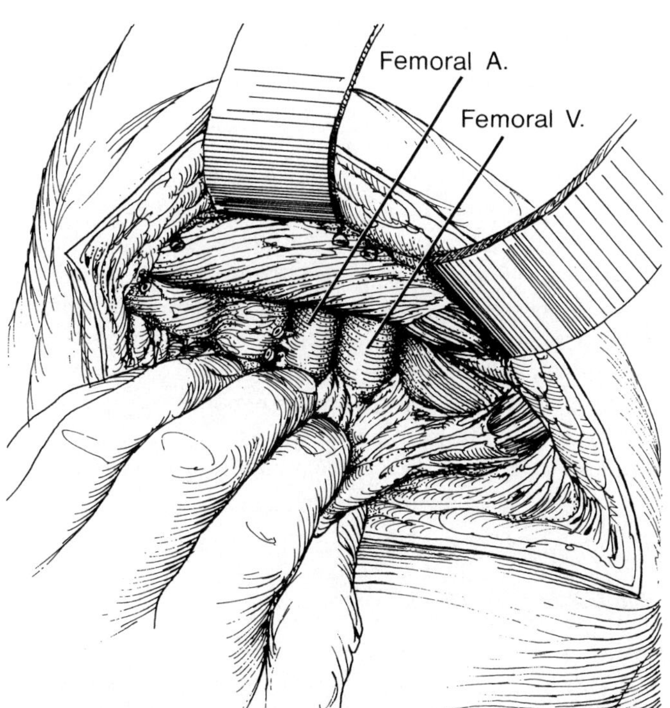

Fig. 40.6. En bloc dissection is continued in the femoral sheath clearing the tissues anterior to the femoral vessels.

rius muscle from the anterior superior iliac spine is exposed. With medial traction on the dissected superior block of tissues, the fibrofatty tissue and fascia covering the sartorius muscle are sharply divided downward to define the lateral boundary of the femoral triangle (Fig. 40.7). With downward traction on the dissected tissues, stripping of the femoral vessels is resumed. All fibrofatty and nodal tissues are meticulously dissected off the anterolateral aspect of the femoral artery and vein. Lifting the vessels and clearing the posterior aspect are not necessary as there are usually no draining lymph nodes behind the vessels. The profunda femoris branch arises from the posterior aspect of the femoral artery at about 3 cm distal to the inguinal ligament. This important arterial branch should be identified and carefully preserved. As the femoral vein is dissected, the termination of the greater saphenous vein is noticed passing through the fossa ovalis. The greater saphenous vein is ligated and divided at its junction with the femoral vein (Fig. 40.8). The edges of the fossa ovalis are divided medially, where it continues as fascia lata covering the adductor longus. All the tissues and fascia lata covering the medial margin of adductor longus are sharply divided downwards until they join the lateral dissection along the medial margin of the sartorius muscle. At the distal limit of the inferior dissection, the greater saphenous vein is encountered again and divided between ligatures (Fig. 40.9). We have proposed that preservation of the greater saphenous vein with meticulous skeletonization may be therapeutically effective with added benefit of reduced chance of postoper-

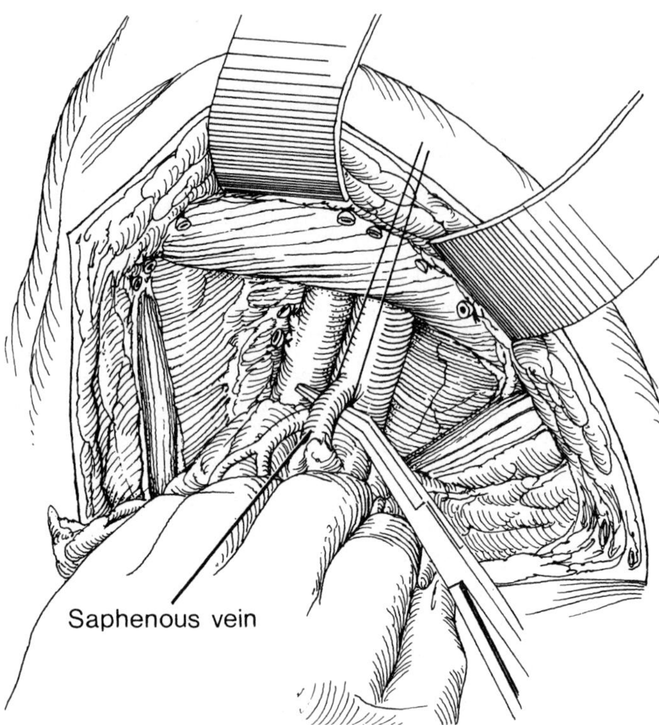

Fig. 40.8. Further dissection in the floor of the femoral triangle. Ligation and division of the greater saphenous vein.

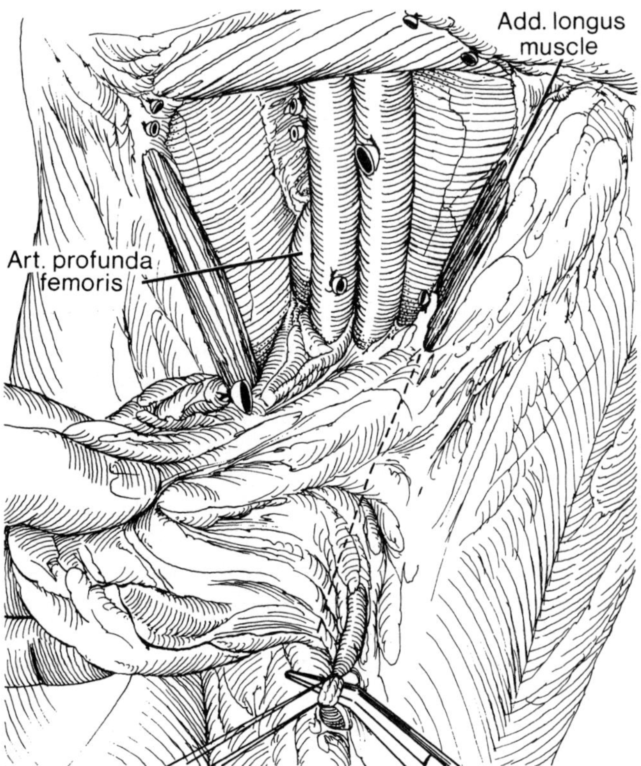

Fig. 40.9. Distal limit of dissection at the apex of the femoral triangle. The greater saphenous vein is again ligated and divided.

ative edema of the lower extremities. There are no controlled studies available in support or against this conjecture. Centrally, the stripping of the anterior aspect of the femoral vessels is continued up to the apex of the femoral triangle, removing the deep inguinal glands en bloc with the rest of the specimen.

WOUND CLOSURE

The wound is irrigated with saline and any visible bleeding or lymphatic oozing is controlled. The inguinal ligament is sutured to the Cooper's ligament with interrupted 2-0 silk sutures to close the empty femoral canal medial to the femoral vein. The sartorius muscle is dissected off its origin from the anterior superior iliac spine. It is partially mobilized medially to cover the femoral vessels and is secured to the inguinal ligament with interrupted 2-0 silk horizontal mattress sutures. The subcutaneous tissue of the lower flap is anchored to the underlying muscles with interrupted 4-0 polyglycolic acid sutures. This eliminates the dead spaces and prevents fluid collections in the wound. A 7 mm Jackson-Pratt suction drain is inserted through the distal flap. Several millimeters of excess skin are removed from the edges of the skin flaps. The use of intravenous fluorescin and Wood's lamp helps delineate viable skin edges. The skin edges are reapproximated with interrupted 4-0 Prolene sutures. So that the vascularity of the skin flaps may not be compromised, sterile dressings are applied and secured loosely to avoid pressure.

POSTOPERATIVE CARE

Patients who undergo ileoinguinal lymphadenectomy are maintained with bedrest, have an indwelling urethral catheter and closed suction drains, and are given prophylaxis for deep venous thrombosis.

Strict bedrest with the legs elevated is maintained for 5 to 7 days. During this period the patient is given minidoses of heparin. The dose of heparin is adjusted according to the value of the partial thromboplastin time (31). Intermittent compression stockings are placed before the procedure and used throughout the patient's hospital stay.

The closed suction drains are not removed until the output is less than 30 mL in 24 hours. Usually, the drainage has decreased to this level within 5 to 7 days. The Foley catheter is removed 48 hours postoperatively.

COMPLICATIONS

Although the operative mortality rate for ileoinguinal node dissection is approximately 1% (17), the morbidity rate is staggering; as many as 82 to 86% of patients experience some morbidity from the procedure (9, 30). It is this high morbidity rate that has resulted in the controversies about the procedure.

Table 40.4. Complications of Groin Dissection

COMPLICATION	% OF CASES	REFERENCES
Flap necrosis	23–82	12, 17, 27, 30
Leg edema	30–50	12, 17, 27, 30
Severe leg edema	15–35	17, 30
Seroma	4–16	17, 27, 30
Scrotal edema	15	30
Wound infection	10–18	12, 17, 27, 30
Lymphocele	9	27, 30
Thrombophlebitis	3–6	12, 30
Death	0–3	12, 17, 30

The complications and their relative frequencies are listed in Table 40.4.

The two most common complications are necrosis of the skin edges and lymphedema. Wound breakdown may occur in 50 to 80% of incisions and may require skin grafting to achieve closure 10 to 40% of the time (27, 30). Approximately 30% of patients experience severe lymphedema of the lower extremity after this procedure. This can be a debilitating complication and is prominent in most reported series. Sometimes the edema will resolve with time, but it is often permanent. The use of support stockings, elevation, and diuretics may ameliorate the symptoms. The routine use of transposition of the sartorius muscle to cover the femoral vessels has almost eliminated the devastating complication of delayed hemorrhage (30, 32).

MODIFICATIONS

Because the morbidity of the procedure is so great, investigators continue to search for modifications that will lower the complication rate of this necessary procedure.

In 1972, Fraley and Hutchens described a technique that uses two incisions on each side. One of the incisions is made above the groin crease and the other is made below. This leaves an intervening bridge of skin. They described an extremely low rate of skin loss in a small series. Other complications were not enumerated (33).

In 1988, Catalona described a modified inguinal lymphadenectomy (28). The operation he proposed is similar to the one described in this text with the following differences.

1. The saphenous vein is preserved throughout its course.
2. The lateral limit of the dissection is the femoral artery.
3. The sartorius muscle is not mobilized and transposed.
4. Iliac node dissection is only performed if the frozen section is positive for malignancy in the inguinal nodal packet.

Using this procedure, only one of six patients experienced a small area of skin slough. All patients experienced at least transient lower extremity edema, but none were debilitated.

Preservation of the saphenous vein to reduce morbidity was also described by Smith and Crawford (34). This represents an attractive alternative in patients with no evidence of disease. In those patients with extensive adenopathy, a complete dissection is warranted because surgical excision is the only proven therapy for metastatic disease.

In 1991, Ornellas described the use of a Gibson incision to perform both the inguinal and iliac lymphadenectomies with a much lower morbidity rate than other incisions used at the same institution (27). His techniques are similar to those described by Fraley and Hutchens (33), but a single incision is used. The wound breakdown rate was only 5%, and the lymphedema rate was 16%. Fraley and Hutchens described a significant infection rate (15%). The sartorius muscle was not transposed. They believed that this was a better incision because the superior flap's vascularity was always preserved. The number of nodes obtained was similar with this incision to that obtained with other approaches. If other surgeons report similar results with this approach, it may gain popularity.

In 1993, two groups from India reported that they have begun the routine use of the removal of the skin overlying the nodal package and immediate reconstruction with an abdominal or tensor fascia lata flap. They report 100% wound healing and 30% lymphedema rates using this technique (9, 17, 35). This is an expansion of the technique described by Prakash in 1982 for treatment of nodes that grossly involved the skin (36). This represents an alternative with which the surgeon should be familiar if the skin is involved or if the patients have received prior radiation therapy, as is used for selected patients in India (17).

SURVIVAL

The nodal status is the most reliable predictor of survival in invasive penile cancer. The presence of any positive nodes, increasing number of positive nodes, presence of extranodal tumor, bilateral positive nodes, and positive iliac nodes all adversely affect long-term survival. The grade of tumor also correlates with survival.

The expected 5-year survival rate for patients with invasive cancer and a negative early lymphadenectomy is 74 to 95% (10, 11, 24,). The recurrence rate after a negative node dissection is 5 to 7% (10, 24). The 5-year survival rate in the face of an early positive node dissection is 29 to 53% (10, 24). Survival correlates with the number of positive nodes at dissection. With one to three positive unilateral inguinal nodes, the 5-year survival rate is approximately 80%. The 5-year survival rate for patients with negative iliac nodes and greater than three positive inguinal nodes is approximately 50%. Bilateral inguinal adenopathy adversely affects 5-year survival rates (12 to 60%). The presence of extranodal tumor is associated with large nodes and an approximate 5-year survival rate of 5% (10, 11). The presence of positive pelvic nodes is believed to portend a poor prognosis (10, 24), with only rare long-term survival (9, 29). Iliac nodes are positive in 30 to 45% of patients with positive inguinal nodes (9, 10).

Multiple publications (9, 16, 23, 24, 26) report a direct

Table 40.5.   Survival Versus Number of Positive Nodes at Lymphadenectomy

NO. OF POSITIVE NODES	NO. OF PATIENTS	5-YEAR SURVIVAL (%)	REFERENCE
1	6	82	11
1–3[a]	58	81	10
1–6	16	54	11
>3[a]	10	50	10
>6	10	40	11

[a] Excludes any patient with positive inguinal and positive pelvic nodes.

Table 40.6.   Survival Versus Nodal Status and Timimg of Lymphadenectomy

NODAL STATUS	NO. OF PATIENTS	5-YEAR SURVIVAL (%)	REFERENCE
Negative (early)	3	100	13
Negative (early)	103	95	10
Negative (early)	65	87	24
Negative (early)	41	74	11
Positive (early)	6	83	13
Positive (early	98	56	10
Positive (early)	55	29	24
Positive (delayed)	1	0	13
Positive (delayed)	37	0	24
Positive (delayed)	8	13	22
Positive (delayed)	16	50	9

Table 40.7.   Poor Prognostic Findings at Lymphadenectomy

FINDING	NO. OF PATIENTS	5-YEAR SURVIVAL (%)	REFERENCE
Positive iliac nodes	30	0	10
Positive iliac nodes	11	0	11
Positive iliac nodes	6	33	9
Perinodal infiltration	17	5.8	10
Perinodal infiltration	22	4.5	11
Perinodal infiltration	22	32	9
Bilateral positive nodes[a]	25	60	10
Bilateral positive nodes	24	12	11
>3 Positive nodes[a]	10	50	10
>6 Positive nodes	10	40	11

[a] Excludes patients with positive inguinal and iliac nodes.

correlation between grade of the primary tumor and the probability of nodal metastases; therefore, there is no place for a watch and wait philosophy when dealing with high-grade tumors and a negative clinical examination of the groin. A patient with a poorly differentiated tumor had a 75% probability of nodal spread in one series (23) and only a 16.7% probability of 5-year survival in another (9).

Patients who die of metastatic penile cancer tend to do so within the first 2 years after diagnosis (88%). All patients in a large series who died of recurrent penile cancer after an early lymphadenectomy did so within 2 years. In that same series, those patients who underwent a palliative dissection were believed to have a better quality of life but no significant survival advantage (24).

Survival with relation to the number of positive inguinal nodes, timing of lymphadenectomy, and in the face of poor prognostic factors is summarized in Tables 40.5, 40.6, and 40.7, respectively.

SUMMARY

Invasive carcinoma of the penis is a surgically curable disease even in the face of regional nodal metastases. Aggressive surgical management, although associated with significant morbidity, affords the patient the best chance for survival.

REFERENCES

1. Murphy L. The history of urology. Springfield, IL: Charles C. Thomas, 1972.
2. MacCormack W. Five cases of amputation of the penis for epithelioma. Br Med J 1886;1:343.
3. Young H. A radical operation for cure of cancer of the penis. J Urol 1931;26:285.
4. Lewis L. Young's radical operation for the cure of cancer of the penis; a report of 34 cases. J Urol 1931;26:295.
5. Daseler E, Anson BJ, Reimann AF. Radical excision of the inguinal and iliac lymph glands. Surg Gynecol Obstet 1948; 87:679.
6. Schellhammer P, Jordan G, Schlossberg S. Tumors of the penis. In: Walsh P, Retik A, Stamey T, et al., eds. Campbell's urology. New York: WB Saunders, 1992:1264.
7. Jackson S. The treatment of carcinoma of the penis. Br J Surg 1966;53:33.
8. American Joint Committee on Cancer. Manual of staging for cancer. 3rd ed. Philadelphia: JB Lippincott, 1988:189.
9. Kamat M, et al. Carcinoma of the penis: the Indian experience. J Surg Oncol 1993;52:50.
10. Ravi R. Correlation between the extent of nodal involvement and survival following groin dissection for carcinoma of the penis. Br J Urol 1993;72:817.
11. Srinivas V, et al. Penile cancer: relationship of extent of nodal metastasis to survival. J Urol 1987;137:880.
12. Beggs J, Spratt J. Epidermoid carcinoma of the penis. J Urol 1964;91:166.
13. McDougal WS, et al. Treatment of carcinoma of the penis: the case for primary lymphadenectomy. J Urol 1986;136:38.

14. Eng T, et al. Lymph node metastasis for carcinoma in situ of the penis: a case report. J Urol 1995;153:432.

15. Seixas A, et al. Verrucous carcinoma of the penis: retrospective analysis of 32 cases. J Urol 1994;152:1476.

16. Solsona E, et al. Corpus cavernosum invasion and tumor grade in the prediction of lymph node condition in penile carcinoma. Eur Urol 1992;22:115.

17. Ravi R. Morbidity following groin dissection for penile carcinoma. Br J Urol 1993;72:941.

18. Vapnek J, et al. Recent advances in imaging studies for staging of penile and urethral carcinoma. Urol Clin North Am 1992;19:257.

19. Luciani L, et al. Value and role of percutaneous regional node aspiration cytology in the management of penile carcinoma. Eur Urol 1984;10:294.

20. Scapini P, et al. Penile cancer: aspiration biopsy cytology for staging. Cancer 1986;58:1526.

21. Cabanas R. An approach for the treatment of penile carcinoma. Cancer 1977;39:456.

22. Johnson D, Lo R. Management of regional lymph nodes in penile carcinoma. Urology 1984;24:308.

23. Ayyappan K, et al. Can regional lymph node involvement be predicted in patients with carcinoma of the penis? Br J Urol 1994;73:549.

24. Ornellas A, et al. Surgical treatment of invasive squamous cell carcinoma of the penis: retrospective analysis of 350 cases. J Urol 1994;151:1244.

25. Perinetti E, et al. Unreliability of sentinel lymph node biopsy for staging penile carcinoma. J Urol 1980;124:734.

26. Fraley E, et al. The role of ilioinguinal lymphadenectomy and significance of histological differentiation in treatment of carcinoma of the penis. J Urol 1989;142:1478.

27. Ornellas A, et al. Analyses of 200 lymphadenectomies in patients with penile carcinoma. J Urol 1991;146:330.

28. Catalona W. Modified inguinal lymphadenectomy for carcinoma of the penis with preservation of saphenous veins: technique and preliminary results. J Urol 1988;140:306.

29. Hardner G, et al. Carcinoma of the penis: analysis of therapy in 100 consecutive cases. J Urol 1972;108:428.

30. Johnson D, Lo R. Complications of groin dissection in penile cancer: experience with 101 lymphadenectomies. Urology 1984;24:312.

31. Leyvraz PF, et al. Adjusted versus fixed-dose subcutaneous heparin in the treatment of deep vein thrombosis after total hip replacement. N Engl J Med 1983;309:954.

32. Barnosky ID. Technique of inguinal node dissection. Surgery 1948;24:555.

33. Fraley E, Hutchens H. Radical ilio-inguinal node dissection: the skin bridge technique: a new procedure. J Urol 1972;108:279.

34. Smith R, Crawford ED. Ilioinguinal lymphadenectomy. Surgical Rounds 1986;9:85.

35. Abraham V, et al. Primary reconstruction to avoid wound breakdown following groin block dissections. Br J Plast Surg 1992;45:211.

36. Prakash S. The use of myocutaneous flaps in block dissections of the groin cases with gross skin involvement. Br J Plast Surg 1982;35:413.

41

Surgical Management of Urethral Carcinoma

Peter R. Carroll

Urethral carcinoma is rare. Although Thiaudierre published the first report in 1834, little more than 1500 cases have been reported in the English language literature since then. It generally arises during the sixth and seventh decades of life, is the only genitourinary cancer that is more common in women than men (0.02% of cancers in women), and occurs more commonly in whites than blacks. Because of the substantial anatomic differences between the male and female urethra, the roles of surgery and radiation in the management of urethral cancers in each sex will be considered separately. However, the chapter will conclude with sections addressing combined modality treatment of locally advanced urethral cancer in men and women and the management of metastatic disease.

Most reports of these rare cancers, even from large referral institutions, include both relatively small numbers and substantial variation among individual tumors because of differences in tissue structure, grade, site, and anatomic extent. Thus, no consensus has been reached on the optimal management. Currently, treatment decisions must be based on the biologic characteristics of the tumor (i.e., stage, grade, and site), the morbidity of each mode of treatment, and its ability to eradicate or control the malignancy.

MALE URETHRAL CARCINOMA

Anatomy

The male urethra is approximately 21 cm long and can be divided into three regional segments—prostatic, membranous, and penile (1). (Fig. 41.1). The prostatic urethra, approximately 3 cm long, is surrounded by prostatic tissue and contains the ejaculatory and prostatic ducts. The membranous urethra, the thickest and shortest segment (averaging between 2 and 2.5 cm), is surrounded by smooth and skeletal muscle, the latter constituting the external urinary sphincter. The penile urethra, the longest segment, is contained within the corpus spongiosum and extends from the pelvic floor musculature to the external urinary meatus (approximately 15 cm). The proximal portion, the bulbar urethra, is expanded in a fusiform fashion and is covered by the bulbospongiosus muscle. As the pendulous

urethra approaches the meatus, it widens once again to form the fossa navicularis. The posterior urethra consists of the prostatic and membranous portions. The anterior urethra is contained in the penile segment (bulbar and pendulous). However, most authors will describe lesions in the bulbar urethra as being posterior lesions because of their similar prognosis to tumors of the membranous urethra.

The epithelial lining of the urethra varies—transitional in the prostatic urethra; pseudostratified or stratified columnar in the membranous, bulbar, and penile segments; and stratified squamous epithelium at the urinary meatus (Fig. 41.1). Paired bulbourethral glands, Cowper's glands, lie within the deep perineal compartment of the urogenital diaphragm surrounding the membranous urethra. The paired ducts of these glands run distally into the corpus spongiosum and open into the bulbar urethra. Numerous submucosal glands, the glands of Littré, can be found along the anterior urethra.

The urethra is surrounded by structures with a rich blood supply. The internal pudendal artery, a branch of the hypogastric artery, gives rise to two arteries that supply the anterior urethra—the bulbar and urethral arteries. The former supplies the bulbar urethra and bulbospongiosum; the latter supplies the corpus spongiosum. The glans penis is supplied by the deep dorsal artery, which lies below Buck's fascia between the dorsal veins and nerves.

A thorough knowledge of regional anatomy and the lymphatic drainage of the urethra is essential to tumor staging and treatment planning. Generally, lesions of the anterior urethra drain into the inguinal lymph nodes and lesions of the posterior urethra drain into the pelvic lymph nodes. The lymphatics of the glans penis and the penile urethra drain into the deep subinguinal lymph node group underneath the fascia lata and medial to the femoral vein. There are generally only one to three lymph nodes in this group (2), which then drain into the external iliac lymph node chain.

If a urethral carcinoma invades the corpus cavernosum or penile or scrotal skin, more extensive inguinal nodal metastases may occur. These structures drain into the superficial inguinal lymph nodes, which are contained (along with the saphenous

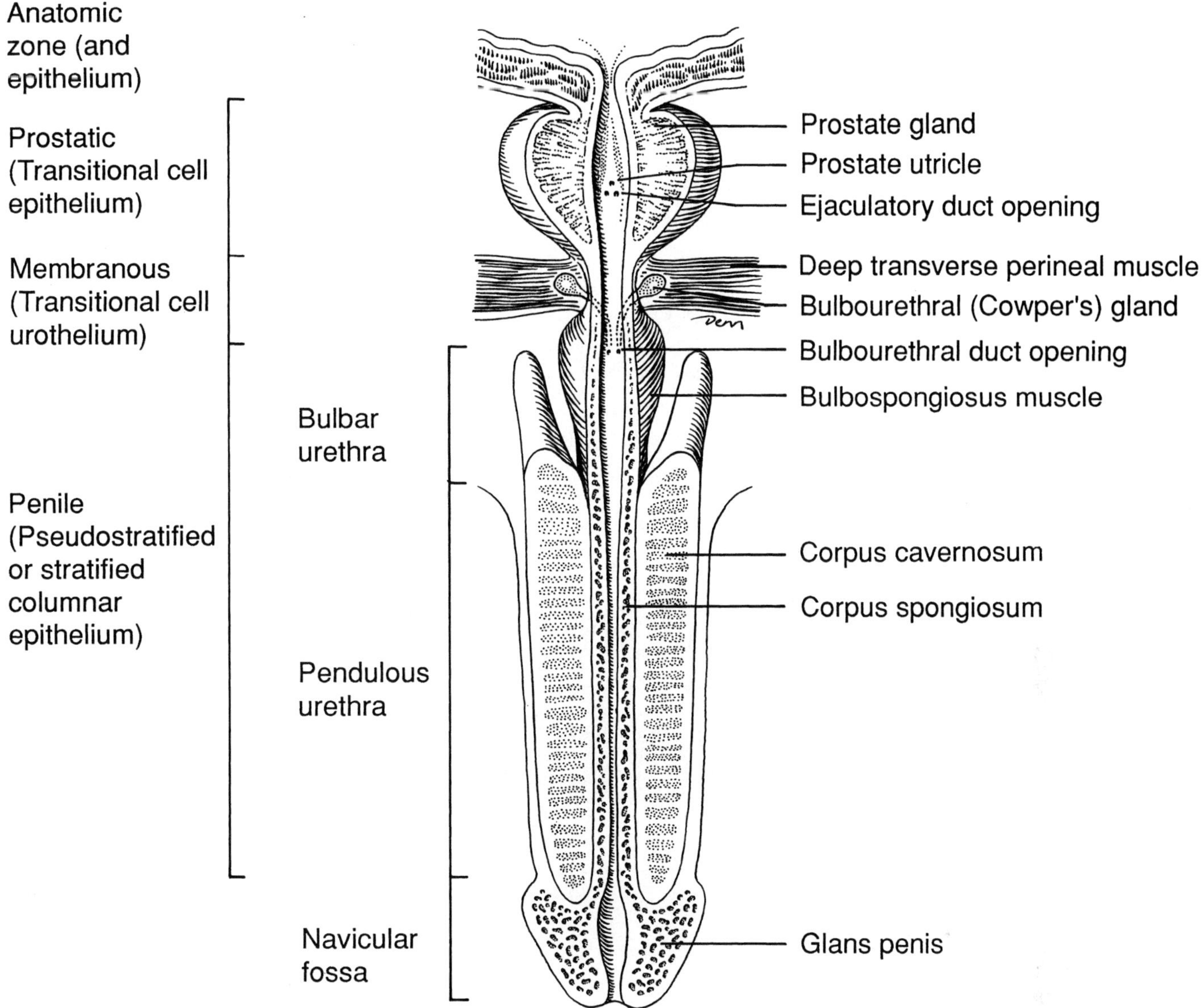

Fig. 41.1. Anatomy of the male urethra.

vein) within the superficial fascia of the thigh in an area bounded by the inguinal ligament, sartorius muscle, and adductor longus muscle. The number of lymph nodes in this group varies considerably, and they can be divided into five groups according to their relationship with the junction of the saphenous and femoral veins (3). Generally, lymphatic channels from the penis and scrotum drain into the central and medial segments.

The bulbar, membranous, and prostatic urethral segments drain into three lymphatic channels (4). One channel travels with the dorsal vein underneath the suspensory ligament to drain into the external iliac lymph node chain (generally 8 to 10 lymph nodes are found in this region); another channel travels along the course of the internal pudendal artery to empty into the obturator lymph node group (4 to 8 lymph nodes); a third channel empties into the presacral lymph nodes. The lymphatic drainage may vary considerably in individual cases depending on the extent of the tumor and whether it obstructs the primary lymphatic drainage system.

The perineum is bounded by the pubic symphysis anteriorly, the ischial tuberosities laterally, and the coccyx posteriorly (Fig. 41.2). The urogenital diaphragm lies anterior to a line drawn between the ischial tuberosities; the anal triangle lies posterior to this line. The posterior urethra is most often approached surgically through the urogenital diaphragm. Deep to the skin and subcutaneous fat is the membranous continuation of the superficial fascia of the anterior abdominal wall, the Colles' fascia. Beneath this fascial layer is the superficial space of the perineum in which are three paired muscles—bulbospongiosus, ischiocavernosus, and transversus perinei superficialis. The

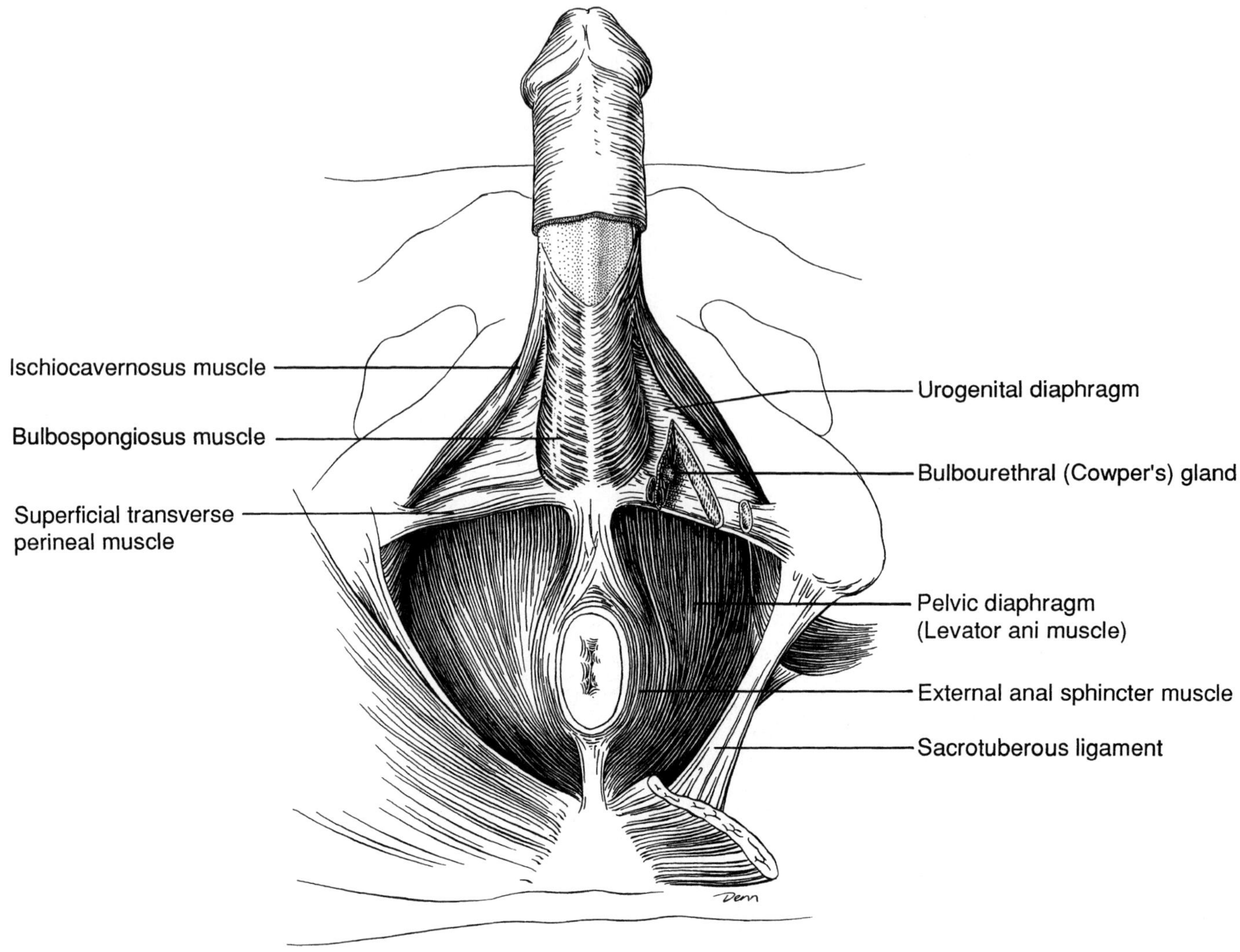

Fig. 41.2. Anatomy of the male perineum.

bulbospongiosus muscle lies in the midline covering the bulb of the penis; laterally, the ischiocavernosus muscle extends from the ischium to the pubic arch covering the crura of the penis; at the base of the superficial space, the paired transverse perinei superficialis muscles extend from the ischium laterally to the perineal body centrally. The deep perineal space is covered by a perineal membrane. Within this space lie striated muscular components of the external urinary sphincter, the transversus perinei profundus muscles, and Cowper's glands. Deep to this region lies a deep fascial layer covering the obturator internus muscles.

Blood to this region is supplied by branches of the internal pudendal artery. An inferior branch, the inferior hemorrhoidal, supplies the anal triangle. Anterior branches supply the urogenital diaphragm. One branch enters the superficial space to supply the superficial perineal musculature and then extends forward as the posterior scrotal artery. Deep branches enter the deep compartment running along the perineal membrane to supply the sphincter muscles of this layer. As mentioned previ-

ously, the internal pudendal artery supplies the bulbar and urethral branches.

Histopathology and Pathophysiology

Because the epithelial lining varies along the course of the urethra, histologic findings will also vary. The most common histologic type is squamous carcinoma (77%) (5–13). Most are moderate and high-grade tumors (6, 8, 11). Primary transitional cell carcinoma accounts for 16% of all urethral carcinomas. Of carcinomas originating in the bulbar, membranous, and prostatic urethras, 85% are squamous cell carcinoma; of all primary carcinomas of the prostatic urethra, 90% are transitional cell. The latter should be differentiated from the more common finding of regional extension of bladder transitional cell carcinoma. Urethral adenocarcinoma is rare (6%) and must be differentiated from extension of a primary adenocarcinoma of the prostate. The exact origin of this histologic type is the subject of some speculation, but it may arise in the periurethral glands of Cowper or Littré or from areas of metaplasia (14, 15). Rarely, it will resemble clear cell adenocarcinoma of the female genital tract (characterized by cells with abundant clear cytoplasm and pleomorphism). These carcinomas must be differentiated from benign, nephrogenic adenomas. Melanoma is a rare tumor of the male urethra (16). The most common site of origin is the meatus or fossa navicularis. Other, usually metastatic, tumor types have been reported. The most common metastatic tumors are from the prostatic, colon, and bladder carcinomas (17, 18).

Approximately 35% of male urethral carcinomas occur in the anterior urethra (meatus, fossa navicularis, and pendulous) and 65% in the posterior urethra (bulbar, membranous, and prostatic). Urethral carcinoma must be differentiated from benign urethral cysts, polyps, and condylomata acuminata.

Metastases to regional lymph nodes occur in approximately 14 to 30% of patients, but have been reported in up to 50% (6, 13, 19). Distant metastases are rare at the time of presentation (10 to 14%) (11, 13). The most common sites include the liver, lung, and skeleton.

Risk factors for urethral carcinoma are not as yet definitive. A high association (27 to 88%) exists with a history of urethral stricture disease or infection. These may promote metaplasia of the urethral epithelium and the subsequent progression to squamous cell malignancy. Alternatively, stricture disease may have been a misdiagnosis in a patient with urethral carcinoma and obstructive voiding symptoms. The relatively high association with a history of venereal disease raises the possibility that a sexually transmitted agent might be responsible for tumor development. Wiener et al. detected oncogenic human papillomavirus type 16 DNA in 29% of squamous cell cancers of the male urethra. Such cancers were more likely to occur in the pendulous urethra and be associated with a more prolonged survival (20). Such viral DNA can be commonly found in condylomata acuminata but has not been thought to be associated with a high rate of carcinogenesis.

Analysis of tumor DNA content by flow cytometry has been used to predict prognosis and progression rates for a variety of urologic tumors, including urethral carcinoma. Those found to have a normal DNA content (diploid) tend to be of lower stage and progress less frequently (18%) than those with an abnormal, higher DNA content (aneuploid) (93%). Patients with diploid tumors have a higher 5-year survival rate than patients with aneuploid tumors (85% versus 20%). Squamous cell carcinomas of the bulbomembranous urethra are more likely to exhibit aneuploidy than tumors of the penile urethra (69% and 29%, respectively) (21). Measurement of DNA content by flow cytometry may add prognostic information not gained by examining individual tumor grade or stage alone.

Diagnosis and Staging

Signs and symptoms of urethral carcinoma can vary widely. More common symptoms include bleeding (34%), obstructive voiding (40%), and dysuria or frequency (28%). The more common signs in men include a palpable mass (40%); the less common, an abscess or fistula of the perineum or genitalia.

A careful evaluation is required to confirm the diagnosis and to assess the anatomic extent. Precise staging will allow selective and appropriate management. Patients with low-stage lesions may be spared extensive surgery, radiation, or chemotherapy with their attendant morbidity, whereas patients with more extensive tumors can be offered early aggressive management. Unfortunately, a staging system based on a TNM classification scheme has not been developed for urethral carcinomas as it has been for other genitourinary malignancies. Currently, most clinicians use those staging systems developed by Ray and associates or Levine (Table 41.1).

Staging begins with a careful physical examination noting the presence of a urethral mass (size, site, and any fixation), fistula formation, infection, and regional or distant lymphadenopathy. Biopsy, preferably under anesthesia, is the most important method of diagnosis and local tumor staging. Tumor size, extent, and location should be carefully estimated. If possible, the bladder and most proximal urethral segments should be examined to note the proximal extent of the tumor and the presence of bladder involvement.

Retrograde urethrography has been the primary imaging technique for local disease (Fig. 41.3). This is now well complemented by magnetic resonance imaging (MRI) (Fig. 41.4),

Table 41.1.   Staging of Male Urethral Carcinoma

RAY (MEMORIAL) STAGING SYSTEM

Stage 0	Confined to the mucosa only (in situ)
Stage A	Into but not beyond the lamina propria
Stage B	Into but not beyond the substance of the corpus spongiosum or into but not beyond the prostate
Stage C	Direct extension into tissue beyond the corpus spongiosum (corpora cavernosa, muscle fat, fascia, skin, direct skeletal involvement) or beyond the prostatic capsule
Stage D1	Regional metastases including inguinal and pelvic lymph nodes (with any primary tumor)
Stage D2	Distant metastases (with any primary tumor)

LEVINE STAGING SYSTEM

Stage 0	In situ (limited to mucosa)
Stage A	Submucosal (not beyond submucosa)
Stage B	Into but not beyond the substance of the corpus spongiosum (corpora cavernosa, muscle, fat, fascia, skin, direct skeletal involvement) or beyond the prostatic capsule
Stage C	Direct extension into tissue beyond the corpus spongiosum (corpora cavernosa, muscle, fat, fascia, skin, direct skeletal involvement) or beyond the prostatic capsule
Stage D	Metastasis 1. Inguinal lymph nodes 2. Pelvic lymph nodes below the bifurcation of the aorta 3. Lymph nodes above the bifurcation of the aorta 4. Distant

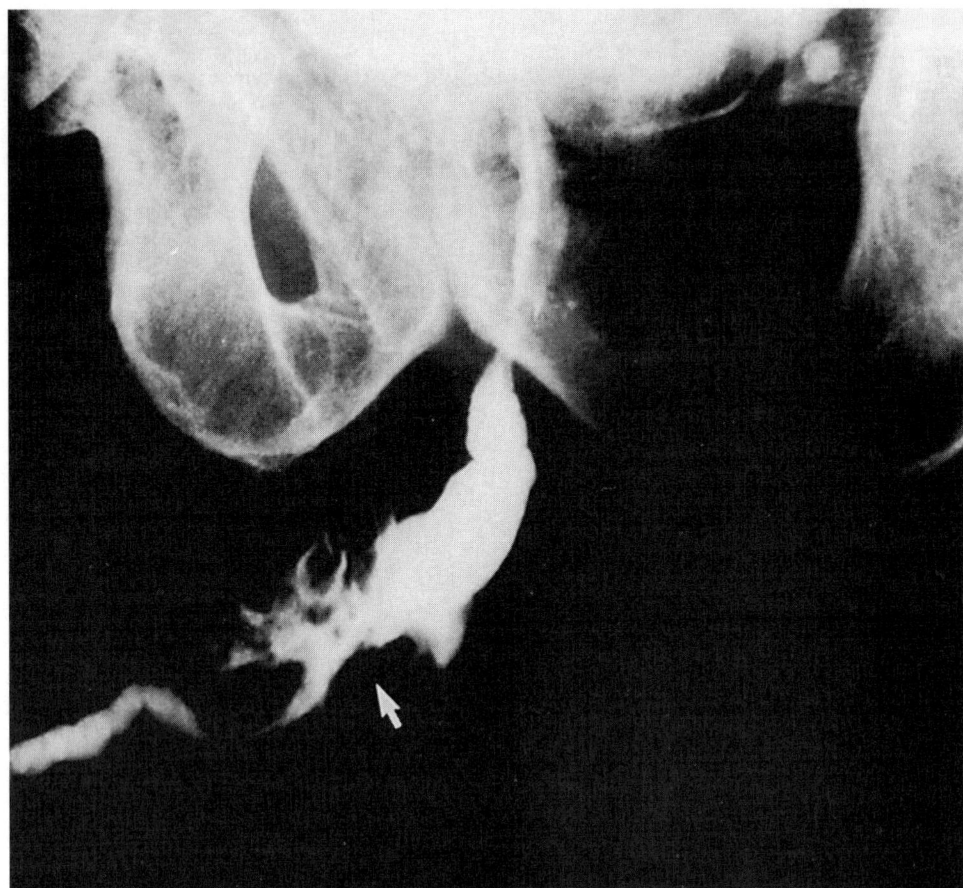

Fig. 41.3. An extensive bulbar urethral carcinoma demonstrated by retrograde urethrography (arrow).

which allows for multiplanar imaging and excellent soft tissue contrast. Regional extension may be better estimated with this technique than with the conventional methods of urethrography or computed tomography (CT). Although cavernosography has been used to assess the extent of primary or metastatic penile carcinomas, its use in urethral carcinoma has been limited (22). Similar information may be gained noninvasively with MRI.

Inguinal lymph node metastases may be assessed with physical examination, CT, or MRI (Fig. 41.5). Pelvic lymphadenopathy is best assessed radiographically with CT or MRI. Chest radiography and bone scan will complete staging in most patients.

Conservative Surgery

Selected low-grade and low-stage urethral malignancies can be managed with local resection. Squamous cell tumors suitable for such an approach would be low-grade squamous papillomas of the meatus or fossa navicularis (23). These may be excised with standard transurethral resection techniques or carbon dioxide or Nd:YAG lasers. Patients managed in such a fashion require careful surveillance, and adjunctive treatment with topical chemotherapy is often warranted. This approach has been successful in patients with low-grade, superficial transitional cell carcinomas of the urethra, usually associated with a history of bladder carcinoma (5, 24).

Radiation Therapy

Invasive, higher-grade lesions of the urethra require more aggressive treatment to cure the malignancy and prevent local progression. Radiation has had variable success (5, 7, 8, 10, 25). Long-term survival is uncommon (approximately 15%), and local recurrence arises in the majority who receive irradiation alone. Radiation seems most effective for small-volume lesions of the anterior urethra that are minimally to moderately invasive. The delivery of interstitial radiation with modern techniques may allow for more accurate treatment with limited morbidity (26). Radiation may be an important palliative therapy in treating patients with unresectable local tumor or symptomatic metastatic disease.

Surgery seems to be more effective than radiation for invasive tumors. In patients with anterior urethral carcinoma, local recurrence has been documented in approximately 8% and 5-year survival in approximately 55% (27). Carcinoma of the posterior urethra frequently presents at an advanced stage and therefore carries a poorer prognosis; the 5-year survival rate is

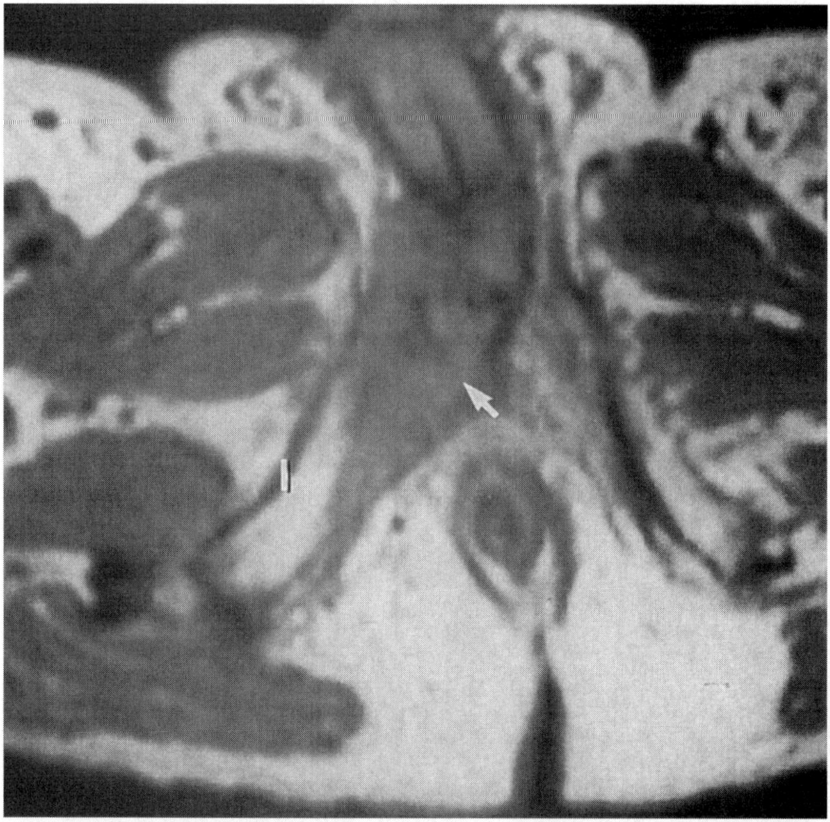

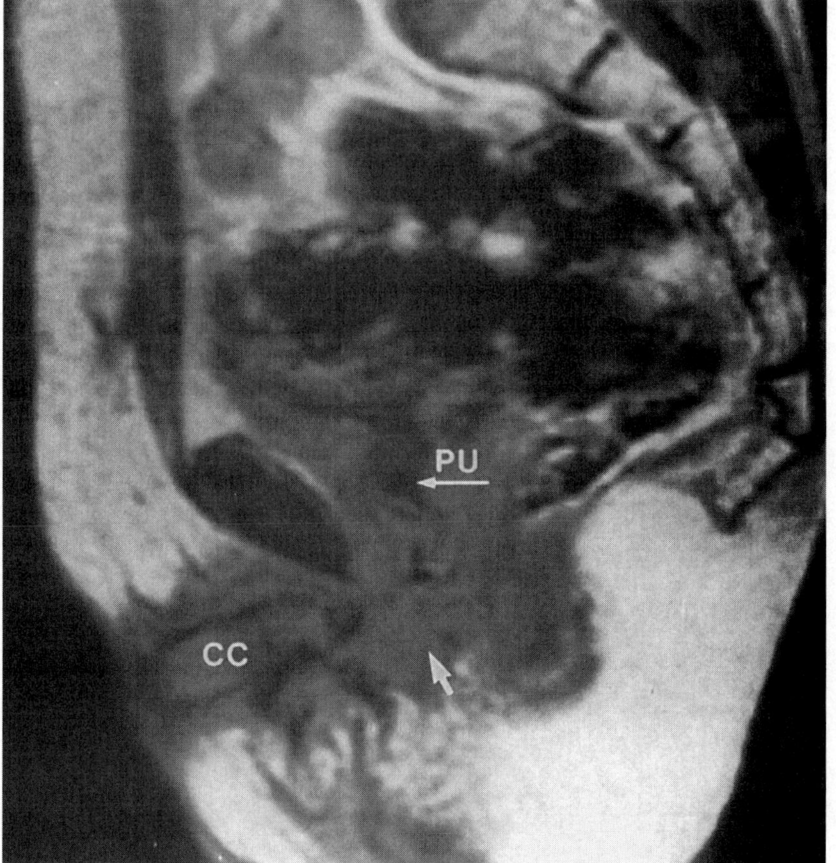

Fig. 41.4. MRI of an extensive bulbomembranous urethral carcinoma. **A.** T1-weighted transaxial view showing invasion of ischium (I). **B.** Sagittal view showing dilated prostatic urethra (PU), large urethral carcinoma (arrow), and corpus cavernosum (CC).

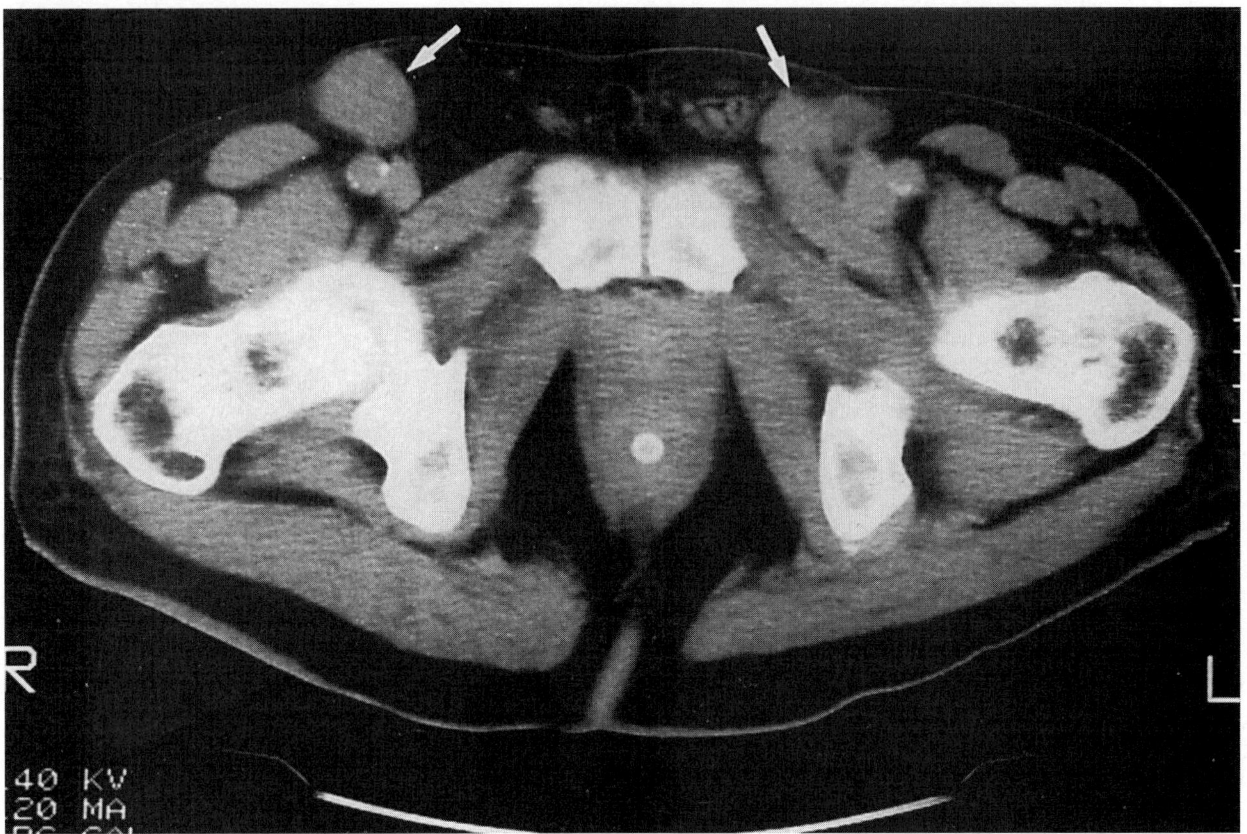

Fig. 41.5.   CT showing bilateral inguinal metastases (arrows) just anterior to the femoral vessels.

approximately 24% (5,7–11, 13, 28, 29) and local recurrence is more common (approximately 20%).

The surgical approach to invasive urethral carcinoma varies with the site, size, and volume of the tumor. Anterior carcinoma often can be excised, preserving an adequate margin of resection with less extensive surgery than that required for posterior tumors.

Surgical Excision of Anterior Urethral Carcinomas

Preoperative preparation should include prophylactic antibiotic therapy in patients with no evidence of infection. A broad-spectrum antibiotic administered perioperatively is usually adequate. With evidence of infection, a broad-spectrum antibiotic combination should initially be followed by specific treatment once culture results are available. Surgery should be delayed until the inflammatory process has resolved or stabilized. A limited bowel-cleansing program is usually instituted the day before surgery.

Patients undergoing distal or segmental urethrectomy alone may be placed in the standard lithotomy position. Those patients requiring excision of the more proximal urethral segments with construction of a perineal urethrostomy or complete urethrectomy after previous cystectomy should be placed in the extreme or exaggerated lithotomy position (Fig. 41.6), with

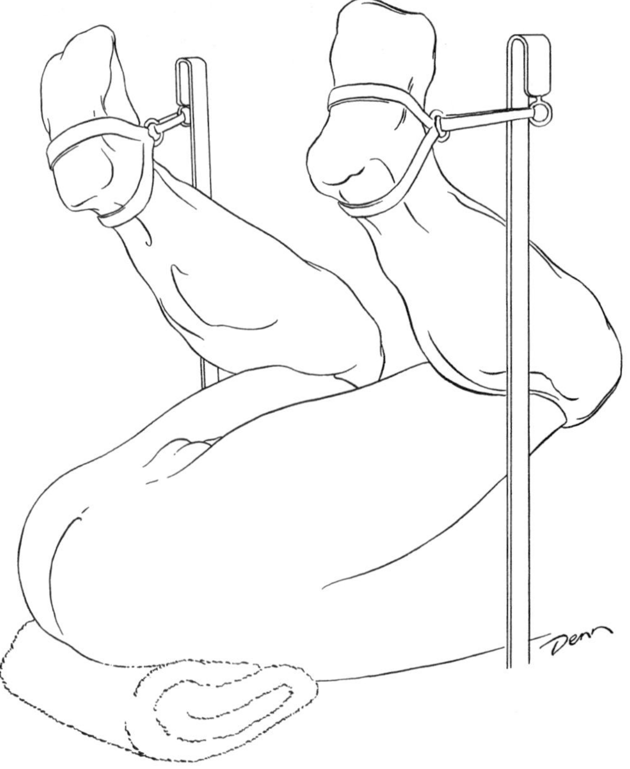

Fig. 41.6.   Extreme or exaggerated lithotomy position.

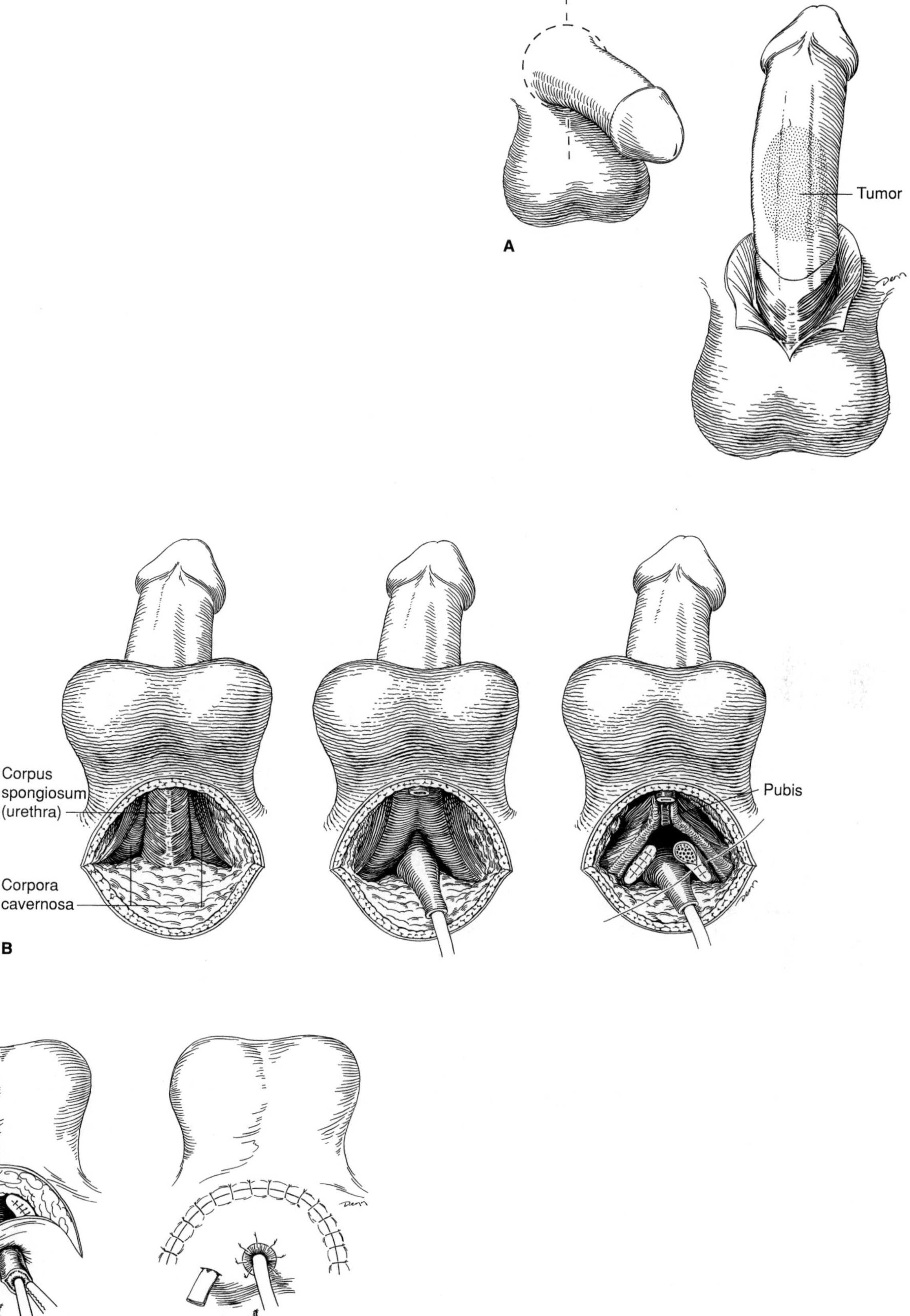

Fig. 41.7. Penectomy, urethrectomy, and creation of a perineal urethrostomy. **A.** Incision around base of penis. **B.** Perineal incision made allowing proximal dissection and easy exposure of the entire bulbar urethra and crura. Urethra incised and dissected free proximally. The corpora cavernosae have been incised and closed underneath the pubis **C.** Perineal urethrostomy completed.

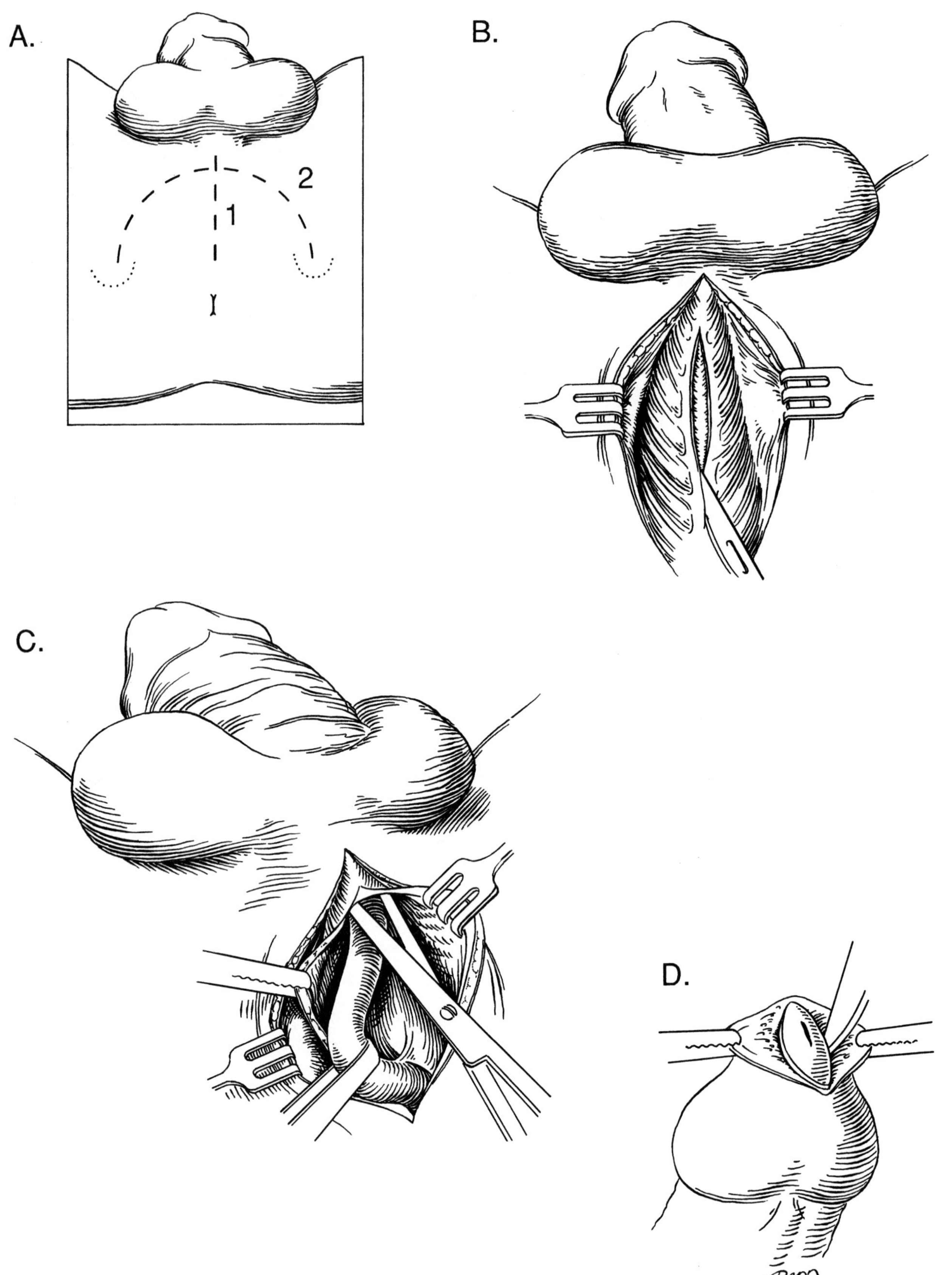

Fig. 41.8. Urethrectomy after previous cystectomy. **A.** Choice of incisions—midline, vertical incision (1), or inverted U incision (2). **B.** Exposure of bulbar urethra. **C.** Dissection along bulbar urethra proceeds anteriorly toward meatus. **D.** Excision of meatus and fossa navicularis.

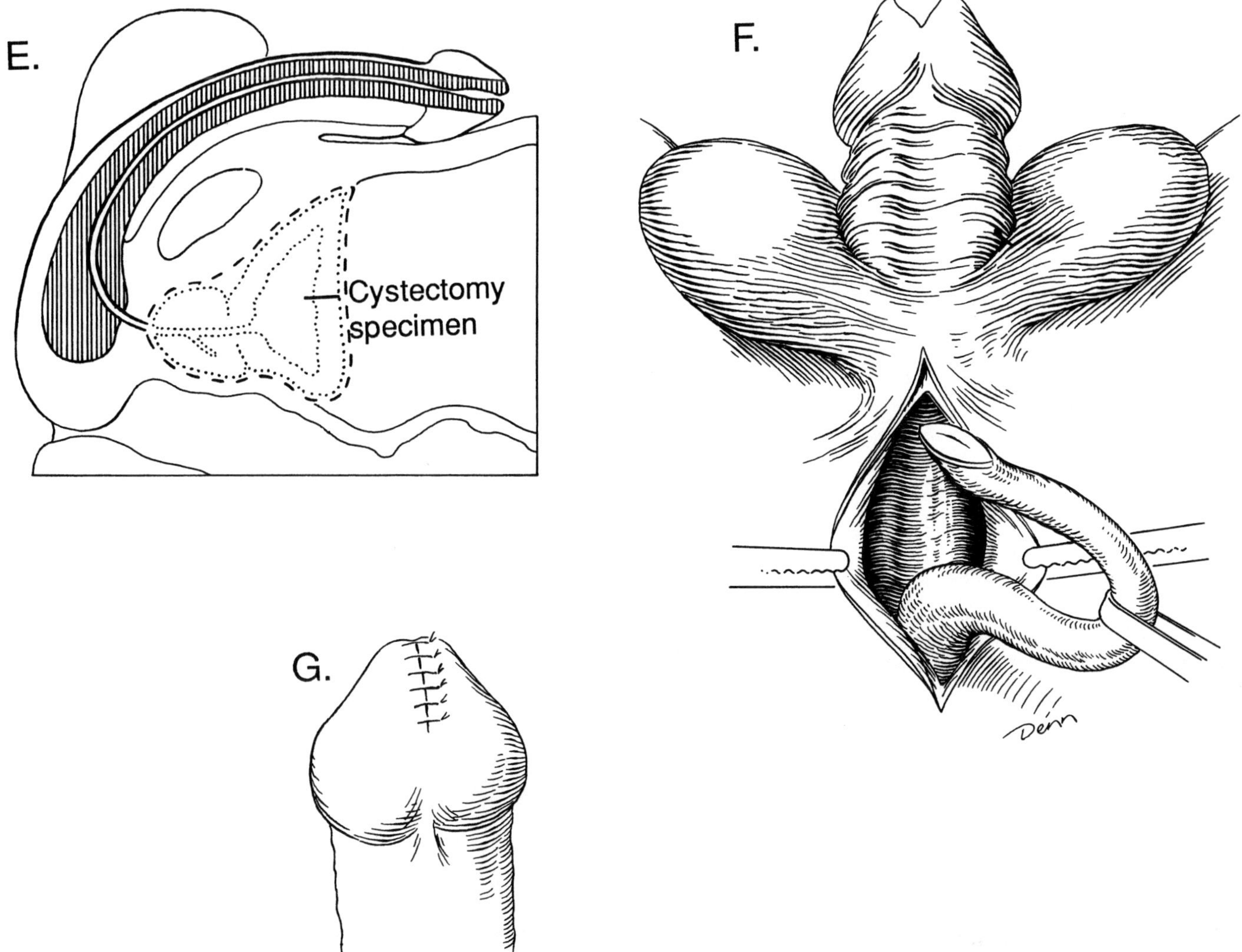

Fig. 41.8.   *(continued)* **E.** Sagittal view of urethra showing its relationship with pelvic floor; previously excised cystectomy specimen outlined. **F.** Excision of distal urethra. **G.** Closure of glans penis.

the legs in stirrups rotated in a cephalad direction. A rolled towel can be placed underneath the sacrum to ensure that the perineum is almost parallel with the floor. All pressure points should be padded carefully.

Rarely, noninvasive lesions may be managed by segmental urethrectomy followed by end-to-end reanastomosis of the proximal and distal urethral segments (which should be examined intraoperatively with frozen sections to ensure complete excision of the carcinoma). A distal urethrectomy alone, with preservation of the corpora cavernosa, is indicated in only those rare patients with superficial or minimally invasive lesions of the anterior urethra. An inverted U, or curvilinear, incision is made extending just medial to and between the ischial tuberosities (Figs. 41-7 and 41-8). For more distal exposure, a midline incision can be added at the apex. The subcutaneous tissue is divided and the bulbocavernosus muscle is incised in the midline. Dissection proceeds along the urethra distally toward the

meatus, with gradual mobilization resulting in inversion of the penis. At the glans, the penis is inverted back to its normal anatomic position. An incision is made around the entire meatus. The meatus and fossa navicularis are separated from the surrounding spongy tissue of the glans, thereby completing dissection of the penile and distal bulbar segments of the urethra. The meatal incision is closed with 3-0 or 4-0 chromic sutures. Glanular drainage usually is not necessary. The most proximal part of the urethral dissection is then completed. The midbulbar urethra should be mobilized proximally, preserving its extensive blood supply. A small ellipse of skin is excised in the midline at the base of the original incision, and a tunnel is created in the subcutaneous tissue by blunt dissection. The urethra is spatulated and anastomosed to the skin with interrupted 3-0 absorbable suture material. A small Penrose or Jackson-Pratt drain is left along the area of dissection and is brought out in a separate lateral skin incision. The subcutaneous layers are brought together with interrupted 2-0 or 3-0 absorbable suture material. The original skin incision is closed similarly, and the drain is left in place for approximately 48 hours or until drainage becomes minimal.

Frankly invasive lesions of the anterior urethra require either partial or total penectomy. Very distal lesions can be managed with partial penectomy, a procedure similar to that for management of primary penile carcinoma (see Chapter 39). For more proximal lesions of the anterior urethra, partial penectomy may not allow for sufficient reconstruction of the penile urethra to direct the urinary stream or ensure a tumor-free margin. These should be managed with total penectomy and creation of a perineal urethrostomy (Fig. 41.7).

The patient should be placed in the extreme lithotomy position. An elliptical incision is made around the base of the penis, and dissection should proceed proximally along the corporal bodies with care to preserve a clear margin of resection. The dorsal vessels are divided at the level of the pubic symphysis after the suspensory ligament has been divided. Dissection should proceed proximally along the corpus spongiosum until a tumor-free margin of approximately 2 cm has been achieved. For more proximal dissection, a separate perineal incision may be necessary. The spongiosum is then dissected free from the corpora cavernosa proximally. The corpus spongiosum and urethra are then divided sharply, and a sample of the proximal margin is sent for frozen section review. The corpora cavernosa are divided sharply underneath the pubic symphysis and closed with interrupted 2-0 absorbable suture material. The proximal urethral segment is brought to the skin as a perineal urethrostomy.

Surgical Excision of Posterior Urethral Carcinomas

Carcinoma of the posterior urethra rarely lends itself to urethrectomy alone; resection of contiguous structures is usually required (30). Because of the advanced nature of these lesions, preoperative radiation or combined radiation and chemotherapy should be considered in the large number of patients in whom surgical resection alone may not allow complete local tumor excision.

Because cystectomy and urinary diversion are required for complete excision of most advanced posterior urethral carcinomas, complete bowel preparation should be performed preoperatively (31, 32). To avoid preoperative dehydration, intravenous hydration should be continued beginning the day before surgery.

Some surgeons have recommended staged procedures in which urinary diversion is performed first, followed in 2 weeks by cystectomy, prostatectomy, urethrectomy, and resection of contiguous structures (10, 33). However, all but the more debilitated patients should undergo a one-stage procedure. Patients requiring cystectomy in combination with urethrectomy should be placed in the low lithotomy position to permit simultaneous abdominal/pelvic and perineal exposure. A midline or paramedian incision extending from the pubic symphysis to

midway between the umbilicus and xiphoid is made. An initial laparotomy with bilateral pelvic lymphadenectomy is performed first to exclude visceral metastases or extensive metastases to the pelvic or retroperitoneal lymph nodes. The bladder and prostate should be mobilized as for excision of invasive bladder carcinoma. Dissection should proceed to that point where the bladder is completely mobilized along its lateral and posterior margins. The puboprostatic ligaments need not be incised because the pubic symphysis will be completely or partially removed later.

After completion of the pelvic lymphadenectomy and preliminary mobilization of the bladder, the perineal dissection should begin. Extensive carcinomas often require en bloc resection of the penis and all or a portion of the scrotum (Fig. 41.8) (34). An elliptical incision is made around the base of the penis and through or around the scrotum (depending on the extent of the tumor). The incision is deepened superiorly, allowing ligation of the dorsal vasculature, incision of the suspensory ligament of the penis, and exposure of the pubic symphysis. The lateral dissection should extend to the fascial covering of the adductor musculature bilaterally. Orchiectomy is often necessary in patients who require complete scrotal excision. The inferior incision should be deepened by incising the muscles of the superficial perineal space—bulbospongiosus, ischiocavernosus, and transverse perinei superficialis—to allow mobilization of the bulbomembranous urethra and visualization of the deep perineal fascia. Those striated muscles attached to the pubic symphysis and medial aspect of the inferior pubic ramus (adductor longus, gracilis, adductor brevis, obturator internus, levator ani, and portions of the adductor magnus) are transected at their insertions with a periosteal elevator and electrocautery tool. All or a portion of the pubic symphysis and inferior pubic rami are then resected with a Gigli saw (Fig. 41.9). A curved Kocher clamp is passed from the perineum just lateral to the inferior pubic ramus through the obturator foramen into the pelvis. The tip of the clamp should be directed medially to prevent damage to the obturator nerve or vessels. One end of a Gigli saw is grasped and brought to the perineum. The Kocher clamp is then passed medial to the inferior pubic ramus and ischium into the pelvis, and the second end of the Gigli saw is grasped and brought to the perineum. A similar procedure is performed on the opposite side. A Gigli saw is then passed around the pubic symphysis. A Kocher clamp is passed through the obturator foramen more anteriorly on either side of the pubic symphysis. Each end of a Gigli saw is grasped and brought to the perineum. Laterally and upwardly beveled osteotomies are made through both inferior pubic rami and the inferior aspect of the pubic symphysis, respectively. Usually only the inferior rim of the pubic symphysis, rather than the entire pubis, need be resected to ensure an adequate margin of resection. This completes the dissection because the bladder and prostate had been mobilized previously. Urinary diversion or, in selected patients, construction of a continent urinary reservoir is then performed.

The perineal wound, which is often large, should be drained

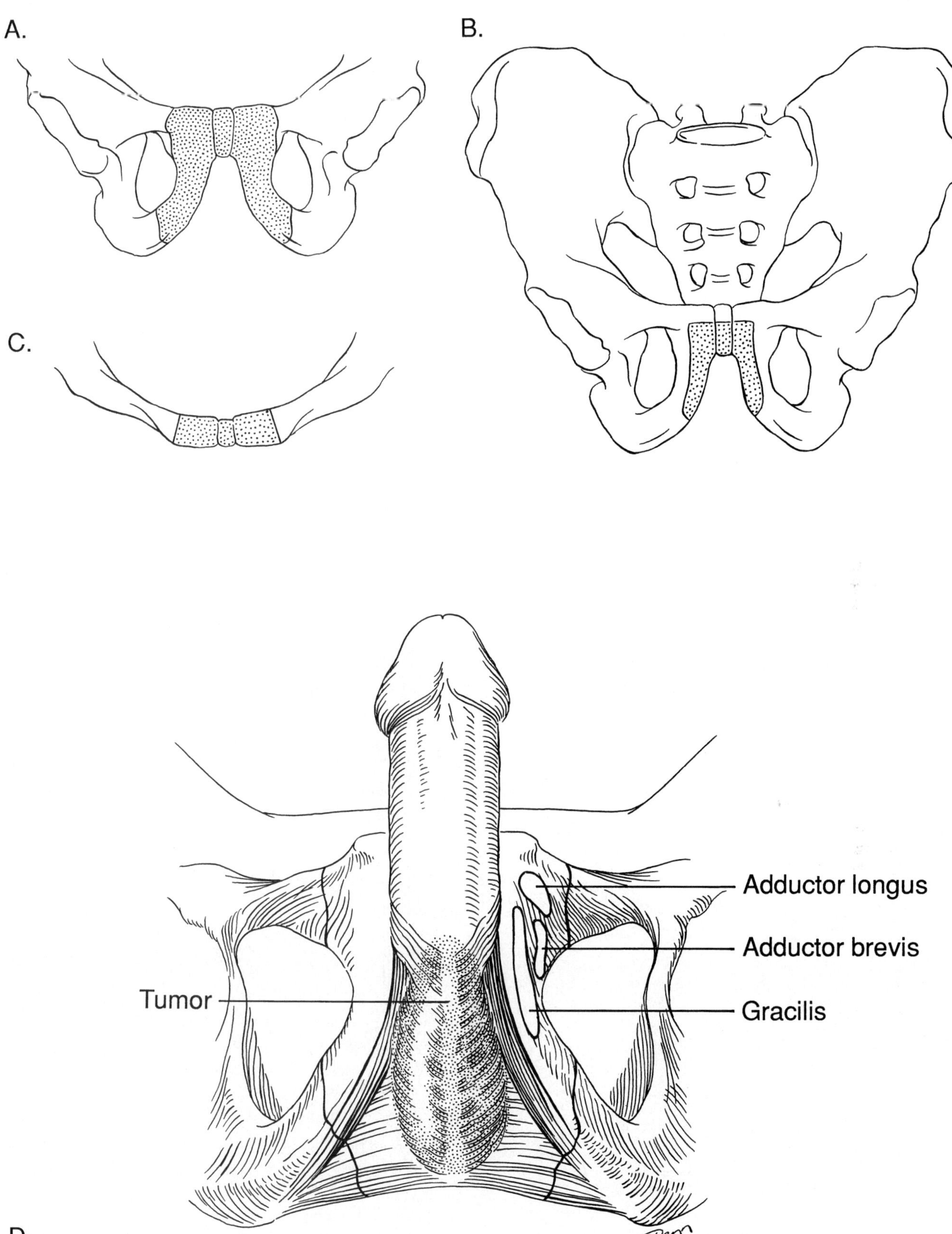

Fig. 41.9.   Excision of high-stage urethral carcinoma. Shaded areas represent portions of pelvis excised for higher (**A**) or lower volume. **B.** Urethral carcinomas. **C.** Cephalad view of pelvis showing beveling of pubic bone incision to allow pubic symphysis to be lifted out. **D.** En bloc excision of posterior urethral carcinoma. Structures to be excised are outlined.

and closed with scrotal skin, if available. Large defects may be closed with gracilis myocutaneous flaps. An omental flap may also be used to fill the pelvis and separate the intestine from the perineal wound.

In selected cases in which the carcinoma is confined to the most proximal portions of the urethra, the corpora cavernosa may be spared and the penis preserved. The abdominal and pelvic portions of the procedure should proceed as described. The perineal dissection would begin with an inverted U incision between and just medial to the ischial tuberosities. The posterior and lateral dissection would be similar to that described; however, anteriorly the corpora cavernosa can be incised at the crura, preserving the overlying skin and dorsal vasculature. The pubic symphysis need not be resected. Segmental resection of the urethra and corpus spongiosum with primary urethral realignment or use of a skin substitute has also been performed in rare cases (35).

Regional Disease

Approximately 14 to 30% of patients will have inguinal lymph node metastases at the time of presentation (6, 11, 13). Although inguinal lymph node metastases are more common with invasive carcinomas of the anterior urethra, they may be present in up to 28% of patients with invasive bulbomembranous tumors (11). A higher rate of distant relapse is to be anticipated, but ileoinguinal lymphadenectomy may be curative for small-volume disease and may be palliative in limited high-stage disease. Extended survival has been reported (11).

The indications for ileoinguinal lymphadenectomy are not as well defined for urethral as for penile carcinoma. However, the procedure seems advisable in those patients with suspected (palpable) or confirmed (biopsied) inguinal lymph node metastases who have no evidence of more distant disease. Patients with no evidence of disease may be followed carefully with periodic physical examination of the inguinal lymph nodes. Should lymphadenopathy develop, more extensive disease must be excluded by bone scan, chest radiograph, and CT or MRI of the pelvis and abdomen before ileoinguinal lymphadenectomy is performed.

Transitional Cell Carcinoma of the Urethra After Cystectomy

Transitional cell carcinoma of the bladder is often a multifocal urothelial disease that may involve the renal pelvis, ureter, or urethra. Cancers are likely to develop in the urethra if it is left in place after cystectomy in patients with cancers at the bladder neck and those in whom preoperative biopsies show cancers in the prostatic urethra and invading the prostatic stroma (36). Transurethral resection biopsies containing both mucosal and prostatic tissue will identify most patients who require urethrectomy at the time of radical cystectomy (37). Approximately 4 to 10% of patients who undergo cystectomy alone will have recurrences in the retained urethral segment (38–45),

most often proximally and rarely in the meatus (46). All such patients should undergo careful surveillance to detect low-volume, low-stage disease amenable to urethrectomy (47, 48). Collection of urethral wash specimens for cytology and perhaps flow cytometry should be performed routinely, along with careful physical examination.

Patients who require urethrectomy should be positioned in the extreme lithotomy position (Fig. 41.6). An inverted curvilinear or midline incision is made between the ischial tuberosities, which are easily palpable (Fig. 41.8). Dissection proceeds through the superficial fascial and subcutaneous layers of the perineum. The bulbocavernosus muscle is incised in the midline. Dissection proceeds along the urethra distally toward the meatus. As the dissection proceeds to the glans, the urethra is gradually mobilized, resulting in inversion of the penis. At this point, the penis is inverted back to its normal anatomic position and the meatus and fossa navicularis are dissected free from the surrounding spongy tissue of the glans. The meatal incision is closed with 3-0 or 4-0 chromic sutures. Attention is then directed at completing the most proximal part of the urethral dissection. The proximal bulbar urethra is further mobilized to the level of the membranous urethra. Because this is often retained after cystectomy, dissection must proceed into the deep perineal compartment of the genitourinary diaphragm. Careful and meticulous dissection along the urethra will allow complete excision without damage to any intestinal segments that may have fallen into the pelvic space above the genitourinary diaphragm after cystectomy. A drain is often left along the area of the dissection, brought through a separate incision, and removed when output becomes minimal. The subcutaneous tissue layers are closed with interrupted 2-0 or 3-0 absorbable suture material. The skin is closed in a similar fashion. A light gauze dressing is applied, reinforced with fluff gauze, and kept in place with a scrotal support.

FEMALE URETHRAL CARCINOMA

Anatomy

The female urethra is approximately 4 to 6 cm long, running from the bladder neck to the external urethral meatus, which lies just anterior to the vaginal hiatus and approximately 2 cm inferior to the glans clitoris (1) (Fig. 41.10). The urethra is rich in collagen and elastic fibers; therefore, it is occluded except during voiding. The mucous membrane is composed of transitional cell epithelium along the proximal third of the urethra and stratified squamous epithelium along the distal two thirds. Submucosal glands, lined by pseudostratified and stratified columnar epithelium, can be found opening along the entire length. The female urethra has a muscular wall composed of an inner longitudinal muscle coat, which is continuous with the inner layer of the detrusor muscle, and an outer semicircular coat, which is continuous with the outer wall of the detrusor muscle. Somewhat arbitrarily, the female urethra can be divided into anterior and posterior segments—the former

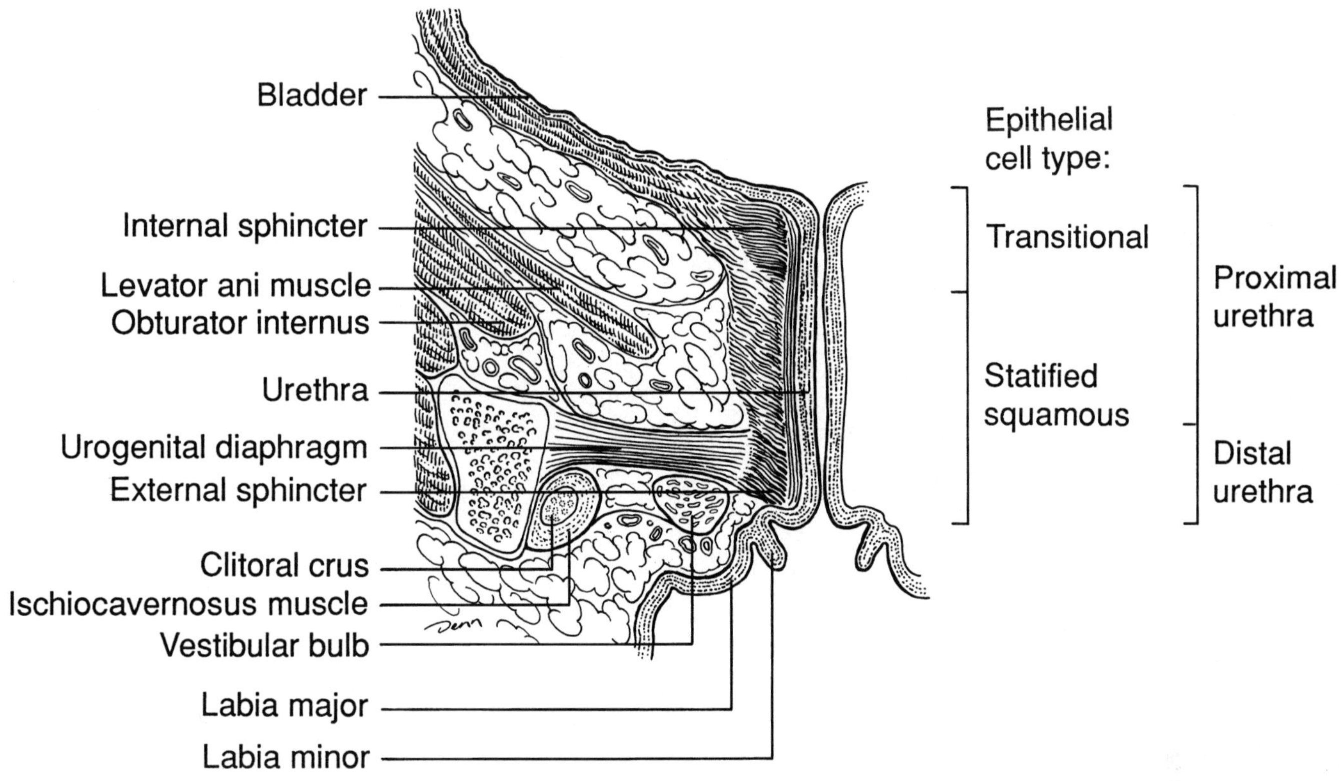

Fig. 41.10.   Anatomy of the female urethra.

representing the most distal third and the latter representing the proximal two thirds.

The boundaries and anatomy of the female perineum are similar to those in the male, with the major exception being that the vaginal canal separates the components of the urogenital triangle in the midline (Fig. 41.11). In addition to the transverse perinei superficialis and ischiocavernosus, the muscles of the superficial space include the sphincter vaginae, which are paired striated muscles surrounding the vagina.

The lymphatics of the distal urethra drain into the superficial and deep inguinal lymph nodes; those of the proximal urethra drain preferentially into the pelvic lymph nodes (external and internal iliac, obturator, and presacral).

Histopathology and Pathophysiology

In women, as in men, the majority of urethral cancers are squamous cell carcinomas (approximately 70%) (49–55). Transitional cell carcinomas account for approximately 15% and must be differentiated from primary bladder carcinoma. Adenocarcinomas are identified in approximately 10 to 13% of women with urethral tumors and appear to be of two histologic types—clear cell and columnar/mucinous (56). The former must be differentiated from clear cell tumors of the female genital tract and are characterized by cells with abundant clear cytoplasm and cellular pleomorphism (57). The latter resembles colonic or endocervical adenocarcinoma, most commonly showing tubular glands with focal papillary areas. The cells are generally columnar with regular nuclei and little pleomorphism. Adenocarcinomas are thought to arise from neoplastic differentiation of transitional cell epithelium of the urethra or glandular epithelium of the paraurethral glands. These tumors present at a higher stage and carry a worse prognosis than squamous carcinomas. In one rather large series, extension to local structures or regional lymph nodes was identified in 82% of patients, and 64% were dead of their disease within 2 years of diagnosis (56). Melanomas account for a small number of urethral carcinomas and most commonly occur along the anterior urethra (58). They also have a poor prognosis because of a higher rate of regional and metastatic disease.

Approximately 45% of urethral tumors in women are located along the anterior urethra alone, 7% in the posterior urethra alone, and 48% located along the entire urethra on clinical examination (50, 51, 53). Seventy-five percent are moderately well-differentiated or poorly differentiated neoplasms (grade 2 or 3) (51, 53). Urethral carcinoma must be differentiated from benign abnormalities including urethral caruncle, cyst, condylomata acuminata, urethral prolapse, and periurethral abscess.

Risk factors are not well documented. A history of significant infection or trauma is not as common in women as in men. Urethral caruncles have been found in a small percentage of women with urethral cancers. Several tumors arising within urethral diverticulae have been reported (59), the majority

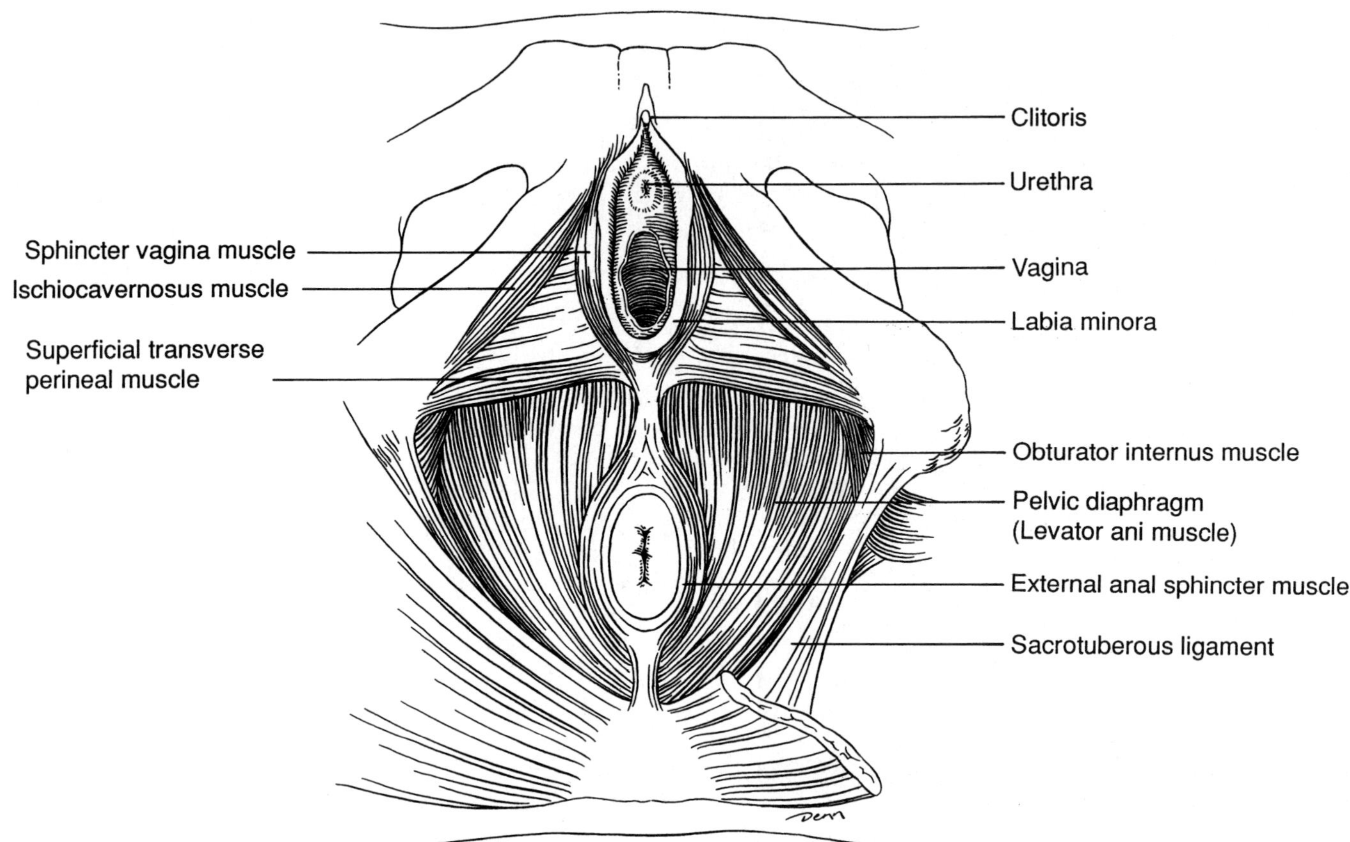

Fig. 41.11.   Anatomy of the female perineum.

being adenocarcinomas. Human oncogenic papillomavirus type 16 DNA has been detected in 47% of invasive cancers occurring in women (60). Types 16 and 18 papillomaviruses have been identified in as many as 70% of invasive cervical carcinomas.

Approximately 28% of women with urethral carcinoma will present with metastases to inguinal lymph nodes. These are more common with high-stage lesions. Distant metastases are rare (10 to 15%) (53). As in men, the most common sites of metastases include the liver, lungs, skeleton, and brain.

Diagnosis and Staging

The most common presenting symptoms and signs of urethral carcinoma in women include bleeding (60 to 75%), obstructive voiding or incontinence (27 to 52%), irritative voiding symptoms (21 to 65%), pain (25 to 40%), and a palpable mass (6 to 40%) (51–53, 56). A careful physical examination should be performed, noting the presence of a mass on inspection or on bimanual palpation. Its size, color, and extent should be assessed, as should the presence of any inguinal or supraclavicular adenopathy. A more accurate examination can be performed under anesthesia, at which time the mass may be excised or biopsied. Cystoscopy should be performed, if possible, noting the proximal extent of the lesion and the presence of bladder involvement. The vaginal vault and cervix should be carefully

examined to assess regional extension to these areas and exclude the possibility that the urethral tumor represents local infiltration by a primary tumor of the genital tract.

As in men, extension to local structures and regional lymph nodes may be assessed with lymphangiography, CT, or MRI (Fig. 41.12). The presence of any pulmonary or bony metastasis may be assessed initially by chest radiograph and nuclear bone scan, respectively. Urethral carcinoma in women is most often staged clinically according to the schemes developed by Grabstald et al. (53) and Prempree et al. (61) (Table 41.2).

Radiation Therapy

In women, the experience with radiation therapy is much more extensive than in men (51, 53, 61–68). The best results have been seen in low-stage, anterior lesions where local control and long-term survival rates are favorable. Such lesions are amenable to an integrated approach whereby patients receive 4000 to 4500 cGy by external beam radiation therapy delivered initially from anteroposterior parallel-opposed fields. This is followed after 3 to 4 weeks with interstitial radiation therapy to bring the total dose to 6500 to 7000 cGy. The dose can be distributed homogeneously with a urethral template attached to a vaginal cylinder. Needle placement and radioactive seed distribution are tailored to the site and size of the tumor.

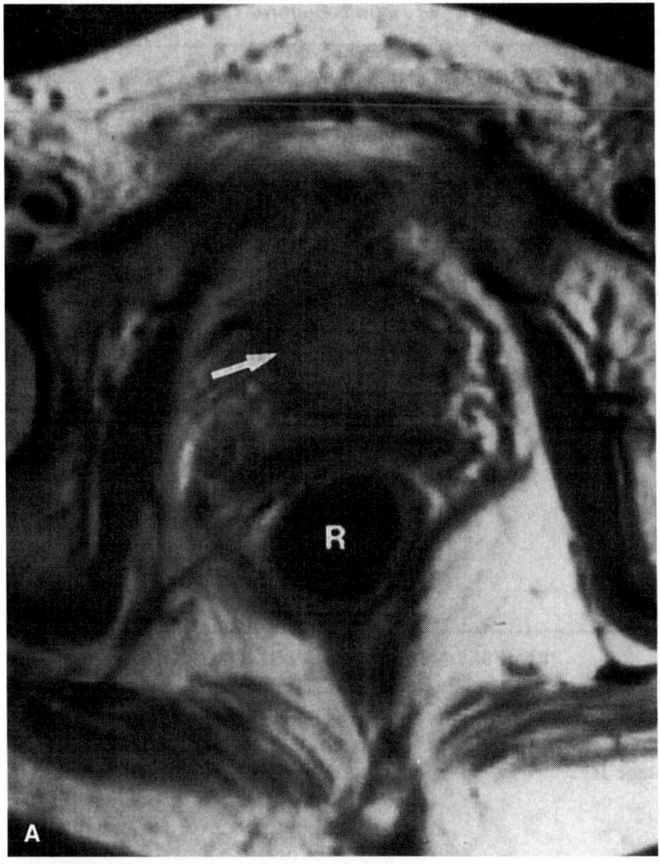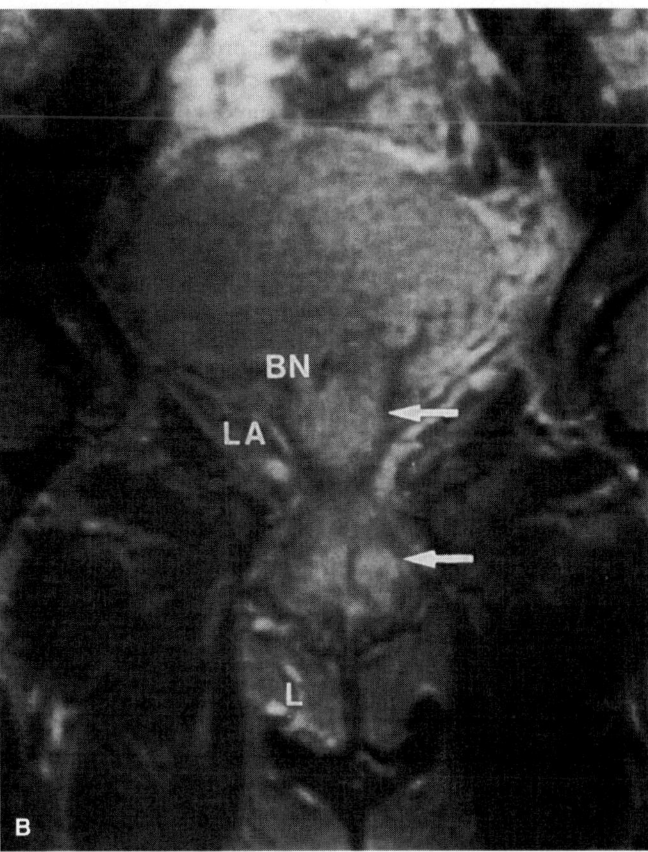

Fig. 41.12. MRI of female urethral melanoma (arrows). **A.** TI-weighted transaxial view of tumor anterior to rectum (R). **B.** Coronal view showing hourglass appearance of tumor (arrows). Tumor involves entire urethra above and below genitourinary diaphragm. Bladder neck (BN), levator ani (LA), and labia (L).

Radiation therapy alone with either external beam radiation therapy or a combination of external beam and interstitial radiation therapy has not been as effective for posterior or higher-stage urethral carcinomas. Local recurrence is common, and survival is limited. Most series report complication rates of approximately 15 to 25% (range, 0 to 42%) (Table 41.3). Complications include urinary incontinence, urethral stricture, local tissue necrosis or ulceration, fistula or abscess formation, and osteomyelitis.

Surgery has been used in all stages of disease, although more often for advanced disease because of the high failure rate of radiation alone. However, the local recurrence rate is often high and survival is limited, even with aggressive surgical management (Table 41.4). Patients treated with radiation therapy followed by anterior exenteration may have fewer local recurrences than those patients treated with either surgery or radiation therapy alone (55, 71). The preoperative use of chemotherapy in addition to radiation may permit better downstaging and more complete surgical excision.

Surgical Techniques

Certain low-volume and low-stage carcinomas (i.e., stages O, A, B, or I) of the anterior urethra may be completely excised with an adequate margin and preservation of urinary continence. The distal one half of the urethra may be excised without risking postoperative continence.

Patients should be placed in the standard lithotomy position. The labia minora should be sutured laterally with silk sutures, and a weighted speculum should be placed in the vagina to allow clear visualization of the periurethral area (Fig. 41.13). A 16F or 18F urethral catheter is inserted to facilitate the dissection. A circumferential incision is made around the urethra inferior to the clitoris. The incision should extend widely around the tumor. The anterior urethra is freed from surrounding tissue by careful, sharp dissection. After a clear margin has been achieved, the urethra may be transected. Frozen sections should be taken on both the proximal and distal margins of resection to ensure complete tumor excision. Bleeding points should be grasped with fine forceps and cauterized. The urethral meatus should be reconstructed with interrupted 3-0 chromic suture material. Postoperative pain and discomfort are usually limited, and the patient is often ready for hospital discharge on the first postoperative day. The catheter is left in place for 5 to 7 days.

Higher-stage tumors (i.e., B, C, or II, III) require more aggressive surgery, and preoperative radiation with or without chemotherapy should be considered in all but the lowest-vol-

Table 41.2. Staging of Female Urethral Carcinoma

GRABSTALD (MEMORIAL STAGING SYSTEM)

Stage 0 (Tis)	In situ (limited to mucosa)
Stage A (T1)	Submucosal (not beyond submucosa)
Stage B (T2)	Muscular (infiltrating periurethral muscle)
Stage C (T3–4)	Periurethral
C1	Infiltrating muscular wall of the vagina
C2	Infiltrating muscular wall of the vagina with invasion of vaginal mucosa
C3	Infiltration of other adjacent structures, such as bladder, labia, and clitoris
Stage D (N+/M+)	Metastasis
D1	Inguinal lumph nodes
D2	Pelvic lymph nodes below the bifurcation of the aorta
D3	Lymph nodes above the bifurcation of the aorta
D4	Distant

PREMPREE MODIFICATION STAGING SYSTEM

Stage I	Disease limited to the distal half of the urethra
Stage II	Disease involving the entire urethra, with extension to the periurethral tissues but not involving the vulva or bladder neck
Stage III	
a	Disease involving the urethra and vulva
b	Disease invading the vaginal mucosa
c	Disease involving the urethra and bladder neck
Stage IV	
a	Disease invading parametrium or paracolpium
b	Metastases
1	Inguinal lymph nodes
2	Pelvic nodes
3	Para-aortic
4	Distant

Table 41.4. Surgery Alone for Female Urethral Carcinoma

AUTHOR	NO. OF PATIENTS	LOCAL RECURRENCE (%)	SURVIVAL* (2–5 YEARS) (%)
Grabstald et al. (53)	26	54	39
Bracken et al (55)	11	64	45
Mayer et al. (63)	10	60	30
Moinuddin et al. (70)	5	40	40
Monaco et al. (54)	5	0	100

* Disease-free survival for patients followed more than 24 months.

ume disease (generally external beam radiation to approximately 4500 cGy). The concurrent administration of chemotherapeutic agents with synergistic antitumor activity (i.e., mitomycin, 5-fluorouracil, and cisplatin) should be considered in locally aggressive lesions. Most high-stage urethral tumors will require complete anterior exenteration. Rarely, a patient may be managed by urethrectomy alone with preservation of the bladder, but they will require a suprapubic catheter or construction of a continent stoma (72).

Preoperative preparation is similar to that in men—complete bowel preparation, intravenous hydration, and antibiotic prophylaxis previously. The patient should be placed in the low lithotomy position, which allows for both abdominal and perineal exposure. A midline incision is made from over the pubic symphysis to midway between the umbilicus and xiphoid. The abdomen and retroperitoneum are inspected for the presence of metastatic disease. A bilateral pelvic lymphadenectomy is then completed. The bladder and uterus (and usually the ovaries) are mobilized and excised. However, the dissection is not completed at this point. The vagina is opened just distal to the cervix, and the incision is extended down either side approximately two thirds of its length. Blood vessels in this posterior pedicle are clamped and ligated sequentially. The entire lateral and anterior segments of the vagina should remain attached to the specimen to preserve a tumor-free margin of

Table 41.3. Radiation Therapy for Female Urethral Carcinoma

AUTHOR	NO. OF PATIENTS	LOCAL RECURRENCE (%)	SURVIVAL (2–5 YEAR) (%)	COMPLICATIONS (%)
Pointon and Poole-Wilson (12)	92	NS	46	0
Desai et al. (51)	14	NS	39	NS
Grabstald et al. (53)	29	69	24	NS
Monaco et al. (54)	8	NS	75	NS
Bracken et al. (55)	50	46	32	42
Prempree et al. (61)	14	36	71	21
Antoniades (62)	20	25	50	30
Mayer et al. (63)	5	100	40	NS
Weghaupt et al. (64)	62	NS	65	NS
Klein et al. (67)	3	0	66	0
Gardin et al. (69)	84	35	64	49

NS, not stated.

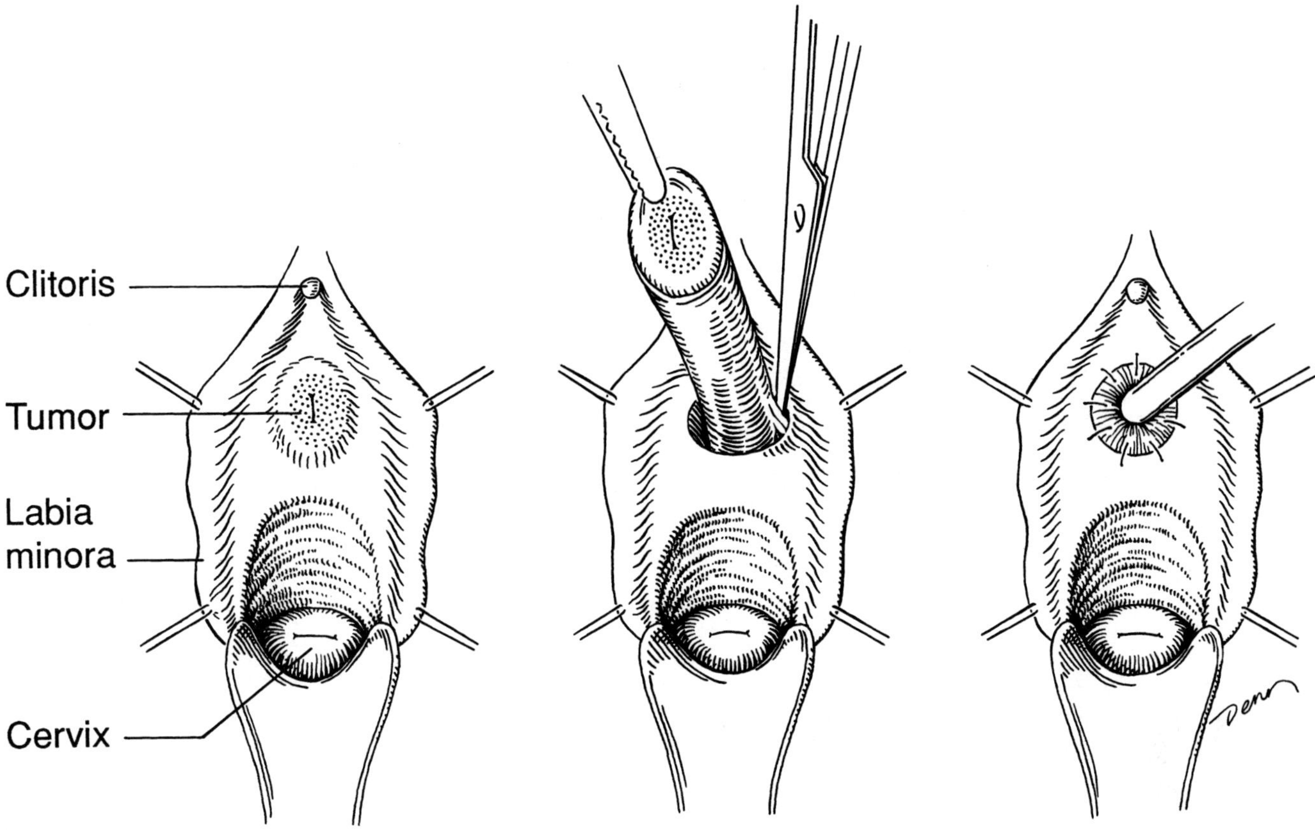

Fig. 41.13. Anterior urethrectomy for female urethral carcinoma.

resection. On occasion, the entire vagina is resected. At this point, attention is directed to the perineal dissection.

A semicircular incision is made beginning at the level of the previous incisions in the posterior vaginal wall. This should extend laterally to include both labia minora (Fig. 41.14). The clitoris should be included within the anterior limits of the incision for removal of large tumors that extend anteriorly. The incision is deepened anteriorly to expose the periosteum of the pubic symphysis and laterally through the muscular elements of the urogenital triangle until the periosteum of the inferior pubic ramus is reached. The insertions of the adductor muscles along the inferior pubic ramus may be incised with the periosteal elevator and electrocautery. The distal third of the vagina may be incised on either side to join with the vaginal incisions made during the pelvic part of the dissection.

The pubic arch resection is completed next in a fashion similar to that for men. Laterally and upwardly beveled osteotomies are made through both inferior pubic rami and the inferior aspect of the pubic symphysis, respectively. Usually only the inferior rim of the pubic symphysis, rather than the entire pubic symphysis, need be resected to ensure an adequate margin of resection. The entire specimen is then removed and hemostasis achieved. An omental flap or polyglycolic acid mesh is placed within the pelvis to separate the intestines from the perineal incision and prevent a future enterocele or fistula. The vaginal remnant, if present, is brought anteriorly and sutured to the vulvae with running or interrupted 2-0 or 3-0 absorbable suture material. The perineal wound can be closed primarily or with myocutaneous gracilis flaps if a large defect is present. In selected patients, bilateral myocutaneous gracilis flaps can be used to create a functional vagina. Closed pelvic and perineal drainage systems are placed, and routine abdominal closure is completed.

Postoperative complications are similar to those described for radical cystectomy. In addition, osteitis pubis and adductor muscle spasms have been reported in a few patients. Rarely, a patient will develop sacroiliac instability secondary to complete pubic arch excision.

Regional Disease

Approximately 28% of women with urethral carcinoma will present with metastases to inguinal lymph nodes (Table 41.5). Management is similar to that described for men. Ileoinguinal lymphadenectomy should be performed for biopsy-proven inguinal metastases or palpably enlarged inguinal lymph nodes. In patients with unresectable inguinal metastases, systemic chemotherapy and radiation should be considered.

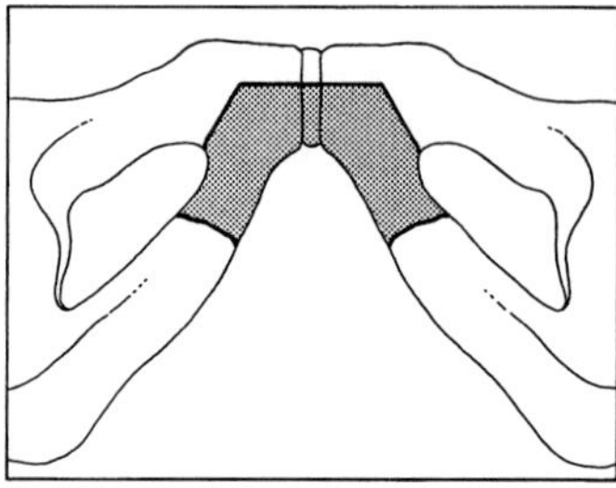

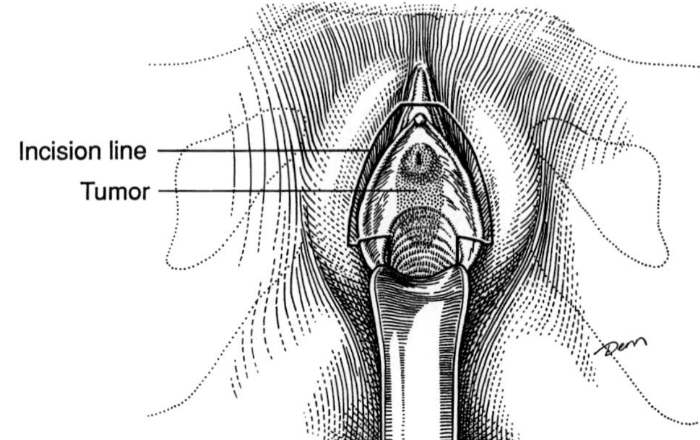

Fig. 41.14. Excision of high-stage urethral carcinoma in women. Skin incision outlined. Exact limits of the skin incision depend on the size and extent of the tumor. Clitoris should be excised when the urethral carcinoma is large or extends anteriorly. Area of pubic arch to be excised is shaded (in box). The entire pubic symphysis can be excised when the tumor is large to ensure an adequate margin of resection.

Combination Therapy for Urethral Carcinoma in Men and Women

Primary chemotherapy has been used in only a small number of patients with localized urethral cancers. Much experience has been gained treating localized and metastatic transitional cell carcinoma of the bladder with cisplatin-based combination chemotherapy (73–75). Pure transitional cell carcinoma of the prostatic and membranous urethra has been treated similarly. A complete clinical response was seen in three of five patients (76).

Because urethral cancers are rare, the use of chemotherapy for their management remains limited. The use of chemotherapy for penile cancers is more extensive. Because both cancers are frequently of the same histologic type, occur in similar anatomical locations, and often share common biologic features, the effect of chemotherapy on one may be applied with justification to the other. Cisplatin, bleomycin, and methotrexate either alone or in combination with 5-fluorouracil and vincristine have been shown to be active drugs for the management of squamous carcinomas of the urethra and penis (77–79). Given the success noted with neoadjuvant chemotherapy followed by radiation and selective surgery for the management of squamous cell carcinomas of the anus, esophagus, and head and neck, many clinicians have evaluated similar regimens for the management of genital squamous cancers in an effort to avoid surgery in some patients, improve surgical margins or allow less extensive surgery in those that require surgery, and improve disease-free survival in all patients.

Radiation and chemotherapy are synergistic, and their use in combination seems likely to be superior to either used alone. Edsmyr et al. treated 42 patients with stages T1 to T3 penile cancers with bleomycin and radiation (80). A complete response to treatment was noted in 39 patients, and the 5-year survival rate for the entire group was 77%. Maiche treated eight patients in a similar fashion and noted a complete response in two of two patients with stage I disease and two of three patients with stage II disease (81). Both Johnson et al. and Baskin and Turzan have described the use of chemotherapy and radiation in the management of locally extensive urethral cancers (82, 83). Significant downstaging occurred in both cases. The case described by Baskin and Turzan was notable for the fact that combined treatment allowed for urethrectomy to be performed without resection of the corpora cavernosa, thereby preserving the penis.

Given the high recurrence rates noted with radiation and surgery for locally advanced urethral cancers in men and women and the extensive nature of the surgery performed in such patients, the use of combination therapy should be considered more often. Specifically, such therapy may allow for organ preservation as it has for squamous cell carcinomas of the larynx and anus. Phase II trials critically evaluating such therapy are needed.

Management of Metastatic Urethral Carcinoma

Relatively few patients with urethral cancer present with distant metastases. Cisplatin-based chemotherapy (methotrexate, vinblastine, doxorubicin, and cisplatin [MVAC] or cisplatin, methotrexate, and vinblastine [CMV]) is effective in metastatic transitional cell carcinoma, but has not been used extensively

Table 41.5. Lymph Node Involvement in Female Urethral Carcinoma

AUTHOR	INGUINAL LYMPH NODES		PELVIC LYMPH NODES
	CLINICALLY POSITIVE	HISTOLOGICALLY POSITIVE	
Grabstald et al. (53)	25/79 (32%)	22/24 (92%)	13/26 (50%)
Weghaupt et al. (64)	19/62 (14%)	7/7 (100%)	
Pointon and Poole-Wilson (12)	46/132 (35%)		
Desai et al. (51)	6/16 (33%)	2/6 (33%)	
Monaco et al. (54)	5/23 (22%)	2/5 (40%)	

for squamous cell carcinoma of the urethra because of the disease's rarity and low rate of metastases (73, 74, 84–86). As mentioned, cisplatin, bleomycin, and methotrexate either alone or in combination with 5-fluorouracil and vincristine have been shown to be active drugs for the management of squamous carcinomas of the urethra and penis (77–79, 87, 88). Patients with unresectable local lesions and/or evidence of metastases should be offered such chemotherapy.

In addition, experience in the management of squamous cell carcinomas of the cervix, cloaca, and head and neck suggests that the use of mitomycin C, doxorubicin, and ifosfamide in combination with the agents mentioned above deserves evaluation (i.e., bleomycin, ifosfamide, and cisplatin or mitomycin C and 5-fluorouracil). Patients with progressive local or metastatic disease who are not candidates for treatment or who have experienced relapse after various forms of treatment should be offered aggressive palliative care including pain medication, emotional and social support, and focal radiation therapy for isolated, painful metastases (89).

CONCLUSION

Urethral carcinomas are rare human malignancies. Low-volume and low-stage tumors can be treated with a variety of surgical or radiotherapeutic techniques designed to preserve genitourinary function. Unfortunately, high-volume and high-stage carcinomas frequently present with advanced local and regional disease not amenable to either excision or radiation alone. An integrated management approach should be considered. The use of neoadjuvant chemotherapy should be investigated in an attempt to increase downstaging and the likelihood of complete tumor excision.

REFERENCES

1. Tanagho EA. Anatomy of the lower urinary tract. In: Walsh PC, Gittes R, Stamey TA, et al., eds. Campell's urology. 5th ed. Philadelphia: WB Saunders, 1986.
2. Johnson DE, Ames FC. Surgical anatomy and lymphatic drainage of the ilioinguinal region. In: Johnson DE, Ames FC, eds. Groin dissection. Chicago: Year Book Medical Publishers, 1985.
3. Daselar EH, Anson BJ, Reimann AF. Radical excision of the inguinal and iliac lymph glands: a study based on 450 anatomical dissections and upon supportive clinical observations. Surg Gynecol Obstet 1948;87:679.
4. Hand JR. Surgery of the penis and urethra. In: Campell MF, Harrison JH, eds. Urology. 3rd ed. Philadelphia: WB Saunders, 1970.
5. Mullin EM, Anderson EE, Paulson DF. Carcinoma of the male urethra. J Urol 1974;112:610.
6. Anderson KA, McAninch JW. Primary squamous cell carcinoma of the anterior male urethra. Urology 1984;23:134.
7. Guinn GA, Ayala AG. Male urethral cancer: report of 15 cases including a primary melanoma. J Urol 1970;107:176.
8. Mandler JI, Pool TL. Primary carcinoma of the male urethra. J Urol 1966;96:67.
9. King LR. Carcinoma of the urethra in male patients. J Urol 1964;91:555.
10. Bracken RB, Henry R, Ordonez N. Primary carcinoma of the male urethra. South Med J 1980;73:1003.
11. Ray B, Canto AR, Whitmore WF. Experience with primary carcinoma of the male urethra. J Urol 1977;117:591.
12. Pointon RCS, Poole-Wilson DS. Primary carcinoma of the urethra. Br J Urol 1968;40:682.
13. Kaplan GW, Bulkley GJ, Grayhack JT. Carcinoma of the male urethra. J Urol 1967;98:365.
14. Sacks SA, Waisman J, Appelbaum HB, et al. Urethral adenocarcinoma (possibly originating in Littre's glands). J Urol 1975;113:50.
15. Bourque J, Chargi A, Gauthier G, et al. Primary carcinoma of Cowper's gland. J Urol 1970;103:758.
16. Pow-Sang JM, Klimberg IW, Hacket RL, et al. Primary malignant melanoma of the male urethra. J Urol 1988;139:1304.
17. Iverson AP, Blackard CE, Schulberg VA. Carcinoma of the prostate with urethral metastases. J Urol 1972;108:901.
18. Selikowitz SM, Olsson CA. Metastatic urethral obstruction. Arch Surg 1973;107:906.
19. Rishes EW, Cullen TH. Carcinoma of the urethra. Br J Urol 1951;2:209.
20. Wiener JS, Liu ES, Walther PJ. Oncologenic human papillomavirus type 16 is associated with squamous cell cancer of the male urethra. Cancer Res 1992;52:5018.
21. Winkler HZ, Lieber MM. Primary squamous cell carcinoma of the male urethra nuclear deoxyribonucleic acid ploidy studied by flow cytometry. J Urol 1988;139:298.
22. Escribano G, Allona A, Burgos FJ, et al. Cavernosography in diagnosis of metastatic tumors of the penis: 5 new cases and a review of the literature. J Urol 1987;138:1174.
23. Konnak JW. Conservative management of low grade neoplasms of the male urethra: a preliminary report. J Urol 1980;123:175.
24. Hillyard RW, Ladaga L, Schellhammer PF. Superficial transitional cell carcinoma of the bladder associated with mucosal involvement of the prostatic urethra: results of treatment with intravesical bacillus Calmette-Guerin. J Urol 1988;139:290.
25. Raghavaiah NV. Radiotherapy in the treatment of carcinoma of the male urethra. Cancer 1978;41:1313.
26. Ticho BH, Perez-Tamayo C, Konnak JW. Primary carcinoma of the distal male urethra: a case treated with lymphadenectomy and interstitial radiation therapy. J Urol 1988;129:1302.
27. Dinney CPN, Johnson DE, Swanson DA, et al. Therapy and prognosis for male anterior urethral carcinoma: an update. Urology 1994;43:506.
28. Marshall VF. Radical excision of locally extensive carcinoma of the deep male urethra. J Urol 1957;78:252.
29. Hotchkiss RS, Amelar RD. Primary carcinoma of the male urethra. J Urol 1954;72:1181.
30. Shuttleworth KED, Lloyd-Davies RW. Radical resection for tumours involving the posterior urethra. Br J Urol 1969;41:739.
31. Condon RE, Bartlett JG, Greenlee H, et al. The efficacy of oral and systemic antibiotic prophylaxis in colorectal surgery. Arch Surg 1983;188:496.

32. Nichols RL, Condon RE, Gorbach SL, et al. Efficacy of preoperative antimicrobial preparation of the bowel. Ann Surg 1972;176:227.

33. Johnson DE, Lo RK. Tumors of the penis, urethra and scrotum. In: deKernion JB, Paulson D, eds. Genitourinary cancer management. Philadelphia: Lea & Febiger, 1987:219.

34. Klein FA, et al. Inferior pubic rami resection with en bloc radical excision for invasive proximal urethral carcinoma. Cancer 1983;51:1238.

35. Jewett HJ, Oesterling JE. A simple substitute for a missing segment of the proximal anterior urethra. J Urol 1987;138: 1241.

36. Tobisu K-I, Tanaka Y, Mizutani T, et al. Transitional cell carcinoma of the urethra in men following cystectomy for bladder cancer: multivariate analysis for risk factors. J Urol 1991;146:1551.

37. Sakamoto N, Tsuneyoshi M, Naito S, et al. An adequate sampling of the prostate to identify prostatic involvement by urothelial carcinoma in bladder cancer patients. J Urol 1993; 149:318.

38. Poole-Wilson DS, Barnard RJ. Total cystectomy for bladder tumors. Br J Urol 1978;43:16.

39. Faysal MH. Urethrectomy in men with transitional cell carcinoma of the bladder. Urology 1980;16:23.

40. Zabbo A, Montie JE. Management of the urethra in men undergoing radical cystectomy for bladder cancer. J Urol 1984; 131:267.

41. Beahrs JR, Fleming TR, Zincke H. Risk of local urethral recurrence after radical cystectomy for bladder cancer. J Urol 1984;131:264.

42. Raz S, McLorie G, Johnson S, et al. Management of the urethra in patients undergoing radical cystectomy for bladder carcinoma. J Urol 1978;120:298.

43. Schellhammer PF, Whitmore WF. Transitional cell carcinoma of the urethra in men having cystectomy for bladder cancer. J Urol 1976;115:56.

44. Sarosdy MF. Management of the male urethra after cystectomy for bladder cancer. Urol Clin North Am 1992;19:391.

45. Freeman JA, Esrig D, Stein JP, et al. Management of the patient with bladder cancer; urethral recurrence. Urol Clin North Am 1994;21:645.

46. Schellhammer PF, Whitmore WF. Urethral meatal carcinoma following cystourethrectomy for bladder carcinoma. J Urol 1976;115:61.

47. Wolinska WH, Melamed M, Schellhammar PF, et al. Urethral cytology following cystectomy for bladder carcinoma. Am J Surg Pathol 1973;1:225.

48. Hermansen DK, Badalament RA, Whitmore WF, et al. Detection of carcinoma in the post-cystectomy urethral remnant by flow cytometric analysis. J Urol 1988;139:304.

49. Johnson DE, O'Connell JR. Primary carcinoma of female urethra. Urology 1983;21:42.

50. Turner A, Hendry WF. Primary carcinoma of the female urethra. Br J Urol 1980;52:549.

51. Desai S, Libertino JA, Zinman L. Primary carcinoma of the female urethra. J Urol 1973;110:693.

52. Srinivas V, Ali Khan S. Female urethral cancer: an overview. Int J Urol Nephrol 1987;19:423.

53. Grabstald H, Hilaris B, Henschke U, et al. Cancer of the female urethra. JAMA 1966;197:835.

54. Monaco AP, Murphy GB, Dowling W. Primary cancer of the female urethra. Cancer 1958;11:1215.

55. Bracken RB, Johnson DE, Miller LS, et al. Primary carcinoma of the female urethra. J Urol 1976;116:188.

56. Meis JM, Ayala AG, Johnson DE. Adenocarcinoma of the urethra in women: a clinicopathologic study. Cancer 1987;60: 1038.

57. Young RH, Scully RE. Clear cell adenocarcinoma of the urethra in women: a clinicopathologic study. Cancer 1987;60: 1038.

58. Katz JI, Grabstald H. Primary malignant melanoma of the female urethra. J Urol 1976;116:454.

59. Gonzalez MO, Harrison ML, Boileau MA. Carcinoma in diverticulum of female urethra. Urology 1985;26:328.

60. Wiener JS, Walther PJ. A high association of oncogenic human papillomaviruses with carcinomas of the female urethra: polymerase chain reaction-based analysis of multiple histological types. J Urol 1994;151:49.

61. Prempree T, Amornmarn R, Patanaphan V. Radiation therapy in primary carcinoma of the female urethra. Cancer 1984;54: 729.

62. Antoniades J. Radiation therapy in carcinoma of the female urethra. Cancer 1969;24:70.

63. Mayer R, Fowler JE, Clayton M. Localized urethral carcinoma in women. Cancer 1987;60:1548.

64. Weghaupt K, Gerstner GJ, Kucera H. Radiation therapy for primary carcinoma of the female urethra: a survey over 25 years. Gynecol Oncol 1984;17:58.

65. Taggart CG, Castro JR, Rutledge FN. Carcinoma of the female urethra. AJR 1972;114:145.

66. Delclos L, Wharton JT, Rutledge FN. Tumors of the vagina and female urethra. In: Fletcher GH, ed. Textbook of radiotherapy. Philadelphia: Lea & Febiger, 1980:812.

67. Klein FA, Moinuddin M, Kersh R. Carcinoma of the female urethra: combined iridium Ir 192 interstitial and external beam radiotherapy. South Med J 1987;80:1129.

68. Nori D, Cain JM, Hilaris BS, et al. Metronidazole as a radiosensitizer and high-dose radiation in advanced vulvovaginal malignancies, a pilot study. Gynecol Oncol 1983; 16:117.

69. Gardin AS, Zagars GK, Delclos L. Primary carcinoma of the female urethra: results of radiotherapy. Cancer 1993;71:3102.

70. Moinuddin M, Klein FA, Harza TA. Primary female urethral carcinoma. Cancer 1988;62:54.

71. Skinner EC, Skinner DG. Management of carcinoma of the female urethra. In: Skinner DG, Lieskovsky G, eds. Genitourinary cancer. Philadelphia: WB Saunders, 1988:490.

72. Hedden RJ, Husseinzadeh N, Bracken RB. Bladder sparing surgery for locally advanced female urethral cancer. J Urol 1993;150:1135.

73. Bosl GJ, Fair WR, Herr HW, et al. Bladder cancer: advances in biology and treatment. Crit Rev Oncol Hematol 1994;16: 33.

74. Logothetis CJ, Dexus FH, Finn L, et al. A prospective randomized trial comparing MVAC and CISCA chemotherapy for patients with metastatic urothelial tumors. J Clin Oncol 1990;8:1050.

75. Schaltz PK, Herr HW, Zhang ZF, et al. Neoadjuvant chemotherapy for invasive bladder cancer: prognostic factors for

survival of patients treated with MVAC with 5-year follow up. J Clin Oncol 1994;12:1394.

76. Scher HI, Yagoda A, Herr HW, et al. Neoadjuvant M-VAC (methotrexate, vinblastine, doxorubicin and cisplatin) for extravesical urinary tract tumors. J Urol 1988;139:475.

77. Eisenberger MA. Chemotherapy for carcinomas of the penis and urethra. Urol Clin North Am 1992;19:333.

78. Hussein A, Benedetto P, Sridhar K. Chemotherapy with cisplatin and 5-fluorouracil for penile and urethral squamous cell carcinomas. Cancer 1990;65:433.

79. Dexus FH, Logethetis CJ, Sella A, et al. Combination chemotherapy with methotrexate, bleomycin and cisplatin for advanced squamous cell carcinoma of the male genital tract. J Urol 1991;146:1284.

80. Edsmyr F, Andersson Esposti PL. Combined bleomycin and radiation therapy in carcinoma of the penis. Cancer 1985;56: 1257.

81. Maiche AG. Combined bleomycin and radiation treatment of penile carcinoma. Acta Oncol 1989;28:548.

82. Johnson DW, Kessler JF, Ferrigni RG, et al. Low dose combined chemotherapy/radiotherapy in the management of locally advanced urethral squamous cell carcinoma. J Urol 1989;41:615.

83. Baskin L, Turzan C. Carcinoma of the male urethra: management of locally advanced disease with combined chemotherapy, radiotherapy and penile-preserving surgery. Urology 1992;39:21.

84. Sternberg CN, Yagoda A, Scher HI, et al. M-VAC (methotrexate, vinblastine, doxorubicin and cisplatin) for advanced transitional cell carcinoma of urothelium. J Urol 1988;139:461.

85. Harker WG, Meyers FJ, Frieha FS, et al. Cisplatin, methotrexate, and vinblastine (CMV): an effective chemotherapy regimen for metastatic transitional cell carcinoma; a Northern California Oncology Group study. J Clin Oncol 1985;3:1463.

86. Kasimis BS. Primary carcinomas of the male and female urethra. In: Spiers ASD, ed. Chemotherapy and urological malignancy. New York: Springer-Verlag, 1982:106.

87. Ahmed T, Sklaroff R, Yagoda A. Sequential trials of methotrexate, cisplatin, and bleomycin for penile cancer. J Urol 1984;132:465.

88. Dexeus FH, Logothetis CJ, Sipahi H. Chemotherapy for advanced squamous carcinoma of the male external genital tract and urethra. In: Johnson DE, Logothetis CJ, Von Eschenbach AC, eds. Systemic therapy for genitourinary cancers. Chicago: Year Book Medical Publishers, 1989:255.

89. Hanks CW, ed. Pain in Cancer. Cancer Surv 1988;7:1.

SCROTUM

Squamous Cell Carcinoma of the Scrotum

Franklin C. Lowe and Lonnie T. Klein

Squamous cell carcinoma of the scrotum was the first environmentally induced cancer identified. In 1775, Sir Percivall Pott noted an increased incidence of scrotal carcinoma among chimney sweepers (1). Because of his work, carcinoma of the scrotum has often been referred as Pott's Cancer or chimney sweepers cancer (2). Subsequently, a high incidence was noted in England among textile factory workers (mule spinners); hence, the eponym mule spinners cancer (3). Various other occupations with high industrial exposure to oils have been associated with scrotal carcinoma (4–7).

ETIOLOGY

Many potential causative agents and risk factors have been associated with scrotal carcinoma. Pott suggested that soot embedded in the rugae of the scrotum was responsible for development of this carcinoma in chimney sweepers. Scrotal skin contact with industrial oils, paraffin wax, and tar can lead to the development of the disease (4, 8). In 1870, Bell, Volkmann, and Ogsden all reported that oil contributed to the development of this cancer (4). In 1900, Passy demonstrated that alkaline ether from chimney soot was an etiologic agent (9). In the same year, Southam and Wilson showed that mechanical irritation, dust, grease, repeated trauma, and poor personal hygiene were causative agents in English textile workers (mule spinners) (10). In 1920, Leitch showed that various oils and their products used in lubricating industrial machinery were carcinogenic (11). Also in 1920, Kennaway and Kennaway showed that high distillation coal tar was more carcinogenic than tar formed at lower temperatures (12). Twort and Fulton firmed these findings and also found that purification of oils with sulfuric acid decreased their carcinogenic potential (13).

The combination of psoralens and ultraviolet light A (PUVA) has recently been shown to increase the incidence of both penile and scrotal malignancy (14). Patients with psoriasis treated with PUVA have a dose-dependent increase in the risk of squamous cell carcinoma on all parts of the body exposed

during therapy (15, 16). In a prospective study by Stern, the risk of PUVA therapy inducing a genital malignancy was 286 times (14). Additionally, the risk of genital malignancy is 5 to 15 times greater than other exposed parts of the body at similar dose levels (14). Stern also determined that ultraviolet B radiation had a 4.6 times higher risk of causing a genital tumor (14). Thus, scrotal shielding is recommended when exposure to PUVA/PUVB is used for therapeutic, recreational, or cosmetic reasons. Many psoriasis patients in whom scrotal cancer later developed had been previously treated with arsenic and tar (17); both of these agents are known carcinogens.

Human papillomavirus (HPV) might be another etiologic factor in the development of scrotal carcinoma. Buschke-Löwenstein tumors, which can occur on the penis and the scrotum, have been linked with HPV subtypes 6 and 11 (18). These subtypes are identified using a polymerase chain reaction assay (19). In the Mayo clinic series, 6 of 14 patients (45%) with squamous cell carcinoma of the scrotum had a documented prior HPV infection (19). Because HPV infection is currently epidemic, an increased incidence of genital malignancies can be expected.

CLINICAL PRESENTATION

Men with scrotal carcinoma usually present during the sixth decade of life and live to a mean age of 61.6 years (20). The initial presentation is usually a solitary lesion. In a study of 19 patients at Memorial Sloan-Kettering Cancer Center, 17 patients (90%) had a solitary lesion (21). The lesion is usually described as a slow-growing pimple, wart, or nodule on the anterolateral aspect of the scrotum that persists for approximately 6 months before ulceration occurs. The subsequent ulcer has raised, rolled edges with seropurulent discharge. The base of the lesion is indurated. Rarely, patients with advanced lesions can have invasion of scrotal contents or the penile shaft (10).

The lesion is usually brought to the attention of a physician about 8 to 12 months after the initial presentation. Patients often treat scrotal lesions with various cleansing agents and ointments before seeking medical assistance.

These lesions are most commonly found on the anterolateral aspect of the scrotum; there is no predilection for a particular side (4, 21). However, in England 60 to 84% of primary lesions occurred on the left side; this reflects the occupational exposure of mule spinners, who rubbed their left side against the machinery and were exposed to carcinogenic oils (22).

Approximately 50 to 60% of patients with scrotal carcinoma have palpable inguinal adenopathy at the time of diagnosis. Half of these men (25% overall) will have metastasis in the surgical specimen on inguinal node evaluation (22). Similar observations have been made in patients with penile carcinoma (23).

DIFFERENTIAL DIAGNOSIS

There are other malignant and benign lesions that need to be differentiated from squamous cell carcinoma of the scrotum. Benign lesions include sebaceous cysts, eczema, nevus, psoriasis, and folliculitis. Other benign diseases include syphilis, tuberculous epididymitis with a draining scrotal sinus, and periurethral abscess. Malignant lesions include basal cell carcinoma, malignant melanoma, Paget's disease, and various sarcomas (24). Biopsy is imperative in distinguishing these lesions.

PATIENT EVALUATION

A careful evaluation of the external genitalia, inguinal lymph nodes, and distant lymph nodes must be undertaken before initiating therapy. Wide local excision of the suspected scrotal lesion should be performed initially. If the patient has palpable inguinal lymphadenopathy, a 4- to 6-week course of broad-spectrum antibiotics should be given to treat inflammatory nodes before inguinal node evaluation. If all palpable nodes resolve, a sentinel node biopsy should be performed. If the initial lesion was near the median raphe or if palpable lymphadenopathy persists despite antibiotic therapy, bilateral sentinel node biopsy is indicated. If the sentinel node biopsy is positive on one side, a contralateral sentinel biopsy and an ipsilateral ilioinguinal lymphadenectomy should be undertaken (25).

Computed tomography (CT) imaging and bipedal lymphangiography have limited applications in assessing the ilioinguinal lymph nodes. The CT scan can show the size of lymph nodes but cannot distinguish inflammatory from metastatic nodes. It can help determine the extent of pelvic involvement with proven bulky inguinal disease. However, the results of a CT scan would not influence the decision of whether to operate on a patient with only minimal or no inguinal disease (26).

TREATMENT OF THE PRIMARY LESION

Wide local excision with a 2-cm margin is the treatment of choice for primary scrotal carcinoma. The skin and underlying dartos muscle should be excised to assure a negative deep margin (10). For small- or medium-sized tumors, the scrotum can be closed primarily. For large scrotal defects, the development of an upper thigh pouch in which the testes are placed while using local thigh flaps or split-thickness skin grafts to cover the scrotum is recommended (25). Local recurrences have been reported adjacent to previously excised lesions. Recurrence rates range from 21 to 40% (6, 21). Unless the primary lesion directly invades the underlying structures, excision of the scrotal contents is rarely necessary.

TREATMENT OF REGIONAL LYMPH NODES

The lymphatic drainage of the scrotum is to the superficial inguinal lymph nodes. In 1911, Morley showed that there was free communication between the superficial lymphatic network on both sides of the scrotum and that the median raphe does not act as a barrier (27). Through his numerous dissections of the scrotal and inguinal lymphatics, Morley noted 10 to 15 lymphatic collecting trunks on each side of the scrotum. He divided them into anterior, lateral, and posterior groups according to the area drained. The anterior trunks are the most important because scrotal carcinomas usually occur in that region. His most important discovery was that the lymphatic drainage of the scrotum drains only into the superficial inguinal nodes and that no trunks bypass the inguinal nodes to drain directly into the pelvic nodes (Fig. 42.1).

Based on Morley's work, Pack and Rekers (28) and Hovnanian (29) recommended bilateral ilioinguinal lymphadenectomy for all patients. Dean was the first to recognize the significant morbidity (lymphedema and wound dehiscence) associated with this procedure and the failure of prophylactic inguinal lymphadenectomy to improve survival (30). Therefore, he advised bilateral ilioinguinal lymphadenectomy only for biopsy-proven inguinal disease (30). Immediate or prophylactic lymphadenectomy was unnecessary for 75% of patients; only 50% had palpable nodes at presentation, and only 50% of these (25% of the overall group) had metastatic disease in the nodes (30). Subsequently, others advocated delaying inguinal lymphadenectomy until metastasis was clinically apparent (21, 31).

Sentinel node biopsy was first described for penile cancer by Riveros et al. in 1967 (32). Although the reliability of this procedure for staging penile cancer has been seriously questioned (33), sentinel biopsy has been recommended for the evaluation of scrotal carcinoma because Morley's work proved that scrotal lymphatics do not bypass the inguinal nodes (25, 34). The Mayo clinic series demonstrated that sentinel biopsy was useful in 5 of 14 patients in diagnosing metastasis (25). The sentinel node was the only positive node in two patients. Also, seven of eight stage A1 patients (86%) avoided inguinal or ilioinguinal lymphadenectomy and its potential significant morbidity by undergoing only sentinel node biopsy (25).

Controversy still exists concerning lymph node management in terms of the following.

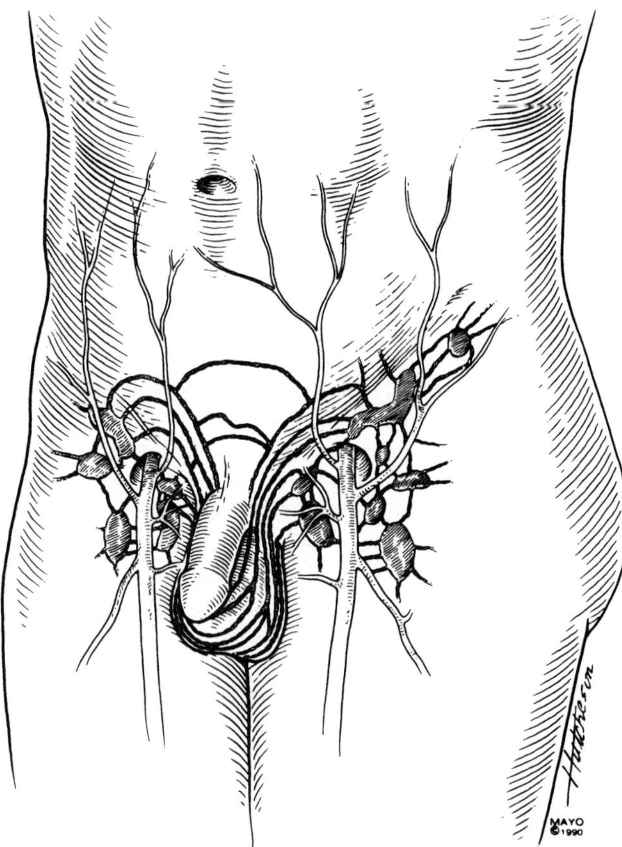

Fig. 42.1.   Lymphatic drainage of the scrotum. (Reprinted with permission of the Mayo Foundation.)

1. Inguinal versus ilioinguinal lymphadenectomy.
2. Unilateral versus bilateral lymphadenectomy.
3. Prophylactic versus delayed lymphadenectomy.

Prior studies have advocated ilioinguinal lymphadenectomy (4, 21, 28, 29, 34–37). McDonald believed that patients with positive pelvic nodes could not be cured; therefore, pelvic dissection was not beneficial (31). Ray and Whitmore previously reported on five patients with pelvic metastasis; none were cured with surgery (21). Therefore, Lowe had recommended that patients with positive pelvic nodes be classified as stage C instead of B2 to reflect this finding (34). Because surgery offers the only possible cure for this disease, ilioinguinal lymphadenectomy is still recommended for those patients with biopsy-proven inguinal disease and minimal or no pelvic lymph node involvement (34, 38).

Because of Morley's work, which demonstrated bilateral cross-over of lymphatic drainage from both sides of the scrotum, authors frequently recommended bilateral lymphadenectomy. However, the Mayo series confirmed the low likelihood (14%) of bilateral disease in patients with stage A1 or B disease (25). Therefore, the current recommendation is for ipsilateral ilioinguinal lymphadenectomy and contralateral sentinel node biopsy when metastatic inguinal disease is found. If the contra-

lateral sentinel node is also positive, then bilateral ilioinguinal lymphadenectomy is undertaken (25, 34).

Prophylactic (immediate) versus delayed (therapeutic) lymphadenectomy is controversial because of the high likelihood for negative nodes (75%) and the significant postoperative morbidity. McDougal et al. have advocated and demonstrated the survival advantage for early lymphadenectomy in patients with penile cancer (39). Similar results have never been shown for scrotal carcinoma. Sentinel lymph node biopsy offers a less-invasive method to ascertain inguinal metastasis and should be performed to determine whether lymphadenectomy is needed (40). Andrews et al. recommended sentinel biopsy only for those patients with palpable nodes after antibiotic therapy (25). The concern with this approach is that patients might not be diligent in their follow-up and nonresectable metastasis might develop before intervention. Therefore, inguinal node evaluation should be undertaken.

SENTINEL NODE BIOPSY

A 5-cm incision is made parallel to the inguinal ligament approximately 4.5 cm lateral and 4.5 cm distal to the pubic tubercle, as described by Cabanas (40). This represents a point overlying the saphenofemoral junction. The sentinel node corresponds to the lymph node associated with the superficial epigastric vein located in Daseler's zone (41). Care must be taken not to devascularize the overlying skin flaps by preserving the subcutaneous adipose tissue. Lymphostasis is crucial, and suction drains are left in at the end of the procedure (40, 42).

If the biopsy specimen of the sentinel node is positive for carcinoma on frozen section, an immediate ipsilateral ilioinguinal lymphadenectomy is recommended. Only if the contralateral biopsy specimen is positive should a bilateral ilioinguinal lymph node dissection be undertaken (25, 34).

TECHNIQUE OF ILIOINGUINAL LYMPHADENECTOMY

The incision that was made for the sentinel node biopsy can be extended laterally and medially to provide adequate exposure for completing the superficial and deep inguinal node dissections. The inguinal dissection must remove all lymph nodes from the area of the saphenofemoral junction and around the femoral vessels. A modified approach to inguinal adenopathy, which includes sparing the saphenous vein, has been recommended (31). This decreases the incidence of postoperative lymphedema. The sartorius muscle is freed from its insertion of the anterior superior iliac spine and is sutured to the inguinal ligament to protect the femoral vessels from exposure and erosion in the event of a wound infection. Closed suction drains are placed to keep the skin flaps adherent to the underlying tissue and to prevent lymphocele formation. Dry sterile dressings are applied without pressure to preserve vascularity of the flaps.

A lower midline abdominal incision is used to gain access

to the pelvic nodes. The pelvic dissection should remove all obturator and external iliac nodes from the bifurcation of the common iliac artery to the entrance to the femoral canal at the node of Cloquet. The femoral space must be closed with a nonabsorbable suture (usually 2-0 Prolene) to prevent herniation (43).

The patient is maintained on bedrest and with intermittent compression stockings for 3 to 7 days. Minidose heparin is given to prevent deep venous thrombosis. Postoperative lymphedema occurs in almost 40% of patients who have had complete dissections. The use of contralateral sentinel node dissection appears to lessen this complication.

ADJUVANT THERAPY

In general, radiation therapy is not an effective treatment for squamous cell carcinoma of the scrotum and is reserved for those cases of recurrence or for poor surgical candidates (25, 34, 44). The use of chemotherapeutic agents has minimal success (32). The successful use of bleomycin in two patients has been reported (45). However, combination chemotherapy with bleomycin in conjunction with cyclophosphamide, vincristine, methotrexate, and 5-fluorouracil has been unsuccessful in advanced disease (31).

STAGING/PROGNOSIS

The recommended staging system for scrotal carcinoma consists of four stages (Table 42.1) (34). Stage A is localized disease (A1 localized to the wall, A2 localized to the genital structures). Stage B is with inguinal nodal metastasis. Previously, stage B included those patients with positive pelvic metastasis who could undergo resection; however, because it is highly unlikely that these patients will be cured, all patients with positive pelvic nodes should be classified as stage C (34). Stage D is distant metastatic disease.

In general, survival is poor for patients with squamous cell carcinoma of the scrotum, with a 5-year survival rate of 30 to 52% (22). Lione and Denholm (6) provided the best 5-year survival rate of 70%. However, when stage-specific survival rates are identified, 70 to 80% of stage A and 40 to 50% of stage B patients have long-term survival. Patients with stage C or D disease rarely survive 5 years (21).

Table 42.1. Staging For Scrotal Carcinoma (34)

STAGE	DESCRIPTION
A1	Localized to scrotal wall
A2	Locally extensive tumor invading adjacent structures (testes, spermatic cord, penis, pubis, perineum)
B	Metastatic disease involving inguinal nodes only
C	Metastases plus positive pelvic nodes; no distal spread
D	Distant metastases beyond pelvic nodes

CONCLUSION

The incidence of squamous cell carcinoma of the scrotum has been declining because of improved hygiene and changes in the work place, but recent identification of HPV as a possible contributing factor could herald further increases in this disease. The basis for treatment depends on wide local excision. Patients should then be treated with 4 to 6 weeks of antibiotics before sentinel node biopsy. Sentinel node biopsy should be performed to rule out micrometastasis and to establish the need for a formal ilioinguinal lymphadenectomy. Careful development and handling of skin flaps will prevent wound complications. Unilateral modified inguinal node dissections and contralateral biopsy will decrease postoperative lymphedema. Adjuvant chemotherapy or radiation therapy is not beneficial. Prognosis is directly related to stage. Those with stage A disease have an excellent prognosis, and even those patients with inguinal metastasis have a good chance for survival.

REFERENCES

1. Pott P. Cancer scroti. In: Howes L, Clark W, Collens R, eds. Chirurgical works. London: Langerman, 1775;5:63.
2. Melicow MM. Percivall Pott (1713–1788); 200th anniversary of 1st report occupation induced cancer of the scrotum in chimney sweepers (1745). Urology 1975;6:745.
3. Brockbank EM. Mule-spinner's cancer. Br Med J 1941;1:622.
4. Graves RC, Flo S. Carcinoma of the scrotum. J Urol 1940;43:309.
5. Cruickshank CND, Squire JR. Skin cancer in engineering industry from the use of mineral oil. Br J Ind Med 1950;7:1.
6. Lione JG, Denholm JS. Cancer of the scrotum in wax pressman; part II: clinical observations. Arch Ind Health 1959;19:530.
7. Avellan L, Breine U, Jacobson B. Carcinoma of the scrotum induced by mineral oil. Scand J Plast Reconstr Surg 1967;1:135.
8. Lee WR. Occupational aspects of scrotal cancer and epithelioma. Ann N Y Acad Sci 1976;271:138.
9. Passy RD. Experimental soot cancer. Br Med J 1922;2:1112.
10. Southam AH, Wilson SR. Cancer of the scrotum; the etiology, clinical features, and treatment of the disease. Br Med J 1922;2:971.
11. Leitch A. Mule spinners cancer and mineral oils. Br Med J 1924;2:941.
12. Kennaway EL, Kennaway NM. The social distribution of cancer of the scrotum and cancer of the penis. Cancer Res 1946;6:49.
13. Twort CC, Fulton JD. Experiments on the nature of carcinogenic agents mineral oils. J Pathol Bacteriol 1929;32:149.
14. Stern RS. Members of the photochemotherapy follow-up study: genital tumors among men with psoriasis exposed to psoralens and ultraviolet A radiation (PUVA) and ultraviolet B radiation. N Engl J Med 1990;322:1093.
15. Stern RS, Lang R. Non-melanoma skin cancer occurring in patients treated with PUVA five to ten years after the first treatment. J Invest Dermatol 1988;91:120.

16. Stern RS, Laird N, Melski J. Cutaneous squamous cell carcinoma in patients treated with PUVA. N Engl J Med 1984;310:1156.

17. De La Brassinne M, Richert B. Genital squamous cell carcinoma after PUVA therapy. Dermatology 1992;185(4):316.

18. Villa L, Lopes A. Human papilloma virus DNA sequences in penile carcinoma in Brazil. Int J Cancer 1986;37:853.

19. Burmer GC, True LD, Krieger JN. Squamous cell carcinoma of the scrotum associated with human papilloma viruses. J Urol 1993;149(2):374.

20. Henry SA. The study of fatal cases of cancer of the scrotum from 1911 till 1935 in relation to occupation, with special references to chimney sweeping and cotton mule spinning. Am J Cancer 1937;31:28.

21. Ray B, Whitmore WF Jr. Experience with carcinoma of the scrotum. J Urol 1977;117:741.

22. Lowe FC. Squamous cell carcinoma of the scrotum. Urol Clin North Am 1992;19:397.

23. Catalona WJ. Role of lymphadenectomy in carcinoma of the penis. Urol Clin North Am 1980;7:785.

24. Hotchkiss RS. Cancer of the skin of the male genitalia. In: Andrade R, Gumport SL, Popkin GL, et al., eds. Cancer of skin: biology, diagnosis, management. Philadelphia: WB Saunders, 1976;2:1409.

25. Andrews PE, Farrow GM, Oesterling JE. Squamous cell carcinoma of the scrotum, long term follow up of 44 patients. J Urol 1991;146:1299.

26. Jing BS, Wallace S, Zoroza J. Metastasis to retroperitoneal and pelvis: computerized tomography and lymphangiography. Radiol Clin North Am 1982;20: 511.

27. Morley, J. The lymphatics of the scrotum in relation to the radical operation for scrotal epithelioma. Lancet 1911;2:1545.

28. Pack GT, Rekers PE. The management of malignant tumors in the groin: a report of 122 groin dissections. Am J Surg 1972;56:545.

29. Hovnanian AP. The evolution and present status of pelvi-inguinal lymphatic excision. Surg Gynecol Obstet 1967;124:851.

30. Dean AL. Epithelioma of the scrotum. J Urol 1948;60:508.

31. McDonald MW. Carcinoma of the scrotum: Urology 1985;25:63.

32. Riveros M, Garcia R, Cabanas R. Lymphadenography of the dorsal lymphatics of the penis: technique and results. Cancer 1967;20:2026.

33. Catalona WJ. Modified inguinal lymphadenectomy for carcinoma of the penis with preservation of the saphenous veins: technique and preliminary results. J Urol 1988;140:306.

34. Lowe FC. Squamous cell carcinoma of the scrotum. J Urol 1983;130:427.

35. Kickham CJE, Dufresne M. An assessment of carcinoma of the scrotum. J Urol 1967;98:108.

36. Coleman MW, Joyce R, Graves RS. Carcinoma of the scrotum; new approach to inguinal node dissection. J Urol 1952;68:534.

37. Tourenc FJ. Le cancer du scrotum chez les decolléteurs (àpropos de 21 cas) Presse Med 1964;72:2009.

38. Lowe FC. Squamous cell carcinoma of the scrotum. Urology 1985;25:63.

39. McDougal WS, Kirchner FK Jr, Edwards RN, et al. Treatment of carcinoma of the penis: the case for primary lymphadenectomy. J Urol 1986;136:38.

40. Cabanas RM. Anatomy and biopsy of sentinel lymph nodes. Urol Clin North Am 1992;19:267.

41. Daseler EH, Anson BJ, Reinman AF. Radical excision of the inguinal and iliac node lymph glands: study based on 450 anatomical dissections and upon supportive clinical observations. Surg Gynecol Obstet 1948;87:679.

42. Crawford DE, Daneshgari F. Management of regional lymphatic drainage in carcinoma of the penis. Urol Clin North Am 1992;19:305.

43. Loughlin KR. Technique of ilioinguinal node dissection for penile and urethral cancer. Contemp Surg 1988;33:33.

44. Higgins CC, Warden JG. Cancer of the scrotum. J Urol 1949;62:250.

45. Ichikawa T, Nakano I, Hirokawa I. Bleomycin treatment of tumors of the penis and scrotum. J Urol 1969;102:699.

XI

PEDIATRIC

43

Pediatric Genitourinary Tumors

An Overview

Laurence S. Baskin

INTRODUCTION

Cancer among children younger than 15 years of age is increasing in incidence in the United States (1). In this age group, cancer is increasingly equal among whites and blacks and among girls and boys. In white children, the increase appears to be largely due to new diagnoses of acute lymphoblastic leukemia, tumors of the brain and nervous system, and not to changes in the incidence of Wilms' tumor, sarcomas, lymphomas, Hodgkin's disease, and neuroblastoma. Despite the increase in incidence, cancer mortality before the age of 15 continues to decline in both sexes and both races. This implies an improved overall survival for childhood cancer. The overall mortality rate for children younger than 15 years of age has decreased 38% from 1973 to 1988, with the overall cure rate being 70 to 90% (1). This group of successfully treated pediatric urologic cancers includes neuroblastoma, Wilms' tumor, rhabdomyosarcoma, and testicular neoplasms. This chapter provides an overview to our current understanding of the biology and treatment strategies of these pediatric urologic malignancies.

Neuroblastoma

Neuroblastoma is the most common malignant tumor of infancy after brain tumors and is the most common intra-abdominal malignancy of childhood. The overall incidence is 8.7 cases per million per year, slightly higher than the incidence of Wilms' tumor, which is 7 cases per million per year (2). More than half the children that have neuroblastoma will present when they are younger than 2 years of age. Approximately 500 new cases are diagnosed in the United States each year. Differential diagnosis includes other causes of abdominal masses in the neonate (Table 43.1). The most common primary sites are in the abdomen, particularly the adrenal gland. Sixty percent of patients with newly diagnosed disease will have metastatic disease. The predominant metastatic sites are the bone marrow, liver, and lymph nodes (2). Unlike patients with Wilms' tumor, patients with neuroblastoma appear sicker at presentation and often manifest pain, malaise, weight loss, anorexia, fever, or neurologic impairment secondary to nerve impingement.

Neuroblastoma remains an enigma. Intensive study into the cellular, molecular, and immunobiology of neuroblastoma has led to an increased understanding of this childhood malignancy. It is now well confirmed that a cytogenic abnormality with a deletion of the short arm of chromosome 1 is typical in primary human neuroblastoma. This has been observed in tumor-derived cell lines and in patients with advanced disease (3). This deletion may represent a loss of the neuroblastoma suppressor gene. Clone cytometric analysis of the DNA content in neuroblastoma specimens also correlates with lower-stage disease and improved response to chemotherapy in patients with a hyperdiploid or near triploid state. In contrast, a normal DNA diploid or near tetraploid DNA content is associated with advanced stage and poorer response to chemotherapy (4).

A strong correlation between amplification of the N-myc proto-oncogene and tumor stage has been demonstrated. Amplification of the N-myc oncogene has been shown to correlate very closely with clinical outcome in advanced-stage disease and to correlate with outcome within each stage (5–7). Amplification of the N-myc oncogene occurs in 30% of untreated patients with advanced-stage disease. It may be that patients with advanced disease who do not show N-myc amplification have development and progression of the neuroblastoma from an overexpression of a single copy of the N-myc oncogene. Other genes commonly implicated in cancers, such as p53 or the ras oncogene family, do not seem to be affected in the neuroblastoma tumor.

The fascinating biology of the neuroblastoma tumor was first studied in 1963 by Beckwith, when he found microscopic clusters of neuroblastoma cells (i.e., neuroblastoma in situ) in the adrenal glands of 1 in every 100 infants younger than 3 months who died of other causes. The clinical incidence of

Table 43.1. Differential Diagnosis of Abdominal Masses in the Child

Malignant tumors
    Neuroblastoma
    Wilms' tumor
    Rhabdomyosarcoma
    Hepatoblastoma
    Lymphoma
    Lymphosarcoma
    Renal cell carcinoma
Benign abdominal masses
    Multicystic dysplastic kidney
    Hydronephrosis
    Polycystic kidney
    Renal abscess
    Congenital mesoblastic nephroma
    Mesenteric cyst
    Choledochal cyst
    Intestinal duplication cyst
    Splenomegaly

neuroblastoma is approximately 1 in 10,000 children. A spontaneous tumor regression typically occurs in the first 6 months of life, which may account for the discordant incidence of clinical versus autopsy neuroblastoma.

Accurate staging of neuroblastoma is important for treatment and prognosis. Although several staging systems have been proposed, it is recommended that the International Neuroblastoma Staging System be universally implemented to facilitate comparisons worldwide (8, 9). This system is based on clinical, radiographic, and surgical evaluation of patients using physical examination, computed tomography (CT) scan or magnetic resonance imaging (MRI), bilateral bone marrow aspirates and biopsy, catecholamine metabolite evaluation of the urine, and serum evaluation for lactate dehydrogenase, ferritin, and neuron-specific enolase (10, 11). Patients with neuroblastoma can be divided into those with favorable and unfavorable features using a criteria of 2-year survival with no evidence of disease as equivalent to cure. A combination of factors can now be used to give a definitive prognosis (12). By combining age, stage, serum ferritin, N-myc amplification, and tumor histology, an accurate assessment can be made at the time of diagnosis (13).

The goal of cancer treatment today is to select those patients who will benefit from aggressive therapy while minimizing the morbidity of treatment in those patients who have a good prognosis at initial diagnosis. As we become more sophisticated in understanding the biology of neuroblastoma, this disease may prove to be a model for this type of approach. Therefore, patients with neuroblastoma can be divided into low-risk, intermediate-risk, and high-risk groups, and therapy can be tailored to these patients' specific needs. Surgical intervention is a treatment of choice for patients who have localized disease. For patients with stage I and II disease in the low-risk group (single copy of N-myc) approximately 95% can be cured by

surgery alone (14). However, debulking of large tumors, which carries a potentially high surgical morbidity, is not indicated because chemotherapy and radiation allow tumor shrinkage and possible resection at a later date (14).

Neuroblastoma is chemoresponsive. Multiple agents—especially cisplatin, doxorubicin, etoposide, and cyclophosphamide—have shown efficacy against this tumor. Radiation therapy, although not curative, can be cytoreductive in anticipation of further surgery or in combination with chemotherapy. Autologous bone marrow transplantation, using a combination of high-dose chemotherapy (melphalan, doxorubicin, and teniposide) and total body irradiation, has been the greatest advance in the treatment of patients who have unfavorable disease at the time of diagnosis (15, 16). Survival in this group has increased from 15% to a more recent optimistic outlook of 50%.

A subset of patients who present with stage IV disease is a unique group, in that spontaneous remission is likely. At birth or within the first year of life, extensive neuroblastoma can develop throughout the liver, subcutaneous fat, and bone marrow in these infants. The metastatic tumor may grow rapidly, and the mechanical effect can cause pulmonary distress from an incapacitating liver enlargement. After this unusual tumor growth spurt, a spontaneous regression typically occurs. Therefore, treatment in stage IV-S neuroblastoma should be directed toward comorbidities, such as massive hepatomegaly, or respiratory compromise where low-dose radiation may reduce organ size until the tumor spontaneously remits (17).

New therapies for neuroblastoma, such as monoclonal antibodies to specific neuronal components (e.g., G_{D2} ganglioside) and approaches using cytokines and interleukin-2 to further stimulate the host immune response, are now undergoing trials. Other approaches using the radioisotope iodine 131 to target neuroblastoma are being combined with cytotoxic antibodies (2). It is hoped that current research will lead to improved outcome in patients with all stages of neuroblastoma, decreased morbidity in low-risk patients, and improved survival in patients who previously had dismal prognoses.

Wilms' Tumor

Wilms' tumor was characterized in 1899 by Max Wilms. Wilms' tumor is the most common malignant neoplasm of the urinary tract and accounts for approximately 8% of all solid tumors in children (18). The peak incidence for Wilms' tumor is between the ages of 3 and 4, slightly later than the peak incidence of neuroblastoma. These tumors are often massive in size at the time of diagnosis.

The evolution of the treatment of Wilms' tumor has been dependent on the cooperative studies that have been carried out by the National Wilms' Tumor Study Group (NWTSG) in the United States and the International Society of Pediatric Oncology (SIOP) in Europe (19–22). Comparing the multimodal approach with surgery, chemotherapy and radiation therapy have improved the survival of patients with Wilms' tumor from 25% in the 1940s to close to 85% for all stages of Wilms' tumor in 1995 (18, 23). The improved survival of patients with Wilms' tumor follows the history of radiation therapy in cancer treatment, with radiation improving the survival to the 50% range. With the advent of chemotherapy, initially actinomycin D in the 1950s at Boston Children's Hospital and subsequently vincristine and cyclophosphamide, survival has further improved.

There have been significant recent developments in the molecular and cellular biology of Wilms' tumor. Areas of excitement have been in the discovery and elucidation of the Wilms' tumor suppressor gene WT1 and characterization of a possible Wilms' tumor growth factor, insulin-like growth factor II (IGF-2). The Wilms' tumor suppressor gene WT1 has been shown to be highly expressed in patients whose Wilms' disease is associated with specific congenital syndromes, such as the Denys-Drash syndrome (early onset of nephropathy, pseudohermaphroditism in males, and high risk of Wilms' tumor). An additional transmutation of WT1 has also been described in the WAGR syndrome (Wilms' tumor, aniridia, genital urinary malformations, and mental retardation) (24). The fact that a DNA mutation in WT1 has not been seen in patients with sporadic Wilms' tumor may be explained by a mutation occurring in a promoter region of the Wilms' WT1 gene. Recent data have shown a single transacting mRNA deletion that can create tumor genesis in sporadic tumors. This mRNA splicing mutant may be the most common mutation in Wilms' tumor biology but needs further confirmation (25).

It is known that a subset of patients with unilateral Wilms' tumor is taller than age-matched cohorts. This may be explained by the expression of IGF-2, which may control both somatic growth and the initiation of Wilms' tumor (26). Further work into IGF-2 expression may help our understanding of this interesting biologic tumor.

Patients with Wilms' tumor should be evaluated for potential congenital syndromes and associated anomalies (24). For example, approximately 3% of Wilms' tumor patients will have hemihypertrophy. Other associated anomalies consist of the Beckwith-Wiedemann syndrome, which consists of visceromegaly involving the adrenocortex, kidney, liver, pancreas, and gonads. Secondary malignant neoplasms such as sarcomas, adenocarcinomas, and leukemias are reported to occur in 15% of long-term survivors of Wilms' tumor (27). This highlights the concept of tailoring treatment to minimize morbidity in hopes of decreasing this rate of secondary malignancies, without influencing long-term survival.

DIAGNOSIS

Discovery of an abdominal mass in a relatively healthy child is the most frequent presenting sign leading to the diagnosis of Wilms' tumor; it occurs in 75% of cases (28). Unlike patients with neuroblastoma, these children are not typically sick due to other symptoms. Differential diagnosis includes other causes of abdominal masses in the newborn, as previously noted (Table 43.1). Ultrasound is an excellent first-line diagnostic technique

to establish the origin of an abdominal mass. In patients with suspected Wilms' tumor, cross-sectional imaging with CT and MRI allows accurate staging (29, 30).

Currently, we may be coming to a crossroads in the staging of patients with Wilms' tumor. Classically, staging had always been performed with intraoperative assessment of the affected kidney, as well as contralateral exploration of the nonaffected kidney. However, with modern imaging techniques, there seems to be excellent correlation with preoperative imaging in respect to surgical outcomes (30). If this proves to be the case, it may be that accurate staging can be performed with cross-sectional CT, MRI, and percutaneous or open biopsy without the need for contralateral exploration in all patients. In theory, this would limit the amount of surgery required for patients with Wilms' tumor, thus avoiding the need to open the peritoneum, which subjects patients to an increased risk of postoperative intestinal obstruction (31).

The most widely accepted clinical pathologic staging system of Wilms' tumor was created by the NWTSG and has been successfully used to compare outcome results worldwide. The most important prognostic factor for patients with Wilms' tumor is the initial histologic type (32). Patients with anaplasia (which is characterized by the presence of mitotic figures, a three-fold enlargement in the nuclei, and a hyperchromatic pattern) have a four-fold higher chance of relapse and a death rate 9 times greater than those without anaplasia (33). This group makes up approximately 5% of all Wilms' tumor cases. The presence of hematogenous metastases, which most commonly occur in the lung but can also occur in the liver, bone, or brain, is an important prognostic determinant. Other prognostic factors are lymph node involvement and tumor extension at the site of the primary tumor. One or more of these features were seen in 100% of patients with stage I favorable histologic type Wilms' tumor who had relapse (32).

The goal of the NWTSG has been to improve survival for all patients, yet to limit intensive therapy for patients who have a favorable prognosis. This has been accomplished by changing the surgical philosophy toward patients with Wilms' tumor. The advent of excellent chemotherapy and radiation has resulted in a new approach of renal preservation at the time of difficult surgery in lieu of attempting heroic resection of all tumor mass. This has decreased the number of complications, such as injury to adjacent organs, that occur when removing large tumors. Most centers are now using chemotherapy for reducing the size of Wilms' tumor preoperatively. The philosophy is to give maximum chemotherapy to patients with an unfavorable prognosis and to minimize chemotherapy in those who will not benefit (34). In highly selected patients in whom conventional therapy fails, some success has been achieved with high-dose lethal chemotherapy followed by autologous bone marrow transplantation.

The SIOP protocols have recommended chemotherapeutic treatment before performing tissue biopsy. This approach has not been embraced by the NWTSG for fear of understaging tumors, not making an exact histologic diagnosis, and missing the biologic inherent potential of the tumor before pretreatment (35, 36). In the NWTSG I, albeit before the modern cross-sectional imaging techniques, 30 of 606 patients (5%) had an incorrect preoperative diagnosis (37). This raises the concern that some of these children with abdominal masses who received chemotherapy before histologic diagnosis may be receiving treatment for a potentially benign disease, emphasizing the need for prechemotherapy histologic confirmation. In prior years, a flank approach was clearly contraindicated because adequate staging of the abdomen and contralateral kidney could not be performed and lymph nodes could not be completely assessed. The retroperitoneal surgical approach has a theoretical advantage of decreasing the incidence of postoperative bowel obstruction. If cross-sectional imaging withstands the test of time for accurate preoperative staging, it may change the surgical approach to Wilms' tumor.

Rhabdomyosarcoma

Rhabdomyosarcoma is the most common soft tissue sarcoma of childhood, with a bimodal age distribution peaking in the first 2 years of life and in adolescence (38). Approximately 20% of rhabdomyosarcomas arises from the genital urinary tract (paratesticular, bladder, prostate, vagina, and uterus). Similar to the improved prognosis in Wilms' tumor patients (a result of the NWTSG), treatment of patients with rhabdomyosarcoma has greatly improved with the Intergroup Rhabdomyosarcoma Study (IRS) (39–43). Although survival has improved with IRS studies I to IV, results have not been as dramatic as with Wilms' tumor. Like Wilms' tumor, however, there have been exciting recent discoveries in the area of molecular and cellular biology.

To confirm the diagnosis of poorly differentiated rhabdomyosarcoma, which can be difficult based on histologic type alone, newer immunohistochemical staining techniques may be useful. For example, the MyoD protein (which is important in early skeletal muscle differentiation) is a specific marker for rhabdomyosarcoma (44). There also is a characteristic translocation in the alveolar histologic subtype of rhabdomyosarcoma involving chromosomes 2 and 13. This translocation results in the formation of a chimeric protein and may lead to transcriptional deregulation in the rhabdomyosarcoma cells (45). Specific probes have been developed for this protein that may help in differential diagnosis. Clarifying the histologic subtype with new biologic markers may improve the prognostic staging of this disease. Currently, the best predictors of outcome are age at diagnosis, tumor invasiveness, metastases, regional lymph node involvement, and histopathologic subtype (38, 46).

Previously, surgery had been the primary treatment modality for rhabdomyosarcoma, with radical excision providing the best hope of survival. Currently, surgery has played a more limited role, with less aggressive pelvic surgery and organ-preserving techniques combined with more effective radiation and chemotherapy (47, 48). Initially, it was thought that the success of organ-sparing surgery might be disappointing; however, recent data from IRS-III suggest that the majority of patients can survive with intact pelvic organs after pelvic radiation and intensive chemotherapy (42). This has been possible with the addition of Adriamycin and cisplatin to the pulse vincristine, actinomycin D, and cyclophosphamide (VAC) regimen, allowing sparing of pelvic organs. The current mortality rate for pelvic rhabdomyosarcoma is less than 10% in patients with disseminated embryonal cell disease.

Patients with paratesticular rhabdomyosarcomas have an overall survival rate of 90%. The relatively high morbidity resulting from radiation and retroperitoneal lymph node dissection is now being questioned. Retroperitoneal lymph node dissection is currently reserved for patients with evidence of disease on CT scan, rather than implementing surgery prophylactically. A recent study has shown that 14% of patients with clinically negative nodes had tumor at the time of retroperitoneal lymphadenectomy. Based on the high relapse-free rates and excellent survival rates, the current recommendation is still to perform retroperitoneal lymphadenectomy only for patients with nodal disease on CT scan. A subgroup of boys older than 16 years of age has been identified with a particularly poor prognosis, and more aggressive therapy needs to be considered. Secondary malignancies have also been reported in patients treated for rhabdomyosarcoma (49).

The emphasis on quality of life without compromising survival continues to be the approach for patients with rhabdomyosarcoma. IRS protocols I through IV have been essential in increasing our knowledge and understanding of this disease. The advent of new biological markers may help in the selection of patients with more favorable prognoses who require less therapy and the selection of patients with more aggressive tumors who need further treatment.

Testis Tumors in Children

Testicular tumors account for 1 to 2% of all pediatric solid tumors (50). Peak incidence occurs at approximately 2 years of age. Yolk sac tumors comprise 80% of all prepubertal germ cell tumors. Although it is not typical that they present in the neonatal period, a recent review of 338 testis tumors from the prepubertal testis tumor registry of the American Academy of Pediatrics showed that 22 cases occurred in the neonatal period, emphasizing the fact that invasive germ cell tumors should be considered in a differential diagnosis of a scrotal mass in a neonate (50). More common causes of a scrotal mass include inguinal hernia, testicular torsion, hydrocele, or hematoma. Treatment of prepubertal testis tumors needs to be tailored to the specific histologic type. Staging with tumor markers, such as alpha-fetoprotein and beta human chorionic gonadotropin, is useful. CT scan and ultrasound can be used to evaluate the retroperitoneum and chest for disseminated disease.

CONCLUSION

The incidence of cancer continues to increase for both children and adults. However, for children the mortality rate decreases;

whereas for adults, there has been an increase. In contemporary series of children in whom cancer was diagnosed, 80% are predicted to be long-term survivors. Childhood cancer is rare and represents only 1% of the total U.S. cancer problem. However, approximately 50% of all children with cancer, but only 2% of all adults, are studied via the National Cancer Institute (NCI) cooperative group mechanism (51). For rhabdomyosarcoma and Wilms' tumor, as many as 70 to 85% of all cases are managed via NCI-sponsored trials. Essentially, all pediatric cancer is treated by combination treatment with radiation, surgical resection, and systemic chemotherapy. This approach has contributed to high cure rates.

Our understanding of the late effects of being a cancer survivor has come from longitudinal studies of children. The most severe long-term effects related to radiation therapy in childhood are adverse effects on growth and development, adverse effects on fertility, and the induction of secondary malignant tumors. Although the effort is great, the number of person-years of potential lives saved annually is rewarding in patients with pediatric cancers.

REFERENCES

1. Bleyer WA. What can be learned about childhood cancer from cancer statistics review 1973–1988. Cancer 1993;71(Suppl): 3229.
2. Matthay KK. Neuroblastoma; a clinical challenge and biologic puzzle. CA Cancer J Clin 1995;45(3):179.
3. Brodeur GM, Fong CT. Molecular biology and genetics of human neuroblastoma. Cancer Genet Cytogenet 1989;41(2): 153.
4. Look AT, et al. Cellular DNA content as a predictor of response to chemotherapy in infants with unresectable neuroblastoma. N Engl J Med 1984;311:231.
5. Schwab M, et al. Enhanced expression of the human gene N-myc consequent to amplification of DNA may contribute to malignant progression of neuroblastoma. Proc Natl Acad Sci 1984;81:4940.
6. Seeger RC, et al. Association of multiple copies of the N-myc oncogene with rapid progression of neuroblastomas. N Engl J Med 1985;313:1111.
7. Brodeur GM, et al. Amplification of N-myc in untreated human neuroblastomas correlates with advanced disease stage. Science 1984;224:1121.
8. Brodeur GM, et al. International criteria for diagnosis, staging, and response to treatment in patients with neuroblastoma. J Clin Oncol 1988;6:1874.
9. Smith EI, et al. A surgical perspective on the current staging in neuroblastoma: the International Neuroblastoma Staging System proposal. J Pediatr Surg 1989;24:386.
10. Hann HW, et al. Prognostic importance of serum ferritin in patients with Stages III and IV neuroblastoma: the Children's Cancer Study Group experience. Cancer Res 1985;45:2843.
11. Zeltzer PM, et al. Prognostic importance of serum neuron specific enolase in local and widespread neuroblastoma. Prog Clin Biol Res 1985;175:319.
12. Brodeur GM, et al. Revisions of the international criteria for neuroblastoma diagnosis, staging, and response to treatment. J Clin Oncol 1993;11:1466.
13. Joshi VV, et al. Evaluation of the Shimada classification in advanced neuroblastoma with a special reference to the mitosis-karyorrhexis index: a report from the Children's Cancer Study Group. Mod Pathol 1991;4:139.
14. Kiely EM. The surgical challenge of neuroblastoma. J Pediatr Surg 1994;29:128.
15. Matthay KK, et al. Allogeneic versus autologous purged bone marrow transplantation for neuroblastoma: a report from the Children's Cancer Group. J Clin Oncol 1994;12:2382.
16. Dini G, et al. Bone marrow transplantation for neuroblastoma: a review of 509 cases. EBMT Group. Bone Marrow Transplant 1989;4(Suppl):42.
17. Matthay KK. An overview on the treatment of neuroblastoma. J Nucl Biol Med 1991;35:179.
18. Ritchey ML, GM Haase, Shochat S. Current management of Wilms' tumor. Semin Surg Oncol 1993;9:502.
19. D'Angio GJ, et al. The treatment of Wilms' tumor: results of the second National Wilms' Tumor Study. Cancer 1981;47: 2302.
20. Sutow WW, et al. Prognosis in children with Wilms' tumor metastases prior to or following primary treatment: results from the first National Wilms' Tumor Study (NWTS-1). Am J Clin Oncol 1982;5:339.
21. Breslow N, et al. Prognostic factors in nonmetastatic, favorable histology Wilms' tumor: results of the third National Wilms' Tumor Study. Cancer 1991;68:2345.
22. Thomas PR, et al. Results of two radiation therapy randomizations in the third National Wilms' Tumor Study. Cancer 1991;68:1703.
23. Shochat SJ. Wilms' tumor: diagnosis and treatment in the 1990s. Semin Pediatr Surg 1993;2:59.
24. Coppes MJ, Huff V, Pelletier J. Denys-Drash syndrome: relating a clinical disorder to genetic alterations in the tumor suppressor gene WT1. J Pediatr 1993;123:673.
25. Haber DA, et al. WT1: mediated growth suppression of Wilms tumor cells expressing a WT1 splicing variant. Science 1993;262:2057.
26. Ogawa O, et al. Constitutional relaxation of insulin-like growth factor II gene imprinting associated with Wilms' tumour and gigantism. Nat Genet 1993;5:408.
27. Blatt J, et al. Second malignancies in very long-term survivors of childhood cancer. Am J Med 1992;93:57.
28. Caty MG, Shamberger RC. Abdominal tumors in infancy and childhood. Pediatr Clin North Am 1993;40:1253.
29. Ritchey ML, et al. Accuracy of current imaging modalities in the diagnosis of synchronous bilateral Wilms' tumor: report from the National Wilms Tumor Study Group. Cancer 1995; 75:600.
30. Koo AS, et al. The necessity of contralateral surgical exploration in Wilms tumor with modern noninvasive imaging technique: part 2; a reassessment. J Urol 1990;144:416. Discussion no. 422.
31. Ritchey ML, et al. Small bowel obstruction after nephrectomy for Wilms' tumor: a report of the National Wilms' Tumor Study-3. Ann Surg 1993;218:654.
32. Green DM, et al. The relationship between microsubstaging variables, age at diagnosis, and tumor weight of children with

stage I/favorable histology Wilms' tumor: a report from the National Wilms' Tumor Study. Cancer 1994;74:1817.

33. Green DM, et al. Treatment of children with stages II to IV anaplastic Wilms' tumor: a report from the National Wilms' Tumor Study Group. J Clin Oncol 1994;12:2126.

34. Ritchey ML, et al. Management and outcome of inoperable Wilms tumor: a report of National Wilms Tumor Study-3. Ann Surg 1994;220:683.

35. Zoeller G, et al. Wilms tumor: the problem of diagnostic accuracy in children undergoing preoperative chemotherapy without histological tumor verification. J Urol 1994;151:169.

36. Zuppan CW, et al. The effect of preoperative therapy on the histologic features of Wilms' tumor: an analysis of cases from the Third National Wilms' Tumor Study. Cancer 1991;68: 385.

37. Ehrlich RM, et al. Wilms tumor, misdiagnosed preoperatively: a review of 19 National Wilms Tumor Study I cases. J Urol 1979;122:790.

38. La Quaglia MP, et al. The effect of age at diagnosis on outcome in rhabdomyosarcoma. Cancer 1994;73:109.

39. Hays DM, et al. Rhabdomyosarcoma of the female urogenital tract. J Pediatr Surg 1981;16:828.

40. Hays DM, et al. Primary chemotherapy in the treatment of children with bladder: prostate tumors in the Intergroup Rhabdomyosarcoma Study (IRS-II). J Pediatr Surg 1982;17: 812.

41. Hays DM, et al. Bladder and prostatic tumors in the Intergroup Rhabdomyosarcoma Study (IRS-I): results of therapy. Cancer 1982;50:1472.

42. Hay DM. Bladder/prostate rhabdomyosarcoma: results of the multi-institutional trials of the Intergroup Rhabdomyosarcoma Study. Semin Surg Oncol 1993;9:520.

43. Raney RB Jr, et al. Primary chemotherapy with or without radiation therapy and/or surgery for children with localized sarcoma of the bladder, prostate, vagina, uterus, and cervix: a comparison of the results in Intergroup Rhabdomyosarcoma Studies I and II. Cancer 1990;66:2072.

44. Parham DM. The molecular biology of childhood rhabdomyosarcoma. Semin Diagn Pathol 1994;11:39.

45. Shapiro DN, et al. Fusion of PAX3 to a member of the forkhead family of transcription factors in human alveolar rhabdomyosarcoma. Cancer Res 1993;53:5108.

46. Tsokos M. The diagnosis and classification of childhood rhabdomyosarcoma. Semin Diagn Pathol 1994;11:26.

47. Verga G, Parigi GB. Conservative surgery of bladder-prostate rhabdomyosarcoma in children: results after long-term follow-up. J Pediatr Surg 1993;28:1016.

48. Hays DM, et al. Partial cystectomy in the management of rhabdomyosarcoma of the bladder: a report from the Intergroup Rhabdomyosarcoma Study. J Pediatr Surg 1990;25: 719.

49. Raney B Jr, et al. Sequelae of treatment in 109 patients followed for 5 to 15 years after diagnosis of sarcoma of the bladder and prostate; a report from the Intergroup Rhabdomyosarcoma Study Committee. Cancer 1993;71:2387.

50. Levy DA, Kay R, Elder JS. Neonatal testis tumors: a review of the Prepubertal Testis Tumor Registry. J Urol 1994;151:715.

51. Donaldson SS. Lessons from our children. Int J Radiat Oncol Biol Phys 1993;26:739.

44

Neuroblastoma

Alfred A. DeLorimier

Neuroblastoma is the most common malignant solid tumor in children and accounts for 17% of all childhood malignancies and 15% of malignancy deaths (1). There are approximately 500 new cases per year in the United States, and an incidence of 8.7 per million per year in the population younger than 15 years (2). In the abdomen, it is second in frequency only to Wilms' tumor.

Neuroblastoma originates from cells arising in the neural crest portion of the neuroectoderm (3). These neuroblasts were destined to form the sympathetic and chromaffin portions of the nervous system. Therefore, neuroblastoma most often arises in any position along the sympathetic chain from the neck to the pelvis. Rarely, it may originate intracranially from the sphenopalatine, ciliary, or otic ganglia. Neuroblastoma may have a primary origin within the spinal canal, but spinal cord compression most often results from a dumbbell tumor that arises from the sympathetic chain and grows through the intervertebral foramen into the spinal canal. This tumor rarely develops in the extremities from major neural structures such as the sciatic nerve or the brachial plexus (4).

Neuroblastoma arising within the olfactory nerves occurs in older age groups, demonstrates an indolent biologic behavior, and does not excrete products of catecholamine metabolism, as do those that have other sites of origin. Therefore, olfactory neuroblastoma is usually called an esthesioneuroblastoma (5).

Some embryonic neuroblasts migrate to regions adjacent to the sympathetic ganglia and condense into clusters of paraganglia. These cells contain enzymes that convert norepinephrine to epinephrine. In histologic sections, epinephrine stains brown with chrome salts, which designates these cells as part of the chromaffin system. Chromaffin cells are typical of the adrenal medulla and may be found in clusters along the abdominal aorta, particularly at the level of the inferior mesenteric artery where they are known as the organ of Zuckerkandl.

PROGNOSTIC CONSIDERATIONS

The biologic behavior of neuroblastoma, and thus the outcome of the disease, is highly variable and correlates with the age of the patient, site of primary origin, stage of the disease, sex, resectability, histologic appearance, biochemical maturity of the tumor, and chromosomal abnormalities in the tumor (6–15). Tumor markers such as serum ferritin, neuron-specific enolase, and chromosome analyses; the presence of N-myc oncogene amplification; identification of aneuploidy; and the proportion of cells in the mitotic phase using flow cytometry are also important prognostic indicators.

To calculate survival rates, the time after which most patients will die of disease should be defined. Collins et al. introduced a concept of tumor doubling time, that is, the length of time in which a given tumor will double in size (16). They proposed that pediatric tumors such as neuroblastoma are congenital in origin; thus, assuming a constant rate of tumor cell division, a period of risk for the recurrence of tumor would be the patient's age at diagnosis plus 9 months (the length of gestation) (16).

Because neuroblastoma is a rapidly growing tumor, some authors have suggested that 14 months are equivalent to a 5-year survival period in adult tumors (7). A review of children who were followed by the California Tumor Registry (before the era of chemotherapy) allows a comparison of the survival rates for the interval as defined by Collins et al., the 14-month interval, and the 2-year interval, as related to patient age (9). Eight percent of the patients died after 14 months and 5% after 2 years; 2 of 212 patients died after the period of risk as defined by Collins et al. Because Collins et al.'s interval is too long for a practical definition of long-term survival, most authors have used the 2-year period to define cure rate. Currently, survival and disease-free survival are usually calculated by life-table analysis using the Kaplan-Meier method, but 2-, 3-, and 5-year intervals remain as reference periods (17).

Neuroblastoma occurs from the newborn period to adulthood. The mean age at diagnosis is 3 years. Two thirds of cases are diagnosed by 2 years of age, 75% by 5 years, and 85% by 10 years. There is no difference in survival in patients between 2 and 4 years of age, 5 and 9 years of age, and in those older than 10 years (8, 12–14). The frequency and survival rates according to age group from data before 1974 are shown in Table 44.1 (13). With better pre-operative and postoperative

Table 44.1. Incidence and Survival Rate by Age for Neuroblastoma Before 1974 (13)

AGE	INCIDENCE (%)	SURVIVAL RATE (%)
0–11 mo	28	55
12–23 mo	19	24
Older than 2–4 yr	53	8

care, the current survival in infants is 96% (18). Age is an important variable in prognosis, and comparison of various series must be corrected for variation in the age distribution of reported cases.

Spontaneous Regression and Maturation

Of all reported cases of spontaneous "cure" of malignant tumor, neuroblastoma is the most frequent (12). Infants with stage IV-S neuroblastoma are typical examples of this phenomenon (19–22). In the era before chemotherapy, there were 20 documented patients with extensive hepatic and subcutaneous metastases who received no treatment because early death was expected (22). On later follow-up, they were found to have no evidence of residual disease. This phenomenon is confined to infants. Regression occurred in 72% of those younger than 6 months of age and in 24% of those who were between 6 months and 1 year, with the oldest patient being younger than 18 months old. The tumors involuted and were replaced by varying amounts of scar tissue.

Spontaneous regression of neuroblastoma may be more common than is clinically recognized. Beckwith and Perrin have noted cells in the adrenal glands similar to neuroblastoma in fetuses and newborns dying of unrelated causes (23). They found an incidence of adrenal "neuroblastoma in situ" occurring once in every 250 newborns, whereas clinically evident neuroblastoma will eventually develop in only 1 in 10,000 live born infants. The "neuroblastoma in situ" is not found after the age of 3 months. The fortyfold decrease in the occurrence of neuroblastoma, confined to young infants, would seem to be further evidence of spontaneous regression. However, the cells suggestive of neuroblastoma in situ may be embryonal neuroblasts and not neoplastic cells, which eventually mature to adrenal medulla (24).

Maturation of neuroblastoma to ganglioneuroma is also described as a mechanism of spontaneous cure in the natural evolution of tumor. This process of spontaneous maturation is rare (25). Although there may be an actual development of neuroblastoma cells into ganglioneuroma, it is likely that the neuroblastoma elements of a ganglioneuroblastoma regress, leaving only the ganglion cells.

It is unclear if ganglioneuromas themselves develop from this mechanism of maturation. Ganglioneuromas are rare in infancy and are most commonly encountered in adults (25). Ganglioneuroma occurs 4 times as frequently in the mediastinum than in any other location, while a retroperitoneal origin for neuroblastoma is twice as common as it is for ganglioneu-

roma. It is possible that this difference in distribution for ganglioneuroma is related to the better prognosis for extra abdominal neuroblastoma and that it is because of spontaneous regression (perhaps maturation) in the mediastinum. It should be noted that in the course of chemotherapy, neuroblastoma usually evolves toward ganglioneuroblastoma in which ganglion-like cells become very prominent.

The unique biologic behavior of neuroblastoma in the young age groups has prompted intense interest in the immune mechanism of tumor control. Cells of the lymphoid series are known to be important in cell-mediated immunity. A retrospective review of the histologic type of neuroblastoma has shown that extensive infiltration of tumor by lymphocytes is seen in patients with longer survival (26). However, these particular tumors also had greater degrees of differentiation than those with poor outcomes.

There has been no correlation between absolute peripheral blood lymphocyte counts and survival in neuroblastoma patients (27). In cell cultures, lymphocytes from some neuroblastoma patients have been shown to have cytotoxic effects against their own tumors and against neuroblastomas from other patients (28, 29). In addition, the lymphocytes from some mothers and siblings of children with neuroblastoma have also shown cytotoxic effects on tissue-cultured neuroblastoma cells (29). However, there has been no correlation between the lymphocyte reactivity against tumor cells and the subsequent prognosis.

More recent studies have demonstrated the existence of enhancing and blocking antibodies that greatly modify the tumoricidal effect of lymphocytes (29). Despite the strong suggestion of an influence by the immune system, there has been no breakthrough in using immunity to control neuroblastoma.

Neonatal Screening

Because infants have a much better survival than older patients, and neuroblastoma is presumed to be congenital in origin, there has been great interest in early detection. A spot test of the urinary catecholamines vanillylmandelic acid (VMA), homovanillic acid (HVA), and vanillacetic acid in 6-month-old infants has been used as a mass screening effort for early detection of neuroblastoma in Japan and Canada (30–33). The occurrence of neuroblastoma was found in 1:15,500 to 1:18,749 cases screened. In the United States, we already mass screen infants for hypothyroidism, phenylketonemia, and galactosemia, and the incidence of neuroblastoma exceeds these diseases. Of the screened infants in Japan, 96% were asymptomatic and 72% had no evidence of a mass. Through the mass screening, they found a higher incidence of favorable stage I and stage II tumors, whereas the distribution of the primary site of origin was the same as that in previously published series. However, there were a number of children in the screened population who did not have abnormal catecholamine values and in whom neuroblastoma then developed after 18 months of age. These children presented with more advanced stage tumors. There-

Table 44.2.   Incidence of Primary Site of Origin

LOCATION	INCIDENCE IN NEONATES (%)	INCIDENCE IN ALL AGE GROUPS (%)	SURVIVAL IN ALL AGE GROUPS (%)
Neck	5.2	3.0	100.0
Mediastinum	33.0	15.8	85.0
Adrenal	36.7	55.0	72.0
Extra Adrenal	18.3	19.9	72.0
Celiac	0.0	4.0	0.0
Pelvis	5.2	4.8	80.0
Unknown	1.6	1.5	—

fore, screening at about 18 months of age is being considered (31, 32). The tumors detected at screening before 1 year of age have been very small and difficult to find. An analysis of the various imaging procedures shows that magnetic resonance imaging has been the most effective.

Site of Origin

The incidence of primary site of origin with comparison between infants and all ages for stage I to III tumors is shown in Table 44.2 (9, 15, 34). The overall survival is shown in the third column. This general distribution seems to be consistent in various geographic areas. However, some centers have reported a disproportionately large number of intraabdominal or mediastinal tumors, which will alter the overall prognosis of these series. The site of primary origin is an important variable in prognosis (9).

Stage of the Disease

Staging of neuroblastoma is important because the prognosis and intensity of treatment will vary depending on the extent of disease. However, because of the vagaries in the natural history of neuroblastoma, there has been no universal agreement of a staging system. The systems of staging that are used most often are those of the Children's Cancer Group (CCG), the Pediatric Oncology Group (POG), and the International Neuroblastoma Staging System (INSS) (14, 18, 19). The CCG, POG, and INSS systems are defined in Table 44.3.

In the POG staging system, the presence of lymph node metastases is considered a variable that adversely affects prognosis. In 1988, the International Criteria for Diagnosis writing committee modified the CCG staging system described here to gain prospective information on the importance of regional metastatic nodes (34). Ninane et al. reviewed 33 children with CCG stage II tumors; of 20 children who had no lymph node metastases, 4 died of toxicity to treatment and the remaining 16 were long-term survivors (35). Thirteen of the 33 children had positive lymph nodes and 7 survived. It was concluded that patients with stage II tumors and no metastatic nodes require only surgical resection, whereas the presence of lymph node metastases was associated with significant mortality and

Table 44.3.   Disease Staging

CHILDREN'S CANCER GROUP

Stage I	Tumor confined to the organ or structure of origin
Stage II	Unilateral tumor extending in continuity beyond the organ or structure of origin but not crossing the midline, which is incompletely excised; ipsilateral and contralateral lymph nodes are microscopically negative or the regional ipsilateral nodes are positive; intraspinous extension of tumor is stage II
Stage III	Tumors infiltrating in continuity beyond the midline; tumor that overlaps the midline and does not infiltrate around midline structures is considered stage II; a unilateral tumor with contralateral or bilateral nodes is stage III
Stage IV	Remote disease involving bone, parenchymatous organ and soft tissues, distant lymph node groups, or bone marrow
Stage IV-V	Infants who would otherwise be stage I or II but who have remote disease confined to one or more of the following sites: liver, skin, or bone marrow (without evidence of bone osteolysis)

PEDIATRIC ONCOLOGY GROUP

Stage A	Complete gross excision of primary tumor, with margins histologically negative or positive; intracavitary lymph nodes not intimately adhered to and removed with resected tumor are histologically free of tumor; if primary is in abdomen (including pelvis), liver is histologically free of tumor by biopsy
Stage B	Incomplete gross resection of primary; the lymph nodes and liver are histologically free of tumor, as in stage A
Stage C	Complete or incomplete gross resection of primary; the intracavitary nodes are histologically positive for tumor; the liver is histologically free of tumor by biopsy
Stage D	Disseminated disease beyond intracavitary nodes (i.e., bone marrow, liver, skin, or lymph nodes beyond the cavity containing the primary tumor)

INTERNATIONAL NEUROBLASTOMA STAGING SYSTEM

Stage 1	Unilateral localized tumor; complete excision with or without microscopic residual disease; ipsilateral (unattached) nodes negative
Stage 2A	Unilateral localized tumor; incomplete excision; ipsilateral and contralateral nodes negative
Stage 2B	Unilateral localized tumor; with complete or incomplete gross resection, ipsilateral (unattached) nodes positive, contralateral nodes are negative
Stage 3	Unresectable localized tumor or tumor infiltrating across the midline, with or without regional lymph node involvement, or unilateral tumor with contralateral nodes positive; or midline tumor (pelvic) with bilateral nodes positive
Stage 4	Distant metastases to lymph nodes, bone, liver, lung
Stage 4S	Localized tumor as in stage I, IIA or IIB; with remote disease confined to skin, liver, and/or bone marrow (infants less than one year of age)

warranted more aggressive treatment. Hayes et al., of St. Jude Children's Research Hospital, described 58 children with stage II tumors; 24 of 25 without lymph node metastases survived, and 24 of 33 with metastatic lymph nodes survived (36). In this group with metastatic nodes, all 5 infants survived, but 7 of 12 children older than 1 year died. In the same St. Jude's series of 36 stage III tumors, in which all were associated with lymph node metastases, 6 of 13 children younger than 1 year old and 19 of 23 older children died. Because of their findings, the POG isolated metastatic lymph nodes as an important prognostic variable that they refer to as stage C, when there is no disseminated disease (19).

By contrast, Evans et al. reviewed 251 cases of localized and regional neuroblastoma (CCG stage I, II, and III) and noted that the survival rate was the same for 15 patients with negative nodes as it was for 93 patients with positive nodes (18). There was no difference in survival if the nodes were attached to the primary tumor or separate from it. However, with stage III tumors in which metastatic nodes were separated from the primary tumor, the survival rate was only 30%. The St. Jude Hospital/POG combined staging system does not recognize the decidedly adverse effect of neuroblastoma extending across the midline, for which the survival rate with unilateral tumors is 80% and the survival rate with tumors extending across the midline is 50%. The POG system is not as discriminating between stages as is the CCG system (Table 44.4) (18). Finally, the POG classification does not recognize the special group of infants with widespread tumor (stage IV-S), for whom the prognosis is excellent.

The INSS was developed to incorporate attributes of both the CCG and POG staging systems. The validity of the INSS was analyzed retrospectively from 424 patients treated by CCG protocols between 1980 and 1992 (37). This system emphasizes the completeness of excision (38). If, for example, a tumor arises on both sides of the midline but is completely excised, it would be stage III in the CCG system but stage 1 in the INSS; the prognosis turns out to be consistent with other stage I primary tumors, with an overall survival rate of 97%. There was little difference in survival between stage 2A and stage 2B, so that lymph node metastases were not a prognostic factor and the survival rate was 86%. The INSS stage 3 tumors had essentially the same survival rates as CCG stage III, at 62% (37). About 23% of all neuroblastoma patients have stage I disease. CCG stage II or INSS 2 neuroblastoma has local extension to adjacent organs or local lymph node metastasis confined to the same

side of the midline as the primary tumor. The tumor has been incompletely excised. Ipsilateral and contralateral nodes should be excised and proved to be negative for metastatic tumor. Intraspinal or dumbbell tumors without lymph node metastases are also classified as stage 2A and have an excellent prognosis unless the extraspinal extent of the tumor infiltrates across the midline. Intraspinal extension of abdominal or thoracic primary sites occurs in 6 to 14% of cases. Stage II may also consist of similar tumor that has been completely or incompletely excised, but ipsilateral nodes contain metastases and contralateral nodes do not. About 13% of neuroblastomas are classified as stage II disease.

CCG stage III and INSS stage 3 neuroblastoma are defined as tumor infiltrating across the midline of the body. A unilateral tumor that overlaps the midline is stage II. A unilateral tumor with contralateral metastatic nodes is stage III. Stage III tumors are almost exclusively intraabdominal in origin, with occasional mediastinal and rare cervical primary tumors. Approximately 9% of neuroblastomas are stage III at diagnosis.

The staging of neuroblastoma arising from pelvic primary origin needs to be clarified because the prognosis of the midline pelvic tumors is better than that of other stage III retroperitoneal primary sites. Pelvic tumors might be staged as follows. Those completely excised are stage 1, and residual gross or microscopic tumor in the area of resection or regional lymph nodes on one side only are stage 2. A pelvic tumor invading both sides of the pelvis or if there are bilateral lymph node metastases is stage 3. The INSS rectifies these scenarios, whereas the CCG staging would characterize all pelvic tumors as midline, stage III.

Stage IV disease consists of either lymphatic or hematogenous metastasis far beyond the area of the primary tumor. Most often, stage IV tumors are characterized by osteolytic bone metastases. Favorite sites for bone disease are the base of the skull and calvarium, metaphyses of the long bones, vertebral bodies, and pelvis. Cervical, mediastinal, and retroperitoneal metastases may become so extensive that confluence of the nodes will produce prominent tumor masses. Rarely, metastases may appear in the liver, lungs, and brain. Approximately 40 to 60% of neuroblastomas are stage IV.

A special form of stage IV metastatic tumor has been designated stage IV-S. This occurs in infants and has an excellent prognosis (20, 21). At birth, or within several months subsequently, extensive neuroblastoma develops throughout the liver and/or in subcutaneous fat throughout the body. These infants may also have neuroblastoma cells in the bone marrow aspirate, but there is no evidence of osteolytic metastases. If osteolytic bone lesions are found on skeletal radiographic survey, however, the biologic behavior of the tumor indicates a poor prognosis and the extent of the tumor is considered stage IV and not stage IV-S. In addition, the presence of tumor markers such as N-myc amplification, indicating a poor prognosis, identifies a stage IV rather than a IV-S condition (see below). In some rare congenital cases, neuroblastoma has been noted in the lung, spleen, kidney, and other sites of metastasis not found in older children. In stage IV-S, the primary tumor is usually small,

Table 44.4. A Comparison of the Influence of Staging On Survival in the Children's Cancer Group, Pediatric Oncology Group, and International Neuroblastoma Staging System (18, 37)

	CCG (%)	POG (%)	INSS (%)
Stage I	100	87	97
Stage II	85	85	(2A + B) 86
Stage III	44	74	62

commonly arising in one or both adrenal glands. The metastatic tumors in these infants may grow rapidly and dramatically, to the extent that there may be almost as much tumor as normal tissue. The mechanical effects of this tumor bulk can be devastating when the enormous enlargement of the liver compromises pulmonary, renal, and gastrointestinal function. There may be severe anemia from hemorrhage in the multiple masses or because of replacement of the bone marrow by tumor. However, a spontaneous regression of all tumor masses after a phase of alarming growth during the first 6 to 9 months of life will occur in most infants.

From a review of 137 infants with stage IV-S disease filed with the Armed Forces Institute of Pathology, Stephanson et al. identified two risk groups (21). The high-risk group was those infants younger than 6 months old with liver involvement alone (29 cases) or those with liver plus bone marrow metastases (9 cases) and no skin metastases. Only 32% survived. The low-risk group was composed of 7- to 12-month-old children with any combination of metastases or those younger than 6 months of age who had skin metastases. The survival rate in the low-risk group was 86%. It has been speculated that all these tumor masses may be multiple primary sites of origin and are not metastases at all (21). Recent studies have shown that the stage IV-S tumors are composed of cells that are predominantly aneuploid. However, the overall cure rate is greater than 70%; death occurs either from aggressive treatment or from physiologic impairment by the tumor masses (20). Only 3% of stage IV-S tumors progressed to stage IV. The incidence and overall survival rates taken from data before 1970 and between 1970 and 1985 for the five CCG stages of neuroblastoma are shown in Table 44.5 (9, 12, 13, 37).

The improved survival is probably related to better overall care of the children, as well as more effective chemotherapy.

Gender

Males are affected slightly more frequently than females, with a ratio of about 1.25:1. Of four series' correlating gender and survival, two suggested and one clearly indicated a better survival rate in females (30%) than in males (18%) (9, 10, 13). Wilson and Draper reported that the females in their series

were younger and had a greater proportion of favorable sites of origin, stage, and histologic grades of tumor (13). More recent studies fail to identify a difference in prognosis based on gender (18).

Resectability

The more localized the tumor, the more likely that it is resectable. Stella et al. noted that of 12 children whose tumors were completely removed, 11 (92%) survived (10). Nineteen of 34 patients (58%) survived when complete surgical excision was accompanied by radiation therapy given preoperatively or postoperatively (10). In contrast, only 12 of 93 patients (13%) survived who had only partial resection or biopsy as surgical treatment, along with radiation and chemotherapy (10).

The degree of residual primary tumor should be noted because it is also a determinant of prognosis (18). Residual disease has been graded as follows (18).

Grade 1—Microscopic residual tumor occurs when there was not a clean resection or metastatic nodes were present.

Grade 2—When less than 5% of the original primary tumor remains.

Grade 3—When there is 5 to 25% residual tumor.

Grade 4—When there is more than 25% residual tumor or only a biopsy has been performed.

More than 90% of patients with stage I, complete excision survived. Patients who had grade 1 residual tumor had an 81% survival rate, and those with grade 2 residual tumor had an intermediate survival of 60 to 75% (18). Grade IV residual disease had a survival rate of 55% (18).

In a review of four CCG protocols for stage III tumors, reclassified by the INSS, complete resection resulted in a 70% survival rate, whereas incomplete resection resulted in only a 50% survival rate (37).

Histologic Differences

Undifferentiated neuroblastoma is characterized by small, round cells containing dark-staining nuclei with little cytoplasm, closely packed together, with abundant vascular channels. With cellular elements lacking any differentiation, it may be impossible to distinguish neuroblastoma from some forms of retinoblastoma, Ewing's sarcoma, rhabdomyosarcoma, extranodal lymphoma, synovial cell sarcoma, Wilms' tumor, germ cell tumor, small cell osteosarcoma, or primitive neuroectodermal tumor (PNET) (39). These cases have been traditionally referred to as "small, round-celled tumors." The differentiation of these various tumors requires electron microscopy, immunocytochemistry, and occasionally more special techniques such as in situ hybridization with DNA or RNA probes or cytogenetics (39).

Shimada et al. have developed a histologic grading system based on schwannian (stroma) and neuronal differentiation, prevalence of mitoses, and age, all of which have prognostic significance (40). This system seems to be reproducible by var-

Table 44.5. Incidence and Survival Rates for Neuroblastoma by Stage of Tumor

STAGE	INCIDENCE	SURVIVAL RATE BEFORE 1970 (%)	SURVIVAL RATE AFTER 1970 (%)
I	23	59	100
II	13	47	78
III	9	19	43
IV	44	5	15–30
IV-S	11	70	91
Total	100	29	

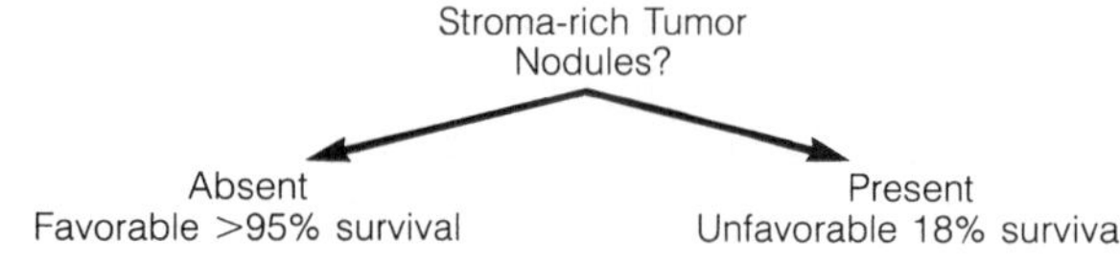

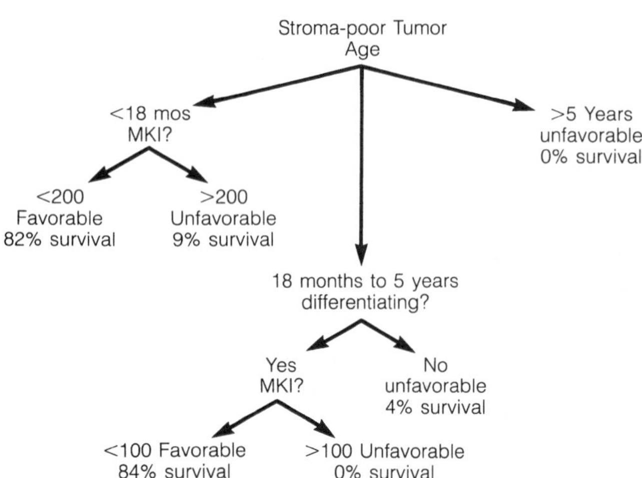

Fig. 44.1. Shimada classification of neuroblastomas.

ious pathologists. The scheme is shown in Figure 44.1. The first dividing criterion that correlates with good prognosis is the predominance of deeply eosinophilic, schwannian spindle cell stroma surrounding the neoplastic cells. The stroma-rich component of schwannian spindle cells should not be confused with neutrophil, which is acellular and contains pale-staining and finely fibrillar or granular areas in the tumor. Stroma-rich tumors usually surround isolated, well-differentiated neuroblastoma cells, or there may be clusters of neuroblastoma cells of microscopic size intermixed with the stroma. The stroma-rich tumors comprise 20% of the total cases reviewed. However, if there are one or more macroscopic nodules or discrete masses of neuroblastoma cells within the stroma-rich tumor, the prognosis is adversely affected (Fig. 44.1).

Of the stroma-poor tumors, the age of the patient is an important determinant. Three age groups are considered—younger than 18 months, 18 months to 5 years, and older than 5 years. Within these age groups, a prognostic factor is the mitotic activity of the tumor. The number of cells in mitosis can be quantitated. It is often difficult to distinguish mitotic figures from karyorrhexis; therefore, the incidence of the two are combined for the total count. This count per 5000 cells is obtained from randomly selected, high-power microscopic fields and is called the mitosis-karyorrhexis index (MKI). In the age group younger than 18 months, an MKI above or below 200 determines prognosis.

Between 18 months and 5 years of age, an MKI below 100 defines a good prognosis; an MKI above 100 is associated with a poor prognosis. In this age group, an additional variable is the degree of differentiation of the nuclei and cytoplasm of the

neuroblasts toward a ganglioneuroma pattern. The tumor is considered to be differentiating when at least 5% of the cells have an enlarged vesicular nucleus and an eosinophilic cytoplasm with a distinct cell border and cell processes. If there is no differentiation of cells occurring, the prognosis is poor. In those stroma-poor tumors showing differentiation, an MKI below 100 defines a good prognosis, whereas an MKI above 100 has a poor prognosis. It should be noted that all stroma-poor specimens from children older than 5 years are associated with a poor prognosis regardless of the MKI or degree of differentiation of the tumor cells.

Shimada et al.'s classification was developed from patients who had not been treated at the time of biopsy or excision and included all stages of disease. Subsequently, Chatten et al. reviewed pathology specimens obtained from patients with CCG stage III and stage IV disease (41). All stage III tumors were reviewed before treatment, whereas many of the stage IV tumor tissues were obtained at various times in the course of chemotherapy or radiation treatment. This study correlated well with Shimada et al.'s original results. In the stage IV patients, the analysis of tumor tissue was just as predictive when the tissue was from the primary site or from a metastatic lesion, and it was predictive for tumor tissues obtained after various forms of treatment. In Chatten et al.'s review, calcification within a tumor was also identified as a favorable histologic finding. The survival was more than 2.75 times greater in patients who had tumors with calcification. Overall, the survival rate for patients with favorable histology was 90%; unfavorable histology dropped the survival rate to 23%.

Chromosome Analysis

Tissue culture of neuroblastoma allows characterization of the chromosome composition and gene abnormalities. In neuroblastoma, variable lengths of deletion in the short arm of chromosome 1 (lp-) have been found beyond band 32 (42). It is speculated that the loss of DNA in this location represents a loss of suppressor or regulator genes that allows the development of neuroblastoma. The lp- is rarely noted in stage I, II, or IV-S tumors, but it is found in most of the stage III and stage IV tumors (42). Poor prognosis is also related to the presence of diploid or hypotetraploid tumor cells, and lp- is found in all of the tumors with these chromosomal anomalies (41). There does not seem to be a relationship between N-myc amplification and lp-, although N-myc is considered to be one of the best identifiers of poor prognosis (see below). The presence of lp- abnormalities may be a more important predictor of prognosis than other abnormal DNA/RNA variables, such as N-myc, described so far (42).

Other abnormalities noted in 20% of cases include additional chromosomal material in the long arm of chromosomes 1 and 17 (43). Loss of a sex chromosome is present in 30% of cases (43). In addition, many neuroblastomas show varying lengths of homogeneously staining regions (HSR) within the short or long arms of various chromosomes (44). DNA is also

Table 44.6. The Relationship of Stage, Frequency of N-myc Amplification, and Survival

STAGE	AMPLIFIED (%)	SURVIVAL (%)
I	0–4	100
II	10–17	85
III	10–40	50
IV	40	10
IV-S	6	95
Ganglioneuromas	0	100

present in the cytoplasm of some neuroblast cells, which are extrachromosomal paired chromatin bodies without centromeres, called double minutes (DM) (44). The finding of DM and HSR has the same connotation as amplified N-myc, predicting a poor prognosis (see below).

The N-myc Oncogene

One of the most important predictors of prognosis is analysis of the N-myc oncogene composition in the DNA of neuroblastoma cells. This proto-oncogene is normally found in the short arm of chromosome 2 (2p23–24) as a single copy in all mammalian cells. Many neuroblastomas demonstrate amplification of the N-myc oncogene where multiple copies are present. Seeger et al. have been able to correlate prognosis with the number of N-myc copies in the tumor (45, 46). Those with one copy of N-myc have an overall survival rate of 65% in all stages of disease. The survival drops to 25% when three N-myc copies are present. There are essentially no survivors when more than 10 copies are found (Table 44.6) (46).

The presence or absence of N-myc amplification and the number of copies seem to be specific for each tumor. There is no evidence that a neuroblastoma can progress from a low number of copies to a many-fold increase, when there has been progression of disease (44, 47).

Amplification of N-myc occurs in 30% of untreated patients with advanced-stage neuroblastoma (44). It is predictive of progressive dissemination when the tumor was originally localized. However, another 30% of patients who have progressive tumor show no amplification of N-myc (46). It is postulated that in these cases, the development and progression of neuroblastoma are caused by overexpression of a single copy of the N-myc oncogene in the absence of amplification, or that there are other oncogenes that may be responsible for the particularly malignant course of many neuroblastomas (45). In an analysis of four CCG protocols staged by INSS, amplified N-myc was found in 4% of stage I tumors and 10 to 17% of stage II and III tumors (37).

DNA Analysis

Flow cytometry provides a method for measuring the DNA content of tumor cells. These studies can be performed on fresh tissue or by processing paraffin blocks. The tumor cells are treated with a fluorescent dye that binds to DNA, and the amount of fluorescence produced from each cell passed through a fluorescent-activated cell sorter is registered to quantitate the total DNA and the mitotic phase of each cell (47–49). Normal cells and some neuroblastoma tumor cells are characterized by the normal number of 48 diploid chromosomes. Many malignant cells are hyperdiploid, that is, replication of DNA occurs by mitosis, in the absence of cellular division, which results in more than 48 chromosomes per cell (aneuploidy). In most adult tumors, excessive DNA content has been associated with poor prognosis. However, in neuroblastoma, aneuploidy is associated with a favorable prognosis. In an analysis of 51 neuroblastomas, Hayashi et al. noted near diploid (42 to 47 chromosomes) in 11 cases, 10 of whom had stage III and IV disease (42). There were three cases with hypotetraploid (80 to 83 chromosomes) that had stage IV tumors. Hyperdiploidy (50 to 60 chromosomes) were found in four tumors, and near triploidy (60 to 77 chromosomes) were present in 33 tumors. With the exception of five stage III tumors, hyperdiploid and near triploid tumors were from stage I, II, and IV-S patients. As many as 100 chromosomes have been found in neuroblastoma cells (41, 50). Gansler et al. reported that euploid cells were present in 36% of survivors and 79% of nonsurvivors (48).

Flow cytometry is also used to detect the proportion of cells in the various phases of the cellular growth cycle; hence, the rate of mitosis (50). When there is a high proportion of cells in the DNA synthetic or S phase, G2, and mitotic M phases (related to the total in the quiescent G0 G1 phases of the cell cycle), the prognosis is poor. Survivors had a mean of 21 to 22% of cells in the S, G2 M phase, whereas 34% of the nonsurvivors had a greater number of cells in the mitotic phases (43). The proportion of cells in the S, G2 and M phase can be substituted for the MKI in the Shimada et al. classification and may be a better predictor of poor prognosis histology (48, 50).

Tumor Cell Markers for Neuroblastoma

Neuroblastoma produces at least seven different metabolic products that can be measured in the plasma or urine. These markers are useful in establishing the diagnosis. Some have prognostic significance, and some can be used to follow the response to treatment and to detect recurrence of tumor. The markers that are particularly effective are serum ferritin, serum neuron-specific enolase, plasma and urine products of catecholamine metabolism, cystathionine, gangliosides, chromogranin, and neuropeptide.

Neuroblastomas (and some hepatomas) secrete ferritins that can be measured in the serum (51). Ferritins are normally iron storage compounds found within the reticuloendothelial cells throughout the body, and normal serum levels range from 7 to 150 μg/L. Ferritins have an adverse effect on host-immune mechanisms such as blocking rosette formation by T lymphocytes with sheep cell erythrocytes, by blocking the lymphocyte response to mitogens, and by depressing some granulocyte functions (51). Elevated serum ferritin levels are found in about 35 to 65% of patients with stage III or stage IV neuroblastoma, while serum ferritin is less commonly elevated in stage I, II, and IV-S tumors. The level of serum ferritin does not seem to be related to the tumor burden. For example, the serum ferritin is elevated in stage IV patients but not in stage IV-S patients in whom the tumor cells themselves contain comparable amounts of ferritin (46). There is a correlation between the level of serum ferritin and ultimate survival in neuroblastoma. Evans et al. noted that a serum ferritin level less than 150 ng/mL was associated with an 83% survival rate, whereas a greater level resulted in only a 19% survival rate (18). Hann et al. found that the survival rate for children with stage III tumors was 76% when ferritin was normal and only 23% when ferritin was elevated (51). In stage IV disease, the survival was 27% with a low serum ferritin and only 3% when the ferritin was elevated. The serum ferritin level is an independent predictor of survival, unrelated to patient age. The level of serum ferritin might also be used as a marker to identify tumor response to treatment.

Neuron-specific enolase is secreted by some neuroblastomas and apudomas (52). The serum levels are highest and most commonly elevated with stage III and IV disease, but they are not raised in stage IV-S tumors. Serum neuron-specific enolase may be elevated when catecholamine excretion is normal. Infants younger than 1 year of age with stage IV disease, and children younger than 2 years of age with stage III tumors and elevated neuron-specific enolase levels have a poor prognosis (52). Neuron-specific enolase is not specific for neuroblastoma because it may be found in medulloblastoma, PNETs, retinoblastoma, Wilms' tumor, Ewing's sarcoma, pancreatic carcinoma, and dysgerminoma. NSE seems to be a reliable tumor marker for following the clinical course of the disease (52).

As might be expected of cells destined to become ganglia, neuroblastomas secrete neurotransmitters. In sympathetic ganglia, tyrosine is converted to dihydroxyphenylalanine (DOPA), which is then metabolized to norepinephrine and, in the adrenal medulla, to epinephrine (Fig. 44.2). There are many metabolites in the degradation of DOPA, norepinephrine, and epinephrine. It is possible to measure each of these metabolites in the plasma and urine (Table 44.7) (53–54). Approximately 10% of neuroblastomas do not excrete catechols, but some produce acetylcholine, and these tumors have a particularly malignant course (55).

Table 44.7. Variations in Levels of Vanillylmandelic Acid and Homovanillic Acid According to Age

AGE	VMA CONCENTRATION (U/mg CREATININE)	HVA CONCENTRATION (U/mg CREATININE)
0–6 mo	1.4–82.7	14.0–36.8
7–11 mo	0.1–21.6	2.0–42.0
1–2 yr	0.7–14.5	1.1–34.1
2–5 yr	1.4–12.4	3.9–33.8
5–10 yr	0.7–10.2	3.0–25.8
10–15 yr	0.8–8.5	1.8–22.2

The more malignant neuroblastomas are deficient in dopamine hydroxylase and do not produce norepinephrine. Therefore, they excrete the degradation products of dopamine, particularly HVA, and low levels of the catecholamines metabolites of norepinephrine VMA. In contrast, a more enzymatically differentiated neuroblastoma will produce norepinephrine, and this will be reflected in a significant excretion of VMA. Therefore, the prognosis can be predicted by the ratio of VMA to HMA; a ratio greater than 1 has a favorable prognosis with an 84% survival, whereas the predominance of HVA is associated with a 44% survival (56). Normal levels for VMA and HVA excretion in the urine are related to urinary creatinine, and are shown in Table 44.7.

Unlike pheochromocytoma, neuroblastoma does not have an erratic secretory rate of catecholamine by-products, and levels in 8-, 12-, or 24-hour urine specimens are adequate. The urine should also be tested for the presence of cystathionine (57). Cystathionine is an intermediate metabolite of methionine metabolism; it is normally found in the brain, with smaller amounts present in the liver, kidney, and muscle. Cystathionine is not present in the urine of healthy individuals but it has been found in children with neuroblastoma who had no VMA excretion. There is no correlation between the presence of cystathionine and the clinical course of the tumor, except that all patients in whom the tumor was completely controlled had no further excretion of cystathionine. However, some children have stopped excreting cystathionine during active tumor spread.

Ganglioside GD2 is present in small quantities on the surface of cell walls of many normal cells, such as neurons, renal glomerulus, testicular and ovarian stroma, myometrium, and lymphoid follicles of the spleen (58–61). More than 95% of neuroblastomas have high concentrations of GD2 on the cell surface, and elevated serum levels are found in 84% of patients with all stages of neuroblastoma. It can be used to follow the clinical course of the disease, as the serum levels are related to tumor burden. If the initial serum GD2 ganglioside level is less than 103 p mol/mL, there is a 70% survival, whereas a level greater than 568 p mol/mL decreases the survival to 24% (58). Monoclonal antibodies to GD2 are available and, when conjugated with radioisotopes, radionuclide scanning may be used to locate the extent of tumor and for following the course of treatment.

Chromogranin A is a protein stored in the same intracellular vesicles as catecholamines and it is released by exocytosis. Plasma chromogranin A is elevated in more than 90% of patients in all stages of neuroblastoma (62). Plasma levels of less than 190 ng/mL are associated with a 2-year survival of 70%, whereas a plasma level greater than 190 ng/mL drops the survival to 30% (62).

Neuropeptide Y is elevated in the plasma of most children with neuroblastoma (63). It can be used to follow the course of treatment. In one study, the nine children who had the plasma neuropeptide Y levels return to normal during treatment survived; three who had levels that did not normalize died (63).

Lactic dehydrogenase (LDH) and plasma carcinoembryonic antigen (CEA) may be elevated in most children with neuro-

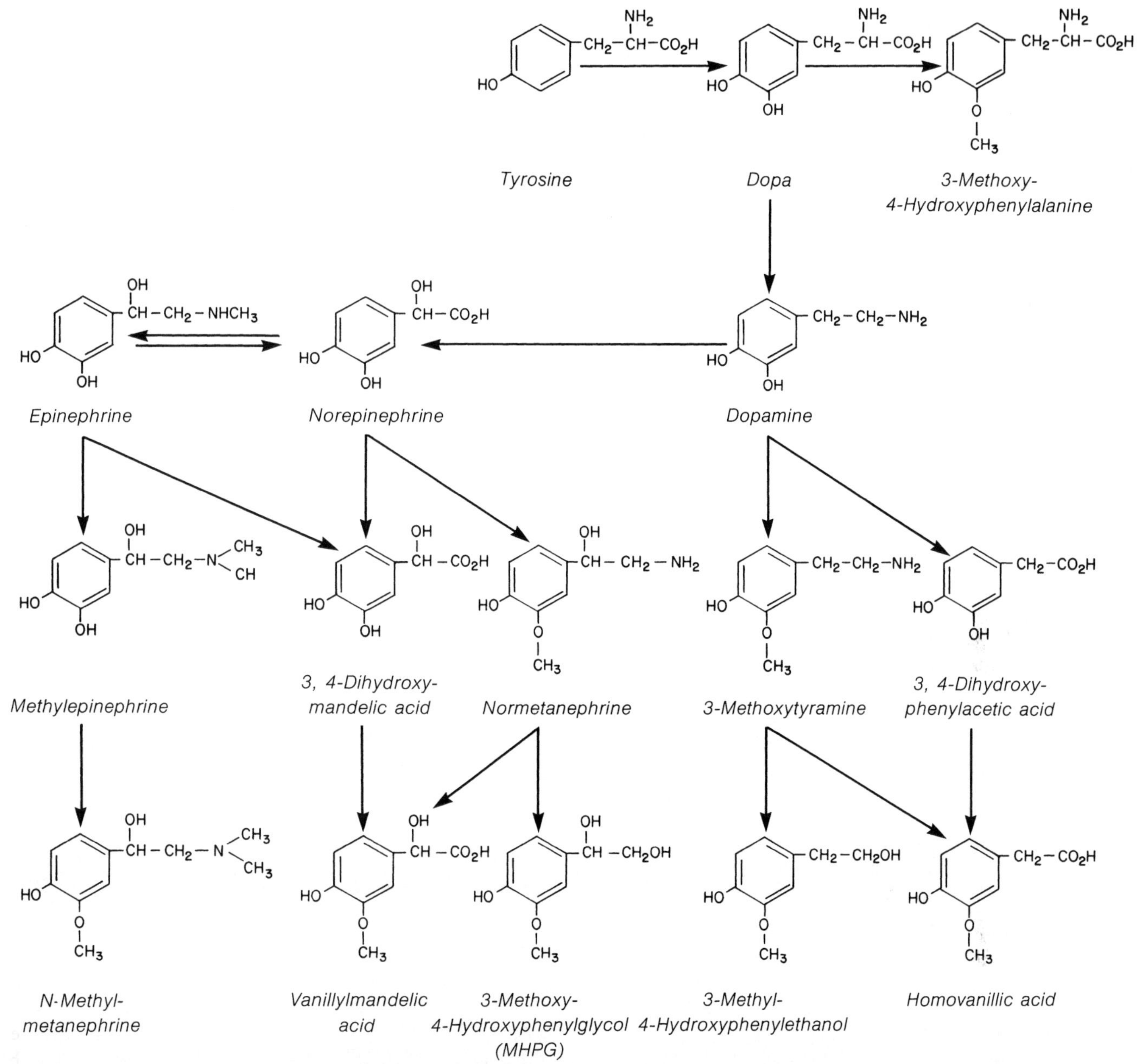

Fig. 44.2. Pathways for metabolism of dopamine, norepinephrine, and epinephrine. Children with neuroblastoma who excrete more homovanillic acid (HVA) than vanillylmandelic acid (VMA) have poorer prognoses. Presumably, this is because biologically primitive (hence more malignant) tumors lack dopamine-B-hydroxylase to convert dopamine to norepinephrine.

blastoma (64, 65). LDH and CEA are elevated in many kinds of tumors (lung, breast, colon, and liver), and serial plasma determinations might be helpful in following the course of disease. A serum LDH level greater than 1500 IU/L is associated with aggressive neuroblastoma (64).

DIAGNOSIS

Symptoms and Physical Findings

In more than half the children with neuroblastoma, the initial manifestation of tumor is the presence of a mass (34, 66). The mass may be asymptomatic, but it is often associated with symptoms secondary to compression of surrounding structures, particularly the lungs, whether from a mediastinal or an intra-abdominal primary site. The mass is usually firm, irregular, and bosselated. Any grossly irregular mass extending across the midline of the abdomen is likely to be a neuroblastoma.

Frequently, the child will have recently had a normal physical examination, only to have the abrupt appearance of the mass. The tumor is often tender, and this seems to be associated with hemorrhage into the mass, which may account for the recent enlargement. High thoracic lesions may encroach on the airway. Tumors arising from the stellate ganglion will produce Horner's syndrome, and if the tumor arises in utero, it will be associated with a lack of pigmentation of the ipsilateral iris (heterochromia) (67). Some masses extend into the intervertebral foramen, producing cord compression manifested by bladder and bowel atony, pain in the lower extremities, or anesthesia and paralysis (68). Tumors arising in the pelvis may obstruct the bladder and rectum. These tumors can extend through the sciatic notch to become evident as masses in the buttocks. Edema and cyanosis of the lower extremities may occur from venous and lymphatic compression.

In approximately one third of patients, the initial presenting symptoms result from metastases rather than from the primary tumor (34, 66). This usually occurs in older children in whom the nonspecific symptoms of listlessness, anorexia, weight loss, fever, vague aches and joint pains, a limp, or an unwillingness to move about develop. The symptoms may be confused with rheumatic fever. The base of the skull is a frequent site for metastases, producing proptosis of one or both eyes, with periorbital ecchymoses. Lymph node metastases are frequent, particularly in the cervical and supraclavicular nodes. Obvious irregularities of the skull or metaphyses of the long bones are caused by osteolytic metastases.

In infants, subcutaneous metastases will have a bluish discoloration, prompting the term "blueberry muffin baby" (69, 70). Spontaneous blanching of the skin overlying the tumor nodules has been described, presumably because of local vasoconstriction from norepinephrine produced and secreted by the tumors (71).

Hypertension occurs in 10 to 50% of children in various reported series (34, 66). Increased catecholamine excretion by these tumors may also produce flushing and sweating. The blood pressure elevation is usually not hemodynamically significant, although there are instances in which hypertensive cardiomyopathy, similar to that occurring in patients with pheochromocytoma, requires the use of preoperative beta-adrenergic blockers to prevent perioperative hemodynamic complications. In these instances, the prognosis for cure of the tumor is excellent. Hypertension is often not caused by catecholamines but by compression of one or both kidneys or their blood supply.

Associated Syndromes

APUD and VIP-Producing Tumors

In addition to producing products of norepinephrine metabolism, some neuroblastomas manufacture polypeptides similar to other amine precursor uptake decarboxylase (APUD) tumors. APUD cells are derived from the neural crest, giving rise to the enterochromaffin cells of the gastrointestinal tract and tracheobronchial tree (72). Neoplasms originating from APUD cells include carcinoid tumors, ACTH-producing bronchogenic carcinoma, islet cell tumors of the pancreas (insulinoma, glucagonoma, gastrinoma, and somatostatinoma), medullary carcinoma of the thyroid (which produces calcitonin), and others.

In common with some APUD tumors, neuroblastoma can secrete vasoactive intestinal peptide (VIP) (73). A syndrome of watery diarrhea, abdominal distention, hypokalemia, and acidosis has been reported in children with ganglioneuroma or ganglioneuroblastoma arising in the neck, mediastinum, and abdomen (74). Approximately 7% of children with neuroblastoma will have persistent watery diarrhea. This syndrome is associated with high levels of VIP in the plasma and tumor. Unlike the more common VIP-producing tumors of pancreatic or bronchial origin, increased catecholamine excretion was found in all VIP-producing ganglioneuroblastomas. VIP is a vasodilator, which may counteract some of the vasopressor effects of catecholamines. However, profound postoperative hypotension can occur after removal of the tumor, presumably because VIP has a longer hemodynamic effect than the catecholamines. Therefore, beta-adrenergic blockage with phenoxybenzamine and inhibition of the synthesis of tyrosine-containing octapeptides with metyrosine have been advocated to avoid postoperative hypovolemia and vasodilator shock (74).

Myoclonus–Opsoclonus Syndrome

Another syndrome occurring in approximately 2% of cases of neuroblastoma is the combination of myoclonus and opsoclonus (75–77). These children have involuntary, uncoordinated, irregular, flickering muscular movements involving the limbs, trunk, head, and eyes that mimic cerebellar ataxia and nystagmus. The neurologic abnormality may resolve before treatment, but it usually persists for many months after resection of the tumor. More than one half of children with myoclonus and opsoclonus will develop mental retardation. The neurologic abnormality is usually the first manifestation, preceding the discovery of the tumor by several weeks to more than 1 year. The neuroblastoma may be difficult to find when the cerebellar dysfunction is recognized. The tumor was located in the mediastinum in 53% of reported cases; cervical, retroperitoneal, and pelvic primary tumor have also been reported. Seventy-one percent were favorable stage I, II, and IV-S cases, with a survival rate of close to 100% (76). However, even patients with stage III and IV disease had a 71% survival rate (76). The better prognosis in children with the myoclonus–opsoclonus syndrome is not related to a predominance in the favorable age group, because only 7% were younger than 2 years old.

The cause for the neurologic disability is unknown, but three mechanisms have been proposed.

1. Neurotropic virus infecting neural crest cells and cerebellum, producing tumor transformation and encephalopathy.
2. Neuroblastoma releasing a neurotoxin.
3. Antibody formation to neuroblastoma antigen producing cross reactions with cerebellar cells.

The last theory is popular. The better prognosis in these patients, even with advanced stage disease, is thought to be related to antibody control of the tumor. No cerebellar lesions have been proven at autopsy, and the immune mechanism has not been established.

Other Associated Diseases

Neuroblastoma has been associated with the clinical picture of myasthenia gravis and Cushing's syndrome, which responded promptly after excision of the tumor (78, 79). Ganglioneuroma and neuroblastoma have also been described in patients with neurofibromatosis (80). The development of malignant pheochromocytoma and subsequent renal cell carcinoma has been reported following treatment of neuroblastoma (81). The familial occurrence of neuroblastoma has also been described (82).

Imaging Studies

The diagnostic evaluation requires clarification of the position of the primary tumor in relation to the surrounding normal structures and an indication of the presence of any metastases. Neuroblastoma metastasizes to local and distal lymph nodes, metaphyses of long bones, basal and parietal areas of the skull, and, in infants, the liver. Pulmonary metastases are rare. Radiologic studies include chest radiograph; intravenous pyelogram; CT or MRI scans of the chest, abdomen, and pelvis; and a skeletal survey (Fig. 44.3). CT and MRI scans of the thoracic, abdominal, and pelvic masses provide clear definition of the tumor. More than 70% of neuroblastomas contain calcifications that can be readily detected on CT scans, thereby providing a further indication of the type of tumor. The disadvantage of the CT scan is the requirement of oral and intravenous contrast and the radiation exposure. CT images are usually in an axial plane only. CT scanners have been improved by abbreviating the time for imaging, using the helical (spiral) CT that also allows three-dimensional reconstruction of the tumor and adjacent structures (83). The distinct advantage of the CT scan is to demonstrate calcification within a tumor.

MRI has become a valuable method for outlining tumors with respect to surrounding normal structures that can be readily accomplished in the coronal, sagittal, and axial planes (84–86). The technique is especially effective in identifying infiltration of tumor within the spinal canal. The disadvantage of the MRI technique is the need for heavy sedation or general anesthesia and the difficulty monitoring completely immobilized small children during the study.

An abdominal or neck mass can also be delineated by sonograms. The sonogram may be the preferred initial study because it is noninvasive and eliminates radiation exposure. It can usually determine the relationship of the mass to surrounding structures and determine whether the mass is cystic or solid.

Isotope scans of the soft tissues and bones using radionuclides such as technetium, gallium, or metaiodobenzylguanidine (MIBG) are essential for determining the extent of tumor (Fig. 44.4). For visualization of the primary tumor and metastases, the gallium (^{67}Ga) scan has been advocated as a prognostic indicator (87). Most neuroblastomas do not take up gallium, but those that do seem to have a poor outcome.

MIBG is a guanethidine derivative resembling norepinephrine that can be labeled with iodine isotopes 123 or 131 (88). For imaging purposes, the 123 isotope is preferred because it emits gamma ray and has a short half-life, which reduces radiation ex-

posure, offers better imaging, and offers the ability to use larger doses (89). When given intravenously, it is bound to norepinephrine binding sites and then stored in neurosecretory granules of the adrenal medulla, pheochromocytoma, and other neural crest tumors. However, uptake in the salivary glands, heart, and liver and excretion in the bladder and colon may obscure tumors (90). MIBG scan is the preferred scanning technique because it identifies metastatic neuroblastoma in soft tissue sites of spread and in bone; it has a greater sensitivity and specificity than other scanning materials. However, it is slightly less sensitive than bone marrow aspiration and biopsy for detecting bone marrow metastases. MIBG will localize in neuroblastoma that does not produce catecholamines, whereas approximately 15% of neuroblastomas do not take up MIBG (91).

Hematologic Studies

The blood count may show anemia either from bleeding into the tumor or from bone marrow replacement by metastases. "Cogwheel" erythrocytes have been described in patients with neuroblastoma (77). All patients with neuroblastoma should have a bone marrow aspiration and biopsy performed to help in identifying any metastatic spread.

Additional blood tests should include platelet count, prothrombin time, and partial thromboplastin time (92). If a coagulation defect is detected, a deficit in specific clotting factors may have to be studied. Neuroblastomas are frequently highly vascular, and hemorrhage into the tumors can deplete coagulation factors. In addition, disseminated intravascular coagulopathy may occur. Blood samples for fibrinogen and fibrin-split products should be determined if coagulopathy seems to be present.

To summarize, the diagnostic evaluation of children with neuroblastoma should include the following.

1. Blood count, platelet count, prothrombin time, and partial thromboplastin time.
2. Serum BUN, creatinine, albumin, SGOT, LDH, alkaline phosphatase, neuron-specific enolase, ferritin, and ganglioside. GD2, plasma chromagranin A.
3. Urine routine analysis, spot or 8-hour collection for VMA, HVA, dopamine measured with total creatinine excretion, and cystathionine.
4. Bone marrow aspiration and biopsy from each iliac crest.
5. Bone scan—MIBG.
6. Skeletal survey.
7. MRI or CT scan or ultrasound of the primary tumor.
8. MRI scan or CT myelogram for paraspinous tumors with possible intraspinous extension.

Bone Marrow Examination

Usually the posterior iliac crest marrow is aspirated and tumor cells will be seen in approximately 30–50% of patients. If bilateral aspirates are performed, there is an increased detection of tumor cells. Bone marrow trephine biopsy increases the yield of finding tumor cells by more than 20% beyond aspiration alone (93).

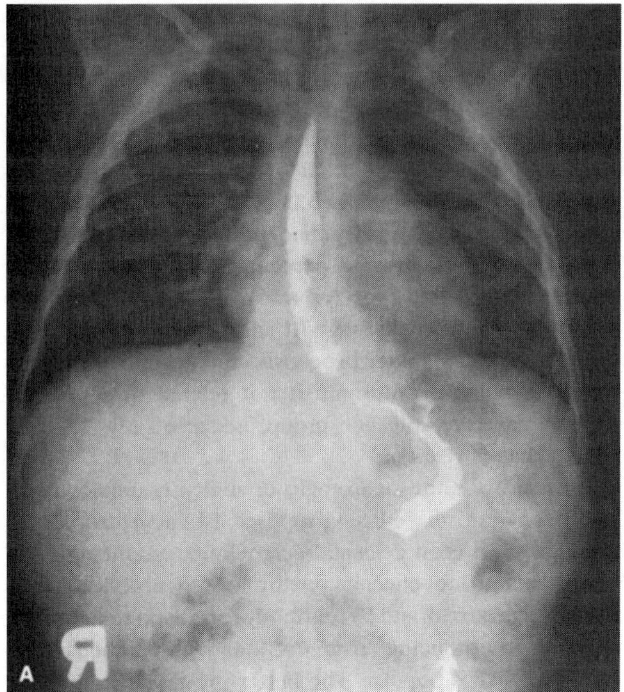
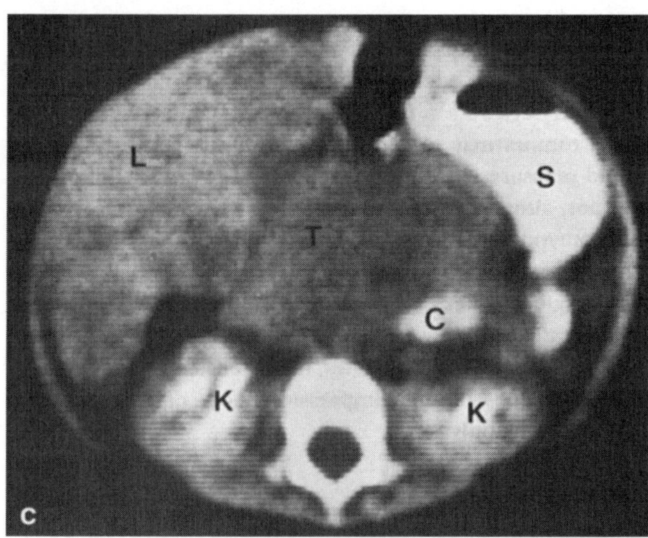
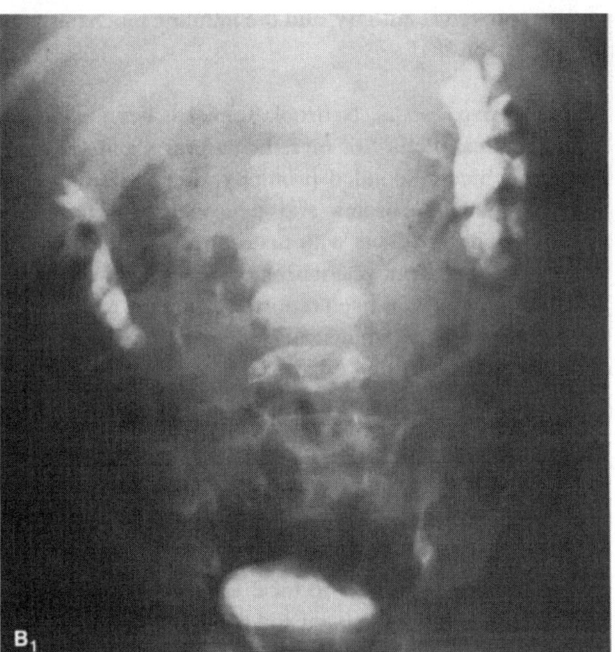
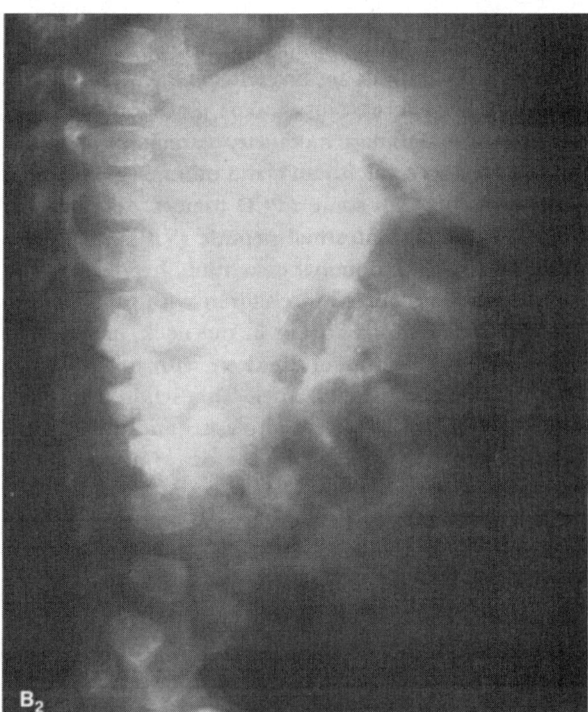

Fig. 44.3.   Radiologic studies showing the appearance of neuroblastoma. **A**, Esophagram shows displacement of esophagus by an adrenal neuroblastoma extending into the posterior mediastinum through the aortic hiatus. **B**, Anterior-posterior (1) and lateral abdominal (2) radiographs of an intravenous pyelogram showing both kidneys displaced laterally by a large neuroblastoma arising from the celiac and superior mesenteric autonomic nerve plexuses. **C**, Computerized axial tomogram at the level of the second lumbar vertebra showing large celiac neuroblastoma (T) containing calcification **(C).** The tumor is anterior to both kidneys (K) containing contrast medium. The liver (L) is visualized, and the stomach (S) and small bowel are outlined by ingested contrast medium.

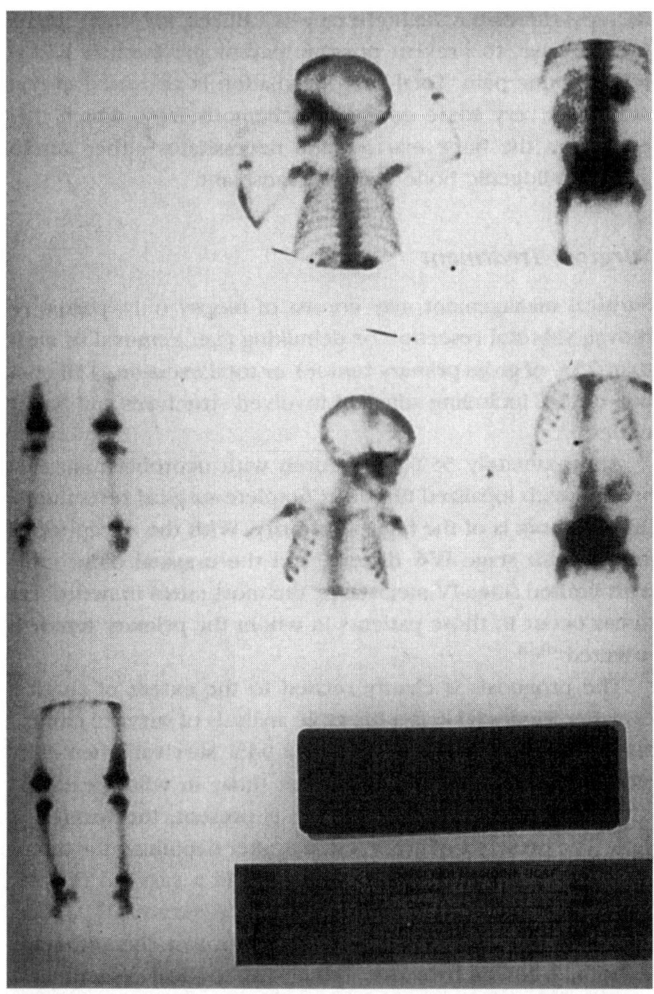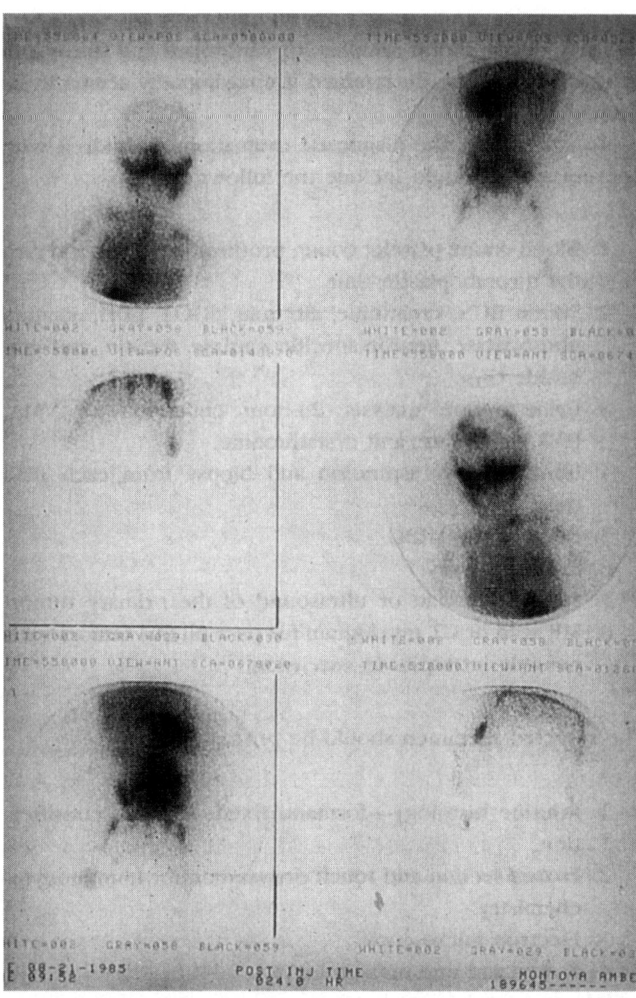

Fig. 44.4. *Left,* Technetium bone scan with uptake into tumor involving the calvarium, base of skull, left mandible, head of the scapulae and humerus bilaterally, the right ulna, thoraco-lumbar spine, retroperitoneal tumor on the left, both proximal femurs, right mid- and distal femurs, and both proximal and distal femurs. Note the concentrated technetium appearing in the right kidney and in the full bladder, which could obscure other tumor masses. *Right,* 131 I MIBG scan showing background uptake in the salivary glands, heart, and liver. There is uptake in the metastases of the calvarium and base of the skull, left clavicle and thoraco-lumbar spine, pelvis, and head of the femurs. A large, left retroperitoneal tumor is also seen. Excretion into a distended bladder obscures the lower lumbosacral spine and pelvis.

The resected specimen should be processed for the following.

1. Routine histology—formalin fixed; Shimada classification.
2. Frozen section and touch preparation for immunocytochemistry.
3. Electron microscopy.
4. N-myc and immunocytology.
   a. Several tumor pieces 0.3 × 1.0 × 1.0 cm should be immersed in isopentane and immediately placed in dry ice and stored at below −20°C for N-myc and immunohistology analysis. This specimen should contain areas of the tumor most likely to be viable and frozen immediately after removal.
   b. The bone marrow aspirate can be processed by differential sedimentation to concentrate any neuroblastoma cells present. By incubating the marrow cells with a panel of monoclonal antibodies for neuroblastoma, one tumor cell in 10^5 normal marrow cells can be identified (94).

TREATMENT

Four modalities of treatment are used to attempt cure of neuroblastoma—surgical resection, chemotherapy, radiation therapy (including radioiodinated MIBG), and intensive chemotherapy with or without total body irradiation, requiring bone marrow transplantation. The initial treatment of neuroblastoma depends on the stage of the tumor and the effect the tumor is having on adjacent structures. Stage I and stage II neuroblastomas are treated primarily, and possibly exclusively, by surgical resection. Stage IV tumors and most stage III neuroblastomas are managed by chemotherapy initially, followed by surgical excision of remaining bulk disease and continued aggressive chemotherapy thereafter. Radiation therapy is used for unresectable bulk disease, or to prevent possible pathologic fracture, and to relieve bone pain. Marrow ablative chemotherapy with or without total body irradiation is also used to kill residual neuroblastoma, but also eradicates the bone marrow and necessitates either autologous or allogeneic bone marrow transplantation.

Surgical Treatment

Surgical management may consist of biopsy only, partial removal, subtotal resection or debulking (i.e., removal of more than 75% of gross primary tumor), or total excision of all obvious tumor, including adjacent involved structures and lymph nodes.

Approximately 55% of children with neuroblastoma first present with localized tumors. Complete surgical resection of these tumors is of the highest priority. With the exception of infants with stage IV-S disease, most cures in neuroblastomas occur in those patients in whom the primary tumor is resected (10, 19, 37, 38).

The prognosis is clearly related to the extent of surgical excision. Figure 44.5 is a life table analysis of survival and extent of surgical excision showing a 94% survival rate when complete excision is accomplished (18). These are stage I tumors. For those in whom excision with microscopic residual disease (stage II) is present, the survival is 81%. The presence of gross residual (INSS stage II or III disease) after debulking the tumor (grade II or III residual disease) results in a survival rate of 79%, whereas those with biopsy only have a 55% survival rate (18, 37). A poor-risk patient should have a course of chemotherapy, followed by a later attempt at surgical resection. The survival rate for patients with stage III tumors who eventually had complete tumor excision was 70%, whereas for those without excision it was 45% (18, 37).

Anesthesia and Intubation

General anesthesia and an endotracheal tube are mandatory in every case in which a neuroblastoma is to be resected. A large-bore cannula should be placed into the superior vena cava or right atrium. This is readily accomplished following general anesthesia with a percutaneous needle puncture of the deep jugular or subclavian vein. Another peripheral extremity vein should be cannulated to provide an additional route for the administration of medication, fluids, or blood. The central venous cannula can be connected to a transducer to monitor the pressure. Central venous pressures above 10 cm of water suggest vascular volume overload or myocardial failure. However, a normal central venous pressure may be recorded in the presence of severe hypovolemia because venous constriction occurs to preserve venous return to the heart. Most anesthetic agents, administered in concentrations that provide muscular relaxation, depress vasomotor tone and myocardial contractility. Therefore, the plane of anesthesia may have to be maintained at a light level, with muscle relaxants used to facilitate surgical exposure. This technique will mask the magnitude of hypovolemia. Thus, the absolute level of central venous pressure must be correlated with the adequacy of perfusion, manifested by the rate of skin capillary refill following compression, by the briskness of bleeding from a fresh wound, and by the volume of urine output. Radial or pedal artery cannulation should be established for sampling of arterial blood for blood gas and pH measurements. The presence of metabolic acidosis indicates inadequate tissue perfusion, most likely because of hypovolemia. It is helpful to place a Foley catheter in the bladder to measure the rate of urine formation. A urine flow of between 1 and 2 mL/kg/hr is desirable.

Control of Blood Loss and Fluid Replacement

Some large neuroblastomas are vascular and friable, and attempted removal produces extensive blood loss. If immediate surgical resection is indicated, rather than radiation and chemotherapy followed by a second-look procedure, the technique of deliberate hemodilution, hypothermia, and hypotension should be considered (95). In this technique, the patient's blood is withdrawn into a citrate-phosphate-dextrose anticoagulant container and replaced with a volume of Ringer's lactate solution and/or hetastarch three times the volume of blood removed. Blood is withdrawn until the hematocrit value is between 15 and 20%. Because this technique greatly diminishes the oxygen-carrying capacity of the blood, it is necessary to reduce the metabolic rate of the tissues. Although anesthesia accomplishes this to some extent, deliberate induction of hypothermia to a core temperature of 32° C reduces the metabolic rate to 50% of normal.

The status of arterial and central venous blood pH, PCO_2, and PO_2 must be monitored closely. Tissue perfusion is maintained by compensatory increased heart rate and cardiac output, lower blood viscosity, and lowered peripheral vascular resistance. Inadequate tissue perfusion is detected by the appearance of metabolic acidosis and requires more fluid volume. The mean blood pressure is lowered to 40 mm Hg by increasing the depth of anesthesia. The operative procedure can thus be accomplished with greatly reduced bleeding. The blood loss is re-

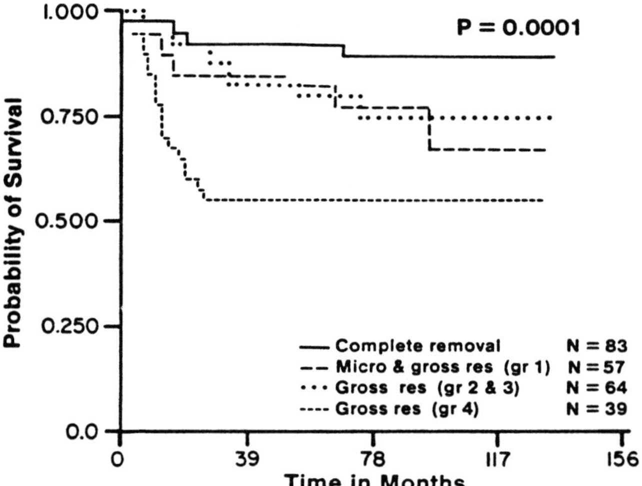

Fig. 44.5. Life-table analysis of survival correlated with the extent of removal of local and regional neuroblastoma (18).

placed with equal or greater volumes of Ringer's lactate solution or hetastarch. Blood is not infused unless the mixed venous oxygen saturation falls below 50% or metabolic acidosis persists despite volume replacement, or the hematocrit falls below 15%.

On completion of the operation, the blood that was withdrawn is warmed and replaced. To avoid the subsequent hypervolemia and cardiac failure, diuresis is induced by giving furosemide (Lasix) at 1 mg/kg intravenously. The patient is rewarmed by the heating mattress, the warmth of the operating room, heated nebulization of anesthetic gases, and irrigation of the abdomen or chest with Ringer's lactate warmed to 38° C. When the core temperature rises to 34 to 36° C, the child may be awakened. However, endotracheal ventilatory support is maintained for approximately 4 hours, until two thirds of the infused Ringer's/hetastarch has been voided and the child has demonstrated adequate spontaneous ventilation. This technique of deliberate hemodilution, hypotension, and hypothermia allows for easier surgical removal of vascular tumors, but it also requires a team of anesthesiologists and surgeons to monitor metabolic responses intensively intraoperatively and during postoperative care.

During the course of the operative procedure, significant third-space fluid losses occur from the wound and serosal surfaces. The composition of this fluid is essentially that of plasma, except for a much lower protein content. This fluid is not only sequestered at the operative site, but capillary integrity seems to be impaired throughout the body for approximately 48 hours postoperatively. Therefore, the fluid replacement should be with Ringer's lactate or acetate solution. Dextrose (5% solution) added to the Ringer's solution is preferred, but because hyperglycemia and osmotic diuresis from glycosuria may occur with large-volume infusions, the urine and blood sugar content should be monitored. Hyperglycemia can be managed by Ringer's solution without dextrose. A large operative dissection may warrant a rate of volume infusion between 8 and 15 mL/kg/hr during the procedure.

When hemodilution and hypothermia are not used, the volume of blood loss must be measured closely. Dry sponges may be used so they can be weighed to identify the volume of blood loss, although this technique tends to underestimate the actual blood loss because of evaporation. The canister used to collect blood suctioned from the wound should be calibrated to measure the volume and should be close to the patient to minimize dead space in the tubing. If the patient was not initially anemic, transfusion is not necessary until blood loss exceeds 10% of blood volume. Blood volume can be calculated as 80 mL/kg of body weight. A difficult surgical resection can result in losses equivalent to 2 or 3 times the patient's blood volume. Because transfused blood is usually refrigerated, it should be rewarmed before administration by being passed through coils of tubing placed in a water bath maintained at a temperature of at least 37° C.

Control of Temperature

When the hemodilution-hypothermia technique is not being used, normal body temperature should be preserved during the operation; this requires measurement of the core temperature with an esophageal or rectal thermometer probe. Although the metabolic rate is depressed with hypothermia under general anesthesia, on termination of the procedure, shivering occurs, accompanied by a significant catecholamine excretion that results in an abrupt increase in the metabolic rate. Under these circumstances, the depressed, hypothermic child may be incapable of adapting to this metabolic demand, and cardiovascular and respiratory failure may occur. The child should be placed on a water mattress where the circulating fluid can be either cooled or warmed to help regulate the desired core temperature. The operating room temperature is initially maintained at approximately 30° C until the sterile preparation and draping are completed. The use of adherent plastic drapes is valuable to minimize heat loss. One of the most effective methods for preventing hypothermia is to use a heated humidifier to convey the anesthetic gases in the tubing connected to the endotracheal tube. This avoids large evaporative heat losses from the lung. If normal body temperature is maintained, postoperative care will be much less intense and there will be little risk of cardiac arrhythmia, respiratory depression, and metabolic acidosis.

Surgical Approach

The approach used in the operative procedure itself will depend on the extent to which the tumor has involved surrounding structures. Neuroblastoma does not arise within an organ that provides a clear demarcation from adjacent normal structures. Each site of origin—in the neck, mediastinum, abdomen, and pelvis—provides unique problems for the surgeon.

Neck Tumors

In the neck, complete surgical resection is feasible for a well-circumscribed tumor of one of the cervical ganglia. However, these tumors commonly extend into the thoracic inlet and involve major vessels and nerves, such as the phrenic, vagus, and recurrent laryngeal nerves and the brachial plexus. A combined neck-and-chest incision may be required. Despite extensive exposure, microscopic residual tumor frequently remains in the vicinity of the major neurovascular structures. The potential for neurologic complications is significant, resulting in such abnormalities as Horner's syndrome, vocal cord or diaphragmatic paralysis, muscle weakness, and focal numbness of the arms and hands.

Mediastinal Tumors

In the mediastinum, complete surgical resection is probably more common than in any other site of origin. The tumor is usually densely adherent to the vertebral body and ribs, with a varying extension along the intervertebral foramen. Excision of these tumors frequently includes the affected intercostal nerves and a portion of the intercostal muscle. Block excision of the ribs or adjacent vertebral body is not indicated because a plane of resection can be accomplished subperiosteally. Rib resections may produce debilitating scoliosis in later years. Frequently, the tumor extends beyond the margin of transection in the intervertebral foramen. An MR scan or a CT myelogram may be indicated to assess the extent of infraspinous involvement.

Retroperitoneal Tumors

Intraabdominal neuroblastoma presents one of the greatest surgical challenges. A well-circumscribed, readily resectable primary tumor may be present in those children in whom the mass is discovered as a result of other symptoms, such as the myoclonus–opsoclonus syndrome. However, children who present with an abdominal mass as the dominant symptom usually have retroperitoneal tumors that are large and difficult to resect. Three types of retroperitoneal masses may be encountered—adrenal, celiac, and nonceliac extraadrenal primary tumors.

Adrenal and Extraadrenal Tumors

Adrenal and extraadrenal tumors may be well circumscribed or may intimately involve the adjacent kidney, aorta, or vena cava and may extend through the crura of the diaphragm into the chest. Upper abdominal tumors should be approached through an incision that can be lengthened into the chest to gain access to a mediastinal extension of tumor. Despite the bulk of growth, most adrenal and extraadrenal neuroblastomas can be resected of all gross tumor. The excision may require removal of the adrenal gland and adjacent kidney. Tumors arising from the lower lumbar area usually have a well-developed plane along the adventitia of the aorta and vena cava.

Celiac Tumors

Neuroblastomas arising from the area of the celiac and superior mesenteric autonomic nerve plexuses are the most difficult to manage. These masses extend across the midline to encircle the aorta and vena cava and the renal, superior mesenteric, and celiac vessels. Commonly, they spread into the hilus of the liver and invade the pancreas and the bowel mesentery. It is easy to underestimate the normal size of the major vessels coursing through these tumors; the vessels may be accidentally ligated, producing infarction of the bowel, liver, or kidneys.

Careful judgement is necessary before undertaking an aggressive resection. Although a kidney may be removed to allow complete excision of tumor, major vessels supplying the bowel, opposite kidney, liver, and spinal cord must not be compromised. If complete resection is not possible, the decision for biopsy or a debulking procedure must be made. Theoretically, removal of as much neoplasm as possible decreases the tumor burden for radiation and chemotherapy and enhances the ability of the patient's immune system to eradicate residual disease effectively. It is often better to remove sufficient tumor for

histology, tumor markers and chromosome analysis and rely on subsequent chemoradiation therapy to reduce the tumor. Second- and third-look operative resection can be effective.

Unlike with many other tumors, wide en bloc resection may not be possible with neuroblastoma, but dissection into the mass does not produce widespread dissemination of tumor with inevitable local recurrence. However, some neuroblastomas are extremely vascular; a fragmented excision and a morsellating or scooping out of the tumor can produce extensive blood loss. If resection seems to be hazardous during this initial exploration, a generous biopsy specimen should be obtained and the procedure should be terminated. The patient would then undergo intensive chemotherapy so that a reexploration in 4 to 5 months might result in a better operative resection.

Pelvic Tumors

Pelvic neuroblastoma tends to be circumscribed and is resectable by way of a lower transabdominal approach. It is often difficult to recognize whether the poor functioning of the bladder is caused by obstruction and compression or if the nervi erigentes are involved with tumor. In males, the presence or absence of sleep erections of the penis may help determine the integrity of the sacral autonomic nerve control. In either instance, a deep-lying tumor that has invaded the pelvic walls, or has extended to the level of the levator musculature, might preferably be treated initially by chemotherapy and possibly irradiation to diminish the size of the tumor. A second-look procedure could result in a smaller risk of autonomic nerve injury. The prognosis for pelvic primary tumors is excellent, and it is important to preserve autonomic nerve function.

Stage IV-S Disease

Resection of the primary tumor in infants with stage IV-S disease has been advocated to accelerate involution of multiple metastases. There is no evidence that this approach is effective because spontaneous regression occurs almost uniformly. However, after apparent complete regression of all gross disease, CT scans should be obtained to detect residual primary tumor. If a tumor mass persists, resection may be justified because some of these tumors later recur and metastasize, with a fatal outcome. Because spontaneous regression and disappearance of all metastatic tumor seem to develop in infants with stage IV-S disease, there is question as to whether radiation and chemotherapy are justified in their management. The only mortality occurring in stage IV-S tumors is because of the massive involvement of the liver producing mechanical encroachment on the lungs, intraabdominal vessels, and kidneys. Almost invariably, this is seen in infants within the first 6 weeks of life, when explosive growth of tumor within the liver develops. Those infants younger than 6 weeks of age who have liver involvement without skin metastases have only a 32% survival, but if there are associated skin metastases, 88% survive. Life-threatening liver enlargement was noted in 75% of the 34 cases analyzed by Suarez et al (96). Cyclophosphamide and vincristine have not been uniformly effective. Therefore, radiation therapy and newer agents such as cisplatin (CDDP), etoposide (VP-16) and teniposide (VM26) might be considered. In desperation, a tense abdominal wall, with a greatly increased intraabdominal pressure, has been treated by making a large abdominal wall hernia. The hernia can then be repaired after the huge liver has regressed in size.

Intraspinous Extension of Neuroblastoma

Intraspinous extension of a cervical, thoracic, abdominal, or pelvic primary tumor usually produces a neurologic deficit. Flaccid paralysis, paresis, sensory deficits, and impaired bladder and anal sphincter function may develop. An MRI scan is the preferred imaging technique to outline the intraspinal and extraspinal extent of the tumor. Resolution of any neurologic deficit takes precedence over attempted control of the extraspinal tumor component. A laminectomy has been indicated in the past for emergency decompression when recent deterioration of nerve function developed. The combination of a laminectomy and postoperative radiation therapy has resulted in severe kyphoscoliosis, often requiring orthopedic correction. The tumor often extends three or more vertebral levels cephalad and caudad to the extension through the intervertebral foramen, and laminectomy at these multiple levels is extremely deforming. Furthermore, return of neurologic function occurs only in 40 to 65% of reported cases with laminectomy. More recently, chemotherapy has become the primary mode of treatment (97). In addition, stress doses of adrenal corticoids are indicated to reduce local edema of the cord adjacent to the tumor. There seems to be prompt response to the tumor with a much greater incidence of return of good neurologic function. Long-term survival and complete control of these tumors are excellent. The amount of persistent neurologic deficit varies, depending on the severity of the original spinal cord compression.

Bad Prognosis—Stage II, III, and IV Disease

Patients who present with obvious, extensive metastatic disease (stage IV) are usually seriously ill and have severe bone pain, ecchymosis, anemia from bleeding and/or replacement of bone marrow by tumor, and emaciation. These patients are not candidates for surgical intervention. It would be tempting to establish the diagnosis by removing a portion of a large primary tumor. However, confirmation of neuroblastoma can be achieved by the typical findings on imaging studies, presence of tumor markers in the blood and urine, bone marrow aspirate showing neuroblastoma cells by routine histology, monoclonal antibodies, and N-myc amplification in the DNA. These patients will initially require intensive chemotherapy, with surgical resection of gross residual disease deferred until maximum regression of the tumor has been achieved, which is usually before 16 weeks into therapy.

Those patients who are not so critically ill, and who do not have bone marrow involvement on bone aspiration or biopsy, require tissue diagnosis by either removal of metastatic nodes or biopsy/excision of the primary tumor. A well-circumscribed primary tumor might be readily resected, but more often there is extensive involvement of normal structures; therefore, only a wedge biopsy is indicated. Immediate primary resection does not improve survival, and delayed primary resection after initial chemotherapy may improve survival. The advantage of initial surgical resection is to obtain tissue that can be studied for all the prognostic indicators. More than 70% of neuroblastomas will have apparent complete or partial response to currently available chemotherapy agents. However, most often, residual tumor is present and resectable. Further, in contrast to the usually friable, very bloody tumors encountered with initial primary resection, most of the tumors, after chemotherapy, become "matured" toward ganglioneuroma and are solid, firm, rubbery, and relatively avascular. After chemotherapy, if total excision is not feasible because of involvement of large visceral blood vessels or organs, a debulking procedure is indicated. The use of an ultrasonic dissector has been helpful in removal of tumor around major blood vessels, avoiding injury to the vessels. Occasionally, a complete resection requires removal of a kidney or a segment of bowel, which is justified if the remaining kidney is healthy or the length of bowel resection will not produce malabsorption.

In some institutions, intraoperative focal irradiation can be given at the time of surgical resection or several days later. After resection, the area of tumor involvement and residual disease may be outlined with metallic clips so that a subsequent plane abdominal radiograph will identify the involved field for external radiation therapy. These clips should be composed of tantalum, which will not produce artifactual scatter when follow-up CT scans are performed. After surgical resection or radiation therapy, aggressive chemotherapy will be required for long-term control of the tumor.

Radiation Therapy

Radiation therapy has had a diminished role in the management of neuroblastoma because it obliterates hematopoiesis in the marrow in the treatment field, thereby limiting the intensity of chemotherapy. It probably has no place in the treatment of stage I and II tumors. However, in low doses (150 cGy/day for 3 days) it may induce regression of life-threatening stage-IV-S extensive liver involvement. It is also useful to treat severe pain and impending fractures in focal areas of bone metastases. Patients with intraspinous extension of neuroblastoma, producing rapidly increasing neurologic deficit, might be treated with radiation. However, there is a risk of subsequent kyphoscoliosis; therefore, chemotherapy is preferable to induce rapid reduction of the mass.

Chemotherapy

During the past two decades, there has been an increasingly aggressive use of chemotherapy to improve survival. Although patients with stage I tumors and most infants are long-term survivors, most of the patients are older children with more advanced stage tumors who do not survive. With the current identification of prognostic factors, the population of patients who should have the most aggressive treatment can be identified. Any patient, in any stage, who has an elevated serum ferritin, elevated neuron-specific enolase, elevated LDH, unfavorable histology, cytogenetic studies showing diploidy or hypotetraploidy, abnormal chromosome 1, homogeneously staining regions (HSR), double minutes (DM), and particularly an amplification of N-myc has a poor prognosis. Aggressive chemotherapy is indicated.

In the 1960s and 1970s, the Children's Cancer Group and Pediatric Oncology Group studied single and combination chemotherapy agents causing regression of neuroblastoma. Complete or partial response rates for single agents were as follows: peptichemio (PTC) 92%, cyclophosphamide (CPM) 59%, cisplatin (CCDP) 46%, Adriamycin (ADR) 41%, epipodophyllotoxins, VP-16, and VM26 30%, vincristine (VCR) 24%, and dacarbazine (DTIC) 14%, (Table 44.8) (19). It became clear that most neuroblastomas were resistant to single agents. In those patients with disseminated disease, in whom there was a good response, almost all subsequently had recurrence of tumor, presumably by clones of cells that developed drug resistance. Therefore, multidrug therapy evolved. Combinations of agents were tried in patients with stage-IV tumors, using varying doses and sequences of the above drugs. The combination of CPM, VCR, and DTIC resulted in survival rates of 10 to 15%. Until 1978, the best results were a 20% overall survival, where 50% of infants, 5% of children between the ages of 1 and 6 years old, and 44% of children older than 6 years of age had complete, long-term regression of tumor (98). Subsequently, Green et al. recognized the importance of aggressive induction to achieve complete responses in the early course of treatment (99). By using CPM daily for 7 days (which kills tumor cells in all phases of the growth cycle), they induced increased mitotic activity in the tumor. At the end of the 7-day period, ADR was given, which is most effective during mitosis. This regimen resulted in a 52% rate of complete remission, with 15 of 35 patients being long-term survivors. Those without complete response then received combinations of VCR and ADR or VP-16, VM 26 and ADR, or VCR and DTIC, or CDDP and VM 26; the complete response rate was improved to 70%. Shafford et al. used pulses of CPM, VCR, CDDP, and VM 26 over a 3-day period repeated every 3 weeks and achieved a complete regression in 78% of patients. The addition of ADR did not improve the response rate (100). However, the eventual survival was 20%, similar to many previous trials.

Many newer agents are being used. Ifosfamide, used alone, has caused partial or complete response in 44% of previously untreated patients. Carboplatin is similar to cisplatin but has less renal, neural, and hearing toxicity than cisplatin. Topotecan is an inhibitor of topoisomerase resulting in DNA breaks, interfering with DNA replication and RNA transcription. It is a semisynthetic analog of camptothecin, an alkaloid derived from the camptothecin tree. Retinoic acid is a synthetic analog of vitamin A, which influences the growth and differentiation of many neoplastic cells.

Intensification of chemotherapy is known to increase the rate of tumor regression, but severe toxicity is the limiting factor. However, a number of agents are used to counteract these side effects. Mesna inhibits the urotoxicity of the oxazaphosphorines ifosfamide and cyclophosphamide. Numerous cytokines that are important in the stimulation, proliferation, and maturation of progenitor hematopoietic cells of the erythroid, myeloid, and megakaryocyte series have been developed through recombinant DNA biotechnology. The severe bone marrow suppression that follows intense chemotherapy can be

Table 44.8. Chemotherapeutic Agents Available for Neuroblastoma

AGENT	INTRAVENOUS DOSE (mg/m^2)	TOXIC EFFECTS
Cyclophosphamide (CPM)	300–750	Nausea, vomiting, alopecia, bone marrow depression, immunosuppression, hemorrhagic cystitis and azotemia
Melphalan (L-PAM)	140	Nausea, vomiting, diarrhea, mucosal ulcers, hemorrhagic cystitis, alopecia, liver enzyme abnormalities and increased ADH secretion
Vincristine (VCR)	1.5	Local tissue necrosis, neurotoxicity and alopecia
Dacarbazine (DTIC)	250	Nausea, vomiting and bone marrow depression
Teniposide (VM-26)	15	Nausea, vomiting, alopecia, bone marrow depression and allergic reactions
Etoposide (VP-16)	100	Nausea, vomiting, alopecia, allergic reactions, hypotension and pancytopenia
Adriamycin (ADM)	35	Local tissue necrosis, nausea, vomiting, bone marrow depression and myocardiopathy with total dose above 500 mg/m^2
Cisplatin (CDDP)	60	Anorexia, nausea, severe vomiting, renal toxicity, hearing loss, pancytopenia, hypocalcemia and hypomagnesemia
Peptichemio (PTC)	1–1.5 mg/kg/day	Leukopenia, thrombocytopenia, alopecia, and phlebosclerosis
Ifosfamide	3000	Bone marrow suppression, nephrotoxicity
Topotecan	1	Bone marrow suppression, nausea, elevated transaminase, alopecia, diarrhea
Taxotere	55–100	Hypersensitivity reactions, neuropathy, bone marrow suppression, arrhythmias, alopecia, mucositis, nausea, vomiting

reversed rapidly using granulocyte colony-stimulating factor (G-CSF), granulocyte-macrophage colony-stimulating factor (GM-CSF), interleukin-3 (IL-3), and erythropoietin individually and in combination to synergistically produce rapid recovery of myelosuppression. Interferon gamma (IFN-γ) is a cytokine that stimulates HLA class I antigen expression on neuroblastoma cells to facilitate autoimmune antitumor effects.

Newer protocols are studying as many as six drugs in combination, including CPM, VCR, DTIC, CDDP, and the podophyllins. In some trials, the doses are being intensified, and continuous infusions are being used to achieve antitumor efficacy and minimize normal cell toxicity. Retrospective analysis of protocols shows that response rate, median survival, and progression-free survival are related to dose intensity of the drugs (99). With the initiation of therapy, the drug doses are intensified to achieve rapid reduction of tumor. This is referred to as the induction phase of therapy. Usually, this involves four courses of a combination of agents within 3 to 4 months. The patient is reassessed at that time, using all of the imaging studies and bone marrow aspiration to identify residual local and metastatic disease. The second phase of treatment is referred to as a consolidation phase. At this time, aggressive resection of residual bulk disease and radiation therapy of residual tumor may be used. When a good response has been achieved, a third phase of therapy is begun, referred to as a maintenance phase, in which a combination of chemotherapy agents is used less intensively than they are in the induction phase. In all previous trials in which aggressive induction and consolidation therapy produced a complete or partial response, relapse developed frequently within 24 weeks of treatment. Therefore, current protocols are aimed at ablation of all tumor within the 24- to 26-week interval, and there has been some deemphasis on the maintenance phase of tumor suppression. When induction has been effective, second-look or delayed primary exploration of the primary tumor is advocated in the consolidation portion of the regimen. Even when imaging studies showed no residual tumor, surgical exploration usually reveals resectable remaining tumor.

Myeloablative Chemotherapy With or Without Total Body Irradiation

The unsatisfactory results of the multiple chemotherapy regimens in poor-prognosis patients have prompted innovative approaches to treatment. Recognizing that a $70 + \%$ complete or partial response of primary and metastatic neuroblastoma can be achieved with combination chemotherapy, and with the realization that recurrence (i.e., tumor resistance) evolves within 24 weeks, massive chemoradiation therapy is being tried. Various combinations of high-dose chemotherapy such as VM26, ADR, melphalan, CDDP with or without total body radiation (TBI) are being added to the consolidation phase following multiagent induction (101). The TBI dose is 1000 cGy, and is fractionated to 333 cGY over 3 days to minimize toxicity to the eyes and lungs. It is known that neuroblastoma cells are less capable of

repairing DNA injury than are normal tissues after sublethal radiation therapy.

As expected, massive chemoradiation treatment produces lethal and irreversible destruction of the bone marrow. Therefore, bone marrow transplantation becomes essential. Both autologous and allogeneic transplantation are being used (101). The advantage of autologous marrow transplantation is the absence of morbidity from graft-versus-host reactions and its treatment. The bone marrow is harvested from the patient at about the 12th week of therapy. Before this, the bone marrow aspirate is analyzed for the presence of metastatic neuroblastoma and to ensure that the myeloid cells have recovered to at least 15×10^6 normal marrow cells.

There is a significant risk of transplanting neuroblastoma cells back to the patient. It is known that 75 to 85% of bone marrow samples from stage-IV patients, in which no obvious neuroblastoma is seen by routine histologic methods, will contain malignant cells by immunocytologic techniques. Methods have been developed to identify as few as 1 neuroblastoma cell per 10^6 marrow cells, and techniques have been developed to purge the harvested bone marrow of neuroblastoma cells for transplantation (101). The technique uses a combination of differential sedimentation, filtration, and tagging of the neuroblastoma cells with a number of monoclonal antibodies. The neuroblastoma monoclonal antibodies can be coated on magnetized beads, and when the antibody-bead neuroblastoma cell conjugate is placed in a magnetic field, the neoplasm is removed while the marrow stem cells are preserved. After purging the marrow, it is cryopreserved until it is required after chemotherapy with or without TBI, at approximately 22 weeks into the treatment program.

Allogeneic bone marrow transplant is possible when there is an HLA-MHC–matched sibling as a donor. However, only approximately 25% of patients are likely to have an available matched donor. Because the neuroblastoma recipient is immunocompromised by the intensive chemo radiation, transfusion with even HLA-matched marrow can result in a graft-versus-host reaction because of a "minor" HLA mismatch (102). There may be a significant advantage of allogeneic marrow transplantation because the transplanted T-cell population may be cytotoxic to residual neuroblastoma. A similar immunologic approach might be a future direction for treatment of metastatic neuroblastoma. The technique of allogeneic bone marrow transplantation after intensive myeloablative therapy has produced survival rates of approximately 50%.

Other Treatment Modalities

When MIGB was found to localize in chromaffin tumors, it was natural to consider its use in the treatment of unresectable neuroblastoma, similar to the treatment of metastatic thyroid carcinoma using ^{131}I (103). The patient takes iodine to minimize uptake of ^{131}I-MIBG in the thyroid gland and must be isolated with precautions to protect both hospital personnel and family from contamination from the isotope. ^{131}I MIBG is injected intravenously over 4 to 6 hours. The drug is excreted in the urine, but the patient can be discharged from the hospital after 5 days. The radiation dose to be given is difficult to estimate because the amount of radiation received in systems such as the bone marrow cannot be measured. Although there is selective uptake in thyroid and salivary glands, heart, and liver, no notable toxicity to these organs has occurred. The limiting factor has been thrombocytopenia, particularly when the patient has had intensive chemotherapy or a previous bone marrow transplant. The results have been disappointing, although one half of patients may subsequently have reduction in tumor size or stable disease; recurrence has occurred almost uniformly. It is possible that a significant problem with these results is that all patients have had multiple trials of other therapy, and the ^{131}I MIBG treatment has been used in a particularly resistant disease (104).

There is great interest in using radioiodinated monoclonal antibodies specific for surface antigens on neuroblastoma cells to achieve control of metastatic disease (105). However, as with MIBG, uptake in healthy tissues and problems providing the appropriate dose have limited the usefulness of these techniques.

CONCLUSION

The aggressiveness of therapy is based on the prognostic factors of stage, age, histology, chromosomal anomalies and tumor markers. The following outline might be a guide for treatment options (Table 44.9).

Not every variable is indicated in this scheme. For example, deletion of the short arm of chromosome 1 may outweigh all other factors such as stage or N-myc in requiring aggressive treatment. Further experience will determine if there is a discordance between the importance of serum ferritin, LDH and histology in stage II and stage III tumors, or between an elevated serum ganglioside and diploidy, which will alter the approach to treatment. Only by pooling these cases in multi-institutional protocols will there be advances made in the diagnostic evaluation and treatment of this highly variable and complex tumor.

Table 44.9. Treatment Strategies Based on Prognostic Factors

Stage	Age	Histology	NSE	Ferritin	N-myc	Treatment
I	All	All	All	All	All	Excision and observation
II	<1	Favorable	<100 μg/mL	<142 μg/mL	<3 copies	Excision and observation
II	<1	All	>100 μg/mL	>143 μg/mL	>3 copies	Excision and chemo
II	>1	All	All	All	>3 copies	Excision and chemo or with bulky disease; chemotherapy, excision + local RT chemo
II	>1	All	All	All	<3 copies	Excision and chemo
III	All	Favorable	All	<142 μg/mL	<3 copies	Excision or debulking local RT
III	>1	Unfavorable	All	>142 μg/mL	<3 copies	Chemo, excision or debulking, local RT chemo
IV	<1	All	<100 μg/mL	All	<3 copies	Excision, aggressive chemo
IV	>1	All	All	All	All	Aggressive chemo, excision + local RT and aggressive chemo or myelolablative chemo with or without TBI
IV-S	All	All	<100 μg/mL	>142 μg/mL	<3 copies	Observation radiation to liver, ventral hernia
IV-S	All	All	>100 μg/mL	>142 μg/mL	>3 copies	Probably IV—not IV-S

NSE, neuron-specific enolase; chemo, chemotherapy; RT, radiation therapy; TBI, total body irradiation.

REFERENCES

1. Bill AH Jr, Hartmann JR, Beckwith JB. The unique biology of childhood tumors. Pac Med Surg 1967;75:281.
2. Young JL, Ries LG. Cancer incidence, survival and mortality for children under 15 years of age. Cancer 1986;58:598.
3. Blande RP. The neurocrestopathies; a unifying concept of disease arising in neural crest maldevelopment. Hum Pathol 1974;5:409.
4. Newbitt KA, Vidone RA. Primitive neuroectodermal tumor (neuroblastoma) arising in sciatic nerve of a child. Cancer 1976;37:1562.
5. Kadish S, Goodman M, Wang CC. Olfactory neuroblastoma. a clinical analysis of 17 cases. Cancer 1976;37:1571.
6. Gross RE, Farber S, Martin IW. Neuroblastoma sympatheticum. a study and report of 217 cases. Pediatrics 1959.15;23:1179.
7. Koop CE, Hernandez R. Neuroblastoma: experience with 100 cases in children. Surgery 1964.6;50:726.
8. Priebe CJ, Clatworthy HW Jr. Neuroblastoma. evaualtion of the treatment of 90 children. Arch Surg 1967;95:538.
9. De Lorimier AA, Bragg KU, Linden F. Neuroblastoma in childhood. Am J Dis Child 1969;117:441.
10. Stella JG, Schweisguth O, Schlienger M. Neuroblastoma. a

study of 144 cases treated in the Institute Gustave-Roussy over a period of 7 years. AJR 1970;108:324.

11. Breslow N, McCann B. Statistical estimation of prognosis for children with neuroblastoma. Cancer Res 1971;31:2098.

12. Koop CE, Johnson DG. Neuroblastoma: an assessment of therapy in reference to staging. J Pediatr Surg 1971;6:595.

13. Wilson LMK, Draper GJ. Neuroblastoma, its natural history and prognosis: a study of 487 cases. Br Med J 1974;3:301.

14. Jaffee N. Neuroblastoma: review of the literature and an examination of factors contributing to its enigmatic character. Cancer Treat Rev 1976;3:61.

15. Grosfeld JL, Bachner RL. Neuroblastoma: an analysis of 160 cases. World J Surg 1980;4:29.

16. Collins VP, Loeffler RK, Tivey H. Observations on growth rates of human tumors. AJR 1956;76:988.

17. Kaplan E, Meier P. Non-parametric estimation from incomplete observations. J Am Stat Assoc 1958;53:457.

18. Evans AE, Diangio GS, Sather HN, et al. A comparison of four staging systems for localized and regional neuroblastoma: a report from the Children's Cancer Study Group. J Clin Oncol 1990;8:678.

19. Hayes FA, Smith EI. Neuroblastoma. In: Pizzo PA, Poplack DG, eds. Principles and practice of pediatric oncology. Philadelphia: JB Lippincott, 1989;607.

20. Evans AE, Baum E, Chard R. Do infants with stage IV-S neuroblastoma need treatment? Arch Dis Child 1981;56:271.

21. Stephanson SR, Cook BA, Mease AD, et al. The prognostic significance of age and pattern of metastases in stage IV-S neuroblastoma. Cancer 1986;58:372.

22. Everson TC, Cole WH. Spontaneous regression of cancer. Philadelphia: WB Saunders, 1966.

23. Beckwith JB, Perrin EV. In situ neuroblastoma: a contribution to the natural history of neural crest tumors. Am J Pathol 1963;43:1089.

24. Turkel SB, Itabashi HH. The natural history of neuroblastic cells in the fetal adrenal gland. Am J Pathol 1974;76:225.

25. Dyke PC, Mulkey DA. Maturation of ganglioneuroblastoma to ganglioneuroma. Cancer 1967;20:1343.

26. Martin RF, Beckwith JB. Lymphoid infiltrates in neuroblastomas: their occurrence and prognostic significance. J Pediatr Surg 1968;3:161.

27. Evans AE, et al. Factors influencing survival of children with non-metastatic neuroblastoma. Cancer 1976;38:661.

28. Hellstrom KE, Hellstrom I. Immunologic defenses against cancer. Hosp Pract 1970;5:45.

29. Hellstrom KE, Hellstrom I. Lymphocyte-mediated cytotoxicity and blocking serum activity to tumor antigens. Adv Immunol 1974;18:209.

30. Sawada T, et al. Mass screening for neuroblastoma in infancy. In: Advances in neuroblastoma research. New York: Alan R. Liss, 1988:525.

31. Naito J, Sasaki M, Yamashiro K, et al. Improvement in prognosis of neuroblastoma through mass population screening. J Pediatr Surg 1990;25:245.

32. Lemieux B, Auray-Blais C, Giguere R, et al. Neuroblastoma screening: the Canadian experience. Med Pediatr Oncol. 1989;17:379.

33. Woods WF, Tuchman M, Robison LL, et al. Screening for neuroblastoma in North America; preliminary results from the Quebec project. Proc Am Soc Clin Oncol 1990;9:294.

34. Brodeur GM, et al. International criteria for diagnosis, staging and response to treatment in patients with neuroblastoma. In: Advances in neuroblastoma research. New York: Alan R. Liss, 1988:509.

35. Ninane J, et al. Stage II neuroblastoma. adverse prognostic significance of lymph node involvement. Arch Dis Child 1982;57:438.

36. Hayes FA, Green A, Huster O, et al. Surgicopathological staging of neuroblastoma: prognostic significance of regional lymph node metastases. J Pediatr 1983;102:59.

37. Haase GM, Atkinson JB, Stram DO, et al. Surgical management and outcome of locoregional neuroblastoma: comparison of the Children's Cancer Group and the International Staging Systems. J Pediatr Surg 1995;30:289.

38. Haase GM, Wong KY, deLorimier AA, et al. Improvement in survival after excision of primary tumor in Stage IV neuroblastoma. J Pediatr Surg 1989;24:194.

39. Triche TJ, Cavazzana AO. Pathology in pediatric oncology. In: Pizzo PA, Poplack DG, eds. Principles and practice of pediatric oncology. Philadelphia: JB Lippincott 1993:93,115.

40. Shimada H, et al. Histopathologic prognostic factors in neuroblastic tumors: definition of subtypes of ganglioneuroblastoma and an age-linked classification of neuroblastomas. J Natl Cancer Inst 1984;73:405.

41. Chatten J, et al. Prognostic value of histopathology in advanced neuroblastoma: a report from the Children's Cancer Study Group. Hum Pathol 1988;19:1187.

42. Hayashi Y, et al. Cytogenetic findings and prognosis in neuroblastoma and emphasis on marker chromosome 1. Cancer 1989;63:126.

43. Gilbert F, et al. Human neuroblastomas and abnormalities of chromosomes 1 and 17. Cancer Res 1984;44:5444.

44. Brodeur GM, Seeger RC. Gene amplification in human neuroblastoma: basic mechanisms and clinical implications. Cancer Genet Cytogenet 1986;19:101.

45. Seeger RC, et al. Association of multiple copies of the N-myc oncogene with rapid progression of neuroblastoma. N Engl J Med 1986;313:1111.

46. Seeger RC, et al. Expression of N-myc by neuroblastoma with one or multiple copies of the oncogene. In: Evans AE, et al., eds. Advances in neuroblastoma research. New York: Alan R. Liss, 1988:41, 57.

47. Kaneko Y, et al. Different karyotypic patterns in early and advanced stage neuroblastomas. Cancer Res 1987;47:311.

48. Gansler T, Chatton J, Vardlo M, et al. Flow cytometric DNA analysis of neuroblastoma. Cancer 1986;58:2453.

49. Look TA, et al. Cellular DNA as a predictor of response to chemotherapy in infants with unresectable neuroblastoma. N Engl J Med 1984;311:231.

50. Oppedal BR, Storm-Mathisen I, Lie So, et al. Prognostic factors in neuroblastoma: clinical, histopathologic, and immunohistochemical features and DNA ploidy in relation to prognosis. Cancer 1988;62:772.

51. Hann HWL, et al. Prognostic importance of serum ferritin in patients with stage III and IV neuroblastoma: the Children's Cancer Study Group experience. Cancer Res 1985;45:2843.

52. Zeltzer PM, Marangos PJ, Evans AE, et al. Serum neuron-specific enolase in children with neuroblastoma: relationship to stage and disease course. Cancer 1986;57:1230.

53. Tsuchida Y, et al. Serial determination of serum neuron-

specific enolase in patients with neuroblastoma and other pediatric tumors. J Pediatr Surg 1987;22:419.

54. Gitlow WE, Dziedzic LB, Dziedzic SW. Catecholamine metabolism in neuroblastoma. In: Pochedly C, ed. Neuroblastoma. Acton: Publishing Sciences Group, 1976.

55. Yokomori K, Tsuchida Y, Saito S. Tyrosine hydroxylase and choline acetyltransferase activity in human neuroblastoma. Cancer 1983;52:263.

56. Alvarado CS, et al. Plasma dopa and catecholamines in the diagnosis and follow-up of children with neuroblastoma. Am J Pediatr Hematol Oncol 1985;7:221.

57. Geiser CF, Efron ML. Cystathioninuria in patients with neuroblastoma or ganglioneuroblastoma. its correlation to vanillylmandelic acid excretion and its value in diagnosis and therapy. Cancer 1968;22:856.

58. Cheung NK, Miraldi FD. Iodine 131 labeled GD2 monoclonal antibody in the diagnosis and therapy of human neuroblastoma. In: Advances in neuroblastoma research. New York: A.R. Liss, 1988:595.

59. Wu ZL, Schwartz E, Seeger R, et al. Expression of GD2 ganglioside by untreated primary human neuroblastomas. Cancer Res 1986;46:440.

60. Ladisch S, Wu ZL, Feig S, et al. Shedding of GD2 ganglioside by human neuroblastoma. Int J Cancer 1987;39:73.

61. Valentino L, Moss T, Olson E, et al. Shed tumor gangliosides and progression of human neuroblastoma. Blood 1990;75:1564.

62. Hsiao RJ, Seeger RC, Yu AL, et al. Chromogranin A in children with neuroblastoma; serum concentration parallels disease stage and predicts survival. J Clin Invest 1990;85:1555.

63. Rascher W, Kremens B, Wagner S, et al. Serial measurements of neuropeptide Y in plasma for monitoring neuroblastoma in children. J Pediatr 1993;122:914.

64. Joshi VV, Cantor AB, Brodeur GM. Correlation between morphologic and other prognostic markers of neuroblastoma. a study of histologic grade, DNA index, N-myc gene copy number, and lactic dehydrogenase in patients in the Pediatric Oncology Group. Cancer 1993;71:3173.

65. Frens DB, Bray PF, Wu JT, Lahey ME. The carcinoembryonic antigen assay: prognostic value in neural crest tumors. J Pediatr 1976;88:591.

66. Fernbach DJ, Williams TE, Donaldson MH. Neuroblastoma. In: Sutow WW, Vietti TJ, Fernbach DJ, eds. Clinical pediatric oncology. 2nd ed. St. Louis: CV Mosby, 1977.

67. Jaffe N, et al. Heterochromia and Horner syndrome associated with cervical and mediastinal neuroblastoma. J Pediatr 1975;87:75.

68. King D, et al. Dumbbell neuroblastomas in children. Arch Surg 1975;110:888.

69. Shown TE, Durfee MJ. Blueberry muffin baby: neonatal neuroblastoma with subcutaneous metastases. J Urol 1970;104:193.

70. Schneider KM, Becker JM, Krasna IH. Neonatal neuroblastoma. Pediatrics 1965;36:359.

71. Hawthorne HC Jr, Nelson JS, Witzleben CL, Giangiacomo J. Blanching subcutaneous nodules in neonatal neuroblastoma. J Pediatr 1970;77:297.

72. Welbourn RB. Current status of the apudomas. Ann Surg 1977;185:1.

73. Trump DL, Livingston JN, Baylin SB. Watery diarrhea syndrome in an adult with ganglioneuroma-hemochromocytoma. Cancer 1977;40:1526.

74. Kaplan SJ, et al. Vasoactive intestinal peptide secreting tumors of childhood. Am J Dis Child 1980;134:21.

75. Altman AJ, Baehner RL. Favorable prognosis for survival in children with coincident opso-myoclonus and neuroblastoma. Cancer 1976;37:846.

76. Berg BO, Albin AR, Wang W, et al. Encephalopathy associated with occult neuroblastoma. J Neurosurg 1974;41:567.

77. Williams TH, House RF Jr, Burgert EO Jr, et al. Unusual manifestations of neuroblastoma: chronic diarrhea, polymyoclonia-opsolonus, and erythrocyte abnormalities. Cancer 1972;29:475.

78. Robinson MH, Howard RN. Neuroblastoma, presenting as myasthenia gravis in a child aged 3 years. Pediatrics 1969;43:111.

79. Kagut MD, Donnell GN. Cushing's syndrome in association with renal ganglioneuroblastoma. Pediatrics 1961;28:566.

80. Bolande RP, Towler SF. A possible relationship of neuroblastoma to von Recklinghausen's disease. Cancer 1970;26:162.

81. Fairchild RS, Kyner JL, Hermreck A, et al. Neuroblastoma, pheochromocytoma, and renal cell carcinoma. JAMA 1979;24:220.

82. Wong K, Hanenson IB, Lampkin BC. Familial neuroblastoma. Clin Nucl Med 1980;5:450.

83. Korobkin M, Helical CT. Principles, techniques, and clinic applications. 1993 primary session: imaging symposium. Radiographics 1994;14:885.

84. Boechat MI, Kangarloo H. MR imaging of the abdomen in children. AJR 1989;152:1245.

85. Dietrich RB, Kangarloo H, Lanarsky C, et al. Neuroblastoma: the role of MR imaging. AJR 1987;148:937.

86. Cohen MD, et al. Efficacy of magnetic resonance imaging in 139 children with tumors. Arch Surg 1986;121:522.

87. Bidani N, et al. Gallium scan as a prognostic indicator in neuroblastoma. Clin Nucl Med 1980;5:450.

88. McEwan AJ, et al. Radioiodobenzylguanidine for the scintigraphic location and therapy of adrenergic tumors. Semin Nucl Med 1985;15:132.

89. Shapiro B, Gross MD. Radiochemistry, biochemistry, and kinetics of ^{131}I-metaiodobenzylguanidine (MIBG) and ^{123}I-MIBG. Med Pediatr Oncol 1988;15:170.

90. Lumbroso JD, et al. Metaiodobenzylguanidine (mIBG) scans in neuroblastoma: sensitivity and specificity: a review of 115 scans. In: Advances in neuroblastoma research. New York: A.R. Liss, 1988:689.

91. Gordon I, Peters AM, Gutman A, et al. Skeletal assessment in neuroblastoma: the pitfalls of iodine—123-MIBG scans. J Nucl Med 1990;31:129–134.

92. McMillan CW, Gaudry CL Jr, Holemans R. Coagulation defects and metastatic neuroblastoma. J Pediatr 1968;72:347.

93. Franklin IM, Pritchard J. Detection of bone marrow invasion by neuroblastoma is improved by sampling at 2 sites with both aspirates and trephine biopsies. J Clin Pathol 1983;36:1215.

94. Moss TJ, Reynolds CP, Sather HN, et al. Immunocytology improves detection of marrow metastases and provides prognostic information for patients with neuroblastoma. N Engl J Med 1991;324:219.

95. Adzick NS, et al. Major childhood tumor resection using normovolemic hemodilution anesthesia and hetastarch. J Pediatr Surg 1985;20:372.

96. Suarez A, Hartmann O, Vassal G, et al. Treatment of stage IV-S neuroblastoma; a study of 34 cases treated between 1982 and 1987. Med Pediatr Oncol 1991;19:473.

97. Hayes FA, et al. Chemotherapy as an alternative to laminectomy and radiation in the management of epidural tumor. J Pediatr 1984;104:221.

98. Finkelstein JZ, et al. Multiagent chemotherapy for children with metastatic neuroblastoma: a report from the Children's Cancer Study Group. Med Pediatr Oncol 1979;6:179.

99. Green AA, Green MD, Hayes A, et al. Sequential cyclophosphamide and doxorubicin for induction of complete remission in children with disseminated neuroblastoma. Cancer 1981;48:2310.

100. Shafford EA, Rogers DW, Pritchard J. Advanced neuroblastoma: improved response rate using a multiagent regimen (OPEC) including sequential cisplatin and VM-26. J Clin Oncol 1984;2:742.

101. Seeger RC, et al. Bone marrow transplantation for poor prognosis neuroblastoma. In: Advances in neuroblastoma research. New York: A.R. Liss, 1988:203.

102. Matthay KK, Atkinson JB, Stram DO, et al. Patterns of relapse after autologous purged bone marrow transplantation for neuroblastomas: a Children's Cancer Group pilot study. J Clinc Oncol 1993;11:2226.

103. Hartmann O, et al. The therapeutic use of ^{131}I meta-iodobenzylguanidine (MIBG) in neuroblastoma: a phase II study in 12 patients. In: Advances in neuroblastoma research. New York: A.R. Liss, 1988:655.

104. Matthay KK, Huberty SP, Hattner RS, et al. Efficacy and safety of (131I) metaiodobenzyl-guanidine therapy for patients with refractory neuroblastoma. J Nucl Biol Med 1991;35:244.

105. Etoh T, Takashi H, Maie M, et al. Tumor imaging by anti-neuroblastoma monoclonal antibody and its application to treatment. Cancer 1988;62:1282.

45

Testicular Tumors in Children

Kirk J. Wojno
David A. Bloom

INTRODUCTION

Prepubertal testis tumors are exceedingly rare (1 per million children per year) (1–5) and account for 1 to 5% of all pediatric solid tumors (6–8). Between 1980 and 1994, the Prepubertal Testicular Tumor Registry accrued only 338 tumors, which emphasizes their rarity (9). There is a bimodal age distribution with a peak in the first 5 years of life and a gradual increase in frequency in adolescence (2). Prepubertal testis tumors are less common in African Americans than whites (8). Even with modern molecular and subatomic treatment options for certain testicular tumors, surgical exploration and inguinal orchiectomy remain the standard of management.

Nongerm cell tumors make up a greater proportion of testis tumors in prepubertal boys than in adults (25% versus 5%) (4). Germ cell tumors (seminoma, embryonal carcinoma, and malignant mixed germ cell tumors) are more common in adults (10) and rarely, if ever, occur in the prepubertal testes (4, 11). Testis tumors in children are more likely to be benign and have a lower incidence of metastasis than their adult counterparts (12). The current classification of prepubertal testis tumors and tumor-like lesions is listed in Table 45.1 (3, 11).

The staging of prepubertal testis tumors is the same as for adults (11). Stage I is tumor limited to the scrotum. Stage IIa is microscopic tumor involvement of retroperitoneal lymph nodes not suspected by imaging or elevated serum alpha-fetoprotein (AFP). Stage IIb is bulky retroperitoneal disease demonstrated either by pathologic examination of the tissue or by imaging. Stage III is distant metastasis outside the retroperitoneum (13). With the success of modern chemotherapy in treating these tumors, extent of disease at diagnosis is the most important independent predictor of survival (14). Although still debated by some, most studies have shown that age at diagnosis is not an independent predictor of prognosis (10).

PATHOGENESIS

Recent studies on the pathogenesis of pediatric germ cell neoplasia indicate that the common pediatric germ cell tumors arise directly from immature germ cells as opposed to progression through intratubular germ cell neoplasia (ITGCN), as is the case with adult tumors (15–17). Figure 45.1 emphasizes this point. There is additional evidence that prepubertal testis tumors are biologically different than their adult counterparts as suggested by the fact that the isochromosome of the short arm of chromosome 12 (i12p), which is present in the majority of adult germ cell tumors (20–22), is not present in pediatric yolk sac tumors (23). Further study is needed to clarify the pathogenesis of these tumors (Figure 45.1).

ITGCN is rare in children (1 to 2% of orchidopexy specimens (24–26) and 2 to 3% of prepubertal testicular biopsies (27–29)) and has only been found adjacent to one pediatric teratoma, whereas ITGCN is commonly seen adjacent to germ cell tumors in adults. Therefore, the preinvasive germ cell lesion may be morphologically different in infants and young children. The characteristic morphology of ITGCN in adults (30–32) and children (28) has been described. ITGCN is morphologically different in the cryptorchid testis in that neoplastic germ cells are haphazardly arranged in the seminiferous tubules as opposed to the usual basal location in the adult form. The need to biopsy the testis at orchipexy is as controversial as is the management of ITGCN if found. For adults, ITGCN conveys a 5-year 50% risk of testicular cancer development (31, 33); the significance of this finding in children has not been defined. Radiation for ITGCN has been proposed by some (29, 31) but not in the pediatric age group. Biopsy may be indicated in specific situations, such as intersex syndromes with dysgenetic gonads and at the time of orchipexy for patients with ambiguous genitalia or 45X/46XY karyotype. The incidence of ITGCN in intersex states is 6% (2% prepubertal and 17% pubertal) (34). Identification of ITGCN in infants cannot rely on immunohistochemical markers like placental alkaline phosphatase (PLAP) because they are often normally expressed in this age group (35). In situ hybridization or ploidy analysis may be useful. The characteristic cytogenetic abnormality seen in adult germ cell tumors (i12p) is not found in ITGCN (23, 36).

Table 45.1. Classification of Prepubertal Testis Tumors and Tumor-like Lesions

Germ cell tumors
  Yolk sac tumor
  Teratoma
  Mixed germ cell tumor
  Seminoma
Sex cord stromal tumors
  Leydig cell tumor
  Sertoli cell tumor
  Juvenile granulosa cell tumor
  Undifferentiated sex cord stromal tumor
Mixed tumors
  Gonadoblastoma
  Mixed sex cord stromal and germ cell tumor
Tumors of supporting tissues
  Adenomatoid tumor
  Leiomyoma
  Hemangioma/lymphangioma
  Fibroma
  Sarcoma
Lymphomas and leukemias
  Tumor-like lesions
    Epidermoid cyst
    Tunica albugenea cyst
    Cystic dysplasia of the testis
  Secondary tumors
    Metastatic neuroblastoma
  Tumors of the adnexa
    Embryonal rhabdomyosarcoma
    Adenomatoid tumor
    Epididymal papillary cystadenoma
    Melanotic neuroectodermal tumor of infancy
  Tumor-like lesions of the adnexa
    Epididymal cysts
    Meconium peritonitis
    Adrenal ectopia and related lesions
    Neurofibromatosis
    Inflammatory myofibroblastic tumor
    Sarcoidosis

The cryptorchid patient has 4 to 11 times the risk of the general population for testicular tumor development (27, 37, 38). Cryptorchidism occurs in 37% of newborns, with the majority spontaneously descending by 3 months of age; the incidence rate subsequently declines to equal that of the general population by 9 months (0.8%) (39). ITGCN is eventually found in 2 to 3% of cryptorchid testes that are examined histologically, but generally germ cell tumors do not occur in the cryptorchid testis until later in life. Orchidopexy by the age of 2 is the currently accepted treatment for cryptorchidism and serves several purposes. It makes the testis available for self-examination, it decreases psychologic damage of an empty scrotum, and it may improve fertility if done before 2 years of age (39). There is no evidence that orchidopexy decreases the malignant potential of a cryptorchid testis. Two-stage endo-

scopic orchidopexy has been successful (40, 41) and has recently increased in popularity.

There appears to be an inherited form of testicular germ cell tumor, as several familial clusters of testis tumors have been reported (42–44). It has also been recently postulated that because the frequency of bilateral testicular tumors is higher than can be explained by chance alone, there must be a hereditarily predisposed subpopulation that accounts for 33% of all cases (45, 46). The 22% risk for a brother to also have a testicular tumor develop can be explained by a single predisposing autosomal recessive gene (45). If the assumption that the malignant phenotype results from a single gene in a homozygous state is correct, then 1 in 10 individuals in the general population would be heterozygous for this allele (45).

GERM CELL TUMORS

A minority of pediatric germ cell tumors occurs in the gonads (47). Extragonadal germ cell tumors arise from totipotent germ cells that migrate aberrantly along midline locations. As is the case in the testis, the yolk sac tumor is the most common malignant pattern in sacrococcygeal teratomas. A right-sided predominance seems to exist for testis tumors, as opposed to the varicocele that tends to occur on the left side (11). Germ cell tumors tend to be less aggressive in infancy compared with the malignant potential in adolescents and adults (20). There appear to be two distinct age-related populations of testicular germ cell tumors—those that occur in infancy (younger than 3 years) and those that occur near puberty. The infantile tumors include yolk sac tumor and teratoma, and the peripubertal tumors have a spectrum similar to the adult testis tumors. Testicular tumors in boys between 4 and 9 years of age are usually not germ cell tumors (19) but some other type of testicular or paratesticular tumor (embryonal rhabdomyosarcoma). A similar racial distribution is seen in adult testis tumors (occurring in more whites than African Americans) (48, 49). Pure choriocarcinoma has never been reported in children (3).

Yolk Sac Tumor

Yolk sac tumor is the most common testicular neoplasm in prepubertal boys, accounting for more than two thirds of cases (3, 9, 11, 50). Its many synonyms include endodermal sinus tumor, juvenile or infantile testicular embryonal carcinoma, adenocarcinoma of the testis, orchidoblastomas, Telium's tumor, Schiller's tumor, and Vitelline tumor. Yolk sac tumor is the current preferred terminology (51) that is accepted by the Prepubertal Testis Tumor Registry (11). It was first described in the medical literature in 1910 by White and was specifically distinguished from embryonal carcinoma in 1951 by Mager and Bryant. The term yolk sac tumor grew out of work by Telium, who first noted the resemblance of this tumor to the endodermal sinus of the rat yolk sac. Subsequent work (16, 17) has shown that this tumor is of germ cell origin and not of yolk sac derivation.

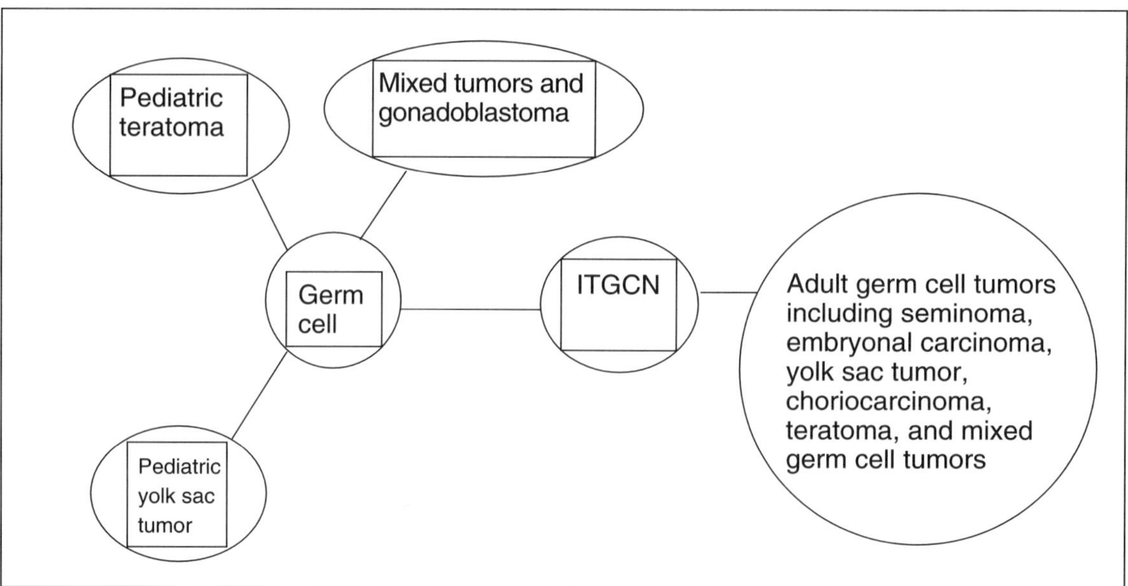

Fig. 45.1.   Pathogenesis of prepubertal germ cell tumors. (Modified from Hawkins (5), Shakkebaek (16), Czaja (17), Ulbright (18), and Visfeldt (19).)

Yolk sac tumor is the most common pure germ cell tumor (87%) and usually occurs in the pediatric age group. Although common as part of adult mixed germ cell tumors (40%), it is rare in pure form in adults (3, 52). These differences in tumor biology between adults and children may be related to age-dependent differentiation (53), cytogenetic distinctions (23), or other differences in tumor pathogenesis (15). Most yolk sac tumors occur before the age of 3, with a median of 17 months (1, 3, 8, 51) and a range of 0 to 11 years (3). They can occur during the first month of life, at which point they are the second most common tumor (second to stromal tumors) (3).

Grossly, these tumors are fairly well circumscribed. On cut section they bulge above surrounding testicular parenchyma with a pale yellow to red coloration, often with a mucoid appearance. Histologically, this tumor often has numerous patterns within the same neoplasm. The most common pattern is reticular and microcystic, characterized by a network of irregularly shaped spaces lined by attenuated cuboidal to columnar cells set in a background of ill-defined primitive mesenchyme. Schiller-Duval bodies, the name given to single epithelial-lined fibrovascular projections into cystic spaces, are characteristic of yolk sac tumors, as are pink hyaline globules. These hyaline globules stain with AFP immunoperoxidase. Other patterns include solid, cystic, vacuolated, glandular, papillary, and festoon, to name a few. The histologic pattern of these tumors has no prognostic implication (54).

Most yolk sac tumors present as painless testicular masses, although 10% present with metastasis, 14% develop subsequent metastasis, and there is a 13% overall mortality rate. Therefore, overall, the prognosis is good, with mean survival of 87% for all stages (11, 48) However, stage IIb and III disease uniformly have a poor prognosis despite aggressive therapy. Some data suggest that metastases are slightly more frequent in children older than 2 years of age, although the numbers are small and not statistically significant (3). In general, it appears that age does not affect prognosis (11), and pure prepubertal yolk sac tumors behave no differently stage for stage than embryonal carcinoma in adults (11).

The majority (84 to 85%) of patients with yolk sac tumors present with stage I disease (55). AFP is elevated in 77% of cases (11), and beta human chorionic gonadotropin is not a useful marker for pure yolk sac tumors (11). Computed tomography (CT) scan has a 60% sensitivity and a 98% specificity in detecting metastatic disease in this age group (11). After CT scan, abdominal ultrasound and chest radiographs add little additional information. As opposed to the adult testis tumors that spread via the lymphatics to retroperitoneal lymph nodes, yolk sac tumors spread with equal frequency hematogenously and via lymphatics (11, 55). Some have used this fact to argue that there is limited value of retroperitoneal lymph node dissection (RPLD), with its associated morbidity, with the relatively high probability of hematogenous metastasis.

Inguinal orchiectomy with close surveillance is the currently accepted initial mode of therapy (9, 56, 57) and is adequate for most stage I yolk sac tumors (11). There is no data to support any adjuvant therapy for stage I disease, including RPLD (11, 48). Because there have been no recurrences after 14 months in large series, a 2-year disease-free interval has been touted as indicative of "cure" (11). Long-term surveillance is, however, still advocated by most, especially with conservative management of stage I disease (Table 45.2).

Although RPLD plays a major role in the management of adult nonseminomatous germ cell tumors, it is currently not advocated for stage I pediatric yolk sac tumors. However, when there is strong evidence for metastatic disease confined to the retroperitoneum (3, 9), RPLD may still play a role. This current

Table 45.2. Current Surveillance Recommendations for Stage I Yolk Sac Tumor

	PHYSICAL EXAMINATION	CHEST AND ABDOMEN CT SCAN	SERUM ALPHA-FETOPROTEIN	CHEST X-RAY
1 mo post orchiectomy	X	X	X	
Year 1 post orchiectomy	Monthly	Every 3 months	Monthly	Monthly
Year 2 post orchiectomy	Every 2 months	Every 6 months	Every 2 months	Every 2 months
Year 3–5 post orchiectomy	Yearly	Yearly	Yearly	Yearly

conservative approach stems from the desire to reduce morbidity (principally ejaculatory failure) in view of the fact that most stage I patients do well with orchiectomy alone. Adequate surveillance to detect recurrent disease early has led to acceptable salvage rates (64%) with aggressive chemotherapy, sometimes combined with radiation therapy or surgery (11). If RPLD is indicated or desired, it should be restricted to the ipsilateral side if there is no gross or micrometastatic disease evident on frozen section at the time of the procedure (48). For those requiring full RPLD, a nerve-sparing procedure should be considered to reduce morbidity (58).

Adjuvant chemotherapy has been used for advanced-stage and recurrent disease. There is limited data on the success of such therapy because most patients present at an early stage. Chemotherapy including vincristine and actinomycin has a 64% response rate (11). Overall chemotherapy-related mortality (4.3%) and morbidity (39%) have been reported for combination chemotherapy in adults (59), but good data are available for children apart from agent-specific toxicities (hemorrhagic cystitis and testicular damage with cyclophosphamide; hypomagnesemia, renal insufficiency, and ototoxicity with cisplatin (59)) as well as infectious and hematologic complications. The effect of chemotherapy on subsequent infertility of the prepubertal patient is not well documented; however, long-term survivors without complications are known (60, 61). Infertility in adulthood should be considered in making decisions regarding chemotherapy. No standard protocol exists, but the Children's Cancer Study Group protocol includes cisplatin, etoposide, and bleomycin (62) for gross metastatic disease or persistent elevated AFP. Other protocols include vincristine, dactinomycin, and cyclophosphamide (63). National protocol entry should be considered so that chemotherapy can be optimized for this disease; however, the individual circumstances of each patient should be given priority in making any therapeutic decision. Morbidity avoiding chemotherapy, radiation, or RPLD and using careful surveillance (51) has become a priority with the realization that the majority of patients are cured with orchiectomy alone. Although effective, the role of radiation therapy is limited by potential injury to spinal cord, bowel, bone marrow, testis, and kidneys in small children (48).

TERATOMA

Teratoma is the second most common germ cell tumor in children and accounts for 14% of prepubertal testis tumors (3,

64). This tumor is benign in children and does not have the malignant potential of the tumor of the same name in adults (65). Median age at diagnosis is 14 months (3), and most occur before the age of 4 years (66). There has been only one reported case in the neonatal period (3). No metastatic pediatric testis teratomas were identified in the literature; therefore, orchiectomy or enucleation are reasonable means of therapy. Rare bilateral cases have been reported (65).

Grossly, these tumors usually combine cystic and solid components. Microscopically, they consist of mature and immature elements of all three germ layers (endoderm, mesoderm, and ectoderm). Germ layers may be represented by gastrointestinal mucosa and liver (endoderm), cartilage and muscle (mesoderm), and skin and adnexa (ectoderm). Endodermal tissue in teratomas stain for AFP (67). Testicular teratoma does not have any biologic significance, as opposed to ovarian teratomas, teratomas in other locations, or presence of immature elements in a testis in adults (68). In the prepubertal age group, these tumors are uniformly benign; in adults, they behave similarly to other malignant nonseminomatous germ cell tumors. Orchiectomy alone is adequate therapy for prepubertal teratoma.

MIXED GERM CELL TUMORS

Five cases of mixed teratoma and embryonal carcinoma with similar behavior to yolk sac tumor have been reported (11). Most of these occurred at the upper end of the pediatric age spectrum. Teratoma and yolk sac tumor are the only mixed tumors in the Prepubertal Testis Tumor Registry and appear to have similar behavior to the pure yolk sac tumors. Therefore, they can be considered together for clinical decision-making.

SEMINOMA AND EMBRYONAL CARCINOMA [ADULT TYPE TUMORS]

Seminoma has a very low incidence in children (3, 69), and most reported cases were adolescents (19, 48, 70–76). These patients should be treated as adults with inguinal orchiectomy and radiation or RPLD as needed (3). Embryonal carcinoma occasionally occurs in older boys in late adolescence and should be regarded as an adult disease.

SEX CORD STROMAL TUMORS

Sex cord stromal tumors are more common in children than adults but can be found at any age. They are the most common testis tumors in newborns younger than 1 month old (3) and are the most common in the prepubertal age group, where they represent 6 to 8% of testicular tumors (3, 77). Those tumors found in infancy are usually benign, but in older children these tumors seem to have metastatic potential and should be watched carefully (3). They may be hormonally active. They can be divided into four main groups—Leydig cell tumor, Sertoli's cell tumor, granulosa cell tumor, and undifferentiated sex cord stromal tumors.

Leydig Cell Tumor

Leydig cell tumors represent about 7% of all prepubertal testicular tumors and tend to occur between 6 and 12 years of age (11). Three percent are bilateral. They are essentially benign and usually present with precocious puberty, gynecomastia, or both (77). In a child, a swollen testis and precocious puberty should suggest a Leydig cell tumor. In contrast to the 10% risk of metastasis in adults, there are only rare reports of metastatic disease in the prepubertal age group (78). Nonsuppressible elevations of plasma and urinary 17-ketosteroids help differentiate Leydig tumors from congenital adrenal hyperplasia. These tumors are usually solid, sharply circumscribed masses ranging from 3 to 5 cm in diameter; they are yellow to brown and can have foci of hemorrhage and necrosis. The neoplastic cells have abundant granular eosinophilic cytoplasm that is occasionally vacuolated. When present, Reinke crystals and lipochrome pigment are useful in diagnosis. Malignant behavior constitutes the diagnosis of malignancy because histologic features are unreliable. Orchiectomy is usually curative, but long-term follow-up is recommended due to reports of late metastasis (79).

Sertoli's Cell Tumor

Sertoli's cell tumors are rare in children and account for less than 1% of testis tumors. Among prepubertal boys, the behavior of Sertoli's tumors is usually benign. As with Leydig cell tumors, malignant behavior is defined by metastasis. Malignant Sertoli's cell tumors have very rarely been reported in children (75, 80). Grossly, these tumors are circumscribed, lobulated, yellow to white masses that can have foci of hemorrhage. The cells are polygonal with finely vacuolated amphophilic cytoplasm and are arranged in tubules, solid nests, or cords of cells. Charcot-Böttcher crystals are characteristic of Sertoli's cell differentiation but usually are only visualized with electron microscopy. An association with Peutz-Jeghers syndrome has been noted (81, 82). Large cell calcifying Sertoli's is a variant of Sertoli's cell tumor with distinct clinicopathologic features that include multifocality, bilaterality, intratubular growth, and calcification. Pituitary adenomas and adrenocortical hyperplasia—along with acromegaly, gigantism, hypercortisolemia, and precocity—have also been associated with this variant (67).

Juvenile Granulosa Cell Tumor

The term juvenile granulosa cell tumor (JGCT) was coined by Lawrence because of the morphologic similarity to the ovarian tumor. Recent evidence, however, suggests that this tumor is composed of immature Sertoli's cells with phenotypic resemblance to granulosa cells (83). It comprises approximately 15% of gonadal stromal tumors. Although the potential for malignant behavior exists based on analogy to the adult variant, there have been no recorded cases of malignant behavior in neonates or children (3, 9, 84, 85). JGCT occurs more frequently in patients with mixed gonadal dysgenesis (X/XY mosaicism) (67). It is the most common sex cord stromal tumor of the testis in the neonatal period (85, 86), with 90% occurring before the age of 6 months (83). Grossly and by ultrasound, it has a multilocular appearance without calcification (87). Orchiectomy and surveillance are adequate therapies based on current limited information.

Undifferentiated Sex Cord Stromal Tumor

Undifferentiated sex cord stromal tumors constitute more than half of prepubertal sex cord stromal tumors (3). They are usually firm, yellow-white nodules without hemorrhage or necrosis. This tumor has a spectrum of histologic patterns ranging from predominately epithelial to predominately spindled stromal cells. No distinct pattern of differentiation dominates to allow classification into one of the stromal tumor categories. As opposed to patients older than 10 years of age, of whom one third have had a malignant course, only two reports of malignancy have occurred before puberty (1, 11, 80).

MIXED TUMORS

Mixed tumors are composed of sex cord stromal cells and immature germ cells.

Gonadoblastoma

Gonadoblastoma is associated with intersex syndromes and occurs mainly in patients with mixed gonadal dysgenesis, 46XY pure gonadal dysgenesis, and dysgenetic male pseudohermaphroditism (67). It is the most common tumor in mixed gonadal dysgenesis (88). Histologically, it contains germ cells (resembling seminoma cells) and sex cord stromal cells (immature Sertoli's cells and sometimes Leydig cells) presenting in a specific pattern (large nests with mixture of germ cells and stromal cells surrounding hyaline nodules, occasionally with foci of calcification). These tumors are usually solid but may be cystic (89). The majority occur after puberty (3), and most are benign if resected. However, there may be an increased risk for invasive germ cell tumors in lesions left in situ (5, 67, 87, 90–93). In the setting of abnormal sexual differentiation, the incidence of gonadal tumors is 44%, with mixed and pure gonadal dysgenesis having the greatest risk; therefore, although it is controversial, consideration should be given to early bilateral prophylactic gonadectomy (90).

Germ Cell Sex Cord Stromal Tumors

These very rare tumors can occur in dysgenetic gonads and very rarely in the normal testis (53, 94). Although these tumors contain a mixture of germ cells and sex cord stromal elements, they are not present in the patterns that are typical of gonadoblastoma. Therefore, they comprise a distinct and morphologically diverse population of tumors, usually in older men. There is only one reported case in the prepubertal testis (95).

TUMORS OF SUPPORTING STRUCTURES

Adenomatoid Tumor

Adenomatoid tumor can present as a testicular mass, where it usually arises from the tunica albuginea and expands into the parenchyma of the testis. It is much more common in the adnexa, especially the epididymis (see the section on tumors of the adnexa in this chapter for a more complete discussion).

Leiomyoma and Fibroma

Of soft tissue tumors, leiomyoma is the second most common after adenomatoid tumor in the testis (1). Only sporadic cases of fibroma have been reported (1). Both of these soft tissue tumors are benign.

Lymphangioma/Hemangioma

Lymphangioma and capillary hemangioma, although common in other sites, rarely occur in the spermatic cord and testis (96, 97). Hemangioma can occur in the scrotal skin, where conservative management is the best approach.

Leukemia and Lymphoma and Pseudolymphoma

Microscopic leukemic infiltrates have been found at autopsy in 64% of patients with acute leukemia (98). The testicle is the first site of relapse in 8 to 36% of boys with acute lymphoblastic leukemia (99, 100). This is probably because optimal concentrations of chemotherapeutic agents are not achieved in the testicle. The leukemic infiltrate usually involves the interstitial space, spares the seminiferous tubules, and presents as painless swelling (101). Relapses can occur during complete marrow remission, and some protocols advise testicular biopsy before discontinuing therapy and then repeated during surveillance. Ultrasound, although useful in screening for leukemic infiltrates, does not replace biopsy (102). Standard open biopsy is performed bilaterally. Aspiration biopsy results may be positive when open biopsy results are negative. The usual treatment for testicular relapse is resumption of chemotherapy with or without local radiation (103, 104).

Although usually a disease of older men, lymphoma may occur occasionally in prepubertal testes. Burkitt's lymphoma, a common pediatric tumor in Africa, comprised 50% of testicular tumors in one report (105). Lymphoma is otherwise rarely mentioned in any other series on pediatric gonadal tumors. When it does occur, it has a poor prognosis because the disease is widely disseminated at that point. Hayes et al reported four children with testicular lymphoma, and all but one died within 4 months of diagnosis (106).

TUMOR-LIKE LESIONS OF THE TESTIS

Intratesticular epidermoid cyst is distinct from teratoma and can be differentiated from teratoma by ultrasound (107). Epidermoid cysts do not contain skin appendages and are probably monophasic teratomas. Monodermal teratoma accounts for 3% of pediatric testis tumors (108) and bilaterality is rare (107). They represent 1.2% of tumors in the Prepubertal Testis Tumor Registry. If stable in size and without elevated tumor markers, testis-sparing operation (enucleation) is indicated (3). In postpubertal males, these are best treated like teratomas.

Dermoid cysts contain skin appendages, and elements of a second germ layer may also be present. These lesions have been described in children 6 months old and have been intrascrotal but extratesticular (109–111). These behave in a benign fashion.

Tunica albuginea cysts are benign, mesothelial-lined retention cysts or may result with capsule formation following resolution of hemorrhage after trauma (112).

Cystic dysplasia of the testis is rare and can occur in diffuse and localized forms (113, 114). It is characterized by multiple cysts lined with cuboidal epithelium (reminiscent of rete epithelium) located in the mediastinum of the testis and adjacent parenchyma. It is thought to represent abnormal cystic dilatations of the rete testis due to abnormal connection to the mesonephric ductules during embryonic development (115). The diffuse form is associated with Potter syndrome (116).

SECONDARY TUMORS

Metastatic Neuroblastoma

Neuroblastoma can rarely metastasize to the testis; 3 to 4% of patients have metastatic disease in the testis, with most also having bone marrow involvement (117). Congenital paratesticular neuroblastomas that present as scrotal masses have also been reported (118).

TUMORS OF THE ADNEXA

Embryonal Rhabdomyosarcoma

Rhabdomyosarcoma is the most common soft tissue sarcoma of childhood (0.5 to 0.7 per million children per year). It is almost as common as Wilms' tumor or neuroblastoma and more common than germ cell tumors or osteosarcoma (63, 119). It accounts for 3 to 10% of all tumors in children younger than

Table 45.3.   Clinical Grouping Classification and Intergroup Rhabdomyosarcoma Study Group IV Treatment Protocols

GROUP	CLASSIFICATION	TREATMENT
I	Localized disease, completely resected (alveolar subtype excluded)	Vincristine and actinomycin D for 1 year (no radiation therapy)
II	Grossly resected tumors with microscopic residual disease or regional nodal metastasis	Vincristine, actinomycin D, and either cyclophosphamide or ifosfamide for 1–2 yr plus conventional radiation therapy
III	Incomplete resection or biopsy with gross residual disease	3–7 drug regimen plus conventional or hyperfractionated radiation therapy
IV	Distant metastasis present at diagnosis	Same as group III

15 years (63, 120) and 13% of nongerm cell tumors in the scrotum of male children (121). There seems to be no racial predisposition as with germ cell tumors. Because they arise from embryonal mesenchyme, they can arise anywhere in the body. However, 15 to 20% of rhabdomyosarcomas involve the genitourinary tract (122), and 4 to 15% arise in the paratesticular region (123–127). Paratesticular rhabdomyosarcomas do better than the same tumors in other locations. The reasons for this are unclear and possibly related to earlier detection (127–129). Survival at 3 years for paratesticular rhabdomyosarcoma is 89% (127). Nonresectable tumors have the highest mortality rate (130). A bimodal age distribution exists with peaks between 2 and 6 and 15 and 19 years of age. Ninety-three percent have embryonal histology (131). A subgroup of paratesticular embryonal rhabdomyosarcomas with spindle cell morphology (27% of paratesticular embryonal rhabdomyosarcomas) has been associated with a very favorable prognosis (131, 132)—a 95% 5-year survival rate compared with 80% for the nonspindle cell type (131).

The tumors are usually firm, white to tan-pink, and rubbery in consistency. They are composed of small oval to spindle-shaped cells with high nucleus/cytoplasm ratios. Occasionally, strap cells with cross-striations are noted. Immunoperoxidase staining for desmin and muscle-specific actin are useful in diagnosis.

Staging includes CT scans of the chest and abdomen, bone scan, skeletal survey, and bone marrow aspirate/biopsy (122). The clinical staging system of the Intergroup Rhabdomyosarcoma Study Group is shown in Table 45.3.

Initial therapy is radical inguinal orchiectomy with proximal vascular control. If biopsy is necessary to establish diagnosis, tumor spillage should be avoided. Nodal involvement occurs in 28 to 38% of patients (127, 133) and is not always evident by CT staging. Because group 2 receives radiation therapy, the status of the retroperitoneal lymph nodes is important for management decisions. Sequelae of multimodality therapy—such as short stature from prepubertal radiation to the spine, esophageal and common bile duct strictures, and inguinal nerve entrapment—are important concerns (134). Ipsilateral retroperitoneal lymph node sampling may preserve sympathetic nerves important in ejaculation (122, 127, 134). However, because this is controversial, some advocate no RPLD with CT negative cases (129, 135, 136) and others suggest RPLD only with CT enlarged lymph nodes. We favor RPLD

as part of staging and management of most group I and II tumors. If there is scrotal contamination in otherwise group 1 disease, then hemiscrotectomy and relocation of the testis with radiation to the area are recommended.

Repetitive pulse vincristine, actinomycin D, and cyclophosphamide have been compared with other combination chemotherapy protocols for all locations, and preliminary data show no significant advantage (137). However, data on only genitourinary tumors have not been published. Cyclophosphamide is avoided in stage I tumors in an effort to try to preserve fertility.

Melanotic Neuroectodermal Tumor of Infancy

Melanocytic neuroectodermal tumor of infancy is generally benign (3 to 4% malignant) (138). This tumor is of neural crest origin (139). Ninety-five percent occur in children younger than 1 year old, usually in the head and neck, with 2% occurring in the epididymal region (140). Only 18 cases in the epididymis have been reported to date (141). They are similar in appearance to embryonal rhabdomyosarcoma but contain pigment and show neural differentiation. It is important to make this distinction so that aggressive therapy (RPLD, chemotherapy) that is usually given to paratesticular sarcomas can be avoided.

PRIMARY EPIDIDYMAL NEOPLASMS

Epididymal tumors account for about 5% of scrotal masses in all age groups (142).

Adenomatoid Tumor

Primary epididymal neoplasms are uncommon in children. The most frequent neoplasm is the adenomatoid tumor (60%). This tumor is derived from mesothelium and is usually benign. It is rare in children. It is typically well circumscribed and composed of solid gray-white tissue. Microscopically, it is composed of varying sized tubules lined by flat to columnar cells. Although malignant degeneration has very rarely occurred after local recurrence in an older age group, there are not enough pediatric cases for valid conclusions (143).

Papillary cystadenomas occur over a wide age range and have been reported in children as young as 7 years of age (peak, 10 to 30 years) (66). Most occur in association with von Hippel-

Lindau disease and may be the initial manifestation of the disease. Most are small solid or cystic nodules less than 2 cm, but lesions as large as 5 or 6 cm have been recorded. Histologically, they are composed of varying sized tubules with papillary enfoldings, lined by cuboidal cells with clear cytoplasm. Rare cases of carcinoma have been reported but not in the pediatric age group. Papillary cystadenoma is benign and strongly associated with von Hippel-Lindau. Of malignant tumors, sarcomas are more common than carcinomas (144).

TUMOR-LIKE LESIONS OF THE ADNEXA

Inflammatory Myofibroblastic Tumor

Inflammatory myofibroblastic tumor mimics epididymal sarcoma (145). In the pediatric age group, some cases are associated with torsion or trauma. The tumors are usually less than 2.5 cm and occur in children younger than 14 months (146). In general, these lesions are thought to be reactive.

Epididymal Cysts

About 33 to 66% of patients with cryptorchidism have associated epididymal anomalies. There is also a strong association of epididymal anomalies with cystic fibrosis, von Hippel-Lindau syndrome, and in utero diethylstilbestrol exposure. These lesions, such as epididymal cysts, usually become symptomatic at puberty when these tubes begin to function (146).

Sarcoidosis

Sarcoidosis is a rare cause of a scrotal mass in children, with only seven reported cases (147).

Meconium Peritonitis

Meconium peritonitis may cause scrotal calcification. Because testicular masses are often evaluated without abdominal radiographs, this diagnosis may be missed. Meconium peritonitis results from in utero perforation of the gastrointestinal tract. The meconium spills into the peritoneum and provokes a sterile inflammatory reaction resulting in calcification and fibrosis. It is often associated with atresia of the bowel, volvulus, or peritoneal bands. It can be asymptomatic and only discovered incidentally. Infants may present with hydroceles at birth; the hydroceles contain serous fluid and meconium. After birth, the meconium calcifies and hardens into a scrotal mass. The presence of abdominal and scrotal calcification may make exploration necessary (148–150).

Adrenal Ectopia

Ectopic adrenal tissues (Marshand's rests) are common microscopic findings (15%) along the spermatic cord and tunica albu-

genia in autopsy series (115). In an abnormal hormonal mileu (Nelson's syndrome, congenital adrenal hyperplasia), hyperplasia of this tissue may present as a mass lesion (140, 151). Pleuripotential cells of the testicular hilum have also formed similar mass lesions with an appearance similar to Leydig cell tumors in adrenogenital syndrome (152).

Genitourinary Neurofibromatosis

Genitourinary neurofibromatosis is rare, with only seven reported cases in children (153). It usually originates from the pelvic autonomic plexus and can occur in the spermatic cord as a mass (154). Other regions of the genitourinary tract have been involved (prostate, perineum, seminal vesicles, penis, and scrotum) (153).

NEONATAL TESTIS TUMORS

Less than 1% of pediatric testis tumors occur in the first month of life (9). Stromal tumors are more common than yolk sac tumors, which comprise only 27% of neonatal tumors (3, 9). Stromal, granulosa, and gonadoblastoma are most frequently seen (9). AFP is not helpful in detecting or diagnosing yolk sac tumor in the neonate because of the wide normal range at this age. Most patients with yolk sac tumor at this age have AFP in the normal range (9). Melanotic neuroectodermal tumor of infancy occurs in the neonatal period (138).

EVALUATION OF SCROTAL MASSES

The incidence of scrotal masses in children is 1 to 5 per 100,000 children per year (1, 155). Therefore, workup of these lesions is common and should begin with consideration of torsion. If there is a strong clinical suspicion of torsion, immediate exploration is warranted. Careful history taking and physical examination can usually distinguish the most common entities such as torsion, hydrocele, varicocele, or hernia. Trauma may bring such a mass to clinical attention but may also cause local irritation, which may cause the lesion to appear more suspicious. Evaluation for precocity is important and may provide significant clues to hormonally active tumors. Careful palpation can usually discern gonadal anatomy even in the presence of a hydrocele or hernia. Ultrasound is a useful adjunct. The differential diagnosis of intrascrotal masses in children always begins with torsion of the spermatic cord. When a tumor is suspected, scrotal incision is avoided and an inguinal approach is used. The likely causes of intrascrotal enlargements are hydrocele, hematoma, and hernia. Trauma may produce a hematocele or may exacerbate a hernia or hydrocele. Varicoceles are sometimes misconstrued as testicular tumors. According to data from the Prepubertal Testis Tumor Registry, a painless scrotal mass is the most common presentation of testicular tumors, occurring in nearly all cases. Trauma and hydrocele make up only a small percentage of clinical presentations (3).

Physical examination, transillumination, ultrasound, and

tumor markers are the principle tools for preoperative evaluation of scrotal masses.

AFP is the most useful tumor marker in children. Beta human chorionic gonadotropin, although useful in the evaluation of adult testis tumors, is not useful before puberty because choriocarcinoma has not been reported in this age range and the rare seminomas have not had syncytiotrophoblastic giant cells (3). Care must be taken when evaluating AFP in the first 8 months of life because this marker is normally elevated in the newborn and may persist for up to 8 months despite its half-life of 5 days (3, 156). Knowledge of this half-life and the nomogram (156) of neonatal AFP levels is essential to understanding both preoperative and postoperative results in the first 8 months of life (157). In a series of 10 patients, AFP levels were within nomogram range during this time, but most were stromal tumors. False-negative AFP levels have been noted despite retroperitoneal nodal metastasis; therefore, a normal AFP does not preclude metastasis (158, 159).

SUMMARY

Scrotal masses in children are occasionally (7%) caused by neoplasms of the testis and paratesticular tissue (155). The distribution of tumor types differs in children compared with adults, with a much lower proportion of germ cell tumors. Yolk sac tumor is the most common neoplasm in the pediatric age group. The primary treatment is radical inguinal orchiectomy. There is still controversy about the appropriate staging (need for RPLD versus advanced imaging) and optimal treatment for more advanced disease. Therefore, decisions about such treatment should be guided by a team of specialists (in the areas of pediatrics, oncology, urology, radiology, and pathology) and be tailored to the particular needs and limitations of the patient. With advances in technology, it will be important to ensure that appropriate measures are taken with imaging, tissue harvest, and analysis to allow optimal staging and prognostication so that adjunctive therapy (with its attendant side effects) is provided only when necessary.

All scrotal masses in children should be considered malignant until proven otherwise. Control of vascular and lymphatic channels before manipulation is optimal and best achieved by an inguinal approach. Once exposed, a mass can be safely examined and biopsied. If the lesion is benign, a testis-sparing procedure can be undertaken to preserve future fertility. Even if the lesion is malignant, cure is still likely with modern therapy although life-long surveillance is still required.

Radical inguinal orchiectomy remains the initial step. Testis-sparing surgery is an option for prepubertal teratoma and epidermoid cyst (12, 160). RPLD is used only when necessary (48). Combination chemotherapy with bleomycin, etoposide, and cisplatin for low-stage disease with elevated markers and advanced-stage disease is superior to previous combinations (161–163). All new testicular tumors in children should be reported to the Prepubertal Testicular Tumor Registry.

REFERENCES

1. Young JL, Ries LG, Silverberg E, et al. Cancer incidence, survival and mortality for children younger than age 15 years. Cancer 1986;58:598.
2. Green DM. Testicular tumors in infants and children. Semin Surg Oncol 1986;2:156.
3. Kay R. Prepubertal testicular tumor registry. J Urol 1993; 150:671.
4. Brosman SA. Testicular tumors in prepubertal children. Urology 1979;13:581.
5. Hawkins EP. Pathology of germ cell tumors in children. Crit Rev Oncol Hematol 1990;10:165.
6. Brown NJ. Teratomas and yolk sac tumors. J Clin Pathol 1976;29:1021.
7. Kaplan GW. Prepubertal testicular tumors. World J Urol 1981;2:238.
8. Li FP, Fraumeni JF Jr. Testicular cancers in children: epidemiological characteristics. J Natl Cancer Inst 1972;48: 1575.
9. Levy DA, Kay R, Elder JS. Neonatal testis tumors: a review of the Prepubertal Testis Tumor Registry. J Urol 1994;151: 715.
10. Sesterhenn IA, Mostofi FK, Davis CJ. Testicular tumors in infants and children. In: Jones WG, Ward AM, Anderson CK, eds. Germ cell tumors. New York: Pergamon Press, 1986;2:173.
11. Kaplan, GW, Cromie WJ, Kelalis PP, et al. Prepubertal yolk sac testicular tumors; report of the Testicular Tumor Registery: part 2. J Urol 1988;140:1109.
12. Rushton HG, Belman BA. Testis-sparing surgery for benign lesions of the prepubertal testis. Urol Clin North Am 1993; 20:27.
13. Boden G, Gibb R. Radiotherapy and testicular neoplasms. Lancet 1951;2:1195.
14. Birch R, Williams SD, Cone A, et al. Prognostic factors for favorable outcome in disseminated germ cell tumors. J Clin Oncol 1986;4:400.
15. Manivel JC, Simonton S, Wold LE, et al. Absence of intratubular germ cell neoplasia in testicular yolk sac tumors in children. Arch Pathol Lab Med 1988;112:641.
16. Skakkebaek NE, Berthelsen JG, Giwercman A, et al. Carcinoma in situ of the testis: possible origin from gonocytes and precursors of all types of germ cell tumors except spermatocytoma. Int J Androl 1987;10:19.
17. Czaja JT, Ulbright TM. Evidence for the transformation of seminoma to yolk sac tumor, with histogenetic considerations. Am J Clin Pathol 1992;97:468.
18. Ulbright TM, Roth LM. Testicular and paratesticular neoplasms. In: Sternberg SS, ed. Diagnostic surgical pathology. 2nd ed. New York: Raven Press, 1994.
19. Visfeldt J, Jorgensen N, Muller J, et al. Testicular germ cell tumors of childhood in Denmark, 1943–1989: incidence and evaluation of histology using immunohistochemical techniques. J Pathol 1994;174:39.
20. Hoffner L, Deka R, Chakravarti A, et al. Cytogenetics and origins of pediatric germ cell tumors. Cancer Genet Cytogenet 1994;74:54.
21. Atkin NB, Baker MC. Specific chromosome marker in

seminoma and malignant teratoma of the testis. Cancer Genet Cytogenet 1983;10:199.

22. Samaniego F, Rodrigues E, Houldsworth J, et al. Cytogenetic and molecular analysis of human male germ cell tumors. Genes Chromosom Cancer 1990;1:289.

23. Perlman EJ, Cushing B, Hawkins E, et al. Cytogenetic analysis of childhood endodermal sinus tumors: a Pediatric Oncology Group study. Pediatr Pathol 1994;14:695.

24. Parkinson MC, Ramani P. Intratubular germ cell neoplasia in an infantile testis. Histopathology 1993;23:99.

25. Rozansky T, Wojno KJ, Bloom DA. The remnant orchiectomy. J Urol 1996;155:712.

26. Parkinson MC, Swerdlow AJ, Pike MC. Carcinoma in situ in boys with cryptorchidism: when can it be detected? Br J Urol 1994;73:431.

27. Giwercman A. Carcinoma in situ of the testis: screening and managemant. Scand J Urol Nephrol Suppl 1992;148:1.

28. Muller J, Skakkebaek NE, Nielsen OH, et al. Cryptorchidism and testis cancer. Atypical infantile germ cells followed by carcinoma in situ and invasive carcinoma in adulthood. Cancer 1984;54:629.

29. MacMahon RA, Cussen LJ. Detection of gonadal carcinoma in situ in childhood and implications for management. Aust N Z J Surg 191;61:667.

30. Sigg, Hedinger. Atypical germ cells in testicular biopsy in male sterility. Int J Androl Suppl 1981;4:163.

31. Skakkebaek NE, Berthelsen JG, Muller J. Carcinoma in-situ of the undescended testis. Urol Clin North Am 1982;9:377.

32. von der Maase H, Giwercman A, Muller J, et al. Management of carcinoma in-situ of the testis. Int J Androl 1987;10:209.

33. Pryor JP, Cameron KM, Chilton CP et al. Carcinoma in-situ in testicular biopsies from men presenting with infertility. Br J Urol 1983;55:780.

34. Ramani P, Yeung C, Habeebu SSM. Testicular intratubular germ cell neoplasia in children and adolescents with intersex. Am J Surg Pathol 1993;17:1124.

35. Hustin J, Gillerot Y, Collette J, et al. Placental alkaline phospahatase in developing normal and abnormal gonads and in germ cell tumours. Virchows Arch A Pathol Anat Histopathol 1990;417:67.

36. Vorechovsky I, Mazanec K. Is isochromosome i(12p) present in gonadal precancerous tissue? Neoplasma 1989;36:697.

37. Farrer JH, Walker AH, Rajfer J. Management of the postpubertal cryptorchid testis: a statistical review. J Urol 1985;134:1071.

38. Benson RC, Beard CM, Kelalis PP, et al. Malignant potential of the cryptorchid testis. Mayo Clin Proc 1991;66:372.

39. Rozanski TA, Bloom DA. The undescended testis: theory and management. Urol Clin North Am 1995;22:107.

40. Bloom DA. Two step orchipexy with pelviscopic clip ligation of the spermatic vessels. J Urol 1991;145:1030.

41. Bloom DA, Semm K. Advances in genitourinary laparoscopy. Adv Urol 1991;4:167.

42. Boiesen PT, Lyrdal F. Testicular malignancy in father and son: a case report. Scand J Urol Nephrol 1987;21:69.

43. Dieckmann KP, Becker T, Jonas D, et al. Inheritance and testicular cancer: arguments based on a report of three cases and a review of the literature. Oncology 1987;44:367.

44. Yonemitsu N, Mori K, et al. Testicular tumors in non-twin

45. Nicholson PW, Harland SJ. Inheritance and testicular cancer. Br J Cancer 1995;71:421.

46. Dieckmann KP, Boeckmann W, et al. Bilateral testicular germ cell tumors: report of nine cases and review of the literature. Cancer 1986;57:1254.

47. Dehner LP. Gonadal and extragonadal germ cell neoplasia of childhood. Hum Pathol 1983;14:493.

48. Leonard MP, Jeffs RD, Levanthal B, et al. Pediatric testicular tumors: the Johns Hopkins experience. Urology 1991;37:253.

49. Forman D, Gallagher, Moller H, et al. Aetiology and epidemiology of testicular cancer report of consensus group. Prog Clin Biol Res 1990;357:245.

50. Jacobsen GK, Jacobsen M. Possible liver cell differentiation in testicular germ cell tumors. Histopathology 1983;7:537.

51. Connolly JA, Gearhart JP. Management of yolk sac tumors in children. Urol Clin North Am 1993;20:7.

52. Mostofi FK, Davis CJ, Sasterhenn IA. The pathologists view of testicular germ cell tumor management. AUA Update 1988;7:18.

53. Talerman A, Haije WG, Baggerman L. Serum α-fetoprotein (AFP) in paatients with germ cell tumors of the gonads and extragonadal sites: correlation between endodermal sinus (yolk sac) tumor and raised serum AFP. Cancer 1980;46:380.

54. Talerman A. The pathology of gonadal neoplasms composed of germ cells and sex cord derivatives. Pathol Res Pract 1980; 170:24.

55. Grady RW, Ross JH, Kay R. Patterns of metastatic spread in prepubertal yolk sac tumor of the testis. J Urol 1995;153: 1259.

56. Jeffs RD. Management of embryonal adenocarcinoma of the testis in childhood: an analysis of 164 cases. In: Gooden JO, ed. Cancer in childhood. New York: Plenum Press, 1973:68.

57. Exelby PR. Testicular cancer in children. Cancer 1980;45: 1803.

58. Jewett MS, et al. Retroperitoneal lymphadenectomy for testis tumor with nerve sparing for ejaculation. J Urol 1988;139: 1220.

59. Moul JW, Robertson JE, George SL, et al. Complications of therapy for testicular cancer. J Urol 1989;142:1491.

60. Holbrook CT, Crist WM, Cain W, et al. Successful chemotherapy for childhood metastatic embryonal cell carcinoma of the testicle: a preliminary report. Med Pediatr Oncol 1980;8:75.

61. Brodeur GM, Howarth CB, Pratt CB, et al. Malignant germ cell tumors in 57 children and adolescents. Cancer 1981;48: 1890.

62. Kay R, Kaplan GW. Testicular tumors in infants and children. AUA Update Series. 1992;9:114.

63. Griffin GC, Raney RB, Snyder HM, et al. Yolk sac carcinoma of the testis in children. J Urol 1987;137:954.

64. Tapper D, Lack EE. Teratomas in infancy and childhood: a 54 year experience at the Children's Hospital Medical Center. Ann Surg 1983;198:398.

65. Carney JA, Kelalis PP, Lynn HB. Bilateral teratoma in the testis in an infant. J Pediatr Surg 1973;8:49.

66. Damjanov I. Tumors of the testis and epididymis. In: Murphy WM, ed. Urologic pathology. Philadelphia: WB Saunders, 1989:341.

brothers from a consanguineous marriage. Acta Pahtol Jpn 1988;38:1077.

67. Young RH, Scully. Testicular tumors. Chicago: American Society of Clinical Pathologists Press, 1990:42.

68. Hudson ME, Konvolinka CW, Deshmukh N. High grade immature teratoma of the testis in infancy. Mil Med 1992; 157:501.

69. Harms D, Janig U. Germ cell tumors of childhood: report of 170 cases including 59 pure and partial yolk sac tumors. Virchows Arch Pathol Anat 1986;409:223.

70. Grechi G, Zampi GC, Selli C, et al. Polyorchidism and seminoma in a child. J Urol 1980;123:291.

71. Maurou C. Hypothyroidism and seminoma in association with Down's syndrome. J Pediatr 1967;70:810.

72. Viprakasit D, Navraoo E, Guarin UK, et al. Seminoma in children. Urology 1977;9:568.

73. Tanini R, Ricci AM. A case of typical seminoma in a 4-year-old boy. Arch De Vecchi Anat Patol 1982;65:103.

74. Perry C, Servadio C. Seminoma in children. J Urol 1980;124: 932.

75. Sharma S, Seam RK, Kapoor HL. Malignant Sertoli cell tumour of the testis in a child. J Surg Oncol 1990;44:129.

76. Naome D, Regnier E. Une cas de seminome chez l'enfant. Acta Urologica Belgica 1993;61:29.

77. Kaplan GW, Cromie WJ, Kelalis PP, et al. Gonadal stromal tumors: a report of the Prepubertal Testicular Tumor Registry. J Urol 1986;136:300.

78. Kapoor HL, Seam RK, Sharma S, et al. Malignant interstitial cell tumour of testis in a child. Indian J Cancer 1988;25:241.

79. Silverberg SG, Thompson JW, Higashi G, et al. Malignant interstitial cell tumor of the testis: case report and review. J Urol 1966;96:356.

80. Rosvoll RV, Woodard JR. Malignant Sertoli cell tumor of the testis. Cancer 1968;22:8.

81. Niewenhuis JC, Wolf MC, Kass EJ. Bilateral asynchronous Sertoli cell tumor in a boy with the Peutz-Jeghers syndrome. J Urol 1994;152:1246.

82. Young S, Gooneratne S, Straus FH, et al. Feminizing Sertoli cell tumor in boys with Peutz-Jeghers syndrome. Am J Surg Pathol 1995;19:50.

83. Groisman GM, Dische MR, Fine EM, et al. Juvenile granulosa cell tumor of the testis: a comparative immunohistochemical study with normal infantile gonads. Pediatr Pathol 1993;13:389.

84. Uehling DT, Smith JE, Logan R, et al. Newborn granulosa cell tumor of the testis. J Urol 1987;138:385.

85. Lawrence WD, Young RH, Scully RE. Juvenile granulosa cell tumor of the infantile testis: a report of 14 cases. Am J Surg Pathol 1985;9:87.

86. Young RH, Talerman A. Testicular tumors other than germ cell tumors. Semin Diagn Pathol 1987;4:342.

87. May D, Shamberg R, Newbury R, et al. Juvenile granulosa cell tumor of an intraabdominal testis. Pediatr Radiol 1992; 22:507.

88. Wallace TM, Levin HS. Mixed gonadal dysgenesis: a review of 15 patients reporting single cases of malignant intratubular germ cell neoplasia of the testis, endometrial adenocarcinoma, and a complex vascular anomaly. Arch Pathol Lab Med 1990; 114:679.

89. Luisiri A, Vogler C, Steinhardt G, et al. Neonatal cystic testicular gonadoblastoma: sonographic and pathologic findings. J Ultrasound Med 1991;10:59.

90. Gourlay W, Johnson HW, Pantzar JT, et al. Gonadal tumors in disorders of sexual differentiation. Urology 1994;43:537.

91. Schellhas HF. Malignant potential of the dysgenetic gonad. Obstet Gynecol 1974;44:455.

92. Troche V, Hernadez E. Neoplasia arising in dysgenetic gonads. Obstet Gynecol Surv 1986;41:74.

93. Scully RE, Gonadoblastoma: a review of 74 cases. Cancer 1970;25:1340.

94. Bolen JW. Mixed germ cell-sex cord stromal tumor: a gonadal tumor distinct from gonadoblastoma. Am J Clin Pathol 1981;75:565.

95. Leake J, Levitt G, Ramani P. Primary carcinoid of the testis in a 10 year old boy. Histopathology 1991;19:373.

96. Arda S, Senocak ME, Buyukpamukcu N, et al. Lymphangioma of the spermatic cord and tunica vaginalis in children. Eur Urol 1992;21:253.

97. Kuraoka T, Uematsu K, et al. A case of capillary hemangioma of the testis of the child. Acta Urologica Japonica 1994;40:361.

98. Givler RL. Testicular involvement in leukemia and lymphoma. Cancer 1969;23:1290.

99. Rosenkrantz JG, et al. Leukemic infiltration of the testis during long term remission. J Pediatr Surg 1978;13:753.

100. Stoffel TJ, Nesbit ME, Levitt SH. Extramedullary involvement of the testis in childhood leukemia. Cancer 1975;35:1203.

101. Shepard BR, Hensle TW, Marboe CC. Testicular biopsy and occult tumor in acute lymphoblastic leukemia. Urology 1983; 22:36.

102. Philipps G, Kumari-Subaiya S, Sawitshki A. Ultrasound evaluation of the scrotum in lymphoproliferative disease. J Ultrasound Med 1987;6:169.

103. Saiontz HI, et al. Testicular relapse in childhood leukemia. Mayo Clin Proc 1978;53:212.

104. Kim TH, et al. Pretreatment testicular biopsy in childhood acute lymphocytic leukemia. Lancet 1981;2:657.

105. Junaid TA. Testicular cancer in children and adolescents in Ibadan Nigeria. Urology 1981;18:510.

106. Hayes MM, Sacks MI, King HS. Testicular lymphoma, a retrospective review of 17 cases. S Afr Med J 1983;64:1014.

107. Price EB. Epidermoid cysts of the testis: a clinical pathologic analysis of 69 cases from the testicular tumor registry. J Urol 1969;102:708.

108. Mansfield JT, Cartwright PC. Bilateral testis tumors in an infant: synchronous teratoma and epidermoid cyst. J Urol 1995;153:1077.

109. Bloom DA, Dipietro MA, Gikas PW, et al. Extratesticular dermoid cyst and fibrous dysplasia of the epididymis. J Urol 1987;137:996.

110. Ford J, Singh S. Paratesticular dermoid cyst in a 6 month old infant. J Urol 1988;139:89.

111. Gupta SK, Gupta S, Khanna S. Dermoid cyst of the scrotal raphe containing calculi. Br J Urol 1974;46:348.

112. Warner KE, Noyes DT, Ross JS. Cysts of the tunica albuginea testis: a report of three cases with review of the literature. J Urol 1984;132:131.

113. Tesluk H, Blackenberg TA. Cystic dysplasia of the testis. Urology 1987;29:47.

114. Nistal M, Regadera J. Cystic dysplasia of the testis. Arch Pathol Lab Med 1984;108:579.

115. Gondos B, Wong T. Non-neoplastic diseases of the testis and epididymis. In: Murphy, ed. Urologic pathology. Philadelphia: WB Saunders, 1989:276.

116. Fisher JE, et al. Ectasia of the rete testis with ipsilateral renal agenesis. J Urol 1982;128:1040.

117. Kushner BH, Vogel R, Hajdu SI. Metastatic neuroblastoma and testicular involvement. Cancer 1985;56:1730.

118. Yamashina M, Kayan H, Katayama I. Congenital neuroblastoma presenting as a paratesticular tumor. J Urol 1988;139:796.

119. Crist WM, Garnsey L, Beltangady M, for the Intergroup Rhabdomyosarcoma Study Committee, et al. Prognosis in children with rhabdomyosarcoma: a report of the Intergroup Rhabdomyosarcoma Studies I and II. J Clin Oncol 1990;8:443.

120. Rodary RB, Hays DM, Lawrence W, et al. Paratesticular rhabdomyosarcoma in childhood. Cancer 1978;42:729.

121. Cromie WJ, Raney RB, Duckett JW. Paratesticular rhabdomyosarcoma in children. J Urol 1979;122:80.

122. Shapiro E, Strother D. Pediatric genitourinary rhabdomyosarcoma. J Urol 1992:148:1761.

123. Debruyne FMJ, Bokkerink JPM, de Vries JD. Current concepts in the management of paratesticular rhabdomyosarcoma. Eur Urol 1985;11:289.

124. Grosfeld JL, Weber TR, Weetman RM, et al. Rhabdomyosarcoma in childhood: analysis of survival in 98 cases. J Pediatr Surg 1983;18:141.

125. Kingston JE, McElwain TJ, Malpas JS. Childhood rhabdomyosarcoma: experience of the Children's Solid Tumor Group. Br J Cancer 1983;48:195.

126. Quesada EM, Diez B, Silva M, et al. Paratesticular rhabdomyosarcoma in children. J Urol 1986;136:303.

127. Raney RB, Tefft M, Lawrence W, et al. Paratesticular sarcoma in childhood and adolescence: a report from the Intergroup Rhabdomyosarcoma Studies I and II, 1973–1983. Cancer 1987;60:2337.

128. Newton WA Jr, Soule EH, Hamoudi AB, et al. Histopathology of childhood sarcomas, Intergroup Rhabdomyosarcoma Studies I and II: clinicopathologic correlation. J Clin Oncol 1988;6:67.

129. Cecchetto G, Grotto P, de Bernardi B, et al. Paratesticular rhabdomyosarcoma in childhood: experience of the Italian Cooperative Study. Tumori 1988;74:645.

130. Laquaglia MP, Ghavimi F, Heller G, et al. Mortality in pediatric paratesticular rhabdomyosarcoma: a multivariant analysis. J Urol 1989;142:473.

131. Leuschner I, Newton WA, Schmidt D, et al. Spindle cell variants of embryonal rhabdomyosarcoma in the paratesticular region: a report of the Intergroup Rhabdomyosarcoma study. Am J Surg Pathol 1993;17:221.

132. Cavazzana AO, Schmidt D, Ninfo V, et al. Spindle cell rhabdomyosarcoma: a prognostically favorable variant of rhabdomyosarcoma. Am J Surg Pathol 1992;16:229.

133. Blyth B, Mandell J, Bauer SB, et al. Paratesticular rhabdomyosarcoma: results of therapy in 18 cases. J Urol 1990;144:1450.

134. Hughes LL, Baruzzi MJ, Ribeiro RC, et al. Paratesticular rhabdomyosarcoma: delayed effects of multimodality therapy and implications for current management. Cancer 1994;73:476.

135. Goldfarb B, Khoury AE, Greenberg ML, et al. The role of retroperitoneal lymphadenectomy in localized paratesticular rhabdomyosarcoma. J Urol 1994;152:785.

136. Olive D, Flamant F, Zucker JM, et al. Paraaortic lymphadenectomy is not necessary in the treatment of localized paratesticular rhabdomyosarcoma. Cancer 1984;54:1283.

137. Maurer H, Gehan E, Crist W, et al. Intergroup Rhabdomyosarcoma Study III: a preliminary report of overall outcome. Proc Am Soc Clin Oncol 1989;8:296.

138. Diamond DA, Breitfeld PP, Bur M, et al. Melanotic neuroectodermal tumor of infancy: an important mimicker of paratesticular rhabdomyosarcoma. J Urol 1992;147:673.

139. Ricketts RR, Majmudar B. Epididymal melanotic neuroectodermal tumor of infancy. Hum Pathol 1985;16:416.

140. Johnson RE, Scheithauer BW, Dahlin DC. Melanotic neuroectodermal tumor of infancy: a review of seven cases. Cancer 1983;52:661.

141. Jurincic-Winkler C, Metz KA, Klippel KF. Melanotic neuroectodermal tumor of infancy in the epididymis. Zentralbl Pathol 1994;140:181.

142. Elasser E. Tumors of the epididymis: recent results. Cancer Res 1977;60:163.

143. Tjandra BS, Daeman MJ, Weil EH. Papillary mesothelioma of the albuginea testis. Urology 1994;43:118.

144. Longo VJ, McDonald JR. Primary neoplasms of the epididymis. JAMA 1951;147:937.

145. Yamashina M, Honma T, Uchijima Y. Myofibroblastic pseudotumor mimicking epididymal sarcoma: a clinicopathologic study of three cases. Pathol Res Pract 1992;188:1054.

146. Wollin M, et al. Aberrant epididymal tissue: a significant clinical entity. J Urol 1987;138:1247.

147. Kohn DB, Horowitz SD, Finlay J, et al. Sarcoidosis presenting as a scrotal mass. Pediatr Infect Dis 1985;4:302.

148. Friedman AP, Haller JA, Goodman JD. Sonography of scrotal masses in healed meconium peritonitis. Urol Radiol 1983;5:43.

149. Ring KS, Axelrod SL, Burbige KA, et al. Meconium hydrocele: an unusual etiology of a scrotal mass in the newborn. J Urol 1989;141:1172.

150. Heetderks DR, Verbrugge GP. Healed meconium peritonitis presenting as a scrotal mass in an infant. J Pediatr Surg 1969;4:363.

151. Franco-Saenz R, et al. Cortisol production by testicular tumors in a patient with congenital adrenal hyperplasia. J Endocrinol Metab 1981;53:85.

152. Rutgers JL, Young RH, Scully RE. The testicular tumor of the adrenogenital syndrome: a report of six cases and review of the literature on testicular masses on patients with adrenocortical disorders. Am J Surg Pathol 1988;12:503.

153. Chung AK, Michels V, Poland GA, et al. Neurofibromatosis with involvement of the prostate. Urology 1995.

154. Ogowa A, Watanabe K. Genitourinary neurofibromatosis in a child presenting with an enlarged penis and scrotum. J Urol 1986;135:755.

155. Macksood MJ, James RE. The scrotal mass: cause and diagnosis. Am J Surg 1983;145:297.

156. Brewer JA, Tank ES. Yolk sac tumors and alpha-fetoprotein in first year of life. Urology 1993;42:79.

157. Wu JT, Book L, Sudar K. Serum alpha-fetoprotein (AFP) levels in normal infants. Pediatr Res 1981;15:50.

158. Homsy Y, Arrojo-villa F, Khoriaty N, et al. Yolk sac tumor of the testicle: is retroperitoneal lymph node dissection necessary? J Urol 1984;132:532.

159. Kramer SA, et al. Yolk sac carcinoma: an immunohistochemical and clinicopathologic review. J Urol 1983;129:350.

160. Rushton HG, Belman BA, Sesterhenn I, et al. Testicular sparing surgery for prepubertal teratoma of the testis: a clinical and pathologic study. J Urol 1990;144:726.

161. Nair R, Pai S, Saikia TK, et al. Malignant germ cell tumors in childhood. J Surg Oncol 1994;56:186.

162. Williams SD, Einhorn LH, Greco FA, et al. VP16-213 salvage therapy for refractory germinal neoplasms. Cancer 1980;46:2154.

163. Einhorn L, Donohue J. Cisplatin, vinblastine, and bleomycin combination chemotherapy in disseminated testicular cancer. Ann Intern Med 1977;70:2568.

46

Wilms' Tumor

Current Perspectives

Hrair-George J. Mesrobian
Pamela I. Ellsworth

INTRODUCTION

The incidence of Wilms' tumor is 1 in 10,000 children, which corresponds to 450 to 500 new cases annually in the United States (1). Despite this apparent low incidence, Wilms' tumor is the most common solid intra-abdominal childhood malignancy. The multiple cooperative national and international study groups have made this one of the most carefully studied tumors (2). These efforts have resulted in an overall 2-year survival rate exceeding 85%. Although the majority of the refinements in treatment protocols have appropriately focussed on chemotherapy and radiation therapy, considerable advances have been made in imaging and in the surgical aspects of the multidisciplinary care of the patient presenting with a Wilms' tumor. These advances are opening new possibilities, and new concepts are being proposed; examples include the possibility of performing partial nephrectomy in highly selected patients with unilateral disease (with maximal renal parenchymal preservation) or deleting adjuvant chemotherapy in select patients with stage I disease (3, 4). This chapter provides an overview of these recent advances while emphasizing the clinical aspects of diagnosis and the principles of treatment.

EPIDEMIOLOGY AND ASSOCIATED ANOMALIES

Wilms' tumor has a bimodal incidence, with sporadic cases occurring at a mean patient age of 3.5 years and hereditary and bilateral cases at 2.5 years. It has now been recognized that the heritable fraction is very uncommon (less than 1% incidence) (5). Numerous epidemiologic studies have been performed, indicating an association with the following risk factors: maternal exposure during pregnancy to cigarettes, coffee or tea, oral contraceptives, hormonal pregnancy tests, or hair coloring products; maternal hypertension; vaginal infection; and higher birth weight of the child. A recent report from the National Wilms'

Tumor Study (NWTS) group has failed to confirm the existence of these maternal risk factors (6). A new association between a history of household insect and pesticide extermination, which is being further investigated, was described. In addition, they concluded that paternal preconceptional exposure may play a more significant role in the etiology of Wilms' tumor. Thus, future studies may result in an enhanced understanding of environmental risk factors.

The occurrence of associated congenital anomalies and their investigation have significantly improved our understanding of the genetic aspects of Wilms' tumors. The most frequent anomalies are congenital genitourinary malformations, sporadic aniridia, and mental retardation (collectively referred to as the WAGR syndrome) (7). These genitourinary anomalies consist of, in order of decreasing frequency, cryptorchidism, renal anomalies (horseshoe kidney, unilateral renal agenesis), and hypospadias. Because the Wilms' tumor gene (WT1) has been shown to be involved in differentiation of the genitourinary tract, it is tempting to speculate on an etiologic association (see following discussion). The discovery of sporadic aniridia, hemihypertrophy, or the Beckwith-Wiedemann syndrome (umbilical hernia, macroglossia, neonatal hypoglycemia, gigantism, and increased risk for Wilms' tumor, adrenocortical carcinoma, and hepatoblastoma) in a patient may herald the development of a Wilms' tumor; hence, periodic monitoring of the kidneys with sonography is essential. There is evidence that a greater number of low-stage tumors may be identified in patients whose tumor is detected only on radiographic screening (8). Wilms' tumors also occur in association with the Drash (pseudohermaphroditism, glomerulonephritis, and Wilms' tumor) and Perlman syndromes as well as with neurofibromatosis.

MOLECULAR BIOLOGY

The knowledge of the molecular biology of Wilms' tumor continues to progress rapidly since the discovery of the WT1 gene and its cloning. The two-step mutational model proposed in 1972 by Knudson and Strong has provided the basis of our current knowledge and understanding of tumor development (8). According to this model, tumor formation is dependent on two genetic events—either a constitutional mutation followed by a somatic mutation (hereditary form) or two somatic mutations (sporadic form). This was followed by the discovery of the WT1 gene, located on chromosome 11p13. It has also become apparent that the WT1 gene is essential for normal kidney and gonadal formation (9). Tumor development is associated with a mutation or deletion on the WT1 gene, thus characterizing this gene as a tumor suppressor gene (10). Developmentally, its expression is restricted to the differentiating metanephric mesenchyme, sex cords, primitive gonad, and coelomic cavity mesenchymal lining. During nephronogenesis, the highest level of WT1 expression is detected during the formation of the S-shaped bodies of the glomerulus. As the nephrons mature, WT1 expression becomes extinct. In Wilms' tumor tissue, it is highly expressed in the blastemal and immature epithelial cells but not in the stromal and differentiated cells (11).

Although WT1 has been cloned, its biologic role has yet to be defined. It does code a zinc finger DNA-binding protein, allowing it to act as a transcription factor, regulating the expression of genes downstream. Some of its possible functions have been shown to include repression of insulin-like growth factor II expression (which is considered a blastemal mitogen) (12) and expression of the platelet-derived growth factor chain A (known to be involved in wound healing). These genes appear to be downstream targets of WT1, but there is a lack of in vivo data assessing their functional significance. In addition to deletions, a number of subtle mutations have been described that convert WT1 from a transcription repressor to an enhancer (13). The majority of mutations occur within the zinc finger domains. Similar mutations have also been described in persistent nephrogenic rests that are thought to represent precursor lesions to Wilms' tumors (14).

Genetic linkage studies on patients with Beckwith-Wiedemann syndrome (known to have a predisposition for Wilms' tumors development) have resulted in the identification of a second gene at the 11p15 locus, referred to as WT2 (15, 16). The relationship between the WT1 and WT2 genes in the genesis of Wilms' tumor is unknown, and several hypotheses are currently being tested. A third locus has also been postulated in familial Wilms' tumor that does not segregate to the short arm of chromosome 11p (17).

It has been shown that mutations of the tumor suppressor gene p53 in Wilms' tumor cells may be associated exclusively with anaplasia. The p53 gene product lies in an adoptotic pathway activated by cytotoxic drugs, and its mutation may confer resistance to these anticancer drugs (18, 19). This finding may partially explain why patients with anaplasia have a poor prognosis.

IMAGING/DIAGNOSIS

Most children with Wilms' tumor present with an abdominal mass, frequently detected by a parent and less commonly by a physician. Abdominal pain and hematuria (gross or microscopic) are less frequent. The mass is typically firm and smooth and does not cross the midline. The tumor might produce symptoms of nausea, vomiting, malaise, and anorexia by virtue of its size or secondary to advanced disease at the time of presentation. Less frequently, patients have been described as presenting with an acute abdomen and/or shock. These symptoms have been ascribed to spontaneous hemorrhage with or without anemia or rupture and urinary extravasation (20). In this age group, abdominal pain or hematuria following mild trauma always raises the suspicion of a renal mass or a congenital renal anomaly and deserves further evaluation. Although malignant hypertension has been described as a rare presenting feature, hypertension is not a usual finding. Other presenting symptoms can be related to intracaval and intracardiac tumor thrombus extension.

The diagnostic studies are aimed at uncovering the origin and nature of the mass and at radiographic and biochemical staging of the extent of disease. When a renal mass is suspected, abdominal sonography is the initial study of choice, replacing the intravenous pyelogram. The sonogram will confirm that the mass is of renal origin and assists in the visualization of the inferior vena cava. Because half the patients with caval tumor extension have no symptoms or signs that would make its presence suspect, routine visualization of the inferior vena cava is desirable (Fig. 46.1) (21). Magnetic resonance imaging (MRI) may, however, be superior to all other modalities combined for inferior vena cava visualization (22). Further experience is necessary to validate this hypothesis.

If the mass is large and/or not clearly of renal origin, computed tomography (CT) is the next study of choice following the initial sonogram. Although staging requires information derived from surgery and pathology, the CT scan can provide valuable insight in terms of what operative findings can be anticipated and the extent of the disease. In addition, the CT will provide some information about kidney function and, in particular, about the normal kidney. Nonvisualization or nonfunction of the affected kidney is further suggestive of renal vein thrombosis or tumor invasion of the renal pelvis (23, 24). Thus, nonvisualization is an indication for retrograde ureteropyelography. CT visualization of the inferior vena cava can be difficult, and false-positive results have been reported.

The CT scan is also useful in the follow-up of patients receiving chemotherapy after the initial surgical exploration. There is controversy regarding the accuracy of CT scanning in detecting contralateral small synchronous lesions; the CT scan is likely to miss small lesions (1 to 3 cm), some of which could harbor tumors with discordant pathologic findings (compared with the main tumor) (25). Therefore, it would appear wise not to rely on the CT scan alone and explore the contralateral kidney at the time of surgery for the presence or absence of synchronous

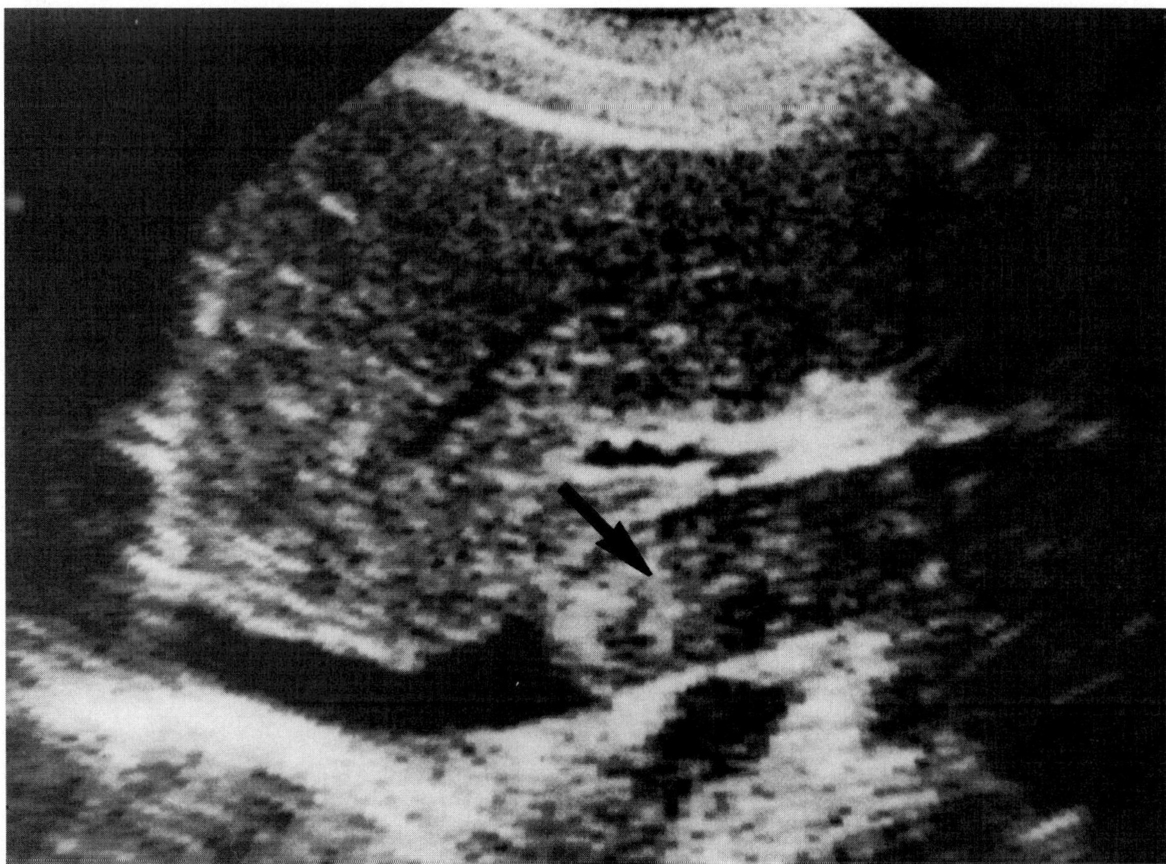

Fig. 46.1. Ultrasound appearance of tumor thrombus in the inferior vena cava (arrow) of a patient with Wilms' tumor.

tumors. Gross or microscopic hematuria are evaluated preoperatively with cystoscopy and retrograde studies as tumor metastases to the ureter, bladder, and urethra have been reported (26).

In addition to the above, a plain radiograph of the chest in four projections is required. The routine performance of a CT scan of the chest does not seem to be warranted when the initial chest radiograph is normal. The need for additional studies depends on the presence of specific signs and symptoms.

Currently, there are several biochemical tumor markers specific for Wilms' tumors that are undergoing scrutiny. Examples of serum markers include renin and neuron-specific enolase (27). Examples of both serum and urine markers include hyaluronic acid, hyaluronidase, and hyaluronic acid stimulating activity (28). The value of these markers in the assessment of response to treatment is an area of intense current interest and investigation.

Follow-up imaging for nonmetastatic disease consists of chest radiographs obtained every 3 months for 2 years, every 6 months for 1 year, and yearly thereafter for another 2 years. An abdominal sonogram is performed yearly and more frequently if the original tumor was associated with nephroblastomatosis. Skeletal surveys of the lumbosacral spine and pelvis are done yearly until full growth. When radiation therapy is used, skeletal surveys are done every 5 years indefinitely to detect second-

ary neoplasms such as osteochondroma. The frequency of these studies is increased for anaplastic tumors. Additional follow-up studies are obtained as clinically indicated.

PATHOLOGY AND STAGING

Treatment and prognosis are determined by tumor stage and histologic type. Staging is done surgically and pathologically. The presence or absence of vascular extension beyond the hilum is carefully ascertained. Staging requires careful exploration of the contralateral normal kidney (see below) and biopsies of any discovered lesions. Although a formal lymph node dissection has not been advocated, it is highly desirable to include a sampling of lymph nodes for microscopic examination in the final pathologic specimen in addition to the primary tumor. The importance of hilar, paraaortic, and paracaval lymph node sampling is best exemplified by the dramatic decrease in mortality between the National Wilms' Tumors Studies 1 and 3 as a result of a more intense regimen of chemotherapy in patients in whom the presence of lymph node metastases was recognized pathologically (29). Beyond the lymph nodes, the renal capsule, hilar fat, and tumor pseudocapsule are carefully examined and evaluated for the presence of metastases (Fig. 46.2). The specimen is also carefully evaluated for the presence of nephrogenic

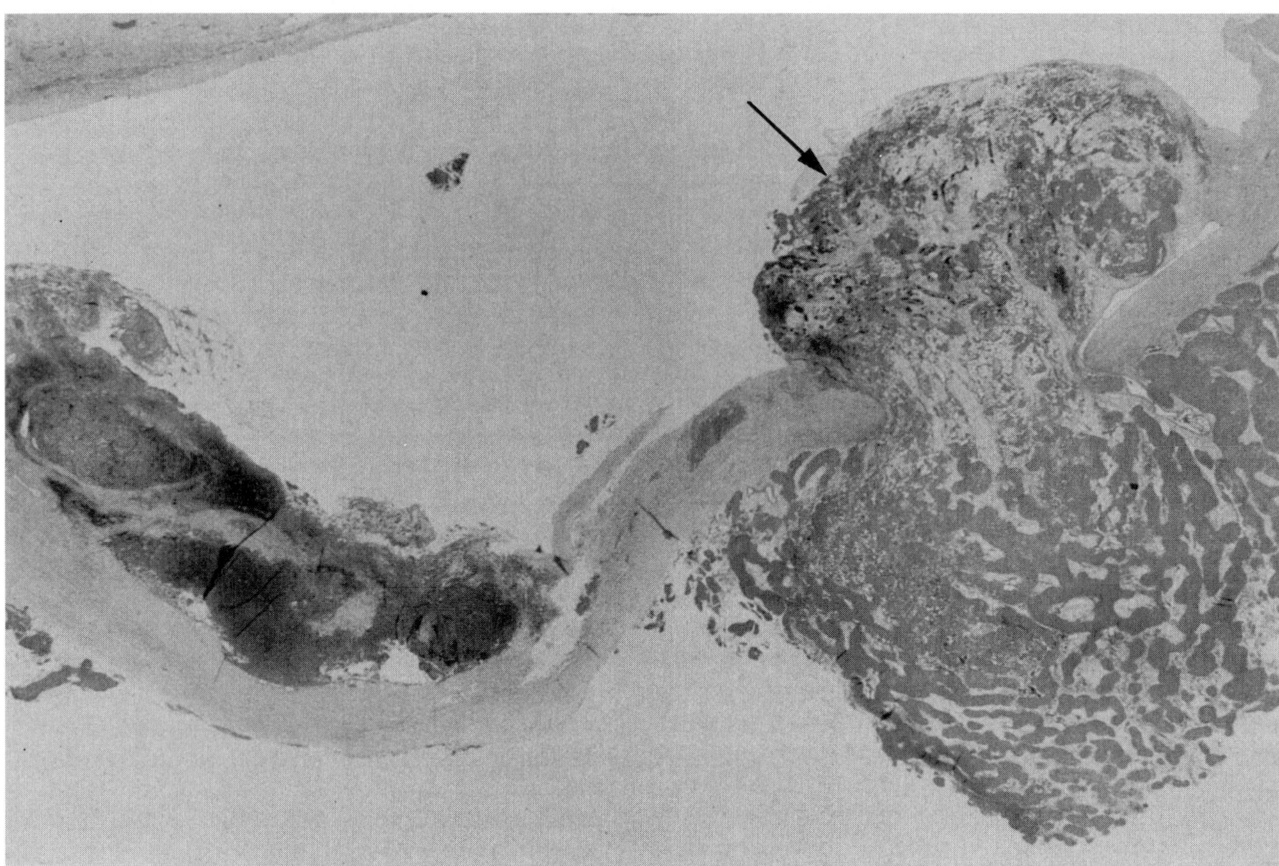

Fig. 46.2. Example of capsular penetration by Wilms' tumor cells (arrow) that was only apparent microscopically and on one section.

rests, previously termed nodular renal blastema or nephroblastomatosis (30). The significance of microstaging in this manner is not fully appreciated at this time. Future studies may allow microstaging to be useful in the identification of patients with tumors of favorable histologic type and low stage, who nevertheless may be at risk for relapse (31). In one study, the following factors were found to be associated with relapse: the presence of an inflammatory pseudocapsule, invasion of the tumor capsule, involvement of the renal sinus, and tumor in intrarenal vessels. Conversely, the absence of these features may help identify patients with stage I disease in whom nephrectomy alone may be curative.

The classic Wilms' tumor has a favorable histologic type and consists of a mixture of blastematous, epithelial, and stromal elements, leading to a triphasic appearance. Heterotopic cell types (adipose tissue, cartilage, muscle cells, and even bone) can be encountered, and biphasic and monophasic architectural appearances are common. Anaplasia occurs in 5% of patients and is a poor prognostic sign, associated with increased rates of relapse and mortality (7). It can be focal or diffuse; therefore, thorough sampling of the tumor is essential. The presence of mitotic figures, nuclear enlargement, and hyperchromasia are the hallmarks of anaplasia. Clear cell sarcoma (CCSK) and rhabdoid tumor of the kidney are now considered variants of Wilms'

tumor, whereas they previously represented unfavorable histologic subtypes. CCSK is also known as the bone metastasizing tumor, and the outcome of its treatment has significantly improved with the addition of doxorubicin (32). Rhabdoid tumor of the kidney can spread to the brain in addition to bone.

The combination of the surgical and pathologic findings allows staging to be completed. This is of utmost importance because treatment is initially driven by tumor stage (Table 46.1). Understaging can result in undertreatment, with potential relapse and mortality; overstaging can result in overtreatment and the potential for increased short-term and long-term morbidity.

SURGICAL ASPECTS

Surgery is the foundation on which so many essential aspects of the overall outcome depend. The surgeon has several objectives to fulfill as part of the multidisciplinary team of specialists caring for the child with a Wilms' tumor. For the purposes of this discussion, these objectives can be separated as follows.

1. Staging of the disease.
2. Extirpation of the tumor.
3. Special objectives/situations.

Table 46.1. Current Staging of Wilms' Tumor

Stage I	Tumor limited to kidney, completely excised; capsular surface intact; no tumor rupture; no residual tumor apparent beyond margins of resection
Stage II	Tumor extends beyond kidney but is completely excised; regional extension of tumor; vessel infiltration; tumor biopsied or local spillage of tumor confined to the flank; no residual tumor apparent at or beyond margins of excision
Stage III	Residual nonhematogenous tumor confined to the abdomen; lymph node involvement of hilus, periaortic chains, or beyond; diffuse peritoneal contamination by tumor spillage or peritoneal implants of tumor; tumor extends beyond surgical margins either microscopically or macroscopically; tumor not completely removable because of local infiltration into vital structures
Stage IV	Deposits beyond stage III, i.e., lung, liver, bone, brain
Stage V	Bilateral renal involvement at diagnosis

To accomplish these objectives, the patient is prepared overnight with adequate hydration. The appropriate amount of blood for size is prepared and made available in the operating room for the day of surgery. If indicated, diagnostic cystoscopic examination with or without retrograde studies is performed following the induction of a general anesthetic. A central venous line is inserted that can subsequently serve as a portal for chemotherapy and blood drawing postoperatively. Our preference is for the external jugular or the anterior facial vein on either side. The choice of catheters is determined by patient age and size and varies from the smaller Broviac catheters to the larger Hickman catheters (33). After insertion of the central line, the patient is positioned for a transverse transperitoneal incision starting at the level of the tip of the 12th rib on the involved side and extending just across the midline. To facilitate exposure, the patient is positioned supine with a rolled towel elevating the involved side. A Foley catheter is inserted to monitor urine output.

Surgical Staging

The abdomen is thoroughly explored. The extent and mobility of the tumor are carefully assessed. The liver and paraaortic and hilar lymph nodes are palpated for size and consistency. At this point and before proceeding with primary excision of the tumor, the contralateral kidney is examined. This is done by opening Gerota's fascia and mobilizing the kidney anteriorly and posteriorly. Both surfaces are palpated and visually inspected. Nephrogenic rests appear grossly as white to pink lesions 2 to 3 cm thick with a rubber-like consistency (Fig. 46.3). When these or any other lesions are present, they are biopsied. If the intraoperative diagnosis of bilateral Wilms' tumor is made, the procedure is terminated (see subsequent discussion). The reported incidence of bilateral synchronous disease is approximately 5% (34). In the more likely event of

a negative contralateral exploration and if the tumor is resectable, one can proceed with complete surgical extirpation (see below). After nephrectomy, the hilar, paraaortic, and paracaval lymph nodes are sampled for subsequent histologic examination. It is worthwhile remembering that when the surgeon is confident that the lymph nodes are negative, the pathologist almost always agrees. However, the converse is confirmed in only 39% of cases (35).

Extirpation of the Tumor

The retroperitoneum is exposed following medial mobilization and reflection of the overlying colon. The tumor is handled very gently to avoid rupture and spillage. Intraoperative spillage upstages the disease and places the patient at risk for intraabdominal recurrence (20). The renal vein is usually splayed over the tumor and deserves careful handling. If the renal artery and vein are free of involvement or encroachment, they are ligated before tumor mobilization. Otherwise, the tumor is mobilized staying outside of Gerota's fascia. Although a radical nephrectomy may not offer any statistically appreciable advantages in terms of patient survival, it may allow for a clean and complete tumor extirpation in the individual patient. Following mobilization of the tumor, the ureter is divided as far distally as possible. If the hilar vessels have not been previously ligated, they are individually ligated at this time. With large tumors, the hilar anatomy may be distorted and it is of vital importance have to identify the contralateral renal vessels, the superior mesenteric artery, and even the aorta before their ligation. The above arteries have been erroneously ligated (36). In addition, the renal vein is carefully palpated before ligation to exclude intravascular tumor extension. Intracaval extension is identified before exploration, allowing for adequate preparation. Although excision of all tumor is desirable, heroic attempts at accomplishing this objective are counterproductive. Small amounts of residual tumor respond well to chemotherapy and do not influence the survival, stage for stage. In addition, significant complications are associated with resection of contiguous visceral organs that may be involved with disease (37). When only a formidable operation can accomplish total extirpation of the tumor, shrinkage with chemotherapy and/or radiation therapy may facilitate removal at a later date and avoid significant morbidity. Residual and nonresectable tumors are outlined with titanium clips for facilitation of subsequent radiation therapy when the latter becomes necessary. This will also facilitate subsequent CT visualization of these areas.

Special Surgical Objectives/Situations

Bilateral Disease at Presentation

The preoperative knowledge of the presence (or suspicion) of bilateral disease as suggested by imaging studies does not preclude a surgical exploration. The purpose of such exploration

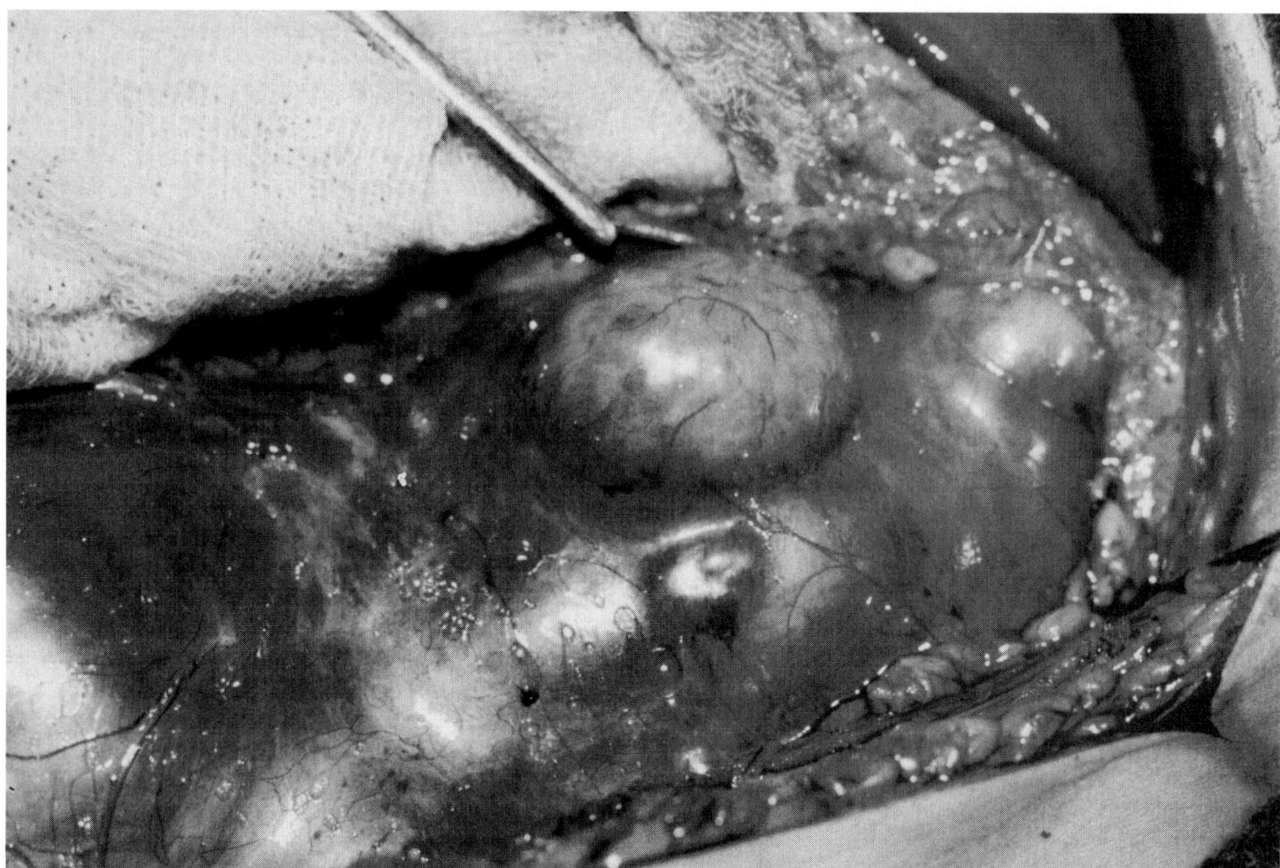

Fig. 46.3.   Contralateral normal kidney that, at exploration, had the typical appearance of nephroblastomatosis.

is for careful staging as outlined previously. In addition, even with current advances in imaging modalities, 7% of patients with synchronous bilateral Wilms' tumor will go unrecognized if formal surgical exploration of the contralateral kidney is omitted (Fig. 46.3) (25).

The exploration includes generous biopsies from both kidney lesions and a sampling of perihilar lymph nodes. Because anticipated chemotherapy may render the lymph nodes negative, their omission from the staging process may result in undertreatment and place the patient at subsequent risk for local recurrence. The former practice of performing a nephrectomy of the more involved side followed by a partial nephrectomy of the least involved side has been abandoned. The current recommendation is initial biopsy only followed by chemotherapy that is guided by the most advanced stage. An interval imaging study (usually a CT) is obtained to monitor the response. As long as there is continuous tumor shrinkage, chemotherapy is continued until the second-look procedure (Fig. 46.4). This approach results in maximal preservation of renal tissue while maintaining an excellent survival rate of 80% and the lowest morbidity (38). Using this approach, nearly 75% of renal units were preserved in the NWTS series. Nephrectomy is performed as a last resort. The timing of the second look procedure depends on the response to chemotherapy.

1. It can be as early as 6 weeks if there is excellent response or, conversely, if the tumor progressively enlarges (40).
2. It can be as late as 6 months as long as progressive response is documented.
3. It can be 3 months, if there is no or minimal response.

The purpose of the second-look procedure is to perform a partial nephrectomy or an excisional biopsy, if all tumor can be removed. If this is not possible, biopsies are obtained and chemotherapy is continued with the addition of radiation therapy to one or both sides. The objective of a third look, the timing of which is dictated by the response to combination therapy, is to extirpate all tumor while preserving as much renal tissue as possible. Bilateral nephrectomy followed by dialysis is an undesirable option, exercised only as a last resort.

Massive Disease at Presentation

Impressive shrinkage of unilateral tumors following chemotherapy is well documented (Fig. 46.5) (40). In addition, as a result of chemotherapy, a thick capsule is produced around the tumor. This decreases the possibility of likely intraoperative spillage and in some cases allows for partial nephrectomy as the definitive treatment. Because the incidence of surgical com-

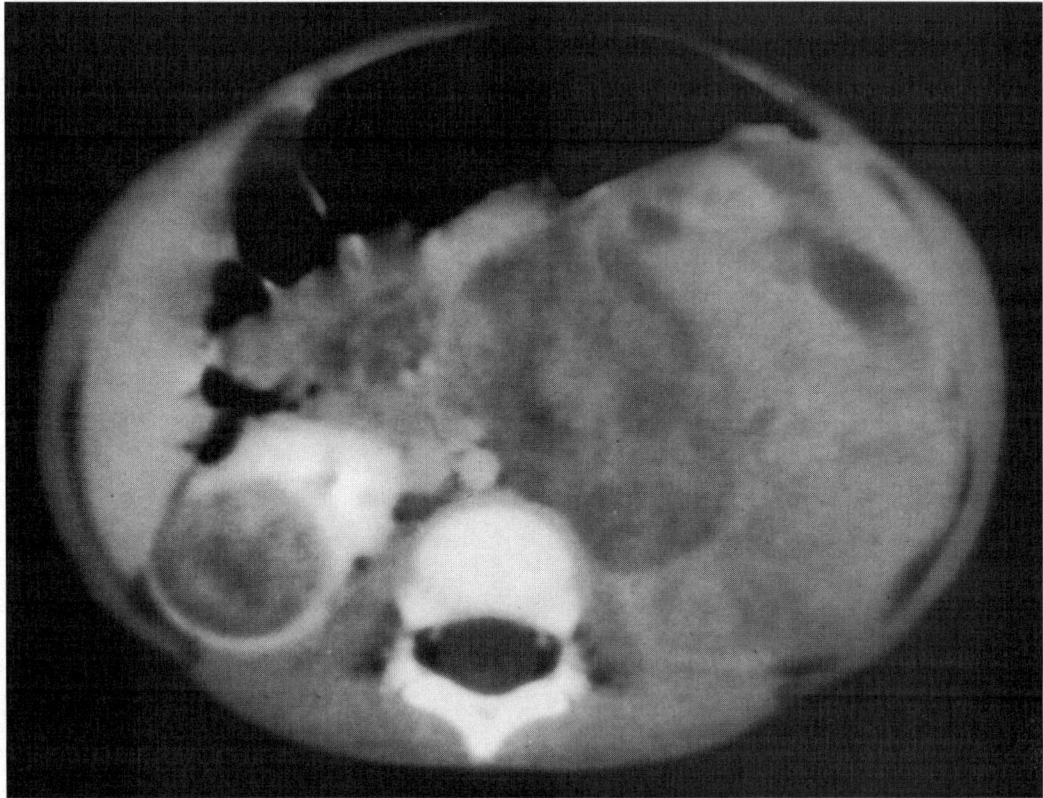

Fig. 46.4.   CT appearance of bilateral Wilms' tumor of favorable histologic type at presentation.

plications increases dramatically when heroic attempts are undertaken to excise large tumors surgically, it would seem prudent to initiate chemotherapy on these patients after the initial exploratory staging procedure as outlined above. Furthermore, when en bloc excision of large tumors is associated with the removal of contiguous visceral organs that appear to be grossly involved, only 17% are subsequently shown to be histologically involved (37). Thus, preoperative shrinkage can potentially spare the removal of adjacent visceral organs. The same guidelines that apply to chemotherapy and radiation therapy in the context of bilateral disease can be followed when massive and unresectable disease is encountered at initial exploration (41, 42).

Tumor Extension Into the Vena Cava/Right Atrium

Tumor extension into the extrarenal renal vein occurs in 11.3% of patients and into the vena cava and right atrium in an additional 4% (43). Renal vein involvement alone is rarely apparent preoperatively, and its presence does not present a formidable intraoperative problem. Involvement beyond the renal vein can consist of a free-floating thrombus that can be extracted even when extending to the right atrium. When tumor thrombus is adherent to the wall of the cava, it can still be extracted, but vena caval infiltration often requires its partial or total resection. Fortunately, involvement of the cava does not alter prog-

nosis or survival. Nevertheless, major complications have occurred in 43% of patients who underwent surgical excision of a vena caval thrombus. Therefore, preoperative chemotherapy as a meaningful alternative has recently received renewed attention (44, 45). Although complete response with resolution of the tumor thrombus cannot be expected in all patients, it does occur in the majority. The major concern revolves around the risk of tumor embolization during chemotherapy and it appears to be minimal. To the contrary, the use of preoperative chemotherapy appears to facilitate tumor resection in the majority of cases and results in a significant decrease in morbidity. As an example, median sternotomy was avoided in 70% of patients with atrial extension in whom preoperative chemotherapy was administered (45). It appears that preoperative chemotherapy following an open biopsy may be indicated in cases in which invasion of the cava is suspected and the tumor thrombus extends above the level of the hepatic veins. It is currently unclear whether a skinny-needle biopsy of the tumor combined with imaging studies is sufficient for the proper selection of the chemotherapeutic regimen and/or whether radiation therapy will be required.

The preceding discussion of the surgical aspects of the treatment of this tumor is the product of two decades of advances. Surgical complications continue to occur, albeit at a lower rate. In their review of 1910 nephrectomies in the NWTS-3, Ritchey et al. have identified a 20% surgical complication rate (37). In

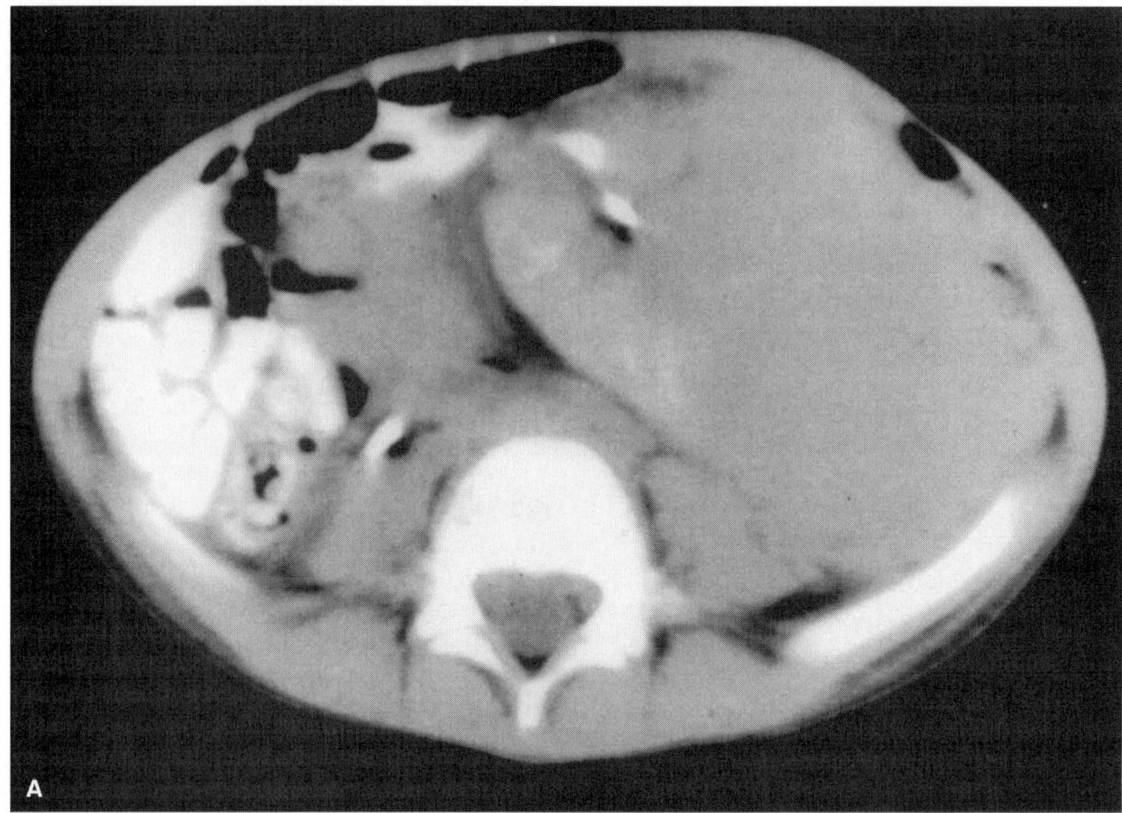

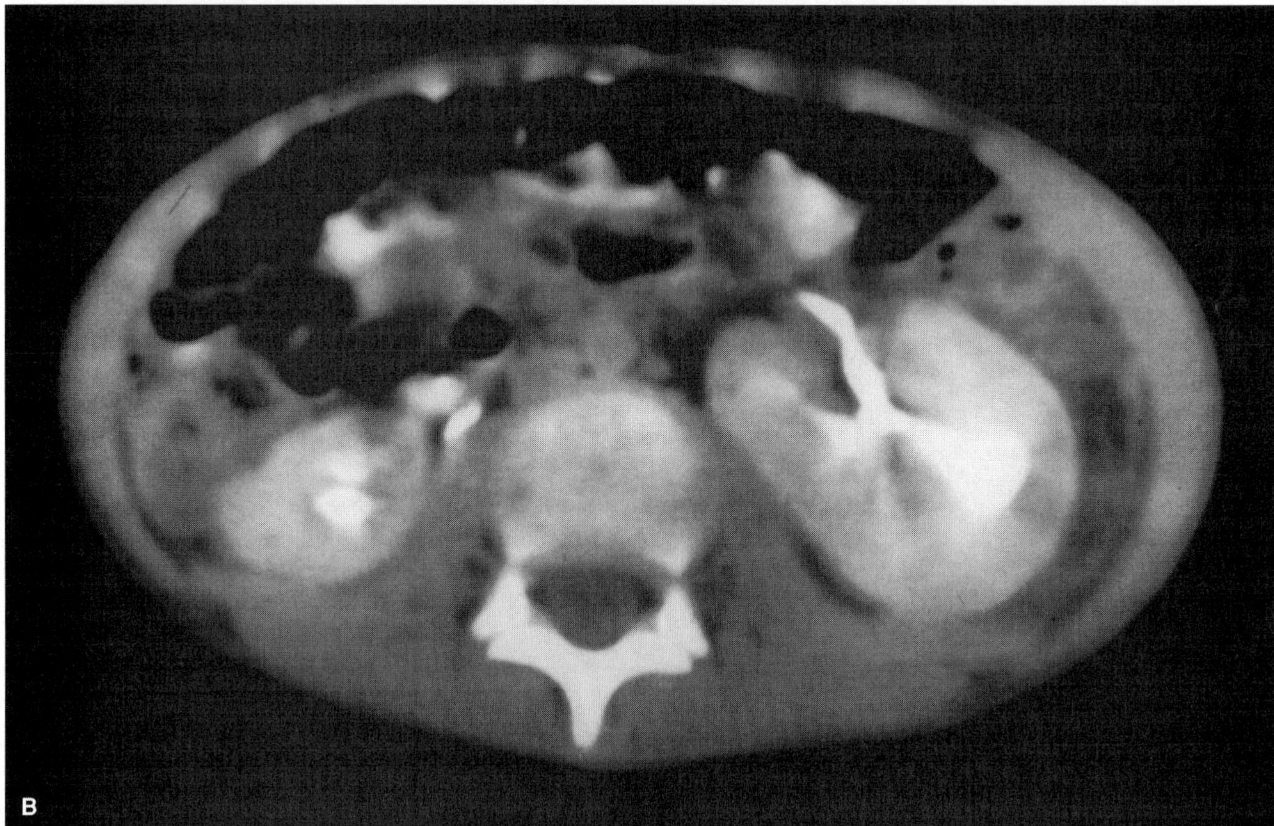

Fig. 46.5.   Dramatic Wilms' tumor shrinkage after chemotherapy. **A.** Before chemotherapy. **B.** After chemotherapy.

Table 46.2.   National Wilms' Tumor Study 4 Protocol

DISEASE	INITIAL THERAPY	RADIATION THERAPY	CHEMOTHERAPY REGIMEN
Stage I/FH	Surgery	None	AMD + VCR (24 wk)
Stage I/anaplastic			Pulsed, intensive AMD + VCR (18 wk)[a]
Stage II/FH	Surgery	None	AMD + VCR (22 and 65 wk)
			Pulsed, intensive AMD + VCR (18 and 60 wk)[a]
Stage III/FH	Surgery	10.8 cGy	AMD + VCR + ADR (26 and 65 wk)
			Pulsed, intensive AMD + VCR + ADR (24 and 54 wk)[a]
High risk (clear cell sarcoma, all stages) and stage IV/FH	Surgery	Yes[b]	AMD + VCR + ADR (65 wk)
			AMD + VCR + ADR + C (65 wk)[a]

From Mesrobian H-GJ. Wilms' tumor: past, present future. J Urol 1988;140:231.

FH, favorable histologic type; AMD, actinomycin D; VCR, vincristine; ADR, doxorubicin; C, cyclophosphamide.

[a] Latest National Wilms' Tumor Study protocol for dosage and length of treatment

[b] Patients with clear cell sarcoma receive 10.8 cGy, and those with stage IV cancer of favorable histologic type are given 10.8 cGy if the primary tumor would qualify as stage III were there no metastasis.

order of decreasing frequency, these complications consisted of small bowel obstruction, major intraoperative hemorrhage, wound infection, vascular injury, and injury to other organs. These complications led to nine deaths, one of which was intraoperative. The factors that were associated with an increased incidence of such complications were advanced tumor stage at diagnosis, intravascular tumor extension, resection of visceral organs at the time of nephrectomy, and thoracoabdominal incisions. The surgical plan of therapy proposed above draws on this experience; it is our belief that as a result, future series will show a significant decrease in surgical morbidity.

POSTOPERATIVE THERAPY

Postoperative therapy principles are geared toward accomplishing improvement in the cure rate while minimizing the intensity and duration of therapy. Significant advances have been made toward this objective by the NWTS group, which has just closed its fourth trial. Treatment results will not be available until at least 2 additional years of follow-up have passed. In the interim, new patients continue to be treated and randomized according to the NWTS-4 guidelines (Table 46.2). It is anticipated that the excellent results obtained with the NWTS-3 will be maintained or enhanced with less hematologic toxicity (Table 46.3).

Conventional therapy consists of combination chemotherapy with actinomycin D (AMD) and vincristine (VCR), which is adequate for stage I favorable histology (FH) and unfavorable histology (UH) and stage II FH. Radiation therapy is not required. Adriamycin (ADR) is added to the regimen for stage III patients with FH in conjunction with radiation therapy. Patients with stage II to IV anaplastic tumors currently receive either the three-drug combination (AMD + VCR + ADR) or in addition receive cyclophosphamide (CPM). They all receive radiation therapy. Stage IV patients with FH are randomized in a similar manner. The intensive chemotherapy protocols have recently been shown to be safe (46).

Table 46.3.   National Wilms' Tumor Study 3 Results

HISTOLOGIC TYPE/STAGE	NO. OF PATIENTS	% RELAPSE-FREE	
		AT 2 YR	AT 4 YR
FH/I	306	90.9	89.0
	301	92.3	91.8
FH/II	70	91.2	87.9
	71	88.5	86.9
	67	89.2	87.4
	70	92.5	90.1
FH/III	68	83.7	82.0
	66	85.9	85.9
	71	71.4	71.4
	70	78.3	76.8
FH/IV	64	71.9	71.9
	56	80.0	77.9
UH/I–III	69	68.7	67.1
	61	70.6	62.4
UH/IV	12	58.3	58.3
	17	52.9	52.9

FH, favorable histologic type; UH, unfavorable histologic type.

Modified from D'Angio GJ, Breslow N, Beckwith JB, et al: Treatment of Wilms' Tumor: results of the Third National Wilms' Tumor Study. Cancer 64:349 1989.

METASTATIC DISEASE

Evidence of hematogenous dissemination at the time of diagnosis is present in 12% of patients (47). These patients have an excellent prognosis, especially if their tumor is of the FH variety. It is the patients who have relapse with metastatic disease, and especially UH, who have a poor prognosis. The majority of these metastases are pulmonary and are treated with chemotherapy and radiation. Surgical resection of pulmonary nodules will rarely be indicated. However, in an attempt to reduce the incidence of postirradiation interstitial pneumonitis, chemotherapy alone followed by resection of residual pulmonary metastases has been used with satisfactory results (48). The presence of singular or multiple hepatic lesions at presentation does not alter the treatment approach to the primary tumor. In this setting, the surprising survival rate is 72% at 4 years when dealing with FH. In contradistinction, relapse to the liver carries a poor prognosis, and surgical resection of residual metastatic disease does not offer any additional advantage.

LATE EFFECTS

As the number of survivors of Wilms' tumor increases, it is expected that the late effects of treatment may become increasingly prominent concerns for patients and physicians alike. Side effects of treatment have virtually included all organs and systems (2, 49–52). Although modern chemotherapeutic regimens may have reduced or eliminated many side effects, late sequelae of treatment may continue to be shown. The effects on renal and pulmonary function, effects on the musculoskeletal system, and appearance of secondary malignancies may become more prominent. It appears that there may be a reduction in overall renal function, with the appearance of diastolic hypertension and proteinuria in some patients. When radiation therapy is used on the solitary kidney, significant renal dysfunction is more likely to appear. The use of radiation therapy for pulmonary metastases may decrease total lung volume and capacity, but not at the expense of normal gas exchange. In addition, radiation therapy is likely to potentiate injury resulting from the use of chemotherapeutic agents such as doxorubicin and actinomycin, especially on the liver and gastrointestinal tract.

Second tumors can occur as early as 1 year after treatment. The most common ones are osteochondroma followed by acute leukemia. Interestingly, WT1 mRNA expression has recently been identified in non-Wilms' malignancies, including 50% of acute leukemias (53). Therefore, it would be desirable to find out if mutations in the WT1 gene play a role in the pathogenesis of these malignancies. If that proved to be the case, then acute leukemias occurring in patients treated for Wilms' tumors would not be considered secondary to treatment, but as another manifestation of a genetic predisposition to malignancies. Thus, survivors of Wilms' tumors require lifelong follow-up.

NEW APPROACHES TO TREATMENT

Partial Nephrectomy

The concerns summarized above regarding the long-term effects of treatment on renal function have appropriately led to the search for methods to maximize renal parenchymal preservation. At the one extreme are patients with bilateral disease at presentation and in whom initial biopsy only, followed by combination therapy, has resulted in preserving renal function while maintaining an excellent cure rate. It was therefore natural to consider partial nephrectomy for unilateral disease. Because most unilateral tumors are too large at presentation for

partial nephrectomy to be feasible, preoperative chemotherapy is administered following an initial biopsy. In their series of partial nephrectomy in patients with unilateral disease, McLorie et al. reported a postchemotherapy mean tumor shrinkage rate of 77% and an 89% survival rate, with a mean follow-up of 24 months (3). Careful and frequent imaging is critical to overall management. The concerns regarding the possibility of undertreatment secondary to the downstaging that is expected to result from preoperative chemotherapy must be addressed on a larger scale. Nevertheless, this approach may further decrease the surgical morbidity by facilitating the performance of the operation and result in better preservation of long-term overall renal function.

Surgery Only

It would seem ironic to consider the elimination of postoperative chemotherapy and radiation therapy from the treatment protocol of patients with Wilms' tumors because historically, it was their sequential addition that improved survival to the contemporary levels (2). Nevertheless, the identification of pathologic features in stage I patients that allows the prediction of a relapse-free recovery, makes such a proposition cogent (32). In addition, the treatment outcome in patients younger than 2 years of age with small stage I and FH tumors is excellent. With this in mind, the desire to minimize the side effects of postoperative chemotherapy (in this instance by eliminating it) makes surgery alone an attractive proposition in this highly select group of patients. Larsen et al. have reported on eight such patients treated by nephrectomy alone who are alive and free of disease, with a mean follow-up of 5 years (54). It is worthwhile emphasizing that these patients were surgically and pathologically staged. With future identification of markers that may help detect patients at risk (who would then be the subjects of a careful screening process), earlier identification of Wilms' tumors might result in the possibility of a more widespread application of this approach.

FUTURE DIRECTIONS

In addition to the above concepts, the future may be enhanced by the identification of molecular and other biologic markers that might further stage the disease and help refine therapy or stimulate the search for newer and more effective modes of therapy. Examples include hyaluronic acid and p53 mutations (55). Tumors that harbor the p53 mutation are anaplastic and less likely to respond to conventional therapy (20), thus emphasizing the need for additional forms of therapy. Alternatively, for the majority of patients, it may be that earlier identification of tumors may lead to the detection of a higher number of individuals with lower-stage disease, the treatment of which may result in lower morbidity. Furthermore, the frequency of relapses may decrease. Efforts directed at the investigation of the etiology of Wilms' tumors and their variable biologic behaviors may ultimately result in prevention.

REFERENCES

1. Young JL, Miller RW. Incidence of malignant tumors in U.S. children. J Pediatr 1975;86:254.

2. Mesrobian H-GJ. Wilms tumor: past, present, future. J Urol 1988;140:231.

3. McLorie GA, McKenna PH, Greenburg M, et al. Reduction in tumor burden allowing partial nephrectomy following preoperative chemotherapy in biopsy proved Wilms' tumor. J Urol 1991;146:509.

4. Larsen E, Perez-Atayde A, Green DM, et al. Surgery only for the treatment of patients with stage I (Cassady) Wilms' tumor. Cancer 1990;66:264.

5. Green DM, Fine NE, Li FP. Offspring of patients treated for unilateral Wilms' tumor in childhood. Cancer 1982;49:2285.

6. Olshan AF, Breslow NE, Falletta JM, et al. Risk factors for Wilms tumor: report from the National Wilms Tumor Study. Cancer 1993;72:938.

7. Kelalis PP, Mesrobian H-GJ. Tumors of the upper urinary tract. In: Kelalis P, King L, Belman A, eds. Clinical pediatric urology. 3rd ed. Philadelphia: WB Saunders, 1992;2:1415.

8. Green DM, Breslow NE, Beckwith JB, et al. Screening of children with hemihypertrophy, aniridia, and Beckwith-Wiedemann syndrome in patients with Wilms' tumor: a report from the National Wilms Tumor Study. Med Pediatr Oncol 1993;21:188.

9. Coppes MJ, Haber DA, Grundy PE. Genetic events in the development of Wilms' tumor of the kidney. N Engl J Med 1994;331:586–590.

10. Call KM, Glaser T, Ito CY, et al. Isolation and characterization of a zinc finger polypeptide gene at the human chromosome 11 Wilms' tumor locus. Cell 1990;60:509–520.

11. Pelletier J. Molecular genetics of Wilms' tumor: insights into normal and abnormal renal development. Can J Oncol 1994;4:262–272.

12. Drummond IA, Madden SL, Rowher-Nutter P, et al. Repression of the insulin-like growth factor II gene by the Wilms' tumor suppressor gene WT1. Science 1992;257:674–678.

13. Park S, Tomlinson G, Nisen P, et al. Altered transactivational properties of a mutated WT1 gene product in a WAGR-associated Wilms' tumor. Cancer Res 1993;53:4757–4760.

14. Park S, Bernard A, Bove K. Inactivation of WT1 in nephrogenic rests, genetic precursors to Wilms' tumour. Nature Genet 1993;5:363–367.

15. Koufos A, Grundy P, Morgan K, et al. Familial Wiedemann-Beckwith syndrome and a second Wilms' tumor locus both map to 11p15.5. Am J Hum Genet 1989;44:711–719.

16. Joy Ping A, Reeve AE, Law DJ, et al. Genetic linkage of Beckwith-Wiedemann syndrome to 11p15. Am J Hum Genet 1989;44:720–723.

17. Schwartz CE, Haber DA, Stanton VP, et al. Familial predisposition to Wilms' tumor does not segregate with the WT1 gene. Genomics 1991;10:927–930.

18. Clarke AR, Purdie CA, Harrison DJ, et al. Thymocyte apoptosis induced by p53-Dependent and independent pathways. Nature 1993;362:849–852.

19. Lowe SW, Ruley HE, Jacks T, et al. p53-Dependent apoptosis modulates the cytotoxicity of anticancer agents. Cell 1993;74:957–967.

20. Ramsay NKC, Dehner LP, Coccia PF, et al. Acute hemorrhage into Wilms' tumor: a cause of rapidly developing abdominal mass with hypertension, anemia and fever. J Pediatr 1977;91:763.

21. Clayman RV, Sheldon CA, Gonzalez R. Wilms' tumor: an approach to vena caval intrusion. Prog Pediatr Surg 1982;15:285.

22. Roubidoux MA, Dunnick NR, Sostman HD, et al. Renal carcinoma: detection of venous extension with gradient-echo MR imaging. Radiology 1992;182:269–272.

23. Johnson KM, Horvath LJ, Gaisie G, et al. Wilms tumor occurring as a botryoid renal pelvicalyceal mass. Radiology 1987;163:385.

24. Canty TG, Nagaraj HS, Shearer LS. Nonvisualization of the intravenous pyelogram: a poor prognostic sign in Wilms' tumor? J Pediatr Surg 1979;14:825.

25. Ritchey M, Pringle K, Breslow N, et al. Accuracy of current imaging modalities in the diagnosis of synchronous bilateral Wilms tumor. Cancer In press.

26. Pagano F, Pennelli N. Ureteral and vesical metastases in nephroblastoma. Br J Urol 1974;46:409.

27. Johnston MA, Carachi R, Lindop GBM, et al. Inactive renin levels in recurrent nephroblastoma. J Pediatr Surg 1991;26:613–614.

28. Stern M, Longaker MT, Adzick NS, et al. Hyaluronidase levels in urine from Wilms' tumor patients. J Natl Cancer Inst 1991;83:1569–1574.

29. Breslow NE, Churchill G, Nesmith B, et al. Clinicopathologic features and prognosis for Wilms' tumor patients with metastases at diagnosis. Cancer 1986;58:2501.

30. Beckwith JB, Kiviat NB, Bonadio JF. Nephrogenic rests, nephroblastomatosis, and the pathogenesis of Wilms' tumor. Pediatr Pathol 1990;10:1–36.

31. Weeks DA, Beckwith JB, Luckey DW. Relapse-associated variables in stage I favorable histology Wilms' tumor: a report of the National Wilms' Tumor Study. Cancer 1987;60:1204.

32. D'Angio GJ, Breslow N, Beckwith JB, et al. Treatment of Wilms' tumor: results of the Third National Wilms' Tumor Study. Cancer 1989;64:349–360.

33. Springer JC, Azizkhan RG, Mesrobian H-GJ. Continuous venous access in children with urological diseases. J Urol 1989;141:364–366.

34 Blute ML, Kelalis PP, Offord KP, et al. Bilateral Wilms' tumor. J Urol 1987;138:968.

35. Leape LL, Breslow NE, Bishop HC. The surgical treatment of Wilms' tumor: results of the National Wilms Tumor Study. Ann Surg 1987;187:351.

36. Ritchey ML, Lally KP, Haase GM, et al. Superior mesenteric artery injury during nephrectomy for Wilms' tumor. J Pediatr Surg 1992;25:1–2.

37. Ritchey ML, Kelalis PP, Breslow N, et al. Surgical complications after nephrectomy for Wilms' tumor. Surg Gynecol Obstet 1992;175:508–514.

38. Shaul DB, Srikanth MM, Ortega JA, et al. Treatment of bilateral Wilms' tumor: comparison of initial biopsy and chemotherapy to initial surgical resection in the preservation of renal mass and function. J Pediatr Surg 1992;27:1009–1015.

39. Kelalis PP. Bilateral tumor: surgical treatment: NWTS recommendations. Dialog Pediatr Urol 1985;8:6.

40. Voute PA, Tournade MF, Delamarre JF, et al. Preoperative

chemotherapy (CT) as 1st treatment in children with Wilms' tumor: results of the SIOP nephroblastoma trials and studies. Med Pediatr Oncol 1987;15:323. Abstract.

41. Gough DCS. Wilms' tumor: trials and tribulation. Prog Pediatr Surg 1985;22:94–105.

42. Bracken RB, Sutow WW, Jaffe N, et al. Preoperative chemotherapy for Wilms' tumor. Urology 1982;19:55–60.

43. Ritchey ML, Kelalis PP, Breslow NE, et al. Intracaval and atrial involvement with nephroblastoma: review of National Wilms' Tumor Study-3. J Urol 1988;140:1113–1118.

44. Kogan SJ, Marans H, Santorineau M, et al. Successful treatment of renal vein and vena caval extension of nephroblastoma by preoperative chemotherapy. J Urol 1986; 136:312.

45. Ritchey ML, Kelalis PP, Haase GM, et al. Preoperative therapy for intracaval and atrial extension of Wilms tumor. Cancer 1993;71:4105–4110.

46. Green DM, Breslow NE, Evans I, et al. The effect of chemotherapy dose intensity on the hematological toxicity of the treatment for Wilms' tumor: a report from the National Wilms' Tumor Study. Am J Pediatr Hematol Oncol 1994;16: 207–212.

47. Breslow NE, Churchill G, Nesmith B, et al. Clinicopathologic features and prognosis for Wilms' tumor patients with metastases at diagnosis. Cancer 1986;58:2501–2511.

48. de Kraker J, Lemerle J, Voute PA, et al. Wilms' tumor with pulmonary metastases at diagnosis: the significance of primary chemotherapy. J Clin Oncol 1990;8:1187–1190.

49. Green DM. Effects of treatment for childhood cancer on vital organ systems. Cancer 1993;71:3299–3305.

50. Attard-Montalto SP, Kingston JE, Eden OB, et al. Late follow-up of lung function after whole lung irradiation for Wilms' tumour. Br J Radiol 1992;65:1114–1118.

51. Levitt GA, Yeomans E, Dicks Mireaux G, et al. Renal size and function after cure of Wilms' tumor. Br J Cancer 1992;66: 877–882.

52. Mpofu C, Mann JR. Urinary protein/creatinine index in follow-up of patients with Wilms' tumor after nephrectomy. Arch Dis Child 1992;67:1462–1466.

53. Miwa H, Beran M, Saunders GF. Expression of the Wilms' tumor gene (WT1) in human leukemias. Leukemia 1992;6: 405–409.

54. Larsen E, Atayde-Perez A, Green DM, et al. Surgery only for the treatment of patients with stage I (Cassady) Wilms' tumor. Cancer 1990;66:264–266.

55. Ritchey ML, Haase G, Shochat S. APSA Newsletter 11/14/ 1994.

56. Lowe SW, Ruley HE, Jacks T, et al. p53-Dependent apoptosis modulates the cytotoxicity of anticancer agents. Cell 1993;74: 957–967.

47

Management of Genitourinary Rhabdomyosarcoma in Children

Richard W. Sutherland
Edmond T. Gonzales, Jr.

Rhabdomyosarcoma is the fifth most common solid malignant tumor in childhood (behind central nervous system tumors, lymphoma, Wilms' tumor, and neuroblastoma) and is the most common soft tissue sarcoma. This tumor ranks seventh as a cause of death from cancer in childhood (1). Although these neoplasms can occur almost anywhere, nearly 20% arise within the true pelvis, primarily from the bladder, prostate, or vagina. In some instances, the tumor can only be classified as arising from an unspecified pelvic or retroperitoneal site. In advanced cases, it may not be possible to define an exact site of origin because these tumors tend to be locally aggressive and readily invade adjacent viscera. A smaller percentage of these tumors occur in the spermatic cord, usually in the immediate paratesticular area. Rhabdomyosarcomas occur at any age, although there are peaks in young childhood (2 to 6 years) and adolescence. Paratesticular lesions occur relatively more often in older age groups.

HISTOLOGIC CHARACTERISTICS AND GROWTH PATTERNS

Rhabdomyosarcomas are thought to arise from embryonic mesenchyme and, when they occur in the genitourinary region, their propensity for developing in the prostate, trigone, vagina, and immediate paratesticular areas suggests that they originate from cells of the urogenital sinus or mesenchymal tissue of the mesonephros (2, 3). Three histologic patterns of rhabdomyosarcoma are classically recognized: (1) embryonal, a pattern seen most commonly in young children; (2) alveolar, described most often in the adolescent and generally in tumors presenting in the extremity; and (3) pleomorphic rhabdomyosarcoma, more common in adults.

The embryonal form of rhabdomyosarcoma is typical of the histologic findings from tumors arising in the pelvic region. Embryonal rhabdomyosarcoma is characterized by a primitive mesenchyme with differentiation of some of the cellular elements to the embryonal rhabdomyoblast. The rhabdomyoblast assumes several different histologic characteristics but, if sufficiently differentiated, may form cross striations (a finding seen in approximately one third of cases). A significant component of mixed cells is also commonly present (4). Sarcoma botryoides is a term used to describe the large, bulky intraluminal polypoid masses growing under an epithelial layer. Sarcoma botryoides is typical of rhabdomyosarcoma of the bladder and vagina. Once thought to represent a separate category, these neoplasms also show a histologically typical embryonal pattern. The alveolar form of rhabdomyosarcoma is characterized by a structural alveolar pattern of spaces surrounded by fibrous stroma lined with neoplastic round cells. A solid variant of alveolar rhabdomyosarcoma that does not show alveolar spaces has also been included in this group (5).

Attempts have been made to classify rhabdomyosarcomas based on other cytologic characteristics. Palmer and Foulkes (6) reviewed the pathologic material from the Intergroup Rhabdomyosarcoma Study (IRS) and proposed that these tumors could be classified as monomorphous, anaplastic, and mixed. In the monomorphous variety, the cells are uniform in size with constant nuclear characteristics throughout the tumor. This particular variety of rhabdomyosarcoma has an unfavorable prognosis. In the anaplastic variety, there are many bizarre and enlarged mitotic figures that also indicate an unfavorable prognosis. Both of these varieties represent only approximately 20% of the total population of tumors studied. The mixed variety represents nearly 80% of all tumors in the IRS study group and bodes a more favorable prognosis. Tsokos and Triche (7) described a solid variant of rhabdomyosarcoma that lacked many of the classical histologic features of rhabdomyosarcomas. They were able to use immunocytochemical staining for muscle markers to identify this more primitive form of rhabdomyosarcoma from other round cell tumors of soft tissue, i.e., Ewing's sarcoma and peripheral neuroepithelioma.

Hawkins and Camacho-Velasquez studied 47 rhabdomyosarcomas from all sites and classified the tumors as either anaplastic or well differentiated (8). Distinction was not made among embryonal, alveolar, or pleomorphic varieties. This simpler histologic classification correlated well with ultimate survival—patients with anaplastic tumors did much worse than those whose tumors were well differentiated.

Recently, the classification of rhabdomyosarcoma by the major oncology groups (5, 9) has emphasized a combination of both cytologic and histologic form. Based on their analysis of patient survival and treatment, they proposed a classification system of the following.

1. BOT: Botryoid rhabdomyosarcoma.
2. SC: Spindle cell rhabdomyosarcoma.
3. E: Embryonal rhabdomyosarcoma.
4. A: Alveolar rhabdomyosarcoma.
5. UND: Sarcoma, undifferentiated.
6. NOS: Sarcoma, not otherwise specified.
7. WRG: Wrong diagnosis—none of the above.

Spindle cell rhabdomyosarcoma has been distinguished from embryonal cell rhabdomyosarcoma because of its high degree of skeletal muscle differentiation and its low malignancy rate.

Growth patterns of rhabdomyosarcoma are somewhat predictable. Lesions of the bladder and vagina tend to spread beneath the mucosa and are seen initially as clusters of intraluminal masses. Distant metastases are infrequent at the time of presentation. Tumors arising within the prostate or from nonvisceral undetermined pelvic sites tend to spread directly along fascial planes and to disseminate early by both hematogenous and lymphatic routes (10). Although the tumors often appear encapsulated, infiltration of malignant cells extends to and beyond the margin of the pseudocapsule. Raney et al. (11) studied the sites of origin for these tumors and correlated the sites with ultimate prognosis. This study demonstrated that tumors of the bladder, prostate, and vagina had a better prognosis than tumors arising from a nonvisceral pelvic wall location. They suggested in this study that this may simply be because the lesions that are easily seen (vaginal introitus tumors), or the lesions that are likely to cause urinary obstruction (bladder and prostate), are diagnosed earlier in the course of the disease than are the deeper pelvic lesions.

Most children initially present with symptoms secondary to local growth—a palpable suprapubic mass, a visible tumor at the vaginal introitus, or obstruction to urinary outflow. The data from IRS-III have shown that the genitourinary rhabdomyosarcomas have a significantly better outcome than rhabdomyosarcomas from other sites. Genitourinary rhabdomyosarcomas that do not involve the bladder neck or prostate (vagina, uterus, bladder dome) have the best outcome for all rhabdomyosarcomas regardless of the site of origin, with tumors that involve the bladder neck and prostate having only slightly worse results. Paratesticular neoplasms are recognized as solid, nontender scrotal masses. Because of local invasion, the testis may be indistinguishable from the mass. Retroperitoneal lymphatic spread can be expected to be present in one third of patients at the time of presentation.

TREATMENT: GENERAL CONSIDERATIONS

The treatment of rhabdomyosarcoma remains one of the more controversial topics in pediatric oncology. Before the now accepted management with multidisciplinary treatment, radical wide surgical excision was the only effective form of management for these tumors. As late as 1972, early radical extirpation was recommended for management of pelvic rhabdomyosarcoma (3). Limited or less aggressive surgical procedures were universally associated with local recurrences.

Chemotherapy

Before 1966, the use of chemotherapy in this disease was limited to individual agents used in the treatment of metastases (12–15). Responses were reported in up to 83% of cases, but these were usually of short duration. In 1966, James et al. first reported improved objective responses in one third of patients treated with a combination of actinomycin D and vincristine (16). In 1969, Grosfeld et al. also combined these agents, but used them in repeated courses, with prolonged survival in 12 of 18 patients (17). Shortly thereafter, several groups reported the use of a combined multidisciplinary approach to embryonal rhabdomyosarcoma arising in a variety of sites and introduced the concept of "reasonable" surgical treatment for this neoplasm: wide excision of the primary tumor, but without gross sacrifice of form or function (18–24). At the same time, Heyn et al. reported on a prospective, controlled, randomized study of 28 patients whose tumors had been completely resected or who had only microscopic residual tumors; 86% of patients were free of disease after 2 years when treated with a multidisciplinary protocol of surgery, radiation therapy, and combination chemotherapy (actinomycin D and vincristine)—a dramatic improvement in survival for this disease (25). A follow-up report of the original 28 children who achieved a complete response demonstrated that 24 (85.7%) remained disease free for at least 3 years (26).

Chemotherapeutic regimens have continued to change as new protocols are initiated and analyzed, and one should refer to the references given at the end of this chapter for dosages, schedules, and lengths of treatment. Most protocols have included both vincristine and actinomycin D (22) or these two agents in addition to cyclophosphamide and Adriamycin (27–29). Exelby has suggested an aggressive, seven-agent chemotherapeutic regimen that includes actinomycin D, cyclophosphamide, bleomycin, vincristine, Adriamycin, methotrexate, and BCNU (carmustine) (30).

Radiation Therapy

Concurrent with the development of effective chemotherapy was the observation of the benefit of radiation therapy for local control of these tumors, which extended the concept of a truly multidisciplinary approach to these lesions (31). Dritschilo et al. have reported that local control of the primary tumor from a variety of sites was achieved in 96% of patients who received radiation therapy, although the majority also received chemotherapy (32). Radiation therapy has become primary therapy for the local lesion of rhabdomyosarcoma of the orbit, head, and neck (27). Dosage at a level of 5000 to 6000 cGy is generally recommended.

Brachytherapy has been studied as an alternative to the external beam radiation that has been used in most protocols. Haie-Meder et al. used this form of radiation in a select group of 15 patients with genitourinary rhabdomyosarcoma. They had survival outcomes comparable to other protocols with minimal complications related to radiation to the bladder (33).

IRS

The IRS was organized in 1972 to evaluate various combinations of surgery, chemotherapy, and radiation therapy. In 1977, IRS-I published a most encouraging report (28). In this study, all patients underwent excision of the primary tumor (or biopsy if the neoplasm was unresectable or involved a vital structure) and were grouped according to the following classification.

- Group I: Localized disease, completely resected.
- Group II: Localized disease, microscopic residual tumor.
- Group IIA: Grossly resected tumor, microscopic residual tumor, no nodal involvement.
- Group IIB: Regional nodal disease, completely resected, no microscopic residual tumor.
- Group IIC: Regional nodal disease, grossly resected, but with evidence of microscopic residual tumor.
- Group III: Incomplete resection or biopsy with gross residual regional disease.
- Group IV: Distant metastases present at time of diagnosis.

We are now in the process of analyzing the data from IRS-III, with IRS-IV underway. IRS-III maintained the previous clinical grouping classification found in IRS-I and IRS-II. Within this classification, there was the incorporation of the tumor histologic type in an attempt to identify patients with a less or more aggressive tumor (favorable versus unfavorable). Rhabdomyosarcoma of the pelvis that was incompletely resected at initial staging has a different prognosis than rhabdomyosarcoma from other sites and has its own clinical group, Group III (special pelvic sites).

IRS-IV is now underway and has changed the clinical staging classification for patients. Staging will now be assessed pretreatment instead of after initial surgical biopsy or resection. One of the possible deficiencies in the classification process of the previous staging system was the fact that a 10- or 15-cm mass with lymph node involvement that was completely resected could be in the same classification group as a 1-cm

Table 47.1. Staging Classification

STAGE	SITES	T	SIZE	N	M
1	Orbit	T1 or T2	a or b	N0 or N1 or NX	M0
	Head and neck (excluding parameningeal)				
	GU-nonbladder/ nonprostate				
2	Bladder/prostate	T1 or T2	a	N0 or NX	M0
	Extremity				
	Cranial parameningeal				
	Other (includes trunk, retroperitoneum, etc.)				
3	Bladder/prostate	T1 or T2	a	N1	M0
	Extremity		b	N0 or N1 or NX	M0
	Cranial parameningeal				
	Other (includes trunk, retroperitoneum, etc.)				
4	All	T1 or T2	a or b	N0 or N1	M0

Definitions
  Tumor
    T(site)1—Confined to anatomic site of origin
      a ≤5 cm in diameter
      b >5 cm in diameter
    T(site)2—extension and/or fixation to surrounding tissue
      a ≤5 cm in diameter
      b >5 cm in diameter
  Regional nodes
    N0 Regional nodes are not clinically involved
    N1 Regional nodes are clinically involved by neoplasm
    NX Clinical status of regional nodes unknown
  Metastasis
    M0 No distant metastasis
    M1 Metastasis present

mass without lymph node involvement that was also completely resected (both group I). Table 47.1 shows the most recent staging classification.

RHABDOMYOSARCOMA OF THE PELVIS

The treatment of rhabdomyosarcoma of the pelvis is generally considered as a single entity, although significant differences exist among tumors in this general location depending on the site of origin. In addition, data gathered by the IRS-I through III, suggest that genitourinary tumors may have a more favorable prognosis than primary tumors in the extremities or in the region of the head and neck (29, 34). Because of the high incidence of local recurrence after limited surgical excision, survival was rare before current concepts of therapy were established (35). With the introduction of more radical surgical procedures (anterior or total exenteration), improved survival was obtained with bladder and vaginal tumors (3, 30, 36, 37), but remained dismal for primary prostatic tumors (38).

Not until the introduction of planned multidisciplinary therapy has significant improvement in survival been realized for all forms of pelvic rhabdomyosarcoma. With improving survival and the appreciation of the effectiveness of combined, cyclic, and long-term chemotherapy, surgeons and medical oncologists began to reevaluate the primary thrust of management of these lesions. In 1975, Rivard et al. suggested using intensive chemotherapy as a primary method of management of pelvic rhabdomyosarcoma. This approach demonstrated a reduction in primary tumor bulk, allowing more limited surgical intervention than originally planned in nine patients (39). Belman and Baum also described a similar, although smaller, series in support of this concept (40). The original series of Rivard et al. was updated by Ortega (41). Thirteen patients were included in this series. Five children had died, although three of these had metastatic disease at the time of presentation and would not have been candidates for radical surgical treatment. Only one child did not have a response to chemotherapy and required an early radical surgical procedure. Eight patients were alive without evident disease at the time of the report, although all but one also had an operation or radiation therapy as well. However, it was the author's opinion then that less surgical intervention was required after chemotherapy than would originally have been necessary without it; and for the group as a whole, only two urinary diversions were necessary.

Other authors also have observed the benefits of initial chemotherapy in the reduction of both tumor bulk and the extent of surgery, thereby improving the quality of life for these children (10, 42). The IRS has recognized this special consideration for primary pelvic tumors and has established a subgroup within the protocol to evaluate chemotherapy as the primary and, perhaps, only therapy after biopsy in initially resectable pelvic tumors, Clinical Group III (special pelvic sites).

Since the development of the IRS, several investigators have assessed their results in an effort to better define the appropriate relationships among chemotherapy, surgery, and radiation therapy to maximize survival. In 1982, Hays et al. reported the initial data from IRS-1 in 64 children with primary bladder or prostatic tumors (43). Most of the patients underwent some initial surgical procedure followed by chemotherapy and radiation therapy, depending on the clinical group as outlined by the IRS. Fifty-three children presented without clinical evidence of metastases. Thirty-seven of these had initial surgery followed by chemotherapy or radiation therapy, and 16 began a primary chemotherapy and radiation therapy program. The number of children in each treatment group and their incidence of recurrence are listed in Table 47.2.

In this initial report from the IRS, those children managed initially by aggressive surgery fared best. The authors con-

Table 47.2. Incidence of Recurrence

INITIAL TREATMENT PROGRAM	NO. OF PATIENTS	RECURRENCE
Primary bladder tumor		
Exenteration	11	2
Partial cystectomy	12	5
Chemotherapy/	5	3
radiation therapy		
Prostatic tumors		
Exenteration	14	0
Chemotherapy/	11	2
radiation therapy		

cluded that pelvic exenteration, when combined with local radiation therapy and appropriate chemotherapy, results in a high rate of survival and contrasts sharply with the dismal survival statistics before multidisciplinary management. They expressed concern, however, that this report had not decreased the mutilative aspect of surgery for pelvic rhabdomyosarcoma and proposed a trial of more intensive primary nonsurgical efforts with frequent biopsies. Surgical excision would be reserved for incomplete responses or recurrence.

Hays et al. subsequently reported on 29 children with bladder or prostatic primaries treated initially with chemotherapy alone in an effort to preserve pelvic organ function ("pulse VAC" at first; addition of Adriamycin when response was inadequate) (44). Radiation therapy and limited surgery were included when clinical response was incomplete or in cases of recurrence. In this series, 38% of the total group of children maintained satisfactory bladder function, although only 2 of 29 achieved this on chemotherapy alone. The mortality rate was 27%. This mortality figure contrasts with a mortality rate of 5% in IRS-I in children treated by exenteration (most often anterior exenteration only).

Scholtmeyer et al. reviewed 16 children (10 boys and 6 girls) with genitourinary rhabdomyosarcoma and reported a 60% overall survival rate (45). However, in each case, surgical management was necessary to achieve a disease-free site. Fleming et al. presented a most encouraging report from the St. Jude Children's Research Hospital (46). Twenty-two children were seen with genitourinary rhabdomyosarcomas (10 vaginal and 12 bladder or prostate) in the pelvis. One patient with a vaginal primary refused surgery and subsequently died despite chemotherapy and radiation therapy. The other nine children with vaginal lesions had preoperative chemotherapy (and subsequent radiation therapy if tumor response was believed to be inadequate) followed by surgical excision. Eight of these children were free of disease: seven after hysterovaginectomy only and one after anterior exenteration. One child had active residual disease after surgery. Twelve children had bladder or prostate lesions. In 11 cases, preoperative chemotherapy and radiation therapy were used. Five of these children had functioning bladders without evidence of disease. Six had active disease or are dead.

Ghavimi et al. reported on their experience with 27 patients at Memorial Sloan-Kettering Cancer Center (47). A combination of surgeries, chemotherapy, and radiation therapy was used. Eighteen patients were alive and well at the time of the report, and nine of these had a functional bladder. Primary chemotherapy failed to achieve satisfactory control of these tumors in the majority (only 2 of 27). They demonstrated that extirpative surgery followed by chemotherapy in their program gave the best overall results.

Broecker et al. reported the results of management for pelvic rhabdomyosarcoma from the Great Ormond Street Hospital in London (48). From a population of 20 children, there was a survival rate of 55% and bladder salvage in half of these. Once again, their conclusion was that complete surgical resection of the tumor combined with chemotherapy and radiotherapy offers the highest chance of cure.

Green summarized the results of the first two Intergroup Rhabdomyosarcoma studies in 1987 (49). The conclusions were as follows.

1. Aggressive, combination chemotherapy is indicated as initial therapy.
2. Patients must be followed carefully at this stage because of a high incidence of progressive disease development despite chemotherapy. Complete response to chemotherapy only is unusual.
3. After a partial response (at 6 weeks after initial therapy), consideration is given to either surgical management or radiation therapy, depending on the extent of residual disease. If total excision is possible (especially if this can be accomplished with organ salvage, i.e., partial cystectomy), surgery would be chosen rather than radiation therapy.
4. Radiation therapy may not be necessary if margins after resection are completely clear of tumor.
5. Chemotherapy must be continued postoperatively.

The results of IRS-III have shown an improvement in the management of patients with genitourinary rhabdomyosarcoma. One of the goals of IRS-III was to reduce the treatment for patients with a favorable prognosis and to increase the treatment for patients with a poor prognosis. Patients in clinical Group I (favorable histologic type) from all sites had cyclophosphamide removed from their regimen used previously in IRS-II. Their 5-year progression-free survival, and survival, did not change. Patients in Group III (special pelvic sites) benefited as much as any individual group in IRS-III. Intensification of treatment, additional chemotherapy, second-look surgery, and early radiation resulted in significant changes in outcome when compared with IRS-II (Table 47.3) (33).

The results of IRS-III show a dramatic improvement in bladder salvage rate that must be attributed to the changes in the treatment protocol from IRS-II. The children with residual disease after initial resection continue to be the largest group of children with pelvic rhabdomyosarcoma. It is in this group of children that bladder salvage must be weighed against survival.

Table 47.3.   Group III (Special Pelvic Sites)

	IRS-II (%)	IRS-III (%)
Complete response	70	81
Progression-free survival	58	74
Survival	72	83
Bladder		
Salvage	25	60

There are many variables that must be considered when comparing IRS-II outcome to IRS-III. The timing of radiation treatment was advanced to week 6 from week 20 in patients with bladder neck or prostate rhabdomyosarcoma. Chemotherapy induction now included doxorubicin in all patients. Patients not in complete remission at 20 weeks underwent a second-look surgery with possible resection of residual tumor. If complete remission was not achieved by surgery, additional chemotherapy and radiation were initiated. Second-look surgery has shown the inadequacy of computed tomography (CT) and magnetic resonance imaging (MRI) scans. Children thought to have residual disease were sometimes found to have only necrotic tissue, while children thought to be in complete response were occasionally noted to have residual microscopic disease.

In England, Atra et al. (50) were able to achieve similar results with their protocols, with an overall survival rate of 73% and an 88% bladder salvage rate in the surviving group. Their improved bladder salvage rate was attributed to their surgical management being done by only two senior surgeons and a thorough understanding of the limitations of CT and MRI scans.

The function of the salvaged bladder must be considered. Subtotal cystectomy with 5000 to 6000 cGy of radiation can have a dramatic effect on the bladder function in a child. Yeung et al. (51) studied the function and renal preservation in children surviving treatment of pelvic rhabdomyosarcoma. In 11 patients with bladder salvage, 7 had undergone some form of radiation treatment to the bladder. All seven patients had reduction in their bladder volumes and abnormal voiding patterns. Four of seven patients had upper tract dilation, of which two required surgical reconstruction. Of the four patients who did not receive radiation treatment, all had normal functional capacity and normal voiding habits.

Other factors that correlate with survival rates are site of origin of the tumor and histologic differentiation. Raney et al. compared survival of children with bladder and prostate tumors (n = 8) with those who had a pelvic tumor arising separate from the bladder (n = 8) (11). In those patients with a bladder or prostate lesion, the tumors were smaller at presentation, showed more histologic differentiation, and demonstrated fewer distant metastases. At the time of their report, six of eight patients having either a bladder or prostate tumor were alive and thought to be free of disease; only three of eight patients with primary pelvic tumors were alive, and only one was apparently tumor free. The authors believed that although there were many factors that might have influenced survival, the most important seemed to be that bladder or prostate tumors caused urinary symptoms early and were picked up sooner than pure pelvic lesions.

Ragab et al. assessed the significance of age in the prognosis for rhabdomyosarcoma (51a). Seventy-eight (5%) of 1561 patients in the IRS as of May 1983 were younger than 1 year of age (7). Except for a slightly greater incidence of undifferentiated histologic type in the infant group (18% versus 7%), the other demographic factors did not differ significantly between the two groups. There was a somewhat higher rate of bladder/prostate/vagina primary site in the infants compared with older children (24% versus 10%). More toxicity to treatment developed in infants. However, overall survival was no different for the two groups. Compared with Wilms' tumor and neuroblastoma, in which younger patients have a more favorable prognosis, age does not affect the prognosis of those with rhabdomyosarcoma.

There has been an increasing amount of data that have attempted to identify some genetic marker that can be correlated with prognosis. The ploidy of the cell is one area of study (52, 53). Pappo et al. (53) found that patients with nonmetastatic unresectable embryonal rhabdomyosarcoma that were hyperploid rather than diploid had marked improvement in complete response (82% versus 42%) and a 5-year progression-free survival rate of 91% versus 11%. IRS-V may include the use of genetic markers when assigning patients to a particular protocol.

It is clear after analyzing these many reports that survival is best with a combination of aggressive multimodal therapy; that chemotherapy alone is only rarely successful in completely controlling the majority of tumors, although some partial response can be expected in most; that local excision may be possible with organ preservation and that this is best assessed after a short course of intensive chemotherapy; and that radiation therapy is effective and essential if residual tumor is left behind.

The principles of management that we prefer, as outlined here, are based on the observations discussed above and parallel the protocol and recommendations of the IRS. It must be emphasized, however, that controversy exists, especially regarding the timing of the surgical procedure and radiation therapy, and that the surgeon must carefully and thoughtfully consider each patient individually in regard to the location and size of tumor and the consequences of radical surgical intervention, radiation therapy, or extensive chemotherapy. At our institution, all rhabdomyosarcoma patients are followed by a team of physicians including surgeons, medical oncologists, and radiation oncologists.

The initial surgical treatment for suspected pelvic rhabdomyosarcoma should be limited: transurethral resection for biopsy of vesical or prostatic lesions, and direct biopsy for intraluminal vaginal lesions. It should be stressed that these polypoid neoplasms (sarcoma botryoides) often have considerable edematous mucosa overlying the submucosal tumor, and deep, "fleshy" biopsies must be obtained. A few cases of rhabdomyosarcoma are not accessible for endoscopic biopsy and are best biopsied via an open surgical approach. At this time, dissection should be limited, and only as much tumor should be excised as can be removed safely without sacrifice of any vital organ, e.g., the bladder, genital system, or rectum. Rarely, a lesion in this area may not involve any viscera, and the biopsy may result in total removal of all grossly identifiable tumor. If laparotomy is performed, iliac and paraaortic node sampling should be done. Any urinary tract obstruction that occurs before or during treatment should be corrected promptly through appropriate means.

After diagnosis is confirmed, chemotherapy is instituted. Protocols vary, as noted previously, but should initially include at least vincristine and actinomycin D. The clinical group and stage will affect which additional chemotherapeutic agent is to be used. Timing and dosage will depend on the protocol followed. We are currently following IRS-IV protocols that use a combination of both the previous group classification and the new TNM stage classification. Group I, stage I and Group I, stage II patients do not undergo radiation treatment. All other stages and groups have a course of radiation included in their treatment. Response to therapy is then monitored initially by radiographic studies.

Reevaluation is carried out at the end of 20 weeks with a second examination under anesthesia including open or endoscopic biopsy. The ability to stage a patient accurately with radiologic studies only should be questioned. Rebiopsy may be the only way to accurately assess response to therapy. If apparently complete or significant partial remission has occurred, chemotherapy is continued per protocol.

If the biopsy result is positive or if progressive disease is identified, intensification of chemotherapy, surgical treatment, or radiation therapy should be included in the therapeutic program. Radiation therapy is attractive because it does not sacrifice any vital structure, but the early and late sequelae of radiation therapy are significant. We prefer limited surgical excision before radiation therapy. However, if on exploration total exenteration appears necessary, the surgeon might consider continued intensive chemotherapy and/or radiation therapy in the hope that further reduction in size might allow for a more limited surgical procedure later. It is also important to emphasize that the best survival results are in those children who have surgical removal of the tumor, even if removal requires anterior (rarely total) exenteration. In our experience, as in that of most other investigators, regression is only partial with primary chemotherapy and additional therapy will be indicated.

Although there has been dramatic improvement in the bladder salvage rate over the past 10 years, many bladder neck lesions and prostatic lesions will require total cystectomy and prostatectomy. A simultaneous pelvic lymphadenectomy should be accomplished to complete the staging of the tumor. The choice of urinary diversion depends on the experience and philosophy of the surgeon. Current continent diversions offer the possibility of avoiding appliances and improving body image for these children (54). In females, pretreatment might reduce the bulk of the tumor so that simultaneous hysterectomy and vaginectomy will not be necessary. Although most vesical neoplasms arise at the level of the bladder neck and trigone, 25% of these tumors presented to the IRS appeared to arise from and to be confined to the dome of the bladder, making partial cystectomy theoretically possible after pretreatment. If the margins of the dissection show tumor or if the nodes are involved with disease, then radiation therapy can be added as the third therapeutic method. Uterine and vaginal tumors have responded well to pretreatment chemotherapy, and a survival rate of 75% can be anticipated with chemotherapy only or with limited surgical treatment (partial vaginectomy or hysterovaginectomy), but without radiation therapy (42, 55).

Tumors arising within the confines of the bony pelvis, but without any obvious relationship to the pelvic organs and without an intraluminal component that is accessible to endoscopic observation and biopsy, constitute a particularly difficult subgroup of pelvic rhabdomyosarcoma. They tend to infiltrate widely and are rarely suitable for primary surgical extirpation when first seen. After initial celiotomy, with removal of as much tumor as is safe, but without exenteration, primary intensive chemotherapy should be instituted. As opposed to bladder and vaginal lesions, we believe radiation therapy should be included as part of the initial therapy because local recurrences in our experience have been common after chemotherapy only and are generally not then amenable to surgical extirpation. After completion of the initial phase of therapy, a second-look celiotomy should be considered for repeated biopsy and excision of any apparent residual tumor.

In summary, the management of pelvic rhabdomyosarcoma is complex and involves the judicious use of surgical procedures, chemotherapy, and radiation therapy. It can no longer be said that primary radical surgical intervention is the preferred approach and that initial chemotherapy is reserved only for unresectable or metastatic lesions. Clinical trials continue to evaluate these concepts, but each case must still be carefully considered individually.

PARATESTICULAR RHABDOMYOSARCOMA

Paratesticular rhabdomyosarcoma is somewhat less common than pelvic lesions and tends to occur in an older age group. In the series of genitourinary rhabdomyosarcoma reported by Exelby, 40% of tumors were paratesticular (30). These lesions are usually seen as firm, nontender, rapidly growing scrotal masses that may be indistinguishable from the testis.

As for any malignant scrotal mass, the initial surgical approach should be inguinal. If the tumor is accidentally approached scrotally, a hemiscrotectomy should be done. Unless the tumor is small and completely excised locally, radiation therapy should be administered to the ipsilateral hemiscrotum and to the inguinal area because, as with all rhabdomyosarcomas, the local recurrence rate is high. If local radiation is to

be used, the surgeon should consider transplantation of the contralateral testis into the thigh.

Paratesticular rhabdomyosarcoma metastasizes widely but does so primarily to the regional lymphatics (56). Approximately one third of patients in the original IRS had metastases to the retroperitoneal nodes at the time of presentation. Because of this, we believe all patients without evidence of hematogenous metastases at the time of presentation should still undergo a retroperitoneal lymphadenectomy. Cromie et al. had previously suggested a complete, bilateral dissection from the level of the renal hila to the bifurcation of the aorta and then along the ipsilateral iliac vessels (57), although others suggested that an adequate node sampling is all that is necessary. The risk of future infertility that might be averted with a more limited dissection appeared justified, in their view, by the improved staging and possible potential therapeutic benefit of a complete dissection.

Subsequent data, including information from IRS-II, suggested that such an aggressive approach may not be necessary. Raney et al. reviewed the cases of 95 boys with paratesticular rhabdomyosarcoma seen in the IRS (58). Seventy-seven of these children were in Group I or II and they achieved a survival rate of more than 90% at 3 years. Twenty-eight percent of these children had positive retroperitoneal nodes, but the authors found no difference in the incidence of positive nodes or overall survival whether unilateral or bilateral retroperitoneal lymphadenectomy was performed. Therefore, it seems that a more limited node sampling, significantly reducing the risk of seminal emission failure, is appropriate. If the retroperitoneal nodes are not involved with disease, radiation therapy can be withheld. When they are involved, radiation therapy should be directed to the retroperitoneal and mediastinal areas.

Olive et al. have suggested that retroperitoneal lymphadenectomy may not be indicated in Group I patients studied by intravenous urography and bipedal lymphangiography (59). In a series of 18 patients (only 16 had lymphangiography), all maintained on chemotherapy, 17 have remained free of disease, most for more than 2 years. It remains unclear just how effective chemotherapy alone is in sterilizing metastatic retroperitoneal nodes. In six patients in IRS-I who had relapses in the paraaortic nodes, all died (60).

Chemotherapy should be continued whether the nodes are involved or not. The chemotherapeutic protocol can be modified according to the extent of recognized residual disease. In the absence of hematogenous metastases or bulk lymphatic disease, a less toxic program using vincristine and actinomycin D alone might be used. This is supported by results from the IRS-III study in which patients in clinical Group II (favorable histologic type) had outcomes similar to patients in the IRS-II studies that included cyclophosphamide. With more extensive bulky disease, an intensive program as described for pelvic lesions would be appropriate. Through a selective, multidisciplinary program, survival can now be anticipated in greater than 80% of these neoplasms.

SEQUELAE OF THERAPY

Although the primary goal of cancer therapy in children is disease-free survival, some publications have drawn attention to the delayed sequelae of successful treatment for the primary lesion (61–63). The effects of radical surgical extirpation are obvious and lifelong. For radical pelvic procedures, these effects include abdominal stomas, sterility, and impotence in males.

Cutaneous urinary diversion in children, especially the ileal conduit, has also been associated with a high long-term complication rate, including atrophic pyelonephritis, calculos disease, delayed loop strictures, ureterointestinal anastomotic strictures, and stomal stenosis (64). More contemporary forms of urinary diversion, including antireflux ureterointestinal anastomoses and continent abdominal stomas, offer an improved quality of life and, possibly, a better outlook for renal preservation. These techniques, however, are technically complex, have a high incidence of immediate postoperative complications, and remain unproven over several decades of follow-ups (54).

The long-term effects of chemotherapy are not yet fully known. The tendency for cyclophosphamide to produce hemorrhagic cystitis is well documented, but its effects on germ cells are less clear. Adriamycin can cause cardiomyopathy and cardiac failure. The most serious sequelae, if the child survives, arise from the use of radiation therapy. Abnormalities in bone growth, scoliosis, chest wall deformities, and soft tissue fibrosis have all been reported. The skeletal abnormalities may be particularly disabling (65). Radiation is oncogenic, and increasing numbers of secondary tumors are being reported. Li et al. have calculated that the risk of a second tumor after radiation therapy for a childhood neoplasm is 17%, with the peak incidence occurring 15 to 19 years after initial therapy (66).

REFERENCES

1. Miller RW. Fifty-two forms of childhood cancer. United States mortality experience, 1960–1966. J Pediatr 1969;75:685.
2. Batsakis JG. Urogenital rhabdomyosarcoma: histogenesis and classification. J Urol 1963;90:180.
3. Tank ES, et al. Treatment of urogenital tract rhabdomyosarcoma in infants and children. J Urol 1972;107:324.
4. Stout AP, Lattes R. Tumor of the soft tissues. In: Atlas of tumor pathology. Fascicle 1. Washington, DC,: AFIP, 1967.
5. Asmar L, et al. Agreement among and within groups of pathologists in the classification of rhabdomyosarcoma and related childhood sarcomas. Cancer 1994;74:2579.
6. Palmer N, Foulkes M. Histopathology and prognosis in the second Intergroup Rhabdomyosarcoma Study. Proc Am Soc Clin Oncol 1983;2:229.
7. Tsokos M, Triche TJ. Primitive, solid variant rhabdomyosarcoma. Lab Invest 1986;54:65. Abstract.
8. Hawkins HK, Camacho-Velasquez JV. Rhabdomyosarcoma in children: correlation of form and prognosis in one institution's experience. Am J Surg Pathol 1987;11:531.
9. Tsokos M, et al. Rhabdomyosarcoma: a new classification scheme related to prognosis. Arch Pathol Lab Med 1992;116:847.
10. Bartholomew TH, Gonzales ET, Starling KA, et al. Changing concepts in management of pelvic rhabdomyosarcoma in children. Urology 1979;13:613.
11. Raney B, et al. Primary site as a prognostic variable for children with pelvic soft tissue sarcomas. J Urol 1986;136:874.
12. Steinberg J, et al. Clinical trials with cyclophosphamide in children with soft tissue sarcoma. Cancer Chemother Rep 1963;28:39.
13. Sutow WW. Chemotherapy in childhood cancer (except leukemia). Cancer 1965;18:1585.
14. Sutow WW, et al. Vincristine sulfate therapy in children with metastatic soft tissue sarcoma. Pediatrics 1966;38:465.
15. Tan CTC, Golbey RB, Yap CL. Clinical experience with actinomycin-D. Ann N Y Acad Sci 1960;89:426.
16. James DH, et al. Childhood malignant tumor: concurrent chemotherapy with dactinomycin and vincristine sulfate. JAMA 1966;197:1043.
17. Grosfeld JL, Clatworthy HW, Newton WA. Combined therapy in childhood rhabdomyosarcoma. Pediatr Surg 1969;4:637.
18. Pratt CB, et al. Coordinated treatment of childhood rhabdomyosarcoma with surgery, radiotherapy and combination chemotherapy. Cancer Res 1972;32:606.
19. Kilman JW, et al. Reasonable surgery for rhabdomyosarcoma: a study of 67 cases. Am Surg 1973;17:346.
20. Ghavimi F, et al. Combination therapy of urogenital embryonal rhabdomyosarcoma in children. Cancer 1973;32:1178.
21. Jaffe N, et al. Rhabdomyosarcoma in children: improved outlook with a multidisciplinary approach. Am J Surg 1973;125:482.
22. Heyn RM, et al. The role of combined chemotherapy in the treatment of rhabdomyosarcoma in children. Cancer 1974;34:2128.
23. Exelby PR. Management of embryonal rhabdomyosarcoma in children. Surg Clin North Am 1974;54:849.
24. Ghavimi F, et al. Multidisciplinary treatment of embryonal rhabdomyosarcoma in children. Cancer 1975;35:677.
25. Heyn RM. The role of combined chemotherapy in the treatment of rhabdomyosarcoma in children. Cancer 1974;34:2128.
26. Heyn RM, Holland R, Joo P. Treatment of rhabdomyosarcoma in children with surgery, radiotherapy, and chemotherapy. Med Pediatr Oncol 1977;3:21.
27. Donaldson SS, et al. Rhabdomyosarcoma of the head and neck in children. Cancer 1973;31:26.
28. Maurer HM, et al. The Intergroup Rhabdomyosarcoma Study: a preliminary report. Cancer 1977;40:2015.
29. Raney BB, Gehan EA, Maurer HM. Evaluation of intensified chemotherapy in children with advanced rhabdomyosarcoma (clinical groups III and IV). Cancer Clin Trials 1979;2:19.
30. Exelby PR, Ghavimi F, Jereb B. Genitourinary rhabdomyosarcoma in children. J Pediatr Surg 1978;13:746.
31. Cassady JR, et al. Radiation therapy for rhabdomyosarcoma. Radiology 1968;91:116.
32. Dritschilo A, et al. The role of radiation therapy in the treatment of soft tissue sarcoma of childhood. Cancer 1978;42:1192.

33. Haie-Meder C, Flamant F, Revillon Y, et al. The role of brachytherapy in the therapeutic strategy of vesico-prostatic rhabdomyosarcoma in children. Ann Urol (Paris) 1994;28:302.

34. Crist W, et al. The Third Intergroup Rhabdomyosarcoma Study. J Clin Oncol 1995;13:610.

35. Ghazali S. Embryonic rhabdomyosarcoma of the urogenital tract. Br J Surg 1973;60:124.

36. Jarman WD, Kenealy JC. Polypoid rhabdomyosarcoma of the bladder in children. Trans Am Assoc Genitourinary Surg 1969; 61:80.

37. Williams DI, Schistad G. Lower urinary tract tumors in children. Br J Urol 1964;36:51.

38. Mackenzie AR, Whitmore WF, Melamed M. Myosarcomas of the bladder and prostate. Cancer 1968;22:833.

39. Rivard GE, et al. Intensive chemotherapy as primary treatment for rhabdomyosarcoma of the pelvis. Cancer 1975;36:1593.

40. Belman AB, Baum ES. Current trends in treatment of childhood rhabdomyosarcoma of lower genitourinary tract. Urology 1976;8:31.

41. Ortega JA. A therapeutic approach to childhood pelvic rhabdomyosarcoma without pelvic exenteration. J Pediatrics 1979;94:205.

42. Hays DM. Pelvic rhabdomyosarcomas in childhood. Cancer 1980;45:1810.

43. Hays DM, et al. Bladder and prostatic tumors in the Intergroup Rhabdomyosarcoma Study (IRS-I). Cancer 1982;50: 1472.

44. Hays DM, et al. Primary chemotherapy in the treatment of children with bladder-prostate tumors in the Intergroup Rhabdomyosarcoma Study (IRS-II). J Pediatr Surg 1982;17: 812.

45. Scholtmeyer RJ, Tromp CG, Hozebroek FWJ. Embryonal rhabdomyosarcoma of the urogenital tract in childhood. Eur Urol 1983;9:69.

46. Fleming ID, et al. The role of surgical resection when combined with chemotherapy and radiation in the management of pelvic rhabdomyosarcoma. Am Surg 1984;199: 509.

47. Ghavimi R, et al. Treatment of genitourinary rhabdomyosarcoma in children. J Urol 1984;132:31.

48. Broecker BH, et al. Pelvic rhabdomyosarcoma in children. Br J Urol 1988;61:427.

49. Green DM. The treatment of advanced or recurrent malignant genitourinary tumors in children. Cancer 1987;60:602.

50. Atra A, Ward HC, Aitken K, et al. Conservative surgery in multimodal therapy for pelvic rhabdomyosarcoma in children. Br J Cancer 1994;70:1004.

51. Yeung CK, Ward HC, Ransley PG, et al. Bladder and kidney function after cure of pelvic rhabdomyosarcoma in childhood. Br J Cancer 1994;70:1000.

51a. Ragab AH, et al. Infants younger than 1 year of age with rhabdomyosarcoma. Cancer 1986;58:2606.

52. Shapiro DN, Parham DM, Douglass EC, et al. Relationship of tumor cell ploidy to the histologic subtype and treatment outcome in children and adolescents with unresectable rhabdomyosarcoma. J Clin Oncol 1991;9:159.

53. Pappo DS, Crist WM, Kuttesch J, et al. Tumor cell DNA content predicts outcome in children and adolescents with clinical group III embryonal rhabdomyosarcoma. J Clin Oncol 1993;11:1901.

54. Decter RM, Gonzales ET. Bladder augmentation in the pediatric age group. J d'Urologie 1988;94:91.

55. Kumar APM, et al. Combined therapy to prevent complete pelvic exenteration for rhabdomyosarcoma of the vagina or uterus. Cancer 1976;37:118.

56. Olney LE, et al. Intrascrotal rhabdomyosarcoma. Urology 1979;14:113.

57. Cromie WJ, Raney RB, Duckett JW. Paratesticular rhabdomyosarcoma in children. J Urol 1979;122:80.

58. Raney RB, et al. Paratesticular sarcoma in childhood and adolescence. Cancer 1987;60:2337.

59. Olive D, et al. Para-aortic lymphadenectomy is not necessary in the treatment of localized paratesticular rhabdomyosarcoma. Cancer 1984;54:1283.

60. Raney EB, et al. Prognosis of children with soft tissue sarcoma who relapse after achieving a complete response: a report from the Intergroup Rhabdomyosarcoma Study I. Cancer 1983;52: 44.

61. Jaffe N. Nononcogenic sequelae of cancer chemotherapy. Radiology 1975;114:167.

62. Jaffe N. Late side effects of treatment: skeletal, genetic, central nervous system, and organic. Pediatr Clin North Am 1977;23: 233.

63. Schein PS, Winokur SH. Immunosuppressive and cytotoxic chemotherapy: long-term complications. Ann Intern Med 1975;82:84.

64. Shapiro SR, Lebowitz R, Colodny AH. Fate of ninety children with ileal conduit urinary diversion a decade later: analysis of complications, pyelography, renal functions, and bacteriology. Urology 1975;114:289.

65. Jaffe N, et al. Childhood urologic cancer therapy-related sequelae and their impact on management. Cancer 1980;45: 1815.

66. Li FP, Cassady JR, Jaffe N. Risk of second tumors in survivors of childhood cancer. Cancer 1975;35:1230.

CHEMOTHERAPY

Treatment of Metastatic Renal Cell Carcinoma

Mitchell H. Sokoloff
Robert A. Figlin
Arie S. Belldegrun

In 1995, 28,800 renal cell carcinomas will be diagnosed in Americans and will account for 3% of all adult malignancies (1). Surgically unresectable disease has a poor outcome because no successful radiation or chemotherapy strategies have been devised (2). The natural history of renal cell carcinoma is not always predictable, and spontaneous regression of metastases after nephrectomy does occur, albeit rarely (less than 1%). Early observations of spontaneous regression, along with the discovery of circulating humoral and cellular elements in such patients, delayed growth of metastatic lesions, and varying tumor doubling times suggested involvement of the immune system in the natural host response to this neoplasm (3). Since then, treatment modalities directed at enhancing antitumor immune responses have been developed, and renal cell carcinoma has become a paradigm for the immunotherapeutic approach to treating solid organ malignancies. This chapter explores the role of immunotherapy in the treatment of advanced renal malignancies. Principles of immunotherapy will be discussed. This will be followed by a review of the evolution of contemporary immunologic-based therapies. Future investigative directions and approaches to patient management will also be outlined.

FUNDAMENTALS OF IMMUNOTHERAPY

The immune system contributes to the surveillance and destruction of tumor cells, primarily through cellular agents (4). Such cellular mediators with antitumor activity include natural killer (NK) cells, lymphokine-activated killer (LAK) cells, and MHC-restricted cytotoxic T cells (Tc). The goal of immunotherapy in the treatment of advanced and recurrent cancers is to sensitize these immune effector cells to tumor antigens, producing a cytolytic response directed at sites of tumor with minimal systemic toxicity. The application of immunotherapy is limited to immunogenic malignancies. These tumors, which include renal cell carcinoma, are vulnerable to immune-mediated cytotoxicity. Modern immunotherapy can be applied to neoplastic disease in one of several manners:

1. By systemic or locoregional infusion of immunostimulatory agents;
2. By passively transferring immune cells with antitumor reactivity (such as LAK cells or tumor-infiltrating lymphocytes [TIL]) to the tumor-bearing host to attack sites of cancerous cells ("adoptive immunotherapy"); or
3. By vaccination with tumor cells transformed with genes or other immune stimulators to generate immune lymphoid cells with antitumor activity, or by systemic or locoregional transfection of tumor cells with genetic material that can induce tumor cell differentiation, cause direct cytolytic activity, produce regional cytokine secretion, or enhance MHC receptor expression ("active immunotherapy").

Adoptive Immunotherapy

Adoptive immunotherapy involves the in vitro growth, expansion, and immune modification of lymphoid cells (NK and T cells) before reinfusion back into the host (5–7). One such example is TIL therapy, which has been shown to cause regression of bulky tumors in a variety of animal tumor models and in humans. TIL are lymphoid cells isolated from fresh solid tumors on coculturing a tumor-cell suspension with interleukin-2 (IL-2). After expansion of these cells in culture, which usually takes 5 to 6 weeks, TIL are reinfused into the patient in the hope that these cytotoxic T lymphocytes will recognize, attach to, and destroy tumor deposits throughout the body (6, 8). At our institution, TIL have been used in patients with advanced renal cell carcinoma and have resulted in a response rate of 34% (9).

Active (Specific) Immunotherapy

Active immunotherapy refers to immunization of patients with agents that increase the host immunologic response against the tumor. The first report dates to 1971 when a patient with metastatic renal cell carcinoma was cured after receiving serum obtained from a relative, also with renal cell carcinoma, but in remission (10). Current research is concentrated on creating tumor vaccines. During the intervening 20 years, the study of immunotherapy has introduced systemic cytokine treatment modalities and the adoptive immunotherapeutic techniques of LAK cells and TIL into the fight against cancer.

Tumor vaccine protocols use the ability of cytokines to enhance tumor cell immunogenicity, thereby increasing the ability of the host immune system to recognize and destroy cancer foci. Autologous tumor cells are transfected in vitro with cytokine-producing genes. These transfected cells, now producing cytokines and expressing increased MHC class I antigens, are retransplanted into the host where they stimulate a tumor-specific immune response. Cytokine production occurs only at the implant site, thereby producing a strong antitumor response without systemic toxicity. The stimulated immune effector agents can then diffuse throughout the host to hunt down and destroy other tumor foci and provide immunologic memory to the host. Studies in animals with subcutaneously placed vaccines have demonstrated potent, specific, and long-lasting antitumor immunity with protection on rechallenge with tumor (11, 12).

Another approach to modulating the host immune response is by increasing the tumor's immunogenicity in vivo by systemic or intralesional injections of genetic elements that will transfect tumor cells and enhance MHC class I expression, stimulate regional cytokine production, or introduce foreign antigenic material (13). Such genetic material includes cytokine, suicide, and suppressor genes. This modality of gene therapy is currently under investigation, and is so far limited by technical difficulties involving efficient and safe gene delivery systems.

Cytokines

Cytokines are important elements in the antitumor response—they are soluble factors that are responsible for communication among cells of the immune system. In addition to direct tumoricidal action, they also activate effector components of the immune system (4, 14–20). The introduction of cytokine genes into tumor cells has been repeatedly proven to enhance antitumor immune responses in both in vitro and in vivo studies. The following are the cytokines that have shown the most promise in treating solid neoplasms.

- Tumor necrosis factor-α (TNF-α) has direct effects on neoplastic cells resulting in cell death.
- Interferon alfa (IFN-α) induces a significant increase in the surface expression of class I MHC antigens in addition to direct antitumor activity. It also upregulates adhesion molecule expression on the surface of tumor cells, aiding the immune response.
- Interferon gamma (IFN-γ) induces a significant increase in the surface expression of class I and II MHC antigens.

- IL-2 is produced by activated T cells and causes proliferation of Tc, NK, and LAK cells capable of lysing autologous, syngeneic, or allogeneic tumor cells, but not normal cells. IL-2 has no direct antitumor effect, but secretion of IL-2 from tumor cells abrogates tumorigenicity by stimulating the activation and proliferation of immune effector cells (21).

MANAGEMENT OF METASTATIC DISEASE

The Role for Surgical Management

When renal cell carcinoma is diagnosed, approximately one third of patients already have metastatic lesions. For these patients, the 5-year survival rate is less than 20% (22). Metastases from renal cell carcinoma are usually multifocal, either within the same organ or to multiple sites. Occasionally (1 to 3% of cases), patients will present with solitary metastasis. The 5-year survival rate after excision of such lesions is approximately 25% (22, 23). In a study at our institution, aggressive therapy of solitary skeletal, central nervous system, and soft tissue lesions produced significant palliation of symptoms and occasionally prolonged survival (22). This is a select group of patients, however, and only those with a definite solitary lesion and no lymphatic involvement have any prospect of benefiting from surgical management. The most favorable lesions for resection are solitary pulmonary masses, which occasionally appear more than 1 year after removal of the primary tumor (24). Unfortunately, a metastatic lesion identified at the time of diagnosis of renal cell carcinoma is seldom an isolated lesion, and more clinically evident lesions invariably appear shortly after surgical excision.

In the past, nephrectomy was advocated in the treatment of metastatic disease as a method of both reducing the growth of the primary lesion and possibly triggering a spontaneous regression of metastatic disease. Unfortunately, this can be expected to occur in less than 1% of cases, the remissions are extremely short lived, and the mortality rate from surgery can approach 15%, depending on patient selection (25). This concept has been abandoned as it is now clear that nephrectomy itself seldom, if ever, has any influence on metastatic disease. Therefore, the routine use of "adjunctive nephrectomy" is unwarranted. Palliation of symptoms is, however, a reasonable rationale for nephrectomy in the face of metastases, provided the primary tumor can be completely removed without undue morbidity. Patients with perineoplastic syndromes will sometimes benefit from palliative nephrectomy, especially if metastatic sites are not large. Repeated hemorrhage and tumor pain can also often be ameliorated by nephrectomy.

The advent of immunotherapy for renal cell carcinoma has once again raised the issue of the role of surgery in patients with metastatic disease. Studies at our institution (24, 25) and elsewhere (26) have documented improved response rates to immunotherapy when given in conjunction with removal of the diseased kidney. Our data indicate that even when considering all the various prognostic factors, patients who receive immunotherapy have a better response rate when nephrectomy is performed before treatment. It is debatable whether nephrectomy is best performed before or after immunotherapy, and it is hoped that a randomized study that is currently being performed will resolve this question.

Other than for palliation, at UCLA our current philosophy is to perform adjunctive nephrectomies in patients with disseminated disease only in conjunction with immunotherapy, either to obtain tissue for TIL and other experimental protocols or to reduce tumor load in very large primary tumors, which are either symptomatic or have a probability of becoming symptomatic in the near future. Conversely, patients with small primary masses and/or multiple small metastatic lesions are first given immunotherapy. Those patients whose metastases respond to the treatment are then subsequently selected for nephrectomy.

The Role of Radiation Therapy

Radiation therapy has been applied to renal cell carcinoma as both an adjuvant to surgical therapy and as a treatment for metastatic lesions. Palliative radiation therapy has been successful in treating painful metastases and is a powerful tool for pain management. Although postoperative adjuvant radiation therapy has been proposed for patients with T3 tumors, no study has demonstrated a distinct survival advantage (27). The role of radiation therapy as a primary treatment for locally extensive renal cell carcinoma has failed to show a beneficial effect, although a possible preoperative role to decrease the size of the primary tumor and delay local recurrence after resection does exist (27, 28).

Hormonal Therapy and Chemotherapy

Hormonal therapy protocols were based on observations that progestinal agents inhibited the growth of renal cell tumors (29). Although early reports were encouraging, no studies have substantiated the initial results, including a study at UCLA in which none of 110 patients treated with progesterone had an objective response (22). Other hormonal agents including tamoxifen have been equally ineffective (30, 31).

Although cytotoxic drugs are the cornerstone of therapy for most solid malignancies, the success of chemotherapy in treating renal cell carcinoma has been poor (32, 33). The most common agents, vinblastine and floxuridine, have response rates of 7% and 16%, respectively. In a review of 72 agents evaluated in phase II trials in more than 3500 patients between 1983 and 1992, an objective response rate of 5.6% was noted, and the response was usually of very short duration.

IMMUNOTHERAPY

Manipulation of the immune system has always been an attractive concept for the management of metastatic disease because of the occasional spontaneous regression of renal cell masses, discovery of circulating humoral and cellular elements in such patients, delayed growth of metastatic lesions, and varying tumor doubling times.

Initial approaches to immunotherapy used nonspecific stimulators such as xenogeneic RNA-treated lymphocytes, bacille Calmette-Guérin, *Corynebacterium parvum*, and transfer factor. Despite early enthusiasm, these approaches ultimately yielded no significant improvement in prognosis and are now mainly of historical interest with regard to treating renal cell carcinoma (34–36). With the advent of the modern era of genetic engineering and the mass production of molecular agents, new opportunities have arisen for immunotherapy of renal cell carcinoma.

Biologic Therapy with Cytokines

The isolation, identification, and molecular cloning of IL-2 revolutionized the field of cancer immunotherapy and significantly altered the treatment of metastatic renal cell carcinoma (37, 38). Since then, other immunostimulatory cytokines have been identified and purified. With the advent of recombinant DNA technology, the ability to produce large quantities of these cytokines has resulted in their widespread use and, in a relatively short period, these agents have become an accepted treatment for metastatic disease. To date, most studies investigating the use of cytokines in the treatment of metastatic renal cell carcinoma have used IFN-α, IL-2, combinations of these cytokines, or adoptive immunotherapy with TIL or LAK cells. The role of a new generation of cytokines such as IL-4, IL-7, IL-12, and granulocyte-macrophage colony-stimulating factor (GM-CSF) is currently under investigation.

IFN-α

Research studies at UCLA in the early 1980s were among the first to demonstrate the effectiveness of IFN-α in the treatment of metastatic renal cell carcinoma (39). Independent studies at the same time confirmed the regression of metastatic disease with objective response rates of 16 to 26%, lasting an average of 8 to 10 months (40, 41). These numbers have not changed significantly in the past decade, despite numerous phase II trials and attempts at modifying doses and dosing schedules (42–53). Table 48.1 summarizes the major studies of the past decade, demonstrating a reproducible response rate of 15 to 20% and a response duration of 8 to 10 months. Responses appear independent of the preparation and dosing used. Improved response rates of 30% and durable clinical responses lasting more than 27 months can be seen in a select subset of patients treated with IFN-α (49, 51). These patients have had a prior nephrectomy, no previous chemotherapy or radiation therapy, good to excellent performance status, and primarily pulmonary metastases. Lung metastases appear more responsive to IFN-α therapy than those of other viscera (47). At UCLA, survival times increased from 49 to 115 weeks in IFN-α–treated patients with these favorable prognostic variables (51).

Table 48.1. Phase II Trials of Interferon Alpha for the Treatment of Metastatic Renal Cell Cancer

AUTHOR	REFERENCE NO.	YEAR	NO. OF PATIENTS	RESPONSE (%)
deKernion et al.	39	1983	43	16.5
Quesada et al.	40	1983	19	26
Neidart et al.	45	1984	33	15
Figlin et al.	52	1985	23	13[a]
Quesada et al.	41	1985	50	26
Kirkwood et al.	42	1985	30	23
Umeda and Niijima	44	1986	226	17.7
Fossa et al.	54	1986	18	33[a]
Muss et al.	49	1987	97	7[b]
Creagan et al.	53	1987	29	34[c]
Sarna et al.	51	1987	43	14[d]
			22	14[a]
Figlin et al.	43	1989	18	26
Minasian et al.	48	1993	159	10[a]
Total			651	20

[a] Addition of vinblastine (0.15 mg/kg).
[b] Select subpopulation (+ prior nephrectomy, − prior chemotherapy, − bone metastases) had 23% response rate.
[c] Aspirin 600 mg by mouth four times a day.
[d] Select subpopulation (+ prior nephrectomy, − prior chemotherapy, − bone metastases) had 24% response rate.

Side effects of IFN-α treatment include fever, chills, myalgia, anorexia, and headache. These are usually associated with the initial dosing and frequently improve spontaneously with continued administration of the drug. Some reversible hematologic and hepatic changes are occasionally noted, but they also usually resolve without necessitating changes in dosing (55, 56).

Combining accessory agents with IFN-α has been investigated as a means of increasing responsiveness and decreasing toxicity. In one study, the addition of aspirin increased response rates to 34%. Few changes in constitutional symptoms, the reason for adding aspirin to the treatment protocol, occurred (53). In vitro, the administration of 5-fluorouracil (5-FU) increases the susceptibility of renal cell carcinoma to LAK cells, and the combined administration of 5-FU and IFN-α for the treatment of bladder cancer has also shown promise (57–59).

Several studies have investigated using different combinations of IFN-α and chemotherapeutic agents to treat renal cell carcinoma and have demonstrated a favorable response rate. At the M.D. Anderson Cancer Center, combinations of IFN-α, mitomycin C, and 5-FU were found to be synergistic and improved the response rate to 35% (60). With the combination of IL-2, IFN-α, and 5-FU, the response rate increased to 45% with only moderate toxicity (61). Clinical trials investigating this combination of biologic and chemotherapeutic agents are currently underway. The addition of other agents such as vinblastine (52, 54), doxorubicin (62), and BCNU (63) do not appear to alter the response rate or the duration of the response, yet result in increased fatigue, hepatotoxicity, and myelosuppression (64).

Several studies have investigated the use of IFN-γ in the treatment of metastatic renal cell carcinoma. The response rates and duration of response were favorable but no better than those of IFN-α or IL-2 (65–69). The toxicities are similar and consist primarily of malaise, fever, anorexia, and headache. As discussed earlier, IFN-α upregulates expression of MHC class I antigens while IFN-γ increases both class I and II expression. Because these two cytokines have different roles in stimulating the immune response, there is speculation that a treatment approach combining both IFN-α and IFN-γ would be complementary and thus more effective. In vitro studies have demonstrated synergistic activity between IFN-α and IFN-γ (70), although preliminary clinical trials have failed to show any additive effects and toxicity was substantial (71–73).

IL-2

IL-2 was the first cytokine demonstrated to mediate antitumor effects via the host immune system. IL-2 has no demonstrable direct antitumor effect but activates immune effector cells, which then target neoplastic lesions (74). IL-2 can generate NK and LAK cells, enhance their function, augment alloantigen responsiveness, stimulate cytotoxic T-cell growth, and mediate the regression of large tumor burdens (Fig. 48.1) (75). In the first large study investigating the therapeutic role of IL-2 in metastatic renal cell carcinoma, 60 patients were treated with IL-2, with an overall response rate of 18% (76). Other researchers have confirmed these results (77, 78) and, when combined with additional studies comprising a total of 255 patients treated with IL-2, an overall objective response rate of 15% and a duration of almost 2 years were demonstrated (79). Rosenberg et al. summarized their experience with high-dose IL-2 therapy and metastatic renal cell carcinoma, noting a 20% overall response rate (80). Table 48.2 lists the major clinical studies of IL-2 on metastatic renal disease. These studies have identified certain patient characteristics associated with a better response to IL-2 therapy such as good to excellent performance scores and either lung, lymph node, or small-volume extrahepatic abdominal disease.

The current "high-dose" IL-2 protocol at our institution consists of 600,000 IU/kg every 8 hours for up to 14 doses. Following a 9-day respite, the same cycle is repeated. Six weeks after initiating therapy, the patient is restaged. If a response is noted, the course is repeated. Tolerance of the IL-2 dosage, with regard to cardiac, renal, and respiratory functions, is reassessed with each treatment cycle. If the patient is unable to tolerate therapy, the doses are held until the toxicity in question is reversed.

The use of IL-2 is associated with significant side effects, the most serious of which is a prerenal azotemia with resultant hypotension, pulmonary edema, renal failure, and fluid retention. Myocardial infarction, gastrointestinal bleeding and perforation, and death may also occur. These major toxicities are dose-related and result from increased membrane permeability and subsequent fluid and colloid loss into viscera and soft tissue

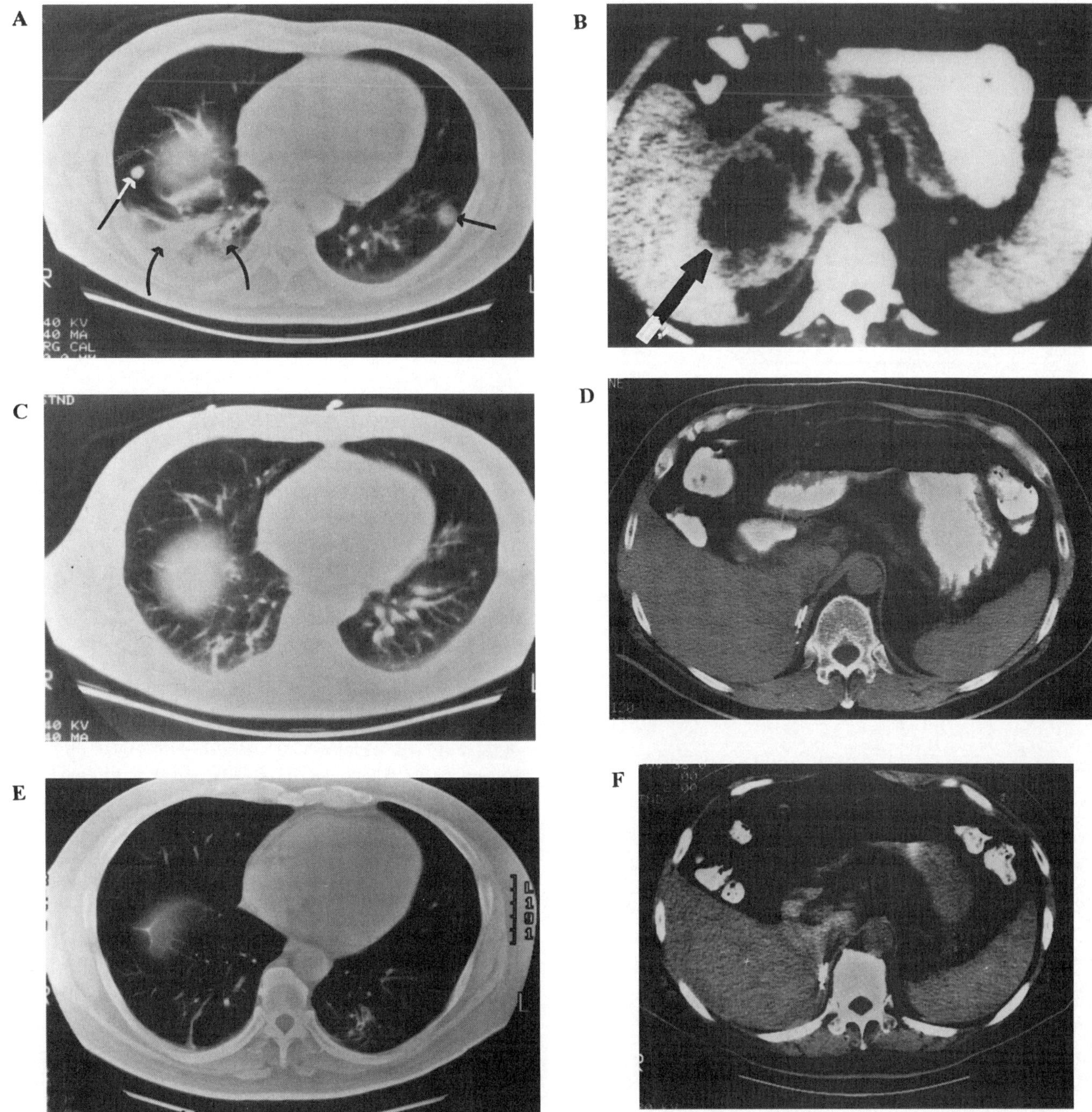

Fig. 48.1. Computed tomography (CT) scans from a patient with complete response to TIL therapy for metastatic renal cell carcinoma. **A and B.** Preoperative films. Thin arrows highlight pulmonary metastasis; thick arrow highlights primary tumor. **C and D.** Scans taken at the completion of TIL therapy. **E and F.** Scans from a 5-year follow-up study.

(86–90). Other common side effects include fever, chills, anorexia, gastrointestinal upset, mental status changes, tachyarrhythmias, and third spacing of fluids. These are reversible and usually resolve within 72 hours of discontinuing therapy. Although the mortality rate from IL-2 therapy was initially 1.5 to 4% (81, 91), more recent data show reduced toxicity as more experience is gained with this treatment modality (80). There have been no deaths in our series.

To prevent these severe yet largely reversible toxicities, alternative infusion schedules and dosing regimens have been devised. Several studies have compared continuous versus bolus IL-2 administration (77, 82–84). Results demonstrate similar response rates of 15 to 20% and equivalent side effects between the two groups, although continuous infusion of IL-2 requires less total drug.

Other researchers have focused on low-dose IL-2 therapy,

Table 48.2. Phase II Trials of Interleukin-2 for the Treatment of Metastatic Renal Cell Cancer

AUTHOR	REFERENCE NO.	YEAR	NO. OF PATIENTS	RESPONSE (%)
West et al.	77	1987	40	32
Fisher et al.	78	1988	35	16
Rosenberg et al.	81	1989	54	22
Bukowski et al.	82	1990	41	12
Geerten et al.	83	1992	30	20
Weiss et al.	84	1992	94	18
Rosenberg et al.	76	1992	60	18
Atkins et al.	85	1993	71	17
Rosenberg et al.	80	1994	143	20
Total			568	20

Table 48.3. Phase II Trials of Combination Cytokine Therapy for Metastatic Renal Cell Cancer

AUTHOR	REFERENCE NO.	YEAR	NO. OF PATIENTS	RESPONSE (%)
Rosenberg et al.	97	1989	35	31[a]
Mittleman et al.	98	1990	18	22
Kirchner et al.	99	1990	17	29
Atzpodien et al.	100	1990	17	36
Atzpodien et al.	101	1990	14	35
Hirsch et al.	102	1990	15	40
Bukowski et al.	103	1990	20	15
Thomas et al.	104	1992	34	6
Spencer et al.	105	1992	22	5
Budd et al.	106	1992	21	10
Figlin et al.	107	1992	52	25
Sznol et al.	108	1992	42	19[a]
Rosenberg	76	1992	41	34
Ilson et al.	109	1992	34	12
Lipton et al.	110	1993	39	33
Atkins et al.	85	1993	28	11
Bermann et al.	111	1993	30	30
Vogelzang et al.	91	1993	42	12
Total			521	22

[a] Includes LAK cells

especially since many metastatic renal cell carcinoma patients are not candidates for high-dose treatment given their age, concomitant disease states, and overall incapacity. The results are inconsistent. Although all studies associated the lower dose with decreased toxicity, some demonstrated similar efficacy between high- and low-dose IL-2 therapy (92, 93), while others (94) failed to observe any objective response with low-dose treatment. Low-dose IL-2 therapy at our institution consists of 18 million IU administered subcutaneously daily for 5 days of the first week. For weeks 2 through 4, 9 million IU are given on days 1 and 2, and 18 million IU are given on days 3 through 5. No doses are given on days 6 and 7. After a 2-week "holiday," restaging is performed at week 6. If disease is stable or improved, therapy is repeated in an identical fashion. The advantage of this regimen is its outpatient delivery and lack of requirement of intensive care unit monitoring. Late cumulative toxicity may occur in patients subjected to many treatment courses.

Combination Therapy: IL-2 and IFN-α

Combining IL-2 infusion with other cytokines has also been investigated as a means of reducing toxicity. Based on in vitro studies demonstrating synergistic activity of IL-2 and IFN-α (95, 96), patients with metastatic renal cell carcinoma were treated in this fashion, demonstrating a 31% response rate (97). Since then, other studies have investigated this combined approach. The results are listed in Table 48.3, with response rates averaging 22%, depending on patient selection and study assessment parameters. At our institution, an outpatient regimen of low-dose continuous infusion IL-2 (6 million IU/M^2/day for days 1 through 4) in combination with subcutaneous IFN-α (6 million IU/M^2/day on days 1 and 4) has produced good results with a notable reduction in toxicity when compared with high-dose IL-2. Since 1988, 52 patients at UCLA have been treated with combination IL-2 and IFN-α, the results comparing favorably with those achieved with high-dose IL-2 alone—the response rate was 25%, the median duration of response was 23 months, and the median duration of survival

was 34 + months (107). Similar studies have corroborated these findings (101, 102), confirming that combination IL-2/IFN-α therapy can be administered successfully and safely on an outpatient basis with results similar to that of high-dose IL-2 alone. The main adverse effects of combination therapy include fever, chills, nausea, anorexia, and hypotension. These are less severe than those of high-dose IL-2 alone, however, and are easily treated on a symptomatic basis.

Cellular Therapy Using TIL

The most engaging application of IL-2 is in conjunction with cellular adoptive immunotherapy, or more specifically, with TIL. Earlier approaches to adoptive immunotherapy used LAK cells. Generated by cultivating peripheral blood cells with IL-2 for 3 to 4 days, LAK are nonspecific NK cells that mediate lysis of tumor in a non-MHC restricted fashion (112) and have a combined response rate of 23.5% (84, 92, 108, 113–117). A randomized study that compared IL-2 alone with IL-2 combined with LAK cells was unable to demonstrate any superiority of combined IL-2/LAK (113), and LAK immunotherapy has subsequently all but been abandoned.

TIL, conversely, are activated cytotoxic T cells that show great specificity in targeting tumor deposits, including those of renal cell carcinoma (118, 119). They are capable of eradicating advanced and bulky tumors against which LAK cells have been unsuccessful. TIL are isolated from solid tumors and are grown by preparing a single cell suspension of tumor tissue and then culturing these cells with IL-2. After in vitro expansion with

IL-2, TIL are reinfused back to the patient in the hope that they will attach to tumor deposits and destroy the neoplastic tissue while leaving normal tissue unscathed.

On a cellular basis, TIL are fiftyfold to one hundredfold more potent than LAK cells in mediating tumor regression (120). The preparation of TIL is well established (88). Under sterile conditions, a radical nephrectomy specimen is mechanically and enzymatically disrupted to obtain a single cell suspension of both lymphoid and tumor cells. Cells are expanded ex vivo by culturing with IL-2. This produces a TIL population with antitumor specificity. After 5 to 6 weeks in culture, 10^{10} to 10^{11} TIL are produced and then infused into the patient along with IL-2.

Few clinical studies have been undertaken with TIL immunotherapy. The UCLA experience includes 48 patients with a response rate of 33%, an average response duration of 14 months, and a mean survival of 22 months (88). Survival is increased in patients with good to excellent performance status, prior nephrectomy, less metastatic sites, and no prior cytotoxic therapy.

An early problem with TIL therapy was the heterogeneity of harvested cells, consisting primarily of noncytolytic CD4+ cells. We have increased our efficacy to 40% by enhancing the proportion of cytolytic CD8 + cells in our TIL population (121, 122). Before nephrectomy, patients at UCLA are "primed" with IL-2 and/or IFN-α to increase the CD8 + fraction to more than 50%. Additionally, recent technologic advances have enabled us to further purify the cytolytic lymphocyte population. Based on our improved response rate, a multicenter randomized trial comparing the results of nephrectomy and IL-2 versus nephrectomy, IL-2, and CD8$^+$/TIL is currently underway.

FUTURE DIRECTIONS

An important new strategy to overcome the poor immunogenicity of some neoplastic lesions is to insert cytokine genes directly into tumor cells. Animal studies of this technique have demonstrated prevention of tumor growth, decreased metastatic spread, and prolonged immunologic memory, resulting in the rejection of subsequent tumor challenges (123–130). This treatment strategy is the "tumor vaccine" eluded to earlier in this chapter. At UCLA, we have transfected the genes for IL-2 and IFN-α into human renal cell carcinoma cell lines. When these cells are implanted subcutaneously into nude mice, cytokine secretion from these cells prevents tumor growth locally and is more effective than systemic IL-2 and IFN-α administration (131). The local production of high concentrations of cytokine may directly alter tumor properties associated with invasion and metastasis. Another approach to cytokine gene therapy is the direct transfection of TIL with cytokine genes. The rationale is that the TIL will traffic directly to tumor deposits, concentrate at these sites, and secrete high levels of cytotoxic cytokines with minimal systemic toxicity. Preliminary studies, including the use of double-gene marking approaches to evaluate the homing properties of renal TIL versus peripheral blood lymphocytes, are currently being performed (132, 133).

CURRENT RECOMMENDATIONS (FIG. 48.2)

Approaching the patient with disseminated renal cell carcinoma is a therapeutic challenge. No effective radiation therapy or chemotherapeutic options are available. Although surgical extirpation is successful in ameliorating pain and hemorrhage, it offers no curative potential. Immunotherapeutic agents offer a potentially curative and durable treatment option, but only when applied to appropriate patient populations within an established immunotherapy center. Such programs must emphasize a cooperative effort among urologic surgeons, medical oncologists, and their support staffs. Likewise, the availability of and a familiarity with an intensive care unit care are essential.

At UCLA, management is tailored to each patient. On initial evaluation, patients are assessed for the ability to receive IL-2–based therapy. This requires adequate cardiac, pulmonary, renal, hepatic, and hematologic function; the presence of central nervous system disease must be excluded; and the performance scale should be low. Younger patients with favorable performance status and organ reserve are stratified to high-dose IL-2–based therapy. All others receive low-dose IL-2–based therapy. Experimental protocols involving other cytokines or chemotherapeutic agents may be offered.

The role of nephrectomy is controversial. At UCLA, pretherapy nephrectomies are performed in cases of disseminated disease in conjunction with immunotherapy or to reduce tumor load in very large primary tumors. Conversely, patients with small primary masses and/or multiple small metastatic lesions are first given immunotherapy. Those patients whose metastases respond to treatment can then subsequently undergo nephrectomy.

Following each course of therapy, the patient is reevaluated and restaged. If a positive response is noted and therapy is well tolerated, treatment is continued until the maximal effect is achieved. Therapy is discontinued for progressive and persistently static disease. After therapy is completed, routine follow-up is essential. The treatment of relapses is also individually tailored with respect to the initial agent and response to that therapy. With such a treatment algorithm, successful clinical responses and significant improvements in the quality and duration of life can be achieved.

CONCLUSIONS

The past two decades have witnessed impressive advancements in the application of immunotherapy to renal cell carcinoma. At UCLA, we have seen a progressive increase in responses to treatment as therapy has evolved from systemic IFN-α administration (16%), to combination IFN-α/IL-2 use (25%), to the current method of bulk TIL (33%) and CD8$^+$/TIL (40%). We have identified patient characteristics that predict improved responsiveness to therapy and have established treatment proto-

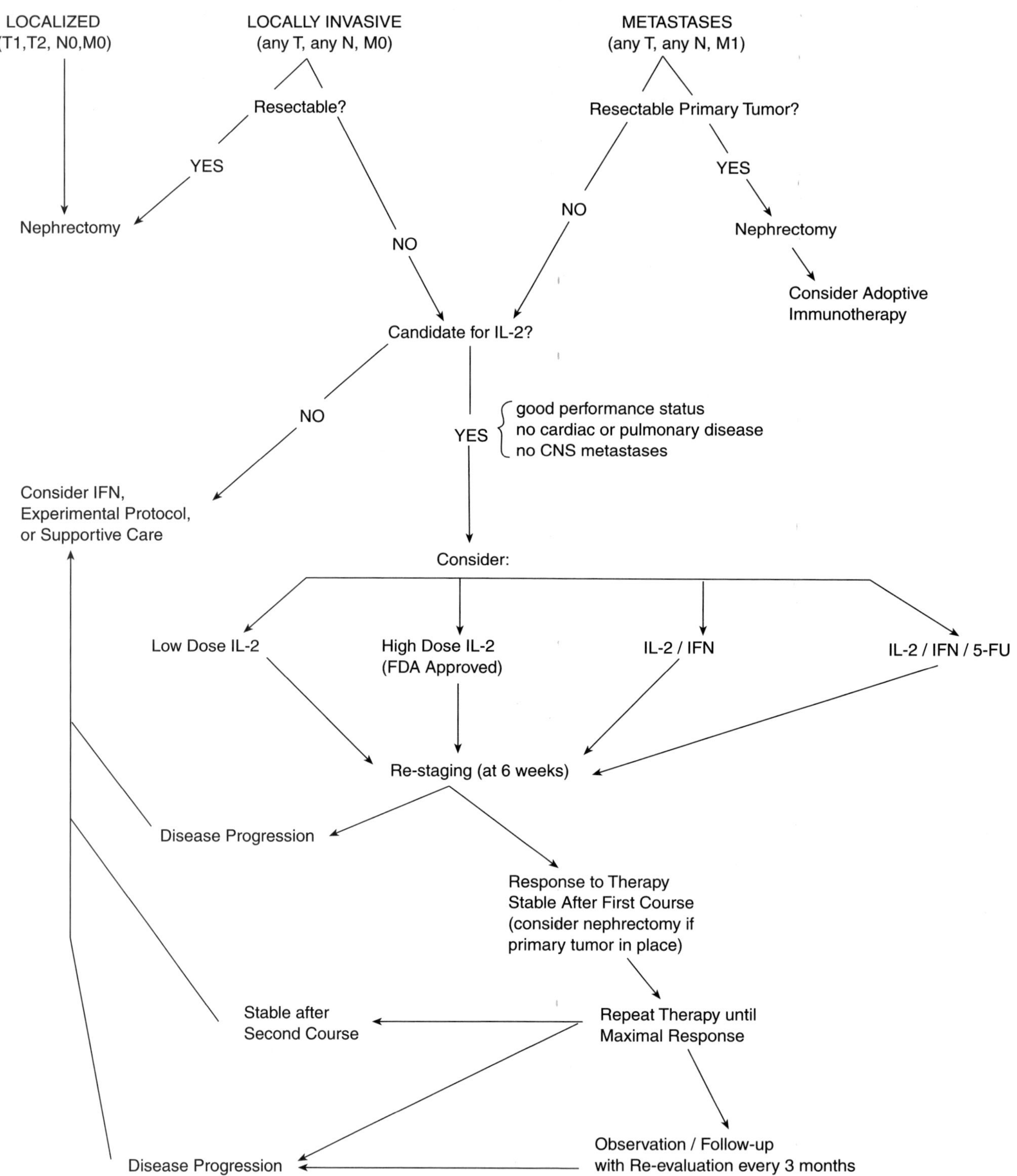

Fig. 48.2. Management algorithm used at UCLA when treating a patient with advanced renal cell carcinoma.

cols that decreased toxicity. The most encouraging results have been the improved rates of complete clinical response, most of which are durable and long lasting. Our current focus is on creating tumor vaccines and furthering systemic gene therapy modalities.

Further refinements in the treatment of renal cell carcinoma with immunotherapy are still needed, yet there is no doubt that current immunotherapeutic protocols produce changes in the natural history of renal cell carcinoma and cause significant and lasting remissions in select patients.

REFERENCES

1. Wingo PA, Tong T, Bolden BA. Cancer statistics, 1995. CA Cancer J Clin 1995;45:8.

2. deKernion JB, Belldegrun A. Renal tumors. In: Walsh PC, et al., eds. Campbell's urology. Philadelphia: WB Saunders, 1993:1053.

3. de Kernion JB. Renal tumors. In: Skinner DG, ed. Genitourinary cancer. Philadelphia: WB Saunders, 1978.

4. Nabel GJ, Chang AE, Nabel EG, et al. Immunotherapy of malignancy by in vivo gene transfer into tumors. Hum Genet Ther 1992;3:399.

5. Belldegrun A, Figlin R, deKernion J. Immunotherapy for renal cell carcinoma. Semin Urol 1992;10:23.

6. Rosenberg SA, Spiess P, Lafreniere R. A new approach to the adoptive immunotherapy of cancer with tumor-infiltrating lymphocytes. Science 1986;233:1318.

7. Belldegrun A, Tso CL, Sakata T, et al. Human renal carcinoma line transfected with interleukin-2 and/or interferon-gamma genes: implications for live cancer vaccines. J Natl Cancer Inst 1993;85:207.

8. Spiess PJ, Yang JC, Rosenberg SA. In vivo anti-tumor activity of tumor-infiltrating lymphocytes expanded in recombinant interleukin-2. J Natl Cancer Inst 1987;79:1067.

9. Pierce W, Belldegrun A, Figlin R. Cellular therapy: scientific rationale and clinical results in the treatment of metastatic renal cell cancer. Semin Oncol 1995;22:74.

10. Horn HJG. Hormone-induced and spontaneous regression of metastatic renal cancer. Cancer 1973;32:1066.

11. Pardoll D. Immunotherapy with cytokine gene-transduced tumor cells the next wave in gene therapy for cancer. Curr Opin Oncol 1992;4:1124.

12. Sanda MG, Ayyagari SR, Jaffee E, et al. Demonstration of a rational strategy for human prostate cancer gene therapy. J Urol 1994;151:622.

13. Pardoll DM. New strategies for enhancing the immunogenicity of tumors. Curr Opin Immunol 1993;5:719.

14. Gansbacher B, Rosenthal FM, Zier K. Retroviral vector-mediated cytokine gene transfer into tumor cells. Cancer Invest 1993;11:345.

15. Hill ADK, Redmond HP, Croke DT, et al. Cytokines in tumor therapy. Br J Surg 1992;79:990.

16. Talmadge JE. Development of immunotherapeutic strategies for the treatment of malignant neoplasms. Biotherapy 1992;4:215.

17. Weidmann E, Bergmann L, Heckler P, et al. Rapid cytokine release in cancer patients treated with Interleukin-2. J Immunol 1992;12:123.

18. Tomita Y, Watanabe H, Kobayashi H, et al. Interferon-gamma but not tumor necrosis factor alpha decreases susceptibility of human renal cell cancer cell lines to lymphokine-activated killer cells. Cancer Immunol Immunother 1992;35:381.

19. Ogasawar M, Rosenberg SA. Enhanced expression of HLA molecules and stimulation of autologous human tumor infiltrating lymphocytes following transduction of melanoma cells with gamma-interferon genes. Cancer Res 1993;35:3561.

20. Gansbacher B, Zier B, Cronin K, et al. Retroviral gene transfer induced constitutive expression of interleukin-2 or interferon-gamma in irradiated human melanoma cells. Blood 1992;80:2817.

21. Smith KA. Interleukin-2: inception, impact, and implications. Science 1988;240:1169.

22. deKernion JB, Ramming KP, Smith RB. Natural history of metastatic renal cell carcinoma: a computer analysis. J Urol 1978;120:148.

23. deKernion JB, Berry D. The diagnosis and treatment of renal cell carcinoma. Cancer 1980;45:1947.

24. Belldegrun A, Koo AS, Bochner B, et al. Immunotherapy for advanced renal cell cancer: the role of radical nephrectomy. Eur Urol 1990;18(Suppl):42.

25. Belldegrun A, Abi-Aad ASB, Figlin R, et al. Renal cell carcinoma: basic and current approaches to therapy. Semin Oncol 1991;18(Suppl):96.

26. Walther MM, Alexander RB, Weiss GH, et al. Cytoreductive surgery prior to IL-2 based therapy in patients with metastatic renal cell carcinoma. Urology 1993;42:250.

27. Rabinovitch RA, Zelefsky MJ, Gaynor JJ, et al. Patterns of failure following surgical resection of renal cell carcinoma: implications for adjuvant local and systemic therapy. J Clin Oncol 1994;12:206.

28. Van der Werf-Messing B. Carcinoma of the kidney. Cancer 1973;32:1056.

29. Bloom HJ. Hormone-induced and spontaneous regression of metastatic renal cancer. Cancer 1973;32:1006.

30. deKernion JB. Treatment of advanced renal cell carcinoma: traditional methods and innovative approaches. J Urol 1982;130:2.

31. Ferrazi E, Salvagno L, Fornasiero A, et al. Tamoxifen treatment for advanced renal cell cancer. Tumori 1980;66:601.

32. Yagoda A. Chemotherapy of renal cell carcinoma: 1983–1989. Semin Urol 1989;7:199.

33. Yagoda A, Abi-Rached B, Petrylak D. Chemotherapy for advanced renal cell carcinoma. Semin Oncol 1995;22:42.

34. deKernion JB, Ramming KP. The therapy of renal adenocarcinoma with immune RNA. Invest Urol 1980;17:378.

35. Morales A, Wilson JL, Pater JL, et al. Cytoreductive surgery and systemic BCG therapy in metastatic renal cancer: a phase II trial. J Urol 1982;127:230.

36. McCune CS, Schapira DV, Henshaw EC. Specific immunotherapy of advanced renal carcinoma: evidence for polyclonality of metastases. Cancer 1981;47:1984.

37. Morgan DA, Ruscetti FW, Gallo R. Selective in vitro growth of T lymphocytes from normal human bone marrow. Science 1976;193:1007.

38. Duckett T, Figlin RA, Belldegrun A. Biological response modifiers in metastatic renal cell carcinoma. Curr Opin Urol 1992;2:339.

39. deKernion J, Sarna G, Figlin RA, et al. The treatment of renal cell carcinoma with human leukocyte alpha-interferon. J Urol 1983;130:1063.

40. Quesada JR, Swanson DA, Trindale A, et al. Renal cell carcinoma: antitumor effects of alpha-interferon. Cancer Res 1983;43:940.

41. Quesada JR, Swanson DA, Gutterman JU, et al. Phase II study of interferon alpha in metastatic renal cell carcinoma. J Clin Oncol 1985;3:1086.

42. Kirkwood JM, Harris JE, Vera R, et al. Randomized study of low and high doses of leukocyte alpha-interferon in metastatic renal cell carcinoma. Cancer Res 1985;45:863.

43. Figlin RA, deKernion JB, Mukamel E, et al. Recombinant interferon alpha-2a in metastatic renal cell carcinoma. J Clin Oncol 1988;6:1604.

44. Umeda T, Niijima I. Phase II study of alpha interferon on renal cell carcinoma: summary of three collaborative trials. Cancer 1986;58:1231.

45. Neidhart JA. Interferon-alpha treatment of renal cancer. Cancer Res 1984;44:4140.

46. Vugrin D, Hood L, Laszlo J. A phase II trial of high dose human lymphoblastoid alpha interferon in patients with advanced renal carcinoma. J Biol Resp Mod 1986;5:309.

47. Vugrin D, Hood L, Taylor W, et al. Phase II study of human lymphoblastoid interferon in patients with advanced renal carcinoma. Cancer Treat Rep 1985;69:817.

48. Minasian LM, Motzer RJ, Glucke L, et al. Interferon alfa-2a in advanced renal cell carcinoma. J Clin Oncol 1993;11:1368.

49. Muss HB, Welander C, Caponera M, et al. Recombinant alfa interferon in renal cell carcinoma: a randomized trial of two routes of administration. J Clin Oncol 1987;5:286.

50. Neidhart JA. Interferon therapy for the treatment of renal cancer. Cancer 1986;57(Suppl):1696.

51. Sarna G, Figlin R, deKernion JB. Interferon in renal cell carcinoma. Cancer 1987;59:610.

52. Figlin RA, deKernion JB, Maldazys J, et al. Treatment of renal cell carcinoma with alpha interferon and vinblastine in combination: a phase I–II trial. Cancer Treat Rep 1985;69: 263.

53. Creagan ET, Kovacs JS, Long HJ, et al. An evaluation of recombinant leukocyte: α-interferon with aspirin in patients with metastatic renal cell cancer. Cancer 1988;61:1787.

54. Fossa SD, de Garis ST, Heier MS, et al. Recombinant interferon α-2a with and without vinblastine in metastatic renal cell carcinoma. Cancer 1986;57:1700.

55. Jones GJ, Itri LM. Safety and tolerance of recombinant interferon 2a in cancer patients. Cancer 1986;57:1709.

56. Taguchi T. Clinical studies of recombinant interferon α-2a in cancer patients. Cancer 1986;57:1705.

57. Logothetis C, Hossan E, Sella A, et al. 5-fluorouracil and interferon-alpha in chemotherapy-refractory bladder carcinoma. Anticancer Res 1994;14:1265.

58. Logothetis C. Treatment of chemotherapy-refractory metastatic urothelial tumors. Urol Clin North Am 1992;19: 775.

59. Tomita Y, Imai T, Katagiri A. 5-fluorouracil increases susceptibility of renal cell cancer cell lines to lymphokine-activated killer cells. Cancer Lett 1993;75:27.

60. Sella A, Logothetis CJ, Fitz K, et al. Phase II study of interferon-alpha and chemotherapy (5-FU and mitomycin-C) in metastatic renal cell carcinoma. J Urol 1992;147:573.

61. Sella A, Zukiwski A, et al. Interleukin-2 with interferon-alpha and 5-fluorouracil in patients with metastatic renal cell cancer. Proc Am Soc Clin Oncol 1994;13:237.

62. Muss HB, Welander C, Coponera M, et al. Interferon and doxorubicin in renal cell carcinoma. Cancer Treat Rep 1985; 69:721.

63. Creagan ET, Kovacs JS, Long HS, et al. Phase I study of recombinant leukocyte α human interferon combined with BCNU in selected patients with advanced cancer. J Clin Oncol 1986;4:408.

64. Homma Y, Aso Y. Effect of alpha-interferon alone and combined with other anti-neoplastic agents on renal cell carcinoma determined by the tetrazolium microculture assay. Eur Urol 1994;25;164.

65. Ellenhorst JA, Kilbourne RG, Amato RJ, et al. Phase II trial of low dose gamma-interferon in metastatic renal cell carcinoma. J Urol 1994;152:841.

66. Rinehart J, Young D, Laforge J, et al. Phase I/II trial of human recombinant beta-interferon serine in patients with renal cell carcinoma. Cancer Res 1986;46:5364.

67. Quesada JR. Phase II studies of recombinant human interferon gamma in metastatic renal cell carcinoma. J Biol Resp Mod 1987;6:20.

68. Rinehart JJ, Laforge J, Young D, et al. Phase I/II trial of recombinant human interferon gamma in renal cell carcinoma. J Biol Resp Mod 1986;5:300.

69. Aulitzski W, et al. Successful treatment of metastatic renal cell carcinoma with a biologically active dose of recombinant interferon-gamma. J Clin Oncol 1989;7:187.

70. Sayers TS, Wiltrout TA, McCormick K, et al. Anti-tumor effects of alpha-interferon and gamma interferon in a murine renal cell carcinoma in vitro and in vivo. Cancer Res 1990; 20:5414.

71. Geboers AD, Mulder PH, Debruyne FM, et al. Alpha and gamma interferon in the treatment of advanced renal cell carcinoma. Semin Surg Oncol 1988;4:191.

72. Nair SG. Phase I/II trial of recombinant interferons alpha and gamma in patients with metastatic renal cell carcinoma. Proc Am Soc Clin Oncol 1988;7:126.

73. Ernstoff MS, Nair SG, Bahnson RR, et al. A phase Ia trial of sequential administration of recombinant DNA-produced interferons. J Clin Oncol 1990;8:1637.

74. Smith KA. Interleukin-2: inception, impact, implications. Science 1988;240:1169.

75. Rosenberg SA. Immunotherapy of cancer using IL-2. Immunol Today 1988;9:58.

76. Rosenberg SA. The immunology and gene therapy of cancer. J Clin Oncol 1992;10:180.

77. West WH, Tauer KW, Yarinelli JR, et al. Constant-infusion recombinant interleukin-2 in adoptive immunotherapy of advanced cancer. N Engl J Med 1987;316:898.

78. Fisher RI. Metastatic renal cancer treated with interleukin-2 and lymphokine-activated killer cells. Ann Intern Med 1988; 108:518.

79. FDA Biological Response Modifiers Advisory Committee Hearings, Washington, DC, 1992.

80. Rosenberg SA, Yang JC, Topalian SL, et al. Treatment of 283 consecutive patients with metastatic melanoma or renal cell cancer using high-dose bolus interleukin-2. JAMA 1994; 271:907.

81. Rosenberg SA, Lotze MT, Yang JC, et al. Experience with the use of high-dose interleukin-2 in the treatment of 652 cancer patients. Ann Surg 1989;210:474.

82. Bukowski RM, Sharfman W, Murthy S, et al. Phase II trial of high-dose intermittent interleukin-2 in metastatic renal cell carcinoma. J Natl Cancer Inst 1990;82:143.

83. Geertsen PF, Hermann GG, van der Maase H, et al. Treatment of metastatic renal cell carcinoma by continuous

intravenous infusion of recombinant interleukin-2: a single center phase II study. J Clin Oncol 1992;10:753.

84. Weiss GR, Margolin KA, Aronson FR, et al. A randomized phase II trial of continuous infusion interleukin-2 or bolus injection interleukin-2 plus lymphokine-activated killer cells for advanced renal cell carcinoma. J Clin Oncol 1992;10:275.

85. Atkins MB, Sparano J, Fischer RI, et al. Randomized phase II trial of high-dose interleukin-2 either alone or in combination with interferon alfa-2b in advanced renal cell carcinoma. J Clin Oncol 1993;11:661.

86. Rosenstein M, Ettinghausen SE, Rosenberg SA. Extravasation of intravascular fluid mediated by the systemic administration of recombinant interleukin-2. J Immunol 1986;137:1735.

87. Siegel JP, Puri RK. Interleukin-2 toxicity. J Clin Oncol 1991;9:694.

88. Belldegrun A, Pierce WC, Kaboo R, et al. Interferon alpha-primed tumor infiltrating lymphocytes combined with interleukin-2 and interferon-alpha as a therapy for metastatic renal cell carcinoma. J Urol 1993;150:1384.

89. Belldegrun A, Webb DA, Austin HA, et al. Effects of interleukin-2 on renal function in patients receiving immunotherapy for advanced cancer. Ann Intern Med 1987;106:817.

90. Webb ED, Austin HA, Belldegrun A, et al. Metabolic and renal effects of IL-2 immunotherapy for metastatic renal cell carcinoma. Clin Nephrol 1988;30:141.

91. Vogelzang NJ, Lipton A, Figlin RA. Subcutaneous IL-2 plus interferon in metastatic renal cell cancer: an outpatient multicenter trial. J Clin Oncol 1993;11:1809.

92. Thompson JA, Shulman KL, Benyunes MC, et al. Prolonged continuous intravenous infusion interleukin-2 and lymphocyte-activated killer cell therapy for metastatic renal cell carcinoma. J Clin Oncol 1992;10:960.

93. Buter J, Sleijfer DT, van der Fgraaf WT, et al. A progress report on the outpatient treatment of patients with advanced renal cell carcinoma using subcutaneous recombinant interleukin-2. Semin Oncol 1993;20(Suppl):16.

94. Koretz MJ, Lawson DH, York RM, et al. Randomized study of interleukin-2 alone vs IL-2 plus lymphokine-activated killer cells for treatment of melanoma and renal cell cancer. Arch Surg 1991;126:898.

95. Rosenberg SA, Schwarz SL, Spiess PJ. Combination immunotherapy for cancer: synergistic antitumor interactions of interleukin-2, alfa interferon, and tumor-infiltrating lymphocytes. J Natl Cancer Inst 1988;80:1393.

96. Brunda MJ, Bellantoni D, Sulich V. In vivo anti-tumor activity of combinations of interferon alpha and interleukin-2 in a murine model. Int J Cancer 1987;40:365.

97. Rosenberg SA, Schwartz SL, Spiess PJ, et al. Combination therapy with interleukin-2 and alpha-interferon for the treatment of patients with advanced cancer. J Clin Oncol 1989;7:1863.

98. Mittelman A, Huberman M, Puccio C, et al. A phase I study of recombinant human interleukin-2 and alpha-interferon-2a in patients with renal cell cancer, colorectal cancer, and malignant melanoma. Cancer 1990;66:664.

99. Kirchner H, Korfer A, Palmer PA, et al. Subcutaneous interleukin-2 and interferon-alpha-2b in patients with metastatic renal cell cancer: the German outpatient experience. Mol Biother 1990;2:145.

100. Atzpodien J, Korfer A, Franks CR, et al. Home therapy with recombinant interleukin-2 and interferon-alpha-2b in advanced human malignancies. Lancet 1990;335:1509.

101. Atzpodien J, Korfer A, Palmer PA, et al. Treatment of metastatic renal cell cancer patients with recombinant subcutaneous human interleukin-2 and alpha-interferon. Ann Oncol 1990;1:377.

102. Hirsch M, Lipton A, Harvey H, et al. Phase I study of interleukin-2 and interferon-alpha-2a as outpatient therapy for patients with advanced malignancy. J Clin Oncol 1990;8:1657.

103. Bukowski RM, Murthy S, Sergi J, et al. Phase I trial of continuous infusion recombinant interleukin-2 and intermittent recombinant interferon-alpha-2a: clinical effects. J Biol Resp Mod 1990;9:538.

104. Thomas H, Barton C, Saini A, et al. Sequential interleukin-2 and alpha-interferon for renal cell carcinoma and melanoma. Eur J Cancer 1992;28:1047. Abstract.

105. Spencer WF, Linehan WM, Walter MM, et al. Immunotherapy with interleukin-2 and alpha interferon in patients with metastatic renal cell carcinoma with in situ primary cancers: a pilot study. J Urol 1992;147:24.

106. Budd GT, Murthy S, Finke J, et al. Phase I trial of high dose bolus interleukin-2 and interferon-alpha-2a in patients with metastatic malignancy. J Clin Oncol 1992;10:804.

107. Figlin RA, Belldegrun A, Moldawer N, et al. Concomitant administration of recombinant human interleukin-2 and recombinant interferon alfa-2a: an active outpatient regimen in metastatic renal cell carcinoma. J Clin Oncol 1992;10:414.

108. Sznol M, Clark JW, Smith JW, et al. Pilot study of interleukin-2 and lymphokine-activated killer cells combined with immunomodulatory doses of chemotherapy and sequenced with interferon alfa-2a in patients with metastatic melanoma and renal cell carcinoma. J Natl Cancer Inst 1992;84:929.

109. Ilson DH, Motzer RJ, Kradin RL, et al. A phase II trial of interleukin-2 and interferon alfa-2a in patients with advanced renal cell carcinoma. J Clin Oncol 1992;10:1124.

110. Lipton A, Harvey H, Givant E, et al. Interleukin-2 and interferon alpha-2a outpatient therapy for metastatic renal cell carcinoma. J Immunother 1993;13:122.

111. Bergmann L, Fenchel K, Weidmann E, et al. Daily alternating administration of high-dose alpha-2b interferon and interleukin-2 bolus infusion in metastatic renal cell cancer. Cancer 1993;72:1733.

112. Grimm EA, Mazumder A, Zhang HZ, et al. Lymphokine-activated killer cell phenomenon. J Exp Med 1993;155:1823.

113. Rosenberg SA, Lotze MT, Yang JC, et al. Prospective randomized trial of high-dose interleukin-2 alone or in conjunction with lymphokine-activated killer cells for the treatment of patients with advanced cancer. J Natl Cancer Inst 1993;85:622.

114. Parkinson DR, Fisher RI, Rayner AA, et al. Therapy of renal cell carcinoma with interleukin-2 and lymphokine-activated killer cells: phase II experience with a hybrid bolus and continuous infusion interleukin-2 regimen. J Clin Oncol 1990;8:1630.

115. Dillman RO, Church C, et al. Inpatient continuous-infusion interleukin-2 in 788 patients with cancer: the National Biotherapy Study Group experience. Cancer 1993;71:2358.

116. Palmer PA, Vinke J, Evers P, et al. Continuous infusion of recombinant interleukin-2 with or without autologous lymphocyte-activated killer cells for the treatment of advanced renal cell carcinoma. Eur J Cancer 1992;28:1038. Abstract.

117. Foon KA, Walther PJ, Bernstein ZP, et al. Renal cell carcinoma treated with continuous-infusion interleukin-2 with ex-vivo activated killer cells. J Immunother 1992;11:184.

118. Belldegrun A, Pierce W, Sayah D, et al. Soluble tumor necrosis factor expression in patients with metastatic renal cell carcinoma treated with interleukin-2-based immunotherapy. J Immunother 1993;13:175.

119. Schendel DJ, Gansbacher B, Oberneder R, et al. Tumor-specific lysis of human renal cell carcinomas by tumor-infiltrating lymphocytes. J Immunol 1993;151:4209.

120. Rosenberg SA, Packard BS, Aebersold PM, et al. Use of tumor-infiltrating lymphocytes and interleukin-2 in the immunotherapy of patients with metastatic melanoma. N Engl J Med 1988;319:1676.

121. Steger GG, Pierce WC, et al. Patterns in cytokine release of unselected and CD8 + selected renal cell carcinoma tumor-infiltrating lymphocytes. Clin Immunol Immunopathol 1994;72:237.

122. Belldegrun A, Pierce W, deKernion JB. Clinical activity of purified CD8 + tumor infiltrating lymphocytes and low dose IL-2 in the treatment of metastatic renal cell carcinoma. J Urol 1994;151:315. Abstract.

123. Watanabe Y, Kuribayashi K, Miyatake S, et al. Exogenous expression of mouse interferon-G cDNA in mouse neuroblastoma C1300 cells results in reduced tumorigenicity by augmented anti-tumor immunity. Proc Natl Acad Sci USA 1989;86:9456.

124. Gansbacher B, Zier K, Daniels B, et al. Interleukin-2 gene transfer into tumor cells abrogates tumorigenicity and induces protective immunity. Exp Med 1990;172:1217.

125. Gansbacher B, Bannerji R, Daniels B, et al. Retroviral vector-mediated gamma-interferon gene transfer into tumor cells generates potent and long-lasting antitumor immunity. Cancer Res 1990;50:7820.

126. Asher AL, Mule JJ, Kasid A, et al. Murine tumor cells transduced with the gene for tumor necrosis factor-alpha: evidence for paracrine immune effects of tumor necrosis factor against tumors. J Immunol 1991;146:3227.

127. Hock H, Dorsch M, Diamantstein T, et al. Interleukin-7 induced CD4 + T-cell dependent tumor rejection. J Exp Med 1991;174:1291.

128. Golumbek PT, Lazenby AJ, Levitsky HI, et al. Treatment of established renal cancer by tumor cells engineered to secrete interleukin-4. Science 1991;254:713.

129. Kirchner H, Anton P, Hanninen EL, et al. Adjuvant treatment of locally advanced renal cell carcinoma with active specific immunotherapy. J Urol 1994;151:316. Abstract.

130. Jaffee EM, Marshall FF, Mulligan RC, et al. Feasibility of human gene therapy for renal cell carcinoma. J Urol 1994;151:486. Abstract.

131. Hathorn RW, Tso CL, Kaboo, et al. In vitro modulation of the invasive and metastatic potentials of human renal cell carcinoma by interleukin-2 and/or interferon-alpha gene transfer. Cancer 1994;74:1904.

132. Hinkel A, Werner TW, deRiese W, et al. Active specific immunotherapy with autologous virus modified tumor vaccines in human renal cell carcinoma. J Urol 1994;151:316. Abstract.

133. Toloza E, et al. In vivo trafficking patterns of human melanoma and renal tumor-infiltrating lymphocytes: results of a double gene marking clinical trial. Society of Surgical Oncology annual meeting, Boston, MA, 1995.

49

Immunotherapy for Bladder Carcinoma

Michael F. Sarosdy

Since the first report of the use of bacille Calmette-Guérin (BCG) in superficial bladder cancer by Morales in 1976 (1), it has been determined that superficial bladder cancer does respond to a variety of immunotherapeutic compounds. The fact that BCG was approved by the Food and Drug Administration (FDA) for the intravesical therapy for carcinoma in situ (CIS), a subpopulation that accounts for approximately 10 to 20% of patients with superficial disease, attests to the solid body of evidence supporting clinical efficacy of BCG. The number of additional immunotherapeutic compounds that have been shown to have efficacy in superficial bladder cancer now exceeds the number of chemotherapeutic drugs instilled intravesically to treat superficial bladder cancer (2). Part of the reason for this is an effort to improve on immunotherapy with BCG. As Morales himself has said regarding BCG, "It is evident that the vaccine will be replaced by different drugs or techniques that will prove to be more effective or devoid of adverse effects" (3).

It is quite reasonable to include a chapter on immunotherapy for bladder cancer in a comprehensive treatise on genitourinary cancer surgery for many reasons. Used effectively through an adequate understanding of the principles of immunotherapy, immunotherapy can act as an extremely powerful adjunct to surgical resection of even high-risk superficial bladder cancers. Also, when used correctly, it can safely spare a large percentage of patients from undergoing cystectomy, at least for a prolonged period. Furthermore, new forms of immunotherapy may further delay cystectomy in patients in whom BCG has failed or, as suggested by Morales, may eventually replace BCG as the preferred adjunct to surgical therapy. Finally, as an in vivo testing ground for nonsystemic therapy for bladder cancer, superficial bladder cancer provides an exciting and safe organ in which to test the delivery and efficacy of new agents such as gene therapy and toxin conjugate compounds, therapies that represent a shift to specific immunotherapy.

It is helpful to keep in mind that immunotherapy may be either active or passive, and that each of those categories may be subdivided into specific and nonspecific. Active immunotherapy is that which induces a change in the state of immune responsiveness in the host animal or patient, whereas passive immunotherapy delivers to the host immunologically active agents that are responsible directly for an antitumor response. Specific subcategories include individual patient tumor-derived vaccine or gene therapy products (active) or monoclonal antibodies (passive). Nonspecific immunotherapy includes the use of agents such as BCG, interferon (IFN), interleukin-2 (IL-2), tumor necrosis factor (TNF), and bropirimine (active) as well as lymphokine-activated killer (LAK) cells expanded by IL-2 incubation (passive).

An additional and important principle to keep in mind is that intravesical therapy should be tailored to the disease process of each patient (2). Table 49.1 outlines disease process characteristics assessable at all hospitals by histopathology, cytopathology, and flow cytometry. Patients presenting with a single favorable tumor do not require either intravesical immunotherapy or chemotherapy, as more than half of such patients will never have a tumor recurrence (4, 5). However, patients with favorable tumor characteristics who have recurrences of the same nature (i.e., nuisance tumors, Table 49.2) might well be treated by intravesical chemotherapy or immunotherapy (6–13). BCG clearly is indicated in patients with frequent, recurrent nuisance (i.e., troublesome) tumors for which prior chemotherapy has failed. A patient presenting with an unfavorable disease process or so-called dangerous tumor should receive intravesical BCG immunotherapy after resection of all visible tumor (14–16). The intent of tailoring the treatment to the disease process is to achieve a beneficial effect in patients who require it and to avoid excessive toxicity in those patients who do not.

BCG

BCG is an attenuated live tuberculosis vaccine subcultured from a virulent strain of *Mycobacterium bovis*. The first clinical application of BCG was in 1921, and the vaccine continues to be used quite effectively to prevent infection with tuberculosis (17).

Pearl reported a possible antineoplastic effect of tuberculosis infection in 1929, marking the initial linkage between the

Table 49.1. Classification by Initial Superficial Tumor Characteristics

FAVORABLE	UNFAVORABLE
Single tumor	Multiple tumors
Stage Ta	Stage T1
Low grade	High grade
No field changes	Atypia or dysplasia
Diploid	Aneuploid
Negative cytology	Positive cytology

Table 49.2. Classification of Transitional Cell Carcinoma of the Bladder

NO.	TRADITIONAL (BY STAGE)	PRACTICAL (BY STAGE AND OCCURRENCE HISTORY)
1	Superficial	Superficial
		Nuisance
		Troublesome
		Dangerous
2	Muscle invasive	Muscle invasive
3	Metastatic	Metastatic

Table 49.3. Bacillus Calmette-Guérin Response Rates in Residual Tumor*

REFERENCE	NO. OF PATIENTS	RESPONSE	PERCENTAGE
Morales et al. (20)	6	4	67
Lamm et al. (21)	23	14	61
Brosman (22)	10	6	60
deKernion et al. (23)	22	8	36
Schellhammer et al. (24)	29	16	55
Kavoussi et al. (25)	27	11	41
Total	97	59	60

* Carcinoma in situ only patients not included.

Table 49.4. Bacillus Calmette-Guérin Response Rates for Carcinoma in Situ

REFERENCE	NO. OF PATIENTS	COMPLETE RESPONSE	PERCENTAGE
Lamm (26)	14	11	79
Herr et al. (27)	47	34	72
Brosman (15)	33	27	82
Schellhammer et al. (24)	6	6	100
deKernion et al. (23)	19	13	68
Kavoussi et al. (25)	50	23	46
Total	169	114	68

immunomodulatory effects of mycobacteria and cancer (3). However, it was not until 1969 that Mathé et al. reported the use of BCG as an adjuvant therapy in acute lymphoblastic leukemia (18). Shortly thereafter, Morton reported the regression of malignant melanoma treated with intralesional injections of BCG (3). Thereafter, the race was on to evaluate BCG in a variety of human carcinomas, including intraperitoneal administration for ovarian cancer and the intrathoracic administration for lung cancers, as well as in a variety of additional human cancers. Unfortunately for most human cancer patients, the majority proved to be unresponsive to immune modulation with BCG. Fortunately for patients with superficial bladder cancer, the results were more encouraging.

During the 1970s, animal studies helped to define under which conditions BCG therapy might be effective against human cancers. These conditions included the following.

1. Close contact between the tumor cells and BCG.
2. An immunocompetent host.
3. Limited tumor burden.
4. An adequate number of viable BCG organisms (19).

Superficial bladder cancer provides a nearly ideal setting and organ system in which to meet these requirements, especially when superficial tumor has been completely or nearly completely resected or the patient has CIS, when the patient can retain the solution adequately, and when the patient is neither debilitated nor taking medications that suppress the immune system.

The evaluation of intravesical BCG therapy for superficial transitional cell carcinoma (TCC) has undergone a sophistication and maturation over the past 20 years. Early clinical trials of intravesical BCG were small, often essentially anecdotal, with poor or inadequate use of control groups. After the efficacy of BCG was recognized through such reports, it was further confirmed and compared with intravesical chemotherapy through randomized prospective trials. It was only through such efforts that BCG was approved by the FDA for CIS. The mechanism of action and factors modulating that have been elucidated over the past 10 years, with application of that knowledge leading toward newer and more promising compounds.

Early BCG Trials

In the early 1980s, BCG was found to be effective in the treatment of residual, unresected papillary disease. Table 49.3 demonstrates that eradication of residual papillary disease can be expected in roughly one third to two thirds of patients so treated.

BCG immunotherapy appears to be even more successful against CIS of the bladder than it is when used for residual papillary disease. Table 49.4 demonstrates that the range of percentages of patients experiencing a complete response is variable, but that roughly 68% of patients can be expected to respond to BCG therapy. It should be noted that higher apparent complete response rates may result from inclusion of patients in clinical trials who carry the diagnosis of CIS, but in whom all existing disease was resected at the time of transure-

Table 49.5. Bacillus Calmette-Guérin Prevention of Papillary Tumor Recurrence

REFERENCE	NO. OF PATIENTS	RESPONSE	PERCENTAGE
Kelley et al. (28)	17	16	94
Haaf et al. (29)	29	26	90
Sarosdy and Lamm (16)	82	73	89
Lamm (26)	31	27	87
Lamm et al. (30)	63	22	35
deKernion et al. (23)	22	15	67
Total	244	179	73

thral resection. None of the listed studies required documentation that existing CIS was still present in the bladder at the time BCG was administered by requiring positive postbiopsy cytologies. Thus, a mixture of patients who still had existing disease in the bladder combined with patients in whom all disease actually had been resected may account for the wide range of apparent complete responses. An additional and potentially important reason for variability in response rates that will be addressed below is the lack of a consistently used regimen for administration of intravesical BCG.

In addition to the prevention of recurrence in a majority of patients (Table 49.5), BCG has been shown to prevent stage progression as well. Using what is now generally recognized as a less than adequate regimen of BCG, i.e., only a single 6-week course, Herr et al. demonstrated a significant reduction in stage progression, the development of T2 disease, development of metastases, percentage of patients going on to cystectomy, and the percentage of patients dying (31). Eure et al. addressed the issue of prevention of progression in T1 tumors and found that among 30 described as high risk, 66% of 26 with positive cytologies normalized after two 6-week courses, and only 6% progressed in stage and 3% to metastatic disease (32).

In a much larger but similarly nonrandomized report of patients undergoing much more intensive BCG therapy, Cookson and Sarosdy reported results in 86 patients with T1 tumors before intravesical BCG therapy (33). Importantly, all patients had at least one occurrence of T1 disease immediately before therapy, and 58 had multiple previous tumors, including a large percentage with concomitant CIS. Overall follow-up from the time of initial therapy ranged from 9 to 149 months (median, 59 months). Recurrences were abolished in 59 of 86 patients (69%) with initial therapy, including some maintenance treatments. Among 27 patients who had recurrences after initial therapy, additional courses of BCG led to the abolishment of recurrences in 19 patients, for an overall recurrence-free status in 91% of patients, with follow-up ranging from 31 to 139 months (median, 47 months). Importantly, progression to T2 or greater disease occurred in only six patients (7%) during this lengthy period of follow-up, and only two patients died of bladder cancer.

BCG Versus Intravesical Chemotherapy

In all but two comparative clinical trials of BCG versus intravesical chemotherapy, BCG has been found to be superior. This includes two comparisons to intravesical thiotepa (34, 35), the Southwest Oncology Group (SWOG) comparison of BCG to intravesical doxorubicin (30), and the SWOG comparison of intravesical BCG to intravesical mitomycin C (36). In the comparison to doxorubicin, 236 patients were randomized, with 109 having CIS and 127 having rapidly recurrent papillary tumors. Complete resolution of CIS was seen in 37 of 52 BCG-treated patients (71%) and in 27 of 57 doxorubicin-treated patients (47%, P < 0.01). Papillary tumor recurrence was seen in 34 of 60 BCG-treated patients (57%) and in 53 of 67 doxorubicin-treated patients (79%, P = 0.005). In the SWOG trial comparing intravesical BCG to intravesical mitomycin, patients with rapidly recurring superficial tumors without CIS received either 50 mg Tice BCG or mitomycin C 20 mg in 20 mL normal saline weekly for 6 weeks and then monthly to complete 1 year. Recurrent tumors were seen in 37 of 190 patients (19.4%) receiving BCG compared with 61 of 187 patients (32.6%) receiving mitomycin C (P = 0.0052).

Two Dutch reports found BCG and mitomycin C to be equivalent, but both used a 30-mg dose of mitomycin C and less-intense BCG consisting of 6 weeks only, with no maintenance (37, 38). With an average follow-up of only 12 months in one study, 30% of BCG-treated patients experienced tumor recurrence compared with 25% of mitomycin-treated patients (37). It is likely that the RIVM preparation that was used has lower efficacy than the preparations used in the United States due to manufacturing properties that decrease fibronectin binding (see below).

Mechanism of Action of BCG

An improved understanding of the mechanism of action of BCG and clinical trial results have culminated in the understanding that intravesical therapy alone is both sufficient and required; i.e., additional percutaneous inoculation is not required. Ratliff et al. have elegantly demonstrated that direct contact of the bacillus organism with binding to the cell surface through fibronectin binding sites is a requirement for activation of the immune response (39). That this binding might be interfered with by medication or fibronolysins may explain in part some of the failures of BCG therapy. Additionally, even with fibronectin-mediated binding, an intact T-cell system is required for the patient to mount a response to the bacillus organism and the bladder cancer cells (40). CD3, CD4, and CD8 T-cell subsets are involved, and the latter two at least are critically required (41, 42). In addition, Prescott et al. have shown in a limited clinical study that the degree of T-cell infiltration of the bladder wall is proportional to the clinical response of patients to BCG therapy, with responders having more infiltrate than nonresponders (42). Thus, exogenous steroids such as prednisone used for arthritis or other conditions of impaired immunity may interfere with the efficacy of BCG administration. A further key factor is that after fibronectin-mediated binding, BCG may have a direct inhibitory effect on tumor cell invasion, although it does not appear to affect proliferation or tumor cell attachment (43).

Because of the success of intralesional therapy for melanoma with direct percutaneous inoculation, and following the lead of Morales in combining percutaneous BCG inoculation with intravesical therapy, early investigators in superficial bladder cancer generally combined intravesical and percutaneous administration. To evaluate the role of percutaneous inoculation at the time of intravesical administration, we performed a prospective randomized comparison (44). Sixty-six patients with rapidly recurrent superficial TCC were randomized, after resection of all visible tumor, to receive intravesical BCG alone or in combination with percutaneous inoculation. All patients received Tice BCG, 50 mg intravesically weekly for 6 weeks, and again at weeks 8, 10, and 12, as well as at 6 months and semiannually thereafter for 4 years. Of 30 evaluable patients receiving intravesical BCG only, 13 (43%) had tumor recurrence at a mean of 5 months. Of 36 patients who in addition received percutaneous BCG, 15 (42%) had tumor recurrence at a mean of 7 months.

How Much or How Many Treatments Should Be Used?

Unfortunately, as Lamm and Sosnowski stated in 1990, it is still true that "the optimal protocol for BCG immunotherapy remains undefined and is somewhat controversial" (45). Despite more than 10 years of fairly systematic investigation at several large centers and despite several large multicenter trials, the course that provides the optimum benefit with the lowest morbidity remains to be defined.

It is clear that although a single 6-week course of therapy is effective in some patients in preventing recurrence and treating CIS, a substantial number of patients require additional BCG. As can be seen from Table 49.6, a variety of reports in the latter part of the 1980s demonstrated that greater success could be achieved when second or third courses of BCG were used in patients in whom an initial course failed. An additional option, used by some, is the use of an initial 6-week course of therapy, with a second course repeated following a 6-week period of rest and after surveillance cystoscopy. This may be the

most agreed on clinical principle in recent years (46). Using weekly therapy continuously in patients with CIS, Brosman reported disease-free status in 18 of 27 patients (67%) at 12 weeks, 24 of 27 patients (89%) at 18 weeks, and 27 of 27 patients (100%) at 24 weeks (15). However, toxicity was high, and six additional patients never made it from week 6 to week 12. The importance of two separate 6-week courses as opposed to 12 consecutive weekly treatments has been noted by Ratliff et al., who found a decreased clinical response rate and a decreased lymphocytic response with the latter course (47).

Despite the very large (660 patients) prospective SWOG study of intense maintenance versus a single 6-week course, the question of the necessity and intensity of maintenance BCG remains unanswered (48). Badalament et al. and Hudson et al. both reported smaller earlier trials in which no advantage was recognized when either monthly or quarterly single treatment maintenance courses were used following an initial 6-week course of therapy, compared with 6 weeks initial therapy alone (49, 50). The SWOG study also used a single 6-week course of therapy in the control arm, whereas the maintenance group received substantially more therapy than in the previous two maintenance studies by Badalament et al. and Hudson et al. This consisted of one half of an induction course or three consecutive weekly treatments at 3 months and 6 months following an initial 6-week course of therapy; this was followed by an additional three weekly treatments semiannually for an additional 2.5 years. Although the maintenance arm has been reported to have demonstrated a highly significant delay in time to recurrence or the development of progression in stage of disease, this was obtained at relatively high toxicity. Of 586 patients receiving 6-week courses of therapy following enrollment into the trial, grade 3 toxicity (requiring cessation, withholding of therapy, reduction in dose, or isoniazid [INH] therapy) was seen in 53 patients (9%). Of 247 patients randomized to additional intense maintenance therapy, 64 (26%) experienced grade 3 toxicity, and at least 10% refused to complete the prescribed course of therapy due to the toxicity they experienced.

Thus, the question continues as to how much therapy is required to achieve a successful outcome yet prevent serious side effects that might potentially cause a patient to stop therapy before achieving success. The potential need for some dose of maintenance treatments was furthered by a recent report

Table 49.6.   Six Weeks of Bacillus Calmette-Guérin is Less Than Optimal

| | | SUCCESS AND NO. OF 6-WEEK COURSES | | |
| | | --- | --- | --- |
REFERENCE	USE	1	2	3
Kelley et al. (28)	BT	11/17 (65%)	6/17 (94%)	
Haaf et al. (29)	BT	20/29 (69%)	26/29 (90%)	
Haaf et al. (29)	CIS	8/19 (42%)	13/19 (68%)	
Sarosdy and Lamm (16)	BT/CIS	64/82 (78%)	70/82 (85%)	73/82 (89%)

BT, prophylaxis for papillary tumor; CIS, carcinoma in situ.

detailing continued late recurrences over long periods following initial success in BCG-treated patients by the Washington University group, with similar long-term late recurrence curves now seen in patients on the older SWOG (51).

Until this question is answered, if ever, it is reasonable to tailor the regimen of BCG to each patient according to the earlier mentioned principles of patient tumor characteristics (2). For the patient with low- or intermediate-grade Ta recurrent nuisance tumors, a single 6-week course of BCG followed by observation may be sufficient. Administration of a second 6-week course of intravesical therapy following an eventual recurrence would be reasonable, and its use following the first cystoscopy, if negative, should be considered potentially beneficial but not mandatory. To the contrary, in a patient who has a dangerous tumor process, consisting of G2 or G3 T1 lesions, CIS alone, or T1 lesions with CIS, aggressive BCG therapy should be used. This should consist of an initial 6-week course following resection of all visible tumor. After a 6-week rest and performance of the 12-week cystoscopy, any recurrent tumor should be resected. After resection, or if no recurrent tumor is present, a second 6-week course of therapy should be administered. Should the patient still have either CIS or recurrent T1 tumors after two 6-week courses of therapy in this fashion, either alternative forms of immunotherapy should be used or the patient should undergo cystectomy, unless the lesions have downgraded and downstaged. For such a dangerous disease process in a patient who appears to have responded to two 6-week courses of therapy, the question of maintenance therapy of some sort should be discussed with the patient. If the patient has tolerated intravesical treatments without severe side effects, it may be reasonable to use some form of maintenance. However, many such patients prefer not to receive additional BCG unless there are clear-cut indications in the form of recurrent disease or positive cytology.

Complications of BCG Therapy

Complications or toxicity of therapy with intravesical BCG occur in almost all patients. This toxicity ranges from mild to moderate in up to 90% of patients and to severe or life-threatening in less than 5%. Therefore, a thorough understanding and familiarity with these side effects is crucial to the safe use of BCG in superficial bladder cancer.

Cystitis and dysuria are the most common side effects, occurring in up to 90% of patients (52, 53). These usually are first seen after the third or fourth treatment with BCG and may worsen in intensity with further treatments. Both are most often short-lived, resolving within 24 hours of BCG administration.

Hematuria as a result of treatment with BCG often accompanies the symptoms of cystitis, seen in 20 to 35% of patients (52). Patients with a severe degree of hematuria should probably not receive additional treatments until the hematuria has resolved; absorption through an ulcerated or bleeding urothelial surface may lead to systemic complications.

Low-grade constitutional symptoms may accompany the local symptoms of cystitis, dysuria, and hematuria (52). Malaise, fatigue, and lethargy are present in approximately 20% of patients and are usually short-lived like cystitis. Low-grade fever elevations to less than 101° occur in approximately 10 to 15% of patients, and like the symptoms above, usually resolve spontaneously in less than 24 hours.

Life-threatening systemic infection with the live bacillus organism can occur. This is heralded by the onset of severe fever, to elevations greater than 103°, occurring in up to 3% of patients (52). This extreme temperature elevation helps distinguish complications that demand aggressive intervention and therapy from the short-lived mild or moderate symptoms that most patients experience. Early intervention with appropriate therapy as outlined below usually results in prompt defervescence and improvement in overall condition (54, 55). Failure to recognize and treat or delayed treatment can result in progressive systemic signs of sepsis, including vascular collapse and organ failure. A number of deaths secondary to BCG sepsis have now been reported (55).

It is possible, and physicians using intravesical BCG should be aware, that the delayed appearance of some infectious complications may occur. Böhle et al. reported the case of a 64-year-old man who experienced "an increased temperature" (although it was not specified) along with malaise and chills at the time of his first dose (56). Responding quickly to 2 days of therapy, the patient completed a 6-week course and did well, although he underwent cystectomy 3 months later for progressive disease. Fourteen months after BCG therapy, he was found to have pulmonitis due to culture-proven infection with BCG during evaluation of a pleural effusion and pulmonary infiltrate. Fortunately, he responded well to triple-drug antituberculosis therapy.

Treatment and Prevention of BCG Toxicity

Patients with mild local or systemic symptoms generally require no support or at most, acetaminophen, pyridium, or anticholinergic therapy (57). It is important, however, to ensure that the patients are not uncomfortable and that their level of concern is understood by the physician.

Patients with local or mild symptomatology that does not resolve in 12 to 24 hours or those in whom symptoms are more severe may receive effective palliation by the use of isoniazid at the time of treatment (57). Although not proven by clinical trials, the empiric therapy used by most investigators is INH 300 mg daily for three consecutive days, commencing therapy the day before subsequent treatments, the same day of treatment, and the day following treatment. Patients will report much improved symptomatology with subsequent therapy, and this avoids the prolonged daily administration of INH for the remaining treatment period. There is no clinical evidence to suggest decreased efficacy of BCG when INH is used in this fashion, although De Boer et al. have reported an impaired immune response to BCG in guinea pigs treated with INH

(58). We have liberally used INH for relief of moderate symptoms in our patients and have not been able to discern a negative effect on our results.

Patients who have fever greater than 103° F should be admitted to the hospital for aggressive monitoring and therapy (54, 55, 58). The usual bacteriologic cultures should be obtained from urine and blood, and appropriate broad-spectrum antibacterial therapy instituted pending culture results. It is unnecessary to culture for acid-fast bacillus or perform urinary acid-fast bacillus stains. These may be positive, and delay of appropriate antituberculosis therapy pending culture outcome may result in mortality. Instead, in addition to antibacterial antibiotics, patients should immediately be given cycloserine at 250 to 500 mg by mouth twice daily. Patients who appear less ill may respond to two-drug therapy with isoniazid 300 mg and rifampicin 600 mg daily. However, this combination of drugs does not exert a significant antibacillus effect for up to 1 week, so cycloserine should be chosen in patients who are seriously ill.

Avoidance of severe systemic toxicity is better than treatment and is possible by paying attention to detail during administration of BCG. Specifically, patients should not receive BCG within 7 days of tumor resection or bladder biopsy, or if gross hematuria following the resection is still present even 1 to 2 weeks after resection or biopsy. Patients frequently have continued microscopic hematuria in the absence of gross hematuria, and it is reasonably safe to administer BCG in those patients after the required 7-day rest period. Additionally, if traumatic catheterization is recognized, BCG should not be administered. BCG should also not be administered through gravity flow, by injecting the BCG solution into a catheter tip syringe attached to a catheter in which the bulb or piston has been removed. "Transurethral push" using a bulb or piston syringe should not be performed because this may result in "IV push," with subsequent systemic signs of infection.

Less common complications include granulomatous prostatitis, usually diagnosed through development of a suspicious digital rectal examination, or subsequent transurethral resection of the prostate with findings of granulomatous foreign bodies in the prostate (52). Symptoms rarely result. Also included are ureteral obstruction and contracted bladder, although it is well known that these may result from repeated transurethral resection alone (52). Very rare complications include immune complex glomerulonephritis, choroiditis and other ocular reactions, nephrogenic adenoma, suppurative lymphadenitis, lupus vulgaris, and, very rarely, intramuscular abscesses at sites distant from the inoculation (59).

Patients who have high fever only should have further BCG treatments withheld until all symptoms have resolved. BCG may be restarted at one half the usual dosage with 3-day INH coverage initiated 1 day before therapy. For patients with life-threatening sepsis and evidence of systemic BCG infection, BCG therapy should not be reinstituted.

OTHER COMPOUNDS IN CLINICAL TRIALS

A wide variety of additional compounds have demonstrated potential for successful immunotherapy for superficial bladder cancer. Included among these are three agents that have each demonstrated efficacy in two or more clinical trials: keyhole-limpet hemocyanin (KLH), IFN, and bropirimine. Other agents have demonstrated potential activity in animal laboratory studies or in studies with minimal power to estimate accurately clinical efficacy. For this reason, most of this discussion will be restricted to the former three agents.

KLH

KLH is a high molecular weight respiratory pigment protein of the mollusk Megathura crenulata. KLH is highly immunogenic among naturally occurring proteins and has been used for many years as an experimental antigen in the evaluation of delayed-type hypersensitivity. It may be used to evaluate cellular and humoral immune response, as most patients have never been exposed to keyhole-limpet.

Olsson first noted a marked reduction in recurrence of superficial tumors in patients immunized with subcutaneous KLH as a test of immunologic responsiveness (60). As a result of this notation, a prospective study was performed in which 19 patients were divided into a KLH immunized group and a nonimmunized control group (60). One tumor recurrence was seen in the KLH-treated group, whereas 7 of 10 patients demonstrated tumor recurrence in the control group (P < 0.005). No toxicity relative to KLH administration was seen.

In a subsequent study, Jurincic et al. compared KLH to mitomycin C, using 1 mg of KLH intradermally followed by 10 mg KLH intravesically monthly for 2 years (61). Mitomycin C was administered 20 mg in 20 mL normal saline on a monthly schedule. Recurrent superficial tumor was seen in 3 of 21 patients (14%) who received KLH, compared with 9 of 23 patients (39%) who received mitomycin C (P < 0.07). The rate of tumor recurrence per 100 patient months was reduced approximately threefold, being 3.26 in the KLH group versus 9.28 in the mitomycin C group. Additionally, 81 patients were treated with KLH without randomization. A tumor recurrence rate of 1.19 per 100 patient months was seen in this group.

A single, limited institution study is underway in the United States, testing a new regimen for toxicity. Widespread access to it is currently not available.

IFN

IFN are naturally occurring glycoproteins with antiviral and antiproliferative properties. The three major IFN include alpha, synthesized by leukocytes; beta, which is synthesized by fibroblasts; and gamma, which is synthesized by T cells and natural killer (NK) cells.

The IFN shown to be most active in human bladder cancer is alpha, which primarily stimulates NK cell maturation. In the presence of IL-2, the NK cells mature and produce IFN-γ. Since IFN-γ is known to peak within 24 hours of administration of BCG intravesically, it made sense to initiate clinical trials using recombinant alpha-2b IFN (r-α2b-IFN) in superficial bladder cancer, the first IFN to be readily available in bulk volume thanks to recombinant technology.

Christophersen et al. reported the successful treatment of superficial bladder tumors with systemic therapy using intramuscular injections of r-α2b-IFN (62). After this, Ikic et al. reported that transurethral injections of r-α2b-IFN into tumor daily for 3 weeks resulted in complete regression in four of eight patients (63).

Complete response in four of eight patients with CIS was reported by Shortliff et al. using intravesical instillation (64). Patients received 50, 100, or 200 mU intravesically weekly for 8 weeks. Several additional small reports indicated a consistency in response to intravesical r-α2b-IFN.

Torti et al. reported a large, escalating dosage phase I/II trial using intravesical r-α2b-IFN at dosages ranging from 50 million to 1 billion units weekly for 8 weeks (65). Six of 17 patients (32%) with CIS had a complete response, and five additional patients (26%) had negative biopsies but continued positive urinary cytology. Furthermore, 4 of 16 patients who had marker papillary tumors in place had complete resolution of tumors.

In an effort to confirm the apparently good response to weekly treatment with r-α2b-IFN for patients with CIS, a large, multicenter, international trial was launched in 1985 (66). Patients with biopsy-proven CIS and positive urinary cytology after biopsy were randomized to receive either 10 million or 100 mU intravesically weekly for 12 weeks. Patients who had a complete response or at least had no progressive disease develop were allowed to continue monthly treatment using the same dosage for an additional 9 months. A complete response consisting of negative biopsies and negative urinary cytology was seen in 20 of 47 patients (45%) receiving 100 mU weekly compared with 2 of 38 patients (5%) receiving 10 mU. Importantly, prior BCG therapy had failed in five patients receiving the higher dosage, with two complete responses seen in those patients.

A further large-scale clinical trial has not been performed with r-α2b-IFN. Critically lacking is a threshold-determining study to find whether 100 mU is really required or if the effective dose might be closer to 10 mU than 100 mU. The primary reason for this has to do with cost of the drug and the potential need for maintenance therapy. Because the drug is FDA-approved for hepatitis, it is commercially available and in many states approved by Medicare for use in patients with CIS of the bladder. Thus, it may prove to be a valuable adjunct for the patient with CIS following adequate BCG therapy and potentially delay or avoid cystectomy in selected patients.

The efficacy of intravesical IFN against existing papillary tumors or its use for prophylaxis of recurrent tumors following resection has not been sufficiently established to recommend its use in those settings. Da Silva has reported some apparent benefit in prophylaxis against resected papillary disease using a dose of 60 mU weekly, but the study thus far lacks power and has other design problems that weaken conclusions of efficacy (67). Further investigation appears warranted.

Bropirimine

Bropirimine is an aryl pyrimidinone, a family of chemically synthesized drugs known as IFN inducers first synthesized in 1976 (68). One of several different pyrimidinone IFN inducers, bropirimine has a wide range of antitumor, antiviral, and immunomodulatory effects. One of its most exciting characteristics, from the patient's perspective, is that it is active when administered orally, avoiding the necessity, inconvenience, cost, and discomfort of intravesical administration.

Simmons et al. and Sidky et al. both reported efficacy of bropirimine against the murine transitional cell cancer MBT-2 (69, 70). In screening several compounds for BCG-like activity against the same tumor, we were most impressed with its ability to engender a more intense, earlier, and longer lasting NK activation than even BCG (71). For this reason, we tested bropirimine in conjunction with BCG against MBT-2 in C3H mice and found that it appeared to cause a synergistic improvement in the efficacy of BCG compared with the use of either agent alone.

Based on the above animal data, a human clinical trial was launched using escalating dosages in patients with either marker papillary tumors present or existing CIS (72). Interestingly, no apparent efficacy was seen against papillary tumors except at the highest dose level, although 5 of 11 patients with CIS had a complete response. Included in this were four of six patients who received bropirimine at an oral dosage of 3 g/day for three consecutive days.

Based on this, a confirmatory phase II trial was launched in patients having CIS with positive cytology still present after biopsy. At a dosage of 3 g/day for three consecutive days repeated weekly for 12 weeks, 20 of 39 evaluable patients (51%) demonstrated a complete response (73). Complete responses were also seen in a subgroup of patients who had disease still present despite previous BCG therapy. In this group, 43% had a complete response. Importantly, with therapy continued to complete 1 year and then stopped, durability of complete response extended to longer than 17 months from the time of complete response. The four patients who experienced therapy failure and who had any form of tumor recurrence had papillary tumor only (two patients) and CIS only (two patients).

Other clinical trials with bropirimine are currently underway throughout the United States, Canada, and Europe. These include a phase II trial in patients with BCG-failed CIS and a phase III randomized comparison of intravesical BCG versus oral bropirimine in patients with newly diagnosed CIS. SWOG is also performing a phase II trial combining oral bropirimine with intravesical BCG in patients with CIS to determine if a heightened response over what has historically been seen with BCG alone might be possible as indicated in the MBT-2 model.

OTHER AGENTS AND NEW DIRECTIONS

A variety of other compounds with immunomodulatory capacity have either been used in the laboratory setting or in clinical efforts too small and underpowered to be called trials. These include agents such as II-2 alone or in combination with BCG, IFN-γ, TNF-alpha, and *Corynebacterium parvum*. At best, no conclusion is possible regarding even speculative comments on potential clinical therapeutic efficacy of these agents at this time.

A new era of "immune-like" therapy is dawning, and that is the era of genetic-based therapy. The areas of tumor suppressor gene replacement and cytokine production codon therapy are currently receiving the most attention, with clinical trials likely in the near future. Genes such as p53 and Rb have been found to be mutated in large percentages of invasive tumors, as well as in some more superficial tumors. As with intravesical chemotherapy and immunotherapy, the bladder provides a great testing ground for nonsystemically administered investigational drugs, and early work in the laboratory has been encouraging (74, 75).

Nongenetic but molecular-based therapy is also on the horizon, and in fact already tested clinically. TP-40 is one of many "bifunctional" compounds, consisting of a fragment of TGF-alpha fused to a segment of the Pseudomonas exotoxin P-40 (76). Serving as a targeting device, the TGF-alpha binds to epidermal growth factor (EGF) receptors that are present in much higher numbers and density on the surfaces of malignant cells than on normal urothelial cells (77, 78). The bound exotoxin is then internalized, poisoning cells positive for EGF receptors but leaving normal cells untouched and unharmed. TP-40 was found to be highly effective against TCC cell lines in vitro (79, 80). A phase I clinical trial has been completed, with some apparent efficacy against CIS reported (81). Further trials with TP-40 and similar engineered compounds that are selectively toxic are likely in the future.

CONCLUSION

Immunotherapy for superficial bladder cancer now plays a major role in the successful treatment of patients with Ta, T1, and Tis. Verification of early results with BCG and a scientific approach to determining its mechanism of action have improved the benefits of surgery alone for such patients. Efforts to improve the efficacy and decrease the toxicity of BCG have resulted in the identification of several compounds that have high potential of replacing or augmenting adjunctive therapy with BCG. The successes in this arena are particularly due to the willingness of both academic and nonacademic urologists to enroll patients collaboratively in clinical trials that are large enough to be able to determine both efficacy and toxicity of new compounds in a reasonable period. Through such efforts, patients with superficial TCC will continue to have a much better potential for bladder preservation at minimal risk and, subsequently, maintenance of a more normal lifestyle.

REFERENCES

1. Morales A, Eidinger D, Bruce AW. Intracavitary bacillus Calmette-Guérin in the treatment of superficial bladder tumors. J Urol 1976;116:180.
2. Sarosdy MF. Principles of intravesical chemotherapy and immunotherapy. Urol Clin North Am 1992;3:509.
3. Morales A, Nickel JC. Immunotherapy for superficial bladder cancer. Urol Clin North Am. 1992;3:549.
4. Heney NM, Ahmed S, Flanagan MJ, et al. Superficial bladder cancer: progression and recurrence. J Urol 1983;130:1083.
5. Rubben H, Lutzeyer W, Fischer N, et al. Natural history and treatment of low and high risk superficial bladder tumors. J Urol 1988;139:283.
6. Flamm J. Long-term versus short-term doxorubicin hydrochloride instillation after transurethral resection of superficial bladder cancer. Eur Urol 1990;17:119.
7. Huland H, Kloppel G, Feddersen I, et al. Comparison of different schedules of cystostatic intravesical instillations in patients with superficial bladder carcinoma: final evaluation of a prospective multicenter study with 419 patients. J Urol 1990;14:68.
8. Koontz WW Jr, Prout GR Jr, Smith W, et al. The use of intravesical thiotepa in the management of non-invasive carcinoma of the bladder. J Urol 1981;125:307.
9. Lum B, Torti F. Adjuvant intravesical pharmaco-therapy for superficial bladder cancer. J Natl Cancer Inst 1991;83:682.
10. Prout GR, Koontz WW Jr, Coombs LJ, et al. Long-term fate of 90 patients with superficial bladder cancer randomly assigned to receive or not to receive thiotepa. J Urol 1983;130:677.
11. Soloway MS, Murphy WM, Defuria MD, et al. The effect of mitomycin C on superficial bladder cancer. J Urol 1981;125:646.
12. Williams R, Sarosdy MF, Catalona W, et al. Randomized trial of high dose vs. low dose intravesical interferon alpha 2-B (IFN-A2B) treatment of bladder carcinoma in situ (CIS). Proc Am Soc Clin Oncol 1988;7:121.
13. Zincke H, Utz DC, Taylor WF, et al. Influence of thiotepa and doxorubicin instillation at time of transurethral surgical treatment of bladder cancer on tumor recurrence: a prospective, randomized double-blind, controlled trial. J Urol 1983;129:505.
14. Althausen AF, Prout GR Jr, Daly JJ. Non-invasive papillary carcinoma of the bladder associated with carcinoma in situ. J Urol 1976;116:575.
15. Brosman SA. Experience with bacillus Calmette-Guérin in the therapy of bladder carcinoma in situ. J Urol 1985;134:36.
16. Sarosdy MF, Lamm DL. Long-term results of intravesical bacillus Calmette-Guérin therapy for superficial bladder cancer. J Urol 1989;142:719.
17. Guerin C. Early history of BCG. In: Rosenthal ER, ed. BCG vaccination against tuberculosis. Boston: Little Brown, 1957:48.
18. Mathé G, Amiel J, Schwartzenberg L, et al. Immunotherapy for acute lymphoblastic leukemia. Lancet 1969;1:697.
19. Zbar B, Rapp WJ. Immunotherapy of guinea pig with BCG. Cancer 1974;34:1532.
20. Morales A, Ottenhof P, Emerson L. Treatment of residual,

non-infiltrating bladder cancer with bacillus Calmette-Guerin. J Urol 1981;125:649.

21. Lamm DL, Thor DE, Stogdill VD, et al. Bladder cancer immunotherapy. J Urol 1982;128:931.

22. Brosman SA. Experience with bacillus Calmette-Guerin in patients with superficial bladder cancer. J Urol 1982;128:27.

23. deKernion JB, et al. The management of superficial bladder tumors and carcinoma in situ with intravesical bacillus Calmette-Guerin. J Urol 1985;133:598.

24. Schellhammer PF, Ladaga LE, Fillion MB. Bacillus Calmette-Guerin for superficial transitional cell carcinoma of the bladder. J Urol 1986;135:261.

25. Kavoussi LR, Torrence RJ, Gillen DP, et al. Results of 6 weekly intravesical bacillus Calmette-Guérin instillations on the treatment of superficial bladder tumors. J Urol 1988;139:935.

26. Lamm DL. BCG in immunotherapy for bladder cancer. J Urol 1985;134:40.

27. Herr HW, et al. Effect of intravesical bacillus Calmette-Guerin on carcinoma in situ of the bladder. Cancer 1983;51:1323.

28. Kelley DR, Ratliff TL, Catalona WJ, et al. Intravesical bacillus Calmette-Guerin therapy for superficial bladder cancer: effect of bacillus Calmette-Guerin viability on treatment results. J Urol 1985;134:48.

29. Haaff EO, Dresner SM, Ratliff TL, et al. Two courses of intravesical Calmette-Guerin for transitional cell carcinoma of the bladder. J Urol 1986;136:820.

30. Lamm DL, Blumenstein B, et al. A randomized trial of intravesical doxorubicin and immunotherapy with bacillus Calmette-Guérin transitional cell carcinoma of the bladder. N Engl J Med 1991;325:1205.

31. Herr HW, et al. B bacillus Calmette-Guerin therapy alters the progression of superficial bladder cancer. J Clin Oncol 1988;6:1450.

32. Eure GR, Ladaga LE, Schellhammer PF. BCG therapy for stage T1 superficial bladder cancer. J Urol 1990;143:341. Abstract.

33. Cookson MS, Sarosdy MF. Management of stage T1 bladder cancer with intravesical BCG. J Urol In press.

34. Brosman SA. Experience with bacillus Calmette-Guerin in patients with superficial bladder cancer. J Urol 1992;128:27.

35. Netto NR Jr, Lemos CGA. A comparison of treatment methods for prophylaxis of recurrent superficial bladder tumors. J Urol 1983;129:33.

36. Lamm DL, Crawford ED, Blumenstein B, et al. SWOG 8795: a randomized comparison of bacillus Calmette-Guerin and mitomycin C prophylaxis in stage Ta and T1 transitional cell carcinoma of the bladder. J Urol 1993;149:282. Abstract.

37. Debruyne FMJ, Van der Meijden APM, et al. BCG-RIVM versus mitomycin C intravesical therapy in patients with superficial bladder cancer. Urology 1988;31(Suppl):20.

38. Witjes JA, Van der Meijden APM, et al. Randomized prospective study comparing intravesical instillations of mitomycin C, BCG-tice and BCG-RIVM in Pta, PT1 tumors and primary CIS of the urinary bladder. Eur J Cancer 1993;29:1672.

39. Ratliff TL, Kavoussi LR, Catalona WJ. Role of fibronectin in intravesical BCG therapy for superficial bladder cancer. J Urol 1988;139:410.

40. Ratliff T, Gillen D, Catalona W. Requirement of a thymus

dependent immune response for BCG-mediated antitumor activity. J Urol 1987;137:155.

41. Prescott S, James K, Hargreave TB, et al. Intravesical Evans strain BCG therapy: quantitative immunohistochemical analysis of the immune response within the bladder wall. J Urol 1992;147:1636.

42. Ratliff TL, Ritchey JK, Yuan JJJ, et al. T-cell subsets required for intravesical BCG immunotherapy for bladder cancer. J Urol 1993;150:1018.

43. Garden RJ, Liu BC-S, Redwood M, et al. Bacillus Calmette-Guerin abrogates in vitro invasion and motility of human bladder tumor cells via fibronectin interaction. J Urol 1992;148:900.

44. Lamm DL, DeHaven JI, Shriver J, et al. A randomized prospective comparison of oral versus intravesical and percutaneous BCG for superficial bladder cancer. J Urol 1982;128:1104.

45. Lamm DL, Sosnowski JT. Immunotherapy of bladder carcinoma. In: Crawford ED, Das S, eds. Current genitourinary cancer surgery. Philadelphia: Lea & Febiger, 1990.

46. Morales A, Nickel JC, Wilson JWL. Dose-response of bacillus Calmette-Guerin in the treatment of superficial bladder cancer. J Urol 1992;147:1256.

47. Ratliff TL, Catalona WJ. Depressed proliferative responses in patients treated with 12 weeks of intravesical BCG: part 2. J Urol 1989;141:230. Abstract.

48. Lamm DL, Crawford ED, Blumenstein B, et al. Maintenance BCG immunotherapy of superficial bladder cancer: a randomized prospective Southwest Oncology Group study. J Urol 1992;147:274. Abstract.

49. Badalament RA, Herr HW, Wong GY, et al. A prospective randomized trial of maintenance versus non-maintenance intravesical bacillus Calmette-Guérin therapy of superficial bladder cancer. J Clin Oncol 1987;5:441.

50. Hudson MA, Ratliff TL, Gillen DP, et al. Single course versus maintenance bacillus Calmette-Guérin therapy for superficial bladder tumors: a prospective, randomized trial. J Urol 1987;138:295.

51. Nadler RB, Catalona WJ, Hudson MA, et al. Durability of the tumor-free response for intravesical bacillus Calmette-Guérin therapy. J Urol 1994;152:367.

52. Lamm DL, Stogdill VD, Stogdill BJ, et al. Complications of bacillus Calmette-Guérin immunotherapy in 1,278 patients with bladder cancer. J Urol 1985;135:272.

53. Lamm DL, Steg A, Boccon-Gibod L, et al. Complications of bacillus Calmette-Guérin immunotherapy: review of 2602 patients with comparison of chemotherapy complications. Prog Clin Biol Res 1989;310:335.

54. DeHaven JI, Traynellis C, Riggs DR, et al. Antibiotic and steroid therapy of massive systemic bacillus Calmette-Guérin toxicity. J Urol 1992;147:738.

55. Rawls WH, Lamm DL, Lowe BA, et al. Fatal sepsis following intravesical BCG administration for bladder cancer: a Southwest Oncology Group study. J Urol 1990;144:1328.

56. Böhle A, Kirsten D, Schröder K-H, et al. Clinical evidence of systemic persistence of bacillus Calmette-Guerin: long-term pulmonary bacillus Calmette-Guerin infection after intravesical therapy for bladder cancer and subsequent cystectomy. J Urol 1992;148:1894.

57. Lamm DL, Meijden APM van der, Morales A, et al. Incidence

and treatment of complications of bacillus Calmette-Guérin intravesical therapy in superficial bladder cancer. J Urol 1992; 147:596.

58. De Boer LC, Steerenberg PA, van Der Meijden PM, et al. Impaired immune response by isoniazid treatment during intravesical BCG administration in the guinea pig. J Urol 1992;148:1577.

59. Lamm DL. Complications of bacillus Calmette-Guerin. Urol Clin North Am 1992;19:565.

60. Olsson C, Chute R, Rao C. Immunologic reduction of bladder cancer recurrence rate. J Urol 1974;111:173.

61. Jurincic CD, Engelman V, Gasch J, et al. Immunotherapy in bladder cancer with keyhole-limpet hemocyanin: a randomized study. J Urol 1988;139:723.

62. Christophersen IS, et al. Interferon therapy in neoplastic disease. Acta Med Scand 1978;204:471.

63. Ikic D, et al. Application of human leukocyte interferon in patients with urinary bladder papillomatosis, breast cancer, and melanoma. Lancet 1981;1:1022.

64. Shortliffe LC, et al. Intravesical interferon therapy for carcinoma in situ and transitional cell carcinoma of the bladder. J Urol 1984;131:171.

65. Torti FM, et al. Alpha-interferon in superficial bladder cancer: a Northern California Oncology Group study. J Clin Oncol 1988;6:475.

66. Glashan R. A randomized controlled study of intravesical-2b-interferon in carcinoma in situ of the bladder. J Urol 1990; 144:658.

67. Da Silva FC. Interferon alpha 2b 60 millions vs 100 millions in intravesical prophylaxis of superficial bladder cancer. J Urol 1993;149:282. Abstract.

68. Wierenga W. Antiviral and other bioactivities of pyrimidinones. Pharmacol Ther 1985;30:67.

69. Simmons WB, Reichert DF, Lucion RM, et al. Pyrimidinone interferon inducers in the treatment of murine transitional cell carcinoma. J Urol 1983;129:169. Abstract.

70. Sidky YA, Borden EC, Wierenga W, et al. Inhibitory effects of interferon-inducing pyrimidinones on the growth of transplantable mouse bladder tumors. Cancer Res 1986;46: 3798.

71. Sarosdy MF, Kierum CA. Combination immunotherapy of murine transitional cell carcinoma using BCG and an interferon-inducing pyrimidinone. J Urol 1989;143:1376.

72. Sarosdy MF, Lamm DL, Williams RD, et al. Phase I trial of oral bropirimine in superficial bladder cancer. J Urol 1992; 147:31.

73. Sarosdy MF, Lowe BA, Schellhammer PF, et al. Bropirimine immunotherapy of bladder CIS: positive phase II results of an oral interferon inducer. J Urol 1994;13:304. Abstract.

74. Griffin KP, Segura L, Kan N, et al. The effects on proliferation, metabolism and tumorigenicity of MBT-2 using a retroviral vector human wild type p53 gene. J Urol 1993; 149:485. Abstract.

75. Connor J, Bannerji R, Saito S, et al. Regression of bladder tumors in mice treated with interleukin 2 gene-modified tumor cells. J Exp Med 1993;177:1127.

76. Siegall CB, Xu Y, Chaudhary V, et al. Cytotoxic activities of a fusion protein comprised of TGF and pseudomonas exotoxin. FASEB J 1989;3:2647.

77. Neal D, Bennet M, Hall R, et al. Epidermal-growth-factor receptors in human bladder cancer: comparison of invasive and superficial tumors. Lancet 1985;1:366.

78. Messing EM. Clinical implications of the expression of epidermal growth factor receptors in human transitional cell carcinoma. Cancer Res 1990;50:2530.

79. Heimbrook D, Stirdivant S, Ahern J, et al. Transforming growth factor α-pseudomonas exotoxin fusion protein prolongs survival of nude mice bearing tumor xenografts. Proc Natl Acad Sci USA. 1990;87:4697.

80. Sarosdy MF, Hutzler DH, Yee D, et al. In vitro sensitivity testing of human bladder cancers and cell lines to TP40: a hybrid protein with selective targeting and cytotoxicity. J Urol 1993;150:1950.

81. Goldberg MR, Heimbrook DC, Russo P, et al. Transforming growth factor α-pseudomonas exotoxin-40 (TP40) phase I clinical study of the recombinant oncotoxin TP40 in superficial bladder cancer. Clin Cancer Res 1995;1:57.

50

Chemotherapy of Bladder Cancer

Harmesh R. Naik
Kenneth J. Pienta

INTRODUCTION

In 1994, bladder cancer developed in approximately 50,000 people in North America and 10,000 died of their disease (1). Approximately 75% of patients will be diagnosed with superficial bladder cancer with relatively good prognosis (2). Approximately 20 to 30% of patients will have muscle-invasive disease and half of them will die within 2 years of metastatic bladder cancer, and 5% of patients will present with metastatic disease that is not curable with currently available chemotherapy (3).

Most of the bladder cancers diagnosed in North America are transitional cell carcinomas that are fairly sensitive to various chemotherapeutic agents. Chemotherapy of bladder cancer has evolved from single-agent therapy to a variety of combination regimens capable of inducing high response rates and some complete remissions. In the past decade, several important trials were conducted to define the incorporation of chemotherapy in the management of bladder cancer patients. These trials will be discussed at length in this chapter. Commonly used response criteria to assess the efficacy of treatment directed at bladder cancer are listed in Table 50.1.

CHEMOTHERAPY FOR METASTATIC DISEASE

Metastatic disease will develop in approximately 40% of bladder cancer patients, most commonly involving the lungs, liver, bones, and lymph nodes (4). Bladder cancer is a chemoresponsive disease; however, the majority of patients remain incurable with currently available regimens. For those patients, the goal of the treatment is palliation.

Single Agents

The effective single-agent chemotherapy agents are listed in Table 50.2. Cisplatin is considered the most effective single agent in the treatment of metastatic disease and is part of virtually all effective combination regimens. Initial studies of cisplatin at Memorial Sloan-Kettering Cancer Center showed an overall response rate of 30% (5). Several other investigators reported similar responses with cisplatin (10); however, in recent phase III trials using cisplatin as a single agent, lower response rates of 9 to 31% have been reported (12–14). The principal toxicities of cisplatin are renal insufficiency, auditory dysfunction, and vomiting. Many older and frail bladder cancer patients with concurrent medical problems are unable to tolerate cisplatin. As an alternative, the platinum analog carboplatin has been tested because it is less nephrotoxic. Response rates with carboplatin have varied from 8 to 20% in phase II trials (4).

Methotrexate is another active agent, with response rates of 23 to 35% (4, 5). Higher doses of methotrexate seem to be slightly more active, but no randomized trial has been conducted comparing low- versus high-dose methotrexate (5, 6, 15). Other active agents with response rates between 10 and 20% include doxorubicin, vinblastine, vincristine, cyclophosphamide, 5-fluorouracil (5-FU), and mitomycin-C (2, 4, 7, 8, 16). Older trials, using variable response criteria, reported high response rates up to 30% with cyclophosphamide and 5-FU as single agents. With modern criteria, only a 7% response rate was seen with cyclophosphamide (5), and a recent trial using 5-FU resulted in 14% overall response rate (9). Recently, 17 to 62% overall response rates have been reported using gallium nitrate in chemorefractory patients (11, 17).

Most of the responses reported with single agents are partial responses and short lived with an occasional complete response of longer duration. A majority of patients with metastatic disease will die within 2 years (2, 3, 5). Despite these shortcomings, early single-agent trials served an important function of identifying active agents against bladder cancer.

Combinations

In hopes of increasing the response rate and achieving higher complete response rates, various combinations of active agents have been developed for metastatic disease. In the early phase II experience with various combinations, cisplatin and metho-

Table 50.1.   Clinical Response Criteria for Bladder Cancer[a]

CR[b]	Complete disappearance of all clinically detectable lesions for > 1 month
PR	> 50% reduction in the sum of products of two largest perpendicular diameters of all measurable lesions
SD	< 50% decrease in tumor size with no new lesions
PD	25% or more increase in size or development of new lesions

CR, complete response; PR, partial response; SD, stable disease; PD, progressive disease.
[a] Criteria used in individual trial may be different.
[b] Includes negative cytology for local tumors.

Table 50.2.   Single-Agent Chemotherapy in Bladder Cancer

DRUG	OVERALL RESPONSE (%)	REFERENCE
Cisplatin	30	Yagoda (5)
Methotrexate	29	Yagoda (5)
Methotrexate, high dose	50	Turner (6)
Doxorubicin	17	Yagoda (5)
Vinblastine	16	Blumenreich (7)
Vincristine	12	Richards (8)
Cyclophosphamide	7	Yagoda (5)
5-Fluorouracil	14	Knight (9)
Mitomycin C	21	Torti (6)
Gallium	17	Seidman (11)

Table 50.3.   Doses in mg/m^2 and Schedule for Methotrexate, Vinblastine, Doxorubicin, Cisplatin Regimen (18)

	DAYS[a]			
DRUG	1	2	15	22
Methotrexate	30	—	30	30
Vincristine	—	3	3	3
Doxorubicin	—	30	—	—
Cisplatin	—	70	—	—

Doses in mg/m^2 and Schedule for Cisplatin, Methotrexate, Vinblastine Regimen (19)

	DAYS[b]		
DRUG	1	2	8
Cisplatin	—	100	—
Methotrexate	30	—	30
Vinblastine	4	—	4

[a] Repeated every 4 weeks.
[b] Repeated every 21 days.

trexate combinations appeared to be superior to other combinations, with overall response rates of more than 40% (5). The newer combinations included methotrexate, vinblastine, and cisplatin with doxorubicin (MVAC) (Table 50.3) or without doxorubicin (CMV) (Table 50.3) and the combination of cisplatin, doxorubicin, and cyclophosphamide (CISCA or CAP).

Table 50.4.   Randomized Trials in Metastatic Bladder Cancer

REFERENCE	AGENTS	OVERALL RESPONSE RATE (%)	MEDIAN SURVIVAL	SIGNIFICANCE
Gagliano (25)	A	19	28 wk	NS
	A + C	43	31 wk	
Hillcoat (14)	C	31	7.2 mo	NS
	C + MTX	45	8.7 mo	
Khandekar (21)	P	17	6 mo	NS
	CAP	33	7.3 mo	
Al-Sarraf (23)	m-AMSA	19	21 wk	NS
	CAP	43	28 wk	
Soloway (12)	P	20	—	NS
	CTX + P	12	—	
Troner (22)	P	16	21 wk	NS
	CAP	21	29 wk	
Loehrer (13)	P	12	8.2 mo	S
	MVAC	39	12.5 mo	
Logothetis (26)	MVAC	65	48.3 wk	S
	CISCA	46	36.1 wk	

A, doxorubicin; NS, no statistically significant difference; C, cisplatin; MTX, methotrexate; CAP, cisplatin, doxorubicin, cyclophosphamide; CTX, cyclophosphamide; S, statistically significant difference; MVAC, methotrexate, vinblastine, doxorubicin, cisplatin; CISCA, cisplatin, doxorubicin, cyclophosphamide.

These combinations have resulted in dramatic increases in partial and complete response rates in metastatic disease. The MVAC, a regimen developed at the Memorial Sloan-Kettering Cancer Center, resulted in significant tumor regression in 72% of patients, including 36% complete responses (18). The highest proportion of complete responses was seen in lymph nodes but responses were seen at all disease sites. Twenty-eight percent of patients had primarily refractory disease to MVAC. Similarly, CMV produced an overall response rate of 56% including 28% complete responses (19). The combination of cisplatin, cyclophosphamide, and doxorubicin (CISCA) induced a 39% complete response rate with an overall response rate of 70% (20). A similar combination, CAP, reported a 20 to 43% response rate (21–23).

Significant single-agent activity of gallium has prompted study of gallium-containing combinations. In previously untreated patients, a combination of gallium, vinblastine, and ifosfamide (VIG) with granulocyte colony-stimulating factor (G-CSF) has resulted in a 68% response rate (24). Ten of 25 treated patients achieved disease-free status, 5 with VIG alone and 5 with VIG followed by surgery. This combination appears active but toxic, resulting in one treatment-related death and one patient with temporary blindness.

In general, combination chemotherapy is considered superior to single-agent therapy for advanced bladder carcinoma; however, only one prospective randomized trial was large enough to demonstrate superiority of cisplatin-containing combination therapy over single-agent cisplatin with regard to responses, duration of responses, and survival (Table 50.4). In this study, MVAC administration resulted in a significantly greater overall response rate (39% versus 12%), progression-free survival (6.6 months versus 2.4 months), and overall survival (12.5 months versus 8.2 months) when compared with cisplatin alone (13). The response rate to MVAC in this inter-group study was lower than originally reported by Memorial investigators (18) and may be related to patient selection. Two additional trials have failed to corroborate the results of the above study favoring a combination over single-agent cisplatin (12, 14). Hillcoat et al. compared cisplatin-methotrexate (CM) combination to cisplatin alone and found no significant differences in overall response (45% versus 31%), complete responses (9% for each arm), or median survival (8.7 months versus 7.2 months) (14). Another randomized trial compared cisplatin with cyclophosphamide (CP) to cisplatin alone and found no differences with respect to response rate or survival between the two arms (12).

A Southwest Oncology Group (SWOG) study, comparing doxorubicin versus doxorubicin-cisplatin combination demonstrated no difference in median survival between the two treatment arms (28 weeks versus 31 weeks) (25). Similarly, all three randomized trials comparing combinations containing doxorubicin, cisplatin, and cyclophosphamide with single-agent chemotherapy have failed to prove the superiority of the combination. In two phase III trials, CAP administration did not result in statistically significant differences in response and survival compared with single-agent cisplatin (21, 22). In a third study, the overall response to CAP was better compared with amascrine (43% versus 19%); however, no significant differences were reported in duration of response or survival times between the two groups (23). In all three trials, combination treatment resulted in greater toxicity than the single-agent arm. The failure of all except one randomized trial (13) to demonstrate superiority of combination over single-agent therapy may be due to the smaller number of patients and the limited efficacy of chemotherapy used in these trials.

In an important randomized study at M.D. Anderson Cancer Center, MVAC was compared with CISCA. MVAC chemotherapy was found to be superior to CISCA, achieving a higher response rate (65% versus 46%) and a longer median survival (48.3 weeks versus 36.1 weeks) (26). No trial comparing MCV with MVAC has been reported, and median survival appears to be similar with both combinations. However, median survival in patients achieving complete response appears to be longer for MVAC than CMV (38 months versus 14 months) (2).

Thus far, MVAC has emerged as a superior combination regimen in the treatment of metastatic bladder cancer, resulting in higher response rates; however, this benefit appears to be gained at the expense of greater toxicity (3).

Dose Escalation Studies

In an attempt to further enhance the response rates obtained by MVAC, various investigators have studied escalated doses with use of hematopoietic growth factor with inconsistent re-sults. Logothetis et al. reported 23% complete response rates and 17% partial response rates using escalated doses of MVAC with granulocyte-macrophage colony-stimulating factor (GM-CSF) in 32 previously treated patients with metastatic urothelial tumors (27). These results were unexpected in a pretreated patient group and suggested a dose-response relationship for cisplatin and doxorubicin. A subsequent randomized study from M.D. Anderson evaluated the role of GM-CSF with escalated MVAC. The patients not receiving GM-CSF achieved a higher complete remission rate (39% versus 26%), questioning the relevance of GM-CSF addition to MVAC (28). Loehrer et al. reported significant marrow toxicity, including 80% of patients developing grade 3 or 4 neutropenia and 23% early deaths. There were no apparent benefits of escalated doses of MVAC with regard to complete responses and survival in 35 patients with previously untreated advanced urothelial cancer (29). In the latter study, doses of all four agents were escalated simultaneously compared with only three in the M.D. Anderson study. Seidman et al. have reported a 69% response rate with 25% complete responses in a feasibility study using escalated doses of MVAC with G-CSF administration in previously untreated patients. Febrile neutropenia developed in 58% of patients (30). Two other smaller studies have confirmed the feasibility of escalated MVAC (31, 32).

Except for the first M.D. Anderson study (27), the results with escalated MVAC appear no better than those with standard dose MVAC. Escalated doses of MVAC therapy are unlikely to improve significantly the outcome for metastatic disease, although only a randomized study comparing standard dose MVAC and selectively escalated doses of MVAC can provide a valid comparison between the two approaches.

Chemorefractory Disease

For patients in whom a cisplatin-methotrexate chemotherapy regimen fails, salvage therapies are limited. At M.D. Anderson, a 30% partial response rate was achieved with a 5-FU/interferon alfa (IFN-α) combination (33). Addition of 13-cisretinoic acid did not enhance the responses (34). High-dose folinic acid with 5-FU failed to produce any significant activity in a Canadian trial (35). A phase I trial of 5-FU, IFN-α, cisplatin, and methotrexate has been completed for chemorefractory patients but no efficacy data are yet available (36). Response rates varying from 17 to 62% have been seen with gallium nitrate (11, 17). In one study, four of eight patients (all with pelvic or abdominal disease) had complete responses; one additional patient achieved a partial response (17). A 50% partial response rate has been seen recently with the combination of gallium and 5-FU (37). Reports of nephrotoxicity and optic neuropathy with gallium administration are a cause for major concern. Paclitaxel (Taxol; Bristol Meyer Squibb, Princeton, NJ) as a single agent has resulted in an objective response rate of 42% with 19% complete responses (38). Docetaxel, a derivative, may also be an active agent and needs further evaluation in bladder cancer (39).

Noncisplatin Regimens

Potential toxicities of cisplatin and doxorubicin regimens can exclude a significant number of bladder cancer patients from receiving chemotherapy. Attempts to reduce the morbidity while maintaining similar response rates have led to development of various carboplatin-containing chemotherapy regimens for bladder cancer. A 48% response rate was reported using a combination of carboplatin, methotrexate, and vinblastine, and the regimen was well tolerated without any renal toxicity (40). A similar regimen containing carboplatin, vinblastine, and methotrexate with leucovorin resulted in a 70% response rate in an early report (41). Another combination containing methotrexate, vinblastine, mitoxantrone, and carboplatin (MVMJ) achieved impressive 27% complete response and 36% partial response rates (42). However, another study using the same combination resulted in 43% objective responses, which were mainly seen in limited stage bladder cancer (43). MVMJ appears to be less toxic and effective; however, the follow-up is short and further confirmation of its efficacy in a larger study is required.

Patient Selection

Before embarking on a combination regimen, pretreatment prognostic factors should be evaluated in patients to determine any potential benefit of the therapy. Geller et al. found Karnofsky performance status and normal alkaline phosphatase to be predictive of survival (44). Patients aged 60 years or older were likely to survive longer, probably indicating stringent selection among the elderly. Nodal disease alone in the absence of metastases elsewhere was significant in univariate analysis; however, it did not emerge as an independent factor in multivariate analysis. In another trial, poor performance status, history of weight loss, and site of metastases (lung, liver, and bones) were associated with poor outcome (13). The variations in dose intensity of MVAC were not associated with response or survival in one analysis (45).

The combination regimens discussed above can contribute to substantial morbidity (18, 19, 46), and treatment-related deaths have been reported in 5% of treated patients (4). The toxicities include nausea, vomiting, nephrotoxicity, myelotoxicity, sepsis, mucositis, and neurotoxicity. The question of quality of life with these combination regimens has not been addressed in a systematic way. Keeping this in mind, careful assessment of associated medical problems and individual patient tolerance to proposed chemotherapy is mandatory. Internal urinary reservoirs, long ileal conduits, and ascites can alter methotrexate kinetics, predisposing the patient to mucositis. Similarly, inability to tolerate fluid and borderline renal function may preclude use of cisplatin in older patients. In the presence of cardiac dysfunction, use of doxorubicin may be contraindicated. Alternative combination regimens containing less toxic agents like carboplatin (42) and epidoxorubicin (47) are under investigation.

The overall effect of combination chemotherapy on survival has been the subject of debate. The median survival of responders treated with MVAC or CMV is better compared with nonresponders; consequently, more central nervous system relapses have been reported in survivors, suggesting a change in the natural history of disease (18, 19). Despite improved responses, only a small percentage of patients are long-term survivors. The available information suggests that combination therapy using three or four agents should be considered standard first-line treatment of metastatic bladder cancer; however, patients should be carefully evaluated for prognostic factors to maximize the benefit and reduce potential toxicities.

Chemotherapy for Locally Advanced Bladder Cancer

No other issue has been more controversial in urologic oncology in recent years than the management of muscle-invasive bladder cancer. Radiation oncologists and urologists have been unable to agree on the relative merits of conventional therapies (radiation and cystectomy) in the treatment of invasive bladder cancer (48). However, modest 5-year survival rates in the range of 50% from conventional treatments (48) have led to investigation of newer approaches targeting the presumed presence of micrometastatic disease at the time of diagnosis. The treatment approach for such patients is based on two basic principles. First, to treat micrometastases with systemic therapy, with the ultimate goal of reducing mortality from metastatic disease. Second, to attempt to preserve bladder function without jeopardizing local control (49). The heterogeneous nature of this disease with variable local invasiveness and metastatic potential, however, requires accurate identification of various prognostic indicators to choose optimal treatment (49, 50). The following discussion will provide insight into current knowledge about adjuvant therapy, neoadjuvant therapy, combined chemoradiation, and finally integration of various modalities.

COMBINED CHEMORADIATION

The principal goal of any treatment designed for muscle-invasive bladder cancer is to increase overall survival. Two currently available therapies, radical cystectomy and radical radiation therapy (RT) with or without chemotherapy, have the same goal. Only RT provides an opportunity for bladder preservation in selected patients. Unfortunately, persistent disease and local failures are common problems after RT alone (2, 51). This knowledge, in combination with physician biases, has made radical cystectomy a preferred treatment for invasive bladder cancer in North America, with RT being used sparingly as treatment in patients who are not considered to be candidates for cystectomy for a variety of reasons (52). In contrast, radical RT is considered standard primary treatment in Europe and Canada, with cystectomy reserved as a salvage modality (51). The selection biases involved in the treatment assignment for invasive bladder cancer make direct comparison of RT and surgery invalid except in a randomized trial. Unfortunately, no direct randomized trial comparing RT and surgery has been conducted. Accepting this major limitation, the following discussion will review recent studies attempting to define the role of RT alone or as part of multimodality regimens in the treatment of muscle-invasive bladder cancer.

RT has been used in the treatment of muscle-invasive bladder cancer for many decades, and a number of trials of definitive RT in muscle-invasive bladder carcinoma have been reported in the literature. Similar to neoadjuvant studies, however, lack of uniform criteria for patient selection, staging, response assessment, and trial endpoints makes comparisons very difficult. Most series have reported initial complete response rates of 40 to 50% and 5-year survival rates of 20 to 40% with RT alone (51–53). Patients who do not have complete response require salvage cystectomy, which carries significant risks because of difficulties in operating in irradiated fields. Even among those having a complete response, one fourth to one third of patients will subsequently have local failure (51). Ultimately, only approximately one third of patients will maintain a tumor-free bladder after definitive RT (51). This is in contrast to 5-year survival rates of 64 to 75% in node-negative patients and 35% in node-positive patients after radical cystectomy (54). Cystectomy is highly effective in local control, as demonstrated by only 9% of patients having pelvic recurrences (55). Despite good local control, many patients will die of distant metastases within 5 years (51). Attempts to improve the results by combining surgery and RT have failed in most instances. Randomized trials of definitive RT with bladder preservation versus preoperative RT followed by cystectomy have shown no significant difference in survival between the two (56, 57). A recent randomized trial failed to show any significant difference between cystectomy versus preoperative RT followed by cystectomy (58). Currently, the role of preoperative RT remains unclear and controversial (2, 52). Both cystectomy and definitive RT resulted in suboptimal long-term survival since neither affects the micrometastases outside the field of treatment. Since the advent of effective chemotherapy, there has been tremendous interest in combined modality treatment protocols.

Attempts to increase the effectiveness of RT and bladder preservation have led to combination of RT with chemotherapy in a variety of ways. Concurrent RT and chemotherapy explore the radiosensitization properties of chemotherapeutic agents like 5-FU and cisplatin. Numerous phase II trials of chemotherapy combined with RT have reported complete responses in 61 to 90% of patients (51–53). In one of the earliest trials, concurrent administration of cisplatin with radical RT resulted in a 77% complete response rate in patients completing RT (59). At 4 years, the survival rate for clinical stage T2 was higher (64%) than that for clinical T3 and T4 (24%). Follow-up phase studies of cisplatin and RT have confirmed these results (53, 60–62). For patients unable to receive cisplatin, alternative agents have been investigated.

Local control rates similar to cisplatin (50 to 70%) have been obtained by combining 5-FU with RT (53, 63, 64). In a

study by Rotman et al., additional transurethral resection of residual disease followed by intravesical mitomycin C or Bacile Calmette-Guérin brought the overall complete response rate to an impressive 89% (63). At 5 years, the survival rate was 62%. Recently, concurrent vinblastine and RT were reported to induce 71% clinical complete responses, with a 3-year progression-free survival rate of 66% (65).

Few trials of RT with concurrent, combination chemotherapy have been reported. In one such trial, a reduced-dose 5-FU/cisplatin administration with bifractionated split course RT resulted in 74% histologic complete responses. The disease-free survival rate at 3 years was 62%, and the regimen was well tolerated (66). In another trial, concomitant cyclic chemoradiation using 5-FU, folinic acid, and cisplatin resulted in a 50% complete response rate in node-positive patients. Six of seven patients achieving complete responses were alive at 14 months, whereas all those achieving less than a complete response died within 12 months (67). Excellent tolerance to the regimen was reported with no grade III or IV toxicity. The results of initial phase II trials have reported higher response rates and local control rates compared with historical controls without a significant increase in toxicity (52, 61, 68). Severe complications develop in less than 10% of patients (53). Assessment of durability of such responses will require longer follow-up of 5 years or more. In addition, a definite advantage of combined chemoradiation must be demonstrated in randomized trials to confirm these data.

Only a limited number of randomized studies have been completed (Table 50.5), and all have been criticized for a variety of reasons. In an early study, adjuvant doxorubicin/5-FU after radiation did not show any survival advantage over no chemotherapy (72). Another study using neoadjuvant and adjuvant methotrexate after radiation reported similar survivals with or without chemotherapy (71). The results of both trials were not surprising because both excluded cisplatin, probably the most active agent.

Another report combined pooled data from two different trials using preradiation single-agent cisplatin and failed to show a survival difference between the treatment and control groups (70). Although there were no major differences between the two arms, RT was delayed by 6 to 9 weeks for cisplatin administration in the treatment arm, which may have allowed metastatic disease to manifest. The last dose of cisplatin was given 3 weeks before RT; therefore, it is likely that it did not provide optimal sensitization.

A recent prospective randomized study conducted by NCI Canada assigned patients to a control versus concomitant cisplatin arm. A significantly lower rate of pelvic recurrence was seen in the cisplatin arm compared with the control arm (67% versus 45%), suggesting improved local control. At 2 years no significant difference has been observed in overall survival; however, there is a trend in favor of the cisplatin arm (69). Additional follow-up is awaited from this trial.

Table 50.5. Randomized Trials of Radiation Therapy and Chemotherapy

REFERENCE	NO. OF PATIENTS	SCHEMA	SURVIVAL AT 3 YR (%)	COMMENT
Coppin (69)	99	C+ RT	61[a]	NS[b] (P = 0.067)
		RT	43	
Wallace (70)	255	C->RT	40	NS
		RT	40	
Shearer (71)	376	MTX->RT->MTX	39	NS
		RT	37	
Richards (72)	129	RT->5-FU/A	35	NS
		RT	37	

C, cisplatin; RT, radiation therapy; NS, no statistically significant difference; MTX, methotrexate; 5-FU, 5-fluorouracil; A, doxorubicin.
[a] Survival at 2 years.
[b] Trend toward significance.

Neoadjuvant Chemotherapy Followed by Concurrent RT and Chemotherapy

Improved local control can translate into survival benefit only for patients in whom uncontrolled local tumor is the cause of death (59). Because chemotherapy used in concurrent radiosensitization protocols has the potential to increase the local control rate but has a minimal effect on distant metastases, improvement in long-term survival may not be a realistic goal. This concept and superior results of combination chemotherapy programs in metastatic disease have led to integration of combination chemotherapy with RT. Phase II studies have demonstrated feasibility of delivering a full dose of definitive RT after neoadjuvant chemotherapy (52, 73). At Massachusetts General Hospital, two courses of MCV chemotherapy were followed by cisplatin plus radiation for treatment of T2 to T4 transitional cell bladder carcinoma. Substantial toxicities were seen, with nausea and vomiting in 73% and significant myelosuppression in 34% of patients. Complete responses at the local site were seen in 58% of patients, and approximately 25% of patients underwent cystectomy. Of the complete responders, 89% maintained a functioning bladder. At a median follow-up of 4 years, 45% of patients were alive and disease free; however, metastases had developed in 42%. Tumor stage and hydronephrosis but not DNA ploidy analysis were found to be of prognostic importance in regard to bladder preservation and survival (73). Of equal importance was the development of superficial bladder carcinoma in 21% of patients who had initial complete response. Based on the results of this pilot trial, a prospective trial has been initiated that randomizes patients between neoadjuvant MCV versus no upfront chemotherapy, followed by cisplatin plus RT (74). Another study reported a 3-year survival rate of 65% using a similar approach of neoadjuvant combination chemotherapy (75). In this trial, 84% of stage T2 patients were alive at 3 years.

From reported trials, no definite conclusions can be drawn regarding superiority of combined chemoradiation over definitive radiation alone and bladder preservation modalities. Before their acceptance as a standard therapy, randomized trials would be required to show effectiveness of such treatments without jeopardizing the survival. It is realized that combined therapy may have a major effect on local control, but a significant effect on distant disease and survival benefit remains elusive. Important observations must not be overlooked while attempting bladder preservation using RT. To achieve a goal of bladder preservation, better prediction of tumor response is required. Histologic grade, DNA ploidy, and similar factors have not been consistent in predicting accurate response (60, 73). Optimal debulking of bladder tumor by transurethral resection (TUR) seems to improve local control (68, 76). In the absence of the ability to identify favorable subgroups in advance, only patients who are complete responders after initial treatment should be selected for bladder preservation. Not all patients respond to combined therapy, and for the nonresponders, salvage cystectomy may offer a chance of cure (68, 76). Adequate follow-up is mandatory after bladder preservation because residual tumor carries a bad prognosis and salvage cystectomy may cure a number of patients (76). Even in patients with complete response, new tumors or recurrences can occur that may be salvageable by additional treatment (73). Currently, there is no evidence that this type of selective bladder-conserving approach can be successful without compromising patient survival (68).

Future directions of combined chemoradiation will involve the use of hyperfractionated or accelerated RT. In one pilot study using a four-drug combination alternating with twice-a-day accelerated RT, there was an 89% complete response rate. One death was reported due to acute hematologic toxicity; acute leukemia developed in another patient 1 year after treatment. No cystectomies were required. The 3-year survival rate was 60%, with metastases developing in 14% of patients (77).

ADJUVANT THERAPY FOR BLADDER CANCER

Chemotherapy given to patients after surgery is referred to as adjuvant therapy. Occasionally, the adjuvant term has been used for chemotherapy given after transurethral removal of bladder tumor (TUR) or RT. The rationale for adjuvant chemotherapy is based on the findings that most patients in whom local control can be achieved by primary therapy still experience relapse due to micrometastases present at the time of diagnosis. Adjuvant therapy is given in the immediate postoperative period in hopes of eradicating micrometastases. The advantages of the adjuvant approach are many.

More precise pathologic staging allows better patient selection for therapy and minimizes unnecessary exposure to chemotherapy for patients who are cured by surgery alone. Potentially curative surgery is applied before chemotherapy, thus reducing the chance of resectable tumor becoming unresectable if chemotherapy should fail. Early administration of chemotherapy in the presence of minimal tumor burden presumably reduces the chance that resistance will develop. In addition, surgical removal of the bladder by cystectomy eliminates the risk of recurrent tumor formation at the primary site. With the availability of newer internal urinary diversions, this approach is more acceptable. However, a major disadvantage of adjuvant therapy is the inability to judge the response in vivo; therefore, an important prognostic tool is lost. No in vitro methods are currently available to assess the efficacy of proposed chemotherapy before the administration of adjuvant chemotherapy. This limitation may lead to administration of ineffective and potentially toxic therapy without any clinical benefit (78). The efficacy is determined by disease-free survival and overall survival.

Early nonrandomized, single-institution adjuvant trials used chemotherapy with limited efficacy in a small number of patients. It is not surprising that they have led to no definite conclusions regarding the usefulness of adjuvant therapy (79, 80). However, these trials proved the feasibility and safety of this approach in a patient population that is often elderly and has compromised renal function. Both single-agent and combination chemotherapies have been investigated in adjuvant settings. In one such large trial at the M.D. Anderson Cancer Center, investigators used the CISCA regimen in patients treated with radical cystectomy. A high-risk group was defined by the presence of vascular or lymphatic invasion, extravesical tumor extension, extension into pelvic viscera, or positive nodal disease. The 5-year disease-free survival rates of the treated high-risk, untreated high-risk, and low-risk group patients were 70%, 37%, and 70%, respectively, suggesting a benefit for CISCA-treated high-risk patients (81). In the adjuvant

group, 62% of patients were alive and disease free for a mean follow-up of 118 weeks. Patients with node-positive, extravesical, and locally advanced disease benefited; however, patients with vascular or lymphatic invasion alone did not. Although results of this trial are interesting, its nonrandomized nature raises a possibility of heavy selection bias and makes it difficult to draw definite conclusions.

In another trial, selected patients received adjuvant MVAC therapy within 1 month after radical cystectomy and were compared with patients not receiving adjuvant MVAC at the same institution. In early results, treated patients with nodal disease appear to have better survival compared with control subjects (82). The benefit for N1 patients appears more dramatic, as evidenced by 8 of 8 patients receiving chemotherapy being alive at 7 months compared with only 2 of 10 patients not receiving chemotherapy being alive at 1 year. However, significant selection differences may exist between treated and untreated patients and follow-up is still short.

A few randomized trials of adjuvant therapy have been reported (Table 50.6). In a Swiss study, 77 patients were randomly assigned to observation or three courses of cisplatin chemotherapy postoperatively (84). The depth of invasion (PT3a) and presence of carcinoma in situ were associated with improved survival (86). At 5 years, 54% of patients in the control group and 57% of patients in the treated group survived. Thus, no significant survival difference was noted from adjuvant cisplatin treatment. The higher 5-year survival rate in the control group may have indicated selection of fit patients and may have masked a small improvement in survival. In addition, the limits of confidence intervals were wide, suggesting a need for a larger number of patients to determine smaller differences in survival between the two groups. Another possibility is that cisplatin alone may not be the most effective adjuvant treatment.

Results of two randomized trials using combination adjuvant therapy are more promising. Skinner et al. assigned pT3, pT4, or pN+ bladder cancer patients to either adjuvant CISCA or observation alone after radical cystectomy (85). At 3 years, disease-free survival was significantly better in the treated group compared with the nontreated group (70% versus 46%). Although chemotherapy prolonged the median time to recur-

Table 50.6. Randomized Trials of Adjuvant Chemotherapy

REFERENCE	NO. OF PATIENTS	SCHEMA	SURVIVAL (%)	COMMENT
Stockle (83)	49	Surgery->MVAC/MVEC	—	S
		Surgery		
Struder (84)	77	Surgery->Cisplatin	57	NS
		Surgery	54	
Skinner (85)	91	Cystectomy-> CISCA	70[a]	NS
		Cystectomy	46	

MVAC, methotrexate, vinblastine, doxorubicin, cisplatin; MVEC, methotrexate, vinblastine, epirubicin, cisplatin; S, statistically significant difference; NS, no statistically significant difference.

[a] Progression-free survival reported.

rence by 14 months, no advantage could be demonstrated by 2 years. The benefit was more apparent in patients with one positive node and node-negative patients, whereas patients with two or more positive lymph nodes derived no benefit. This study invited significant criticism for a variety of reasons. Out of 229 patients with pT3, pT4, or pN+ disease, only 160 were considered eligible. Of 160 patients invited to participate, 37% refused, leading to a possibility of selection bias. In the chemotherapy group, 25% of randomized patients elected not to receive it and only 61% completed the planned four cycles. Not all patients received CISCA due to the modification in chemotherapy based on a clonogenic sensitivity assay in 28% of patients. Despite all criticism, this was the first prospective randomized study to demonstrate any potential benefit in favor of adjuvant therapy.

A recent German trial reported similar observations (83). In this trial, 49 patients were randomized to three cycles of adjuvant treatment with MVAC/MVEC or no adjuvant treatment after cystectomy. An additional 20 patients received adjuvant therapy off the protocol. The 38 total patients receiving adjuvant therapy (18 on randomized trial and 20 off trial) were compared with 45 patients not receiving adjuvant chemotherapy. A significant prognostic advantage was reported in favor of adjuvantly treated patients. Patients with 0 or 1 node involvement appeared to benefit more than those with a higher number of nodes. A considerable number of patients had problems tolerating all three cycles. Once again, the results are not without controversies. This trial was only partly randomized because of the early conclusion by the authors in favor of adjuvant treatment from an interim analysis, which led to early closure. Consequently, more patients were selected in a nonrandomized fashion to receive adjuvant therapy (20 versus 18). In patients randomized to receive chemotherapy, 8 of 28 patients did not receive protocol treatment. However, the authors concluded that there was significant prolongation of progression-free and overall survival with three cycles of adjuvant MVAC/MVEC. The authors are currently comparing MVEC versus a methotrexate/cisplatin combination in a randomized fashion.

Most urologists consider TUR alone to be insufficient therapy for invasive bladder cancer. However, Herr has reported 82% survival in selected patients who underwent TUR alone, but most of these patients had only superficially invasive tumors (87). A small study using three cycles of MVAC after TUR has been reported. At a median follow-up of 36 months, 11 of 51 patients had progressive disease, for which 8 patients required cystectomy (88). Six patients died of progressive bladder cancer. Hall et al. have reported the use of high-dose methotrexate with leucovorin rescue following TUR or partial cystectomy for T3 transitional cell carcinoma. The bladder was free of tumor in 84% at 1 year and 79% at 2 years (89). In the absence of controlled studies, it is impossible to make any judgment about this approach.

The data from these adjuvant trials are certainly provocative. However, larger studies with longer follow-up are required to confirm the benefit of adjuvant therapy before it can be recommended as a standard therapy for muscle-invasive bladder cancer. The patient group that would benefit from adjuvant chemotherapy remains to be better defined. From the above results it appears that patients with higher number of nodal involvement may derive no or minimal benefit from adjuvant therapy. Difficulties encountered in the drug administration in reported trials are a reminder for careful patient selection to avoid serious morbidity. Currently, adjuvant therapy can still be considered investigational, and individual patients should be entered on adjuvant clinical trials whenever possible. A randomized trial comparing neoadjuvant versus adjuvant MVAC is currently ongoing (90) and will provide an interesting comparison of two different approaches to invasive bladder cancer.

NEOADJUVANT THERAPY FOR BLADDER CANCER

A limited number of cures achieved by definitive surgery and/or RT and improved success rates in advanced disease with combination chemotherapy programs have led to extensive investigations of chemotherapy as part of integral therapy for muscle-invasive disease. Despite significant advances, muscle-invasive disease remains incurable for most patients. As an alternative to adjuvant therapy, chemotherapy can be given upfront or in a preemptive fashion as part of multimodality therapy. This type of neoadjuvant chemotherapy has been used for preserving bladder and treating micrometastases believed to be present at the time of treatment; however, the ultimate goal is still to improve survival. The principal advantage of neoadjuvant therapy is the ability to assess in vivo response in the bladder lesion and thus provide valuable prognostic information. Decreasing size (downstaging) may allow an unresectable lesion to be resectable or, in the case of complete response, may allow bladder preservation. Micrometastases are treated early in the course of the disease, thus reducing the chance of developing resistance. Because chemotherapy is delivered before any surgery or radiation, patient tolerance is expected to be superior (91).

Despite several advantages, the following pitfalls must be kept in mind before selecting the neoadjuvant approach. Not all patients require systemic therapy. Because clinical staging is inaccurate and generally upstages a higher number of patients, neoadjuvant therapy may not be of any real benefit for some patients. In addition, the absence of any reliable biologic markers makes it more difficult to delineate patients who will benefit from neoadjuvant therapy. The difficulty in accurate assessment of response or false interpretation may delay the curative surgical therapy. Importantly, patients with successful bladder preservation continue to be at risk for new tumors (92). In elderly patients, concurrent medical conditions may preclude the use of agents like cisplatin or doxorubicin, making the neoadjuvant approach difficult.

Phase I–II Neoadjuvant Trials

Reported phase I–II trials have yielded a wide range of results in regard to responses, survival, and toxicity. While reviewing the results, it is important to realize that methodologic differences in eligibility, patient selection, staging procedures, prognostic factors, chemotherapy agents, dose intensity, and trial endpoints are too great to allow direct comparison of various clinical trials (93). The differences in methodology also could explain the disparities in the results of various trials. No definite conclusions can be drawn from comparison of results from nonrandomized trials for the same reasons (94). Randomized trials are required to establish the true effect of neoadjuvant therapy on survival (91, 94).

Chemotherapy can induce significant responses in the bladder primarily. Using MVAC as an example, a 48% complete response rate was noted at cystoscopy (92). Intraarterial administration of neoadjuvant chemotherapy has also been found to be equally effective in inducing complete remissions (95, 96). The clinical evaluation for response uniformly shows higher proportions of responses when compared with pathologic evaluations. Using the same MVAC series as an example, the complete response rate dropped to 23% based on pathologic examination of the bladder by partial or radical cystectomy (92). Clinical understaging was found in 30% of patients (92). The findings of clinical understaging create significant problems in accurate assessment of response and determination of eligibility for bladder preservation. Generally, response inversely correlates with stage of disease and depth of invasion. After MVAC therapy, 100% of T2 patients achieved downstaging compared with only 42% with T4 disease (97).

Transitional histology responds better compared with other histologies (97). The number of complete responses has varied between different combinations and even with the same combination in different trials (91). With different combination chemotherapy regimens, pathologic complete responses have been seen in 22 to 43% of patients (91). The rate of pathologic complete responses demonstrates that for the majority of patients, neoadjuvant chemotherapy alone is inadequate treatment and additional surgery/radiation is necessary for optimal local control (91). The subsequent treatment, aimed at bladder preservation in the form of concurrent chemoradiation or less radical surgery, is currently under study. The response in the primary is of prognostic significance and may be useful in determining the type and extent of additional treatment (91, 98).

In one of the most extensive experiences, survival in a group of 111 patients who received neoadjuvant MVAC appeared similar to reported cystectomy series (99). The 5-year survival rates were 60%, 58%, 45%, and 32% for T2, T3a, T3b, and T4a patients, respectively. However, initial response does not always correlate with survival (93). Long-term tumor control with MVAC may be disappointing as recently demonstrated by Connor et al., who reported that only one of six patients treated with neoadjuvant MVAC was alive at 45 months (100). Similarly, only one of five patients receiving adjuvant MVAC was alive at 45 months. In selected patients, bladder preservation can be obtained (99). For T4 patients, bladder preservation may not be a realistic goal (it is considered an achievable goal for T2–T3a patients) (91).

Currently, the optimal neoadjuvant chemotherapy combination, route of administration (intravenous versus intraarterial), number of cycles, schedule and timing of integration with RT/surgery, optimal response evaluation, and many other parameters remain less defined. Further delineation of these parameters will help in the design of integrated multimodality approaches. Combined efforts of the medical oncologist, urologist, radiation oncologist, and pathologist are mandatory for bladder preservation.

Randomized Trials of Neoadjuvant Approaches

Despite encouraging data from phase II neoadjuvant trials, randomized comparisons are needed to evaluate survival and the true role of neoadjuvant therapy for invasive bladder cancer. One trial comparing neoadjuvant cisplatin/doxorubicin followed by cystectomy with RT and cystectomy without chemotherapy has shown a significantly higher overall survival for chemotherapy treated T2–T4a patients (P = 0.018) (101). Responders survived longer than nonresponders in this study.

An ongoing Spanish study compares cystectomy with three courses of preoperative cisplatin followed by cystectomy. A response rate of 44% and a complete response rate of 17% were achieved with preoperative cisplatin. The median follow-up of 24.5 months' actuarial survival appears to be slightly better in the cisplatin arm compared with surgery alone (79% versus 67%) (102). An Italian randomized study comparing neoadjuvant MVAC with MVEC (doxorubicin replaced by epirubicin) showed no differences in complete response rates between the two groups (19% versus 16%). However, MVEC appears less toxic compared with MVAC. In both groups responders have longer survival than nonresponders (103). In another trial comparing neoadjuvant MVEC plus cystectomy to cystectomy alone, no differences were observed between the two groups (104).

The reported results from the above trials are encouraging, but early and longer follow-up is awaited before definite conclusions can be drawn. The Southwest Oncology Group initiated a trial comparing cystectomy versus three cycles of neoadjuvant MVAC and cystectomy in patients with locally advanced bladder cancer (105). Another trial randomizes patients between three cycles of CMV versus no chemotherapy before definitive treatment (cystectomy or radiation) for T2, T3, and T4a bladder cancers. The primary endpoint is survival, and the expected recruitment of 1000 patients will be able to detect a 10% improvement in survival at 2 years (106). Until the definite results of randomized trials become available, neoadjuvant therapy should be considered experimental (Table 50.7).

Selection of Primary Therapy for Invasive Bladder Cancer

Considering the treatment options available today for patients with invasive bladder cancer, therapy selection can be difficult. The available approaches include radical cystectomy with or

Table 50.7. Randomized Trials of Neoadjuvant Therapy

REFERENCE	SCHEMA	OVERALL RESPONSE (%)	COMPLETE RESPONSE (%)	COMMENT
Passalacqua (103)	MVAC->Surgery	48	19	NS
	MVEC->Surgery	45	16	
Pellegrini (104)	MVEC->Surgery	—	—	NS
	Surgery	—	—	
Rintala (101)	A + C->Surgery	—	—	S*
	Surgery	—	—	
Shipley (74)	CMV->C + RT	—	—	NA
	C + RT	—	—	
M. Pinerio (102)	C->Surgery	79	—	NS
	Surgery	67	—	
Hall (106)	CMV->Local therapy	—	—	NA
	Local therapy	—	—	
Crawford (105)	MVAC->Surgery	—	—	NA
	Surgery	—	—	

MVAC, methotrexate, vinblastine, doxorubicin, cisplatin; MVEC, methotrexate, vinblastine, epirubicin, cisplatin; NS, no statistically significant difference; A, doxorubicin; C, cisplatin; S, statistically significant difference; CMV, cisplatin, methotrexate, vinblastine; RT, radiation therapy; NA, not avaiable.
[a] P = 0.018.

without adjuvant chemotherapy, radical RT, combined chemoradiation, or neoadjuvant therapy followed by bladder preservation or cystectomy as evaluated by response. The selection of any modality and integration of the various multimodality treatments may be different at different institutions. Currently, the inability to identify in advance patients who will benefit from bladder preservation versus poor-risk patients limits the general applicability of bladder-preservation treatment approaches. In the future, better understanding of tumor biology and molecular aspects of bladder cancer may provide improved patient selection. Availability of internal bladder reservoirs has made cystectomy followed by adjuvant chemotherapy an attractive option. Concomitant chemoradiation provides improved local control without added toxicity. Neoadjuvant chemotherapy followed by less radical surgery, as pioneered by the Memorial investigators, or neoadjuvant therapy followed by concurrent chemoradiation, as pioneered by the Massachusetts investigators, appears promising. All these approaches are currently being evaluated in randomized trials; until the results from those trials are available, they should be administered only in the setting of a clinical trial.

NONTRANSITIONAL BLADDER CANCER

Nontransitional bladder cancers are considered less responsive to chemotherapy (2, 97). Occasional cases of small cell and adenocarcinoma have been reported to respond to MVAC, CMV, or cisplatin/etoposide combinations (2, 107). For squamous cell bladder cancer, responses were seen using a combination of 5-FU and mitomycin C with concurrent RT (108). Recently, successful bladder preservation with CMV chemotherapy followed by RT has been reported (109). Because of the limited experience with chemotherapy in the treatment of nontransitional bladder cancer, no definite recommendations can be made regarding its use in nontransitional bladder cancer.

CONCLUSIONS

The past few years have seen a tremendous amount of information becoming available, using a variety of combined modality approaches for the treatment of invasive bladder carcinoma. The challenge remains to determine the best way of integrating two or more of the available treatment modalities to achieve the ultimate goal of cure for invasive bladder cancer. Significant progress has been made in combination chemotherapy for metastatic cancer; however, cure of metastatic bladder cancer remains elusive. Various ongoing investigations should provide valuable new information to move us in the direction of a cure for bladder cancer.

REFERENCES

1. Boring CC, et al. Cancer statistics, 1994. CA Cancer J Clin 1994;44:7.
2. Fair WR, et al. Cancer of the bladder. In: De Vita VT, et al., eds. Cancer: principles and practice of oncology. Philadelphia: JB Lippincott, 1993:1052.
3. Steinberg GD, Trump DL, Cummins KB. Metastatic bladder cancer: natural history, clinical course and consideration for treatment. Urol Clin North Am 1992;19:735.
4. Kantoff PW, Scher HI. Chemotherapy for metastatic bladder cancer. Hematol Oncol Clin North Am 1992;6:195.
5. Yagoda A. Chemotherapy for urothelial tract tumors. Cancer 1987;60:574.
6. Turner AG. Methotrexate in advanced bladder cancer. Cancer Treat Rep 1981;65:183.
7. Blumenreich MS, et al. Phase II trial of vinblastine sulfate for metastatic urothelial tumors. Cancer 1982;50:435.
8. Richards R, et al. Vincristine in advanced bladder cancer: An EORTC phase II trial. Cancer Treat Rep 1983;67:575.
9. Knight EW, et al. Comparison of 5FU and doxorubicin in the treatment of carcinoma of the bladder. Cancer Treat Rep 1983;67:514.

10. Torti FM, et al. Chemotherapy of advanced transitional cell carcinoma. Cancer Chemother Pharmacol 1983;11(Suppl):1.

11. Seidman AD, et al. Continuous infusion gallium nitrate for patients with advanced refractory urothelial tract tumors. Cancer 1991;68:2561.

12. Soloway MS, et al. A comparison of cisplatin and the combination of cisplatin and cyclophosphamide in advanced urothelial cancer. Cancer 1983;52:767.

13. Loehrer PJ Sr, et al. A randomized comparison of cisplatin alone or in combination with methotrexate, vinblastine and doxorubicin in patients with metastatic urothelial carcinoma: a cooperative group study. J Clin Oncol 1992;10:1066.

14. Hillcoat BL, et al. A randomized trial of cisplatinum versus cisplatinum plus methotrexate in advanced cancer of the urothelial tract. J Clin Oncol 1989;7:706.

15. Oliver RTD, et al. Methotrexate in the treatment of metastatic and recurrent primary transitional cell carcinoma. J Urol 1984;131:483.

16. Yagoda A. Phase II trials with urothelial tract tumors: the Memorial Sloan-Kettering Cancer Center. Cancer Chemother Pharmacol 1983;2(Suppl):9.

17. Seligman PA, Crawford ED. Treatment of advanced transitional cell carcinoma of the bladder with continuous infusion gallium nitrate. J Natl Cancer Inst 1991;83:1582.

18. Sternberg CN, et al. M-VAC for advanced transitional cell carcinoma of the urothelium: efficacy, and patterns of response and relapse. Cancer 1989;64:2448.

19. Harker WG, et al. Cisplatin, methotrexate and vinblastine (CMV); an effective chemotherapy regimen for metastatic transitional cell carcinoma of the urinary tract: a Northern California Oncology Group study. J Clin Oncol 1985;3:1463.

20. Logothetis CJ, et al. Cisplatin, cyclophosphamide and doxorubicin chemotherapy for unresectable urothelial tumors. J Urol 1989;141:33.

21. Khandelkar JD, et al. Comparative activity and toxicity of cis-diamminodichloroplatinum (DDP) and a combination of doxorubicin, cyclophosphamide and DDP in disseminated transitional cell carcinomas of the urinary tract. J Clin Oncol 1985;3:539.

22. Troner MD. Cyclophosphamide (C), Adriamycin (A) and platinol (P) in the treatment of urothelial malignancy. Proc Am Soc Clin Oncol 1985;4:106.

23. Al-Sarraf M, et al. Phase II trial of cyclophosphamide, doxorubicin and cisplatinum (CAP) versus amascrine in patients with transitional cell carcinoma of the urinary bladder: a Southwest Oncology Group study. Cancer Treat Rep 1985;69:189.

24. Einhorn LH, et al. Vinblastine, ifosfamide and gallium (VIG) combination chemotherapy in urothelial carcinoma. Proc Am Soc Clin Oncol 1994;13:229.

25. Gagliano R, et al. Adriamycin versus Adriamycin plus cis-diamminodichloro-platinum in advanced transitional cell bladder carcinoma: a Southwest Oncology Group study. Am J Clin Oncol 1983;6:215.

26. Logothetis CJ, et al. A prospective randomized trial comparing MVAC and CISCA chemotherapy for patients with metastatic urothelial tumors. J Clin Oncol 1990;8:1050.

27. Logothetis CJ, et al. Escalated therapy for refractory urothelial tumors: methotrexate-vinblastine-doxorubicin-cisplatin plus

28. Logothetis CJ, et al. Escalated (Esc) M-VAC + rhGM-CSF (Schering-Plough) in metastatic transitional cell carcinoma: (TCC): preliminary results of a randomized trial. Proc Am Soc Clin Oncol 1992;11:202.

29. Loehrer PJ, et al. Escalated doses of methotrexate, vinblastine, doxorubicin and cisplatin plus recombinant human granulocyte colony-stimulating factor in advanced urothelial carcinoma: an Eastern Cooperative Oncology Group trial. J Clin Oncol 1994;12:483.

30. Seidman AD, et al. Dose intensification of MVAC with recombinant granulocyte macrophage colony stimulating as initial therapy in advanced urothelial cancers. J Clin Oncol 1993;11:408.

31. Moore MJ, et al. Princess Margaret Hospital and Toronto Bayview Cancer center, Toronto, Canada: a phase II study of methotrexate, vinblastine, doxorubicin and cisplatin (MVAC) + GM-CSF in patients (pts) with advanced transitional cell carcinoma. Proc Am Soc Clin Oncol 1992;11:199.

32. Sternberg CN, et al. Escalated MVAC chemotherapy and recombinant human granulocyte-macrophage colony stimulating factor (GM-CSF) in patients with advanced urothelial tract tumors. Ann Oncol 1993;4:403.

33. Logothetis CJ, et al. Fluorouracil and recombinant human interferon alfa-2a in the treatment of metastatic chemorefractory urothelial tumors. J Natl Cancer Inst 1991;83:285.

34. Recondo G, Kilbourn RG, Logothetis CJ. Evidence for synergistic antitumoral effect of 5-fluorouracil (5-FU) with α-interferon (IFN) and 5-FU with 13-cis retinoic acid (RA) or 4-hydroxyphenyl-retinamide (4-HPR) in human transitional cell carcinoma cell lines. Proc Am Soc Clin Oncol 1991;10:341.

35. Huan S, et al. Biochemical modulation using 5-fluorouracil (5-FU) and high dose folinic acid (FA) in metastatic bladder cancer after MVAC failure. Proc Am Soc Clin Oncol 1994;13:753.

36. Phillip P, et al. 5-fluorouracil, α-interferon, cisplatin (FAP) and methotrexate (MTX) in patients with transitional cell carcinoma (TCC). Proc Am Soc Clin Oncol 1994;13:796.

37. Schultz P, et al. Combination gallium nitrate and 5-fluorouracil for platinum resistant metastatic transitional cell carcinoma of the bladder. Proc Am Assoc Cancer Res 1991;34:1209. Abstract.

38. Roth BJ, et al. Paclitaxel in previously untreated, advanced transitional cell carcinoma of the urothelium: a phase II trial of the Eastern Cooperative Oncology Group. Proc Am Soc Clin Oncol 1994;13:230.

39. Sadan S, et al. Docetaxel in patients with advanced transitional cell cancer (TCC) who failed cisplatin based chemotherapy. Proc Am Soc Clin Oncol 1994;13:761.

40. Bellmunt J, et al. Carboplatin, methotrexate and vinblastine in patients with bladder cancer who were ineligible for cisplatin based chemotherapy. Cancer 1992;70:1974.

41. Small EJ, et al. Treatment of advanced transitional cell carcinoma (ATCC) in elderly patients: the use of carboplatin (CBDCA) instead of cisplatin (CDDP). Proc Am Soc Clin Oncol 1994;13:243.

42. Waxman J, et al. New combination chemotherapy program for bladder cancer. Br J Urol 1989;63:68.

43. Frassoldati A, et al. Are old age or concurrent illness still contraindications to chemotherapy for bladder cancer? a pilot study with MVMJ (Methotrexate, vinblastine, mitoxantrone and carboplatin) regimen. Proc Am Soc Clin Oncol 1994;13:889.

44. Geller NL, et al. Prognostic factors for survival of patients with advanced urothelial tumors treated with methotrexate, vinblastine, doxorubicin and cisplatin chemotherapy. Cancer 1991;67:1525.

45. Scher HI, et al. Effect of cumulative dose intensity on survival of patients with urothelial cancer treated with methotrexate, vinblastine, Adriamycin and cisplatin (MVAC). Proc Am Soc Oncol 1991;10:165.

46. Tannock I, et al. M-VAC chemotherapy for transitional cell carcinoma: the Princess Margaret Hospital experience. J Urol 1989;142:289.

47. Goldfarb A, et al. Methotrexate, vindesine, epidoxorubicin and cisplatin (M-VEC) for stage III-IV bladder cancer: final results. Proc Am Soc Clin Oncol 1992;11:210.

48. Raghavan D, et al. Biology and management of the bladder cancer. N Engl J Med 1990;322:1129.

49. Scher HI, Kantoff PW. Chemotherapy for muscle-infiltrating bladder cancer. Hematol Oncol Clin North Am 1992;6:169.

50. Scher HI. Systemic chemotherapy in regionally advanced bladder cancer: theoretical considerations and results. Urol Clin North Am 1992;19:747.

51. Zietman AL, Shipley WU, Kaufman DS. The combination of cisplatin based chemotherapy and radiation in the treatment of muscle invading transitional cell cancer of the bladder. Int Radiat Oncol Biol Phys 1993;27:161.

52. Gospodarowicz MK, Warde PR. A critical review of the role of definitive radiation therapy in bladder cancer. Semin Urol 1993;11:214.

53. Porter AT. Radiotherapy combined with chemotherapy in treatment of muscle-invasive bladder carcinoma. Semin Oncol 1990;17:583.

54. Skinner DG, et al. Contemporary cystectomy with pelvic node dissection compared to preoperative radiation plus cystectomy in management of invasive bladder cancer. J Urol 1984;131:1069.

55. Montie JE, et al. Radical cystectomy without radiation therapy for carcinoma of the bladder. J Urol 1984;131:477.

56. Bloom HJ, et al. Treatment of T3 bladder cancer: controlled trial of pre-operative radiotherapy and radical cystectomy versus radical radiotherapy. Br J Urol 1982;54:136.

57. Sell A, et al. Treatment of advanced bladder cancer category T2, T3 and T4a. Scand J Urol Nephrol 1993;138:193.

58. Crawford ED, Das S, Smith JA. Preoperative radiation therapy in the treatment of bladder cancer. Urol Clin North Am 1987;14:781.

59. Shipley WU, et al. Treatment of invasive bladder cancer by cisplatin and radiation in patients unsuited for surgery. JAMA 1987;258:931.

60. Tester W, et al. Combined modality program with possible organ preservation for invasive bladder carcinoma: results of RTOG protocol 85-12. Int J Radiat Oncol Biol Phys 1992;25:783.

61. Saur R, et al. Radiotherapy with and without cisplatin in bladder cancer. Int J Radiat Oncol Biol Phys 1990;19:687.

62. Jaske G, Frommhold H, Nedden DZ. Combined radiation and chemotherapy for locally advanced transitional cell carcinoma of the urinary bladder. Cancer 1985;55:1659.

63. Rotman M, et al. Treatment of advanced transitional cell carcinoma of the bladder with irradiation and concomitant 5-fluorouracil infusion. Int J Radiat Oncol Biol Phys 1990;18:1131.

64. Russell KJ, et al. Combined 5 fluorouracil and irradiation for transitional cell carcinoma of the urinary bladder. Int J Radiat Oncol Biol Phys 1990;19:693.

65. Kragelj B, et al. Concurrent vinblastine and radiation therapy in bladder cancer. Cancer 1992;70:2885.

66. Housset M, et al. Combined radiation and chemotherapy for invasive transitional cell carcinoma of the bladder: a prospective study. J Clin Oncol 1993;11:2150.

67. Di Palma M, et al. Concomitant cyclic radiochemotherapy for node positive bladder carcinoma. A phase I–II study. Proc Am Soc Clin Oncol 1994;13:250.

68. Shipley WU, et al. Radiochemotherapy for invasive carcinoma of the bladder. Rec Cancer Res 1993;126:207.

69. Coppin C, et al. Improved local control of invasive bladder cancer, concurrent cisplatin, and preoperative or radical radiation. Proc Am Soc Clin Oncol 1992;11:198.

70. Wallace DMA, et al. Neo-adjuvant (pre-emptive) cisplatin therapy in invasive transitional cell carcinoma of the bladder. Br J Urol 1991;67:608.

71. Shearer RJ, et al. Adjuvant chemotherapy in T3 carcinoma of the bladder: a prospective trial; preliminary report. Br J Urol 1988;62:558.

72. Richards B, et al. Adjuvant chemotherapy with doxorubicin (Adriamycin) and 5-fluorouracil in T3, Nx, MO bladder cancer treated with radiotherapy. Br J Urol 1983;55:386.

73. Kaufman DS, et al. Selective bladder preservation by combination treatment of invasive bladder cancer. N Engl J Med 1993;329:1377.

74. Shipley WU, et al. The integration of chemotherapy, radiotherapy and transurethral surgery in bladder sparing approaches for patients with invasive tumors. Prog Clin Biol Res 1990;353:85.

75. Rifkin MN, et al. Systemic chemotherapy followed by radiation therapy and adjuvant cisplatin: a 3 year follow up. Proc Am Soc Clin Oncol 1992;11:606.

76. Dunst J, et al. Organ sparing treatment of advanced bladder cancer: a 10 year experience. Int J Radiat Oncol Biol Phys 1994;30:261.

77. Vikram B, et al. A pilot study of chemotherapy alternating with twice a day accelerated radiation therapy as an alternative to cystectomy in muscle infiltrating (Stages T2 and T3) cancer of the bladder: preliminary results. J Urol 1994;151:602.

78. Scher HI. Chemotherapy for invasive bladder cancer: neoadjuvant versus adjuvant. Semin Oncol 1990;17:555.

79. Tannock I. The current status of adjuvant chemotherapy for bladder cancer. Semin Urol 1990;8:291.

80. Sternberg CN. Adjuvant chemotherapy following radical cystectomy. World J Urol 1993;11:169.

81. Logothetis CJ, et al. Adjuvant cyclophosphamide, doxorubicin

and cisplatin chemotherapy for bladder cancer: an update. J Clin Oncol 1988;6:1590.

82. Fradet Y, et al. Adjuvant MVAC chemotherapy after radical cystectomy for invasive bladder cancer. J Urol 1992;147:446. Abstract.

83. Stockle M, et al. Adjuvant polychemotherapy of nonorgan-confined bladder cancer after radical cystectomy: long term results of a controlled prospective study and further clinical experience. J Urol 1995;153:47.

84. Struder UE, et al. Adjuvant cisplatin chemotherapy following cystectomy for bladder cancer: results of a prospective randomized trial. J Urol 1994;152:81.

85. Skinner DG, et al. The role of adjuvant chemotherapy following cystectomy for invasive bladder cancer: a prospective comparative trial. J Urol 1991;145:459.

86. Mazzucchelli L, et al. Invasion depth is the most important prognostic factor for transitional-cell carcinoma in a prospective trial of radical cystectomy and adjuvant chemotherapy. Int J Cancer 1994;57:15.

87. Herr H. Conservative management of muscle infiltrating bladder cancer: a prospective experience. J Urol 1987;138: 1162.

88. Rubben H, et al. Adjuvant systemic chemotherapy after complete transurethral resection of superficially invasive bladder carcinoma. Urol Int 1990;45:78.

89. Hall RR, et al. Treatment of invasive bladder cancer by local resection and high dose methotrexate. Br J Urol 1984;56: 668.

90. Logothetis CJ, et al. A prospective randomized trial comparing neoadjuvant to adjuvant MVAC in patients with high stage (vascular invasion, T3b, T4a) bladder carcinoma. Proc Am Soc Clin Oncol 1991;10:166.

91. Scher HI. Chemotherapy for invasive bladder cancer: neoadjuvant versus adjuvant. Semin Oncol 1990;17:555.

92. Scher HI, et al. Neoadjuvant chemotherapy for bladder cancer: experience with M-VAC regimen. Br J Urol 1989;64: 250.

93. Raghvan D, et al. Preemptive; neoadjuvant chemotherapy: can analysis of eligibility criteria, prognostic factors and tumor staging from different trials provide valid or useful comparisons? Semin Oncol 1990;17:613.

94. Geller NL, et al. Can we combine available data to evaluate the effects of neoadjuvant chemotherapy for invasive bladder cancer? Semin Oncol 1990;17:628.

95. Chechile G, et al. Neo-adjuvant intra-arterial chemotherapy in locally advanced bladder cancer. Prog Clin Biol Res 1990; 353:153.

96. Sumiyoshi Y, et al. Neoadjuvant intra-arterial doxorubicin chemotherapy in combination with low dose radiotherapy for the treatment of locally advanced transitional cell carcinoma of the bladder. J Urol 1994;152:362.

97. Scher HI, et al. Neoadjuvant MVAC: effect on the primary bladder lesion. J Urol 1988;139:470.

98. Splinter TAW, et al. The prognostic value of the pathological response to combination chemotherapy before cystectomy in patients with invasive bladder cancer. J Urol 1992;147:606.

99. Schultz PK, et al. Neoadjuvant chemotherapy for invasive bladder cancer: prognostic factors for survival of patients treated with MVAC with a 5 year follow-up. J Clin Oncol 1994;12:1394.

100. Connor JP, et al. Long term follow-up in patients treated with methotrexate, vinblastine, doxorubicin and cisplatin (MVAC) for transitional cell carcinoma of urinary bladder: cause for concern. Urology 1989;34:353.

101. Rintala E, et al. Neoadjuvant chemotherapy in bladder cancer: a randomized study. Nordic Cystectomy Trial I. Scand J Urol Nephrol 1993;27:355.

102. Martinez-Pineiro JA, et al. Neo-adjuvant cisplatin in locally advanced urothelial bladder cancer: a prospective randomized study of the group CUETO. Prog Clin Biol Res 1990;353: 95.

103. Passalacqua R, et al. Neoadjuvant chemotherapy for locally invasive bladder cancer: a prospective randomized trial comparing the M-VAC and M-VEEC combinations. Eur J Cancer 1991;27(Suppl):104.

104. Pellegrini A, et al. Neoadjuvant treatment for locally advanced urothelial bladder cancer: a randomized prospective clinical trial. Proc ECCO Eur J Cancer 1991;27(Suppl):107.

105. Crawford ED, Natale RB, Burton H. Southwest Oncology Group Study 8710: trial of cystectomy alone versus neo-adjuvant M-VAC and cystectomy in patients with locally advanced bladder cancer (intergroup trial 0080). Prog Clin Biol Res 1990;353:111.

106. Hall RR, Parmar MKB. Randomized intercontinental trial of loco-regional therapy with or without neoadjuvant chemotherapy. Prog Clin Biol Res 1990;353:105.

107. Davis MP, et al. Successful management of small cell carcinoma of the bladder with cisplatin and etoposide. J Urol 1989;142:817.

108. Patterson JM, et al. A new treatment for invasive squamous cell bladder cancer; the Nigro regimen; preoperative chemotherapy and radiation therapy. J Urol 1988;140:379.

109. Oblon DJ, et al. Bladder preservation and durable complete remission of small cell carcinoma of the bladder with systemic chemotherapy and adjuvant radiation therapy. Cancer 1993;71:2581.

51

Hormonal Therapy for Advanced Carcinoma of the Prostate

Edward P. DeAntoni
E. David Crawford

INTRODUCTION

More than 50 years ago, Charles Huggins confirmed the androgen dependence of carcinoma of the prostate (1). In the half century since Huggins' landmark study, hormonal therapy has solidified its status as the mainstay for the management of advanced carcinoma of the prostate. Many of the same clinical issues raised 50 years ago continue to be debated today, but clinical and basic science have uncovered much of the basic biologic behavior of this neoplasm. Spectacular palliative advances have been achieved; however, curative therapy for systemic disease remains forever elusive.

SURGICAL ABLATION OF TESTOSTERONE, THE MAJOR ANDROGEN SOURCE

Initial enthusiasm for Huggins' breakthrough led clinicians to embrace bilateral orchiectomy as the surest solution to androgen ablation and disease control (2). The growth of prostatic tissue is dependent on androgenic stimulation, and testosterone (90 to 95% of which is produced in the Leydig cells of the testes) is the primary circulating androgen (3). The usual serum concentration of testosterone is approximately 600 ng/dL. Orchiectomy achieves prompt castrate levels of testosterone (43 ± 32 ng/dL) within 2 to 3 hours (4–6). The reduction of serum testosterone level yields effective tumor regression and appreciable symptomatic improvement (7). Response has been consistently noted in 60 to 80% of patients. Patient compliance is assured with the procedure, morbidity and mortality are low, and compared with contemporary therapeutic alternatives orchiectomy may be considered highly cost-effective. Side effects are not inconsiderable—loss of libido, impotence, and hot flashes. When offered an alternative, patients today may not choose orchiectomy (8). Contraindications for the procedure are chronic infection, immunosuppression, and bleeding dyscrasia. Orchiectomy has conventionally been labeled the gold standard against which all subsequent hormonal therapies have been compared (5, 6).

MEDICAL CASTRATION

Concurrent with Huggins' discovery, results appeared on the use of estrogenic substances to control prostate cancer (9). Estrogens block the release of luteinizing hormone (LH) from the anterior pituitary. LH has the primary role in controlling the synthesis of androgens by the Leydig cells. With estrogen therapy, castrate levels of androgen synthesis are reached within 10 to 14 days and remain so throughout the course of treatment.

Estrogens stimulate the production of increased levels of sex steroid binding globulin, thereby increasing the proportion of bound and metabolically inactive testosterone. Secondary immunoregulatory effects, including stimulation of phagocytic activity with a rise in gammaglobulin levels, may contribute to the therapeutic profile of estrogens. Estrogens also promote prolactin release from the pituitary. Prolactin is known to enhance androgen utilization and transport into the prostatic cells. Prolactin effect of estrogen may prove deleterious to the patient in enhancing the utilization of the available androgen by the androgen-dependent carcinoma prostate cells.

Side effects of estrogen therapy can be categorized under feminizing effects, cardiovascular complications, gastrointestinal disturbances, and edema. The feminizing effects include atrophy of genitalia, loss of libido, impotence, azoospermia and gynecomastia associated with hypersensitivity, breast tenderness, and hyperpigmentation of the nipples.

The earliest and one of the most commonly used estrogens in the hormonal therapy for carcinoma of the prostate has been diethylstilbestrol (DES). In the 1960s, the Veterans Administration Cooperative Urologic Research Group (VACURG) conducted randomized trials with DES as primary treatment of advanced carcinoma of the prostate. A dose of 5 mg/day resulted in significant cardiovascular complications. The VACURG study concluded that a 3 mg/day dose was effective in reducing mortality from carcinoma of the prostate (10). However, DES therapy has fallen out of favor with most urologists because of the serious cardiovascular complications that often accompany this regimen (11, 12).

Alternative natural synthetic estrogens, although less clinically effective than DES, can also reduce serum testosterone levels and have unique, individual therapeutic indications.

Premarin and ethinyl estradiol are as effective as DES in suppressing serum testosterone, but neither offers any significant advantage over DES. Chlorotrianisene (TACE), a synthetic estrogen, has produced clinical responses in patients without completely suppressing LH or testosterone levels. A dose of 12 mg twice a day, orally, yields a 40 to 60% suppression of serum testosterone. The drug is structurally different from DES and has fewer side effects; however, it is not therapeutically superior (13).

Estramustine phosphate (Emcyt) is a cytotoxic combination of the estrogen estradiol phosphate with nitrogen mustard. The drug has the estrogen effects of suppressing testosterone with the cytotoxic effects of an alkylator. Estramustine therapy in previously untreated patients results in response rates similar to those seen with orchiectomy or DES (14). Approximately 50% of patients with disseminated disease that are resistant to estrogen therapy have been reported to respond favorably to this drug (15). This agent, however, does not appear to offer any survival advantage either in previously untreated patients or patients in whom prior hormonal therapy failed; the drug is rarely used as initial therapy.

With the almost simultaneous appearance of these two therapeutic advances—orchiectomy and estrogen therapy—the question of comparability of surgical versus medical treatment of advanced carcinoma of the prostate was immediately joined, as were questions of early versus deferred hormonal treatment, the appropriate design and interpretation of clinical studies, and, most basically, whether any survival benefit was evidenced from hormonal manipulation of advanced carcinoma of the prostate (16, 17). For half a century, these questions have framed (or constricted) the debate and most of the subsequent clinical research in the treatment of advanced prostate cancer (18). No standard treatment of the disease has ever been adapted unanimously (19). In fact, just 5 years after Huggins published his landmark studies, a rather comprehensive list of "problems and results" of hormonal therapy for prostate cancer appeared (16). Many of these "issues" remain unresolved; some have never been adequately addressed (Table 51.1).

With experience, the limitations of androgen ablation became readily apparent. Orchiectomy or oral DES affected long-term local control and significant palliation of metastatic disease, but these methods proved unable to cure disseminated prostate cancer (16). More than 85% of patients with stage D1 disease will have disease progression within 5 years (20). Patients with stage D2 disease have a median survival of only

Table 51.1. Identification of Issues of Hormonal Therapy for Prostate Cancer, 1946 (16)

Symptomatic improvements
  Relief from pain for varying periods
  Relief of symptoms of urinary tract obstruction to a varying degree (bleeding, residual urine, improvement of infection)
  Improvement of general well-being (strength, vigor, appetite, weight, anemia)
Value of hormone control therapy in producing regression of local and metastatic growth of prostatic cancer
Value of serum acid and alkaline phosphatases as diagnostic and prognostic guides
Histologic changes in the cancerous tissue after hormone control therapy
Therapeutic effects relative to grade or differentiation of cancer
Changes in the "hormone excretion pattern" in the urine from both quantitative and qualitative standpoints
Response to orchiectomy in patients of different age groups
Results of treatment when compared with duration of disease before the treatment was instituted
Evaluation of orchiectomy as prophylaxis against local growth, extension of the tumor, and metastases
Consideration of the results in so-called prophylaxis cases or those with early nonmetastatic cancer compared with those having metastases
Value of castration versus estrogenic therapy
Value of the various estrogenic substances alone, before, with, or after castration
Effect of various estrogenic substances on tissues other than the prostatic cancer
Effect of radiation therapy directly to the adrenals and pituitary in combination with other "hormonal control" methods
Life expectancy or survival after hormone control therapy compared with the many other therapeutic procedures that have been used to combat this disease

30 months and a 5-year survival rate of 20%. Progression to hormone-refractory disease usually occurs 12 to 18 months after the initiation of hormonal therapy (21). After progression, half of patients die within 6 months of relapse. Mean survival of patients presenting with metastatic disease is less than 2 years (22).

ENDOCRINOLOGY OF PROSTATIC TISSUE GROWTH AND DIFFERENTIATION

The endocrine axis responsible for androgen production and control has been well-characterized since the halcyon days of Huggins (Fig. 51.1) (23). The production of androgens by the testes and the adrenal glands is controlled by the hypothalamus and the anterior pituitary gland. The hypothalamus releases gonadotrophin-releasing hormone (GnRH, also known as luteinizing hormone-releasing hormone, or LHRH) and corticotrophin-releasing factor to the anterior pituitary via the hypothalamus-pituitary portal venous system in a pulsatile fashion. The anterior pituitary responds with production and secretion

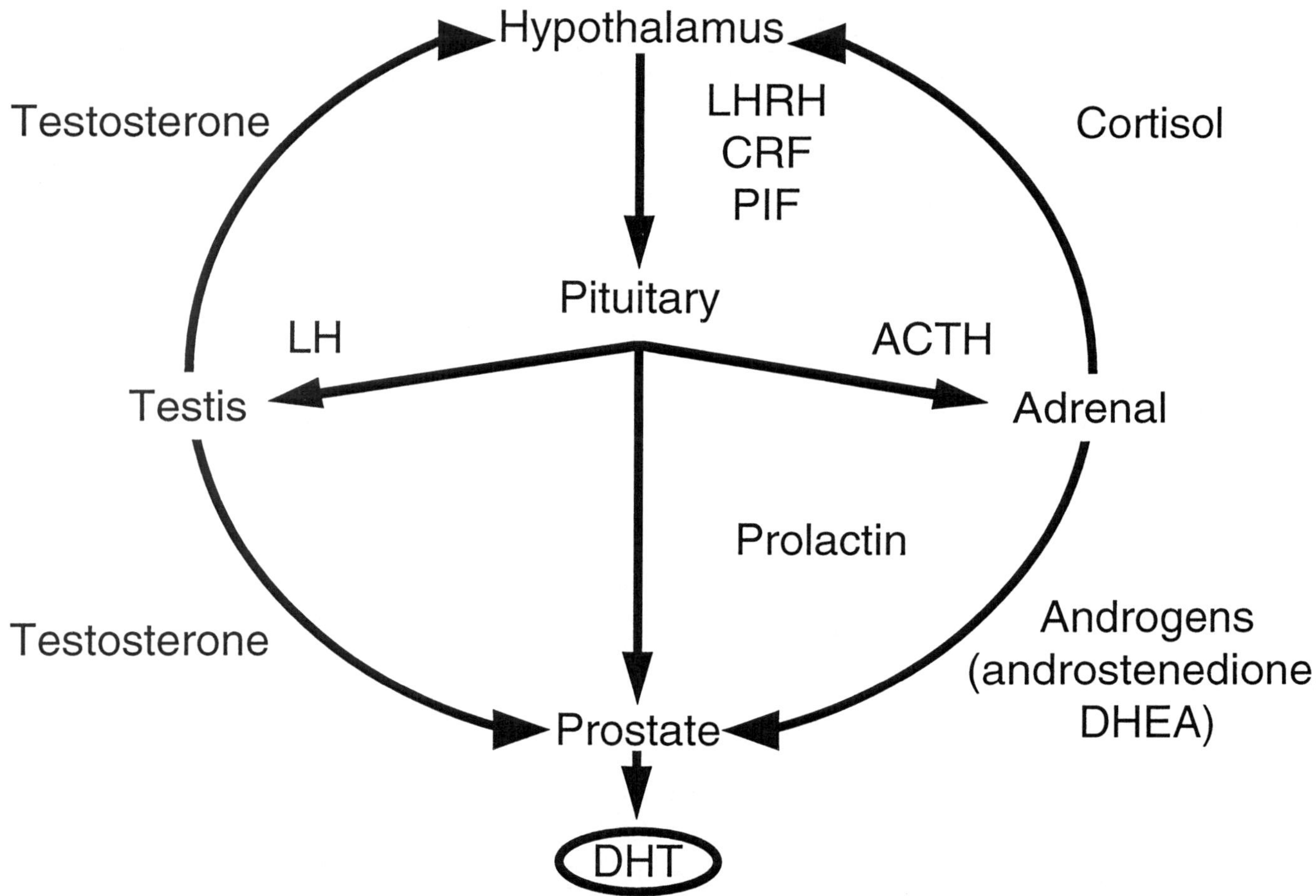

Fig. 51.1. Endocrine axis in hormonal regulation of prostate growth. LHRH: Luteinizing hormone-releasing hormone; CRF: corticotropin-releasing factor; LH: luteinizing hormone; ACTH: adrenocorticotropic hormone; DHEA: dihydroepiandrosterone; DHT: dihydrotestosterone.

of LH and adrenocorticotropic hormone (ACTH) to the testes and adrenal cortices, respectively. LH stimulates the testicular production of testosterone, and ACTH stimulates the adrenocortical production of androstenedione and dihydroepiandrosterone (DHEA), which are subsequently converted to testosterone. The relatively weak adrenal androgens comprise less than or equal to 10% of the normal circulating androgen pool. As with most hormonal axes, these androgen pathways are under negative-feedback inhibition; circulating androgens from the testes and adrenals regulate the releasing mechanisms of the hypothalamus (Fig. 51.1).

Within androgen-sensitive cells of the prostate, testosterone is converted to the more potent dihydrotestosterone (DHT) via the enzyme 5-α-reductase. DHT is internalized into the nucleus and causes transcription of novel mRNA, with the ultimate translation of key proteins necessary in the maintenance of androgen responsiveness. DHT has threefold the potency of testosterone, which in turn is 5 to 10 times more potent than the adrenal androgens (24). DHT is the greatest stimulant to both benign and malignant prostatic growth.

Adrenal androgens are less potent than testosterone and comprise a small percentage of the circulating androgen pool.

Nevertheless, their importance in stimulating (or aggravating) the progression of metastatic prostatic carcinoma is becoming increasingly evident. After surgical or medical castration, approximately 50% of intraprostatic DHT persists (25), and adrenal androgens are responsible for approximately 20% of this residual (26). Advocates of combined testicular-adrenal androgen ablation argue that it is likely that the seemingly innocuous adrenal androgens are responsible for the inexorable development of androgen insensitivity, hormone-refractory disease, and death (27). Adrenal androgens have provided the impetus behind innovative hormonal therapies for advanced carcinoma of the prostate and remain the lightning rod of intense debate.

LHRH ANALOGS

The introduction of LHRH analogs provided an alternative, equally effective monotherapeutic model to orchiectomy and estrogens in the hormonal management of advanced carcinoma of the prostate (22, 28). The significantly better side effect profile of LHRH analog therapy accounts for its widespread use. In a randomized trial of leuprolide acetate or DES, no significant difference in 1-year survival was observed but fewer cardiovascular complications and less gynecomastia occurred in the leuprolide arm (22). Administration of LHRH analogs does result in atrophy of the reproductive organs, loss of libido, and impotence. The chief disadvantages relate to cost and the necessity of monthly parenteral administration. The medications do not cause many of the side effects associated with estrogen, namely gynecomastia, gastrointestinal disturbances, or cardiovascular and thromboembolic complications.

LHRH analog administration initially causes stimulation of LH and follicle stimulating hormone production, with a transient rise in the level of testosterone to 140 to 170% of basal levels within several days (29). The number of GnRH receptors in the pituitary diminishes with resultant pituitary depletion of LH and follicle stimulating hormone (30). The end result is a chemically selective hypophysectomy causing the suppression of testicular synthesis of testosterone. Testosterone begins to fall within 1 to 2 weeks, and castrate levels are reached in approximately 1 month. Continuous drug administration maintains castrate levels. The therapy has been considerably enhanced by the development of depot preparations of 1- and 3-month injections (31). The Food and Drug Administration has approved both Depo Lupron (TAP Pharmaceuticals, Deerfield, IL) and Zoladex (Zeneca Pharmaceuticals, Wilmington, DE) for sustained-release intramuscular or subcutaneous injection.

However, the initial surge of testosterone and a worsening of clinical symptoms, referred to as the "flare phenomenon," that occur in approximately 10% of patients may have serious clinical consequences (32, 33). Temporary increases in the degree of bone pain and obstructive voiding symptoms have been noted within the first 72 hours of therapy. The presumed cause is stimulation of prostatic tumor cells by the transiently raised level of testosterone (22). Two approaches have been studied for preventing this disease flare. The first is to reduce the surge of testosterone by inhibiting the secretion of gonadotropin with DES or cyproterone acetate (CPA) (34, 35). The administration of either of these drugs for 1 week before the start of LHRH agonist therapy and of both drugs concomitantly for 1 week does limit the increase in plasma testosterone levels, but not completely (34). The second approach is to antagonize the effect of testosterone on its receptors, so that the response of the tissue to the testosterone peak is blocked (36). The result is no rise in prostatic tumor markers and no increase in bone pain, urinary obstruction, or neurologic symptoms.

Nonsteroidal antiandrogens will also block this flare. The purpose of this approach is to antagonize the effect of testosterone on its receptors, so that the response of the tissue to the testosterone peak is blocked. In one study, men receiving an LHRH analog were randomized to receive either an antiandrogen or a placebo (37). Despite similar changes in plasma testosterone levels in both groups, the concentration of plasma prostatic acid phosphatase decreased almost immediately in the group receiving the antiandrogen but did not decrease for 2 weeks in the group receiving the placebo. Median prostate-specific antigen (PSA) levels decreased immediately in the anti-

androgen arm, but in men receiving placebo PSA levels did not decrease until day 8. A significantly lower occurrence of bone pain was also observed in the antiandrogen arm (37).

OTHER MONOTHERAPY FORMS OF HORMONAL MANAGEMENT FOR ADVANCED CARCINOMA OF THE PROSTATE

Orchiectomy, estrogen therapy, and LHRH agonists are the most common monotherapeutic forms of hormonal management of advanced carcinoma of the prostate in men with newly diagnosed disease. Other monotherapies have been researched and many are widely used in Europe, but none has been shown in randomized trials to be superior to these three basic monotherapeutic modalities. These other hormonal monotherapies include progestational agents, prolactin antagonists, and antiandrogens.

Progestational Agents

Progestational agents, including Depostat and megestrol acetate (Megace; Bristol Meyer Squibb, Princeton, NJ), act primarily by suppressing pituitary secretion of LH while directly inhibiting steroidogenesis and weakly binding to androgen receptors in the prostate gland. With therapy, there is a transient reduction in plasma testosterone followed, however, by a gradual rise with chronic use. The mechanism of this escape is poorly understood. Progestational agents are usually administered concomitantly with other agents, such as DES, to prevent the escape (38).

Prolactin Antagonists

As prolactin promotes pituitary-mediated androgen activity, prolactin antagonists (including levodopa and bromocriptine) have demonstrated efficacy in relieving symptoms, especially pain, in some patients no longer responsive to standard hormonal therapy (39).

Antiandrogens

Antiandrogens are either steroidal or nonsteroidal compounds. Steroidal antiandrogens include CPA, currently not available in the United States but widely used in Europe, and Megace, which is available but not indicated for treatment of carcinoma of the prostate in the United States. CPA and Megace are synthetic steroids with pronounced progestational and antiandrogenic properties. As steroidal antiandrogens, they block gonadotrophin release from the pituitary. In addition, they inhibit both the formation of DHT-receptor complex in the prostatic cells and the C21-19 desmolase enzyme, which is key to the synthesis of adrenal androgens. Synthesis of testosterone in the Leydig cells of the testes is also inhibited. CPA is well tolerated but requires reinforcement with low-dose DES to maintain serum testosterone levels in the castrate range (40, 41). Reports of European studies attest to the effectiveness of steroidal anti-androgens, although they are no more effective than the standard estrogen therapy (42).

Nonsteroidal antiandrogens are drugs that are neither hormone nor hormonal analogs. Because their action does not result in a reduction of serum testosterone levels, a major advantage of nonsteroidal antiandrogens as monotherapy is the preservation of potency. These compounds block the cellular action of androgens at the target organ by inhibiting the nuclear uptake of DHT (43). The negative feedback of testosterone on the hypothalamus no longer registers, resulting in higher levels of LHRH and LH. The testes are thus stimulated to produce higher levels of testosterone. The high serum level of testosterone will overcome the blockade. Higher levels of estrogen also result from the LHRH and LH stimulus. In contrast to the steroidal compounds, these drugs are not associated with cardiovascular toxicity, fluid retention, or adverse effect on carbohydrate and lipid metabolism (44). Three nonsteroidal antiandrogens currently in use are flutamide, nilutamide, and bicalutamide.

Flutamide, a nonsteroidal anilide, has not been extensively studied as monotherapy and is approved only in combination with an LHRH analog. One study of previously untreated stage D patients who were given flutamide monotherapy reported that most (85%) had a favorable response lasting 2 to 56 months (mean, 12.5 months) (45). Randomized trials of flutamide alone or estrogens showed flutamide to be as effective as estrogens but without loss of libido and potency (46, 47). A recent U.S. randomized trial of DES (1 mg) or flutamide (250 mg), three times a day, reported similar overall response rates (62% and 50%, respectively; median survival was greater in the DES arm—43.2 months versus 23.2 months; P = 0.007) (48).

Nilutamide has similar efficacy as flutamide and, as with flutamide, is usually given in combination with an LHRH analog (49). Nilutamide does cause impaired adaptation to darkness in up to 90% of patients (less than 5 minutes in duration) and, rarely, interstitial pneumonitis (1 to 3%) (50).

Bicalutamide is a new drug that, because of a long half-life, allows once-daily dosing (51). In animal studies, bicalutamide was shown to have a fourfold greater affinity for the prostate androgen receptor than 2-hydroxyflutamide, the active metabolite of flutamide (52). In a recent randomized controlled trial of bicalutamide versus flutamide, each in combination with an LHRH analog, in patients with advanced prostatic carcinoma, bicalutamide was reported to have superior efficacy over flutamide (53). Time to treatment failure was significantly better for the bicalutamide plus LHRH group than for the flutamide plus LHRH group. The hazard ratio for treatment failure of bicalutamide plus LHRH to flutamide plus LHRH was 0.749, indicating that patients in the flutamide plus LHRH group were 34% more likely to experience treatment failure. Results for secondary endpoints (survival, quality of life, subjective response) were similar in both treatment arms; gastrointestinal distress (diarrhea) was significantly greater in the flutamide

plus LHRH arm (24%) than in the bicalutamide arm (10%). Currently, this drug appears similar to flutamide in overall efficacy.

Gynecomastia (20 to 50%) is a common effect of these nonsteroidal antiandrogens, as is diarrhea (10 to 15%), flushing (15 to 30%), and, rarely, liver function abnormalities. In today's cost-conscious health-care system, expenses related to this therapy are also major concerns.

COMBINED ANDROGEN BLOCKADE

In Huggins' day, orchiectomy or estrogen therapy brought significant palliation to patients with advanced carcinoma of the prostate, but the effects were transitory. Disease progression and death were measured in months after therapeutic intervention. Recognizing that after orchiectomy any residual androgen would be of adrenal origin, Huggins initially attempted total androgen blockade in 1945. Performing bilateral adrenalectomy in four patients in whom initial endocrine manipulation had failed, Huggins reported disappointing results. Without adequate adrenal hormone replacement therapy, the patients survived only 1.5, 1.5, 11, and 116 days, respectively, after surgery (54). With the availability of cortisol replacement, adrenalectomy became feasible. Cortisone (50 mg orally 4 times daily and then titrated to effect) showed early promise (55).

Aminoglutethimide was one of the first therapies to suppress adrenal steroid production by potently inhibiting several P-450 mediated hydroxylation steps. A 40% response rate and subjective improvement were reported by early studies in hormone refractory patients (56, 57). The use of aminoglutethimide required the coadministration of physiologic doses of hydrocortisone to avert adrenal escape of suppression by pituitary override. A number of patients treated with this regimen for hormone-refractory prostate cancer had to discontinue therapy due to its side effects of lethargy, nausea, vomiting, and ataxia. A medical adrenalectomy had been achieved with minimal side effects. From these initial attempts at total androgen ablation, the question remained whether blocking the production of adrenal androgens would add significantly to any of the monotherapies for advanced prostate cancer.

Two separate studies added to the controversy. Labrie et al. demonstrated that as high as 50% of intraprostatic DHT remains after surgical or medical castration (58). Harper et al. showed that the adrenal androgens were responsible for roughly 20% of the total intraprostatic DHT (59). These data, when combined with the hypothesis of tumor cell heterogeneity and the variability of hormonal sensitivity of prostate cancer cells, form the basis for the rationale of combined androgen blockade (CAB) in treating metastatic prostate cancer.

The search for a safe and effective means of ablating or blocking the adrenal androgens ended with the introduction of the nonsteroidal antiandrogens nilutamide and flutamide. With experience came the realization that these drugs represented the ideal agent for utilization in total androgen blockade regimens.

In the early 1980s, Labrie et al. reported their results with combination therapy for stage C and D prostate cancer, demonstrating a remarkably enhanced survival time in patients treated with combination therapy (60). The trials lacked appropriate control arms as comparisons were made to historical controls. Nevertheless, the trials generated considerable interest and several groups set out to test their hypothesis.

INT 0036 and Demonstrated Effect of CAB

The first study to document clearly the benefits of CAB was the National Cancer Institute Intergroup Study (INT 0036). The premise of this randomized controlled trial was based on the observation that monotherapy (surgical or medical testicular androgen ablation) for metastatic prostatic carcinoma invariably progresses to a hormone-refractory state. When this condition is reached, death follows quickly. The study hypothesis was that the addition of an antiandrogen (flutamide) to an LHRH analog (leuprolide) for the suppression of adrenal and testicular androgens would enhance "total" androgen ablation and maximize the benefits of hormonal therapy.

The study of leuprolide plus flutamide or placebo demonstrated statistically significant improvements in both time to progression and survival in favor of CAB (Figs. 51.2 and 51.3) (61). A 26% increase in median survival of patients receiving combination therapy was observed when compared with monotherapy with leuprolide. This represents an average survival advantage of 7 months. For patients with good prognosis (minimal disease and good performance status) the survival advantage is even greater, approaching 2 years (Figs. 51.4 and 51.5).

The study was prescient in stratifying patients by Eastern Cooperative Oncology Group performance status (0 to 2 versus 3) and by extent of disease (minimal versus severe) (Table 51.2). The trial demonstrated superior outcomes for patients with better prognostic profiles. It emphasized the importance of carefully stratifying patients by means of a range of prognostic factors before the initiation of trial accrual (62). Such patient evaluation has become codified to determine an accurate prognosis for treatment response (63).

A recent review and statistical update of INT 0036 reported that anemia, anorexia, weight loss, bone pain, use of analgesics, number of metastatic lesions on bone scan, and elevated alkaline phosphatase are all of significant prognostic value and are

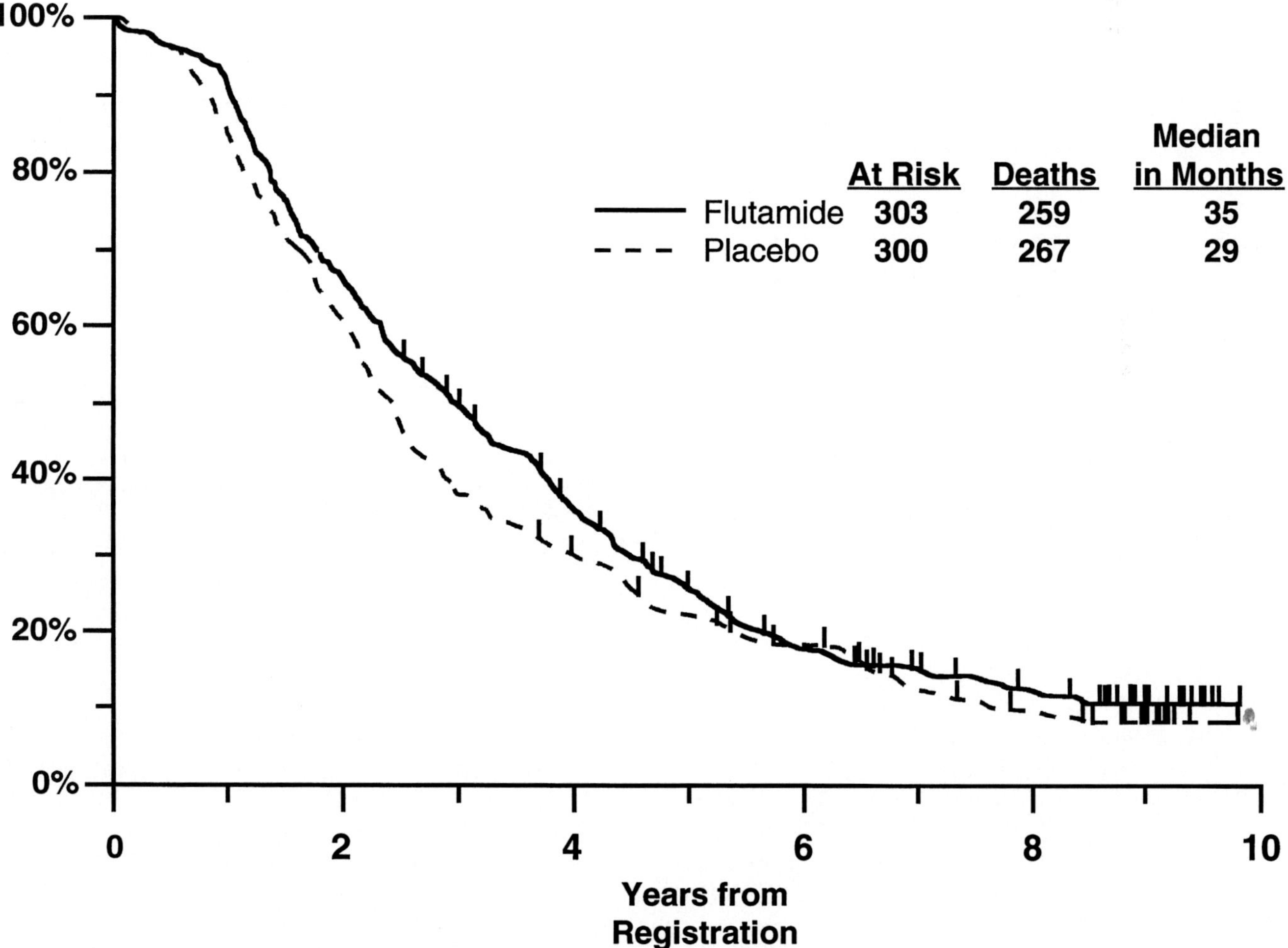

Fig. 51.2.   National Cancer Institute Intergroup Protocol 0036. Leuprolide and flutamide or placebo. Overall survival on April 20, 1995.

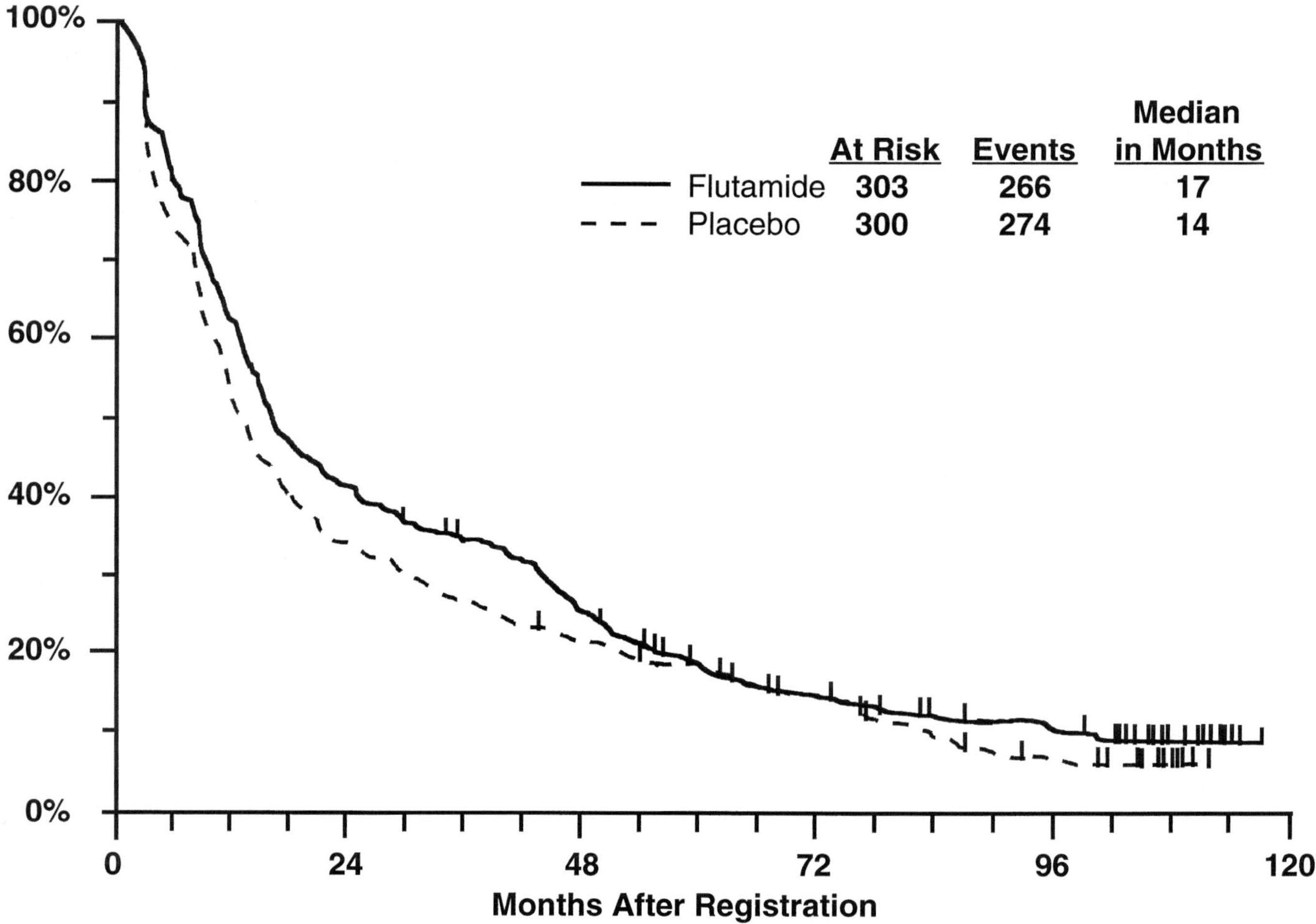

Fig. 51.3. National Cancer Institute Intergroup Protocol 0036. Leuprolide with flutamide or placebo. Progression-free survival on April 20, 1995.

Table 51.2. Definition of Extent of Disease (All Stage D2)

Minimal disease
   pelvis/axial skeleton only
     and/or
   soft tissue nodal (locoregional and/or distant) only
Severe disease
   pelvis/axial skeleton and/or ribs, skull, long bones
     and/or
   soft tissue visceral (with or without nodal involvement)

strongly associated with extent of disease (64). Nearly all patients experienced benefit from CAB, but patients with minimal disease receiving CAB experienced disease progression significantly later than patients receiving monotherapy (Fig. 51.6). Quality of life would seem to be enhanced by this longer disease-free period, which is longer in fact than the mean survival time of patients receiving monotherapy. Patients receiving CAB also have a shorter terminal period of disease progression.

Because PSA is being used more extensively as a diagnostic tool, prostatic carcinoma is being diagnosed earlier in the course of disease across all stages. Consequently, a majority of patients with advanced disease do not present with widespread painful osseous metastases, as most patients did a decade ago. Most prostatic carcinomas are now diagnosed with very minimal metastatic deposits in the patient's skeleton. The INT 0036 study results should be considered the gold standard for hormonal manipulation.

Controversy surrounding the value of CAB is exacerbated by issues of cost-effectiveness. Hillner et al. applied a decision analysis model to hypothetical cohorts of 70-year-old men presenting with metastatic prostate cancer; anticipated survival and incremental cost per life-year gain were calculated (65). Time to progression and survival rate were taken from the INT 0036 trial. Flutamide was estimated to reduce the relative risk of progressive disease by 25%, and costs and survival benefits were discounted at a 5% annual rate. For the minimal disease group, median survival increased from 42.3 to 49.4 months with flutamide and average survival by 5.2 months at an incremental cost of $25,300. If the efficacy were 50%, the benefit would be 12 months at a cost of $13,700 per life-year gained. This study concluded that flutamide has an incremental cost-effectiveness more favorable than most accepted therapies.

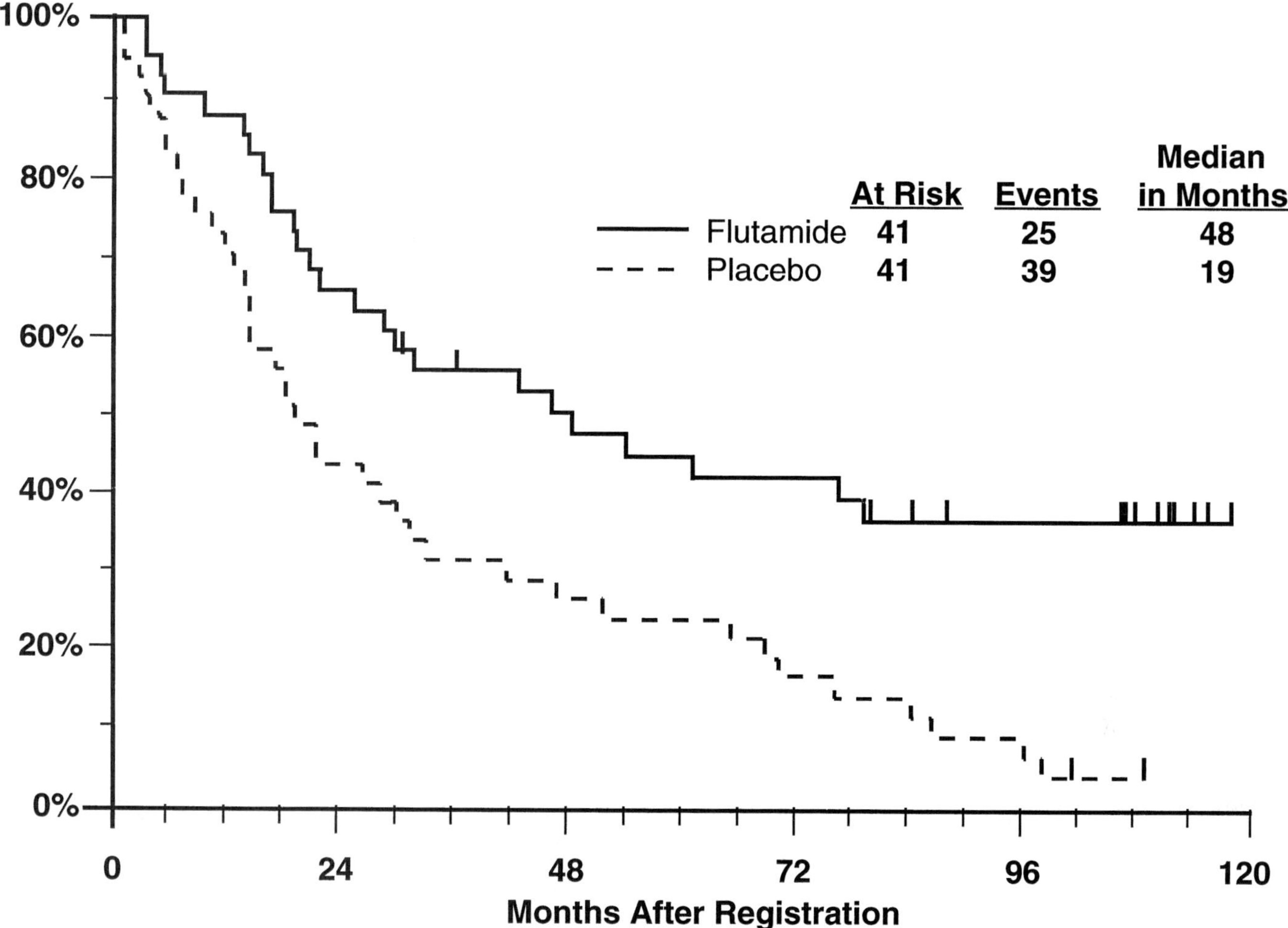

Fig. 51.4. National Cancer Institute Intergroup Protocol 0036. Leuprolide with flutamide or placebo. Overall survival on April 20, 1995. Good prognosis subset.

These authors recommend that if drug costs are covered by health insurance, flutamide should be initiated and covered for all good performance status patients.

CLINICAL TRIALS OF CAB AND THE INTERPRETATION OF DATA

A similar study undertaken by the European Organization for Research and Treatment of Cancer (EORTC) compared depot goserelin acetate plus flutamide with bilateral orchiectomy. Initially, the study showed no statistically significant differences in survival. However, a recent analysis of the more mature data has documented the benefits of maximal androgen ablation in metastatic prostate cancer (66). The premature results of this study have been used on many occasions to discredit CAB. They were presented at the annual American Urological Association meeting as a negative study and even published as a negative study (67). Initially negative results became positive because the early reporting of results, before enough events (i.e., disease progression and deaths) occurred, showed no difference. It is

unusual to see differences early in such a clinical trial, because differences in survival will not appear for 2 to 3 years. Early reporting of clinical trial results is not appropriate, unless some very important statistical difference emerges early in a study, and should be discouraged.

A recent meta-analysis shows only a slight benefit to CAB (68). Unfortunately, the majority of trials included in the analysis lack adequate power to confirm or disprove results of the U.S. Intergroup (SWOG) trial, use different antiandrogens, and employ different methods of castration. An excellent statistical critique of clinical trials in advanced prostate cancer documents these shortcomings (69).

Several trials have used bilateral orchiectomy with an antiandrogen as the modality for CAB. Jankenegt et al. (70) reported on 457 patients with metastatic prostate cancer who were randomized to receive bilateral orchiectomy and placebo or to receive the antiandrogen nilutamide. A 7.3 month survival advantage was noted. This study answers yet another criticism of CAB, namely whether it is effective with bilateral orchiectomy.

Currently, all clinical trials with sufficient patients to dem-

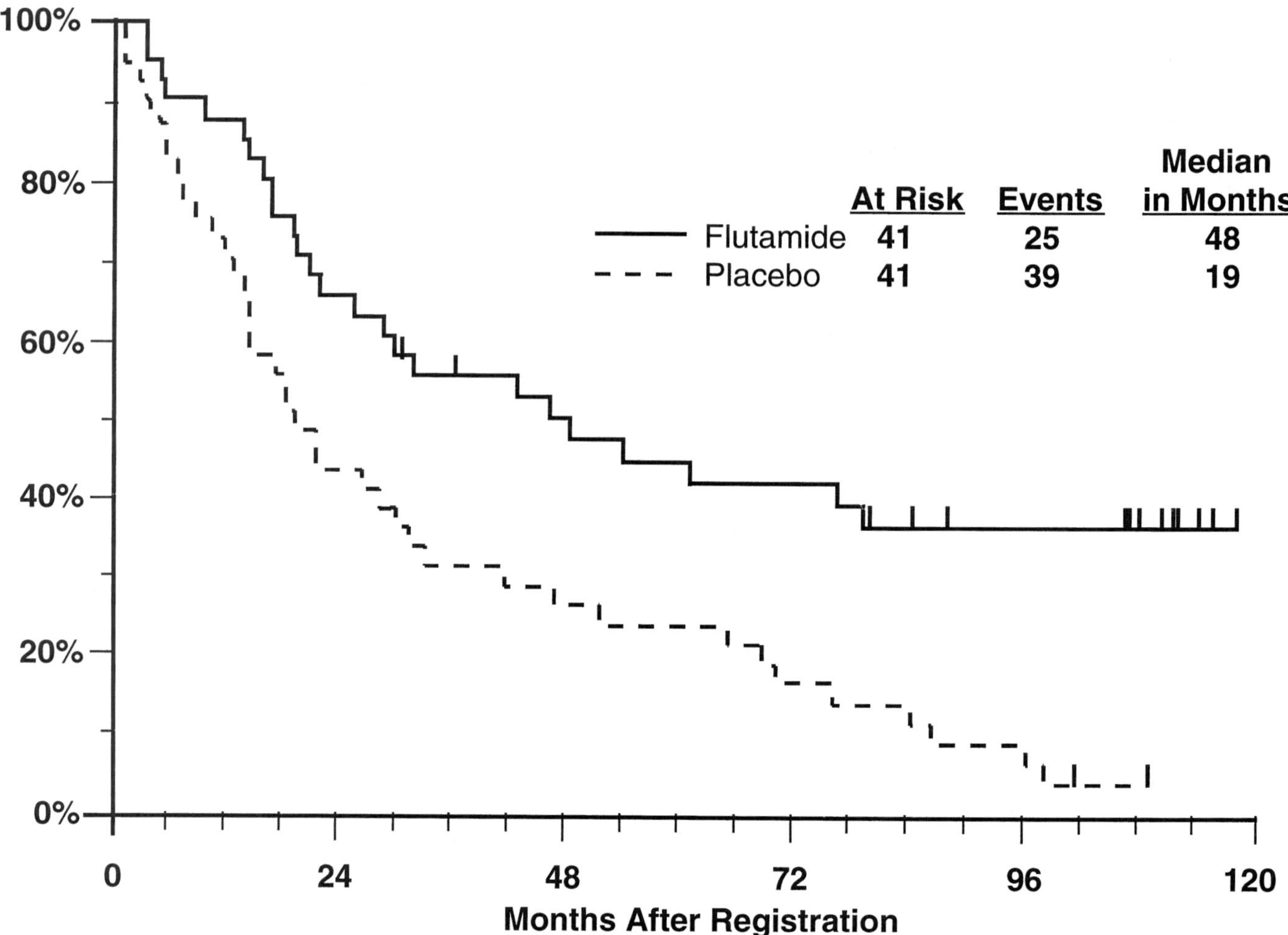

Fig. 51.5.   National Cancer Institute Intergroup Protocol 0036. Leuprolide with flutamide or placebo. Progression-free survival on April 20, 1995. Good prognosis subset.

onstrate a difference have supported a survival advantage for CAB. Nearly all patients will experience benefit. Although controversy continues whether CAB should be initiated in asymptomatic patients, this therapy may be considered the new gold standard of hormonal management of advanced prostatic carcinoma. All trials subsequent to INT 0036 have considered it the reference point for assessing patient response, overall survival, and disease-free survival.

Flutamide Withdrawal and Intermittent Androgen Blockade

Several observations have been reported that withdrawal of flutamide results in a significant PSA decline and symptomatic relief (72–75). In two studies (73, 74), flutamide was stopped when patients who had initially responded to CAB (LHRH agonist or bilateral orchiectomy and flutamide) began to show disease progression. Serum PSA decreased by greater than or equal to 80% in most patients. Sartor et al. have hypothesized that prolonged exposure to flutamide results in the selective proliferation of cancer cells containing a mutant androgen receptor that aberrantly recognizes flutamide metabolites and nonandrogenic steroids as androgenic stimuli (75).

Research is currently being conducted on this phenomenon in the form of a follow-up study to a randomized controlled trial of orchiectomy with or without flutamide trial. Eligible patients are those randomized to flutamide as their initial hormonal therapy but who show evidence of disease progression while participating in the trial. Evidence of progression includes a rising PSA greater than 20 ng/mL. Flutamide therapy will be stopped for these patients to test their response.

Intriguing exploration is also underway into phenomena that can delay progression to androgen independence. This research is based on observations that progression is associated with the activation of previously androgen-repressed genes, some of which may code for autocrine or paracrine growth factors that substitute for androgens in maintaining the viability of the tumorigenic stem cells (76). Therefore, replacing androgens before the initiation of progression should cause the surviving stem cells to give rise to an androgen-dependent

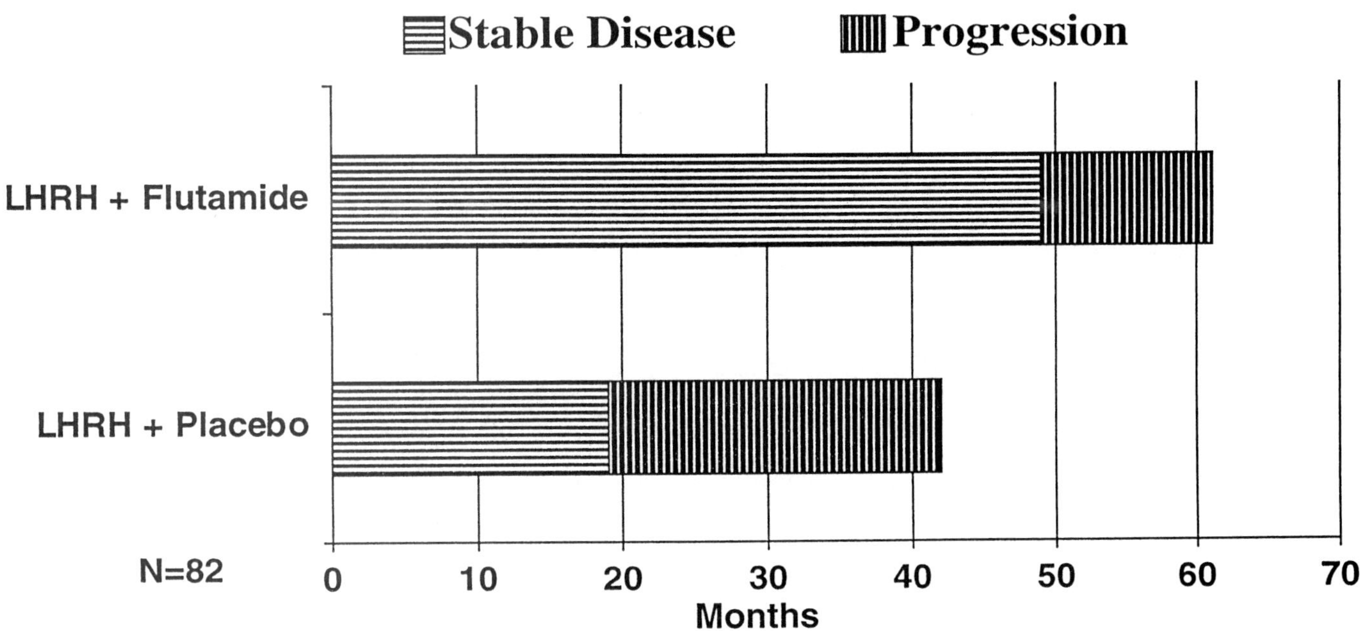

Fig. 51.6. National Cancer Institute Intergroup Protocol 0036 update on survival and progression, minimal disease subset.

tumor amenable to retreatment by androgen withdrawal. This provides the rationale for "intermittent androgen deprivation." In experimental models, this approach resulted in threefold prolongation of the duration of androgen dependence (76). Although clinical data are limited, studies done using variable methods of intermittent androgen deprivation suggest that this intriguing concept should be further investigated (76–78). In addition to delaying progression and potentially improving survival, this approach is attractive in that it is associated with improved quality of life and potentially reduced cost of therapy.

CRITERIA FOR INITIATING HORMONAL THERAPY

For more than 40 years, the indication for hormonal therapy was the confirmation of advanced metastatic disease, usually with clinical presentation of various symptoms—urinary retention, lower pelvic bone pain, bowel disorders, or anemia. Hormonal ablation palliates symptoms quickly. Hormonal therapy is also indicated on disease recurrence after radical prostatectomy or radiation, even being preemptively initiated after signs of chemical relapse, i.e., a rising PSA, which precedes physical symptoms by 6 to 18 months. Hormonal therapy has also been used adjuvantly after surgery or radiation therapy and as primary treatment of older men who are not candidates for radical treatment. Neoadjuvant hormonal therapy has been attempted to downsize locally advanced prostatic carcinomas; however, reports of its efficacy are mixed (79, 80).

PROGNOSTIC EVALUATION OF CANDIDATES FOR HORMONAL THERAPY

After a diagnosis of advanced carcinoma of the prostate is confirmed, prognostic factors are assessed and a recommendation

for the most suitable hormonal therapy is made. Assessment of prognostic factors has significantly increased knowledge of the natural history of the disease and has identified those factors that will influence a patient's outcome. The intensity of therapy can also be gauged by a patient's prognosis. Studies of prognostic factors have progressively expanded to include more subjective areas such as functional status, pain, and comorbid conditions.

An elaborate mathematical model to predict survival among patients with advanced prostate cancer was first developed from analysis of the clinical trial of the VACURG (81). The model used pain, acid phosphatase, ureteral dilation, metastases, functional status, weight, hemoglobin, and age to categorize patients for prognosis and survival. A hierarchy of risk groups was based on the accumulation of negative prognostic factors in patients—the greater the accumulation, the lower the survival. The only factor that was not significantly related to survival time was pain due to cancer.

Univariate and multivariate analyses were conducted for clinical trials of the National Prostatic Cancer Project on a broader range of prognostic variables for advanced prostate cancer (82). The important, independent prognostic factors for objective response to treatment were (in order of importance) previous hormone response status, analgesics, pain, elevated acid phosphatase, and anemia. For survival time, the significant factors were (in order of importance) previous hormone response status, anorexia, elevated acid phosphatase, pain, elevated alkaline phosphatase, obstructive symptoms, tumor grade, performance status, anemia, and age. Previous hormone response status was the most important prognostic factor in both analyses, demonstrating that patients with newly diagnosed cancers will have more favorable responses and longer survival times than patients whose cancers were diagnosed previously.

The European Organization for Research on Treatment of Cancer Genitourinary Group (EORTC-GU) conducted similar analyses and identified (in order of importance) performance status, acid phosphatase, alkaline phosphatase, tumor category, and comorbidity as the critical prognostic factors (83). De-Voogt and Smith (11) concluded that additional, expensive laboratory tests to measure hormonal levels, glycoproteins, cholesterol, triglycerides, and other biologic parameters were unnecessary.

The introduction and widespread use of PSA as an independent marker of treatment response and disease progression has provided physicians with a much more sensitive prognostic tool (84, 85). Previous studies were unable to link clinical chemistry, subjective assessments of pain and functional status, and degree of metastatic spread into an effective prognostic algorithm of treatment and response. PSA has now become the basis for prognosis with which other factors are tested to find a suitable algorithm (86–88).

In addition to the importance of its initial level, PSA may be the best intermittent prognostic factor. Patients with a posttreatment PSA nadir of less than 4 ng/mL have a significantly longer remission duration than those whose posttreatment nadir PSA remained elevated (87). Periodic PSA measurements from the initial pretreatment level indicate both response to therapy and disease-free survival until the inevitable onset of hormone-refractory disease (85, 89, 90). Consecutively rising PSA measurements are predictive of an increase in the number of skeletal lesions appearing on a bone scan and indicative of extent of disease (89, 91). A recent schema to evaluate prognostic factors combines initial bone scan results, performance status, and PSA in an attempt to capture the best of prior research, provide physicians with an efficient and effective prognostic methodology, and integrate objective and subjective measures of prognosis (92).

CONCLUSIONS

Like ceaseless tides against the sand, unflagging attempts to make significant progress against advanced carcinoma of the prostate have continued for a half century. Gains in time to progression and in survival have been made, scientific understanding has increased, but the disease remains incurable and leads inexorably to a painful death. The clinician has many more therapeutic options to offer men with advanced prostatic carcinoma, but subtle therapeutic distinctions are easily blurred. If the past 50 years have taught us anything, we have learned to respect this killer and to explore any means by which it can be halted, neutralized, disarmed, and even eliminated. The undying hope is that another 50 years will not elapse before this is achieved.

Whatever the immediate future will bring—with regard to stage migration, the identification of novel prognostic factors able to predict progression, or the development of palliative strategies aimed to further improve a patient's quality of life—today's clinician must continue to integrate a tremendous amount of clinical and scientific information to make informed recommendations to a broad, diverse group of patients. The results of scientific studies and clinical trials discussed in this chapter can only suggest; they cannot with assurance predict. The physician's judgment can only be informed, never replaced.

REFERENCES

1. Huggins C, Hodges CV. Studies on prostatic cancer: part 1. the effect of castration, of estrogen, and of androgen injection on serum phosphatases in metastatic carcinoma of the prostate. Cancer Res 1941;1:293.
2. Whitmore WF. Hormone therapy in prostate cancer. Am J Med 1956;21:697.
3. Coffey DS, Issacs JT. Control of prostate growth. Urology 1981;17:17.
4. Young HH, Kent JR. Plasma testosterone levels in patients with prostatic carcinoma before and after treatment. J Urol 1968;99:788.
5. Robinson MR, Thomas BS. Effects of hormonal therapy on plasma testosterone levels in prostatic carcinoma. Br Med J 1971;4:391.
6. Seftel AD, Spirnak JP, Resnick MI. Hormonal therapy for advanced prostatic carcinoma. J Surg Oncol 1989;1:14.
7. Grayhack JT, Keeler TC, Kozlowski JM. Carcinoma of the prostate: hormonal therapy. Cancer 1987;60:589.
8. Cassileth BR, Soloway MS, Vogelzang NJ, et al. Patients' choice of treatment in stage D prostate cancer. Urology 1989;33:57.
9. Herbst WP. Effects of estradiol dipropionate and diethylstebestrol on malignant prostatic tissue. Trans Am Assoc Genitourin Surg 1941;34:195.
10. Veterans Administration Cooperative Urologic Research Group. Treatment and survival of patients with cancer of the prostate. Surg Gynecol Obstet 1967;124:1011.
11. deVoogt HJ, Smith PH, European Organization for Research on Treatment of Cancer Urological Group, et al. Cardiovascular side effects of diethylstebestrol, cyproterone acetate, medroxyprogesterone acetate and estramustine phosphate used for the treatment of advanced prostatic cancer: results from European Organization for Research on Treatment of Cancer Trials 30761 and 30762. J Urol 1986;135:303.
12. Henriksson P, Edhag O. Orchidectomy versus oestrogen for prostatic cancer: cardiovascular effects. Br Med J 1986;293:413.
13. Resnik MI. Hormonal therapy in prostatic carcinoma. Urology 1984;24(Suppl):18.
14. Foss SD, Miller A. Treatment of advanced carcinoma of the prostate with estramustine phosphate. J Urol 1976;115:406.
15. Benson RC, Wear JB, Gill GM. Treatment of stage D hormone resistant carcinoma of the prostate with estramustine phosphate. J Urol 1979;121.
16. Vest SA, Frazier TH. Survival following castration for prostatic cancer. J Urol 1946;56:97.
17. Nesbit RM, Baum WC. Endocrine control of prostatic carcinoma. JAMA 1950;143:1317.
18. Scott WW. Historical overview of the treatment of prostatic cancer. Prostate 1983;4:435.

19. Denis L, Mahler C. Prostatic cancer: an overview. Rev Oncol 1990;29:665.

20. Kozlowski JM, Grayhack JT. Carcinoma of the prostate. In: Gillenwater JY, Grayhack JT, Howards SS, et al., eds. Adult and pediatric urology. 2nd ed. Chicago: Year Book Medical Publishers, 1991:1277.

21. Blackard CE, Byar DP, Jordan WP Jr. Veterans Administration cooperative urological research group: orchiectomy for advanced carcinoma: a re-evaluation. Urology 1973;1:553.

22. Leuprolide Study Group. Leuprolide versus diethylstilbestrol for metastatic prostate cancer. N Engl J Med 1984;311:1281.

23. Daneshgari F, Crawford ED. Endocrine therapy of advanced carcinoma of the prostate. In: Das S, Crawford ED, eds. Cancer of the prostate. New York: Marcel Dekker, 1993:333.

24. Walsh PC. Physiologic basis for hormonal therapy in carcinoma of the prostate. Urol Clin North Am 1975;2:125.

25. Labrie F, Luthy I, Veillux R, et al. New concepts on the androgen sensitivity of prostate cancer. Prog Clin Biol Res 1987;243:145. Abstract.

26. Harper ME, Pike A, Peeling WB, et al. Steroids of adrenal origin metabolized by human prostate tissue both in vivo and in vitro. J Endocrinol 1984;60:117.

27. Crawford ED, DeAntoni EP. Current status of combined androgen blockade: optimal therapy for advanced prostate cancer. J Clin Endocrin Metab 1995;80:1062.

28. Klioze SS, Miller MF, Spiro TP. A randomized, comparative study of buserelin with DES/orchiectomy in the treatment of stage D2 prostatic cancer patients. Am J Clin Oncol 1988; 2(Suppl):5176.

29. Wenderoth UK, Jacobi GH. Gonadotropin-releasing hormone analogues for palliation of carcinoma of the prostate. World J Urol 1983;1:40.

30. Glode LM, Smith JA, The Leuprolide Study Group. Long-term suppression of luteinizing hormone, follicle-stimulating hormone and testosterone by daily administration of leuprolide. J Urol 1987;137:57.

31. Sharife R, Soloway M, The Leuprolide Study Group. Clinical study of leuprolide depot formulation in the treatment of advanced prostate cancer. J Urol 1990;143:68.

32. Kahan A, Delrieu F, Amor B, et al. Disease flare induced by D-Trp6-LHRH analogue in patients with metastatic prostatic cancer. Lancet 1984;1:971.

33. Waxman J, Man A, Hendry WF, et al. Importance of early tumour exacerbation in patients treated with long acting analogues of gonadotropin releasing hormone for advanced prostatic cancer. Br Med J 1985;291:1387.

34. Stein BS, Smith JA Jr. DES lead-in to use of luteinizing hormone releasing hormone analogs in treatment of metastatic carcinoma of prostate. Urology 1985;25:350.

35. Bocon-Gibod L, Laudat MH, Dugue MA, et al. Cyproterone acetate lead-in prevents initial rise of serum testosterone induced by luteinizing hormone-releasing hormone analogs in the treatment of metastatic carcinoma of the prostate. Eur Urol 1986;12:400.

36. Moguilewshy M, Fiet J, Tournemine C, et al. Pharmacology of an antiandrogen, anadron, used as an adjuvant therapy in the treatment of prostate cancer. J Steroid Biochem 1986;24:139.

37. Kuhn J-M, Billebaud T, Navratil H, et al. Prevention of the transient adverse effects of a gonadotropin-releasing hormone analogue (buserelin) in metastatic prostatic carcinoma by administration of an antiandrogen (nilutamide). N Engl J Med 1989;321:413.

38. Geller J, Albert J, Yen SSC, et al. Medical castration of males with megestrol acetate and small doses of diethylstilbestrol. J Clin Endocrinol Metab 1981;52:576.

39. Von Eschenbach AC. Cancer of the prostate. Curr Prob Cancer 1981;5:12.

40. Bracci U. Antiandrogens in the treatment of prostatic cancer. Eur Urol 1979;5:303.

41. Schroeder FH, et al. Metastatic cancer of the prostate managed with buserelin versus buserelin plus cyproterone acetate. J Urol 1987;137:912.

42. Pavone-Macaluso M, de Voogt HJ, Viggiano G, et al. Comparison of diethylstilbestrol, cyproterone acetate and medroxyprogesterone acetate in the treatment of advanced prostatic cancer: final analysis of a randomized phase III trial of the European Organization for Research on Treatment of Cancer Urologic Group. J Urol 1986;136:624.

43. Neri R, Kassem N. Biological and clinical properties of antiandrogens. In: Bresciani F, King RJB, Lippman ME, et al., eds. Progress in cancer research and therapy. New York: Raven Press, 1984:507–518.

44. Neri RO, Monahan M. Effects of a novel nonsteroid antiandrogen on canine prostatic hyperplasia. Invest Urol 1972;10:123.

45. Sogani PC, Vagaiwala MR, Whitmore WF Jr. Experience with flutamide inpatients with advanced prostate cancer without prior endocrine therapy. Cancer 1984;54:744.

46. Lund F, Rasmussen F. Flutamide versus silboestrol in the management of advanced prostatic cancer: a controlled prospective study. Br J Urol 1988;61:140.

47. Jacobo E, Schmidt JD, Weinstein SH, et al. Comparison of flutamide (SCH-13521) and diethylstilbestrol in untreated advanced prostatic cancer. Urology 1976;8:231.

48. Chang A, Yeap B, Blum R, et al. A double blind randomized study of primary treatment for stage D2 prostate cancer: diethylstilbestrol (DES) versus flutamide. Proc Am Soc Clin Oncol 1992;11:202.

49. Raynaud JP, Bonne C, Moguilewshy M, et al. The pure antiandrogen RU 23908 (anadron), a candidate of choice for the combined antihormonal treatment of prostatic cancer: a review. Prostate 1984;5:299.

50. Crawford ED, Smith JA, Soloway MS, et al. A randomized controlled clinical trial of leuprolide and anadron versus leuprolide and placebo for advanced prostate cancer. J Urol 1990;143:221. Abstract.

51. Kennealey GT, Furr BJ. Use of the nonsteroidal anti-androgen casodex in advanced prostatic carcinoma. Urol Clin North Am 1991;18:99.

52. Furr BJ. Casodex (ICI 176,334): a new, pure, peripherally-selective anti androgen: preclinical studies. Horm Res 1989; 32(Suppl):69.

53. Schellhammer P, Sharifi R, Blick N, et al. A controlled trial of bicalutamide versus flutamide, each in combination with luteinizing hormone-releasing hormone analogue therapy, in patients with advanced prostate cancer. Urology 1995;45:745.

54. Huggins C, Scott WW. Bilateral adrenalectomy in prostatic cancer: clinical features and urinary excretion of 17-ketosteroids and estrogens. Ann Surg 1945;122:1031.

55. Miller GM, Hinman F Jr. Cortisone treatment in advanced carcinoma of the prostate. J Urol 1954;72:485.

56. Drago JR, Santen RJ, Lipton A, et al. Clinical effect of aminoglutethimide medical adrenalectomy in the treatment of 43 patients with advanced prostatic carcinoma. Cancer 1984; 53:1447.

57. Crawford ED, Ahmann FR, Davis MA, et al. Aminoglutethimide in metastatic adenocarcinoma of the prostate. Prog Clin Biol Res 1987;243:283. Abstract.

58. Labrie F, Luthy I, Veilleux R, et al. New concepts on the androgen sensitivity of prostate cancer. Prog Clin Biol Res 1987;243:145. Abstract.

59. Harper ME, Pike A, Peeling WB, et al. Steroids of adrenal origin metabolized by human prostatic tissue both in vivo and in vitro. J Endocrinol 1974;60:117.

60. Labrie F, Dupont A, Belanger A, et al. New approach in the treatment of prostate cancer: complete instead of partial withdrawal of androgens. Prostate 1983;4:579.

61. Crawford ED, Eisenberger MA, McLeod DG, et al. A controlled trial of leuprolide with and without flutamide in prostatic carcinoma. N Engl J Med 1989;321:419.

62. Eisenberger MA, Crawford ED, Wolf M, et al. Prognostic factors in stage D_2 prostate cancer; important implications for future trials: results of a cooperative intergroup study (INT.0036). Semin Oncol 1994;21:613.

63. DeAntoni EP, Crawford ED. Pretreatment of metastatic disease: prostate cancer in the older male. Cancer 1994;74: 2182.

64. Hussain M, Wolf M, Marshall E, et al. Effects of continued androgen-deprivation therapy and other prognostic factors on response and survival in phase II chemotherapy trials for hormone-refractory prostate cancer: a Southwest Oncology Group report. J Clin Oncol 1994;12:1868.

65. Hillner BE, McLeod DG, Crawford ED, et al. Estimating the cost effectiveness of total androgen blockade with flutamide in M1 prostate cancer. Urology 1995;45:633.

66. Denis LJ, Whelan P, De Moura JL, et al. Goserelin acetate and flutamide versus bilateral orchiectomy: a phase II EORTC trial (30853). Urology 1993;42:119.

67. Denis L, Smith JL, De Moura JL, et al. Orchidectomy vs. zoladex plus flutamide in patients with metastatic prostate cancer. Eur Urol 1990;18(Suppl):34.

68. Denis L, Murphy GP. Overview of phase III trials on combined androgen treatment in patients with metastatic prostate cancer. Cancer 1993;72:3888.

69. Blumenstein BA. Some statistical considerations for the interpretation of trials of combined androgen therapy. Cancer 1993;72:3834.

70. Jankenegt RA, Abbou CC, Bartoletti R, et al. Orchiectomy and nilutamide or placebo as treatment of metastatic prostatic cancer in a multinational double-blind randomized trial. J Urol 1993;149:77.

71. Ahmnann FR, Dalkin BL. Controversies in the management of newly diagnosed metastatic prostate cancer. In: Dawson NA, Vogelzang NJ, eds. Prostate cancer. New York; Wiley-Liss, 1994;215.

72. Kelly K, Scher HI. Prostate specific antigen decline after antiandrogen withdrawal: the flutamide withdrawal syndrome. J Urol 1993;149:607.

73. Scher HI, Kelly WK. Flutamide withdrawal syndrome: its impact on clinical trials in hormone-refractory prostate cancer. J Clin Oncol 1993;11:1566.

74. Dupont A, Gomez J-L, Cusan L, et al. Response to flutamide withdrawal in advanced prostate cancer in progression under combination therapy. J Urol 1993;150:908.

75. Sartor O, Cooper M, Weinberger M, et al. Surprising activity of flutamide withdrawal, when combined with aminoglutethimide in treatment of hormone-refractory prostate cancer. J Natl Cancer Inst 1994;86:222.

76. Akakura K, Bruchovsky N, Goldenberg SL, et al. Effects of intermittent androgen suppression on androgen-dependent tumors. Cancer 1993;71:2782.

77. Klotz LH, Herr HW, Morse MJ, et al. Intermittent endocrine therapy for advanced prostate cancer. Cancer 1986;58:2546.

78. Vahlensieck W, Wegner G, Lehmann HD, et al. Comparison between continuous and intermittent administration of estracyt in the treatment of carcinoma of the prostate. Urol Res 1985; 13:209.

79. Labrie F, Cusan L, Gomez J-L, et al. Down-staging of early stage prostate cancer before radical prostatectomy: the first randomized trial of neoadjuvant combination therapy with flutamide and a luteinizing hormone-releasing hormone agonist. Urology 1994;44(Suppl):29.

80. Pummer K, Crawford ED, Daneshgari F, et al. Hormonal pretreatment does not affect the final pathologic stage in locally advanced prostate cancer. Urology 1994;44(Suppl):38.

81. Byar DP, Huse R, Bailar JC III. An exponential model relating censored survival data and concomitant information for prostatic cancer patients. J Natl Cancer Inst 1974;52:321.

82. Emrich LJ, Priore RL, Murphy GP, et al. Prognostic factors in patients with advanced stage prostate cancer. Cancer Res 1985; 45:5173.

83. de Voogt HJ, Suciu S, Sylvester R, et al. Multivariate analysis of prognostic factors in patients with advanced prostatic cancer: results from 2 EORTC trials. J Urol 1989;141:883.

84. Cooper EH, Armitage TG, Robinson MRG, et al. Prostatic specific antigen and the prediction of prognosis in metastatic prostatic cancer. Cancer 1990;66:1025.

85. Petros JA, Andriole GL. Serum PSA after antiandrogen therapy. Urol Clin North Am 1993;20:749.

86. Arai Y, Yoshiki T, Yoshida O. Prognostic significance of prostate specific antigen in endocrine treatment for prostatic cancer. J Urol 1990;144:1415.

87. Miller JI, Ahmann FR, Drach GW, et al. The clinical usefulness of serum prostate specific antigen after hormonal therapy of metastatic prostate cancer. J Urol 1992;147:956.

88. Mulders PFA, del Moral PF, Theeuwes AGM, et al. Value of biochemical markers in the management of disseminated prostatic cancer. Eur Urol 1992;21:2.

89. Fossa SD, Waehre H, Paus E. The prognostic significance of prostate specific antigen in metastatic hormone-resistant prostate cancer. Br J Cancer 1992;66:181.

90. Matzkin H, Soloway MS. Response to second-line hormonal manipulation monitored by serum PSA in stage D2 prostate carcinoma. Urology 1992;40:78.

91. Soloway MS. The importance of prognostic factors in advanced prostate cancer. Cancer 1990;66:1017.

92. Newling DWW, McLeod D, Soloway M, et al. Distant disease. Cancer 1992;70:365.

52

Systemic Treatment of Hormone-Refractory Prostate Cancer

Mario A. Eisenberger

Conventional systemic treatment of patients with metastatic prostate cancer focuses primarily on the use of various endocrine manipulations designed to lower the amount of circulating androgens. This effective approach is usually temporary because the disease eventually progresses to a hormone-independent status. Data accumulated from prospective clinical trials conducted over the past few decades involving various endocrine approaches tested in patients with stage D2 disease have shown modest progress in duration of disease control (time to disease progression) and survival. The median time to progression and median survival in cohorts of stage D2 patients entered onto prospective randomized comparisons of various endocrine manipulations have ranged between 12 and 18 months and between 24 and 36 months, respectively (1–7).

Progress in cell and molecular biology over the past decade has provided new insight on fundamental mechanisms of tumor cell growth, differentiation, and metastasis. This knowledge has expanded our understanding of prostate cancer pathophysiology and provided new opportunities for developing therapeutic approaches targeted at mechanisms studied specifically in this disease.

Following androgen ablation, prostate cancer cells enter a swift, self-destructive, programmed cell death cascade that clinically is expressed by dramatic tumor responses and rapid declines of serum prostate-specific antigen (PSA) levels (8). As the tumor progresses, however, there is decreased response to apoptotic stimuli and at the same time tumor cell proliferation rates begin to exceed cell death (8, 9). This phenomenon largely reflects a progressive and selective growth of endocrine independent cells that eventually will characterize the predominant cell population and constitute what is perceived as a "hormone-refractory" state (10).

Contrary to previous belief, evolving experience also suggests that in some cases the progression from a hormone-sensitive to insensitive state represents a gradual, crescendo, movement that includes a series of intermediary biologic events, some of which may still operate under endocrine control. This consideration has evolved from the observations of gene mutations that result in a functionally altered androgen receptor (11). In vitro studies have shown that the active metabolite of flutamide, hydroxyflutamide, and progestational and estrogenic compounds may stimulate the growth of the hormone-sensitive prostate cancer cell line, LNCAP, which is known to contain the mutant form of androgen receptor (12). Although a definite cause-effect relationship has not been clearly documented, the observation of a paradoxical response after discontinuation of the nonsteroidal antiandrogen in patients demonstrating evidence of disease progression who are receiving a combined androgen blockade regimen (with flutamide) suggests that this mechanism could be involved. Ongoing prospective studies should provide more information regarding the incidence, magnitude, and significance of the antiandrogen withdrawal effects.

Changes in the differentiation pathway (13); mutations of tumor suppressor genes (14); expression of oncogenes that are able to affect cell growth, proliferation, and apoptosis (15); possibly overexpression of autocrine growth factors (16); and enhanced tumor angiogenesis (17) are among other biologic events identified in association with tumor progression following androgen ablation.

In addition to the important preclinical information, much has been learned about the clinical characteristics of advanced prostate cancer. Information derived from careful analyses of well-studied parameters within the organized environment of clinical trials has enhanced our knowledge of the clinical behavior of this disease. This knowledge can be applied in the evaluation and testing of new treatments and in the daily care of these patients.

CLINICAL AND METHODOLOGIC CONSIDERATIONS

Recognition of the inherent prognostic role of clinical, pathologic, laboratory, and biologic parameters is a critical element in the evaluation of new treatment programs in patients with metastatic prostatic carcinoma. Table 52.1 illustrates various parameters that have been shown to have prognostic significance with regard to disease outcome. Among those that consistently have a significant prognostic role in multivariate analysis are baseline performance status, hemoglobin values, alkaline and acid phosphatase, presence of liver metastasis, and extent of bone disease. Highly anaplastic lesions and those with small cell elements in the pathologic specimen usually represent part of an aggressive subset usually unresponsive or poorly responsive to androgen deprivation.

The majority of patients present exclusively with bone metastasis. Soft tissue and visceral involvement is exceedingly uncommon. The distribution of involved disease sites as reported in various chemotherapy series is shown in Table 52.2. Most commonly, bone metastases are expressed by osteoblastic lesions that cannot be measured reliably by currently available in imaging technology. Furthermore, the selection of patients, with bidimensionally measurable soft tissue or visceral disease

with or without concomitant bone metastasis, continues to be the subject of controversy. This is due to the uncertainties regarding the significance of measurable soft tissue response in the context of a vastly predominant bone involvement that cannot be assessed reliably with regard to response to therapy. It is also likely that patients with bulky visceral or nodal involvement are more representative of a subgroup with an aggressive phenotype that has distinct clinical, pathologic, and biologic properties from the common variety of adenocarcinoma of the prostate. Evolving data suggest that identification of these patients may have important value in the selection of treatment.

The significance of the extent of prior endocrine treatment is evolving as a potentially important factor with regard to response to treatment. As mentioned above, the recently described response following withdrawal of antiandrogens, albeit relatively uncommon and likely of short duration, is a good example of the importance of a well-defined prior treatment profile. In 1993, Scher and Kelly (23) and Dupont et al. (24) reported their retrospective observations of a flutamide withdrawal effect, manifested mostly by declines in serum PSA values in 30% and 75% of patients, respectively, and at times with subjective and measurable disease improvements. In the Dupont et al. series (24), the mean duration of response appeared to be relatively long (approximately 58 months), whereas the median duration was approximately 5 months in the Scher and Kelly experience (23).

In a prospective evaluation of a larger series reported by Small and Srinivas (25), the incidence of a response to flutamide withdrawal using the same parameters was quite low (15%) and the median duration was only approximately 3 months, which most likely reflects an accurate description of the actual frequency and duration of this effect. Although it is unlikely that this maneuver produces clinical benefits of sufficient magnitude to have a major effect on time to disease progression and survival, this aspect requires further study. Furthermore, the same clinical observations have now been reported with other nonsteroidal and steroidal antiandrogens.

Another important consideration regarding the antiandrogen withdrawal effect may be related to the fundamental underlying biologic significance of this event. As mentioned above, the underlying mechanism of disease progression following initial androgen deprivation may not always reflect a selective

Table 52.1. Parameters of Prognostic Significance Reported by Chemotherapy Studies

CATEGORY	PARAMETERS	RESPONSE
Clinical	Performance status	Measurable response
	Extent of bone metastasis	
	Liver involvement	Bulky soft tissue
	Severity of pain[a]	
	Number of prior endocrine treatments[a]	Predominantly lytic metastasis[a]
	Time from endocrine treatment to chemotherapy[a]	
	Permanent androgen suppression[a]	
Laboratory	Elevated baseline: PSA,[a] LDH,[a] hemoglobin, alkaline phosphatase, acid phosphatase	Subsequent PSA decline ($\geq$4 wk) by $\geq$50%
Pathology	Degree of cell differentiation	
	Small cell anaplastic pattern	
	Transitional cell elements	
Other	p53[a]	
	Neuroendocrine markers[a]	

[a] Reported by some studies (but not all).

Table 52.2. Metastatic Sites Reported in Various Chemotherapy Series

REFERENCE	TOTAL	BONE %	LIVER %	LUNG %	SOFT TISSUE OR LYMPH NODES %
Hudes (18)	36	36 (100)	2 (5.5)	0 —	7 (19)
Pienta (19)	42	42 (100)	5 (12)	3 (7)	13 (31)
Sella (20)	39	36 (92)	3 (8)	3 (8)	9 (23)
Moore (21)	27	22 (81)	2 (7.0)	2 (7.0)	10 (37)
Eisenberger (22)	109	108 (99)	4 (4)	6 (5.5)	15 (14)
Total	253	244 (96)	16 (6.5)	14 (5.5)	54 (21)

growth of exclusively hormone independent cells, but instead a clonal expansion of cells with a dysfunctional, mutant, androgen receptor (11). Most of the mutations have been reported to occur in the hormone binding domain of the androgen receptor gene, and this may raise the possibility of a change in hormonal sensitivity rather than complete loss of hormone dependence or development of a hormone-refractory state (11). Subsequent responses to second-line endocrine maneuvers primarily reported with corticosteroids, aminoglutethimide, and the antifungal compound ketoconazole in this group of patients could further support this hypothesis (26–29). This issue is also of critical importance in the evaluation of the therapeutic benefits reported with various new combination regimens that contain one or more hormonal compounds.

Another critical issue relates to the use of PSA as a marker to establish therapeutic responses. Despite the frequency of elevated serum PSA levels, the usefulness of this marker as a surrogate endpoint for clinical trials remains to be determined. Kelly et al. (30) suggested that a 50% or more decline in serum PSA levels lasting longer than 4 weeks has significant prognostic importance with regard to survival, and this prompted a widespread utilization of this parameter for phase II trials testing new drugs. More recently, Sridhara et al. (31) failed to define a measure of PSA decline that could be relied on with sufficient specificity as a treatment response criterion in uncontrolled trials. These authors have argued against the use of this marker as the sole indicator of therapeutic efficacy for new drug trials. To add further complexity to this issue, recent reports suggest that the expression of PSA may be altered by various commonly used agents, without a concomitant change in tumor growth (32, 33). Other markers, such as serum acid phosphatase and alkaline phosphatase, have not proven to be sufficiently reliable (34).

For several years, a group of investigators proposed criteria for response that include a category of disease stabilization (SD) as evidence of response to treatment (35). In their definition, SD reflects no evidence of disease progression (or worsening) during the initial 12 weeks of treatment. Survival analysis of SD patients appeared to be comparable to survival analysis of those who had evidence of tumor regression (partial responses [PR]) during that same 12-week period; SD and PR patients lived significantly longer than those who did not respond (NR). These observations prompted the considerations of SD in the category of "responding" patients together with those who demonstrated evidence of PR. What remains unproven, however, is that stabilization of disease was caused by treatment. Similarly, it is possible that SD patients have a relatively indolent biology and slow progression rate, which is inherent to their disease and unrelated to treatment. It is conceivable that those who have not demonstrated evidence of disease progression at 12 weeks will live for a shorter time than those patients whose disease is progressing slower. With the advent of PSA, it also remains possible that some of the SD patients who demonstrate improvement of symptoms and performance status without other objective changes can be otherwise characterized

as responders if they demonstrate major declines in serial measurements of this marker.

THE EXPERIENCE WITH CHEMOTHERAPY

Most chemotherapeutic agents available in clinical practice have been applied or systematically tested in patients with endocrine-resistant disease (36, 37). The evaluation of the experience with chemotherapy, however, needs to take into consideration the time in which the trials have been reported. Much has to do with the availability of the PSA test and, to a lesser extent, the development of instruments to measure quality of life. It is likely that early recognition of disease progression following androgen suppression is now accomplished by routine serial monitoring of serum PSA levels. Recent reports suggest that a PSA rise may precede other evidence of disease progression by approximately 6 months (38). This should indicate that patients currently referred to an oncologist for chemotherapy may have less advanced and symptomatic disease and potentially are better candidates for treatment. This factor is also important when the survival of patients with hormone-refractory prostate cancer is evaluated in phase II studies. Previous experience suggested that the survival of patients with hormone-refractory disease ranged between 6 and 12 months (36, 37); however, if survival is measured from time of "PSA progression," this is likely to be a few months longer (38). Table 52.3 illustrates the experience with various single agents, and Table 52.4 illustrates the experience with commonly used combinations.

Because of the methodologic problems alluded to above, it is difficult to estimate the exact level of antitumor activity of most drugs. This is particularly evident for drugs frequently used in this disease, such as doxorubicin (Adriamycin) and others. Frequently, a disturbing divergence in response rates is reported with the use of this drug. This variability most likely reflects differences in key issues such as criteria used for establishing response, patient selection factors, and the number of patients included in individual trials.

Scher et al. (39), using doxorubicin every 3 weeks, evaluated 39 patients with measurable disease and reported a 50% or more decrease in tumor mass in only 2 patients. Torti et al. (40) reported 21 of 25 responses using the National Prostatic Cancer Project (NPCP) criteria for response with a weekly "low-dose" schedule of the same drug (the total dose over a 3-week period was approximately the same as that used by Scher et al.); however, only 4 patients had complete response (CR) or PR by conventional criteria. Cisplatin was reported by Merrin (41) to produce responses in 24 of 54 evaluable patients, 17 of which fulfilled the investigator's criteria for objective responses. Unfortunately, these initial, encouraging results with this drug have not been reproduced by others (42–45). The true level of activity of cisplatin in this disease is most likely less than 20% (Table 52.3). Several years ago, Lerner and Malloy (46) reported CR plus PR in 15 of 30 patients treated with

Table 52.3.   Single-Agent Activity Reported Without the Use of PSA

DRUG	RESPONDERS/EVALUABLE (%)	RESPONSE CRITERIA AND COMMENTS
Cyclophosphamide	8/57 (14)	Response criteria not specified; this represented a review of multiple doses and schedules in broad phase II trials
Estramustine phosphate	15/86 (17)	Various response criteria; included are only more sizeable and clearly reported studies
Doxorubicin	13/88 (14.5)	Review of 4 studies including Memorial Sloan-Kettering response criteria, National Prostate Cancer Project, and standard phase II criteria for responses
Cisplatin	24/146 (13.5)	As above; doses ranged from 50–80 mg/m^2 every 3 wk with hydration.
Mitoxantrone	3/64 (5)	Southwest Oncology Group and WHO response criteria; 13 additional patients had improvements in quality-of-life parameters
Vinblastine	NR (8)	Review of multiple trials, with various dose/schedules; response criteria are unclear
	8/39 (21)	Administration by continuous infusion
5-Fluorouracil	<20	Total number is unclear; however, there were no positive trials

NR, not reported.
Modified from Eisenberger et al. (36,37).

Table 52.4.   Most Commonly Used Combinations Reported Without PSA Data

COMBINATION	RESPONDERS/ EVALUABLE (%)
Cyclophosphamide + doxorubicin	12/93 (13)
Estramustine + 5-fluorouracil	3/25 (12)
Carmustine (BCNU) + cyclophosphamide + doxorubicin	7/27 (25)
Cyclophosphamide + prednisolone	7/83 (8)
Doxorubicin + 5-fluorouracil + mitomycin C	31/92 (34)[a]
Melphalan + methotrexate + 5-fluorouracil + vincristine + prednisone	28/84 (32)[b]

Modified from Eisenberger et al. (36,37).
[a] 30/31 patients had responses according to M.D. Anderson response criteria (76).
[b] 24 responders had a 50% decline in acid phosphatase and 3/7 had measurable responses.

single-agent hydroxyurea. Subsequent trials by Loening et al. (47) and Stephens et al. (48) failed to substantiate these initial findings and, in fact, demonstrated the inefficacy of this drug.

In an attempt to improve the therapeutic results with single agents and based on observations in other tumor types suggesting the superiority of drug combinations over single agents, various multidrug regimens have been developed. The development of such treatment regimens was based on various concepts, ranging from kinetic to pharmacologic to simply additive effects. The incidence of actual CR plus PR with the combinations shown has been disappointingly low. In general, such programs are more toxic than single agents, which limits their use in patients with extensive prior radiation and bone marrow involvement by tumor. Tables 52.5 and 52.6 describe the experience in more recent studies involving single agents and combinations with the use of serial PSA evaluations in the criteria for response. Mitoxantrone, a semisynthetic anthracenedione derivative that has shown modest subjective benefits with

otherwise minimal evidence of objective antitumor effects, is among the single agents or combinations that have been reported as showing some activity (52, 53). This agent was subsequently tested in combination with low-dose prednisone (10 mg/day orally) and was reported to produce significant, again mostly palliative, benefits (21). In a prospective randomized trial, Canadian investigators reported a significant improvement in various quality-of-life parameters with the combination of mitoxantrone plus prednisone compared with prednisone alone (60). This study represents the first randomized comparative trial designed to evaluate primarily quality-of-life endpoints in patients with hormone-refractory prostate cancer. The significance of their findings requires confirmation in carefully designed trials conducted by other groups using the same or comparable instruments to measure quality of life.

An interesting observation relates to the conflicting experience reported with some drugs before and after the availability of the PSA test. For example, there is a fairly modest overall activity with bifunctional alkylating agents, such as cyclophosphamide, with reported objective clinical benefits before PSA use ranging between 10 and 20%. Nonetheless, as seen in Table 52.5, this same compound has shown higher response rates in more contemporary studies, especially if one incorporates a PSA decline in the response criteria (49–51).

Estramustine phosphate is a nitrogen mustard derivative of estradiol-17 β phosphate, which has demonstrated limited single-agent activity in this disease (Tables 52.3 and 52.4). This drug has been shown in more recent preclinical evaluation to exert its cytotoxic activity through microtubular inhibition (18) and binding to nuclear matrix (61). In an attempt to enhance the cytotoxicity of estracyt, investigators combined this agent with other drugs, such as vinblastine and Taxol (Bristol Meyer Squibb, Princeton, NJ), that also exert their cytotoxic effects at the level of the microtubule (18, 58, 61). Similarly, it has been shown that etoposide acts synergistically with estracyt in affecting the nuclear matrix (19). Clinical trials testing

Table 52.5. Contemporary Single-Agent Phase II Studies Using PSA Determinations

DRUG	DOSE (REFERENCE)	RESPONSES (%)	COMMENTS
Cyclophosphamide	75–150 mg/day (49)	4/12 (30)	Mostly PSA decline but measurable responses reported
	100 mg/m^2/day + 14 d every 2 weeks × 3 (50)	6/20 (30)	
	1.5–4.5 m/m^2 + GM-CSF + mesna (51)	6/10	
Taxol	135–170 mg/m^2 every 3 wk over 24 hr (52)	1/23	
Mitoxantrone	12–14 mg/m^2 IV (52,53)	0/14	One patient had a measurable decrease in tumor mass; 0/14 had PSA declines
Estramustine phosphate	14 mg/kg/day orally (TID) (54)	9/42 (21)	≥50% PSA decline
5-Fluorouracil	1000 mg/m^2/day by continuous infusion for 5 days, every 28 days (20)	0/18	
Etoposide	50 mg/m^2/day orally for 21 days, monthly (55)	2/24 (8)	One had 50% PSA decline and one had a measurable response (without a ≥50% PSA decline)
Carboplatin	150 mg/m^2 IV weekly (56)	3/25 (12)	3 had ≥50% PSA decline and 2 also had measurable response
Losoxantrone	50 mg/m^2 IV every 21 days (57)	5/29 (25)	17/29 had subjective improvements

Table 52.6. Phase II Trials With Combinations Using PSA Measurements

TREATMENT REGIMEN	REFERENCE	≥50% PSA DECLINE (%)	MEASURABLE RESPONSE (%)
Estramustine + vinblastine	Seidman (58)	13/24 (54)	2/5
	Hudes (18)	22/36 (61)	1/7
Estramustine + etoposide	Pienta (19)	29/42 (69)	9/18 (50)
Estramustine + Taxol	Hudes (58)	10/17 (59)	3/6
Doxorubicin + cyclophosphamide + G-CSF	Small (59)	12/29 (41)	4/12
Suramin + hydrocortisone	Review of 9 studies; Eisenberger (22)	128/338 (38)	25/85 (29)
Mitoxantrone + prednisone	Moore (21)	5/23 (21.5)	1/7
Ketoconazole + doxorubicin + hydrocortisone	Sella (20)	21/39 (55)	7/12

the combination of estramustine plus vinblastine or etoposide or Taxol have resulted in promising preliminary evidence of antitumor activity (Table 52.6). As with estracyt, etoposide, vinblastine, and Taxol all have minimal single-agent activity in patients with hormone-resistant prostate cancer (Tables 52.3–52.5). This suggests that the mechanistic preclinical observations may be clinically pertinent and are worth pursuing further.

Suramin is a new investigational drug currently in active development for the treatment of various solid tumors. Phase I/II trials have thus far resulted in encouraging preliminary evidence of antitumor activity in patients with hormone-refractory adenocarcinoma of the prostate; further testing in phase III trials is underway in this disease (62–64).

Suramin is a polysulfonated naphthylurea with a unique chemical structure that includes several aromatic rings and three sulfonic radicals on each side of the molecule (six in total). These sulfonic radicals are responsible for the intensely charged chemical reactivity of the drug, and this explains its affinity to various proteins of the extracellular matrix. Suramin has been shown to inhibit binding of various growth factors such as transforming growth factor-β (65), platelet-derived growth factor (PDGF) (66), fibroblast growth factor (FGF) (67), insulin-like growth factor (IGF) (68), and epidermal growth factor (EGF) (69). Other proteins that appear to be affected by suramin are protein-kinase-C (70), tumor necrosis factor (71), interleukin-2 (72), transferrin (73), apolipoprotein-β (74), interleukin-6, and nuclear DNA topoisomerase II (75). In addition, suramin has been shown to reduce bone resorption in a neonatal mouse calvarium bone resorption model (76). This effect has been considered as a possible explanation for the dramatic relief of bone pain previously observed in clinical trials by independent investigators (2, 3).

Suramin may suppress gonadotropin function, decrease circulating testosterone levels in rats (77), and produce significant suppression of adrenal steroidogenesis probably through enzymatic inhibition of the P450 enzymatic pathway (78). Adrenal insufficiency remains a potential irreversible toxicity of suramin, although the incidence of severity of this side effect has not been extensively studied nor have the drug's effects on the synthesis and release of sex hormones been appropriately investigated.

Table 52.7.   Therapeutic Efficacy Reported With Suramin in Hormone-Refractory Patients

REFERENCE	NO. OF PATIENTS	RESPONSE $\geq$50% $\downarrow$ PSA[a]	$\geq$75% $\downarrow$ PSA	MEASURABLE	SUBJECTIVE
Petrylak (79)	30	13/28	7/28	2/11	NR
Mendoza (80)	26	5/10	NR	2/11	NR
Wilding (81)	38	3/18	1/18	NR	NR
Reyno (82)	40	20/38	19/38	0/4	12/23
Kobayashi (83)	54	13/43	—	NR	NR
Eisenberger (84)	69	36/67	27/67	7/18	36/49
Myers (63)	38	21/38	13/38	6/17	15/21
Memorial Sloan-Kettering (85)	28	9/19	NR	1/9	NR
Ahman (86)	15	7/15	NR	7/15	NR

Modified from Eisenberger et al. (73).
NR, not reported.
[a] 50% $\downarrow$ in PSA over $\geq$4 weeks.

Current clinical experience with this novel compound is shown in Table 52.7. Much of the drug's pharmacologic properties, spectrum of toxicity, characterization of dose-limiting toxicity, and documentation of antitumor activity have been studied and reported in the recent literature (62–64, 84). The toxicity of the drug is expressed primarily by a syndrome of malaise and fatigue, which may be severe in approximately 5% of patients if treatment does not exceed a 3-month period with a widely used schedule designed to maintain plasma concentrations between 150 and 250 μg/mL. Other less common toxicities are modest elevations of BUN and creatinine, paresthesias, dermatitis, and at high doses a syndrome of progressive motor-sensory deficit that resembles a Guillain-Barré syndrome. With lower doses and limited treatment duration, treatment is safe and toxicities are almost always reversible (22). Despite this, a number of important issues still require careful and better definition. These issues range from a careful study of inherent clinical-pharmacologic properties of the drug to a more definitive proof that the antitumor activity thus far reported actually represents a significant advance in the treatment of prostate cancer.

RANDOMIZED TRIALS

Table 52.8 shows the results reported in randomized trials in the literature. The NPCP has tested single agents and combinations for patients with hormonally resistant disease in a series of randomized phase II studies (Table 52.8). By using response as the main study endpoint, the NPCP investigators initially compared single agents with a "standard treatment" in two separate trials. This standard treatment arm consisted of a variety of palliative therapies, including radiation therapy and/or an alternate hormonal treatment, including corticosteroids and/or analgesics (Studies 100 and 200, Table 52.8). The higher rate of "objective responses" (CR + PR + SD) on the chemotherapy arms was not associated with survival advantages compared with the control arms (36, 37). Nevertheless, these initial studies served as the foundation for the continuing evaluation of other single agents and combinations without further comparisons to a control arm, as illustrated on Table 52.8. A total of 258 objective responders was reported on the 9 trials shown; however, 230 (89%) were in the stable disease category.

Because NPCP chemotherapy trials were not designed to use survival as their main endpoint, the sample sizes of each study provide us with sufficient power to rule out only 70 to 80% improvement in median survivals between treatment arms. Nevertheless, smaller improvements would only reflect prolongation of survival by a few months, which probably does not represent any significant therapeutic achievement.

Because NPCP studies involved the use of a cross-over treatment, it may be argued that such salvage therapy could have influenced survival. However, the generally poor results with any chemotherapy in this disease make it highly unlikely that additional benefits can be expected with second-line treatment. Furthermore, in NPCP Studies 100 and 200, the survival of patients initially receiving chemotherapy was not superior to that of patients receiving standard treatment, although the former group received cross-over therapy while the latter were followed until death or no other salvage treatment.

In a randomized phase II trial reported by Smalley et al. (87), 5-fluorouracil (5-FU) and the combination of cyclophosphamide, doxorubicin, and 5-FU produced similar response rates and median survivals of 34 weeks and 25 weeks, respectively (differences were not statistically significant). The Eastern Cooperative Oncology Group (ECOG) compared doxorubicin and 5-FU (75). A 7% response rate observed in the initial 56 patients randomized to the 5-FU arm prompted the early termination of that arm and the assignment of patients directly to the doxorubicin arm. Responses in patients with measurable disease were more frequently observed in those receiving doxorubicin (25%) than in those receiving 5-FU (7%) (P < 0.05). Median survival for all doxorubicin patients was 29 weeks compared with 24 weeks for 5-FU patients. These differences are

Table 52.8.   National Prostatic Cancer Project: Randomized Trials in Prostatic Carcinoma

TREATMENT	NO. EVALUABLE/ ENTERED	CR + PR	SD	MEDIAN SURVIVAL (wk)
NPCP Study 100				
CTX	41	4	20	47
5-fluorouracil	33	4	14	44
Standard (A)	36	0	7	38
NPCP Study 200				
Estramustine phosphate	46/54	3	11	26
Streptozotocin	38/46	0	12	25
Standard (A)	21/25	0	4	24
NPCP Study 300				27
CTX	35/39	0	9	40
DTIC	55/68	2	13	31
Procarbazine	39/58	0	5	
NPCP Study 400				
Estramustine phosphate + Prednimustine	54	1	6	37
Prednimustine	62	0	8	36
NPCP Study 700				
CTX	43/47	3	12	41
MeCCNU	27/38	1	7	22
Hydroxyurea	28/40	2	2	19
NPCP Study 800				26
Estramustine phosphate	27/38	1	6	22
Vincristine	29/42	1	4	32
a + b	34/41	0	7	
NPCP Study 1100				
Estramustine phosphate	50/63	1	16	43
MTX	58/67	3	21	37
DDP	50/59	2	16	33
NPCP Study 1200				
Estramustine phosphate	40/50	0	7	38
DDP	42/51	0	9	28
a + b	42/48	0	14	40

Modified from Eisenberg et al. (36,37).

CR, complete response; PR, partial response; SD, disease stabilization; A, radiation therapy, prednisone, TACE, dexamethasone, testosterone, DES, Stilphostrol, Aldactone, cryosurgery, Dicorvin, Estinyl.

not statistically significant. However, by adjusting for prognostic variables (performance status, weight loss, protein aversion, and bone metastasis), this difference became significant at a P level of 0.03 (30 weeks adjusted median survival for doxorubicin versus 22 weeks for 5-FU).

The Southwest Oncology Group has compared the combination of cyclophosphamide and doxorubicin to hydroxyurea alone in patients with hormone-resistant disease (48). Of the 137 patients evaluable for analysis, 18 of 68 (26%) on the combination arm and 9 of 69 (13%) on the single-agent arm had symptomatic improvements. In patients with measurable disease, 6 of 19 (32%) and 1 of 24 (4%) responded to the combination and single agent, respectively (P = 0.06, Fisher's exact test). Median survival times for both groups were virtually the same (28 and 27 weeks). The authors concluded that, although more responses resulted from this combination, no effect on survival was achieved. Moreover, they suggest that cy-

clophosphamide and doxorubicin were not sufficiently effective and stress the need for more effective agents to be developed.

SYSTEMIC USE OF RADIOPHARMACEUTICALS FOR THE TREATMENT OF BONE METASTASIS

A major morbidity of metastatic prostate cancer relates to progressive bone involvement, which results in pain and bone destruction with pathologic fractures. The conventional management of these patients involves the use of external beam radiation, which represents an effective form of local palliation.

The use of radiopharmaceutical compounds capable of binding to bone matrix without marrow cells' affinity has been explored for many years for systemic use and treatment of diffuse bone pain caused by metastasis. The initial experience with phosphorus-32 suggested moderate benefits but at the cost of significant hematologic toxicity in a substantial proportion of

Table 52.9.   Radiopharmeaceuticals

AGENT	HALF-LIFE (DAYS)	TYPE OF EMISSION
$^{32}P-$Orthophosphate	14.3	Beta
Strontium-89	50.5	Beta
^{186}Rhenium-HEDP	3.8	Beta, gamma
^{153}Samarium-EDTMP	1.9	Beta
^{113m}Sn(tin) - DTPA	13.6	Gamma

patients (86). More recently, a number of newer radiopharmaceuticals have been used in the clinic. Among the most extensively used is strontium-89 chloride, which is preferentially retained by bone sites with enhanced osteogenesis. Strontium-89 decays by beta emission with a physical half-life of 50.5 days. The maximum range of the beta energy in tissue is approximately 8 mm (88). The drug behaves similarly to other drugs that clear rapidly from the blood into the bone mineral. The pharmacokinetics of this agent may vary substantially, depending on the extent and type of bone involvement. Extensive osteoblastic disease is associated with a much longer retention time compared with relatively limited focal skeletal involvement (89). It also appears that toxicity may be enhanced with a longer retention time in patients with more extensive bone metastasis (89).

Clinical trials with single or repeated intravenous administration of strontium-89 have demonstrated that effective palliation can be accomplished in approximately 30% of patients (range, 20 to 50%). The usual dose recommended is 4 mCi given intravenously. If repeated administrations are needed, these are usually given at 3-month intervals (89). However, current experience suggests that cumulative toxicity (myelosuppression) is a significant problem with repeated administration.

Experience with strontium-89 was reported by Blake et al. and Porter et al. (90, 91). In a prospective, randomized, placebo-controlled study, these investigators demonstrated that the addition of the radiopharmaceutical to local field radiation therapy reduces the progression of symptoms related to prostate cancer bone metastasis. Toxicity was primarily hematologic and delayed as well as cumulative when repeated administrations were given.

Other radiopharmaceutical compounds in development in the United States are shown in Table 52.9. Current data do not allow us to select one compound over another. Appropriate questions that remain unanswered include best schedule, doses, effects of repeated administrations and their effects on the natural history of the disease, and response/toxicity when given in combination with other systemic approaches such as cytotoxic chemotherapy.

REFERENCES

1. Byar DP. Review of the Veterans Administration studies of cancer of the prostate and new results concerning treatment of stage I and II tumors. In: Pavone-Malacuso M, Smith PH, Edsmyr F, eds. Bladder tumors and other topics in urological oncology. New York: Plenum-Press, 1980:471.

2. Crawford ED, Eisenberger MA, McLeod DC, et al. A controlled randomized trial of leuprolide with and without flutamide in prostatic cancer. N Engl J Med 1989;321:419.

3. Denis L, Whetan P, Carneiro De, et al. Goserelin acetate and flutamide versus bilateral orchiectomy: a phase III EORTC study (30853). Urology 1993;42:119.

4. Eisenberger MA, O'Dwyer PJ, Friedman MA. Gonadotropin hormone releasing analogues: a new therapeutic approach for prostate cancer. J Clin Oncol 1986;4:414.

5. McLeod D. Hormonal therapy in the treatment of carcinoma of the prostate. Cancer 1995;75:1914.

6. The Leuprolide Study Group. Leuprolide versus diethylstilbestrol for metastatic prostate cancer. N Engl J Med 1984;311:1281.

7. Turkes AO, Peeling WB, Griffith H. Treatment of patients with advanced cancer of the prostate: phase III trial, Zoladex against castration: a study of the British prostate group. J Steroid Biochem 1987;27:543.

8. Isaacs JT, Lundmo PI, Berges R, et al. Androgen regulation of programmed cell death of normal and malignant prostatic cells. J Androl 1992;13:457.

9. Berges RR, Vukanovic J, Epstein J, et al. Implications of cell kinetic changes during the progression of human prostatic cancer. Clin Can Res 1995;1:473.

10. Isaacs JT, Wake N, et al. Genetic instability coupled to clonal selection as a mechanism for tumor progression in the Dunning R-3327 rat prostatic adenocarcinoma system. Cancer Res 1982;42:2353.

11. Taplin ME, Bubley GJ, Shuster TD, et al. Mutation of the androgen-receptor gene in metastatic androgen-independent prostate cancer. N Engl J Med 1995;332:1393.

12. Wilding G, Chen M, Gelmann EP. Aberrant response in vitro of hormone-responsive prostate cancer cells to antiandrogens. Prostate 1989;14:103.

13. diSant'Agnese PA. Neuroendocrine differentiation in prostatic carcinoma: recent findings and new concepts. Cancer 1995; 75(Suppl):1850.

14. Thompson TC, Kadmon D, Timme TL, et al. Experimental oncogene induced prostate cancer. In: Isaacs JT, ed. Prostate cancer; cell and molecular mechanisms in diagnosis and treatment: cancer surveys. New York: Cold Spring Harbor Laboratory Press, 1991;1155.

15. Berges RR, Furuya Y, Remington L, et al. Cell proliferation, DNA repair and p-53 are not required for programmed cell death of prostatic glandular cells induced by androgen ablation. Proc Natl Acad Sci USA 1993;90:8910.

16. Story MT. Polypeptide modulators of prostatic growth and development. In: Isaacs JT, ed. Prostate cancer cell and molecular mechanisms in diagnosis and treatment. New York: Spring Harbour Laboratory Press, 1991;11:123.

17. Weidner N, Carroll PR, Faux J, et al. Tumor angiogenesis correlates with metastasis in invasive prostate cancer. Am J Pathol 1993;143:401.

18. Hudes G, Greenberg R, Krigel RL. Phase-II study of estramustine and vinblastine, two microtubule inhibitors, in

hormone-refractory prostate cancer. J Clin Oncol 1992;10: 1754.

19. Pienta K, Redman B, Hussain M, et al. Phase-II study of estramustine and oral etoposide in hormone-refractory adenocarcinoma of the prostate. J Clin Oncol 1994;12:2005.

20. Sella A, Kilbourn R, Amato R, et al. Phase-II study of ketoconazole combined with weekly doxorubicin in patients with androgen-independent prostate cancer. J Clin Oncol 1994;12:683.

21. Moore MJ, Osoba D, Murphy K, et al. Use of palliative endpoints to evaluate the effects of mitoxantrone and low-dose prednisone in patients with hormonally resistant prostate cancer. J Clin Oncol 1994;12:689.

22. Eisenberger MA, Reyno L, Sinibaldi V, et al. The experience with suramin in advanced prostate cancer. Cancer 1995; 75(Suppl):1927.

23. Scher HI, Kelly KW. Flutamide withdrawal syndrome: its impact on clinical trials in hormone refractory prostate cancer. J Clin Oncol 1993;11:1566.

24. Dupont A, Gomez JL, Cusan L, et al. Response to flutamide withdrawal in advanced prostate cancer in progression under combination therapy. J Urol 1993;150:908.

25. Small E, Srinivas S. The antiandrogen withdrawal syndrome: experience in a large cohort of unselected advanced prostate cancer patients. Proc Am Urol Assoc 1995;153:448. Abstract no. 878.

26. Sartor O, Myers C. The influence of amino-glutethimide and corticosteroids on the therapeutic benefits of flutamide withdrawal. Proc Am Soc Clin Oncol 1995;14:245.

27. Sartor O, Cooper M, Weinberger M, et al. Surprising activity of flutamide withdrawal, when combined with aminoglutethimide in the treatment of hormone-refractory prostate cancer. J Natl Cancer Inst 1994;86:222.

28. Tannock I, Gospodarowicz M, Meakin W, et al. Treatment of metastatic prostatic cancer with low-dose prednisone: evaluation of pain and quality of life as pragmatic indices of response. J Clin Oncol 1989;7:590.

29. Herrada J, Hossan B, Amato R, et al. Adrenal androgens predict for early progression to flutamide withdrawal in patients with androgen independent prostate cancer. Proc Am Soc Clin Oncol 1994:237.

30. Kelly K, Scher HI, Mazumbar M. Prostate specific antigen as a measure of disease outcome in hormone-refractory prostate cancer. J Clin Oncol 1993;11:607.

31. Sridhara R, Eisenberger MA, Sinibaldi VJ, et al. Evaluation of prostate specific antigen as a surrogate marker for response of hormone refractory prostate cancer to suramin therapy. J Clin Oncol 1995;13:2944.

32. Steiner MS, Seckin B, Anthony CT, et al. Can prostate specific antigen be used as a valid endpoint for chemotherapy efficacy in advanced prostate cancer? Proc Am Assoc Cancer Res 1995; 36:209. Abstract no. 1245.

33. Larocca RV, Danesi R, Cooper MR, et al. Effect of suramin on human prostate cancer cells in vitro. J Urol 1991;145:393.

34. Yagoda A. Response in prostate cancer: an enigma. Semin Urol 1984;1:311.

35. Slack N, Mittleman A, Brady MF, et al. The importance of the stable category for chemotherapy treated patients with advanced and relapsed prostate cancer. Cancer 1980;46:2393.

36. Eisenberger MA. Chemotherapy for prostate carcinoma. NCI Monogr 1988;7:151.

37. Eisenberger MA, Simon R, O'Dwyer P, et al. A re-evaluation of non-hormonal cytotoxic chemotherapy in the treatment of prostate cancer. J Clin Oncol 1985;3:827.

38. Eisenberger M, Crawford ED, McLeod D, et al. The prognostic significance of prostate specific antigen in stage D2 prostate cancer: interim evaluation of intergroup 0105. Proc Am Soc Clin Oncol 1995;14:236. Abstract no. 613.

39. Scher H, Yagoda A, Watson R, et al. Phase II trial of Adriamycin in bidimensionally measurable prostatic adenocarcinoma. J Urol 1984;13:1099.

40. Torti F, Aston D, Lum BL, et al. Weekly doxorubicin in endocrine refractory carcinoma of the prostate. J Clin Oncol 1983;1:477.

41. The Leuprolide Study Group. Leuprolide versus diethylstilbestrol for metastatic prostate cancer. N Engl J Med 1984;311:1281.

42. Yagoda A, Watson RC, Natale RB, et al. A critical analysis of response criteria in patients with prostatic cancer treated with cis-diamminedichloro platinum II. Cancer 1979;44:1553.

43. Rossof AH, Talley RW, Stephens R, et al. Phase II evaluation of cis-dichloro diammine platinum (II) in advanced malignancies of the genitourinary and gynecological organs: a Southwest Oncology Group study. Cancer Treat Rep 1979;63: 1557.

44. Qazi R, Khandekar J. Phase II study of cisplatin for metastatic prostatic carcinoma: an Eastern Cooperative Oncology Group study. Am J Clin Oncol 1983;6:203.

45. Moore MR, Troner MB, DeSimone P, et al. Phase II evaluation of cisplatin for metastatic prostatic carcinoma: an Eastern Cooperative Oncology Group study. Am J Clin Oncol 1983;6: 203.

46. Lerner JH, Malloy TR. Hydroxyurea in stage D carcinoma of the prostate. Urology 1977;10:35.

47. Loening SA, Scott WW, deKernion J, et al. A comparison of hydroxyurea, methyl-chloroethyl-chlorohexyl-nitrosourea and cyclophosphamide in patients with advanced prostate cancer. J Urol 1981;125:812.

48. Stephens RL, Vaughn C, Lane M, et al. Adriamycin and cyclophosphamide versus hydroxyurea in advanced prostatic cancer: a randomized Southwest Oncology Group study. Cancer 1984;53:406.

49. Von Roemeling R, Fisher HAG, Horton J. Daily oral cyclophosphamide is effective in hormone-refractory prostate cancer: a phase-I/II pilot study. Proc Am Soc Clin Oncol 1992; 11:213. Abstract no. 665.

50. Abell FL, Wilkes JD, Divers L, et al. Oral cyclophosphamide for hormone-refractory prostate cancer. Proc Am Soc Clin Oncol 1995;14:213. Abstract no. 646.

51. Smith DC, Vogelzang N, Goldberg HL, et al. High-dose cyclophosphamide with granulocyte-macrophage colony stimulating factor in hormone-refractory prostate cancer. Proc Am Soc Clin Oncol 1992;11:213. Abstract no. 666.

52. Rearden TP, Small EJ, Valone F, et al. Phase II study of

mitoxantrone for hormone refractory prostate cancer. Proc Am Soc Clin Oncol 1995;14:218. Abstract no. 688.

53. Raghavan D, Bishop J, Woods I. Mitoxantrone a non-toxic, moderately active agent for hormone resistant prostate cancer. Proc Am Soc Clin Oncol 1986;5:102. Abstract.

54. DeWys WD, Begg CB, Brodowsky H, et al. A comparative clinical trial of Adriamycin and 5-fluorouracil in advanced prostatic cancer: prognostic factor and response/prostate. 1983; 4:1.

55. Logothetis CJ, Samules ML, Von Eschenback AC, et al. Doxorubicin, mitomycin-C and 5-fluorouracil (DMF) in the treatment of metastatic hormonal refractory adenocarcinoma of the prostate, with a note on the staging of metastatic prostate cancer. J Clin Oncol 1983;1:368.

56. Hussain M, Pienta K, Redman BG, et al. Oral etoposide in the treatment of hormone refractory prostate cancer. Cancer 1994;74:100.

57. Canobbio L, Guarneri D, Miglietta L, et al. Carboplatin in advanced hormone-refractory prostatic cancer patients. Eur J Cancer 1993;29:2094. Abstract.

58. Seidman AD, Scher HI, Petrylak D, et al. Estramustine and vinblastine: use of prostatic specific antigen as a clinical trial endpoint for hormone refractory prostatic cancer. J Urol 1992; 147:931.

59. Small EJ, Srinivas S, Madhavan S, et al. Use of doxorubicin and dose-escalated cyclophosphamide with granulocyte colony stimulating factor in the treatment of hormone refractory prostate cancer. Proc Am Soc Clin Oncol 1995;14:243. Abstract no. 648.

60. Tannock I, Osoba D, Ernst S, et al. Chemotherapy with mitoxantrone palliates patients with hormone-resistant prostate cancer: results of a Canadian randomized trial. Proc Am Soc Clin Oncol 1995;14:245. Abstract no. 353.

61. Hudes G, Nathan F, Chapman A, et al. Combined antimicrotubule therapy of metastatic prostate cancer with 96-Hr paclitaxel and estramustine: activity in hormone-refractory disease. Proc Am Soc Clin Oncol 1995;14:236. Abstract no. 622.

62. Stein CA, LaRocca R, McAtee N, et al. Suramin, an anti-cancer drug with a unique mechanism of action. J Clin Oncol 1988;7:499.

63. Myers C, Cooper M, Stein C, et al. A novel growth factor antagonist with activity in hormone-refractory metastatic prostate cancer. J Clin Oncol 1992;10:881.

64. Eisenberger MA, Reyno LM, Jodrell DI, et al. Suramin, an active drug for prostate cancer: interim observations in a phase I trial. J Natl Cancer Inst 1993;85:611.

65. Wade T, Kasid A, Stein C, et al. Suramin interference with transforming growth factor-B inhibition of human renal cell carcinoma in culture. J Surg Res 1992;53:195.

66. Huang S, Huang J. Rapid turnover of the platelet derived growth factor receptor in sis-transformed cells and reversal by suramin. J Biol Chem 1988;263:12608.

67. Yayon A, Klagsbrun M. Autocrine transformation by chimeric signal peptide-basic fibroblast growth factor: reversal by suramin. Proc Natl Acad Sci USA 1990;87:5346.

68. Pollak M, Richard M. Suramin blockade of insulinlike growth factor 1-stimulated proliferation of human osteosarcoma cells. J Natl Can Inst 1990;82:1349.

69. Cardinali M, Sartor O, Robbins K. Suramin, an experimental chemotherapeutic drug, activates the receptor for epidermal growth factor and promotes growth of certain malignant cells. J Clin Invest 1992;89:1242.

70. Hensey C, Boscoboinik D, Assi A. Suramin, anti-cancer drug, inhibits protein kinase C and induces differentiation in neuroblastoma cell clone NB2A. FEBS Lett 1989;258:156.

71. Grazioli L, Alzani R, Ciomei M, et al. Inhibitory effect of suramin on receptor binding and cytotoxic activity of tumor necrosis factor. Int J Immunopharmacol 1992;14:637.

72. Mills G, Zhang N, May C, et al. A suramin prevents binding of interleukin 2 to its cell surface receptor: a possible mechanism for immunosuppression. Cancer Res 1990;50: 30306.

73. Rossi M, Zetter B. Selective inhibition of prostatic carcinoma cell by transferrin. Proc Natl Acad Sci USA 1992;89:6197.

74. Schneider W, Beisiegel U, Goldstein J, et al. Purification of the low density lipoprotein receptor, an acidic glycoprotein of 164,000 molecular weight. J Biol Chem 1982;257:2664.

75. Bojanowski K, Lelievre S, Markovitz J, et al. Suramin is an inhibitor of DNA topoisomerase II in vitro and in Chinese hamster fibrosarcoma cells. Proc Natl Acad Sci USA 1992;89: 3025.

76. McClellan MW, Kragel PJ, Trahan E, et al. Suramin inhibits bone resorption and reduces osteoblast number in a neonatal mouse calvarial bone resorption assay. Endocrinology 1992; 131:2263.

77. Marzouk H, Hoflandl L, denHolder F, et al. Effects of suramin on hormone release by culture rat anterior pituitary cells. Mol Cell Endocrinol 1990;72:95.

78. Levine A, Gill P, Cohen J, et al. Suramin antiviral therapy in the acquired immunodeficiency syndrome. Ann Intern Med 1986;105:32.

79. Petrylak DP, Yagoda A, O'Connor J, et al. Phase-II trial of suramin in hormone refractory prostate cancer. Proc Am Soc Clin Oncol 1994;780:249.

80. Mendoza E, Belldegrun A, Landaw E, et al. Suramin efficacy and toxicity in hormone refractory prostate cancer. Proc Am Soc Clin Oncol 1994;801:254.

81. Wilding G, Rago R, Hutsons P, et al. Phase-I trial of a six week intermittent bolus schedule of suramin. Proc Am Soc Clin Oncol. 1994;717:233.

82. Reyno L, Eisenberger M, Sridhara R, et al. Safety and efficacy of a pharmacologically derived fixed schedule of suramin. Proc Am Soc Clin Oncol 1994;729:236.

83. Kobayashi K, Vokes E, Janish L, et al. Suramin is safe and active in prostate cancer without adaptive control. Proc Am Soc Clin Oncol 1994;353:140.

84. Eisenberger MA, Reyno L. Suramin. Cancer Treat Rev 1994; 20:259.

85. Scher HI. Suramin: here to stay? J Natl Cancer Inst 1993;85: 594.

86. Ahmann FR, Schwartz J, Dorr R. Suramin in hormone resistant prostate cancer: significant activity by unanticipated toxicity. Proc Am Soc Clin Oncol 1991;10:178.

87. Smalley RV, Bartolucci A, Hemstreet G, et al. A phase II

evaluation of a three drug combination of cyclophosphamide, doxorubicin and 5-fluorouracil and of 5-fluorouracil in patients with advanced bladder carcinoma or stage D prostatic carcinoma. J Urol 1981;125:191.

88. Burnet NG, Williams G, Howard N. Phosphorus-32 for intractable bony pain from carcinoma of the prostate. Clin Oncol 1990;220.

89. Blake GM, Gray JM, Zivanovic MA. Strontium-89 radionuclide therapy: a dosimetry study using impulse response function analysis. Br J Radiol 1987;60:685.

90. Blake GM, Zivanovic MA, McEwan AJ. Strontium kinetics in disseminated carcinoma of the prostate. Eur J Nucl Med 1986; 12:447.

91. Porter AJ, McEwan AJB, Powe JE, et al. Results of a randomized phase III trial to evaluate the efficacy of strontium-89 adjuvant to local field external beam irradiation in the management of endocrine resistant metastatic prostate cancer. Inst J Radiat Oncol Biol Phys 1993;25:805.

92. Huan SD, Natale RB, Stewart DJ, et al. A phase-II multicenter trial of losoxantrone (DUP-941) in patients with metastatic hormone-refractory prostate cancer. Proc Am Soc Clin Oncol 1995;14:238. Abstract no. 626.

53

Chemotherapy for Stage I and II Testicular Cancer

Robert J. Amato
Christopher J. Logothetis

STAGE I

With the 5-year survival rate approaching 100% in patients with stage I germ cell tumors, recent emphasis has been on reducing the short- and long-term toxicities of therapy (1–5). One of the most important refinements in the treatment of these tumors is the use of prognostic factors to indicate risk-adapted treatments (6–10). The accuracy of current staging procedures and the assumption that tumor recurrence can be treated effectively with chemotherapy or the combination of chemotherapy and surgical therapy have led investigators to reconsider what may be unnecessarily aggressive surgical therapy for patients with clinical stage I disease.

Clinical stage I disease is defined as tumor confined to the testis. To define clinical stage, the patient undergoes physical examination, chest x-ray, computed tomography scan of the abdomen and pelvis, and biochemical serum analysis of alpha-fetoprotein, beta human gonadotropin, and lactate dehydrogenase isoenzyme I. The current management options following orchiectomy, the standard primary treatment, are retroperitoneal lymphadenectomy or surveillance. Although the mortality rate after retroperitoneal lymph node dissection (RPLND) is negligible, its morbidity cannot be overlooked. Surveillance can be a disconcerting option to the patient. Thus, a third option to consider for the management of clinical stage I non-seminomatous germ cell tumor of the testis (NSGCTT) is chemotherapy (11).

Chemotherapy for pathologic and clinical stage I germ cell tumor has not been widely accepted. Using the information obtained by evaluation of prognostic factors, investigators have advocated adjuvant chemotherapy for selected patients with stage I disease, the rationale being to find a more effective modality than RPLND and to eliminate the uncertainty of surveillance. Because risk stratification is not perfect, a proportion of the high-risk group is overtreated as not all would relapse even without chemotherapy.

Published reports of patients receiving adjuvant chemotherapy in clinical and pathologic stage I NSGCTT are few. The studies are composed of small numbers of patients and mixed pathologic and clinical stage I disease; the earlier reports use a variety of ineffective chemotherapeutic agents. No randomized studies have been published. These studies are reviewed in some detail in the following paragraphs.

Ansfield et al. treated 13 patients following orchiectomy, including 6 patients who had a lymph node dissection performed (4 with positive nodes). Chemotherapy consisted of chlorambucil, methotrexate, and actinomycin D. The median follow-up was 32 months (range, 3 to 65 months). There were two relapses after adjuvant chemotherapy, with both patients dying of tumor. Two patients at the time of the report were still receiving chemotherapy (12).

Skinner treated 30 patients following RPLND regardless of whether disease was confined to the testis or positive nodes were found. The chemotherapy used was single-agent actinomycin D in the majority of cases. The author concluded that the 5-year survival rate was more than 90% for patients with negative nodes or minimal retroperitoneal metastases (13).

Ekman and Edsmyr treated 28 patients with mithramycin and orchiectomy after RPLND (25 restricted to the tumor side, 3 bilateral). No metastatic spread was demonstrated by histologic examination. Twenty-three patients (93%) remained disease free after 2 to 6 years of follow-up (14).

Sandeman and Yang treated 16 patients with chemotherapy. Histologic review of the primary orchiectomy specimen showed vascular invasion in all 16. Nine patients also received abdominal radiation therapy after orchiectomy. Five patients had persistent elevated serum biochemical markers after orchiectomy. Chemotherapy consisted of either vinblastine and bleomycin or cisplatin, vinblastine, and bleomycin. The median follow-up was 60 months (range, 24 to 120 months). There were two relapses after adjuvant chemotherapy and one before starting. Only one patient died of disease. A 94% overall survival rate was attained (15).

Gimmi et al. treated 28 high-risk patients after orchiectomy. High risk was defined as the presence of embryonal carcinoma (23 patients), pT stage of 2 or greater (18 patients), or both (16 patients). Chemotherapy consisted of cisplatin and bleomycin plus either vinblastine or etoposide. At a median follow-up of 30 months (range, 7 to 74 months), all patients were alive and free of disease (16).

Pont et al. started a prospective study in 1985 in which patients with vascular invasion were assigned to two courses of adjuvant chemotherapy with cisplatin, etoposide, and bleomycin. Patients free of vascular invasion after orchiectomy were placed in a surveillance program. At a median follow-up of 30 months (range, 3 to 50 months), there was one relapse in the surveillance group of 22 patients (4.5%) and two relapses in the adjuvant chemotherapy group of 18 patients (11%). Two patients in the chemotherapy group died, one of lung cancer and one of progressive germ cell cancer. The overall survival rate was 100% in the surveillance group and 91% in the chemotherapy group. The authors concluded that low- and high-risk clinical stage I NSGCTT can be identified by the presence of vascular invasion. The presence of embryonal carcinoma and vascular invasion was interrelated. In 94% of patients with blood vessel invasion, the invading histologic element was embryonal carcinoma. Pont et al. concluded that two courses of adjuvant chemotherapy appeared to decrease the relapse rate in high-risk patients but was not entirely preventive (17).

From 1984 to 1988, Made and Pawinski treated 72 patients with clinical stage I NSGCTT. Thirty patients were selected for adjuvant chemotherapy because of vascular or lymphatic invasion or involvement in the rete testis or epididymis. Chemotherapy consisted of three courses of cisplatin, vinblastine, and bleomycin. The other 42 patients were managed by surveillance. One of 42 patients in the surveillance arm had a relapse at 16 months but was free of disease after chemotherapy and remained so for longer than 32 months. No relapses occurred in the adjuvant chemotherapy arm. All 72 patients were alive and disease-free for a follow-up period of 12 months to longer than 60 months (18). As in the study by Pont et al., it must be emphasized that these studies were not randomized—patients were selected because of the poor prognostic features evident in the primary tumor specimen.

Oliver et al. also selected patients with clinical stage I NSGCTT for adjuvant chemotherapy. Twenty-two patients with a high or intermediate risk of relapse according to the medical research council (United Kingdom) prognostic factor analysis were treated with two courses of adjuvant chemotherapy. The chemotherapy consisted of etoposide, bleomycin, and cisplatin. An additional 19 patients with a low relapse risk were observed after orchiectomy. With a median follow-up of 43 months, one patient (5%) in the adjuvant chemotherapy arm had a relapse at 6 months and later died of disease, despite achieving a 4-month complete remission following salvage chemotherapy. Three patients (6%) in the surveillance group had relapses; all were successfully treated with chemotherapy. The survival rates were 95% and 100%, respectively (19).

Studer et al. treated 41 patients with high-risk clinical stage I NSGCTT with one or more risk factors (embryonal carcinoma, 39; vascular invasion, 18; and testicular capsular penetration,

5). Patients were treated with two courses of adjuvant chemotherapy consisting of cisplatin, bleomycin, and either etoposide or vinblastine. With a median follow-up of 39 months, there was one relapse (2%) of mature teratoma in the iliac region after 2 years. After subsequent surgical excision, the patient remained free of disease for 2 years. The survival rate was 100% (20).

Cullen et al. treated 115 high-risk patients after orchiectomy. High risk was defined as the presence of any three or all four of the following: vascular invasion, lymphatic invasion, undifferentiated cells, and absence of endodermal sinus tumor. This risk predicted a 50% or more chance of recurrence. Patients received two courses of chemotherapy consisting of bleomycin, etoposide, and cisplatin. At a median follow-up of 25 months (range, 0 to 6 years), two relapses (2%) have occurred. The authors concluded that two courses of adjuvant chemotherapy reduced the risk of relapse to 2% from an expected 50% or more in this high-risk clinical stage I NSGCTT group (21). As in the previous studies mentioned, it must again be emphasized that this study was not randomized; patients were selected because of the poor prognostic features evident in the primary tumor specimen.

The adjuvant chemotherapy strategy should be evaluated more extensively in the academic medical setting as an alternative to the standard options for patients with clinical stage I NSGCTT. This is true even though no randomized trials have been performed. Results of adjuvant chemotherapy appear to be as good as those after RPLND, and adjuvant chemotherapy may reduce the need for strict patient compliance associated with surveillance programs. Phase III randomized trials may be indicated.

STAGE II

Traditional management of clinical stage II NSGCTT of the testis, defined as a retroperitoneal mass smaller than 10 cm in maximum transverse diameter, has been RPLND. This has served not only as a therapeutic modality, but also as a staging technique to identify those patients who would benefit from additional therapy. Historically, when used as the sole therapeutic modality, RPLND effectively controls local disease in more than 95% of patients with microscopic stage II disease and cures up to 65% of patients with stage IIB (less than or equal to 2 cm) and 40% of patients with stage IIC (greater than 2 and less than or equal to 5 cm) disease (22, 23).

Relapse rates after RPLND alone increased with increasing bulk of retroperitoneal disease, ranging from 25 to 50% for stage IIB and IIC to almost 80% for stage IID (greater than 5 cm and less than or equal to 10 cm) disease. RPLND is an inadequate therapeutic procedure for many patients with clinical stage II disease; when used as the primary treatment modality, most patients require additional chemotherapy. Optimal management would be to use one form of therapy without the need for a subsequent modality. However, the question remains, which primary therapy?

Adjuvant Chemotherapy

The clinical staging system used at the M. D. Anderson Cancer Center for patients with stage II NSGCTT covers the spectrum, ranging from elevated and rising serum biomarkers after an orchiectomy to viable retroperitoneal disease of less than 10 cm in diameter (24). Patients in the clinical stage II category share the following characteristics: a high cure rate with combination chemotherapy and surgery, curative potential for a portion of the patients with surgery, and a common therapeutic dilemma. The therapeutic options for these patients include the use of surgery only, surgery and chemotherapy, or chemotherapy only.

Stage II NSGCTT has traditionally been treated with primary retroperitoneal lymphadenectomy. In this setting, RPLND dissection has served not only as a therapeutic technique, but also as an indicator of the need for additional therapy.

A multiinstitutional trial by the Intergroup Testicular Cancer Study between May 1979 and October 1984 entered 195 evaluable patients who had pathologic stage II testicular cancer into a randomized, controlled clinical trial comparing two strategies of management. One strategy involved monthly examination plus chemotherapy if there was evidence of recurrent disease (control group). The other strategy involved administering two cycles of multiagent chemotherapy beginning 2 to 4 weeks after completion of surgery (adjuvant therapy group). The adjuvant chemotherapy was either cisplatin, vinblastine, and bleomycin (CVB) or cisplatin, cyclophosphamide, dactinomcyin, bleomycin, and vinblastine (VAB-6 regimen) (23, 25, 26). The patients had been monitored for a minimum of 2.5 years. At entry into the study, the randomized groups were comparable regarding surgical treatment, extent of disease, pathologic data, and serum biomarkers. Tumor recurred in 48 of 98 patients (49%) in the control group, and 5 patients died (3 of tumor). Tumor recurred in 6 of 97 patients (6%) in the adjuvant therapy group. Five of these six patients, however, had not received adjuvant therapy either because of refusal (one patient) or because disease recurred between assignment and the initiation of therapy (four patients).

The disease-free survival rates for the two groups were significantly different. However, the difference between the overall survival rates was not. Similarly, the difference in death due to testicular cancer was not significant. Most recurrences in the control arm were categorized as small volume disease. Recurrence appeared more frequently in the lungs, which is more easily monitored, than in the retroperitoneum. Patients who had relapses responded well to chemotherapy, achieving a complete remission in more than 90% of cases. In this study, the data demonstrated that in selected patients close observation following RPLND is as safe as administering two immediate postoperative courses of chemotherapy.

From another multinstitutional trial by the Testicular Tumor Study Group, Hartlapp et al. published the results of a randomized trial of the necessity and extent of adjuvant chemotherapy in stage IIA and IIB patients (27). A total of 210 patients were evaluated (48 stage IIA patients and 162 stage IIB patients). In stage IIA disease, there were no relapses in 32 patients after two cycles of vinblastine, bleomycin, and cisplatin (VBP) and only one relapse in 16 patients (6%) who were assigned to the surveillance group after RPLND. Patients with stage IIB disease were randomized to two versus four courses of VBP chemotherapy. Of the 87 patients randomized to two cycles, 3 (3%) had relapses, whereas 1 of 75 patients (1%) given four courses of chemotherapy had relapses. Of the patients randomized to two cycles, 85% received chemotherapy as planned, whereas only 48% of those who were to have received four courses finished therapy.

Motzer et al. treated 51 patients with pathologic stage II disease who had a predicted recurrence rate of more than 50% with observation. Criteria included more than five lymph nodes involved, any involved lymph node greater than 2 cm in diameter, or extranodal involvement. Chemotherapy consisted of two courses of etoposide and cisplatin. Fifty of 51 patients completed the two cycles of adjuvant chemotherapy. One patient had a marker surge during the first course of chemotherapy and successfully completed four courses. With a median follow-up of 30 months (range, 5 to 68 months), all patients are alive and relapse free. The survival rate was 100% (28).

The combination of retroperitoneal lymphadenectomy and adjuvant chemotherapy can cure virtually all patients with pathologic stage II disease. In the Intergroup study, no difference in survival in the two arms was appreciable. Survival was not impaired by close observation and treatment on relapse. The observation approach appears to be as safe as administering two immediate postoperative courses of chemotherapy. Treatment at relapse required the use of three or four courses of chemotherapy, with the possibility of surgical resection of residual disease.

The results of the Intergroup trial have been widely accepted. However, the trial did not really clarify the approach to the treatment with clinical stage II NSGCTT for various reasons. The median numbers of pathologically positive nodes were three in the control arm and two in the adjuvant arm. To identify patients with such small numbers of pathologically positive nodes, the investigators must have routinely required RPLND for patients presenting with clinical stage I disease. If the endpoint of the study is a reduction in complications, it would be important to incorporate into the analysis the influence of using a therapeutic approach normally used in stage II disease for patients with clinical stage I disease.

The Intergroup study did not demonstrate that RPLND performed on patients with clinical stage II disease can reduce the total amount of chemotherapy. Clinically defined stage II disease is likely to have a higher volume of retroperitoneal disease than the median of two pathologically positive nodes identified in the adjuvant arm of the Intergroup study. Such a misinterpretation of the data may result in a higher relapse rate than that achieved with the Intergroup study if only two courses of adjuvant chemotherapy are used.

Two earlier trials from the Memorial Sloan-Kettering Cancer Center illustrate the high curability of early stage II disease managed according to surgical staging (29, 30). Ten percent of the surgical stage IIA tumors recurred with pulmonary metastases, emphasizing the need for close follow-up and the prompt institution of aggressive combination chemotherapy. None of the patients with surgical stage IIA disease treated with mini-VAB had recurrence and none of the 17 patients with surgical stage IIB tumor treated aggressively with VAB-3 had recurrence, compared with a recurrence rate of 37% among the 24 patients treated adjunctively by actinomycin D plus chlorambucil or mini-VAB. Factors influencing the relapse rate were the nodal category and chemotherapy used. Based on this, the recommendation was for patients with resected stage IIB disease, particularly those with extranodal extension of tumor, to receive aggressive adjuvant chemotherapy.

Pizzocaro and Monfardini concluded that patients with pathologic stages IIA and IIB disease could be treated safely at the time of recurrence, while adjuvant chemotherapy would be reserved for those with stage IIC cancer (31). In a retrospective analysis by Richie and Kantoff, a similar conclusion was reached, i.e., that RPLND alone is adequate treatment for the majority of patients with pathologic stage IIA testicular cancer. Adjunctive chemotherapy should be reserved for recurrence (32).

In patients with pathologic stage II nonseminomatous testicular cancer, judicious use of prognostic factors may help select those who may benefit from chemotherapy after retroperitoneal lymphadenectomy. In most cases, adjuvant chemotherapy requires only two cycles of drugs. Observation is a satisfactory approach; however, follow-up must be meticulous and compliance is crucial.

Primary Chemotherapy for Clinical Stage II Disease

With the success in treating stage III nonseminomatous germ cell tumors with chemotherapy at the University of Texas M. D. Anderson Cancer Center, we questioned whether patients with stage II NSGCTT would benefit from receiving chemotherapy rather than surgery as the primary treatment modality. We therefore began a protocol of primary chemotherapy for clinical stage II disease (retroperitoneal mass smaller than 10 cm in maximum transverse diameter). We based the trial on the hypothesis that some patients may be cured without the need for subsequent surgery; therefore, these patients would be spared the morbidity of double therapy. From 1982 to 1985, 50 patients with clinical stage II NSGCTT of the testis were evaluated; 7 patients underwent primary RPLND and 43 received primary chemotherapy consisting of cisplatin, cyclophosphamide, and doxorubicin, alternating with vinblastine and bleomycin (CISCA-II, VB-IV) (Fig. 53.1) (33, 34). Chemotherapy was delivered in a flexible number of courses, according to individual patient response. Patients received two additional courses of chemotherapy after achieving either a complete remission (defined as normal serum biomarker levels and a radiographically negative abdomen) or stable radiographic mass and normal serum markers. The latter patients then underwent RPLND. Of the 50 patients, 48 achieved long-term disease-free survival and 39 were spared RPLND. Histologic tumor type was the most important predictor of the need for postchemotherapy node dissection. Eleven patients with embryonal

plus teratomatous elements required RPLND, whereas only two patients with embryonal and/or seminomatous elements required retroperitoneal lymphadenectomy.

We concluded from this experience that aggressive chemotherapy delivered to patients with clinical stage II NSGCTT can achieve a very high complete remission rate. This complete remission rate is equivalent to that of patients with pathologically defined stage II disease.

Experience with primary chemotherapy in stage II NSGCTT at other centers has resulted in similar excellent survival rates. Peckham treated 52 clinical stage II patients with bleomycin, etoposide, and cisplatin (PEB) or etoposide and cisplatin (EP). Ninety-six percent of the patients were alive and disease free for a median follow-up of 36 months (range, 12 to 82 months). Approximately 25% required postchemotherapy RPLND (51% with teratomatous elements versus 20% without) (35).

Socinski et al. treated 19 patients who had low-volume clinical stage II disease with four courses of cisplatin, vinblastine, and bleomycin. All were free of disease at a median follow-up of 22 months (range, 6 to 59 months); 13 patients (68%) after chemotherapy alone and 6 patients (32%) after postchemotherapy retroperitoneal lymphadenectomy (36).

Vugrin and Whitmore treated 17 patients with stage II disease using VAB-4, VAB-5, or VAB-6. A complete remission was obtained in 13 patients (76%), and 4 patients required a retroperitoneal lymphadenectomy to obtain complete remission (37). The most consistent predictor of need for postchemotherapy RPLND was the presence of teratomatous elements in the primary tumor.

Oliver et al. treated 44 patients with clinical stage II disease with three or four courses of BEP or PVB chemotherapy. Seventy-seven percent of patients achieved a complete remission with chemotherapy alone, whereas six patients (14%) required a postchemotherapy retroperitoneal lymphadenectomy (38).

In summary, stage II NSGCTT of the testis can be effectively treated with either primary RPLND with or without adjuvant chemotherapy or with primary chemotherapy with selected postchemotherapy resection of residual masses. The goal is to avoid unnecessary double therapy. When treating patients with clinical stage II NSGCTT, our purpose is to maintain the present high cure rate and simultaneously to reduce the frequency of unnecessary therapy. Extent of tumor burden and histologic type of the primary tumor allow for rational selection. At the M. D. Anderson Cancer Center, patients with embryonal carcinoma receive primary chemotherapy for stage II disease, whereas those with teratomatous elements and limited stage II tumors undergo primary RPLND.

CONCLUSION

To minimize morbidity and increase the likelihood of tumor-free survival, we must evaluate and stage patients carefully, paying particular attention to the histologic assessment of the primary tumor. To do this, we evaluate the relative proportion of different tumor cell types, presence of vascular and lymphatic invasion, pretreatment tumor markers, and T stage of the pri-

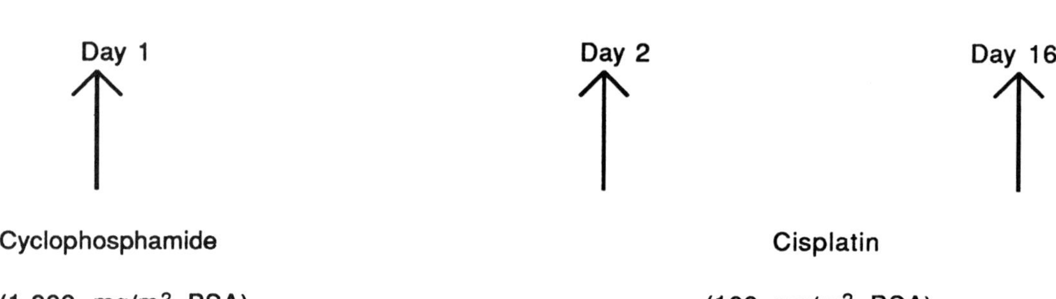

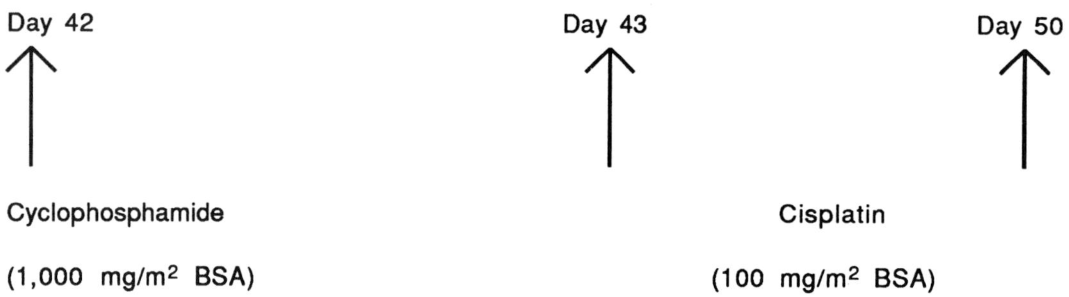

Fig. 53.1. Cyclophosphamide plus sequential cisplatin. BSA: Body surface area.

mary tumor. Patients are then stratified for specific treatment regimens. For those in whom the disease is confined to the testis and who have no risk factors, we consider surveillance after radical orchiectomy to be safe and effective therapy and will spare these patients the morbidity of RPLND. In our experience, approximately one third of stage I patients make up this group, which thus far has a relapse rate of 0%. For those patients with stage I disease and any risk factors, the relapse rate is approximately 50%. If there are teratomatous elements in the primary tumor, relapse is most likely to occur in the retroperitoneum, and these patients are treated primarily with RPLND. For those patients with predominant embryonal carcinoma (greater than or equal to 80%), 50% relapse; the recurrences are distributed equally between the retroperitoneum and chest. Choice of treatment for these patients is less obvious. Retroperitoneal lymphadenectomy or surveillance both lead to excellent survival rates. The third option (based on prognostic factor analysis), adjuvant chemotherapy after orchiectomy, has proven to be effective in a number of phase II trials.

For those patients with clinical stage II disease and embryonal carcinoma, we may well be able to omit lymphadenec-tomy because primary chemotherapy can totally eradicate retroperitoneal disease. Approximately 80% of these patients will not require RPLND and will not experience the morbidity of combined treatments. Further, cure rates are equivalent to those achieved with primary RPLND and adjuvant chemotherapy. However, for those patients with stage II disease and teratomatous components in the primary tumor, the higher incidence of postchemotherapy residual mass makes primary retroperitoneal lymphadenectomy the best choice for initial therapy. For those patients who have had minimal retroperitoneal disease completely resected and a favorable histologic type, we can thus avoid extensive chemotherapy.

Overall, our experience with strategies to avoid RPLND indicates that we can stratify patients to receive appropriate therapy, which minimizes morbidity and preserves a high level of tumor-free survival.

REFERENCES

1. Raghavan D, Colls B, Levi J, et al. Surveillance for stage I nonseminomatous germ cell tumours of the testis: the optimal protocol has not yet been defined. Br J Urol 1988;61:522.

2. Fung CY, Garnick MB. Clinical stage I carcinoma of the testis: a review. J Clin Oncol 1988;6:734.

3. McLeod DG, Weiss RB, Stablein DM, et al. Staging relationships and outcome in early stage testicular cancer: a report from the Testicular Cancer Intergroup study. J Urol 1991;45:1178.

4. Scher HI, Sternberg CN. Chemotherapy of urologic malignancies. Semin Urol 1985;3:239.

5. Sternberg CN, Bosl G. Advances in testicular cancer: role of chemotherapy. Prog Clin Biol Res 1988;277:79.

6. Freidman LS, Parkinson MC, Jones WG, et al. Histopathology in the prediction of relapse of patients with stage I testicular teratoma treated by orchiectomy alone. Lancet 1987;2:294.

7. Fung CY, Kalish LA, Brodsky GL, et al. Stage I nonseminomatous germ cell testicular tumor: prediction of metastatic potential by primary histopathology. J Clin Oncol 1988;6:1467.

8. Mead GM, Stenning SP, Parkinson MC, et al. The second medical research council study of prognostic factors in nonseminomatous germ cell tumors. J Clin Oncol 1992;10:85.

9. Hesketh PJ, Krane RJ. Prognostic assessment in nonseminomatous testicular cancer: implications for therapy. J Urol 1990;144:1.

10. Dunphy CH, Ayala AG, Swanson DA, et al. Clinical stage I nonseminomatous and mixed germ cell tumors of the testis. Cancer 1988;62:1202.

11. Sternberg CN. Role of primary chemotherapy in stage I and low-volume stage II nonseminomatous germ-cell testis tumors. Urol Clin North Am 1993;20:93.

12. Ansfield FJ, Korbitz BC, Davis HL Jr, et al. Triple drug therapy in testicular tumors. Cancer 1969;24:442.

13. Skinner DG. Nonseminomatous testis tumors: a plan of management based on 96 patients to improve survival in all stages by combined therapeutic modalities. J Urol 1976;115: 65.

14. Ekman EP, Edsmyr F. Chemotherapy in nonseminomatous testicular tumours stage I. Br J Urol 1981;53:184.

15. Sandeman TF, Yang C. Results of adjuvant chemotherapy for low-stage nonseminomatous germ cell tumors of the testis with vascular invasion. Cancer 1988;62:1471.

16. Gimmi C, Sonntag R, Brunner K, et al. Adjuvant treatment of high risk (HR) clinical stage I testicular carcinoma (TC) with cisplatin (C), bleomycin (B) and vinblastine (V) or etoposide (E). Proc Am Soc Clin Oncol 1990;9:140.

17. Pont J, Wolfgang H, Kosak D, et al. Risk-adapted treatment choice in stage I nonseminomatous testicular germ cell cancer by regarding vascular invasion in the primary tumor: a prospective trial. J Clin Oncol 1990;8:16.

18. Made JG, Pawinski A. Risk-related adjuvant chemotherapy for stage I non-seminoma of the testis. Clin Oncol 1991;3:270.

19. Oliver TRD, Raja MA, Ong J, et al. Pilot study to evaluate impact of a policy of adjuvant chemotherapy for high risk stage I malignant teratoma on overall relapse rate of stage I cancer patients. J Urol 1992;148:1453.

20. Studer UE, Fey MF, Calderoni A, et al. Adjuvant chemotherapy after orchiectomy in high-risk patients with clinical stage I nonseminomatous testicular cancer. Eur Urol 1993;3:444.

21. Cullen MH, Stenning SP, Parkinson MC, et al. Short course adjuvant chemotherapy in high risk stage I non-seminomatous germ cell tumours of the testis (NSGCTT). Proc Am Soc Clin Oncol 1995;1679.

22. Donohue JP, Einhorn LH, Perez JM. Improved management of nonseminomatous testis tumors. Cancer 1978;42:2903.

23. Williams SD, Stablein DM, Einhorn LH, et al. Immediate adjuvant chemotherapy versus observation with treatment at relapse in pathological stage II testicular cancer. N Engl J Med 1987;317:1433.

24. Logothetis CJ. The case of relevant staging of germ cell tumors. Cancer 1989;65:709.

25. DeWys WD. Basis for adjuvant chemotherapy for stage II testicular cancer. Cancer Treat Rep 1979;63:1693.

26. DeWys WD, Green SB, Einhorn LH, et al. Adjuvant chemotherapy for testicular cancer. In: Jones SE, Salmon SE, eds. Adjuvant therapy of cancer. Orlando, FL: Grune & Stratton, 1984;4:529.

27. Hartlapp JH, Weissbach L, Bussar-Maatz R. Adjuvant chemotherapy in nonseminomatous testicular tumour stage II. Int J Androl 1987;10:277.

28. Motzer RJ, Bajorin DF, Bosl GJ, et al. Etoposide (E) and Cisplatin (P) is effective adjuvant chemotherapy (CT) in patients (PTS) with stage II nonseminomatous germ cell tumors (NSGCT) following retroperitoneal lymph node dissection (RPLND). Proc Am Soc Clin Oncol 1995:313.

29. Bredael JJ, Vugrin D, Whitmore WF Jr. Selected experience with surgery and combination chemotherapy in the treatment of nonseminomatous testis tumors. J Urol 1982;129:985.

30. Vugrin D, Whitmore WF Jr, Cvitkovic E, et al. Adjuvant chemotherapy in nonseminomatous testis cancer: Mini-VAB regimen: long-term follow-up. J Urol 1980;126:49.

31. Pizzocaro G, Monfardini S. No adjuvant chemotherapy in selected patients with pathologic stage II nonseminomatous germ cell tumors of the testis. J Urol 1983;131:677.

32. Richie JP, Kantoff PW. Is adjuvant chemotherapy necessary for patients with stage B1 testicular cancer? J Clin Oncol 1991;9:1393.

33. Logothetis CJ, Samuels ML, Selig DE, et al. Primary chemotherapy followed by a selective retroperitoneal lymphadenectomy in the management of clinical stage II testicular carcinoma: a preliminary report. J Urol 1985;134: 127.

34. Logothetis CJ, Swanson DA, Dexeus F, et al. Primary chemotherapy for clinical stage II nonseminomatous germ cell tumors of the testis: a follow-up of 50 patients. J Clin Oncol 1987;5:906.

35. Peckham MJ, Hendry WF. Clinical stage II nonseminomatous germ cell testicular tumours: results of management by primary chemotherapy. Br J Urol 1985;57:763.

36. Socinski MA, Garnick MB, Stomper PC, et al. Stage II nonseminomatous germ cell tumors of the testis: an analysis of treatment options in patients with low volume retroperitoneal disease. J Urol 1988;140:1437.

37. Vugrin D, Whitmore WF. The role of chemotherapy and surgery in the treatment of retroperitoneal metastases in advanced nonseminomatous testis cancer. Cancer 1984;55: 1874.

38. Oliver RTD, Dhaliwal HS, Hope-Stone HF. Short-course etoposide, bleomycin and cisplatin in the treatment of metastatic germ cell tumours: appraisal of its potential as adjuvant chemotherapy for stage I testis tumours. Br J Urol 1988;61:53.

54

Chemotherapy and Radiation Therapy for Wilms' Tumor

Marilyn H. Duncan
Stuart S. Winter

Wilms' tumor was first described in 1899 and is a malignant neoplasm of the kidney. It commonly presents as a fixed, bulging, and painless flank mass in toddlers and young children. Wilms' tumor can occasionally present with constitutional symptoms of fever and malaise. Anemia and hematuria may result from tumor extension into the renal pelvis, whereas local obstruction of the renal vasculature may cause hypertension (1). Wilms' tumor arises from nephrogenic blastemal cells and is characterized by a triad of microscopic findings—blastema, stroma, and nephrogenic epithelial tissue.

Wilms' tumor can occur in both sporadic and heritable forms. In 1972, Knudson initially proposed that the syndromes associated with Wilms' tumor represent a "two hit" mechanism of oncogenesis (2). Heritable forms of Wilms' tumor were hypothesized to involve a second mutation in an inherited gene defect, whereas sporadic cases involved two acquired gene mutations resulting in a "loss of heterozygosity." Beckwith-Wiedemann syndrome, hemihypertrophy, and aniridia have been associated with Wilms' tumor, as well as syndromes involving urogenital malformations, including WAGR syndrome (Wilms' tumor, aniridia, genital malformations, and mental retardation), Denys-Drash syndrome, and Perlman syndrome (3). Several tumor suppressor genes are involved in the pathogenesis of Wilms' tumor, two of which are located on 11p13 and 11p15.5 (3, 4). The suppressor gene located on 11p13 (WT1) has been recently cloned (5). The gene product is a zinc finger DNA-binding protein that is involved in the control of human genitourinary development (4, 5). Loss of heterozygosity at 16q and 1p has been associated with adverse outcomes in Wilms' tumor (6). Research efforts to understand the significance of these genes are currently underway.

Major contributions to success in the treatment of Wilms' tumor have come from the organized study of multidisciplinary cancer treatment, including surgery, radiation therapy, and chemotherapy. Over the past 4 decades, the discovery of effective treatment of Wilms' tumor has dramatically improved long-term survival rates. The decreasing mortality rate observed among children with all stages of Wilms' tumor has resulted from the use of more effective chemotherapy rather than from earlier detection of the disease or a change in incidence (7, 8). The long-term survival rate among children with Wilms' tumor has risen from approximately 30% with surgery alone to greater than 80% with current therapeutic regimens (9–21).

The first National Wilms' Tumor Study (NWTS) trials began in 1969 (10). Participation in NWTS protocols is currently the standard management for most children with Wilms' tumor diagnosed in the United States. Sequential prospective randomized clinical trials conducted by the NWTS have addressed important questions regarding epidemiology (22), histopathology (18, 19, 23–27), and combined modality treatment including surgery, chemotherapy, and radiation therapy (9–13, 17–19, 28–34). Information gained from the NWTS trials has made significant contributions to the multidisciplinary management of patients with Wilms' tumor. Cooperative trials in Europe have also addressed important aspects of Wilms' tumor management (14–16, 20, 21). The successful treatment of Wilms' tumor requires multidisciplinary cooperation among urologic surgeons, pathologists, pediatric oncologists, and radiation therapists. Chemotherapy has routinely been given in all stages of Wilms' tumor to supplement surgery and to achieve control of both microresidual and overt metastatic disease.

CLINICAL STAGING AND HISTOLOGY TYPE (NWTS)

Patients entering NWTS trials have been categorized by clinical stage and histologic type at the time of surgery (10–13, 17–19, 23, 27, 29, 31, 32). Clinical staging of Wilms' tumor must be accurate at the time of initial diagnosis because this information is necessary for optimal therapy and prediction of

STAGE I

Tumor is limited to kidney and is completely excised.

The surface of the renal capsule is intact. Tumor was not ruptured before or during removal. There is no residual tumor apparent beyond the margins of resection.

STAGE II

Tumor extends beyond the kidney but is completely excised.

There is regional extension of the tumor, i.e., penetration through the outer surface of the renal capsule into the perirenal soft tissues. Vessels outside the kidney substance are infiltrated or contain tumor thrombus. The tumor may have been biopsied or there has been local spillage of tumor confined to the flank. There is no residual tumor apparent at or beyond the margins of excision.

STAGE III

Residual nonhematogenous tumor confined to abdomen.

Any one or more of the following occur:

  a. Lymph nodes on biopsy are found to be involved in the hilus, the periaortic chains, or beyond.

  b. There has been diffuse peritoneal contamination by tumor such as by spillage of tumor beyond the flank before or during surgery, or by tumor growth that has penetrated through the peritoneal surface.

  c. Implants are found on the peritoneal surfaces.

  d. The tumor extends beyond the surgical margins either microscopically or grossly.

  e. The tumor is not completely resectable because of local infiltration into vital structures.

STAGE IV

Hematogenous metastases.

Deposits beyond stage III, e.g., lung, liver, bone, and brain.

STAGE V

Bilateral renal involvement at diagnosis.

An attempt should be made to stage each side according to the above criteria on the basis of extent of disease before biopsy.*

* The clinicopathologic stage is determined by the surgeon and the pathologist, who also determines whether the histologic features are favorable or unfavorable.

prognosis. Clinical stage is ascertained by the surgeon in the operating room and by the pathologist, who further establishes whether the histologic type is favorable (FH) or unfavorable (UH). Wilms' tumor types with unfavorable histology, currently treated on NWTS protocols, include those with focal or diffuse anaplasia and sarcomatous features (18, 23, 26, 27). The current NWTS clinicopathologic staging system is summarized in Table 54.1 (13).

HISTOPATHOLOGIC CONSIDERATIONS AND PROGNOSIS

The histologic classification system derived from analysis of NWTS data has good correlation with clinical outcome (13,

18, 19, 29, 31, 32). In NWTS-1, 11% of children had renal tumors with unfavorable histologic features. These children had a much higher tumor-related mortality rate than the children with favorable histologic characteristics (57% versus 7%) (23). Other pathologic findings that correlated with the increased risk of local and/or distant relapse included the following: large tumor mass, capsule penetration, direct extension to adjacent organs, and involvement of regional lymph nodes (29). On the basis of these findings, staging and treatment protocols for subsequent NWTS trials have been modified to intensify therapy for high-risk histologic types, regardless of stage, and to reduce therapy for patients with localized disease and favorable histologic types (9–13, 17–19, 31, 32).

IMAGING STUDIES

A child found to have an abdominal mass requires a plain radiograph of the abdomen. Wilms' tumor usually does not cross the midline and typically does not exhibit intraparenchymal calcification (in contrast to neuroblastoma). Abdominal ultrasonography should always be performed. The procedure is safe and can yield important information about tumor extension into regional vessels, including the renal veins, inferior vena cava, and right atrium. Abdominal computed tomography (CT) studies can guide the surgeon to biopsy suspicious regional lymph nodes and areas suggestive of tumor extension. Because distant metastatic disease commonly involves the lungs, a preoperative chest radiograph must be obtained. In the event the chest radiograph is normal, a chest CT is not currently recommended preoperatively (35). Patients with advanced disease or UH, e.g., malignant rhabdoid tumor of the kidney or clear cell sarcoma of the kidney, should have more extensive postoperative imaging. Depending on the stage and histologic type, additional studies including CT of the chest and abdomen, skeletal survey, radionuclide bone scan, and cranial imaging may be necessary to evaluate distant sites for metastatic disease and to complete the staging workup (19, 35, 36).

ACTIVE CHEMOTHERAPY AGENTS

Current therapy for most children with Wilms' tumor includes radical nephrectomy, followed by combination chemotherapy with or without postoperative radiation therapy (9–21). Three drugs constitute first-line therapy against Wilms' tumor—actinomycin D, vincristine, and doxorubicin (Adriamycin). The development of effective chemotherapeutic regimens using these drugs has led to dramatic improvement in the overall survival rate from Wilms' tumor (7–21).

A number of other chemotherapy agents have activity against Wilms' tumor and are being tested in the treatment of children with high-risk or recurrent tumors.

Actinomycin D (Dactinomycin)

In the late 1950s, Farber reported that the antibiotic actinomycin D showed clinical activity against Wilms' tumor. Dramatic tumor regressions were observed in children with advanced metastatic disease. A prospective trial demonstrated improved survival in patients with Wilms' tumor who received nephrectomy followed by postoperative chemotherapy with actinomycin D and radiation therapy. Pulmonary metastases were also curable by chemotherapy and radiation (37). Following confirmation of these results by other investigators (38), cooperative group studies using standardized protocols were organized to answer questions systematically regarding therapy (39–41). The NWTS-3 and NWTS-4 have shown that actinomycin D is efficacious when given on a "pulse-intensive" schedule using single-day doses given more frequently than the standard divided-dose schedule (17).

Vincristine

Vincristine was identified as an active antitumor agent for the treatment of Wilms' tumor in the early 1960s (42, 43). When used as adjuvant chemotherapy following surgery and postoperative radiation therapy, vincristine produced survival rates comparable to those reported for actinomycin D (43). Southwest Oncology Group investigators found that vincristine combined with radiation therapy was an effective treatment of metastatic disease in patients unresponsive to actinomycin D (44).

Adriamycin

The anthracycline antibiotic Adriamycin is active against Wilms' tumor. Early clinical trials of Adriamycin demonstrated regression of metastatic disease in advanced, refractory Wilms' tumor (45, 46). The potential for cardiac toxicity in patients receiving Adriamycin has required that it be used cautiously in the management of children with Wilms' tumor. The NWTS-2 found that surgery and radiation therapy combined with three-agent chemotherapy (Adriamycin, actinomycin D, and vincristine) were better than two-agent chemotherapy (actinomycin D and vincristine) for patients with stages II, III, and IV (FH) tumors (11).

In NWTS-3, the survival for stage III (FH) patients and all stages of clear cell sarcoma was best when three-agent chemotherapy with Adriamycin, actinomycin D, and vincristine was combined with low-dose radiation therapy (13, 19).

Other Drugs

Cyclophosphamide and its chemical analog ifosfamide have activity against Wilms' tumor in patients with high-risk and recurrent disease (47–49). Because cyclophosphamide was useful in the treatment of soft tissue sarcomas, the NWTS-3 added the drug to the combination chemotherapy regimen for patients with UH tumors.

On both NWTS-3 and NWTS-4, patients with stages II to IV diffuse anaplasia had a much better 4-year relapse-free survival rate (55% versus 27%) when a four-drug regimen including cyclophosphamide, Adriamycin, actinomycin D, and

vincristine was compared with the same three-drug regimen without cyclophosphamide (18).

Studies of both high-dose cyclophosphamide and ifosfamide with mesna bladder protection and hyperhydration have demonstrated promising antitumor activity (49, 50). High-dose ifosfamide regimens have been associated with more nephrotoxicity, especially Fanconi renal syndrome, than cyclophosphamide-based regimens when administered to patients with only one kidney. Lower ifosfamide doses, however, may be highly effective and tolerable when used in combination regimens (50). Etoposide has also shown good activity against high-risk and recurrent Wilms' tumors both as a single agent and in combination with cyclophosphamide and ifosfamide (50–52). Carboplatin, an analog of cisplatin, is also an active agent in relapsed disease. This drug is relatively well tolerated in patients with a single kidney, especially if dosing is tailored to renal function and the patient is carefully monitored and supported during treatment (50, 53).

COMBINATION CHEMOTHERAPY REGIMENS

The use of effective front-line combination chemotherapy has had a major effect on the relapse-free survival rates of children with Wilms' tumor. NWTS-1, completed in 1974 (Table 54.2), showed that combination chemotherapy with actinomycin D and vincristine was superior to either agent used alone in children with locally advanced tumors (stages II and III) (10).

NWTS-2, finished in 1979 (Table 54.2), demonstrated that double-agent chemotherapy (vincristine and actinomycin D) improved the relapse-free survival for stage I patients by reducing the frequency of flank and distant recurrences. Furthermore, the length of treatment could be reduced from 15 months to 6 months without worsening the excellent (greater than 90%) survival rate. Triple-agent chemotherapy (Adriamycin, vincristine, and actinomycin D) was superior to double-agent chemotherapy (actinomycin D and vincristine) in stages II, III, and IV FH patients (11, 12).

The British Medical Research Council trial reported that maintenance chemotherapy with intensive vincristine was better than single-agent intermittent actinomycin D (54).

The NWTS-3, completed in 1985, found that survival (above 90%) for stage I FH patients was similar whether double-agent chemotherapy (vincristine and actinomycin D) was given for 6 months or 10 weeks. Patients with stage II FH tumors had excellent (approximately 90%) survival with double-agent chemotherapy (vincristine and actinomycin D) given for 15 months without radiation therapy. The addition of a third drug (Adriamycin) or radiation therapy (2000 cGy) made no difference in outcome. In stage III FH patients, three-agent chemotherapy (vincristine, actinomycin D, and Adriamycin), with either 1000 cGy or 2000 cGy radiation therapy, gave slightly better relapse-free survival (84%) than double-agent chemotherapy (74%). For all high-risk patients (stage IV FH or all stages UH), the addition of cyclophosphamide to standard

Table 54.2. Survival Rates, National Wilms' Tumor Studies I–III

| | | SURVIVAL RATE AT 4 YEARS (%) | |
| | | RELAPSE FREE | ALIVE |
GROUP/STAGE	THERAPY		
NWTS-1			
I(<2 y)	AMD × 15 mo, RT	89	94
	AMD × 15 mo, no RT	88	90
I(≥2 y)	AMD × 15 mo, RT	76	98
	AMD × 15 mo, no RT	57	81
II/III	AMD, RT	56	71
	VCR, RT	57	71
	AMD + VCR, RT	79	84
NWTS-2			
I	AMD + VCR × 6 mo, no RT	96	97
	AMD + VCR × 15 mo, no RT	90	91
II/III/IV	AMD + VCR × 15 mo, RT	65	74
	AMD + VCR + ADR × 15 mo, RT	79	84
NWTS-3 +			
I FH	AMD + VCR × 10 weeks vs. 6 months, no RT	90	97
II FH	AMD + VCR ± ADR × 15 months, ± RT (2000 cGy)	88	92
III FH	AMD + VCR ± ADR × 15 months, RT (1000 vs. 2000 cGy)	79	87
IV FH	AMD + VCR + ADR × 15 mo versus AMD + VCR + ADR + CPM × 15 mo, RT[a]	75	83
I/II/III/UH	Same	65	68
IV UH	Same	56	55
All Patients		83	89

RT, radiation therapy; AMD, actinomycin D; VCR, vincristine; ADR, Adriamycin; CPM, cyclophosphamide; FH, favorable histology; UH, unfavorable histology; cGy, centiGray (1 rad).
All patients received nephrectomy and cyclic chemotherapy.
[a] All stage IV FH patients received 2000 cGy flank RT and RT to other sites.
UH patients of all stages received age-adjusted flank RT and RT to other sites.
+ Chemotherapy Dosage:
AMD = 15 mcg/kg/d × 5d (IV) VCR = 1.5 mg/m^2/week (IV)
ADR = 20 mg/m^2/d × 3d (IV) CPM = 10 mg/kg/d × 3d (IV)

three-agent chemotherapy (vincristine, actinomycin D, and Adriamycin) did not improve the survival rate. Patients with stages II through IV for all anaplastic tumors did better (4-year survival rates, 82% versus 37%) on the four-agent regimen (cyclophosphamide plus Adriamycin, vincristine, and actinomycin D) than on the same three-agent regimen without cyclophosphamide. The subset of UH patients with stage I anaplastic and clear cell sarcoma tumors did relatively well (4-year survival rates, 89% and 75%, respectively) receiving three-agent chemotherapy (Adriamycin, vincristine, and actinomycin D) and radiation therapy (13, 18, 19).

The NWTS-4, a randomized, prospective clinical trial, was open from 1985 through 1994 and had the following objectives.

1. To simplify, shorten, and refine treatment methods for all children.
2. To test treatment hypotheses relating to chemotherapy dose intensity, schedule, and duration of treatment.
3. To collect epidemiologic data.
4. To correlate outcome with clinicopathologic stage and histologic type.

5. To evaluate long-term effects of treatment.

Patients were randomized both by stage and by whether the histologic type was FH or UH (either diffuse or focal anaplasia or clear cell sarcoma of kidney). Patients with stage I FH and anaplastic tumors received postoperative double-agent chemotherapy (actinomycin D and vincristine) for either 18 or 24 weeks without radiation therapy. In stage II FH tumors, postoperative double-agent chemotherapy (actinomycin D and vincristine) was given for a short course (18 or 22 weeks) or a longer course (60 or 65 weeks) without radiation therapy. Stages III and IV FH and stages I through IV clear cell sarcoma of the kidney received postoperative triple-agent chemotherapy (actinomycin D, vincristine, and Adriamycin) given for a short (26 weeks) or longer (65 weeks) course plus radiation therapy. Stages II through IV anaplastic tumors received postoperative three- or four-agent chemotherapy (actinomycin D, vincristine, Adriamycin ± cyclophosphamide) for 65 weeks plus radiation therapy. Adriamycin and actinomycin D, drugs given in a "pulse-intensive" manner, allowed higher doses of chemotherapy to be administered without greater hematologic toxicity (17, 18). Preliminary data from NWTS-4 show an almost 90%

overall survival rate for all patients treated for Wilms' tumor, suggesting that pulse-intensive therapy has not compromised the excellent progress made in earlier trials (DM Green, personal communication, 1995).

Early in the course of the NWTS-4, severe hepatic toxicity developed in a few patients receiving the pulse-intensive regimen. The dose of actinomycin D was modified and resulted in hepatic toxicity that was similar to that of the standard regimens (55).

NWTS-5 opened in mid-1995. The objectives of this trial are as follows.

1. To increase the survival rates for children with Wilms' tumor.
2. To decrease the acute and long-term morbidity of treatment associated with Wilms' tumor.
3. To determine if the loss of heterozygosity of 16q in tumor tissue is associated with a poorer prognosis.
4. To establish a tissue bank available for scientific analysis.
5. To develop guidelines for radiographic evaluation of previously undiagnosed patients.
6. To provide uniform treatment guidelines for children with relapsed Wilms' tumor (6, 35).

The NWTS-5 will also evaluate the role of surgery alone in children younger than 24 months of age with very favorable stage I FH tumors weighing less than 550 g. These patients will not routinely receive chemotherapy after nephrectomy but will be followed carefully with surveillance clinical examinations and imaging studies. Patients with unresectable abdominal tumors, intrahepatic, vena cava, or atrial extension of tumor at initial diagnosis will receive 6 weeks of prenephrectomy chemotherapy followed by reevaluation, surgery, and additional postoperative treatment. Patients having only diffuse intraoperative tumor spill and no other upstaging findings will be classified as having stage II instead of stage III disease. Patients who experience relapse after initial therapy will receive site- and histology-specific treatment including chemotherapy with cyclophosphamide, etoposide, and carboplatin followed by surgery and radiation therapy for sites of residual disease. Patients achieving a partial or complete remission will be considered for high-dose chemotherapy followed by autologous bone marrow transplantation, which has shown promise for a few patients with relapsed disease (56).

SPECIAL MANAGEMENT PROBLEMS

Bilateral Tumors

The prognosis for children with bilateral Wilms' tumors entered on the NWTS trials has been good. These children have had nearly 80% 3-year survival rates when managed with various treatment regimens including surgery, chemotherapy, and radiation therapy (57, 58). Treatment should be individualized to preserve as much renal parenchyma and function as possible

while obtaining tumor control. Current recommendations for the management of bilateral tumors on NWTS are individualized to the histologic type, stage, and response to treatment. General guidelines include the following.

1. Initial surgical exploration and complete excision when possible, bilateral biopsies and staging, and postoperative chemotherapy.
2. Second-look operation and complete tumor excision when possible or biopsies of remaining tumor followed by postoperative chemotherapy.
3. If persistent tumor is identified at the second-look operation, postoperative radiation therapy and more intensive chemotherapy are given.
4. Additional surgical procedures may be undertaken if there is evidence of persistent tumor and permitted by the clinical condition of the patient.

Inoperable Tumors

Experience in NWTS trials and European studies has shown that preoperative chemotherapy and radiation therapy can reduce tumor bulk and the risk of tumor rupture during nephrectomy (10, 11, 13–16, 59–61). Preoperative chemotherapy has proven benefit in cases where extensive intracaval and intraatrial tumor thrombus are found at diagnosis. Tumor shrinkage can lessen the likelihood of intraoperative tumor spillage and lessen the risk of tumor embolization; however, the tumor tissue can become quite fibrotic, making its removal more difficult (61).

Overall survival rates have not been significantly influenced by preoperative therapy, and accurate surgical staging information may be lost (60). For these reasons, current recommendations for the management of inoperable tumors after biopsy are as follows.

1. Initiate two-agent chemotherapy (vincristine and actinomycin D) for approximately 6 weeks while observing for tumor shrinkage, then
2. Reevaluate.

When adequate shrinkage has occurred, surgery should be performed. The NWTS studies have assumed that all patients receiving preoperative chemotherapy have stage III disease and require treatment with postoperative radiation therapy and chemotherapy (35, 61).

The International Society of Pediatric Oncology (SIOP) studies have not routinely given radiation therapy if the tumor is confined to the kidney (14, 15, 20, 21, 59).

RADIATION THERAPY

In the past, age-adjusted postoperative radiation therapy was given routinely to all children with Wilms' tumor, but its role in management has gradually been refined.

The results of the first three NWTS trials were as follows.

1. Routine, postoperative radiation therapy for the flank is not necessary for children with stage I FH or anaplastic tumors or for stage II FH tumors when postoperative two-drug chemotherapy with vincristine and actinomycin D is administered.
2. The prognosis for stage III FH patients is best when three-drug chemotherapy with actinomycin D, vincristine, and Adriamycin is combined with low-dose (1000 cGy) radiation therapy to the flank (10, 11, 13).

Radiation therapy is routinely delivered to distant sites of metastatic disease.

Sequential SIOP trials have evaluated both preoperative and postoperative radiation therapy in combined modality management of Wilms' tumor (14, 15, 20, 21, 59).

TOXICITY

In general, standard therapeutic regimens currently used in the treatment of Wilms' tumor are well tolerated. The most significant toxicities have been noted in children receiving both chemotherapy and radiation therapy and include myelosuppression, hepatic toxicity, and enhanced radiation reaction from actinomycin D and Adriamycin (17, 28, 33, 34, 55). The frequency of toxic deaths on the first three NWTS trials has been approximately 1 to 2% (10, 11–13, 30). Infants younger than 12 months of age are especially sensitive to chemotherapy and related toxicity. The chemotherapy dose given to infants is routinely decreased by 50%, an adjustment that has significantly reduced toxicity without apparent loss of therapeutic efficacy (33).

Radiation sequelae have resulted in cosmetic deformities and increased disease morbidity (20, 28, 34). The potential for the development of radiation-associated second malignancies is being evaluated in long-term follow-up studies of NWTS patients.

The current management of children with suspected or confirmed Wilms' tumor is complex. After diagnosis, these patients should be treated by a multidisciplinary team of trained oncologists familiar with all aspects of surgery, radiation, and chemotherapy.

REFERENCES

1. Kobrinsky NL, et al. Wilms' tumor. Hematol Oncol Ann 1993;1:173.
2. Knudson AG Jr. Introduction to the genetics of primary renal tumors in children. Med Pediatr Oncol 1993;21:193.
3. Clericuzio CL. Clinical phenotypes and Wilms tumor. Med Pediatr Oncol 1993;21:182.
4. Coppes MJ, Haber DA, Grundy PE. Genetic events in the development of Wilms' tumor. N Engl J Med 1994;331:586.
5. Call KM, et al. Isolation and characterization of a zinc finger polypeptide gene at the human chromosome 11 Wilms' tumor locus. Cell 1990;60:509.
6. Grundy PE, et al. Loss of heterozygosity for chromosomes 16q and 1p in Wilms' tumors predicts an adverse outcome. Cancer Res 1994;54:2331.
7. Everson RB, Fraumeni JF Jr. Declining mortality and improving survival from Wilm's tumor. Med Pediatr Oncol 1975;1:3.
8. Young JL Jr, et al. Cancer incidence, survival and mortality for children younger than age 15 years. Cancer 1986;58:598.
9. D'Angio GJ, et al. Wilms' tumor: an update. Cancer 1980;45:1791.
10. D'Angio GJ, et al. The treatment of Wilms' tumor: results of the National Wilms' Tumor Study. Cancer 1976;38:633.
11. D'Angio GJ, et al. The treatment of Wilms' tumor: results of the Second National Wilms' Tumor Study. Cancer 1981;47:2302.
12. D'Angio GJ. Wilms' tumor. Curr Concepts Oncol 1982;4:3.
13. D'Angio GJ, et al. Treatment of Wilms' tumor: results of the Third National Wilms' Tumor Study. Cancer 1989;64:349.
14. Lemerle J, et al. Effectiveness of preoperative chemotherapy in Wilms' tumor: results of an International Society of Paediatric Oncology (SIOP) clinical trial. J Clin Oncol 1983;1:604.
15. Burger D, et al. The advantages of preoperative therapy in Wilms' tumor: a summarized report on clinical trials conducted by the International Society of Paediatric Oncology (SIOP). Z Kinderchir 1985;40:170.
16. Pritchard J, et al. Results of the United Kingdom Children's Cancer Study Group First Wilms' Tumor Study. J Clin Oncol 1995;13:124.
17. Green DM, et al. The effect of chemotherapy dose intensity on the hematological toxicity of the treatment for Wilms' tumor: a report from the National Wilms' Tumor Study. Am J Pediatr Hematol Oncol 1994;16:207.
18. Green DM, et al. Treatment of children with stages II to IV anaplastic Wilms' tumor: a report from the National Wilms' Tumor Study Group. J Clin Oncol 1994;12:2126.
19. Green DM, et al. Treatment of children with clear-cell sarcoma of the kidney: a report from the National Wilms' Tumor Study Group. J Clin Oncol 1994;12:2132.
20. Tournade MF, et al. Results of the Sixth International Society of Pediatric Oncology Wilms' Tumor Trial and Study: a risk-adapted therapeutic approach in Wilms' tumor. J Clin Oncol 1993;11:1014.
21. Jereb B, et al. Radiotherapy in the SIOP (International Society of Pediatric Oncology) nephroblastoma studies: a review. Med Pediatr Oncol 1994;22:221.
22. Breslow NE, Beckwith JB. Epidemiological features of Wilms' tumor: results of the National Wilms' Tumor Study. J Natl Cancer Inst 1982;68:429.
23. Beckwith JB, Palmer NF. Histopathology and prognosis of Wilms' tumor: results from the First National Wilms' Tumor Study. Cancer 1978;41:1937.
24. Haas JE, et al. Ultrastructure of malignant rhabdoid tumor of the kidney. Hum Pathol 1981;12:646.
25. Beckwith JB. Wilms' tumor and other renal tumors of childhood: a selective review from the National Wilms' Tumor Study Pathology Center. Hum Pathol 1983;14:481.
26. Haas JE, Bonadio JF, Beckwith JB. Clear cell sarcoma of the kidney with emphasis on ultrastructural studies. Cancer 1984;54:2978.
27. Bonadio JF, et al. Anaplastic Wilms' tumor: clinical and pathologic studies. J Clin Oncol 1985;3:513.

28. Tefft M. Radiation related toxicities in National Wilms' Tumor Study Number 1. Int J Radiat Oncol Biol Phys 1977; 2:455.

29. Breslow NE, et al. Wilms' tumor: prognostic factors for patients without metastases at diagnosis—results of the National Wilms' Tumor Study. Cancer 1978;41:1577.

30. Jones B, Breslow NE, Takashima J. Toxic deaths in the Second National Wilms' Tumor Study. J Clin Oncol 1984;2:1028.

31. Breslow NE, et al. Prognosis for Wilms' tumor patients with nonmetastatic disease at diagnosis—results of the Second National Wilms' Tumor Study. J Clin Oncol 1985;3:521.

32. Breslow NE, et al. Clinicopathologic features and prognosis for Wilms' tumor patients with metastases at diagnosis. Cancer 1986;58:2501.

33. Morgan E, et al. Chemotherapy-related toxicity in infants treated according to the Second National Wilms' Tumor Study. J Clin Oncol 1988;6:51.

34. Thomas PRM, et al. Acute toxicities associated with radiation in the Second National Wilms' Tumor Study. J Clin Oncol 1988;6:1694.

35. D'Angio GJ, et al. Position paper: imaging methods for primary renal tumors of childhood: costs versus benefits. Med Pediatr Oncol 1993;21:205.

36. Cohen MD. Review: staging of Wilms' tumour. Clin Radiol 1993;47:77.

37. Farber S. Chemotherapy in the treatment of leukemia and Wilms' tumor. JAMA 1966;198:826.

38. Fernbach DJ, Martyn DT. Role of dactinomycin in the improved survival of children with Wilms' tumor. JAMA 1966;195:1005.

39. Burgert EO Jr, Glidewell O. Dactinomycin in Wilms' tumor. JAMA 1967;199:464.

40. Wolff JA, et al. Single versus multiple dose dactinomycin therapy of Wilms' tumor. N Engl J Med 1968;279:290.

41. Wolff JA, et al. Long-term evaluation of single versus multiple courses of actinomycin D therapy of Wilms' tumor. N Engl J Med 1974;290:84.

42. Sutow WW, Thurman WG, Windmiller J. Vincristine (leurocristine) sulfate in the treatment of children with metastatic Wilms' tumor. Pediatrics 1963;32:880.

43. Sullivan MP. Vincristine (NSC-67574) therapy for Wilms' tumor. Cancer Chemother Rep 1968;52:481.

44. Vietti TJ, et al. Vincristine sulfate and radiation therapy in metastatic Wilms' tumor. Cancer 1970;25:12.

45. Tan C, et al. Adriamycin: an antitumor antibiotic in the treatment of neoplastic diseases. Cancer 1973;32:9.

46. Pratt CB, Shanks EC. Doxorubicin in treatment of malignant solid tumors in children. Am J Dis Child 1974;127:534.

47. Haddy TB, et al. Clinical trials with cyclophosphamide (Cytoxan) in children with Wilms' tumor: preliminary report. Cancer Chemother Rep 1962;25:81.

48. Sutow WW. Cyclophosphamide (NSC-26271) in Wilms' tumor and rhabdomyosarcoma. Cancer Chemother Rep 1967; 51:407.

49. Tournade MF, et al. Ifosfamide is an active drug in Wilms' tumor: a phase II study by the French Society of Pediatric Oncology. J Clin Oncol 1988;6:793.

50. Marina NM, et al. Refining therapeutic strategies for patients with resistant Wilms' tumor. Am J Pediatr Hematol Oncol 1994;16:296.

51. Pein F, et al. Etoposide in relapsed or refractory Wilms' tumor: a phase II study by the French Society of Pediatric Oncology and the United Kingdom Children's Cancer Study Group. J Clin Oncol 1993;11:1478.

52. Pein F, et al. Etoposide and carboplatin: a highly effective combination in relapsed or refractory Wilms' tumor: a phase II study by the French Society of Pediatric Oncology. J Clin Oncol 1994;12:931.

53. de Camargo B, et al. Phase II study of carboplatin as a single drug for relapsed Wilms' tumor: experience of the Brazilian Wilms' Tumor Study Group. Med Pediatr Oncol 1994;22:258.

54. Morris-Jones PH, Pearson D, Johnson AL. Medical Research Council's Working Party on Embryonal Tumors in Childhood: management of nephroblastoma in childhood. Arch Dis Child 1978;53:112.

55. Green DM, et al. Severe hepatic toxicity after treatment with vincristine and dactinomycin using single-dose or divided-dose schedules: a report from the National Wilms' Tumor Study. J Clin Oncol 1990;8:1525.

56. Garaventa A, et al. Autologous bone marrow transplantation for pediatric Wilms' tumor: the experience of the European Bone Marrow Transplantation Solid Tumor Registry. Med Pediatr Oncol 1994;22:11.

57. Bishop HC, et al. Survival in bilateral Wilms' tumor: review of 30 National Wilms' Tumor Study cases. J Pediatr Surg 1977;12:631.

58. Blute MI, et al. Bilateral Wilms' tumor. J Urol 1987;138:968.

59. Voute PA, et al. Preoperative chemotherapy as first treatment in children with Wilms' tumor: results of the SIOP nephroblastoma trials and studies. Proc Ann Meet Am Soc Clin Oncol 1987;6:880. Abstract.

60. D'Angio GJ. SIOP and the management of Wilms' tumor. J Clin Oncol 1987;1:595. Editorial.

61. Ritchey ML, et al. Preoperative therapy for intracaval and atrial extension of Wilms' tumor. Cancer 1993;71:4104.

XIII

Radiation Therapy

Introduction to Radiation Therapy in the Management of Genitourinary Cancer

Jeffrey D. Forman

BACKGROUND

X rays were discovered by Wilhelm Roentgen in 1895. Within 2 years of this discovery, the therapeutic application of radiation for the eradication of tumors was implemented. In 1889, Henri Becquerel discovered radioactivity in the form of radium. It has therefore been a little more than a century since the discovery of radiation.

Early in this century, radiobiology experiments demonstrated the important role of oxygen, protracted fractionation, mitotic rate, and dose-rate effects. Since World War II, there have been rapid developments in treatment planning computers, treatment delivery systems, and the understanding of physics and biologic systems pertaining to radiation therapy.

TYPES OF RADIATION

Radiations of clinical significance in the treatment of cancer are ionizing radiations that cause the localized release of large quantities of energy. Ionizing radiation causes biologic effects by breaking chemical bonds within critical tissues. X rays are a form of indirect ionizing that produce biologic effects through the release of electrons. X rays are produced when an electrical device accelerates electrons against a high Z target (e.g., tungsten). This kinetic energy is then converted into X rays or photons.

Other forms of radiation used clinically in genitourinary malignancies include neutrons and protons produced from cyclotrons. Photons are positively charged particles with a mass 2×10^3 times larger than electrons. Neutrons have a mass similar to protons with no charge. Neutrons are produced when a charged particle (such as a deuteron) is accelerated against a target (e.g., beryllium). Neutrons are also indirectly ionizing in that the recoil particles formed after neutrons collide with atoms are what mitigate for the biologic effect. The biologic properties of neutrons that make them different from X rays include less dependence on oxygen for biologic effects, de-creased repair of sublethal and potentially lethal damage, and less variation in the radiation sensitivity across the cell cycle. Neutrons have been most effective in tumors that are bulky, hypoxic, and slow growing.

The biologic effects of protons do not differ from X or gamma rays. Their major benefit is not biologic but physical, based on the accurate dose localizations that can be obtained. Both protons and neutrons have been the subject of randomized trials in prostate cancer.

RADIATION DOSE

The biologic effects of radiation correlate well with the absorbed dose in tissue. This is most commonly expressed as the energy per unit mass of tissue. Until recently, the unit of dose most used was the rad. This has recently been replaced by the gray (Gy). One gray is equivalent to 100 rad and 1 cGy is equal to 1 rad. The goal in achieving a satisfactory therapeutic ratio is to deliver a dose that is sufficient to eliminate the malignancy but is tolerated by the surrounding normal tissues. Successful treatment is judged by the probability of uncomplicated local control and/or uncomplicated survival. Thus, a broad knowledge of the natural history of the disease, radiobiology, and physics is essential to the successful management of malignancy.

RADIOBIOLOGIC PRINCIPLES

A familiarity with the biologic principles of radiation therapy can provide a better appreciation of the merits of differing therapeutic approaches and a rationale to develop new techniques. Radiobiology has clarified the mechanisms that explain the preferential effect of radiation on a tumor vis-a-vis the surrounding normal tissues. For example, protraction of treatment can circumvent the problem of hypoxic cells by allowing the hypoxic cells to become more sensitive, a process called reoxygenation. In addition, normal cells have a greater ability to repair sublethal radiation damage than do tumors, allowing for a net therapeutic gain in many situations.

The primary targets for radiation damage in human tumors appear to be the nuclear DNA and membrane. The DNA-induced damage may occur from the indirect action of free radicals (e.g., X rays) or from the direct action of recoil particles (e.g., neutrons). This action is the principle process for high linear energy transfer (LET) radiation such as neutrons. In humans, healthy tissues vary considerably in their sensitivity to varying doses of ionizing radiation. With respect to genitourinary malignancies, whole organ tolerance doses for the kidney (2500 cGy) and bladder (6500 cGy) vary tremendously.

The benefits of modern fractionated radiation therapy may be best understood in terms of the radiobiologic principles of repair, reassortment within the cell cycle, reoxygenation, and repopulation. Normal tissue complication probabilities and tumor control probabilities can be modified by small changes in the time-dose relationships of delivered radiation. Examples of this are hyperfractionation and accelerated fractionation. In both strategies, multiple daily treatments are used. Hyperfractionation maintains the overall treatment time but attempts to separate the early from the late effects. Late effects are mediated by the fractional dose, but tumor control is mediated by total dose; therefore, local control rates will increase with increased dose. In accelerated fractionation, multiple standard fractional doses are used in a shorter period. This approach is used to reduce the problem of repopulation seen in rapidly dividing tumors.

DEFINITIVE RADIATION THERAPY IN UROLOGIC MALIGNANCIES

Definitive irradiation implies the curative treatment of intact tumor. This treatment is most commonly applied to adenocarcinoma of the prostate followed by transitional cell carcinoma of the bladder. Penile and urethral carcinomas are rarely irradiated due to both the low incidence and frequent use of surgery.

Definitive radiation therapy for prostate cancer has been used for decades, with survival rates that rival surgically treated patients. However, recent advances in assessing the success of radiation therapy—including PSA levels, transrectal ultrasound, and postradiation biopsies—point out deficiencies in certain subgroups that have been and still are being addressed by clinical trials. The high rate of locally persistent disease in patients with locally advanced disease has led to the successful implementation of three-dimensional treatment planning, radiation dose escalation, neutron or proton irradiation, brachytherapy boosts, and neoadjuvant hormonal therapy. The use of

neutron irradiation has twice been found to result in improved local control and survival in phase II randomized trials. Avoiding unacceptable late toxicities, such as rectal or bladder injuries and impotence, remains an important concomitant factor in the treatment of nonmetastatic prostate cancer with radiation.

Bladder cancer is only rarely treated definitively with radiation alone. However, success rates of 20 to 40% have been reported and are affected by stage, grade, and volume of disease present at the time of treatment. Strategies that incorporate simultaneous and/or neoadjuvant chemotherapy have been tested with improved outcomes. In an era of orthotopic neobladders, the role of radiation in bladder preservation schemes needs to be further assessed.

Preoperative irradiation in bladder cancer has fallen out of favor due to the lack of proven survival benefit in a phase III randomized trial. However, preoperative irradiation for bladder and renal cancers has been reported to improve local control and may help render tumors resectable that would otherwise be unresectable. Preoperative radiation for genitourinary malignancies is rarely applied today.

Adjuvant or postoperative irradiation is commonly used after radical prostatectomy, orchiectomy for stage I and stage IIa seminoma, and, rarely, cystectomy or nephrectomy. Postoperative irradiation is used for patients at high risk of having residual disease after definitive surgery.

Palliative irradiation is used for the relief of symptoms, often in advanced or metastatic disease. The most common symptom palliated is pain, such as from osseous metastasis. Local and systemic radiation approaches have been used and will be reviewed in the chapter on palliative treatments. However, radiation can also treat hematuria from renal and bladder primaries, with most patients experiencing a benefit.

RADIATION PHYSICS AND TREATMENT PLANNING

Although an understanding of the molecular and radiobiologic principles of radiation-induced damage is critical, careful treatment planning and delivery of the prescribed dose are essential. The extreme importance of encompassing all the tumor in the volume of treatment is evidenced by that fact that if even a 1 mm^3 volume is underdosed within a 5×5 cm mass, a recurrence is inevitable.

Therefore, the use of radiation in urologic malignancies requires a thorough understanding of the natural history of the disease, radiobiology, and physics. This knowledge ensures that this local treatment will be applied to patients who will benefit most. These principles of radiobiology and physics can be exploited to improve the therapeutic ratio between local control and complications.

56

The Role of Radiation Therapy Alone or as an Adjunct to Surgery in Muscle-Invasive Bladder Carcinoma

James T. Parsons
Robert A. Zlotecki

In many centers in the United States, the role of radiation therapy in the treatment of bladder cancer has diminished during the past 10 to 15 years. There are still many situations, however, in which radiation therapy may prove beneficial to the patient with bladder cancer. This is particularly true if any serious attempt is going to be made to conserve the bladder. This chapter reviews the rationale and results of radiation therapy alone (external beam, interstitial, intraoperative), radiation therapy plus radical or partial cystectomy (preoperative radiation therapy), and radiation therapy combined with chemotherapy for patients with muscle-invasive bladder cancer.

RADIATION THERAPY ALONE

Full-dose external beam radiation therapy (with cystectomy reserved for salvage) is a common treatment scheme in Canada (1) and Great Britain (2, 3). In the United States, initial surgery is more commonly used; external beam radiation therapy is usually administered by default, that is, if the patient is medically unfit, refuses cystectomy, or has disease too advanced for surgery. Patients treated by radical radiation therapy ideally should have an adequate bladder capacity without substantial voiding symptoms or incontinence.

The rate of complete response at first follow-up cystoscopy after full-dose external beam radiation therapy is 45 to 55% in most reported series (4). Subsequent bladder relapse occurs in 40 to 50% of those patients in whom a complete remission was attained, leading to permanent local control in only 25 to 35% of patients (5). Multiple series have shown that long-term survival is correlated to a highly significant degree with initial complete response after radiation therapy.

Other factors generally believed to predict clinical outcome are T stage, tumor morphology (papillary more favorable than nonpapillary), completeness of transurethral resection, tumor site, ureteral obstruction, hemoglobin level, performance status, and dose of radiation.

Five-year survival rates after external beam radiation therapy in a number of studies are approximately 40% for stage T2, 20 to 25% for T3, and 10% for T4 tumors (4–6). The 5-year survival rates are only slightly affected by salvage cystectomy; most patients who have a recurrence after radiation therapy are not suitable candidates because of advanced disease, old age, poor medical condition, or refusal.

RADIATION THERAPY AS AN ADJUNCT TO SURGERY

Radiation Therapy Plus Total Cystectomy

For patients with clinical stage T2 disease, radical cystectomy is commonly used. Most patients do not need preoperative radiation therapy. We recommend preoperative radiation therapy for patients with large (greater than or equal to 4 cm) or high-grade T2 lesions because the risk of serious understaging in these situations is high, as shown by Marshall (7) 40 years ago and more recently by many other investigators. In the University of Iowa series, patients with stage B (T2) cancer measuring greater than 3 cm had a 5-year survival rate of 50% when treated by preoperative radiation therapy and cystectomy versus 16% after radical cystectomy alone (8).

The role of preoperative radiation therapy in T3 bladder cancer has already been extensively reviewed (6, 9) and recently confirmed in a study of 570 patients with muscle-invasive bladder cancer at the M.D. Anderson Cancer Center (10). Between 1960 and 1985, patients routinely received preoperative radiation therapy; after 1985, radical cystectomy alone was used. In a multivariate analysis of factors affecting local control in patients with T3b disease, only one treatment type (preoperative radiation therapy versus cystectomy alone) significantly predicted outcome (P = 0.008). Survival, freedom from distant metastasis, and freedom from disease rates were all better in the preoperative radiation therapy group, although the differences did not reach statistical significance (10). In the recently published randomized trial by the Danish Vesical Cancer Group (DAVECA) (11), 183 patients with T2 to T4a transitional cell carcinoma were randomized to preoperative radiation therapy (4000 cGy) versus radiation therapy followed by salvage cystectomy. Survival favored the preoperative radiation therapy group (P = 0.08).

RADIATION THERAPY PLUS PARTIAL CYSTECTOMY

Carefully chosen patients with muscle-invasive disease or superficial disease not suitable for transurethral surgery may be treated by segmental resection (partial cystectomy). Failure to observe very narrow indications for the procedure leads to local recurrence rates of 50 to 75% in T2 lesions (12–17) and even higher rates in T3 disease.

The presence of circumferential submucosal tumor extensions in the muscle planes and lymphatic vessels within the muscularis deep to adjacent normal mucosa—as described in whole organ sections 35 years ago (18)—and the fact that most recurrences occur at the margins of resection rather than elsewhere within the bladder justify the use of either preoperative radiation therapy (19–21) or an interstitial implant adjacent to the bladder suture line at the time of segmental resection (22). Bladder capacity is not adversely affected by preoperative radiation therapy (19, 23).

INTRAOPERATIVE RADIATION THERAPY (INTERSTITIAL IMPLANTATION OR INTRAOPERATIVE ELECTRON BEAM TREATMENT)

In the past, permanent gold or radon seed implants were performed in the United States and abroad (24–26). In more recent years, interstitial therapy for bladder cancers has been largely discontinued in the United States. In those institutions that still perform implants, removable sources (radium, cesium, iridium, or tantalum) are used. Although the technique is infrequently used in the United States today, the excellent results obtained at an increasing number of institutions abroad should prompt U.S. trials.

The 5-year bladder relapse rate in 700 patients with T2 disease treated by interstitial or intraoperative therapy was 20 to 25%. The 5-year survival rate was 55 to 60% (Table 56.1) (22–32). Two thirds of the relapses in one series were at the site of initial disease (29). The rate of development of new (second) primary cancers elsewhere in the bladder was 7% in both the French and the Dutch experiences (22, 29).

Matsumoto et al. (27) reported a 5-year recurrence rate of 18% and a 5-year survival rate of 62% in 28 patients with T2 cancer when treated with intraoperative electrons plus external beam radiation therapy. These results compare very favorably with those reported after radical cystectomy, the major difference being that the irradiated patients in whom cure is achieved maintain their bladder function.

EXTERNAL BEAM RADIATION THERAPY: TECHNIQUE AND COMPLICATIONS

Technique

At the University of Florida, a four-field box technique is used (Fig. 56.1) (33). The treatment is simulated with 30 to 50 mL

Table 56.1. T2 Bladder Carcinoma: Results of Treatment With Intraoperative or Removable Interstitial Sources—5-Year Bladder Relapse Rates (Same Site or Elsewhere in the Bladder) and Survival Rates (6)

REFERENCE	TREATMENT	NO. OF PATIENTS	BLADDER RELAPSE (%)	SURVIVAL (%)
Matsumoto et al. (27)	Intraoperative electrons (25–30 Gy) plus EB (30–40 Gy)	28	18	62
Williams et al. (28)	Tantalum-182	76	30	41
Van der Werf-Messing et al. (29)	EB (10.5 Gy) plus radium	328	23	56
Battermann and Tierie (30)	EB (10.5–30 Gy) plus radium	89	26	55
Mazeron et al. (22)	EB (8.5 Gy) plus partial cystectomy plus iridium-192	30	7	55
Boiteux et al. (31)	EB (10.5 Gy) plus partial cystectomy plus iridium-192	66	18*	63
Van der Werf-Messing and van Putten (32)	EB (40 Gy) plus radium (within 1 wk)	48	12	73

[a] 51 months mean follow-up.

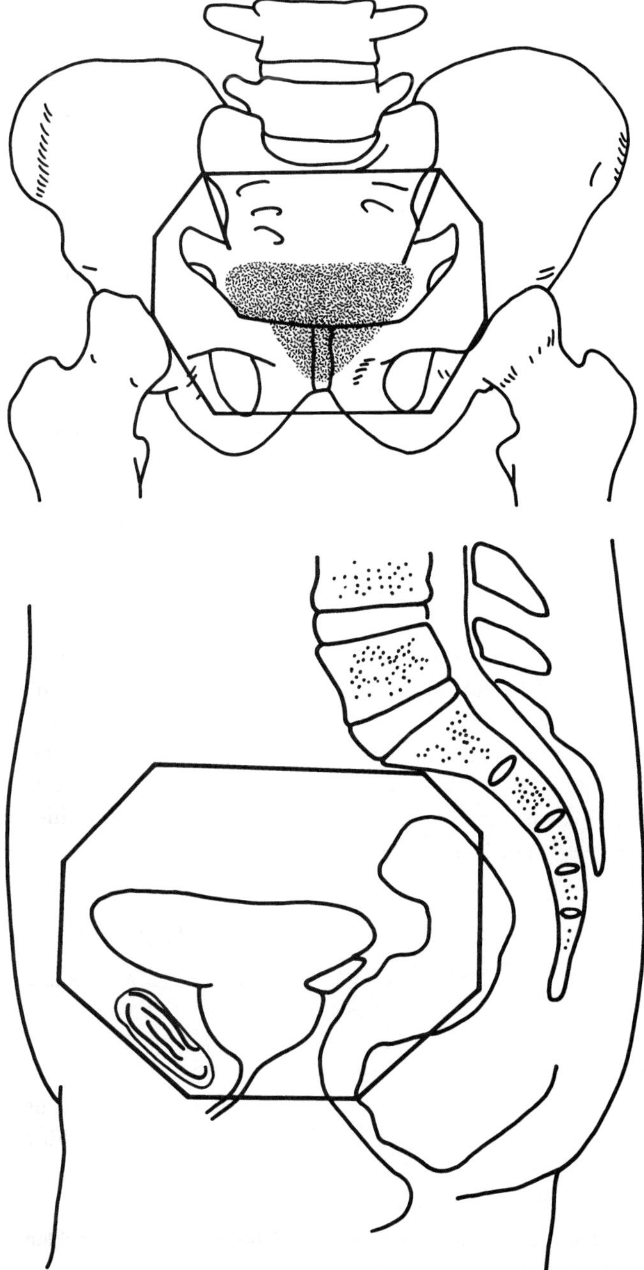

Fig. 56.1. Radiation treatment portals for bladder cancer. **A.** Anterior and posterior portals. **B.** Lateral portals. Modified from Shipley WU. (33).

of contrast medium and a small amount of air in the patient's bladder and dilute barium in the rectum. Treatment is usually with 20-MV X rays. The cephalad margin is usually at the middle of the sacroiliac joint or sometimes at L5-S1, depending on the extent of disease. The caudal margin is at the bottom of the obturator foramen unless there is diffuse involvement of the bladder neck or prostatic urethra with carcinoma in situ, in which case the portals are extended to the bottom of the ischial tuberosities. The bony pelvic side walls are treated with approximately a 1.5-cm margin by the anterior and posterior

portals. On the lateral portals, the posterior margin is set at least 3 cm behind the most posterior extent of the tumor or the posterior bladder wall (whichever is most posterior) as determined by palpation or computed tomography (CT). The size of the portals is reduced after 4500 to 5040 cGy (180 cGy per fraction). The total dose is 6480 to 6840 cGy in patients treated by radiation therapy alone. In most patients, the reduced portals exclude at least a portion of the uninvolved bladder. When preoperative radiation therapy is used, we deliver a dose of 4400 cGy in 22 fractions over 4.5 weeks followed by cystectomy in approximately 3 weeks.

Complications

The morbidity of radical external beam radiation therapy mainly relates to complications of the bladder (8 to 10%), rectum (3 to 4%), and small bowel (1 to 2%) (2, 34). The mortality rate attributable to late radiation therapy complications was 1% (2). The rates of severe morbidity are strongly correlated with radiation therapy technique (5). Using a modified bladder symptom score, Lynch et al. (35) addressed the concern that postradiation therapy cystitis and diarrhea so severely affected the quality of life that cure by radiation therapy was not worth the price. When irradiated patients were compared with a control group matched for sex and age, there was no significant difference between the two groups.

COMBINED RADIATION THERAPY AND CHEMOTHERAPY

Several recent studies involving aggressive transurethral resection and cisplatin-based chemoradiation therapy have shown that roughly equivalent survival rates can be achieved (compared with historical controls of patients treated by radical cystectomy alone). These studies have also shown that a gratifying proportion of the survivors have maintained an adequately functioning bladder, greatly strengthening the argument for a conservative approach for selected patients with muscle-invasive bladder cancer.

Neoadjuvant Chemotherapy Plus Radiation Therapy and Cisplatin

Between May 1986 and July 1990, 94 patients with T2 to T4NXM0 (T2, 28; T3, 42; T4, 24) transitional cell carcinoma of the bladder were treated at the University of Florida with as complete a transurethral resection as possible, followed by two to three cycles of cisplatin, methotrexate, and vinblastine (CMV) chemotherapy with or without doxorubicin, followed by restaging by CT, cystoscopy, cytology, and deep bladder biopsies. Forty percent of patients had a complete response (CR) (no radiographic, cystoscopic, or pathologic evidence of cancer); 19% had a partial response (PR) (downstaging to Ta, Tis, or T1 disease or positive cytology); and 41% showed no response (NR) (persistent muscle-invasive disease) to chemotherapy. CR rates were higher in T2 than in T3 and higher in T3 than in T4 disease. One patient withdrew from the study during chemotherapy, and three patients died during chemotherapy.

Of 90 patients who completed chemotherapy, 49 subsequently received 6480 cGy (180 cGy per fraction) along with concomitant cisplatin (10 mg/m^2 per week for 7 weeks). Of 49 patients who received radiation therapy, 33 had a PR or CR previously. Of 16 patients who had NR to chemotherapy, 9 (56%) had CR after radiation therapy and cisplatin.

Of 41 patients who did not receive radiation therapy, 22 underwent cystectomy (4 after CR and 18 after NR) and 8 underwent partial cystectomy. Four patients died before further treatment was administered, and seven patients received follow-up only after chemotherapy.

Of 30 patients in whom recurrent disease developed in the bladder after CR (following chemotherapy and radiation therapy, with or without partial cystectomy), there were 8 patients (27%) whose recurrences invaded muscle, and 22 (73%) whose recurrences were superficial (Ta, Tis, T1) and were treated by transurethral resection and bacille Calmette-Guérin (BCG) or mitomycin C.

The 5-year absolute survival rate (endpoint, death due to any cause) using Kaplan-Meier analysis (36, 37) was 51% (T2, 80%; T3, 56%; T4, 11%). The 5-year survival rate was 37% in those who had hydronephrosis compared with 60% in those who did not (P = 0.03). Of 39 patients who are currently alive with recent follow-up, 41% have intact functioning bladders. It is concluded that the overall 5-year survival rates equal or surpass the 5-year results after radical cystectomy, the main difference being that almost half of the survivors in the current series maintained bladder function.

Kaufman et al. (38) at the Massachusetts General Hospital reported similar results for 53 consecutively treated patients with T2 to T4 disease who underwent transurethral surgery, then CMV chemotherapy, followed by radiation therapy plus cisplatin. The 5-year survival rate was 48%, with 20 patients surviving with bladders apparently free of tumor. As in the University of Florida series, 75% of patients in whom local recurrence was observed had superficial recurrences that could usually be successfully treated by transurethral surgery and intravesical drug therapy.

The results of the Radiation Therapy Oncology Group (RTOG) protocol 85-12, in which patients with T2 to T4 bladder cancer were treated with radiation therapy plus concomitant cisplatin (100 mg/m^2 on days 1 and 22 of radiation therapy), were reported by Tester and colleagues (39). No attempt was made to resect all tumor at cystoscopy. The CR rate after cisplatin plus 4000 cGy was 66%. Patients with CR received a third dose of cisplatin plus an additional 2400 cGy. Patients with residual tumor were assigned radical cystectomy. The 3-year overall survival rate was 64%. As in the University of Florida and Massachusetts General Hospital studies, most of the relapses were noninvasive.

Concomitant Cisplatin/5-Fluorouracil Plus Radiation Therapy

Housset et al. (40) designed an interesting prospective study using a combination of 5-fluorouracil (5-FU) plus cisplatin and concomitant radiation therapy followed by either cystectomy or additional chemotherapy and radiation therapy. Fifty-four patients with stage T2 to T4 were treated by transurethral resection, followed by 2400 cGy in 8 fractions over 17 days with 2 fractions of 300 cGy each on days 1, 3, 15, and 17, and cisplatin (15 mg/m^2/day) and 5-FU (400 mg/m^2/day) as a short infusion over 2 hours on days 1, 2, 3, 15, 16, and 17. A control cystoscopy with deep biopsies was performed 6 weeks after completion of chemoradiation therapy. Those with incomplete responses underwent radical cystectomy. Patients with CR underwent either additional chemoradiation therapy or cystectomy. The boost dose in patients who underwent further chemoradiation therapy was 2000 cGy administered in a 250-cGy twice-a-day scheme on days 64, 66, 78, and 80 (to a total dose of 4400 cGy in 16 fractions over an 11.5-week interval) plus the same chemotherapy as previously administered.

At control cystoscopy, 40 of 54 patients (74%) had a CR histologically. Among the 40 patients, 22 underwent concomitant chemoradiation therapy and 18 underwent cystectomy. All 18 of the latter patients were found to have pT0 disease after cystectomy, and none had nodal involvement. Pelvic recurrence subsequently developed in only 1 of 18 patients; distant metastases developed in 3 patients. The 7-year survival rate in the cystectomy group was 77%.

Of 22 patients with CR who underwent further chemoradiation therapy, invasive bladder recurrence (1 pT3) or superficial bladder recurrences (1 Ta, 1 T1) developed in 3 patients. The patient with invasive recurrence and the one with Ta recurrence were salvaged by cystectomy. The patient with a T1 recurrence was salvaged by transurethral resection (TUR) plus intravesical BCG. Distant metastases developed in three patients. The 3-year survival rate was 81%.

Of 14 patients with NR, 12 underwent cystectomy. The two who refused cystectomy were treated with further chemoradiation therapy. Distant metastases developed in 10 of 14 patients (71%). The 3-year survival rate was 23%.

The overall 3-year survival rate for all 54 patients was 59%; the 3-year disease-free survival rate was 62% (66% in T2 and 53% in T3 to T4 patients).

No small bowel obstruction or bladder contracture occurred in any patients, and surgical morbidity was tolerable.

CONCLUSIONS

During the past 20 years, multimodality organ-sparing treatment has become widely accepted therapy for many patients with soft tissue sarcoma, head and neck cancer, breast cancer, anal canal cancers, and rectal cancer. Standard therapy for muscle-invasive bladder cancer in the United States remains radical cystectomy. Patients who are not considered good candidates for radical cystectomy, either through refusal or medical inoperability, are generally offered external beam radiation therapy alone, a treatment that offers unsatisfactory survival rates. New bladder-conserving protocols should focus on either interstitial therapy or combination chemotherapy and radiation therapy, both of which appear to hold considerably greater promise than external beam radiation therapy alone.

ACKNOWLEDGMENT

The authors thank the research support staff of the Department of Radiation Oncology, University of Florida College of Medicine, for their help with statistics, editing, and manuscript preparation.

REFERENCES

1. Goodman GB, Hislop TG, Elwood JM, et al. Conservation of bladder function in patients with invasive bladder cancer treated by definitive irradiation and selective cystectomy. Int J Radiat Oncol Biol Phys 1981;7:569.
2. Duncan W, Quilty PM. The results of a series of 963 patients with transitional cell carcinoma of the urinary bladder primarily treated by radical megavoltage x-ray therapy. Radiother Oncol 1986;7:299.
3. Hope-Stone HF, Oliver RTD, England HR, et al. T3 bladder cancer: salvage rather than elective cystectomy after radiotherapy. Urology 1984;24:315.
4. Fosså SD, Woehre H, Aass N, et al. Bladder cancer definitive radiation therapy of muscle-invasive bladder cancer: a retrospective analysis of 317 patients. Cancer 1993;72:3036.
5. Pollack A, Zagars GK, Swanson DA. Muscle-invasive bladder cancer treated with external beam radiotherapy: prognostic factors. Int J Radiat Oncol Biol Phys 1994;30:267.
6. Parsons JT, Million RR. The role of radiation therapy alone or as an adjuvant to surgery in bladder carcinoma. Semin Oncol 1990;17:566.
7. Marshall VF. The relation of the preoperative estimate to the pathologic demonstration of the extent of vesical neoplasms. J Urol 1952;68:714.
8. Henry K, Miller J, Mori M, et al. Comparison of transurethral resection to radical therapies for stage B bladder tumors. J Urol 1988;140:964.
9. Parsons JT, Million RR. Planned preoperative irradiation in the management of clinical stage B2-C (T3) bladder carcinoma. Int J Radiat Oncol Biol Phys 1988;14:797.
10. Cole CJ, Pollack A, Zagars GK, et al. Local control of muscle-invasive bladder cancer: preoperative radiotherapy and cystectomy versus cystectomy alone. Int J Radiat Oncol Biol Phys 1994;30(Suppl):200. Abstract.
11. Sell A, Jakobsen A, Nerstrøm B, et al. Treatment of advanced bladder cancer category T2 T3 and T4a: a randomized multicenter study of preoperative irradiation and cystectomy versus radical irradiation and early salvage cystectomy for residual tumor. Danish Vesical Cancer Group Protocol 8201. Scand J Urol Nephrol Suppl 1991;138:193.
12. Cummings KB, Mason JT, Correa RJ Jr, et al. Segmental resection in the management of bladder carcinoma. J Urol 1978;119:56.
13. Masina F. Segmental resection for tumours of the urinary bladder: ten-year follow-up. Br J Surg 1975;114:391.
14. Novick AC, Stewart BH. Partial cystectomy in the treatment of primary and secondary carcinoma of the bladder. J Urol 1976;116:570.
15. Resnick MI, O'Conor VJ Jr. Segmental resection for carcinoma of the bladder: review of 102 patients. J Urol 1973;109:1007.
16. Schoborg TW, Sapolsky JL, Lewis CW Jr. Carcinoma of the bladder treated by segmental resection. J Urol 1979;122:473.
17. Utz DC, Schmitz SE, Fugelso PD, et al. A clinicopathologic evaluation of partial cystectomy for carcinoma of the urinary bladder. Cancer 1973;32:1075.
18. Baker R. Correlation of circumferential lymphatic spread of vesical cancer with depth of infiltration: relation to present methods of treatment. J Urol 1955;73:681.
19. Ojeda L, Johnson DE. Partial cystectomy: can it be incorporated into integrated therapy program? Urology 1983;22:115.
20. Skinner DG, Lieskovsky G. Management of invasive and high-grade bladder cancer. In: Skinner DG, Lieskovsky G, eds. Diagnosis and management of genitourinary cancer. Philadelphia: WB Saunders, 1988:295.
21. Zingg EJ, Plowman PN, Wallace DMA, et al. Treatment of muscle-invasive bladder cancer. In: Zingg EJ, Wallace DMA, eds. Bladder cancer. Berlin: Springer-Verlag, 1985:189.
22. Mazeron JJ, Crook J, Chopin D, et al. Conservative treatment of bladder carcinoma by partial cystectomy and interstitial iridium 192. Int J Radiat Oncol Biol Phys 1988;15:1323.
23. Skinner DG, Kaufman JJ. Management of invasive and high grade bladder cancer. In: Skinner DG, deKernion JB, eds. Genitourinary cancer. Philadelphia: WB Saunders, 1978:269.
24. Barringer BS. Radium therapy of bladder cancer, retrospect and prospect. J Urol 1952;68:280.
25. Carver JH. Interstitial radiation in the treatment of selected cases of cancer of the bladder. Br J Urol 1959;31:313.
26. Dix VW, Shanks W, Tresidder GC, et al. Carcinoma of the bladder; treatment by diathermy snare excision and interstitial irradiation. Br J Urol 1970;42:213.
27. Matsumoto K, Kakizoe T, Mikuriya S, et al. Clinical evaluation of intraoperative radiotherapy for carcinoma of the urinary bladder. Cancer 1981;47:509.
28. Williams GB, Trott PA, Bloom HJG. Carcinoma of the bladder treated by interstitial irradiation. Br J Urol 1981;53:221.
29. Van der Werf-Messing BHP, Menon RS, Hop WCJ. Cancer of the urinary bladder category T2, T3, (NXM0) treated by interstitial radium implant: second report. Int J Radiat Oncol Biol Phys 1983;9:481.
30. Battermann JJ, Tierie AH. Results of implantation for T1 and T2 bladder tumours. Radiother Oncol 1986;5:85.
31. Boiteux JP, Rozan R, Giraud B, et al. Interstitial iridium-192 therapy for bladder cancer: a multicentric survey. J Urol 1988;139:181. Abstract.
32. Van der Werf-Messing BHP, van Putten WLJ. Carcinoma of the urinary bladder category T2,3 NXM0 treated by 40 Gy external irradiation followed by cesium-137 implant at reduced dose (50%). Int J Radiat Oncol Biol Phys 1989;16:369.
33. Shipley WU. Radiation therapy for patients with bladder carcinoma: rationale, results, techniques, and possible

innovations. In: Bonney WW, Prout GR Jr, eds. AUA monographs: bladder cancer. Baltimore: Williams & Wilkins, 1982:243.

34. Miller LS. Bladder cancer: superiority of preoperative irradiation and cystectomy in clinical stages B2 and C. Cancer 1977;39:973.

35. Lynch WJ, Jenkins BJ, Fowler CG, et al. The quality of life after radical radiotherapy for bladder cancer. Br J Urol 1992; 70:519.

36. Kaplan EL, Meier P. Nonparametric estimation from incomplete observations. J Am Stat Assoc 1958;53:457.

37. SAS Institute. SAS technical report P-179, additional SAS/ STAT procedures, release 6.03. Cary, NC: SAS Institute, 1988: 49.

38. Kaufman DS, Shipley WU, Griffin PP, et al. Selective bladder preservation by combination treatment of invasive bladder cancer. N Engl J Med 1993;329:1377.

39. Tester W, Porter A, Asbell S, et al. Combined modality program with possible organ preservation for invasive bladder carcinoma: results of RTOG protocol 85–12. Int J Radiat Oncol Biol Phys 1993;25:783.

40. Housset M, Maulard C, Chretien Y, et al. Combined radiation and chemotherapy for invasive transitional-cell carcinoma of the bladder: a prospective study. J Clin Oncol 1993;11:2150.

57

Radiation Therapy for Prostate Carcinoma

Steven L. Hancock

INTRODUCTION

Radiation therapy includes several highly effective means of treating primary prostatic cancer—conventional external beam irradiation, neutron beam irradiation, and temporary or permanent interstitial implants (1–5). These approaches are capable of achieving survival and cause-specific survival rates similar to those reported with radical prostatectomy in early stages of disease, durable local control for the majority of patients with more advanced tumors, and effective palliation of metastatic disease. When properly administered, prostatic irradiation has a low frequency of serious side effects and a lower probability of urinary incontinence and erectile impotence than is generally achieved with radical prostatectomy (6–8). Preliminary reports of a national cooperative trial suggest that adding transient androgen deprivation for a brief period before and during prostatic irradiation may improve the outcome of irradiation with locally advanced prostatic tumors (9). The development of monoclonal antibodies that have a high, specific affinity for prostatic cancers and may be labeled with radioisotopes offers a new avenue for delivering radiation as an agent against disseminated prostatic cancer (10).

BACKGROUND

The use of radiation to produce significant regression of prostatic cancer was first reported by two European groups within 20 years of the discovery of radium (11, 12). Hugh Hampton Young, the urologist at Johns Hopkins Hospital, brought these techniques to the United States and reported his early experience with transurethral irradiation using radium in 1917 (13). Two groups reported response of prostatic cancer to externally applied, high-energy X-rays in the early 1930s, and Flocks et al. reported favorable responses following interstitial application of radioactive colloidal gold in the 1950s (14–17). The ability to irradiate the prostate gland uniformly using external sources required the development of megavoltage X-ray (linear accelerator) or gamma ray (^{60}cobalt) sources. The results of early experiences with such treatments were reported by Bagshaw et al., George et al., and del Regato in the late 1960s (18–20).

Modern linear accelerators have become preferred to ^{60}cobalt therapy because they have higher energy beams that increase depth of penetration and dose homogeneity, and have less penumbra, which allows more rapid attenuation of dose in adjacent normal tissues, such as the bladder and rectum. Most of the following discussion will focus on the long-term outcome of external beam irradiation conducted with modern linear accelerators because it has more general applicability and longer sequential experience than other radiation approaches.

PATIENT SELECTION

Radiation can be used to treat a broader range of patients with primary prostatic cancer than radical prostatectomy and is also useful in the management of persisting or recurring disease after radical prostatectomy. The tolerance of normal tissues to irradiation is well established, and most normal tissues repair radiation injury unless they have been treated to unacceptable dose levels or have been compromised by prior surgery or vascular disease. Radiation can safely treat broader margins around clinically or radiologically identifiable tumor than are achievable with radical prostatectomy. Patients whose prostatic cancer extends beyond the capsule of the prostate or involves seminal vesicles or regional lymph nodes may be appropriately treated with irradiation, with a moderately high probability of clinical local control and a modest probability of cure. Because external beam irradiation is well-tolerated, noninvasive therapy that requires no general anesthesia, advanced age and intercurrent medical illnesses are not strict contraindications for therapy in reasonably functional individuals. Therefore, series of patients treated with prostatic irradiation frequently include patients with more clinically advanced disease, higher average age, and more intercurrent disease than is typical for surgical series. Radiation series also lack pathologic evaluation of lymph nodes and of the actual extent of disease within the prostate—both of which are frequently underestimated by clinical staging (21, 22). Similarly, potential selection biases must be considered when comparing the results of prostatic implantation with external beam irradiation.

Potential candidates for prostatic irradiation should have

careful clinical palpation of the prostate gland and transrectal ultrasound examination with multiple prostatic biopsies to delineate the extent of disease. A TNM staging system has proven to be useful in estimating prognosis after irradiation for more than 20 years at Stanford, and a similar system has been defined in the current, fourth edition of the American Joint Committee on Cancer (AJCC) staging manual (AJCC-4) (23). As will be demonstrated below, the summed major and minor histologic pattern scores proposed by Gleason are useful in assessing prognosis after irradiation (24). The summed Gleason score has also correlated with the risk of lymph node metastases identified in series of patients who underwent staging lymphadenectomies. A simple formula predicting the probability of pelvic or paraaortic lymph node involvement is: % probability of involved nodes = (summed Gleason score − 4) × 15 (25).

All potential candidates for prostatic irradiation should have measurement of the serum level of prostate-specific antigen (PSA) at a time when the prostate gland is undisturbed by extensive examination, biopsy procedures, or other instrumentation. High PSA values have correlated with an increased risk of lymph node involvement by prostatic cancer (26). The risk of lymph node metastases correlated well in one series when the factors of pretreatment PSA and summed Gleason pattern score were considered together according to the equation: % probability of involved nodes = 2/3 × (PSA) + (summed Gleason score − 6) × 10 (27). Most potential candidates for prostatic irradiation should undergo a chest radiograph and bone scan either as a baseline for future comparison or to rule out distant metastases if local disease is clinically extensive, summed Gleason score exceeds 6, or PSA exceeds 15 ng/mL. For such patients, who have a moderate to high risk of disease beyond the prostate, imaging the abdomen and pelvis by magnetic resonance imaging (MRI) or computed tomography (CT) scanning is useful for evaluating lymph nodes, defining the extent of prostatic disease and seminal vesicle involvement, and planning radiation fields (28).

PLANNING FOR RADIATION THERAPY

Modern prostatic irradiation features treatments that are given 5 times each week with fields shaped to conform to prostatic and periprostatic tissues. All fields are treated each day to maximize dose homogeneity and minimize the daily dose to uninvolved normal tissues.

Prostatic irradiation is planned by obtaining initial, orthogonal localizing radiographs after the instillation of a radiologic contrast reagent (Hypaque; Sanofi Winthrop, New York, NY)

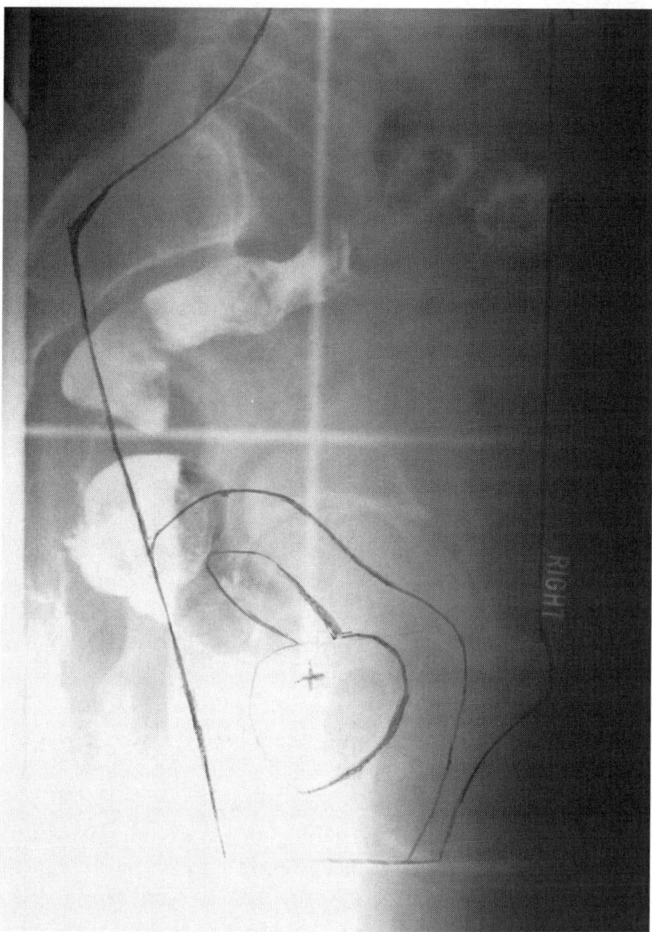

Fig. 57.1. Example of a lateral pelvic radiograph used to plan treatment of the prostate gland and pelvic lymph nodes. Radiopaque contrast has been inserted in the rectum and the urethra. The contours of the prostate gland and seminal vesicles have been transposed from a treatment-planning CT scan. A small boost field conforms to the CT, designed to provide an approximately 1.5-cm margin around the prostate and seminal vesicles. This margin allows buildup of dose adjacent to the blocks and accommodates some variation in the position of the prostate during daily therapy.

into the urethra (for anteroposterior and posteroanterior images) and into the rectum (for lateral images) (Fig. 57.1). A treatment planning CT scan is used to design protective blocking by defining field widths at various regions through the gland and by showing the location and superior extent of the seminal vesicles. A treatment planning computer is used to adjust the array and weighting of beams to produce dose homogeneity through the tumor volume and to assist in designing blocks that conform to the prostate gland. Patients who have

Fig. 57.2. Anteroposterior (**A**) and lateral (**B**) linear accelerator port films showing typical focal treatment of the prostate gland and periprostatic tissues. Both fields are opposed to matching posteroanterior and lateral fields to produce typical four-field treatment. Anteroposterior (**C**) and lateral (**D**) port films show typical fields used to treat the prostate and regional lymph nodes. The stepped field edges are generated from initial planning radiographs and positioned for each field, using a computerized multileaf collimator on the linear accelerator. The actual dose distribution within tissue achieved with multileaf collimation closely approximates that obtained with poured metal alloy (Cerrobend) blocks. The large pelvic fields are typically treated at 180 to 200 cGy to 4500 to 5000 cGy and combined with a focal boost to treat the prostate gland to 7000 cGy.

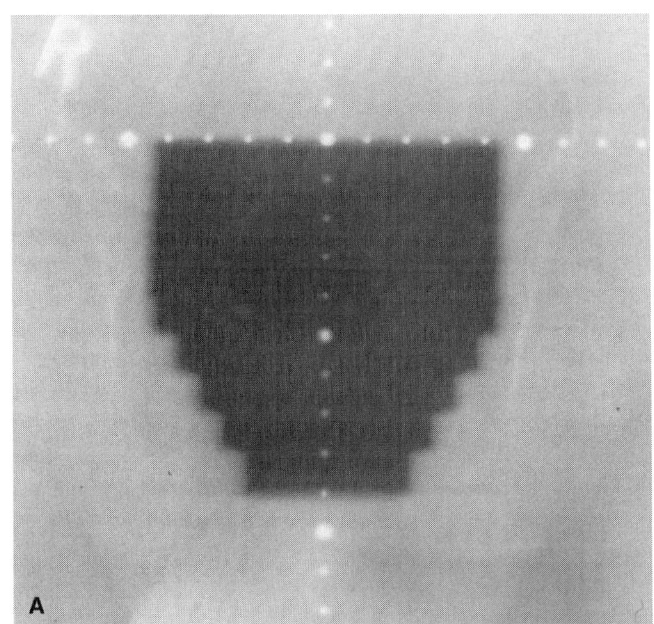

A

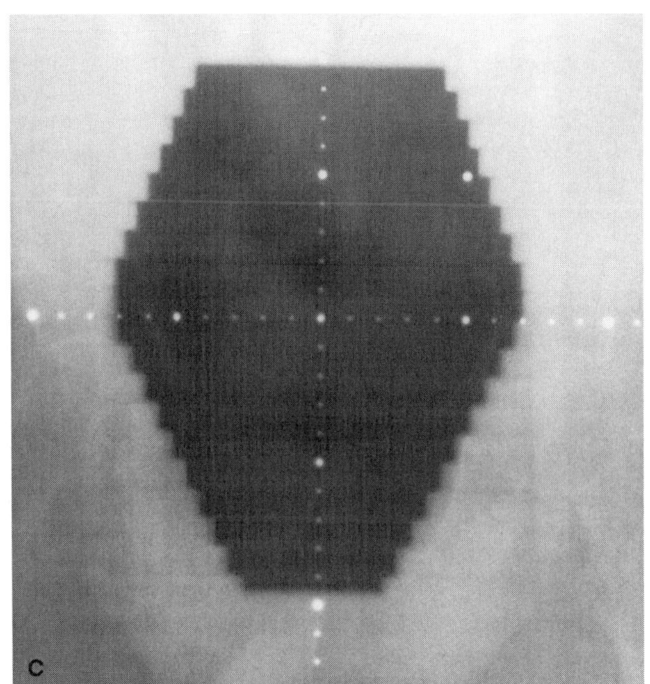

C

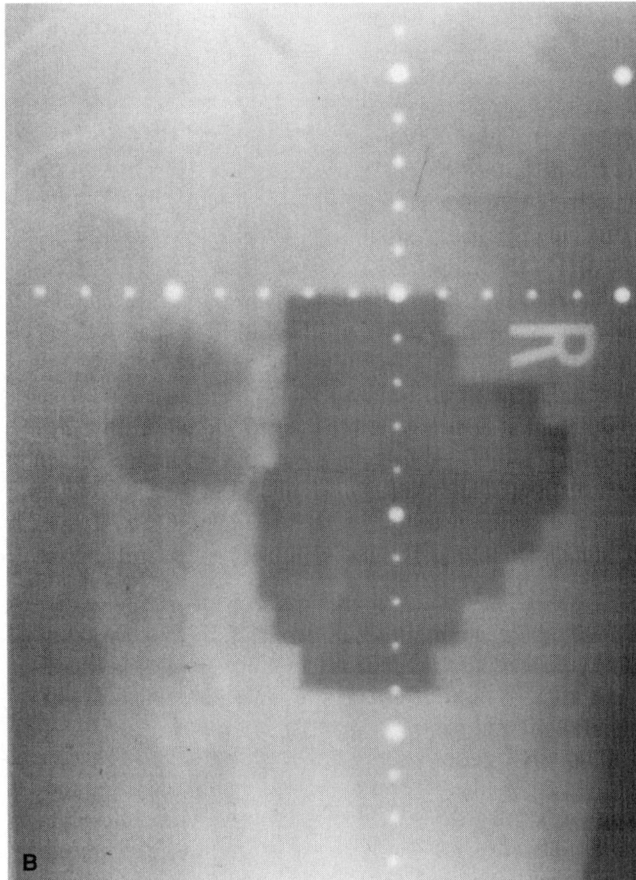

B

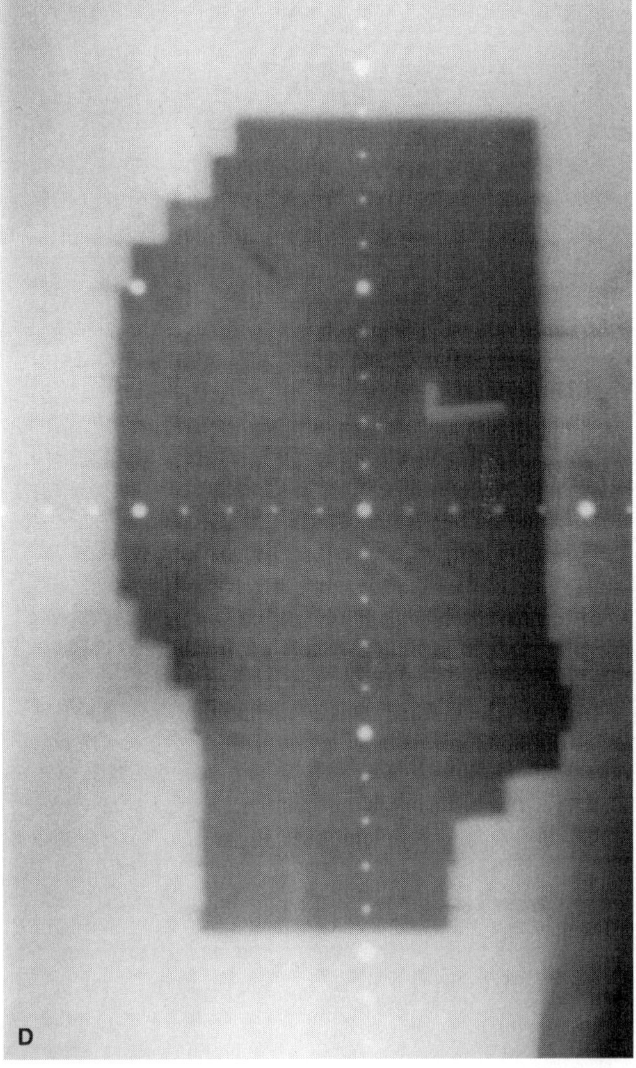

D

a low probability of lymph node involvement (Gleason score below 7, primary stage T1b or less, and PSA below 15 ng/mL) are generally treated to the prostate gland alone with four to six small, highly focused fields that conform to the contours of the prostate and periprostatic tissues. Prostate doses up to 7000 to 7600 cGy administered over 7 to 8 weeks are commonly administered using these small, shaped fields at a dose rate of 180 to 200 cGy per day. Some investigators have escalated the radiation dose to prostatic tissue to 8100 cGy using three-dimensional, conformal techniques that produce a dose gradient through the posterior prostate without exceeding the tolerance dose limit to the anterior rectal wall (29). Whether such dose escalation approaches will significantly improve local control and survival in locally confined prostatic cancer will be determined by future studies.

Field shaping may be accomplished by manufacturing poured, metallic alloy (Cerrobend; Atlantic Metals and Alloys Inc., Old Greenwich, CT) blocks or by using computer-defined multileaf collimators that achieve similar dose contours within tissue but allow more efficient treatment of multiple fields through less direct manipulation of blocks.

Patients who have a moderate or high risk of pelvic lymph node metastases are usually treated to four opposed anteroposterior and lateral fields that encompass the prostate gland and draining lymph nodes to the upper aspect of the fifth lumbar vertebra. The lateral treatment fields are shaped to exclude the posterior rectum and anus to minimize acute and late radiation proctitis. All four fields that encompass the prostate and lymph nodes are treated 5 days each week to achieve a total dose of 180 to 200 cGy per day. The total dose administered to the pelvic lymph nodes generally ranges between 4500 and 5000 cGy over 5 weeks. The prostate gland is treated further by small, conformal fields to a total dose of 7000 cGy. Examples of anterior and lateral port films obtained on the linear accelerator with multileaf collimation are shown in Figure 57.2.

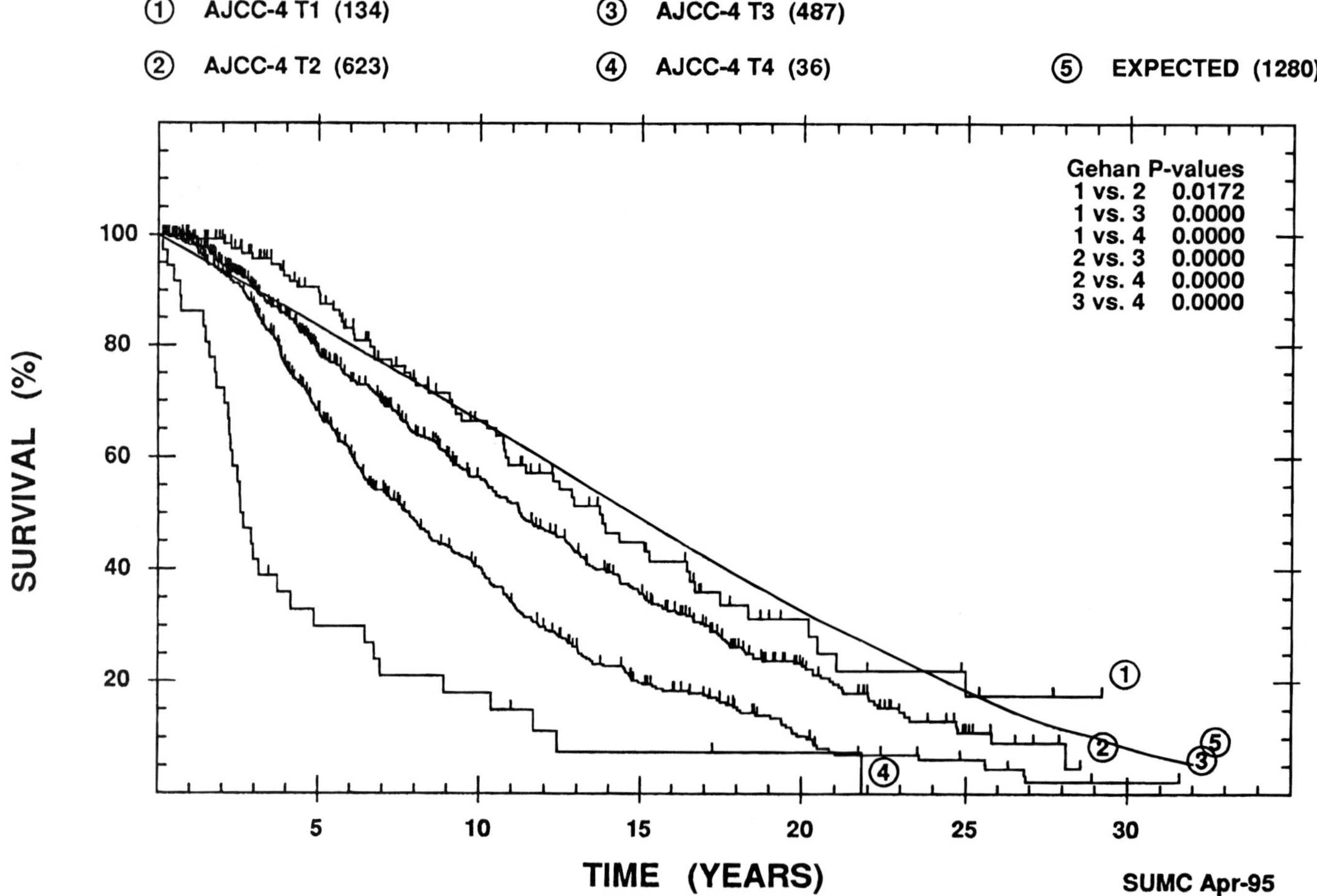

Fig. 57.3. Survival according to primary tumor stage before irradiation (lymph node status unknown). Downward steps represent deaths from any cause; tick marks above the lines denote patients who were alive at last contact and are censored at that interval after therapy. Curve 5 denotes the survival expected for an age and racially matched male population (n = 1280) based on general rates.

RESULTS OF PROSTATIC CANCER IRRADIATION

Since 1956, 1280 men have received external beam irradiation for prostatic cancer in the Department of Radiation Oncology at Stanford. The results of treatment according to the clinical stage of the primary tumor are shown in Figures 57.3 to 57.6. The tumor stages were assigned retrospectively according to the AJCC-4 guidelines by review of TNM stages previously designated according to the Stanford staging system (23, 30). Results are depicted using Kaplan-Meier plots with tick marks denoting patients who were censored at their last follow-up (31). P values assessing the significance of differences between curves were calculated by the Gehan test (32).

In Figure 57.3, curve 5 depicts the survival expected in a general population that is calculated by compiling person-years of observation for each of the 1280 patients from the date of initial treatment of prostatic cancer to the last follow-up date or date of death and multiplying by age- and race-specific, annualized mortality rates for men in the San Francisco Bay area using the techniques of Monson (33). As shown in Figure 57.3, the survival of patients irradiated for stage T1 disease approximated that expected in the general population, but survival decreased significantly with advancing clinical tumor stage.

Figure 57.4, which depicts cause-specific survival by censoring deaths from diseases other than prostatic cancer, shows 20-year prostatic cancer survival rates of 76% for patients with T1, 58% for T2, 32% for T3, and 20% for T4 primaries. Freedom from relapse of prostatic cancer at any site is depicted in Figure 57.5 and was 71% for T1, 40% for T2, and 22% for T3 primary tumors at 20 years after treatment. Durable local control (as judged by periodic digital rectal examination) was achieved in 94% of patients with T1 primaries and approximately 60% of patients with more clinically advanced primary disease (Fig. 57.6). Distant metastases developed in the majority of patients who had recurrences (Fig. 57.7).

Figure 57.8 demonstrates the effect of the summed Gleason histologic pattern score on outcome, showing significant differ-

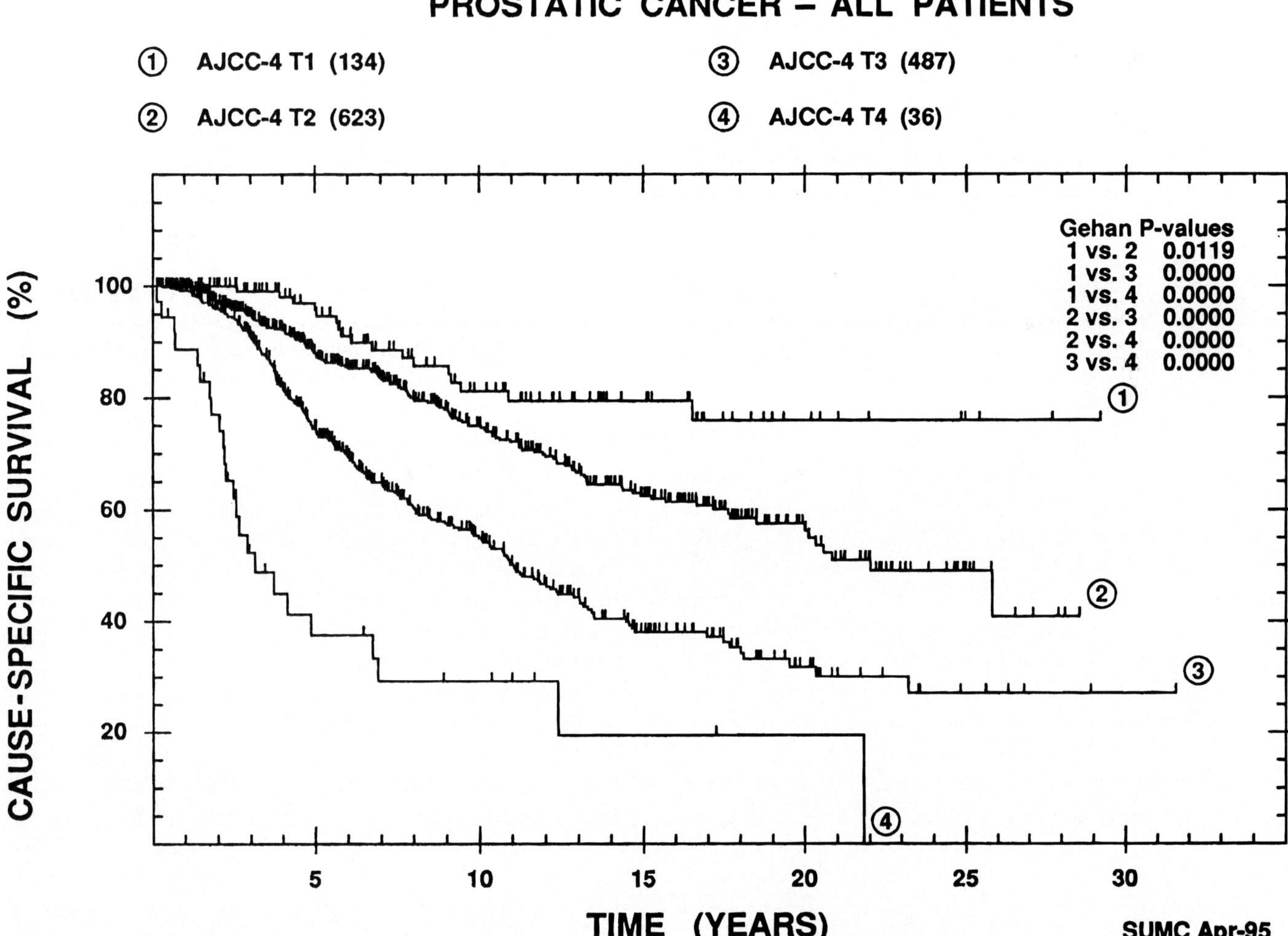

Fig. 57.4. Survival specific for prostatic cancer. Downward steps denote deaths due to prostatic cancer; tick marks above the lines are patients censored at their last contact or their death due to intercurrent disease.

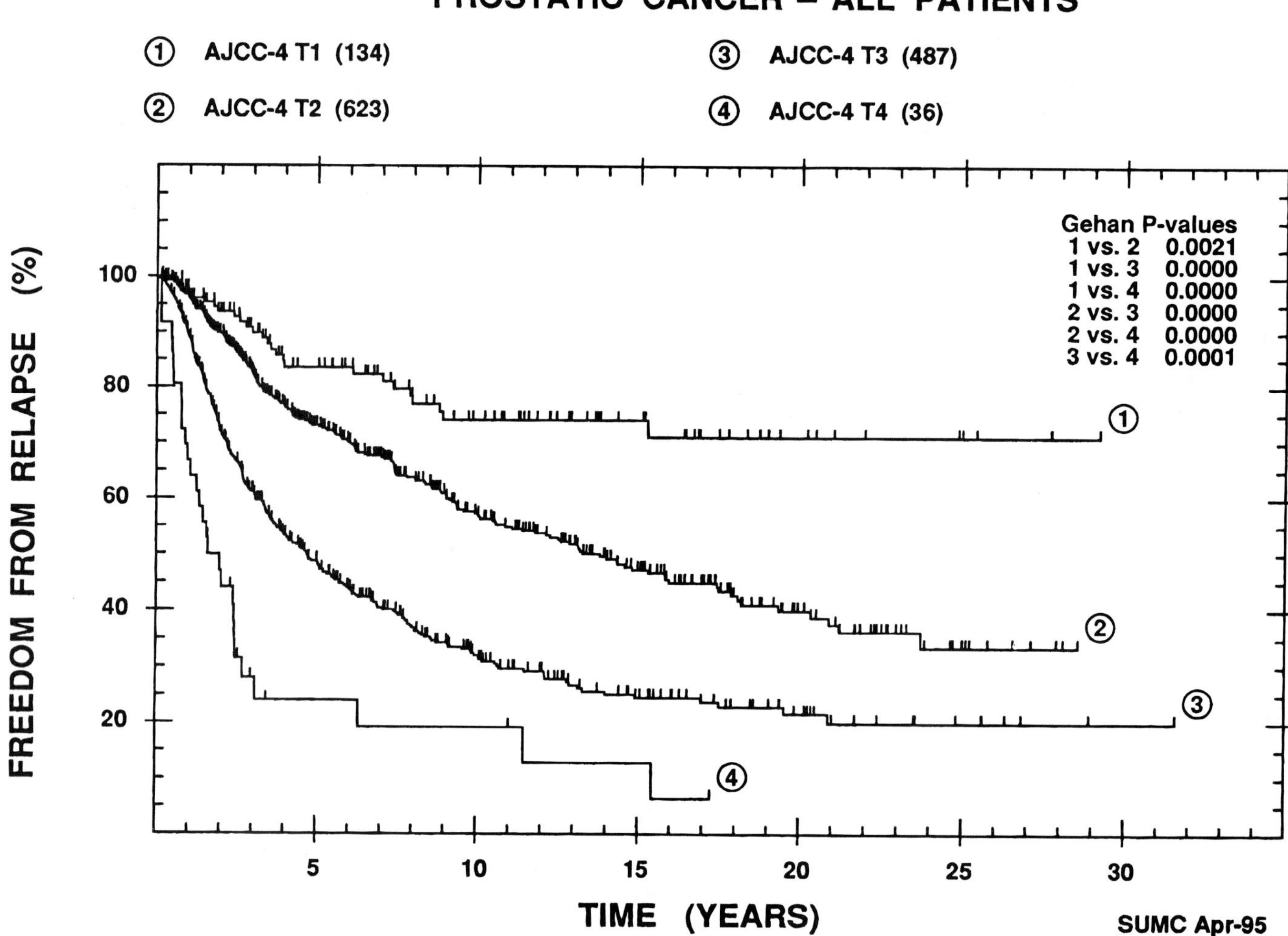

Fig. 57.5.   Freedom from relapse of prostatic cancer after prostatic irradiation. Downward steps denote first recurrence of prostatic cancer, either within the prostate gland or at a distant site; tick marks above the lines show patients who were disease free at the specified interval after therapy or who died without clinical relapse.

ences in survival from prostatic cancer for Gleason scores less than or equal to 5, 6, or 7 and greater than or equal to 8. Outcome did not vary significantly for patients with summed Gleason scores that ranged from 2 to 5 or from 8 to 10. The summed Gleason pattern score had a similar effect on the other clinical endpoints as well, significantly affecting survival, freedom from relapse, local control, and freedom from metastasis (data not shown). Similar long-term outcome after prostatic irradiation has been reported from national patterns of care studies and from several other centers (34, 35).

Measurement of the serum PSA has provided a new ability to detect prostatic cancer, evaluate clinically the extent of disease, and monitor response to various forms of therapy (26, 36–38). Recently, Stamey et al. have asserted that irradiation controls only 20% of prostatic cancers as assessed by PSA levels that remain at or below 1.0 ng/mL (Hybritech assay) or 1.7 ng/mL (Yang assay) (39). They also suggested that control was independent of clinical tumor stage and Gleason histologic

score and that 80% of patients who were not cured experienced accelerated tumor growth after irradiation. Their study was based on 113 irradiated patients who had a serum PSA measurement between April 1985 and January 1988 and had, at least, one subsequent serum PSA measurement. Some of these patients had been treated by [125]iodine implantation and others by external beam therapy.

When the same entry criteria were applied to the population of patients treated with external beam irradiation in the Stanford Department of Radiation Oncology, 110 patients were identified, 42 of whom (38%) had stable, normal PSA values from 4.4 to 25 years after irradiation (average, 12.4 years) (40). PSA control rates varied significantly by primary tumor stage: T1, 13 of 18 (72.2%); T2, 19 of 51 (37.3%); T3, 9 of 32 (28.1%); and T4 or biopsy-proven lymph node disease, 1 of 9 (11.1%) (P = 0.000001). Pretreatment PSA also affected outcome: 8 of 12 patients (67%) with PSA less than 20 ng/mL remained free of PSA relapse; all 18 patients with pretreat-

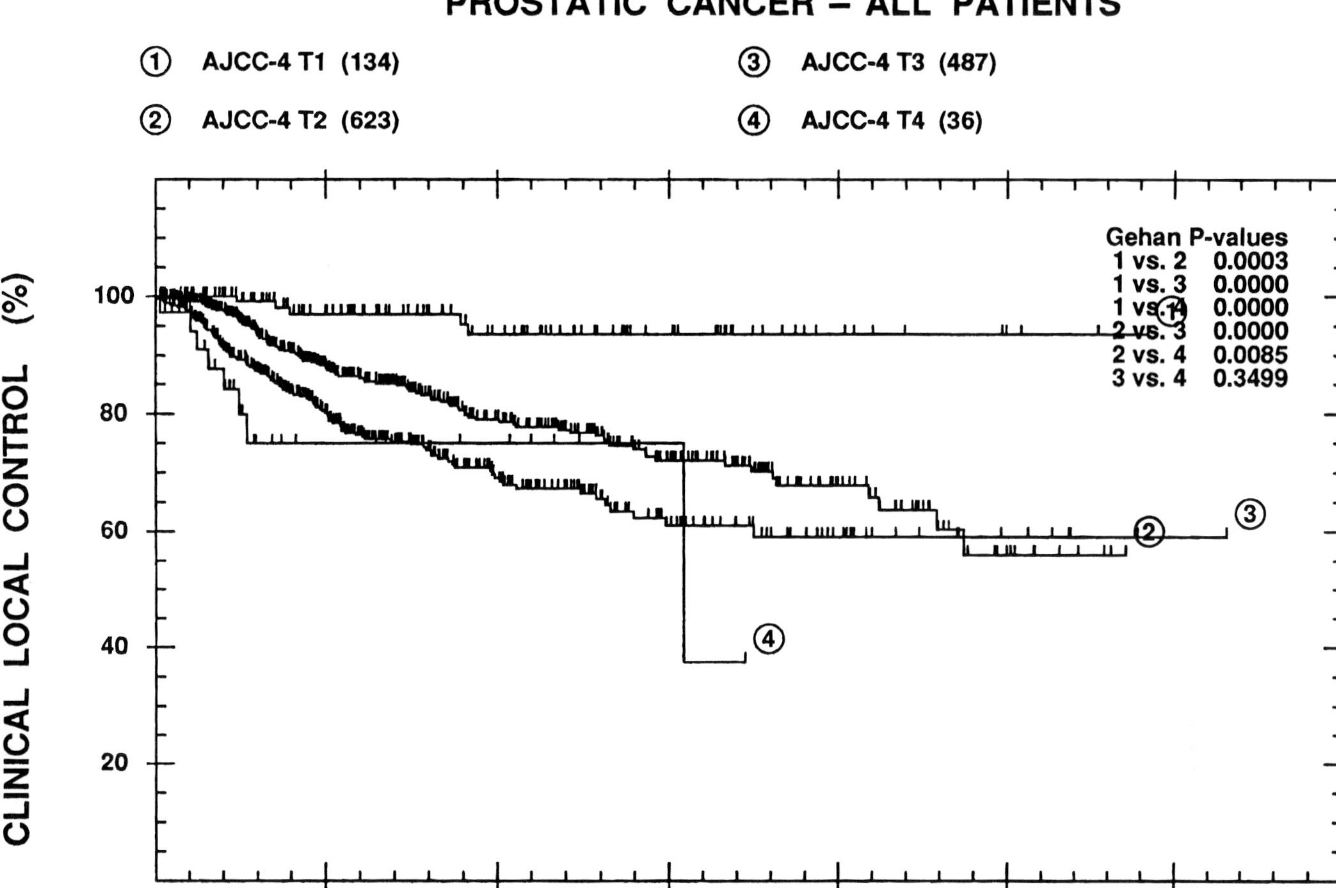

Fig. 57.6. Local control of prostatic cancer after irradiation. Downward steps indicate recurrence of prostatic cancer within the prostate gland based on findings on digital rectal examination; patients who were without evidence of recurrent disease in the prostate at their last follow-up or who died of intercurrent disease or metastatic prostate cancer without clinical local recurrence are censored and are denoted by upward tick marks.

ment PSA greater than or equal to 20 ng/mL had PSA rises compatible with relapse. PSA doubling times at recurrence after irradiation tended to be relatively long in patients who had locally recurrent prostatic cancer alone (average, 11.3 months) and short in patients who had disseminated metastases (average, 3.3 months), as was also demonstrated by analyses by Cox et al. (41). However, patients in whom disseminated metastases developed following prostatic fossa irradiation for PSA elevation or clinical recurrence after radical prostatectomy tended to have very short PSA doubling times (average, 2.2 months); it is unlikely that irradiation for microscopic residual or minimally recurrent disease played a determinant role in these PSA doubling times. Partin et al. have also observed that low PSA velocity correlated with local recurrence and high PSA velocity with distant metastasis in a large series of patients followed after radical prostatectomy (42). None of these findings support the assertion that radiation increases the aggressiveness of uncured prostatic cancer to produce a less favorable outcome.

Because the prostate gland remains intact after irradiation and clinically applicable radiation doses do not curtail protein synthesis, it is unclear what PSA level is compatible with freedom from active prostatic cancer in irradiated patients. Stamey et al. required that the PSA level remain at or below 1.0 mg/mL (Hybritech) after irradiation to consider a patient cured (39). Some authors have reported that a PSA nadir at or below 1.0 within 1 year after irradiation is necessary for a patient to have a high likelihood of remaining free of relapse (43, 44). However, occasional patients have persistently declining PSA values for as long as 30 months after irradiation and should not be considered as having biochemical evidence for treatment failure without an established, exponentially rising serum PSA level. Similarly, patients who have stable, follow-up PSA values that are within the normal range but exceed 1.0 ng/mL years after irradiation should probably not be regarded or managed as having active prostatic cancer (39, 40).

Radiation can be administered safely after radical prostatectomy for suspected or proven residual disease in the prostatic

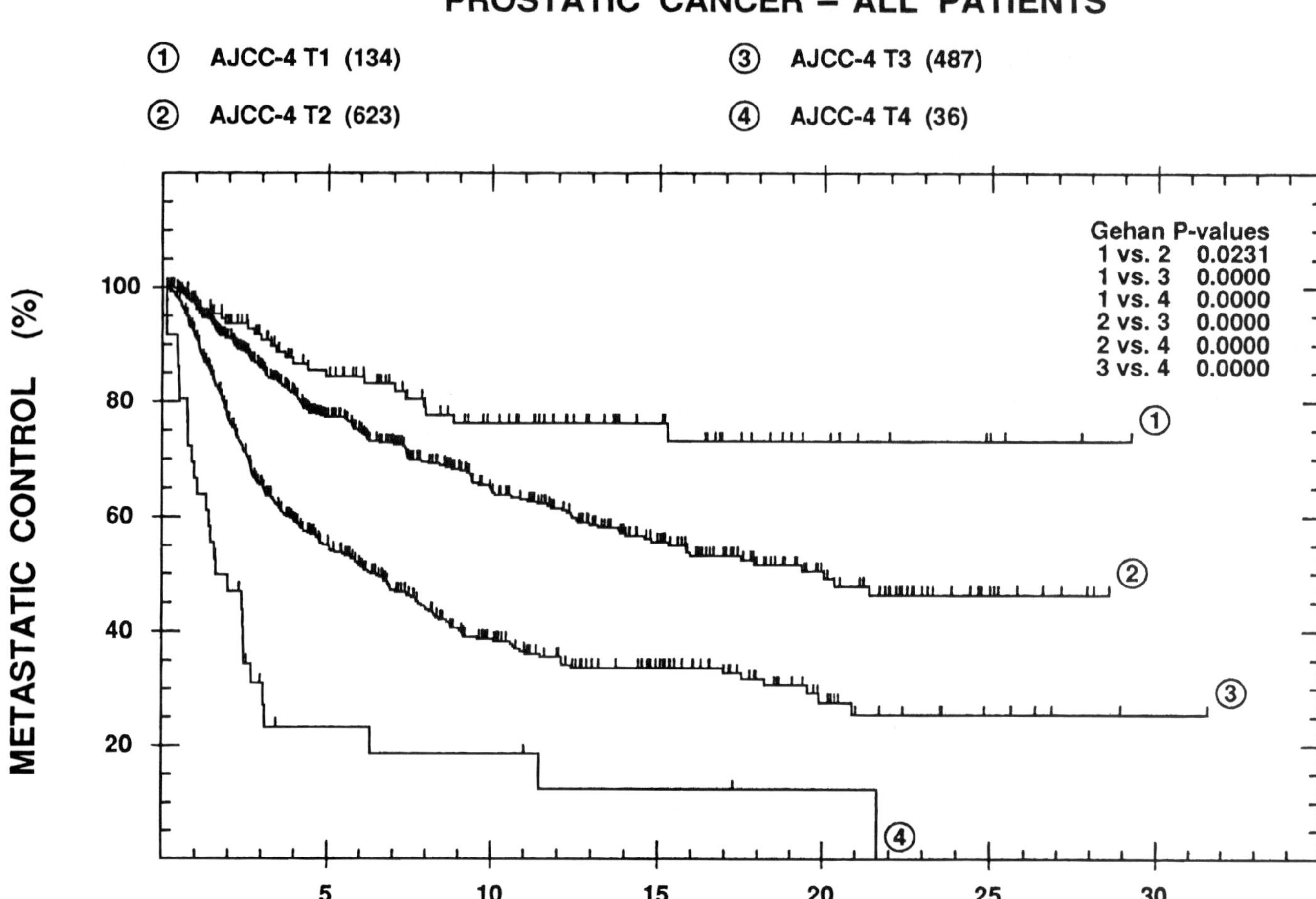

Fig. 57.7. Freedom from distant metastases after prostatic irradiation. Downward steps denote patients in whom distant metastases developed; tick marks denote patients who were censored at their last follow-up or date of death with or without recurrent disease within the prostate gland.

fossa or pelvic lymph nodes or for persisting or recurring serum PSA values after prostatectomy. The techniques of irradiation are similar to those described above for the treatment of an intact prostate gland, and similar radiation doses have been used. With limited experience reported thus far, the results suggest that such treatment reduces the incidence of clinical relapse within the pelvis but may not dramatically reduce the rates of subsequent biochemical recurrence, as evidenced by detectable and rising serum PSA values (45, 46).

SEQUELAE OF PROSTATIC IRRADIATION

During pelvic and prostatic irradiation, patients commonly report mild to moderate diarrhea and some have increased frequency of urination and dysuria. Such symptoms are readily managed by simple, symptomatic medications and typically resolve within several weeks after the conclusion of therapy. Acute side effects are generally minimal among patients who receive focal irradiation of the prostate gland. Recent analyses

summarizing the late effects of external beam irradiation administered in conventional doses to several thousand patients confirm an incidence of severe bowel or bladder complications of less than 1.9% (47, 48). The incidence of either transient hematuria or transient rectal bleeding was approximately 5%. Erectile potency varied from 33 to 60% beyond 5 years from irradiation. These low rates of significant complications and moderate chance of retaining sexual potency are similar to those reported earlier from the Stanford series, in which half of patients who reported erectile potency before prostatic irradiation remained potent at 7 years after treatment (30).

SUMMARY

Radiation therapy remains a viable alternative to radical prostatectomy for the management of organ-confined prostatic cancer and is the standard therapy for patients with locally advanced disease, including those with large primary tumors or disease that extends beyond the capsule of the prostate, into seminal

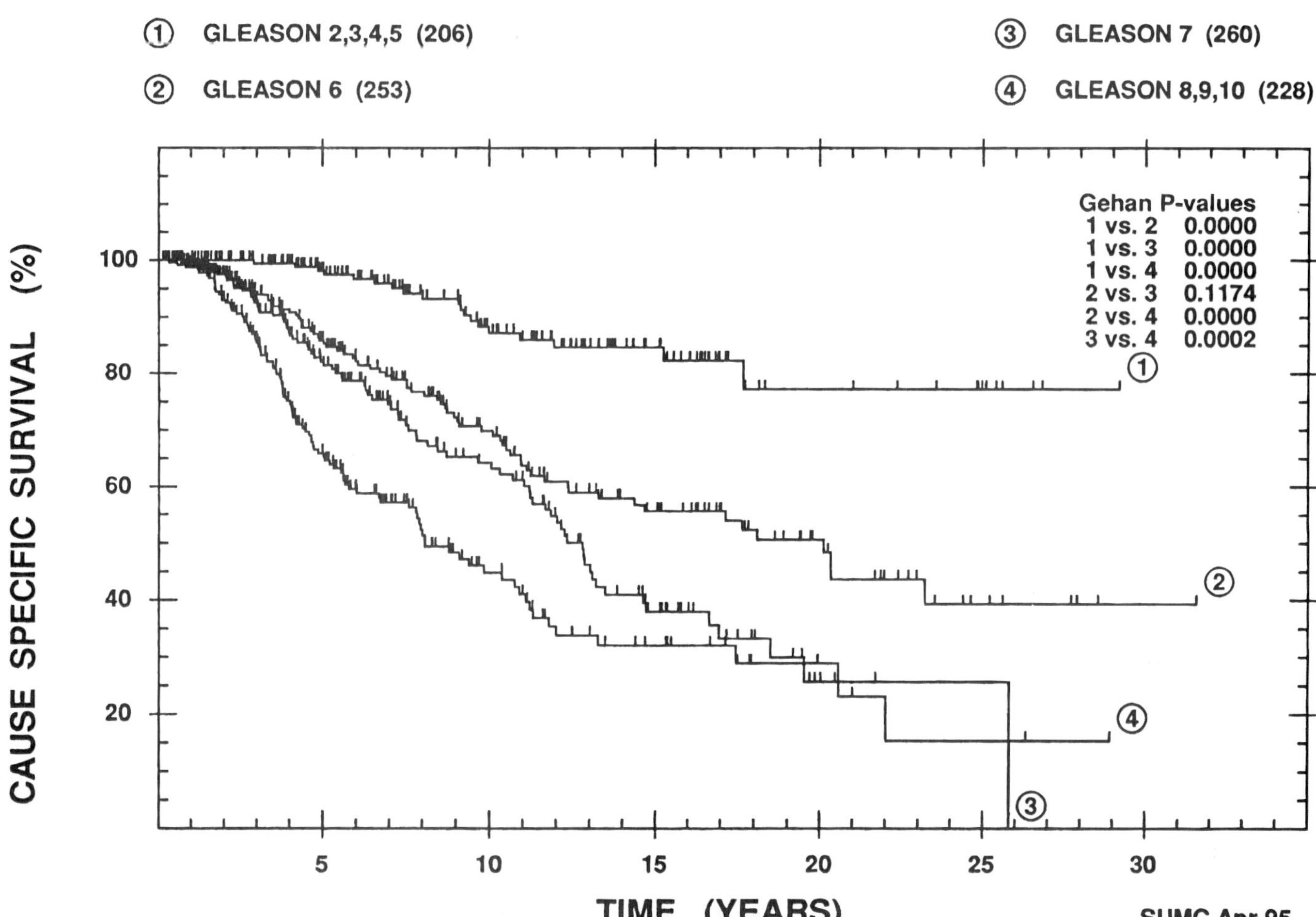

Fig. 57.8. Survival specific for prostate cancer according to the sum of the Gleason major and minor histologic pattern scores. Downward steps denote death from prostate cancer; tick marks above the lines denote patients censored at their last contact or their death due to intercurrent disease.

vesicles, or into regional lymph nodes. There are preliminary reports that transient or permanent androgen deprivation may improve the outcome of irradiation for patients with poor prognosis prostate cancer, although studies are not yet sufficiently mature to judge whether adjuvant hormonal therapy will contribute to improved survival.

Long-term follow-up in large populations of men has confirmed that local control can be achieved in the majority of patients with irradiation, with a low incidence of serious complications. Radiation may be given safely following radical prostatectomy for involved surgical margins, local recurrence, or a rising PSA that suggests local recurrence in the absence of clinically discernible distant disease. Overall, approximately 40% of patients irradiated for prostatic cancer appear to remain free of a subsequent rise in the PSA at long follow-up intervals. The probability of remaining free from biochemical recurrence correlates with the primary tumor stage and Gleason histologic score and parallels the various clinical endpoints of survival, cause-specific survival, local control, and development of distant metastases.

External beam irradiation has achieved prostate cancer-specific survival rates of 76% for T1 disease, 58% for T2 disease, 32% for T3 disease, and 20% for T4 disease at 20 years of follow-up after irradiation at Stanford. Occasional patients are now seen who have remained free of recurrent prostatic cancer for more than 30 years after irradiation.

Several alternate strategies for irradiating the prostate have been advocated in recent years. Excellent local control rates have been reported when standard external beam irradiation of the pelvis (with or without staging lymphadenectomy) has been combined with temporary [192]iridium (alone or with radiofrequency-induced hyperthermia), permanent [103]palladium, or fast neutron beam boosts to the prostate gland (3–5, 49). These approaches achieve higher total radiation doses to the prostatic tumor than have been routinely administered with conventional external beam irradiation.

Multifield conformal therapy derived from computerized three-dimensional treatment planning also escalates prostatic radiation doses using external beam irradiation (29). Differences in patient selection may complicate comparisons among older external beam irradiation series and more recent approaches. Several factors may predispose to better outcomes in more recent series. Patients who are candidates for invasive treatments may fare better than a more general population. Lymph node involvement has major prognostic significance, and studies that include lymphadenectomy allow more accurate segregation of stage or exclusion of node-positive patients, which has major prognostic importance. Pretreatment serum PSA levels may influence patient selection. Clinical staging may be more accurate due to transrectal ultrasonography and improvements in technetium bone scans. CT and MRI scanning have improved both staging and the accuracy of radiation dose delivery. As has been observed in some of the above studies, dose escalation may achieve apparently better local control at the expense of greater morbidity.

Neither radical prostatectomy nor these strategies to improve the local or regional irradiation of prostatic cancer are likely to have a major effect on the survival of the many patients who have clinically apparent or occult metastases from prostatic cancer. More effective means of eradicating distant disease will be required to achieve substantially higher survival and cure rates.

REFERENCES

1. Bagshaw MA, Cox RS, Hancock SL. Control of prostate cancer with radiotherapy: long-term results. J Urol 1994;152:1781.
2. Hanks GE. Radiotherapy or surgery for prostate cancer: ten and fifteen-year results of external beam therapy. Acta Oncol 1991;30:231.
3. Russell KJ, Caplan RJ, Laramore GE, et al. Photon versus fast neutron external beam radiotherapy in the treatment of locally advanced prostate cancer: results of a randomized prospective trial. Int J Radiat Oncol Biol Phys 1994;28:47.
4. Khan K, Thompson W, Bush S, et al. Transperineal percutaneous iridium-192 interstitial template implant of the prostate: results and complications in 321 patients. Int J Radiat Oncol Biol Phys 1992;22:935.
5. Blasko JC, Grimm PD, Ragde H. External beam irradiation with palladium-103 implantation for prostate carcinoma. Int J Radiat Oncol Biol Phys 1994;30(Suppl):219. Abstract.
6. Fowler FJ, Barry MJ, Lu-Yao G, et al. Patient-reported complications and follow-up treatment after radical prostatectomy. Urology 1993;42:622.
7. Jonler M, Ritter MA, Brinkmann R, et al. Sequelae of definitive radiation therapy for prostate cancer localized to the pelvis. Urology 1994;44:876.
8. Bagshaw MA, Ray GR, Cox RS. Complications associated with radiotherapy of prostate cancer. In: Smith RB, Ehrlich RM, eds. Complications of urologic surgery: prevention and management. Philadelphia: WB Saunders, 1990:88.
9. Pilepich MV, Caplan R, A1-Sarraf M, et al. Phase III trial of hormonal cytoreduction in conjunction with definitive radiotherapy in locally advanced prostate carcinoma: the emerging role of PSA in the assessment of outcome. Int J Radiat Oncol Biol Phys 1993;27(Suppl):246. Abstract.
10. Wynant GE, Murphy GP, Horoszewicz JS, et al. Immunoscintigraphy of prostatic cancer: preliminary results with ^{111}In-labeled monoclonal antibody 7E11-C5.3 (CYT-356). Prostate 1991;18:229
11. Paschkis R, Tittinger W. Radiumbehandlung eines prostatasarkoms. Wien Klin Wochenschr 1910;13:1715.
12. Pasteau O, Degrais J. De L'emploi du radium dans le traitement des cancers de la prostate. J d'Urol Paris 1913;4:341.
13. Young HH. Use of radium in cancer of the prostate and bladder. JAMA 1917;68:1174.
14. Smith GS, Pierson EL. The value of high voltage x-ray therapy in carcinoma of the prostate. J Urol 1930;23:331.
15. Widmann BP. Cancer of the prostate: the results of radium and roentgen-ray treatment. Radiology 1934;22:153.
16. Flocks RH, Kerr HD, Elkins HB, et al. Treatment of carcinoma of the prostate by interstitial radiation with radioactive gold: preliminary report. J Urol 1952;68:510.
17. Flocks RH, Culp DA, Elkins HB. Present status of radioactive gold therapy in management of prostatic cancer. J Urol 1959;81:178.
18. Bagshaw MA, Kaplan, HS, Sagerman RH. Linear accelerator supervoltage VII: carcinoma of the prostate. Radiology 1965;85:121.
19. George FW, Carlton CE, Dykhuizen RF, et al. Cobalt 60 teletherapy in definitive treatment of carcinoma of the prostate: a preliminary report. J Urol 1965;93:102.
20. del Regato JA. Radiotherapy in the conservative treatment of operable and locally inoperable carcinoma of the prostate. Radiology 1967;88:761.
21. Ennis RD, Flynn SD, Fischer DB, et al. Preoperative serum prostate-specific antigen and Gleason grade as predictors of pathologic stage in clinically organ confined prostate cancer: implications for the choice of primary treatment. Int J Radiat Oncol Biol Phys 1994;30:317.
22. Epstein JI, Walsh PC, Carmichael M, et al. Pathologic and clinical findings to predict tumor extent of nonpalpable (stage T1C) prostate cancer. JAMA 1994;271:368.
23. American Joint Committee on Cancer: Manual for staging of cancer. 4th ed. Philadelphia: JB Lippincott, 1992:181.
24. Gleason DF, Mellinger GT, Veterans Administration Cooperative Urological Research Group. Prediction of prognosis for prostatic adenocarcinoma by combined histological grading and clinical staging. J Urol 1974;111:58.
25. Woo S, Kaplan I, Roach M, et al. Formula to estimate risk of pelvic lymph node metastasis from the total Gleason score for prostate cancer. J Urol 1988;140:387.
26. Partin SW, Yoo J, Ballentine Carter H, et al. The use of prostate specific antigen, clinical stage and Gleason score to predict pathological stage in men with localized prostate cancer. J Urol 1993;150:110.
27. Roach M, Marquez C, Yuo H, et al. Predicting the risk of lymph node involvement using the pre-treatment prostate specific antigen and Gleason score in men with clinically localized prostate cancer. Int J Radiat Oncol Biol Phys 1994;28:33.
28. Wolf JS, Cher M, Dall'era M, et al. The use and accuracy of cross-sectional imaging and fine needle aspiration cytology for detection of pelvic lymph node metastases before radical prostatectomy. J Urol 1995;153:993.
29. Leibel SA, Zelefsky MJ, Kutcher GJ, et al. Three-dimensional

conformal radiation therapy in localized carcinoma of the prostate: interim report of a phase 1 dose-escalation study. J Urol 1994;152:1792.

30. Bagshaw MA, Cox RS, Ray GR. Status of radiation treatment of prostate cancer at Stanford University. NCI Monogr 1988;7: 47.

31. Kaplan EL, Meier P. Nonparametric estimation from incomplete observations. J Am Stat Assoc 1958;53:457.

32. Gehan EA. A generalized Wilcoxon test for comparing arbitrarily singly-censored samples. Biometrika 1965;52:203.

33. Monson RR. Analysis of relative survival and proportional mortality. Comput Biomed Res 1974;7:325.

34. Hanks GE, Krall JM, Hanlon AL, et al. Patterns of care and RTOG studies in prostate cancer: long-term survival, hazard rate observations, and possibilities of cure. Int J Radiat Oncol Biol Phys 1994;28:39.

35. Perez CA, Hanks GE, Leibel SA, et al. Localized carcinoma of the prostate (stages T1B, T1C, T2, and T3): review of management with external beam radiation therapy. Cancer 1993;72:3156.

36. Catalona WJ, Smith DS, Ratliff TL, et al. Detection of organ-confined prostate cancer is increased through prostate-specific antigen-based screening. JAMA 1993;270:948.

37. Stamey TA, Kabalin JN, McNeal JE, et al. Prostate specific antigen in the diagnosis and treatment of adenocarcinoma of the prostate: part 2. radical prostatectomy treated patients. J Urol 1989;141:1076.

38. Kleer E, Larson-Keller JJ, Zincke H, et al. Ability of pre-operative serum prostate specific antigen value to predict pathologic stage and DNA ploidy. Urology 1993;41:207.

39. Stamey TA, Ferrari MK, Schmid HP. The value of serial prostate specific antigen determinations 5 years after radiotherapy: steeply increasing values characterize 80% of patients. J Urol 1993;150:1856.

40. Hancock SL, Cox RS, Bagshaw MA. Prostate specific antigen after radiotherapy for prostate cancer: a re-evaluation of long term biochemical control and the kinetics of recurrence in patients treated at Stanford. J Urol 1995;154:1412.

41. Cox RS, Kaplan ID, Bagshaw MA. Prostate-specific antigen kinetics after external beam irradiation for carcinoma of the prostate. Int J Radiat Oncol Biol Phys 1994;28:23.

42. Partin AW, Pearson JD, Landis PK, et al. Evaluation of serum prostate-specific antigen velocity after radical prostatectomy to distinguish local recurrence from distant metastases. Urology 1994;43:649.

43. Zietman AL, Coen JJ, Shipley WU, et al. Radical radiation therapy in the management of prostatic adenocarcinoma: the initial prostate specific antigen value as a predictor of treatment outcome. J Urol 1994;151:640.

44. Zagars GK. Prostate specific antigen as an outcome variable for T1 and T2 prostate cancer treated by radiation therapy. J Urol 1994;152:1786.

45. Zietman AL, Coen JJ, Shipley WU, et al. Adjuvant irradiation after radical prostatectomy for adenocarcinoma of the prostate: analysis of freedom from PSA failure. Urology 1993;42:292.

46. Kaplan ID, Bagshaw MA. Serum prostate-specific antigen after post-prostatectomy radiotherapy. Urology 1992;39:401.

47. Shipley WU, Zietman AL, Hanks GE, et al. Treatment related sequelae following external beam radiation for prostate cancer: a review with an update in patients with stages T1 and T2 tumor. J Urol 1994;152:1799.

48. Lawton CA, Won M, Pilepich MV, et al. Long-term treatment sequelae following external beam irradiation for adenocarcinoma of the prostate: analysis of RTOG studies 7506 and 7706. Int J Radiat Oncol Biol Phys 1991;21:935.

49. Bagshaw MA, Prionas SD, Goffinet DR, et al. External beam irradiation combined with the use of 192-iridium implants and radiofrequency-induced hyperthermia in the treatment of prostatic carcinoma. Prog Clin Biol Res 1991;370:275.

58

Management of Stage I and II Seminoma

Stephen R. Smalley
Mark L. Davidner
Richard S. Evans

The management of patients with early stage seminomas has become increasingly complex as therapeutic modalities and understanding of the biologic behavior of this disease have improved. Controversy exists regarding the management of virtually every stage of disease, a situation that mandates detailed understanding of the disease, therapeutic alternatives, and close collaboration of all members of the oncologic team charged with these patients' care.

Seminoma is the most common single histologic type of testicular carcinoma and accounts for 35 to 40% of all testis cancer (1–6). Seminoma most frequently presents in the third to fourth decades of life as a painless enlargement of the testicle. When compared with nonseminomatous germ cell tumors (NSGCT), the mean age of seminomas is almost one decade later (1, 2, 6). The majority, approximately 60 to 80%, present with stage I disease, whereas 10 to 20% present with stage II disease; the remainder manifest stage III to IV presentations (1–6).

Histologically, seminomas are divided into three types. By far the most frequent is classic histologic type, which accounts for 85 to 90% of seminomas (5, 7, 8). Anaplastic seminomas constitute 5 to 15% of seminomas (5, 7–10). Several series have documented that anaplastic seminomas more frequently present with advanced disease when compared with those with classic seminomas (7, 8, 10). Several groups (8, 9, 10) have observed no difference in survival between classic and anaplastic seminomas when evaluated stage for stage. However, others (7), chiefly reporting data from the era before cisplatin (CDDP), reported inferior relapse-free or overall survival with anaplastic histologic type. Spermatocytic type occurs in only 2 to 10% of seminomas (11–13). It is distinguished from the more common histologic types by its absence of lymphocytic and granulomatous host reaction as well as its infrequent but well-recognized association with sarcomas of the testis (11, 12). Spermatocytic seminomas have an exceedingly favorable prognosis, with only

a few case reports in the literature (13) of metastatic disease developing out of a pure seminoma. In the rare instance when spermatocytic seminomas are associated with a sarcoma, the sarcomatous elements may well metastasize (11, 12). Seminomas are frequently associated with a brisk host reaction characterized by dense lymphocytic and granulomatous giant cell features. At times, the lymphocytic and granulomatous reaction can be so dramatic that it confuses histologic identification or produces hypercalcemia mediated via a sarcoidosis-like hyperhydroxylation of vitamin D precursors (14, 15).

Patients with pure seminomas will not produce alpha-fetoprotein (AFP) (3, 6, 10). Those with detectable AFP should be managed as having NSGCT regardless of whether these nonseminomatous germ cell elements can be identified histologically. In contradistinction, 8 to 12% of pure seminomas have detectable elevation of beta human chorionic gonadotropin (β-hCG), which appears to arise from syncytiotrophoblastic giant cells within the seminoma tissue (16–21). Some controversy exists regarding the significance of β-hCG in those with histologically pure seminomas. The majority of series find no adverse prognostic association of β-hCG elevation with outcome (16, 17, 20, 21). Others report those with very high β-hCG levels or advanced tumors have a somewhat adverse outcome when compared with β-hCG–negative tumors (22, 23). It is the authors' admittedly somewhat arbitrary practice to consider those otherwise characteristic seminoma presentations with modest β-hCG elevations (less than or equal to 2 to 5 times institutional upper limits of normal) as having pure seminomas. However, atypical presentations, suspicious histologic features, or β-hCG elevations greater than this are managed as NSGCT. A variety of other biochemical markers have been or are currently being evaluated, including neuron-specific enolase, placental alkaline phosphatase, and others (24). The development of a reliable biochemical marker would be of great value in those with metastatic seminomas because the majority of these are β-hCG negative.

MANAGEMENT OF STAGE I SEMINOMA

Seminoma is one of the most radiosensitive malignancies. Because of this extreme radiosensitivity and historical data indicating a 20 to 30% retroperitoneal relapse rate following radical orchiectomy alone in clinical stage I disease, radiation therapy has been used for decades as adjuvant therapy following orchiectomy. Radiation therapy results spanning several decades are shown in Table 58.1 (4, 25–37). Relapse rates range from 0 to 5%, a result encouraging enough to query whether this standard policy should be further evaluated. Indeed, treatment has failed due to inadequate execution or marginal misses in many patients who have had relapses in these series. It is likely that modern radiation therapy series—with improved staging, treatment planning, imaging modalities, and ability to exclude NSGCT—would have even better relapse-free survivals. Even so, a sizable percentage of patients who have had relapses in these series have undergone salvage therapy. Very few of these series occurred in the CDDP chemotherapy era; therefore, patients underwent salvage radiation therapy. It is likely that in the current era of CDDP salvage therapy, the overwhelming majority of patients would have undergone salvage therapy in the very unusual event that treatment would fail.

Despite the manifest success of adjuvant radiation therapy in stage I seminoma, many investigators are currently evaluating alternative management philosophies in stage I seminoma. Primarily, these considerations flow from an evaluation of long-term treatment sequelae. Acutely, infradiaphragmatic radiation therapy is extremely well tolerated. Approximately half of patients experience some mild nausea and vomiting that are usually effectively addressed by antiemetic therapy. Although some mild myelosuppression can occur, grade 3 or greater toxicity is exceedingly rare (30, 31, 33, 37).

Some reports have documented a small increased risk of

Table 58.1.   Stage I Radiation Therapy Results

REFERENCE	NO. RELAPSE/NO. TREATED (%)	5-YR SURVIVAL (%)
Peckham and McElwain (25)	4/121 (37)	96[a]
Earle et al. (26)	1/78 (1)	100
Werf-Messing (27)	0/91	100
Hamilton et al. (28)	5/232 (2)	94[b]
Dosoretz et al. (29)	7/135 (5)	97
Hunter and Peschel (30)	1/81 (2)	96
Fossa et al. (31)	13/365 (4)	99
Zablow et al. (4)	0/31	100
Giacchetti et al. (32)	4/184 (2)	98
Steinfeld and Newall (33)	0/51	100
Tombolini et al. (34)	2/84 (2)	100
Lai et al. (35)	2/95 (2)	100
Sommer et al. (36)	0/133	100
Glanzman et al. (37)	0/128	100
Total	39/1681 (2)	

[a] 4 intercurrent and 1 second primary deaths.

[b] All deaths due to intercurrent illness.

chronic peptic ulcer disease after infradiaphragmatic radiation therapy. However, these series used larger doses than are used today. Series analyzing this issue have documented excellent long-term gastrointestinal tolerance with less than or equal to 3000 to 3400 cGy conventionally fractionated (31, 36, 38–41). Almost half of those presenting for consideration of adjuvant radiation therapy will have oligospermia or azoospermia (41). Some oligospermia after adjuvant radiation therapy is common due to scattered radiation to the contralateral testicle. However, the oligospermia is almost universally transient, lasting 1 to 1.5 years after radiation therapy with return of sperm counts to normal in 2 to 3 years. It is imperative to use a variety of radiation therapy techniques, including testicular shielding that reduces testicular dose to less than 0.5% of the treatment dose (40–42). The risk of other vascular, renal, or blood pressure chronic toxicity is extremely low (40, 41, 43).

In the past decade, however, an increasing number of reports have raised concerns regarding the incidence of second malignancy in those treated with radiation therapy. Several series have documented an increase in relative risk, ranging from 1.3 to 7.5, of second malignancies in those treated with radiation therapy for testicular carcinoma (44–49). There are several important factors to recognize insofar as radiation-induced second malignancy is concerned. The first is that patients with seminomas or other testicular malignancies appear to be at increased risk of tumor development whether or not they receive radiation. For example, Kleinerman et al. (50) compared irradiated versus nonirradiated patients in a large cohort and found similar increases in second malignancies in both groups. Although a higher risk of sarcoma development in patients with seminomas receiving radiation therapy has been conjectured, the actual incidence of such occurrences is rare.

In addition, the increasing risk of second malignancy is usually not apparent for 5 to 10 years after radiation therapy, and many series (32, 37) have documented that the median time to second malignancy is in excess of 10 years after radiation. Therefore, although the incidence of second malignancy in the Glanzmann et al. series (37) (which showed no increased relative risk in those radiated) was only 0.4% at 4 years, by 24 years this risk had increased to 7.5%; at 35 years, a second malignancy had developed in 24%. Giacchetti et al. (32) reported that second malignancy had developed in 21% of patients at 20 years in their series.

Many of these series have simply evaluated the risk of second malignancy in all testicular cancer patients who have received radiation therapy. Several series (44, 46, 51) have documented that the largest second malignancy risk was in NSGCT patients who received extensive, high-dose radiation therapy in the era before CDDP. These series showed no increased risk in the seminoma patients who were treated with low doses of radiation to the infradiaphragmatic areas only. There are some who have also evaluated this issue and have found no increased risk of subsequent development of tumors (52).

To summarize, although the risk of developing second malignancies appears to be directly proportional to high doses and volumes of radiation therapy that are increasingly eschewed (vide infra), it is probable that patients treated with adjuvant radiation therapy will suffer some increased risk of second malignancies that, although quantitively quite small in absolute terms, will be sustained over the remainder of their lifetimes. Clearly, patients who are contemplating adjuvant radiation therapy must be informed of this significant risk of treatment. Additionally, investigators will be evaluating alternative radiation therapy field and dose fractionation schemes in an effort to diminish the risk of serious harm.

SURVEILLANCE SERIES

During the past decade, several factors led numerous investigators to evaluate the concept of close surveillance in patients with stage I seminomas. These factors included the following.

- The development of highly effective chemotherapy that could salvage the few who had relapses.
- The recognition that those who had relapse with nonbulky stage II disease would receive identical radiation therapy as would be administered with adjuvant treatment, with an extremely high prospect of cure.
- The hope that improved imaging and tumor marker studies would allow more effective diagnosis of early stage II disease, producing a lower relapse rate in those thought to have clinical stage I seminomas.

Surveillance series results are shown in Table 58.2. Surprisingly, relapse following orchiectomy in clinical stage I seminoma remains 15 to 25% even with modern imaging modalities, which would have been expected to produce stage migration in a significant percentage of patients diagnosed in earlier decades. However, 95% of those who have relapses are treated with either salvage radiation therapy or chemotherapy. The frequency with which chemotherapy is used as salvage therapy varies according to the philosophic persuasion of the institution performing surveillance. However, in those series that have a policy of using radiation therapy for nonbulky stage II relapse (55, 58), approximately 20 to 40% of those who relapse will require chemotherapy at the time of first or second relapse. The fact that virtually all patients are cured of their disease establishes close surveillance as a safe management policy for clinical stage I disease.

If surveillance is offered, several principles must be borne in mind. The first is that although the majority of relapses will occur within the first 2 years, a significant percentage will occur from 2 to 4 years after orchiectomy. Therefore, surveillance must be maintained at least 4 to 5 years. Patients must also be suitable candidates for surveillance. Not only must they be reliable for follow-up, but they must also be willing to accept both the risk of relapse and the added expense of frequent follow-up imaging and tumor marker studies. Finally, several series have defined factors that describe a group at higher risk of relapse in those electing surveillance. Patients with a high T stage (53), lymphatic and/or vascular invasion (55), and increasing size of primary testicular tumor (56) have all been reported to have substantially and statistically significant increased risk of tumor relapse. These patients or patients with anaplastic carcinoma should be evaluated very circumspectly insofar as surveillance is concerned.

ADJUVANT CHEMOTHERAPY FOR STAGE I SEMINOMA

Other investigators have evaluated the use of adjuvant chemotherapy for clinical stage I tumors. Oliver et al. have conducted several phase II trials using platinum-based analog in those with clinical stage I seminoma (58, 59). A total of 78 patients received single-agent therapy with a median follow-up of 25 months. Initially, CDDP was used (50 mg/m^2, days 1 and 2 every 3 weeks for two cycles). Subsequently, carboplatin was used. Carboplatin dosage was calculated according to the area under the curve formula (7 × [GFR + 25] mg). Fifty-three of 78 patients receiving single-agent chemotherapy received a total of two courses (median follow-up, 34 months), and 25 received only one course (median follow-up, 19 months). Only one patient relapsed and this patient was salvaged with additional therapy. Although this experience requires corroboration in other centers, the toxicity and low expense justify efforts to obtain further experience with this regimen.

Table 58.2. Surveillance in Stage I Seminoma

REFERENCE	MEDIAN FLU (MO)	NO. RELAPSE/NO. OF PATIENTS (%)	NO. SALVAGED/NO. RELAPSE	NO. NED/NO. OF PATIENTS
Allhoff et al. (53)	48	3/33 (10)	3/3	33/33
Ramakrishnan et al. (54)	44	13/72 (18)	13/13	72/72
Horwich et al. (55)	60	17/103 (17)	17/17	103/103
von der Maase et al. (56)	48	49/261 (19)	46/49	258/261
Warde et al. (57)	47	23/148 (16)	22/23	147/148
Oliver et al. (58)	61	18/67 (27)	16/18	65/67[b]
Total		123/684 (18)	117/123 (95%)	678/684 (99%)

NED, patients with no evidence of disease at last follow-up.

[a] Actuarial risk of relapse at 5 years = 19%.

[b] One of these 65 committed suicide.

MANAGEMENT OF STAGE II SEMINOMA

Seminoma does not frequently present with metastasis confined to the infradiaphragmatic lymphatics (stage II). Approximately 10 to 20% of seminomas present with stage II disease (1, 60–63). Bulky stage II disease accounts for a variable proportion of stage II disease, ranging from one fourth to two thirds of stage II patients (62–66). Our improvements in understanding the natural history of seminoma, its imaging, and radiotherapeutic and chemotherapeutic advances over the past two decades have had a dramatic effect on stage II seminoma management (1, 45, 67). Therefore, it is appropriate to critically assess current therapy and areas of controversy and to identify potential areas of future investigation.

Stage II seminoma is variously substaged on the basis of tumor width. Staging systems reported to separate stage II disease into separate meaningful categories include the following: less than 2 cm versus 2 to 5 cm, versus greater than 5 cm (64, 66); less than or equal to 5 cm versus greater than 5 cm (63, 68); less than 10 cm versus greater than or equal to 10 cm (65, 69); and palpable versus nonpalpable disease (70, 71). Although all these systems have merit, for the purposes of this discussion, stage II disease will be separated into bulky versus nonbulky categories. As will be shown, the prognosis of seminoma that is less than 10 cm in width is so favorable when treated with radiation therapy initially that it is most useful to concentrate on the worse substage that is reported. Therefore, the convention followed here is to classify the largest substage of stage II seminoma as bulky.

Several principles regarding stage II seminoma should be emphasized.

1. Importance of long follow-up. Seminomas commonly relapse 2 years or longer after completion of therapy (63, 72–79). Relapses more than 5 to 10 years apart are rare (74, 75, 77, 78). MacVicar and Horwich have reported that the mean time to relapse after chemotherapy is 28 months (79). Similarly, three separate series (71–73) observed that one fourth to one third of the relapses were more than 2 years following radiation therapy. This predisposition of seminomas to develop late recurrence makes comparison of radiation therapy and chemotherapy results problematic. Because radiation therapy was, until recently, the only reliably curative treatment modality for stage II seminomas, the radiation therapy series tabulated in Tables 58.3 and 58.4 have far more mature follow-up than those of the chemotherapy experiences tabulated in Table 58.5. Therefore, the CDDP-based chemotherapy series may underestimate the true incidence of relapse because of less than optimal follow-up duration.

2. Stage migration as a result of modern imaging modalities. Modern evaluation of stage II seminomas should include a computed tomography (CT) scan of the chest, abdomen, and pelvis. CT scans much more reliably define the extent and location of the infradiaphragmatic tumor and will detect with much greater accuracy the presence or absence of mediastinal, pulmonary intraparenchymal, or other visceral disease. Several radiation therapy series report mediastinal or visceral progression within weeks of initiation of infradiaphragmatic radiation (65, 70, 83), bearing testimony to the fact that many staged in the pre-CT era had stage III or IV seminoma at the time of diagnosis. Because only a significant minority of patients included in the radiation therapy reports had the benefit of modern imaging modalities as opposed to the CDDP-based chemotherapy reports (all of which occurred in the CT scan era), it is probable that stage migration has occurred in the more recent chemotherapy series. Such stage migration will improve the results of stage II seminoma management regardless of the therapeutic modality used.

3. The importance of tumor markers. The issue of β-hCG elevation in pure seminomas has been discussed. It is the authors' recommendation that strong consideration be given to primary chemotherapy in the unusual patient presenting with extreme elevations of β-hCG. More important than β-hCG is AFP. The presence of elevated AFP indicates NSGCT components, and all patients with such elevations should be managed with chemotherapy. Many radiation therapy series (66, 69, 75, 81, 90–93) have reported a significant frequency of patients with apparently pure seminoma relapsing as NSGCT. Peckham et al. (92) and Bredael et al. (93) have reported that 40% of relapsing seminoma patients had NSGCT. Because only a minority of those included in the radiation therapy series (Tables 58.3 and 58.4) were diagnosed during a time that AFP determination was available, it may be assumed that some of those included in these pre-AFP series had undiagnosed NSGCT.

4. The importance of modern therapeutic modalities. Radiation therapy has substantially improved over what was available from 1940 to 1980. These improvements have not only resulted in a diminution of toxicity but also an improvement in treatment efficacy. Likewise, CDDP-based salvage therapy did not exist for patients treated with radiation therapy from 1940 to 1980. Therefore, the overall survival of stage II seminoma treated with radiation therapy, as summarized in Tables 58.3 and 58.4, is clearly a minimal estimate of the survival that would be achieved in today's era of CDDP-based salvage therapy. For all these reasons, the results of radiation therapy and chemotherapy series cannot be considered reliably comparable.

Radiation Therapy for Stage II Seminoma

The results of series spanning a number of decades and using radiation therapy for nonbulky and bulky stage II seminoma are shown in Tables 58-3 and 58-4. In nonbulky stage II disease, initial radiation therapy will cure 90% or more. This

Table 58.3.   Radiation Therapy Results in Nonbulky Stage II Seminomas

REFERENCE	SIZE CRITERIA (CM)	DISEASE-FREE SURVIVAL (%)	SALVAGE (%)	OVERALL SURVIVAL (%)	MEDIAN FOLLOW-UP (YR) (RANGE)
Bayens et al. (72)	<5	22/29 (76)	4/7 (57)*	26/29 (90)	7.5 (0.8–13)
Lindeman and Tiver (80)	<5	8/9 (89)	1/1 (100)	9/9 (100)	4.2 (1.2–9)
Thomas et al. (71)	Nonpalpable	37/40 (93)	0/3 (0)	37/40 (93)	NS
Mason and Kearsley (65)	<5	24/25 (96)	0/1 (0)	24/25 (96)	6.2 (3–19.6)
Mason and Kearsley (65)	5–10	10/12 (87)	0/2 (0)	10/12 (87)	6.2 (3–19.6)
Hunter and Peschel (30)	<5	15/15 (100)	—	15/15 (100)	9 (1–24)
Evenson et al. (66)	<5	23/24 (96)	1/1 (100)	24/24 (100)	6.2 (2–13)
Sagerman et al. (81)	<5	19/21 (90)	2/2 (100)	21/21 (100)	8.5 (0.5–20)
Ball et al. (64)	<5	28/33 (85)	2/5 (40)	30/33 (91)	7.5 (3–17)
Ellerbroek et al. (63)	<5	7/8 (88)	0/1 (0)	7/8 (88)	Minimum 2
Jackson et al. (82)	Nonpalpable	26/29 (90)	0/3 (0)	26/29 (90)	NS
Lai et al. (35)	<5	31/33 (94)	1/2 (50)	32/33 (97)	6.7 (1–24)
Tombolini et al. (34)	<5	20/20 (100)	—	20/20 (100)	3.5 (2–11.6)
Lederman et al. (68)	<5	24/25 (96)	0/1 (0)	24/25 (96)	6 (1–17)
Andrews et al. (83)	<5	16/17 (94)	1/1 (100)	17/17 (100)	8.6 (0.5–12)
Total		310/340 (91)	12/30 (40)	322/340 (95)	

NS, not stated.

[a] Treated with CDDP-based salvage chemotherapy.

Table 58.4.   Radiation Therapy Results in Bulky Stage II Seminomas

REFERENCE	YEARS OF STUDY	SIZE CRITERIA (CM)	DISEASE-FREE SURVIVAL (%)	SALVAGE (%)	OVERALL SURVIVAL (%)	MEDIAN FOLLOW-UP (YR) (RANGE)
Jackson et al. (82)	42–78	Palpable	13/16 (83)	0/3 (0)	13/16 (83)	NS
Doornbos et al. (84)	44–71	>10	11/22 (50)	3/11 (27)	14/22 (61)	NS
Laukkanen et al. (85)	48–83	Palpable	17/23 (74)	3/6 (50)	21/23 (91)[a]	7.6 (2–26 yrs)
Ellerbroek et al. (63)	56–83	>5	8/15 (53)	1/7 (14)	9/15 (60)	Minimum 2
Thomas et al. (71)	58–76	Palpable	22/46 (48)	7/24 (29)	29/46 (63)	NS
Read et al. (73)	60–78	Palpable	30/67 (45)	8/37 (22)	(63)[b]	Minimum 4
Herman et al. (86)	60–81	Palpable	—	—	100/109 (92)[d]	
Zagars and Babaian (69)	60–82	Palpable	7/10 (70)[c]	0/3 (0)	7/10 (70)[c]	6.6
Andrews et al. (83)	62–84	>5	3/4 (75)	1/1 (100)[e]	4/4 (100)	8.6 (0.5–21)
Ball et al. (64)	63–79	>5	14/23 (61)	3/9 (33)	17/23 (74)	7.5 (3–17)
Hunter and Peschel (30)	64–84	>5	3/3 (100)	—	3/3 (100)	9 (1–24)
Martinelli (87)	65–85	Palpable	4/4 (100)	—	4/4 (100)	3.5 (15)
Sagerman et al. (81)	66–85	>5	10/11 (91)	1/1 (100)	11/11 (100)	8.5 (0.5–20)
Mason and Kearsley (65)	68–85	>10	8/12 (67)	1/4 (25)[e]	9/12 (75)	6.2 (3–19.6)
Green et al. (88)	69–80	>6	17/18 (94)	0/1 (0)	17/18 (94)	4 (1–11)
Evensen et al. (66)	71–81	>5	38/48 (79)	5/10 (50)	42/48 (88)	6.2 (2–13)
Smalley et al. (89)	71–82	>5	16/20 (80)	4/4 (100)	20/20 (100)	4.6 (24)
Bayens et al. (72)	75–85	>5	7/9 (78)	1/2 (50)	8/9 (89)	7.5 (0.8–13)
Lindeman et al. (80)	80–87	>5	4/5 (80)	1/1 (100)	5/5 (100)	4.2 (1.2–9)
Total			232/356 (65)	39/124 (31)	375/465 (81)	

NS, not stated.

[a] Disease-specific survival.

[b] Estimated from actuarial survival curves.

[c] One patient relapsing with choriocarcinoma with hCG elevation excluded.

[d] Cause-specific survival.

[e] CDDP or carboplatin used in salvage therapy.

Table 58.5. Mediastinal/Supraclavicular Failure as a Function of Prophylactic Mediastinal Irradiation

	STAGE II NONBULKY	
	NO. OF FAILURES[a]/TOTAL NO.	
REFERENCE	WITH PMI	WITHOUT PMI
Andrews (80)	0/16	1/5
Steinfeld (67)	0/22	0/6
Willan (70)	0/7	2/13
Lai (35)	0/25	0/8
Bayens (72)		3/29
Dosmann (94)	0/36	3/19
Mason (65)	0/22	1/15
Thomas (71)		0/40[b]
Herman (90)		8/197
Total	0/128	18/332 (5.4%)

	STAGE II BULKY	
	NO. OF FAILURES[a]/TOTAL NO.	
	WITH PMI	WITHOUT PMI
Ellerbroek (63)	0/7	1/6
Laukkanen (89)	0/8	4/15
Thomas (71)		10/46[b]
Smalley (93)	1/16	2/4
Herman (90)		20/109
Total	1/31 (3%)	37/180 (21%)

PMI, prophylactic mediastinal irradiation.

[a] Failures in mediastinum and/or supraclavicular areas as a component of failure.

[b] Only sites of initial recurrence reported; subsequent mediastinal/supraclavicular failures not reported.

disease-free survival is quite reliable in view of the long follow-up. Forty percent of those in whom treatment failed underwent salvage therapy, for an overall cure of 95%. The majority of those who underwent salvage therapy received radiation therapy for mediastinal failure. Only a small minority of these series occurred in the modern era of CDDP-based chemotherapy. Most modern chemotherapy series report disease-free and overall survivals well in excess of 70% when CDDP-based treatment follows infradiaphragmatic-only radiation therapy (vide infra). Therefore, using modern radiation therapy and salvage CDDP-based chemotherapy should result in overall survivals well in excess of 95%. These excellent results are achievable even in series that use generous tumor volumes (nonpalpable disease, less than 10 cm disease or 5 to 10 cm tumor widths) to define their nonbulky stage II substage (65, 71, 82, 94). Such excellent results with all stage II seminomas up to 10 cm support the contention that only those with very large seminomas (greater than or equal to 10 cm or palpable disease) should be considered bulky.

Those with large-volume, bulky stage II disease treated with radiation therapy fared considerably less well, as depicted in Table 58.4. These series, spanning several decades, have reported disease-free survival rates of only 65% with radiation therapy as initial management. Only 31% of those reported in

Table 58.4 were salvaged with subsequent therapy, with an overall survival of 77%. Although these very mature data seem somewhat comparable to the results achieved by CDDP-based chemotherapy (Table 58.5), it is somewhat disappointing and seems somewhat inferior to that achieved by modern chemotherapy. However, closer examination reveals that modern radiation therapy results are considerably better than in previous decades. For example, series initiating accrual from 1965 onward (series no. 11 to 18) reported much better disease-free survival (82%) with radiation therapy alone as initial management for large-volume, stage II disease. Only three of these series occurred recently enough to allow the use of CDDP or carboplatin salvage chemotherapy. Nevertheless, some of these patients underwent salvage therapy with mediastinal recurrence by the use of radiation therapy, and the overall survival rate was 91%. It seems likely, therefore, that the improvements in modern radiation therapy will result in a disease-free survival rate of 75 to 80%, with salvage chemotherapy curing the considerable majority of those who have relapses.

Radiation Therapy Treatment Considerations

Standard radiation therapy for seminoma consists of megavoltage irradiation to the paraaortic and ipsilateral pelvic lymph nodes. Treatment volumes that are usually recommended include a superior border at the top of the T-10 vertebral body, lateral borders that will encompass the greater of either the tumor volume or renal hila, and the ipsilateral pelvic lymph nodes down to an inferior margin of the superior portion of the obturator foramen. These treatment fields should be blocked individually to ensure adequate coverage of the important nodal/tumor structures and to spare maximally normal structures from unnecessary radiation. Both the anteroposterior and posteroanterior fields should be treated daily using linear accelerator beams of greater than or equal to 6 MV energies. Daily doses of 150 to 180 cGy/day, 5 fractions per week, should be used. Prophylactic antiemetics are often prescribed in an effort to minimize the risk of gastrointestinal difficulty during therapy. Although these recommendations provide acceptable results in the overwhelming majority, all these treatment volume recommendations bear careful consideration.

The superior border of the infradiaphragmatic field is commonly placed at the superior border of T-10 (68, 69, 71, 95), although many of the series summarized in Tables 58-3 and 58-4 used either variable or different superior margins. The rationale for adopting a uniform policy of placing the superior margin at the top of the T-10 vertebral body consists of an evaluation of the lymphatic flow of the testicle and an evaluation of the failure patterns following either radiation therapy for stage I or II disease or observation for stage I disease. Testicular lymphangiograms (96–100) show that the primary lymphatic drainage of the testes is to the upper paraaortic lymph nodes. Contralateral communication is frequent.

Furthermore, these nodes communicate freely with each other and often extend from T11-L4, with heaviest concentration in the area of the renal hila insofar as pelvic/inguinal lymph node drainage is concerned; one report demonstrated that 2 of 10 right testicles demonstrated drainage to the external iliac lymph nodes (97). However, other reports show no iliac or inguinal lymph node opacification except when there had been previous inguinal or scrotal surgery. The extensive intercommunication of the draining lymphatics to the level of T11 has provided some of the rationale for setting the superior margin of the infradiaphragmatic field at the top level of the 10th vertebral body in an effort to give margin to the known lymphatic drainage to the vertebral body immediately inferior to this. Sagerman et al. (81) have clearly documented failure at the T9-10 paravertebral lymph node sites in 6% of patients treated with radiation therapy. These patients had recurrence in the area of the gap between the paraaortic and mediastinal fields. Pretreatment lymphangiograms in both of these patients showed normal-appearing opacified lymph nodes superior to the cisterna chyli up to the level of the documented relapse site. This lymphangiographic pattern was present in 10% of patients reviewed. Indeed, the retrocrural lymph nodes that lie anterior to the T10-12 vertebral bodies have been well documented to be a site of seminoma failure (63, 69, 81). These lymph nodes exist in the usual location of the gap between the infradiaphragmatic radiation therapy field and the superior diaphragmatic field in those stage II series that use prophylactic mediastinal irradiation. Retrocrural failure was also documented in the Royal Marsden stage I surveillance series. Retrocrural disease was documented in 36% before carboplatin therapy relapse.

The lymphangiogram and failure pattern data clearly support inclusion of the retrocrural lymph nodes anterior to the 10th vertebral body as a reasonable superior margin of the infradiaphragmatic field. However, there is some reason to evaluate this margin carefully on an individual basis. The data collected in the prophylactic mediastinal irradiation series (vide infra) indicate that cardiac irradiation may be associated with a higher risk of subsequent myocardial infarctions. Routine prophylactic mediastinal/supraclavicular irradiation (PMI) has been abandoned, in part, because of the concerns regarding cardiac toxicity. Extension of the radiation therapy field to include retrocrural lymph nodes will necessitate radiation to a variable volume of heart in some patients. The risk of cardiac toxicity as a result of radiation via the infradiaphragmatic portals has not been fully assessed. However, the heart volume irradiated in the infradiaphragmatic fields may be substantial and should be evaluated carefully, especially in individuals who may be at higher risk of cardiac disease development. Such individuals include those with known cardiac disease and those older than 40 years of age (45). Many institutions (30, 34, 66, 70, 72, 85) have adopted a lower superior border of the infradiaphragmatic field, usually the top of either T12 or T11, although sometimes as low as the top of L1, without any definite evidence of diminution in treatment efficacy.

The importance of modern radiation therapy treatment planning cannot be overemphasized. CT-based treatment planning now allows the reliable design of treatment fields to include all infradiaphragmatic disease. Failure at the margin of the radiation therapy fields has been well documented (29, 30, 63, 65, 69, 84, 89, 101). Five series have documented that marginal misses account for 25 to 50% of all local failures observed (29, 63, 65, 69, 101). Only a few stage II series have used CT-based treatment planning to ensure adequate coverage of the entire infradiaphragmatic disease. The Mayo Clinic series (93) and a small series from Royal Marsden (102) used either staging laparotomy or CT-based treatment planning to delineate carefully the infradiaphragmatic tumor volume for purposes of radiation treatment planning. These series, using modern treatment planning techniques, resulted in an initial cure rate with radiation therapy alone of 81% and an overall survival rate (with salvage) of almost 95%.

The role of iliac and/or inguinal radiation therapy has also become a matter of some controversy. The lymphangiogram data previously discussed document that lymphatic drainage to the inguinal or iliac lymph nodes is uncommon (96–100). Some groups report that inguinal failures account for 5 to 10% of failures in patients who have relapses (55, 56, 63, 73, 75, 103, 104). The absolute number of inguinal and/or iliac lymph node failures in those with stage I disease is, however, quite low and occurs in less than or equal to 5 to 10% of those whose pelvic or inguinal lymph nodes are not treated with stage I disease. At the Norwegian Radium Hospital, Evensen et al. (66) treated 73 stage II seminoma patients and administered inguinal irradiation, in general, only when there were previous inguinal surgeries; when the tumor infiltrated the tunica vaginalis, spermatic cord, epididymis or scrotal wall; or when there was transcrotal orchiectomy. No inguinal recurrences occurred. This experience and the low absolute incidence of inguinal node recurrence suggest that inguinal irradiation is unnecessary in otherwise uncomplicated stage I or II seminoma. Prior inguinal surgeries; invasion of the tunica vaginalis, spermatic cord, or scrotal wall; or transcrotal orchiectomy have been documented to increase the risk of inguinal nodal recurrence (60, 61), although even in these unusual circumstances, the risk of inguinal failure in absolute terms is less than 10% (71, 104). Therefore, in this select group of patients, individualization of therapy is appropriate. If inguinal irradiation is administered, particular attention to steps to diminish the contralateral testicular dose is important.

Pelvic lymph nodes are uncommonly involved in stage I seminoma, and some researchers (96, 105) have reported that omission of pelvic radiation therapy is safe in this early stage. However, there are no large series that have systematically investigated the omission of pelvic radiation therapy in stage II seminoma. The Royal Marsden experience with iliac lymph node involvement suggested that bulky paraaortic disease (greater than or equal to 5 cm tumor diameter) predicted for a much greater risk of iliac node involvement than the risk for those without bulky paraaortic disease. Those with documented paraaortic metastasis have been postulated to have altered, retrograde spread from their metastatic disease that accounts for their higher than expected rate of pelvic metastasis. Given the increased risk of pelvic lymph nodes in those with stage II disease, and in the absence of any clinical data supporting its omission, ipsilateral pelvic radiation is recommended. Some have suggested that the contralateral pelvic lymph nodes are also at risk because of the theoretic problem of retrograde, aberrant, lymphatic drainage. However, the incidence of contralateral iliac node disease is less than 1% even in those with bulky stage II disease or factors that might predispose them to inguinal failures (104). In view of the need to conserve bone marrow for the minority of those who will subsequently experience treatment failures, the contralateral pelvic nodes should not receive prophylactic adjuvant therapy.

The role of PMI in stage II disease has dramatically changed with the development of effective chemotherapy (Table 58.5). The overall incidence of mediastinal/supraclavicular failure without PMI is approximately 5 to 10% for nonbulky stage II disease and 20 to 25% in those with bulky infradiaphragmatic metastasis. The overwhelming majority of supradiaphragmatic failures will occur in the left supraclavicular area (94, 106). The recent M.D. Anderson experience with nonbulky stage II disease is noteworthy (94). Patients with stage IIA disease treated in 1984 or after were systematically given infradiaphragmatic radiation alone. Supradiaphragmatic failure only in the left supraclavicular region developed in 3 of 19 patients (16%). Those who did not receive PMI had an inferior disease-free survival compared with those who did receive such therapy (P = 0.02). The M.D. Anderson group now administers prophylactic radiation therapy to the left supraclavicular fossa alone. This approach, which theoretically obviates many of the problems with PMI, will bear close scrutiny. In bulky stage II disease, the risk of supradiaphragmatic failure is higher. Although left supraclavicular failure is almost twice that of mediastinal relapse (106), the risk of visceral relapses also significantly increases in bulky stage II disease. Although the risk of supradiaphragmatic failure increases as the bulk of the diaphragmatic tumor increases, there are three compelling reasons why PMI should not be routinely administered to patients with stage II seminoma.

1. Cardiac risk. PMI increases the risk of serious functional or structural cardiac disease by approximately 5%. Interpretation of this data is problematic for several reasons. Series that span long periods have recently omitted PMI in stage II patients, which results in longer follow-up of those with PMI. Because cardiac disease takes, in general, longer than 5 years from PMI to become manifest (45, 107), those who have received PMI will be more likely to have manifested cardiac disease simply by the longer duration of their follow-up. Additionally, none of these reports has prospectively set out to evaluate cardiac disease, which predisposes these analyses to recall bias. This may account for some institutions reporting completely disparate results in the same group of patients (64, 108). Nevertheless, the data on PMI seem to correlate with the cardiac risk seen in other clinical settings such as Hodgkin's disease. PMI, in all likelihood, exposes patients to the added risk of serious cardiac disease. This increased risk of cardiac disease almost certainly mitigates any potential advantage in prevention of mediastinal/supraclavicular relapse in nonbulky stage II disease.

2. Increased toxicity with salvage chemotherapy. The issue of chemotherapy toxicity after radiation is extensively discussed below. However, whereas prior infradiaphragmatic radiation may have some modest effect on subsequent salvage chemotherapy toxicity, inclusion of both infradiaphragmatic and supradiaphragmatic radiation dramatically increases the risk of salvage chemotherapy toxicity (vide infra).

3. Overall survival considerations. Several groups (63, 66, 94) have evaluated overall survival, including salvage therapy with and without PMI. These series consistently demonstrate that although relapse-free survival may be beneficially affected by the addition of PMI, overall survival is no different.

Therefore, although PMI may improve relapse-free survival by decreasing supradiaphragmatic failure, the substantial risks involved with PMI provide a compelling rationale for its omission in the usual patient with stage II disease. The potential value of supraclavicular radiation alone, as suggested by the M.D. Anderson group, is intriguing.

Dose–Response

The majority of series summarized in Tables 58-1 and 58-3 report no in-field abdominal failures in stage I or nonbulky stage II disease. The occasional series that have observed in-field abdominal failures (65, 69, 71, 94, 109) have reported that this unusual circumstance occurs in less than or equal to 5%. The incidence of in-field abdominal failure may increase to 5 to 10% in stage II if the abdominal disease is 5 to 10 cm in width (65, 70). Lester et al. (110) have reported improved local control with 6500 cGy for stage II disease. It is not unreasonable to use a dose of 2000 to 3000 cGy for stage I disease and 3000 to 3500 cGy for nonbulky stage II disease in view of the well-documented increased risk of acute gastrointestinal toxicity and long-term peptic ulcer disease when doses greater than 3600 cGy are used (39). Doses of less than or equal to 3500 cGy are only very rarely associated with long-term peptic ulcer or other morbidity (37). For bulky stage II seminomas, in-field recurrence has been reported in 20 to 30% (64, 68, 69, 111). Although many of these in-field recurrences may, in fact, have been marginal misses, others are probably due to an inadequate dose. The Mayo Clinic reported in-field control in 20 radiation therapy fields in which seminoma greater than 5 cm was treated. In-field relapse was not observed with greater than 3600 cGy, although it was observed in 14% of fields treated to less than or equal to 3600 cGy (89). In patients who are selected for initial radiation therapy for bulky stage II disease, the initial 1500 to 2000 cGy is often sufficient to produce significant tumor volume reduction. Following the initial 1500 to 2000 cGy, tumor volume can be reevaluated with shrinking fields used to their substantial volumes of normal tissue. The final boost volume dose, however, should probably be greater than 3600 to 4000 cGy.

Seminoma Chemotherapy

Highly effective CDDP-based chemotherapy has dramatically improved survival for advanced seminoma. The results of several CDDP-based chemotherapy reports of advanced seminoma are summarized in Table 58.6 (74–76, 90–92, 112–124). Although follow-up of some chemotherapy series is insufficient to detect all relapses reliably, disease-free survival rates of 75 to 85% have been reported. No prospectively randomized trials have clearly identified which of the several chemotherapy regimens is optimal, especially insofar as overall survival is concerned. Single-agent CDDP or carboplatin produces substantial relapse rates in the area of previous microscopic disease (75, 79, 90, 124). However, series that have used consolidative radiation therapy after carboplatin (75, 79) have observed excellent overall survival. Furthermore, CDDP-based multiagent chemotherapy and/or radiation therapy is capable of salvaging the majority of those in whom single-agent chemotherapy fails.

The volume of seminoma is also important in terms of chemotherapy prognosis. Oliver et al. reported a disease-free survival rate of 77% in those with bulky stage II disease versus 100% with nonbulky stage II disease. Furthermore, relapse-free survival of all nonbulky stage II, III, and IV patients was superior to that of bulky stage II subgroup (90). Tjulandin et al. reported that minimal metastatic disease, defined by the Indiana Prognostic System, had a 75% survival rate when compared with either moderate or advanced disease (approximately 57%) (76). Wilkinson et al. reported that 5-year overall survival was 71% with small-volume disease versus 38 to 44% for larger tumor burdens (119). Most other series have also observed poor outcomes with bulkier disease (74, 113, 116, 117, 122). Because the chemotherapy series listed in Table 58.5 includes all patients with nonbulky tumor burdens (including some with favorable prognoses), the results of these overall series may not truly reflect what could be expected in bulky stage II disease.

Several series have evaluated the efficacy of chemotherapy when administered as initial treatment versus outcome when chemotherapy is used as salvage therapy after radiation therapy failure. A few series (92, 112) show poor survival and inferior disease-free survival when chemotherapy is used as salvage following radiation therapy failure. However, most reports showed no significant difference whether chemotherapy is administered at the time of original diagnosis versus after radiation therapy relapse (74, 91, 113, 116, 118, 119, 125, 126). Consistently, the results of initial chemotherapy appear equiva-

Table 58.6. Cisplatin-Based Chemotherapy for Seminoma

REFERENCE	DISEASE-FREE SURVIVAL (%)[a]	SALVAGE	OVERALL SURVIVAL (%)[b]	MEDIAN FOLLOW-UP (MO) (RANGE)
Clemm et al. (112)	20/24 (83)	1/4	21/24 (87)	30 (3–64)
Loehrer et al. (113)	37/62 (60)	2/22	39/62 (63)	NS
Roth et al. (114)[c]			14/26 (54)	102 (73–144)
Nichols et al. (115)	13/21 (62)	NS	NS	24 (NS)
Williams et al. (116)	30/41 (73)	NS	NS	23 (NS)
Srougi et al. (117)	10/13 (77)	3/3	13/13 (100)	24 (8–38)
Pizzocaro et al. (118)	23/31 (74)	4/7	24/31 (78)	34 (12–77)
Fossa et al. (74)	39/55 (71)	8/16	43/55 (78)	50
Wilkinson et al. (119)			19/37 (51)	50
Berkmen (120)	32/36 (89)	0/4	30/36 (83)	26 (9–60)
Gietema et al. (121)	26/33 (79)	1/3	26/33 (79)	28 (16–88)
Tjulandin et al. (76)	35/59 (61)	0/7	43/59 (73)	>24 (4–70)
Mencel et al. (122)	121/142 (85)	NS	125/142 (88)	43 (3–153)
Logothetis et al. (91)	44/52 (85)	4/8	48/52 (92)	37 (7–109)
Oliver et al. (90)	35/43 (81)	3/7	38/43 (88)	NS
Friedman et al. (123)	15/20 (75)	0/2	15/20 (75)	22 (6–85)
Peckham et al. (92)	35/39 (90)	1/4	36/39 (92)	36 (12–73)
Horwich et al. (75)[d]	54/70 (77)	12/16	60/70 (90)	36 (8–101)
Schmoll et al. (124)[d]	30/43 (70)	10/12	40/43 (93)	31 (NS)
Total	599/784 (76)	49/115 (43%)	634/785 (81)	

NS, not stated.

[a] Following chemotherapy alone without salvage therapy (events include both disease relapse and treatment deaths).

[b] Includes intercurrent deaths when data given in article.

[c] Includes some of same patients in Loehrer.

[d] Single-agent CDDP or carboplatin.

lent to those of chemotherapy salvage if limited infradiaphragmatic-only fields were used before chemotherapy.

The toxicity of chemotherapy does appear somewhat worse when used as radiation therapy salvage. Several groups have reported poor tolerance when chemotherapy is used as salvage treatment (112, 113, 125). However, particularly germane to the issue of stage II seminoma, several groups have reported similar toxicity with initial chemotherapy when compared with salvage chemotherapy after limited, infradiaphragmatic-only radiation therapy (74, 113, 119, 121).

Initial Chemotherapy Versus Radiation Therapy for Bulky Stage II Seminoma

In view of the literature summarized above, the vagaries of treatment comparisons, and the generally similar results reported, it is impossible to make scientifically valid conclusions regarding which modality of treatment is superior for bulky stage II seminomas. In a large series from the Norwegian Radium Hospital, Fossa et al. reported that survival appeared extremely similar whether patients with bulky stage II seminoma received initial chemotherapy versus radiation therapy (74). In view of the fact that CDDP-based chemotherapy was not available for those who had relapses after radiation therapy in this historical control series, and in view of the substantial toxicity and occasional death associated with initial chemotherapy (74, 113, 116, 121, 122), it was the authors' view that initial radiation therapy should be considered for all bulky stage II patients. In those with a high likelihood that radiation therapy will fail, such as stage III or extragonadal primary tumors, treatment with chemotherapy is clearly preferred. Those whose disease is so massive that radiation therapy would require inclusion of the overwhelming majority of both kidneys should also receive initial chemotherapy. Usually, it is possible to treat even bulky infradiaphragmatic disease plus margin and spare the majority of both kidneys. Additionally, following the initial 1500 to 2000 cGy, tumor regression will occur over the next few weeks; this can facilitate shrinking field techniques.

Management of Residual Tumor Following Treatment

Seminoma presents unique problems insofar as the management of residual masses after treatment is concerned. The overwhelming majority of those treated for seminomas will have residual disease (75, 90, 113, 119, 120, 123, 126). Several groups have described the slow resolution of residual tumor masses, which may take several years to fully develop following therapy (90, 123, 127). Several groups report that a true, complete normalization of CT scan findings occurs in only the distinct minority (75, 90, 113, 119, 120, 123). Data regarding the frequency of residual mass lesions after radiation therapy are not as readily available because the majority of these series occurred in the pre-CT era. However, Evensen et al. (66) report that 10 of 45 of those with bulky stage II seminoma had resid-

ual tumor after radiation therapy. These tumors often regress slowly over several years.

In NSGCT, it is standard therapy to resect residual tumor masses. However, there are significant problems with such an approach as a routine management philosophy in seminoma therapy. The overwhelming majority of those with residual masses who undergo exploratory procedures will be found to have fibrotic, nonviable tumors (74, 92, 117–119, 123, 125). The overall likelihood that residual tumor masses will represent tumor is approximately 10%. The fact that surgical resection is often technically difficult because of the dense fibrosis and desmoplasia that occur following regression of seminoma further dampens enthusiasm for routine residual mass resection; this makes resection often incomplete, technically extremely difficult, and associated with a high morbidity (111, 123). Three groups have reported a substantial increase in residual tumor when the tumor mass is greater than 3 cm (121, 128, 129). The observation of increased local failure after chemotherapy for residual masses greater than or equal to 3 cm has prompted several authors (128–132) to recommend either surgical exploration or adjuvant radiation therapy in this situation.

Alternatively, Schultz et al. at Indiana University were unable to corroborate any increase in relapse rate on the basis of postchemotherapy residual mass volume (133). A policy of subjecting all patients to either exploration or adjuvant radiation therapy when residual tumor masses are greater than or equal to 3 cm necessitates a policy of additional toxic therapy to a group of patients who, in the overwhelming majority of cases, are already cured. A practical policy is to carry out very close follow-up with serial CT scanning in those with residual masses of any size. The high rate of local relapse after single-agent CDDP or carboplatin (75, 79, 90) might suggest that those with residual masses in this setting be treated with adjuvant radiation therapy.

Finally, there is intriguing early data that gallium scans are avidly taken up in metastatic seminoma (70, 134). The possibility of using gallium scans before and at the completion of therapy to assess the presence or absence of residual tumor has been suggested. Further experience in additional treatment centers is eagerly awaited.

REFERENCES

1. Kennedy B, Schmidt J, Winchester D, et al. National survey of patterns of care for testis cancer. Cancer 1987;60:1921.
2. Vogelzang N, Fremgen A, Guinan P, et al. Insurance status as a prognostic factor for stage and survival of testicular cancer patients in Illinois. Adv Biosci 1994;91:223.
3. Warner-Efrati E, Sulkes A, Gez E, et al. Testicular seminoma: the Hadassah University Hospital experience. Isr J Med Sci 1988;24:584.
4. Zablow A, Erba P, Sanfilippo L. Early stage pure seminoma testis. New Jersey Med 1989;86:800.
5. Smith R, Dekernion J, Skinner D. Management of advanced testicular seminoma. J Urol 1979;121:429.

6. Horwich A, Dearnaley D. Treatment of seminoma. Semin Oncol 1992;19:171.

7. Bobba V, Mittal B, Hoover S, et al. Classical and anaplastic seminoma: difference in survival. Radiology 1988;167:849.

8. Cockburn A, Vugrin D, Batata M, et al. Poorly differentiated (anaplastic) seminoma of the testis. Cancer 1984;53:1991.

9. Rossai J, Heyderman E, Mostafi F, et al. Mouse teratocarcinoma and oncofetal proteins. International symposium on human testis cancer, University of Minnesota Medical School, 1980.

10. Hanks G, Herring D, Kramer S. Patterns of care outcome studies: results of the national practice in seminoma of the testis. Int J Radiat Oncol Biol Phys 1981;7:1413.

11. True L, Otis C, Delprado W, et al. Spermatocytic seminoma of testis with sarcomatous transformation: a report of five cases. Am J Surg Pathol 1988;12:75.

12. Floyd C, Ayala A, Logothetis C, et al. Spermatocytic seminoma with associated sarcoma of the testis. Cancer 1988; 61:409.

13. Matoška J, Ondruš D, Horňak M. Metastatic spermatocytic seminoma: a case report with light microscopic, ultrastructural, and immunohistochemical findings. Cancer 1988;62:1197.

14. Lehmann D, Temminck B, Litmanen K, et al. Autoimmune phenomena and cytogenetic findings in a patient with carcinoma (seminoma) in situ. Cancer 1986;58:2013.

15. Mostofi F. Testicular tumors: epidemiologic, etiologic, pathologic features. Cancer 1973;32:1186.

16. Mirimanoff R, Sinzig M, Krüger M, et al. Prognosis of human chorionic gonadotropin-producing seminoma treated by postoperative radiotherapy. Int J Radiat Oncol Biol Phys 1993;27:17.

17. Mauch P, Weichselbaum R, Botnick L. The significance of positive chorionic gonadotropins in apparently pure seminoma of the testis. Int J Radiat Oncol Biol Phys 1979;5: 887.

18. Paus E, Fossa A, Fossa S, et al. High frequency of incomplete human chorionic gonadotropin in patients with testicular seminoma. J Urol 1988;139:542.

19. Mann K, Siddle K. Evidence for beta-subunit secretion in so-called human chorionic gonadotropin-positive seminoma. Cancer 1988;62:2378.

20. Dieckmann D, Düe W, Bauer H. Seminoma testis with elevated serum beta-hCG: a category of germ-cell cancer between seminoma and nonseminoma. Int Urol Nephrol 1989;21:175.

21. Swartz D, Johnson D, Hussey D. Should an elevated human chorionic gonadotropin titer alter therapy for seminoma? J Urol 1984;131:63.

22. Herman J, Sturgeon J, Gospodarowicz M, et al. A prospective clinical trial for testicular seminoma and serum markers. Am J Clin Oncol 1983;6:153.

23. Lange P, Nochomovitz L, Rosai J, et al. Serum alpha-fetoprotein and human chorionic gonadotropin in patients with seminoma. J Urol 1980;124:472.

24. Kuzmits R, Schernthaner G, Krisch K. Serum neuron-specific enolase: a marker for response to therapy in seminoma. Cancer 1987;60:1017.

25. Peckham M, McElwain T. Radiotherapy for testicular tumors. Proc Roy Soc Med 1974;67:300.

26. Earle J, Bagshaw M, Kaplan H. Supervoltage radiation therapy of the testicular tumors. AJR 1973;117:653.

27. van der Werf-Messing B. Radiotherapeutic treatment of testicular tumors. Int J Radiat Oncol Biol Phys 1976;1:235.

28. Hamilton C, Horwich A, Easton D, et al. Radiotherapy for stage I seminoma testis. Radiol Oncol 1986;6:115.

29. Dosoretz D, Shipley W, Blitzer P, et al. Megavoltage irradiation for pure testicular seminoma: results and patterns of failure. Cancer 1981;48:2184.

30. Hunter M, Peschel R. Testicular seminoma: results of the Yale University experience, 1964–1984. Cancer 1989;64: 1608.

31. Fossa S, Aass N, Kaalhus O. Radiotherapy for testicular seminoma stage I: treatment results and long-term post-irradiation morbidity in 365 patients. Int J Radiat Oncol Biol Phys 1989;16:383.

32. Giacchetti S, Raoul Y, Wibault P, et al. Treatment of stage I testis seminoma by radiotherapy: long-term results: a 30-year experience. Int J Radiat Oncol Biol Phys 1993;27:3.

33. Steinfeld A, Newall J. Controversies in management of stages I and II testicular seminomas. Urology 1988;31:202.

34. Tombolini V, Capua A, Grapulin L, et al. Ruolo della radioterapia nel trattamento del seminoma del testicolo. Radiol Med 1991;82:334.

35. Lai P, Bernstein M, Kim H, et al. Radiation therapy for stage I and II: a testicular seminoma. Int J Radiat Oncol Biol Phys 1993;28:373.

36. Sommer K, Brockmann W, Hübener K. Treatment results and acute and late toxicity of radiation therapy for testicular seminoma. Cancer 1990;66:259.

37. Glanzmann C, Schultz G, Lütolf U. Long-term morbidity of adjuvant infradiaphragmatic irradiation in patients with testicular cancer and implications for the treatment of stage I seminoma. Radiother Oncol 1991;22:12.

38. Yeoh E, Razali M, O'Brien P. Radiation therapy for early stage seminoma of the testis: analysis of survival and gastrointestinal toxicity in patients treated with modern megavoltage techniques over 10 years. Aust Radiol 1993;37: 367.

39. Aass N, Fossa S, Høst H. Acute and subacute side effects due to infra-diaphragmatic radiotherapy for testicular cancer: a prospective study. Int J Radiat Oncol Biol Phys 1992;22: 1057.

40. Thomas G. Refining the therapy of testicular seminoma. Eur Urol 1993;23(Suppl):24.

41. Horwich A. Questions in the management of seminoma. Clin Oncol 1990;2:249.

42. Schlappack O, Kratzik C, Schmidt W, et al. Response of the seminiferous epithelium to scattered radiation in seminoma patients. Cancer 1988;62:1487.

43. Goodman M, Lalka S, Reddy S. Static and dynamic vascular impact of large artery irradiation. Int J Radiat Oncol Biol Phys 1993;26:305.

44. van Leeuwen F, Stiggelbout A, van den Belt-Dusebout A, et al. Second cancer risk following testicular cancer: a follow-up study of 1,909 patients. J Clin Oncol 1993;11:415.

45. Hanks G, Peters T, Owen J. Seminoma of the testis: long term beneficial and deleterious results of radiation. Int J Radiat Oncol Biol Phys 1992;24:913.

46. Bokemeyer C, Schmoll H. Secondary neoplasms following

treatment of malignant germ cell tumors. J Clin Oncol 1993;
11:1703.

47. Jacobsen G, Mellemgaard A, Engelholm S, et al. Increased incidence of sarcoma in patients treated for testicular seminoma. Eur J Cancer 1993;29:664. Abstract.

48. Kaldor J, Day N, Band P, et al. Second malignancies following testicular cancer, ovarian cancer or Hodgkin's disease: International Collaborative Group Study among cancer registries. Int J Cancer 1987;39:571.

49. Hay J, Duncan W, Kerr G. Subsequent malignancies in patients irradiated for testicular tumors. Br J Radiol 1984;57:597.

50. Kleinerman R, Lieberman J, Li F. Second cancer following cancer of the male genital system in Connecticut, 1935–1982. NCI Monogr 1985;68:139.

51. Fossa S, Langmark F, Aass N, et al. Second non-germ cell malignancies after radiotherapy of testicular cancer with or without chemotherapy. Br J Cancer 1990;61:639.

52. Coleman M, Bell C, Fraser P. Second primary malignancy after Hodgkin's disease, ovarian cancer and cancer of the testis: a population-based cohort study. Br J Cancer 1987;56:349.

53. Allhoff E, Liedke S, De Riese W, et al. Stage I seminoma of the testis: adjuvant radiotherapy or surveillance? Br J Urol 1991;68:190.

54. Ramakrishnan S, Champion A, Dorreen M, et al. Stage I seminoma of the testis: is post-orchidectomy surveillance a safe alternative to routine postoperative radiotherapy? Clin Oncol 1992;4:284.

55. Horwich A, Alsanjari N, A'Hern R, et al. Surveillance following orchidectomy for stage I testicular seminoma. Br J Cancer 1992;65:775.

56. von der Maase H, Specht L, Jacobsen G, et al. Surveillance following orchidectomy for stage I seminoma of the testis. Eur J Cancer 1993;29:1931. Abstract.

57. Warde P, Gospodarowicz M, Goodman P, et al. Results of a policy of surveillance in stage I testicular seminoma. Int J Radiat Oncol Biol Phys 1993;27:11.

58. Oliver R, Edmonds P, Ong J, et al. Pilot studies of 2 & 1 course carboplatin as adjuvant for stage I seminoma to assess if there are enough advantages to justify testing it in a randomised trial against radiotherapy. Int J Radiat Oncol Biol Phys 1994;29:3.

59. Oliver R, Dhaliwal H, Hope-Stone H, et al. Short-course etoposide, bleomycin and cisplatin in the treatment of metastatic germ cell tumours: appraisal of its potential as adjuvant chemotherapy for stage I testis tumours. Br J Urol 1988;61:53.

60. Smith R, Dekernion J, Skinner D. Management of advanced testicular seminoma. J Urol 1979;121:429.

61. Stutzman, R. Management of seminoma. Prog Clin Biol Res 1988;277:63.

62. Thomas G. Controversies in the management of testicular seminoma. Cancer 1985;55:2296.

63. Ellerbroek N, Tran L, Selch M, et al. Testicular seminoma. Am J Clin Oncol 1988;11:93.

64. Ball D, Barrett A, Peckham M. The management of metastatic seminoma testis. Cancer 1982;50:2289.

65. Mason B, Kearsley J. Radiotherapy for stage 2 testicular seminoma: the prognostic influence of tumor bulk. J Clin Oncol 1988;6:1856.

66. Evensen J, Fossa S, Kjellevold K, et al. Testicular seminoma: analysis of treatment and failure for stage II disease. Radiother Oncol 1985;4:55.

67. Steinfeld A, Diamond J, Hanks G. Stage II testicular seminoma evolution of radiotherapeutic practice in the United States. Clin Oncol 1990;2:14.

68. Lederman G, Herman T, Jochelson M. Radiation therapy of seminoma: 17-year experience at the Joint Center for Radiation Therapy. Radiother Oncol 1989;14:203.

69. Zagars G, Babaian R. The role of radiation in stage II testicular seminoma. Int J Radiat Oncol Biol Phys 1987;13:163.

70. Willan B, McGowan D. Seminoma of the testis: a 22-year experience with radiation therapy. Int J Radiat Oncol Biol Phys 1985;11:1769.

71. Thomas G, Rider W, Dembo A, et al. Seminoma of the testis: results of treatment and patterns of failure after radiation therapy. Int J Radiat Oncol Biol Phys 1982;8:165.

72. Bayens Y, Helle P, Van Putten W, et al. Orchidectomy followed by radiotherapy in 176 stage I and II testicular seminoma patients: benefits of a 10-year follow-up study. Radiother Oncol 1992;25:97.

73. Read G, Robertson A, Blair V. Radiotherapy in seminoma of the testis. Clin Radiol 1983;34:469.

74. Fossa S, Borge L, Aass N, et al. The treatment of advanced metastatic seminoma: experience in 55 cases. J Clin Oncol 1987;5:1071.

75. Horwich A, Dearnaley D, A'Hern R, et al. The activity of single-agent carboplatin in advanced seminoma. Eur J Cancer 1992;28:1307.

76. Tjulandin S, Khlebnov A, Nasirova R, et al. VAB-6 and cisplatin-cyclophosphamide combinations in the treatment of metastatic seminoma patients: the U.S.S.R. experience. Ann Oncol 1991;2:667.

77. DeLeo M, Greco F, Hainsworth J, et al. Late recurrences in long-term survivors of germ cell neoplasms. Cancer 1988;62:985.

78. Borge N, Fossa S, Ous S, et al. Late recurrence of testicular cancer. J Clin Oncol 1988;6:1248.

79. MacVicar D, Horwich A. Sites of relapse in seminoma treated with single agent carboplatin chemotherapy: implications for further management. Clin Oncol 1992;4:209.

80. Lindeman G, Tiver K. Management of testicular seminoma at Westmead Hospital from 1980–1987. Aust N Z J Surg 1991;61:211.

81. Sagerman R, Kotlove D, Regine W, et al. Stage II seminoma: results of postorchiectomy irradiation. Radiology 1989;172:565.

82. Jackson S, Olivotto I, McLoughlin M, et al. Radiation therapy for seminoma of the testis: results in British Columbia. Can Med Assoc J 1980;123:507.

83. Andrews C, Micaily B, Brady L. Testicular seminoma. Am J Clin Oncol 1987;10:491.

84. Doornbos J, Hussey D, Johnson E. Radiotherapy for pure seminoma of the testis. Radiology 1975;116:401.

85. Laukkanen E, Olivotto I, Jackson S. Management of seminoma with bulky abdominal disease. Int J Radiat Oncol Biol Phys 1988;14:227.

86. Herman J, Sturgeon J, Thomas G. Mediastinal prophylactic irradiation in seminoma. Proc Am Soc Clin Oncol 1983:133. Abstract.

87. Martinelli D. La radioterapia dei seminomi in secondo stadio. Acta Biomedica de 1989;60:279.

88. Green N, Broth E, George F, et al. Radiation therapy in bulky seminoma. Urology 1983;21:467.

89. Smalley S, Earle J, Evans R, et al. Modern radiotherapy results with bulky stages II and III seminoma. J Urol 1990;144:685.

90. Oliver R, Lore S, Ong J. Alternatives to radiotherapy in the management of seminoma. Br J Urol 1990;65:61.

91. Logothetis C, Samuels M, Ogden S, et al. Cyclophosphamide and sequential cisplatin for advanced seminoma: long-term follow-up in 52 patients. J Urol 1987;138:789.

92. Peckham J, Horwich A, Hendry W. Advanced seminoma: treatment with cisplatinum-based combination chemotherapy or carboplatin (JM8). Br J Cancer 1985;52:7.

93. Bredael J, Vugrin D, Whitmore W. Autopsy findings in 154 patients with germ cell tumours of the testis. Cancer 1982;50:548.

94. Dosmann M, Zagars G. Postorchiectomy radiotherapy for stages I and II testicular seminoma. Int J Radiat Oncol Biol Phys 1993;26:381.

95. Thomas G, Williams S. Testis. In: Perez C, Brady L, eds. Principles and practice of radiation oncology. Philadelphia: JB Lippincott, 1992:1117.

96. Brunt A, Scoble J. Para-aortic nodal irradiation for early stage testicular seminoma. Clin Oncol 1992;4:165.

97. Jamieson J, Dobson J. The lymphatics of the testicle. Lancet 1910;1:493.

98. Busch F, Sayegh E, Chenault O. Some uses of lymphangiography in the management of testicular tumors. J Urol 1965;93:490.

99. Sayegh E, Brooks T, Sacher E, et al. Lymphangiography of the retroperitoneal lymph nodes through the inguinal route. J Urol 1966;95:102.

100. Herr H, Silber I, Martin D. Management of inguinal lymph nodes in patients with testicular tumors following orchiopexy, inguinal or scrotal operations. J Urol 1973;110:223.

101. Cionini L, Ciatto S, Pirtoli L, et al. Radiotherapy of seminoma of the testis: report on 129 patients. Tumori 1978;64:183.

102. Paulson D, Einhorn L, Peckham M. Cancer of the testis. In: DeVita V, Hellman S, Rosenberg S, eds. Cancer principles and practice of oncology. Philadelphia: JB Lippincott, 1982:786.

103. Thomas G. Alternative management options to radiation therapy for stage I and IIA testicular seminoma. Int J Radiat Oncol Biol Phys 1994;28:547.

104. Mason M, Featherstone T, Olliff J, et al. Inguinal and iliac lymph node involvement in germ cell tumours of the testis: implications for radiological investigation and for therapy. Clin Oncol 1991;3:147.

105. Read G, Johnston R. Short duration radiotherapy in stage I seminoma of the testis: preliminary results of a prospective study. Clin Oncol 1993;5:364.

106. Friedman M, Purkayastha M. Recurrent seminoma: the management of late metastasis, or a second primary tumor. AJR 1960;83:25.

107. Lederman G, Sheldon T, Chaffey J, et al. Cardiac disease after mediastinal irradiation for seminoma. Cancer 1987;60:772.

108. Peckham M, McElwain T. Radiotherapy of testicular tumors. Proc Roy Soc Med 1974;67:300.

109. Marks L, Anscher M, Shipley W. Radiation therapy for testicular seminoma: controversies in the management of early-stage disease. Oncology 1992;6:43.

110. Lester S, Morphis J, Hornback N. Testicular seminoma: analysis of treatment results and failures. Int J Radiat Oncol Biol Phys 1986;12:353.

111. Anscher M, Marks L, Shipley W. The role of radiotherapy in patients with advanced seminomatous germ cell tumors. Oncology 1992;6:97.

112. Clemm C, Hartenstein R, Willich N, et al. Combination chemotherapy with vinblastine, ifosfamide and cisplatin in bulky seminoma. Acta Oncol 1989;28:231.

113. Loehrer P, Birch R, Williams S, et al. Chemotherapy of metastatic seminoma: the Southeastern Cancer Study Group experience. J Clin Oncol 1987;5:1212.

114. Roth B, Greist A, Kubilis P, et al. Cisplatin-based combination chemotherapy for disseminated germ cell tumours: long-term follow-up. J Clin Oncol 1988;6:1239.

115. Nichols C, Williams S, Loehrer P, et al. Randomized study of cisplatin dose intensity in poor-risk germ cell tumors: a Southeastern Cancer Study Group and Southwest Oncology Group protocol. J Clin Oncol 1991;9:1163.

116. Williams S, Birch R, Einhorn L, et al. Treatment of disseminated germ-cell tumors with cisplatin, bleomycin, and either vinblastine or etoposide. N Engl J Med 1987;316:1435.

117. Srougi M, Simon S, Menezes de Goes G. Vinblastine, actinomycin D, bleomycin, cyclophosphamide and cis-platinum for advanced germ cell testis tumors: Brazilian experience. J Urol 1985;134:65.

118. Pizzocaro G, Salvioni R, Piva L. Cisplatin combination chemotherapy in advanced seminoma. Cancer 1986;58:1625.

119. Wilkinson P, Read G, Magee B. The treatment of advanced seminoma with chemotherapy and radiotherapy. Br J Cancer 1988;57:100.

120. Berkmen F. Reduced dose PVB treatment of stage IIC-IV testicular seminoma. Eur J Surg Oncol 1993;19:24.

121. Gietema J, Willemse P, Mulder N, et al. Alternating cycles of PVB and BEP in the treatment of patients with advanced seminoma. Eur J Cancer 1991;27:1376.

122. Mencel P, Motzer R, Mazumdar M, et al. Advanced seminoma: treatment results, survival, and prognostic factors in 142 patients. J Clin Oncol 1994;12:120.

123. Friedman E, Garnick M, Stomper P, et al. Therapeutic guidelines and results in advanced seminoma. J Clin Oncol 1985;3:1325.

124. Schmoll H-J, Harstrick A, Bokemeyer C, et al. Single-agent carboplatinum for advanced seminoma. Cancer 1993;72:237.

125. Motzer R, Bosl G, Geller N, et al. Advanced seminoma: the role of chemotherapy and adjunctive surgery. Ann Intern Med 1988;108:513.

126. Horwich A. Chemotherapy of seminoma. Eur Urol 1993;23:26.

127. Horwich A. Questions in the management of seminoma. Clin Oncol 1990;2:249.

128. Fossa S, Kullmann G, Lien H, et al. Chemotherapy of advanced seminoma: clinical significance of radiological findings before and after treatment. Br J Urol 1989;64:530.

129. Motzer R, Bosl G, Heelan R, et al. Residual mass: an indication for further therapy in patients with advanced seminoma following systemic chemotherapy. J Clin Oncol 1987;5:1064.

130. Bajorin D, Herr H, Motzer R, et al. Current perspectives on the role of adjunctive surgery in combined modality treatment for patients with germ cell tumors. Semin Oncol 1992;19:148.

131. Ellison M, Mostofi F, Flanigan R. Treatment of the residual retroperitoneal mass after chemotherapy for advanced seminoma. J Urol 1988;140:618.

132. Kamat M, Kulkarni J, Tongaonkar H, et al. Value of retroperitoneal lymph node dissection in advanced testicular seminoma. J Surg Oncol 1992;51:65.

133. Schultz S, Einhorn L, Conces D, et al. Management of postchemotherapy residual mass in patients with advanced seminoma: Indiana University experience. J Clin Oncol 1989; 7:1497.

134. Jackson F, Dierich H, Lentle B. Gallium-67 citrate scinti-scanning in testicular neoplasia. J Can Assoc Radiol 1976;27: 84.

59

Radiation Therapy for Penile, Urethral, and Renal Cell Carcinoma

Steve W. Waxman
Susan M. Smith

CARCINOMA OF THE PENIS

Penile carcinoma is relatively rare in western countries, with an estimated incidence of 1 case per 100,000 per year in the United States (1). Higher rates have been associated with lack of circumcision, phimosis and resulting poor hygiene, and socioeconomic status. The lesion arises from the glans, prepuce, or coronal sulcus and is nearly always of epidermoid (squamous cell) type. This histologic type accounts for 95% of reported cases (2).

In the United States, surgical management of the primary lesion has been the preferred method of therapy. Surgical therapy ranges from circumcision to micrographic excision to partial and total penectomy (3–7). There have been patient and physician concerns regarding the disfigurement involved with primary excision or partial penectomy. Various surgical alternatives have been investigated including Mohs micrographic surgery and laser therapy to the penile neoplasms (8, 9). Primary squamous cell carcinoma of the penis has been treated with radiation therapy for many years at several institutions. Benefits of this approach include decreased cosmetic and functional morbidity associated with primary excision or partial penectomy. The radiation can be delivered via external beam, surface molds, or brachytherapy. If radiation is chosen as the method of treatment, circumcision is required before the initiation of therapy. This will minimize the associated morbidity of swelling, irritation of the skin, moist desquamation, and secondary infection (10). External beam therapy has become the prevalent form of treatment of primary carcinoma of the penis, although surface molds and interstitial implants are still used at some institutions. Radiation therapy with modern techniques and proper dosages has yielded comparable results to surgery at several institutions.

Local control rates for treatment of the primary lesion with brachytherapy range from 78 to 94% (2). External beam radia-

tion therapy for primary carcinoma of the penis has a local control rate ranging from 52 to 100% (10). This compares to local control with surgery, which ranges from 25 to 80%. The ability of interstitial or external beam radiation therapy to control the primary penile lesion is closely linked to the stage of disease. The London Hospital found a recurrence rate of 70% for external beam radiation therapy compared with 22% for iridium mold therapy when treating stage I tumors (11). Only 10 patients were treated with external beam therapy consisting of cobalt only, which may not have been adequate treatment. Conversely, Grabstald and Kelly treated another group of 10 patients with stage I disease with external beam therapy and achieved 100% local control (12). Recurrence rates for T1, T2, and T3 lesions treated with 192 iridium wires were 11%, 22%, and 29%, respectively (13). Twenty-six percent of patients in the series required subsequent partial penectomy due to failure of iridium to control the local lesion. It is difficult to compare prospectively radiation therapy with surgical excision for primary penile cancer lesions due to the relative rarity of the tumor. Radiation therapy does provide a method for treating primary lesions of the penis while preserving its cosmetic and functional capabilities.

Elective radiation to regional nodes for advanced tumors or poorly differentiated primaries has been undertaken by some institutions. Ekstrom and Edsmyr (14) and Engelstad (15) have shown improved 5-year survival compared with historical controls with the use of elective nodal radiation therapy. The value of this technique has not been tested in a randomized manner for penile carcinoma but has been demonstrated for other tumor sites such as vagina, cervix, testis, and head and neck primaries, where elective therapy for patients at high risk of microscopic nodal metastases results in high probability of tumor control (10).

Irradiation for clinically involved inguinal and pelvic nodes can result in local control and even cure. Staubitz et al. showed that 5 of 13 patients (38%) with documented positive nodes survived 5 years after regional radiation therapy (16). This study predated modern megavoltage machinery, and details of the techniques used were not given. The probability of tumor control is proportional to extent of disease and proper radiation therapy technique.

CARCINOMA OF THE URETHRA

Primary urethral carcinomas in males are rare, with only approximately 600 cases having been reported in the literature (17). In the male, one half to three fourths of these malignancies originate in the bulbar urethra, with the rest being found in the anterior urethra (18). The majority of urethral carcinomas in males are squamous cell type, accounting for 69 to 90%, with transitional cell carcinoma making up 10 to 15% of tumors (mainly in the posterior urethra).

Carcinoma of the urethra in females, although more common than in males, is still relatively rare with only 1500 cases being reported in the literature (19). Squamous cell carcinoma accounts for 70% of all malignant neoplasms of the female urethra, with transitional cell carcinoma and adenocarcinoma making up 10 to 20% (20, 21).

Prognosis for distal urethral carcinomas in males is similar to that of carcinoma of the penis. The primary mode of therapy for carcinoma of the anterior male urethra is either primary excision or partial/total penectomy depending on the location and extent of the primary lesion. Due to the relative rarity of the lesion and very few patients who have undergone this form of therapy, results are scarce. The most common radiation technique for distal urethral lesions is a cross-fire technique using parallel opposed fields with the penis suspended vertically with a urethral catheter (22). Kaplan et al. reported a 5-year survival rate of 16% in 71 patients treated for tumors in the distal urethra by all treatment methods (23). For males with posterior urethral carcinoma, superficial lesions may be treated with endoscopic resection; however, invasive lesions into the prostatic, membranous, or bulbar urethra are best treated with exenterative surgery with or without adjuvant irradiation. In the same series, 5-year survival rates of 10% in patients with bulbomembranous lesions and 4% in patients with prostatic urethral lesions were reported (23).

In females, lesions involve the anterior urethra in 30% of all cases (24–26). Tumor size and location are the two most important factors in determining prognosis and survival (19). Meatal carcinomas are usually treated with interstitial implant using 192 iridium (27). External beam radiation combined with implant is recommended for large tumors extending into the labia, vagina, or entire urethra. Success rates of 70 to 90% have been reported in the treatment of meatal tumors with irradiation alone (28). Tumors involving the entire urethra or involving the urethra and vulva are harder to treat, and the overall local control rate is less, ranging from 20 to 30% (29, 30). Klein et al. reported 5-year survival rates of 40% in women

treated with preoperative radiation combined with radical surgery (31).

Carcinoma of the urethra is rare in both males and females, and its treatment and prognosis are largely dependent on the location, size, and extent of the primary lesion. Local control rates and 5-year survival rates are relatively similar when comparing surgical excision versus radiation therapy.

RENAL CELL CARCINOMA

Renal cell carcinoma has proved to be relatively radiation resistant when radiation is used as a primary treatment modality. Treatment of renal cell carcinoma with radiation therapy alone has not resulted in impressive results. This is mainly due to the inability to deliver high doses to large masses in the upper abdomen. Studies have instead looked at the possible therapeutic advantage of postoperative or preoperative radiation therapy combined with radical nephrectomy in an effort to improve local control, overall survival, and, in the case of preoperative therapy, resectability.

The role of postoperative radiation remains to be elucidated. For patients with pathologic T1 and T2 tumors (i.e., tumors confined to the renal parenchyma), surgery alone can provide 5- to 10-year survival rates of 80% (32–34). Postoperative radiation would not be expected to improve survival in these patients. For patients with residual tumor in the renal fossa, extension into the perinephric fat, regional lymph node involvement, or spillage of tumor, postoperative radiation therapy may be considered to have theoretic advantages. Support for this modality comes from one nonrandomized study by Rafla, in which overall survival and local control were enhanced with postsurgical therapy (35). Two prospective randomized trials by Finney (36) and Kjaer et al. (37) found no overall survival benefit. However, Finney's study lacked staging information, and both trials reported high complication rates including several fatalities attributable to high total dose and high dose per fraction radiation. This may have obscured a survival benefit. With standard fraction size and care to limit dose to less than 30% of the liver parenchyma, complication rates today should be much less.

Three studies have evaluated preoperative radiation therapy in a randomized fashion. van der Werf-Messing performed a trial in which 141 patients with angiographic evidence of renal cell carcinoma were randomized to preoperative radiation with 3000 cGy followed by immediate nephrectomy versus nephrectomy alone (38). Five-year survival was identical in both groups; however, the incidence of residual tumor and tumor recurrence in the fossae was less with the addition of radiation. Resectability for stage III tumors was increased from 50% with surgery alone to 72% in the radiation therapy arm. It should be noted that 34% of patients had stage I disease and would not be expected to necessarily show a survival benefit. In the second study from Finland, 70% of patients had stage I disease, and again no survival benefit was demonstrated (39). Local control and resectability were not stated. Rubin et al. showed no advantage for stage I patients but did show improved 2-year survival for stage II patients with the addition of preoperative radiation (40). Only 21 of 55 patients were believed to have received adequate radiation therapy to the regional nodes. Again, local control and resectability were not addressed.

Patients with clinically localized renal cell carcinoma are best treated with radical nephrectomy alone, with adjuvant radiation reserved for those cases where tumors are incompletely resected or where there is tumor spillage at the time of the operation. The role of preoperative and postoperative radiation currently is best confined to the protocol setting. Satisfactory clarification of this issue will require multiinstitutional randomized trials. Palliative radiation therapy can be helpful in those patients with symptomatic bony metastases or in those patients with vertebral lesions that are encroaching on the spinal canal (potentially causing cord compression).

REFERENCES

1. Crawford ED, Dawkins CA. Cancer of the penis. In: Skinner DG, Lieskovsky G, eds. Diagnosis and management of genitourinary cancer. Philadelphia: WB Saunders, 1988:549.
2. Gerbaulet A, Lambin P. Radiation therapy of cancer of the penis, indications, advantages, and pitfalls. Urol Clin North Am 1992;19:325.
3. Kossow JM, Hotchkiss RS, Morales PA. Carcinoma of the penis treated surgically: analysis of 100 cases. Urology 1973; 11:169.
4. Kurwilla JT, Garlick FH, Mammon KE. Results of surgical treatment of carcinoma of the penis. Aust N Z J Surg 1971; 41:157.
5. Merrin CE. Cancer of the penis. Cancer 1980;45:1973.
6. Narayana AS, Olney LE, Loening AS, et al. Carcinoma of the penis: analysis of 219 cases. Cancer 1982;49:2185.
7. Wajsman Z, Moore R, Merrin C, et al. Surgical treatment of penile cancer: a follow-up report. Cancer 1977;40:1697.
8. Mohs FE, Snow SN, Larson PO. Mohs micrographic surgery for penile tumors. Urol Clin North Am 1992;19:219.
9. Bandieramonte G, Lapera P, Marchesini R, et al. Laser microsurgery for superficial lesions of the penis. J Urol 1987; 138:315.
10. Perez CA, Pilepich MV. Penis and male urethra. In: Perez CA, Brady LW, eds. Principles and practice of radiation oncology. 2nd ed. Philadelphia: JB Lippincott, 1992:1131.
11. El-Demiry MIM, Oliver RTD, Hope-Stone HF, et al. Reappraisal of the role of radiotherapy in surgery and the management of carcinoma of the penis. Br J Urol 1984;56: 724.
12. Grabstald H, Kelley CD. Radiation therapy of penile cancer: 6–10 year follow-up. Urology 1980;15:575.
13. Mazeron JJ, Langlois D, Lobo PA, et al. Interstitial radiation therapy for carcinoma of the penis using iridium 192 wires: the Henri Mondor experience (1970–1979). Int J Radiat Oncol Biol Phys 1984;10:1891.
14. Ekstrom T, Edsmyr F. Cancer of the penis: a clinical study of 229 cases. Acta Chir Scand 1958;115:25.
15. Engelstad RB. Treatment of cancer of the penis at the Norwegian Radium Hospital. Radiology 1948;60:801.
16. Staubitz WJ, Lent MH, Oberkircher OJ. Carcinoma of the penis. Cancer 1955;8:371.
17. Hopkins SE, Grabstald H. Benign and malignant tumors of the male and female urethra. In: Walsh P, Gittes RF, Perlmutter AD, et al., eds. Campbell's urology. 5th ed. Philadelphia: WB Saunders, 1986:1441.
18. Mostofi FK, Davis CJ, Sesterhemn IA. Carcinoma of the male and female urethra. Urol Clin North Am 1992;19:347.
19. Grigsby PW. Female urethra. In: Perez CA, Brady LW, eds. Principles and practice of radiation oncology. 2nd ed. Philadelphia: JB Lippincott, 1992:1059.
20. Meis JM, Ayala AG, Johnson DE. Adenocarcinoma of the urethra in women: a clinicopathologic study. Cancer 1987;60: 1038.
21. Sailer SL, Shipley W, Wang CC. Carcinoma of the female urethra: a review of results with radiation therapy. J Urol 1988;140:1.
22. Haysek R, Parsons JT, Drille DM, et al. Carcinoma of the male urethra. J Urol 1985;134:753.
23. Kaplan GW, Bulkley GH, Grayhack JT. Carcinoma of the male urethra. J Urol 1967;98:365.
24. Antoniades J. Radiation therapy in carcinoma of the female urethra. Cancer 1969;24:70.
25. Grabstald H, Hilaris B, Henschke U, et al. Cancer of the female urethra. JAMA 1966;197:835.
26. Taggart CG, Castro JR, Rutledge FN. Carcinoma of the female urethra. AJR 1972;114:145.
27. Johnson DE, O'Connell JR. Primary carcinoma of the female urethra. Urology 1983;21:42.
28. Prempree T, Amornmarn R, Patanaphan V. Radiation therapy in primary carcinoma of the female urethra: part 2. an update on results. Cancer 1984;54:729.
29. Bracken RB, Johnson DE, Miller JS, et al. Primary carcinoma of the female urethra. J Urol 1976;116:188.
30. Turner AG, Hendry WF. Primary carcinoma of the female urethra. Br J Urol 1980;52:549.
31. Klein FA, Ali MM, Kersh R. Carcinoma in the femal urethra: combined iridium 192 interstitial and external beam radiotherapy. South Med J 1987;80:1129.
32. Shipley WU. Genitourinary cancer. In: Wang CC, ed. Clinical radiation oncology: indications, techniques, and results. Littleton, MA: PSG Publishing Co., 1988:262.
33. Siminovitch JMP, Montie JE, Straffon RA. Prognostic indicators in renal adenocarcinoma. J Urol 1983;130:20.
34. Bassil B, Dosoretz DE, Prout GR. Validation of the tumor, nodes and metastasis classification of renal cell carcinoma. J Urol 1985;134:450.
35. Rafla S. Renal cell carcinoma: natural history and results of treatment. Cancer 1970;25:26.
36. Finney R. An evaluation of postoperative radiotherapy in hypernephroma treatment: a clinical trial. Cancer 1973;32: 1332.
37. Kajer M, Frederiksen PL, Engelholm SA. Postoperative radiotherapy in stage II and III renal adenocarcinoma: a randomized trial by the Copenhagen Renal Cancer Study Group. Int J Radiat Oncol Biol Phys 1987;13:665.
38. van der Werf-Messing B. Carcinoma in the kidney. Cancer 1973;32:1056.
39. Juusela H, Malmio K, Alfthan O, et al. Preoperative irradiation in the treatment of renal adenocarcinoma. Scand J Urol Nephrol 1977;11:227.
40. Rubin P, Keller BO, Cox C, et al. Preoperative irradiation in renal carcinoma: evaluation of radiation treatment plans. Cancer 1975;123:114.

60

Palliative Radiation Therapy for Genitourinary Carcinomas

Arthur T. Porter
John Leung
Marie Duclos
Jeffrey D. Forman

INTRODUCTION

As physicians, our first instinct is to treat cancer with a curative intent. However, despite some dramatic improvements in the treatment of cancer in young people, the overall mortality and curability of solid tumors have changed little in the past half century (1). The majority of cancer patients will eventually die of their cancer, and more than half of these patients will require some form of palliative therapy during their lifetime. Thus, the indications, techniques, and results of noncurative but symptom-relieving therapy are becoming increasingly important.

In the United States, the incidence of genitourinary (GU) cancers is estimated to exceed 285,000 cases (2). Approximately two thirds of the cases are attributed to prostate cancer and the rest to tumors of the urinary tract. Despite improvements in radical surgery, radiation, and chemotherapy, the cancer death rates have increased for prostate and kidney and have decreased for bladder cancers. The fact remains that definitive therapy will eventually fail in a substantial number of patients.

Simply defined, palliation is the alleviation of symptoms in a patient usually with active, progressive disease for whom the prognosis is limited and the focus of care is preserving quality of life. The basic tenets of palliation are to do good, minimize harm, and foster patient autonomy. Due consideration is given to the condition of the patient, the chances of effecting palliation, and, of course, the patient's wishes. Palliative radiation therapy can be highly useful, delivered in a relatively short time, and will cause few side effects when the tolerance of normal tissues is respected. The ability of radiation to decrease pain, prevent hemorrhage and obstruction, and to improve organ function has been well documented. Treatment can usually be completed in 1 to 3 weeks or less.

NATURAL HISTORY

To administer effective palliation, a thorough understanding of the cancer is required.

Prostate

Prostate cancer is the most common GU carcinoma, with an incidence of 250,000 new cases per year. At diagnosis, 50% of patients have disease confined to the prostate gland or vicinity (T1 to T4), 20% have lymph node metastasis, and 30% have distant metastasis (3).

Regional lymph node involvement follows a predetermined pattern. Periprostatic and obturator nodes are involved first, followed by external iliac, hypogastric, common iliac, and peri-aortic nodes (4). The number and magnitude of lymph node involvement correlates well with prognosis. Prout et al. have demonstrated that in patients with solitary lymph node involvement, 20% experience disease progression compared with 75% who have multiple lymph node involvement (5).

Of all patients diagnosed with prostate cancer, more than 50% will die of their disease and more than two thirds will suffer local and/or systemic progression before their death. Prostate carcinoma metastasizes distantly to skeleton, liver, lungs, and occasionally the brain and other sites. Approximately 50% of patients will experience bone metastases at some time during their lifetime. The mechanism of preferential dissemination to the spine and pelvic bones by the vertebral veins was initially proposed by Batson (6). Recently, this concept has been disputed by Dodds et al., who described an equal distribution of skeletal metastases from prostate cancer compared with non-prostatic cancers. The mechanism of dissemination to spine, pelvic bone, and long bones is a function of the regional arterial blood supply rather than the venous drainage (7).

Bladder

Bladder cancer represents the second most common GU malignancy. At presentation, 75 to 85% of bladder carcinomas are superficial and 15 to 25% are muscle invading. However, muscle invasion will eventually develop in many of those with superficial presentation, resulting in approximately 25 to 50% of patients with muscle-invading disease. Regional or distant metastases will eventually develop in two thirds of patients (8).

Bladder cancer metastasizes by direct extension, lymphatic, or hematogenous spread. Skinner et al. have correlated the incidence of pelvic lymph node involvement to the depth of tumor invasion in the bladder wall (9). Babatan correlated the incidence of lymph node involvement to tumor grade (10). In an autopsy study, lymph node involvement was the most frequent site of metastases, being present in 78% of cases. Liver, lung, and bone metastases are the most frequent sites of distant disease and occur in approximately equal frequency (11).

Kidney

The natural history of renal cell carcinoma is not always predictable. This cancer may remain clinically occult for most of its course. This tumor may spread by local infiltration through the renal capsule or by direct extension through the venous channels to the renal vein. It may also spread by lymphatic or hematogenous routes. At diagnosis, 30% of patients will have metastatic disease, 25% will be locally advanced, and only 45% localized (12, 13). Lung is the most common site of metastases (75%), followed by soft tissue (36%), bone (20%), liver (18%), subcutaneous tissue (8%), and central nervous system (8%) (14). Of those with lung metastases, 1 to 3% have solitary metastases (15). Spontaneous regression of metastatic renal cell cancer, primarily to the lung, has been documented in less than 1% (16).

Testis

Both seminomatous and nonseminomatous cancers have the capability to metastasize to lymph nodes (predominantly retroperitoneal lymph nodes) or by the hematogenous route to the lung. The propensity for spread is higher for nonseminomatous cancer and for anaplastic seminoma compared with pure or spermatocystic seminomas.

In a postmortem study, Bredael et al. reported dissemination to the lung in 89%, liver in 73%, and brain and bone in 30% (17).

Others

Upper urinary tract carcinoma has a tendency to be a multifocal process. Dissemination may occur by direct extension, lym-

phatic dissemination (22 to 41%), or hematogenous dissemination. Renal pelvis carcinomas are reported with a higher rate of lymph node dissemination at diagnosis (37 to 82%) (18). Those patients are also at high risk (30 to 50%) of bladder cancer development (19).

Carcinomas of the urethra and penis mainly spread to adjacent structures or lymph nodes. Distant metastases can also occur via hematogenous routes to lungs or liver.

BONE METASTASES

In GU cancers, bone metastases are a common problem. It is estimated that osseous metastases develop in 50 to 70% of prostate and 25 to 50% of kidney cancer patients (20, 21). Many therapies are available for bone metastases, including surgery, medical management, and radiation. Radiation therapy can treat most patients, with highly effective symptom relief.

The hallmark of osseous metastases is localized pain that is many times continuous and unrelenting regardless of the site. The pain caused by bone metastases is not well understood. Some investigators have hypothesized that irritation of the periosteal membrane or the release of biologic mediators is responsible for bony pain. The most serious complication of osseous metastases is spinal cord compression, which is discussed in the next section.

Most bony metastases can be diagnosed by physical examination, plain radiographs, and a bone scan. Plain radiographs are highly accurate in detecting metastatic lesions particularly when associated with pain; however, the sensitivity is poor. The radiographic pattern is typically blastic for prostate cancer and almost always lytic for kidney cancer. Bone scanning is a useful adjunct to plain films. 99mTc-Disphosphonate is taken up in areas of bone production and can be used for detection of bony metastases and following response to therapy. Bone scintigraphy is approximately 50 to 80% more sensitive than plain radiographs (22). It can frequently show metastatic lesions long before changes on plain films are appreciated. Several investigators have estimated that this may be 2 to 6 months (23, 24). Plain films and bone scans are frequently used to plan radiation fields and define technique. Computed tomography (CT) and magnetic resonance imaging (MRI) are sometimes required if there is suspicion of bone involvement but radiographs and bone scan are negative, or if there is soft tissue involvement.

Most clinical situations, including pain management and preservation of bone integrity, can be managed by the judicious use of radiation therapy. Planning radiation requires a clear understanding of the patient's disease and the intent of treatment. Although radiation has been shown to be highly effective, actual treatment delivery, dose, fractionation, and volume can vary greatly from center to center without any apparent effect on efficacy. Therefore, treatment can be customized to the patient's needs. Certainly, a patient with a painful bony lesion and a poor prognosis will most likely have a different

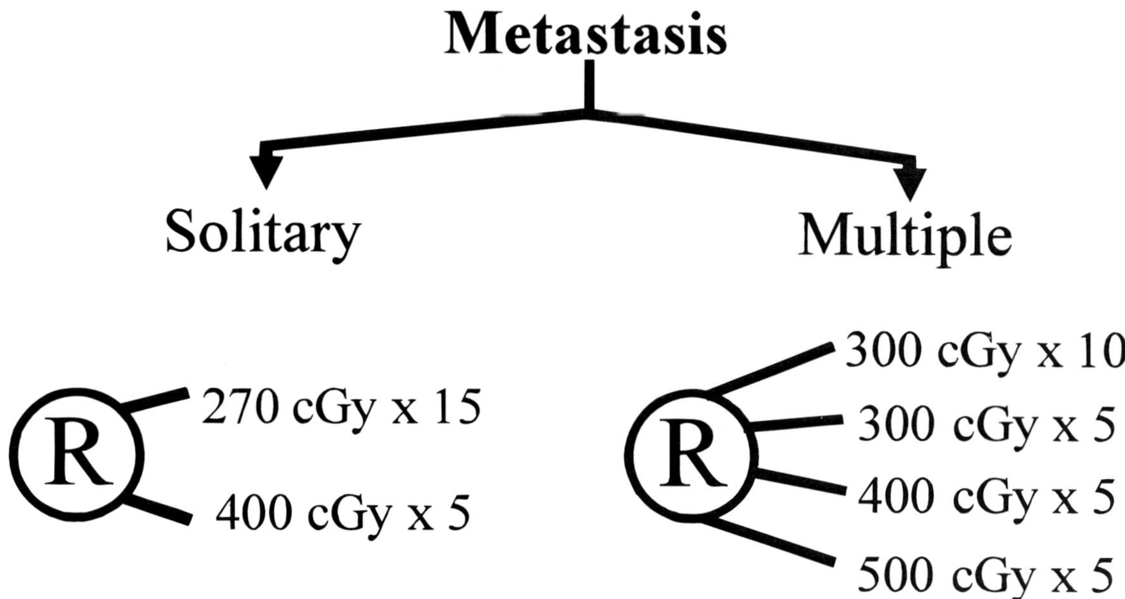

Fig. 60.1. Radiation Therapy Oncology Group Study 74-02 design.

treatment regimen than a patient with a good prognosis. In GU cancer patients, it is likely for patients with bone metastases from prostate cancer to have many useful years of life.

The most widely quoted bone metastases study is the Radiation Therapy Oncology Group (RTOG) trial 74-02 reported by Tong et al. (25). This study analyzed 759 patients. All patients had at least one painful bony site, most required narcotic medications, and 56% described their pain as being constant and severe. These patients were randomized to receive several different radiation therapy regimens (Fig. 60.1). Eighty-three percent of patients had a partial response and 54% had a complete response, usually within 2 to 4 weeks of treatment. Pain relief was influenced by the site and pain status before irradiation. More than 70% of patients who experienced some pain relief did not have a relapse before death. There were no significant differences in the frequency of pain relief among the various treatment arms.

A reanalysis of this RTOG study by Blitzer, however, concluded that the two high-dose protracted programs (270 cGy × 15 and 300 cGy × 10) had significantly better complete responses and decreased narcotic use, and that patients treated to higher doses required fewer re-treatments (Table 60.1) (26). Reviewing the data from currently available prospective studies has shown overall response rates ranging from 85 to 100% using various treatment schedules (27–29). Single-fraction regimens (800 cGy × 1) appear to be as effective as the other more protracted regimens but are also associated with increased acute morbidity, particularly to the abdominal organs. A frequently used regimen in the United States is 3000 cGy given in 10 divided fractions. This dose is adequate for most GU cancers including prostate, bladder, and especially seminoma. Metastatic renal cell cancer, however, has historically been regarded as radioresistant. Several studies, including that of Onu-

frey and Mohiuddin who retrospectively reviewed 125 patients with metastatic renal cancer, have recommended doses of at least 4000 to 4500 cGy (30). A report by Halperin and Harisiadis did not show a dose-response relationship to palliation in 35 patients (31). These authors, however, are in agreement with Onufrey and Mohiuddin and recommend at least 4000 cGy for renal cell metastases.

A metastasis to a weight-bearing region certainly raises many concerns. A pathologic fracture can be painful and disabling both functionally and psychologically. Certain radiographic and clinical factors that warrant consideration of prophylactic surgical fixation include the following.

1. An intramedullary lytic lesion greater than or equal to 50% of the cross-sectional diameter of the bone.
2. A lytic lesion involving a length of cortex greater than or equal to the cross-sectional diameter of the bone or greater than 2.5 cm in axial length (32).

These patients should be evaluated by an orthopedic surgeon.

Table 60.1.   Reported Results for Pain Relief After Local Field Radiation Therapy for Bone Metastasis

	NO. OF PATIENTS	DOSE/ FRACTIONS	OVERALL RESPONSE (%)	COMPLETE RESPONSE (%)
Tong et al. (25)	72	20/5	90	53
	74	40.5/15	92	61
	613	15–30/5–10	89	53
Madsen (27)	27	20/2	48	—
	30	24/6	47	—
Price et al. (28)	140	8/1	85	27
	148	30/10	85	27

If a pathologic fracture has occurred in a weight-bearing region, surgical fixation is required for pain control and to promote adequate healing. In all situations, postoperative radiation is required. Because prostate cancer produces primarily blastic metastases, pathologic fracture is correspondingly infrequent. In addition to being lytic, renal cell bone metastases are also very vascular and are associated with extraosseous extension. CT, angiography, and possible embolization are recommended before surgical manipulation.

SPINAL CORD COMPRESSION

Spinal cord compression is a medical emergency. Failure to diagnose and treat promptly can lead to significant morbidity including paraplegia and autonomic dysfunction. In a study by Bruckman and Bloomer, GU tumors (especially majority prostate and kidney) accounted for 13% of spinal cord compres-sions (33). Approximately 18,000 cases of spinal cord compression occur in the United States every year (34).

The predominant symptom of cord compression is that of pain in approximately 95% of patients (Fig. 60.2) (35). Pain usually precedes a diagnosis of spinal cord compression by approximately 4 months. Symptoms, however, can progress rapidly to neurologic dysfunction in a matter of hours to days. When a patient has progressed to paraplegia, return of function is infrequent. Therefore, early diagnosis and therapy are critical.

Diagnostic tools include radiographs, bone scan, CT, MRI, and myelogram. Plain films are positive in approximately 80% of patients with epidural compression but are neither specific nor sensitive (36). A major limitation of plain films is that the bone requires at least 50% decalcification before radiologic changes can be appreciated. As mentioned earlier, bone scans are more sensitive but not specific. Plain films and bone scans with physical examination can detect most spinal cord compres-

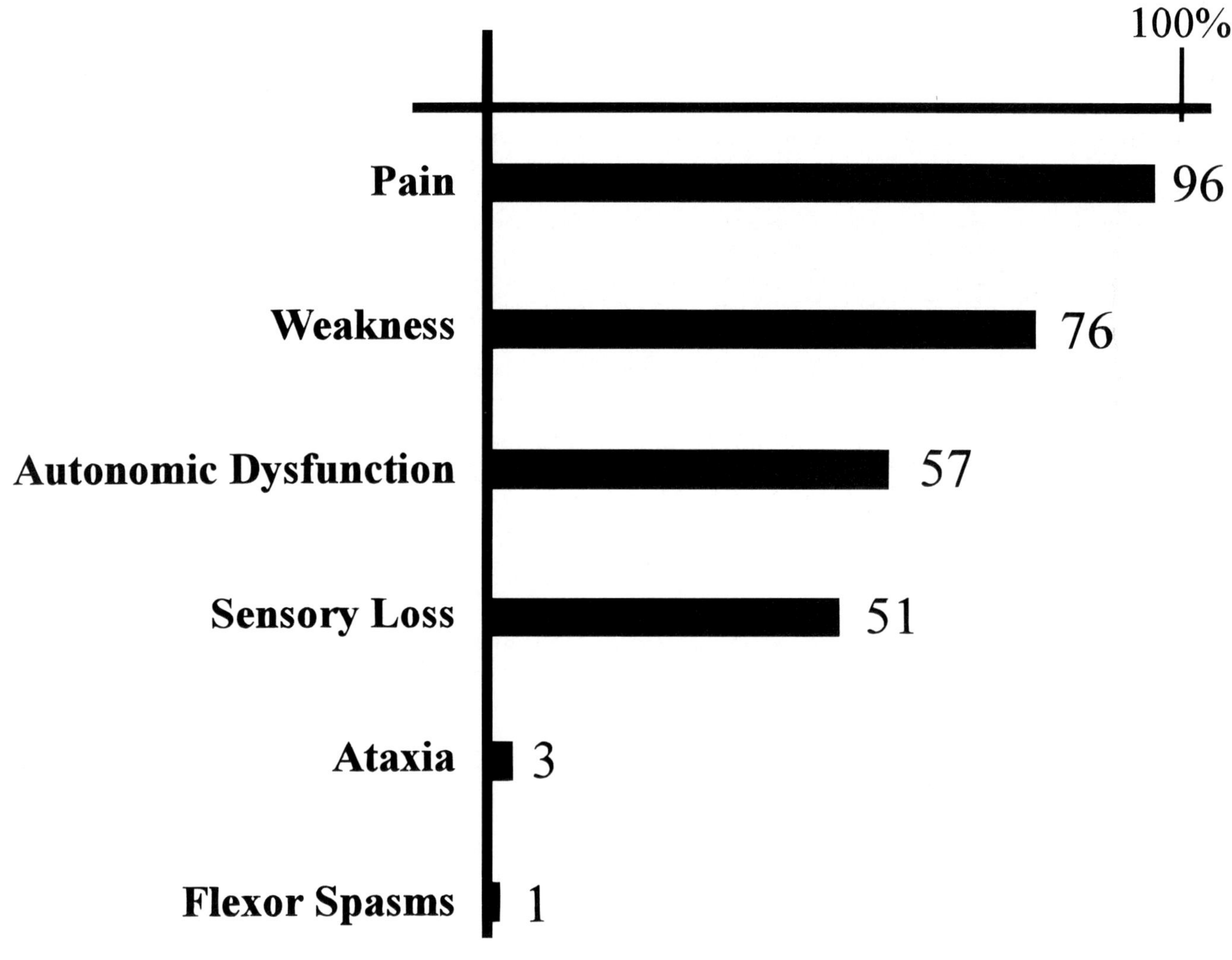

from Gilbert et al.[35]

Fig. 60.2. Signs and symptoms of cord compression at diagnosis.

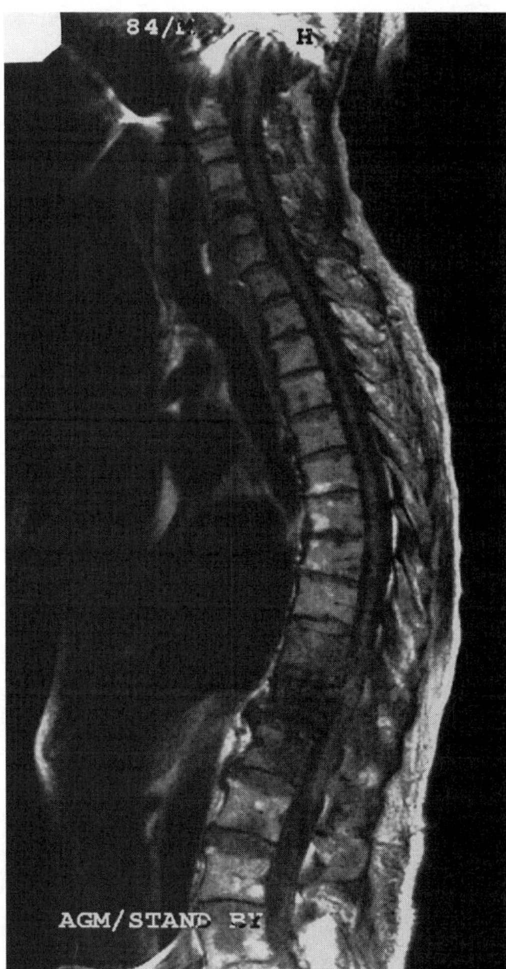

Fig. 60.3. Sagittal image of the cervical, thoracic, and upper lumbar spine of an 84-year-old black man who presented with paresthesias and weakness in bilateral extremities. Prostate-specific antigen level was 1000 ng/mL. Abnormal signal is seen throughout T10 and T11 vertebral bodies. There is deformity and loss of the adjacent subarachnoid space consistent with compression of the lower spinal cord. Numerous other sites of abnormal signal are seen within the vertebrae, consistent with multiple bony metastases.

sions (85 to 90%) (37). The gold standard for diagnosis has traditionally been the myelogram. The sensitivity and specificity are approximately 95% and 88% (38). However, this test is invasive, and several investigators have shown MRI to be of similar if not superior accuracy (39, 40). MRI has the added benefit of imaging the entire spine (Fig. 60.3).

After the diagnosis of spinal cord compression is made, the physician is left with the dilemma of how to treat it. Effective regimens include surgery, radiation, or both. In most instances, radiation therapy suffices and obviates the need for surgery. Several retrospective series have shown equivalent results between radiation alone and laminectomy, plus radiation in terms of pain control, and functional improvement. The most widely quoted study evaluating this issue is that of Gilbert et al. (41). In general (despite the therapy instituted), if a patient is ambu-

latory, there is an 85% chance that he or she will remain ambulatory. If nonambulatory, there is a less than 50% chance of regaining ambulation; if paraplegic, there is a less than 5% chance of becoming ambulatory. Again, this emphasizes the need for early diagnosis and treatment. Successful improvement of pain is analagous to results obtained with radiation therapy for other bone metastases (41).

Radiation therapy can be instituted quickly and efficiently. Results of MRI or other diagnostic tests together with physical examination can help determine the appropriate treatment volume. Multiple epidural lesions can be treated in one continuous field or by multiple treatment fields. The volume treated is usually the level of cord involvement together with two vertebral bodies above and two below the epidural lesion. However, with the accuracy of MRI, many centers use one vertebral body above and one below the area of cord compression. The optimal radiation dose and fractionation scheme have not been firmly established. However, different from the treatment of other bony metastases, the goal is not only pain relief but also tumor reduction. It is for this reason that protracted fractionation for spinal cord compression is recommended.

Friedman et al. demonstrated a good response in 71% of patients who received more than 2500 cGy for epidural compression versus 34% for patients receiving less than 2500 cGy (42). The patients in this study had the diagnosis of lymphoma, which is usually more radiosensitive than other tumor histologic types. Commonly used doses are 3000 to 4000 cGy over 2 to 4 weeks. In all cases, spinal cord tolerance to radiation should be respected. Often, initial doses of 300 to 500 cGy are given for the first two to three treatments to attempt quicker symptom palliation, but there are no firm data to support this.

There are a few instances in which surgery should be considered as an option before radiation. They include pathologic fracture with spine instability or compression of the spinal cord by bone, unknown tissue diagnosis, a history of previous radiation to the same area, and a radiation-resistant tumor with neurologic deficits. As mentioned previously, renal cell carcinoma has been thought by some to be radioresistant. This relative radioresistance does not necessarily support the use of surgery. Hypernephromas are usually well vascularized and often have an extensive extraosseous soft tissue component. Radiation therapy is often safer than surgery and as effective with recommended doses of approximately 4000 to 4500 cGy.

After the diagnosis of cord compression is made or even suspected, all patients should be given steroid therapy. Steroids can decrease edema and provide striking analgesic benefit. The loading dose of dexamethasone is 4 to 100 mg followed by maintenance doses of 4 to 24 mg every 6 hours.

BRAIN METASTASES

Brain metastases are common and devastating complications of systemic cancer. Intracranial metastases will eventually develop in approximately 24% of all cancer patients (43). The parenchymal brain is involved in 15% of all patients, and leptomeningeal and dural metastases occur in 9% (44). GU carcinomas account for 10% of brain metastases.

The clinical presentation of brain metastases is broad and depends primarily on their location within the brain. Headache, hemiparesis, seizures, confusion, and ataxia are some of the clinical symptoms that may lead to the suspicion of brain metastases. Only functional status and age have been shown to affect survival. The available data suggest that histologic type is not a prognostic variable (45). Clinical series indicate that almost half of all patients present with solitary brain metastasis.

In addition, 20% of patients have only two lesions and only 10% have more than five lesions. Certain types of cancer are more likely to be associated with single metastasis like renal cell carcinoma as contrasted to those usually presenting with multiple lesions like seminomas (46). The mechanism of development of brain metastases is through hematogenous dissemination.

The diagnosis of brain metastases usually requires CT or MRI. An MRI scan with gadolinium is superior to CT and performed to exclude multiple metastases if local treatment is

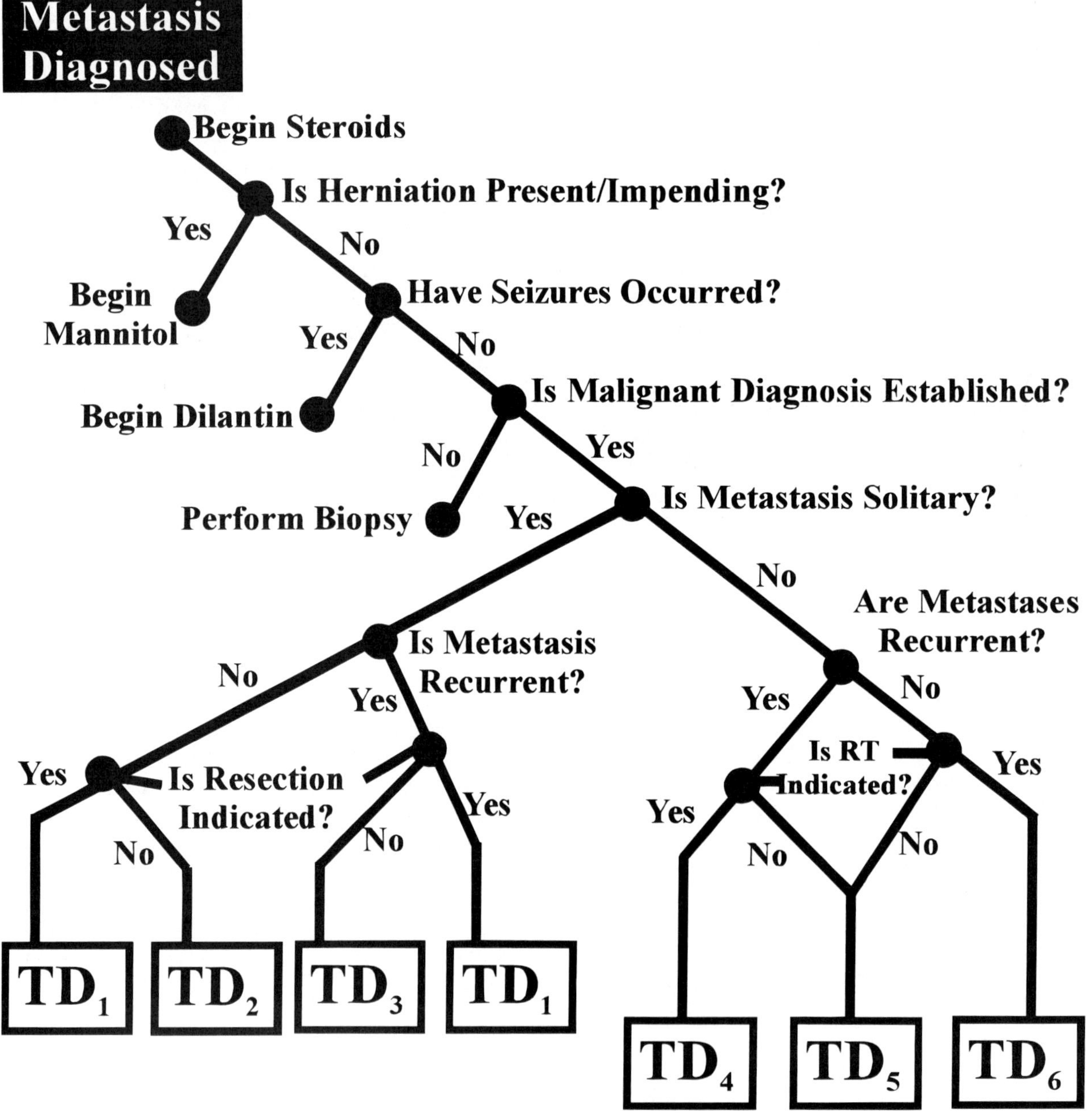

Fig. 60.4. Brain metastasis decision-making. TD1: Surgical excision plus whole-brain radiation therapy; TD2: whole-brain radiation therapy plus boost; TD3: RE-RT/implant; TD4: RE-RT; TD5: no further radiation therapy; TD6: whole-brain radiation therapy.

considered (47). Lumbar puncture with cerebrospinal fluid analysis is essential in the diagnosis of leptomeningeal infiltration by the tumor but not helpful for brain lesions.

The management of brain metastases involves the use of corticosteroids and radiation therapy, with or without surgical resection. A decision tree format has been suggested by the consensus workshop panel on the management of brain metastases in 1992 (Fig. 60.4).

Corticosteroid administration will lead to symptom improvement in 60 to 75% of patients, particularly those with poor neurologic status (48). Most groups recommend its initiation at least 24 hours before the start of radiation. We recommend dexamethasone in a dose of 16 mg daily. Higher doses can be used if no improvement occurs (49). Steroids can be tapered during or following the radiation treatment. Other medications (mannitol or phenytoin) may be used to prevent brain herniation or seizures.

Although almost 50% of patients present with solitary brain metastasis, less than half of these will be candidates for surgical resection based on their performance status (less than 70) or the location of the lesion in the brain. Whole brain radiation remains the primary treatment modality for the majority of patients presenting with brain metastases. Many radiation therapy regimens have been studied by the RTOG, including 3000 to 3600 cGy/10 to 12 fractions, 2000 cGy/5 fractions, 4000 cGy/15 to 20 fractions. None of them have been proved to be superior, with median survivals ranging between 17 and 21 weeks (50). Large fraction sizes, such as 500 to 600 cGy per fraction, have been proven to be less effective (51).

The response to radiation varies according to the different signs or symptoms of presentation and also according to the severity of the neurologic impairment. A general rule is that 70 to 90% improvement is expected within 4 weeks of the initiation of treatment and 50% of patients will achieve a complete response. The severity of neurologic dysfunction affects the response rate, with 35 to 40% of patients with advanced neurologic symptoms achieving a complete response compared with 60 to 70% for those with less neurologic dysfunction. The median duration of improvement is 10 to 14 weeks (52). Survival time varies from 1 month when the patient receives no treatment, to 2 months with corticosteroids alone, to 3 to 6 months with cranial irradiation. The 1-year survival rate is 10 to 30%. Approximately 30 to 50% of patients will die as a direct result of uncontrolled brain metastases (50).

The management of solitary brain metastasis may be different. There is no clear indication for surgical excision. General criteria like performance status (greater than 70) or tumor location are generally used. Surgery alone has been compared with surgery plus adjuvant whole brain radiation therapy in both a retrospective and a randomized study. The results showed an improvement in median survival from 11.5 to 21 months in the radiation group and a decrease in brain relapse from 85% to 21%. These studies also showed that 60% of patients in the surgery group eventually received whole brain radiation therapy for symptomatic recurrence (53, 54). The median duration

of functional independence also improved from 8 to 38 weeks (54). A recent nonrandomized intergroup study showed similar results in favor of their surgical treatment arm (55). Radiation alone has also been evaluated using whole brain radiation alone (3500 cGy) or combined with a boost (1500 cGy). No improvement in local control, palliation of symptoms, or survival was demonstrated (56).

An ongoing intergroup study, SWOG/RTOG 9021, is evaluating the role of complete excision alone, without whole brain radiation, in solitary brain metastasis. Complications from radiation treatment are rare, mainly because of the short survival in this group of patients and, when they occur, they tend to be mild to moderate. Most patients will subsequently have mild to moderate atrophic change on CT without symptoms. A few patients will experience memory loss with or without neuropsychologic dysfunction. Dementia and brain necrosis are rare sequelae (57).

HEMORRHAGE, PAIN, AND OBSTRUCTIVE UROPATHY

Massive GU hemorrhage may occur in patients with locally advanced cancer at diagnosis (renal cell cancer, bladder cancer, and less often, prostate cancer), with recurrent or progressive disease despite treatment. Radiation therapy is the common, primary, palliative treatment modality. A variety of regimens have been studied (58, 59). The usual regimen used consists of 3000 cGy/10 fractions, which leads to complete response of the macroscopic hematuria in 4 weeks in more than 80% of patients. However, other concurrent symptoms such as pain or obstipation are rarely palliated by the irradiation. The proposed mechanism for hemostasis is in increasing the reepithelialization and scarring formation on the mucosa by decreasing the tumor bulk with radiation (60).

Pelvic pain by local extension of the disease may be treated with radiation therapy, using the same regimen of 3000 cGy/ 10 fractions. The results are poor (50%) and short in duration. Higher doses (4000 to 5000 cGy/20 to 25 fractions) have been used with minimal improvement in the response. In the case of locally advanced prostate cancer, hormonal therapy with consideration of radiation therapy may be the first treatment option.

Obstructive uropathy by locally advanced GU carcinoma can be effectively treated using 4000 to 5000 cGy/20 to 25 fractions with a greater than 80% response. The use of surgical stents may be warranted in the case of a nonresponsive ureteral obstruction. Ureteral or bladder neck dilatation may also be used. Radiation should be considered in the case of hormone-resistant, locally advanced prostate cancer.

GYNECOMASTIA

Gynecomastia is usually a side effect related to the use of hormonal therapy. More often associated with the use of estrogen, gynecomastia rarely develops with the use of the newer antiandrogen or luteinizing hormone releasing hormone agonists. Treatment consists of 1000 to 1500 cGy/3 to 5 fractions using an electron beam aimed directly to the nipple-areolar complex. It should be started within 1 month of the appearance of gynecomastia and is well tolerated (61).

Gynecomastia may also develop in 5% of patients with testicular germ cell tumors as a systemic endocrine manifestation of the cancer. Treatment of the primary cancer usually corrects the problem. Radiation therapy is rarely used.

PALLIATIVE SYSTEMIC RADIATION THERAPY

Hemibody Irradiation

The concept of palliative systemic radiation therapy has interested physicians since 1905 (62). Over the years, the techniques and applications of this form of treatment have continued to progress. Before the 1970s, experience in systemic radiation therapy was primarily in the form of total body irradiation. Its use was mostly in the treatment of hematologic diseases. The main limitation of this form of treatment was bone marrow toxicity, which limited the maximal dose that can be given, i.e., 225 to 300 cGy.

Fitzpatrick and Rider began using hemibody irradiation (HBI) to circumvent the shortcomings associated with total body irradiation in the early 1970s. In 1976, they published a landmark paper on their experiences with HBI (63). Using single fractions of 500 to 1000 cGy, they treated 140 patients with symptomatic bone metastases and reported the results of 82 patients. HBI was tolerable and effective in achieving palliation of pain, often within 48 hours of treatment. Deaths from radiation pneumonitis and hematopoietic failure were few. The study also showed that systemic radiation therapy can be effective in treating solid tumors. After this publication, several articles evaluating their retrospective data on HBI for palliation of bony metastases were reported (64, 65). Results were encouraging and prompted the RTOG to evaluate this modality.

The final analysis of RTOG 78-10 was published in 1986 by Salazar et al. (66). The protocol explored increasing single doses of half body irradiation in patients with multiple symptomatic osseous metastases. The doses used were 600 to 800 cGy in the upper hemibody and 800 to 1000 cGy in the lower or middle hemibody. The most common histologic types treated were prostate (40%), breast (29%), and lung (18%) cancers. Pain relief was experienced in 73% of patients. Fifty percent of patients achieved pain relief within 48 hours and 80% within 1 week. There were no fatalities and treatment was considered tolerable. The most effective and safest dosages were 600 cGy for the upper hemibody and 800 cGy for the lower and middle hemibody. When compared with RTOG 74-02 (local irradiation for palliation of bone metastases), HBI achieved a similar number of patients experiencing pain relief; however, local irradiation achieved twice the number of complete responses. Another important finding was that recurrences of pain within irradiated fields were 4 times lower with HBI than with local irradiation. This indicated that prophylactic irradiation to bones can decrease the rate of disease involvement. Studies by Jacobsson (67) and Kaplan et al. (68) showed that prostate cancer patients who received periaortic irradiation subsequently had significantly less lumbar metastases than those who had whole pelvis irradiation alone.

RTOG 82-06 was designed based on the results of RTOG 78-10 and on the preliminary data on prophylactic irradiation. This prospective randomized study evaluated the effect of adjuvant systemic radiation therapy (HBI) in delaying the onset of bony metastases (69). A total of 499 patients with painful bony metastases were randomized to either local radiation or local radiation and HBI 800 cGy. Those patients who received HBI had an increased progression-free survival, 12.6 months versus 6.3 months, and fewer re-treatments. Overall, the incidence of toxicities was 5 to 15%. There were no fatalities or radiating pneumonitis; lung shields were used. The authors of the study concluded that 800 cGy of HBI can cause micrometastases to regress and that HBI has the potential to be used to treat systemic and occult metastases and improve quality of life for these patients.

HBI is delivered by external beam irradiation. The field arrangements have changed little since the conception of this treatment and are shown in Figure 60.5. Because of the long treatment fields, the source to skin distance is usually greater than 180 cm. Shielding is used for the oral cavity and all sites of previous irradiation. Lung blocks are used to reduce lung dose to 600 cGy corrected for lung transmission. The typical dose is 600 cGy to upper hemibody and 800 cGy to the middle and lower hemibody given in a single fraction.

The major chronic toxicity associated with HBI is radiation pneumonitis. Without lung correction, the incidence of radiation pneumonitis is estimated to be 18 to 35% for doses of 600 to 1000 cGy; these figures are less than 10% if corrected for lung transmission (70). Approximately 50% of patients will have depression of their hematologic profile, and 10% of patients may require transient hematologic support. Irradiation of the head can cause xerostomia and cataract formation. If the head and brain have a low incidence of metastatic involvement, then exclusion of the head from the upper hemibody irradiation is acceptable. The most troublesome acute complication is nausea and vomiting, which occurs in 80% of patients, particularly with upper and middle HBI. With the use of premedication programs using prednisone, odansetron, and hydration, the incidence of emesis is less than 5% (71). HBI should be considered in any patient with multiple bony disease sites that are not responsive to hormone or chemotherapy maneuvers and adequate bone marrow function.

Strontium-89

In 1941, a new tool in the treatment of skeletal metastases was introduced—the radionuclide, strontium-89. Strontium-89 is a calcium analog that emits beta irradiation. It has a half-life

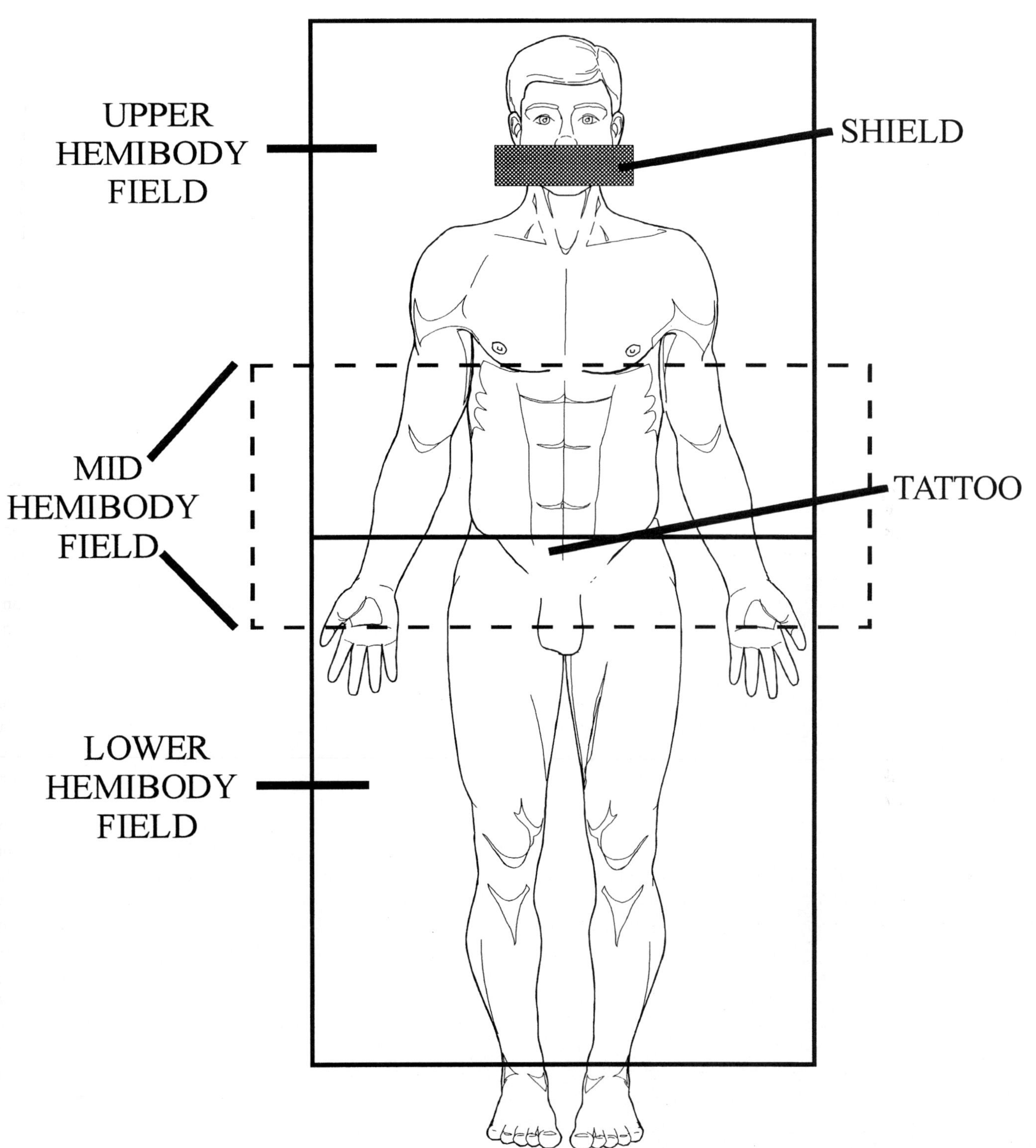

Fig. 60.5. General radiation field arrangement for hemibody irradiation.

of 50.6 days, and the average beta energy is 1.46 MeV. Because of strontium's physical and chemical characteristics, it has the following advantages.

1. Selective uptake in areas of active bone formation.
2. Irradiation of normal tissues is limited; therefore, tolerance is high.
3. Strontium-89 can be administered quickly and easily.
4. The patient is not a radiation hazard to family members or hospital staff.

Strontium-89 has several advantages over HBI, including better patient tolerance and ease of administration, with similar efficacy at least for prostate cancer.

Pecher was first to demonstrate the effectiveness of strontium-89 for the palliation of painful bone metastases in the early 1940s (72). During the following years, numerous studies have confirmed the efficacy and safety of this form of treatment in palliating painful bony metastases, particularly blastic metastases (73–75). Several phase II trials have shown complete pain relief in 6 to 50% of patients and a reduction of analgesic use by 50%. Overall response rates in prostate patients is approximately 80%. Prospective randomized studies looking at this issue have also been completed.

Porter et al. reported the findings of a phase III (TransCanadian) trial evaluating the efficacy of palliative strontium-89 therapy in the management of hormone-resistant metastatic prostate cancer (76). There were 126 patients randomized to strontium therapy versus placebo after local field radiation for symptomatic lesions. Those patients who received strontium had significant reduction in analgesic intake at 3 months (17% versus 2.4% not requiring analgesics), progression of new painful sites (58.7% versus 34% free of new painful sites at 3 months), and need for re-treatment (51 weeks versus 23 weeks' time to re-treatment). The levels of prostate-specific antigen were also significantly reduced with strontium-89 therapy. The results of this study are provocative.

The United Kingdom Metastron Investigators' Group Study is another prospective study evaluating the efficacy of strontium-89 after external beam radiation therapy (77). Entry criteria were similar to the TransCanadian Study. External beam irradiation consisted of either local field or HBI. The dose of strontium-89 was 5.4 mCi. A total of 284 patients were treated according to protocol. Median follow-up was 12 weeks. There were no significant differences in survival or overall pain relief with strontium-89, local field, or hemibody therapy. However, patients receiving strontium-89 were significantly less likely to have new sites of pain develop or to require re-treatment.

Pain relief with strontium-89 usually begins at 10 to 20 days after treatment, and the response lasts approximately 4 to 15 months. Some patients experience a pain flare 1 to 2 weeks after strontium injection, and this usually indicates a better outcome. The recommended dosage of strontium-89 is 4 mCi or 40 to 60 μCi/kg. The drug is administered by slow intravenous injection. Strontium-89 is cleared by the kidneys (two thirds) and by the gastrointestinal tract (one third). All patient excretions can be flushed away without special monitoring. Strontium therapy is well tolerated. The major toxicity is hematologic, especially thrombocytopenic. Most patients show a 24 to 50% decrease in platelet count from pretreatment levels (78). The platelet nadir occurs 4 to 8 weeks after therapy; however, medical intervention or hematologic support is rarely needed. Platelet recovery is gradual and expected. Strontium should be used with caution in patients with platelet counts less than 100,000/cc and leukocyte counts less than 2400/cc. Repeated administrations of strontium are possible based on individual patient response but are generally not recommended at intervals of less than 90 days.

Strontium-89 and HBI are effective systemic tools in palliating and decreasing the incidence of painful bony metastases, particularly for prostate cancers. Several studies have shown benefit for both modalities when used in addition to or adjuvantly with external beam irradiation.

NEW TREATMENT MODALITIES

Altered Fractionation for Treatment of Brain Metastases

The purpose of an altered fractionation regimen is to increase tumor control by increasing the radiation dose without compromising the late effects of irradiation. In a phase I/II study, RTOG-8528 used 160 cGy/fraction twice a day to different dose levels—4800 versus 5440 versus 6400 versus 7040 cGy—and showed an improvement in survival, tumor clearance, and neurologic status for all regimens greater than or equal to 5440 cGy (79).

Hypoxic Radiosensitizers

Many studies have been done to enhance the effect of radiation by using different compounds. Misonidazole, a hypoxic cell sensitizer, and BUDR, a pyrimidine analog that potentiates the lethal effects of radiation, have not yet been proven to increase the response to radiation (80).

Stereotactic External Beam Irradiation and Brachytherapy

These techniques use either linear accelerators or radioactive seed implants to deliver high-dose radiation therapy to a very restricted volume, sparing the normal surrounding structures. These techniques may act like surgical ablation and allow an increase in local control by increasing the local dose in patients who are not candidates for surgery or have lesions that are not surgically accessible (81, 82).

New Radionuclides

Radionuclides currently under investigation include rhenium-189 HEDP and samarium-153 EDTMP for the systemic treat-

Table 60.2. Radiopharmaceuticals for Bone Pain

RADIONUCLIDE	HALF-LIFE	ENERGY (MeV)	ANALGESIC EFFECT (%)	TOXICITY
^{32}P	14 (days)	1.7	50–90	+ +
^{89}Sr	51 (days)	1.5	50–90	+
^{117m}Sn	14 (days)	0.2	—	−
^{186}Re	91 (hr)	1.1	80	+
^{153}Sm	46 (hr)	0.9	80	+

ment of bone metastases. Both radioisotopes have shown the ability to localize in bone lesions and to palliate bony pain (65 to 80%). Furthermore, both agents emit gamma radiation and can therefore be imaged to show their biodistribution (Table 60.2).

REFERENCES

1. Doyle D, Hanks GWC, MacDonald N, eds. Oxford textbook of palliative medicine. New York: Oxford University Press, 1993.
2. American Cancer Society. Cancer facts and figures 1994. American Cancer Society: Atlanta: GA, 1994.
3. Scardino PT, Weaver R, Hudson MA. Early detection of prostate cancer. Hum Pathol 1992;23:211.
4. Pistenma DA, Bagshaw MA, Feiha FS. Extended field radiation therapy for prostatic adenocarcinoma: status report of a limited prospective trial. In: Johnson DE, Samuels ML, eds. Cancer of the genitourinary tract. New York: Raven Press, 1979.
5. Prout GR, Heaney JA, Griffin P, et al. Nodal involvement as a prognostic indicator in patients with prostatic carcinoma. J Urol 1980;124:226.
6. Batson OV. The role of the vertebral veins in metastatic processes. Ann Intern Med 1942;16:38.
7. Dodds PR, Caride VJ, Lytton B. The role of vertebral veins in the dissemination of prostatic carcinoma. J Urol 1981;126:753.
8. Heney NM, Nocks BN, Daly JJ, et al. TA and T1 bladder cancer: occasion, recurrence, and progression. Br J Urol 1982; 54:152.
9. Skinner DG, Tift JP, Kaufman JJ. High dose, short course preoperative radiation therapy and immediate single stage radical cystectomy with pelvic node dissection in the management of bladder cancer. J Urol 1982;127:671.
10. Babaian RJ. Metastases from transitional cell carcinoma of urinary bladder. Urology 1980;16:142.
11. Fetter TR. Carcinoma of the bladder: sites of metastases. J Urol 1959;81:746.
12. Golimbu M, Joshi P, Sperber A, et al. Renal cell carcinoma: survival and prognostic factors. Urology 1986;27:291.
13. Silverberg E. Cancer statistics. Cancer 1981;31:13.
14. Maldazys JD, deKernion JB. Prognostic factors in metastatic renal carcinoma. J Urol 1986;136:376.
15. Sufrin G, Chasan S, Golio A, et al. Paraneoplastic and serologic syndromes of renal adenocarcinoma. Semin Urol 1989;7:158.
16. Montie JE, Stewart BH, Stroffon RA, et al. The role of adjunctive nephrectomy in patients with metastatic renal cell carcinoma. J Urol 1977;117:272.
17. Bredael JJ, Vugrin D, Whitmore WF Jr. Autopsy findings in 154 patients with germ cell tumors of the testis. Cancer 1982; 50:548.
18. Shipley WU. Genitourinary cancer. In: Wang CC, ed. Clinical radiation oncology: indications, techniques, and results. Littleton, MA: PSG Publishing Co., 1988:262.
19. Babaian RJ, Johnson DE. Primary carcinoma of the ureter. J Urol 1980;123:357.
20. Abrams HL, Spiro R, Goldstein N. Metastases in carcinoma: analysis of 1000 autopsied cases. Cancer 1950;3:74.
21. Gilbert HA, Dagan AR. Metastases: incidence, detection, and evaluation. In: Weiss L, ed. Fundamental aspects of metastases. Amsterdam, North Holland: Elsevier Excerpta Medica, 1976.
22. Pagani JJ and Libshitz HI. Imaging in bone metastases. Radiol Clin North Am 1982;20:545.
23. Glasko CSB. Skeletal metastases. Clin Orthop 1986;210:18.
24. Wilner D. Cancer metastasis to bone. In: Wilner D, ed. Radiology of bone tumors and allied disorders. Philadelphia: WB Saunders, 1982:3641.
25. Tong D, Gillick L, Hendrickson FR. The palliation of symptomatic osseous metastases: final results of the Radiation Therapy Oncology Group. Cancer 1982;50:893.
26. Blitzer PH. Reanalysis of the RTOG study of the palliation of symptomatic osseous metastases. Cancer 1985;55:1468.
27. Madsen EL. Painful bone metastases: efficacy of radiotherapy assessed by the patient; a randomized trial comparing 4 Gy $\times$ 6 vs 10 Gy $\times$ 2. Int J Radiat Oncol Biol Phys 1983;9:1775.
28. Price P, Hoskin PJ, Easton D, et al. Low dose single fraction radiotherapy in the treatment of metastatic bone pain: a pilot study. Radiother Oncol 1988;12:297.
29. Cole DJ. A randomised trial of a single treatment versus conventional fractionation in the palliative radiotherapy of painful bone metastases. Clin Oncol 1989;1:59.
30. Onufrey V, Mohiuddin M. Radiation therapy in the treatment of metastatic renal cell carcinoma. Int J Radiat Oncol Biol Phys 1985;11:2007.
31. Halperin EC, Harisiadis L. The role of radiation therapy in the management of renal cell carcinoma. Cancer 1983;51:614.
32. Lane JM, Sculo TP, Zolan S. Treatment of pathologic fractures of the hip by endoprosthetic replacement. J Bone Joint Surg 1980;62:954-959.
33. Bruckman JE, Bloomer WD. Management of spinal cord compression. Semin Oncol 1978;5:135.
34. Black P. Spinal metastases: current status and recommended guidelines for management. Neurosurgery 1979;5:726.
35. Gilbert RW, Kim JH, Posner JB. Epidural spinal cord compression from metastatic tumor: diagnosis and treatment. Ann Neurol 1978;3:40.
36. Rodichok RD, Ruckdeschel JC, Harper GR, et al. Early detection and treatment of spinal epidural metastases: the role of myelography. Ann Neurol 1986;20:696.
37. Portenoy RK, Galer BS, Salamon O, et al. Identification of epidural neoplasm: radiography and bones cintigraphy in the symptomatic and asymptomatic spine. Cancer 1989;64:2207.
38. Carmody RF, Yang PJ, Seely GW, et al. Spinal cord

compression due to metastatic disease: diagnosis with MR imaging versus myelography. Radiology 1989;173:225.

39. Sze G, Krol G, Zimmerman RD. Malignant extradural spinal tumors: MR imaging with Gd-DTPA. Radiology 1988;167:217.

40. Li KC, Poon PY. Sensitivity and specificity of MRI in detecting malignant spinal cord compression and in distinguishing malignant from benign compression fractures of vertebrae. Magn Reson Imaging 1988;6:547.

41. Gilbert RW, Kim JH, Posner JB. Epidural spinal cord compression from metastatic tumor: diagnosis and treatment. Ann Neurol 1978;3:40.

42. Friedman M, Kim TM, Panahon AM. Spinal cord compression in malignant lymphoma. Cancer 1976;37:1485.

43. Pickern J, Lopez G, Tsuhiaki Y, et al. Brain metastases: an autopsy study. Cancer Treat Symp 1983;2:295.

44. Posner JB, Chernik NL. Intracranial metastases from systemic cancer. Adv Neurol 1978;19:579.

45. Zimm S, Wampler GL, Stablein D, et al. Intracerebral metastases in solid tumors patients: natural history and results of treatment. Cancer 1981;48:384.

46. Sze G, Shin J, Krol G, et al. Intraparenchymal brain metastases: MR imaging versus contrast-enhanced CT. Radiology 1988;168:187.

47. Posner JB. Management of central nervous system metastasis. Semin Oncol 1977;4:81.

48. Renaudin J, Fewla D, Wilson CB. Dose dependency of decadron in patients harboring brain tumors. J Neurosurg 1973;39:302.

49. Borgelt B, Gelber RD, Kramer S, et al. The palliation of brain metastases: final results of the first studies by the Radiation Therapy Oncology Group. Int J Radiat Oncol Biol Phys 1980;6:1.

50. Borgelt B, et al. Ultra-rapid high dose irradiation schedule for the palliation of brain metastases: final results of the first two studies by the Radiation Therapy Oncology Group. Int J Radiat Oncol Biol Phys 1981;7:1633.

51. Coia LR. The role of radiation therapy in the treatment of brain metastases. Int J Radiat Oncol Biol Phys 1992;23:229.

52. Diener-West M, Dobbins T, Phillips T, et al. Identification of an optimal subgroup for treatment evaluations of patients with brain metastases using the Radiation Therapy Oncology Group Study 7916. Int J Radiat Oncol Biol Phys 1989;16:669.

53. Smalley S, Schray M, Lans E, et al. Adjuvant radiation therapy after surgical resection of solitary brain metastases: association with pattern of failure and survival. Int J Radiat Oncol Biol Phys 1987;13:1611.

54. Patchell R, Tibbs P, Walsh P, et al. A randomized trial of surgery in the treatment of single metastases to the brain. N Engl J Med 1990;322:494.

55. Sause WT, Crowley JJ, Townsend JJ, et al. Solitary brain metastases: results on an RTOG/SWOG protocol evaluation of surgery and radiation therapy versus radiation alone. Am J Clin Oncol 1990;13:427.

56. Hoskin P, Crow J, Ford H. The influence of extent and local management on the outcome of radiation therapy for brain metastases. Int J Radiat Oncol Biol Phys 1990;19:111.

57. Sheline G, Wara W, Smith V. Therapeutic irradiation and brain injury. Int J Radiat Oncol Biol Phys 1980;6:1215.

58. Spanos WJ, Wasserman T, Meoz R, et al. Palliation of advanced pelvic malignant disease with large fraction pelvic radiation and misonidazole: final report of RTOG Phase I/II study. Int J Radiat Oncol Biol Phys 1987;13:1479.

59. Spanos WJ, Clery M, Perez C, et al. Late effect of multiple daily fraction palliation schedule for advanced pelvic malignancies (RTOG 8502). Int J Radiat Oncol Biol Phys 1994;29:961.

60. Richter MP, Cox LR. Palliative radiation therapy. Semin Oncol 1985;12:375.

61. Larsson LG, Sendbom CM. Roentgen irradiation of the male breast. Acta Radiol 1962;58:253.

62. Dessauer F. Eine neue Anordung mur Roentgen bestrahlung. Archiven fur Physiche Medezin und Technologie (Leipzig) 1905;2:218-223.

63. Fitzpatrick PJ, Rider WD. Halfbody radiotherapy. Int J Radiat Oncol Biol Phys 1976;1:197.

64. Salazar OM, Rubin P, Keller B, et al. Systemic (half-body) radiation therapy: response and toxicity. Int J Radiat Oncol Biol Phys 1978;4:937.

65. Epstein LM, Stewart BH, Antung AR, et al. Half and total body irradiation for carcinoma of the prostate. J Urol 1979;12:330.

66. Salazar OM, Rubin P, Hendrickson FR, et al. Single-dose half-body irradiation for palliation of multiple bone metastases from solid tumors: final Radiation Therapy Oncology Group report. Cancer 1986;58:29.

67. Jacobsson H, Naslund I. Reduced incidence of bone metastases in irradiated areas after external beam radiation therapy of prostate cancer. Int J Radiat Oncol Biol Phys 1991;20:1297.

68. Kaplan ID, Valdagni R, Cox RS. Reduction of spinal metastases after preemptive irradiation in prostate cancer. Int J Radiat Oncol Biol Phys 1990;18:1019.

69. Poulter CA, Cosmatos D, Rubin P, et al. A report of RTOG 82-06: a phase III study of whether the addition of single dose hemi-body irradiation to standard fractionated local field irradiation alone in the treatment of symptomatic osseous metastases. Int J Radiat Oncol Biol Phys 1992;23:207.

70. Rubin P, Scarantino CW. Hemibody irradiation. In: Mouch PM, Loeffler JS, eds. Radiation oncology: technology and biology. Philadelphia: WB Saunders, 1994.

71. Scarantino CW, Ornitz RD, Hoffman LG, et al. On the mechanism of radiation-induced emesis (RIE): the role of serotonin. Int J Radiat Oncol Biol Phys 1994;30:825.

72. Pecher C. Biological investigations with radioactive calcium and strontium: preliminary report on the use of radioactive strontium in treatment of metastatic bone cancer. University of California Publications Pharmacology 1942;11:117.

73. Silberstein EN, Williams C. Strontium-89 therapy for the pain of osseous metastases. J Nucl Med 1985;26:345.

74. Tenvall J, Darte L, Lundgren R, et al. Palliation of multiple bone metastases from prostate carcinoma with strontium-89. Acta Oncol 1988;27:365.

75. Laing AH, Ackery DM, Bayly RJ, et al. Strontium-89 chloride for pain palliation in prostate skeletal malignancy. Br J Radiol 1991;64:816.

76. Porter AT, McEwan AJB, Powe JE, et al. Results of a randomized phase III trial to evaluate the efficacy of strontium-89 adjuvant to local field external beam irradiation in management of endocrine resistant metastatic prostate cancer. Int J Radiat Oncol Biol Phys 1993;25:805.

77. Quilty PM, Kirk D, Bolger JJ, et al. A comparison of the palliative effects of strontium-89 and external beam radiotherapy in metastatic prostate cancer. Radiother Oncol 1994;31:33.

78. Porter AT, Davis LP. Systemic radionuclide therapy of bone metastases with strontium-89. Oncology 1994;8:93.

79. Sause WT, Scott C, Krisch B, et al. RTOG 8528: accelerated fractionation in the treatment of patients with supratentorial brain metastases. Am Radium Soc 1991. Abstract.

80. Phillips T, Diegner M, Wasserman T, et al. Hypofractionated radiation therapy with or without misonidazole for the treatment of brain metastases. Int J Radiat Oncol Biol Phys 1984;10:145.

81. Loeffler J, Kooy H, Wen P, et al. The treatment of recurrent brain metastases with stereotactic radiosurgery. J Clin Oncol 1990;8:576.

82. Coffey R, Flickinger JL, Lunsford LD. Boost radiosurgery for solitary brain metastases: results in 23 consecutive patients. Int J Radiat Oncol Biol Phys 1990;19:148. Abstract.

Imaging Evaluations

Imaging of Urologic Neoplasms

Zoran L. Barbaric

PARENCHYMAL RENAL MASS

Detection

Most renal masses are serendipitous discoveries on computed tomography (CT) or sonography. Detection rates for sonography and for the old standby, intravenous urography, are not very good for renal masses less than 3 cm in diameter. Detection rates are 79% for ultrasound and 67% for urography. These numbers are relatively low because sonography is operator dependent, parts of the kidney may be obscured by overlying structures, or a solid tumor may be isoechoic to the renal parenchyma and thus invisible. Detection of small renal masses on urography depends on subtle changes in renal contour, enhancement, or barely noticeable pelvocalyceal system effacement. By contrast, detection rates for such small lesions are well above 90% on a well-executed, contrast-enhanced, thin section, helical (spiral) CT scan (Fig. 61.1) (1).

Classification After Discovery

In the simplest terms and using all imaging criteria available, a parenchymal renal mass is a (1) simple cyst, (2) minimally complex cyst, (3) complex cyst (likely a neoplasm), (4) solid tumor with fatty tissue, (5) solid tumor, (6) pseudotumor, or (7) indeterminate.

Simple Cyst (Bosniak I) (2)

Imaging criteria that define a simple cyst have not changed over the years and are as follows.

A. Pencil thin wall.
B. Smooth base.
C. Lack of enhancement after contrast injection (CT, intravenous pyelography [IVP], magnetic resonance imaging [MRI]).
D. Anechoic (ultrasonography [US]).
E. Through transmission (US).

F. No septations.
G. No calcification (Fig. 61.2).

Minimally Complex Cyst (Bosniak II)

A septum or small amount of wall or septal calcification would make one pause and consider restudying the lesion in 6 months, preferably by CT. This is to make sure things are stable and the lesion is not a cystic carcinoma. Interim changes, such as increased septal thickness, thickening of the cyst wall, or increased nodularity at the base, indicate malignancy.

A benign cyst may also hemorrhage or contain highly proteinaceous material (3). Hemorrhagic cysts are common in polycystic kidney disease but are also frequently seen in the healthy population. They rarely present with acute pain and are almost always asymptomatic. Characteristically, the cysts are either hyperdense or isodense compared with renal parenchyma on precontrast CT scan (Fig. 61.3). Settling cellular debris within the cyst may be detected on real-time sonography after the patient changes position (4). On MRI, the hemorrhagic cyst is commonly of high signal intensity (bright) on T1- and T2-weighted sequences, although there are variations depending on ratio of hemoglobin and deoxyhemoglobin in the cyst content. If all other criteria point toward a simple cyst, the workup is completed.

Percutaneous aspiration of minimally complex renal cyst is not recommended because clear fluid and absence of malignant cells in the aspirate have also been found in cystic renal carcinoma (5). Therefore, the final arbiter as to whether the cyst is malignant or benign is CT, followed closely by renal ultrasound (Fig. 61.4).

Complex Cyst (Bosniak III)

This is just a fancy name for renal cancer. What else would one suspect if the cystic mass has a thick wall, nodule at the base, numerous and focally thick septa, septal enhancement, or heavy calcification (Fig. 61.5)? It is likely that the lesion is a simple cyst with an ingrowing renal cancer, a cystic renal

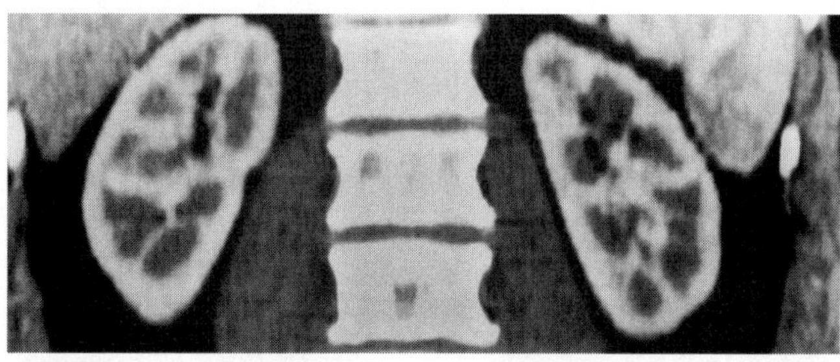

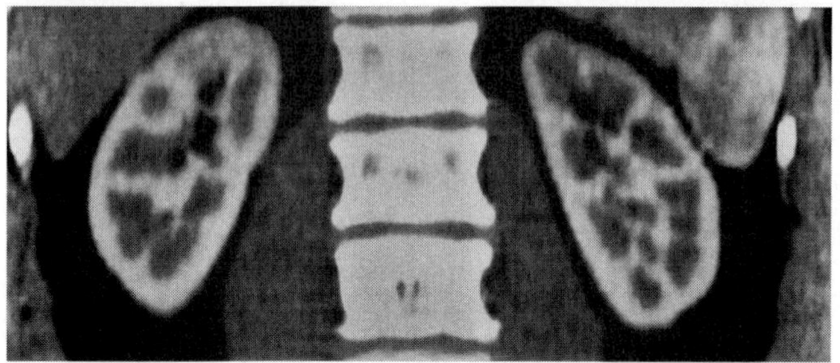

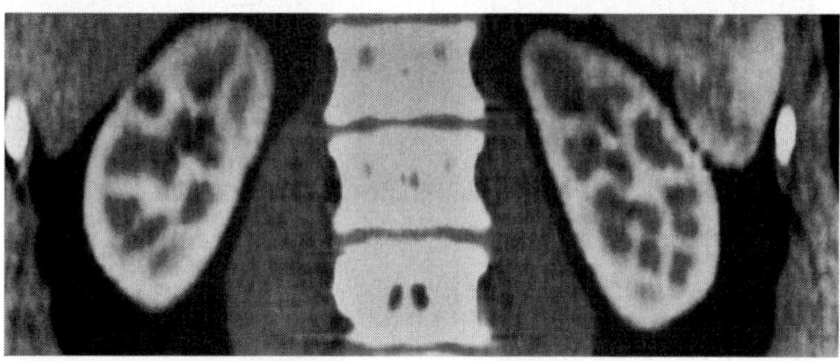

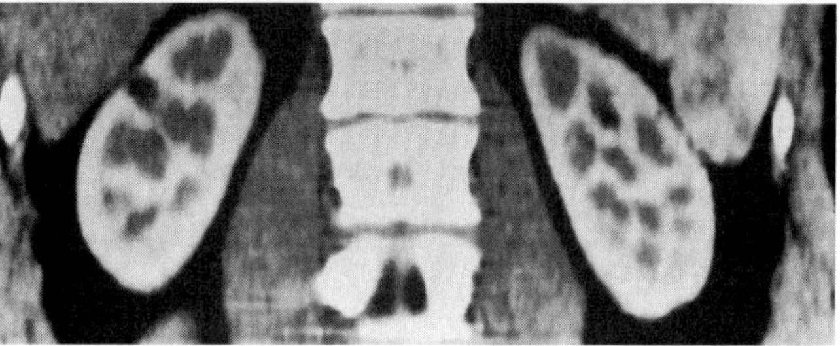

Fig. 61.1. Helical CT scan is a technique where the tabletop and patient are moved inside the CT gantry during continual x-ray tube rotation and exposure. This paints a helical x-ray pathway in the body. If the slices are thin, final images may be reconstructed in any plane, such as in this patient, where on reconstructed coronal images there is a low-attenuation right cortical cyst. On such an early corticomedullary phase of contrast transit, tumors located in unopacified medulla may be missed.

carcinoma, or a necrotic renal carcinoma. Occasionally one will encounter a cystic oncocytoma, an oncocytoma arising from the cyst wall (6), or localized infundibular dysgenesis, but the odds are very high that such a complex cyst is a renal carcinoma.

Solid Renal Tumor With Fatty Tissue

Both MR and CT can detect even small amounts of fatty tissue in a tumor (Fig. 61.6). Presence of fatty tissue in an otherwise solid tumor is a characteristic signature of an angiomyolipoma,

with one notable exception. If any dystrophic calcification is found, the fat tissue containing tumor is most likely a carcinoma and should be treated accordingly (7, 8). Areas of dystrophic calcification are practically impossible to detect on MRI. For this reason, CT remains the gold standard.

Because of fatty tissues, most angiolipomas are hyperechoic on ultrasound. There is a tendency to dismiss a small hyperechoic lesion as a benign angiomyolipoma. This is a mistake because small renal carcinomas can also be hyperechoic (Fig. 61.7).

Angiomyolipomas may be found in the lymph nodes and liver (9, 10), and rarely they can extend into the renal vein and inferior vena cava (11).

Well-circumscribed tumors may be selectively embolized (12). Angiomyolipomas larger than 3.5 cm have a 1 in 3 chance of bleeding (13).

In children, a fat-containing tumor should not be considered benign, particularly in patients without tuberous sclerosis. A fat-containing Wilms' tumor has been described (14).

Solid Renal Tumor

There is little doubt that a mass lesion is solid when it enhances with iodinated contrast (Fig. 61.2), contains dystrophic calcification, has areas of tumor necrosis (Bosniak IV), and shows no through transmission (US). To be sure, a solid mass may also represent any 1 of more than 50 rare solid renal lesions, ranging from obscure rheumatoid granuloma to more common oncocytoma. However, the probability that the solid mass is malignant, and most likely a renal carcinoma, is greater than 85%. Diagnostic effort is appropriately concentrated on the staging process.

Efforts to differentiate a multitude of rare benign renal masses from renal carcinoma have not met with universal success. Renal oncocytoma is one of the most common benign renal tumors, and quite an effort has been made to try to increase specificity of current imaging technology in diagnosis of this tumor (15–18).

There are several radiologic findings suggestive, but not diagnostic, of oncocytoma. These are homogeneous enhancement and central scar (CT), homogeneous pattern (US), spoke wheel sign (angiography), and, possibly, a pseudocapsule (MRI) (19–21). Although not diagnostic, such signs may prompt a urologist to consider an alternate operation instead of radical nephrectomy.

Thin-needle aspiration biopsy did not gain wide support because finding benign cells in the aspirate does not exclude malignancy. Pathologic criteria for diagnosing this tumor are not only the presence of oncocytes in the aspirate, but also the absence of malignant cells on multiple sections. At times, thin-needle aspiration may influence further management, as in a case of bilateral tumors, some of which exhibit imaging criteria suggestive of oncocytoma (22).

Because more than 85% of solid renal masses are malignant, attention is appropriately directed toward staging. This includes lesion size, bilaterality (5 to 10%), multicentricity (up

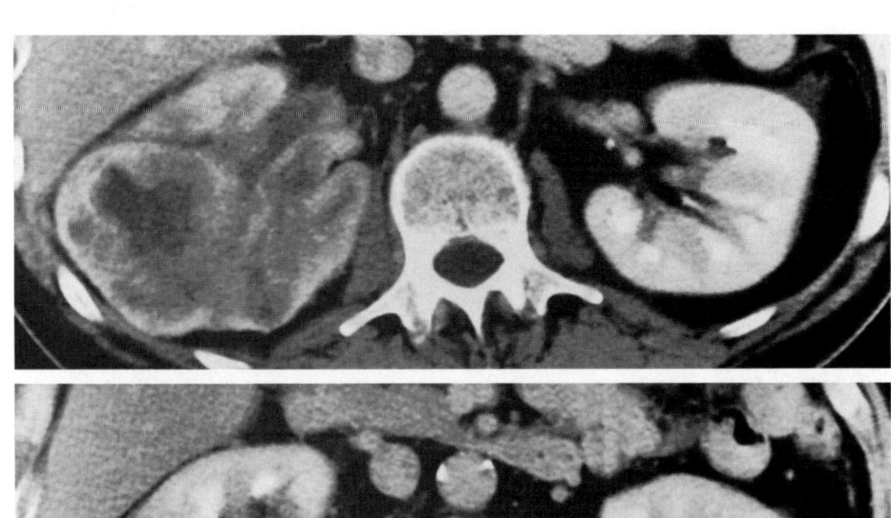

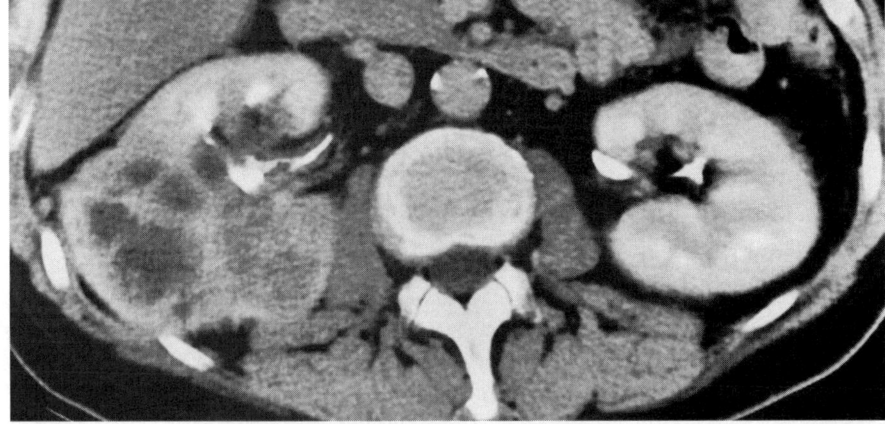

Fig. 61.2. The left cyst has all the characteristics of a benign cyst except for a pencil-thin wall. This is because a deep-seated cyst needs to be much larger to expand and thin out overlying cortex. In contrast to the simple cyst, there is a large, enhancing, heterogeneous tumor in the opposite kidney. Enhancement denotes vascularity. Statistically, the most likely diagnosis is renal carcinoma.

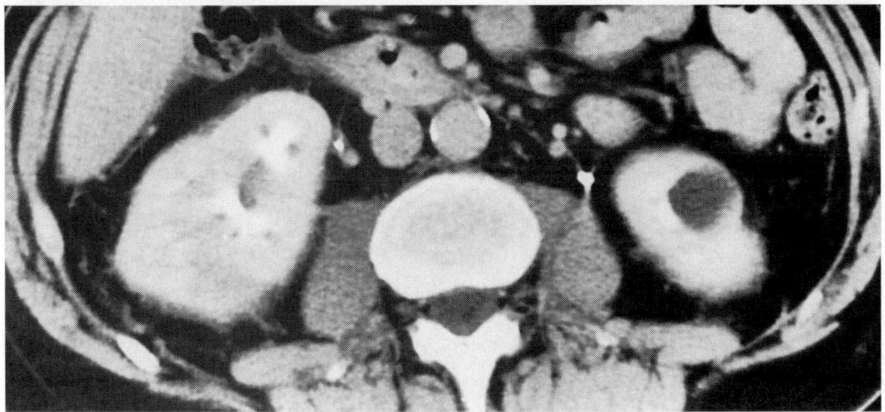

to 13%) (23), renal vein and caval extension, regional lymph node metastases, adrenal metastases, psoas and liver invasion, and distant metastases.

Caval Tumor Thrombus

In most instances, a caval tumor thrombus is seen on initial contrast-enhanced CT study (Fig. 61.8). Cephalad extension can also be determined in most instances. MRI does have some advantages over CT regarding detection, cephalad extension, and size (24). Using special MR sequencing techniques, it is possible to image major vessels in different orthogonal planes. This technique is now widely available and is referred to as MR angiography (MRA). In general, MRA is used in those instances in which CT did not provide convincing information regarding tumor thrombus presence or its cephalad extension. MRA does have some drawbacks. It requires patient cooperation and may require respiratory and cardiac gating to reduce degrading motion artifacts during imaging time, which is measured in minutes.

Intraoperative (25) and transesophageal (26) sonography have also been recommended.

Adrenal Glands and Regional Lymph Node Metastases

Both CT and MR are well suited for estimating local extension. Currently, CT has the advantage of detecting smaller tumors (e.g., contralateral lesion), lymph node involvement, and extension through renal fascia. MR has a slight edge in detection of muscle invasion and differentiating nodes from vessels in those

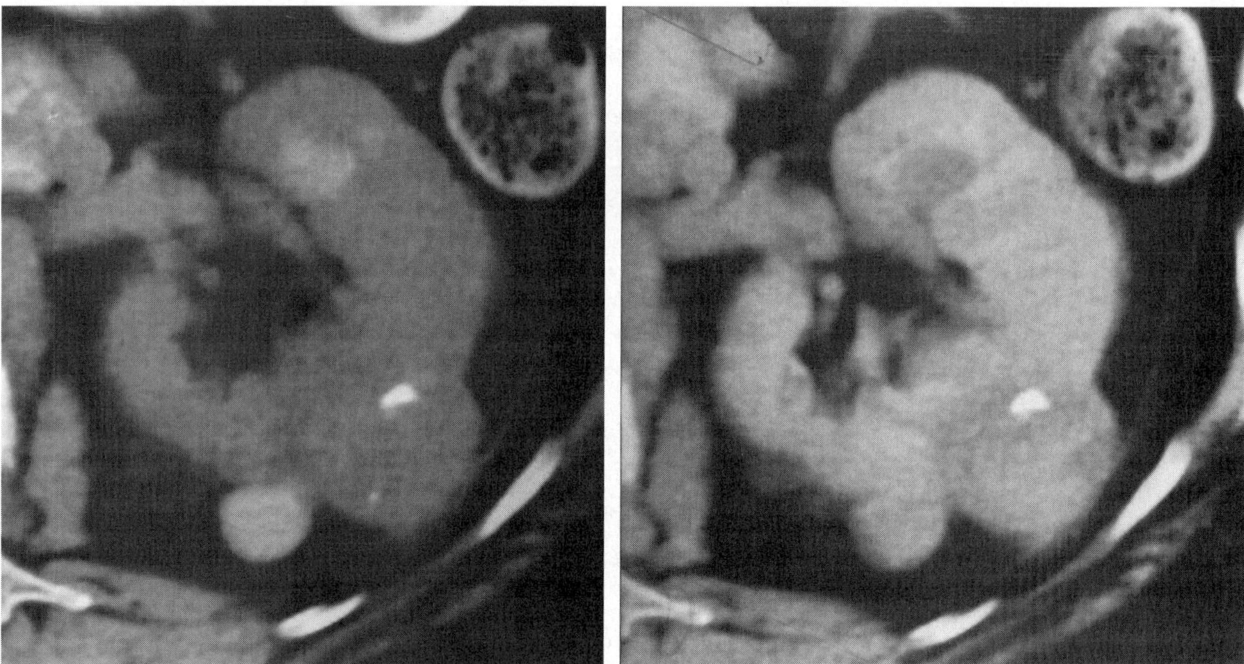

Fig. 61.3.   There are two small hyperdense benign hemorrhagic renal cysts in the left kidney that are clearly seen on precontrast scan (left). These two cysts are not enhanced on the postcontrast scan (right) but become isodense or somewhat hypodense compared with renal parenchyma. In contrast, a solid renal mass with calcification in it was enhanced 30 Hounsfield units (HU) after contrast injection and proved to be a renal carcinoma.

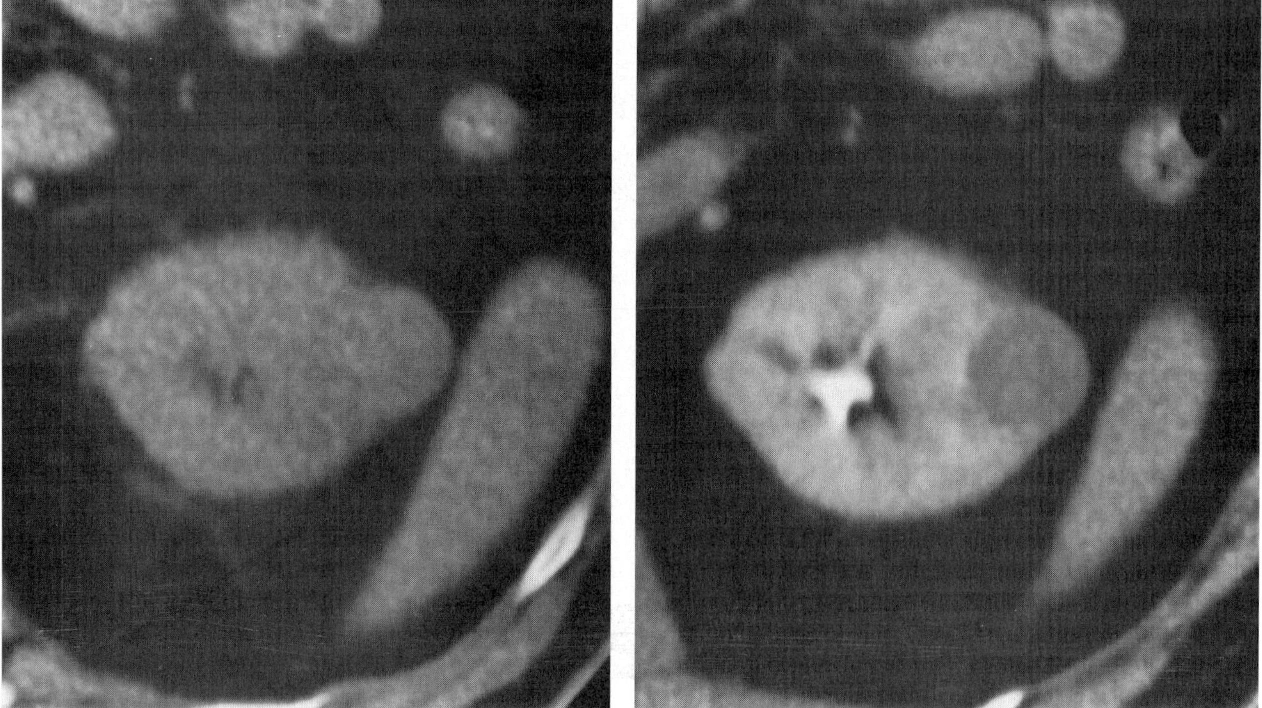

Fig. 61.4.   This is a good example of how a noncontrast CT scan can miss a lesion and cannot differentiate hemorrhagic cyst from tumor. Hemorrhagic cysts can be isodense to renal parenchyma on precontrast scan (left); thus, they become visible only after intravenous injection of contrast. The human eye, however, cannot perceive 15 to 20 HU enhancement in this lesion (right), which proved to be a renal carcinoma. This is why such measurements must be done using electronic means.

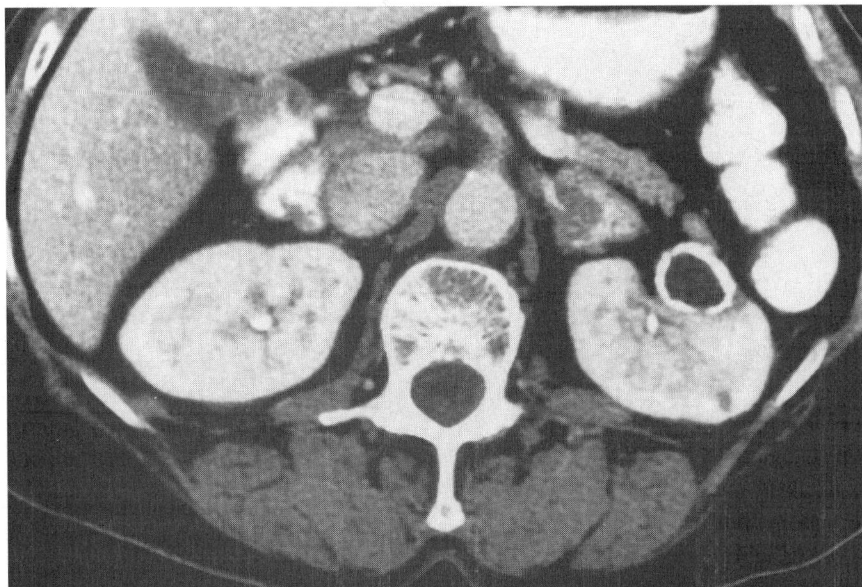

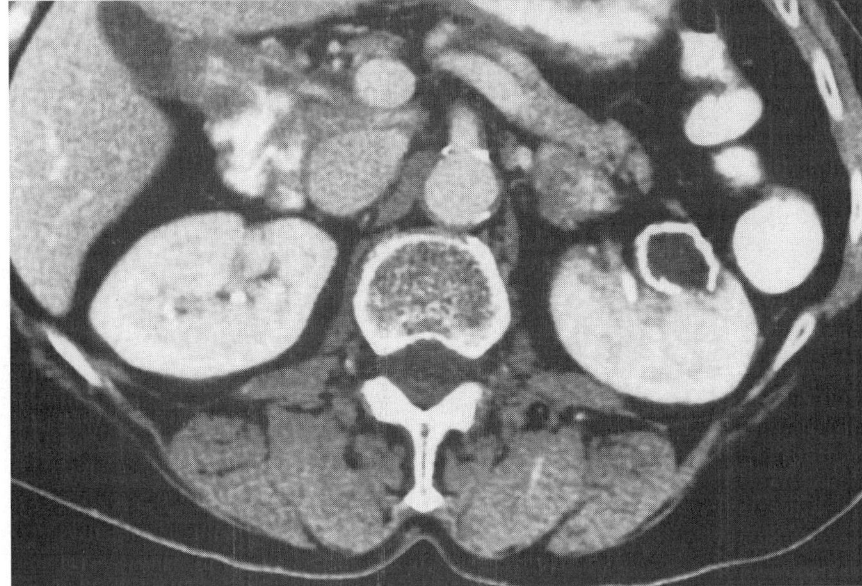

Fig. 61.5. Heavy calcification in the cyst wall raises the odds that this is a renal mass with malignant potential. Just superior to the left kidney and lateral to the aorta is an adrenal mass, which shows heterogeneous enhancement and also must be considered malignant.

patients who are allergic to iodinated contrast. Also, CT is excellent for predicting ipsilateral adrenal gland involvement, either by direct extension or as distant metastases. If the ipsilateral adrenal gland appears normal on preoperative CT, it is likely tumor free (27).

Distant Metastases and Follow-up

CT is the imaging method of choice for detecting pulmonary metastases. The study should be reviewed as it is done, and any suspicious area should be immediately restudied with high-resolution CT. High-resolution CT refers to thin cuts, usually 2 to 3 mm, compared to standard 10-mm slice thickness.

As chemotherapy and immunotherapy are increasingly used, there is a need to gauge tumor response accurately. This usually involves follow-up of pulmonary and osseous metastases, contralateral renal lesion, and retroperitoneal lymphadenopathy. Again, CT is an obvious choice.

Cavernous hemangioma in the liver is a frequent finding and needs to be differentiated from liver metastasis. Tc 99m red blood cell scan or MRI of the liver may help establish the diagnosis (28). Biopsy is also a reasonable alternative.

Other Solid Renal Malignant Parenchymal Tumors

This diverse group includes neoplasms such as sarcomas (29), leukemia, lymphoma, and metastases (30, 31). Secondary lymphoma is suspected if a retroperitoneal tumor extends into the renal sinus and into the perinephric space. Venous propagation with lymphoma and other tumors has been described (32).

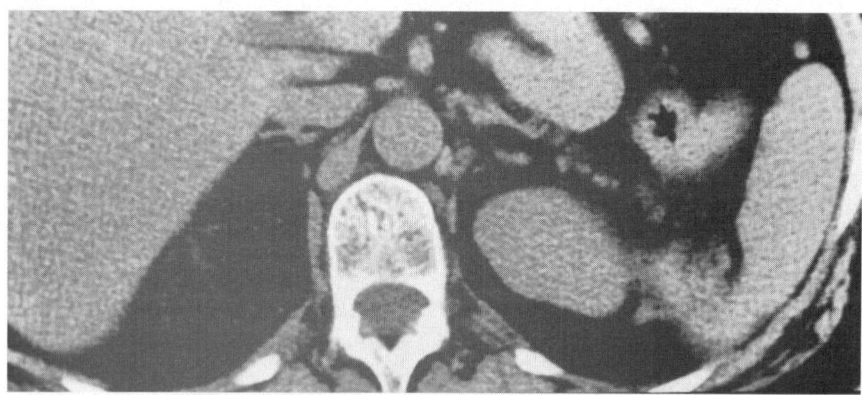

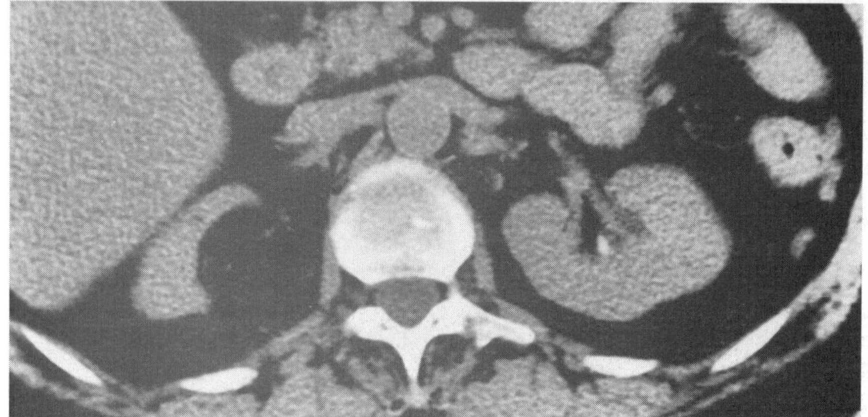

Fig. 61.6. There are two fatty tumors in the right kidney. That they contain fat is obvious just by comparing their density to that of retroperitoneal fat. Both are benign angiomyolipomas.

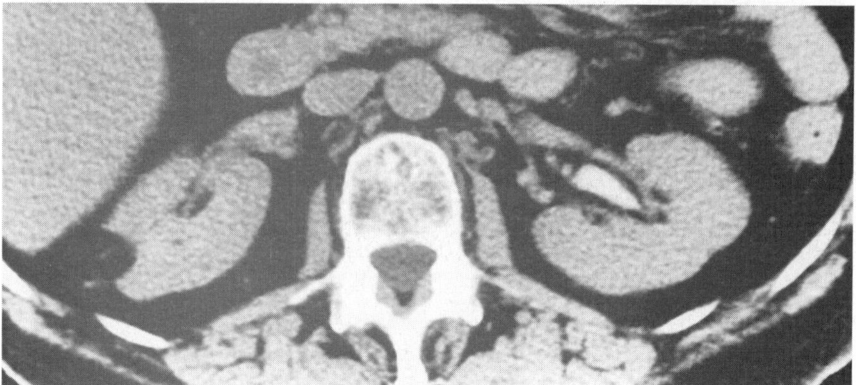

Other renal neoplasms have no distinguishing features to differentiate them from renal carcinoma, except for renal melanoma, which may be moderately hyperdense and mimic a hemorrhagic renal cyst (33).

When metastases to the kidney are suspected, fine-needle aspiration biopsy is indicated if the results will alter the course of therapy (34). Seeding of renal cell carcinoma along the needle tract is very rare (35).

Pseudotumors

The old hypertrophied septum (column) of Bertin comes to mind. New terminology refers to it as junctional parenchyma, which is cortical septum between fused embryonic upper and lower kidney (36). Other pseudotumors should not be confused with renal carcinoma. They are renal abscess, acute focal pyelonephritis, acute renal infarct, arteriovenous malformation, and renal artery aneurysm. CT is the method of choice for sorting out these diagnostic possibilities. Ultrasound runs second best.

Indeterminate Renal Masses

With the advent of CT, MRI, and ultrasound, a fair number of small, less than 1.5 cm, renal lesions are being discovered that are difficult to characterize and classify into any of the above groups. As expected, most are simple renal cysts; however, because differentiation from small renal carcinoma is im-

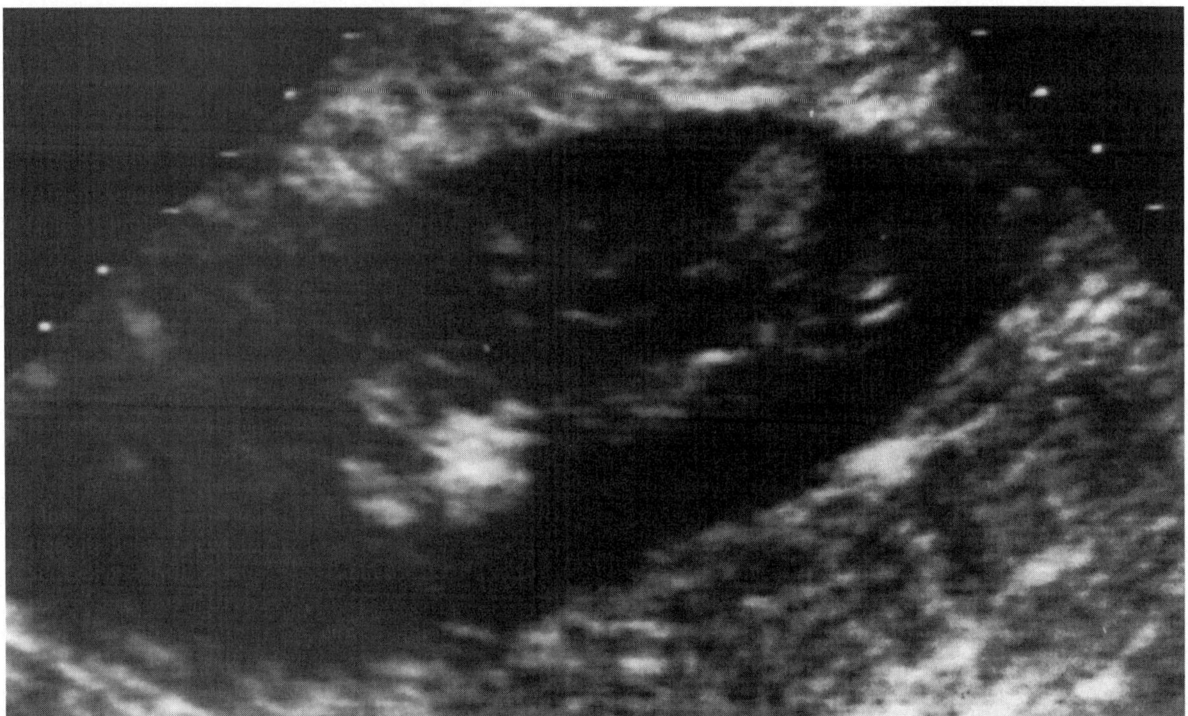

Fig. 61.7. A small hyperechoic tumor in the lower pole is a renal carcinoma, rather than angiomyolipoma. In a situation like this, it is better to obtain several nonenhanced thin cuts through the lesion to confirm or exclude the presence of fatty tissue. If no fat is found and the lesion is another type of solid tumor, it is probably a renal carcinoma.

possible, they present a significant management problem. Currently, it is recommended to obtain a follow-up limited CT scan of the kidneys within 6 months, using thin cuts (3 mm) and precontrast and postcontrast technique. On high-resolution cuts, it is possible to measure Hounsfield unit (HU) values before and after contrast and thus determine if the lesion enhances. An enhancement of 10 to 20 HU units is indicative of a solid tumor. If the enhancing lesion grows to 2 cm, partial nephrectomy should be considered (37).

Many small renal masses are discovered by serendipity on cross-sectional studies done for unrelated diseases (38).

Enhancement can be determined even in patients who are in renal failure, in those for whom the use of iodinated contrast is contraindicated, and in those patients allergic to contrast. In such patients, MRI with intravenous injection of paramagnetic contrasts, such as gadolinium DTPA, can display tumor enhancement (Fig. 61.9) (39–41).

IMAGING IN SPECIFIC SITUATIONS

Von Hippel-Lindau Disease

This rare familial disease presents with a spectrum of findings. Most prominent among these are cerebellar hemangioblastoma, retinal angiomas, multicentric renal carcinomas and cysts, and pancreatic cysts. There is also a high incidence of pheochromocytoma (42). Death is usually caused by intracranial hemor-

rhage, but death due to metastatic renal carcinoma is also frequent. Small renal carcinomas may be excised in an attempt to preserve renal function (43).

Because of such high frequencies of both renal carcinoma and renal cysts, detection of small solid tumor in this patient population requires the best possible imaging technique. Currently, it is suggested that patients with von Hippel-Lindau disease undergo yearly CT of the kidneys, preferably using helical (spiral) CT, thin sections, and precontrast and postcontrast technique. The kidney may appear bizarre on cross-sectional imaging after excision of a renal carcinoma or after partial nephrectomy, so that it is more difficult to appreciate a new solid tumor. Renal angiography has no advantage over properly executed CT (44).

Acquired Cystic Disease of the Kidneys

After 5 years, cysts and neoplasms will have developed in native, end-stage kidneys in 80 to 90% of dialysis patients. The prevalence for renal carcinoma is 1 to 2.6% (45); it is 0.5% for distant metastases (46, 47). In the past, routine yearly CT or sonography was commonly performed to detect an early neoplasm. This is no longer deemed necessary (48). Symptomatic patients are best examined by CT.

Renal Transplants

Malignancy in transplant patients is twice as common as in the general population (49, 50). There is also increased incidence of some cancers, such as Kaposi's sarcoma and lymphoma-like lesions (51).

RENAL NEOPLASMS IN CHILDREN

Parenchymal renal neoplasms in children are mesoblastic nephroma, nephroblastomatosis, and Wilms' tumor. Also, Burkitt's lymphoma commonly involves the kidneys in children.

Mesoblastic Nephroma

Mesoblastic nephroma is usually large (52), and the diagnosis may be suggested if functioning renal parenchyma is seen within the tumor (53, 54).

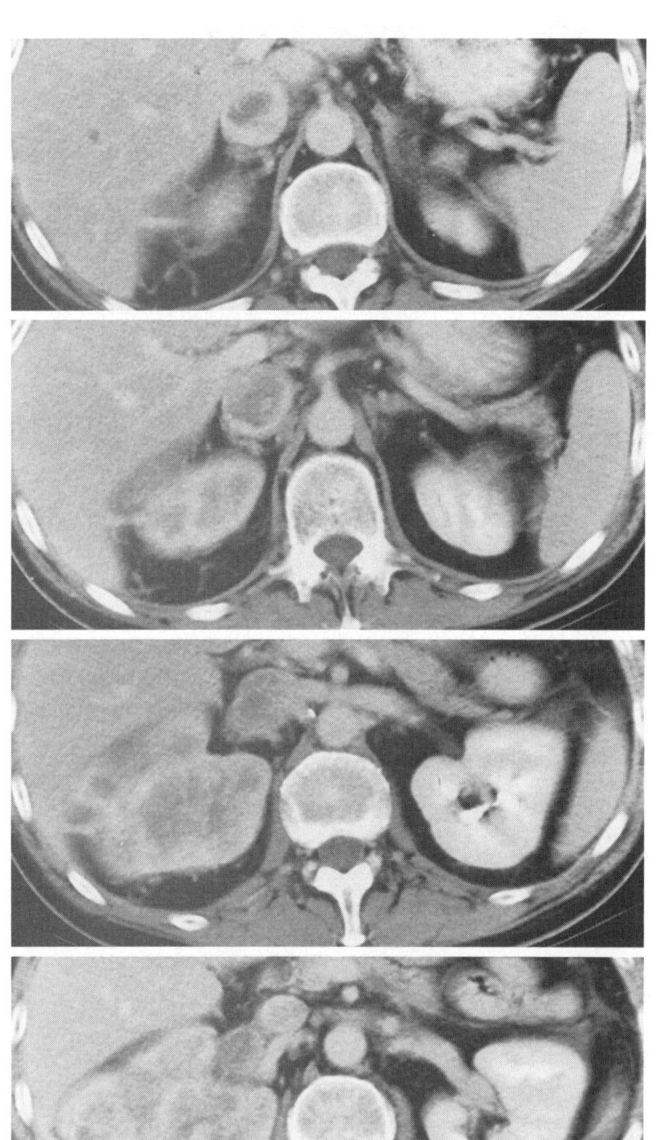

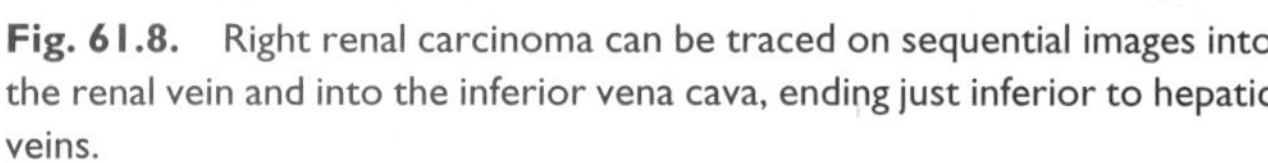

Fig. 61.8.   Right renal carcinoma can be traced on sequential images into the renal vein and into the inferior vena cava, ending just inferior to hepatic veins.

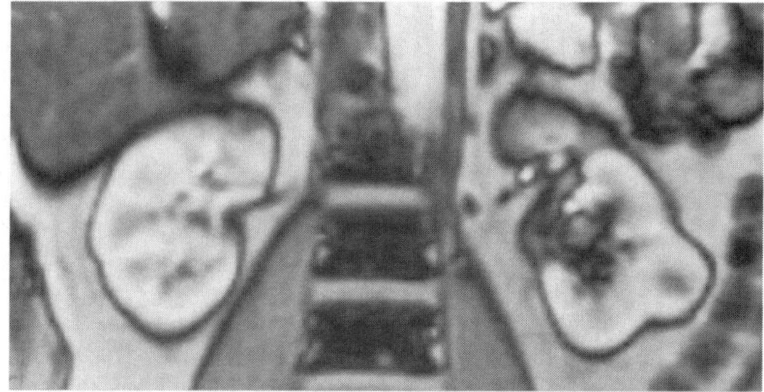

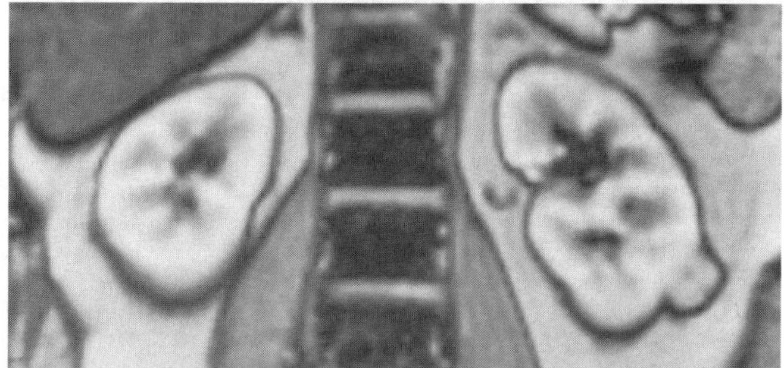

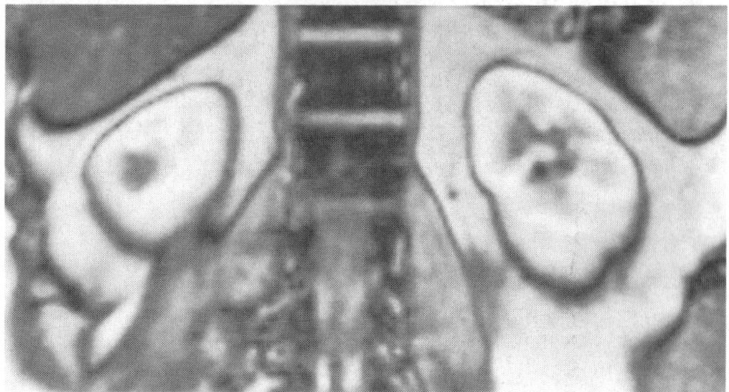

Fig. 61.9.   Enhancement of left lower pole indeterminate renal mass on MRI after intravenous administration of gadolinium DTPA, a paramagnetic contrast material. (Courtesy Dr. Alim Awoni).

Nephroblastomatosis

Nephroblastomatosis, particularly deeply seated cortical and multifocal, is a precursor of Wilms' tumor. Usually, subcapsular hypoechoic tumor nodules are seen on ultrasound, which is the examination of choice for follow-up. The mass lesions are better seen on contrast-enhanced CT, which is the examination of choice (55). Low-attenuating, nonenhancing masses are found (56). Imaging is done to (1) exclude preoperatively contralateral disease in patients with Wilms' tumor, (2) follow up known microscopic or macroscopic disease, and (3) screen patients with syndromes associated with nephroblastomatosis and Wilms' tumor (57).

Wilms' Tumor (Nephroblastoma)

Wilms' tumor is the most common abdominal malignancy in children. Congenital anomalies, such as genitourinary, hemihypertrophy, aniridia, neurofibromatosis, Drash, and Beckwith-Wiedemann syndrome, are present in 15% of patients (58). Also, Wilms' tumor is more common in horseshoe kidney (59, 60). Patients usually present with a symptomatic abdominal mass (61). US is the screening examination of choice. MRI (62) or CT are the preferred imaging modalities. Both can demonstrate tumor size, regional lymph node involvement, and caval tumor thrombus (Fig. 61.10).

Five percent of patients with Wilms' tumor have bilateral

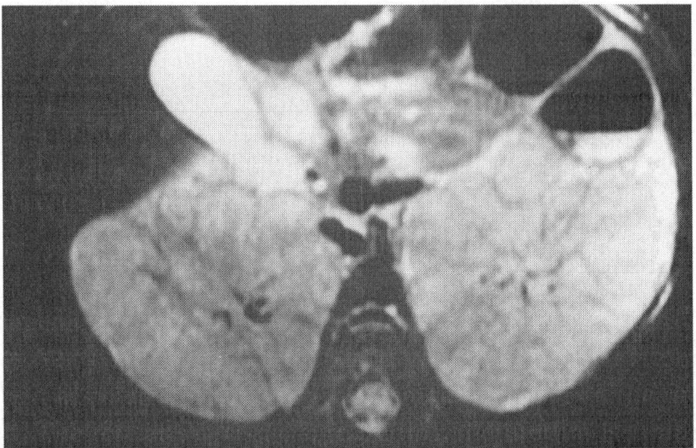
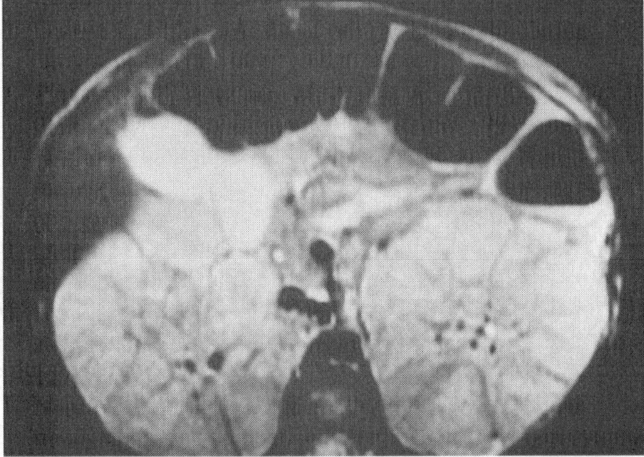
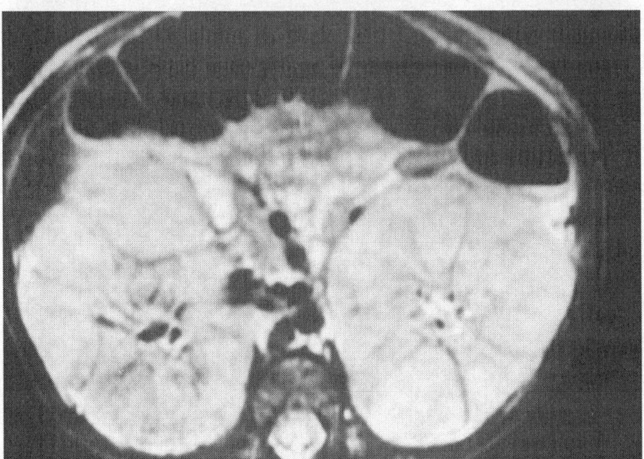

Fig. 61.10. Bilateral Wilms' tumors evaluated by MRI. One can easily recognize this as a T2-weighted sequence because of high-signal (bright) spinal fluid and low-signal (dark) liver. The kidneys are significantly enlarged and replaced by high-signal septated tumor. Great vessels appear dark on this sequence, and one can be assured there is no venous tumor thrombus.

disease. Even with the best imaging with CT, sonography, and MRI, synchronous bilateral Wilms' tumor is unrecognized in 7% of patients if formal exploration of the contralateral kidney is omitted (63).

Renal Cell Carcinoma in Children

Half of all malignant renal tumors in children between 10 and 19 years of age are renal cell carcinoma. Prognosis is worse than for Wilms' tumor but more favorable compared with adult renal cell carcinoma (64).

TRANSITIONAL CELL CARCINOMA OF THE RENAL PELVIS, URETER, AND BLADDER

Transitional cell carcinoma (TCC) is a multicentric, polychronotopic (multiple recurrences in different areas and at different times), and hypovascular neoplasm. Distant metastases are to bone (lytic and mixed), lung, and lymph nodes. TCC develops elsewhere in the urinary tract in 40 to 80% of patients with upper tract tumor, whereas upper tract tumors develop in 3% of patients with bladder TCC.

A classic finding on any imaging study is a filling defect in the collecting system, ureter, or bladder. Differential diagnosis includes a blood clot, radiolucent calculus, fungus ball, sloughed papilla, fibroepithelial polyp, vessel impression, metastases, invasion by renal cell carcinoma, arteriovenous malformation, and cavernous hemangioma (65). The filling defect is usually first detected on an excretory urogram, retrograde pyelogram, or CT. More specific radiographic findings differ in upper and lower tract TCC.

Imaging of Upper Tract TCC

Kidney

In addition to the filling defect, radiographic findings depend on tumor size and stage. When the tumor invades an infundibulum, it may produce infundibular obstruction and hydrocalyx. A nonfunctioning hydrocalyx is called an amputated calyx. In addition to TCC, hydrocalyx can be caused by calculus and stricture. Renal tuberculosis is the prime example.

As renal sinus fat and renal parenchyma become involved, CT will show a soft tissue mass that obliterates renal sinus fat. Staging is best done with CT (Fig. 61.11), which will identify invasion of periureteral, peripelvic or renal sinus fat or renal parenchyma (stage T3), or invasion of adjacent organs, lymph nodes, or transcapsular invasion of perirenal fat (stage T4) (66).

Extension of TCC tumor thrombus in the vena cava is less frequent than renal cell carcinoma, but it does occur (67, 68).

The most frustrating part of imaging is, when in the setting of hematuria and positive urine cytology, no tumor is discovered on repeated radiologic studies. Retrograde pyeloscopy is becoming increasingly popular.

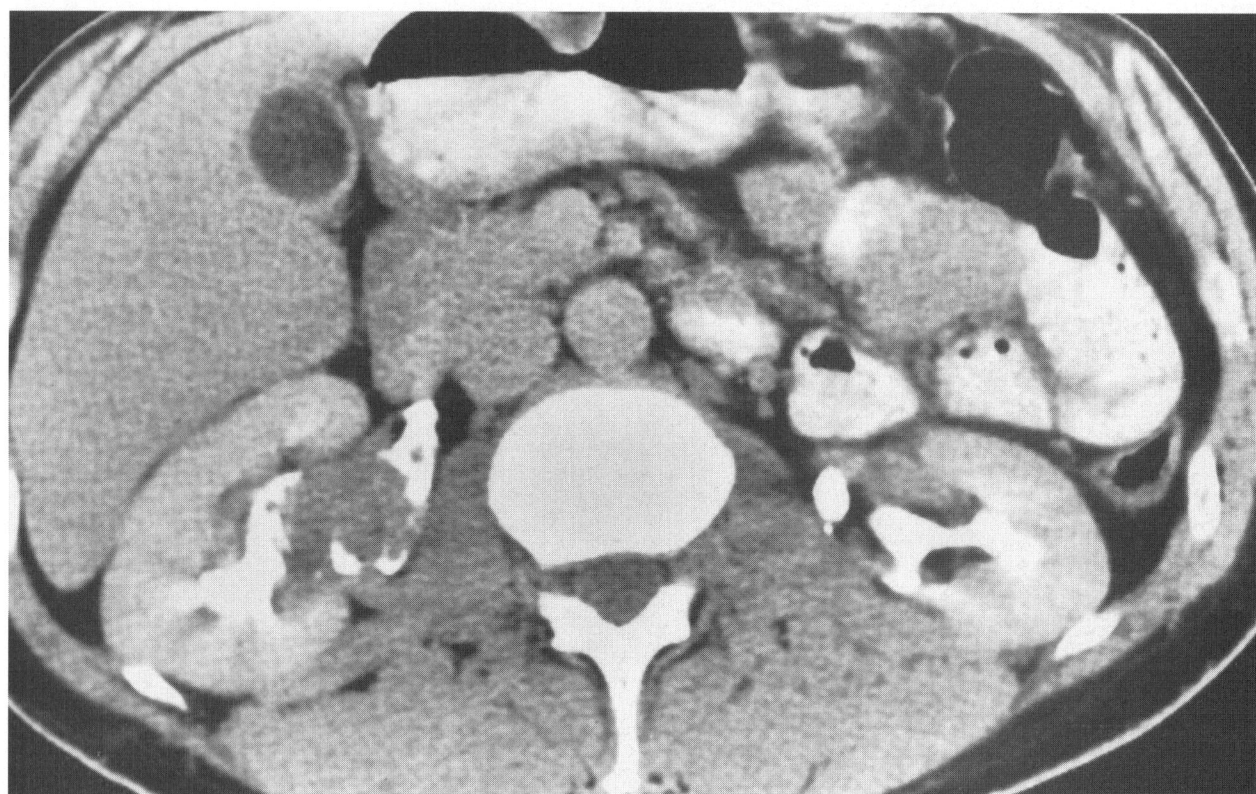

Fig. 61.11. CT scan of renal transitional cell carcinoma. There is an irregular filling defect in the right renal pelvis, seemingly affixed to the pelvis. The left kidney is scarred along its posterior surface. There is no evidence of lymph node enlargement.

Differential diagnosis in invasive TCC includes squamous cell carcinoma and adenocarcinoma of the renal pelvis (69).

Ureter

A filling defect in the ureter is the principal finding. The slowly expanding tumor affects the ureter in a very characteristic way. Marginal cupping develops immediately above and below the lesion (chalice sign). The proximal ureter need not be dilated and is frequently normal in appearance. Often, the retrograde catheter may coil within a somewhat expanded ureter just distal to the tumor (Bergman sign) (70). TCC is more common in the distal ureter.

CT shows nonspecific ureteral wall thickening. CT is very useful to differentiate radiolucent stones from soft tissue intraluminal filling defect (71, 72).

Pseudodiverticulosis is the result of reactive hyperplasia of transitional epithelium secondary to inflammation and represents downward proliferation of epithelium into the loose connective tissue of the lamina propria, producing outpouchings (Fig. 61.12) (73, 74). There is a strong association between ureteral TCC and ureteral pseudodiverticulosis. Because of that, interval follow-up is suggested (75).

Differential diagnosis of a ureteral filling defect also includes inverted papilloma (76), polyp (77, 78), adenoma, squamous cell carcinoma, adenocarcinoma, fibroma, hemangioma, myoma, lymphangioma, sarcoma, angiosarcoma, and carcinosarcoma (mixed) (79).

The most common metastases to the ureter are from the breast, colon, thyroid, prostate, cervix, rectum, melanomas, and renal cancer (80, 81).

Ureteral Stump

In some instances, after nephrectomy and ureterectomy, the very distal ureter is left behind for technical reasons. Recurrence of TCC within the stump is common, and these patients require periodic cystoureteroscopy for follow-up. Primary TCC may also occur in the ureteral stump (82). Retrograde ureterography is the method of choice for demonstrating the presence of a recurrent tumor (83). If retrograde ureterography proves impossible for technical reasons, CT or MRI is indicated (84).

Imaging of Lower Tract TCC

Bladder TCC

For nonurologists, it is important to remember that the diagnosis of bladder TCC is made by cystoscopy and transurethral resection, which provides diagnosis, cellular type, differentiation, grading, number of lesions, morphologic characteristics, and depth of wall invasion. Imaging, as far as diagnosis is con-

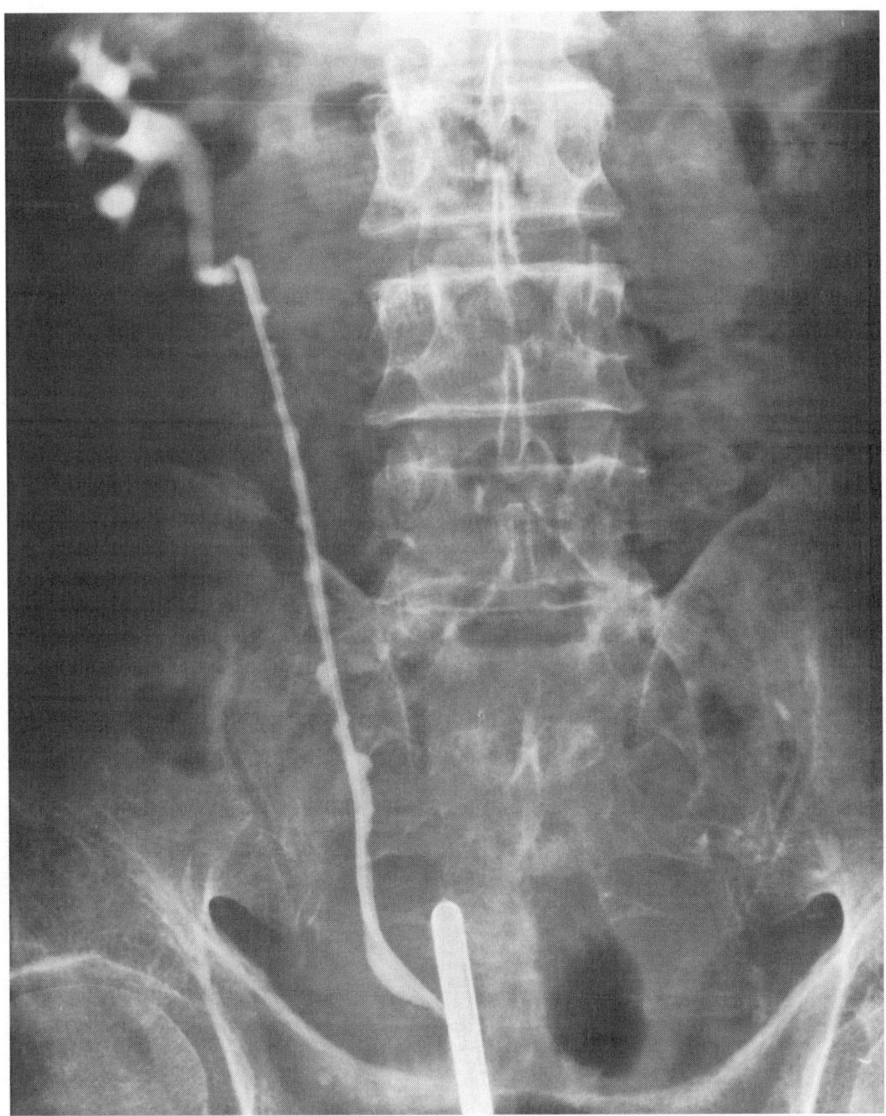

Fig. 61.12. Ureteral pseudodiverticulosis. Retrograde pyelogram demonstrates many small diverticular pouches. Because these do not extend outside the smooth muscle, they are not true diverticula; hence the name pseudodiverticula. Some have found a high association with transitional cell carcinoma and suggest follow-up studies.

cerned, is ancillary and much more important in the staging process. Besides the well-known filling defect, radiographic findings also include bladder asymmetry and pseudoureterocele (85, 86).

In the majority of cases, transurethral resection defines the depth of muscular invasion as superficial (PT2) or deep (PT3a). On CT and MRI, a pedunculated tumor is assumed to be pT1, whereas a sessile tumor is pT2. Thickening of the bladder wall assumes pT3a lesion. Perivesical density implies extension outside the bladder wall or pT3b lesion. Both CT and MRI are fairly accurate in distinguishing pT3a from pT3b lesions, particularly on thin sections with contrast (Fig. 61.13) (87).

MRI has a slight advantage because on T2-weighted sequence, the tumor appears relatively bright (hyperintense) compared with dark (hypointense) detrusor muscle (88, 89). MRI using T1-weighted sequence with Gd-DTPA enhancement demonstrates the tumor even better (90). The most recent MRI technique is dynamic (imaging an area repeatedly at 20-sec

intervals), using T1-weighted sequence and intravenous bolus Gd-DTPA. The tumor, mucosa, and submucosa enhance and become bright before the muscle, which remains dark. For the first time it is possible to differentiate between superficial (PT2) and deep (PT3a) muscle invasion with greater accuracy (91). Local invasion into prostate, seminal vesicles, rectum (T4a), or pelvic wall (T4b) is again best seen on MRI. Staging accuracy using MRI and CT hover around 80 to 85%. The difficulty seems to stem from associated inflammatory component, which tends to overstage some tumors. It is expected that the use of newer sequences, surface coils, and appropriate imaging planes will push MRI staging accuracy above 90% in the near future. MRI is becoming cheaper and will probably become the imaging modality of choice.

It is important to remember that TCC is multicentric and that an intravenous urogram is very useful in evaluating the upper urinary tract for presence of synchronous lesions.

Positron emission tomography (PET) shows increased tumor

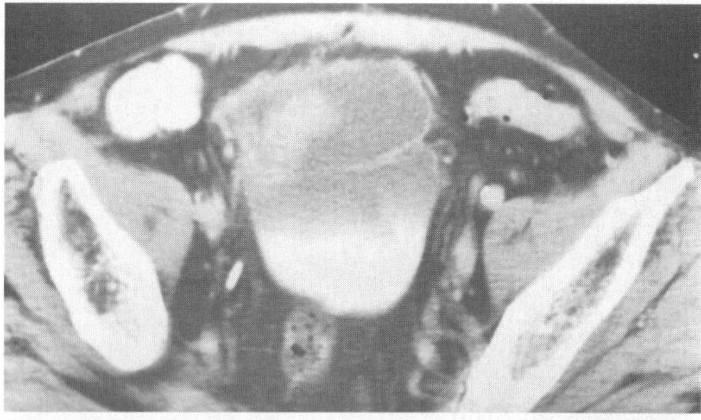
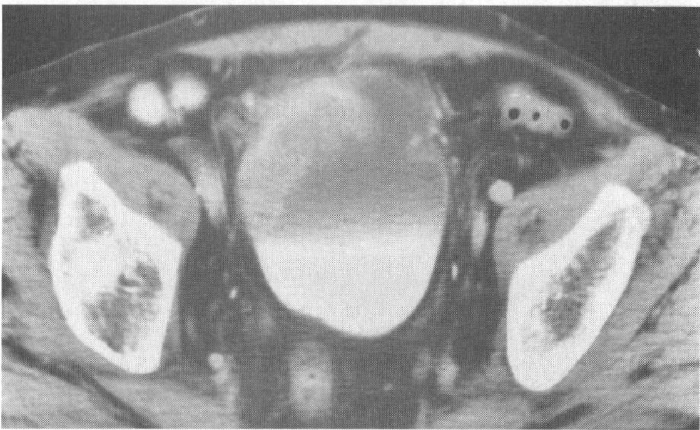
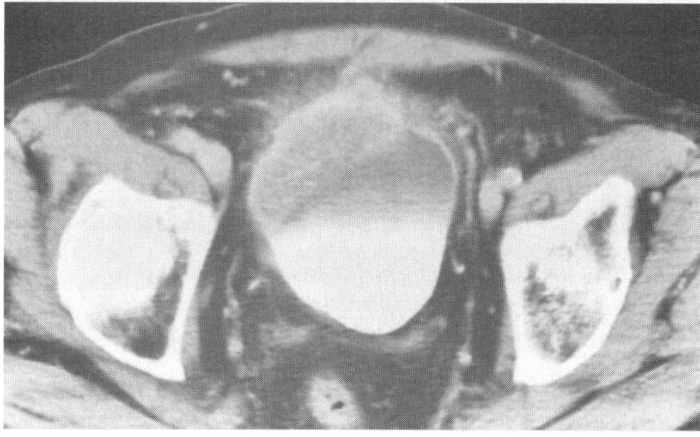

Fig. 61.13. Transitional cell carcinoma of the bladder on CT scan. A space-occupying mass is in the bladder. There seems to be infiltration of the fat tissues along the anterior bladder wall, which would suggest pT3b lesion. The false-positive results stem from an associated inflammatory reaction that is currently impossible to differentiate by imaging.

uptake of fluoro-deoxy-glucose (FDG). FDG excretion and concentration in the pelvocalyceal system, ureters, and bladder make it difficult to judge the presence of tumor within the urinary tract or periureteral lymph nodes, but it may become very useful for detecting distant metastases (92).

Recurrence After Cystectomy

Lymph node, liver, and osseous metastases and local recurrence are best evaluated by CT or MRI. The tumor is of moderate signal intensity and will enhance with Gd-DTPA (93).

Recurrence in the upper tract is best seen on excretory urogram. Some suggest a urogram every 2 years after cystectomy (94), whereas others believe this is unnecessary in asymptomatic patients (95).

Other Bladder Tumors

Squamous cell carcinoma (96, 97) and adenocarcinoma (98, 99) constitute up to 6% of malignant bladder tumors. There are no radiologic features that can distinguish these two malignancies from TCC, except that pelvic lipomatosis is sometimes associated with adenocarcinoma of the bladder (100).

Bladder lymphoma and a variety of rare benign tumors can also present as a filling defect in the bladder. These include bladder hemangioma (101), leiomyoma (102), and nephrogenic adenoma (103) as well as nonneoplastic entities such as ureterocele and endometriosis (104, 105).

Urachal Neoplasms

Urachal cyst is the most common tumor arising from hindgut remnant. Rarely, the cyst may become infected or form an abscess (106, 107). Diagnosis is easily made with CT or sonography.

The most common urachal malignant tumor is mucinous adenocarcinoma followed by nonmucinous-producing adenocarcinoma, sarcomas, squamous cell carcinoma, and TCC. The tumors are rather small (several centimeters in diameter), cystic or solid midline masses close to the bladder dome. Frequently, linear wall calcification is present (108–110). CT is the study of choice because it is best in displaying wall calcification. MRI shows a soft tissue mass (111).

ADRENAL MASS

Adrenal Adenoma Versus Metastases

Most adrenal masses are either a benign adrenal adenoma or a metastasis to the adrenal gland. Benign adenomas are a common CT finding (prevalence, 8%) in patients without malignancy. This becomes a problem in patients with a newly discovered malignancy elsewhere because the adrenal gland is a common site for secondary metastases. Therefore, differentiating these two entities is a major goal of adrenal gland imaging.

In the past, a number of imaging criteria were used but all were only marginally successful in attaining this goal. These include tumor size (112), bilaterality, enhancement (113), heterogeneity (114), calcification, presence of fluid, and hemorrhage (Fig. 61.14). As expected, although imaging was relatively good in depicting these findings, specificity was lacking.

Only recently it was recognized that benign adenomas have a relatively high triglyceride content that makes them relatively hypodense on CT scan. On CT, density is displayed in HU or CT numbers. In general, water is assigned a density value of

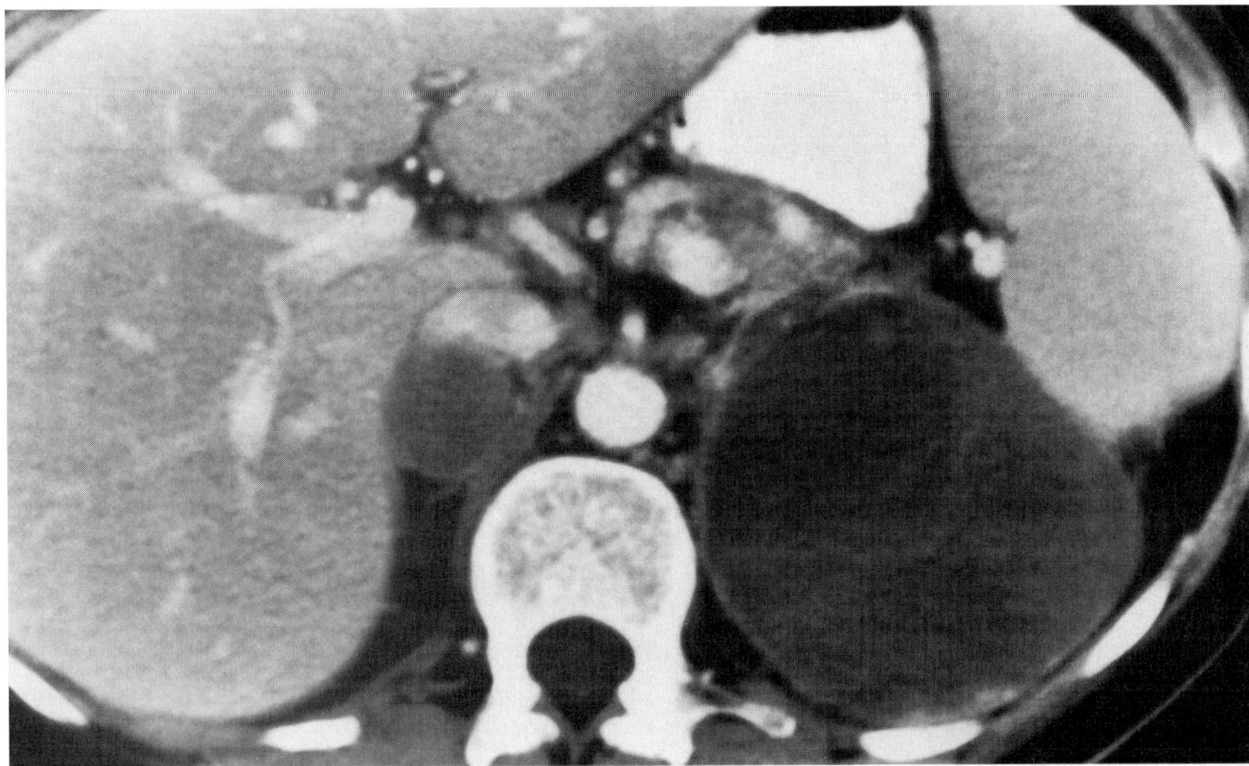

Fig. 61.14. Bronchogenic carcinoma metastatic to adrenal glands seen on CT scan. Bilaterality and heterogeneous enhancement favor neoplasm, but specificity using these criteria is lacking.

0 HU; air, -1000 HU; and cortical bone, $+1000$ HU. Any HU value less than water implies presence of fat or triglycerides. The current criterion for benign adrenal adenoma is that on noncontrast CT using thin (3-mm) sections, values between -10 and 0 HU are diagnostic for benign adenoma (or adrenal cyst) and values between 0 and $+10$ HU are 95% specific for benign adenoma (or adrenal cyst) (115).

Fat or high triglyceride content can also be demonstrated on MRI using various forms of fat suppression imaging (116) or chemical shift FLASH sequences (117, 118). This is also indicative of a benign adenoma.

The current recommendation regarding a newly discovered adrenal tumor is to begin with thin section CT without contrast. Approximately 50% of cases will be resolved using this method. Another 40% can be resolved with various MRI methods for fat imaging. The last 10% that fall in the gray zone are biopsied (119).

Adrenal Carcinoma

Adrenal adenocarcinoma is usually large when first discovered. A large proportion is hormonally active (120). CT is the examination of choice followed by MRI if venous extension is suspected. Heterogeneous areas of tumor necrosis and dystrophic calcification are common. Extension into renal vein, inferior vena cava, and even the right atrium is common (121, 122). Metastases to the adrenal gland can also form a tumor throm-

bus. This should be kept in mind when trying to differentiate an adrenal carcinoma from a metastasis to the adrenal from another site (123).

Pheochromocytoma

Approximately 10% of pheochromocytomas are malignant, and another 10% are extraadrenal (124). MR is considered the imaging method of choice for benign and malignant pheochromocytoma because it has very high signal intensity (bright) on T2-weighted sequences, which is easily contrasted with relatively dark background (Fig. 61.15) (125). Because pheochromocytoma is often bilateral or extraadrenal, the entire abdomen and pelvis can be examined by MRI without the need for intravenous contrast (126, 127). This has some relevance because hypertensive crisis has been observed in patients undergoing routine contrast-enhanced CT, urography, and particularly angiography. Extraadrenal pheochromocytoma (paraganglioma) is more likely to be malignant (128). All patients with pheochromocytoma should be screened for multiple endocrine neoplasia (129).

Scintigraphy using new medullary agent ^{131}I MIBG (methyliodobenzylguadinine) is specific for detecting primary and metastatic pheochromocytoma and neuroblastoma. Because whole body imaging can be easily obtained, scintigraphy has the potential of becoming the primary method for searching for this frequently multicentric tumor.

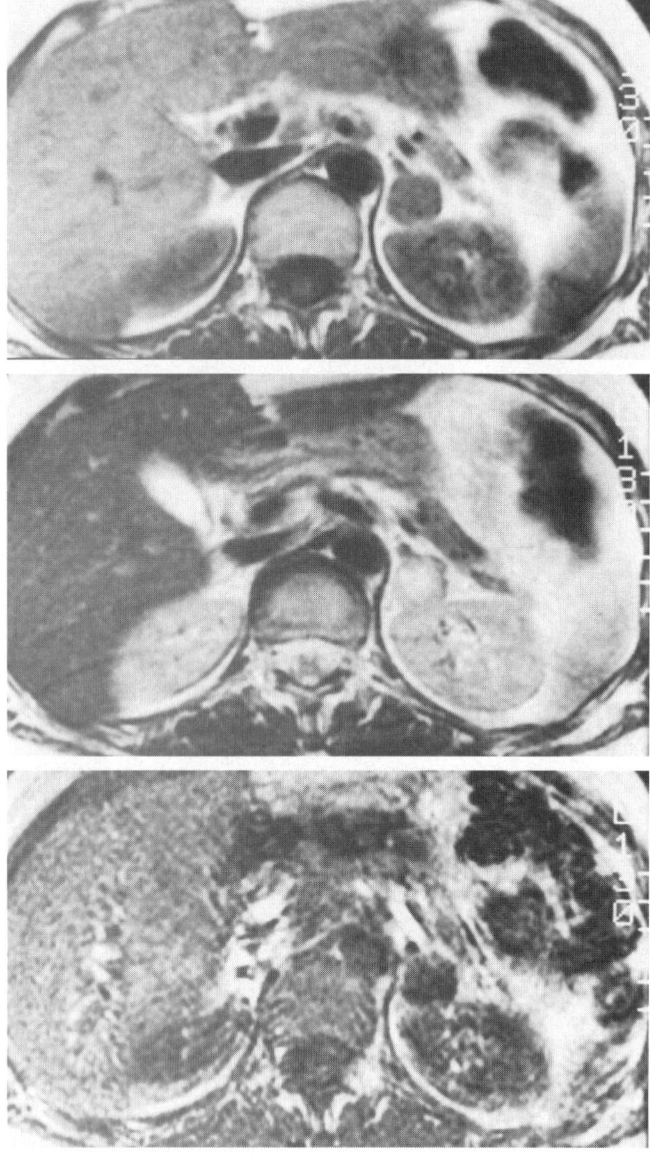

Fig. 61.15. Pheochromocytoma seen on three MRI sequences. The middle sequence is T2-weighted, in which pheochromocytoma usually exhibits a very intense (bright) signal. This is not true in this case. One should expect departures from the norm.

Other Adrenal Tumors

Other tumors and tumor-like masses that originate from adrenal glands are adrenal lymphoma, myelolipoma, adrenal cyst, tuberculous granuloma, and hemorrhage. Of these, myelolipoma has a characteristic signature because it mostly contains fat. Hounsfield value -10 HU to -50 HU is diagnostic (Fig. 61.16) (130, 131). At times, bulky tumors may present with flank pain and nausea (132). Calcification and hemorrhage may also be present and be identified as such on cross-sectional imaging (133).

Adrenal cysts are sonolucent on US and exhibit through transmission just like renal cysts. Adrenal hemorrhage is typically hyperdense on noncontrast CT (134).

In patients with Cushing's syndrome, one may discover bilateral adrenal hyperplasia. In ectopic adrenocorticotropic hormone (ACTH) syndrome, hyperplasia is caused by ACTH produced by a malignant tumor such as carcinoid, oat cell carcinoma, islet cell carcinoma (135), medullary thyroid carcinoma, and pheochromocytoma. Adrenals are usually larger compared with patients with ACTH-producing pituitary adenoma (136). CT is the modality of choice when searching for or evaluating size and resectability of such a malignant ACTH-secreting tumor.

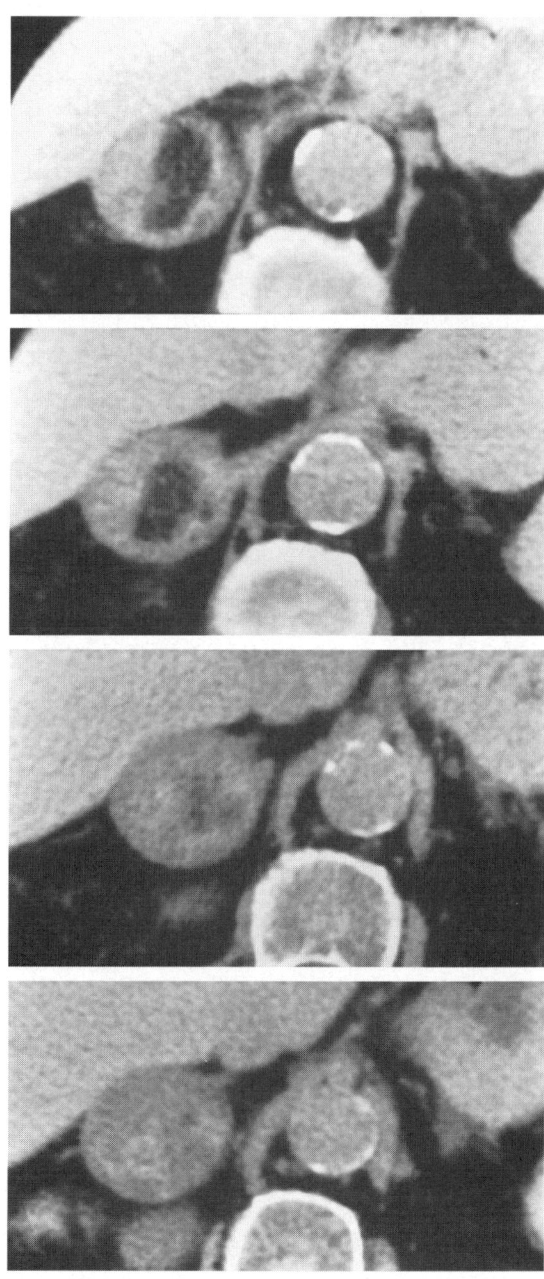

Fig. 61.16. Myelolipoma in the right adrenal gland. On CT scan, there are low-attenuation areas similar to that of retroperitoneal fat. There are also enhancing solid components in this unusual tumor.

Adrenal lymphomas are usually secondary non-Hodgkin's type and are present in one third of patients with systemic disease. Primary adrenal lymphoma is rare (137). Giant lymph node hyperplasia (Castelman disease) has been reported in the adrenals (138).

Neuroblastoma

Neuroblastoma is the most common solid malignant tumor in childhood. It usually presents as a large palpable abdominal mass.

US will quickly determine if the palpable mass is solid or cystic and differentiate it from hydronephrosis, multicystic kidney, and renal cyst. Thereafter, imaging efforts are directed toward staging. Because vascular encasement and spinal cord involvement are crucial in staging, MRI is the examination of choice (139).

The tumor is of high intensity (bright) on T2-weighted sequences. Renal involvement, secondary hydronephrosis, lymph node enlargement, and bone metastases may all be identified. Neuroblastoma must be differentiated from Wilms' tumor (140).

CT is very close to MRI, although it requires intravenous contrast to visualize major abdominal vessels and their relation to the tumor.

RETROPERITONEAL TUMORS

Lymphadenopathy

The only visible expression of lymph node metastases is the lymph node's abnormal size. This is unfortunate because microscopic and many small macroscopic metastases are likely to escape detection. Certainly, technology has come a long way from the days when the only means for detecting enlarged nodes were indirect signs, such as ureteral displacement on urography or bowel displacement on barium studies.

CT is the modality of choice. Lymph nodes are considered pathologically enlarged when crural nodes exceed 0.6 cm, periaortic and aortocaval nodes 1 cm, and pelvic nodes 1.5 cm. These numbers are under scrutiny and are constantly revised. For example, in patients with prostatic carcinoma metastatic nodes are often normal in size. Therefore, even 6-mm pelvic lymph nodes should be suspect if they are asymmetrical on opposite sides (141). It is safe to assume that newer studies will define probability of nodal metastases associated with a particular size for a specific disease.

Nonetheless, when nodes enlarge above the preset values, positive predictive value for metastatic disease is high (Fig. 61.17). Otherwise, some suggest CT-guided biopsy, laparoscopic lymphadenectomy, or open lymphadenectomy.

PET is the latest attempt to image metastatic disease. Tagged FDG is included in the high rate glycolysis process common in tumors and thereby renders the tumor visible on the

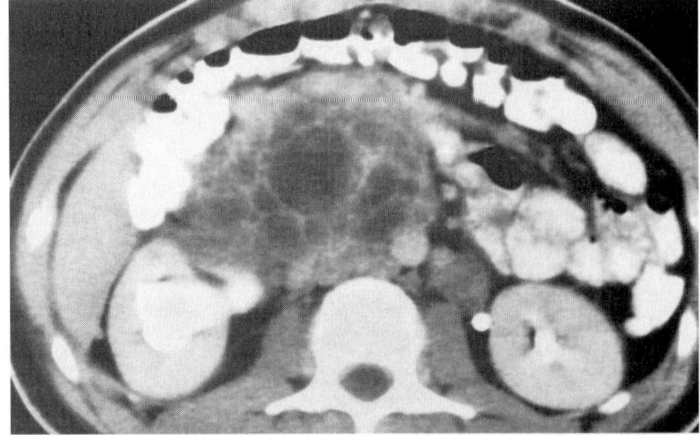

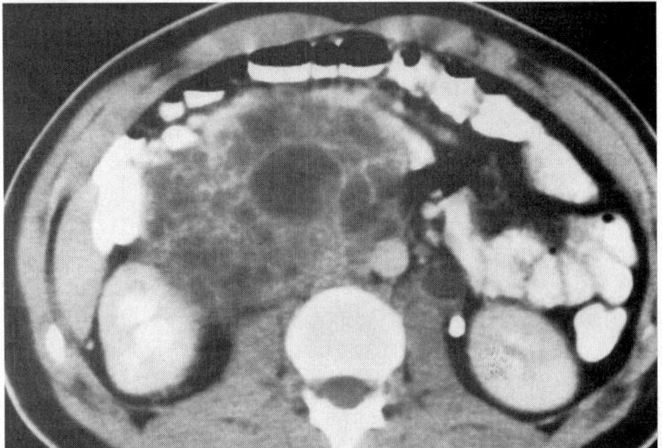

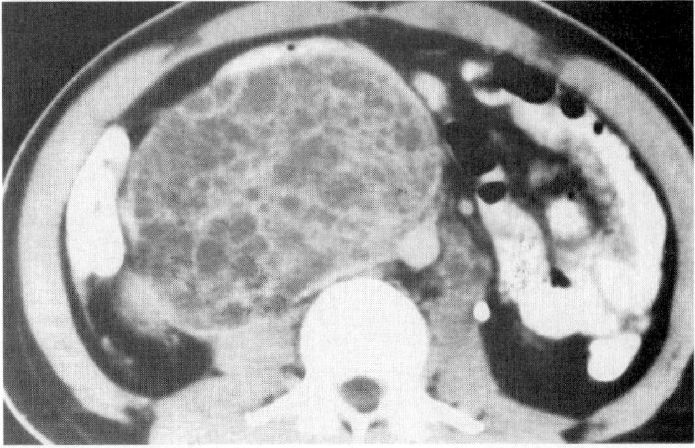

Fig. 61.17. Teratocarcinoma of the testis metastatic to the retroperitoneal lymph nodes. Heterogeneous enhancement and cystic component can be easily seen in the larger of the two metastases. The smaller metastasis is in the left periaortic area.

PET scan (142). There are some disadvantages of PET imaging regarding urinary tract metastatic disease. In addition to high cost, urinary excretion of FDG makes the collecting system, ureters, and bladder "hot," which may interfere with detection of adjacent pathologic nodes.

Malignant Retroperitoneal Fibrosis

Retroperitoneal fibrosis refers to the inflammatory process in the retroperitoneum. When an inflammatory mass cicatrizes and retracts, the ureters and inferior vena cava may become obstructed. One of the causes of retroperitoneal fibrosis is retroperitoneal metastatic disease, which invokes desmoplastic reaction and sclerosis in the retroperitoneum.

On CT, a soft tissue mass may be identified causing ureteral obstruction. MRI may be the study of choice. If the retroperitoneal soft tissue mass is homogeneous, exhibits low-signal intensity both on T1-weighted and T2-weighted sequences, and is well marginated, it is probably a benign retroperitoneal fibrosis. If the mass is heterogeneous, with areas of increased signal intensity (bright) on T2-weighted images, and has ill-defined margins, it may be malignancy, malignant retroperitoneal fibrosis (143), or the inflammatory stage of benign retroperitoneal fibrosis (144).

Short of exploratory surgery, biopsy may be the only means of establishing diagnosis.

Primary Retroperitoneal Tumors

The most common primary retroperitoneal tumors are malignant fibrous histiocytoma, liposarcoma, leiomyosarcoma, paraganglioma, neurofibroma, and neurilemoma (145, 146).

CT and MRI are the imaging methods of choice. Both can detect retroperitoneal tumors and at times be very specific regarding diagnosis, defining local extension and relation to major vessels and other organs (147).

Primary retroperitoneal tumors are usually large when first discovered (Fig. 61.18). Heterogeneous appearance and some enhancement are common such as in malignant fibrous histiocytoma, hemangiopericytoma, and leiomyosarcoma (148). Dystrophic calcifications may be present in fibrous histiocytoma and mature teratoma (148a). Some tumors present with systemic symptoms such as hypoglycemia associated with hemangiopericytoma, or hypertension associated with paraganglioma (extraadrenal pheochromocytoma) (149, 150). Others may contain moderate amounts of fat, such as liposarcoma and mature teratoma.

Specific diagnosis is often impossible, and some recommend CT-guided core biopsy for definitive preoperative diagnosis (151).

BENIGN PROSTATIC HYPERTROPHY

Indications for imaging a patient with benign prostatic hypertrophy (BPH) are as follows.

1. To prove significant postvoid residual (US).
2. To evaluate the upper urinary tract system in symptomatic patients (hematuria, flank pain) (US, IVP).
3. To measure prostatic volume and to judge treatment response or to plan surgery (transrectal ultrasound [TRUS]).
4. To differentiate stromal from nonstromal hyperplasia when pharmacotherapy is planned (MRI).

MRI is 94% accurate in differentiating stromal from non-

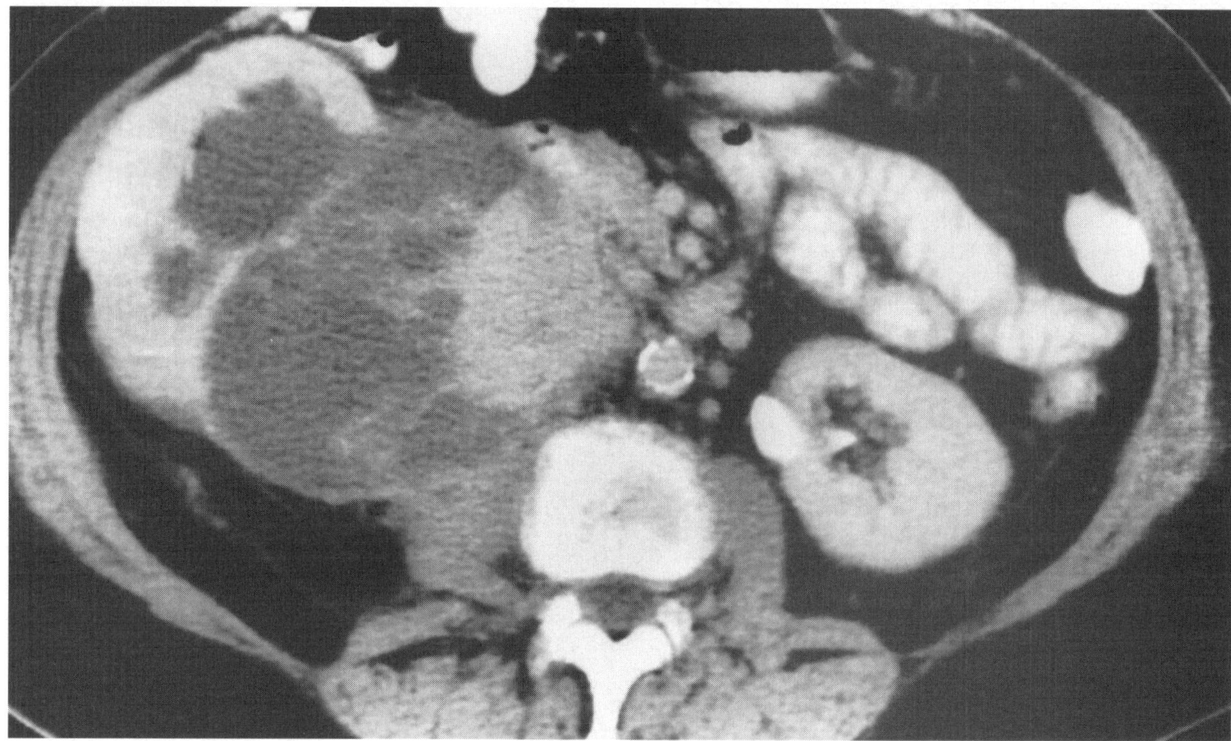

Fig. 61.18.   Spindle cell sarcoma probably originating from inferior vena cava. In this case, it is very difficult to determine if the tumor originates from the kidney (claw sign, parenchymal replacement, hydronephrosis) or from the retroperitoneum, secondarily invading and displacing the kidney.

stromal hyperplasia. In nonstromal hyperplasia, hyperplastic nodules have:

A. Heterogeneous high signal on T2-weighted images;
B. Peripheral enhancement on Gd-enhanced T1-weighted images;
C. A distinct surgical capsule; and
D. An inner gland volume/total volume (inner gland ratio) greater than 0.75.

If none of these findings is discovered, stromal hyperplasia is present (152). This is an excellent noninvasive method for selecting appropriate pharmacotherapy.

IMAGING CARCINOMA OF THE PROSTATE

Detection and Local Staging

TRUS

Echotexture of prostatic carcinoma is usually hypoechoic compared with normal prostatic tissues. Because of different quantities of stromal fibrosis in individuals, carcinoma of the prostate (CAP) may also be isoechoic or hyperechoic compared with the normal prostate. In addition, benign diseases such as infarcts, inflammation, and BPH also have a spectrum of echogenic findings. For these reasons, TRUS is not used as a primary diagnostic tool (153, 154).

This inability of TRUS to detect CAP is also reflected in its poor performance in staging B versus C disease if used as a sole means for staging (155). Used together with elevated prostate-specific antigen (PSA), and if visible tumor volume is less than 3 cc, and if no capsular irregularity is detected, the negative predictive value regarding stage C is reported to be high (156). The main use for TRUS is in guiding systemic prostatic biopsy or a biopsy of a hypoechoic lesion (157).

The newest use for TRUS is in calculating PSA density, which is ratio of PSA values to prostate volume (PSA/P_{cc}) (158), or serum PSA and transition zone volume ratio (PSA/TZ_{cc}) (159), which is considered to be a good method for cancer detection.

CT

CT lacks soft tissue contrast necessary to separate carcinoma from prostatic tissue. Only large carcinomas that are clinically obvious out of capsule can be diagnosed with this method. Therefore, CT is useless for diagnosing or staging local disease. Nor is CT cost-effective in screening for comorbid disease that would affect treatment in patients with newly discovered prostatic carcinoma (160).

MRI

Imaging of the prostate using a body coil failed to improve detection and local staging or accurate tumor volume measurement (161–164).

An MRI surface coil dramatically improves resolution. The endorectal coil was introduced several years ago, initially offering great hopes for improved tumor detection, differentiation, and most importantly local staging (B versus C lesions) (165–167).

As seen on T2-weighted sequence, the tumor is low-signal (dark) compared with relatively high-signal (bright) peripheral zone (Fig. 61.19). A lesion larger than 1 cm and abutting the capsule was thought always to be transcapsular. Also, normal seminal vesicles are of high signal intensity on T2-weighted sequences. Tumor invasion reduces the signal, making the affected seminal vesicle darker.

The newest multiinstitutional studies are not as encouraging as early reports. Overall staging sensitivity, specificity, and accuracy hover around a low 60% (168–170). Although results concerning capsular penetration are poor, the negative predictive value for seminal vesicle involvement is rather high (92.6%) (171).

Detection and local staging, particularly detection of capsular penetration, still elude the most modern imaging techniques.

Metastatic Disease

Pelvic and abdominal lymph node metastases are discussed in the section on retroperitoneal lymphadenopathy. In clinical stage A2, 3% of nodes are already metastatic; in stage B1, approximately 5%; in B2, approximately 10% (172, 173).

Osteoblastic metastases are to vertebrae, ribs, pelvis, long bones, and skull (174). Plain film radiography is too insensitive. Tc 99m HMDP bone scan is the imaging method of choice but must always be correlated to plain radiograph or CT to exclude other causes of increased uptake, such as degenerative bone disease.

Bone scan is likely to upstage 17% of patients from stage B to D (Fig. 61.20). Bone scans are predominately positive in patients with high Gleason grade (175). Without bone pain and normal alkaline and acid phosphatase, the bone scan is more than likely normal (176). Also, PSA serum level below 20 ng/mL suggests absence of skeletal metastases with negative predictive value of 99.7% (177). It is not clear if such a high negative predictive value can be reproduced in other studies (178).

If after radical prostatectomy PSA is normal, a bone scan will more than likely be normal. If PSA is on the rise and there is bone pain, the bone scan will most likely be positive (179).

Metastases to lung present as a reticulonodular pattern. Pleural fluid and mediastinal adenopathy are also common. Metastases to extradural areas in the spine are probably via the Batson's venous plexus. The most serious consequence, cord compression, should be promptly evaluated by MRI. At autopsy, clinically silent metastases to liver and adrenal are fairly common (180).

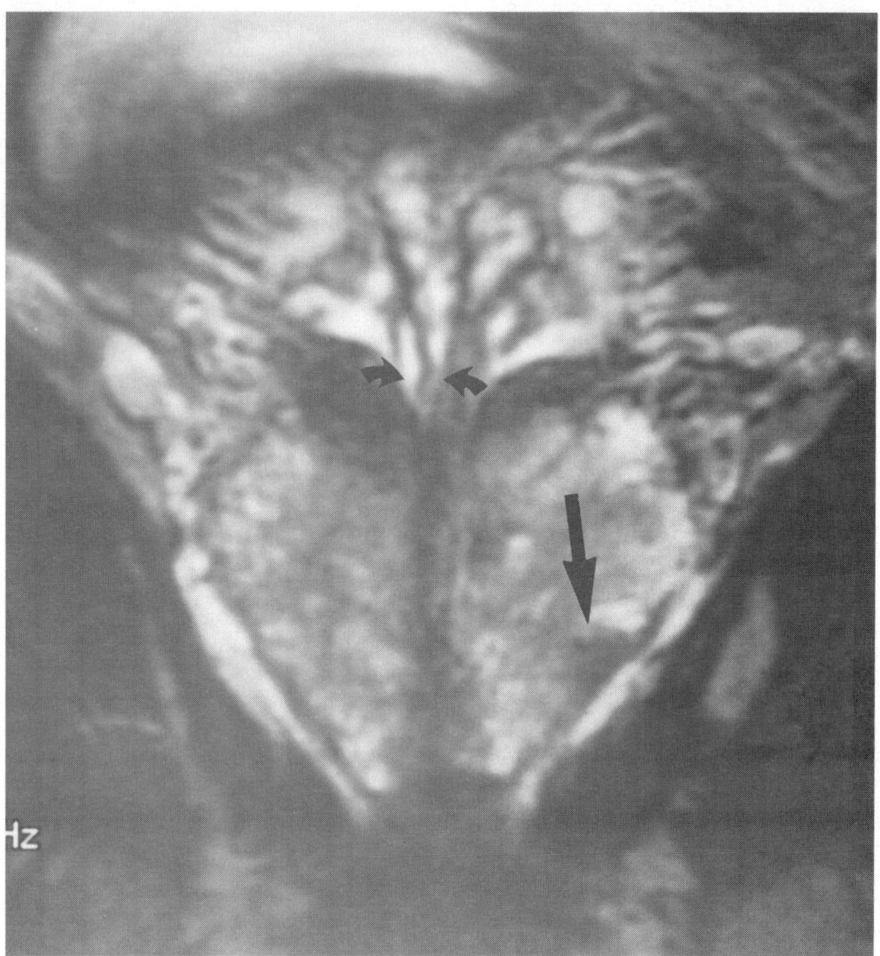

Fig. 61.19.   Prostate carcinoma on coronal T2-weighted sequence obtained with endorectal surface coil. Cancer is the small dark area in the left peripheral zone, adjacent to the prostatic capsule (arrow). Extension into seminal vesicle is excluded. On this particular cut, it is possible to see the junction of the right seminal vesicle and ampullary portion of vas deferens, forming the ejaculatory duct (curved arrows).

Other Prostatic Malignancies

All other prostatic malignancies are rare, and imaging does not differ from that of CAP. These include endometrioid carcinoma (papillary carcinoma), sarcoma, and primary and secondary lymphoma.

Rhabdomyosarcoma of the Bladder (Sarcoma Botryoides)

This is the most common soft tissue sarcoma in children. In addition to the bladder, rhabdomyosarcoma may originate from prostate, vagina, and uterus. A polypoid form of embryonal rhabdomyosarcoma has the morphologic appearance of a grape cluster projecting into the bladder and urethra and is called sarcoma botryoides. Typical large intravesical masses (filling defects) may be seen on CT and MRI, sometimes with local invasion of periprostatic tissues and ischiorectal fossa (181, 182).

URETHRAL CARCINOMA

Squamous cell carcinoma is the most common in the anterior urethra and TCC in the posterior urethra. Adenocarcinoma and melanoma constitute the rest of these rare tumors.

MRI may prove useful in determining tumor extension and in separating neoplastic tissues (bright) from fibrous strictures (dark). The same is true in penile cancer (183). Carcinoma of Cowper's gland is rare and probably best studied with MR (184). Carcinoma and sarcoma of the seminal vesicle are very rare.

Hematospermia is most likely a benign phenomenon or related to prostatic biopsy (Fig. 61.21).

IMAGING OF SCROTAL NEOPLASMS

Testicular Microlithiasis

These polytopic intratubular calcifications are mentioned here because there is high association with germ cell tumors. A speckled pattern of multiple echogenic intratesticular bodies is seen on sonography (185). Yearly screening of patients (20 to 50 years old) with bilateral microlithiasis is advocated. Unilateral speckled pattern is indicative of diseases other than microlithiasis, and biopsy should be considered.

Extratesticular Tumors

Extratesticular solid tumors or tumor-like conditions are usually benign and usually hyperechoic on sonography. The most

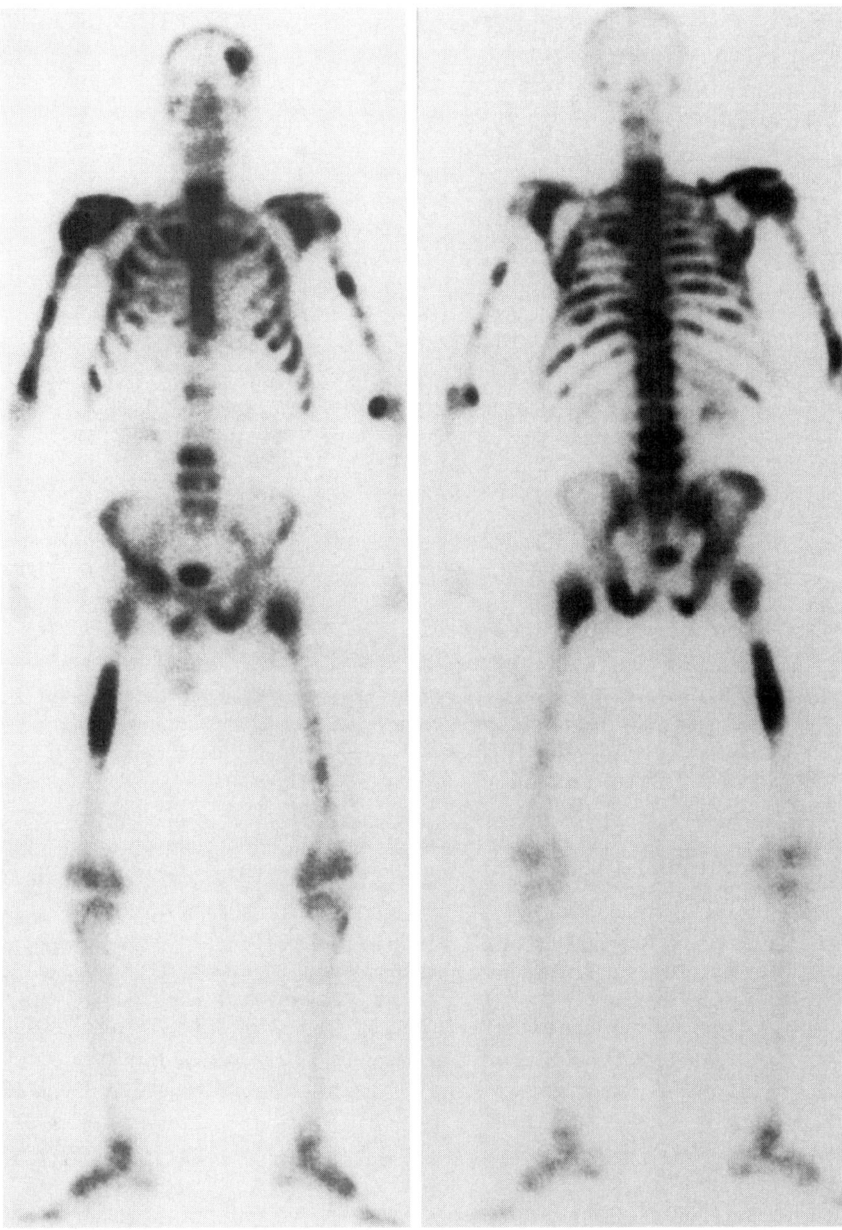

Fig. 61.20. Osseous metastases from prostate cancer. On bone scan, there are diffusely scattered hot areas including metastases to the skull, ribs, humeri, vertebra, pelvis, and femurs.

common are spermatic granuloma, benign mesothelioma, lipoma, myxoma (186), sarcoidosis (187), and adenomatoid tumors of the epididymis, testicular tunic, and spermatic cord (188).

Epididymal cyst is seen as an extratesticular hypoechoic mass and should readily be differentiated from intratesticular pathology.

Benign Intratesticular Tumors

Benign intratesticular cysts are hypoechoic with through transmission (189). They may be differentiated from cystic testicular neoplasms by using strict imaging criteria together with a thorough physical examination and follow-up examination. Epidermoid cysts of the testis have also been described (190).

Intratesticular benign hypoechoic tumors are present in up to 30% of patients with adrenogenital syndrome or Cushing's syndrome. These are either ectopic adrenal tissues or Leydig cells (191).

Malignant Testes Tumors

Most tumors are palpable at the time of discovery. Imaging helps to differentiate extratesticular lesions and to prove the opposite testis normal.

On US, almost all malignant tumors are moderately to mildly hypoechoic compared with normal testis. Seminomas in particular tend to be moderately hypoechoic and homogeneous (192, 193). Nonseminomatous tumors tend to be more hetero-

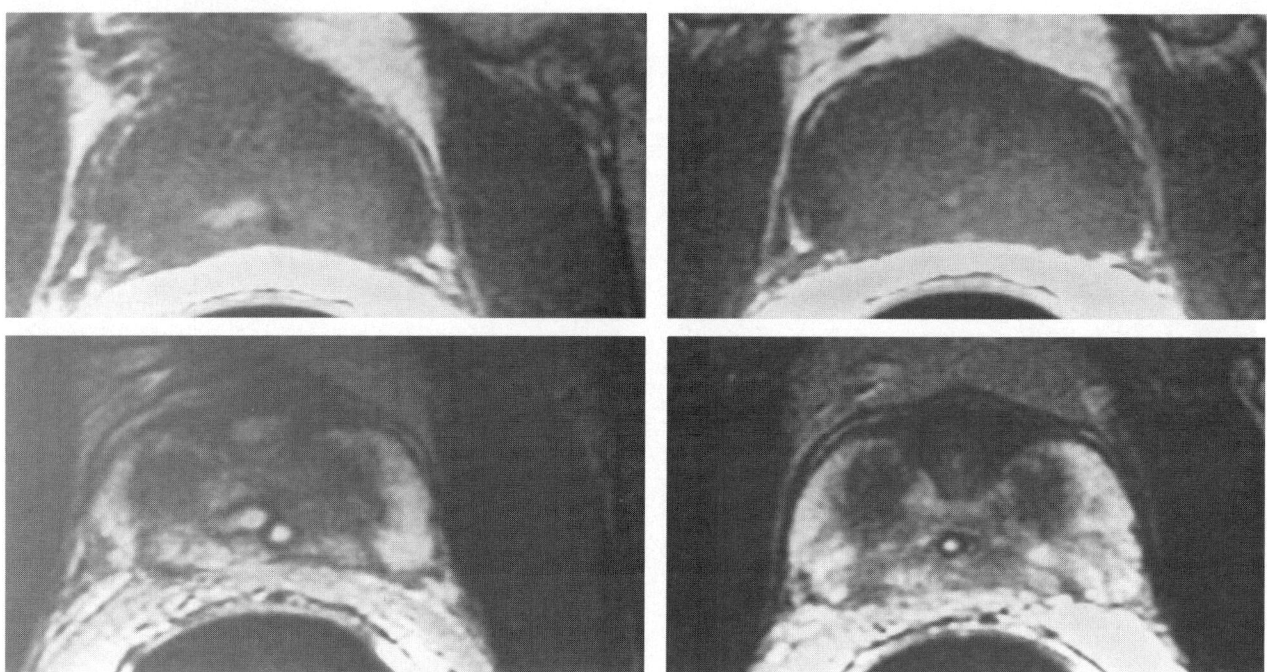

Fig. 61.21.   Hematospermia after prostatic biopsy. An endorectal surface coil was used to obtain these MRI images. The upper row shows T1-weighted sequences, and the lower row shows corresponding T2-weighted sequences. On T1-weighted sequences, the prostate is of uniform, medium-signal intensity (gray). The very distal seminal vesicle contains blood because it is of high signal (bright) on both T1-weighted and T2-weighted sequences. Dark areas on T2-weighted sequences within the peripheral zone of the prostate are more disturbing. This is typically a finding associated with prostatic carcinoma, which this patient does not have. It is more likely that this appearance is due to prostatic biopsy. Therefore, the MRI for local staging of the prostate carcinoma should not be done for some time after prostatic biopsy.

geneous, and the majority have cystic components, or areas of hemorrhage. Bright echogenic foci are seen in the presence of focal calcification, immature bone elements, cartilage, and scarring.

Color Doppler US has a limited role in the evaluation of testicular tumors (194).

Lymphoma infiltrates are also seen as hypoechoic areas. Sometimes infiltration is so diffuse that it may be difficult to appreciate widespread echogenicity (195).

On MRI, testes tumors are usually of lower signal (darker) on T2-weighted sequence compared with the bright normal parenchyma. Superb images may be obtained using a surface coil.

Both ultrasound and MRI are too inaccurate to be used for local (intrascrotal) staging. This in no way influences management because inguinal orchiectomy is done regardless of local tumor stage (196).

Extrascrotal disease is best staged by CT (197). As discussed previously, a pathologic lymph node may be diagnosed only if it is enlarged. Small metastatic deposits are unrecognized. Intracaval extension has been described (198). Overall accuracy of CT staging is approximately 80%.

REFERENCES

1. Cohan RH, Sherman LS, Korobkin M, et al. Renal masses: assessment of corticomedullary phase and nephrographic phase CT scans. Radiology 1995;196:445.

2. Bosniak MA. The current radiological approach to renal cysts. Radiology 1986;158:1.

3. Fishman MC, Pollack HM, Arger PH, et al. High protein content: another cause of CT hyperdense renal cyst. J Comput Assist Tomogr 1983;7:1103.

4. Gooding GAW. Sonography of hemorrhagic cysts with computed tomographic correlation. J Ultrasound Med 1986; 5:699.

5. Amis ES, Cronan JJ, Pfister RC. Needle puncture of cystic renal masses: a survey of the Society of Uroradiology. AJR 1987;148:297.

6. Selzman AA, Hampel N, Hassan MO. Renal oncocytoma arising from a renal cyst: a case report and review of the literature. J Urol 1994;151:1610.

7. Strotzer M, Lehner KB, Becker K. Detection of fat in a renal cell carcinoma mimicking angiomyolipoma. Radiology 1993; 188:427.

8. Helemon O, Chretien Y, Paret F, et al. Renal cell carcinoma containing fat: demonstration with CT. Radiology 1993;188: 420.

9. Sant GR, Ucci AA, Meares EM. Multicentric angiomyolipoma: renal and lymph node involvement. Urology 1986;28:111.

10. Tallarigo C, Baldassarre R, Bianchi G, et al. Diagnostic and therapeutic problems in multicentric renal angiomyolipoma. J Urol 1992;148:1880.

11. Umeyama T, Saitoh Y, Tomaru Y, et al. Bilateral renal angiomyolipoma associated with bilateral renal vein and inferior vena caval thrombi. J Urol 1992;148:1885.

12. Earthman WJ, Mazer MJ, Winfield AC. Angiomyolipomas in tuberous sclerosis: subselective embolotherapy with alcohol, with long-term follow-up study. Radiology 1986;160:437.

13. Van Baal JG, Smits NJ, Keeman JN, et al. The evolution of renal angiomyolipomas in patients with tuberous sclerosis. J Urol 1994;152:35.

14. Williams MA, Schropp KP, Noe HN. Fat containing renal mass in childhood: a case report of teratoid Wilms tumor. J Urol 1994;151:1662.

15. Davidson AJ, Hayes WS, Hartman DS, et al. Renal oncocytoma and carcinoma: failure of differentiation with CT. Radiology 1993;186:693.

16. Endress C, Chita MA. Renal cell carcinoma simulating oncocytoma. AJR 1992;158:920. Letter.

17. Tikkakoski T, Paivansalo M, Alanen A, et al. Radiologic findings in renal oncocytoma. Acta Radiol 1991;32:363.

18. Defosses AM, Yoder IC, Papanicolaou N, et al. Nonspecific magnetic resonance appearance of renal oncocytomas: report of 3 cases and review of the literature. J Urol 1991;145:552.

19. Quinn MJ, Hartman DS, Friedman AC, et al. Renal oncocytoma: new observations. Radiology 1984;153:49.

20. Sos TA, Gray GF Jr, Baltaxe HA. The angiographic appearance of benign renal oxyphilic adenoma. AJR 1976;127:717.

21. Neisius D, Braedel HU, Schindler E, et al. Computed tomographic and angiographic findings in renal oncocytoma. Br J Radiol 1988;61:1019.

22. Gupta RK, Delahunt B, Wakefield J. Preoperative diagnosis of bilateral renal oncocytoma by needle aspiration cytology: a case report. Acta Cytol 1991;35:742.

23. Cheng WS, Farrow GM, Zincke H. The incidence of multicentricity in renal cell carcinoma. J Urol 1991;146:1221.

24. Roubidoux MA, Dunnick NR, Sostman HD, et al. Renal carcinoma: detection of venous extension with gradient-echo imaging. Radiology 1992;182:269.

25. Harris DD, Ruckle HC, Gaskill DM, et al. Intraoperative ultrasound: determination of the presence and extent of vena caval tumor thrombus. Urology 1994;44:189.

26. Treiger BFG, Humphrey LS, Peterson CV Jr, et al. Transesophageal echocardiography in renal cell carcinoma: an accurate diagnostic technique for intracaval neoplastic extension. J Urol 1991;145:1138.

27. Gill IS, McClennan BL, Kerbl K, et al. Adrenal involvement from renal cell carcinoma: predictive value of computerized tomography. J Urol 1994;152:1082.

28. Birnbaum BA, Noz ME, Chapnick J, et al. Hepatic hemangiomas: diagnosis with fusion of MR, CT, and Tc-99m-labeled red blood cell SPECT images. Radiology 1991;181:469.

29. Ochiai K, Onitsuka H, Honda H, et al. Leiomyosarcoma of the kidney: CT and MR appearance. J Comput Assist Tomogr 1993;17:656.

30. Sampaio CA, McLain D, Klein E, et al. Renal masses simulating primary renal cell carcinoma in patients with advanced malignancies. J Urol 1994;151:1505.

31. Devasia A, Nath V, Abraham B, et al. Hematuria, renal mass and amenorrhea: indicators of a rare diagnosis. J Urol 1994;151:409.

32. Wagner JR, Honig SC, Siroky MB. Non-Hodgkin's lymphoma can mimic renal adenocarcinoma with inferior vena cava involvement. Urology 1993;42:720.

33. Fujimoto H, Chitose K, Tobisu KI, et al. Solitary renal melanoma? a case with long survival after initial treatment. J Urol 1995;153:1887.

34. Nicoforo JR, Coughlin BF. Diagnosis of renal cell carcinoma: value of fine-needle aspiration cytology in patients with metastases or contraindications to nephrectomy. AJR 1993;161:1303.

35. Newmark JR, Newmark GM, Epstein JI, et al. Solitary rare recurrence of renal cell carcinoma. Urology 1994;43:725.

36. Yeh HC, Halton KP, Shapiro RS, et al. Junctional parenchyma: revised definition of hypertrophied column of Bertin. Radiology 1992;185:725.

37. Bosniak MA. The small (>3.0 cm) renal parenchymal tumor: detection, diagnosis, and controversies. Radiology 1991;179:307.

38. Aso Y, Homma Y. A survey on incidental renal cell carcinoma in Japan. J Urol 1992;147:340.

39. Rominger MB, Kenney PJ, Morgan DE, et al. Gadolinium-enhanced MR imaging of renal masses. Radiographics 1992;12:1097.

40. Rofsky NM, Weinreb JC, Bosniak MA, et al. Renal lesion characterization with gadolinium-enhanced MR imaging: efficacy and safety in patients with renal insufficiency. Radiology 1991;180:85.

41. Semelka RC, Hricak H, Stevens SK, et al. Combined gadolinium-enhanced and fat-saturation MR imaging of renal masses. Radiology 1991;178:803.

42. Neuman HPB, Berger DP, Sigmund G, et al. Pheochromocytomas, multiple endocrine neoplasia type 2, and von Hippel-Lindau disease. N Engl J Med 1993;329:1531.

43. Frydenberg M, Malek RS, Zincke H. Conservative renal surgery for renal cell carcinoma in von Hippel-Lindau's disease. J Urol 1993;149:461.

44. Miller DL, Choyke PL, Walther McM, et al. Von Hippel-Lindau disease: inadequacy of angiography for identification of renal cancers. Radiology 1991;179:833.

45. Terasawa Y, Suzuki Y, Morita M, et al. Ultrasonic diagnosis of renal cell carcinoma in hemodialysis patients. J Urol 1994;152:846.

46. Chandhoke PS, Torrence RJ, Clayman RV, et al. Acquired cystic disease of the kidney: a management dilemma. J Urol 1992;147:969.

47. Chung WY, Nast CC, Ettinger RB, et al. Acquired cystic renal disease in chronically rejected renal transplants. J Am Soc Nephrol 1992;2:1298.

48. Levine E. Renal cell carcinoma in uremic acquired renal cystic disease: incidence, detection, and management. Urol Radiol 1992;13:203.

49. Feldman JD, Jacobs SC. Late development of renal carcinoma in allograft kidney. J Urol 1992;148:395.

50. Nakamoto T, Igawa M, Mitani S, et al. Metastatic renal cell carcinoma arising in a native kidney of a renal transplant recipient. J Urol 1994;152:943.

51. Honda H, Franken EA Jr, Barloon TJ, et al. Hepatic lymphoma in cyclosporine-treated transplant recipients: sonographic and CT findings. AJR 1989;152:501.

52. Chan HS, Cheng MY, Mancer K, et al. Congenital

mesoblastic nephroma: a clinicoradiologic study of 17 cases representing the pathologic spectrum of the disease. J Pediatr 1987;111:64.

53. Kirks DR, Kaufman RA. Function within mesoblastic nephroma: imaging-pathologic correlation. Pediatr Radiol 1989;19:136.

54. Rieumont MJ, Whitman GJ. Mesoblastic nephroma. AJR 1994;162:76.

55. Fernbach SK, Feinstein KA, Donaldson JS, et al. Nephroblastomatosis: comparison of CT with US and urography. Radiology 1988;166:153.

56. Schreiber MH, Cavallo FM, Dominquez VE, et al. Image interpretation session: 1992. Radiographics 1993;13:169.

57. White K, Kirks DR, Bove K. Imaging of nephroblastomatosis: an overview. Radiology 1992;182:1.

58. Andrews MW, Amparo EG. Wilms' tumor in a patient with Beckwith-Wiedemann syndrome: onset detected with 3-month serial sonography. AJR 1993;160:139.

59. Mesrobian HGJ. Wilms tumor: past present, future. J Urol 1988;140:231.

60. Mesrobian HGJ, Kelalis PP, Harabovsky E, et al. Wilms tumor in horseshoe kidneys: a report from the National Wilms Tumor Study. J Urol 1985;133:1002.

61. Siegel MJ, Shackelford GD. Wilms tumor in children: abdominal CT and ultrasound evaluation. Radiology 1986;160:501.

62. Kangarloo H, Dietrich RB, Erlich RM, et al. Magnetic resonance imaging of Wilms tumor. Radiology 1987;163:291.

63. Ritchey ML, Green DM, Breslow NB, et al. Accuracy of current imaging modalities in the diagnosis of synchronous bilateral Wilms' tumor. a report from the National Wilms Tumor Study Group. Cancer 1995;75:600.

64. Broecker B. Renal cell carcinoma in children. Urology 1991;38:54.

65. Motley RC, Patterson DE, Weiland LH. Ureteroscopic visualization of a cavernous hemangioma of the renal pelvis. J Urol 1990;143:788.

66. McCoy JG, Honda H, Reznicek M, et al. Computerized tomography for detection and staging of localized and pathologically defined upper tract urothelial tumors. J Urol 1991;146:1500.

67. Goldfarb DA, Lorig R, Zelch M, et al. Right renal mass with vena caval thrombus. J Urol 1990;143:574.

68. Leo ME, Petrou SP, Barrett DM. Transitional cell carcinoma of the kidney with vena caval involvement: report of 3 cases and a review of the literature. J Urol 1992;148:398.

69. Nativ O, Reiman HM, Lieber MM, et al. Primary squamous cell carcinoma of the upper tracts. Cancer 1991;68:2575.

70. Bergman H, Friedenberg RM, Sayegh V. New roentgenologic signs of carcinoma of the ureter. AJR 1961;86:707.

71. Kenney PJ, Stanley RJ. Computed tomography of ureteral tumors. J Comput Assist Tomogr 1987;11:102.

72. Parienty RA, Ducellier R, Pradel J, et al. Diagnostic value of CT numbers in pelvocalyceal filling defects. Radiology 1982;145:743.

73. Cochran ST, Waisman J, Barbaric ZL. Radiographic and microscopic findings in multiple ureteral diverticula. Radiology 1980;137:631.

74. Wasserman NF, Posalaky IP, Dykoski R. The pathology of ureteral pseudodiverticulosis. Invest Radiol 1988;23:592.

75. Wasserman NF, Zhang G, Posalaky IP, et al. Ureteral pseudodiverticula: frequent association with uroepithelial malignancy. AJR 1991;157:69.

76. Nadel S, St.Amour TE, Kyriakos M. Asymptomatic woman with unilateral urethelial lesions. Urol Radiol 1987;9:57.

77. MacFarlane MT, Stein A, Layfield L, et al. Preoperative endoscopic diagnosis of fibroepithelial polyp of the renal pelvis: a case report and review of the literature. J Urol 1991;145:549.

78. Gleason PE, Kramer SA. Genitourinary polyps in children. Urology 1994;44:106.

79. Fleming S. Carcinosarcoma (mixed mesodermal tumor) of the ureter. J Urol 1987;138:1234.

80. Esrig D, Kanellos AW, Freeman JA, et al. Metastatic renal cell carcinoma to the contralateral ureter. Urology 1994;44:278.

81. Mitty HA, Droller MJ, Dikman SH. Ureteral and renal pelvic metastases from renal cell carcinoma. Urol Radiol 1987;9:16.

82. Cher ML, Milchgrub S, Sagalowsky AI. Transitional cell carcinoma of the ureteral stump 23 years after radical nephrectomy for adenocarcinoma. J Urol 1993;149:106.

83. Pollack HM, Banner MP, Popky GL. Radiologic evaluation of ureteral stump. Radiology 1982;144:225.

84. Jaffe J, Friedman AC, Seidmon EJ, et al. Diagnosis of ureteral stump transitional cell carcinoma by CT and MR imaging. AJR 1987;149:741.

85. Mitty HA, Schapira HE. Ureterocele and pseudoureterocele: cobra versus cancer. J Urol 1977;117:557.

86. Thornbury JR, Silver TM, Vinson RK. Ureteroceles vs. pseudoureteroceles in adults: urographic diagnosis. Radiology 1977;122:81.

87. Koss JC, Arger PH, Coleman BG, et al. CT staging of the bladder carcinoma. AJR 1981;137:359.

88. Fisher MR, Hricak H, Tanagho EA. Urinary bladder MR imaging. part II. neoplasm. Radiology 1985;157:471.

89. Rholl SK, Lee JKT, Heiken JP, et al. Primary bladder carcinoma: evaluation with MR imaging. Radiology 1987;163:117.

90. Neuerburg JM, Bohndorf K, Sohn M, et al. Urinary bladder neoplasms: evaluation with contrast-enhanced MR imaging. Radiology 1989;172:739.

91. Tanimoto A, Yuasa Y, Imai Y, et al. Bladder tumor staging: comparison of conventional and gadolinium-enhanced dynamic MR imaging and CT. Radiology 1992;185:741.

92. Harney JV, Wahl RL, Liebert M, et al. Uptake of 2-deoxy, 2-(18F) fluoro-d-glucose in bladder cancer: animal localization and initial patient positron emission tomography. J Urol 1991;145:279.

93. Ellis JH, McCullough NB, Frands HB, et al. Transitional cell carcinoma of the bladder: patterns of recurrence after cystectomy as determined by CT. AJR 1991;157:999.

94. Smith H, Weaver D, Barienbruch OBA, et al. Routine excretory urography in follow-up of superficial transitional cell carcinoma of the bladder. Urology 1989;34:193.

95. Hastie KJ, Hamdy FC, Collins MC, et al. Upper tract tumors following cystectomy for bladder cancer. is routine intravenous urography worthwhile? Br J Urol 1991;67:29.

96. Wyman A, Kinder RB. Squamous cell carcinoma of the bladder associated with intrapelvic foreign bodies. Br J Urol 1988;61:460.

97. Stein JP, Skinner EC, Boyd SD, et al. Squamous cell carcinoma of the bladder associated with cyclophosphamide therapy for Wegener's granulomatosis: a report of 2 cases. J Urol 1993;149:588.

98. Abenoza P, Manivel C, Fraley EE. Primary adenocarcinoma of urinary bladder. Clinicopathologic study of 16 cases. Urology 1987;29:9.

99. Blute ML, Engen DE, Travis WD, et al. Primary signet ring cell adenocarcinoma of the bladder. J Urol 1989;141:17.

100. Heyns CF. Pelvic lipomatosis; a review of its diagnosis and management. J Urol 1991;146:267.

101. Pakter R, Nussbaum A, Fishman EK. Hemangioma of the bladder: sonographic and computerized tomography findings. J Urol 1988;140:601.

102. Golubof ET, O'Toole K, Sawczuk IS. Leiomyoma of bladder: report of case and review of literature. Urology 1994;43:238.

103. Heffernan JP, Huisman TK. Nephrogenic adenoma in a bladder diverticulum. J Urol 1994;152:1208.

104. Habuchi T, Okagaki T, Miyakawa M. Endometriosis of bladder after menopause. J Urol 1991;145:361.

105. Posner MP, Fowler JE Jr, Meeks GR. Vesical endometriosis 12 years after a cesarean section. Urology 1994;44:285.

106. Goldman IL, Caldamone AA, Gauderer M, et al. Infected urachal cysts: a review of 10 cases. J Urol 1988;140:375.

107. Wan YL, Lee TY, Tsai CC, et al. The role of sonography in the diagnosis of urachal abscesses. J Clin Ultrasound 1991;19:203.

108. Fiter L, Gimeno F, Martin L, et al. Signet-ring cell adenocarcinoma of bladder. Urology 1993;41:30.

109. Brick HS, Friedman AC, Pollack HM, et al. Urachal carcinoma: CT findings. Radiology 1988;169:377.

110. Henly DR, Farrow GM, Zincke H. Urachal cancer: the role of conservative surgery. Urology 1993;42:635.

111. Maeda H, Kinukawa T, Kuhara H, et al. MR findings in urachal carcinoma. AJR 1992;158:1171. Letter.

112. Bernardino ME. Management of the asymptomatic patient with unilateral adrenal mass. Radiology 1988;166:121.

113. Krestin GP, Steinbrich W, Friedmann G. Adrenal masses: evaluation with fast gradient-echo MR imaging and Gd-DTPA-enhanced dynamic studies. Radiology 1989;171:675.

114. Berland LL, Koslin DB, Kenney PJ, et al. Differentiation between small benign and malignant adrenal masses with dynamic incremented CT. AJR 1988;151:95.

115. Lee MJ, Hahn PF, Papanicolau N, et al. Benign and malignant adrenal masses: CT distinctions with attenuation coefficients, size and observer analysis. Radiology 1991;179:425.

116. Mitchell DG, Crovello M, Matteucci T, et al. Benign adrenocortical masses: diagnosis with chemical shift MR imaging. Radiology 1992;185:345.

117. Tsushima Y, Ishizaka H, Matsumoto M. Adrenal masses: differentiation with chemical shift, fast low-angle shot MR imaging. Radiology 1993;186:705.

118. Francis IR, Gross MD, Shapiro B, et al. Integrated imaging of adrenal disease. Radiology 1992;184:1.

119. Welch TJ, Sheedy PF, Stephens DH, et al. Percutaneous adrenal biopsy: review of a 10-year experience. Radiology 1994;193:341.

120. Nader S, Hickey RC, Selin RV, et al. Adrenal cortical carcinoma: a study of 77 cases. Cancer 1983;52:707.

121. Concepcion RS, Koch MO, McDougal WS, et al. Management of primary nonrenal parenchymal malignancies with vena caval thrombus. J Urol 1991;145:243.

122. Siegelbaum MH, Moulsdale JE, Murphy JB, et al. Use of magnetic resonance imaging scanning in adrenocortical carcinoma with vena caval involvement. Urology 1994;43:869.

123. Gollub MJ, Bosniak MA, Schlossberg P, et al. Extension of a secondary adrenal neoplasm into inferior vena cava. Abdom Imaging 1994;19:359.

124. Hayes WS, Davidson AJ, Grimley PM, et al. Extraadrenal retroperitoneal paraganglioma: clinical, pathologic, and CT findings. AJR 1990;155:1247.

125. Fink IJ, Reining JW, Dwyer AJ, et al. MR imaging of pheochromocytomas. J Comput Assist Tomogr 1985;9:454.

126. Quint EL, Glazer GM, Francis IR, et al. Pheochromocytoma and paraganglioma: comparison of MR imaging with CT and I-131 MIBG scintigraphy. Radiology 1987;165:89.

127. Grenberg M, Moawad AH, Wieties BM, et al. Extraadrenal pheochromocytoma: detection during pregnancy using MR imaging. Radiology 1986;161:475.

128. Whalen RK, Althausen AF, Daniels GH. Extra-adrenal pheochromocytoma. J Urol 1992;147:1.

129. Neuman HPB, Berger DP, Sigmund G, et al. Pheochromocytomas, multiple endocrine neoplasia type 2, and von Hippel-Lindau disease. N Engl J Med 1993;329:1531.

130. Musante F, Derchi LE, Zappasodi F, et al. Myelolipoma of the adrenal gland: sonographic and CT features. AJR 1988;151:961.

131. Meaglia JP, Schmidt JD. Natural history of an adrenal myelolipoma. J Urol 1992;147:1089.

132. Sanders R, Bissada N, Curry N, et al. Clinical spectrum of adrenal myelolipoma: analysis of 8 tumors in 7 patients. J Urol 1995;153:1791.

133. Palmer WE, Gerard-McFarland EL, Chew FS. Adrenal myelolipoma. AJR 1991;156:724.

134. Sakamoto I, Nakahara N, Fukuda T, et al. Atypical appearance of adrenal pseudocysts. J Urol 1994;152:150.

135. Doppman JL, Neiman LK, Cutler JB Jr, et al. Adrenocorticotropic hormone-secreting islet cell tumors: are they always malignant? Radiology 1994;190:59.

136. Doppman JL, Miller DL, Dwyer AJ, et al. Macronodular adrenal hyperplasia in Cushing disease. Radiology 1988;166:347.

137. Alvarez-Castelas A, Pedraza S, Tallada N, et al. CT of primary bilateral adrenal lymphoma. J Comput Assist Tomogr 1993;17:408.

138. Debatin JF, Spritzer CE, Dunnick NR. Castelman disease of the adrenal gland: MR imaging features. AJR 1991;157:781.

139. Westra SJ, Zaninovic AC, Kangarloo H, et al. Imaging of the adrenal gland in children. Radiographics 1994;14:1323.

140. Rosenfield NS, Leonidas JC, Barwick KW. Aggressive neuroblastoma simulating Wilms tumor. Radiology 1988;166:165.

141. Oyen RH, Poppel HPV, Ameye FE, et al. Lymph node

staging of localized prostatic carcinoma with CT and CT-guided fine-needle aspiration biopsy: prospective study in 285 patients. Radiology 1994;190:315.

142. Newman JS, Francis IR, Kaminski MS, et al. Imaging of lymphoma with PET with 2-[F-18]-fluoro-2-deoxy-d-glucose: correlation with CT. Radiology 1994;190:111.

143. Arrivé L, Hricak H, Tavares NJ, et al. Malignant versus nonmalignant retroperitoneal fibrosis: differentiation with MR imaging. Radiology 1989;172:139.

144. Amis ES Jr. Retroperitoneal fibrosis. AJR 1991;157:321.

145. Lane R, Stephens DH, Reiman HM. Primary retroperitoneal neoplasms: CT findings in 90 cases with clinical and pathologic correlation. AJR 1989;152:83.

146. Goldman SM, Hartman DS, Weiss SW. Varied radiographic manifestations of retroperitoneal malignant fibrous histiocytoma revealed through 27 cases. Radiology 1986;135:33.

147. Hartman DS, Hayes WS, Choyke PL, et al. Leiomyosarcoma of the retroperitoneum and inferior vena cava: radiologic pathologic correlation. Radiographics 1992;12:1203.

148. Alpern MB, Thorsen MK, Kellman GM, et al. CT appearance of hemangiopericytoma. J Comput Assist Tomogr 1986;10:264.

148a. Schey WL, Vesely JJ, Radkowski MA. Shard-like calcifications in retroperitoneal teratomas. Pediatr Radiol 1986;16:82

149. Whalen RK, Althausen AF, Daniels GH. Extra-adrenal pheochromocytoma. J Urol 1992;147:1.

150. Hayes WS, Davidson AJ, Grimley PM, et al. Extra-adrenal retroperitoneal paraganglioma: clinical, pathologic, and CT findings. AJR 1990;155:1247.

151. Storm FK, Mahvi DM, Hafez GR. Retroperitoneal masses, adenopathy, and adrenal glands. Surg Oncol Clin North Am 1995;4:175.

152. Ishida, J, Sugimura K, Okizuka H, et al. Benign prostatic hyperplasia: value of MR imaging for determining histologic type. Radiology 1994;190:329.

153. Coffield KS, Speights VO, Brawn PN, et al. Ultrasound detection of prostate cancer in postmortem specimens with histological correlation. J Urol 1992;147:822.

154. Palken M, Cobb OE, Simons CE, et al. Prostate cancer: comparison of digital rectal examination and transrectal ultrasound for screening. J Urol 1991;145:86.

155. Rifkin M, et al. Comparison of magnetic resonance imaging and ultrasonography in staging early prostatic cancer. N Engl J Med 1990;323:621.

156. Gerber GS, Goldberg R, Chodak GW. Local staging of prostate cancer by tumor volume, prostate-specific antigen, and transrectal ultrasound. Urology 1992;40:311.

157. Terris MK, McNeal JE, Stamey TA. Detection of clinically significant prostate cancer by transrectal ultrasound-guided systemic biopsies. J Urol 1992;148:829.

158. Littrup PJ, Kane RA. Williams CR, et al. Determination of prostate volume with transrectal US for cancer screening. Radiology 1991;178:573.

159. Kalish J, Cooner WH, Grahm SD Jr. Serum PSA adjusted for volume of transition zone (PSAD) is more accurate than PSA adjusted for total gland volume (PSAD) in detecting adenocarcinoma of the prostate. Urology 1994;43:601.

160. Forman HP, Heiken JP, Brink JA, et al. CT screening for comorbid disease in patients with prostatic carcinoma: is it cost effective? AJR 1994;162:1125.

161. Rifkin M, et al. Comparison of magnetic resonance imaging and ultrasonography in staging early prostatic cancer. N Engl J Med 1990;323:621.

162. Schiebler ML, Yankaskas BC, Tempany C, et al. MR imaging in adenocarcinoma of the prostate: inter-observer variation and efficacy for determining stage C disease. AJR 1992;158:559.

163. Quint LE, Van Erp JS, Bland PH, et al. Carcinoma of the prostate: MR images obtained with body coils do not accurately reflect tumor volume. AJR 1991;156:551.

164. Quint LE, Van Erp JS, Bland PH, et al. Prostate cancer: correlation of MR images with tissue optical density at pathological examination. Radiology 1991;179:837.

165. Martin JF, Hajek P, Baker L, et al. Inflatable surface coil for MR imaging of the prostate. Radiology 1988;167:268.

166. Schnall MD, Lenkinski RE, Pollack HM, et al. Prostate: MR imaging with an endorectal surface coil. Radiology 1989;172:570.

167. Schnall MD, Imai Y, Tomaszewski J, et al. Prostate cancer: local staging with endorectal surface coil MR imaging. Radiology 1991;178:797.

168. Tempany CM, Zhou X, Zerhouni EA, et al. Staging of prostate cancer: results of radiology diagnostic oncology group project comparison of three MR imaging techniques. Radiology 1994;192:47.

169. Quinn SF, Franzini DA, Demlow TA, et al. MR imaging of the prostate cancer with an endorectal surface coil technique: correlation with whole-mount specimens. Radiology 1994;190:323.

170. Outwater EK, Petersen RO, Siegelman ES, et al. Prostate carcinoma: assessment of diagnostic criteria for capsular penetration on endorectal coil MR images. Radiology 1994;193:333.

171. Chelsky MJ, Schnall MD, Seidmon EJ, et al. Use of endorectal surface coil magnetic resonance imaging for local staging of prostate cancer. J Urol 1993;150:391.

172. Petros JA, Catalona WJ. Lower incidence of unsuspected lymph node metastases in 521 consecutive patients with clinically localized prostate cancer. J Urol 1992;147:1574.

173. Spencer JA, Golding SJ. Patterns of lymphatic metastases at recurrence of prostate cancer: CT findings. Clin Radiol 1994;49:404.

174. Knudson G, Grinis G, Lopez-Majano V, et al. Bone scan as a stratification variable in advanced prostate cancer. Cancer 1991;68:316.

175. Shih WJ, Mitchell B, Wierzbinski B, et al. Prediction of radionuclide bone imaging findings by Gleason histologic grading of prostate carcinoma. Clin Nucl Med 1991;16:763.

176. Gerber G, Chodak GW. Assessment of value of routine bone scans in patients with newly diagnosed prostate cancer. Urology 1991;37:418.

177. Chybowski FM, Keller JJL, Bergstralh EJ, et al. Predicting radionuclide bone scan findings in patients with newly diagnosed, untreated prostate cancer: prostate specific antigen is superior to all other clinical parameters. J Urol 1991;145:313.

178. Andriole GL, Catalona WJ, Becich M. Predicting radionuclide bone scan findings in patients with newly diagnosed, untreated prostate cancer: prostate specific antigen

is superior to all other clinical parameters. J Urol 1992;147:
474.

179. Terris MK, Klonecke AS, McDougall IR, et al. Utilization of
bone scans in conjunction with prostate-specific antigen levels
in the surveillance for recurrence of adenocarcinoma after
radical prostatectomy. J Nucl Med 1991;32:1713.

180. Saitoh H, et al. Metastatic patterns of prostate cancer:
correlation between the sites and number of organs involved.
Cancer 1984:54:3078.

181. Baker ME, Silverman PM, Korobkin M. Computed
tomography of prostatic and bladder rhabdomyosarcomas. J
Comput Assist Tomogr 1985;9:780.

182. Shapiro E, Strother D. Pediatric genitourinary
rhabdomyosarcoma. J Urol 1992;148:1761.

183. Kawada T, Hashimoto K, Tokunaga T, et al. Two cases of
penile cancer: magnetic resonance imaging in the evaluation
of tumor extension. J Urol 1994;152:963.

184. Small JD, Albertsen PC, Graydon RJ, et al. Adenoid cystic
carcinoma of Cowper's gland. J Urol 1992;147:699.

185. Backus ML, Mack LA, Middelton WD, et al. Testicular
microlithiasis: imaging appearances and pathologic
correlation. Radiology 1994;192:781.

186. Schiff SF, Lachman MF, Hammers L. Paratesticular myxoma:
case report and review. J Urol 1993;149:132.

187. Rayan DM, Lesser BA, Crumley LA, et al. Epididymal
sarcoidosis. J Urol 1993;149:134.

188. Tammela TLJ, Karttunen TJ, Mäkäräinen HP, et al.
Intrascrotal adenomatoid tumors. J Urol 1991;146:61.

189. Gooding GAW, Leonhardt W, Stein R. Testicular cysts: US
findings. Radiology 1987;163:537.

190. Grunert RT, Van every MJ, Uehling DT. Bilateral
epidermoid cysts of the testicle. J Urol 1992;147:1599.

191. Vanzulli A, DelMaschio A, Paesano P, et al. Testicular masses
in association with adrenogenital syndrome. Radiology 1992;
183:425.

192. Grantham JG, Charboneau JW, James EM, et al. Testicular
neoplasms studied by high-resolution US. Radiology 1985;
157:775.

193. Schwimer SR, Jacobson E, Lebovic J. Seminoma in an
atrophic testis: ultrasound evaluation. J Ultrasound Med
1987;6:97.

194. Horstman WG, Melson GL, Middleton WD, et al. Testicular
tumors: findings with color Doppler US. Radiology 1992;
185:733.

195. Moorjani V, Mashankar, Goel S, et al. Sonographic
appearance of primary testicular lymphoma. AJR 1991;157:
1225.

196. Thurnher S, Hricak H, Carroll PR, et al. Imaging the testis:
comparison between MR imaging and US. Radiology 1988;
167:631.

197. Williams MP, Husband JE, Heron CW. Stage I
nonseminomatous germ cell tumors of the testis: radiologic
follow-up after orchidectomy. Radiology 1987;164:671.

198. Kwok CK, Horowitz MD, Livingstone AS, et al. Mature
testicular teratoma with vena caval invasion presenting as
pulmonary embolism. J Urol 1993;149:129.

62

Transrectal Ultrasonography

Katsuto Shinohara

INTRODUCTION

Transrectal ultrasonography (TRUS), first clinically used for prostate imaging in 1968 (1), has greatly aided the diagnosis of prostate cancer. It is now widely used for detecting, monitoring, and staging prostate cancer. It is also used to guide a biopsy needle accurately in a suspected area. This chapter explains the current role of TRUS in prostate cancer management.

EQUIPMENT AND PROCEDURE

Generally a 5 to 7.5-MHz transducer is used for transrectal prostate imaging. Axial, mechanical sector, linear, or phased array scanners are available. Current equipment generally has either a biplane or end-firing probe to obtain both transverse and longitudinal images. With each type, images are slightly different, and sonographers must be familiar with both (Figs. 62.1 and 62.2). This chapter explains the anatomy of the gland, the biopsy procedure, and diagnosis and staging of prostate cancer on the basis of images obtained with the biplane probe.

Placing the patient in either the right or left lateral position makes the procedure easier than if he is in the lithotomy position. The transducer is inserted through the anus, and images of the prostate, seminal vesicles, and bladder neck are obtained through the rectal wall. To obtain better images, a water bath is often used (i.e., 30 to 50 mL water in a balloon around the probe tip). Before imaging, a Fleet enema (Lynchburg, VA) should be given to minimize artifacts.

PROSTATE ANATOMY

Historically, the prostate gland was believed to be composed of five lobes (2). However, it is essential to understand the zonal anatomy described by McNeal to interpret ultrasound images (3, 4).

The normal prostate gland is divided into three zones: transition, peripheral, and central. In addition, the fibromuscular stroma is positioned anterior to the prostatic urethra (Fig. 62.3). The transition zone lies on both sides of the prostatic urethra. Normally this occupies only a small portion of the

prostate gland, but it may increase with age (benign prostatic hyperplasia). The central zone surrounds the ejaculatory duct. At the gland's base, it occupies the greatest part of the cross-sectional image, but diminishes at the level of the verumontanum where the ejaculatory ducts merge into the urethra. At the midportion and the apex, the peripheral zone occupies the majority of the gland. In benign prostatic hyperplasia, this zone is compressed posterolaterally by the enlarged transition zone and becomes the so-called surgical capsule. A group of glands at the level of the bladder neck in the midline underneath the trigone may get hyperplasia and grow into the bladder lumen. This is so-called median lobe hyperplasia on cystoscopy finding (5). McNeal et al. reported that 68% of prostate cancers arise from the peripheral zone, whereas only 24% and 8% of cancers arise from the transition and central zones, respectively (6). The prostatic urethra passes through the anterior half of the prostate and changes direction anteriorly about 45° at the level of the verumontanum. The ejaculatory ducts are the continuation of the ampulla of the vasa deferentia and seminal vesicles and penetrate the prostate gland from the posterocranial aspect; they change direction anteriorly near the level of the verumontanum to open into the urethra.

NORMAL PROSTATE

Transverse Plane

The echogenic, relatively homogeneous peripheral zone surrounds the posterolateral aspect of the urethra at the apex (below the verumontanum) (Fig. 62.4). The transition zone begins to be visualized as a relatively coarse area of lower echogenicity on both sides of the urethra above the verumontanum. The verumontanum is often seen as an inverted V-shaped structure in the middle of the gland. The ejaculatory duct complex (composed of the paired ejaculatory ducts and sometimes the utricle surrounded by a fibrous tissue layer) is seen in the midline posterior to the urethra as a small hypoechoic area. The peripheral and the central zone are not clearly differentiated on ultrasonography and are seen as a relatively fine, homogeneous,

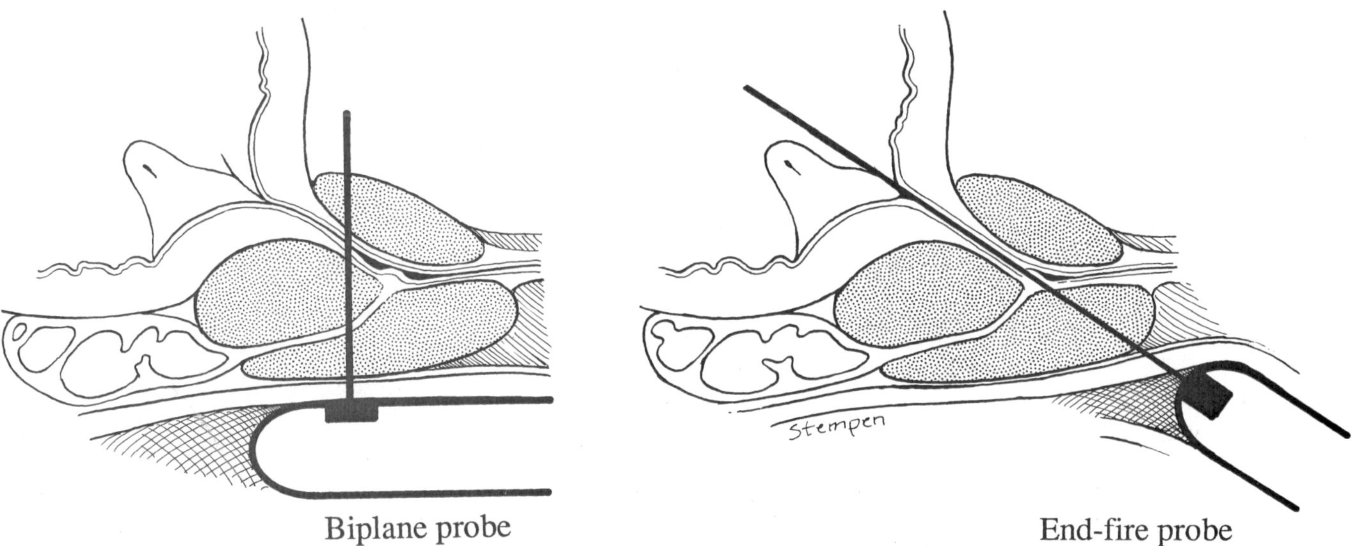

Fig. 62.1. **Left.** Diagram showing scanning plane of the biplane probe. Transverse scanning plane is perpendicular to the rectal wall. **Right.** Transverse scanning plane with end-fire probe is actually oblique frontal section. The plane is almost parallel to the proximal part of the prostatic urethra.

echogenic area surrounding the transition zone and the urethra (Fig. 62.5). At the base of the gland, the fibromuscular stroma is seen as an area of very low echogenicity anterior to the urethra. The rest of the tissue surrounding the urethra is mainly central zone, which exhibits relatively homogeneous, fine echogenicity (Fig. 62.6).

The neurovascular bundle is seen at the posterolateral aspect of the gland on both sides. Anteriorly, the dorsal vein complex and Santorini venous plexus are seen as anechoic fluid-filled structures. The vascular pedicle of the prostate is seen between the seminal vesicle and the base of the gland. Further outside, the levator ani, obturator internus, and pubic bone are seen. Posterior to the prostate, adventitia and muscularis propria of the rectum are seen. The ampullae of the vasa deferentia are seen behind the bladder trigone as two round hypoechoic structures. The seminal vesicles extend posterolaterally from the ampullae. The vascular pedicle of the prostate is seen anterior to the seminal vesicle on both sides (Fig. 62.7).

Sagittal Plane

In the midline image, the bladder neck, prostatic urethra, ejaculatory duct complex, and membranous urethra are visible. The tissue between the urethra and the ejaculatory duct complex is the central zone; the hypoechoic tissue anterior to the urethra is the anterior fibromuscular stroma; and the rest of the tissue

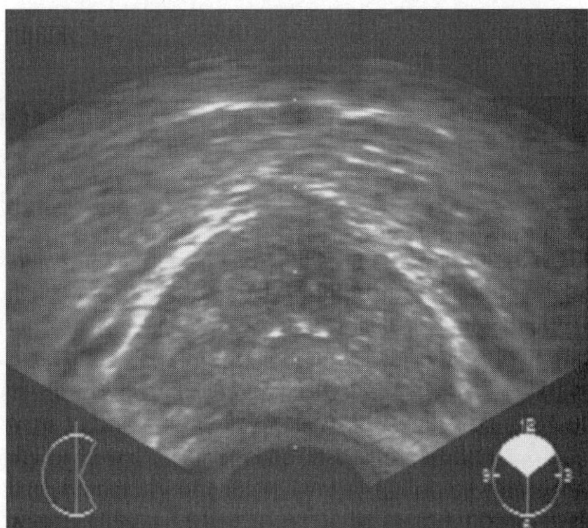

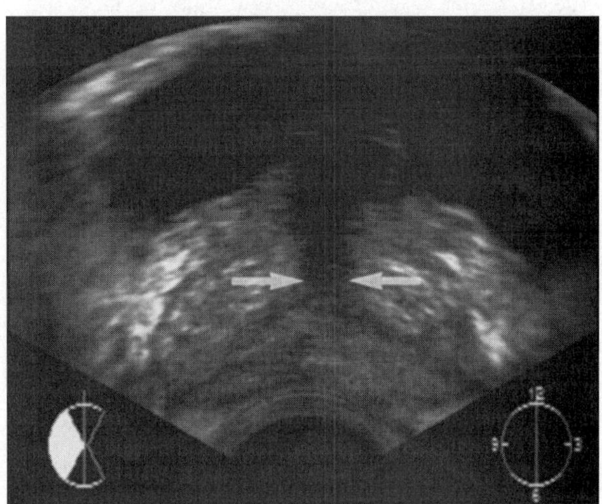

Fig. 62.2. **A.** Transverse scan of the midprostate gland by biplane probe. **B.** Same case with end-fire probe. The verumontanum and the urethra form Eiffel tower sign (arrow), since the scanning plane is parallel to the urethra.

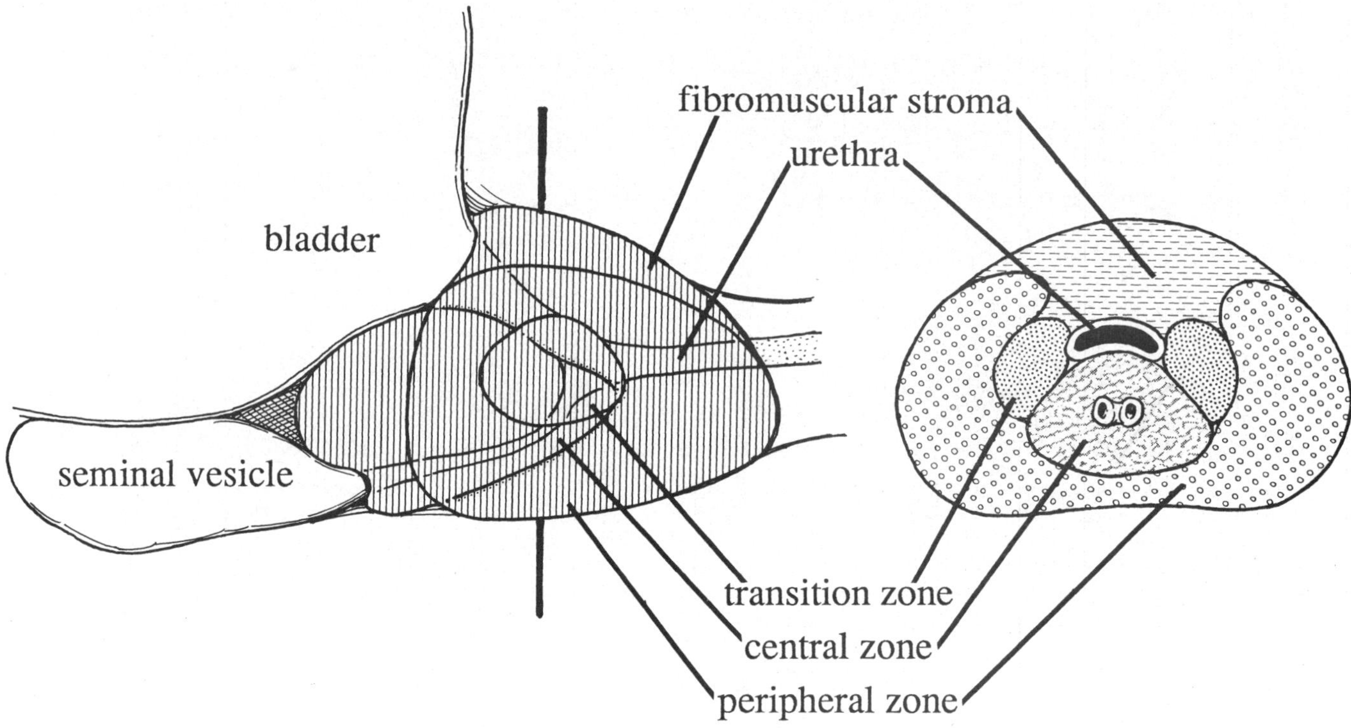

Fig. 62.3.   Diagrams showing the anatomy of the prostate.

is the peripheral zone (Fig. 62.8). In the midline image, the transition zone is not seen. At slightly off the midline, the sagittal image shows the transition zone surrounded by the peripheral and central zones (Fig. 62.9). Further laterally, the sagittal section shows only the peripheral and central zones (Fig. 62.10). The bladder trigone muscle and the ureteral orifices are often appreciated on this view. At the apex, the dorsal vein complex is seen anterior to the membranous urethra. The corpus spongiosum is seen as a structure of low echogenicity caudal to the apex of the prostate. The membranous urethra originates at the apex and enters into the corpus spongiosum and becomes the bulbar urethra. The shape of the apex varies significantly among individuals. Sometimes prostate apical tissue extends behind the membranous urethra. Knowing the

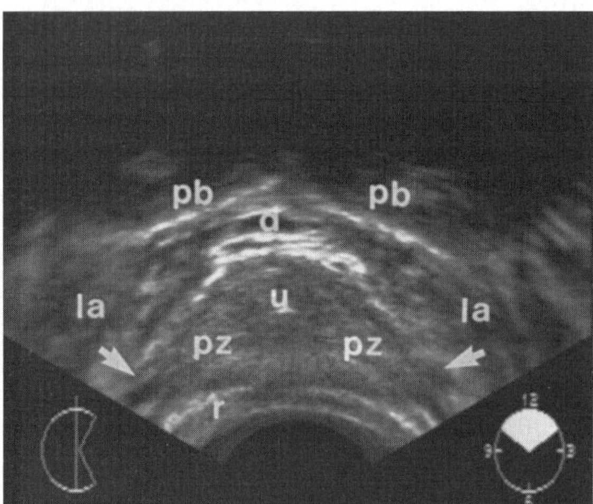

Fig. 62.4.   Transverse scan of the prostate at the apex. Urethra (u) surrounded by peripheral zone (pz) is visible. Neurovascular bundle is seen at the posterior lateral aspect of the gland as a hypoechoic structure (arrows). Pubic bone (pb), levator ani (la), dorsal vein (d), and muscularis propria of rectum (r) are also seen.

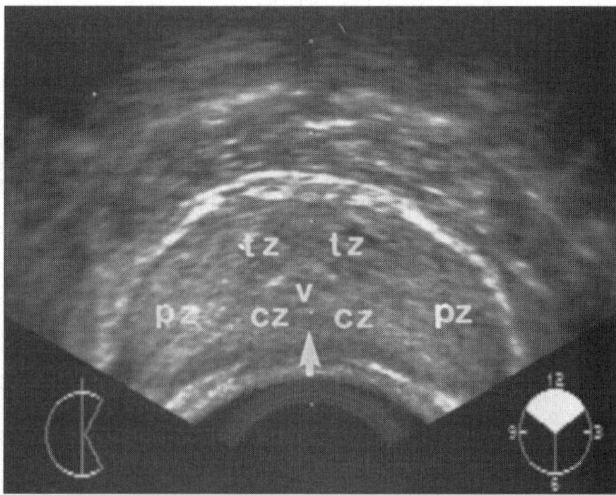

Fig. 62.5.   Transverse scan of the midgland. Transition zone (tz) is visible on both sides of the urethra. Verumontanum (v) is seen as an inverted V-shaped structure. Peripheral zone (pz) is the area with fine homogeneous echo surrounding the transition zone. Central zone (cz) is the area surrounding the ejaculatory duct complex; however, it is not differentiated from the peripheral zone sonographically.

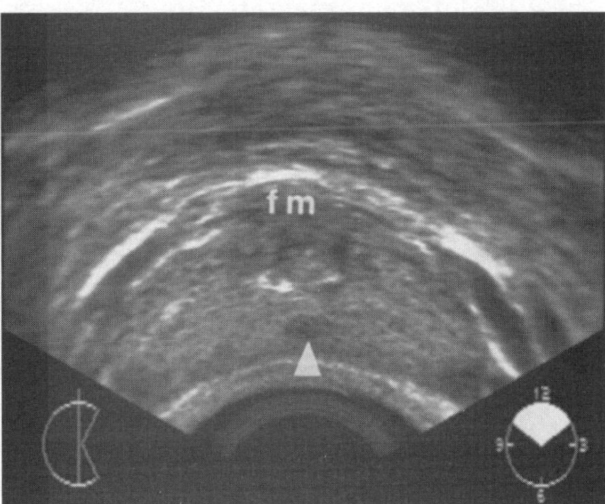

Fig. 62.6. Transverse scan at the base of the gland. Anterior fibromuscular stroma (fm) is seen as a hypoechoic area anterior to the urethra. Central zone occupies the majority of this section. However, central zone and peripheral zone cannot be differentiated. The ejaculatory duct complex is seen as a small hypoechoic area posterior to the urethra.

shape before a radical prostatectomy helps clear dissection of the apex (Fig. 62.11).

BENIGN PROSTATIC HYPERPLASIA

The anatomy of the prostate gland is usually altered significantly by various conditions in elderly men. In the clinic setting, the population is usually elderly with prostates that are rarely normal but are often hyperplastic or atrophied or contain calcifications or cystic degeneration. In a prostate with benign hyperplasia, the transition zone is enlarged and the fibrous tissue dividing it from the peripheral zone is often clearly seen as a hypoechoic layer. The peripheral and central zones are

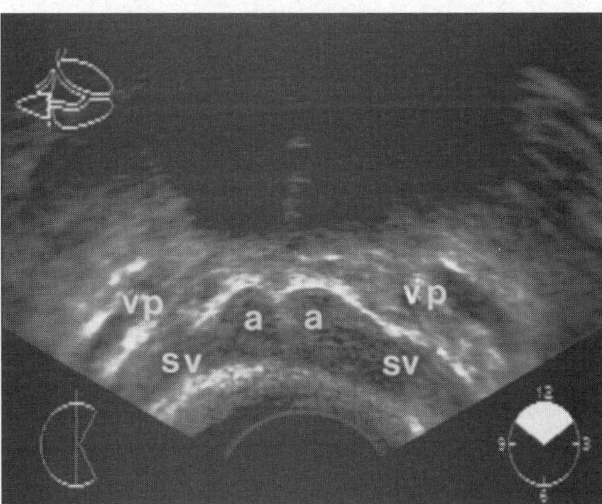

Fig. 62.7. Transverse scan of the seminal vesicles. Ampullae of vasa deferentia (a) are seen anteromedially and seminal vesicles (sv) are seen posterolaterally. Vascular pedicle (vp) of the prostate is seen anterior to the seminal vesicle as multiple hypoechoic structures.

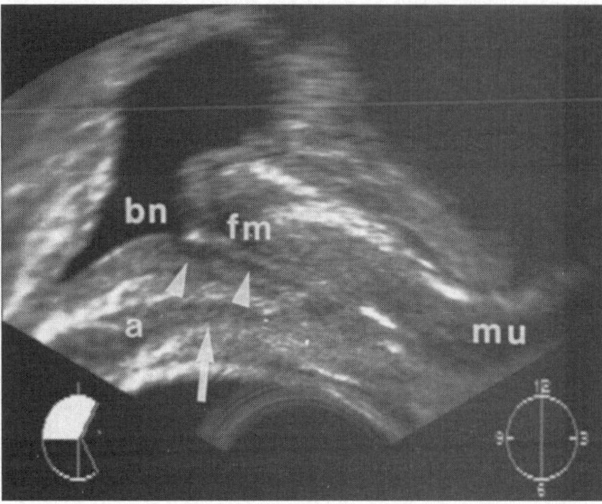

Fig. 62.8. Longitudinal scan of the normal prostate in the midline. Bladder neck (bn) surrounded by fibromuscular stroma (fm) is seen. Prostatic urethra and periurethral sphincter are seen as a parallel linear structure (arrowheads). Ejaculatory duct complex (arrow) is seen as a continuation of the ampulla (a). Membranous urethra (mu) is seen distal to the apex.

compressed posteriorly and laterally and become very thin (Fig. 62.12). Arcuate linear calcifications are often seen at the posterior aspect of the transition zone; these represent prostatic calculi in the terminal portion of the prostatic ducts. Small degenerative cysts are also quite common with benign prostatic hyperplasia (Fig. 62.13). The echogenicity of the transition zone is generally heterogeneous and relatively low, which makes diagnosis of malignancy in this zone very difficult.

PROSTATE VOLUME MEASUREMENT BY TRUS

The prostate volume measurement is important in cancer management. Serial follow-up TRUS after hormone or radiation therapies may determine efficacy of the treatment. Prostate

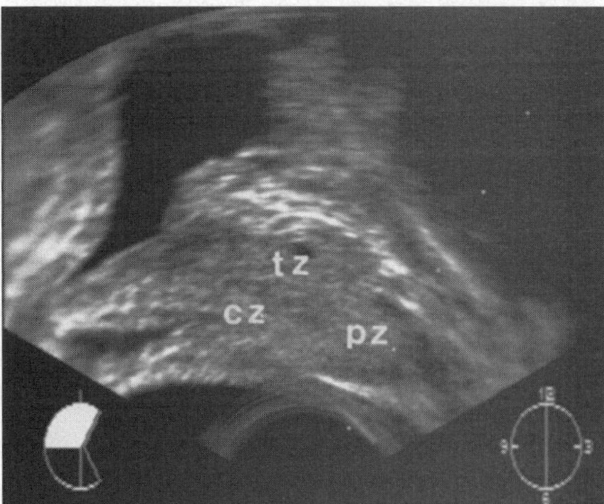

Fig. 62.9. Longitudinal scan of the prostate slightly off the midline. Transition zone (tz) is seen as a slightly low and coarse echoic area surrounded by peripheral (pz) and central zone (cz).

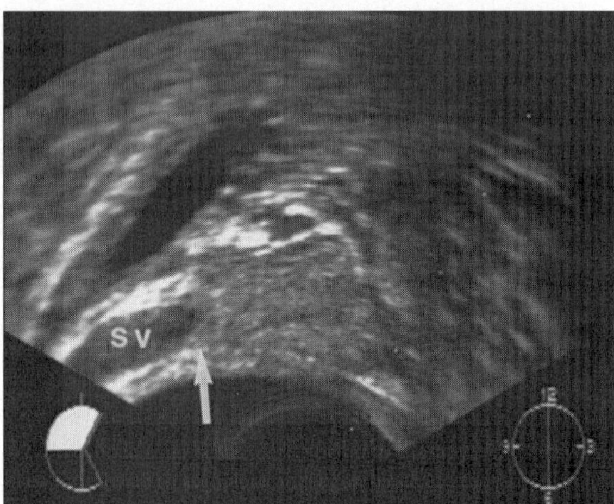

Fig. 62.10. Longitudinal scan of the gland at further lateral area. On this section, peripheral zone occupies the majority of the gland. Seminal vesicle (sv) is seen separated from the gland by a fat plane (arrow).

volume change generally represents the effectiveness of treatment. Prostate-specific antigen (PSA) density is an important adjunct for cancer detection. PSA density can be calculated by serum PSA value divided by prostate volume.

A planimetric technique with serial step sectioning (7) or a prorated ellipsoid method is used to calculate prostate volume. Generally, the prorated ellipsoid method (8) is easier and probably more reproducible than the planimetric method and is commonly used (Fig. 62.14). A prostate volume is calculated by the following formula using the prorated ellipsoid method.

$$V = A \times B \times C \times \pi/6 \text{ (approximately 0.52)}$$

Where A = transverse diameter, B = anterior-posterior diameter, and C = superior-inferior diameter.

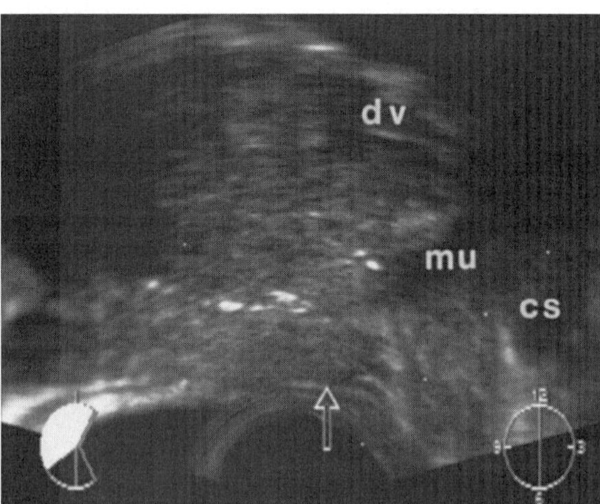

Fig. 62.11. Longitudinal scan of apex of the gland at midline. Membranous urethra (mu) is seen as a hypoechoic curved linear structure. This enters into the corpus spongiosum (cs). The prostate gland extends behind the membranous urethra and is often observed, as seen in this case (arrow). A dorsal vein complex (dv) is seen anterior to the urethra.

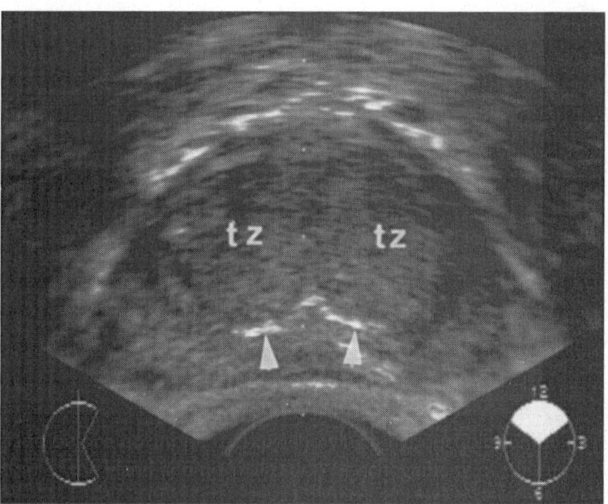

Fig. 62.12. Transverse scan of a BPH gland. Enlarged transition zone (tz) occupies the majority of the gland. Peripheral zone and central zone are compressed laterally. A hypoechoic fibrous tissue layer (arrowheads) separates transition zone from central and peripheral zone. Linear arcuate bright echoes represent prostatic calculi formed inside the distal part of the prostatic ducts.

Sometimes, the superior-inferior diameter measurement can be difficult and cannot be accurately obtained. In that case, V = $A^2 \times B \times \pi/6$ can be used to estimate the volume alternative to the prorated ellipsoid method (9).

DIAGNOSIS OF PROSTATE CANCER

Tumor Echogenicity

In the past, there was some confusion regarding the characteristic findings of prostate cancer, especially its echogenicity. In early studies, it was believed that malignancy characteristically exhibited high echogenicity; but since 1985, many studies have

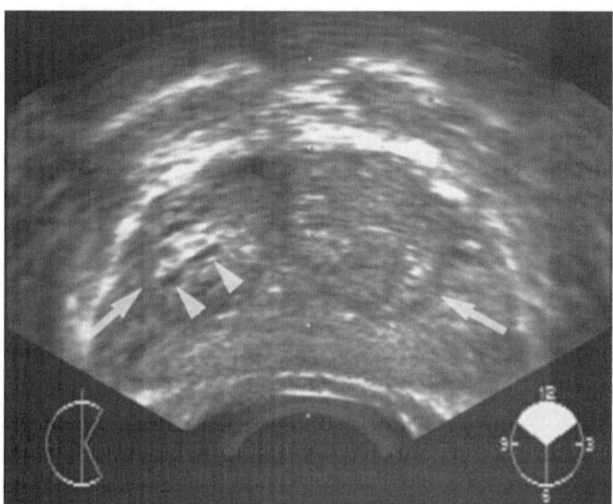

Fig. 62.13. Transverse scan of a BPH gland. Degenerative cysts (arrowheads) are also common findings in the gland in older men.

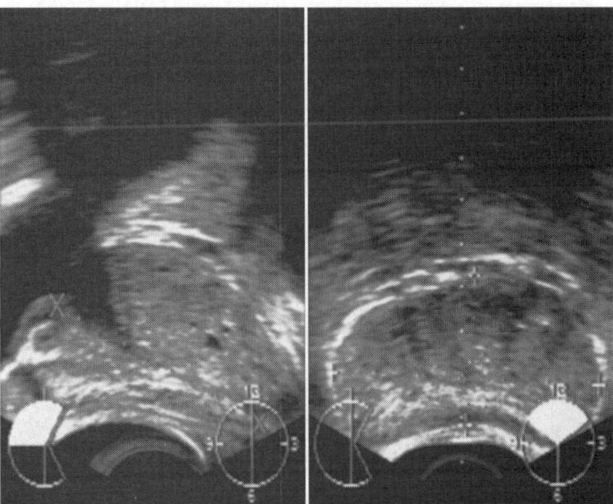

Fig. 62.14. Prostate volume measurement using prorated ellipsoid method. Three dimensions of the gland are measured, and the volume is calculated on the screen.

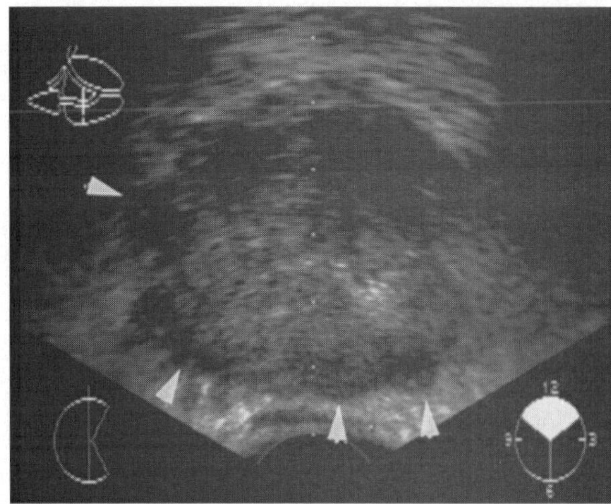

Fig. 62.16. Transverse sectional image of advanced prostate cancer. The gland shape is asymmetrical and distorted. The prostate outline is irregular and disrupted in many areas (arrowheads). The echogenicity of the gland is diffusely heterogeneous and low.

correlated the ultrasound images with pathologic findings on surgical specimen and have shown a hypoechoic area to be more characteristic (Fig. 62.15) (10–12). However, not every cancer is hypoechoic. Approximately 25 to 30% of clinically detectable prostatic cancers are reportedly isoechoic and nearly invisible on TRUS (13). The size and shape of the tumor, its histologic type, the amount of benign glandular tissue remaining in the tumor area, and the echogenicity of surrounding tissue all influence the echogenicity of the tumor (14). Prostate cancer showing hyperechogenicity is rare but has been reported (15).

In advanced cancer, the diagnosis is relatively easy by noting the irregularity, asymmetry, and disruption of the gland's outline (Fig. 62.16). In early cancer, however, the existence of a hypoechoic area may be the only sign. However, in the prostate gland, there are many hypoechoic areas that could be normal anatomic structures, artifacts, or benign conditions (Table 62.1). In many cases, a hypoechoic tumor is associated with a

mass effect (e.g., bulging of the prostate outline or distortion of the internal anatomic structure) that differentiates tumor from a benign condition or artifact.

Diagnosis of Isoechoic Tumor

Approximately 25 to 30% of prostate cancers are isoechoic and cannot be differentiated from the normal tissue on ultrasonography (Table 62.2). These tumors are detected by digital rectal examination or by elevated PSA. Although the tumor area is not visible, its existence is often suspected on ultrasound because of the deformity of the gland, such as asymmetry, bulge, or loss of roundness of the contour (Fig. 62.17).

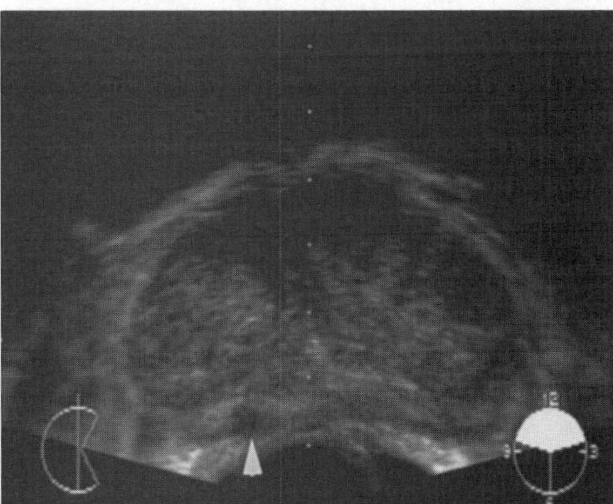

Fig. 62.15. Transverse scan of a prostate with typical hypoechoic tumor (arrowhead).

Table 62.1.   Conditions That May Produce Hypoechoic Areas in the Prostate

Normal Anatomical Structure
   Urethra
   Anterior fibromuscular stroma
   Ejaculatory duct complex
   Prostate capsule
   Seminal vesicles and ampullae
   Periprostatic veins
   Neurovascular bundle
Benign Disease
   Hyperplasia
   Granulomatous and non-specific prostatitis
   Cysts
   Hematoma
Artifacts
   Inappropriate use of DGC adjustment
   Acoustic shadowing
   Edge effect (reflection and refraction)
   Reverberation artifact

Table 62.2.   Sonographic Appearance of Confined (stage A, B or T1, T2) and Not Confined (Stage C or T3, T4) Prostate Cancer

SONOGRAPHIC APPEARANCE

FEATURES	CONFINED	NOT CONFINED
Prostate shape	• symmetrical • semilunar • concave posterior outline	• asymmetrical • distorted • convex posterior outline
Echogenicity	• homogeneous ± focal hypoechoicity	• diffusely heterogeneous • large hypoechoic area
Internal anatomy	• preserved	• distorted
Prostate boundary	• clear, • smooth • round	• fuzzy • irregular • bulging • loss of roundness • disruption
Seminal vesicles	• symmetrical • clear appreciation of ampullae • concave shape • fat plane between prostate and seminal vesicle	• asymmetrical in shape and echogenicity • unclear ampullae • thickened base • convex shape • loss of fat plane between prostate and seminal vesicle • abnormal tissue posterior to the ampullae

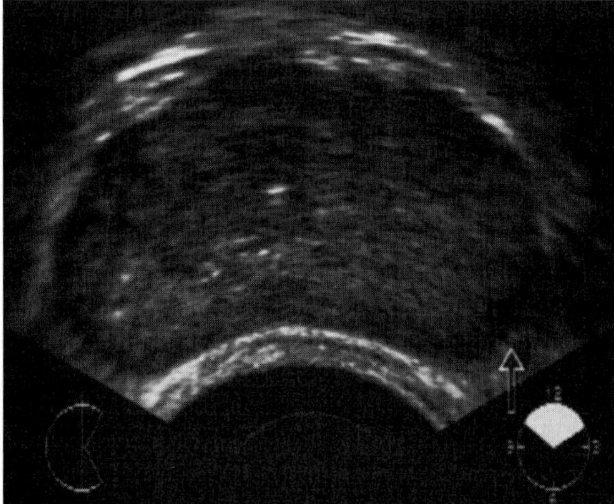

Fig. 62.17.   Transverse scan of the midgland shows a loss of roundness in the left lobe, although the echogenicity of the area is unremarkable (arrow). Biopsy of this area revealed Gleason 3 + 3 adenocarcinoma.

PROSTATE BIOPSY

Indication

Biopsy of the prostate gland is indicated if PSA is elevated, a palpable prostate nodule is detected, or an abnormal hypoechoic lesion is found. Biopsy is the definitive diagnostic procedure, and it is very important to guide the needle into the suspicious area accurately and obtain a good amount of tissue. In an early cancer, tumor volume may be small, and random biopsy may easily miss it. The maximum effort in detecting the suspicious area to perform a lesion directed biopsy is always recommended. Ultrasound-guided biopsy is more accurate than finger-guided biopsy in directing the needle into the suspected area, even when the lesion is clearly palpable. However, if the palpable nodule is not clearly seen on TRUS, at least one biopsy must be done under finger guidance. One cannot rely on ultrasound to guide the needle into the nodule in that case. If an elevated PSA is the only abnormal finding, multiple random biopsies, as described by Hodge et al., are indicated (16). PSA density can help differentiate a PSA elevation caused by benign tissue from that caused by a malignancy (17).

Current positive biopsy rates among patients referred for prostate biopsy to our clinic are presented in Table 62.3 according to PSA, digital rectal examination, and TRUS findings.

Preparation

A Fleet enema and antibiotics, commonly fluoroquinolones, are recommended before prostate biopsy to prevent sepsis. Patients with a history of heart valve disease or knee or hip replacement (or any prosthesis) require antibiotic coverage as recommended by the American Heart Association (AHA) guidelines (18). Patients receiving anticoagulation therapy must not undergo biopsy without their dosage first being adjusted to bring the coagulation status to normal.

Procedure

An 18-gauge biopsy needle loaded in a spring-action automatic biopsy device is commonly used. Prostate biopsy can be done transrectally or transperineally under ultrasound guidance. Because the former approach requires no anesthesia, it can be done with the same patient positioning as for prostate imaging and more easily accesses multiple sites; this has generally been preferred over transperineal biopsy.

The patient is placed in the right or left lateral position. After the prostate images are obtained, a biopsy guideline is placed onto the suspicious lesion. With the biplane probe, the biopsy is done on the sagittal view. If the suspicious lesion is not clearly appreciated, it can first be found on transverse image. With the end-fire probe, biopsy can be done on either transverse or sagittal view. Once the biopsy guide is aligned on the suspicious area, a biopsy needle is inserted into the guide (Fig. 62.18). The needle tip must be placed right at the

Table 62.3. Positive Biopsy Rate According to Digital Rectal Examination (DRE), Prostate Specific Antigen (PSA), and Transrectal Ultrasonography (TRUS) Findings

					Findings				
DRE*	+	+	+	−	+	−	−	−	
PSA**	+	+	−	+	−	+	−	−	
TRUS	+	−	+	+	−	−	+	−	Total
No.	217	57	140	83	75	126	39	29	766
Positive	150	9	40	33	3	28	5	0	268
%	69	16	29	40	4	22	13	0	35

* Asymmetry of the gland is considered to be negative finding.

** PSA less than 4.0 ng/mL by IMX assay is considered to be negative.

boundary of the suspicious lesion before triggering the biopsy device to obtain the tissue from the lesion accurately. If the prostate capsule is "tented up" by the needle tip, tissue may be taken from too deep inside the gland and a tumor located in the periphery may be missed.

For a systematic random biopsy, biopsy of the apex, midportion, and base of the gland in both lobes (sextant biopsy) is commonly performed. However, with bigger glands, the number of biopsies should theoretically be increased (if more than 50 mL, transition zone biopsy—at least—should be added to increase cancer detection) (19).

STAGING WITH TRUS

It has been reported that TRUS is superior to digital rectal examination in staging prostate cancer; however, recent reports have shown discouraging results (20–23). Although papers clearly stating the criteria for differentiating stage A and B (T1, T2) from stage C (T3, T4) are few, disappearance or disruption of the prostate capsule, irregularity, and asymmetry of the prostate or seminal vesicle are generally used (Figs. 62.19 and 62.20) (24). With these criteria, microscopic tumor extension cannot be diagnosed, although gross tumor extension can be picked up. Rosen et al. have reported that a significant number of clinically localized tumors will be shown to be unconfined on surgical pathology. They found extracapsular extension and seminal vesicle invasion in up to 85% and 35%, respectively, of stage T2c tumors. A positive surgical margin was found in 40% of these patients (25). Clearly, detecting microscopic focal tumor extension is important for reducing positive surgical margins. Ohori et al. have shown that, even if the prostate capsule appears intact, focal tumor extension should be suspected if the hypoechoic area bulges out from the boundary, the boundary is irregularly serrated, or the prostate contour loses its roundness (Figs. 62.21 and 62.22) (26).

Asymmetry of the seminal vesicles has been said to be the sign of seminal vesicle invasion (27, 28). However, early on, the shape does not change dramatically. In addition, asymmetrical seminal vesicles are not rare in the healthy population. Salo et al. and Pontes et al. have reported the specificity of TRUS in seminal vesicle invasion to be very high, but the sensitivity to be only 25 to 29% because of overlooked early invasion (29, 30). Three routes of seminal vesicle invasions are known.

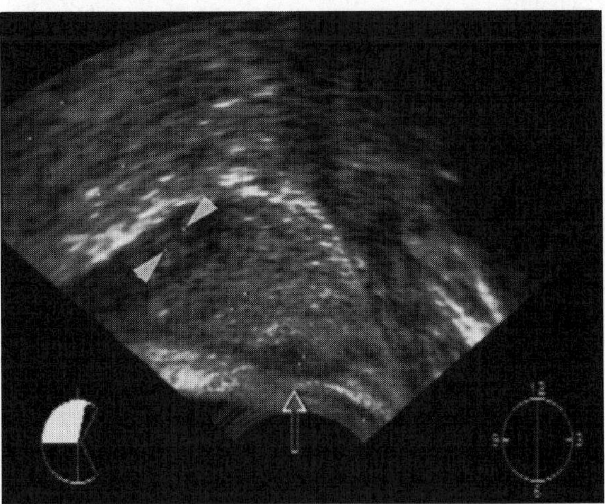

Fig. 62.18. Biopsy guide line (arrow) is aligned on the suspected hypoechoic area (arrowheads).

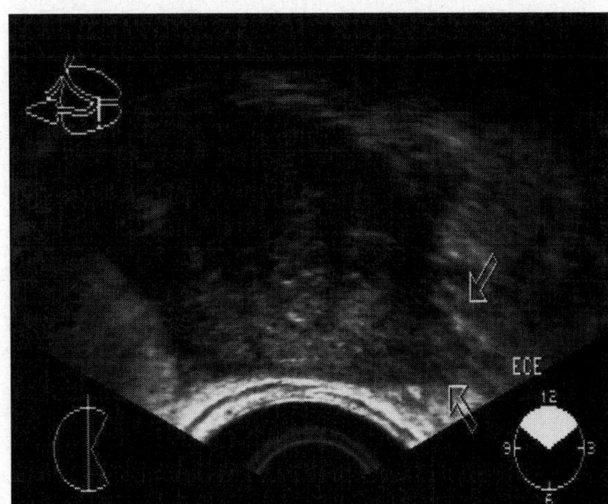

Fig. 62.19. Transverse scan of the prostate showing gross tumor extension through the capsule, noted by a disruption of capsule and tumor extension outside the gland (arrows).

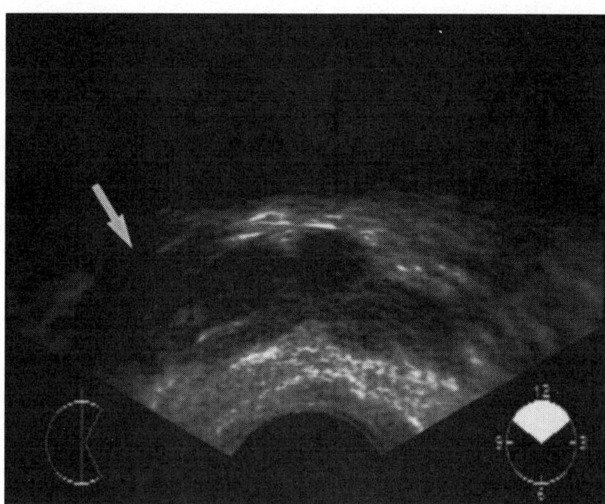

Fig. 62.20.   Transverse scan of the seminal vesicle grossly involved by cancer. The seminal vesicle is asymmetrical with hypoechoic and thickened right side (arrow).

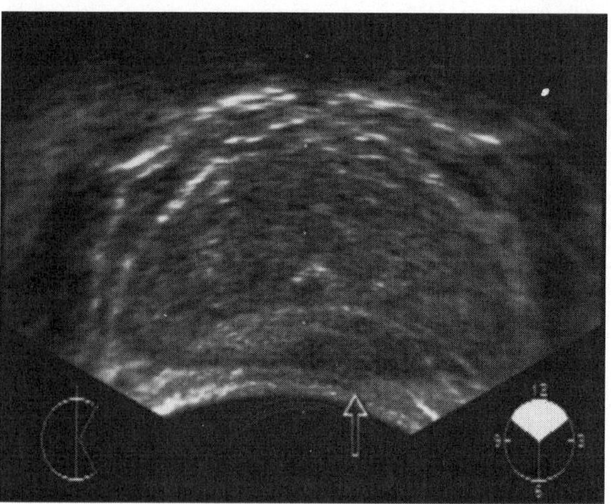

Fig. 62.22.   Transverse scan at the midgland. A hypoechoic area is seen in the left lobe (arrow) with a slight bulge and fuzzy outline. Tumor extension through the prostatic capsule is found in this area.

1. Along the ejaculatory ducts with medial invasion into ampulla and seminal vesicles.
2. Lateral invasion via the vascular pedicle of the prostate with external entry into the seminal vesicle.
3. Metastasis without communication between the prostate and seminal vesicle lesion (31).

In the first case, the seminal vesicle may retain symmetry, but the base of the seminal vesicle thickens and shows convexity toward the rectum (Fig. 62.23). In the second case, cancer is located in the lateral aspect of the prostate. Widening of the angle between the prostate and seminal vesicle, a bridge of hypoechoic tissue between them, and disappearance of the intervening fat plane are the characteristic signs (Fig. 62.24) (32). Careful observation of the junction of the seminal vesicle and

the prostate—not the body of the seminal vesicle—is important in diagnosing early invasion. If suspicion arises on the basis of these findings, the base of the seminal vesicle must be biopsied (33). The procedure is the same as in the prostate biopsy, and the specimen can easily be obtained transrectally. The biopsy specimen must be obtained at the junction of the prostate and the seminal vesicle, as tumor invasion always begins from the gland.

A comparison of reported results of staging accuracy by TRUS and radical prostatectomy specimen is listed in Table 62.4. (23, 34–38). These reports, however, used different equipment, criteria, and histologic methods and were based on the highly selected group of patients who were candidates for radical prostatectomy. Wolf et al. and Gerber et al. reported enhanced TRUS staging results by including PSA value, tumor volume measurement, and Gleason grade (39, 40). Careful examination with good knowledge of early signs of tumor spread should increase the accuracy of TRUS in staging.

TRUS MONITORING AFTER TREATMENT

Follow-up TRUS After Hormone Manipulation

TRUS has been used to monitor changes in local tumor after hormone manipulation. Its clinical use is limited, but TRUS can demonstrate significant volume reduction of the prostate size after these treatments. Approximately 30 to 40% volume reduction is generally observable 3 months after initiation of hormone treatment (Fig. 62.25). In addition to prostate volume reduction, normalization of tumor echogenicity and disappearance of the characteristic sign of extracapsular extension or seminal vesicle invasion are sometimes observed after hormone treatment (41, 42). In our study, reduction in size of the tumor area was more significant than a reduction in prostate size, but disappearance of extracapsular extension or seminal vesicle

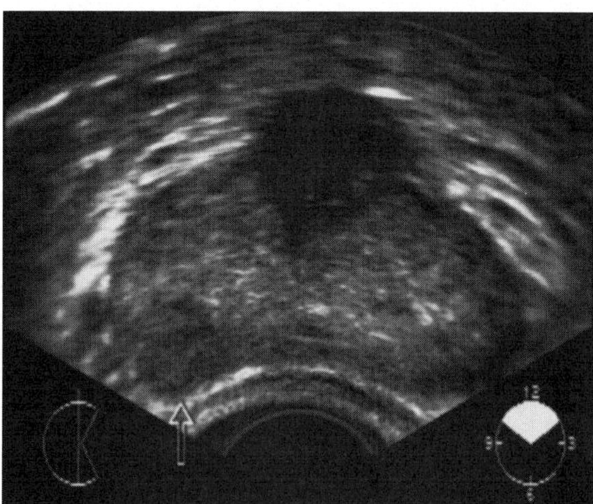

Fig. 62.21.   Transverse scan at the midgland. A hypoechoic area bulges out from the prostate outline, and the boundary of the gland loses normal roundness in the area (arrow). Periprostatic tumor extension is found in this area on histologic study of the radical prostatectomy specimen.

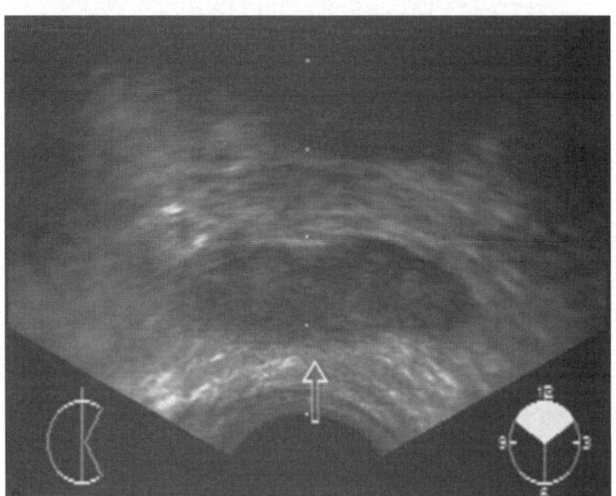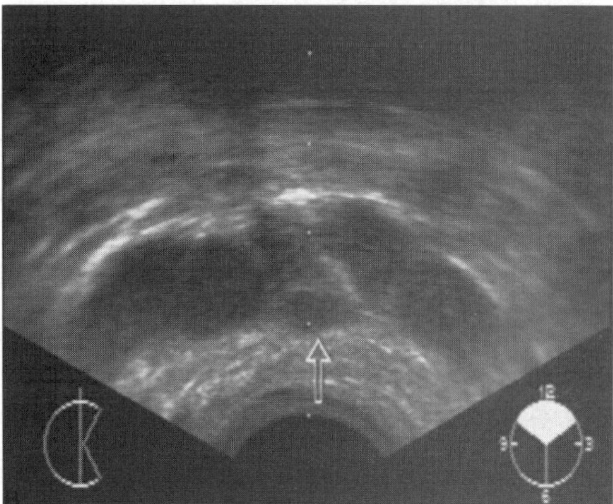

Fig. 62.23.   Seminal vesicle invasion type I. **A.** Transverse scan of the base of the seminal vesicle showing posterior convexity of the outline (arrow). **B.** Transverse section of the base of the seminal vesicle showing abnormal hypoechoic tissue extending behind the ampullae (arrow).

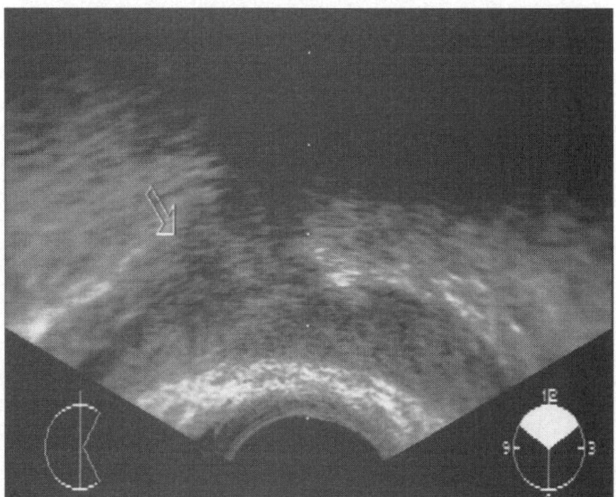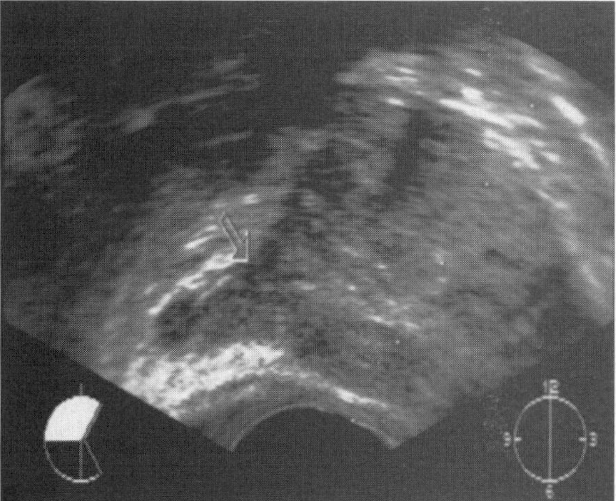

Fig. 62.24.   Seminal vesicle invasion type II **A.** Transverse scan of the base of the seminal vesicle showing hypoechoic tissue anterior to the right seminal vesicle (arrow). **B.** Longitudinal scan of the right seminal vesicle and right lobe in same case. Hypoechoic tissue bridges the prostate and seminal vesicle, and a fat plane normally seen between the prostate and seminal vesicle is lost (arrow).

Table 62.4.   Overall Staging Accuracy of TRUS in Published Studies

	NO.	SENSITIVITY (%)	SPECIFICITY (%)	PPV (%)	NPV (%)	ACCURACY (%)
Perrapato et al., 1989 (34)	25	71	100	100	90	92
Andriole et al., 1989 (35)	64	38	90	55	81	77
Rifkin et al., 1990 (36)	219	66	46	63	49	58
McSherry et al., 1991 (23)	25	29	88	83	37	48
Hamper et al., 1991* (37)	125	68	91	80	85	83
Wolf et al., 1993 (38)	155	48	84	71	59	64

* Prediction of extracapsular extension only.

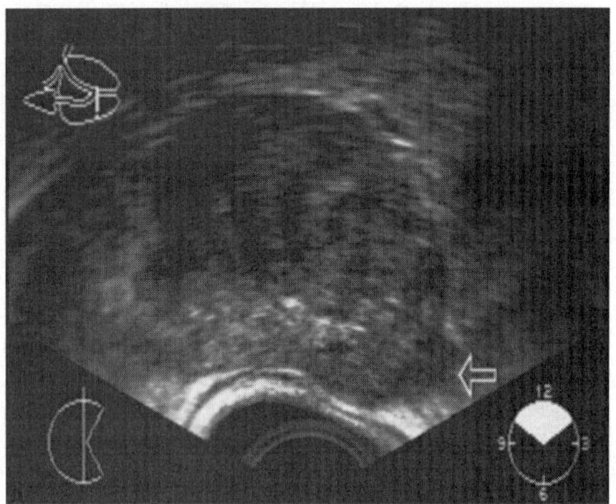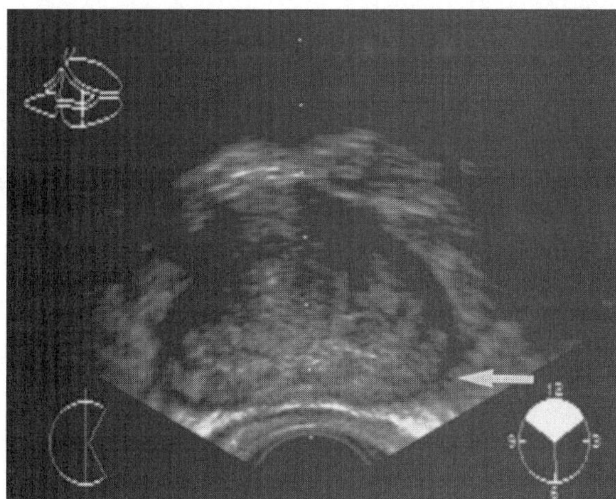

Fig. 62.25.   Follow-up scans after hormone therapy. **A.** Transverse scan of the midgland before hormone therapy showing a hypoechoic tumor (arrow). **B.** Three months after complete androgen blockade therapy. Significant volume reduction of the gland and normalization of echogenicity of the tumor area are noted (arrow).

invasion was rare after 3 months of combined androgen block-ade in stage T3 tumor (43).

Follow-up TRUS After Radiation Treatment

After radiation therapy, findings are similar to those with hor-mone therapy. Prostate gland volume reduction, normalization of echogenicity in the tumor area, and disappearance of extra-capsular extension or seminal vesicle invasion have been re-ported (Fig. 62.26). Volume reduction, however, is found to be less significant and to take longer than after hormone treatment (44). Rectal wall thickening, echo scattering, and subsequent blurring of the prostate boundary are often observed in the irradiated prostate gland (Fig. 62.27). In patients who undergo radioactive seed implantation, bright echo spots associated with the comet sign (reverberation of the seeds) are seen at seeding

locations (Fig. 62.28). Persistence of hypoechoic area at 18 months after radiation treatment (45) and repeat elevation of PSA after its nadir has been reached warrant suspicion of tumor recurrence. Biopsy of the prostate is indicated in these cases.

Detection of Local Recurrence After Radical Prostatectomy

After radical prostatectomy, the anatomy is completely differ-ent. Usually, sagittal section describes the anatomy well (46, 47). The bladder neck, tubularized segment of the bladder wall, anastomotic site, membranous urethra, and corpus spongiosum are clearly visible on this view (Fig. 62.29). The anastomotic site is usually seen as the area where the hypoechoic membra-nous urethra becomes the echogenic tubularized segment of the bladder wall. Sometimes small calcifications are seen at

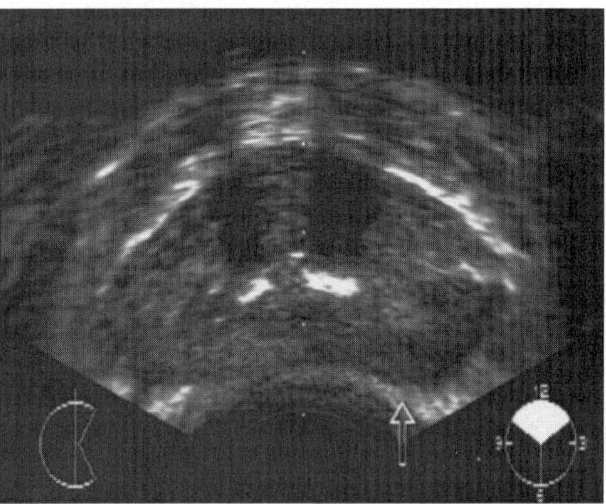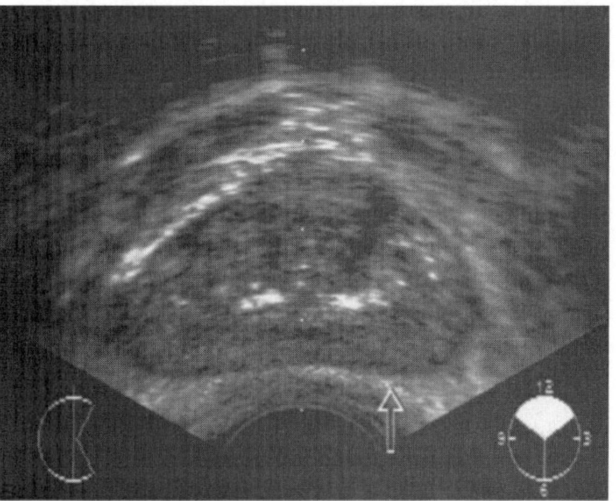

Fig. 62.26.   Follow-up scans after radiation therapy. **A.** Transverse scan of the base of the gland before radiation therapy. A large hypoechoic tumor is seen in the left lobe (arrow). **B.** Nine months after radiation therapy. Significant volume reduction of both prostate and tumor area is noted.

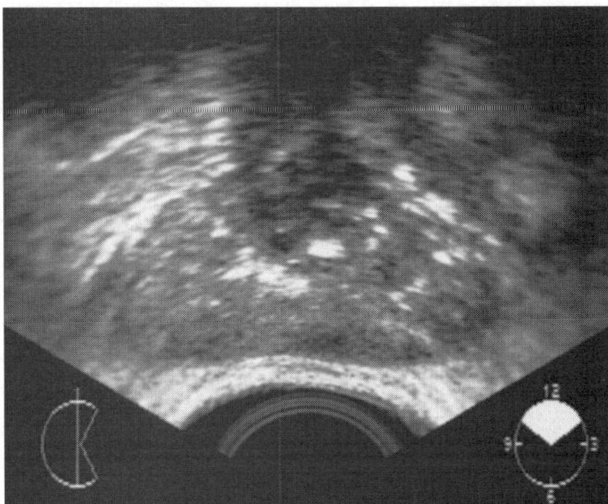

Fig. 62.27. Transverse scan of the irradiated prostate gland. The rectal wall is thickened and more echogenic. The entire image is blurred because of strong scatterings of the ultrasound.

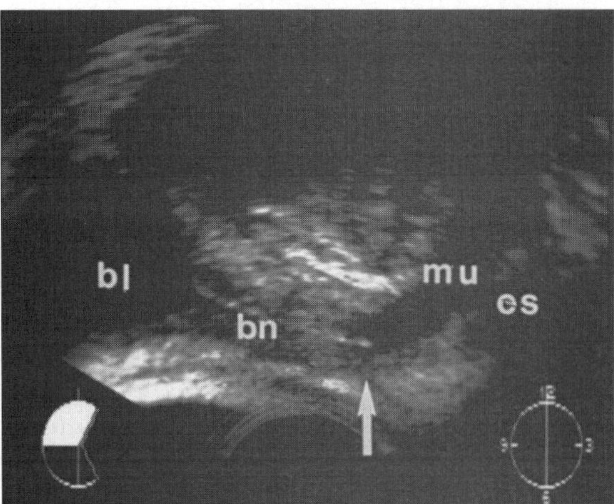

Fig. 62.29. Normal anatomy after radical prostatectomy. Longitudinal scan showing anastomotic site (arrow). Note that the echogenicity changes at the junction between the bladder neck and the membranous urethra. Bladder neck (bn); membranous urethra (mu); bladder (bl); corpus spongiosum (cs).

the site early after radical prostatectomy, probably indicating anastomotic sutures. Local recurrence is frequently seen at the posterior and lateral aspect of the anastomotic site, although it can occur anterior to it, at the level of the bladder neck, or in the retrovesical space (Fig. 62.30) (48). It is never seen distal to the anastomotic site. Understanding the postoperative anatomy and localizing the anastomotic site are therefore very important. Local recurrence is generally seen as a hypoechoic mass or thickening of the tissue around the anastomotic site. Detectable PSA usually suggests possible local recurrence; even 0.1 ng/mL may be a sign. Palpable nodules in the prostatic fossa only account for 29% of local recurrence detected in our experience. The biopsy procedure for local recurrence is the same as described previously. Gross hematuria after biopsy of the anastomotic site is more common than after regular biopsy, as the needle frequently traverses the urethra and bladder.

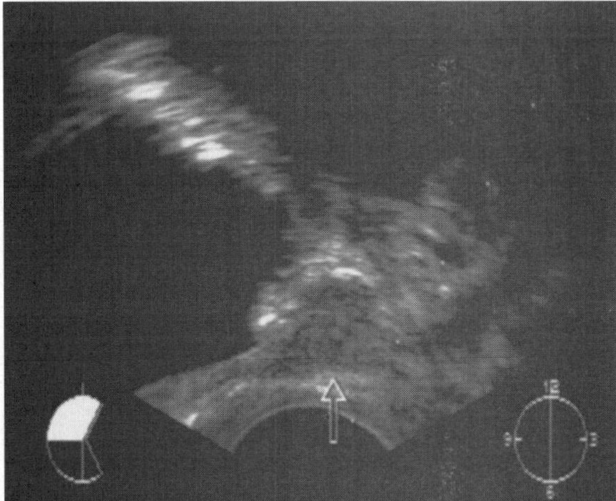

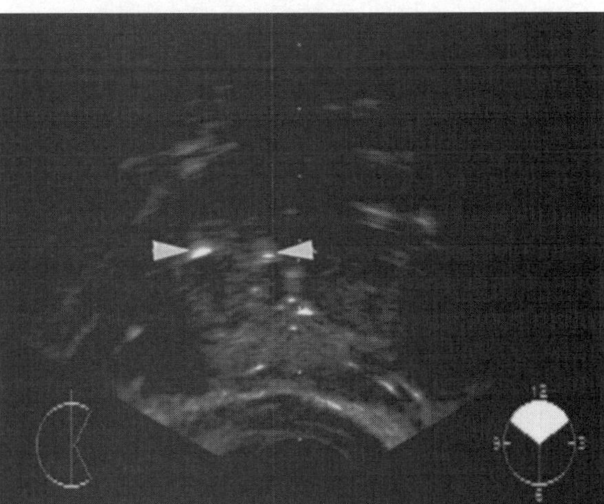

Fig. 62.28. Transverse scan at the base after implantation of radioactive seeds. Some bright echoes with reverberations behind them (comet sign) are seen (arrowheads).

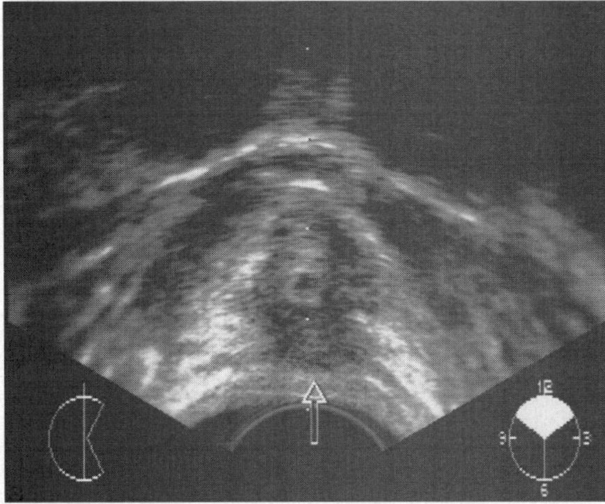

Fig. 62.30. Typical local recurrence after radical prostatectomy. **A.** Longitudinal scan at the anastomotic site. A hypoechoic mass is seen around the anastomotic site (arrow). **B.** Transverse scan slightly proximal to the anastomosis. A hypoechoic mass is seen mainly posterior to the bladder neck (arrow).

REFERENCES

1. Watanabe H, Kato H, Kato T, et al. Diagnostic application of ultrasonotomography for the prostate. Jpn J Urol 1968;59:273.

2. Lawsley OS. The development of the human prostate gland with reference to the development of other structure at the neck of the urinary bladder. Am J Anat 1912;13:299.

3. McNeal JE. Regional morphology and pathology of the prostate. Am J Clin Pathol 1968;49:347.

4. McNeal JE. The prostate and prostatic urethra: a morphologic study. J Urol 1972;107:1008.

5. McNeal JE. Origin and evolution of benign prostatic enlargement. Invest Urol 1978;15:340.

6. McNeal JE, Redwine EA, Freiha FS, et al. Zonal distribution of prostatic adenocarcinoma, correlation with histologic pattern and direction of spread. Am J Surg Pathol 1988;12:897.

7. Watanabe H, Igari D, Tanahashi Y, et al. Measurement of size and weight of prostate by means of transrectal ultrasonotomography. Tohoku J Exp Med 1974;114:277.

8. Littrup PJ, Williams CR, Egglin TK, et al. Determination of prostate volume with transrectal US for cancer screening. part II. accuracy of in vitro and in vivo techniques. Radiology 1991;52:49.

9. Terris MK, Stamey TA. Determination of prostate volume by transrectal ultrasound. J Urol 1991;145:984.

10. Lee F, Gray JM, McLeary RD, et al. Transrectal ultrasound in the diagnosis of prostate cancer: location echogenicity, histopathology, and staging. Prostate 1985;7:117.

11. Dähnert WF, Hamper UM, Eggleston JC, et al. Prostatic evaluation by transrectal sonography with histopathologic correlation: the echogenic appearance of early carcinoma. Radiology 158:97.

12. Shinohara K, Wheeler TM, Scardino PT. The appearance of prostate cancer on transrectal ultrasonography: correlation of imaging and pathological examinations. J Urol 1989;142:76.

13. Ellis WJ, Brawer MK. The significance of isoechoic prostatic carcinoma. J Urol 1994;152:2304.

14. Shinohara K, Scardino PT, Carter SSC, et al. Pathologic basis of the sonographic appearance of the normal and malignant prostate. Urol Clin North Am 1989;16:675.

15. Egawa S, Wheeler TM, Greene DR, et al. Unusual hyperechoic appearance of prostate cancer on transrectal ultrasonography. Br J Urol 1992;69:169.

16. Hodge KK, McNeal JE, Terris MK, et al. Random systematic versus directed ultrasound-guided biopsies of the prostate. J Urol 1989;142:71.

17. Shinohara K, Wolf JS Jr, Narayan P, et al. Comparison of prostate specific antigen with prostate specific antigen density for 3 clinical applications. J Urol 1994;152:120.

18. Dajani AS, Bisno AL, Chung KJ, et al. Prevention of bacterial endocarditis. recommendations by the American Heart Association. JAMA 1990;264:2919.

19. Lui PD, Terris MK, McNeal JE, et al. Indication for ultrasound guided transition zone biopsies in the detection of prostate cancer. J Urol 1995;153:1000.

20. Rorvik J, Halvorsen OJ, Servoll E, et al. Transrectal ultrasonography to assess local extent of prostatic cancer before radical prostatectomy. Br J Urol 1994;73:65.

21. Lorentzen T, Nerstrom H, Iversen P, et al. Local staging of prostate cancer with transrectal ultrasound: a literature review. Prostate Suppl 1992;4:11.

22. Ebert T, Schmitz-Drager BJ, Burrig KF, et al. Accuracy of imaging modalities in staging the local extent of prostate cancer. Urol Clin North Am 1991;18:453.

23. McSherry SA, Levy F, Schiebler ML, et al. Preoperative prediction of pathological tumor volume and stage in clinically localized prostate cancer: comparison of digital rectal examination, transrectal ultrasonography and magnetic resonance imaging. J Urol 1991;146:85.

24. Scardino PT, Shinohara K, Wheeler TM, et al. Staging of prostate cancer: value of ultrasonography. Urol Clin North Am 1989;16:713.

25. Rosen MA, et al. Frequency and location of extracapsular extension and positive surgical margin in radical prostatectomy specimens. J Urol 1992;148:331.

26. Ohori M, Egawa S, Shinohara K, et al. Detection of microscopic extracapsular extension prior to radical prostatectomy for clinically localized prostate cancer. Br J Urol 1994;74:72.

27. Spirnak JP, Resnick MI. Clinical staging of prostatic cancer: new modalities. Urol Clin North Am 1984;11:221.

28. Griffith GJ, Clements R, Jones DR, et al. The ultrasound appearances of prostate cancer with histological correlation. Clin Radiol 1987;38:219.

29. Salo JO, Kivisaari I, Rannikko S, et al. Computerized tomography and transrectal ultrasound in assessment of local extension of prostatic cancer before radical retropubic prostatectomy. J Urol 1987;137:435.

30. Pontes JE, Eisenkraft S, Watanabe H, et al. Preoperative evaluation of localized prostatic carcinoma by transrectal ultrasonography. J Urol 1985;134:289.

31. Ohori M, Scardino PT, Lapin SL, et al. The mechanism and prognostic significance of seminal vesicle involvement by prostate cancer. Am J Surg Pathol 1993;17:1252.

32. Ohori M, Shinohara K, Wheeler TM, et al. Ultrasonic detection of non-palpable seminal vesicle invasion: a clinicopathological study. Br J Urol 1993;72:799.

33. Terris MK, McNeal JE, Freiha FS, et al. Efficacy of transrectal ultrasound-guided seminal vesicle biopsies in the detection of seminal vesicle invasion by prostate cancer. J Urol 1992;148:829.

34. Perrapato SD, Carothers GG, Maatman TJ, et al. Comparing clinical staging plus transrectal ultrasound with surgical-pathologic staging of prostate cancer. Urology 1989;33:103.

35. Andriole GL, Coplen DE, Mikkelsen DJ, et al. Sonographic and pathological staging of patients with clinically localized prostate cancer. J Urol 1989;142:1259.

36. Rifkin MD, Zerhouni EA, Gatsonis CA, et al. Comparison of magnetic resonance imaging and ultrasonography in staging early prostate cancer: results of a multi-institutional cooperative trial. N Engl J Med 1990;323:621.

37. Hamper UM, Sheth S, Walsh PC, et al. Capsular transgression of prostatic carcinoma: evaluation with transrectal US with pathologic correlation. Radiology 1991;178:791.

38. Wolf JS Jr, Shinohara K, Carroll PR, et al. Combined role of transrectal ultrasonography, Gleason score, and prostate-specific antigen in predicting organ-confined prostate cancer. Urology 1993;42:131.

39. Wolf JS Jr, Shinohara K, Narayan P. Staging of prostate

cancer. accuracy of transrectal ultrasound enhanced by prostate-specific antigen. Br J Urol 1992;70:534.

40. Gerber GS, Goldberg R, Chodak GW. Local staging of prostate cancer by tumor volume, prostate-specific antigen, and transrectal ultrasound. Urology 1992;40:311.

41. Voges GE, Mottrie AM, Stockle M, et al. Hormone therapy prior to radical prostatectomy in patients with clinical stage C prostate cancer. Prostate Suppl 1994;5:4.

42. Pinault S, Tetu B, Gagnon J, et al.Transrectal ultrasound evaluation of local prostate cancer in patients treated with LHRH agonist and in combination with flutamide. Urology 1992;34:254.

43. Cher ML, Carroll PR, Small EJ, et al. Neoadjuvant androgen deprivation before radical prostatectomy: current status and trial design. In: Dawson NA, Vogelzang NJ, ed. Current clinical oncology: prostate cancer. New York: Wiley-Liss, 1994.

44. Fujino A, Scardino PT. Transrectal ultrasonography for prostatic cancer: its value in staging and monitoring the response to radiotherapy and chemotherapy. J Urol 1985;133:806.

45. Egawa S, Carter SS, Wheeler TM, et al. Sonographic monitoring of prostate cancer after definitive radiotherapy. Urology 1992;40:230.

46. Wasserman NF, Kapoor DA, Hildebrandt WC, et al. Transrectal US in evaluation of patients after radical prostatectomy: part 1. normal postoperative anatomy. Radiology 1992;185:361.

47. Foster LS, Jajodia P, Fournier G, et al. The value of prostate specific antigen and transrectal ultrasound guided biopsy in detecting prostatic fossa recurrences following radical prostatectomy. J Urol 1993;149:1024.

48. Shinohara K, Presti J Jr, Ingerman A, et al. Local recurrence after radical prostatectomy: characteristics in size, location and PSA. J Urol 1994;151:256. Abstract.

XV

ANCILLARY

63

Pelvic Exenteration in the Female Patient

Ely Brand

Even in medicine, though it is easy to know what wine, hellibore, cautery and surgery are, to know how and to whom and when to apply them so as to effect a cure is no less an undertaking than to be a physician.

ARISTOTLE NICHOMACHEAN
ETHICS IX

Few operations demand as much of the surgeon in skill and judgment as pelvic exenteration. Often the patient and physician have exhausted all therapeutic modalities in treating a pelvic malignancy, leaving extended surgery as the only hope of cure. Occasionally, a patient may require exenteration to extend the quality of remaining life although the hope of cure has passed (1). The operation is technically demanding and requires constant vigilance for many hours. Anterior exenteration consists of removal of the paraaortic and pelvic lymph nodes, bladder, distal ureters, vagina, uterus, Fallopian tubes, ovaries, and tumor with adjacent parametria and levator muscles. Posterior exenteration is rare and requires removal of the anus and rectosigmoid, while sparing the bladder and ureters. Total exenteration encompasses all the pelvic viscera and may occasionally include the vulva and inguinal lymph nodes (2). Often, the most challenging reconstructive phase begins only after a long day removing the tumor and adjacent viscera. Therefore, the procedure should be performed by two experienced surgeons operating in tandem. The well-thought-out exenteration begins with appropriate selection and counseling of the patient.

SELECTION OF THE PATIENT

The major indication for pelvic exenteration is centrally recurrent carcinoma of the cervix, particularly after pelvic irradiation but occasionally after radical hysterectomy and irradiation. The central recurrence rate for stage I disease after radiation is only 2%, but this increases to 17% for stage III disease. Stage IVA disease involving the bladder or rectal mucosa is not usually suitable for exenteration because of the high incidence of extrapelvic disease. After radiation or chemotherapy, some patients with residual disease in stage IVA may be salvaged by exenteration or they may require urinary or fecal diversion because of fistulae. Although the use of hydroxyurea (or cisplatin/5-fluorouracil) as radiosensitizers for advanced cervical carcinoma may improve survival, in a large Gynecologic Oncology Group study, the incidence of central pelvic recurrence was not diminished (3). Persistence of cervical carcinoma 8 to 12 weeks after radiation therapy is generally considered an indication for exenteration. The use of radical hysterectomy after full pelvic irradiation is fraught with complications, particularly fistulae requiring diversions that the physician sought to avoid by performing the radical hysterectomy (4).

Primary carcinomas of the vagina or urethra are best managed by radiation therapy but may occasionally require exenteration. Extensive vulvar carcinoma (stages III and IV) may require pelvic exenteration, although recent advances in preoperative radiation therapy, with or without chemotherapy, often allow more conservative surgery. Sarcoma botryoides is no longer managed by exenteration because of excellent response rates to vincristine, actinomycin D, and cyclophosphamide. Recurrent uterine sarcoma has been treated by exenteration. Recurrent carcinoma of the endometrium is best treated with radiation therapy and progestational agents, although a rare patient may be managed surgically. Extensive or recurrent carcinoma of the bladder, anus, or rectum may also be managed by pelvic exenteration.

Occasionally, carcinoma of the lower genital tract develops following pelvic irradiation. For instance, the patient radiated for cervical carcinoma in whom a vaginal primary develops many years later will require exenteration. Advanced stage diethylstilbestrol-related clear cell carcinoma of the vagina or cervix may require exenteration. Vulvovaginal or urethral melanoma may require exenteration and radical vulvectomy as a primary procedure because of the lack of effective chemotherapy or radiation therapy. By far, the majority of exenterations are undertaken for centrally recurrent postradiation cervical cancer.

After reviewing the initial histology and treatment, including radiation dosage, the surgeon should confirm that recurrent carcinoma is indeed present. The classic triad of sciatica, leg edema, and hydronephrosis is virtually pathognomonic for inoperability. In general, the shorter the interval from primary treatment to recurrence, the lower the likelihood of survival after exenteration. A diligent metastatic survey should follow. As a minimum, this includes computed tomography (CT) scans of the abdomen and pelvis with fine-needle cytology of any suspicious lymph nodes, chest radiographs, and liver function tests. CT scanning of the chest may disclose occult lesions in patients with adenocarcinoma or sarcoma. Magnetic resonance imaging (MRI) may be helpful in assessing whether tumor extends to the pelvic sidewall, although retroperitoneal detail is not necessarily improved with this modality. Preoperative intravenous pyelogram and barium enema facilitate surgical planning and rule out coexistent pathology. Hydronephrosis implies pelvic disease that is not resectable, but occasionally it results from obstruction of the distal or intravesical ureter and may allow exenteration. An upper gastrointestinal series with small bowel follow-through is important if small intestinal anastomosis or continent ileal diversion is planned.

The next step is counseling the patient about therapeutic options. This should not be undertaken in one session but is best staged to guide the patient through the defenses that accompany the diagnosis of recurrent carcinoma. We have found that women who have previously undergone exenteration are among the best support sources in newly diagnosed patients. Frank discussion of sexual rehabilitation is essential, and even abstinent patients are recommended a neovagina because of decreased postoperative morbidity in the reconstructed pelvis.

The patient should understand that a decision to complete the exenteration and the final decision as to type of exenteration can only be made intraoperatively. Approximately 50% of patients undergoing exploration will be found to be unresectable. The mortality from exenteration remains approximately 5% in most centers; however, the major morbidity is as high as 60%. The patient should have the psychologic fortitude to undergo a postoperative program of close follow-up and long-term rehabilitation.

PREOPERATIVE PREPARATION

Advanced age alone is not a contraindication to surgery, but careful selection of patients free from significant cardiopulmonary or renal disease is required. Routine spirometry and a baseline arterial blood gas are suggested. A chest radiograph and electrocardiogram are mandatory. Patients with serum albumin less than 3.0 or other signs of malnutrition benefit from preoperative parenteral hyperalimentation. Central venous access, at least 12 hours before surgery, will reduce the operative time and enable detection of complications, such as pneumothorax, while the patient is still awake. Pulmonary artery catheterization is preferred over central venous catheters because left atrial pressure correlates poorly with left ventricular end-diastolic pressure after pelvic exenteration.

Some authors routinely remove scalene nodes at a separate operation before laparotomy, but the yield of this approach in most hands remains relatively low. A 3-day bowel preparation is undertaken with clear liquids, enemas, and cathartics. Polyethylene glycol (Go-Lytely), 2 to 3 L on the afternoon before surgery, is an excellent cathartic that results in minimal electrolyte imbalance. Neomycin and erythromycin base (1 g) at 1:00 PM, 2:00 PM, and 11:00 PM are given orally. An enema of 2% neomycin (200 mL) is given on the morning of surgery. Potential stoma sites should be marked with methylene blue the day before surgery, with the patient both supine and sitting upright. Broad-spectrum prophylactic antibiotics are administered at least 1 hour before the skin incision, reinfused after 4 hours of surgery, and continued for 24 to 48 hours postoperatively. The patient takes hexachlorophene showers for 3 nights before surgery to reduce the bacterial skin count and uses a Betadine douche as well. Subcutaneous heparin, 5000 U every 8 hours, is started the night before surgery and timed so that no dose is given within 2 hours of surgery. It is helpful to begin intravenous fluids the day before surgery to allow slight hemodilution at the time of operation. The preoperative hematocrit should exceed 35%, with transfusion if needed.

POSITIONING THE PATIENT

After satisfactory induction of general anesthesia, the patient should be positioned by the surgeon in Allen stirrups allowing exposure of the perineum, vagina, and abdomen. Pneumatic compression stockings are placed. The abdomen is prepared to the nipple line, and the thighs should be prepared to the knees for access to gracilis myocutaneous flaps or split-thickness skin grafts. Great care is taken to avoid pressure on the peroneal nerves at the fibulae and to pad the soles of the foot, avoiding excessive dorsiflexion at the ankles (5). The hips should be flexed at approximately 30 to 35° and abducted no more than 45°. The knees can be extended or slightly flexed and the hips internally rotated (Fig. 63.1).

SELECTION OF THE TYPE OF EXENTERATION

Examination under anesthesia is the first critical test of operability. The tumor should be free from the pelvic sidewall. At times, it may be difficult to distinguish radiation fibrosis from recurrent tumor, although the former tends to be smooth, regular, and symmetric. If there is a possibility of resectability, the patient should be explored. Cystoscopy and proctosigmoidoscopy are performed to visualize tumor spread and as a last check if bladder or rectal conservation is planned. Bullous edema of the bladder heralds muscular infiltration and mandates cystectomy. Very low rectal anastomosis can be accomplished if 3 to 5 cm of tumor clearance is possible above the anal sphincter. Involvement of the lower vagina will require a wider perineal phase (vulvectomy) and levator resection. Urethral or labial

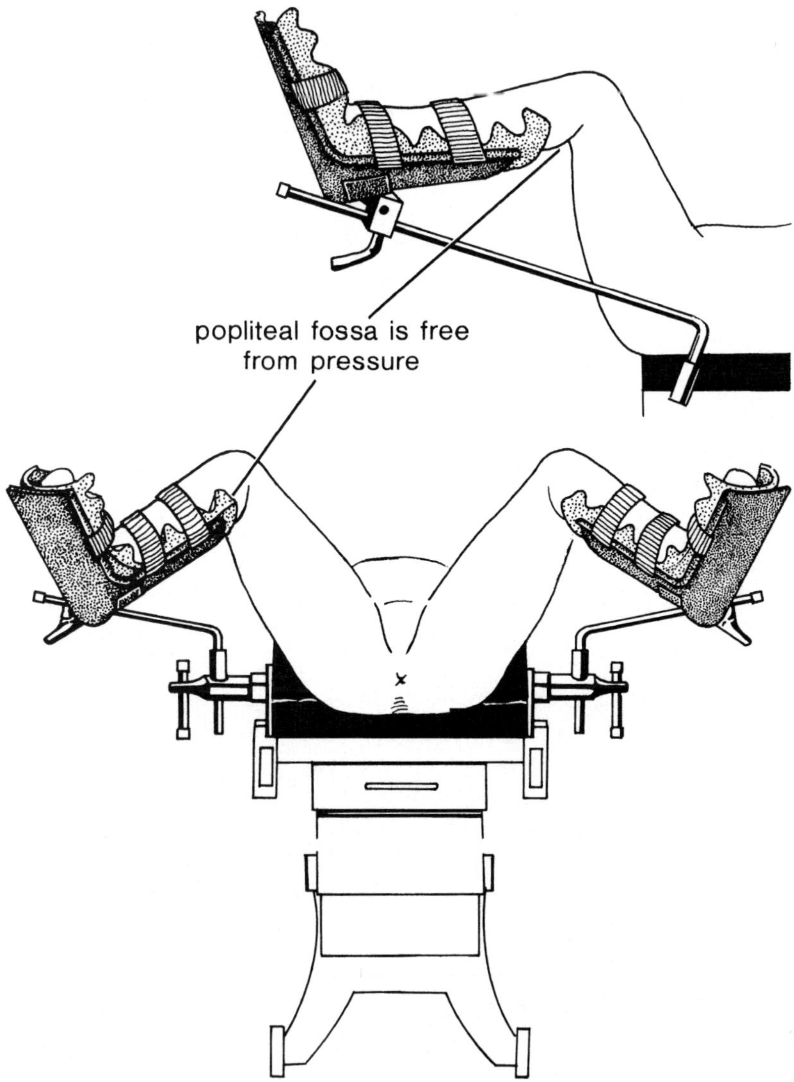

Fig. 63.1. Proper positioning of the patient in stirrups for the combined abdominoperineal approach.

involvement will require vulvectomy as well. Having assessed the gross spread of tumor and the degree of resection required, the surgeons prepare for exploratory laparotomy.

OPERATIVE PROCEDURE

Exploratory Laparotomy

Most surgeons favor a midline incision for adequate exposure and exploration of the upper abdomen, high paraaortic lymphadenectomy, use of a transverse colon conduit, and omental lid. However, a midline incision does not provide as much exposure in the pelvis, especially at the sidewalls, as does a transverse incision. Our preference is to use a Cherney incision (division of the rectus muscles at their tendinous insertion into the pubic symphysis) or Mallard (rectus cutting) incision. This allows for more facile pelvic surgery at the expense of limiting the aortic node sampling to below the inferior mesenteric takeoff.

After thorough evaluation of the upper abdomen for metastatic spread, the paraaortic nodes are palpated and any enlarged nodes are submitted for frozen section histology. Metastatic disease in the paraaortic nodes is an absolute contraindication to pelvic exenteration. In the absence of suspicious lymph nodes, formal paraaortic lymphadenectomy is begun.

Paraaortic Lymphadenectomy

The retroperitoneum is entered by dividing the round ligaments bilaterally. The incision extends cephalad, parallel to the infundibulopelvic ligaments. Usually, the cecum is mobilized along the line of Toldt and the ureter retracted medially. This will expose the common iliac vessels and lower inferior vena cava. Some surgeons continue lymphadenectomy to the level of the renal vessels. This may be easier to accomplish by a transmesenteric approach. Paraaortic node metastases contraindicate further surgery. Patients with centrally recurrent cervical carcinoma will have aortic node metastases in approximately 15% of cases, with no long-term survivors in this group.

Pelvic Exploration

To ascertain resectability in the pelvis, the pararectal and paravesical spaces are developed bluntly. Inability to develop free spaces at the pelvic sidewalls contraindicates pelvic exenteration, except in highly selected cases performed for palliation. After suture ligation and division of the round ligament near the canal of Nuck, the paravesical space can be developed with the back of a long DeBakey forceps or a straight Heaney retractor. Two forceps are placed against each other at the pelvic sidewall below the external iliac vessels, caudad to the round ligament and lateral to the ureters and the superior vesical artery. The angle of inclination is approximately 30°, pointing toward the apex of the vagina. With gentle spreading motions, the avascular potential space develops, pushing the vagina and bladder medially and the cardinal ligament posteriorly. In approximately 10% of patients, an aberrant obturator artery or vein arising from the external iliac will be noted and avoided. Exposure of the obturator nerve requires dissection more medially to avoid the obturator vein. The levator ani muscles form the floor of the paravesical space with the obturator internus muscle inferolaterally.

Next, the pararectal space is developed posterior to the cardinal ligament and lateral to the rectum. Staying close to the hypogastric vessels laterally will prevent incidental injury to the sigmoid and hemorrhoidal vessels medially on the left side. Inferiorly, the middle hemorrhoidal vessels should be avoided because they traverse the floor of the pararectal space. Aiming slightly caudally will avoid the gluteal branches of the hypogastric vessels. The intervening tissue between the pararectal and paravesical spaces constitutes the cardinal ligament, referred to as the vascular "web" by Meigs (Fig. 63.2). Although tumor extending to the levator or obturator muscles at the sidewall contraindicates exenteration, a frozen section is necessary to distinguish between radiation fibrosis and carcinoma.

Anterior Exenteration

The patient in whom anterior instead of total exenteration can encompass the tumor is one with a small central recurrence confined to the cervix and/or bladder. Parametrial extension is generally a contraindication to rectal preservation. The posterior vaginal fornices and posterior vagina should be free of disease on biopsy. Results of sigmoidoscopy and barium enema should be normal. Lesions larger than 3 cm are generally treated by total exenteration. Paradoxically, in a review from the University of Alabama, patients who had bladder invasion had only a 23% 5-year survival compared with 70% if disease was confined to the cervix (6). This may simply reflect the inadvisability of modified exenteration in patients with large lesions.

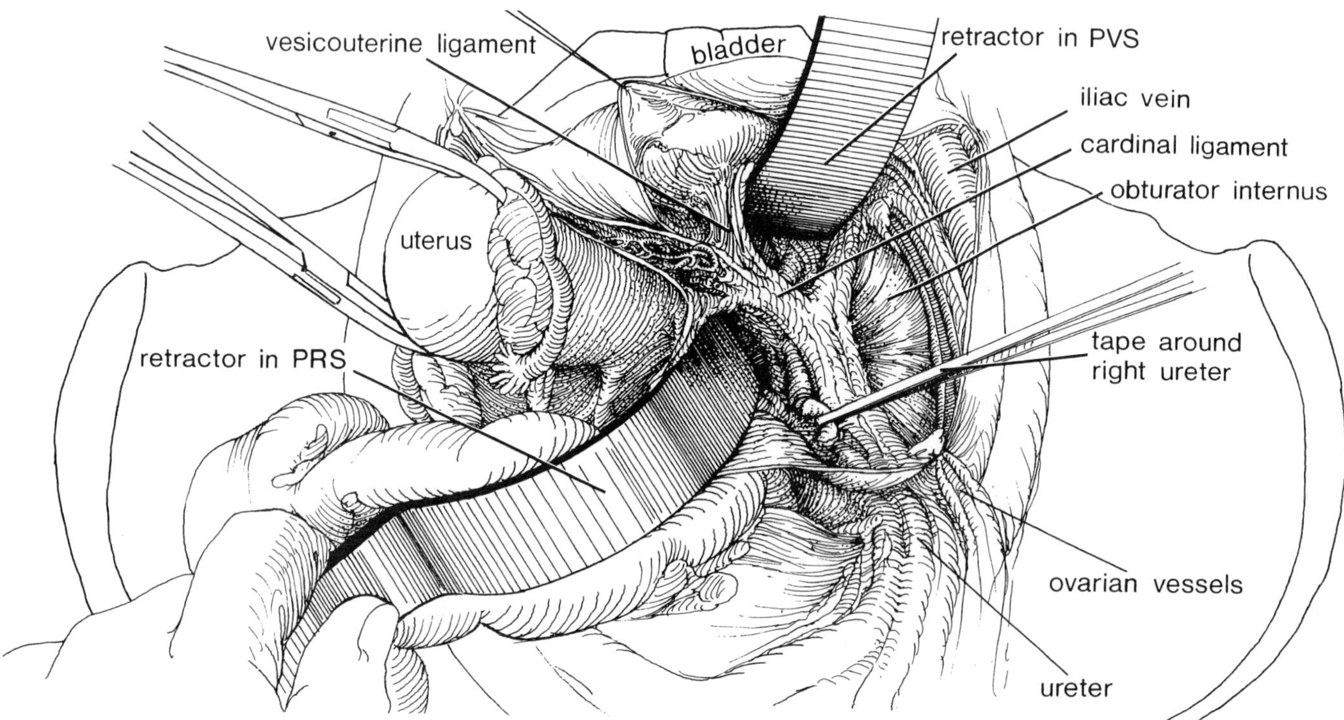

Fig. 63.2. Development of the paravesical (PVS) and pararectal (PRS) spaces with the intervening cardinal ligament between the spaces.

Anterior exenteration begins by ligating the uterine arteries at their origin from the hypogastric or superior vesical arteries. The superior vesical artery, the first branch of the anterior division of the hypogastric artery, is also ligated. Next the rectovaginal septum is developed by incising the peritoneum across the posterior cul-de-sac below the ureters. With firm elevation and caudal retraction of the uterus, the operator places a hand above the rectum and gently pushes it posteriorly in the midline. The volar surfaces of the fingers hold the vagina anteriorly. The dissection continues toward the inferior pubic ramus with the hand parallel to the floor. Induration or gross cancer here necessitates total exenteration. The uterosacral ligaments are divided between Heaney or Zeppelin clamps and suture ligated near the sacrum, taking care to avoid the rectum medially (Fig. 63.3). The ureters may be divided before or after this step. The lower the ureteral division, the greater mobility for later anastomosis, but the higher the radiation dose to the ureter. The ureters should not be dissected out of the cardinal ligaments. The ureters are mobilized with preservation of a sheath of peritoneum and then divided. Vascular clips may be placed to prevent drainage of urine in the operative field, or ureters may be stented, with the ends placed in a bag, to measure urine output until a conduit is formed. If significant bleeding is encountered, the hypogastric arteries can be isolated and ligated. Because most patients have received pelvic irradiation, the nonfunctioning ovaries should be removed. The infundibulopelvic ligaments are isolated above the ureters at the pelvic brim, ligated, and divided.

The bladder is detached from the lateral vesical ligaments in the space of Retzius using electrocautery. The filmy retropubic

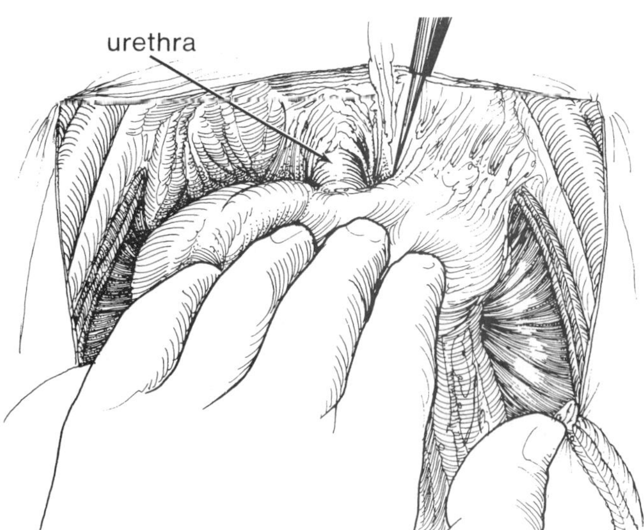

Fig. 63.4. Anteriorly, the urethra is defined and the bladder is detached by division of the lateral vesical ligaments.

attachments are lysed and the urethra is exposed for resection from below (Fig. 63.4).

The cardinal ligaments are divided between serial clamps at the pelvic sidewall avoiding the hypogastric veins (Fig. 63.5). In a fully irradiated pelvis, resection of the pelvic lymph nodes is controversial because disease here is unlikely to allow survival. Some surgeons remove the common, external, and internal iliac and obturator nodes for frozen section, proceeding with exenteration only if the nodes are negative. However, in a subgroup of patients with only unilateral microscopic involvement, lymphadenectomy may have therapeutic benefit, with up to 25% of patients alive at 5 years (7). Clearly, morbidity increases after pelvic lymphadenectomy in a radiated pelvis, whereas the benefit is debatable. The availability of intraoperative radiation therapy may improve the prognosis in patients with sidewall disease.

Perineal Resection

The perineal phase of surgery can be started during this time. The second surgical team makes an incision below the clitoris if possible and extending circumferentially around the vagina (Fig. 63.6). Resection of the vulva requires a larger circumference. With Allis clamps at 4-o'clock and 8-o'clock positions, an incision is made at the mucocutaneous border of the vagina and perineum. The rectovaginal septum is developed sharply with Metzenbaum scissors. Moderate bleeding is common because of vascular attachments between the lower vagina and rectum. The internal pudendal vessels are ligated in Alcock's canal. The vagina is mobilized laterally and then anteriorly to expose the urogenital diaphragm. Detachment of the vagina and urethra from the pubic bone is one of the last steps because bleeding from the inferior pubic ramus may be difficult to control with the specimen in place. The inferior fascia of the

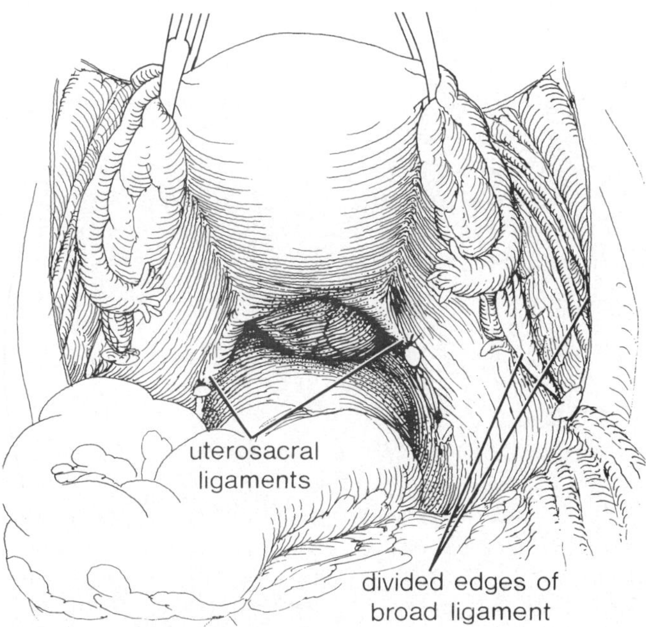

Fig. 63.3. Development of the rectovaginal septum and division of the uterosacral ligaments.

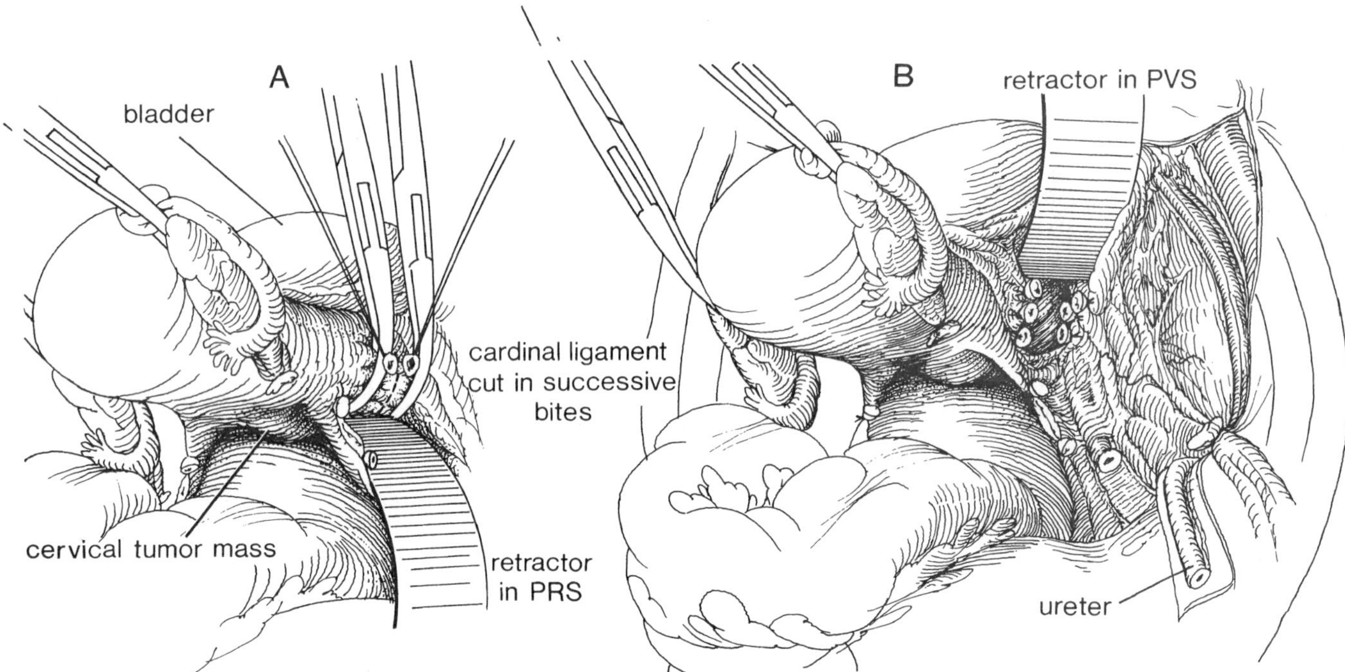

Fig. 63.5.   The uterus is retracted laterally, and the cardinal ligament is divided and ligated in successive pedicles at the pelvic sidewall.

urogenital diaphragm is divided with electrocautery. The intervening superficial transverse perineal muscles are clamped laterally near the ischium below the pubic rami. If the abdominal surgeons divide the superior fascia of the urogenital diaphragm, this guides the perineal team. The pubococcygeus portions of the levator ani can be divided by either team. Lastly, the urethra is freed from ligamentous attachments to the pubis. If bleeding is difficult to control, a 2-0 polyglactin suture on a Keith needle is passed from below under the pubis and back again on the

opposite side. The puborectalis portion of the levators is then approximated with 2-0 polyglactin sutures to support the perineum.

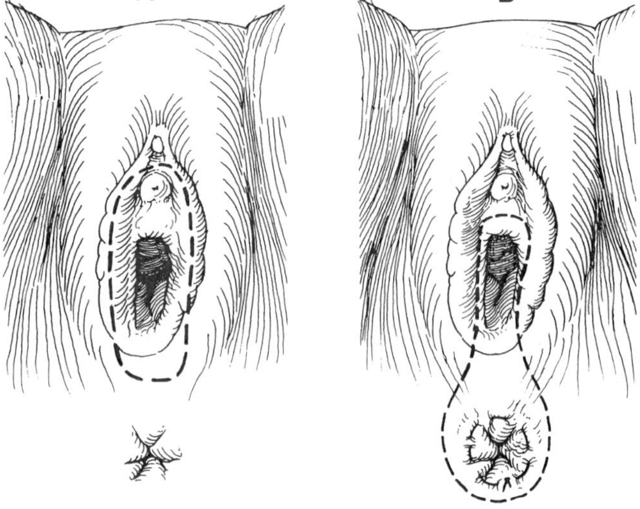

Posterior Exenteration

Posterior exenteration is performed for recurrent cervical cancer in the posterior vagina or rectovaginal septum. The operation is not appropriate if disease extends to the anterior vagina. In cases with cervical involvement or parametrial extension, total exenteration should be chosen because of occult spread anteriorly into the bladder pillars and to avoid any ureteral dissection in the parametria. Although the ureters could be divided at the pelvic brim and reimplanted into the bladder, this is not advisable because parametrial extension often goes hand in hand with vesicouterine extension. The posterior exenteration proceeds as described for anterior exenteration except that the rectovaginal septum is not dissected. Because the bladder is conserved, the anterior peritoneal incision extends from the round ligaments along the vesicouterine reflection in the anterior culde-sac. With the uterus firmly retracted cephalad, the bladder is developed sharply off the cervix and upper vagina. This is best done in the relatively avascular midline. The uterine vessels are ligated, and the superior vesical artery is preserved. The ureter is dissected from the parametria using a right-angle clamp and gently spreading directly on top of the ureter. The dissection continues to free the ureter in the vesicouterine pillar or "tunnel" as it enters the bladder. The smaller posterior vesicouterine ligament beneath the ureter is ligated separately. The ureters are then retracted laterally to allow resection of the

Fig. 63.6.   Perineal incision for anterior **(A)** and posterior **(B)** exenteration.

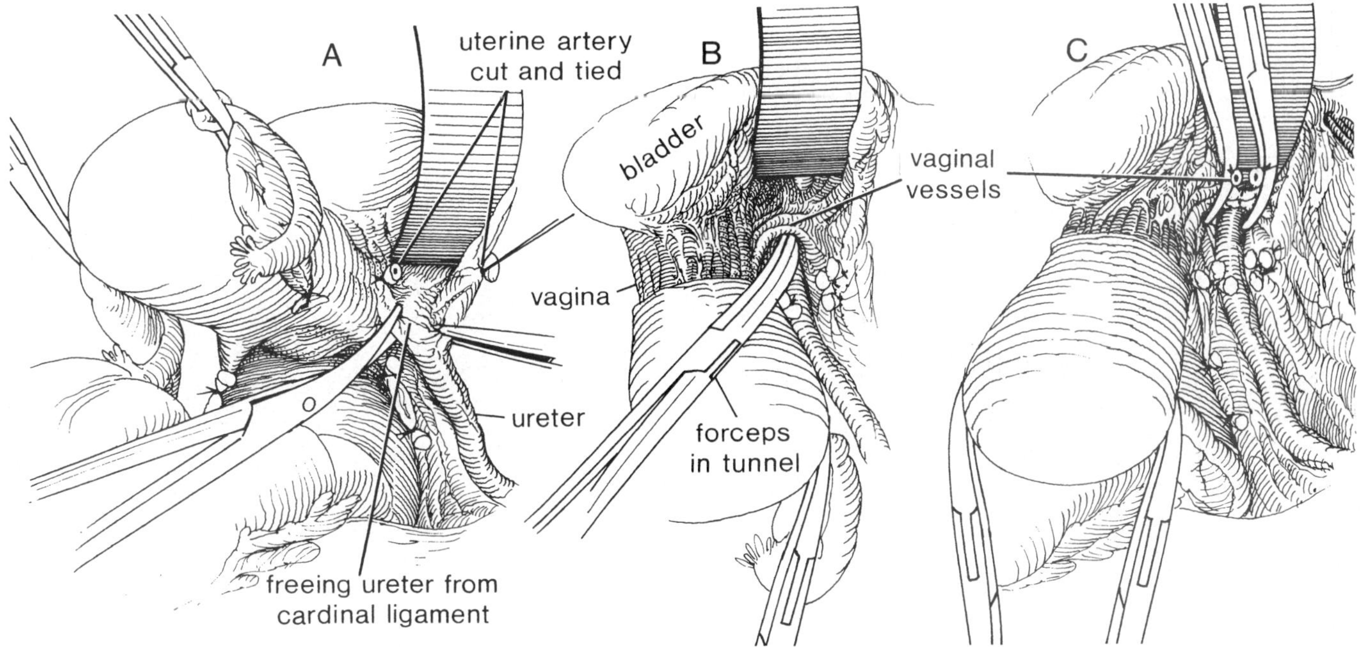

Fig. 63.7.   The ureter is dissected successively from the cardinal ligament and the vesicouterine ligament.

lateral cardinal and uterosacral ligaments in successive pedicles replaced with 0 polyglactin sutures (Fig. 63.7). To this point, the technique resembles that of a radical hysterectomy, except for more careful attention to ureteral vascularity after irradiation.

The mesentery of the sigmoid colon is divided in an avascular area and the colon divided below the pelvic brim using the GIA stapler. The mesentery and inferior sigmoid vessels are then serially ligated. The surgeon separates the rectosigmoid from loose retrorectal attachments to the sacrum with the electrocautery. Care is taken not to injure the middle sacral vessels. The rectal stalks and proximal uterosacral ligaments are divided close to the sacrum. The rectum is freed from the puborectalis muscle posteriorly by blunt dissection with the hand insinuating toward the pubis in the presacral space (Fig. 63-8). The middle rectal artery is sacrificed near the hypogastric artery. The anococcygeal ligament is ligated and divided. The perineal phase of the procedure encompasses the rectum as in an abdominoperineal resection and continues anteriorly to circumscribe the vagina (Fig. 63.8).

The disadvantage of posterior exenteration is the high degree of bladder atony and neurogenic incontinence because of sacrifice of the nervi erigentes in the uterosacral and rectal stalks. In addition, the ureteral dissection in the parametria, when the patient has received pelvic irradiation, is associated with a fistula rate of at least 5 to 10%. For these reasons, posterior exenteration is uncommonly performed for recurrent cervical carcinoma but may be used in certain cases of vaginal carcinoma not amenable to, or failing, radiation therapy. Occasionally, modified posterior exenteration is used to clear the pelvis for optimal tumor reduction of ovarian carcinoma.

Total Exenteration

Total pelvic exenteration is required in at least half the cases of recurrent cervical carcinoma. The technique combines procedures outlined in the sections on anterior and posterior exenteration and may be performed with resection of the levator plate (Fig. 63.9) or in a supralevator fashion (Fig. 63.10). As in posterior exenteration when the rectosigmoid colon is resected, the proximal sigmoid can be used for a urinary conduit to avoid use of the small bowel and enteroenterostomy. The perineal phase of total pelvic exenteration encompasses the urethra, vagina, perineum, and anus. The gracilis myocutaneous flap with an overlying omental pedicle is the procedure of choice for vaginal and pelvic floor reconstruction (8). Extended resections, as have been performed by Pearlman et al. for recurrent rectal carcinoma, may have a role in selected patients with symphysis and sacral recurrences (9). These cases should be highly individualized. As experience accumulates with internal sacral resections, the pelvic surgeon may wish to consider these procedures.

Supralevator Exenteration

In certain patients with carcinoma above the lower vagina, the perineal phase of the operation may be omitted and the surgery undertaken abdominally to the levator plate (Fig. 63.10). The levator ani are preserved. The vagina is resected as low as possible without division of the urogenital diaphragm or distal puborectalis at the pelvic floor. The vaginal cuff is closed with interrupted sutures of 2-0 polyglactin. The rectum is transected at the levator muscles using the thoracoabdominal stapler with a rotating head to facilitate acute angulation in the pelvis (TA-

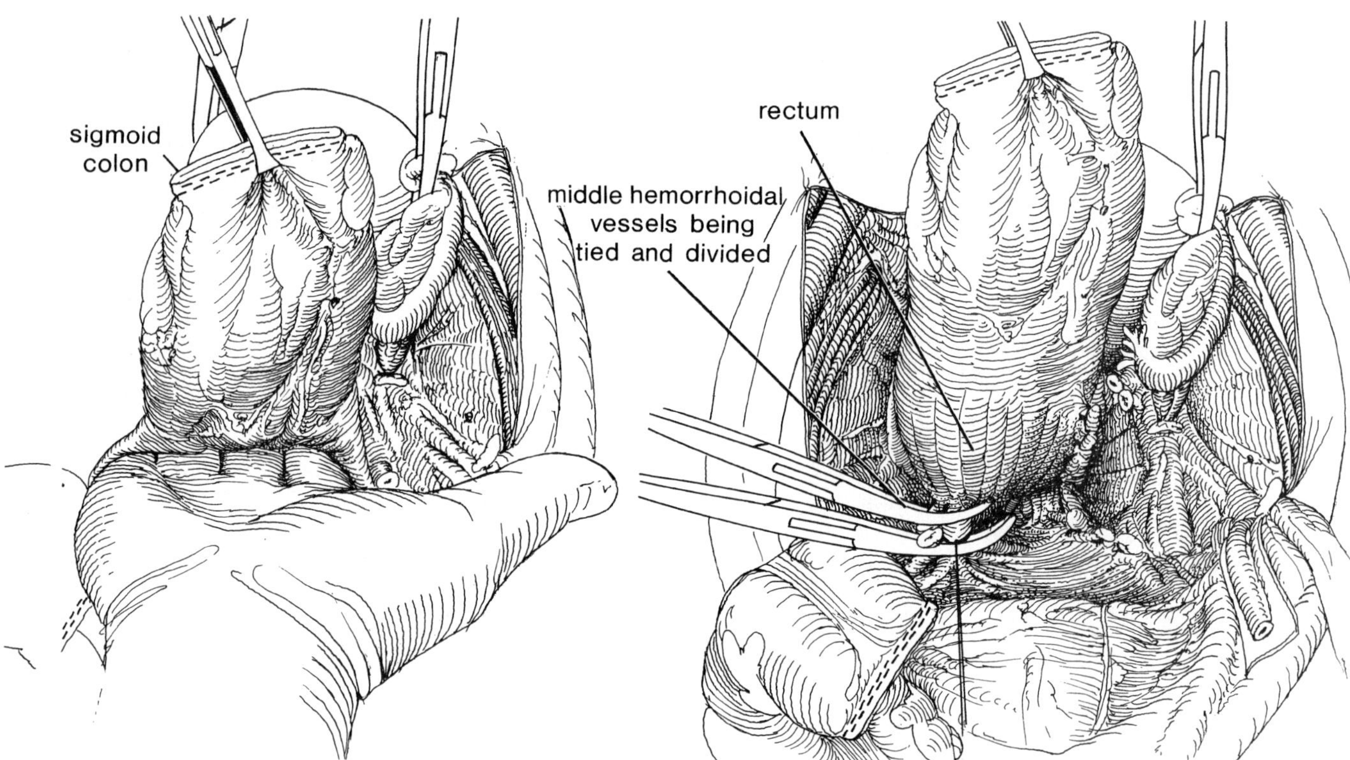

Fig. 63.8. **A.** Sigmoid colon is divided and the retrorectal space is developed. **B.** Rectal stalks are divided and ligated close to the sacrum.

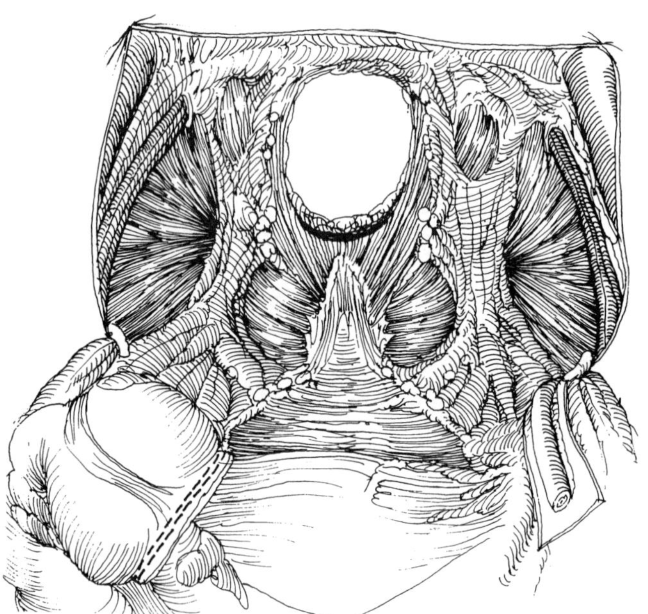

Fig. 63.9. Pelvis, viewed from above, following total exenteration.

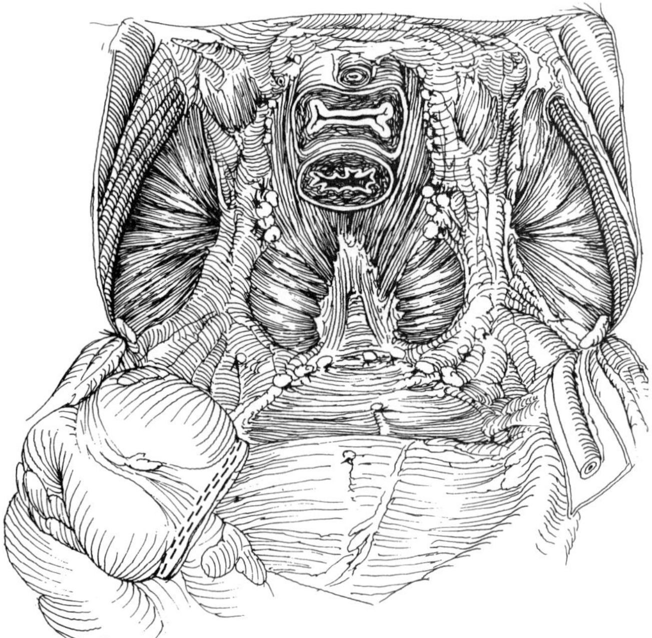

Fig. 63.10. Pelvis, viewed from above, following supralevator total exenteration.

55). Preservation of the puborectalis and rectum allows reanastomosis of the rectosigmoid colon to the rectum using the end-end stapler (EEA) because carcinoma of the cervix rarely involves the anus or distal 5 cm of rectum. The distal urethra is not excised but resected at the superior fascia of the urogenital diaphragm. The supralevator exenteration usually does not require a perineal resection and allows the greatest flexibility in reconstructive options, although only small recurrences are appropriate for this type of exenteration. Frozen sections of the vaginal, urethral, and rectal margins are important in supralevator exenteration. Occasionally, a perineal resection facilitates total vaginectomy and still allows preservation of the urogenital diaphragm or puborectalis in selected cases.

Pelvic Reconstruction

After removal of the tumor, the surgeon begins the more arduous phase of attempting to minimize morbidity and allow functional restoration for the patient. The most common form of urinary diversion is the Bricker pouch or ureteroileal conduit (10, 11). This procedure is described in Chapter 30. If the patient has undergone total exenteration, the sigmoid colon provides a conduit that may eliminate the need for small bowel anastomosis. However, because the sigmoid colon and ileum have often received significant irradiation, the transverse colon conduit may have to be considered. As surgical technique has improved, several centers have adopted techniques of continent urinary diversion such as the modified Kock pouch or the ileocolonic pouch. Any grey-white discoloration of the small bowel that might signify radiation enteritis would preclude the use of these segments of bowel. Technical details can be found in Chapters 31–33.

Coloproctostomy

If the distal 3 to 8 cm of rectum are preserved, low or very low rectal anastomosis allows the patient to avoid colostomy (12). However, in the heavily irradiated patient, the surgeon should opt for a temporary diverting colostomy. If possible, the anastomosis should be checked by filling the pelvis with saline and injecting air through a Toomey syringe placed in the anus. If bubbles are seen, there is a leak. The anastomosis should be repaired or taken down entirely and redone. If there is tension on the anastomosis or inadequate repair, a diverting colostomy is necessary.

Most of the defects in low rectal anastomosis are posterior because of the difficulty in directly observing this part of the bowel. This can be checked by rotating the EEA stapler after firing and before releasing it. A newer type of stapler (CEEA, Autosuture; U.S. Surgical Corp., Norwalk, CT) allows a simpler solution because the head is easily detached. If there is enough mobility of the sigmoid colon, an end-to-side anastomosis (Strasbourg-Baker) may allow the formation of a rectal pouch that serves as a reservoir, as in the normal rectal ampulla (13). The distal TA-55 staple line can be punctured with the shaft of

the EEA. The proximal sigmoid is punctured using an adapter (CEEA) along the antimesenteric side 5 to 7 cm from the previously resected end (Fig. 63.11). The head of the CEEA is replaced onto the shaft through the colotomy in the proximal bowel segment. No purse-strings are needed, and firing of the stapler creates the end-side anastomosis. The proximal sigmoid is then closed with the TA-55 stapler. Although all these maneuvers can be accomplished directly by hand, the use of the automatic stapling device shortens operative time, decreases complications, and allows for improved blood flow to the anastomosis (13).

Neovagina

After rectal anastomosis, the vagina is reconstructed using a split-thickness skin graft. A myocutaneous flap is generally not required because the rectum forms a suitable posterior vaginal plate. The Brown air-driven dermatome or Padgett dermatome is then set to $^{12}/_{1000}$ to $^{16}/_{1000}$ of an inch and the donor site prepared with mineral oil. Generally the anteromedial thigh is most accessible, although some patients prefer a lateral buttock site. The size of the graft should be 10 to 15 cm. The donor site is dressed with scarlet red and loose fluffy gauze.

The split-thickness skin graft is meshed at a 2:1 or 3:1 ratio and sewn over a loose obturator such as a Heyer-Schulte stent or large syringe barrel that has been opened at both ends, using interrupted 4-0 polyglactin. The end that will become the proximal vagina is closed over the end of the stent (Fig. 63.12). The graft is then inserted into the vaginal cavity. Meticulous hemostasis is imperative because bleeding will separate the graft from the neovaginal bed. Evans et al. have suggested the use of topical thrombin sprayed on the graft bed (14). Serum will escape without separating the graft if it has been properly meshed or "pie-crusted." Several interrupted sutures are used to anchor the skin graft to the rectum and circumferentially to the labia at the introitus. As one team prepares the neovagina, the omental J-pexy is then brought into the pelvis anteriorly to support the neovagina and is sewn to the anterior and lateral rectum and the inferior pubic symphysis. The neovagina is then snugly packed, withdrawing the plastic obturator as the packing is laid. A Heyer-Schulte stent need not be removed at surgery. At 7 days, the packing or stent is removed and the vagina examined for percent engraftment.

Gracilis Myocutaneous Neovagina

If the levator plate has been resected and a colostomy performed, the capacious space in the pelvis is best filled with bilateral gracilis myocutaneous flaps. Unlike skin grafts, this type of neovagina achieves excellent sensation for coitus and, using omentum, prevents small bowel from adhering to the pelvic floor with possible perineal herniation or obstruction.

A line is drawn with a sterile surgical marker from the pubic tubercle to the medial tibial epicondyle using a straight edge. The gracilis muscle is just inferior to this line where a pedicle

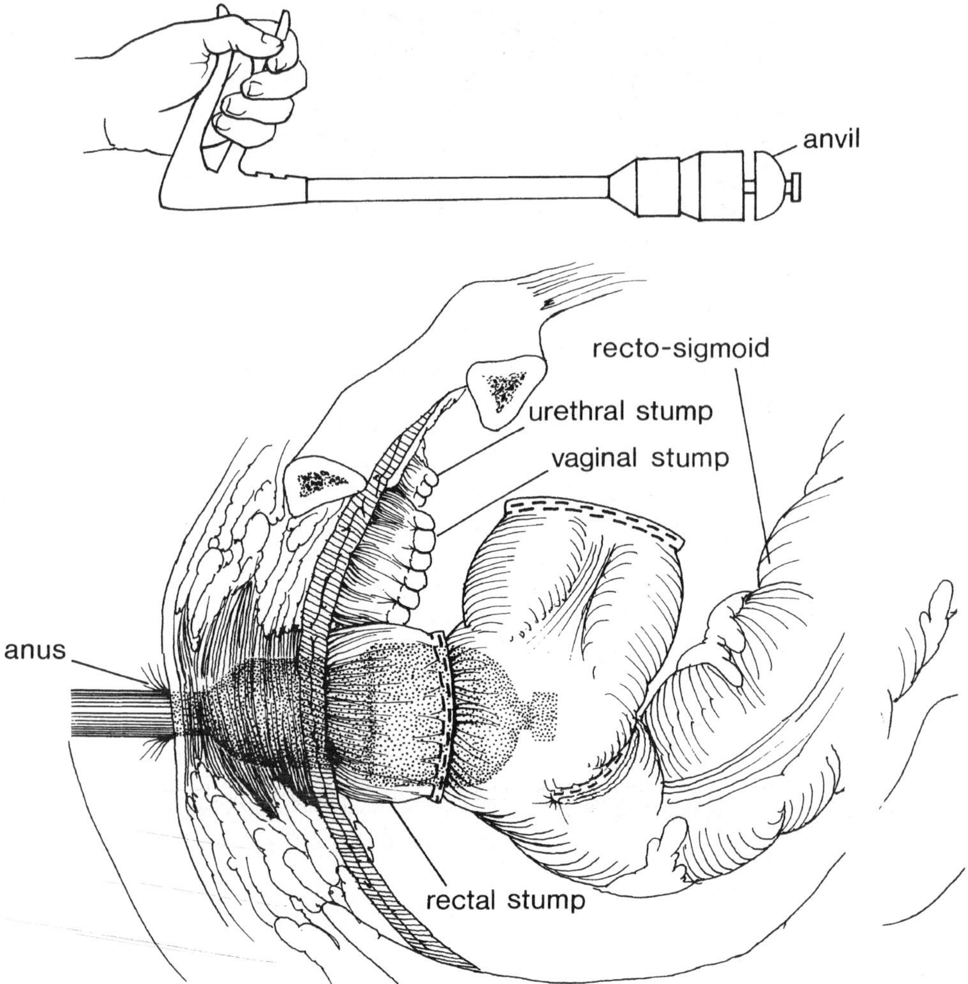

Fig. 63.11.   Anastomosis of the rectal stump to the side of sigmoid colon using the CEEA stapler.

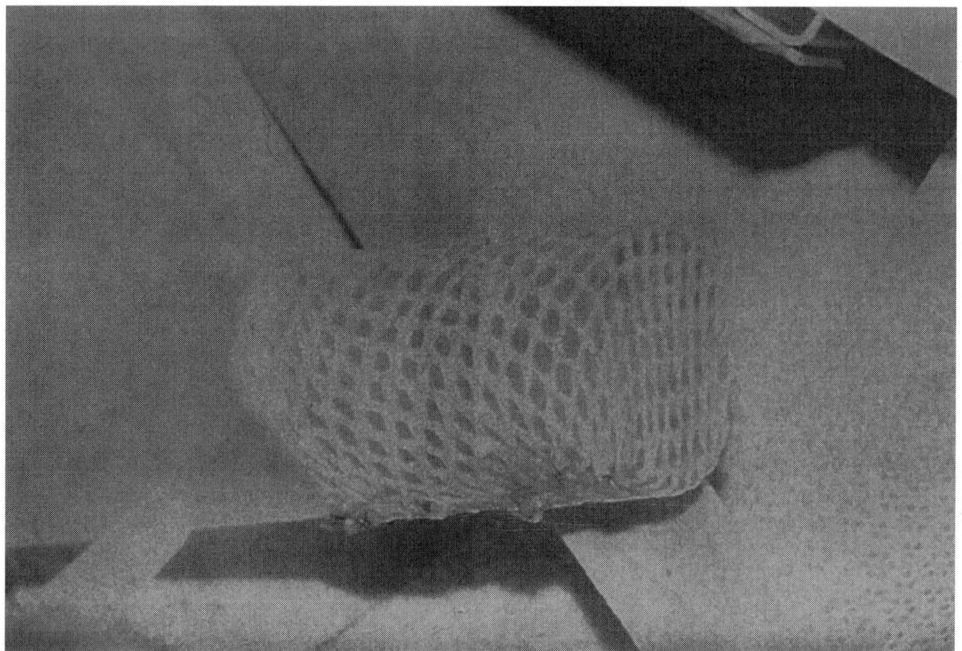

Fig. 63.12.   Split-thickness skin graft draped on a syringe barrel and sewn over one end.

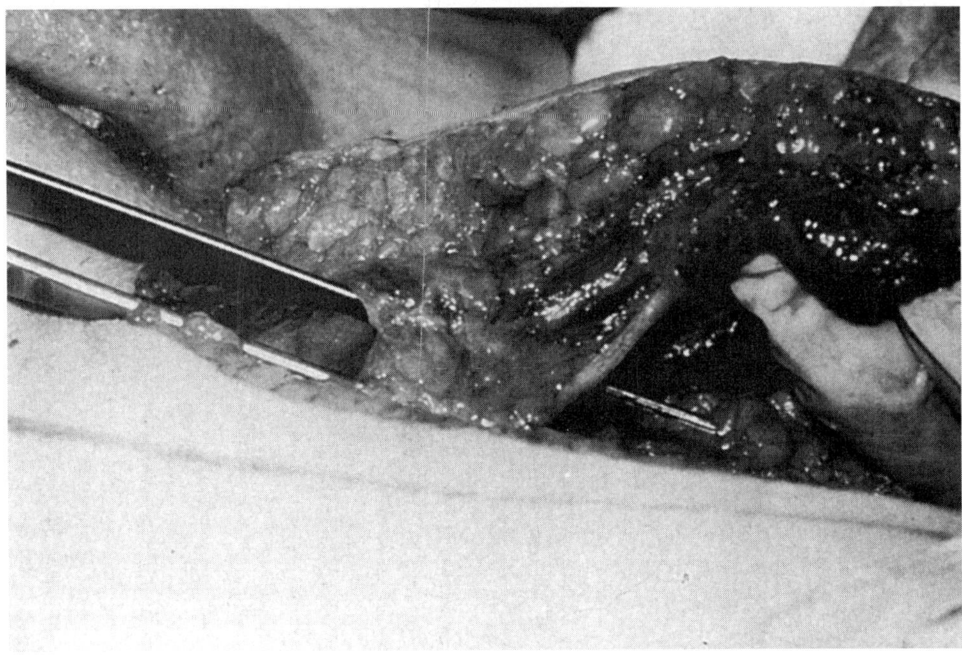

Fig. 63.13.   Gracilis myocutaneous flap dissected with its intact neurovascular supply.

10- to 15-cm long, and half as wide, is outlined in elliptical fashion. The myocutaneous flap is supplied by a neurovascular bundle emerging from the adductor longus muscle, superior to the adductor magnus. The neurovascular bundle is usually 6 to 9 cm from the pubic tubercle. Injury to this narrow and precarious pedicle may result in flap necrosis. Dissection of the pedicle flap continues, with care not to separate the skin from the underlying gracilis. The skin and gracilis are transected distally using electrocautery. It is not advisable to divide the gracilis near its insertion at the pubis. The skin and muscle are mobilized, and the areolar attachments are divided parallel to the neurovascular bundle (Fig. 63.13). It is usually necessary to secure the skin to the gracilis with interrupted 2-0 polyglactin proximally and distally. The pedicle flap is then rotated using Babcock clamps and brought under the skin bridge consisting of the superomedial thigh and vulva to lie perpendicu-

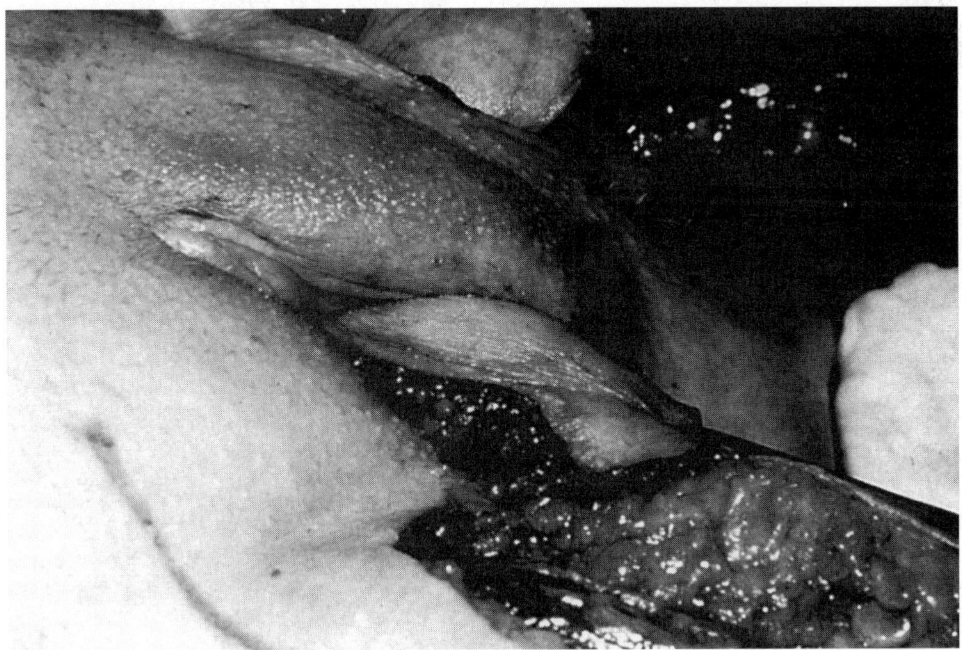

Fig. 63.14.   The myocutaneous flap is brought onto the perineum underneath the bridge of the medial thigh and labia.

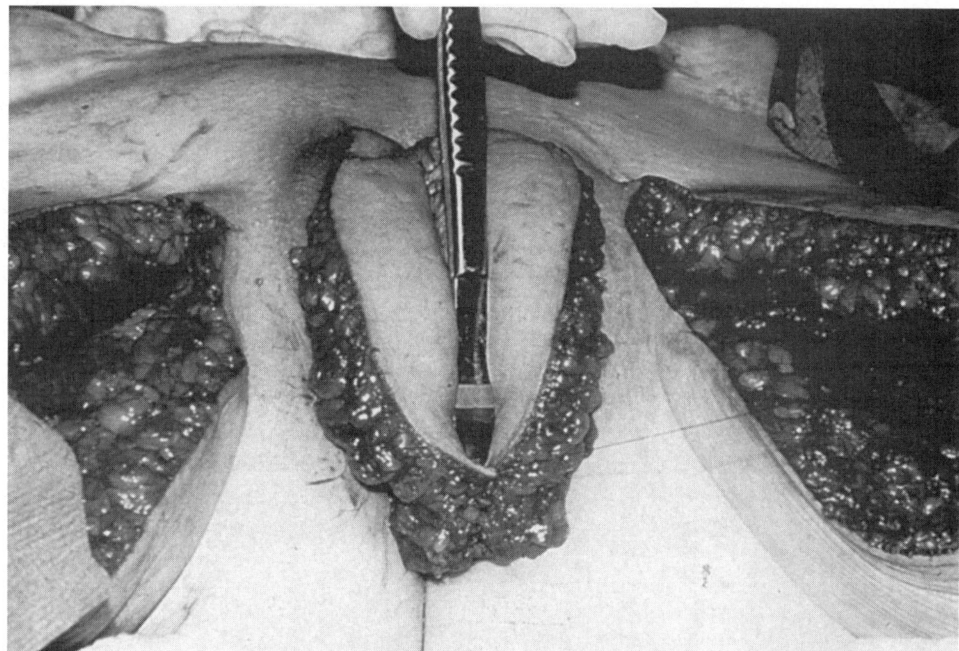

Fig. 63.15.   The myocutaneous flap from both sides is brought onto the vulva and is sewn together from above downward.

larly at the introitus (Fig. 63.14). A continuous suture of 3-0 polyglactin is started superiorly and attaches the right and left flaps. This continues to the distal flap and then up to the proximal portions to form a pouch with skin inside and fatty tissue on the outside (Figs. 63.15 and 63.16). The grafts are then rotated 90° to fill the vaginal bed. The superior portion is attached by the abdominal team to the sacral periosteum, pubis, levator muscles, and, finally, from below, to the introitus at the labia using 2-0 interrupted polyglactin sutures (Fig. 63.17). A stent or pack is usually unnecessary. The incisions on the thigh are closed in two layers, the first with continuous 3-0 polyglactin and the skin with metal clips or mattress sutures. Closed suction drains are placed in the incision, exiting through stab wounds on the thigh. Other methods of neovaginal construction have been described, such as the use of the vascular but short vulvobulbocavernosus pedicle or a pedicle of rectus abdominis muscle.

Pelvic Floor

The omentum is detached from the transverse colon in the avascular plane and divided using the LDS stapler below the greater curvature of the stomach from the right side. The branches of the right gastroepiploic vessels are sacrificed, and the J-shaped lid is fashioned with the left gastroepiploic vessels intact (Fig. 63.18). The pedicle flap is carpeted over the pelvis to exclude the small bowel and is attached to the pelvis at the sidewalls and over the neovagina (Fig. 63.18). If the omentum is not available or is inadequate, then a pelvic lid is fashioned with a double layer of absorbable mesh (15). The major morbidity of exenteration remains small intestinal fistulae and obstruc-

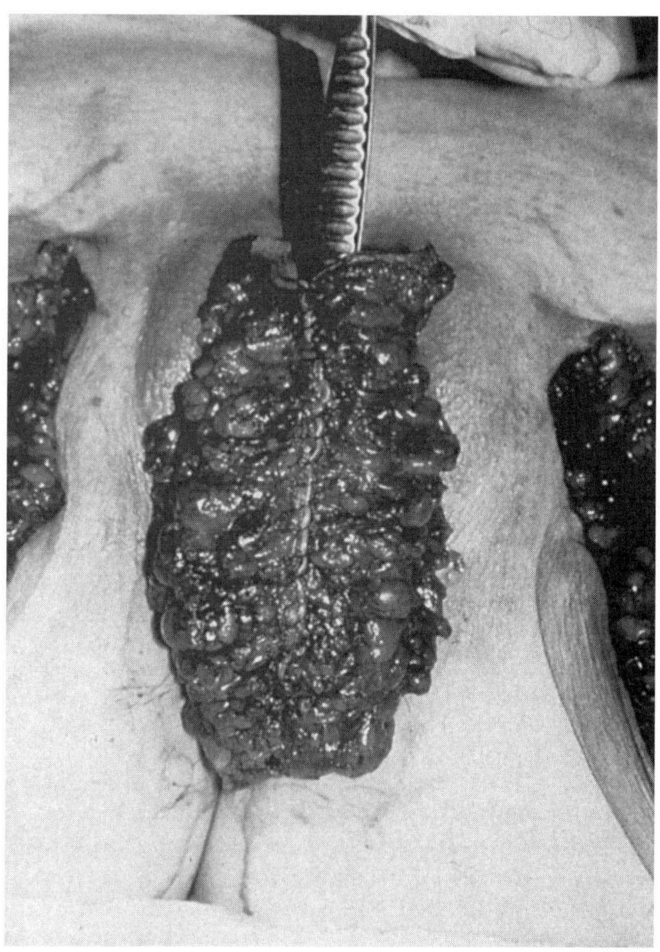

Fig. 63.16.   The suturing is continued upward to create the neovaginal pouch.

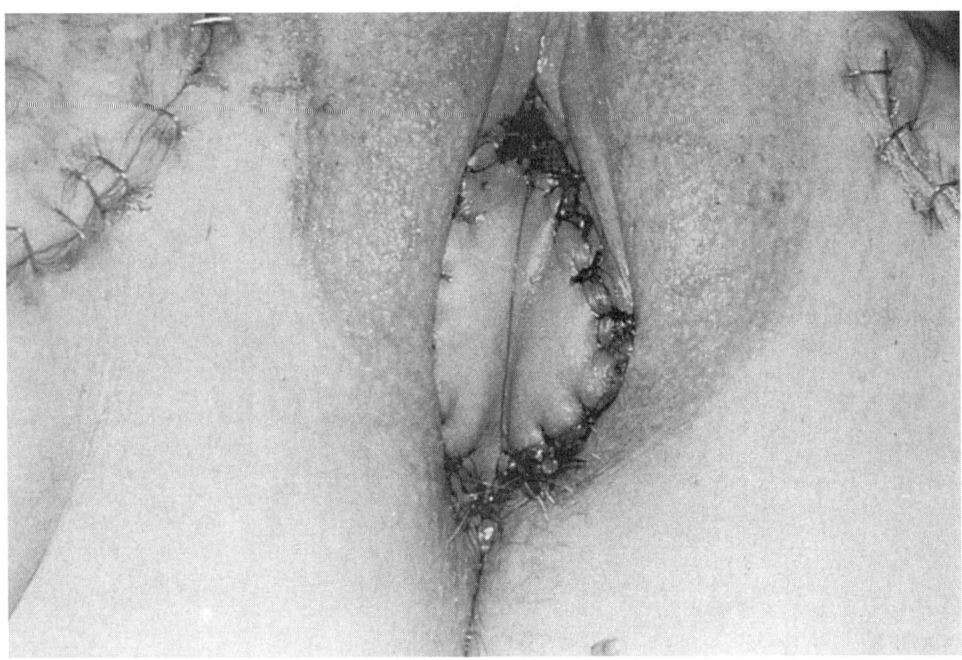

Fig. 63.17. The neovagina is rotated into the vaginal bed and sutured to the labia.

tion (16, 17). Therefore, thoughtful pelvic floor reconstruction can avert disaster.

With the use of reconstructive procedures for the bladder, vagina, and rectum, it is possible for the first time to perform total pelvic exenteration without the use of any stomata except the continent urostomy stoma, thereby avoiding external appliances. Furthermore, vaginal reconstruction enables the preservation of sexual function and limits the psychologic debilitation that accompanies such radical resections.

POSTOPERATIVE CARE AND COMPLICATIONS

In modern series, intraoperative mortality rates should be less than 2%. The total postoperative death rate remains between 3 and 5% in the first 90 days after surgery. The typical exenteration patient requires 3 to 5 days of intensive care, during which massive fluid and electrolyte shifts, hemorrhage, cardiopulmonary instability, and nutritional imbalance are corrected. The average blood loss is approximately 1500 to 2500 mL in the first 5 days. Even the young and otherwise healthy patient is best managed with Swan-Ganz catheterization for 48 to 72 hours. When third space fluids reenter the intravascular and intracellular compartments, one must vigilantly watch for pulmonary edema. This most commonly occurs between the second and fourth postoperative day.

Major operative morbidity is high after pelvic exenteration. Approximately one third to one half of patients who undergo exenteration will experience some complications (3, 12). By far, the majority of these will need a blood transfusion or experience postoperative fever. Life-threatening postoperative complications are much less common, with fistulas and bowel obstruction leading the list (16, 18). Pelvic cellulitis and pelvic abscess are usual.

Febrile morbidity is the rule after exenteration (19). However, rather than use broad-spectrum triple antibiotics reflexively, a careful search for underlying causes, often pulmonary or renal, is more rewarding. The injudicious use of antibiotics may mask intraabdominal abscess formation, delaying life-saving drainage. Supervening candidemia after prolonged courses of multiple antibiotics may be fatal. The use of CT scanning or labeled white blood cell scans has not been particularly helpful in diagnosing abscesses because of the extensive anatomic changes and inflammation. Fungal blood cultures should be obtained in patients receiving broad-spectrum antibiotics. Often, colonization of the urinary tract with Candida may be the first clue to fungal sepsis.

Occasional deleterious events include stomal necrosis or prolapse, urinary leakage from the conduit or ureter, hematoma, perineal or incisional hernia or dehiscence, and cardiovascular events such as myocardial infarction and pulmonary embolism. Persistent sinus tachycardia is common, and EKG will rule out treatable supraventricular arrhythmias.

Prolonged ileus is managed with intestinal intubation, and there may be difficulty ruling out a small bowel obstruction. If the patient's condition remains stable, continued expectant care is preferable to a hasty return to the operating room. In patients undergoing total exenteration with multiple small and large intestinal anastomoses, a gastrostomy tube placed in a Witzel fashion at surgery avoids the discomfort of 7 to 21 days

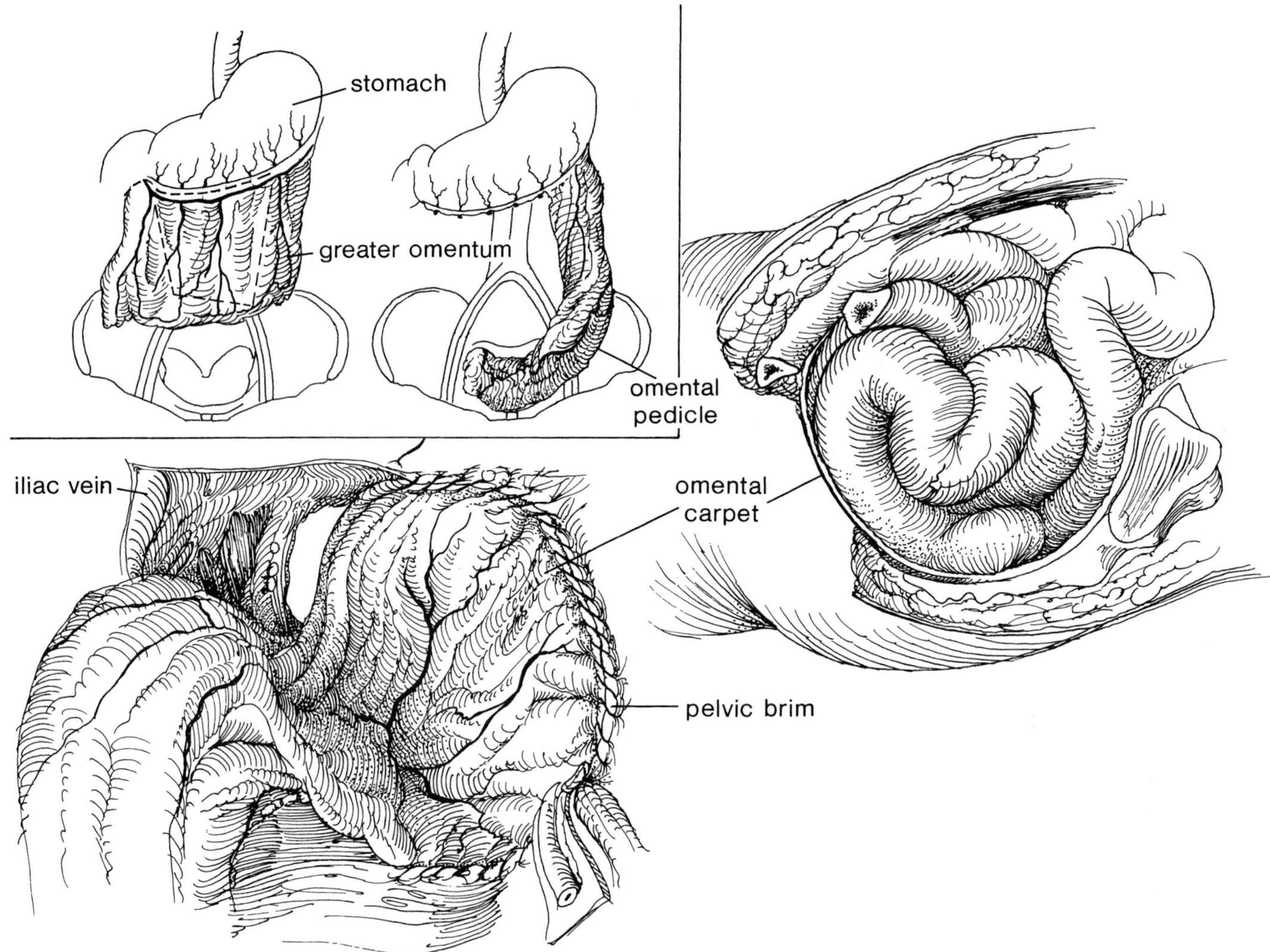

Fig. 63.18.   Construction of the greater omental carpet. The greater omentum is detached from the transverse colon and the greater curvature of stomach by ligature and division of the right gastroepiploic vessels (inset). The detached omentum is fashioned into a J-shaped lid with intact left gastroepiploic vessels (left). The pedicled flap is carpeted over the neovagina in the pelvis and attached to the pelvic parities (right).

of nasogastric intubation. If a fistula is suspected, Gastrografin (Bristol Meyer Squibb, Evansville, IN) gastrointestinal series are used to define the anatomy. Ureteral obstruction should be evaluated with renal ultrasound or intravenous pyelogram. Most of these serious complications will resolve with continued parenteral nutrition. Obstructed ureters often result from edema at the anastomosis, and temporary nephrostomies or antegrade endoscopic stents will often obviate surgical repair. Elective reoperations should be delayed for 4 to 6 weeks to allow the patient's condition to improve and the associated edema and inflammation to subside.

Long-term complications include recurrent pyelonephritis, hyperchloremic acidosis, intestinal stricture or fistula, lymphedema, and lymphocysts. Lymphocysts can be avoided by drainage of the pelvic and paraaortic lymphadenectomy sites until the daily output is less than 30 mL. Chronic lymphedema occurs in less than 5% of patients. The risks of lymphatic compli-

cations must be weighed in deciding whether to perform a thorough pelvic lymphadenectomy at the time of exenteration in the irradiated pelvis.

PROGNOSIS AND LONG-TERM FOLLOW-UP

Of patients explored for pelvic exenteration, approximately one half will be candidates for completion of the operation. Between 30 and 60% of exenteration patients will become long-term survivors (20–23). Approximately 80% of recurrences manifest in the first 2 years. Progressive radiation fibrosis may be difficult to distinguish from recurrent tumor, although asymmetry in the pelvis suggests tumor. Fine-needle aspiration is often definitive. Tumor markers, including carcinoembryonic antigen and squamous cell carcinoma antigen, are useful adjuncts to clinical examination. A chest radiograph is obtained every 6 months for 2 years. CT or MRI scanning is relatively insensitive and nonspecific but may be helpful on an annual basis, particularly to rule out progressive hydronephrosis because of strictures. If native vagina remains, annual cytologic smears are indicated. In at least nine cases, squamous cell carcinoma has developed in a neovagina. Adenocarcinoma and transitional cell carcinoma have occurred in the urinary conduits. The treatment of recurrent disease remains unrewarding, with a mean survival of 3 to 6 months. Meticulous follow-up and continuing psychologic support allow most patients to resume healthy and productive lives free from disease.

ACKNOWLEDGMENTS

Great appreciation is extended to Dr. Leo D. Lagasse for thoughtful and constructive review of this manuscript.

REFERENCES

1. Stanhope CR, Symmonds RE. Palliative exenteration: what, when, and why? Am J Obstet Gynecol 1985;152:12.
2. Brunschwig A. Complete excision of the pelvic viscera for advanced carcinoma. Cancer 1948;1:177.
3. Hreschyshyn MM, et al. Hydroxyurea or placebo combined with radiation to treat stages IIIB and IV cervical cancer confined to the pelvis. Int J Radiat Oncol Biol Phys 1979;5:317.
4. Rubin SC, Hoskins WJ, Lewis JL. Radical hysterectomy for recurrent cervical cancer following radiation therapy. Gynecol Oncol 1987;27:316.
5. Hoffman MS, Roberts WS, Cavanaugh D. Neuropathies associated with radical pelvic surgery for gynecologic cancer. Gynecol Oncol 1988;31:462.
6. Hatch KD, et al. Anterior pelvic exenteration. Gynecol Oncol 1988;31:205.
7. Rutledge FN, McGuffee VB. Pelvic exenteration: prognostic significance of regional lymph node metastasis. Gynecol Oncol 1987;26:374.
8. Berek JS, Hacker NF, Lagasse LD. Vaginal reconstruction performed simultaneously with pelvic exenteration. Obstet Gynecol 1984;63:318.
9. Pearlman NS, et al. Pelvic and sacropelvic exenteration for locally advanced or recurrent anorectal cancer. Arch Surg 1987;122:537.
10. Bricker EM, Kraybill WG, Lopez MJ, et al. The current role of ultraradical surgery in the treatment of pelvic cancer. Curr Probl Surg 1986;23:871.
11. Orr JW, Shingleton HM, Hatch KD. Urinary diversion in patients undergoing pelvic exenteration. Am J Obstet Gynecol 1982;142:883.
12. Lagasse LD, et al. Use of sigmoid colon for rectal substitution following pelvic exenteration. Am J Obstet Gynecol 1973;116:106.
13. Wheeless CR, Dorsey JH. Use of the automatic stapler for intestinal anastomosis associated with gynecologic malignancies. Gynecol Oncol 1981;11:1.
14. Evans TN, Poland ML, Boving RL. Vaginal malformations. Am J Obstet Gynecol 1981;141:910.
15. Clarke-Pearson DL, Soper JT, Creasman WT. Absorbable synthetic mesh (polyglactin 910) for the formation of a pelvic lid after radical pelvic resection. Am J Obstet Gynecol 1988;198:158.
16. Lipshitz S, Johnson R, Roberts JA, et al. Intestinal fistula and obstruction following pelvic exenteration. Surg Gynecol Obstet 1981;152:630.
17. Symmonds RE, Pratt JH, Webb MJ. Exenteration operations: experience with 198 patients. Am J Obstet Gynecol 1975;121:907.
18. Orr JW, et al. Gastrointestinal complications associated with pelvic exenteration. Am J Obstet Gynecol 1983;145:325.
19. Morgan LS, Daly JW, Monif GRG. Infectious morbidity associated with pelvic exenteration. Gynecol Oncol 1980;10:318.
20. Averette HE, Lichtinger M, Sevin BU, et al. Pelvic exenteration. A 15-year experience in a general metropolitan hospital. Am J Obstet Gynecol 1984;150:179.
21. Barber HRK. Pelvic exenteration. Cancer Invest 1987;5:331.
22. Curry SL, et al. Pelvic exenteration: a 7-year experience. Gynecol Oncol 1981;11:119.
23. Morley GW, Lindenaur SM. Pelvic exenterative therapy for gynecologic malignancy: an analysis of 70 cases. Cancer 1976;38:581.

64

Intestinal Surgery for the Urologic Oncologist

Robert A. Read
Greg Van Stiegmann

This chapter focuses on selected aspects of intestinal surgery as they relate to urologic oncology. An overview of intestinal physiology and anatomy is discussed in the context of bowel operations germane to urologic disease. Several techniques for the repair, resection, and reestablishment of bowel continuity will be described as well as standard principles of perioperative management for patients undergoing intestinal surgery.

PHYSIOLOGY OF THE INTESTINAL TRACT

Digestion

The primary functions of the small and large intestine are digestion and absorption of water, nutrients, vitamins, and minerals. Fluid and electrolyte transport occurs along the entire length of the small intestine. The net driving force for the movement of water and electrolytes represents the combined effects of active, passive, and solvent drag transport processes (1). The majority of the estimated 9 L of daily intestinal fluid is absorbed in the jejunum by passive and solvent drag processes secondary to monosaccharide absorption (2). Using these mechanisms, the jejunum absorbs large volumes of essentially isotonic fluid. The duodenum and ileum, although essential for the digestion and absorption of nutrients, play a relatively minor role in the balance of fluid and electrolytes and serve mainly to alter the qualitative composition of intestinal fluid.

The digestion and absorption of nutrients and vitamins, unlike the absorption of fluids and electrolytes, are complex and rely on sequential processes throughout the intestine, which are unique for each major nutrient category (3). The majority of these processes occur in the proximal small bowel; however, bile salts are conserved through a high-efficiency reabsorption system in the distal ileum. The enterohepatic circulation recycles the entire bile salt pool approximately 6 times each day and limits the daily bile salt losses in the feces to only 500 mg (4). With distal ileal resections of less than 100 cm, hepatic synthesis is usually able to adequately compensate for the re-

sultant bile salt losses; however, the unabsorbed bile salts that pass to the colon often lead to a net colonic fluid secretion and bile salt diarrhea. Ileal resections greater than 100 cm may result in both bile acid malabsorption and steatorrhea (fecal fat greater than 20 g/day). If the resultant steatorrhea exceeds 40 g/day, patients suffer from significant nutritional deficiencies and weight loss (5). The majority of fat, carbohydrate, and protein digestion and absorption occur in the duodenum and jejunum. The ileum appears to be responsible for only a limited amount of normal nutrient digestion and absorption (6–8).

The absorption of vitamins depends on their lipid solubility. Fat-soluble vitamins (A, D, E, and K) are metabolized and absorbed in the proximal intestine in a manner similar to the absorption of dietary fat. Water-soluble vitamins, with the exception of vitamin B_{12}, are metabolized and transported across the intestinal brush border by way of vitamin-specific transport mechanisms. Vitamin B_{12} absorption is a complex process that requires gastric pepsin, intrinsic factor, pancreatic proteases, optimum intestinal pH, and ileal receptors specific for intrinsic factor-cobalamine complexes (9).

Motility

Intestinal motility influences many aspects of intestinal function. At rest, the intestine displays a periodic pattern of bursts of propagated contractions. These begin in the stomach (sometimes as high as the distal esophagus) and migrate slowly through the length of the intestine approximately every 90 minutes (10). Oral feedings temporarily abolish these "migrating motor" complexes and induce a series of irregular contractions that persist for 3 to 4 hours after each meal. The irregular pattern of contraction then slowly reverts to the migrating pattern as digestion proceeds (11, 12).

Paralytic ileus, a relatively common form of functional intestinal obstruction that may follow abdominal operations, is thought to represent an imbalance between the sympathetic and parasympathetic nervous systems (i.e., a relative sympathetic hyperactivity). Animal studies have demonstrated elevated systemic catecholamine levels associated with paralytic ileus (13). Postoperative ileus may be prevented in animals by chemical sympathectomy (13, 14). The clinical causes of paralytic ileus include all forms of peritonitis, retroperitoneal hematomas, ureteral colic, pneumonia, rib fractures, and myocardial infarction. The current mainstays of treatment are elimination of the cause, nasogastric decompression, and time.

Microbiology

The rate of postoperative infectious complications following abdominal operations increases significantly if the intestine is opened. Although the polymicrobial nature of the intestinal microflora was described as early as the 1930s (15), only recently, with improvements in collection and culture techniques, has the importance of anaerobic microflora been appreciated (Table 64.1).

The normal microflora of saliva includes aerobic streptococci, staphylococci, *Neisseria*, *Haemophilus*, and many anaerobes at a concentration of approximately 10^6/mL to 10^8/mL. Large quantities of bacteria are ingested daily, but few survive the acidic environment of the normal human stomach. The bacterial population of the stomach is directly related to its acidity, and patients taking H_2 antagonists or those who have undergone antiulcer procedures have a consistently higher bacterial load (16). The proximal small intestine normally contains few gram-negative and anaerobic organisms. Except in disease states causing bacterial overgrowth, the bacterial count in the proximal small intestine is between 10^1/mL and 10^2/mL (17). The distal small bowel is a transition zone between the relatively sterile proximal bowel and the colon. Here, under normal conditions, there are relatively equal numbers of aerobic and anaerobic organisms (approximately 10^4/mL to 10^7/mL). In contrast, the colon contains predominantly anaerobic organisms (10^9/mL to 10^{11}/mL). Disease states or alterations in the normal continuity of the bowel may result in dramatic alterations in the quality and quantity of intestinal microflora.

ANATOMY OF THE INTESTINAL TRACT

The entire small bowel, with the exception of the duodenum and occasionally the last few centimeters of ileum, is anchored to the posterior peritoneum by a mesentery that extends from the ligament of Treitz inferolaterally to the ileocecal valve in the right iliac fossa. The length of this segment of bowel measures 600 to 800 cm at autopsy. In the living state, however, this figure is closer to 300 cm, the discrepancy representing a reflection of the smooth muscle tone of the intestinal wall. The small bowel is supplied by the superior mesenteric artery (SMA), which originates from the abdominal aorta approximately 1 to 1.5 cm inferior to the celiac trunk. The initial branches of the SMA are the middle colic and inferior pancreaticoduodenal arteries; however, numerous aberrant branches have been described including right hepatic (16%), gastroduodenal (10%), and common celiomesenteric trunk (1%) (18) (Fig. 64.1). The superior mesenteric vein drains the jejunum, ileum, cecum, and ascending and transverse colon. Its branches roughly parallel the branches of the SMA.

The length of the colon is variable, measuring approximately 90 cm. The partial circumferences of both the ascending and descending colon are retroperitoneal, whereas the transverse and sigmoid colon are intraperitoneal. The transverse mesocolon extends from the junction of the first and second portion of the duodenum and across the pancreas and forms the inferior wall of the lesser peritoneal sac. Anteriorly, the transverse colon is covered by the omentum, which extends from the greater

Table 64.1. Human Endogenous Gastrointestinal Microflora

REGION	PREDOMINANT MICROFLORA	CONCENTRATION (per g or mL of aspirate)		AEROBES	ANAEROBES
		AEROBES	ANAEROBES		
Oropharynx	Slight predominance of anaerobic organisms	10^4–10^5	10^5–10^7	*Streptococcus, Haemophilus, Neisseria,* diphtheroids	*Peptostreptococcus, Fusobacterium, Bacteroides melaninogenicus, Bacteroides oralis, Peptococcus*
Esophagus	Slight predominance of anaerobic organisms	10^4–10^5	10^5–10^7	Same as oropharynx	
Stomach	Both aerobic and anaerobic organisms	Microflora is absent or minimal if normal gastric acidity and motility are present		*Streptococcus, Escherichia coli, Klebsiella, Enterobacter, Enterococcus*	*Peptostreptococcus, Bacteroides oralis, Bacteroides melaninogenicus*
Proximal small intestine	Slight predominance of aerobic organisms	10^2	10–10^2	*Streptococcus, Escherichia coli, Klebsiella, Enterobacter, Enterococcus*	*Peptostreptococcus, Bacteroides oralis, Bacteroides melaninogenicus*
Distal ileum	Slight predominance of aerobic organisms	10^4–10^6	10^5–10^7	*Escherichia coli, Klebsiella, Enterobacter, Enterococcus*	*Bacteroides fragilis, Peptostreptococcus, Clostridium*
Colon	Great predominance of anaerobic organisms	10^5–10^8	10^9–10^{11}	Same as distal ileum	

From Adinolfi MF, Cerise EJ, Nichols RL. Microbiology of the small intestine. In: Nelson RL, Nyhus LM, eds. *Surgery of the small intestine.* East Norwalk, CT: Appleton-Lange, 1987.

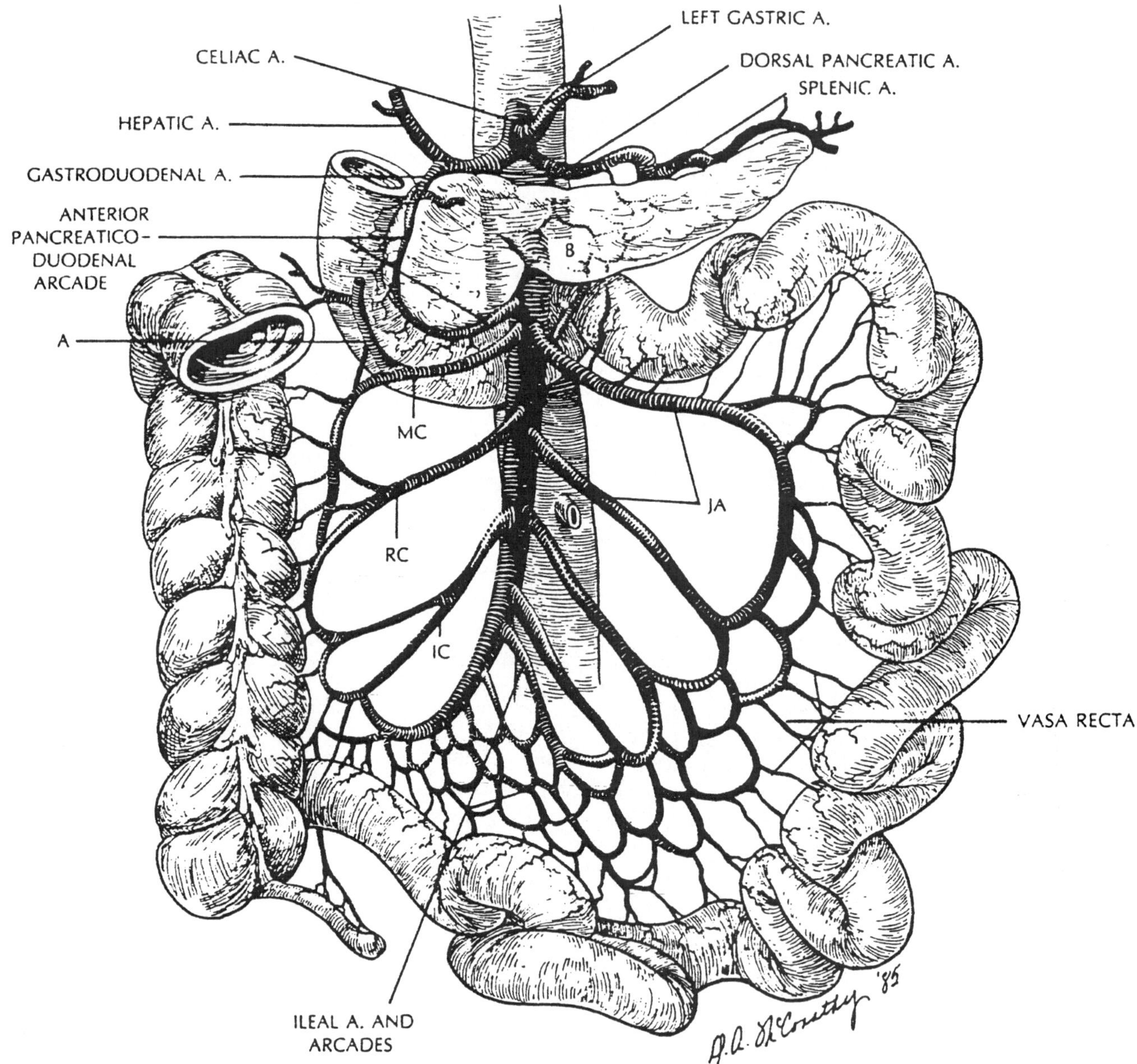

Fig. 64.1.   Superior mesenteric artery and branches. A: Left branch of middle colic artery; IC: ileocolic artery; JA: jejunal arteries; MC: middle colic artery; RC: right colic artery. (Reprinted with permission from Monsen H. Anatomy of the jejunum and ileum. In: Nelson RL, Nyhus LM, eds. Surgery of the small intestine. East Norwalk, CT: Appleton-Lange, 1987.)

curvature of the stomach, draping the bowel, and forms the anterior wall of the lesser sac. Unlike the small bowel, the longitudinal muscle layer of the colon forms three distinct longitudinal bands, the tenia coli. These bands foreshorten the colon, drawing it into a series of sacculi or haustra along its length (Fig. 64.2).

The arterial supply of the colon arises from both the inferior and superior mesenteric arteries. A rich network of anastomoses between all the principal vessels provides abundant collateral blood flow. Occasionally the anastomotic network is incomplete, most frequently at the watershed area of the splenic flex-

ure between the left colic and branches of the middle colic arteries (Fig. 64.2).

PERIOPERATIVE MANAGEMENT

Both mechanical and chemical methods have been developed for the preoperative preparation of the intestinal tract. These have resulted in lowered postoperative infectious complication rates. The methods available for debulking intestinal stool include prolonged preoperative fasting on elemental diets, magnesium citrate, mannitol, and polyethylene glycol cathartics,

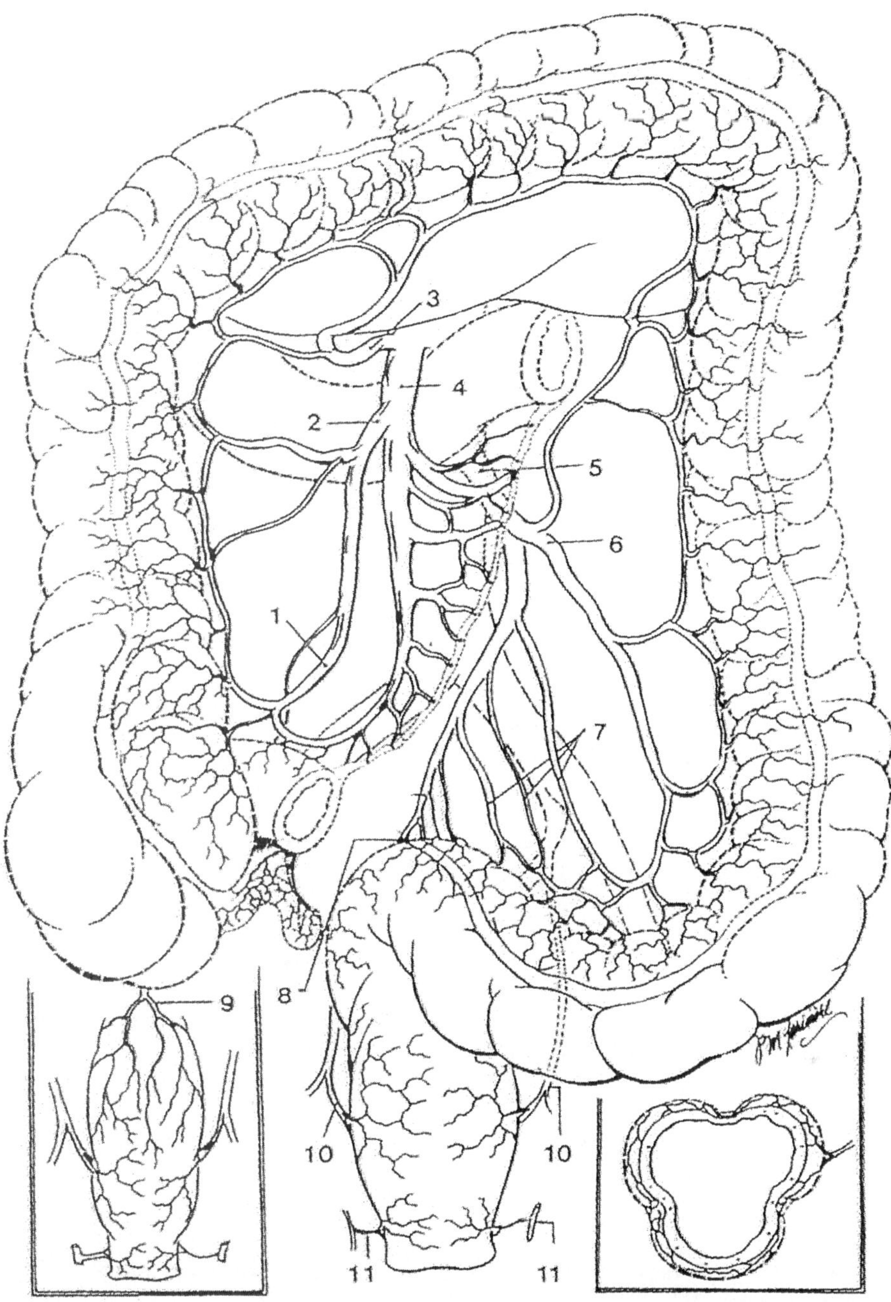

Fig. 64.2. The arterial supply of the colon and rectum. 1: ileocolic; 2: ileocolic artery giving off the right colic artery; 3: middle colic artery; 4: superior mesenteric artery; 5: inferior mesenteric artery; 6: left colic artery; 7; sigmoidal branches of the inferior mesenteric artery; 8 and 9: superior hemorrhoidal artery; 10: middle hemorrhoidal artery; 11: inferior hemorrhoidal artery. (Reprinted with permission from Ellis H. Resection of the colon. In: Schwartz S, Ellis H, eds. Maingot's abdominal operations. East Norwalk, CT: Appleton-Lange, 1985.)

in addition to various laxatives and enemas. Most of these methods are effective and can be used in combination, depending on the nature of the proposed operation and the tolerance of the patient. Antibiotic preparations, if used properly, reduce the bowel microflora to a minimum. Such regimens include oral administration of nonabsorbable neomycin and erythromycin before the planned operation. The typical large bowel preoperative regimen used at the University of Colorado consists of the oral administration of polyethylene glycol, with or without oral antibiotics, the day before the planned operation augmented as necessary with tap water enemas.

Nutritional Support

Many patients presenting with long-standing disease are physiologically malnourished. The key to optimal perioperative management is appropriate nutritional assessment and support. Consultation from a nutrition team should be sought early.

Adequate nutrition can be delivered by either enteral or parenteral routes. Feeding should begin 7 to 14 days preoperatively in the patient who has lost more than 10% of his or her lean body mass. The choice of delivery route depends on the functional integrity of the bowel and the relative risks of potential aspiration and intravenous line complications. Various enteral formulas differ in protein, residue, fat, and caloric content. Parenteral formulas are complex mixtures of concentrated dextrose solutions together with amino acids, vitamins, and minerals, supplemented with hydrolyzed vegetable oils. These solutions are considerably more expensive than enteral formulas but are useful in patients with limited bowel function or severe nutritional deficits.

PERIOPERATIVE COMPLICATIONS

Complications unique to intestinal operations occur with an overall frequency of 6% (19). Perioperative antibiotics together with meticulous operative technique have reduced the wound infection rate of abdominal operations without enterotomy to less than 2%. Enterotomies and resections without gross spillage (clean contaminated) are associated with a wound infection rate of approximately 6%, and gross spillage of intestinal contents increases this rate to 20 to 50% (19).

Most postoperative intraabdominal abscesses result from errors in surgical technique, commonly spillage of intestinal contents. The detection of an abscess is based on clinical suspicion supplemented with diagnostic studies. Most patients with intraperitoneal abscesses subsequently have fever and leukocytosis and a progressive paralytic ileus. The diagnosis is confirmed with ultrasonography, computed tomography, or exploratory laparotomy. Therapy consists of aggressive drainage, antibiotics, and physiologic support. The mortality associated with an ineffectively treated intraabdominal abscess remains high.

Enterocutaneous fistula may occur as a result of Crohn's disease or cancer; however, most follow abdominal operations in which the bowel is injured or an anastomosis fails. Management of a controlled fistula consists of skin protection and fluid and electrolyte replacement. Complete bowel rest and parenteral alimentation may be needed. Fistulas associated with inflammatory bowel disease, cancer, distal obstruction, foreign bodies, or abscesses rarely resolve with conservative therapy and usually require operative intervention (20).

Paralytic ileus occurs frequently after intestinal operations and usually lasts for 24 to 72 hours. Prolonged paralytic ileus may result from ongoing peritonitis and mesenteric or retroperitoneal hematomas following extensive dissections. Prolonged or recurrent ileus typically produces silent, painless distention, whereas mechanical bowel obstruction is associated with colicky abdominal pain and characteristic high-pitched bowel sounds. Frequently, the distinction between prolonged ileus and mechanical obstruction is difficult. A meglumine diatrizoate (Gastrografin; Bristol Meyer Squibb, Evansville, IN) contrast study may be helpful in delineating slow bowel transit from mechanical obstruction.

Anastomotic leaks are uncommon following properly conducted bowel operations. Colonic anastomoses are more prone to leakage because of the presence of virulent bacteria, the thin muscle wall, and less luxuriant blood supply of the colon. Rectal anastomoses may be associated with a nearly 20% leakage rate, although only approximately 5% of these are clinically significant. The latter may manifest as intraabdominal abscesses and require laparotomy with a colostomy and wide drainage (21).

OPERATIVE TECHNIQUES

Inadvertent Enterotomy

Inadvertent bowel lacerations may occur during lysis of adhesions commonly associated with previous operations or peritonitis. Multiple full-thickness bowel lacerations in close proximity are best treated by segmental resection of the affected bowel and primary reanastomosis. Small enterotomies in healthy bowel can be treated by primary repair. The edges of the enterotomy are debrided of any nonviable tissue. The enterotomy is then closed transversely using a two-layer technique with a running 3-0 absorbable suture full-thickness inner layer followed by an outer layer of interrupted 3-0 silk or absorbable suture material and Lembert inverting seromuscular sutures (Fig. 64.3).

End-To-End Anastomosis

Segmental bowel resections are usually completed with primary end-to-end reanastomosis. Many techniques have been described. The most widely used in the United States is a two-layer open technique. Following placement of noncrushing bowel clamps proximal and distal to the limits of resection, the bowel is divided along with the intervening mesentery. The edges of the bowel are carefully inspected for adequacy of blood supply and viability and approximated to ensure that an anastomosis can be constructed under no tension.

The initial step involves placement of a series of interrupted 3-0 Lembert sutures to approximate the posterior wall beginning with the corner sutures. Next, the inner layer is begun using two full-thickness 3-0 running absorbable sutures starting at the midpoint of the posterior wall and continued around the circumference of the bowel using a Connell or baseball stitch on the anterior wall. The anastomosis is then completed with a series of interrupted Lembert sutures forming the outer layer of the anterior wall. The patency of the lumen is checked, and the mesenteric defect is closed (Fig. 64.4).

Side-to-Side Anastomosis

The chief use of the side-to-side anastomosis is to bypass areas of obstruction secondary to malignant disease or radiation, re-

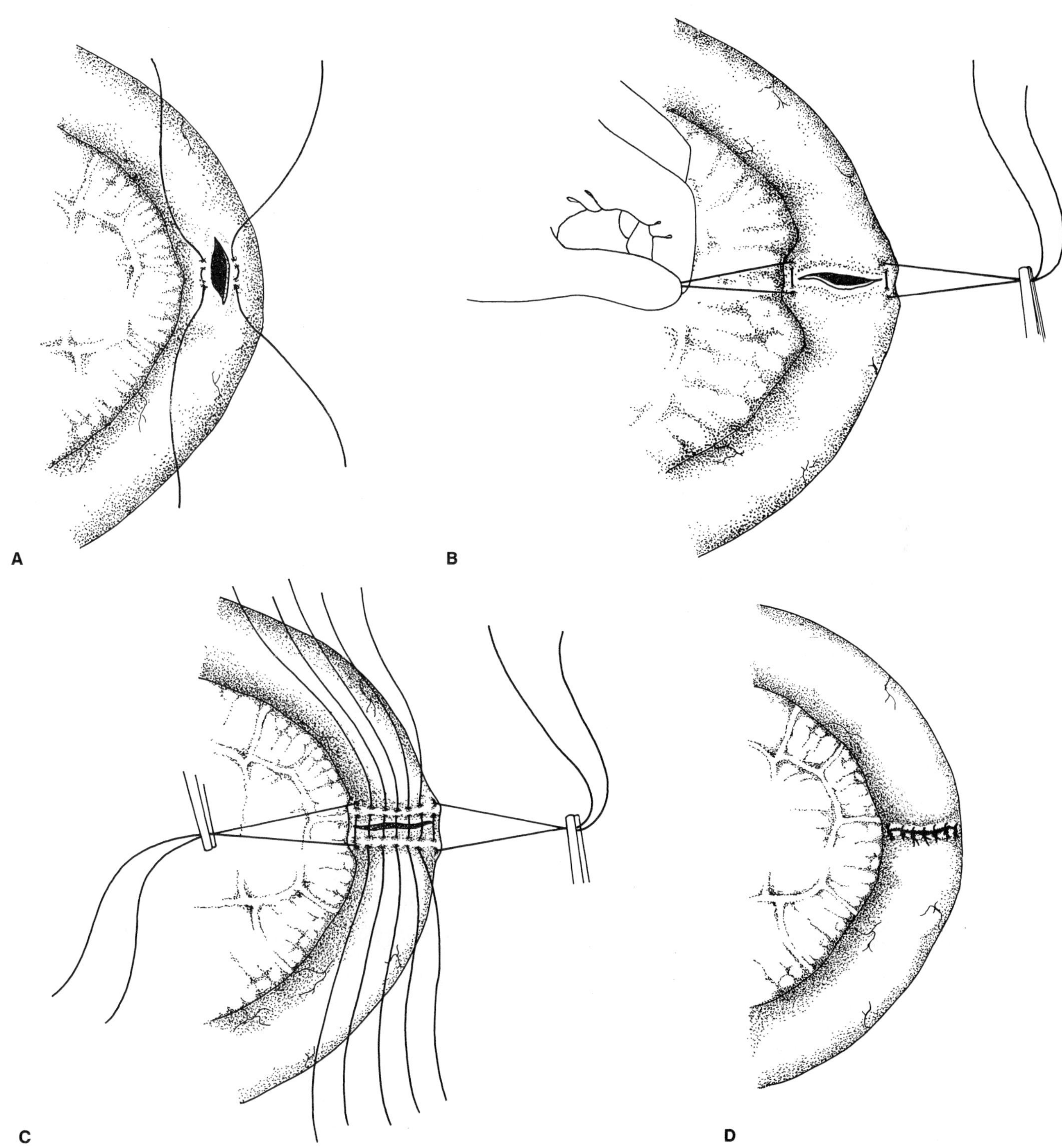

Fig. 64.3. Closure of inadvertent enterotomy. **A.** Seromuscular Lembert sutures placed on the mesenteric and antimesenteric aspects of the enterotomy. **B.** Tension applied to sutures to set up a transverse closure. **C.** The closure is completed with the placement of additional Lembert sutures between the initial corner sutures. **D.** The sutures are tied and cut; the enterorrhaphy is completed.

section of which would involve extensive or prolonged dissection. To use this technique, normal areas of bowel proximal and distal to the point of obstruction are identified and arranged in an isoperistaltic fashion before the construction of the anastomosis. The common hand-sewn form of this technique uses two layers in a manner similar to the end-to-end anastomosis. Initially, 3-0 silk corner sutures are placed at either end of the proposed stoma, halfway between the mesenteric and antimes-

enteric borders of the bowel. The outer layer of the posterior row is then constructed with a series of interrupted 3-0 silk Lembert sutures. Longitudinal enterotomies twice the diameter of the bowel are made in each loop of bowel along the posterior row of sutures. The running inner layer of full thickness 3-0 absorbable suture is started at the midpoint of the posterior row and continued anteriorly with a Connell or baseball stitch. The anterior wall of the anastomosis is completed with a series

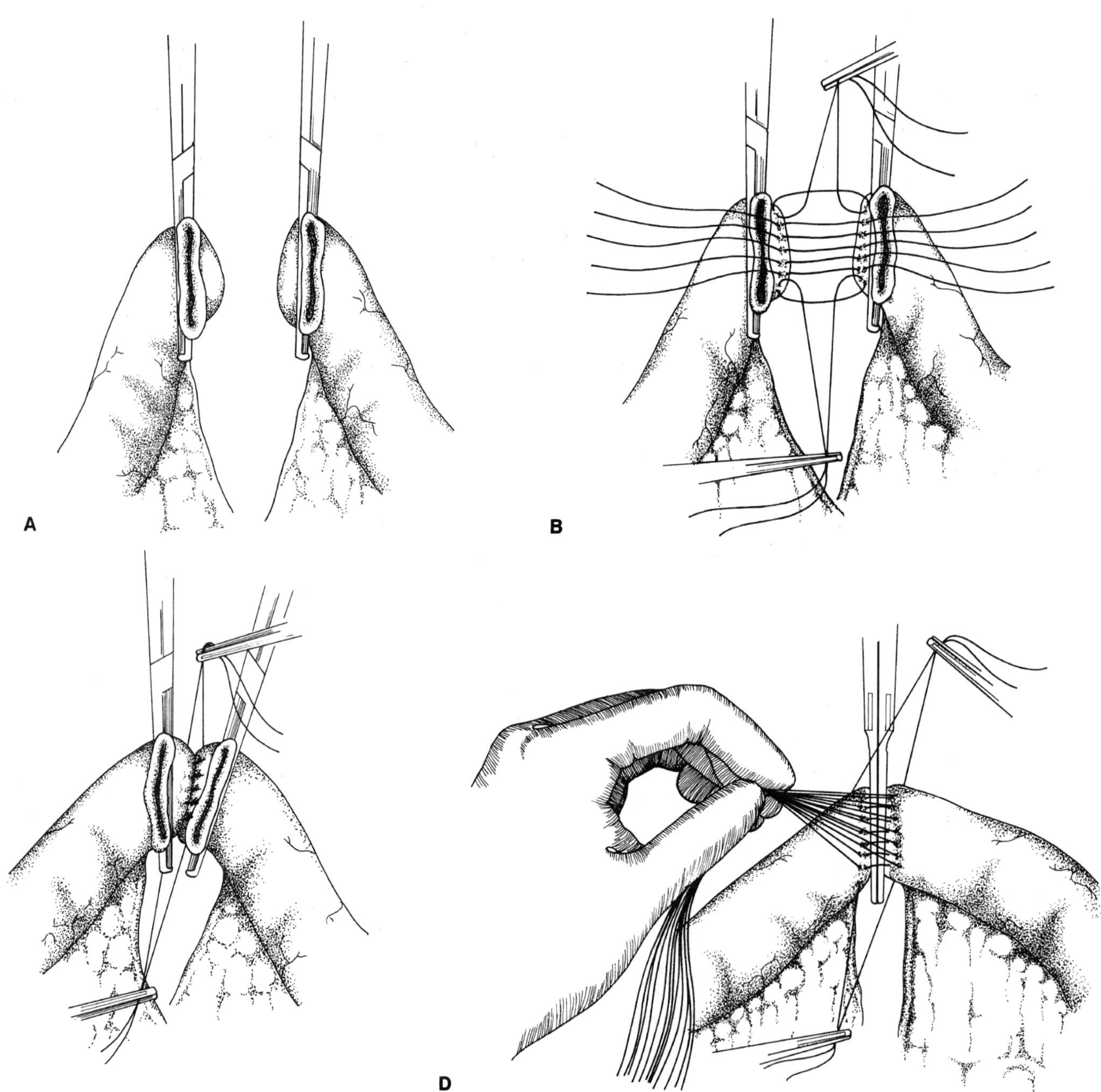

Fig. 64.4.   Closed end-to-end anastomosis. **A.** The divided intestine is held by noncrushing bowel clamps. **B.** Corner sutures are placed in the mesenteric and antimesenteric edges and tagged. The back row of seromuscular Lembert sutures is placed. **C.** The posterior row is completed; the sutures are tied and cut. **D.** The anterior row of seromuscular Lembert sutures is placed after the excess bowel has been trimmed and the clamps approximated under no tension.

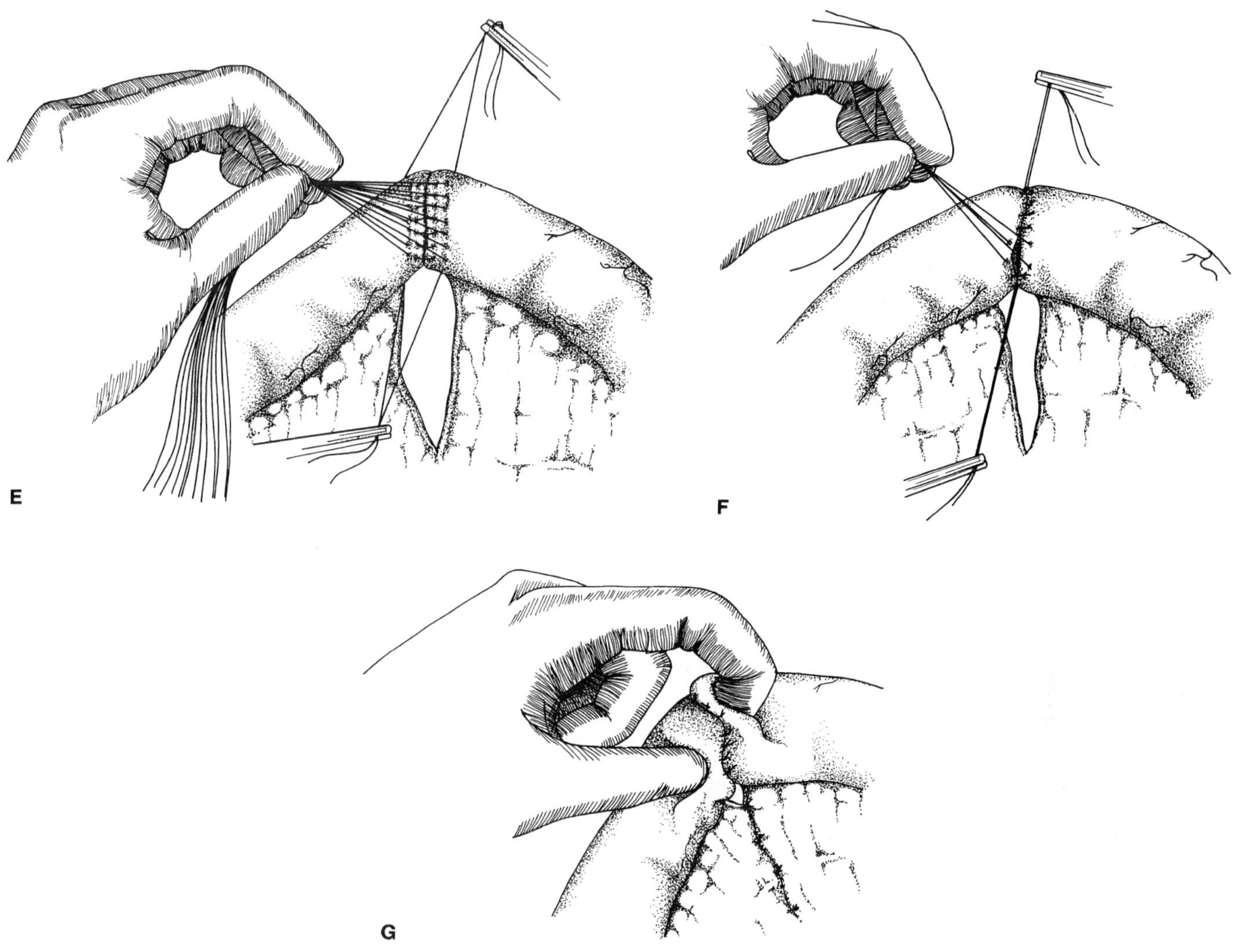

Fig. 64.4. *(continued)* **E** and **F.** The bowel clamps are removed, and the anterior row of sutures is tied. **G.** The patency of the anastomosis is checked by palpation. The mesenteric defect is closed with interrupted sutures.

of interrupted 3-0 silk Lembert sutures. The patency of the lumen is checked and the mesentery is closed to prevent internal herniation of bowel (Fig. 64.5).

End Colostomy

A colostomy may be necessary when the colon or rectum is inadvertently entered, for decompression of distal obstruction, or diversion of the fecal stream from a segment of previously irradiated or otherwise compromised bowel. The colon is divided between bowel clamps or with a GIA stapling device, and the mesentery is mobilized to allow approximately 5 cm of viable bowel to extend through the abdominal wall at the site selected for the colostomy. The distal colonic segment is resected and closed in two layers and, if possible, sutured to the anterior abdominal wall near the colostomy site to facilitate future mobilization for colostomy takedown. A circle of skin 2 to 3 cm in diameter is excised at the site selected for the

colostomy. The abdominal wall muscles are divided, and the fascia opened widely to avoid constriction of the bowel. The colon, still closed, is then passed through the abdominal wall defect and anchored to the external fascia with four quadrant seromuscular 3-0 absorbable sutures. Any internal hernia is closed by attaching the colonic mesentery to the anterior and lateral abdominal wall, and the operation is completed and the incision closed before maturing the colostomy. The colostomy can be matured following closure of the abdomen or 24 to 48 hours later with a series of interrupted full-thickness 3-0 sutures between the cut edge of the colon and the skin edge of the colostomy (Fig. 64.6).

Staple Techniques

The ease and speed of stapling devices for bowel operations have increased their popularity in recent years. The principles governing intestinal anastomoses are the same for staple and

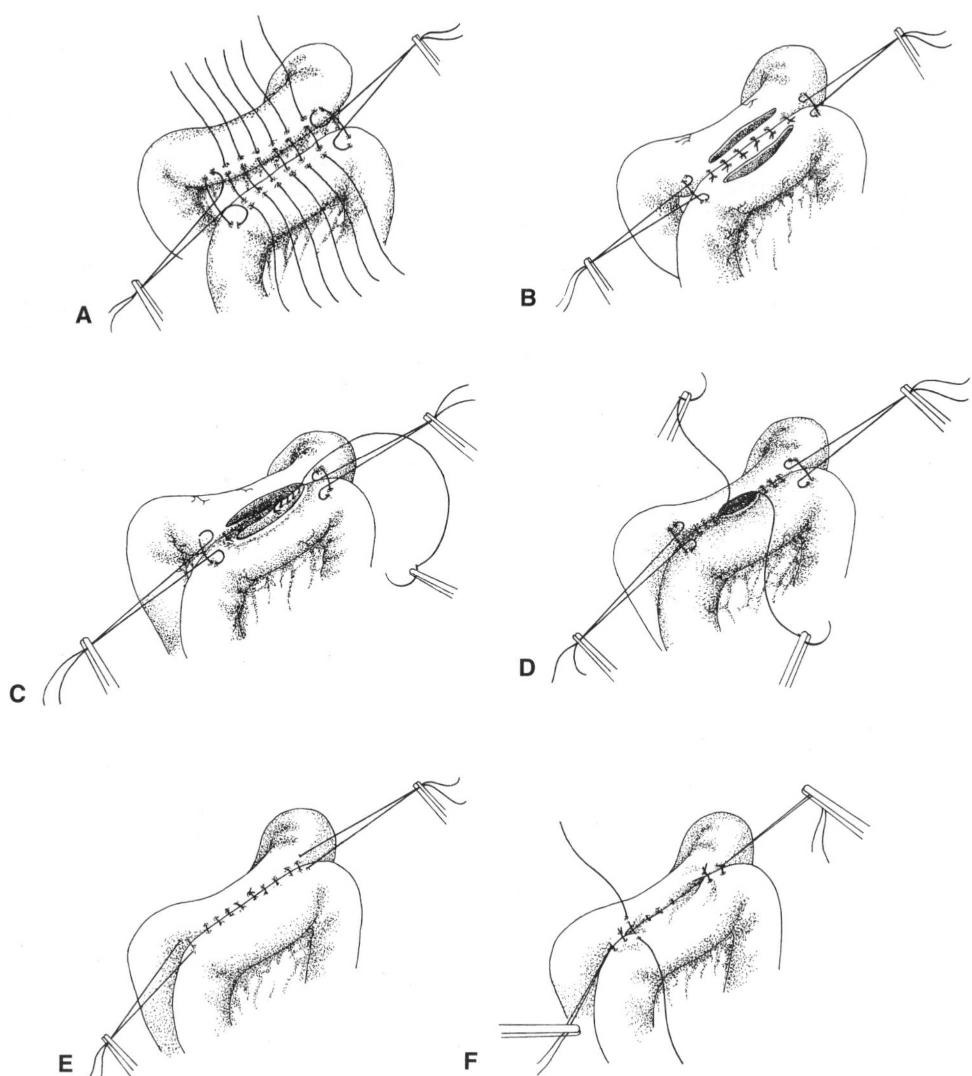

Fig. 64.5. Side-to-side two-layer anastomosis. **A.** The posterior layer of seromuscular Lembert sutures is placed first. **B.** The posterior sutures are tied and cut. The enterotomies are made, and hemostasis is secured with electrocautery. **C.** The inner layer of 3-0 absorbable suture is begun at the center of the posterior row and run as an over-and-over stitch toward each corner. **D.** and **E.** The anterior inner layer is completed with a Connell or baseball stitch. **F.** The anastomosis is completed with the anterior outer layer of seromuscular Lembert sutures.

suture techniques. Adequate blood supply, meticulous anastomotic technique, and lack of tension are essential for the success of any bowel anastomosis. Common errors in staple techniques include failure to overlap suture lines, leaving gaps in the anastomotic line, and failure to include the full thickness of the bowel wall within the jaws of the stapler, creating weak points in the anastomosis and potentiating leaks.

A standard staple technique for an end-to-end anastomosis is the triangulation method. Preparation of the intestine for anastomosis includes mesenteric clearance of a more liberal margin of intestine at the points to be anastomosed to ensure that staples are placed through full thickness of the entire circumference of the bowel. Because excess bowel is ultimately excised, there is usually adequate vascularity to ensure healing of the anastomotic site.

With the aid of full-thickness stay sutures at the mesenteric and antimesenteric edges of the bowel to be anastomosed and with an Allis clamp grasping the full thickness of both bowel walls, the posterior row of staples is applied to the full thickness of both bowel walls; the excess is excised from within the lumen. An additional stay suture placed anteriorly triangulates the bowel, and two additional applications of staples are made anteriorly to include the full thickness of the bowel wall. The lines of staples should overlap to avoid gaps in the anastomotic lines. The mesenteric defect is then closed (Fig. 64.7).

The use of the GIA stapling instrument provides a quick method of side-to-side anastomosis to bypass obstructed intestine. The loops are arranged in isoperistaltic fashion and approximated with full-thickness stay sutures placed a distance of 2 to 3 cm greater than the proposed stoma. One fork of the

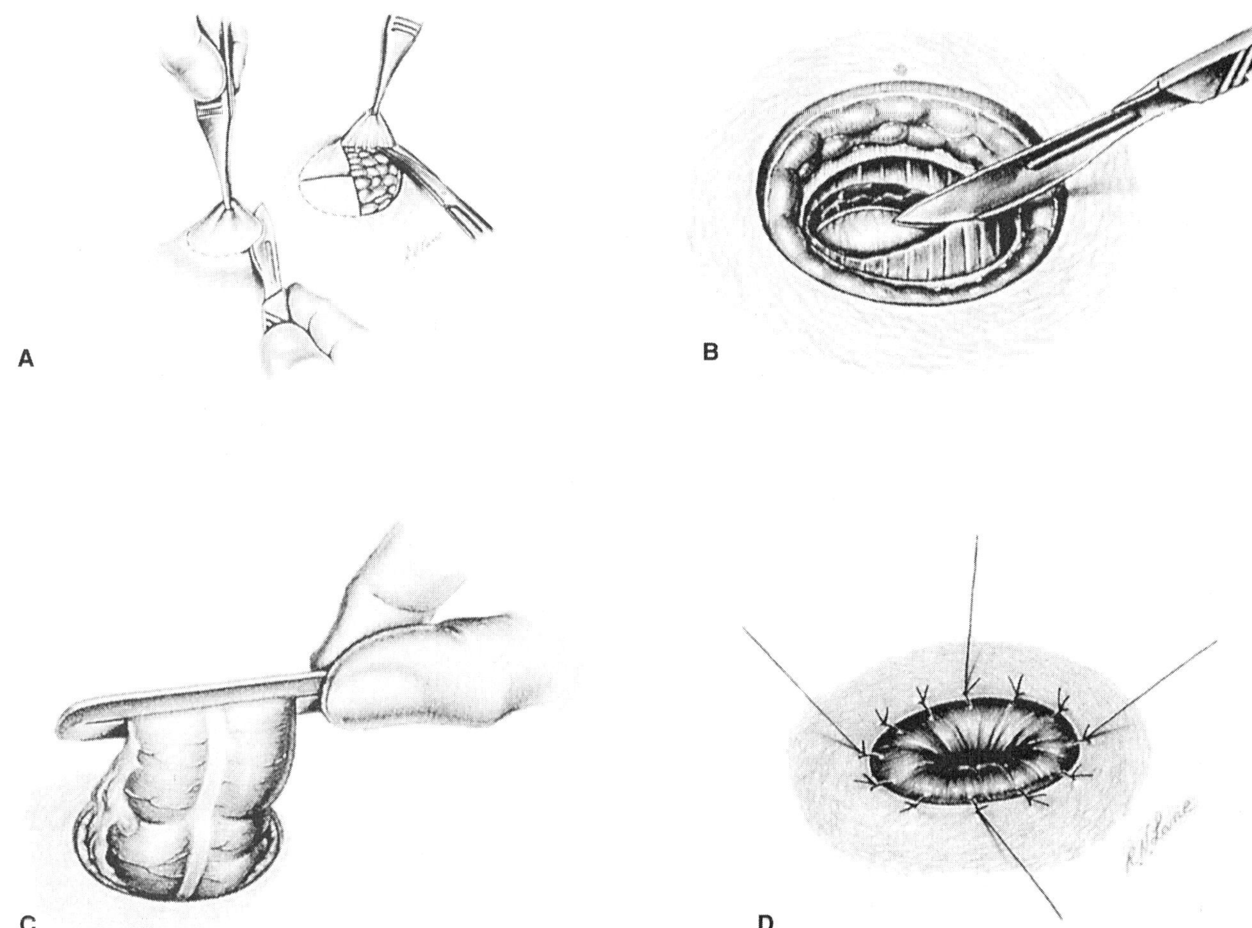

Fig. 64.6.   End colostomy. **A.** The exact site for the colostomy should be selected to ensure that an appliance will fit satisfactorily away from the umbilicus. **B.** Fascia, muscle, and peritoneum are divided to create a generous opening for the colostomy. **C.** The colon is delivered through the anterior abdominal wall. **D.** After the abdominal incision has been closed, a mucocutaneous suture is used to mature the colostomy. (Reprinted with permission from Thomson JPS. Colostomy: end iliac and loop transverse. In: Todd IP, Fielding LP, eds. Rob and Smith's operative surgery: alimentary tract and abdominal wall, colon, rectum, and anus. London: Buttersworth, 1983.)

GIA instrument is inserted into each loop via an enterotomy; the instrument is fired, thus making the entire anastomosis. After removal of the GIA, the twin enterotomies are closed with the TA 30, taking care that no gaps remain (Fig. 64.8).

Gastrostomy

The Stamm gastrostomy is one of several techniques commonly used to establish tube enterostomy access to the gastrointestinal tract for decompression or long-term enteral feeding.

A site in the body of the stomach along the greater curvature of the stomach is selected. Two concentric purse-string sutures are placed in the anterior surface of the stomach. The stomach is opened in the center of the purse-string sutures. The gastrostomy tube (usually a 24F or larger Foley catheter) is placed within the stomach, and the inner purse-string suture secured. A portion of the stomach wall is invaginated as the second purse-string suture is tied. The gastrostomy tube is brought

out the abdominal wall through a separate incision. Several interrupted sutures are placed to fix the stomach to the abdominal wall and skin at the catheter exit site. Malecot, Foley, and mushroom catheters have all been used successfully as gastrostomy tubes. One advantage of the Stamm gastrostomy technique is that once the need for enterostomy feeding has passed, the tube can simply be removed and the ostomy will generally seal promptly without the need for operative closure (22) (Fig. 64.9).

Needle-Catheter Jejunostomy

Another commonly used technique for enteral feeding is the needle-catheter jejunostomy. A thin-wall, 14-gauge needle is used to make a 3- to 5-cm seromuscular tunnel along the antimesenteric border of the jejunum 15 to 20 cm distal to the ligament of Treitz. A 16-gauge polyvinyl catheter is inserted through the thin-wall needle and fed 10 to 20 cm distally in

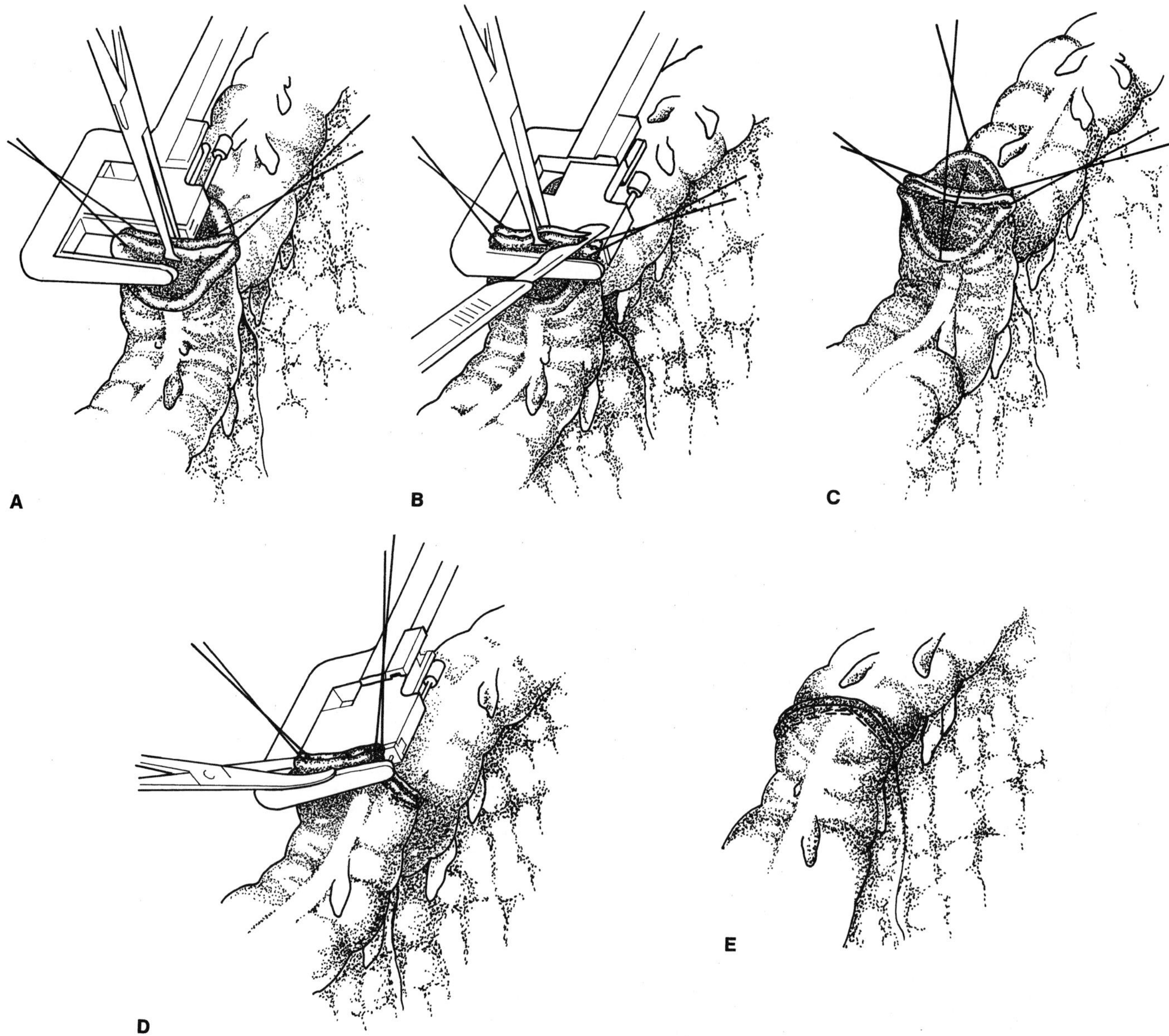

Fig. 64.7. End-to-end anastomosis, staple technique. **A.** Approximately 1 cm of bowel should be cleared of mesentery. This length will allow secure application of staples with the TA 55 and is not excessive because the excess bowel will be trimmed. Full-thickness sutures of 2-0 silk are placed at the mesenteric and antimesenteric edges of the bowel to be anastomosed, and the full thicknesses of both posterior walls are held in the center with an Allis clamp. The jaws of the TA 55 are placed to include the full thickness of both posterior walls beneath the sutures and clamp. **B.** After the posterior row of staples is placed, the excess bowel is shaved above the TA 55 between the stay sutures, which are retained. **C.** An additional full-thickness stay suture of 2-0 silk is placed anteriorly, midway between the corner sutures. **D.** Taking care to overlap the previously placed posterior row of staples, the full thickness of each remaining half of the anterior wall is alternately placed between the jaws of the TA 55, and the anterior rows of staples are placed. The excess is shaved above the instrument, retaining the center suture until the final anterior row of staples has been placed. Retention of the suture at the midpoint anteriorly ensures that the rows of staples overlap and that no gap exists between the anterior lines of staples. **E.** The anastomosis is completed, and the mesenteric defect is closed. The anastomosis should be checked again to ensure that no gaps exist between the line of previously placed staples.

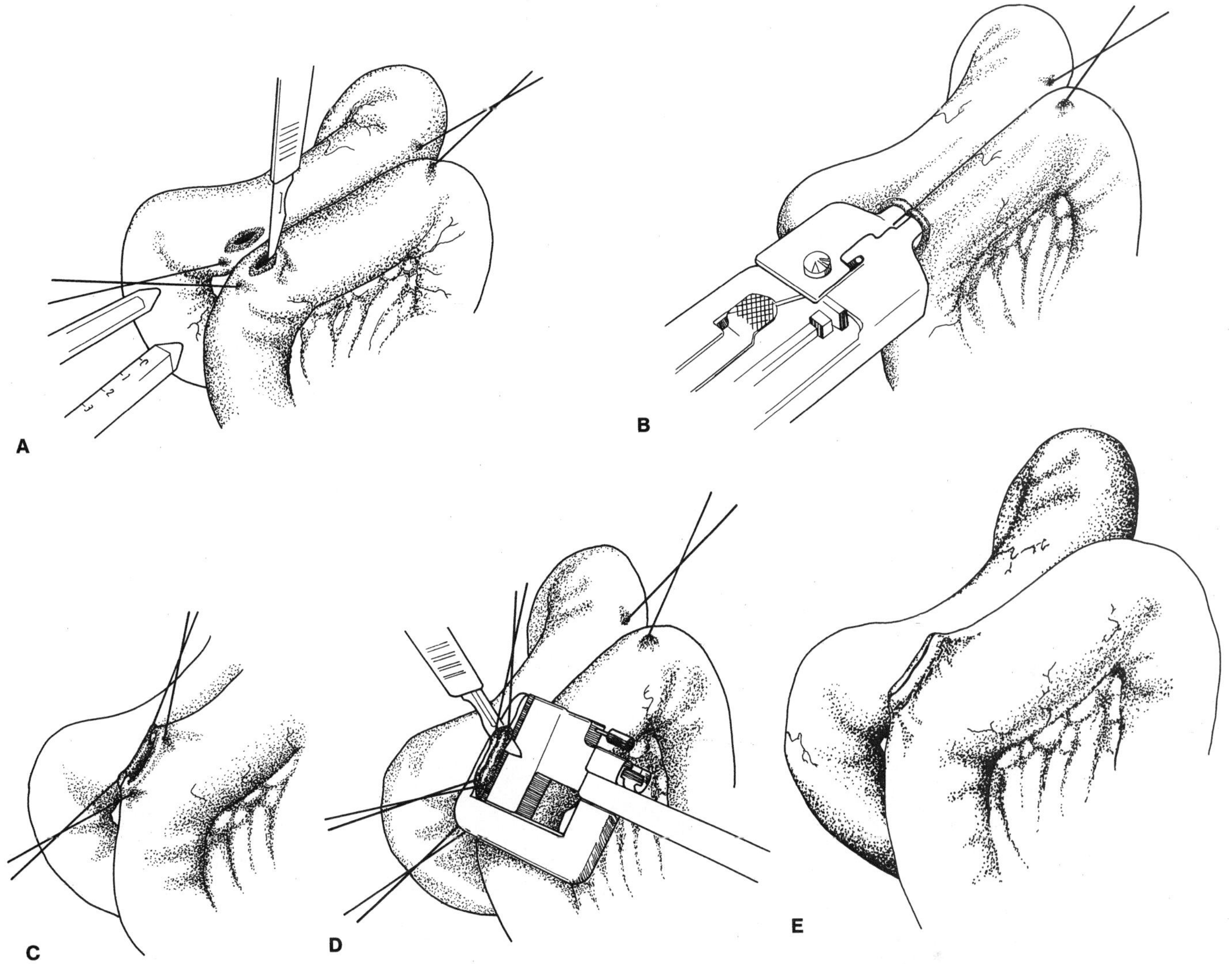

Fig. 64.8. Stapled side-to-side anastomosis. **A.** Stay sutures are used on the bowel. Small enterotomies are made to allow insertion of the GIA instrument. **B.** The side-to-side anastomosis is performed with the GIA instrument. **C.** The edges of the now common enterotomy are separated with stay sutures. **D.** The enterotomy is closed with a TA instrument in line with the longitudinal axis of the intestine. **E.** The completed side-to-side stapled anastomosis.

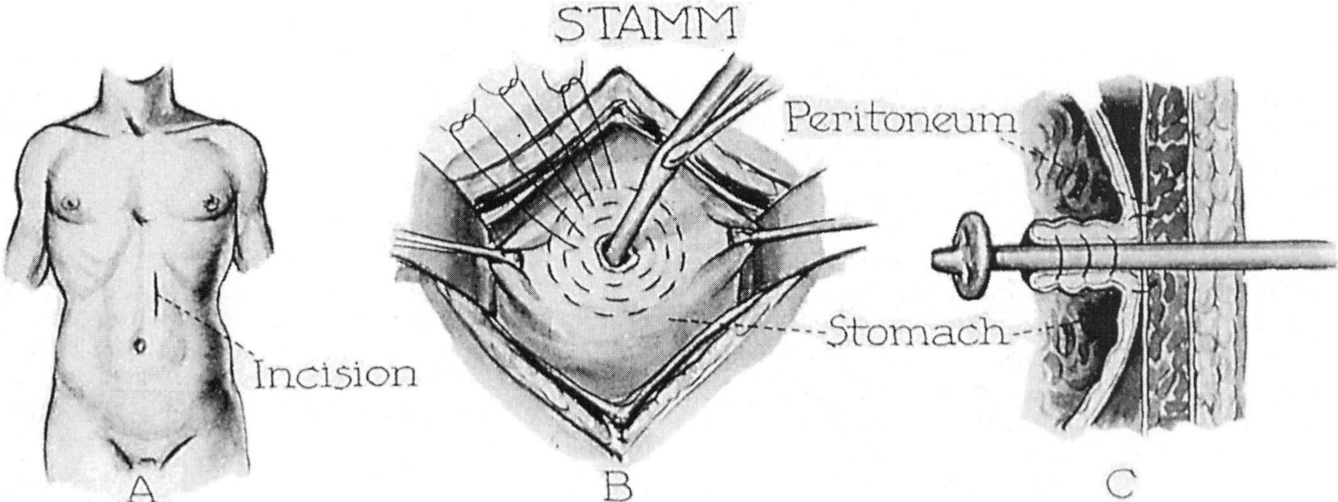

Fig. 64.9. Stamm gastrostomy. **A.** Insertion site identified in the body of the stomach through abdominal incision. **B.** A Foley or mushroom catheter is inserted within concentric purse-string sutures. **C.** Stomach sutured to the peritoneum after purse-string sutures are tied. (Reprinted with permission from Thorek P. Atlas of surgical techniques. Philadelphia: JB Lippincott, 1970.)

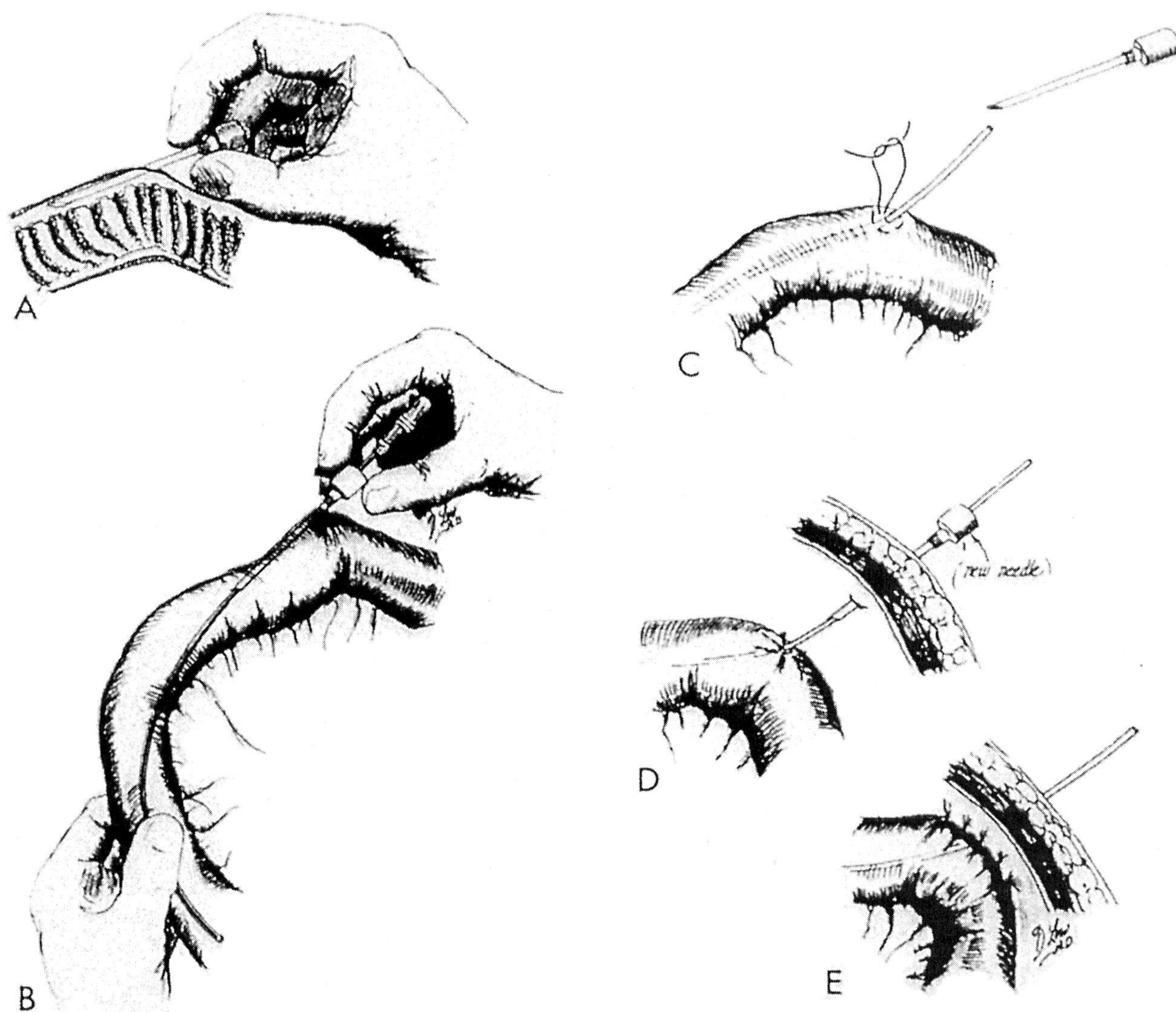

Fig. 64.10. Needle-catheter jejunostomy. **A.** Insertion of the needle within the jejunal wall. **B.** Insertion of the catheter with stylet through the needle into the jejunal lumen. **C.** Removal of the needle and placement of anchoring suture. **D.** Insertion of the needle through the abdominal wall for the catheter's exit. **E.** Jejunopexy. (Reprinted with permission from Rombeau JL, Barot LR, Low DW, et al. Feeding by tube enterostomy. In: Rombeau JL, Caldwell MD, eds. Enteral and tube feeding. Philadelphia: WB Saunders, 1984;1.)

the jejunum. The catheter is secured to the jejunal wall with a single 3-0 purse-string suture. A separate 14-gauge needle is passed through the abdominal wall, and the catheter is fed outside the abdomen. The jejunum, 5 to 10 cm proximal and distal to the insertion site, is secured to the abdominal wall; the catheter is secured to the skin (23) (Fig. 64.10). Feeding may start at 24 to 48 hours after the operation.

REFERENCES

1. Binder HJ. Absorption and secretion of water and electrolytes by small and large intestine. In: Sleisenger MH, Fordtran JS, eds. Gastrointestinal disease: pathophysiology, diagnosis, management. 3rd ed. Philadelphia: WB Saunders, 1983:844.

2. Fordtran JS. Stimulation of active and passive sodium absorption by sugars in the human jejunum. J Clin Invest 1975;55:728.

3. Gray GM. Mechanisms of digestion and absorption of food. In: Sleisenger MH, Fordtran JS, eds. Gastrointestinal disease pathophysiology, diagnosis, management. 3rd ed. Philadelphia; WB Saunders, 1983:844.

4. Hofmann AF, Poley JR. Role of bile acid malabsorption in the pathogenesis of diarrhea and steatorrhea in patients with ileal resection. Gastroenterology 1972;62:918.

5. Hofmann AF. Bile acid malabsorption caused by ileal resection. Arch Intern Med 1972;130:597.

6. Gray GM. Carbohydrate digestion and absorption: role of the small intestine. N Engl J Med 1975;292:1225.

7. Fordtran JS, Rector FC, Carter W. The mechanisms of sodium absorption in the human small intestine. J Clin Invest 1968; 47:884.

8. Adibi SA, Kim YS. Peptide absorption and hydrolysis. In: Johnson LR, ed. Physiology of the gastrointestinal tract. New York: Raven Press, 1981:325.

9. Donaldson RM. Intrinsic factor and the transport of cobalamin. In: Johnson LR, ed. Physiology of the gastrointestinal tract. New York: Raven Press, 1981.

10. Dent J, et al. Interdigestive phasic contractions of the human lower esophageal sphincter. Gastroenterology 1983;84:452.

11. Wever ID, et al. Disruptive effect of test meals on interdigestive motor complex in dogs. Am J Physiol 1978;235:661. Editorial.

12. Wood JD. Intrinsic neural control of intestinal motility. Ann Rev Physiol 1981;43:33.

13. Smith J, Kelly KT, Weinshilboum RM. Pathophysiology of postoperative ileus. Arch Surg 1977;112:203.

14. Heimbach DM, Crout JR. Treatment of paralytic ileus with adrenergic neuronal blocking drugs. Surgery 1971;69:582.

15. Altemier WA. The bacterial flora of acute perforated appendicitis with peritonitis. Ann Surg 1938;107:517.

16. Brooks JR, Smith HE, Pease FB. Bacteriology of the stomach immediately following vagotomy; the growth of *Candida Albicans*. Ann Surg 1974;179:859.

17. Bornside GH, Welsh JS, Cohn I. Bacterial flora of the human small intestine. JAMA 1966;196:109.

18. Derrik JR, Fadhli HA. Surgical anatomy of the superior mesenteric artery. Am Surg 1965;31:545.

19. McGuire HH. Complications of intestinal surgery. In: Greenfield LJ, ed. Complications in surgery and trauma. Philadelphia: JB Lippincott, 1984:447.

20. Reber HA, et al. Management of external gastrointestinal fistulas. Ann Surg 1978;188:460.

21. Beart RW, Kelly KA. Randomized prospective evaluation of the EEA stapler for colorectal anastomoses. Am J Surg 1981;141:143.

22. Randall HT, Caldwell MD. Enteral nutrition: nasoenteric and ostomy feeding. In: Scott HW, Sawyers JL, eds. Surgery of the stomach, duodenum, and small intestine. Boston, MA: Blackwell Scientific Publications, 1987.

23. Delany HM, Carneval NJ, Garvey JW. Jejunostomy by a needle catheter technique. Surgery 1973;73:786.

XVI

MEDICAL AND PSYCHIATRIC

65

Perioperative Nutritional Care of Genitourinary Cancer Patients

Robert C. Flanigan
Robert R. Isacksen

Malnutrition is a common finding in hospitalized surgical patients in general and in cancer patients in particular (1, 2). It occurs in 40 to 50% of patients with advanced pelvic malignancies, including urothelial cancer (3).

Malnutrition is essentially an imbalance between the intake of nutrients and their expenditure. Decreased intake may be secondary to anorexia or dysphagia; impaired digestion, external nutrient loss, competition for nutrients by tumor, and increased energy expenditures by the host may also contribute to malnutrition. Circulating factors in cancer patients may also be contributory. It has been proposed that tumor-host interactions may lead to an inflammatory response mediated by various cytokines that prevent nutritional repletion in some cancer patients, thereby promoting cachexia (4).

ALTERATIONS IN METABOLISM

Cancer patients have consistently been shown to have an elevated resting energy expenditure (5). In contradistinction to the situation with healthy subjects, this increased metabolic rate is maintained despite decreased alimentation (6, 7). Most patients fail to respond appropriately by increasing their intake of nutrients, and malnutrition results. Additionally, specific alterations in metabolism have been identified in cancer patients.

Carbohydrate Metabolism

Insulin resistance is a common development in cancer patients and may necessitate the use of exogenous insulin. Some tumors consume excessive amounts of glucose, contributing to caloric wasting. The tumor-bearing host may also exhibit increased whole body glucose utilization and turnover. Increased gluconeogenesis and Cori cycle activity are seen in patients with progressive weight loss (8). Tumors may consume glucose by

anaerobic glycolysis, producing lactic acid that requires reconversion to glucose by the host (an energy-losing cycle) (7).

Lipid Metabolism

The net effect of altered lipid metabolism is progressive depletion of body fat (7). Fat breakdown, serum lipid levels, and serum triglycerides are all increased. This loss of body lipid, caused by mobilization of free fatty acids from adipose tissue, occurs in the cancer patient at a time of increased caloric expenditures, resulting in an unbalanced caloric deficit (9).

Protein Metabolism

Cachexia and negative nitrogen balance have been shown to result in a loss of skeletal muscle mass in patients with cancer (9). Alterations in protein metabolism in cancer patients represent a failure to adapt appropriately to increased energy requirements at a time when nitrogen intake is frequently reduced. Starvation-adapted individuals typically reduce protein utilization to 5% or less of their energy requirements. In contrast, protein metabolism may account for 15 to 20% of energy expenditures in cancer patients.

NUTRITIONAL ASSESSMENT

Nutritional status has been shown to be predictive of a cancer patient's ability to withstand therapy and overall survival. The association between improving nutritional status and reduced perioperative morbidity, although intuitively sensible, is not convincingly supported by the available data. Assessment of nutritional status is nevertheless an integral part of the evaluation of cancer patients.

Anthropometrics, immune competence, and visceral protein status are commonly used for nutritional assessment (Table

Table 65.1.   Tests Commonly Used for Nutrition Assessment

TEST	MILD	MODERATE	SEVERE
Weight loss/last 3 months (lb)	10	10–20	>20
Lymphocyte count (/mm^3)	1200–2000	800–1200	<800
Albumin (g/dL)	3–3.5	2.5–3	<2.5
Skin recall antigens	—	—	Unresponsive
Transferrin (mg/dL)	150–200	100–150	<100

65.1). Anthropometric parameters are used to assess fat stores and muscle mass by measuring triceps skinfold thickness, mid-arm circumference, creatinine-height index, and weight-to-height ratio. Cell-mediated immunity may be evaluated by total lymphocyte count and skin testing for delayed hypersensitivity to recall antigens such as *Candida* and mumps. Serum albumin, transferrin, and prealbumin are useful measurements of visceral protein status. These measurements are useful for comparison to normal values and for serial evaluation during therapy. Nutritional assessment based on these factors demonstrates that approximately 20% of hospitalized patients are moderately malnourished and 5% are severely malnourished. This number approaches 40% in patients with advanced urothelial cancers (10).

The high incidence of malnutrition and anorexia in cancer patients necessitates early dietary assessment and intervention. Improved patient care is possible when the counseling and assessment skills of a dietitian are added to the oncology team.

NUTRITIONAL REQUIREMENTS

An important goal of nutritional therapy is to supply all caloric requirements in the form of nonprotein calories. This avoids use of endogenous proteins for energy and allows exogenous proteins to be used in anabolic processes. Therefore, it is necessary to determine caloric and protein requirements and provide these needs using appropriate amounts of carbohydrate, lipids, and proteins.

There are several ways to determine a patient's caloric requirements. Basal energy expenditure can be estimated by the Harris-Benedict equation, which takes into consideration age, weight, and height. A rough estimate for healthy individuals is 25 kcal/kg/day or 900 kcal/m^2 of body surface area/day. The actual resting energy expenditure can be estimated by considering the disease state and clinical condition. These estimates represent multiples of baseline energy requirements and increase with the severity of the patient's clinical condition.

A more accurate method of assessment, indirect calorimetry, involves measuring the net amount of oxygen absorbed into the pulmonary circulation over a given period. This can be calculated by determining the oxygen content of arterial blood and subtracting the oxygen content of blood obtained from the pulmonary artery (a mixed venous sample). This is assumed to be equal to the amount of oxygen consumed by metabolic processes. With this information, caloric needs (approximately 5 kcal/L of oxygen consumed) can be calculated.

It is also possible to measure the amount of carbon dioxide produced in relation to the amount of oxygen consumed by metabolic processes. This ratio is known as the respiratory quotient and can be used to tailor therapy to avoid overfeeding with carbohydrates. Conversion of excess carbohydrates to fat produces large amounts of carbon dioxide (i.e., has a high respiratory quotient), which may hamper efforts in weaning critically ill patients from ventilator support or worsen carbon dioxide retention in patients with pulmonary disease. By providing such patients with lipid calories in greater proportion, carbon dioxide production may be reduced.

Daily protein needs are approximately 1.2 to 1.5 g/kg body weight/day. Protein requirements can be more accurately determined by measuring urinary nitrogen excretion. Assuming that urea accounts for 85% of total nitrogen excretion, urinary urea excretion can be compared with the amount of protein ingested or administered, and therapy can be adjusted to maintain positive nitrogen balance.

In addition to basic caloric and protein requirements, essential fatty acids, vitamins, and free elements must be considered. Essential fatty acid deficiency can occur within 1 week in patients receiving total parenteral nutrition (TPN). Fat emulsions provide a concentrated source of calories in addition to preventing essential fatty acid deficiency. Vitamins are supplied by adding a multivitamin formulation to the standard TPN solution daily. Trace elements such as zinc, copper, magnesium, chromium, and selenium are similarly supplied on a daily basis.

NUTRITIONAL INTERVENTION

Enteral Nutrition

Nutritional support should be delivered enterally whenever possible. The cost-savings of enteral nutrition over TPN are substantial. In addition, by using the alimentary tract, gut mucosa remains intact and bacterial translocation can be minimized, thereby reducing the risk of sepsis. Complications associated with obtaining and maintaining central venous access are also avoided.

Malnourished patients with a functioning gastrointestinal tract who are unable to adjust their regular diet to meet nutritional needs may benefit from a variety of commercially available supplements. Patients who are physically unable to ingest the required amount may benefit from placement of a small nasogastric feeding tube through which supplements may be administered. Gastric overdistention, gastroesophageal reflux, and aspiration can be avoided by adjusting feeding schedules and serially measuring retained gastric volumes. Continuous nasogastric infusion is more readily tolerated than bolus feedings. Diarrhea may be controlled by adding pectin to the formula (Table 65.2).

Table 65.2. Enteral Formulas[a]

PRODUCT	CALORIC DENSITY (kcal/mL)	% PROTEIN	% CARBOHYDRATE	% FAT	OSMOLALITY (mOsm/L)
Criticare HN	1.06	14.0	81.5	4.5	650
Ensure Plus HN	1.50	16.7	53.3	30.0	650
Glucerna	1.0	16.7	33.3	50.0	375
Netro	2.0	14.0	43.0	43.0	635
Osmolite	1.06	14.0	54.6	31.4	300
Osmolite HN	1.06	16.7	53.3	30.0	300
Pediasure	1.0	12.0	43.5	44.5	310
Peptamen	1.0	16.0	51.0	33.0	380
Portagen	1.0	14.0	40.0	46.0	310
Pulmocare	1.5	17.0	28.0	55.0	490
Replete	1.0	25.0	45.0	30.0	380
Suplena	2.0	6.0	51.0	43.0	600
Twocal HN	2.0	16.7	43.2	40.1	690
Ultracal	1.06	17.0	46.0	37.0	310

[a] Manufacturer's data.

Parenteral Nutrition

Parenteral solutions that use carbohydrates as the primary energy source are of high osmolarity and have a sclerotic effect on veins, necessitating central venous administration. Because fat is a more efficient energy source, providing 9 kcal/g compared with 4 kcal/g for carbohydrates, lipid solutions are less concentrated and can be administered peripherally. It should be noted that peripheral hyperalimentation alone is rarely adequate to achieve positive caloric balance because the peripheral delivery of carbohydrates is limited by the hypertonicity of the solution (Table 65.3).

The most common complication of TPN is infection related to the access catheter. Hyperglycemia is also common, affecting 15 to 25% of patients. Other complications include electrolyte abnormalities, elevation of liver function studies, and complica-

Table 65.3. Amino Acid Formulas

MIXED AMINO ACID FORMULATION		
Amino acids (4.25%)	42.5 g/L 250 g/L	Approximate volume 1050 mL
Dextrose (25%)	4.5 mEq/L	1825 mOsm/L
Calcium	5 mEq/L	1020 kcal/L
Magnesium	40 mEq/L	6.7 g nitrogen/L
Potassium	35 mEq/L	Calorie : nitrogen ratio
Sodium	74.5 mEq/L	127 : 1
Acetate	52.5 mEq/L	
Chloride	12 mM/L	
Phosphorus	1000 units/L	
Heparin sodium	10 mL	
*Multivitamins	1 mL	
*Trace elements		

ESSENTIAL AMINO ACID FORMULATION		
Essential amino acids (2%)	15.7 g 350 g	Approximate volume 800 mL
Dextrose (43%)	1.6 mEq	1935 mOsm/L
Potassium	31.5 mEq	1253 kcal
Acetate	1000 units	2.5 g Nitrogen
Heparin sodium	10 mL	
Multivitamins		

* Daily additives
Modified from Parenteral and enteral nutrition manual, 6th ed. University of Michigan Medical Center, 1990.

Table 65.4. Complications

COMPLICATION	CAUSE
Sepsis	*Staphylococcus aureus*
	Candida albicans
	Gram-negative (rare)
Metabolic	Blood glucose 800–1500 mg/100
Hyperosmolar nonketotic coma	mL secondary to glucose intolerance (present in 15–25% of patients)
Hyperchloremic metabolic acidosis	Excess Cl⁻ in solution
	Renal failure resulting in inability to excrete acid urea
	Gastrointestinal or renal losses of base
Hyponatremia	Mild inappropriate ADH secretion with water retention
Abnormal liver functions (SGOT, SGPT, alkaline phosphatase, bilirubin)	Essential fatty acid deficiency
	Excess carbohydrate administration
Catheter insertion Pneumothorax Hemothorax Arterial injuries Air embolism	Incorrect technique

Table 65.5.   Variables to be Monitored

VARIABLE	INITIAL	DAILY	TWICE WEEKLY	WEEKLY	AS INDICATED
Urine					
Glucose		x			
Specific gravity		x			
24° UUN	x				x
Blood					
Hgb, WBC	x			x	
BUN, creat., lytes	x		x		
Ca, PO$_4$	x		x		
Glucose	x		x		
Liver function tests	x		x		
Triglycerides	x			x	
Mg	x			x	

tions associated with obtaining central venous access (Table 65.4). Many centers have designated nutrition support teams that frequently provide specific recommendations for monitoring serum electrolytes, glucose, and renal and liver function studies on a regular basis in patients receiving TPN (Table 65.5).

RESULTS OF THERAPY

Although the idea that perioperative nutritional support would benefit cancer patients by reducing perioperative morbidity and mortality is appealing, existing data are mixed. Many reports are hampered by poor study design, such as including well-nourished and malnourished patients in the same treatment groups and treating patients with nonstandardized regimens for variable treatment periods. Although many of these studies showed improvement in parameters used to assess nutritional status, few have shown improvement in clinically important endpoints.

Klein and Koretz have provided an excellent review of prospective randomized clinical trials of nutritional therapy in surgical patients with cancer (11). Of 22 prospective trials evaluating perioperative TPN, only 5 studies found statistically significant differences in clinical endpoints. One study reported decreased mortality and perioperative complications (wound infections, anastomotic leak, bowel obstruction, abscess, and prolonged ileus) in the treatment group (12). Two studies reported decreased incidence of postoperative complications and no significant difference in mortality (13, 14). In contrast, a large multicenter Veterans Administration study reported similar complication rates in TPN and control groups, but an increased incidence of infections was observed in the TPN group (15). Six of seven studies reporting length of hospitalization showed no significant difference between treatment and control groups. A single study by Askanazi et al. involving 35 patients with bladder cancer demonstrated a significant decrease in length of hospitalization from 24 to 17 days in TPN-treated patients (16). Combined data from 10 studies that pro-

vided at least 7 days of preoperative TPN showed a decrease in the absolute complication rate of 5%.

Seven prospective randomized trials that evaluated preoperative and postoperative enteral nutrition showed no significant difference in mortality or length of hospitalization, but did demonstrate a 15% decrease in perioperative complications in the treatment group (17–23). This difference was even greater if only studies involving malnourished patients were considered.

Neither TPN nor enteral nutrition has been shown to provide obvious benefits related to survival, tumor response, or chemotherapeutic toxicity in patients undergoing chemotherapy or radiation therapy (11).

In summary, these data suggest that perioperative nutritional support will be beneficial to malnourished surgical patients by preventing approximately 5 to 15% of major postoperative complications. Malnourished patients should be identified preoperatively by nutritional assessment and should receive a minimum of 7 days of preoperative support, continued postoperatively until adequate oral intake resumes. Nutritional support should also be initiated postoperatively in those patients in whom a lengthy period of fasting or inadequate intake is anticipated.

Nutrition and Renal Failure

The urologic oncologist is occasionally confronted with patients whose renal function is impaired. This may necessitate modification of nutritional support, with specific attention to volume status, protein source, and the administration of glucose and electrolytes.

Patients with chronic renal insufficiency require a reduced protein diet to minimize production of nitrogenous waste. Essential amino acid requirements can be met while providing 0.6 g protein/kg body weight/day. Caloric (energy) requirements are not specifically altered in patients with renal insufficiency.

In a landmark work, Rose and Wixoni not only established

and characterized the amino acids as either essential or nonessential, but also observed that in healthy patients, as little as 1.42 g of essential amino acids along with small amounts of nonessential acids were capable of establishing nitrogen equilibrium (24). Further research indicated that in patients fed predominantly essential amino acids, the nitrogen by-products of urea could serve as a source of synthesis of nonessential amino acids (25). In this setting, urea must be broken down into ammonia and carbon dioxide by intestinal bacteria, recycled in the biliary system, and transformed into nonessential amino acids (26).

This concept has been incorporated into current intravenous renal formula TPN solutions. These solutions typically contain 2.5 g of nitrogen as essential amino acid and 43% dextrose in 750 mL of solution. Flow rates for this solution should begin at approximately 30 mL/hr to a maximum of 75 to 80 mL/hr.

Although the rationale for the use of essential amino acids in renal failure is to reduce the rate of urea production by eliminating nonessential amino acids, much controversy still exists regarding whether the use of essential amino acid solutions in this patient population is necessary. Formulas containing both essential and nonessential amino acids in reduced quantities have also been tested in patients with renal failure. Freiend and Fischer demonstrated a decreased BUN and creatinine as well as decreased mortality in patients receiving only essential amino acids (27). Conversely, in a prospective randomized trial, Mirtallo et al. found no difference in serum creatinine or survival (28). For this reason, the use of essential amino acid solutions in patients with renal failure remains questionable. Certainly, if patients are receiving dialysis, these solutions are not mandatory.

NUTRIENT MODULATION

There is increasing evidence suggesting that specific individual nutrients may be beneficial to cancer patients (29). Amino acids such as arginine and glutamine have been studied most intensively. Effects of arginine-enhanced diets may include retarding tumor growth, modulating immune function, and improving wound healing (30–32). Other studies have investigated nutrients such as branched-chain amino acids, omega-3 fatty acids, and nucleic acids. The effect of such nutrient modulation on clinical outcomes remains to be shown.

CONCLUSION

Malnutrition is a common finding in genitourinary cancer patients that should be sought through careful assessment and treated appropriately by the enteral or parenteral route. Appropriate intervention may prevent perioperative morbidity and contribute to better all-around patient care.

REFERENCES

1. Meguid MM, Meguid V. Preoperative identification of the surgical cancer patient in need of postoperative supportive total parenteral nutrition. Cancer 1985;55:258.

2. Bristrian BR, et al. Protein status of general surgical patients. JAMA 1974;230:858.

3. Mohler JL, Flanigan RC. The effect of nutritional status and support on morbidity and mortality of bladder cancer patients treated by radical cystectomy. J Urol 1987;137:404.

4. Espat NJ, Moldawer LL, Copeland EM. Cytokine-mediated alterations in host metabolism prevent nutritional repletion in cachectic cancer patients. J Surg Oncol 1995;58:77.

5. Theologides A. Cancer cachexia. Cancer 1979;43:2004.

6. Grande F, Anderson JT, Keyes A. Changes of basal metabolic rate in men in semi-starvation and re-feeding. J Appl Physiol 1958;12:230.

7. Theologides A. Cancer cachexia in nutrition and cancer. In: Winick M, ed. Current concepts in nutrition. New York: John Wiley & Sons, 1977;6:75.

8. Holroyade CP, et al. Altered glucose metabolism in metastatic carcinoma. Cancer Res 1975;35:3710.

9. Kralovic RC, Zepp EA, Cenedella RJ. Studies of the metabolism of carcass fat depletion in experimental cancer. Eur J Cancer 1977;13:1071.

10. Flanigan RC, Rapp RP, McRoberts JW. Nutritional assessment and therapy in advanced urothelial cancer. Urol Clin North Am 1984;11:671.

11. Klein S, Koretz R. Nutrition support in patients with cancer: what do the data really show? Nutr Clin Pract 1994;9:91.

12. Müller JM, Brenner U, Dienst C, et al. Preoperative parenteral feeding in patients with gastrointestinal carcinoma. Lancet 1982;1:68.

13. Heatley RV, Williams RH, Lewis MH. Preoperative intravenous feeding: a controlled trial. Postgrad Med J 1979;55:541.

14. Woolfson AM, Smith JA. Elective nutritional support after major surgery: a prospective randomized trial. Clin Nutr 1989;8:15.

15. The Veterans Affairs Total Parenteral Nutrition Cooperative Study Group. Perioperative total parenteral nutrition in surgical patients. N Engl J Med 1991;325:525.

16. Askanazi J, Hensle TW, Starker PM, et al. Effect of immediate postoperative nutritional support on length of hospitalization. Ann Surg 1986;203:236.

17. von Meyenfeldt MF, Meyerink WJ, Soeters PB, et al. Perioperative nutritional support results in a reduction of major postoperative complications especially in high risk patients. Gastroenterology 1991;100:553. Abstract.

18. Sagar S, Harland P, Shields R. Early postoperative feeding with elemental diet. Br Med J 1979;1:293.

19. Ryan JA, Page CP, Babcock L. Early postoperative jejunal feeding of elemental diet in gastrointestinal surgery. Am Surg 1981;47:393.

20. Shukla HS, Rao RR, Banu N, et al. Enteral hyperalimentation in malnourished surgical patients. Indian J Med Res 1984;80:339.

21. Smith RC, Hartemink RJ, Hollinshead JW, et al. Fine bore jejunostomy feeding following major abdominal surgery: a controlled randomized clinical trial. Br J Surg 1985;72:458.

22. Foschi D, Cavagna G, Callioni F, et al. Hyperalimentation of jaundiced patients on percutaneous transhepatic biliary drainage. Br J Surg 1986;73:716.

23. Flynn MB, Leightty FF. Preoperative outpatient nutritional

support of patients with squamous cancer of the upper
aerodigestive tract. Am J Surg 1987;154:359.

24. Rose WC, Wixoni RL. The amino acid requirements of man:
part XVI. the role of the nitrogen intake. J Biol Chem 1955;
217:997.

25. Mahler JF, Schreiner GE. Metabolic problems related to
prolonged dialytic maintenance of life in oliguria. JAMA
1961;176:399.

26. Schboerb PR. Essential L-amino acid administration in uremia.
Am J Med Sci 1960;252:650.

27. Freiend HR, Fischer JE. Parenteral nutrition in acute renal
failure using essential and non-essential amino acids. Presented
at the fourth clinical congress of the American Society of
Parenteral and Enteral Nutrition, Chicago, 1980.

28. Mirtallo MS, et al. A comparison of Nephramine and
Freamine-II in the nutritional support of patients with
compromised renal function. Presented at the fourth clinical
congress of the American Society of Parenteral and Enteral
Nutrition, Chicago, 1980.

29. Lind DS, Cendan JC, Copeland EM. Nutrition for the cancer
patient. Contemp Surg 1995;47:17.

30. Reynolds JV, Daly JM, Shou J, et al. Immunologic effects of
arginine supplementation in tumor-bearing and nontumor-
bearing hosts. Ann Surg 1990;211:202.

31. Lieberman MD, Nishioka K, Redmond HP, et al.
Enhancement of interleukin-2 immunotherapy with L-arginine.
Ann Surg 1992;215:157.

32. Kirk SJ, Hurson M, Regan MC, et al. Arginine stimulates
wound healing and immune function in elderly human beings.
Surgery 1993;114:155.

66

Psychosexual Support for Genitourinary Cancer Patients

Marilyn Davis

The most fundamental principle of medicine is love.
PARACELSUS (1493–1541)

With the increasing life expectancy patterns of men and women, the incidence of genitourinary cancers will continue to escalate propelled by high-incidence tumors of older adulthood such as bladder and prostate cancer. Scientific concentration and discovery in the fields of basic and clinical cancer research have illuminated new pathways for earlier diagnosis, multimodality treatment, and continuing care with corresponding benefits as measured by decreased morbidity and prolonged survival. Coincident with the revolutionary discoveries in science and technology has been the growing acknowledgment of psychosocial issues globally referred to as quality of life, incorporating physical, mental, and social well-being components. This chapter reviews principles and practices in facilitating communication and incorporating supportive maneuvers in the management of urologic malignancies, with special emphasis on psychosexual concerns and interventions.

GENERAL CONSIDERATIONS

Rehabilitative Process

With the growing number of individuals experiencing extended survival after a cancer diagnosis and institution of therapy designed to cure, control, or palliate malignancy, measures to facilitate the rehabilitative process have been developed in the decades since the passage of the National Cancer Act in 1971. Rehabilitation goals as defined by the National Cancer Institute's 1972 objectives included the following.

- Provision of psychological support at diagnosis.
- Achievement of optimal physical functioning after diagnosis.
- Application of vocational counseling as appropriate.
- Promotion of social functioning (1).

Because human beings are inherently sexual from the time of birth through death, maintenance of an optimal level of psychosexual functioning is implicit in the Institute's stated objectives. An interdisciplinary approach to promote optimal physical, psychological, and social functioning throughout the diagnostic, therapeutic, continuing care, and surveillance phases is suggested to achieve the rehabilitation objectives and to assist the individual with a genitourinary malignancy to develop and achieve realistic rehabilitative goals.

Psychological Preparation

Continuous acknowledgment of the unique individuality of the patient, maintenance of the patient rather than the disease as the focal point, and finally recognition of predictable points throughout the cancer continuum that are associated with either precipitation or exacerbation of stress are suggested. These trigger points for stress include the diagnostic phase, initiation of therapy, completion of therapy, evaluation of response, introduction of a treatment modality new to the patient, demonstration of locally recurrent or metastatic disease, exacerbation of symptoms, and exhaustion of all viable options. The degree and intensity of stress may be directly proportional to the time interval between achievement of a complete response and subsequent recurrence (2).

Anxiety-arousing events that may intensify stress include:

A. Diagnostic procedures;
B. Staging extent of disease;
C. Treatment phase—surgery, radiation therapy, chemotherapy, hormonal manipulation, and biologic response modifiers;
D. Increasing supportive care needs—pain control, nutritional supplementation, mobility assistance, and dependency interventions;
E. Financial impact;
F. Spirituality;
G. Socialization.

Psychological preparation, defined as "the emotional perspective that the patient and family will adopt to manage the diagnosis, treatment, and related deficits," is fundamental to a positive rehabilitative process (3). The following suggestions in initial and subsequent health-care provider/patient discussions are offered to promote and maintain an optimal degree of psychological preparation.

1. Focus on the individuality of each patient and uniqueness of the situation.
2. Set a specific place and time for discussion.
3. Encourage the presence of support individual(s) as requested or permitted by the patient.
4. Allow ample time, encourage questions, and assure privacy.
5. Review anatomic structure and physiologic function through models or diagrams.
6. Provide written material about planned procedures and treatments.
7. Elicit degree of comprehension by a technique such as asking for the patient's recall of information previously reviewed.

A discussion of universal concerns and emotions tailored to the stage of disease, although time-intensive, may be beneficial in the psychological preparation necessary for a functional emotional outlook. Universal concerns include body image, self-esteem, loss of body parts and function, loss of independence, impact on loved ones, uncertainty, and financial costs associated with disease and treatment. Anger, confusion, guilt, fear of pain, loneliness, grief, and anticipation of disease-related death are commonly experienced. Also, the global perception of cancer is a negative one. Establishment of the universality of concerns and emotions frequently sets the stage for the individual and his or her loved ones to discuss personal concerns.

AGE CONSIDERATIONS

Developmental Issues and Challenges

Predictable, developmental tasks in early adulthood include gaining work expertise, selecting and adapting to a mate, starting a family, and fulfilling community and civic roles (4). A diagnosis of cancer such as a testicular tumor in early adulthood may affect timely achievement of the tasks and one's view of self as a sensual and sexual individual.

The individual from 35 to 55 years of age is mastering an occupation, achieving civic and social mastery, experiencing physiologic changes, and adjusting to aging parents and older children while developing leisure and volunteer activity patterns (4). Clearly, a diagnosis of a genitourinary malignancy such as prostate cancer in middle age will have a powerful effect on task accomplishment. The middle-aged adult's self-image and self-esteem as a worker, parent, mate, and community member will be pivotal in the process of adapting to the diagnosis of cancer and internalization of living with a chronic disease that may affect individual longevity.

The transition from mid-life to older adulthood is characterized by role changes precipitated by a gradual shift in family responsibilities, retirement, and a decline in economic opportunities. The major developmental challenge is achievement of ego integrity or a comfortable acceptance of one's limitations (5). The aging adult's tasks are adjusting to the process of physiologic aging, retirement, reduced income, loss of spouse, and deaths of relatives and friends, while affiliating with one's age group and maintaining a safe and solvent environment (4). The older adult's tasks, although conceptually more compatible with adaptation to the additional challenge of living with a chronic disease, may be colored by a magnitude of changes associated with loss of familiar work, home, and community routines, particularly if relocation at retirement has occurred. Timing of a cancer diagnosis may be particularly devastating for the older adult who has extended the mastery of work tasks for additional years to achieve a personal goal in retirement (6).

Genitourinary cancers are estimated to account for 24% of all new cancer cases in the United States (7). The majority of new malignancies are diagnosed in individuals older than age 50 (8). Before age 50, the incidence of cancer is higher in women, whereas after age 60, the incidence of cancer is significantly higher in men; this reflects tumor/age distributions for high-incidence genitourinary cancers, most notably prostate cancer (9). More than half of all cases of cancer are diagnosed after the age of 65, although this population accounts for approximately 12% of the U.S. population (10, 11). In contrast to a probability of 1 in 700 of developing cancer within 5 years at age 25, the probability is 1 in 14 at age 65 (9). Thus, common values of the aging population are considered.

The older person is generally concerned about finances, losing independence, and placing a burden on family or society. The senior adult is more likely to approach the health-care system dreading a potentially negative outcome and avoiding the practitioner from a passive perspective, not wanting to inconvenience the provider with a litany of symptoms and complaints. An individual with Medicare has acute care coverage but may not have comprehensive coverage for early detection, including screening, and oral medications. Because the aggressive pursuit of symptoms may not be undertaken vigorously in the older adult, delay in diagnosis may result. Although intellectual function is usually maintained in older adulthood, short-term memory may gradually decline, reinforcing the need for application of recall and repetitive techniques. The older adult needs special interdisciplinary consideration in the establishment of a framework for open communication to identify components of his or her dilemma that may be modified or alleviated to facilitate psychosexual rehabilitation and maintain psychological preparation.

SEXUAL CONSEQUENCES

Awareness of the effect of cancer on the individual is essential not only in the early, diagnostic phase, but also throughout the therapeutic, continuing care, and surveillance phases to recognize frustrations and challenges peculiar to one's inability to fulfill general age-specific developmental tasks and to maintain a unique perspective as a sensual, sexual human being. Sexuality, defined as the "physical, emotional, intellectual, and social aspects of an individual's personality, which expresses maleness or femaleness," is inextricably woven into the fabric of one's profile of developmental tasks, goals, and achievements (12). For example, the young adult with cancer may experience an exaggerated sense of guilt, particularly with respect to a sense of abandoning one's spouse or children, whereas the older adult may grieve the loss of intimacy with a spouse. Clarification of the sexual issues unique to the individual will greatly enhance adjustment to disease and treatment and support the foundation of psychological preparation.

Self-Image and Self-Esteem

The closely related concepts of self-image (defined as a mental mirror image of oneself) and self-esteem (how valuable a person feels individually to self and others) are affected by the physiologic processes associated with aging as well as physical and emotional changes precipitated by a life crisis such as cancer. The actual or potential change in a body part or function such as that manifested by malignancy will have negative connotations from both self-image and self-esteem perspectives. The actual loss of body tissue, an organ, or function will have a unique meaning for the individual as he or she strives to incorporate the loss into the evolving self-image. Expression of grief associated with the loss is likely. Persistence or intensification of a grief reaction or escalation to severe depression signals the need for psychological intervention. Inability to incorporate the physical changes into one's self-image within 6 months to 1 year after surgery suggests the need for professional counseling. A feeling of relief or hope on removal or eradication of the malignancy often occurs and may provide the impetus for the individual to set new goals and master new challenges, thereby expanding internal resources and revitalizing self-image.

In addition to the challenge of adjusting self-image to accommodate the loss or change precipitated by a genitourinary malignancy, the individual has an equally complex task of maintaining self-esteem. Enhancement or support of one's self-esteem is facilitated by encouraging the individual to accept his or her uniqueness and value. Self-esteem may be promoted by encouraging the individual to do the following.

1. Share anxieties, fears, and hopes with others and permit others to share their anxieties, fears, and hopes.
2. Respond to the challenges of tumor diagnosis and treatment with courage and dignity.
3. Take responsibility for what is happening to oneself by being knowledgeable and interactive in seeking medical attention, reporting symptoms, and participating in therapy decisions.

McKenna recommends the following guidelines for maintaining an individual-focused perspective in treatment and support.

- Treat a patient individually, respecting his or her right to accept or refuse offered therapy.
- Permit the individual's choice in degree of willingness to discuss his or her cancer experience.
- Avoid labeling the individual by diagnosis.
- Accept the individual as he or she is and was before the cancer diagnosis (1).

Sexuality

Closely associated with the concepts of self-image and self-esteem is the more global construct of sexuality, which is an integral part of every individual's nature. Nonreproductive sexuality with its key component, sensuality, or the awareness and appreciation of the messages delivered to us by our senses—sights, sounds, touches, smells, tastes, and rhythms in life—is a continuing need in human beings throughout life. Psychosexual stages of development as summarized in Table 66.1 are exquisitely sensitive to influence by a crisis such as the diagnosis of cancer and the ongoing stresses precipitated and aggravated by therapy and continuing concerns regarding response and relapse. In keeping with the individualization of a patient-centered approach to disease and treatment, knowledge of the basic psychosocial tasks and sexual tasks common to chronologic development facilitates a discussion of universal concerns to promote identification, discussion, and resolution of the individual's unique concerns. Because the genitourinary tract exists in tandem with the reproductive system in men and women, cancer treatment often affects sexual function and threatens the individual's sense of maleness or femaleness. Correspondingly, changes chemically mediated by chemotherapy, hormonal therapy, and medications designed to alleviate the side effects of therapy may alter mood, diminish libido, and induce fatigue and lethargy; thus, the capacity for optimal sensual and sexuality expression is indirectly modulated. Sexual concerns are not gender-specific or age-specific. Expressions of sexuality do not exist in a vacuum, but rather in a dynamic equilibrium with pain, fatigue, worry, debility, and other symptoms profoundly affecting libido and sexual performance. Sexual function as a component of sexuality is often overlooked or avoided by physicians based on the clinician's discomfort or perceptions of the insignificance of sexuality in the presence of life-threatening disease. Medical, radiotherapeutic, and surgical interventions with a direct disease focus may be highlighted and psychosexual concerns deemphasized or not acknowledged by the clinician. In general, any time an individual's self-image or self-concept has been challenged or modified by treatment modalities, sexuality has been affected.

Quality of Life

Although disease-free and overall survival are the classic endpoints for therapeutic clinical trials in cancer, the effects of

Table 66.1.   Psychosexual Stages of Development

STAGE	BASIC PSYCHOSOCIAL TASK	SEXUAL TASKS
Infancy (0–2 yr)	Acquiring basic trust, learning to walk, talk	Gender identity
Childhood (2–12 yr)	Acquiring a sense of autonomy versus shame and doubt; entering and adjusting to school	Pleasure-pain associated with sexual organs and eliminative functions; masturbation takes place with resulting shame and acceptance; secondary sex characteristics become evident
Adolescence (13–20 yr)	Acquiring sense of identity versus role confusion	Mastery over impulse control, acceptance of conflict between moral proscription and sexual urges, handling new physiologic functions (menses for girls and ejaculate for boys)
Young adulthood (20–45 yr)	Acquiring a sense of intimacy versus isolation; vocational effectiveness; interpersonal security; "sexual adequacy"	Sexual adequacy and performance plus fertility concerns and questions related to parenting
Middle adulthood (50–70 yr)	Acquiring a sense of self-esteem versus despair; adjusting to diminution of one's energy and competence; "empty nest syndrome" plus care of aging parents or their death; adjusting to change in physique and evidence of aging	For the female, menopause and resulting vasomotor changes, atrophy of breasts, clitoral size, and vaginal lubrication; for the male, delay on attaining an erection, a reduced compulsion to ejaculate, episodic impotence, possible prostatitis
Old age	Adjusting to loss of friends, family, confrontations with old age and dying, painful joint conditions, reduced hearing and visual acuity; adjustment to social stigmatization of being "old"	Reduced vitality, fear of incompetence or injury (coital coronary); fear of being viewed as "dirty old person"; unavailability of a partner (widow/widower); limited physical capacity and reduced options

treatment on physical, mental, and social well-being components of quality of life (as gauged by the patient) are increasingly being systematically measured. Assessments of physical functioning at serial points over time have been applied historically in the clinical setting, as exemplified by the Karnofsky scale, with a percentage score assigned based on the clinician's judgment of the patient's performance status. Subsequent studies have demonstrated that the physician's perception of the patient's quality of life can differ significantly from the patient's perception (13). The standardization of methods has allowed the systematic monitoring of physical function, psychological dimensions, and social dimensions. This may ultimately allow comparison among patients and evaluation of different modalities with equivalent survival expectations; it may also allow adjuvant therapy for patients at risk of recurrence (14). Quality-of-life data may help in the assessment of risk-to-benefit ratios while promoting an integrated patient-focused approach to care and evaluation.

Baseline Sexual Evaluation

Genitourinary cancer and healthy sexuality are not mutually exclusive. In general, a satisfactory pattern of sexuality before cancer diagnosis facilitates the continuation of an equally or acceptably satisfactory pattern after diagnosis. A troubled pattern of sexuality before diagnosis is predictive of trouble after diagnosis. Assessment of the individual's pattern of sexuality before diagnosis greatly enhances the clinician's ability to assess the effect of therapy and recommend interventions that may optimize continuation of a satisfactory sexual pattern. Guidelines for obtaining a brief sexual history include the following.

- Provide privacy for discussion and assure confidentiality.
- Set the stage for the discussion by addressing general themes associated with age, gender, and tumor type.
- Review treatment-associated changes in organ and physiologic function.
- Encourage expression of individual's pattern of libido and sexual performance.
- Concentrate on the individual's perception of cancer and its effect on sexuality.
- Allow for the possibilities of celibacy, a nontraditional partner, or nontraditional expression of sexuality.
- Recognize sexuality issues in need of professional assessment and intervention.

The following questions as suggested by Kolodny et al. focus on sexual function and assist in developing the baseline assessment (15).

Are you sexually active? If "yes," then ask:
What is the frequency of your sexual activity?
Are you satisfied with your sex life? If "no," why not? followed by:
Do you have difficulty obtaining or maintaining an erection?
Do you have difficulty with control of ejaculation?

Masters and Johnson describe the physiologic changes of vasoconstriction and myotonia that are essential to the process of arousal and maintenance of physical capacity for sexual intercourse (16). Therapeutic modalities have varying degrees of influence on these processes either temporarily or permanently. The sexual response cycle for men and women incorporates excitement, plateau, orgasm, and resolution. Components of the male sexual response, including desire, subjective arousal,

Table 66.2.   Elements of Brief Sexual Counseling

Educating patient
   Illustrate genital and pelvic anatomy using models or pictures
   Explain the normal sexual response cycle
   Explain the impact of specific treatments on sexual function
   Give advice on options for sexual rehabilitation:
      Sex therapy
      Vaginal dilators
      Hormone replacement
      Water-based lubricants
      Vacuum erection device
      Home penile injections
      Penile prostheses
      Changes in medication
Minimizing physical handicaps
   Time sex to avoid pain and fatigue
   Learn to cope with ostomy appliance, limb prosthesis, laryngec-
      tomy, and so forth
   Find comfortable positions
   Female dyspareunia can benefit from lubricants and dilators
   Erectile dysfunction can be treated appropriately
   Use open sexual communication, verbal and nonverbal
Changing attitude
   Debunk myths on cancer and sex:
      Venereal contagion of cancer
      Cancer as punishment for sins
      Resuming sex is unhealthy
   Accept noncoital sex when coitus not possible
   Sex cannot always be spontaneous
   Sex is not just for the young and healthy
Giving advice on resuming sex
   Either partner can initiate sex
   Increase expression of nonsexual affection
   Start slowly using sensate focus format
   Discuss how to deal with physical attractiveness (mastectomy, os-
      tomy, and so forth): desensitize to reality versus camouflage
Resolving couple conflict
   Make private time for each other
   Discuss fears and sadness
   Negotiate illness-related changes in marital roles (wage earning,
      childcare, budgeting, and so forth)
   Act as team in dealing with conflict in extended family

erection, emission, ejaculation, and orgasm, have separate mechanisms of control that can be affected independently. Female sexual response incorporating desire, subjective arousal, vaginal expansion, and lubrication may be affected similarly. Elements of brief sexual counseling including education, minimizing physical handicaps, attitude change, advice on resuming sex, and resolving couple conflict are summarized in Table 66.2.

CANCER SITE CONSIDERATIONS

Specific disease sites including bladder, prostate, testis, penis, and kidney are reviewed with particular emphasis on psychosex-

ual concerns and support. Table 66.3 provides an overview of effects of surgery for pelvic or genitourinary cancer on male sexual physiology.

Bladder Cancer

Men and women with a history of recurrent superficial bladder cancer have undergone repetitive cytoscopies frequently accompanied by biopsies along with local therapies including tumor resection, laser therapy, and intravesical instillation of chemotherapeutic and biologic agents to prevent recurrence. In addition to therapeutic results, these procedures and treatments may also have nontherapeutic sequelae including decreased interest in intimate sexual expression. Because superficial bladder cancer may progress to invasive disease, the chronicity of followup and fear of progression may adversely affect sexuality and self-image. Some men report pain with erection or ejaculation, and women may experience pain with intercourse. Additionally, the partners of individuals undergoing therapy for superficial bladder cancer may have concerns regarding tumor contagion and transfer of side effects of therapy. Erectile capacity may also be affected in the population of generally older adults with superficial bladder cancer, due to conditions unrelated to cancer such as cardiovascular diseases and being treated with antihypertensive medications.

Radical cystectomy involves the removal of the urinary bladder, prostate, and seminal vesicles along with pelvic lymphadenectomy. Complete urethrectomy is performed if tumor extension to the urethral mucosa is suspected. Urinary diversion is managed with the creation of an ileal conduit or, when appropriate, a continent urinary reservoir. Resumption of sexual activity favoring continent urinary reservoir has been reported (17). In general, candidates for bladder reconstruction are younger and in overall good health, thus making it difficult for the older adult to contrast quality-of-life issues with comorbid factors. Nerve-sparing radical cystectomy has been reported to result in an 83% recovery of erection with a drop to 40% in men who had complete urethrectomy (18). In a series of 112 men interviewed before cystectomy, 35% reported at least mild erectile dysfunction unrelated to their cancer diagnoses and 20% were no longer sexually active with a partner. In the 73 men from the same original series who provided follow-up data on sexual function after cystectomy, 50% remained sexually active, although 91% experienced some degree of erectile dysfunction. Intensity of orgasm was unchanged for 35%, reduced for 53%, and reported as more pleasurable for 11%. Twelve percent of the original sample elected to have surgical implantation of a penile prosthesis (19). The recent surgical techniques in continent urinary diversion and cavernous nerve-sparing cystoprostatectomy have greatly contributed to the achievement of optimal rehabilitation in many men who wish to remain potent and sexually active.

Women undergoing radical cystectomy experience the removal of the urinary bladder, urethra, uterus, adjacent ligaments, cervix, ovaries, Fallopian tubes, and anterior wall of the

Table 66.3. Effects of Surgery for Pelvic or Genital Cancer on Male Sexual Physiology

SURGICAL PROCEDURE	HORMONAL BASIS OF SEXUAL DESIRE	CAPACITY FOR PLEASURE WITH GENITAL TOUCH	CAPACITY FOR ERECTION	SENSATION OF ORGASM	EJACULATION	DYSPAREUNIA
Radical prostatectomy	Unchanged	Unchanged	Usually impaired.[a] Men younger than 60 are more likely to recover; full recovery takes 6 months	Unchanged or mild loss of intensity	No semen produced; dry orgasm	Rare
Radical cystectomy	Unchanged	Unchanged	Usually impaired.[a] Men younger than 60 are more likely to recover; full recovery takes 6 months	Unchanged or mild loss of intensity	No semen produced; dry orgasm	Rare but is more likely after complete urethrectomy
Abdominoperineal resection	Unchanged	Unchanged	Often impaired, but recovery rates are higher than for radical prostatectomy or cystectomy	Unchanged or mild loss of intensity	Dry orgasm is common because of damage to presacral sympathetic nerves	Rare but some perineal pain or phantom rectal sensations
Total pelvic exenteration	Unchanged	Unchanged	Almost always permanently impaired	Unchanged or mild loss of intensity	No semen produced; dry orgasm	Occasional
Partial penectomy	Unchanged	Erotic sensations still occur in remaining genital area	Unchanged. Penile shaft lengthens to permit coitus and (often) female orgasm	Unchanged	Unchanged	Rare; genital edema after groin dissection
Total penectomy	Unchanged	Erotic sensations still occur in remaining genital area	None	Unchanged but need to relearn erotic zones	Unchanged but semen is expelled through perineal urethrostomy	Occasional; genital edema after groin dissection

[a] With the development of new nerve-sparing surgical techniques, rates of erectile recovery are higher. However, a 6-month recovery period is still necessary.

vagina, with the posterior wall used to retubularize the vagina. Oophorectomy decreases circulating estrogen, which—coupled with removal of the anterior vaginal wall—decreases vaginal lubrication and elasticity. If the woman's postoperative expression of sexuality includes penile-vaginal intercourse, initial dyspareunia may be alleviated with water-soluble vaginal lubricants or estrogen creams. Continent urinary diversion and new techniques to spare more of the anterior vaginal wall may facilitate sexual rehabilitation in sexually active women. Because radical cystectomy does not damage the pudendal nerve in either males or females, orgasmic capacity is retained.

Prostate Cancer

Radical prostatectomy has traditionally resulted in modest to complete erectile dysfunction in the majority of preoperatively potent men. With the refinement of surgical technique to spare one or both neurovascular bundles of the prostatic nerve plexus, gradual recovery of erectile ridigity resulting in erections sufficient for vaginal penetration was reported in 69 to 74% of cases (18). In this same series of patients, in the men for whom one neurovascular bundle was spared, of the 69% who achieved erections sufficient for vaginal penetration, only 32% reported recovery of normal erectile rigidity. Candidates for preservation of neurovascular bundles most likely to achieve functional erection postoperatively are middle-aged men with lower-stage tumors (20). Radical pelvic surgery does not adversely influence libido. Sensory nerves are not damaged during radical prostatectomy. Thus, men can reach orgasm postoperatively, although without any ejaculation of semen, even in the absence of a firm, sustained erection.

Erectile dysfunction after external beam radiation therapy has been estimated to range from 22 to 84%. Interstitial radiotherapeutic implantation is reported to have less impact on erectile function. Goldstein et al. hypothesized that radiation therapy accelerated arteriosclerotic changes in pelvic arteries, thereby reducing blood flow to the penis (21). Subsequent studies using baseline and serial penile blood pressures and flow examinations have not confirmed this hypothesis. Neither external beam nor interstitial irradiation adversely affects libido or sensation on genital skin.

Hormonal therapy designed to provide benefit through reduction of circulating testosterone to castrate levels influences both libido and potency. Sexual dysfunction including loss of libido, difficulty achieving and maintaining erection, reduced semen, and diminished pleasure often results from estrogens, progestins, luteinizing hormone-releasing hormone analogs, and bilateral orchiectomy. Among the available hormonal therapies, the antiandrogen agents that block the prostatic cell androgen receptors do not adversely affect sexual function.

Available therapeutic options for the management of established iatrogenic impotence in the individual who seeks restoration of potency include a broad range of interventions. Vacuum erection devices, which act on a negative pressure principle, offer a noninvasive mechanism for achieving erectile capacity. Pharmacologic erection programs using self-injections of vasodilator substances such as papaverine, phentolamine, or prostaglandin can be tailored to the individual's needs. Finally, a variety of rigid, mechanical, and inflatable penile prostheses present a surgical option for appropriate candidates. For some patients, loss of libido or inability to achieve and maintain erections sufficient for coital sex is not troubling. Instead of provocation or allurement of such patients into a quandary of irrational choices, the physician should carefully explore and inquire about their true needs through pragmatic and sensitive dialogue.

Testis Cancer

The effects of therapy, including surgery, radiation, and chemotherapy, on fertility have been extensively addressed. Reviews have indicated that combination chemotherapeutic regimens as used in the management of testicular cancer do affect fertility; most patients are rendered azoospermatic, with a high degree of recovery of spermatogenesis occurring within 3 to 5 years after initiation of therapy. In a prospective study of 41 testis cancer patients, 77% were oligospermatic and 17% azoospermatic before initiation of any therapy. In the same series, only 6.6% met the requirements for sperm banking (22).

Dysfunction in the testosterone-producing Leydig cells has been suggested. After surgical removal of the involved testicle, congenital abnormality in the remaining testicle may result in a hypogonadal state that can be managed with replacement testosterone (23). Men who have received retroperitoneal irradiation report higher rates of erectile dysfunction, difficulty reaching orgasm, and reduction in the intensity of orgasm. The higher dose of irradiation to the periaortic field in men with seminoma was predictive of problems with erection and orgasm. Several major centers no longer perform routine retroperitoneal lymphadenectomy for men with stage I nonseminomatous tumors to preserve antegrade ejaculation. Loss of seminal emission and/or retrograde ejaculation from damage to retroperitoneal sympathetic innervation following node dissection often results in infertility. Modification of the retroperitoneal lymphadenectomy to preserve the sympathetic ganglia and preaortic plexus retains antegrade ejaculation in 45 to 81% of men. After standard retroperitoneal lymphadenectomy, 18% of men can be anticipated to recover antegrade ejaculation.

Because testicular cancer is the leading cancer in males in young adulthood, psychosexual assaults of disease and therapy strike a particularly vulnerable population. Interdisciplinary efforts to plan and implement strategies to achieve an optimal state of rehabilitation are particularly valuable in this population to enhance quality of life in individuals, many of whom can anticipate achieving a normal life span, recovery of spermatogenesis, and successful parenthood. No fetal abnormalities have been detected in the children of men who have undergone therapy for testis tumors.

Cancer of the Penis

The primary disease and the mutilating effects of various therapies can be devastating for self-image and sexuality in individuals with cancer of the penis. Because the majority of penile cancers occur distally on the penis, a functional phallus for the purpose of coitus and micturition in standing posture can often be realized without compromising cancer excision. Whenever feasible, partial penectomy with or without penile-lengthening procedures should be considered. After partial penectomy, the majority of men will continue to experience erection, ejaculation, and orgasm (24). For invasive, localized malignancy occurring on the proximal penis, total penectomy is performed with the creation of a perineal urethrostomy. Because the internal sphincter is intact, control of urination can be achieved. Orgasm has also been reported in individuals after total penectomy. Human papillomavirus has been associated with promotion of cancers of the penis, thus underscoring the need for screening of partners; the virus has also been associated with cervical, vulvar, and anal cancer. A patient with an inadequate phallus after partial or total penectomy may be considered for phallic reconstruction, which may promote optimal sexual rehabilitation.

Renal Cell Cancer

Although the average age at diagnosis of kidney cancer is 55, many younger patients are encountered in clinical practice. Rapid progression of metastatic disease is the hallmark of kidney cancer; however, some individuals survive for long periods. Historically, the poor prognosis has been associated with the lack of effective systemic therapies for inhibiting progression and extending survival in patients with metastatic disease not amenable to surgical excision. Recently, biologic response modifying therapies—most notably interleukin-2, which received Food and Drug Administration approval for appropriate candidates with metastatic renal cell cancer—have demonstrated clinical benefit (25, 26). With the demonstration of enduring complete responses in a small percentage of patients treated with interleukin-2, the fields of clinical investigation in biotherapy and cellular therapies have been energized, with a corresponding new optimism among clinicians and, most importantly, among patients. In individuals for whom long-term survival and objective response to local or systemic therapies are unlikely, emphasis on improving quality of survival is paramount. Symptom control and promotion of intimacy may offer patients and their partners the opportunity to give and receive pleasure while communicating deeply with one another.

CONCLUSION

Because all patients are capable of deriving joy and satisfaction from everyday messages that are delivered through the senses, life is made infinitely more enjoyable through these messages, which are inherently sensual and often sexual. The urologist plays a pivotal role in supporting patients in the promotion and maintenance of this healthy expression of sexuality.

> To the bee a flower is a fountain of life, And to the flower a bee is a messenger of love, And to both, bee and flower, the giving and receiving of pleasure is a need and an ecstasy.
> KAHLIL GIBRAN

REFERENCES

1. McKenna RJ. Supportive care and rehabilitation of the cancer patient. In: Holleb AI, Fink DJ, Murphy JP, eds. American cancer society textbook of clinical oncology. Atlanta: American Cancer Society, 1982:545.
2. Dansak DA. Psychiatric oncology. In: Crawford ED, Borden TA, eds. Genitourinary cancer surgery. Philadelphia: Lea & Febiger, 1982:517.
3. Cassileth BR, Steinfield AD. Psychological preparation of the patient and family. Cancer 1987;60:547.
4. Havighurst R. Developmental tasks and education. 3rd ed. New York: David McKay, 1972.
5. Erikson E, ed. Adulthood. New York: WW Norton, 1978.
6. Green RL. Psychosocial consequences of prostate cancer: my father's illness and review of literature. Psychiatr Med 1987;5:323.
7. Boring CC, et al. Cancer statistics, 1994. CA Cancer J Clin 1994;44:18.
8. Silverberg E, Lubera JA. Cancer statistics, 1989. CA Cancer J Clin 1989;39:3.
9. Kennedy BJ. Aging and cancer. J Clin Oncol 1988;6:1903.
10. Sondik EJ, et al. 1986 annual cancer incidence review: USPHS National Cancer Institute, NIH publication no. 87-2789, 1987.
11. Yancik R. Frame of reference: old age as the context for prevention and treatment of cancer. In: Yancik R, ed. Perspectives on prevention and treatment of cancer in the elderly. New York: Raven, 1983:5.
12. Cornelius DA, et al. Who cares? a handbook on sex education and counseling services for disabled people. Baltimore: University Park Press, 1982.
13. Slevin JL, Plant H, Lynch D, et al. Who should measure quality of life, the doctor or the patient? Br J Cancer 1988;57:109.
14. Moinpour CM, et al. Quality of life end points in cancer clinical trials, review and recommendations. J Natl Cancer Inst 1989;81:485.
15. Kolodny R, et al. Textbook of human sexuality. Boston: Little, Brown & Co., 1979.
16. Masters WH, Johnson V. Sexual response. Boston; Little, Brown & Co., 1966.
17. Boyd SD, et al. Quality of life survey of urinary diversion patients: comparison of ileal conduits versus continent Kock ileal reservoirs. J Urol 1987;138:1386.
18. Walsh PC, Schlegel PN. Radical pelvic surgery with preservation of sexual function. Ann Surg 1988;208:391.
19. Schover LR, et al. Sexual rehabilitation of the ostomy patient. In: Smith DB, Johnson DE, eds. Ostomy care and the surgical patient: surgical and clinical considerations. Orlando: Grune & Stratton, 1986:103.
20. Quinlan DM, et al. Sexual function following radical prostatectomy: influence of preservation of neurovascular bundle. J Urol 1991;145:998.
21. Goldstein I, et al. Radiation-induced impotence: a clinical study of its mechanism. JAMA 1989;251:903.
22. Draga RE, et al. Fertility after chemotherapy for testicular cancer. J Clin Oncol 1983;1:37.
23. Fossa SD, et al. Testicular function after unilateral orchiectomy for cancer and before further treatment. Int J Androl 1982;5:179.
24. Schover LR, et al. Sexual rehabilitation of urologic cancer patients: a practical approach. CA Cancer J Clin 1984;34:3.
25. Parkinson DR, Sznol M. High-dose interleukin-2 in the therapy of metastatic renal-cell carcinoma. Semin Oncol 1995;22:61.
26. Stadler WM, Vogelzang NJ. Low-dose interleukin-2 in the treatment of metastatic renal-cell carcinoma. Semin Oncol 1995;22:67.

67

Supportive Care for the Patient With Terminal Genitourinary Cancer

S. Lawrence Librach

INTRODUCTION

Patients with advanced genitourinary cancer require a palliative and supportive approach to their care. It is often difficult to determine when a patient becomes "terminally ill." For those patients who have advanced genitourinary cancer, treatment with radiation and/or chemotherapy is usually palliative, i.e., not designed to cure but only to control disease and prolong life. Many of these patients have a steady downhill course leading to death. They are dying but not terminal. Unfortunately, these patients are often deprived of adequate early supportive palliative care that could improve the quality of their life and that of their families. Figure 67.1 illustrates a model of palliative care that includes early interventions. Considerations for a palliative approach governed by concern for quality of life may be forgotten in the pressure to prolong life and to cure. Many studies have documented unmet psychosocial and physical needs of dying patients. This chapter reviews a comprehensive, supportive approach for patients with advanced and terminal cancer and their families, an approach best embodied by palliative or hospice care.

WHAT IS PALLIATIVE OR HOSPICE CARE?

There is no universally accepted definition of palliative care or hospice care. A recent Canadian Palliative Care Standards task force developed the following definition (1):

> Palliative care as a philosophy of care is the combination of active and compassionate therapies intended to comfort and support the patient and family who are living with a life threatening illness, during the illness and bereavement periods. Palliative care strives to meet their physical, psychological, social and spiritual expectations and needs with sensitivity to their personal, cultural and religious values, beliefs and practices. Palliative care can be combined with therapies aimed at reducing or curing the illness or it may be the only focus of care.

Palliative care is planned and delivered through the collaborative efforts of an interdisciplinary team that includes the patient and family, caregivers and service providers. It should be available to the patient and family at any time during the illness trajectory and bereavement. While many service providers may be able to deliver some of the therapies that provide support and comfort, as the degree of distress, discomfort and dysfunction increases, the services of a specialized palliative care program may be required.

Integral to effective palliative care is the provision of opportunity and support for the caregivers and service providers to work through their own emotions and grief related to the care they are providing.

CARE FOR PHYSICAL NEEDS

Pain and Symptom Control

The patient with advanced genitourinary cancer will present a variety of physical symptoms for management. Pain and other symptoms need to have as high a priority for treatment as the disease itself. Many patients have died suffering needlessly from uncontrolled symptoms. Pain and many other symptoms can be controlled or at least ameliorated significantly if the physician uses an active and comprehensive approach.

General Guidelines

An adequate history is the important first step in attempting to control symptoms. The list of symptoms is often forgotten in the quest to obtain information about the tumor. The history of symptoms should be detailed, particularly in regard to pain, because such a comprehensive history may provide significant clues to the cause of pain and, therefore, specific treatment. Other important symptoms such as constipation should not be

The Continuum of Palliative Care

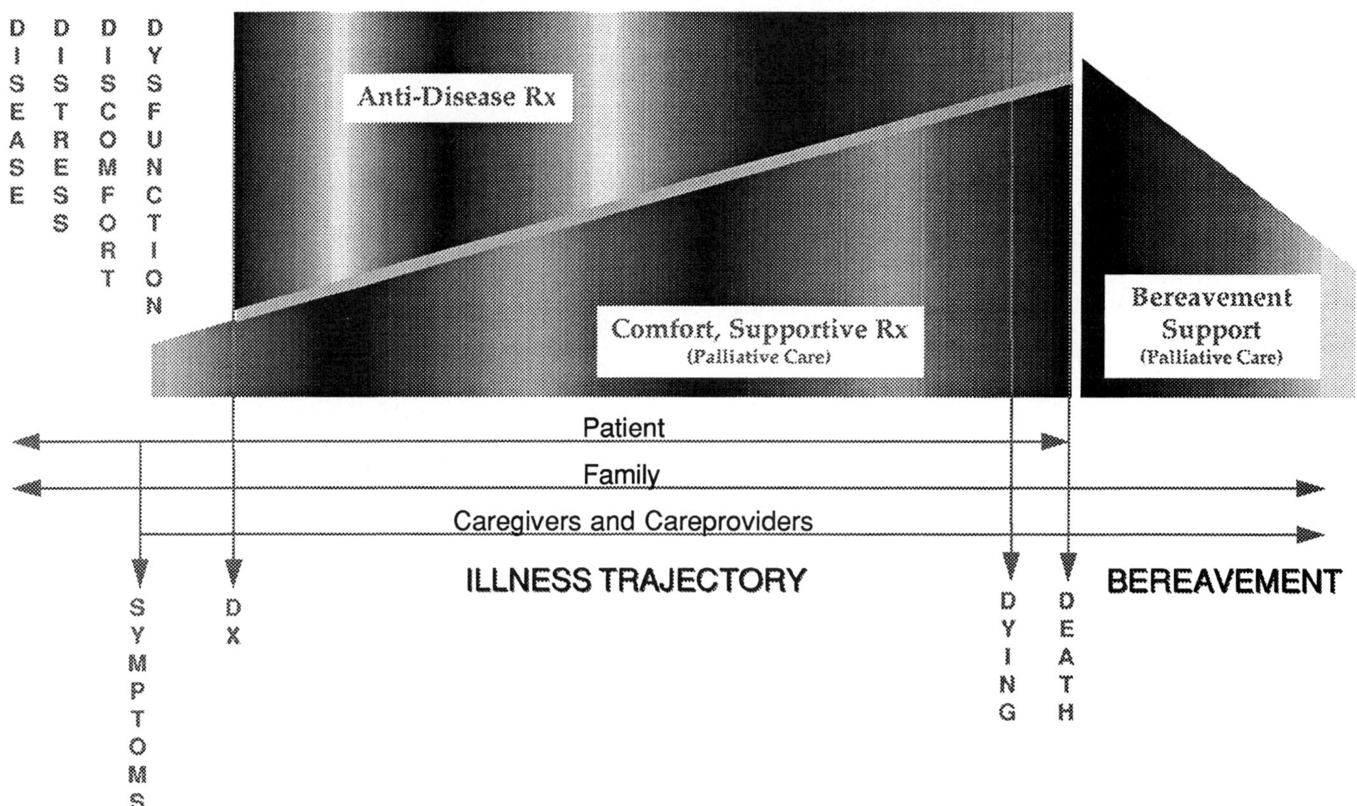

Fig. 67.1.   The continuum of palliative care.

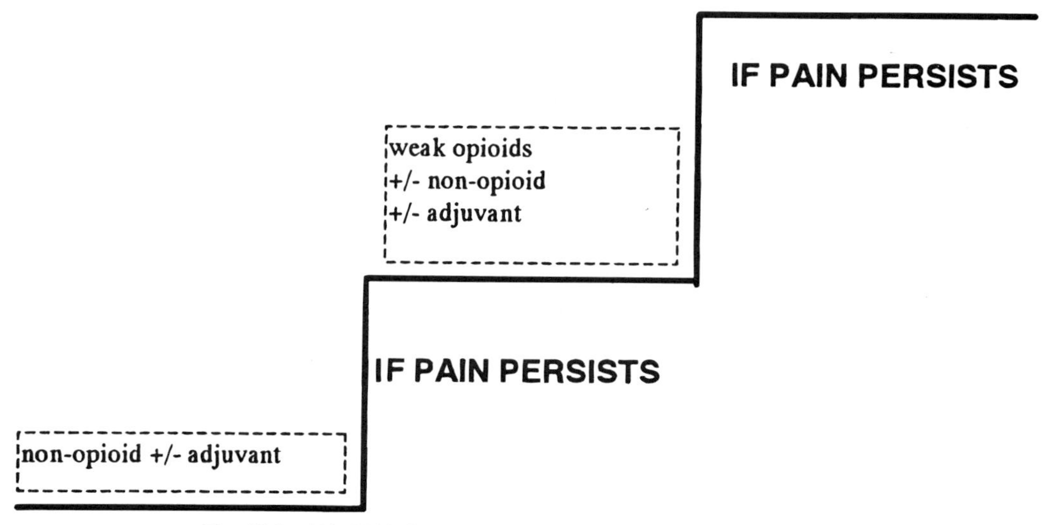

Fig. 67.2.   World Health Organization stepped approach in cancer pain.

dismissed as insignificant because they often contribute greatly to patient suffering.

A pain history should cover the development of pain and the usual questions of location, radiation, quality, duration, severity, timing, and aggravating and relieving factors. The physician should also inquire about analgesic use, the effects and side effects of those medications, and the fears the patient and family have in regard to the pain and its treatment. Many cancer patients have more than one type of pain, and not all pain reported by cancer patients is directly related to the tumor. Pain can be measured subjectively in a patient using an analog scale, verbal or visual, to quantify the pain in that patient. This is also the time to ensure that a psychosocial history is done; psychosocial issues may be a factor in the expression and treatment of pain.

The assessment of pain remains an unclear area for many physicians. Failure to take into account the differences in the manifestations of acute and chronic pain, worry about addiction, and a variety of other biases lead to a mistrust in patient reports of pain. There is no direct way to measure pain. The best judge of a patient's pain is the patient.

Pain Control

Pain is common in advanced cancer of any type. Approximately 65 to 85% of such patients in a number of studies were found to have pain (2). Genitourinary cancers, particularly prostatic and renal cancers, have high incidences of pain.

The Causes of Pain in Advanced Genitourinary Cancer

Pain can be classified into two different types: nociceptive and neuropathic. Nociceptive pain results from tissue damage to somatic or visceral structures. Neuropathic pain is due to injury of peripheral or central nervous system structures. It is important clinically to try and distinguish pain according to this classification because treatment options will vary according to the type of pain. There are a number of causes of pain in genitourinary cancer (Table 67.1).

The World Health Organization's Stepped Approach to Cancer Pain Control

In 1990, the World Health Organization (2) recommended a stepped approach to cancer pain management. A version of this is detailed in Figure 67.2 (3). This approach has been validated in several studies (4, 5).

Nonnarcotic Analgesics

The most useful nonnarcotic (nonopioid) analgesics are acetaminophen, acetylsalicylic acid, and nonsteroidal antiinflammatory drugs (NSAIDs).

These drugs are appropriate for mild to moderate pain, but have little use in more severe pain unless there are specific

Table 67.1.   Causes of Pain in Genitourinary Cancer

	MECHANISM	COMMENTS OR EXAMPLE
Nociceptive pain		
Bone pain	Direct invasion of bone	Sacral erosion from a large pelvic mass
	Bone metastases	Especially with prostatic cancer
	Pathologic fractures	
Visceral pain	Pelvic tumors invading pain-sensitive structures	Usually a combined nociceptive and neuropathic pain
	Liver metastases	Due to expansion of liver capsule
	Brain metastases with raised intracranial pressure	
	Peripheral edema	From lymphatic and/or venous obstruction in the pelvis
Superficial somatic pain	Skin metastases ± ulceration	
Neuropathic pain		
Plexopathy	Invasion, pressure, or destruction of nerves	Lumbosacral plexopathy very common with all pelvic tumors
	Spinal cord compression	From bone or intraspinal metastases
	Postoperative	Surgery to excise tumors may inadvertently damage nerves
Peripheral neuropathy	Invasion, pressure, or destruction of single peripheral nerves	Lateral cutaneous nerve of the thigh may be involved by tumor
	Postchemotherapy	With certain agents, neuropathy is common
	Postradiation neuritis	
	Phantom limb pain	
	Postherpetic neuropathy	

indications for their use in combination with other drugs for conditions such as bone pain. Acetylsalicylic acid should be given in enteric-coated formats. Acetaminophen should be used in full doses of 1000 mg every 4 hours. Both these agents are used in combination with codeine, but no added analgesic effect is seen above the base drug until 60 mg of codeine is added.

A variety of NSAIDs are available. All may have some analgesic effect, but they are most useful as adjuncts in the treatment of pain due to bony metastases or in other cases of nociceptive pain where inflammation may be a factor.

THE USE OF OPIOIDS IN THE TREATMENT OF CANCER PAIN

Opioid drugs (formerly called narcotics or narcotic analgesics) are the most effective drugs in relieving cancer pain. Unfortunately, the proper use of these analgesics is clouded by groundless fears and myths. Addiction is not a problem in cancer patients receiving opioids. Inadequate understanding of the origin and management of the predictable side effects of these agents also contributes to their underuse and consequent undertreatment of pain. It is worthwhile to note that most pain suffered by cancer patients is severe pain; therefore, treatment should begin with potent drugs except in circumstances in which the patient says the pain is mild. The following section will describe a practical approach to the use of opioids.

General Principles for the Use of Opioids

Opioids and other analgesics are just one part of a comprehensive pain-treatment plan. The term "total pain" (6) has been used to describe the pain experience of cancer patients and others with chronic pains. Pain and suffering involve many emotional, familial, spiritual, and cultural factors that need to be addressed by a multidisciplinary team. There should be no hesitation in involving others to help in addressing those needs.

Match the Severity of the Pain to the Strength of the Drug

There is little point in starting with weak drugs for severe pain. The stepped approach from weaker to stronger agents just leaves the patient suffering unnecessarily for a longer period. Do not persist in giving weak opioids if the pain is not rapidly controlled.

Give Medication Orally Whenever Possible

In most patients, opioids can be given orally to control pain. The physician must be aware of the parenteral to oral ratios as demonstrated in Table 67.2, but the approach must be flexible.

Give Medication Regularly and Never As Circumstances Require

Cancer pain, particularly severe pain, is constant. Such constant pain requires continuous around-the-clock administration of analgesics. The medication chosen should be given according to the duration of its analgesic effect. A double dose of the medication may be given at bedtime to avoid waking the patient in the middle of the night. This will not have any detrimental effect on the patient.

Anticipate and Prevent Side Effects

Opioids have a number of frequent and predictable side effects. The best approach to these is a preventive one.

Table 67.2. Useful Strong Opioid Analgesics

DRUG	SUBCUT DOSE (mg)	ORAL DOSE (mg)
Most useful		
Morphine	10	20
Hydromorphone	2	4
Diamorphine (heroin)	6	n/a
Methadone	10	20
Oxycodone	n/a	10
Fentanyl	n/a	25 μg/hr[a]
Possibly useful		
Oxymorphone	1.5	5 (suppository)
Levorphanol	2	4
Not recommended[b]		
Meperidine	75	2
Anileridine	25	75
Pentazocine	60	180

[a] Transdermal.

[b] Not recommended because of poor oral potency or because of unacceptable side effects with chronic administration.

1. Constipation is almost universal among patients who are taking opioids. The approach to this side effect often requires regular administration of larger-than-normal doses of stool softeners such as docusate combined with bowel stimulants such as senna or bisacodyl.
2. Nausea and associated vomiting may occur in up to 70% of patients taking opioids, particularly when the medication is first administered or the dose is increasing. Treatment of this side effect is covered in the section on Other Symptoms.
3. Sedation is the other common side effect, one that usually improves quickly on chronic administration of the opioid. The best treatment of this is to ignore it for the first few days.
4. Although many patients say they are allergic to opioids, true allergy is quite rare. Patients often interpret previous encounters with opioid side effects, such as nausea, as an allergy.
5. Other side effects including confusion, pruritus, urinary retention, and dry mouth are less common and easily treated.
6. Respiratory depression. This most feared of potential side effects of opioids is, in fact, rarely seen with appropriate oral regimens.

Always Leave an Order for a "Breakthrough" Dose

The order for constant regular administration of an opioid should always be accompanied by an "as required" dose to handle any uncontrolled pain. Monitoring of the number of breakthrough doses will indicate the need for an adjustment in the regular dose.

Explain What You Are Doing to Patient and Family and Give Them Some Control

Careful explanation about the opioid medication, its purpose, effects, and side effects is important. This is also an opportunity to explore the patient and family's fears about taking "narcotics." Patients and families should be trusted to monitor medication use and response and be given a range of dosage over which they can exercise some control.

Be Flexible

There is no one dosage of medication that will suit all patients when it comes to treating severe pain with opioids. Fixed dosage limits will only promote uncontrolled pain. In fact, there seems to be no firm upper limit to the amount of opioid required, and dosages of morphine greater than 100 mg every 4 hours are common. A high dose is not an indicator of addiction.

Use Adjuvant Drugs and Other Pain-Relieving Modalities as Appropriate

In bone pain, physicians should also consider the use of NSAIDs. Pain as a result of nerve compression and destruction may respond to corticosteroids and tricyclic antidepressants. These drugs are rarely effective alone and should be given with opioids. Radiation therapy and chemotherapy may also provide relief from pain, but patients should be covered with opioids until those modalities have demonstrated effect. Hypnotherapy, relaxation therapy, and other modalities of pain control of that type are rarely effective when used alone but can be of value in combination with analgesic medication.

Monitor Response to Treatment Frequently

Severe pain requires at least daily monitoring until pain is controlled. Pain diaries are useful to monitor response to analgesics, record doses, and list side effects.

The Most Appropriate Parenteral Route Is the Subcutaneous Route

If parenteral opioids must be administered, use them subcutaneously and not intramuscularly. This is more comfortable for patients, especially those who are quite cachectic. If long-term parenteral opioids are required, then constant subcutaneous infusion of opioids should be considered.

Do Not Be Afraid to Ask for Help From Palliative Care or Hospice Consultants

For difficult pain problems or in cases in which the physician is unsure of the use of particular analgesics, palliative care or pain consultants should be involved early in the management of pain.

Weak Opioids

Useful weak opioid analgesics are codeine and oxycodone. Codeine is the drug of choice in this class because of the flexibility of its dosage forms. Oxycodone is available either in fixed combinations with acetaminophen or acetylsalicylic acid or in tablets of pure oxycodone. In combination formats, it is probably no more effective than codeine combination formulations. Used in pure preparations, it may be equivalent to oral morphine in lower dosage ranges. Dextropropoxyphene should not be used because of inconclusive evidence of its potency over placebo.

Strong Opioids

Table 67.2 lists the strong opioids. Morphine is the gold standard and, for many, the drug of choice. Although other drugs such as hydromorphone and methadone are more potent on a milligram-per-milligram basis, they are not more effective. Long-acting, slow-release preparations of morphine are available and reduce the need for longer-acting drugs such as methadone. Hydromorphone and diamorphine (heroin), if available, are the best choices as a parenteral agent if high opioid doses are required. Meperidine (Demerol; Sanofi Winthrop, New York, NY) is a good choice for patients with acute postoperative pain but is a poor choice for chronic pain because of its poor oral absorption and short duration of action. Pentazocine also has limited usefulness because of poor oral absorption and frequent psychotomimetic side effects.

A recent potentially exciting advance has occurred with the introduction of a fentanyl transdermal delivery system. Fentanyl is a potent opioid, and the transdermal delivery route has been shown to be reliable and effective. Physicians should have skill in using opioids such as morphine before using fentanyl patches because of the more complex pharmacokinetics of the transdermal delivery system. This technique of opioid administration has value in patients who cannot take oral medication and who have a life expectancy beyond a few hours or days and in patients who cannot tolerate oral opioids because of intractable side effects. A plateau level of the drug after the patch is applied is not seen for 12 to 24 hours. There is also a skin depot of medication so that removing the patch results in very gradual elimination of the drug, taking up to 24 hours to reach 50% of the plateau level. This may lead to prolonged side effects for some time after the patch is removed. Each patch is effective for 72 hours, and it is recommended that dosage be changed only every 72 hours. Breakthrough pain in the 72-hour interval must be handled using a short-acting opioid such as immediate release morphine or hydromorphone (7).

The initial oral dose of a potent opioid depends on the severity of the pain, previous daily amount of parenteral opioid administered, and cause of the pain. However, a usual starting dosage of morphine in patients receiving as-required doses of opioids or patients who have not received potent opioids is 10 to 15 mg every 4 hours with a 5 mg breakthrough dose. The dose can be increased every 12 hours if necessary. The dose can be increased by 5-mg increments initially, but as the dose goes above 50 to 60 mg, increments of 10 mg are appropriate. Many patients' pain will be controlled with doses of morphine less than 30 mg every 4 hours, but there are patients—particularly those with nerve compression or destruction—who will require much higher doses. Again, a flexible approach is required. Some adjustment of the dose may be required after the first 2 or 3 weeks to account for drug tolerance, but many patients remain on a stable dose for a long time.

Morphine is available as an oral liquid in a variety of concentrations up to 100 mg/mL or in immediate release tablets in a variety of dosages. Once the dose of morphine is stabilized, then a switch may be indicated to the long-acting, slow-release forms on an every 12 hours or every 8 hours basis. Breakthrough doses should be in the immediate-release liquid or tablet form. Rectal suppositories are available as well, although there is limited flexibility in dosage.

Opioid-Resistant Pain

Certain types of pain may be resistant to opioids. Pain resulting from nerve destruction and damage may not respond to opioids or may only respond to large doses of opioids. Such patients often require a combination of drugs and analgesic modalities as discussed later in this chapter.

Other Methods of Administering Opioids

There are other methods of controlling pain using opioids administered by a number of other techniques.

1. Parenteral. There are patients who may require parenteral administration of opioids on a chronic basis because of the following:

- Intractable side effects with oral medication;
- Inability to swallow;
- Absorption problems, e.g., bowel obstruction;
- Very high doses of opioids;
- Last few hours or days of life because of a combination of the above.

There are a number of useful ways of giving opioids parenterally such as the following.

a. Intermittent subcutaneous preferably using a Butterfly needle with an injection port and covered with a transparent dressing.
b. Continuous subcutaneous infusion using a pump (e.g., Pharmacia CADD Pump), syringe driver (Graseby), or special injector such as the Edmonton Injector. This method of administering opioids should be reserved for the above indications and not used indiscriminately for its high-tech approach. The choice of opioid for continuous subcutaneous infusion relates to potency and solubility. Morphine is less soluble than hydromorphone or diamorphine; therefore, it has limited use in this technique unless patients are receiv-

ing relatively small doses of morphine. Hydromorphone seems to be the preferred drug if large doses of opioids are required.
c. Continuous intravenous infusions are rarely indicated.

2. Buccal membrane administration. Morphine and hydromorphone will be absorbed through oral mucous membranes. The best site is probably the buccal membranes of the cheek and not sublingually. Obviously, immediate release forms of these drugs should be used.

3. Rectal. Use of this technique should be limited, especially in the home setting. Patients may find it distressing and embarrassing. Family members may also have difficulty with this route of administration. This is also not suitable for patients who require large doses of opioids.

4. Epidural opioids. Continuous or intermittent infusions of potent opioids by the epidural route may have particular application in some patients. Epidural administration of opioids may be needed for pelvic pain that is resistant to large doses of analgesics (8). The epidural catheter needs to be permanently implanted for best results. Resistance to epidural opioids may develop rapidly.

Use of Analgesic Adjuncts

There are a number of agents that can be used as adjuncts in the treatment of cancer pain.

A. Bone pain from metastases should usually involve the use of NSAIDs unless there are contraindications to these agents. These drugs should be used at full dose.
B. The pain of nerve compression may respond to corticosteroids such as prednisone 20 to 60 mg per day or dexamethasone 4 to 16 mg daily.
C. The deafferentation pain of nerve destruction may respond to tricyclic antidepressants such as amitriptyline and to anticonvulsants such as carbamazepine or valproic acid. These drugs have a constellation of frequent side effects, which may limit use. Small doses should be tried at first, and the dose gradually increased until pain relief is improved or side effects intervene.
D. If anxiety and depression are thought to be factors in the production of pain, then psychotropic drugs such as the benzodiazepines, phenothiazines. and antidepressants may be used to supplement the effects of analgesics. Caution must be used in using these psychotropic drugs as substitutes for analgesics like opioids.
E. For the patient in overwhelming pain that does not respond to opioids well, high doses of dexamethasone up to 100 mg daily for 3 or 4 days may be effective in helping to control pain.

The Use of Other Modalities of Pain Control

Neurosurgical lysis of spinal cord pathways is best reserved for patients with unilateral lower limb pain. Hypnosis and acupuncture are rarely effective for any length of time as sole measures. Hypnosis or relaxation techniques may be used as adjuncts with good effect in some patients. Transcutaneous electrical nerve stimulation can be effective, particularly using the new types of stimulator, which stimulate a larger number of points randomly (9).

Nerve blocks such as caudal blocks using neurolytic agents like phenol or alcohol may be helpful in patients with pelvic pain that is resistant to other measures (8).

The use of radiation as a palliative treatment for pain should not be ignored. However, treatment with analgesics should not be delayed and should be maintained until the full effect of the radiation is obtained. This may take more than 2 weeks.

OTHER SYMPTOMS

Constipation

Constipation is a common symptom in patients who are terminally ill. There are a number of causes of constipation as outlined in Table 67.3. Untreated constipation may lead to other problems such as nausea and vomiting and may increase pain, particularly if patients have to strain considerably. The approach to treatment of constipation depends, to an extent, on the cause.

Dietary manipulation to include more fiber and fruits may be successful depending on the cause of constipation. However, this regimen is rarely sufficient alone in patients because high-fiber diets may be unpalatable for ill and anoretic patients and because the mild peristaltic stimulation provided may not be sufficient to counteract the cause of constipation. This is particularly true of opioid-induced constipation. Bulk-forming agents such as psyllium mucilloids may not be effective for similar reasons.

It is safe to make the assumption that constipation will develop in every patient taking opioids. This constipation usually requires the use of a combination of larger-than-usual doses of laxatives including a stool softener (e.g., docusate sodium 100 mg twice a day) and stimulant laxatives (e.g., senna, cascara, or bisacodyl or osmotic agents [e.g., lactulose]).

The dose range for these agents in treating constipation induced by opioids is often considerably higher than normal.

Table 67.3. Causes of Constipation

General weakness and debility	Inability to sit on a toilet or use a commode
Poor nutrition	Decreased intake, low fiber diet, and poor fluid intake
Medications	Opioids, antidepressants, and many others
Metabolic	Hypercalcemia, dehydration, and hypothyroidism
Intestinal obstruction	

Table 67.4. Causes of Nausea in Patients with Cancer

Treatment related	Radiation and chemotherapy
Abdominal cancer	Gastric or pancreatic cancer with gastric outlet obstruction
	Diffuse abdominal carcinomatosis
	Intestinal obstruction
	Involvement of celiac plexus
Hypomotility disorders	Secondary to cancer
	Secondary to drugs
	Preexisting
Hepatic enlargement	Secondary to metastases
Drugs	Opioids
	NSAIDs
	Many other drugs
Constipation	Frequent and overlooked
Metabolic	Renal failure
	Hypercalcemia

The aim should be for a bowel movement every 2 or 3 days. It is prudent to use suppositories or enemas if there is no movement after this period. It may also be prudent to keep the stools of a patient with widespread cancer in the pelvis soft to prevent constipation, possible obstruction from fecal material, and increased pain.

Nausea and Vomiting

The physician needs to understand the physiology and cause of nausea and vomiting in patients with cancer. The vomiting center located in the reticular formation of the medulla close to the respiratory center receives input from the gastrointestinal nervous system afferents, chemoreceptor trigger zone, cerebral cortex, and vestibular nucleus. The complex reflex that leads to vomiting may involve inputs from one or more of these sites. The action of antiemetics also differs as to site of action, and this must be taken into account. Table 67.4 lists the causes of nausea in patients with cancer.

For opioid-induced nausea, the best drugs are those that bind to dopamine receptor sites in the chemoreceptor trigger zone where opioids mainly act to produce nausea. Haloperidol, a butyrophenone drug, is particularly useful in such nausea. It can be given once daily orally in a dose up to 15 mg daily but most patients require only 1 or 2 mg daily. It is relatively free of side effects at these low dosages. Phenothiazine drugs such as prochlorperazine are also quite useful in opioid-induced nausea. For prochlorperazine, the dose is 5 to 10 mg every 4 to 6 hours. In the higher dose ranges, there may be considerable sedation and extrapyramidal side effects may limit use. Chlorpromazine in a dose of 25 mg every 4 to 6 hours may also be effective.

Antihistamine drugs, such as dimenhydrinate, that act on the vomiting center have little use in opioid-induced nausea despite the popularity of use of these drugs. They may be effective if there is a distinct but uncommon vestibular component of the nausea, but they should not be used routinely.

Opioids and the cancer itself may induce gastric and bowel hypomotility leading to nausea and vomiting. If this is suspected, drugs such as metoclopramide and domperidone that stimulate gastric emptying and bowel motility are useful. Domperidone in a dose of 10 to 30 mg 4 times a day or cisapride in a dose of 10 to 20 mg 4 times a day are probably the drugs of choice because of a more favorable side effect profile compared with metoclopramide.

If patients have overwhelming nausea and the cause is not evident or resistant to usual therapy, then dexamethasone in a dose of 16 to 60 mg daily for 3 or 4 days may be useful.

If the cause of nausea and vomiting is from bowel obstruction, as it may be in patients with pelvic and abdominal disease from genitourinary cancer, then therapeutic options must be carefully considered. Surgery should still be considered as the first option if the patient's general condition warrants this. Long-term use of nasogastric suction and intravenous fluids beyond 2 weeks should be avoided because of patient discomfort. In many cases obstruction may be intermittent and temporary. Loperamide can be given in a dose of 4 to 8 mg every 4 to 6 hours to control cramps and nausea. Other opioids and antispasmodics can be given by subcutaneous infusion to reduce pain and nausea. Antiemetics can be given to reduce nausea. Two or three episodes of vomiting can be tolerated without panic by the patient, family, or staff if they are given considerable support and education.

Anorexia and Cachexia

Many patients with advanced cancer have anorexia and cachexia. As the disease progresses toward its terminal phase, these symptoms become almost universal. Anorexia is distressing to the patient, family, and staff because of the symbolic importance of food and eating. "If only he would eat, he would feel better," is a common complaint. Anorexia and cachexia develop in a patient with cancer for a number of complex and interrelated factors related to the cancer itself, cancer treatment, and psychological effect of cancer on the patient.

Expensive, commercial nutritional supplements are often promoted as the answer to anorexia and cachexia, but there is little evidence to support their extensive use. The use of small frequent feedings that cater to the patient's food preferences and that make use of high-calorie foods may be enough to maintain caloric intake at a reasonable level. Prednisone at a dose of 15 to 20 mg daily may help to stimulate appetite. Careful counseling and support of the patient, family, and health-care staff may help to minimize unnecessary pressure on the patient.

When the patient stops taking oral fluids, there is always a temptation to start intravenous therapy so that the patient does not become dehydrated. Dehydration by itself is not terribly uncomfortable as long as mouth care is rigorous. Intravenous therapy provides no nutrients of any significance and may be prolonging suffering rather than helping to prevent it. Patients and families need to be counseled and supported appropriately if the decision is made not to start intravenous therapy. If parenteral fluids are to be administered, consider hypodermoclysis, subcutaneous infusion of fluids, instead of intravenous therapy.

Dry and Sore Mouth

A dry and sore mouth is a relatively common symptom that is often multifactorial. It may be caused by decreased fluid intake; drug side effects from agents such as opioids, anticholinergics, and antidepressants; chemotherapeutic agents; and a variety of infections. Oral candidiasis is a commonly overlooked infection. It rarely presents with the classic findings of the thrush seen in infants but often presents as generalized hyperemia. Candidiasis will respond to oral nystatin administered as a mouth rinse; in stubborn cases, it will respond to a short 1-week course of ketoconazole. In patients with dry and sore mouths, mouthwashes containing alcohol (most commercial mouthwashes) should be avoided. Frequent mouth cleansing with aqueous solutions containing salt and sodium bicarbonate are effective and much less irritating.

Other Symptoms

There are many other symptoms that can be problematic for the patient with advanced genitourinary cancer. A number of references are available for further information (10).

CARE FOR PSYCHOLOGICAL, SOCIAL, AND SPIRITUAL NEEDS

Care for Psychological Needs

Patients with advanced cancer and their families have psychological needs that must be addressed. Patients and families should be assessed early on in the course of the illness by the multidisciplinary team. Such assessment is not only important as a prelude to supporting persons who are undergoing tremendous stress and suffering, but is also important to help physicians plan for care appropriately.

Dying patients and their families present a host of emotional reactions including sadness, guilt, anger, and anxiety related to the losses incurred in dealing with a terminal illness. Families require help from understanding health-care professionals who can help mobilize the family's own resources to deal with this time of crisis and loss and who can provide continuing support. Such support is critical to the task of improving the quality of the remaining life for the patient. The physicians should be able to provide such support at times, but most surgeons usually rely on their colleagues in other professions such as social work and psychology to provide such support. The family physician should not be forgotten as an important resource in managing patients and families. Dying is not a psychiatric illness, and psychiatric consultation for such patients should be reserved for those patients and families with serious dysfunction.

Although psychotropic agents such as anxiolytics and antidepressants, particularly the newer serotonin reuptake inhibiting drugs, can be very useful in managing psychological distress, they should be used as adjuncts to adequate support and counseling provided by knowledgeable caregivers.

The unit of care in palliative care is the family. Support can be provided to family members on an individual basis as needed, but emphasis should be placed on working with the family. The patient and family must have sufficient information about the illness to cope with the tasks engendered by this life crisis. Truth-telling is important but the truth must be communicated with sensitivity and with repetition so that the patient and family understand clearly what is happening. The patient and family have an absolute right to participate in decision-making regarding the illness. The onus is on the physician to present information clearly and honestly and to avoid pressuring the patient unnecessarily to accept suggested treatment. The patient and family should be given time to make decisions because few treatment options can be considered emergency situations.

Patients with genitourinary cancers may be very susceptible to psychological problems induced by altered body-image and self-image and loss of function (11, 14). All surgical and chemotherapeutic procedures in patients with genitourinary cancer should be explained carefully and fully to the patient and then to the family. Sensitive areas of urinary function, disfigurement, or loss of sexual organs and sexuality should be sensitively and confidentially probed by the physician and other team members.

In patients with genitourinary cancers, sexuality is a topic that must be raised with patients and their partners. Sexual counseling of these patients requires adequate knowledge and sensitivity. Many of the surgical and hormonal treatments may be detrimental to sexual functioning. Patients must be informed that there are options available to them regarding sexual functioning and fulfillment that extend beyond the act of intercourse. Care should be taken to involve the usual sexual partner in the counseling. One should also avoid assuming that the elderly patient is not interested in sexual functioning.

After the patient dies, the family may require assessment and support during the period of bereavement. Families should be clearly informed of the resources available for such support.

Care for Social Needs

Dying patients and their families also present with a variety of social needs that require exploration. The physician should ensure that these needs are adequately explored by social workers on the team.

Care for Spiritual Needs

In facing the crisis of dying, all patients and families will have spiritual concerns and needs. Religious issues are not the same as spiritual issues. Although patients and their families may profess that religion is not important to them, they may have significant spiritual questions about the meaning and purpose of life and death. These concerns can best be dealt with by chaplains or clergy who have special training and expertise. Spiritual support must be individualized and recognize differences in faith and culture. Physicians need to be aware of this important area and ensure that spiritual counseling is available to their patients.

CARE AT HOME

A cornerstone of palliative care is home care. Patients have a need and right to be maintained at home as long as possible. Home care requires a dedicated multidisciplinary team with a flexible approach and 24-hour service. The aim is to keep patients at home as long as possible and to allow patients to die at home if that is their wish. Often patients are maintained in hospitals far too long because adequate consideration has not been given to home care. Community-based palliative care or hospice programs can provide this home-care expertise. The patient's family physician should play a key role in home management.

CONCLUSION

All patients with advanced genitourinary cancer should receive multidisciplinary care that emphasizes quality of life. Control of pain and other symptoms is of prime importance if this goal is to be achieved. The physician also needs to be aware of the variety of psychosocial and spiritual needs of patients and families and to ensure appropriate treatment so that patients can live and die with support, love, and dignity.

REFERENCES

1. Palliative care: towards a consensus in standardized care. Ottawa, Ontario, Canada: Canadian Palliative Care Association, 1995.
2. World Health Organization. Cancer pain relief and palliative care: a report of a WHO expert committee. World Health Organization technical report series 804. Geneva. 1990.
3. Librach SL. The pain manual: principles and issues in cancer pain management. Toronto: Pegasus Healthcare, 1991:28.
4. Ventafridda V, Tamburini M, Caracenia, et al. A validation study of the WHO method for cancer pain relief. Cancer 1987; 59:850.
5. Walker VA, Hoskin PJ, Hanks GW, et al. Evaluation of WHO guidelines for cancer pain in a hospital-based palliative care unit. J Pain Symp Manage 1988;3:145.

6. Librach SL. The pain manual: principles and issues in cancer pain management. Toronto: Pegasus Healthcare, 1991:11.
7. Mosser KH. Transdermal fentanyl in cancer pain. Am Fam Physician 1992;45:2289.
8. Shetter AG, et al. Administration of intraspinal morphine sulfate for the treatment of intractable cancer pain. Neurosurgery 1986;18:740.
9. Librach SL, Rapson L. TENS: its role in palliative care. Palliat Med 1988;2:15.
10. Levy M, Catalano RB. Control of common physical symptoms other than pain in patients with terminal disease. Semin Oncol 1985;12:411.
11. Mount BM. Psychological impact of urologic cancer. Cancer 1980;45:223.

68

The Genetic Basis for Urologic Malignancy

Diagnosis and Therapy

Michael J. Manyak

INTRODUCTION

Correction of the aberrant genetic code as a means of therapy has been a dream since the first discoveries more than a century ago of an abnormal genetic link to expression of certain disorders. The role of genetic changes in neoplasia has been a controversial subject since the observation of frequent aberrant mitoses in cancer cells by von Hansemann in 1890 (1). The suggestion that neoplasia might result from this observed disturbance in genetic cellular content was first offered 25 years later (2). However, it took nearly 50 years before the technology was available to evaluate critically this hypothesis of cancer arising in a single cell from an acquired genetic change. This somatic theory of mutation is still the predominant paradigm for carcinogenesis and is supported by a wide variety of experimental evidence.

The stem cell concept of cancer genetics, first introduced in 1930, was refined in the 1950s and provided a model of Darwinian selection for cancer pathogenesis. In this model, a dynamic equilibrium maintained by selective pressures can be upset by environmental changes. During this time, many investigators contributed to the understanding of tumor cell proliferative mechanisms (3). This period was also remarkable for the confirmation that both structural and numeric chromosomal abnormalities were associated with both human and experimental animal tumors.

The first consistently noted chromosomal abnormality in a human malignancy was reported in 1960 in patients with chronic myeloid leukemia (4). The discovery of the Philadelphia chromosome gave a significant boost to the field of cancer cytogenetics, which became tempered by the realization that this aberration was an exception in human tumors (Fig. 68.1). The variability in aberrant chromosomal expression in other tumors was viewed as an interesting phenomenon acquired during malignant progression with no pathogenetic significance.

Interest in cancer cytogenetics was revived by the introduction of chromosome banding techniques in the early 1970s.

This revolutionary advance allowed each chromosome to be identified precisely, and more exact conclusions could be drawn from the unique banding patterns associated with each chromosome. Banding analyses have led to the description of consistent chromosomal aberrations and, in some cases, very specific cancer-associated genetic changes in all human tumor types studied in sufficient number to draw conclusions (3). The rapid accumulation of cytogenetic information is stored in a computerized data base that has now grown to more than 20,000 reported cases from the 3144 neoplasms characterized since its establishment in 1983. Cytogenetic analysis is now an important diagnostic component of patient evaluation for hematologic malignancies, an area where more is known about chromosomal abnormalities. This information is used for both prognosis and selection of appropriate therapy. Although cytogenetic information about solid tumors lags behind hematologic neoplasms, corresponding breakthroughs are being reported for solid human tumors.

GENETIC BASIS OF MALIGNANCY

The genetic basis for carcinogenesis is supported by a tremendous amount of evidence that mutations can cause cancer (5). A mutation is defined as any change in the genome, and classification of mutations occurs according to the genetic aberration. These abnormalities can be numeric, where whole chromosomes are added or deleted, or they can manifest as point mutations, insertions, partial deletions, translocations, and amplifications. The genetic origin of malignancy is supported by the observations that nearly all carcinogens induce mutations and that an increased risk of cancer is associated with deficiencies in enzymes that repair DNA. In addition, several inherited disorders with increased chromosome breakage demonstrate an increased incidence of cancer. It is also known that certain hereditary forms of cancer are linked with mutations in every cell in the body, with transfer of the aberrant genome to the next generation. However, cancer appears to arise more commonly from a

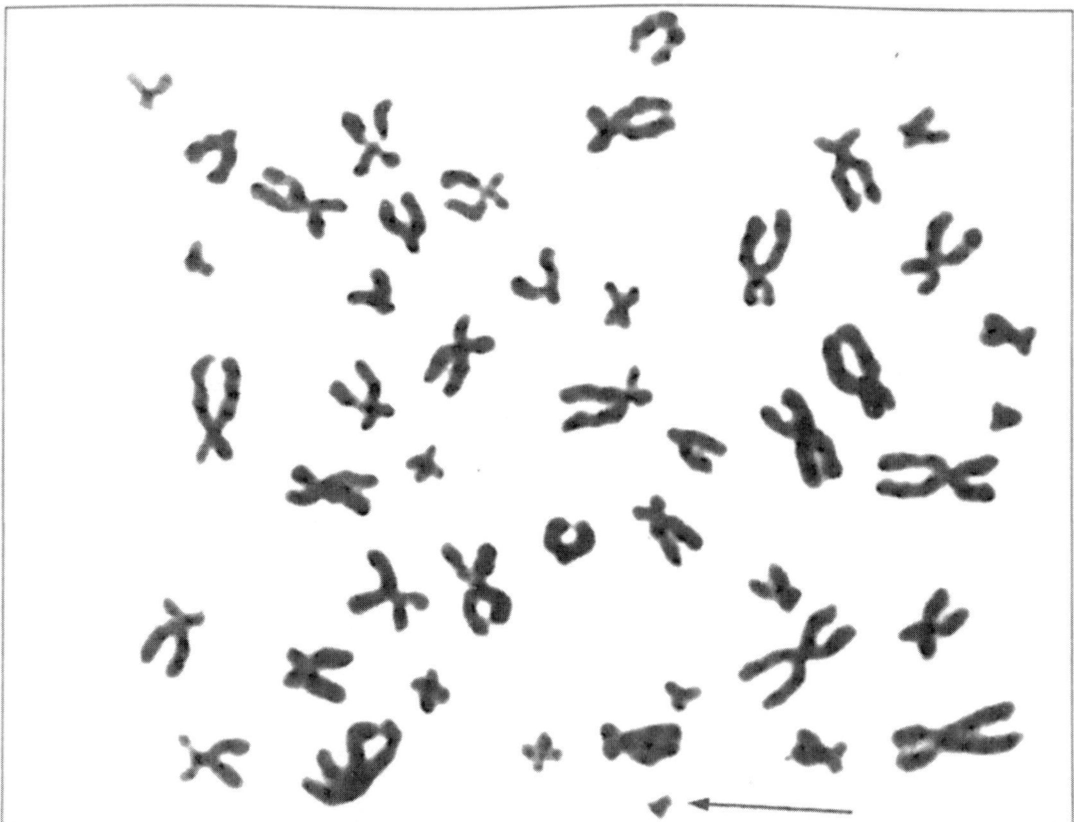

Fig. 68.1.   Classic gene translocation known as the Philadelphia chromosome (arrow) in marrow cell of patient with chronic myelocytic leukemia. (Reprinted with permission from Sandberg AA. Cancer cytogenetics for clinicians. CA Cancer J Clin 1994;44:136.)

single somatic cell with tumor development by clonal proliferation.

Mutational Theory

The mutational theory of carcinogenesis is complex. Although many studies support multiple mutational events as a requirement to change a normal cell into one that is malignant, simple mathematical consideration of cancer data suggests problems with that theory. Because most cancers show a dramatic increase in incidence with age (6), it is estimated that five to seven mutational events are required for transformation of a normal cell to one that is malignant. Multiple mutation theorists must assume an unusually high frequency of mutation in target cells presumed to be present for the lifetime of the individual to create the age-incidence curves that occur for most cancers. The dynamics of normal cell proliferation must be considered in such an equation, and both the small proportion and limited life span of stem cells—the most probable targets of transformation—make the multi-hit theory of mutational transformation less probable. Furthermore, most organs and tissues demonstrate significant variability in proliferation during the lifetime of an individual. Therefore, it has been proposed that rate of cell transformation is more dependent on the growth

kinetics of the tissue and that cell-cell interactions and programmed cell death are important components of the development of malignancy. Because these mechanisms are also susceptible to alteration due to a defective genome, mutations or loss of key genetic sequences in genes regulating these mechanisms may not require multiple events before derailing normal growth. Detailed discussions of these concepts are beyond the scope of this chapter, and the interested reader is referred to the extensive molecular biologic literature available about these subjects.

Defects in Cell Repair Mechanisms

The ability of a cell to repair damaged or mutated DNA may also play a role in carcinogenesis. Mutant cells with a deficiency of enzymes involved in one or more of the steps in the DNA repair process render those cells susceptible to ionizing radiation or chemical agents. Many of the genes involved with these processes have been identified through experiments with yeasts and bacteria (7). There are at least four well-characterized autosomal recessive nonurologic human diseases with defects in the DNA repair process that predispose the individual to malignancy development. Clearly, the mechanisms of DNA repair and various other host resistance capabilities are an important component of the defenses against development of malignancy.

Chromosomal Abnormalities in Tumors

Common chromosomal abnormalities are found in many neoplasms, and this observation suggests the involvement of common genetic mechanisms in the initiation and progression of specific malignancies. One observable manner in which the deviations of normal genetic mechanisms associated with cancer can manifest is by numeric or structural chromosomal changes. Frequently, a variety of chromosomal changes are found in tumors. Although the mechanisms by which chromosomal changes occur largely remain unknown, many chromosomes have fragile sites where they are more susceptible to breakage. Chromosomal rearrangement may also occur at these fragile sites.

Chromosomal changes generally fall into three broad categories, and this structural alteration of genetic material can result in aberrance or loss of gene expression. Reciprocal translocation occurs with no loss of genetic material and results in simple exchange of portions of the chromosomes. Translocation may be balanced or unbalanced and can be diagnostic for the disease related to their expression (Fig. 68.2) The resultant placement of genes from one chromosome near the genes of another often leads to creation of a hybrid gene with expression of an abnormal protein. These types of genetic abnormalities are common in different types of leukemia and sarcoma. Less common are chromosomal inversions (Fig. 68.3) with an abnormal juxtaposition of genetic material within the chromosome that can also result in a chimeric gene.

Nonreciprocal genetic exchanges in chromosomes result in either deletion or addition of chromosomal regions. Deletions of chromosomal material (Fig. 68.4) are common in epithelial adenocarcinomas such as those arising from the colon, breast, lung, and prostate. The multiple deletions frequently noted in these cancers may represent the cumulative process of genetic changes that lead to malignant transformation (8). The growing importance of genetic deletions in carcinogenesis arises from the identification of tumor suppressor genes and the effects of their loss through deletion. Chromosomal insertions (Fig. 68.5) are less common, although their occurrence can lead to aberrant gene expression.

The third general category of chromosomal changes involves an increase in DNA in a specific chromosomal region. These abnormally banding regions represent gene amplification and are commonly associated with oncogenes and drug resistance (5). Gene amplification occurs when several rounds of DNA are synthesized unscheduled during a single cell cycle. Curiously, these occurrences can be located at any site in the genome and are often found at sites other than the usual chromosomal location of the gene amplified. The role of gene amplification in tumor development and its biology is not yet clear, but gene amplification has been reported in several tumors. One example involves the *ras* protein where excessive levels resulting from overexpression of normal *ras* gene have been correlated with development of a malignant phenotype (9).

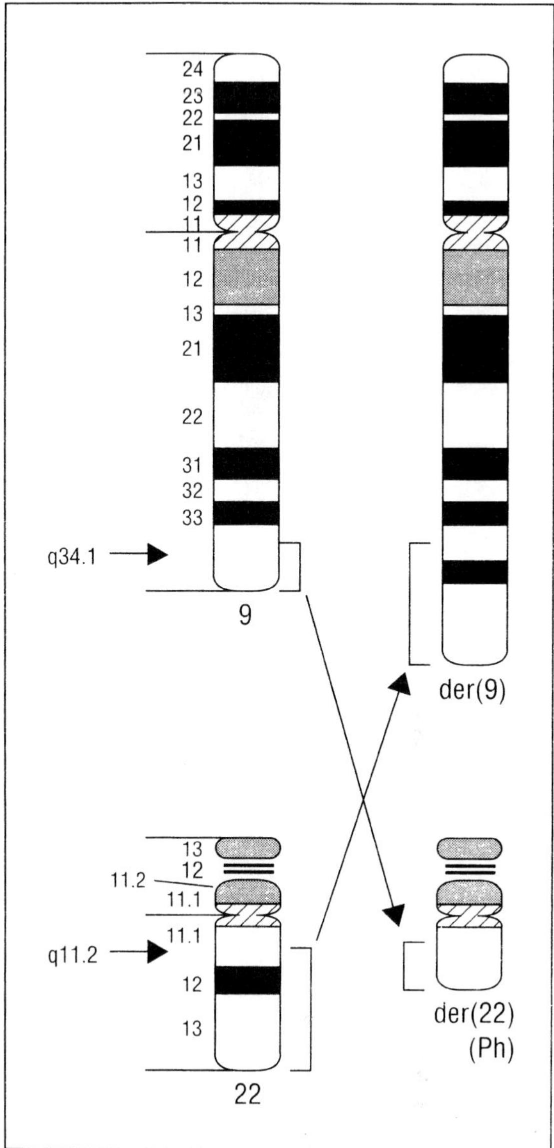

Fig. 68.2. The translocation responsible for the Philadelphia chromosome found in chronic myelocytic leukemia. (Reprinted with permission from Sandberg AA. Cancer cytogenetics for clinicians. CA Cancer J Clin 1994;44:136.)

ALTERED GENES AND CARCINOGENESIS

The possibility that damaged cellular genes may contribute to the induction and progression of cancer has also become more clear since the development and refinement of molecular genetic techniques. These tools have so far uncovered two distinctly different cancer-related gene classes—oncogenes and tumor suppressor genes. As our knowledge about these aberrant genes increases, it is clear that we are on the threshold of significant diagnostic advances and therapeutic applications relating to the genome.

Significant evidence had accumulated by the mid-1970s that cancer had some relationship to damaged genes and that

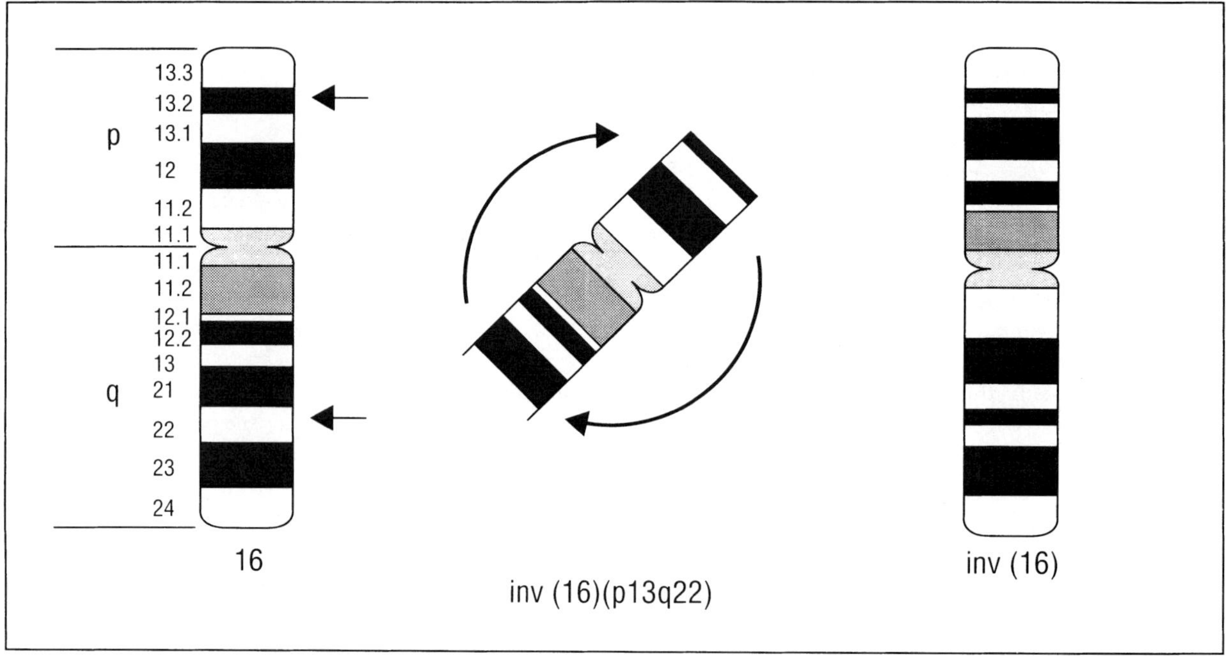

Fig. 68.3. Chromosomal inversion is an uncommon event. This aberration is noted in acute nonlymphocytic leukemia. (Reprinted with permission from Sandberg AA. Cancer cytogenetics for clinicians. CA Cancer J Clin 1994;44:136.)

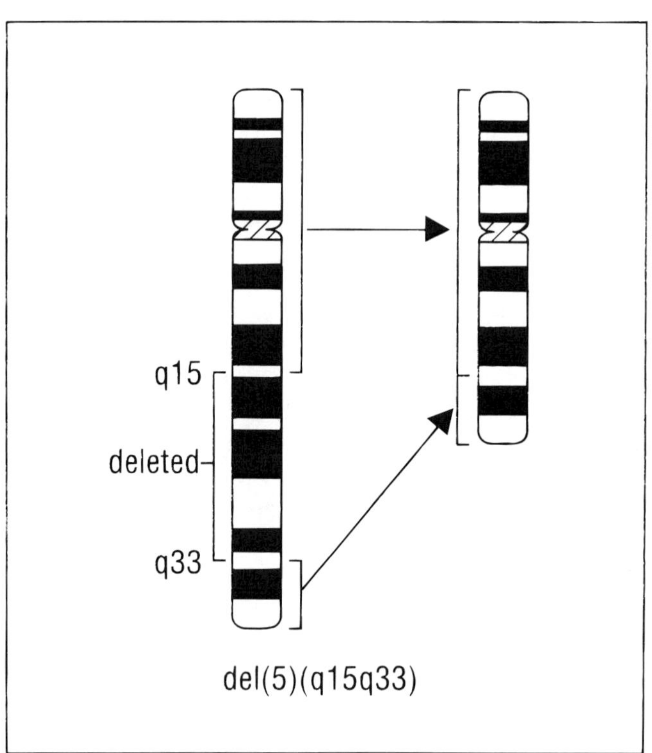

Fig. 68.4. Deletion of chromosomal material is the defect most often associated with loss of tumor suppressor gene function. (Reprinted with permission from Sandberg AA. Cancer cytogenetics for clinicians. CA Cancer J Clin 1994;44:136.)

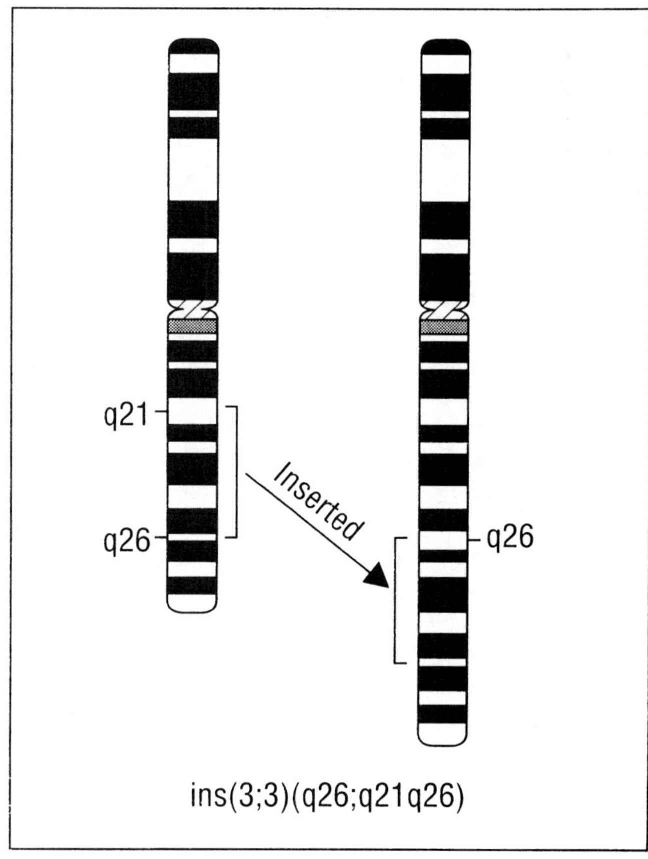

Fig. 68.5. Chromosomal insertion is less commonly seen in urologic malignancies. (Reprinted with permission from Sandberg AA. Cancer cytogenetics for clinicians. CA Cancer J Clin 1994;44:136.)

carcinogenic agents were often able to inflict damage on DNA. It became apparent that tumor cells carried some aberrant form of normal cellular genes that sustained damage during carcinogenesis, although the characterization of these target genes remained elusive (10). The alternative theory of a viral causation of cancer that was in vogue during that time was not borne out when it became evident that the majority of cancers in the Western industrialized countries had no connection to viral involvement. The tumors that have known viral causes, such as cervical cancer, some hepatomas, adult T-cell lymphomas, Burkitt's lymphoma, nasopharyngeal carcinoma, and perhaps Kaposi's sarcoma, really represent a small percentage of the known cancer incidence in this country.

Proto-oncogenes

Although interest waned about the primary viral cause in carcinogenesis because no direct link could be shown, research on animal RNA tumor viruses began to provide a glimpse of the identity of damaged cellular genes that might be present in cancer. These retroviruses have no ability to cause human cancer but were extremely tumorigenic in chickens, cats, rodents, and monkeys. The Rous sarcoma virus, first described in 1911 in chickens, was found to carry a specific gene that transforms infected normal cells to neoplastic ones (11). The transforming gene of this avian sarcoma was termed a viral oncogene because the development of malignancy was directly traced to this single piece of genetic material. Further investigation turned up striking evidence that the Rous sarcoma oncogene was not truly a viral gene but had arisen from a preexisting cellular gene that had been pirated by the ancestor of the avian sarcoma. The ancestor of the Rous sarcoma virus had been able to replicate in infected cells but only became capable of transforming them after it had captured the normal cellular gene. This normal cellular gene was termed a proto-oncogene (11).

This discovery was extremely important because it identified a normal cellular gene with potent transforming capability once activated. This suggested that there was at least one gene that served as a potential target for nonviral carcinogenic chemical agents and ionizing radiation. These nonviral agents could convert the proto-oncogene to an active oncogene by simulating the effects of the retroviruses. The cell containing such an altered gene might respond by altering its growth characteristics and transforming into a malignant cell.

Although the proto-oncogene (*src*) identified by this research on this avian sarcoma has never been found in damaged form in human tumors, this work led to the characterization of a dozen other oncogenes associated with animal retroviruses (10). Because all vertebrates contain nearly identical genes, identification of other proto-oncogenes in the genome of avian and other mammal models would lead to the discovery of its counterpart in human DNA. Therefore, the proto-oncogenes named for the virus in which it was first discovered are targets of human genetic cancer research and do not denote viral transformation in humans. Some of the more commonly studied proto-oncogenes include avian myelocytomatosis virus (*myc*), rat sarcoma virus (*ras*), and avian erythroblastosis virus (*erb*B-1).

Oncogenes

The information gained about retrovirus-associated oncogenes was not initially useful because these species do not infect humans. However, this work became very important in the 1980s when mutant proto-oncogenes were discovered in human tumor DNA. This supported the theory that activation of proto-oncogenes may occur when DNA incurs a mutation from an alternative chemical or physical source. In these cases, the conversion from a proto-oncogene to an active oncogene could be traced to a change in the gene sequence. Since that time, it has been discovered that at least 20 different cellular genes could be transformed by various mutations to become oncogenes (10).

Many types of mutated genes can be found in tumors, however, and the majority of these do not appear to have any dysfunctional capacity. A gene cannot be identified as an oncogene unless it can be introduced into a normal cell and induce some of the attributes of a cancer cell in the recipient (12). There are nearly 100,000 genes in the human genome, but only slightly more than 60 of them to date have been identified as having this capability (13). These genes play an essential role in normal cellular activity but also become a liability because of their potential to transform to an oncogene by mutation. However, only approximately 20 of these proto-oncogenes have been identified in a mutant oncogene form in human tumors. Whether the other candidates will prove to be true oncogenes remains to be elucidated.

Oncogene Function

Normal cell growth is controlled by a complex series of interactions that are controlled primarily by its surrounding environment. The stimulus to proliferate is provided by the adjacent tissues that supply stimulatory or inhibitory information through various growth factors. There is a complex mechanism of proteins to receive and then transmit such signals (Fig. 68.6). In the case of growth stimulation, the cell receives the signal at the surface through a receptor and transmits the message internally. In the cytoplasm, signal transducers become activated by this message and, in turn, activate nuclear transcription factors that activate large groups of cellular genes. These large groups of genes act in concert to coordinate the complex events of cell growth and division. Normal cells will not activate this cascade without the external stimulus provided by its external environment.

Proto-oncogenes play an essential role because they encode many of the proteins involved in the complex circuits that respond to the exogenous growth signals. Oncogenes are dominant over the normal allele and alter this function by changing one or more proteins and creating an aberrant signal. This

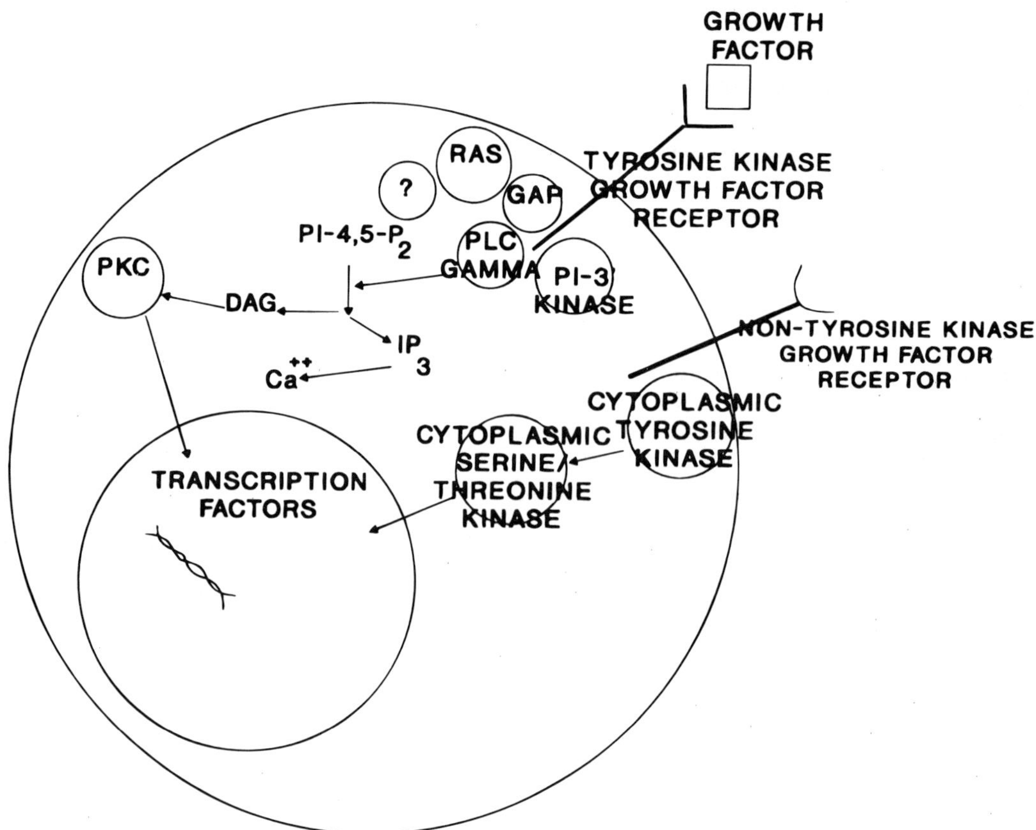

Fig. 68.6.   Signal transduction pathways that govern cell function. Commonly found aberrations of tumor suppressor genes such as p53 exert their influence on key enzymes controlling these functions. The ? represents the as yet unknown target of the ras oncogene. (Reprinted with permission from Minden MD, Pawson AJ. Oncogenes. In: Tannock IF, Hill RP, eds. The basic science of oncology. 2nd ed. New York: McGraw-Hill, 1992:41.)

stimulatory signal is transmitted even in the absence of the exogenous growth factors that would normally stimulate the signal cascade. Therefore, the cell is forced to grow in the absence of its normal regulatory mechanisms. This autonomous growth results in the mass of tissue that we call a tumor.

Tumor Suppressor Genes

It has become clear that the hyperactive growth of cells resulting from oncogene stimulation is only a portion of the complex interactions governing tumor development. In the past few years, another system that inhibits rather than promotes tumor growth has begun to be identified, with realization that its role in carcinogenesis may be at least equally important to that of oncogenes. Whereas oncogenic behavior may be likened to an accelerator for growth, containment of this growth also occurs through the signalling processes produced from the normal presence of genes that have now been termed tumor suppressor genes. It appears that a delicate balance is struck in the normal cell between growth promotion and growth constraint. When the negative influence on abnormal cell growth is lost because of deletion or alteration of tumor suppressor genes, unopposed abnormal growth stimulation overrides normal control mechanisms. Because multiple genetic changes are required before a

normal cell can convert to malignant behavior, it is very likely that both gain of oncogenic function and loss of tumor suppression must occur. Tumors, therefore, result from both a stuck accelerator and a defective braking system (10).

Less than 20 tumor suppressor genes have been identified since 1989, although cytogenetic studies have demonstrated other consistent genetic losses that strongly suggest that other tumor suppressor genes will be identified. As with nearly all genes, two copies of these genes are present in the genome per cell. Inactivation or loss of one copy still maintains normal cell growth provided the remaining copy is not defective. This differs from the dominant function of oncogenes. However, if the second copy is deleted or sustains a mutation, suppressive function is lost and abnormal proliferation is unchecked. When an inactivated form is inherited along with the intact gene, the chance of tumor development is greatly increased. Such is the case in patients who inherit one defective retinoblastoma gene (*RB*) and have a 90% probability of having a retinal tumor by age 7 (14). The *RB* gene is the first tumor suppressor gene identified that on further study may have a role in the development of other tumors as well.

Tumor suppressor gene function can also be lost when one copy of the gene mutates and is able to interfere actively with suppressor function of the remaining normal gene. The importance of this interaction is significant because it appears to be one of the mechanisms by which the p53 tumor suppressor gene function may be lost. Mutant p53 genes have been found in more than 50% of the human tumors examined for their presence, and their central role in cellular function is continually strengthened by experimental discoveries. Because the well-known *ras* oncogenes have been found in less than one quarter of these tumors, p53 tumor suppressor gene alteration is the genetic abnormality most commonly associated with human tumor formation.

Although the identification and characterization of both oncogenes and tumor suppressor genes are an exciting development in neoplastic molecular biology, there are other components to this complex biologic puzzle. Other mechanisms of growth constraint also appear to have a role in tumorigenesis. Strong evidence supports the concept that most cell types have a preprogrammed number of cell divisions before entering senescence and death in a process called apoptosis. However, tumor cell populations appear to have circumvented this limitation through various mechanisms including p53 gene mutation. These findings strengthen the implication that malignant transformation involves a series of successive genetic changes with recognized intermediate steps along the route from normal tissue to neoplasia and metastasis.

UROLOGIC MALIGNANCY AND ITS GENETIC COMPONENT

It has been estimated that in the past decade nearly 75% of urologic procedures and practices have changed dramatically. This frantic pace of change has also been evident in the molecular biologic arena, with advances in our understanding of normal and abnormal cellular mechanisms rapidly accelerating. The technical advances in molecular biology have allowed many investigators to scrutinize various aspects of the molecular basis for malignancy. As with other solid tumors, genetic information about urologic carcinogenesis has lagged behind knowledge gained about hematopoietic malignancies. However, recent developments have shed a great deal of light on the genetic components of some of these most common human tumors.

PROSTATE CANCER

Prostate cancer is now the most common nonepidermal tumor in humans but, until recently, very little attention has been directed to the molecular mechanisms surrounding prostate carcinogenesis. Considering the effects of this disease on public health, it is surprising that so little molecular biologic data exist about prostate cancer. Compounding the clinical significance of this disease is the realization that not all histologically detected prostate cancers progress to cause a clinical problem. Detection of a molecular marker to separate patients destined for progression from those whose tumors will remain clinically insignificant now has become an important ethical and economic quest.

Chromosomal analysis of genetic involvement in prostate cancer has been hindered by the difficulty of culturing prostate cancer cells, but loss of chromosomes 1, 2, 5, and Y and the gain of chromosomes 7, 14, 20, and 22 have been reported in prostate cancer (15). Rearrangements on portions of other chromosomes suggest multiple areas that may be significant in prostate carcinogenesis.

Proto-oncogenes and Oncogenes

Despite identification of more than 60 oncogenes, very few of them have been evaluated for their role in prostate carcinoma (16). Many other structural, cytoplasmic, and secretory proteins with possible relationships to carcinogenesis have been studied to some extent in prostate cancer, as have the cellular morphologic characteristics and intercellular interactions of prostate cancer. But evaluation of the relationship of oncogenes and tumor suppressor genes to these proteins and characteristics is in its infancy.

ras

The *ras* group of genes have received the most attention for their role in prostate cancer. The *ras* gene product p21 was first reported to be overexpressed in prostate cancer in 1986 (17), but subsequent reports have shown wide variability of expression in both primary and metastatic tumors (16). Studies of mRNA among the *ras* family of oncogenes have shown correlation with tumor progression for the Harvey (H)-*ras* gene but no correlation for either the Kirsten (K)-*ras* or Neuroblastoma (N)-*ras* genes (18, 19). Mutations in *ras* genes are infrequent in human prostate neoplasms despite being common in other human tumors (16). This rarity is also observed in the human prostate cancer cell lines tested for *ras* gene mutation (16, 20). A higher incidence of *ras* gene mutations has been reported in Japanese patients by various authors, with a preponderance of these noted in patients with advanced disease (16).

C-*myc* and C-*erb*B-2

Other groups of oncogenes have been evaluated in prostate cancer with variable results. Animal studies have demonstrated the malignant potential of these genes in several instances, but poor correlation exists in human prostate cancers. These oncogenes and their products have also been registered in benign prostatic hyperplasia. The c-*myc* and c-*erb*B-2 genes have been studied in particular partially because of reports of overexpression of their oncoproteins in some prostate cancer cell lines and specimens of prostate tumors (21). Although no correlation appears to exist between c-*erb*B-2 expression and grade or pathologic stage of the prostate tumors evaluated, both recurrence and survival may be adversely affected by the presence of this oncogene (22). It has been pointed out that variations of technique, specimen preparation, and interpretation of results have resulted in different rates of oncogenic expression that need to be clarified in further investigation (16).

Others

Similar variable results have been reported for preliminary studies of other proto-oncogenes. Some of the more intriguing candidates for evaluation include growth-factor–related genes such as c-*sis*, key intracellular signal transduction genes like c-*fos*, tyrosine kinase membrane receptor genes exemplified by c-*kit*, and *Bcl*-2, which circumvents programmed cell death mechanisms (16). The relationship of androgens to these proto-oncogenes is an area of research that has just begun.

Tumor Suppressor Genes

The relationship of tumor suppressor genes to prostate carcinogenesis is an area of research that is now beginning to command deserved interest. Tumor suppressor genes differ from oncogenes because normal function of both alleles must be interrupted before the suppressive effect on tumorigenesis is lost. The previously mentioned *RB* gene, identified as the cause of retinoblastoma and the first tumor suppressor gene reported, and the p53 gene are the most studied of this type of gene. There have been less than 20 tumor suppressor genes reported, but many tumors possess other areas of consistent genetic loss that could harbor tumor suppressor genes.

RB

Potential tumor suppressor genes have been evaluated on chromosomes 8, 10, and 16 following reports of nonrandom frequent deletions in those loci from cytogenetic studies (23). Deletions in these same areas have been pinpointed for other tumor types (24). The *RB* gene has drawn interest because of results from experiments replacing the defective *RB* gene in the DU 145 human prostate cancer cell line. Expression of the mutated dysfunctional *RB* gene was restored with retrovirus-mediated gene transfer, and the DU 145 cells with stable *RB* gene lost the ability to form tumors in animal models (25). A review of *RB* gene alteration in prostate cancer specimens suggests that this abnormality is found in 10 to 20% of the tumors examined (16).

p53

The p53 gene was originally believed to be an oncogene but now is judged to be a tumor suppressor gene. The p53 gene appears to be an important regulatory gene involved with modulation of genes that are activated by DNA-damaging agents (26). Its deletion, in these cases, would constitute the second significant mutation that removes the brake on the uncontrolled growth caused by the activated oncogenes. The p53 gene has also been implicated in the normal function of preprogrammed cell death (apoptosis), and its deletion allows circum-

vention of this mechanism of controlled growth (27). Alterations of p53 appear to occur late in the development of cancer and are located in 6 to 20% of specimens in most reports (16). However, p53 mutations have recently been described in much higher percentages of specimens in three studies (28–30). Furthermore, at least two investigators report a much higher incidence of p53 alterations in patients refractory to hormonal therapy (16, 31). This supports the theory of the late appearance of p53 mutations in tumorigenesis, but further evaluation is required to determine the role of p53 in androgen-insensitive prostate cancer.

Others

Other candidates for tumor suppressor genes related to prostate carcinogenesis are in the early stages of evaluation. Decreased expressions of E-Cadherin and α-catenin, proteins that interact in cell adhesion, have been implicated as being involved with an invasive phenotype of prostate cancer (32, 33). Loss of loci on chromosomes 8, 10, 16, and 17 also suggests the presence of new tumor suppressor genes related to prostate cancer (16). Allelic losses of DCC (deleted in colon carcinoma) on chromosome 18 and decreased expression of nm23-H2 may also be related to prostate carcinoma development.

The uteroglobin (UG) gene is a potential tumor suppressor gene that may have a significant contribution to the prevention of metastasis in prostate cancer and other tumors. UG protein is a potent antiinflammatory protein found in the prostate that inhibits phospholipase A2, the key enzyme necessary for the activation of arachidonic acid (34). UG was discovered recently in the prostate (Fig. 68.7) and found to inhibit significantly the ability of prostate cancer cells to invade extracellular matrix, the first step in metastasis (35). Expression of UG mRNA is absent or aberrant in all human prostate cancer cell lines but is present in normal prostate tissue, and invasion is inhibited in these cell lines from 60% to nearly 100%. Because UG expression is steroid dependent in other epithelial tissues, it has been suggested that hormonal inhibition may downregulate UG expression in the prostate and remove protection against invasion. As with other potential tumor suppressor genes, further understanding of UG mechanisms may have implications for other tumors because UG is currently known to be present in the epithelia of organs that give rise to more than two thirds of human cancers.

BLADDER CARCINOMA

Carcinoma of the bladder is the fifth most common type of cancer in the United States and the second most common urologic malignancy. Approximately 95% of these tumors have a transitional cell origin, and nearly 75% of these initially present as superficial, papillary, well-differentiated, or moderately differentiated lesions. Higher grade and stage correlate with multifocal involvement, recurrence, and progression. Carcinoma in situ (CIS) is a diffuse, high-grade, intraepithelial transitional

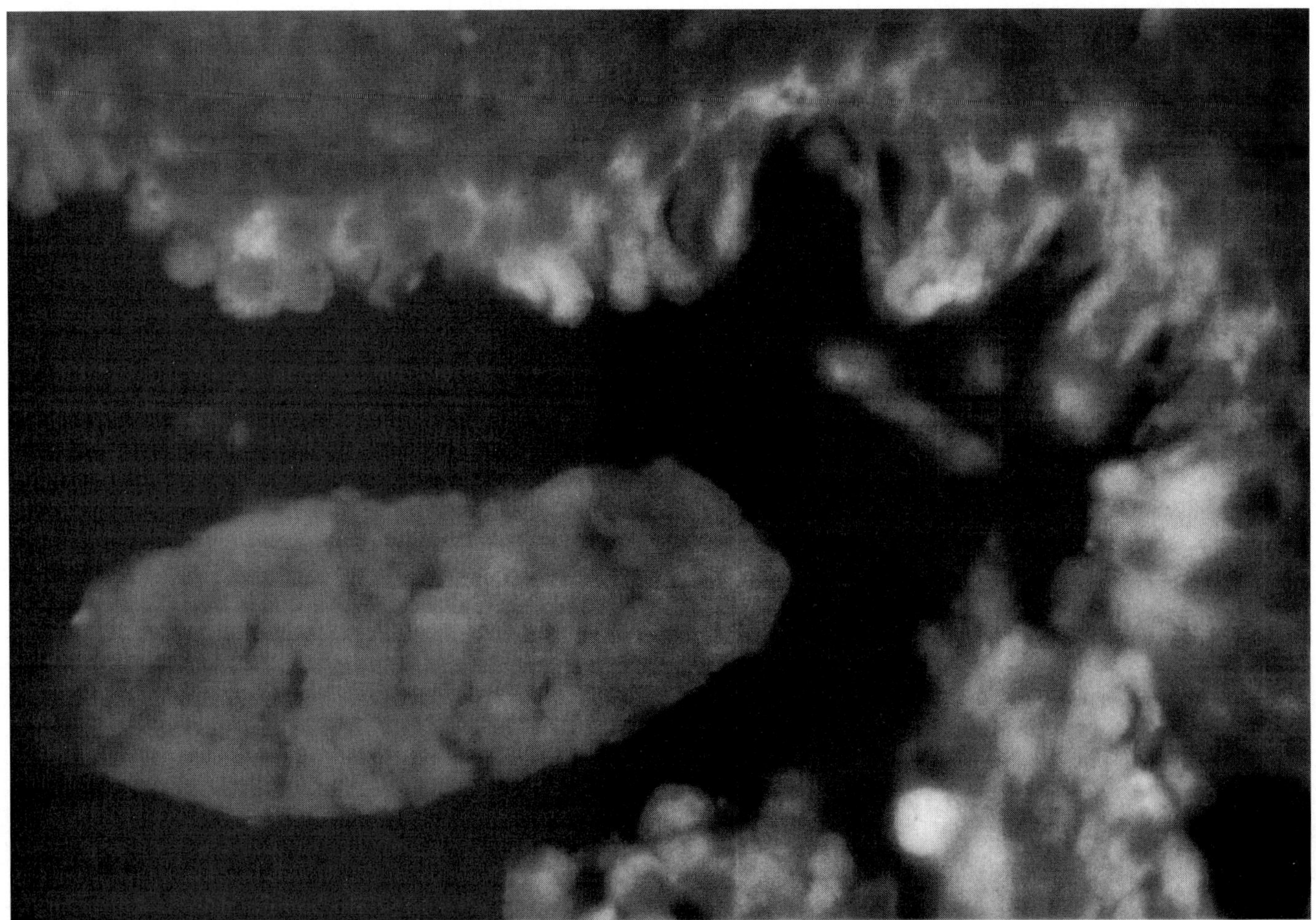

Fig. 68.7. Immunofluorescence of uteroglobin in epithelial cells of prostatic acini demonstrating a high degree of immunoreactivity. (Reprinted with permission from Manyak MJ, Kikukawa T, Mukherjee AB. Expression of uteroglobin-like protein in human prostate. J Urol 1988;140:176.)

cell malignancy of unpredictable, although frequently aggressive, behavior. Cytogenetic and molecular genetic studies have been used to elicit information about the natural history of this disease given its variability in presentation and prognosis. These studies have been almost exclusively directed to transitional cell malignancies, so very little is known about the molecular biology and cytogenetics of the uncommon bladder carcinoma types.

Some of the interesting clinical characteristics presented by transitional cell carcinoma are now becoming clearer because of cytogenetic and molecular genetic information. The multifocal nature of transitional cell carcinoma is well known, with an association of CIS in areas surrounding sites of primary or recurrent tumors in approximately 20% of patients. It is estimated that approximately 25% of bladder tumors in the male population result from occupational exposure (36). The concept has arisen of a diffuse epithelial change ("field change") because of a chemical carcinogen that initiates simultaneous proliferation of many clones, resulting in either synchronous or metachronous tumor formation. Therefore, multiclonal oncogene activation and/or tumor suppressor gene inactivation would result

in multiple tumor formation with malignant characteristics varying with the genetic change sustained in each clone.

However, a monoclonal theory of bladder carcinogenesis with intraepithelial or intravesical spread of viable tumor cells possibly abetted by growth factors and cytokines is supported by several findings (37). First, upper tract transitional cell carcinoma is an uncommon occurrence accounting for approximately 5% of these tumors. Patients with these tumors have an approximately 40% risk of bladder carcinoma development but only a 2% risk of a contralateral upper tract transitional cell tumor. Because upper tract tumors develop in patients with bladder tumors only approximately 1% of the time, monoclonal tumorigenesis with a downstream implantation or intraepithelial spread of viable cells is suggested. This theory is supported by cytogenetic and molecular genetic studies of multiple bladder tumors that have shown within each patient the exact inactivation of the same chromosome in the tumor cells but random inactivations in the normal cells (38). A recent study of one patient with an invasive renal transitional cell tumor, an ipsilateral ureteral tumor, and a concurrent bladder tumor demonstrated identical amplification of c-*erb*B-2 and p53 mutations in all tumors, highly suggestive of a monoclonal origin (39). This tantalizing evidence of a monoclonal origin for transitional cell carcinoma will need further studies to corroborate this theory.

CYTOGENETIC STUDIES OF TRANSITIONAL CELL CARCINOMA

Cytogenetic studies have revealed a large number of structural and numeric chromosomal changes associated with bladder cancers, which may account for their biologic variability (37). It has become apparent after several years of study that no one particular marker chromosome or genetic change is associated

with bladder carcinogenesis. Bladder tumors nearly always have multiple cytogenetic changes (Fig. 68.8). As a predictor of progression, cytogenetic studies in general have shown that an increase in chromosome number (hyperploidy) is associated with aggressive tumor invasion. Low-grade, low-stage tumors are nearly always diploid with less propensity for progression, especially in the absence of an abnormal chromosome.

Structural changes are relatively common in bladder carcinoma, with deletion of part or all of chromosome 9 generally being considered the most common (40). Although more often detected in superficial tumors, abnormalities of chromosome 9 are reported in greater than 50% of tumors regardless of stage and grade in some studies and may be associated with a loss

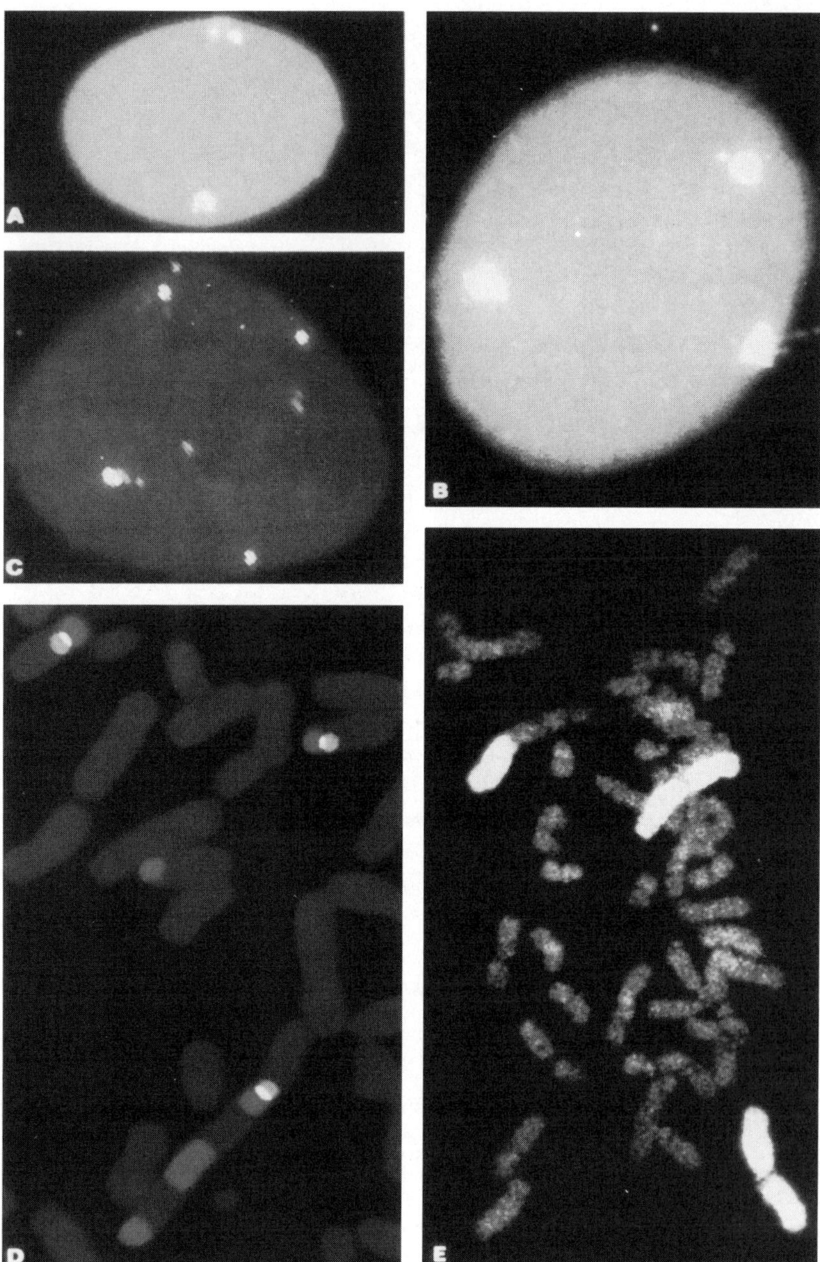

Fig. 68.8. Fluorescence in situ hybridization analysis of **A.** normal bladder cell, **B.** bladder transitional cell carcinoma with three centromeric probes present for chromosome 7, **C.** multiple centromeric probes in bladder transitional cell carcinoma for chromosomes 7 and 8, **D.** multiple abnormalities of chromosome 12 in a germ cell testicular tumor, and **E.** extra chromosome 1 material in a patient with a myelodysplastic syndrome. (Reprinted with permission from Sandberg AA. Cancer cytogenetics for clinicians. CA Cancer J Clin 1994;44:136.)

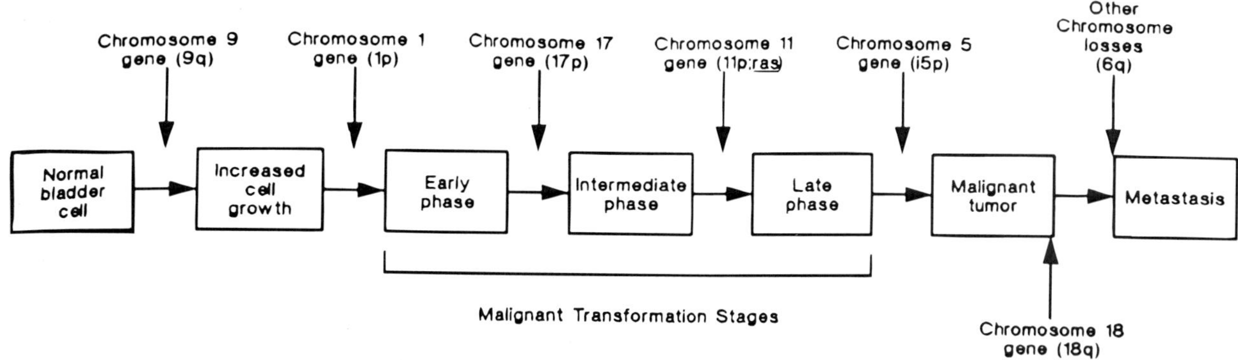

Fig. 68.9. Possible pathway for development of bladder carcinoma demonstrating multiple genetic abnormalities of both oncogenes and tumor suppressor genes. Acquisition of each successive mutation makes a cell less responsive to normal growth control mechanisms and signal transduction pathways. (Reprinted with permission from Sandberg AA, Berger CS. Review of chromosome studies in urological tumors: part 2. cytogenetics and molecular genetics of bladder cancer. J Urol 1994;151:545.)

of a tumor suppressor gene (37). Other structural changes that appear frequently include aberrations of chromosomes 1, 5, 7, and 11.

Loss of portions of chromosomes 17 and 18 is associated with invasive malignancies and may be a relatively late event in tumor biologic progression (Fig. 68.9). Translocations are also relatively common in association with other genomic abnormalities, with more than 25% of bladder tumors presenting with this type of chromosomal change.

Numeric chromosomal changes also occur in bladder carcinoma. Deletion of chromosome 9 is the most common, as stated above, and has been reported as the sole genetic abnormality in all stages and grades. Trisomy of chromosome 7 is also a common change and can be the only anomaly in these epithelial tumors (37) (Fig. 68.8). Loss of chromosome Y has been reported in up to 50% of male patients with bladder cancer (37). Although there have been reports of chromosome Y loss as a consequence of aging, this did not appear to be an age-related phenomenon in this study. Chromosome Y deletion was also associated with more complex karyotypes and poorer clinical prognosis. The loss of chromosome Y could be related to the rapid cellular turnover noted with more aggressive tumors (37).

There are few cytogenetic studies of CIS but, in the absence of karyotypic changes or loss of sex chromosomes, CIS does not usually become invasive although it is recurrent (41). CIS associated with structural abnormalities of chromosomes 1, 5, 8, and 11, however, recurred and was often invasive. Further evaluation is required to determine whether these genetic characteristics are of prognostic value.

Proto-oncogenes and Growth Factors

Some of the earliest work on oncogenes occurred in human bladder carcinoma cell lines, and urothelial malignancies consequently have been some of the most extensively studied human neoplasms (23). The cellular H-*ras* homologue (C-H-*ras*) of the viral oncogene v-H-*ras* was first isolated in bladder cancer cell lines. Overall, approximately 10% of transitional cell tumors

studied contain an abnormal *ras* proto-oncogene. There are at least four different mechanisms by which the *ras* family of genes can manifest. Increased expression of the supposedly normal p21 gene protein has been associated with increased tumor grade (42). Because the *ras* group of genes has a significant role in cellular signal transduction, it is interesting to note that overexpression of one of its downstream products, c-*fos*, may be an important step in cell transformation to the malignant cell type (23). Expression of another *ras* product, p55, has been detected in the urine of more than 50% of bladder cancer patients in one study with inconclusive association with tumor grade and stage (43). One report has related tumor progression in schistosomal-related squamous cell carcinoma to the increased expression of either normal or mutant c-H-*ras* (44).

Less is known about the role of other proto-oncogenes and growth factors in bladder carcinogenesis. There is some correlation of tumor grade, progression, and lower survival with overexpression of epidermal growth factor receptor (EGFR) and HER2/neu (also known as c-*erb*B-2) (23). Because EGF stimulates clonal growth of transitional cell carcinoma cells in vitro, the decreased excretion of EGF in the urine of patients with bladder tumors has been suggested to be related to an increased extraction of EGF by bladder cancer cells (37). Amplification of three other proto-oncogenes (fibroblast growth factors int-2 and hst-1 and apoptosis-related bcl-1) located in chromosome 11 has been noted in 7 to 20% of bladder cancer patients without correlation to tumor grade (45).

Tumor Suppressor Genes

As with nearly all other tumors, p53 mutation has been evaluated for its role in bladder malignancies. Abnormalities of p53 have been associated with high-grade malignancies, higher recurrence rates, and poorer survival rates, although this association is not absolute. p53 resides in chromosome 17 and exhibits the classic signature of a tumor suppressor gene with loss of a normal allele and mutation of the remaining before its effect is noted (23). A study that compared p53 mutations in smokers and nonsmokers concluded that cigarette smoke exposure may not alter the kinds of p53 mutations that occur but may increase the extent of the damage sustained by the DNA (46).

The *RB* gene has also been investigated for its presence and effect in bladder carcinoma. Introduction of *RB* into cell lines devoid of *RB* expression has inhibited in vitro tumor cell growth and tumorigenesis (47). Loss or inactivation of the *RB* gene has been reported in 6 of 17 bladder carcinoma cell lines tested and in specimens from patients (23). *RB* alteration may be more important as a prognosticator in patients who present with muscle-invasive disease because of a relatively high incidence compared with superficial tumors. This statistically significant finding was correlated with a poorer prognosis than patients who retained *RB* expression.

There are a myriad of other candidates for tumor suppressor genes because of the frequency and variety of chromosomal aberrations found in transitional cell carcinomas. The clinical variability of bladder tumors suggests that their description may allow subclassification of urothelial malignancies. Their influence on bladder carcinogenesis awaits further investigation of these genetic abnormalities.

RENAL CANCER

Primary malignant neoplasms of the kidney account for approximately 6% of all adult malignancies, with 85% of these arising from the renal parenchyma. Transitional cell carcinoma involving the kidney is responsible for approximately 8% of renal tumors, with adult Wilms' tumor and sarcomas found in approximately 4%. It is estimated that more than 28,000 new cases of kidney cancer were diagnosed in 1995 and that more than 11,000 deaths occurred due to renal malignancy (48). The reasons for a rising incidence of renal cancer are unclear.

This section concentrates on the genetic abnormalities associated with primary renal parenchymal cancer. Genetic origins of transitional cell carcinoma have been discussed previously and apply to those tumors arising in the kidney.

The evaluation of various proto-oncogenes and growth factors as a contributor to renal carcinogenesis has turned up little evidence of involvement to date. The *ras* family of genes and the c-*erb*B-2 and *mdm*-2 proto-oncogenes do not appear to play a role in this disease (49). Known tumor suppressor genes such as the *RB* gene and p53 also appear to make little contribution to the development of renal cancer, although p53 alterations have been found in one third of cell lines tested (50).

Inherited Renal Cancer

Until recently, there have been two relatively well-defined types of inherited renal cancer that accounted for a relatively small portion of renal malignancy diagnoses. The first genetic clue for renal cancer came from the karyotypic analysis of a family in which cancer developed by the age of 60 in 90% of family members (51). Subsequent description of two other familial clusters a few years later confirmed this unusual occur-

rence (52, 53). The genetic abnormality common to all three groups involved a translocation of the short arm of chromosome 3 with another chromosome (6, 9, 11).

The second form of renal cancer with a genetic component occurs in a syndrome known as von Hippel-Lindau (VHL) disease. VHL disease is characterized by a propensity for the development of multiple tumors of the eye, central nervous system, chromaffin tissue, epididymis, pancreas, and kidney in various combinations often peculiar to each family (54). Patients with VHL disease have characteristic abnormalities of chromosome 3, with deletion being the only detectable genetic aberration in more than 50% of 40 patients studied in one series (55). This pattern suggests deletion of a tumor suppressor gene located on chromosome 3 that is supported by molecular genetic analysis demonstrating loss of the normal allele in each case of a patient who had inherited the other defective allele from one parent (56). That gene has now been identified in a specific area of chromosome 3 (57).

Sporadic, Nonfamilial Renal Cancer

The involvement of chromosome 3 in these relatively rare forms of kidney cancer provided a glimpse of the possibility for a genetic origin of sporadic, nonfamilial renal neoplasms. A high percentage of chromosome 3 abnormalities had been reported in a small series of clear cell carcinoma patients nearly a decade ago (58). This cytogenetic work was confirmed and expanded to include chromosome 3 deletion by molecular genetic techniques (59). Specific chromosome 3 mapping of deleted regions then localized the genomic defect to the precise area of deletion in VHL disease (60). Since that discovery, confirmation of a mutated inactive gene at that locus has been reported in 57% of a larger series of sporadic, nonfamilial renal cell carcinomas (61). When one includes the probable genetic basis for transitional cell carcinoma, it is evident that nearly two thirds of cancers originating from the kidney in adults have a genetic association.

Nephroblastoma (Wilms' Tumor)

One of the most frequent neoplasms found in childhood arises in the kidney. In most cases Wilms' tumor occurs sporadically, although rare instances of a hereditary form are reported (62). Cytogenetic studies have strongly correlated deletions of chromosome 11 with the development of Wilms' tumor in both sporadic and hereditary forms (23). Molecular genetic studies have also demonstrated various genetic abnormalities located on chromosome 11. So far, no involvement of the known proto-oncogene families, such as *ras* or *myc*, has been detected.

Strong evidence for the existence of one or more tumor suppressor genes on chromosome 11 led to the identification of an altered or deleted gene, now termed WT1 (63). It appears that WT1 is involved in DNA binding that represses growth and that this ability is lost with mutation (23). Therefore, WT1 is necessary for controlled growth in the fetal kidney and its loss would promote tumorigenesis. Recent evidence suggests the possibility of at least one or two other regions that may harbor tumor suppressor genes involved with Wilms' tumor development.

TESTICULAR NEOPLASMS

Although testicular malignancies are the most common tumors found in males between the ages of 15 and 35, these neoplasms are relatively uncommon and account for 7000 cases per year. Testicular tumors represent one of the few real triumphs of combined surgical and chemotherapeutic intervention, with survival rates approaching 100% in patients with early stages of the disease. The rapid cellular turnover of germinal tissue has directed attention to a genetic basis of the disease spectrum.

Cytogenetic studies have demonstrated a high incidence of an abnormal chromosome 12 that appears to be an early event in tumorigenesis (23) (Fig. 68.8). Chromosomes 1, 11, X, and Y have also been reported to contain occasional alterations or deletions in germ cell tumors. Molecular genetic studies have shown several altered proto-oncogenes on chromosomes 1, 11, and 12 (*ras, myc, src,* and insulin-like growth factors). Both c-*kit* and *hst*-1 proto-oncogenes have altered expression in germ cell tumors with a high incidence of inverse expression for seminoma (c-*kit* expressed, *hst*-1 absent) and nonseminomatous tumors (*hst*-1 expressed, c-*kit* rarely) (23).

Molecular genetic studies have suggested presence of tumor suppressor genes on chromosome 12. Only the *RB* gene and p53 have been studied to any extent in germ cell neoplasms. Although there is loss of the *RB* gene product in some of the less-differentiated tumors, no *RB* gene alteration has been detected (23). Recent reports of increased p53 protein noted in a high proportion of germ cell tumors suggest that increased expression is associated with decreasing differentiation of embryonal cell carcinoma (64). However, the increased expression of the p53 protein does not appear to correlate with any mutations of p53 (65).

PENILE CARCINOMA

Several premalignant conditions are included in the spectrum of superficial penile cancer in addition to squamous cell carcinoma. Invasive penile carcinoma is usually of the squamous variety and appears to arise in similar fashion to the superficial lesions. Penile carcinoma is rare in the United States and other countries that practice circumcision and have generally good hygienic practices. However, in other parts of the world they comprise some of the most common urologic malignancies.

Investigation into the genetic basis of penile malignancy has followed the theory of human papillomavirus as the causative agent. There appears to be a dichotomy between the viruses associated with benign lesions and those associated with premalignant and malignant lesions (23). Human papillomavirus type 16 has been detected in approximately 50% of penile tumors, with type 18 associated in another 10%. However, human papillomavirus types 6, 11, 42, 43, 44, and 55 are almost exclusively associated with benign condylomata. Neither proto-oncogenes nor tumor suppressor genes have been evaluated to any extent in penile carcinoma.

GENE THERAPY

The possibility of gene therapy represents one of the biggest potential returns on the investment in molecular biologic research over the past several years (66). The first patient was treated with gene therapy for severe combined immunodeficiency in 1990, and the therapy proved to be labor-intensive and expensive. Since then, more than 60 protocols of human gene therapy have been approved by the National Institutes of Health Recombinant DNA Advisory Committee. At least five of these involve urologic malignancies (renal cancer), with others in various stages of approval (67). Although to date expectations have decidedly outweighed results, the rapid acquisition of molecular genetic information and increasingly sophisticated technology have decreased the time and labor required for such treatments.

The use of genetic products for therapy evolved from the initial practical use of recombinant technology to produce massive amounts of a normal gene product to thwart a disease process or to augment standard therapies. Examples of this industrial production include the recombinant human insulin used for diabetes and erythropoietin used for anemia associated with chronic renal failure. Other uses of recombinant technology have resulted in vaccine development such as that provided for hepatitis B. It is only recently that the development of somewhat efficient vehicles has allowed direct transfer of recombinant genetic material into patients.

Cellular Destruction With Gene Therapy

The two general approaches that have been used for clinical application of gene therapy involve selective destruction of cells or replacement of defective genes (67). Cytoreductive gene therapy selectively targets malignant cells for destruction through various avenues. The most popular approach for tumor destruction has involved boosting the host immune response against the tumor through vaccination with genetically altered tumor cells. In this method, tumor cells are removed from the patient and stimulated to produce an immunogenic protein. After irradiation to prevent proliferation in the patient, the reinjected cells enhance the host immune response because of the increased immunogenicity of the treated cells. Several cytokines have been shown to have activity in animal models and are the basis for current clinical trials (68). One major limitation has been the relatively small tumor burden destroyed in the preclinical models, which suggests that the role for this therapy may be as an adjunct to standard therapy. However, researchers are optimistic that identification of tumor antigens will lead to the direct genetic engineering of vaccines that promote an immune response (67).

Cytoreductive therapy can also be used to transfer genes of drug susceptibility into patients. This approach requires less than 100% efficiency of transduction to destroy tumors after drug administration, suggesting that the cytotoxic effect can now have an impact on surrounding neoplastic cells. In another variation of cytoreductive gene therapy, selective cell destruction could also be accomplished by stimulating tissue-specific expression of drug susceptibility. This would require tissue-specific recognition by the injected therapeutic agent.

Genetic Replacement

The other broad avenue of approach involves correction of a defective or deleted gene by introduction of the normal wild-type gene. Localization and characterization of both oncogenes and tumor suppressor genes furnish targets for this method of gene-directed therapy. Urologic malignancies have generated some of the most interest as targets for gene therapy with tantalizing evidence for potential application. The identification of specific gene defects in renal cell carcinoma, Wilms' tumor, VHL disease, bladder carcinoma, and prostatic neoplasms has provided candidates that heighten interest in this approach.

Vectors for Gene Therapy

Both corrective and cytoreductive gene therapy are dependent on the vehicles used to insert the genetic product into the recipient. These vehicles, known as vectors, are engineered portions of DNA or RNA capable of receiving the therapeutic gene for delivery into the patient. Each one contains a promoter sequence that enables the recipient cells to express the inserted gene.

For a vector to be therapeutically successful it must have the ability to insert the desired gene at a high rate into the target cells. There are three ways available today by which this high-efficiency transduction can occur, ranging from a nonspecific genetic transfer to all cells to very tissue-specific exposure only (67). All vectors currently available use a virus for transduction but have limitations to their attractiveness. The vectors are all either retroviruses or DNA viruses that have been genetically altered so that they cannot replicate within human cells. The limitations of these replication-defective vectors vary. For instance, retroviruses are generally characterized by stable expression of the inserted gene and are effective in their transfer but require target cell mitoses. Their use may be limited at this time to tumors with rapid proliferation or require multiple exposures to eventually expose all tumor cells during mitotic activity. Adenoviral vectors, not known for stable gene expression but that can effectively transfer genes and can accept large DNA segments, have been plagued by the potential for development of immunity in the patient receiving the therapy. This limits the ability to transfer the gene frequently, something that is envisioned as probably necessary for durable success. Other stable vectors appear to sustain genetic deletions on transfer, again limiting applicability. The reader is referred elsewhere for more thorough discussions of the attributes and drawbacks of viral vectors (67, 69).

Clinical Application

Renal cell carcinoma has received the most initial attention as a candidate for gene therapy because of the modest success with adoptive immunotherapy using interleukin (IL) cytokines. Plasmid vectors for IL-2 and α-interferon are being evaluated as human renal cell carcinoma vaccines for adjuvant therapy in patients with high risk of relapse after nephrectomy (66). Attention is now being directed to both bladder and prostate malignancies, with successful transfer in animal models now being followed by pilot studies in humans. In one intriguing study, autologous prostate cancer cells have been reintroduced into the patient following radical prostatectomy after they have been transfected with a retroviral vector containing granulocyte-macrophage colony-stimulating factor (GM-CSF) (70). Each of the patients in this small series had increased secretion of GM-CSF with sequential doses, demonstrating that it is possible to have sustained expression of an introduced gene. The bladder is also an interesting target for gene therapy because of the possibility of direct viral introduction into the bladder (71). The simple intravesical approach would circumvent some problems of administration.

Given the rapid evolution of molecular genetic techniques and the amount and breadth of knowledge that is being accumulated, it is reasonable to aspire for a practical use of this information. In addition to detection of high-risk individuals for development of cancer and prognostication about clinical course, molecular biologic advances may be able to provide a therapeutic approach for several malignant states for which treatment is currently limited. It is highly likely that advances toward these ends will be reported before publication of this text. This chapter was designed to provide an overview of this exciting field and to make some sense out of seemingly disparate molecular genetic discoveries. Although it is still safe to say that gene therapy is not yet ready for prime time, it is also evident that synergistic research efforts on several fronts have delineated some very clear urologic targets for gene therapy in the near future. If advances continue at the current pace, gene therapy will indeed progress from the bench to the bedside.

REFERENCES

1. von Hansemann D. Ueber asymmetrische zelitheilung in epithelkrebsen und deren biologische bedeutung. Virchows Arch A pathol Anat 1890;119:299.
2. Boveri T. Zur Frage der Entstehung maligner Tumoren. Jena: Gustav Fischer, 1914.
3. Mitelman F. Chromosomes, genes, and cancer. CA Cancer J Clin 1994;44:133.
4. Nowell PC, Hungerford DA. A minute chromosome in human chronic granulocytic leukemia. Science 1960;132:1497.
5. Squire J, Phillips RA. Genetic basis of cancer. In: Tannock IF,

Hill RP, eds. The basic science of oncology. 2nd ed. New York: McGraw-Hill, 1992:41.

6. Steele GD, Osteen RT, Winchester DP, et al. Clinical highlights for the National Cancer Data Base: 1994. CA Cancer J Clin 1994;44:71.

7. Thompson LM. Somatic cell genetic approach to dissecting mammalian DNA repair. Environ Mol Mutagen 1989;14:264.

8. Sandberg AA. Cancer cytogenetics for clinicians. CA Cancer J Clin 1994;44:136.

9. Kumar R, Sukumar S, Barbacid M. Activation of ras oncogenes preceding the onset of neoplasia. Science 1990;248:1101.

10. Weinberg RA. Oncogenes and tumor suppressor genes. CA Cancer J Clin 1994;44:160.

11. Stehelin D, Varmus HE, Bishop JM, et al. DNA related to the transforming gene(S) of avian sarcoma viruses is present in normal avian DNA. Nature 1976;260:170.

12. Bishop JM. Viral oncogenes. Cell 1985;42:23.

13. Bishop JM. Molecular themes in oncogenesis. Cell 1991;64:235.

14. Hollingsworth RE Jr, Hensey CE, Lee WH. Retinoblastoma protein and the cell cycle. Curr Opin Genet Dev 1993;3:55.

15. Brothman AR, Peehl DM, Patel AM, et al. Frequency and pattern of karyotypic abnormalities in human prostate cancer. Cancer Res 1990;50:3795.

16. Moul JW, Gaddipati J, Srivastava S. Molecular biology of prostate cancer: oncogenes and tumor suppressor genes. In: Dawson NA, Vogelzang NJ, eds. Prostate cancer. New York: Wiley-Liss, 1994:19.

17. Viola MV, Fromowitz F, Oravez S, et al. Expression of ras oncogene p21 in prostate growth. J Endocrinol 1991;131:5.

18. Cooke DB, Quarmby VE, Petrusz P, et al. Expression of ras proto-oncogenes in the Dunning R3327 rat prostatic adenocarcinoma system. Prostate 1991;13:273.

19. Bussemakers MIG, Isaacs JT, Debruyne FMJ, et al. Oncogene expression in prostate cancer. World J Urol 1991;9:58.

20. Carter BS, Epstein JT, Isaacs WB. ras oncogene mutations in human prostate cancer. Cancer Res 1990;50:6830.

21. Zhau HE, Wasn DS, Zhou J, et al. Expression of c-ErbB-2 neu proto-oncogene in human prostatic cancer tissues and cell lines. Mol Carcinog 1992;5:320.

22. Kuhn EJ, Kurnot RA, Sesterhenn IA, et al. Expression of the c-ErbB-2 neu (HER-2/Neu) oncoprotein in human prostate carcinoma. J Urol 1993;150:1427.

23. Strohmeyer TG, Slamon DJ. Proto-oncogenes and tumor suppressor genes in human urological malignancies. J Urol 1994;151:1479.

24. Collins VP, Kunimi K, Bergerheim U, et al. Molecular genetics and human prostatic carcinoma. Acta Oncol 1991;30:181.

25. Bookstein R, Shew JY, Chen PL, et al. Suppression of tumorigenicity of human prostate carcinoma cells by replacing a mutated RB gene. Science 1990;247:712.

26. Kastan MB, Zhan Q, El-Deiry WS, et al. A mammalian cell cycle checkpoint pathway utilizing p53 and GADD45 is defective in ataxia-telangiectasia. Cell 1992;71:587.

27. Clarke AR, Purdie CA, Harrison DJ, et al. Thymocyte apoptosis induced by p53-dependent and independent pathways. Nature 1993;302:844.

28. Van Veldhuizen PJ, Sadasivan R, Garcia F, et al. Mutant p53 expression in prostate carcinoma. Prostate 1993;22:23.

29. de Vere White RW, Gumerlock PH, Chi SG, et al. p53 tumor suppressor gene abnormalities are frequent in human prostate tissues. J Urol 1993;149:654. Abstract no. 376.

30. Chi SG, de Vere White RW, Meyers FJ, et al. p53 in prostate cancer: frequent expressed transition mutations. J Natl Cancer Inst 1994;86:926.

31. Hamdy CF, Thurrell W, Lawry J, et al. p53 mutant expression correlates with hormone sensitivity and prognosis in human prostatic adenocarcinoma. J Urol 1993;149:658. Abstract no. 377.

32. Bussemakers MJG, van Moorselaar RJA, Giroldi LA, et al. Decreased expression of E-cadherin in the progression of rat prostate cancer. Cancer Res 1992;52:2916.

33. Morton R, Ewing C, Nagafuchi A, et al. Expression of a-catenin in human prostate cancer cell lines. Proc Am Assoc Cancer Res 1993;34:198.

34. Manyak MJ, Kikukawa T, Mukherjee AB. Expression of uteroglobin-like protein in human prostate. J Urol 1988;140:176.

35. Leyton J, Manyak MJ, Mukherjee AB, et al. Recombinant human uteroglobin inhibits the in vitro invasiveness of human metastatic prostate tumor cells and the release of arachidonic acid stimulated by fibroblast-conditioned medium. Cancer Res 1994;54:3696.

36. Silverman DT, Levin LI, Hoover RN, et al. Occupational risks of bladder cancer in the United States; part 1: white men. J Natl Cancer Inst 1989;81:1472.

37. Sandberg AA, Berger CS. Review of chromosome studies in urological tumors; part 2: cytogenetics and molecular genetics of bladder cancer. J Urol 1994;151:545.

38. Sidransky D, Frost P, Von Eschenbach A, et al. Clonal origin of bladder cancer. N Engl J Med 1992;319:737.

39. Lunec J, Challen C, Wright C, et al. c-ErbB-2 amplification and identical p53 mutations in concomitant transitional carcinomas of renal pelvis and urinary bladder. Lancet 1992;339:439. Letter.

40. Knowles MA, Cairns JP, Williamson MP, et al. Identification of multiple molecular genetic alterations in bladder cancer. Cancer Genet Cytogenet 1992;63:140. Abstract.

41. Tyrkus M, Powell I, Fakr W. Cytogenetic studies of carcinoma in situ of the bladder: prognostic implications. J Urol 1992;148:44.

42. Viola MV, Fromowitz F, Oravez S, et al. ras oncogene p21 expression is increased in premalignant lesions and high grade bladder carcinoma. J Exp Med 1985;161:1213.

43. Stock LM, Brosman SA, Fahey JL, et al. ras related oncogene protein as a tumor marker in transitional cell carcinoma of the bladder. J Urol 1987;137:789.

44. Fujita J, Nakayama H, Onoue H, et al. Frequency of active ras oncogenes in human bladder cancers associated with schistosomiasis. Jpn J Cancer Res 1987;78:915.

45. Proctor AJ, Coombs LM, Cairns JP, et al. Amplification at chromosome 11q13 in transitional cell tumours of the bladder. Oncogene 1991;6:789.

46. Spruck CH III, Rideout WM III, Olumi AF, et al. Distinct pattern of p53 mutations in bladder cancer: relationship to tobacco usage. Cancer Res 1993;53:1162.

47. Takahashi R, Hashimoto T, Xu HJ, et al. The retinoblastoma gene functions as a growth and tumor suppressor in human bladder carcinoma cells. Proc Natl Acad Sci 1991;88:5257.

48. Wingo PA, Tong T, Bolden S. Cancer statistics, 1995. CA Cancer J Clin 1995;45:8.

49. Reiter RE, Zbar B, Linehan WM. Molecular genetic studies of renal cell carcinoma: potential biologic and clinical significance for genitourinary malignancy. In: Walsh PC, Retik AB, Stamey TA, et al., eds. Campbell's urology. 6th ed. Philadelphia: WB Saunders, 1993:1

50. Reiter RE, Gnarra J, Anglard P, et al. Chromosome 17p deletions and p53 mutations in renal cell carcinoma. Cancer Res 1993;53:3092.

51. Cohen AJ, Li FP, Berg S, et al. Hereditary renal-cell carcinoma associated with a chromosomal translocation. N Engl J Med 1979;301:592.

52. Kovacs G, Frisch S. Clonal chromosome abnormalities in tumor cells from patients with sporadic renal cell carcinomas. Cancer Res 1989;49:651.

53. Pathak S, Strong LC, Ferrell RE, et al. Familial renal cell carcinoma with a 3:11 chromosome translocation limited to tumor cells. Science 1982;217:939.

54. Glenn GM, Daniel LN, Choyke P, et al. von Hippel-Lindau disease: distinct phenotypes suggest more than one mutation allele at the vhl locus. Hum Genet 1991;87:207.

55. Kovacs G, Emanuel A, Neumann HP, et al. Cytogenetics of renal cell carcinomas associated with von Hippel-Lindau disease. Genes Chromosom Cancer 1991;3:256.

56. Tory K, Brauch H, Linehan WM, et al. Specific genetic change in tumors associated with von Hippel-Lindau disease. J Natl Cancer Inst 1989;81:1097.

57. Latif A, Tory K, Gnarra J, et al. Identification of the von Hippel-Lindau disease tumor suppressor gene. Science 1993;260:1317.

58. Yoshida MA, Ohyashiki K, Ochi H, et al. Cytogenetic studies of tumor tissue from patients with nonfamilial renal cell carcinoma. Cancer Res 1986;46:2139.

59. Zbar B, Brauch H, Talmadge C, et al. Loss of alleles of loci in the short arm of chromosome 3 in renal cell carcinoma. Nature 1987;327:721.

60. Anglard P, Trahan E, Liu S, et al. Molecular and cellular characterization of human renal cell carcinoma cell lines. Cancer Res 1992;52:348.

61. Long JP, Anglard P, Gnarra JR, et al. The use of molecular genetic analysis in the diagnosis of renal cell cancer. World J Urol 1994;12:69.

62. Matsunga E. Genetics of Wilms' tumor. Hum Genet 1981;57:231.

63. Cowell JK, Wadey RB, Haber DA, et al. Structural rearrangements of the WT1 gene in Wilms' tumour cells. Oncogene 1991;6:595.

64. Lewis DJ, Sesterhenn IA, McCarthy WF, et al. Immunohistochemical expression of p53 tumor suppressor gene protein in adult germ cell testis tumors: clinical correlation in stage 1 disease. J Urol 1994;152:418.

65. Schenkman NS, Sesterhenn IA, Washington L, et al. Increased p53 protein does not correlate to p53 gene mutations in microdissected human testicular germ cell tumors. J Urol 1995;154:617.

66. Manyak MJ. The clinical relevance of gene therapy. J Urol 1994;152:292.

67. Sanda MG, Simons JW. Gene therapy for urologic cancer. Urology 1994;44:617.

68. Dranoff G, Jaffee E, Lazenby A, et al. Vaccination with irradiated tumor cells engineered to secrete murine granulocyte-macrophage colony-stimulating factor stimulates potent, specific, and long-lasting antitumor immunity. Proc Natl Acad Sci 1993;90:3539.

69. Benchimol S. Viruses and cancer. In; Tannock IF, Hill RP, eds. The basic science of oncology. 2nd ed. New York; McGraw-Hill, 1992:88.

70. Sanda MG, Ayyagari SR, Jaffee EM, et al. Demonstration of a rational strategy for human prostate cancer gene therapy. J Urol 1994;151:622.

71. Morris BD Jr, Drazan KE, Csete ME, et al. Adenoviral-mediated gene transfer to bladder in vivo. J Urol 1994;152:506.

Index

Note: Page numbers in italic indicate figures; page numbers followed by *t* indicate tables.